Complete Review of

Medicine
for NBE

Covering 4200+ Qs with Explanations, 100+ IBQs & 1000+ Colored Illustrations/Images

• **Fifth Edition** •

Includes Recently Changed AIIMS Pattern Questions Review 2019

Special Feature
First Book Covering Sample Video Questions

Deepak Marwah

Director
Medicine Buster Classes
New Delhi, India

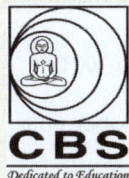

CBS
Dedicated to Education

CBS Publishers & Distributors Pvt Ltd

• New Delhi • Bengaluru • Chennai • Kochi • Kolkata • Mumbai
• Hyderabad • Nagpur • Patna • Pune • Vijayawada

> **Disclaimer**
>
> This book contains questions based on topics asked in previous years' State and National Level PG Entrance and Medical Officer Examinations in India. Often repeated topics and sub-topics have been included for students' benefit. We do not claim that these questions are exact or similar to questions asked in any recent examinations in India. If any such similarity is found, it is purely coincidental and by chance. The questions given in this book is self made and for practice purpose.

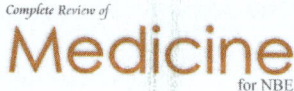

Complete Review of
Medicine
for NBE

ISBN: 978-93-88725-88-0

Copyright © Author & Publishers

Fifth Edition: 2019-20
Fourth Edition: 2018

All rights reserved. No part of this book may be reproduced or transmitted in any form or by any means, electronic or mechanical, including photocopying, recording, or any information storage and retrieval system without permission, in writing, from the author and the publishers.

Published by **Satish Kumar Jain** and produced by **Varun Jain** for

CBS Publishers & Distributors Pvt Ltd
4819/XI Prahlad Street, 24 Ansari Road, Daryaganj, New Delhi 110 002, India.
Ph: +91-11-23289259, 23266861, 23266867   Website: www.cbspd.com
Fax: 011-23243014
e-mail: delhi@cbspd.com; cbspubs@airtelmail.in

Corporate Office: 204 FIE, Industrial Area, Patparganj, Delhi 110 092
Ph: +91-11-4934 4934   Fax: 4934 4935
e-mail: feedback@cbspd.com; bhupesharora@cbspd.com

Branches

- **Bengaluru:** Seema House 2975, 17th Cross, K.R. Road,
  Banasankari 2nd Stage, Bengaluru 560 070, Karnataka
  Ph: +91-80-26771678/79   Fax: +91-80-26771680   e-mail: bangalore@cbspd.com

- **Chennai:** 7, Subbaraya Street, Shenoy Nagar, Chennai 600 030, Tamil Nadu
  Ph: +91-44-26680620, 26681266   Fax: +91-44-42032115   e-mail: chennai@cbspd.com

- **Kochi:** Ashana House, No. 39/1904, AM Thomas Road, Valanjambalam, Ernakulam 682 018, Kochi, Kerala
  Ph: +91-484-4059061-65   Fax: +91-484-4059065   e-mail: kochi@cbspd.com

- **Kolkata:** 6/B, Ground Floor, Rameswar Shaw Road, Kolkata-700 014, West Bengal
  Ph: +91-33-22891126, 22891127, 22891128   e-mail: kolkata@cbspd.com

- **Mumbai:** 83-C, Dr E Moses Road, Worli, Mumbai-400018, Maharashtra
  Ph: +91-22-24902340/41   Fax: +91-22-24902342   e-mail: mumbai@cbspd.com

Representatives

- **Hyderabad** +91-9885175004
- **Pune**   +91-9623451994
- **Patna**   +91-9334159340
- **Vijaywada** +91-9000660880

Printed At : Goyal Offset Printers

Dedications

*I would like to thank my mom and dad for all the values they imbibed in me,
my dear wife Renuka for all the love and patience,
my dear son Abhimanyu for being my stress buster.*

Deepak Marwah

Preface

I am overwhelmed while penning down the preface to the Fifth edition of Complete Review of Medicine. Your stupendous response for the book has always inspired me to thoroughly update the content every year and not simply rewrap the old stuff in new covering. I admire and acknowledge your ardent support and I hope it remains my motivation for many years to come.

The fifth edition of the Complete Review of Medicine unveils an updated approach to tackle the one liner mind teaser MCQs asked in the recent exams and recently changed AIIMS examinations pattern.

As always, I have tried to ensure that this book is not voluminous, and has the right proportion of theory, questions, explanations and ready reckoners presented in most effective manner to aid your journey to your desired college. My intent is to guide you how to optimally utilize this book to prepare for your PGME exams. The approach is to complete a cover to cover first reading of the book in 3 weeks. On every page, mark features which either appear new to you or that you were unaware or were not fully aware of.

I want you to internalize this fact, *"If your conceptual understanding of the subjects is rock solid, no examination is difficult to crack in the first attempt"*. Read the theory and explanations carefully even if you feel you know the topic, because this methodology will help you answer 70-80% of the questions of Internal Medicine based on sound logic. Revise the critical points before the examination and I am confident that you will score well.

As they say "The proof of the pudding is in eating it". Many students who have successfully cracked the NEET 2019 exam have appreciated the fact that as there is no repetition of information, the book is concise and to-the-point which has given them sufficient opportunity to read the book end to end, and still have time before the examination to revise the crucial points highlighted as "Memory Joggers".

Some of the exam toppers who have given heartfelt reviews on my Facebook page, have highlighted another salient feature of this book that the explanations to questions are comprehensive and a thorough study of the theory and explanations has helped them to answer the questions logically and with confidence.

This book has been written for doctors like you whose strength lies in working hard every single day with the same zeal and passion as the day before. I want you to imbibe this simple mantra *"Motivation comes from within and inspiration from outside"*.

Deepak Marwah

Acknowledgements

Heartfelt thanks to my teachers at MAMC, New Delhi who laid the foundation for shaping my career.

Special thanks to my parents for the work ethics they made me imbibe, my loving wife **Renuka** for her time and patience and my loving son **Abhimanyu** for being my stress buster.

Special thanks to:
- All our students in India and abroad for their continuous feedbacks, appraisal and critics, which helped in shaping this book
- All our previous batch students of test and discussion as well as regular batch for their continuous feedbacks and helps needed in compiling the questions
- Our parents whose prayers and blessings has given us the strength to keep working
- Our teachers whose valuable lessons and teachings are always with us at each and every step
- Dr Manoj Kumar Bhoomigari, MS Anatomy for his worthy support and contribution
- Dr Shravan Kumar MD Pediatrics
- Dr Pawan Kumar Kandhari MS Surgery for his precise surgical inputs
- Dr Vaidehi MS (Obs and Gyne) and first female robotic surgeon of India for her critical inputs
- Dr Asma for spinning her PSM magic on our students
- Dr Pallavi MD Dermatology
- Dr Shanthan, MD Biochemistry for taking out time being there whenever needed
- Dr Ankit Goel MD Psychiatry for his valuable suggestions and contribution in psychiatry
- Dr Yusuf Tyagi, MS Orthopaedics, for his priceless suggestions and round the clock availability in shaping this book
- Dr Pallavi Pradeep, Dr Cinderella B, RML New Delhi
- Dr Bushra S Khan and Dr Nida D Rizvi, MD Pharmacology for their outstanding helpful tips and jolliness which were always remarkable
- Dr Shamshi Azmi and Dr Prerna Singh who were always there in need with their best effort round the clock
- MAMC Batch of 1993
- NJMS Batch 2005 (the best ever)
- FMGE Solutions office staffs Mr Naveen, Mr Alam, Mr Soumen, Ms Prachi for always being there and available to help whenever needed.

I would like to thank **Mr Satish Kumar Jain** (Chairman) and **Mr Varun Jain** (Managing Director), M/s CBS Publishers and Distributors Pvt Ltd for providing me the platform in bringing out the book. I have no words to describe the role, efforts, inputs and initiatives undertaken by **Mr Bhupesh Arora,** (Vice President- Publishing and Marketing, PGMEE and Nursing Division) for helping and motivating me.

I sincerely thank the **entire CBS team** for bringing the book colourful with utmost care and presentation. I thank Dr Mrinalini Bakshi (Editorial Head and Content Strategist) for her editorial support and Ms Nitasha Arora (Production Head & Content Strategist), Dr Anju Dhir (Senior Scientific Coordinator/Editor), Mr Nitish Dubey (Senior Editor) and all the production team members Mr Ashutosh Pathak, Mr Chaman Lal, Mr Prakash Gaur, Mr Phool Kumar, Mr Bunty Kashyap, Ms Tahira Parveen, Ms Babita Verma, Mr Chander, Mr Raju Sharma, Mr Manoj Chaudhary, Mr Vikram Chaudhary, Mr Manoj Malakar, Mr Arun Kumar and Ms Manorama for devoting laborious hours in designing and typesetting of the book.

Contents

AIIMS New Pattern 2019 Model Questions VIII
Most Recent Questions (AIIMS May 2019) XXXII
Video Questions XXXVIII

1 Cardiology   1–161

- Theory 2
- Image-based Questions 44
- Answers of Image-Based Questions 52
- Conceptual Diagnostic Algorithm 60
- Multiple Choice Questions 63
- Answers with Explanations 91

2 Neurology   163–321

- Theory 164
- Image-based Questions 193
- Answers of Image-Based Questions 198
- Conceptual Diagnostic Algorithm 203
- Multiple Choice Questions 205
- Answers with Explanations 237

3 Endocrinology   323–408

- Theory 324
- Image-based Questions 341
- Answers of Image-Based Questions 342
- Conceptual Diagnostic Algorithm 343
- Multiple Choice Questions 345
- Answers with Explanations 363

4 Respiratory System   409–506

- Theory 410
- Image-based Questions 429
- Answers of Image-Based Questions 432
- Conceptual Diagnostic Algorithm 435
- Multiple Choice Questions 436
- Answers with Explanations 460

5 Hepatology — 507–557

- Theory 508
- Image-based Questions 517
- Answers of Image-Based Questions 518
- Multiple Choice Questions 519
- Answers with Explanations 531

6 Gastroenterology — 559–607

- Theory 560
- Image-based Questions 570
- Answers of Image-Based Questions 571
- Multiple Choice Questions 572
- Answers with Explanations 583

7 Rheumatology — 609–673

- Theory 610
- Image-based Questions 621
- Answers of Image-Based Questions 623
- Conceptual Diagnostic Algorithm 625
- Multiple Choice Questions 626
- Answers with Explanations 641

8 Disorders of Kidney — 675–741

- Theory 676
- Image-based Questions 692
- Answers of Image-Based Questions 693
- Conceptual Diagnostic Algorithm 694
- Multiple Choice Questions 697
- Answers with Explanations 710

9 Hematology — 743–827

- Theory 744
- Image-based Questions 763
- Answers of Image-Based Questions 764
- Conceptual Diagnostic Algorithm 765
- Multiple Choice Questions 766
- Answers with Explanations 784

10 Fluids and Electrolytes — 829–863

- Theory 830
- Image-based Question 838
- Answer of Image-Based Question 838
- Conceptual Diagnostic Algorithm 839
- Multiple Choice Questions 842
- Answers with Explanations 848

11 Nutrition — 865–876

- Theory 866
- Multiple Choice Questions 868
- Answers with Explanations 871

12 Tumors — 877–900

- Theory 878
- Multiple Choice Questions 882
- Answers with Explanations 887

13 Genetics — 901–910

- Multiple Choice Questions 902
- Answers with Explanations 905

14 Infection — 911–952

- Theory 912
- Conceptual Diagnostic Algorithm 916
- Multiple Choice Questions 917
- Answers with Explanations 926

AIIMS NEW PATTERN 2019 MODEL QUESTIONS

EXTENDED MATCHING QUESTIONS

1. Causes of chest pain
a. Aortic dissection
b. Myocardial infarction
c. Angina pectoris
d. Pericarditis
e. Pulmonary embolism
f. Costochondritis
g. Gastroesophageal reflux disease
h. Spontaneous pneumothorax
i. Mediastinitis
j. Enlarging aortic aneurysm
k. Tension pneumothorax
l. Pleural Effusion
m. Pleurisy

For each presentation below, choose the SINGLE most likely cause from the above list of options.

(i) A 57-year-old man presents with sudden onset of severe and central chest pain radiating to the back. ECG shows ST segment elevation in lead V1-V6, I, aVL. The chest X-ray shows a widened mediastinum

Ans. (a) Aortic dissection

(ii) A 43-year-old 190 cm man post a flight to Chennai presents with left-sided chest discomfort and dyspnea. On chest X-ray, there is a small area devoid of lung markings in the apex of the left lung.

Ans. (h) Spontaneous pneumothorax

Spontaneous pneumothorax occurs from a rupture of an apical pleural bleb and is associated with tall, young males and also with aeroplane ascent.

(iii) A 52-year-old businessman with nephrotic syndrome after a non-stop flight from New York to New Delhi presents with sudden onset of breathlessness, haemoptysis, and chest pain. He is brought into Casualty in shock. His chest X-ray is normal. The ECG shows sinus tachycardia.

Ans. (e) Pulmonary embolism

Long distance air travel is contraindicated in patients with hypercoagulable state. Patients of nephrotic syndrome has a hypercoagulable state. This patient has developed pulmonary embolism. *Pulmonary embolism can present without the classic $S_1Q_3T_3$ ECG strain pattern. Leg findings may also present later and not initially.*

(iv) A 42-year-old man presents with central, crushing chest pain that radiates to the jaw. The pain occurred while jogging around the local park. The pain was alleviated with rest. The ECG is normal.

Ans. (c) Angina pectoris

Angina is aggravated by cold, by anxiety, and by exercise. In the case of a normal resting ECG, an exercise ECG should be obtained.

(v) A 53-year-old woman with ovarian tumor presents with breathlessness and right-sided chest pain. The chest X-ray shows obliteration of the right costophrenic angle.

Ans. (l) Pleural effusion

Ovarian carcinoma can be associated with a right-sided pleural effusion (Meigs syndrome).

2. The treatment of cardiac arrhythmias
a. Atropine 1 mg IV push
b. Implantable cardioverter defibrillator
c. CPR until a defibrillator is present
d. CPR, adrenaline 1:1000 IV push
e. Transvenous pacemaker
f. Defibrillate at 200 Joules
g. External pacemaker
h. Rescue PCI
i. Lignocaine IV
j. Morphine IM

For each patient below, choose the SINGLE most appropriate treatment from the above list of options. *The same option can be used twice.*

(i) A 62-year-old man presents with chest pain and shortness of breath. His ECG shows sinus bradycardia of 45 beats/min.

Ans. (a) Atropine 1 mg IV push

Atropine is given to patients with symptomatic bradycardia.

(ii) A 57-year-old woman is noted to have a slow heart rate. She is asymptomatic. ECG shows no relation between atrial and ventricular rhythm. The ventricular rhythm is 40 beats/min. the QRS complex is wide.

Ans. (e) Transvenous pacemaker

Third-degree AV block is managed with a transvenous pacemaker.

(iii) A 62-year-old man collapses in the street. The event is unwitnessed. He has no pulse.

Ans. (c) CPR until a defibrillator is present

(iv) A 32-year-old man involved in a high-speed RTA is found unconscious at the scene. He is breathing spontaneously. In Accident and emergency, the ECG monitor now shows an irregular rhythm and no P, QRS, ST, or T waves. The rate is rapid.

Ans. (c) CPR until a defibrillator is present

The patient is in ventricular fibrillation.

(v) A 53-year-old man presents to Casualty with severe chest pain. He has a history of angina. ECG shows ST elevation of 4 mm in leads V_1–V_4. Thrombolysis has been done but pain and ECG findings are persisting 90 minutes after start of thrombolysis

Ans. (h) Rescue PCI

3. **The treatment of Emergency admission**
   a. Intramuscular adrenaline
   b. Emergency tracheostomy
   c. Urgent endotracheal intubation
   d. Type and cross match blood
   e. Transfuse O negative blood and apply external fixator
   f. Transfer to burn unit
   g. Tetanus prophylaxis
   h. Intravenous antibiotics
   i. Intravenous dexamethasone
   j. Oxygen and nebulized salbutamol
   k. Take patient straight to theater

   For each case below, choose the SINGLE most likely diagnosis from the above list of options.

   (i) A 42-year-old pedestrian has been struck by a speeding car driven by a juvenile. She is brought into emergency wearing a pneumatic anti-shock garment for an extensive injury to her pelvis which is distorted. She is intubated with fluids running via two grey color cannulas. Her blood pressure is 120/60.

   Ans. (e) Transfuse O negative blood and apply external fixator

   This patient's chief concern will be massive blood loss. No delay should be taken to cross match blood. Blood should be transfused immediately. The blood pressure may be misleading, as she is wearing an anti-shock garment. An external fixator applied by the surgeons will aid in pelvic fracture stabilization and stem blood loss.

   (ii) A 10-year-old boy with smoke inhalation is brought into Casualty with worsening stridor. A face mask with 100% oxygen is covering his face, but his oxygen saturation continues to fall.

   Ans. (b) Emergency tracheostomy

   Due to hot smoke probably both the nasopharynx and oropharynx are compromised, and a tracheostomy to achieve an airway is essential.

   (iii) A 4-year-old girl asthmatic child is brought to casualty. She is not speaking and has fast shallow breathing with pulsus paradoxsus. ABG shows respiratory acidosis.

   Ans. (c) Urgent endotracheal intubation

   The child is having impending respiratory arrest due to severe exacerbation of asthma. Carbon dioxide narcosis will necessitate elective intubation and ventilation.

   (iv) An 18-year-old man presents with fever, drooling of saliva and stridor. His breathing becomes labored with use of accessory muscles. He becomes cyanotic. He initially presented to his GP with a sore throat a few days ago.

   Ans. (c) Urgent endotracheal intubation

   Glandular fever can present as acute airway obstruction. Death from glandular fever/Infectious mononucleosis occurs from failed endotracheal intubation. It is wise to have an ENT surgeon at hand to perform an emergency tracheostomy if necessary.

   (v) A 13-year-old known asthmatic presents with severe wheezing and a respiratory rate of 40. Her pulse rate is 120.

   Ans. (j) Oxygen and nebulized salbutamol

   An acute asthmatic attack is treated initially with oxygen and salbutamol. If necessary IV hydrocortisone is added.

4. **Causes of neurological signs**
   a. Middle cerebral artery infarction
   b. Anterior cerebral artery infarction
   c. Posterior cerebral artery infarction
   d. Vertebrobasilar ischemia
   e. Subacute combined degeneration of the cord
   f. Syringomyelia
   g. Cord compression
   h. Tabes dorsalis

   For each patient below, choose the SINGLE most likely cause from the above list of options.

   (i) A 52-year-old man presents with severe stabbing pains in his chest and limbs. He walks with a wide-based gait. On examination, he has ptosis and small, irregular pupils that react to accommodation but not to light. He has absent deep tendon reflexes and position sense.

   Ans. (h) Tabes dorsalis

   Tabes dorsalis is a manifestation of syphilis occurring 10-25 years after primary infection and results from degeneration of the dorsal columns and nerve roots. Argyll Robertson pupils are associated with syphilis.

   (ii) A 62-year-old man presents with urinary incontinence and contralateral paresis of the foot, leg and shoulder. He is awake but silent.

   Ans. (b) Anterior cerebral artery infarction

   Abulia, contralateral lower limb paresis, and urinary incontinence are all signs associated with the carotid system, i.e. involving the anterior cerebral artery.

   (iii) A 72-year-old man presents with contralateral hemisensory loss and paresis of conjugate gaze to the opposite side.

   Ans. (a) Middle cerebral artery infarction

   (iv) A 70-year-old man presents with dysarthria and intractable hiccups. On examination, he has nystagmus and is noted to have an ataxic gait.

   Ans. (d) Vertebrobasilar ischemia

   (v) A 42-year-old alcoholic man presents with numbness and tingling sensation in his feet. He is noted to have loss of vibration and position senses in his legs with loss of deep tendon reflexes. Full blood count reveals a macrocytic anemia.

   Ans. (e) Subacute combined degeneration of the cord

   Subacute combined degeneration of the cord is associated with vitamin B_{12} deficiency.

5. The management of head injuries
   a. Admit for neurological observation
   b. Assess adequacy of breathing
   c. Removal of penetrating object
   d. Discharge with head injury advice
   e. Detailed neurological assessment
   f. Airway assessment with cervical spine control
   g. Assess circulation and maintain adequate perfusion
   h. Neurosurgical consultation
   i. Obtain urgent CT scan of the head
   j. Intubate the patient
   k. Pronounce the patient as Brain dead

For each case below, choose the SINGLE most appropriate form of management from the above list of options.

(i) A 33-year-old cyclist is struck by a car in a head-on collision and arrives intubated to Emergency department. Upon arrival, his Glasgow Coma Scale is 3. He has fixed and dilated pupils with absent gag reflex and with absence of spontaneous breathing efforts. EEG shows isolated bursts along a flat line.

Ans. (k) Pronounce the patient as brain dead.
A Glasgow Coma Scale of 3 is the lowest score possible.

(ii) A 62-year-old man is brought to Accident and emergency following assault and battery to the head. He has a face mask and reservoir bag delivering 15 L/min of oxygen, a stiff cervical collar and is attached to an intravenous drip. He has no spontaneous eye opening except to pain, makes incomprehensible sounds, and does not obey commands. He demonstrates flexion withdrawal to painful stimuli. On suction, he has no gag reflex.

Ans. (j) Intubate the patient
A GCS of 8 or less or absence of a gag reflex are both indications for intubation.

(iii) A 22-year-old man involved in an RTA presents to Accident and Emergency with a large open scalp wound, multiple facial injuries and a deformed right tibia.

Ans. (f) Airway assessment with cervical spine control
No mention of airway management has been made and therefore should be included in the initial assessment of this patient.

(iv) A 42-year-old man is brought to Casualty with a knife impaled in his occiput.

Ans. (f) Airway assessment with cervical spine control
Penetrating objects should be left in situ until surgery. Again, airway assessment is always the first priority in management of head injuries.

(v) A 32-year-old female involved in an RTA with multiple injuries is brought to casualty intubated with adequate oxygen delivery. Her blood pressure is noted to be 80/50 with a pulse of 120.

Ans. (g) Assess circulation and maintain adequate perfusion
Hypotension should not be assumed to be caused by brain injury.

6. Theme: Investigation of Neurological illness
   a. Blood culture
   b. Blood glucose
   c. Lumbar puncture
   d. CT scan of head
   e. Mantoux test
   f. Electroencephalogram
   g. Complete blood count
   h. Chest X-ray
   i. Urea and electrolytes
   j. Blood alcohol level
   k. Toxicology
   l. Skull X-ray

For each presentation below, choose the SINGLE most ACCURATE investigation from the above list of options.

(i) A 56-year-old man who is a known case of Chronic kidney disease presents with sweating, tremors, drowsiness alternating with agitation. His wife denies any history of alcoholism.

Ans. (b) Blood glucose
The presentation is one of hypoglycemia.

(ii) A 12-year-old girl is brought to the emergency Department by her parents complaining of a persistent rash, photophobia, and neck pain. What is the first investigation to be performed?

Ans. (a) Blood culture
Lumbar puncture is the investigation of choice for meningitis. However, intravenous antibiotic therapy should not be delayed to secure a diagnosis and a blood culture should be taken prior to it. The first investigation in suspected bacterial meningitis is blood culture.

(iii) A 17-year-old college student has recurrent myoclonic jerks. He has no history of drug abuse

Ans (f) Electroencephalogram

(iv) A 40-year-old Known case of ADPKD is having bradycardia and ECG shows broad QRS complexes with absent P waves.

Ans. (i) Urea and electrolytes
The broad qRS complex with absent P waves in a patient of renal failure points to diagnosis of hyperkalemia. Hence KFT and serum electrolytes should be checked.

(v) A 35-year-old professional boxer presents with headache, drowsiness, seizures, and a rising blood pressure.

Ans. (d) CT scan of head

7. Investigation of F.U.O
   a. Hemoglobin
   b. Full blood count
   c. Erythrocyte sedimentation rate
   d. Lymph node biopsy
   e. HRCT
   f. Stool cultures

g. Mantoux test
  h. Monospot
  i. Echocardiography for vegetations
  j. CT Guided Chest Biopsy
  k. HIV antibody titers

For each presentation below, choose the SINGLE most ACCURATE investigation from the above list of options.

(i) A 17-year-old boy presents with a 2-week history of fever, malaise, and cervical lymphadenopathy. On examination, he has tenderness in the right upper quadrant of his abdomen and has yellow sclera.

Ans. (h) Monospot

Infectious mononucleosis is associated with hepatitis.

(ii) A 28-year-old male drug addict presents with a low-grade fever, malaise, a change in heart murmur and pea shaped nodes in the finger pulp.

Ans. (i) Echocardiography for vegetations

This is a case of subacute bacterial endocarditis.

(iii) A 57-year-old man presents with a 2-month history of unilateral enlargement of his right tonsil, fluctuating pyrexia, and multiple neck nodes.

Ans. (d) Lymph node biopsy

Unilateral enlargement of the tonsil may either be associated with quinsy, lymphoma, or carcinoma. Fluctuating fever and the absence of pain suggest a diagnosis of lymphoma.

(iv) A 27-year-old woman presents with fever, malaise, erythema nodosum, and polyarthralgia. Chest X-ray reveals mediastinal hilar lymphadenopathy.

Ans. (j) CT Guided Chest Biopsy

The patient is having classical features of sarcoidosis for which CT Chest Guided Biopsy is useful.

(v) A 31-year-old intravenous drug abuser presents with fever and a neck node discharging a cheesy, malodorous substance.

Ans. (g) Mantoux test

Scrofula is a sign of tuberculosis for which the Mantoux test is diagnostic.

8. The treatment of meningitis
  a. Benzylpenicillin
  b. Chloramphenicol
  c. Ampicillin
  d. Isoniazid, Rifampicin, Ethambutol and Pyrazinamide
  e. Amphotericin B and flucytosine
  f. Gentamicin
  g. Erythromycin
  h. Ceftriaxone plus Vancomycin
  i. Oral Ciprofloxacin
  j. Vancomycin
  k. Supportive

For each case below, choose the SINGLE most appropriate treatment from the above list of options.

(i) A 3-year-old girl presents with acute onset of pyrexia, nausea, and vomiting. Lumbar puncture reveals high protein and polymorph count and low glucose. Gram-negative bacilli are present in the smear and culture.

Ans. (h) Ceftriaxone Plus Vancomycin

Children under 5 are at risk as they do not develop specific antibodies against *H. influenzae* until after the age of 5.

(ii) A 43-year-old man presents with fever and meningeal signs. His lumbar puncture reveals 200 mononuclear cells/mm^3, 2 g/l of protein and a glucose level half his plasma level.

Ans. (d) Isoniazid, Rifampicin, Ethambutol and Pyrazinamide

- Tuberculous meningitis
- Meningeal signs and presence of mononuclear cells with elevated protein indicates tubercular etiology.

(iii) A 17-year-old girl presents with fever, odd behavior, purpura, and conjunctival petechiae. Her lumbar puncture reveals gram-negative cocci.

Ans. (h) Ceftriaxone plus Vancomycin

The clinical diagnosis is Meningococcal meningitis and empirical ceftriaxone is started with vancomycin.

Indication	Antibiotic
Preterm infants to infants <1 month	Ampicillin + cefotaxime
Infants 1-3 months	Ampicillin + cefotaxime or ceftriaxone
Immunocompetent children >3 months and adults <55 years	Cefotaxime, ceftriaxone, or cefepime + vancomycin
Adults >55 years and adults of any age with alcoholism or other debilitating illnesses	Ampicillin + cefotaxime, ceftriaxone or cefepime + vancomycin
Hospital-acquired meningitis, post-traumatic or postneurosurgery meningitis, neutropenic patients, or patients with impaired cell-mediated immunity	Ampicillin + ceftazidime or meropenem + vancomycin

(iv) A 24-year-old man presents with fever, headache, and drowsiness. His lumbar puncture reveals 1000 mononuclear cells/mm^3, 0.5 g/l of protein and a glucose greater than 2/3 of his plasma glucose level. Organisms are absent.

Ans. (k) Supportive

Viral meningitis

(v) The 28-year-old husband of a patient admitted with pyogenic meningococcal meningitis admits to having oral contact with his wife and is anxious.

Ans. (i) Oral Ciprofloxacin

Oral Ciprofloxacin is the recognized prophylactic treatment for close contacts.

9. Investigation of autoimmune disorders
a. Antinuclear antibody
b. Gastric parietal cell antibody
c. Smooth muscle antibody
d. Antibody to mitochondria
e. Thyroglobulin antibodies
f. Antiacetylcholine receptor antibodies
g. Antinuclear cytoplasmic antibody
h. Antibody to reticulin
i. Antibody to platelets
j. Rheumatoid factor

For each presentation below, choose the SINGLE most ACCURATE investigation from the above list of options.

(i) A 46-year-old woman presents with stiff, deformed fingers, and MCP joint swelling worse in the morning.

Ans. (j) Rheumatoid factor

Rheumatoid arthritis

(ii) A 25-year-old woman presents with diplopia, ptosis, and is unable to count to 50 without her voice tiring. She complains of muscle fatigue.

Ans. (f) Antiacetylcholine receptor antibodies

The clinical diagnosis is myasthenia gravis.

(iii) A 22-year-old woman presents with a plethora of signs and symptoms. She complains of arthralgia, depression, alopecia, fits, oral ulceration, and facial rash. She is found to have proteinuria and a normocytic normochromic anemia.

Ans. (a) Antinuclear antibody

Systemic lupus erythematosus

(iv) A 43-year-old man presents with a septal perforation, proteinuria, and hypertension.

Ans. (g) Antinuclear cytoplasmic antibody

Wegener's granulomatosis.

(v) A 52-year-old man presents with vitamin B_{12} deficiency and peripheral neuritis.

Ans. (b) Gastric parietal cell antibody

Pernicious anemia.

10. Diagnosis of Cardiac conditions
a. Anterolateral myocardial infarction
b. Left ventricular failure
c. Atrial fibrillation
d. Acute pulmonary embolism
e. Acute pericarditis
f. Mitral stenosis
g. Right ventricular failure
h. Hypokalemia
i. Hypocalcemia
j. Aortic regurgitation
k. Inferolateral myocardial infarction

For each presentation below, choose the SINGLE most likely diagnosis from the above list of options.

(i) A 62-year-old man presents with chest pain radiating down the left arm. His 12-lead electrocardiogram reveals Q waves in II, III and aVF with T wave changes in V5 and V6.

Ans. (k) Inferolateral myocardial infarction

The T wave changes in V5 and V6 suggest a lateral component to the inferior MI.

(ii) A 53-year-old woman presents with a fast rate with an irregular rhythm. There are no P waves on the electrocardiogram. She states that she has lost weight recently and is feeling nervous all the time.

Ans. (c) Atrial fibrillation

Atrial fibrillation is associated with hyperthyroidism.

(iii) On auscultation, a patient is noted to have a rumbling diastolic murmur at the apex. The murmur is accentuated during exercise.

Ans. (f) Mitral stenosis

(iv) A 62-year-old man on digitalis and diuretics presents with weakness and lethargy. His electrocardiogram shows flat T waves and prominent U waves.

Ans. (h) Hypokalemia

Hypokalemia is a recognized complication of diuretic use.

(v) A 67-year-old man with chronic bronchitis presents with a raised jugular venous pressure, hepatomegaly, ankle and sacral edema.

Ans. (g) Right ventricular failure

11. Investigation of a collapsed patient
a. Blood glucose
b. Full blood count
c. Computed tomography scan of the head
d. Electrocardiogram
e. Chest X-ray
f. Lumbar puncture
g. Urea and electrolytes
h. Pelvic ultrasound
i. Thyroid function tests
j. Ultrasound abdomen
k. Urine pregnancy test

For each presentation below, choose the SINGLE most ACCURATE investigation from the above list of options.

(i) A 22-year-old college student presents to the Emergency Department after collapsing at school. Her last menstrual period was 3 weeks ago and lasted 3 days. She is anxious. Her pulse is irregular and rapid.

Ans. (i) Thyroid function tests

The diagnosis is likely to be hyperthyroidism.

(ii) A 16-year-old female presents to her GP after collapsing she is noted to be febrile with a purpuric rash that does not blanch on pressure.

Ans. (f) Lumbar puncture
- Meningococcal meningitis is the most likely cause for this girl's collapse.

(iii) A 24-year-old female presents to her GP after collapsing at home. She reports nausea which gets worse in the morning. Her last menstrual period was 5 weeks ago.

Ans. (k) Urine pregnancy test

(iv) A 62-year-old female is brought into the Emergency Department after collapsing at home. Her thighs show evidence of lipoatrophy and her shins of necrobiosis lipoidica.

Ans. (a) Blood glucose

(v) A 33-year-old man presents to Casualty after collapsing on the cricket pitch. He takes carbamazepine. There is a hematoma over his right temple.

Ans. (c) Computed tomography scan of the head
- An urgent CT scan is required to exclude intracranial haemorrhage.

12. **Investigation of acute abdomen**
    a. Ultrasound abdomen
    b. Rectal examination
    c. Upper GI endoscopy
    d. Barium meal
    e. Sigmoidoscopy
    f. Colonoscopy
    g. Computed tomography scan of the abdomen
    h. KUB X-ray
    i. Pelvic ultrasound
    j. Laparoscopy
    k. Erect chest X-ray

For each presentation below, choose the SINGLE most ACCURATE investigation from the above list of options.

(i) A 63-year-old man complains of severe colicky pain from his right flank radiating to his groin. His urine analysis reveals trace blood cells.

Ans. (h) KUB X-ray
- The presentation is suggestive of ureteric colic.

(ii) A 28-year-old woman complains of severe lower abdominal pain and increasing abdominal girth. Her urine hCG is negative.

Ans. (i) Pelvic ultrasound
- The presentation is suggestive of ovarian cyst.

(iii) A 62-year-old obese man complains of severe epigastric pain which is relieved by eating and is worse at night.

Ans. (c) Upper GI endoscopy
- The presentation is suggestive of peptic ulcer disease.

(iv) A 67-year-old hypertensive man presents with lower abdominal pain and back pain. An expansive abdominal mass is palpated lateral and superior to the umbilicus.

Ans. (a) Ultrasound abdomen
- The presentation is suggestive of abdominal aortic aneurysm. The size should be evaluated by ultrasound and surgical repair is advisable if the aneurysm is greater than 5 cm in diameter.

(v) An 83-year-old woman suffering from rheumatoid arthritis presents with severe epigastric pain and vomiting. She also complains of shoulder tip pain.

Ans. (k) Erect chest X-ray
- Steroid usage for rheumatoid arthritis puts this woman at risk for a perforated peptic ulcer.

13. **Causes of hypertension**
    a. Coarctation of the aorta
    b. Cushings syndrome
    c. Pheochromocytoma
    d. Primary hyperaldosteronism
    e. Polyarteritis nodosa
    f. Polycystic kidneys
    g. Acromegaly
    h. Preeclampsia
    i. Essential hypertension
    j. Renal artery stenosis
    k. Chronic glomerulonephritis

For each presentation below, choose the SINGLE most likely cause from the above list of options.

(i) A 47-year-old obese woman presents with hypertension and muscle cramps. She is noted to have proximal myopathy, and osteoporosis. She has Hypokalemia with elevated blood sugar levels.

Ans. (b) Cushings syndrome

(ii) A 37-year-old man presents with development of thick speech, hypertension and Spade like hands. His glucose tolerance curve is diabetic.

Ans. (g) Acromegaly
- Spade like hands are a characteristic feature of acromegaly along with impaired glucose tolerance.

(iii) A 48-year-old woman with disproportionately long limbs presents with hypertension. Her blood pressure is different on both arms and lower in the legs.

Ans. (a) Coarctation of the aorta

(iv) A 42-year-old man post thyroidectomy for medullary thyroid carcinoma presents with hypertension and complains of attacks of severe headache and palpitations. He is noted to have glycosuria.

Ans. (c) Pheochromocytoma

(v) A 53-year-old man presents with hypertension, haematuria, and abdominal pain. A large kidney is palpated on exam, and the diagnosis is confirmed on ultrasound.

Ans. (f) Polycystic kidneys

14. **Causes of peripheral neuritis**
    a. Carcinomatous neuropathy
    b. Side-effect of drug therapy
    c. Diabetic neuropathy
    d. Vitamin B_{12} deficiency
    e. Vitamin B_1 deficiency
    f. Polyarteritis nodosa
    g. Guillain-Barré syndrome
    h. Amyloidosis
    i. Sarcoidosis

For each patient below, choose the SINGLE most likely diagnosis from the above list of options.

(i) A 53-year-old man presents with distal sensory neuropathy affecting the lower limbs in a 'stocking' distribution and is noted to have Charcot's joints. The ankle reflex is absent.

Ans. (c) Diabetic neuropathy

(ii) A 57-year-old man who drinks heavily presents with numbness and paresthesia in his feet. He complains of 'walking on cotton wool'.

Ans. (e) Vitamin B_1 deficiency

(iii) A 42-year-old man, who is being treated with chemotherapy for lymphoma, presents with peripheral paresthesia, loss of deep tendon reflexes, and abdominal bloating.

Ans. (b) Side-effect of drug therapy

(iv) A 47-year-old woman presents with peripheral neuropathy. She is noted to have bilateral hilar gland enlargement on chest X-ray and a negative mantoux test. She also suffers from polyarthralgia and has tender red, raised lesions on her shin.

Ans. (i) Sarcoidosis

(v) A 27-year-old man presents with paresthesia followed by a flaccid paralysis of his limbs and face. He has a history of a recent upper respiratory tract infection. Bladder is spared.

Ans. (g) Guillain-Barré syndrome

15. **Diagnosis of Lung diseases**
    a. Pneumoconiosis
    b. Cystic fibrosis
    c. Mycoplasma pneumonia
    d. Adult respiratory distress syndrome
    e. Pulmonary contusion
    f. Carcinoma of the bronchus
    g. Pancoast tumor
    h. Bilateral bronchopneumonia
    i. Sarcoidosis
    j. Tuberculosis

For each case below, choose the SINGLE most likely diagnosis from the above list of options.

(i) A 33-year-old woman presents with fever, pharyngitis, and cough. The chest X-ray shows widespread, bilateral, patchy consolidation. Cold agglutinins are detected.

Ans. (c) Mycoplasma pneumonia

Cold hemagglutinins are associated with 50% of untreated Mycoplasma pneumoniae infection and a titer of 1:64 supports the diagnosis.

(ii) A 42-year-old alcoholic presents with repeated small hemoptysis and cough with mucoid sputum. His chest X-ray shows right upper lobe consolidation and a large central cavity. His Mantoux test is strongly positive.

Ans. (j) Tuberculosis

(iii) A 62-year-old man presents with dyspnea and cough. The X-ray shows extensive pulmonary fibrosis, bilateral pleural thickening, and pleural calcification.

Ans. (a) Pneumoconiosis

(iv) A 14-year-old boy presents with repeated lower respiratory infections. On examination he is noted to have finger clubbing and suffers from weight loss and steatorrhea. The X-ray shows bronchial wall thickening, ring shadows of bronchiectasis, and wide-spread ill-defined shadowing.

Ans. (b) Cystic fibrosis

(v) A 44-year-old man presents with cough and haemoptysis. The X-ray shows a right hilar mass and a patch of consolidation in the right upper lobe laterally.

Ans. (f) Carcinoma of the bronchus

16. **The treatment of hypertension**
    a. Atenolol
    b. Thiazide
    c. Furosemide
    d. Methyldopa
    e. Amlodipine
    f. Nifedipine
    g. Hydralazine
    h. Captopril
    i. Sodium nitroprusside
    j. Lisinopril
    k. D.A.S.H (Dietary approaches to stop Hypertension)

For each patient below, choose the SINGLE most appropriate treatment from the above list of options.

(i) A 63-year-old man presents with a BP of 165/95. He is asymptomatic, and all his investigations are normal.

Ans. (k) (D.A.S.H) Dietary approaches to stop Hypertension

Weight loss and salt restriction are advocated initially.

(ii) A 47-year-old insulin-dependent diabetic presents to his GP with a BP of 170/110. His blood pressure is consistently high on subsequent visits despite conservative measures. His blood tests are normal.

Ans. (j) Lisinopril

(iii) A 60-year-old patient with bronze diabetes presents to his GP with a BP of 180/120. Which drug is absolutely contraindicated for this patient?

Ans. (a) Atenolol

Beta blockers are *contraindicated* in diabetics.

(iv) A 62-year-old man is brought into ER complaining of severe headaches. On arrival he has a seizure. His BP is noted to be 220/140, and on fundoscopic exam, there is papilledema.

Ans. (i) Sodium nitroprusside

(v) A 68-year-old man on atenolol 100 mg OD continues to have a diastolic blood pressure of 115. He also takes allopurinol. Which is absolutely contraindicated?

Ans. (b) Thiazides

Since the patient is on allopurinol, diuretics can trigger attack of acute gout.

17. The treatment of respiratory diseases
a. Erythromycin
b. Tetracycline
c. Vancomycin
d. Azithromycin
e. Cefotaxime
f. Prednisolone
g. Rifampicin, isoniazid, pyridoxine and ethambutol
h. Isoniazid alone
i. Cotrimoxazole
j. Salbutamol inhaler
k. Ciprofloxacin

For each case below, choose the SINGLE most appropriate treatment from the above list of options.

(i) A 23-year-old woman presents with a week's history of fever, rigors, and productive, rusty cough. The X-ray shows a left lower lobe consolidation.

Ans. (d) Azithromycin

First line drug for community acquired pneumonia is Azithromycin. The decision to give OPD or IPD treatment is based on CURB-65 Score.

(ii) A 12-year-old boy with cystic fibrosis presents with a persistent productive cough. The X-ray shows a spherical shadow containing a central lucency. An air-fluid level is also seen.

Ans. (c) Vancomycin

(iii) A 52-year-old man presents with shortness of breath and dry cough. The X-ray shows wide-spread pulmonary shadowing. He takes azathioprine for resistant rheumatoid arthritis.

Ans. (i) Cotrimoxazole

Due to intake of azathioprine, his immunity is reduced and therefore he has high risk of developing Pneumocystis Jiroveci pneumonia.

(iv) A 23-year-old female presents with malaise, cough and progressive shortness of breath. The X-ray shows symmetrical lobulated bilateral hilar gland enlargement.

Ans. (f) Prednisolone

Sarcoidosis is treated with steroid therapy.

(v) A 50-year-old diabetic presents with a productive cough and malaise. The X-ray shows right upper lobe consolidation and hilar lymphadenopathy.

Ans. (g) Rifampicin, isoniazid, pyridoxine and ethambutol

18. Diagnosis of Hepatobiliary disorders
a. Cholestatic jaundice
b. Hepatitis A
c. Haemolytic jaundice
d. Criggler-Najjar syndrome
e. Gilbert's syndrome
f. Chronic active hepatitis
g. Hepatitis B
h. Alcoholic hepatitis
i. Leptospirosis
j. Primary biliary cirrhosis

For each patient below, choose the SINGLE most likely diagnosis from the above list of options.

(i) A 22-year-old man presents with mild jaundice following an upper respiratory tract infection. On fasting, his bilirubin level is high.

Ans. (e) Gilbert's syndrome

High bilirubin on fasting is diagnostic of Gilbert's syndrome, an inherited metabolic disorder leading to increased unconjugated hyperbilirubinemia.

(ii) A 35-year-old woman presents with photosensitivity, abdominal pain, increasing jaundice, and arthralgia. She is noted to have hepatosplenomegaly. She recently donated blood. She is found to have an increase in both conjugated and unconjugated bilirubin.

Ans. (f) Chronic active hepatitis

The presence of photosensitivity in a female with joint pains is suggestive of autoimmune process. Lupoid Chronic Hepatitis presents in young females with inflammation of the liver for at least 3-6 months.

(iii) A 38-year-old IVDA has developed cellulitis and was prescribed Amoxicillin Clavulanic acid by the intern. He now presents with jaundice, pale stools, and dark urine.

Ans. (a) Cholestatic jaundice
- Amoxicillin Clavulanic is associated with cholestatic jaundice.

(iv) A 47-year-old woman presents with pruritis, jaundice and pigmentation. Both the liver and spleen are palpable. Investigations reveal a high alkaline phosphatase and a high bilirubin.

Ans. (j) Primary biliary cirrhosis
- Primary biliary cirrhosis is a progressive nonsuppurative cholangiohepatitis with destruction of the small interlobular bile ducts.

(v) A 57-year-old man presents with pale stool and jaundice. Three days earlier he had fever, malaise, vomiting, and upper abdominal discomfort associated with tender enlargement of the liver.

Ans. (b) Hepatitis A
- The presentation is one of hepatitis A which can be acquired through the fecal-oral route.

19. Causes of arthritis
a. Gout
b. Rheumatoid arthritis
c. Psoriatic Arthropathy
d. Pyrophosphate arthropathy
e. Ankylosing spondylitis
f. Reiter's syndrome
g. Systemic lupus erythematosus
h. Hyperparathyroidism
i. Osteoarthritis
j. Hemochromatosis
k. Gonococcal arthritis

For each patient below, choose the SINGLE most likely cause from the above list of options.

(i) A 22-year-old man after a casual sexual encounter presents with urethritis and a swollen painful wrist.

Ans. (k) Gonococcal arthritis
- Gonococcal arthritis has predilection for upper extremity joints. This helps differentiate between Reiter's syndrome, which predominantly affects the lower extremity joints.

(ii) A 27-year-old man returning from Bangkok after a sex tourism trip presents with urethritis, conjunctivitis, and a swollen left knee.

Ans. (f) Reiter's syndrome
- The triad of symptoms are classic for Reiter's syndrome one of the spondyloarthritides.

(iii) A 53-year-old woman complains of stiffness in her fingers worse at the end of the day. The DIP joints and the first metacarpophalangeal joints are affected.

Ans. (i) Osteoarthritis
- Osteoarthritis is also associated with Heberden nodes of the DIP joints.

(iv) A 23-year-old man presents with morning stiffness, sacroiliitis, and iritis.

Ans. (e) Ankylosing spondylitis

(v) A 24-year-old man presents with a red, hot, swollen metatarsal phalangeal joint, sacroiliitis, and onycholysis.

Ans. (c) Psoriatic Arthropathy
- Psoriatic Arthropathy also has predilection for the upper extremity joints. It can present in the toes and fingers as sausage digits. However, the skin and nail changes help to differentiate this condition from gout or rheumatoid arthritis.

20. Investigation of vomiting
a. Complete blood count
b. Chest X-ray
c. Plasma cortisol level
d. CT scan of head
e. Serum calcium
f. Urea and electrolytes
g. Ultrasound abdomen
h. Urinary porphobilinogen and δ-Aminolevulinic acid
i. Thyroid function tests

For each presentation below, choose the SINGLE most ACCURATE investigation from the above list of options.

(i) A 62-year-old man on insulin presents with itching, nausea, and vomiting. He is noted to have peripheral edema and normocytic anemia.

Ans. (f) Urea and electrolytes
- Chronic renal failure.

(ii) A 52-year-old woman with known breast carcinoma presents acutely with nausea, vomiting, polydipsia, confusion, and drowsiness.

Ans. (e) Serum calcium
- Hypercalcemia associated with bone metastases.

(iii) A 33-year-old man with Hodgkin's disease presents with an insidious onset of weakness, weight loss, nausea, and vomiting. He is noted to have hyperpigmented hand creases.

Ans. (c) Plasma cortisol level
- Chronic adrenal insufficiency

(iv) A 32-year-old woman started on oral contraceptives presents acutely with abdominal pain, vomiting, tachycardia, hypertension and peripheral neuropathy.

Ans. (h) Urinary porphobilinogen and δ-Aminolevulinic acid
- Acute intermittent porphyria from ingestion of the oral contraceptive pill.

(v) A 33-year-old man involved in a RTA presents acutely with severe epigastric pain, left shoulder pain, vomiting and has no bowel sounds on abdominal examination.

Ans. (b) Chest X-ray
- Perforated peptic ulcer with peritoneal signs.

21. Causes of pneumonia
   a. Chlamydia Psittaci
   b. Pneumocystis carinii
   c. Mycoplasma pneumoniae
   d. Tuberculosis
   e. Coxiella burnetii
   f. Aspergillosis
   g. Actinomycosis
   h. Streptococcus pneumoniae
   i. Staphylococcus aureus
   j. Pseudomonas aeruginosa
   k. Legionella pneumophila

For each presentation below, choose the SINGLE most likely causative organism from the above list of options.

(i) A 37-year-old pet-shop owner presents with high fever, excruciating headache, and a dry hacking cough. The X-ray shows patchy consolidation.

Ans. (a) Chlamydia psittaci

(ii) A 43-year-old man who works in an abattoir presents with a sudden onset of fever, myalgia, headache, dry cough, and chest pain. The X-ray shows patchy consolidation of the right lower lobe, giving a ground-glass appearance.

Ans. (e) Coxiella burnetii

(iii) A 47-year-old travelling insurance salesman presents with high fever, myalgia, abdominal pain, and haemoptysis. The X-ray shows diffuse, patchy, lobar shadows. The cough progresses from a modest non-productive cough to producing mucopurulent sputum. The fever persists for 2 weeks.

Ans. (k) Legionella pneumophila

(iv) A 33-year-old man with HIV presents with a productive cough and haemoptysis. The X-ray shows a round-ball in the right upper lobe surrounded by a dome of air.

Ans. (f) Aspergillosis

(v) A 72-year-old woman presents with confusion and productive cough. The X-ray shows right lower lobe consolidation.

Ans. (h) Streptococcus pneumoniae

22. Causes of splenomegaly
   a. Typhoid
   b. Gaucher's disease
   c. Malaria
   d. Schistosomiasis
   e. Lymphoma
   f. Leishmaniasis
   g. Idiopathic thrombocytopenic purpura
   h. Polycythaemia Rubra Vera
   i. Felty's syndrome
   j. Leptospirosis
   k. Chronic myeloid leukaemia

For each case below, choose the SINGLE most likely cause from the above list of options.

(i) A 2-year-old child with recurrent nose bleeds is found to have massive splenomegaly

Ans. (b) Gaucher's disease

At onset, patients with type 1 Gaucher disease commonly present with painless splenomegaly, anemia, or thrombocytopenia. They may also have chronic fatigue, hepatomegaly (with or without abnormal liver function test findings), bone pain, or pathologic fractures and may bruise easily because of thrombocytopenia.

(ii) A 23-year-old man presents acutely with fever, jaundice, purpura, injected conjunctiva, and painful calves after swimming outdoors.

Ans. (j) Leptospirosis

(iii) A 27-year-old man from Bihar presents with intermittent fevers, cough, diarrhoea, epistaxis and massive splenomegaly.

Ans. (f) Leishmaniasis

(iv) A 22-year-old female presents with epistaxis and easy bruising. Her spleen is noted to be enlarged.

Ans. (g) Idiopathic Thrombocytopenic purpura

(v) A 63-year-old female with rheumatoid arthritis presents with splenomegaly. Her full blood count shows a white count of 1500/mm^3.

Ans. (i) Felty's syndrome

Felty's syndrome is the triad of Rheumatoid arthritis, splenomegaly, and leucopenia.

23. Causes of haematuria
   a. Ureteric calculus
   b. Acute pyelonephritis
   c. Benign Prostatic hypertrophy
   d. Acute cystitis
   e. Malaria
   f. Renal cell cancer
   g. Bladder carcinoma
   h. Bilharzia
   i. Prostate carcinoma
   j. Renal vein thrombosis
   k. Acute intermittent porphyria

For each of the cases below, choose the SINGLE most likely cause from the above list of options.

(i) A 62-year-old man presents with intermittent colicky loin pain and night sweats. He is noted to have a left sided varicocele and peripheral edema. He admits to loss of energy and weight loss.

Ans. (f) Renal cell Cancer

(ii) An 20-year-old female started on oral contraceptives complains of colicky abdominal pain, vomiting and fever.

Her urine is positive for red blood cells and protein. She develops progressive weakness in her extremities.

Ans. (k) Acute intermittent porphyria

(iii) A 27-year-old woman presents with fever and tachycardia. On examination the renal angle is very tender. Her urine is cloudy and blood-stained.

Ans. (b) Acute pyelonephritis

(iv) A 42-year-old man complains of severe colicky loin pain that radiates to his scrotum. He is noted to have microscopic haematuria. No masses are palpated.

Ans. (a) Ureteric calculus

(v) A 63-year-old man complains of increased frequency of micturition with suprapubic ache. The urine is cloudy and mahogany brown in color.

Ans. (d) Acute cystitis

24. Causes of haematemesis
a. Chronic peptic ulceration
b. Gastritis
c. Oesophageal varices
d. Mallory-Weiss syndrome
e. Carcinoma of the oesophagus
f. G.I.S.T
g. Haemophilia
h. Epistaxis
i. Angiodysplasia
j. Peutz-Jegher syndrome
k. Ehlers-Danlos syndrome

For each case below, choose the SINGLE most likely cause from the above list of options

(i) A 67-year-old man presents with haematemesis. He is noted to have an enlarged liver with irregular borders

Ans. (f) G.I.S.T

Gastrointestinal stromal tumour presents with hematemesis and if malignant can spread to liver leading to hepatomegaly with irregular liver borders.

(ii) A 42-year-old obese man presents with projectile haematemesis after ingestion of a five-course meal and wine.

Ans. (d) Mallory-Weiss syndrome

(iii) A 53-year-old man presents with massive haematemesis. He is noted to have freckles on his lower lips.

Ans. (k) Ehlers-Danlos syndrome

(iv) A 62-year-old alcoholic man presents with massive haematemesis and shock. He is noted to have finger clubbing and ascites.

Ans. (c) Oesophageal varices

(v) A 73-year-old man with chronic hoarseness presents with retrosternal chest pain and haematemesis. He has a history of achalasia and has lost 10 kg weight

Ans. (e) Carcinoma of the oesophagus

25. Causes of abnormal ECG
a. Hypokalemia
b. Hyperkalaemia
c. Hypocalcemia
d. Hypercalcemia
e. Myocardial ischemia
f. Inferior myocardial infarction
g. Acute pulmonary embolism
h. Acute pericarditis
i. Atrial fibrillation
j. Myxedema
k. Digitalis intoxication
l. Inferolateral myocardial infarction

For each cases below, choose the SINGLE most likely cause of ECG changes from the above list of options.

(i) A 63-year-old woman taking frusemide is noted to have 'U' waves in leads V3 and V4.

Ans. (a) Hypokalemia

Hypokalemia is associated with the use of loop diuretics.

(ii) A 52-year-old man presents with fever and chest pain. He has a history of angina. His ECG reveals concave elevation of the ST segments in leads II, V5 and V6.

Ans. (h) Acute pericarditis

ST elevation with Convexity is seen in MI, whereas here the elevation is concave which is associated with acute pericarditis.

(iii) A 57-year-old man presents with chest pain and dyspnea. His ECG reveals deep Q waves in leads III and aVF and inverted 'T' waves in leads V1-3.

Ans. (g) Acute pulmonary embolism

The ECG shows classical findings of $S_1Q_3T_3$ seen in cases of pulmonary embolism.

(iv) A 58-year-old woman who has undergone thyroidectomy is noted to have an ECG with a QT interval of 0.50

Ans. (c) Hypocalcemia

Hypocalcemia is a recognised complication of thyroidectomy.

(v) A 63-year-old woman presents with hoarseness. She is a smoker and is on Prozac. Her pulse rate is 44/min, and her ECG is noted for sinus bradycardia and reduced amplitude of P, QRS and T waves in all leads.

Ans. (j) Myxedema

The presence of low voltage ECG with bradycardia and hoarseness of voice points to clinical diagnosis of myxedema.

26. The treatment of medical emergencies
   a. Cardioversion
   b. Cricothyroidotomy
   c. Needle thoracocentesis
   d. Needle pericardiocentesis
   e. Insertion of chest drain
   f. Endotracheal intubation
   g. Defibrillation
   h. Needle aspiration
   i. Intravenous heparin
   j. Intramuscular adrenaline
   k. Intravenous aminophylline

For each of the cases below, choose the SINGLE most appropriate treatment from the above list of options.

(i) A 47-year-old woman after eating a pain killer tablet presents with acute dyspnea and stridor. Her tongue is swollen.

Ans. (j) Intramuscular adrenaline

- Anaphylaxis is treated with a prompt injection of 1 ml of 1:1000 adrenaline intramuscularly. This may need to be repeated.

(ii) A 22-year-old student presents with respiratory distress and pleuritic pain. On examination, he has distended neck veins and no breath sounds over the right lung field.

Ans. (c) Needle Thoracocentesis

- Tension pneumothorax requires emergency needle decompression.

(iii) A 32-year-old man presents with chest pain. He has distended neck veins and muffled heart sounds. His blood pressure is 80/50.

Ans. (d) Needle pericardiocentesis

- Cardiac tamponade requires swift needle pericardiocentesis.

(iv) A 53-year-old woman presents with stridor and difficulty swallowing following thyroidectomy. On examination, she has a tense swelling over the surgical site.

Ans. (h) Needle aspiration

- This woman presents with a postoperative hematoma that needs urgent drainage, as it is now compressing her trachea.

(v) A 32-year-old female presents with acute dyspnea and pleuritic pain. Her regular medications include salbutamol inhaler and an oral contraceptive. Her respiratory rate is 30, with a small volume rapid pulse rate of 110 and a blood pressure of 80/50. She has a raised jugular venous pressure. The chest X-ray is normal. Her electrocardiogram shows sinus tachycardia.

Ans. (i) Intravenous heparin

- This woman is at risk for a deep venous thrombosis and pulmonary embolism. Occasionally the signs of deep venous thrombosis appear after the pulmonary embolism which can make diagnosis difficult.

27. Diagnosis of named syndromes
   a. Pendred syndrome
   b. Patterson-Kelly syndrome
   c. Plummer-Vinson syndrome
   d. Reiter's syndrome
   e. Waterhouse-Friderichsen syndrome
   f. Sheehan syndrome
   g. Peutz-Jeghers syndrome
   h. Fanconi syndrome
   i. Zollinger-Ellison syndrome
   j. Reye's syndrome
   k. Mallory-Weiss syndrome
   l. Sjögren's syndrome
   m. Felty's syndrome

For each patient below, choose the SINGLE most likely diagnosis from the above list of options.

(i) A 52-year-old man presents with a low white count and anemia. He is noted to have splenomegaly. He takes diclofenac for his arthritis.

Ans. (m) Felty's syndrome

(ii) A 57-year-old man is noted to have freckles on his lips and occasional rectal bleeding.

Ans. (g) Peutz-Jeghers syndrome

- Peutz-Jeghers syndrome is melanosis of the lips and mucosa associated with jejunal polyposis.

(iii) A 22-year-old man presents with bone pain, polyuria, and polydipsia. He is noted to have glycosuria and aminoaciduria.

Ans. (h) Fanconi syndrome

- Fanconi syndrome is an autosomal recessive renal tubular disorder that presents with rickets, glycosuria, phosphaturia, and aminoaciduria.

(iv) A 27-year-old man presents with arthritis, urethritis, conjunctivitis, and keratoderma blenorrhagicum.

Ans. (d) Reiter's syndrome

(v) A 52-year-old woman with rheumatoid arthritis complains of diminished lacrimation and salivation.

Ans. (l) Sjogren's syndrome

- Sjogren's syndrome presents here with rheumatoid arthritis, keratoconjunctivitis sicca and xerostomia.

28. Investigation of liver disease
   a. Mitochondrial antibodies
   b. Serum iron and total iron-binding capacity
   c. Serum copper and ceruloplasmin
   d. Serum bilirubin and liver function tests
   e. HBs antigen
   f. Antibodies to HCV
   g. Antibodies against nuclei and actin
   h. Antibodies to HAV
   i. Gamma-glutamyl transferase level
   j. Alpha-L-antitrypsin

For each presentation below, choose the SINGLE most ACCURATE investigation from the above list of options.

(i) A 62-year-old man with emphysema presents with liver disease.

Ans. (j) Alpha-L-antitrypsin

- Alpha-L-antitrypsin deficiency is often associated with emphysema and liver disease. Liver biopsy gives a definitive diagnosis.

(ii) A 52-year-old woman presents with pruritus and jaundice. She complains of dry eyes and mouth. On examination she has xanthelasma and hepatosplenomegaly.

Ans. (a) Mitochondrial antibodies

- Primary biliary cirrhosis is associated with hepatomegaly and a high alkaline phosphatase. Antibodies to mitochondria (AMA) are found in 95% of cases.

(iii) A 53-year-old well-bronzed man presents with a loss of libido. He is noted to have hepatomegaly. He takes humulin and Glargine bed time.

Ans. (b) Serum iron and total iron-binding capacity

- The classic triad for idiopathic haemochromatosis is bronze skin pigmentation, diabetes mellitus, and hepatomegaly.

(iv) A 24-year-old man presents with tremor and dysarthria. On examination, he is noted to have a greenish-brown pigment at the corneoscleral junction.

Ans. (c) Serum copper and ceruloplasmin

- Kayser-Fleischer rings are a specific sign for Wilson's disease, a rare inborn error of copper metabolism that leads to a failure of copper excretion.

(v) A 32-year-old woman presents with acute hepatitis. She is pyrexial, jaundiced, with hepatosplenomegaly, bruising, and migratory polyarthritis. She is noted to have a goitre.

Ans. (g) Antibodies against nuclei and actin

- This combination of autoimmune disease and hepatitis is suggestive of autoimmune chronic active hepatitis.

29. Diagnosis of renal failure
a. Goodpasture's syndrome
b. Amyloidosis
c. Systemic lupus erythematosus
d. Polyarteritis nodosa
e. Granulomatosis with angiitis
f. Systemic sclerosis
g. Post-streptococcal glomerulonephritis
h. Multiple myeloma
i. Diabetic glomerulosclerosis
j. Drugs causing nephrotic syndrome
k. Haemolytic Uremic syndrome
l. Acute tubuleinterstitial nephritis

For each cases below, choose the SINGLE most likely diagnosis from the above list of options.

(i) A 4-year-old boy presents to your practise with renal failure after a bout of acute dysentery. His full blood count reveals a leucocytosis, haemolytic anemia, and thrombocytopenia.

Ans. (k) Haemolytic uremic syndrome

- This multisystem disorder of thrombosis of microvasculature with acute glomerulonephritis is the most common cause of childhood acute renal failure.

(ii) A 52-year-old woman presents with fever, polyarthralgia, a skin rash and oliguria. She is a diabetic and suffers from arthritis. She takes insulin and allopurinol.

Ans. (l) Acute tubuleinterstitial nephritis

- Acute tubulo-interstitial nephritis occurs most commonly as a hypersensitivity reaction to allopurinol, penicillins, NSAIDs, phenindione and sulphonamides.

(iii) A 52-year-old man with a history of heart failure now presents in renal failure. On examination, he has an enlarged tongue and pinch purpura. He has 3+ proteinuria with hypoalbuminemia.

Ans. (b) Amyloidosis

- Amyloidosis presents with nephrotic range proteinuria and cardiac failure due to amyloid deposition in the heart. Pinch purpura is again a pointer.

(iv) A 57-year-old man presents in acute renal failure. He suffers from rhinitis. Round lung shadows are noted on chest X-ray.

Ans. (e) Granulomatosis with angiitis

- Granulomatosis with angitis is a generalized vasculitis that involves the upper respiratory tract, lungs and kidneys.

(v) A 22-year-old man presents with rapidly progressive renal failure. He describes a recent history of cough, fatigue, and occasional haemoptysis. His chest X-ray reveals blotchy shadows.

Ans. (a) Goodpasture's syndrome

- Goodpasture's syndrome is a proliferative glomerulonephritis associated with recurrent haemoptysis.

30. The treatment of renal disease
a. Cyclophosphamide
b. Thiazide
c. Haemodialysis
d. Renal transplantation
e. Immunosuppressive treatment and plasmapheresis
f. Fluid and protein restriction
g. Continuous arteriovenous hemofiltration
h. Withdrawal of offending drug
i. Albumin infusion with mannitol
j. Salt-restriction with furosemide
k. Peritoneal dialysis
l. Corticosteroids

For each case below, choose the SINGLE most appropriate treatment from the above list of options.

(i) A 22-year-old man presents with dyspnea, haemoptysis, and acute renal failure. He has serum anti-glomerular basement membrane antibodies.

Ans. (e) Immunosuppressive treatment and plasmapheresis

The treatment for Good pasture's syndrome is plasmapheresis and aggressive immunosuppressive therapy. Prognosis is poor.

(ii) A 57-year-old man is noted to have a nasal septal perforation, hypertension and glomerulonephritis. The chest X-ray reveals multiple nodules.

Ans. (a) Cyclophosphamide

The treatment for granulomatosis with angiitis is cyclophosphamide.

(iii) A 62-year-old man presents with fits confusion, pulmonary edema and anuria. His serum urea is 50 mmol/L, and his potassium is 8 mmol/L. He has previous history of MI and previous bowel resection.

Ans. (g) Continuous arteriovenous hemofiltration

Dialysis is warranted here in view of the progressive uraemia due to development of cardio-renal syndrome.

(iv) A 5-year-old boy presents with generalised edema. On examination, he is noted to have facial edema, ascites, and scrotal edema. His urine is frothy with the presence of proteins and hyaline casts. His serum albumin is 24 g/L, and the serum cholesterol is raised.

Ans. (l) Corticosteroids

Nephrotic syndrome most likely due to minimal change disease and is managed here with a short course of prednisolone.

(v) A 3-year-old boy is brought with bright red urine and edema of the eyelids. His blood pressure is noted to be high. The urine reveals white cells, red cells, granular casts, and protein.

Ans. (f) Fluid and protein restriction

Acute nephritic syndrome most likely due to post-streptococcal glomerulonephritis can be managed with conservative treatment with fluid and protein restriction. Penicillin is given for 3 months to reduce the risk of recurrence.

31. **Causes of Digital Clubbing**
    a. Bronchial carcinoma
    b. Bronchiectasis
    c. Lung abscess
    d. Empyema
    e. Cryptogenic fibrosing alveolitis
    f. Mesothelioma
    g. Cyanotic heart disease
    h. Subacute bacterial endocarditis
    i. Cirrhosis
    j. Inflammatory bowel disease
    k. Coeliac disease
    l. Gut Lymphoma

For each presentation below, choose the SINGLE most likely associative cause from the above list of options.

(i) A 37-year-old drug peddler presents with fever, night sweats and haematuria. On exam he is noted to have a heart murmur and finger clubbing.

Ans. (h) Subacute bacterial endocarditis

(ii) A 52-year-old farmer is noted to have a dry cough, exertional dyspnea, weight loss, arthralgia, and finger clubbing. On X-ray, there are bilateral diffuse reticulonodular shadowing at the bases.

Ans. (e) Cryptogenic fibrosing alveolitis

(iii) A 62-year-old man presents with severe chest pain, dyspnea, and finger clubbing. He admits to asbestos exposure 20 years ago. He denies smoking. The chest X-ray reveals a unilateral pleural effusion.

Ans. (f) Mesothelioma

(iv) A 32-year-old woman presents with fever, diarrhoea, and crampy abdominal pain. She is noted to have finger clubbing, anal fissures, and a skin tag.

Ans. (j) Inflammatory bowel disease

(v) A 52-year-old man presents with haematemesis. He is noted to have finger clubbing, gynaecomastia, and spider nevi.

Ans. (i) Cirrhosis

32. **Causes of headache**
    a. Meningitis
    b. Migraine headache
    c. Cluster headache
    d. Tension headache
    e. Subarachnoid haemorrhage
    f. Sinusitis
    g. Benign intracranial hypertension
    h. Cervical spondylosis
    i. Giant-Cell arteritis

For each case below, choose the SINGLE most appropriate treatment from the above list of options.

(i) A 27-year-old female presents with episodes of unilateral; throbbing headache, nausea, and vomiting. She states that it is aggravated by light. The episodes seem to occur prior to her menstruation.

Ans. (b) Migraine headache

(ii) A 42-year-old man presents with severe pain around his right eye, with eyelid swelling lasting 20 minutes. He has had several attacks during the past weeks. The attacks are worse at night.

Ans. (c) Cluster headache

(iii) A 10-year-old boy presents with fever, headache, left eye pain, and swelling. He described his vision as blurry. He has recently recovered from a cold.

Ans. (f) Sinusitis

(iv) A 65-year-old female presents with bitemporal headache, unilateral blurry vision, and pain on combing her hair. Her ESR is 100 mm fall in 1st hour.

Ans. (i) Giant-Cell Arteritis

(v) A 62-year-old obese female presents with headache and diplopia. On examination, she has papilledema. She is alert with no focal symptoms and signs.

Ans. (g) Benign intracranial hypertension

33. Causes of facial nerve palsy
a. Bell's palsy
b. Parotid tumour
c. Ramsay Hunt syndrome
d. Multiple sclerosis
e. Facial nerve schwannoma
f. Sarcoidosis
g. Temporal bone fracture
h. Suppurative otitis media
i. Guillain-Barre syndrome
j. Cerebrovascular accident
k. Longitudinal temporal bone fracture
l. Malignant otitis externa

For each case below, choose the SINGLE most likely cause from the above list of options.

(i) A 42-year-old man presents with facial pain, a droop to the side of his face, and a preauricular facial swelling.

Ans. (b) Parotid tumour

(ii) A 35-year-old man who has sustained a blow to the back of his head presents with facial nerve palsy and hemotympanum.

Ans. (g) Temporal bone fracture

(iii) A 57-year-old woman presents with a right-sided lower motor neuron facial nerve palsy and sensorineural hearing loss. She is noted to have vesicles in her right ear.

Ans. (c) Ramsay Hunt syndrome

(iv) A 52-year-old diabetic man presents with a unilateral facial nerve palsy and severe earache. On examination, he has granulation tissue deep in the external auditory meatus.

Ans. (l) Malignant otitis externa

(v) A 43-year-old woman presents with unilateral optic neuritis and a facial nerve palsy.

Ans. (d) Multiple sclerosis

34. Diagnosis of liver disease
a. Budd-Chiari syndrome
b. Cholestasis
c. Haemolytic jaundice
d. Hepatocellular failure
e. Acute hepatitis C
f. Acute hepatitis B
g. Acute hepatitis A
h. Primary biliary cirrhosis
i. Alcoholic hepatitis
j. Haemochromatosis
k. Wilson's disease
l. Hepatocellular carcinoma

For each patient below, choose the SINGLE most likely cause from the above list of options.

(i) A 25-year-old woman presents with right upper quadrant abdominal pain and ascites. On examination, she has hepatomegaly. Diagnostic liver scinti-scan shows maximum uptake in the caudate lobe alone. Her regular medications include the oral contraceptive pill and antidepressant medication.

Ans. (a) Budd-Chiari syndrome

Budd-Chiari syndrome results from thrombosis of the major hepatic veins and is associated with the contraceptive pill.

(ii) A 53-year-old woman presents with hepatomegaly and darkened skin pigmentation. She admits to drinking heavily she is noted to have glycosuria.

Ans. (j) Haemochromatosis

Bronzed diabetes or haemochromatosis is an autosomal recessive error of metabolism. Women present later as menstruation recues the iron load.

(iii) A 42-year-old man presents with jaundice. He was started on chlorpromazine for intractable hiccups three weeks ago.

Ans. (b) Cholestasis

Chlorpromazine is associated with obstructive jaundice.

(iv) A 52-year-old man presents with tender hepatomegaly and fever. His blood tests reveal an elevated MCV and an elevated SGOT

Ans. (i) Alcoholic hepatitis

SGOT is specific for alcoholic hepatitis.

(v) A 43-year-old woman presents with tender hepatomegaly and weight loss. She takes the oral contraceptive and atenolol. She is noted to have a raised alpha-fetoprotein.

Ans. (l) Hepatocellular carcinoma

35. Diagnosis of cardiovascular disease
a. Aortic regurgitation
b. Mitral stenosis
c. Mitral regurgitation
d. Aortic stenosis
e. Atrial myxoma

f. Tricuspid regurgitation
   g. Pulmonary stenosis
   h. Atrial septal defect
   i. Ventricular septal defect
   j. Pink Tet
   k. Patent ductus arteriosus
   l. Coarctation of the aorta
   m. Eisenmenger's syndrome

For each patient below, choose the SINGLE most likely diagnosis from the above list of options.

(i) A 20-year-old guy with history of wearing woollen socks in summer season. The doctor notices thin legs and notes blood pressure is elevated in both arms and is lower in the legs.

Ans. (l) Coarctation of the aorta

(ii) A 2-year-old child with finger clubbing and squatting episodes.

Ans. (j) Pink Tet

(iii) A preterm baby presents with expiratory grunting. The baby is noted to have continuous murmur in the second left intercostal space.

Ans. (k) Patent ductus arteriosus

(iv) A 33-year-old woman with Marfan's syndrome is noted to have a fixed wide split of the second heart sound. The ECG shows a partial right bundle block with right axis deviation and right ventricular hypertrophy.

Ans. (h) Atrial septal defect

(v) A 42-year-old drug addict is noted to have a pansystolic murmur. Giant 'cv' waves are present in the jugular venous pulse.

Ans. (f) Tricuspid regurgitation

36. Causes of pneumonia
   a. Chlamydia psittaci
   b. Streptococcus pneumoniae
   c. Mycoplasma pneumoniae
   d. Haemophilus influenza
   e. Staphylococcus aureus
   f. Legionella pneumophila
   g. Coxiella burnetii
   h. Pseudomonas aeruginosa
   i. Pneumocystis Jiroveci
   j. Aspergillus fumigatus
   k. Cytomegalovirus
   l. Actinomyces israelii
   m. Klebsiella pneumoniae

For each case below, choose the SINGLE most likely cause from the above list of options.

(i) A pet-shop owner presents with high, swinging fever, cough, and malaise. The chest X-ray reveals diffuse pneumonia.

Ans. (a) Chlamydia Psittaci

This is transmitted via inhalation from infected parrots.

(ii) A 72-year-old alcoholic man presents with sudden onset of purulent productive cough. The chest X-ray shows consolidation of the left upper lobe.

Ans. (m) Klebsiella pneumoniae

(iii) A 10-year-old boy with cystic fibrosis presents with pneumonia.

Ans. (h) Pseudomonas aeruginosa

(iv) A 33-year-old man with AIDS presents with fever, dry cough, and dyspnea. The X-ray shows diffuse, bilateral, alveolar, and interstitial shadows beginning in the perihilar regions and spreading outward.

Ans. (i) Pneumocystis jiroveci

(v) A 22-year-old male IVDA presents with breathlessness and cough. The X-ray reveals patchy areas of consolidation with abscess formation.

Ans. (e) Staphylococcus aureus

37. Investigation of dementia
   a. Chest X-ray
   b. Serum calcium level
   c. TSH levels and serum T_4
   d. Full blood count and film
   e. Electroencephalogram
   f. Lumbar puncture
   g. Serum Urea
   h. Liver function tests
   i. CT Head
   j. Plasma beta hydroxybutyrate
   k. VDRL
   l. HIV serology
   m. Serum copper and ceruloplasmin
   n. Dietary history
   o. Drug levels

For each case below, choose the SINGLE most ACCURATE investigation from the above list of options.

(i) A 52-year-old woman who underwent thyroidectomy a week prior now presents with dementia. She also complains of perioral tingling.

Ans. (b) Serum calcium level

Hypoparathyroidism may occur following thyroid or neck surgery.

(ii) A 72-year-old man presents with progressive dementia and tremor. On examination, he has extensor plantar reflexes and Argyll Robertson pupils.

Ans. (k) VDRL

(iii) A 42-year-old man with a history of epilepsy presents with progressive dementia with fluctuating levels of consciousness. On examination, he has unequal pupils.

Ans. (l) HIV serology

This is a case of subdural haemorrhage. The elderly and epileptics are at risk. Head trauma may have gone unnoticed.

(iv) A 33-year-old homosexual man presents with weight loss, chronic diarrhoea and progressive dementia. On examination, he has purple papules on his legs.

Ans. (l) HIV serology

The purple papules are most likely Kaposi's sarcoma associated with HIV.

(v) A 32-year-old man post- binge drinking presents with sweating, agitation, tremors and drowsiness. He was admitted and ABG shows anion gap of 24 mEq/L

Ans. (j) Plasma beta hydroxybutyrate levels

Alcoholic ketoacidosis should also be considered when encountering patients with unexplained high anion gap metabolic acidosis with hypoglycemia and fatty liver

38. Diagnosis of intracranial lesions
a. Subdural hematoma
b. Cerebral abscess
c. Astrocytoma
d. Acoustic neuroma
e. Meningioma
f. Pituitary tumour
g. Secondary tumour
h. Cerebral aneurysm
i. Cerebral angioma
j. Subarachnoid haemorrhage
k. Extradural hematoma
l. Medulloblastoma

For each case, choose the SINGLE most likely diagnosis from the above list of options.

(i) A 52-year-old man presents with unilateral tinnitus and dizziness. He also complains of difficulty swallowing and loss of taste.

Ans. (d) Acoustic neuroma

Acoustic neuroma is a cerebellopontine angle tumour and causes cranial nerve palsies via direct compression

(ii) A 47-year-old woman presents with sudden onset of headache, neck stiffness, and double vision. She lapses into a coma. She had a similar episode 2 weeks prior that was not as severe and resolved spontaneously. She has a history of hypertension and no history of head trauma.

Ans. (h) Cerebral aneurysm

Subarachnoid haemorrhage results from a cerebral aneurysm with rebleed peaking at 14 days.

(iii) A 10-year-old boy presents with headache, blurry vision, and vomiting. He is noted to have an ataxic gait, nystagmus and past pointing. His CT scan of the head shows enlarged cerebral ventricles and a cerebellar mass.

Ans. (l) Medulloblastoma

Medulloblastoma occurs in the cerebellum and accounts for the patient's cerebellar signs. It also leads to obstructive hydrocephalus of the fourth ventricle.

(iv) A 42-year-old woman post radical mastectomy now presents with sudden onset of severe headache and confusion. She is afebrile and shows no signs of head trauma. The CT scan of the head shows a space – occupying lesion.

Ans. (g) Secondary tumour

A space-occupying lesion in a woman treated for breast carcinoma is most likely due to a cerebral metastasis.

(v) A 32-year-old cricketer presents in a coma. He had been struck by a cricket ball earlier that day and had been fine until now. On examination he has asymmetrical pupils.

Ans. (k) Extradural hematoma

39. Investigation of haemoptysis
a. Complete Blood counts
b. Clotting studies
c. Bronchography
d. Chest X-ray
e. 12 lead ECG
f. Antinuclear antibodies and free DNA
g. Anti-glomerular basement antibody in the serum
h. Computerised tomography of the chest
i. Mantoux test
j. Urine-analysis
k. CT angiography
l. Tissue biopsy
m. Sputum cytology

For each case below, choose the SINGLE most ACCURATE investigation from the above list of options.

(i) A 42-year-old man presents with recurrent epistaxis, haemoptysis, and haematuria. On examination, he has a nasal septal perforation and nodules on chest X-ray.

Ans. (l) Tissue biopsy

Wegener's granulomatosis is confirmed by biopsy of the involved tissue.

(ii) A 32-year-old man presents with haemoptysis, dyspnea and haematuria. Chest X-ray reveals bilateral alveolar infiltrates. Urine analysis reveals the presence of protein and red cell casts.

Ans. (g) Anti-glomerular basement antibody in the serum

Good pasture's syndrome is confirmed by detecting anti-glomerular basement antibody.

(iii) A 62-year-old man presents with a chronic cough and mild haemoptysis. On examination, he has digital clubbing. Chest X-ray reveals a single nodule.

Ans. (l) Tissue biopsy

Bronchial carcinoma is suggested by the presence of hypertrophic pulmonary osteoarthropathy and a solitary lung nodule. Tissue biopsy is required for a definitive diagnosis

(iv) A 45-year-old cancer pancreas presents with dyspnea and haemoptysis. His chest X-ray is unremarkable, and the ECG shows a sinus tachycardia with a mean P axis shift to the right. Blood gas shows a low PCO_2 and an elevated pH.

Ans. (k) CT angiography

Malignancy is a hypercoagulable state and clinical presentation of patient is suggestive of development of pulmonary embolism. Due to hyperventilation he is having metabolic alkalosis. The IOC is CT angiography.

(v) A 52-year-old man presents with occasional haemoptysis and chronic productive cough. He has history of recurrent pneumonia. Chest X-ray reveals peribronchial fibrosis.

Ans. (c) Bronchography

Bronchiectasis is suggested here and can be confirmed by bronchography if the patient is stable.

40. **Causes of proteinuria**
    a. Alport syndrome
    b. Minimal change disease
    c. Lupus nephritis
    d. F.S.G.S
    e. Membranoproliferative glomerulonephritis
    f. Mesangial proliferative glomerulonephritis
    g. Membranous glomerulopathy
    h. Idiopathic crescentic glomerulonephritis
    i. Diabetic nephropathy
    j. Henoch-Schönlein purpura
    k. Goodpasture's syndrome
    l. Postinfectious glomerulonephritis

For each case below, choose the SINGLE most likely cause from the above list of options.

(i) A 43-year-old man presents with proteinuria, haematuria, and progressive renal failure. He is noted to have a high frequency sensorineural hearing loss. He has a sister who was noted to have microscopic haematuria but is asymptomatic.

Ans. (a) Alport syndrome

(ii) A 7-year-old boy presents with generalised edema and proteinuria. Electron microscopy reveals fusion of the epithelial foot processes and normal appearing capillary and basement membranes.

Ans. (b) Minimal change disease

(iii) A 32-year-old heroin addict presents with hypertension, edema, oliguria, and is noted to have heavy proteinuria. Renal biopsy specimen reveals loss of glomerular cellularity and collapse of capillary loops. Adhesions between portions of the glomerular tuft and Bowman's capsule are also seen.

Ans. (d) F.S.G.S

(iv) A 12-year-old boy presents with sudden onset of haematuria and edema. Further investigations reveal proteinuria and low C_3. Sub-epithelial humps and foot process fusion are seen by electron microscopy.

Ans. (l) Postinfectious glomerulonephritis

(v) A 4-yer-old boy presents with a faint leg rash, bloody diarrhoea, and oliguria. Further investigations reveal heavy proteinuria and an elevated serum IgA.

Ans. (j) Henoch–Schönlein purpura

41. **Investigation of rheumatic diseases**
    a. HLA B27 antigen
    b. Bone scan
    c. Antibody to ds DNA
    d. Anti-nuclear antibody
    e. Rheumatoid factor
    f. HLA-DR4 antigen
    g. Synovial fluid analysis with polarised-light microscopy
    h. X-ray
    i. Anti-centromere antibody
    j. Anti-Jo-1 antibody
    k. Serum uric acid
    l. Anti-Ro antibody

For each case below, choose the SINGLE most ACCURATE investigation from the above list of options.

(i) A 62-year-old alcoholic man presents with a hot, swollen first metatarsophalangeal joint and a lesion on the rim of his left pinna.

Ans. (g) Synovial fluid analysis with polarised-light microscopy

For the diagnosis of gout, serum uric acid is not as specific as joint fluid analysis for negatively birefringent crystals.

(ii) A 67-year-old woman with a history of hypothyroidism presents with a warm, painful swollen knee with effusion. The serum calcium is normal. X-ray reveals chondrocalcinosis.

Ans. (g) Synovial fluid analysis with polarised-light microscopy

With pseudo gout or calcium pyrophosphate Arthropathy the crystals are positively birefringent.

(iii) A 42-year-old woman presents with flexion deformities of her fingers. She has soft-tissue swelling of her digits. She also complains of difficulty swallowing and is noted to have a beaked nose and facial telangiectasia.

Ans. (d) Anti-nucleolus antibody

Anti-nucleolus antibody is detected in up to 60% of patients with systemic sclerosis.

(iv) A 33-year-old woman presents with painful digits worse in the cold and difficulty swallowing. She is noted to have tapered fingers and a fixed facial expression with facial telangiectasia. X-ray reveals calcium around her fingers.

Ans. (i) Anti-centromere antibody

CREST syndrome, a variant of systemic sclerosis is associated with anti-centromere antibody.

(v) A 25-yr-old woman presents with dry eyes, arthralgia, dysphagia, and Raynaud's phenomenon.

Ans. (l) Anti-Ro antibody

Primary Sjogren's syndrome is associated with anti-Ro antibody in 70% of cases.

42. **Risk factors for oncological diseases**
    a. Nasopharyngeal carcinoma
    b. Colorectal carcinoma
    c. Non-Hodgkin's lymphoma
    d. Sino-nasal tumours
    e. Gastric carcinoma
    f. Lung carcinoma
    g. Salivary gland carcinoma
    h. Carcinoma of the pancreas
    i. Thyroid carcinoma
    j. Hodgkin's dise3ase
    k. Esophageal carcinoma

For each case below, choose the SINGLE most likely associated carcinoma from the above list of options.

(i) A 52-year-old man from Nepal presents with unilateral conductive hearing loss. He is noted to have the Epstein-Barr virus.

Ans. (a) Nasopharyngeal carcinoma

(ii) A 43-year-old woman with Sjögren's disease now presents with painless neck nodes.

Ans. (c) Non-Hodgkin's lymphoma

(iii) A 52-year-old woman with blood group A and a history of pernicious anemia now presents with weight loss and epigastric discomfort.

Ans. (e) Gastric carcinoma

(iv) A 42-year-old man presents with hoarseness and dysphagia. He has a prior history of suicidal attempt with lye ingestion.

Ans. (k) Esophageal carcinoma

(v) A 73-year-old woman presents with stridor and a neck mass. She has a prior history of radiation to the neck as a child.

Ans. (i) Thyroid carcinoma

43. **Diagnosis of haematological diseases**
    a. Acute lymphoblastic leukaemia
    b. Multiple myeloma
    c. Acute myeloid leukaemia
    d. Idiopathic thrombocytopenic purpura
    e. Chronic lymphocytic leukaemia
    f. Thrombotic Thrombocytopenic purpura
    g. Chronic Myeloid leukaemia
    h. Polycythaemia Vera
    i. Amyloidosis
    j. Aplastic anemia
    k. Primary myelofibrosis

For each case below, choose the SINGLE most likely diagnosis from the above list of options.

(i) A 72-year-old woman presents to her GP with weakness and bone pain. She also complains of blurry vision. She is noted to be anaemic with increased calcium and uric acid levels. X-ray reveals osteolytic bone lesions.

Ans. (b) Multiple myeloma

(ii) A 4-year-old boy presents with sternal tenderness, bone pain, gum bleeds and weakness.

Ans. (a) Acute lymphoblastic leukaemia

(iii) A 63-year-old man presents with malaise. He is noted to have gum hypertrophy and skin nodules.

Ans. (c) Acute myeloid leukaemia

(iv) A 52-year-old man presents with epistaxis. On examination, he has enlarged non tender neck nodes. His blood count reveals a lymphocytosis, anemia and thrombocytopaenia.

Ans. (e) Chronic lymphocytic leukaemia

(v) A 42-year-old man presents with fever, sweats, and weight loss. He also suffers from gout. On examination, he has an enlarged spleen. Blood tests reveal a lymphocytosis and anemia. The Philadelphia chromosome is detected.

Ans. (g) Chronic myeloid leukaemia

The presence of the Philadelphia chromosome gives the patient a poor prognosis.

44. **Diagnosis of childhood respiratory disease**
    a. Bronchiolitis
    b. Croup
    c. Asthma
    d. Cystic fibrosis
    e. Epiglottitis
    f. Obstructive sleep apnea
    g. Chlamydia trachomatis infection
    h. Pneumonia
    i. Allergic rhinitis
    j. Influenza
    k. Retrotonsillar abscess
    l. Gonorrhoeal infection

For each case below, choose the SINGLE most likely diagnosis from the above list of options.

(i) A 2-year-old boy presents with coughing and wheezing. Other members of the family are also suffering from an upper respiratory tract infection. On examination, he has flaring of the nostrils and audible expiratory wheezes.

Ans. (a) Bronchiolitis

Intrathoracic airway obstruction is either caused by respiratory syncytial virus or by asthma. With a history of other family relations afflicted, bronchiolitis is more likely.

(ii) A 10-year-old thin boy presents with chronic cough. Chest X-ray reveals bronchiectasis. He also suffers from steatorrhea.

Ans. (d) Cystic fibrosis

(iii) A 4-year-old boy presents to the GP for night terrors and loud snoring. On examination, he is a mouth breather with large tonsils that meet at the midline.

Ans. (f) Obstructive sleep apnea

(iv) A 2-week-old infant presents with staccato cough and purulent conjunctivitis. On examination, he is apyrexial with diffuse rales on auscultation of the chest.

Ans. (g) Chlamydia trachomatis infection

(v) A 2-year-old boy presents with a 3-day history of noisy breathing on inspiration and a barking cough worse at night. He has a low-grade fever and is hoarse.

Ans. (b) Croup

Viral croup is most likely. Although epiglottitis should also be considered.

45. Diagnosis of cardiovascular diseases in children
   a. Kawasaki disease
   b. Hereditary angiedema
   c. Congenital nephrotic syndrome
   d. Myocarditis
   e. Pericarditis
   f. Primary pulmonary hypertension
   g. Juvenile rheumatoid arthritis
   h. Acute rheumatic fever
   i. Congestive heart failure
   j. Aortic stenosis
   k. Systemic lupus erythematosus
   l. Paroxysmal atrial tachycardia
   m. Mitral stenosis

For each patient below, choose the SINGLE most likely diagnosis from the above list of options.

(i) A 10-year-old boy presents with stridor. He has history of recurrent swelling of the hands and feet with abdominal pain and diarrhoea. His sister also suffers from similar attacks.

Ans. (b) Hereditary angiedema

This is an autosomal dominant inherited condition. The stridor is caused by laryngeal edema.

(i) A 6-year-old girl presents with spiking fevers. On examination, she has spindle-shaped swellings of the finger-joints.

Ans. (g) Juvenile rheumatoid arthritis

The combination of spiking fevers and spindle-shaped swelling of the finger-joints is suggestive of JRA.

(ii) A 12-year-old boy presents with polyarthritis and abdominal pain. He had a sore throat a week ago. On examination, he is noted to have an early blowing diastolic murmur at the left sternal edge.

Ans. (h) Acute rheumatic fever

Acute rheumatic fever may present with migratory polyarthralgia and carditis. This can manifest as a new murmur, in this instance of aortic regurgitation.

(iii) A 10-year-old boy presents to Casualty following a seizure during gym. On examination, he has a loud systolic ejection murmur with a loud systolic ejection murmur with a thrill.

Ans. (j) Aortic stenosis

Aortic stenosis may give rise to syncope and be mistaken for a seizure.

(iv) A 12-year-old girl presents with pallor, dyspnea, and a pulse rate of 190. She is noted to have cardiomegaly and hepatomegaly.

Ans. (i) Congestive heart failure

46. Causes of ascites
   a. Tuberculous peritonitis
   b. Meigs syndrome
   c. Budd–Chiari syndrome
   d. Constrictive pericarditis
   e. Portal vein thrombosis
   f. Compression of the portal vein by lymph nodes
   g. Cirrhosis
   h. Right heart failure due to mitral stenosis
   i. Pseudomyxoma peritonei
   j. Protein-losing enteropathies

For each patient below, choose the SINGLE most likely cause from the above list of options.

(i) A 42-year-old woman presents with ovarian fibroma, right hydrothorax and ascites.

Ans. (b) Meigs syndrome

(ii) A 25-year-old woman develops nausea, vomiting, and abdominal pain. On examination, she has tender hepatomegaly and ascites. She was recently started on oral contraceptives.

Ans. (c) Budd–Chiari syndrome

Budd-Chiari syndrome occurs from thrombosis of the major hepatic veins and has been associated with oral contraceptives.

(iii) A 32-year-old man develops ascites and right iliac fossa pain. The ascitic fluid is viscous and mucinoid in nature.

Ans. (i) Pseudomyxoma peritonei

Rupture of a mucocele appendix can give rise to pseudomyxoma peritonei.

(iv) A 42-year-old woman presents with ascites. On examination, she has dominant 'a' wave in the pulmonary second sound and a low volume peripheral artery pulse volume. She has history of rheumatic fever.

Ans. (h) Right heart failure due to mitral stenosis

(v) A 52-year-old woman presents with fatigue and ascites. She is noted to have a rapid, irregular pulse rate with small volume. The chest X-ray reveals a small heart with calcification seen on the lateral view. The 12-lead ECG demonstrates low QRS voltage and T wave inversion.

Ans. (d) Constrictive pericarditis

47. Causes of dysphagia
a. Scleroderma
b. Pharyngeal pouch
c. Diffuse oesophageal spasm
d. Globus pharyngeus
e. Plummer-Vinson syndrome
f. Carcinoma of the esophagus
g. Peptic stricture
h. Myasthenia gravis
i. Swallowed foreign body
j. Caustic stricture
k. Retrosternal goitre

For each presentation below, choose the SINGLE most likely cause from the above list of options.

(i) A 34-year-old female presents with hypertension, pinched facies and progressive dysphagia with decreased tone of L.E.S

Ans. (a) Scleroderma

Pinched facies with hypertension point to presence of scleroderma. The tone of LES is reduced in scleroderma due to fibrosis.

(ii) A 73—year-old man presents with a 8 week history of progressive dysphagia, weight loss, and has palpable neck nodes on examination.

Ans. (f) Carcinoma of the esophagus

(iii) A 29-year-old man with a history of depression presents with acute dysphagia. He has a prior history of repeated suicide attempts. There are associated burns in his oropharynx.

Ans. (j) Caustic stricture

(iv) A 62-year-old woman presents with progressive dysphagia. On exam she has a smooth tongue, koilonychias and suffers from iron deficiency anemia.

Ans. (e) Plummer-Vinson syndrome

(v) A 70-year-old man presents with regurgitation of food, dysphagia, halitosis, and a sensation of 'lump in the throat'.

Ans. (b) Pharyngeal pouch

48. Investigation of weight loss
a. Stool for cysts, ova and parasites
b. Urea and electrolytes
c. Chest X-ray
d. Full blood count
e. Serum glucose
f. Urinalysis
g. Thyroid function tests
h. Ultrasound of abdomen
i. Barium swallow
j. Blood cultures
k. Plasma ACTH and cortisol

For each presentation below, choose the SINGLE most ACCURATE investigation from the above list of options.

(i) A 63-year-old man recently treated for renal tuberculosis presents with weight loss, diarrhoea, anorexia, hypotension, and is noted to have hyperpigmented buccal mucosa and hand creases.

Ans. (k) Plasma ACTH and cortisol

This patient has Addison's disease.

(ii) A 26-year-old man presents with steatorrhoea, diarrhoea and weight loss after eating contaminated food.

Ans. (a) Stool for cysts, ova and parasites

Viable protozoon cysts are ingested in contaminated food.

(iii) A 66-year-old man presents with a sudden onset of diabetes, anorexia, weight loss, epigastric and back pain.

Ans. (h) Ultrasound of abdomen

This patient presents with pancreatic cancer. Sudden onset of diabetes in the elderly is also suggestive.

(iv) A 53-year-old woman presents with weight loss, increased appetite, sweating, palpitations, and preference for cold weather, hot, moist palms, and tremors.

Ans. (g) Thyroid function tests

This patient presents with classic signs and symptoms of hypothyroidism.

(v) A 73-year-old woman presents with progressive dysphagia, weight loss, and a sensation of food sticking in her throat.

Ans. (i) Barium swallow

Barium swallow followed by upper GI endoscopy are needed to exclude oesophageal pathology.

49. The treatment of diabetic complications
   a. Insulin sliding scale and 0.9% normal saline
   b. Insulin sliding scale and 0.45% normal saline
   c. Insulin sliding scale, 0.9% normal saline and potassium replacement
   d. Insulin sliding scale, 0.45% normal saline and potassium replacement
   e. 50 ml of 50% dextrose IV
   f. Sugary drink
   g. Chest X-ray
   h. Measure C-peptide levels

For each case below, choose the SINGLE most appropriate treatment from the above list of options.

(i) A 69-year-old man is noted to have a glucose of 600mg% and a Na of 163 mmol/L. he has no prior history of diabetes and has been on intravenous fluids for a week. His other medications include Iv cefuroxime, metronidazole, and dexamethasone.

Ans. (b) Insulin sliding scale, heparin and 0.45% normal saline

This is the treatment for hyperglycaemic hyperosmolar non-ketotic coma.

(ii) A 63-year-old man is brought into Accident and emergency in an unconscious state. His glucose is 350 mg%. His arterial blood gas shows a pH 7.2 and a paCO$_2$ of 2. Serum Na is 140, K is 3.0 Cl is 100, and the HCO$_3$ is 5 mmol/L.

Ans. (c) Insulin sliding scale, 0.9% normal saline and potassium replacement

This is the treatment for diabetic ketoacidosis. The anion gap is 38.

(iii) A 55-year-old woman presents with tachycardia, sweating and agitation. Her husband is a diabetic. She has a history of Munchausen's syndrome.

Ans. (h) Measure C-peptide levels

This patient has factitious hypoglycemia and has probably self-injected her husband's insulin.

(iv) A 42-year-old diabetic actor is started on propranolol for stage-fright. He collapses after a day shooting. He has not changed his insulin regime. His glucose is 40mg%.

Ans. (e) 50 ml of 50% dextrose IV

Propranolol has been known to induce hypoglycemia.

(v) A 53-yr-old diabetic presents in a coma. He is febrile with diminished breath sounds on auscultation. He has warm extremities. His glucose is 20 mmol. His white count is with increased neutrophils.

Ans. (g) Chest X-ray

This patient is most likely septic from a chest infection.

MULTIPLE TRUE/FALSE TYPE QUESTIONS

Multiple options are given below following a statement. Mark the options with either True or False:

50. Consider the following statements regarding drug induced lupus?
1. Isoniazid is an important cause
2. Anti-histone antibodies are characteristically present
3. Kidney involvement is frequent
4. Genetic factors are important in the predisposition to this disorder

Of these statements:
   a. 1, 2 and 4 are correct
   b. 2, 3 and 4 are correct
   c. 1, 2 and 3 are correct
   d. 1, 3 and 4 are correct

Ans. (a) 1, 2 and 4 are correct

51. Which of the following statements are true of cytomegalovirus?
1. It is myxovirus
2. The clinical manifestations of the disease appear when the CD4 count is below 50 mm^3
3. Its infection most commonly presents with choroidoretinitis
4. It may cause polyradiculopathy

Select the correct answer using the codes given below:

Codes
   a. 1 and 2
   b. 3 and 4
   c. 1, 3 and 4
   d. 2, 3 and 4

Ans. (d) 2, 3 and 4

52. The first heart sound is loud in which of the following conditions?
1. Mitral regurgitation
2. Pregnancy
3. Anemia
4. Mitral stenosis

Select the correct answer using the codes given below:

Codes
   a. 1 and 4
   b. 1, 2 and 4
   c. 3 and 4
   d. 2, 3 and 4

Ans. (d) 2, 3 and 4

53. Consider the following statements regarding thyroid hormones:
1. Majority of the circulating T3 remains in bound form
2. TSH estimation is not a sensitive test for diagnosis of primary hypothyroidism
3. Only 50% of the circulating T3 is secreted by thyroid
4. Fetal pituitary-thyroid axis is dependent to a large extent on material pituitary-thyroid axis.

Which of the statements given above is/are correct:
   a. 1 only
   b. 1 and 3 only

c. 3 and 4 only
d. 2, 3 and 4

Ans. (a) 1 only

54. Practice of evidence-based medicine

Options:
a. True
b. False

For each statement below, choose the correct response.

(i) Evidence-based medicine involves using individual clinical expertise or the best available external evidence to treat a patient.

Ans. (b) False

Evidence-based medicine involves using *both* individual clinical expertise and the best available external evidence to determine patient's care.

(ii) Evidence-based medicine is an attempt to lower the cost of patient's care.

Ans. (b) False

(iii) Evidence-based medicine involves using individual clinical skills and the best available external evidence to treat a patient

Ans. (a) True

(iv) Evidence-based medicine is the conscientious, explicit, and judicious use of evidence in making decisions about the care of individual patients.

Ans. (a) True

(v) Evidence-based medicine suggests that the standard for judging the efficacy of a treatment should be based on the systematic review of several randomised trials.

Ans. (a) True

REASON ASSERTION TYPE QUESTIONS

55. **Assertion (A):** Administration of phenobarbitone along with coumarin drugs reduces the anticoagulant effects of coumarin.
    Reason (R): Phenobarbitone acts as enzyme inducer of cytochrome P-450 system.
    a. Both assertion (A) and reason (R) are individually true and (R) is the correct explanation of (A).
    b. Both assertion (A) and reason (R) are individually true and (R) is not the correct explanation of (A).
    c. If (A) true; (R) false
    d. If (A) false; (R) true

Ans. (a) Both assertion (A) and reason (R) are individually true and (R) is the correct explanation of (A)

56. **Assertion (A):** In a patient with raised intracranial tension, lumber puncture should be avoided.
    Reason (R): It may result in severe headache.
    a. Both assertion (A) and reason (R) are individually true and (R) is the correct explanation of (A).
    b. Both assertion (A) and reason (R) are individually true and (R) is not the correct explanation of (A).
    c. If (A) true; (R) false
    d. If (A) false; (R) true

Ans. (b) Both assertion (A) and reason (R) are individually true and (R) is not the correct explanation of (A)

57. **Assertion (A):** Angiotensin converting enzyme (ACE) inhibitors are inhibited for patients of acute myocardial infarction with <40% left ventricular ejection fraction.
    Reason (R): ACE inhibitors counteract ventricular remodeling and improve survival in patients with reduced left ventricular ejection fraction.
    a. Both assertion (A) and reason (R) are individually true and (R) is the correct explanation of (A).
    b. Both assertion (A) and reason (R) are individually true and (R) is not the correct explanation of (A).
    c. If (A) true; (R) false
    d. If (A) false; (R) true

Ans. (a) Both assertion (A) and reason (R) are individually true and (R) is the correct explanation of (A)

58. **Assertion (A):** Preferred thrombolytic regimen for treatment of pulmonary thromboembolism is 100 mg of tPA administered as continuous peripheral intravenous infusion over 2 hours.
    Reason (R): Patients appear to respond to thrombolysis for up to 7 days after the pulmonary thromboembolism has occurred.
    a. Both assertion (A) and reason (R) are individually true and (R) is the correct explanation of (A).
    b. Both assertion (A) and reason (R) are individually true and (R) is **not** the correct explanation of (A).
    c. If (A) true; (R) false
    d. If (A) false; (R) true

Ans. (c) If (A) true; (R) false

MATCH THE FOLLOWING TYPE QUESTIONS

59. Match List-I with List-II and select the correct answer using the codes given below:

List-I	List-II
A. Janeway lesion	1. Coarctation of aorta
B. Rib notching	2. Peripheral pulmonary stenosis
C. Rubella	3. Bacterial endocarditis
D. Pulse deficit	4. Atrial fibrillation

Codes:
a. A-3 B-2 C-4 D-1   b. A-2 B-1 C-4 D-3
c. A-4 B-2 C-3 D-1   d. A-3 B-1 C-2 D-4

Ans. (d) A-3 B-1 C-2 D-4

60. Match List-I with List-II and select the correct answer using the codes given below:

List-I (Syndromes)	List-II (clinical conditions)
A. Leber's disease	1. Optic neuropathy
B. Whipple's triad	2. CBD stone
C. Charcot's triad	3. Rupture of lower esophagus
D. Boerhaave's syndrome	4. Insulinoma

   Codes:
   a. A-1 B-4 C-3 D-2
   b. A-4 B-1 C-2 D-3
   c. A-3 B-2 C-1 D-4
   d. A-1 B-4 C-2 D-3

   Ans. (a) A-1 B-4 C-3 D-2

61. Match List-I (Symptoms) with List-II (Diagnosis) and select the correct answer using the codes given below the lists:

List-I	List-II
A. Hemoptysis	1. Allergic broncho-pulmonary aspergillosis
B. Shortness of breath without wheeze	2. Bronchiectasis
C. Snoring	3. Hammam Rich syndrome
D. Audible wheeze	4. Sleep apnea syndrome

   Codes:
   a. A-2 B-3 C-4 D-1   b. A-2 B-4 C-3 D-1
   c. A-1 B-4 C-3 D-2   d. A-1 B-3 C-4 D-2

   Ans. (a) A-2 B-3 C-4 D-1

62. Match List-I (Nodes) with List-II (Disease) and select the correct answer using the codes given below:

List-I (Nodes)	List-II (Disease)
A. Osler's nodes	1. Sarcoidosis
B. Heberden's nodes	2. Infective endocarditis
C. Erythema nodosum	3. Osteo arthritis
D. Subcutaneous nodules	4. Rheumatic fever

   Codes:
   a. A-2 B-3 C-1 D-4
   b. A-4 B-1 C-3 D-2
   c. A-2 B-1 C-3 D-4
   d. A-4 B-3 C-1 D-2

   Ans. (a) A-2 B-3 C-1 D-4

MOST RECENT QUESTIONS (AIIMS MAY 2019)

1. The given pattern of EEG is found in?

   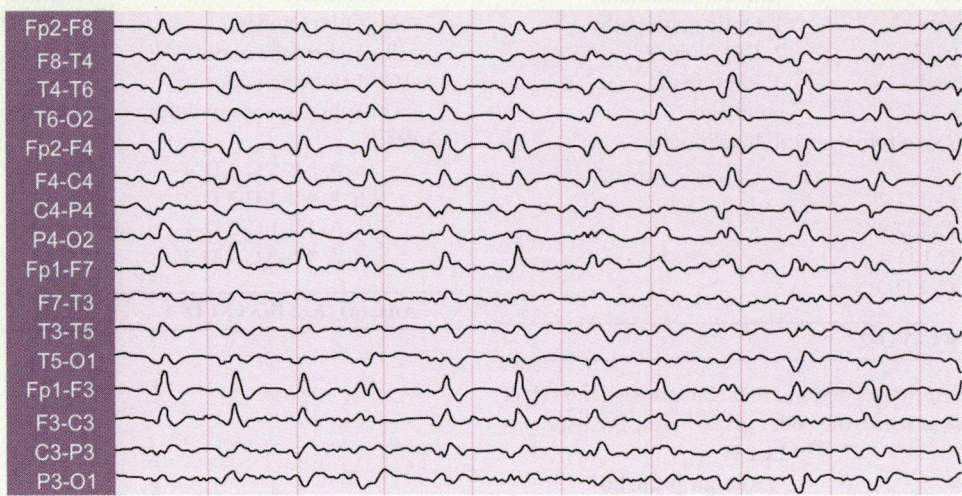

   a. Hepatic encephalopathy   b. Creutzfeldt-Jakob Disease   c. GTCS   d. Herpes simplex encephalitis

2. A patient presents with recent onset breathlessness and ECG was done. The diagnosis is?

   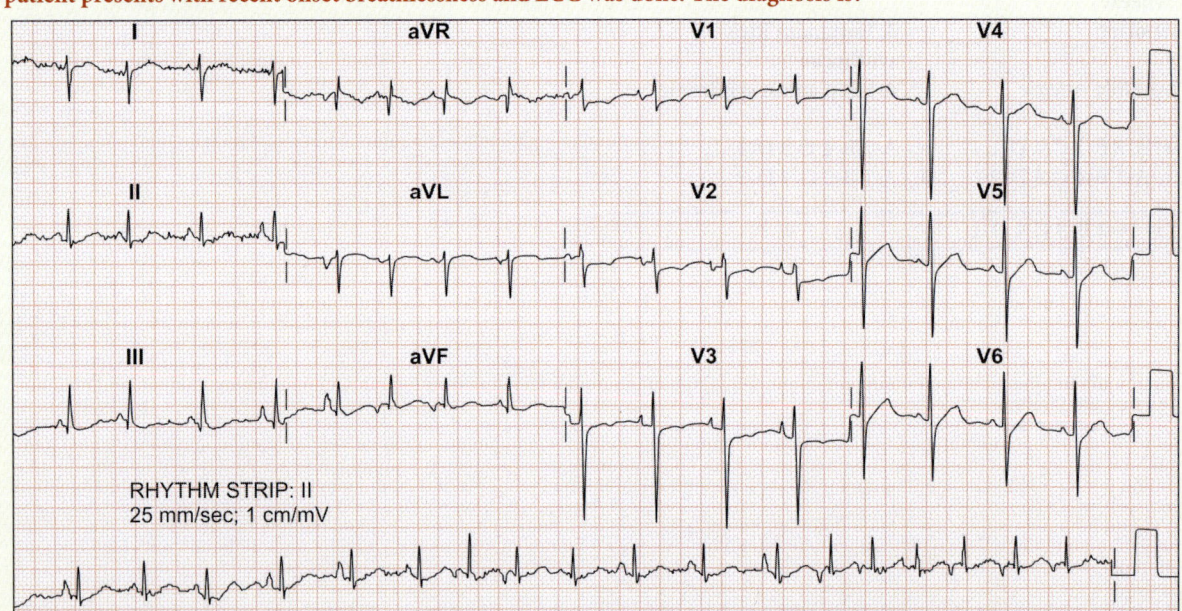

   a. Atrial fibrillation
   b. Paroxysmal supraventricular tachycardia
   c. Acute myocardial infarction
   d. Multi-focal atrial tachycardia

3. Calculate the anion gap from the following information:
   Na^+ = 137 mmol/L
   K^+ = 4 mmol/L
   Cl^- = 110 mmol/L
   HCO_3^- = 15 mmol/L
   a. 22 mmol/L   b. 16 mmol/L
   c. 10 mmol/L   d. 12 mmol/L

4. Berry aneurysm most commonly occurs due to:-
   a. Endothelial injury of vessel due to HTN
   b. Muscle intimal elastic lamina layer defect
   c. Endothelial layer defect
   d. Adventitia defect

5. True/False regarding a Patient who presents with right sided hemiparesis and aphasia since 1 hour
   a. Tenecteplase not started if CT scan normal
   b. Tenecteplase not started before MRI if CT scan normal
   c. rtPA given when BP>150/80
   d. rAtPA given in a patient taking warfarin with INR 1.4
   e. Antiplatelet therapy is given in A.I.S

6. True about Postural Hypotension?
   a. Decrease in Systolic blood pressure 20 mmHg within 6 mins of postural change
   b. Decrease in Systolic blood pressure 20 mmHg within 3 min of postural change
   c. Decrease in Diastolic blood pressure 20 mmHg within 6 mins of postural change
   d. Decrease in Diastolic blood pressure 20 mmHg within 3mins of postural change

7. All of the following characteristics are found in pleural effusion fluid of a rheumatoid arthritis patient except:
   a. RA factor positive
   b. High glucose
   c. Cholesterol crystals
   d. High LDH

8. Most common pulmonary manifestation of SLE:
   a. Shrinking Lung
   b. Pleuritis
   c. Intra alveolar hemorrhage.
   d. Interstitial inflammation

9. Deep Y descent in JVP is seen in all except?
   a. Cardiac tamponade
   b. RCM
   c. Constrictive pericarditis
   d. Tricuspid regurgitation

10. A patient had recurrent optic neuritis of both eyes with extensive transverse myelitis. Visual acuity in right eye is 6/60 & visual acuity in Left eye 6/18. Patient showed 50% response to steroids. Diagnosis is:
    a. NMO (Neuromyelitis optica)
    b. SACD (Subacute combined degeneration of spinal cord)
    c. Posterior cerebral artery stroke
    d. Neurosyphilis

11. Which of the following is most associated with respiratory alkalosis: *(AIIMS May 2019)*
    a. Assisted control mode ventilation
    b. Non-invasive ventilation
    c. Pressure controlled
    d. SIMV

12. Tigroid white matter on MRI is seen in?
    a. Pantothenate kinase deficiency *(AIIMS May 2019)*
    b. Pelizaeus-merzbacher disease
    c. Neuroferritinopathy
    d. Aceruloplasminemia

13. A 40 year male complains of hot flushes each time he bathes. Hb: 20 gm%, Platelet: 1,89,000/μL, WBC: 30,000/μL, Investigation revealed JAK2 mutation. What is the most likely diagnosis?
    a. Progressive massive fibrosis
    b. Chronic myeloid leukemia
    c. Polycythemia vera
    d. Essential thrombocytosis

14. A patient with thalassemia with need of recurrent transfusion, develops transfusion reaction like fever and chills. What can be done to the blood decrease the rate transfusion reactions?
    a. Leucocyte depletion
    b. Antibiotics
    c. Deglycerolization
    d. Washed RBCs

15. A CKD patient had to undergo dialysis. His Hb was 5.2gm% so two blood transfusions were to be given. First bag was completed in 2 hours. Second was started and midway he developed shortness of breath, hypertension. Vitals: BP 180/120 mm Hg and pulse rate 110/min. What is the cause?
    a. Allergic
    b. Transfusion related circulatory overload (TACO)
    c. TRALI
    d. FNHTR

16. Most common functional neuroendocrine tumor of pancreas?
    a. Gastrinoma
    b. Somatostatinoma
    c. Insulinoma
    d. VIPoma

17. A patient presented to emergency after RTA with multiple rib fractures. He is conscious, speaking single words. On examination, respiratory rate was 40/min and BP was 90/40 mm Hg. What is immediate next step?
    a. Urgent IV fluid administration
    b. Intubate the patient
    c. Chest –ray
    d. Needle insert in in 2nd intercostal space

18. Device shown in the image is used for what purpose?

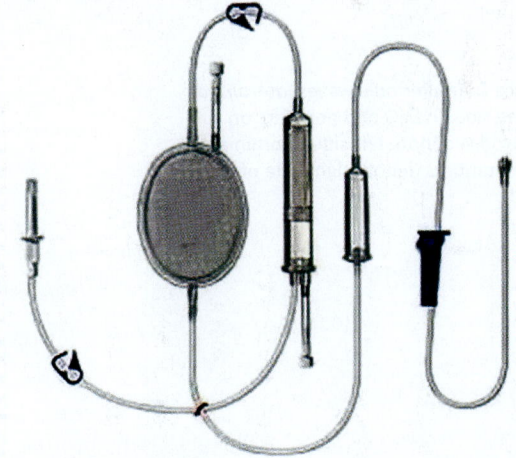

    a. Prevent viral infections
    b. Prevent transfusion related reactions
    c. Prevent infection
    d. All of the above

19. On 5th postoperative day of CABG, patient develops tachypnea and hypertension. What is the most probable cause?
    a. Sepsis
    b. Acute Kidney failure
    c. Acute Respiratory failure
    d. Acute Cardiac Failure

ANSWERS WITH EXPLANATIONS

1. Ans. (b) Creutzfeldt-Jakob Disease

(Ref: Harrison 20th edition, page 3059)

- The EEG shows presence of high voltage bursts present periodically in both left and right sided leads. These are described as **periodic sharp waves complexes** and are a feature of variant Creutzfeldt Jakob disease.

- Choice A has triphasic waves and is hence ruled out.
- Notice the positive red deflections preceded and followed by negative blue deflections. They are called triphasic waves.

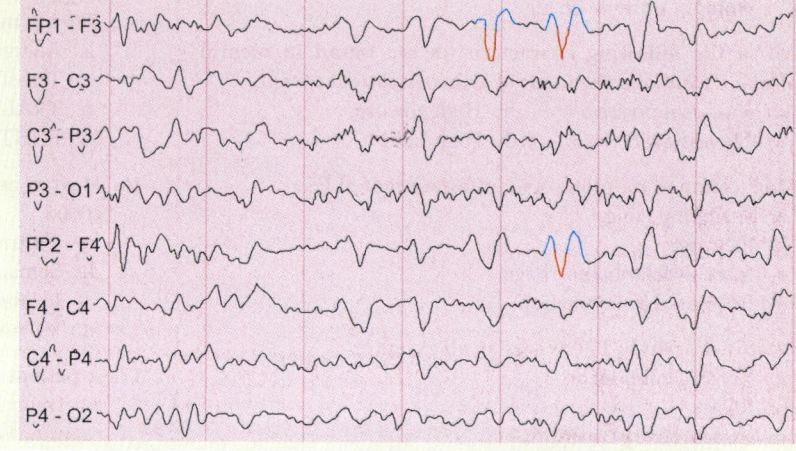

- Choice C has high voltage bursts in all the leads

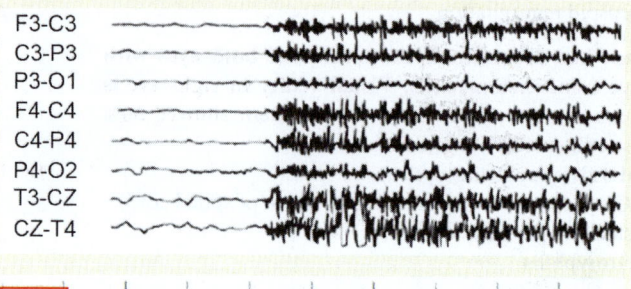

- Choice D has Periodic waves *lateralized* to one side. In EEG odd numbers on electrodes denote left side of brain and even numbers denote right side of brain.

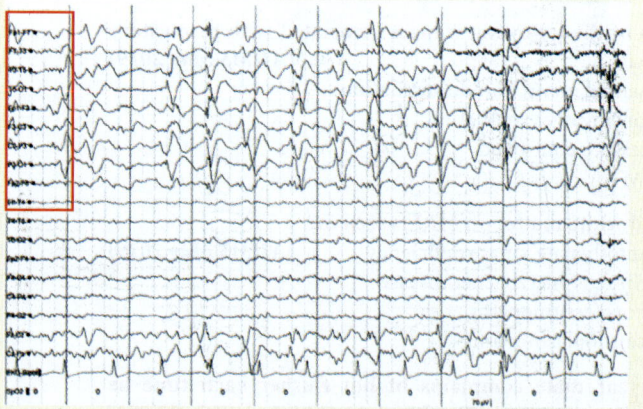

2. Ans. (d) Multi-focal atrial tachycardia

(Ref: Harrison 20th edition, page 1547)

- The heart rate is irregular. Notice the horizontal rhythm strip markings.

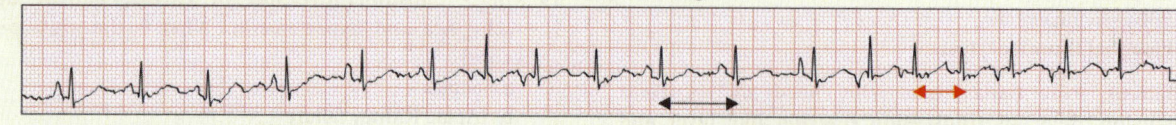

- Right axis deviation is present.

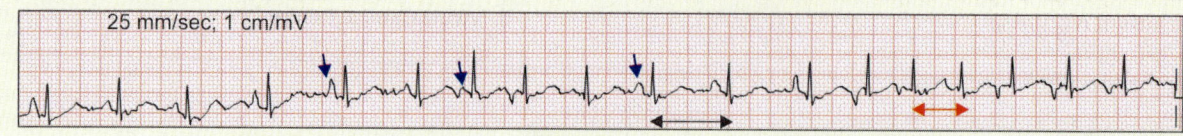

P wave is present and is showing different morphologies. The vertical markings highlight the different shapes of P waves.

- The presence of P waves automatically rules out atrial fibrillation and Paroxysmal supraventricular tachycardia.
- qRS complexes are of normal duration. ST segment is normal.
- Progression of R wave as we move to lateral chest leads is abnormal. Deep S waves in lateral leads point to a possible RV enlargement.
- The given findings point to diagnosis of multifocal atrial tachycardia.

3. Ans. (d) 12 mmol/L

(Ref: Harrison 20th edition, page 317)
- The anion gap formula is $Na^+ - (Cl^- + HCO_3^-) = 137 - (110 + 1(v)) = 12$ mmol/L. The value of potassium is not considered in anion gap

4. Ans. (b) Muscle intimal elastic lamina layer defect

(Ref: Harrison 20th, page 2084)
- As an aneurysm develops, it typically forms a neck with a dome. The length of the neck and the size of the dome vary greatly and are important factors in planning neurosurgical obliteration or endovascular embolization. *The arterial internal elastic lamina disappears at the base of the neck.* The media thins, and connective tissue replaces smooth-muscle cells. At the site of rupture (most often the dome), the wall thins, and the tear that allows bleeding is often ≤0.5 mm long. Aneurysm size and site are important in predicting risk of rupture. Those >7 mm in diameter and those at the top of the basilar artery and at the origin of the posterior communicating artery are at greater risk

5. Ans. (a) False: CT scan is done to rule out hemorrhagic stroke. If CT is normal it implies thrombolysis should be started since findings of ischemic stroke will take some time to evolve. By that we may bypass the actual window period; (b) False: Since there is no need to perform MRI if CT scan is normal; (c) True: Thrombolysis can be done if BP is above 150/80; (d) True: rtPA can be given if patient is having INR of <1.7; (e) True: Antiplatelet therapy has proven to be effective in management of Acute ischemic stroke.

(Ref: Harrison 20th edition, page 3082).

Table: Administration of Intravenous Recombinant Tissue Plasminogen Activator (rPA) for Acute Ischemic Stroke (AIS)

Indication	Contraindication
• Clinical diagnosis of stroke • Onset of symptoms to time of drug administration ≤4.5 h • CT scan showing no hemorrhage or edema of >1/3 of the MCA territory • Age ≥18 years	• Sustained BP > 185/110 mm Hg despite treatment • Bleeding diathesis • Recent head injury or intracerebral hemorrhage • Major surgery in preceding 14 days • Gastrointestinal bleeding in preceding 21 days • Recent myocardial infarction

6. Ans. (b) Decrease in Systolic blood pressure 20 mm Hg within 3 min of postural change

(Ref: AHA clinical Cardiac consult, page 280)
- Orthostatic hypotension is defined as decrease of BP > 20 mm Hg systolic and Diastolic >10 mm Hg accompanied with symptoms of cerebral hypoperfusion.

- *Postural orthostatic tachycardia syndrome* (POTS) is characterized by symptomatic sinus tachycardia that occurs with postural change from a supine position to standing. The sinus rate increases by 30 beats/min or to >120 beats/min within 10 min of standing and in the absence of hypotension.

7. Ans. (b) High glucose

(Ref: Harrison 20th edition, page 2007)
- Since rheumatoid arthritis is an exudate it will have low sugar values. Cholesterol crystals are seen in long standing pleural effusion of rheumatoid arthritis. High LDH is explained by Light's criteria.
- Differentials if glucose in pleural fluid is less than 60 mg/dl

Glucose <60 mg/dL
- Consider: Malignancy
- Bacterial infections
- Rheumatoid pleuritis

8. Ans. (b) Pleuritis

(Ref: Harrison 20th edition, page 2520)
- The most common lung manifestation of SLE is pleuritis with or without pleural effusion. It may respond to NSAIDS or may require steroids. Life threatening manifestations include interstitial inflammation and shrinking lung syndrome.

9. Ans. (a) Cardiac tamponade

(Ref: Harrison 20th edition, page 1843)
- Y descent in JVP occurs due to ventricular diastole. In cardiac tamponade the intrapericardial pressure exceeds the ventricular end diastolic pressure leading to inability of heart to relax and get filled with blood. Hence due to impaired diastolic filling, the y descent disappears from JVP.

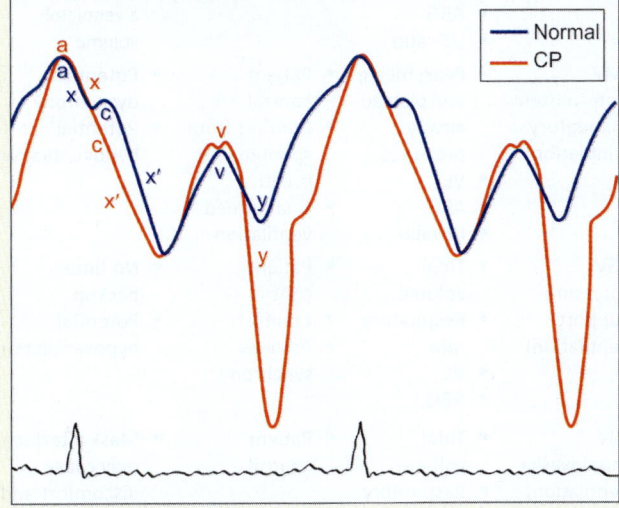

Causes of steep Y descent
1. Constrictive pericarditis
2. Restrictive cardiomyopathy
3. Tricuspid regurgitation

10. Ans. (a) NMO (Neuromyelitis optica)

(Ref: Harrison 20th edition, page 3202)
- The combination of transverse myelitis and optic neuritis is a diagnosis of neuromyelitis optica.
- Choice B has only spinal cord involvement. Choice C is Choice D is ruled out due to response to steroids.

Clinical features in Neuromyelitis Optica

Core clinical characteristics
1. Optic neuritis
2. Acute myelitis
3. Area postrema syndrome: episode of otherwise unexplained hiccups or nausea or vomiting
4. Acute brainstem syndrome
5. Symptomatic narcolepsy or acute diencephalic clinical syndrome with NMOSD-typical diencephalic MRI lesions
6. Symptomatic cerebral syndrome with NMOSD-typical brain lesions

11. Ans. (a) Assisted control mode ventilation

(Ref: Harrison 20th edition, page 2036)
- In assisted controlled mechanical ventilation, the programming is done to initiate ventilator associated breaths for example every 5 seconds. However in between this 5-second interval, if there is a spontaneous breathing effort on part of patient, then ventilator will kick in and aid the patient in taking a breath. This can lead to hyperventilation and development of respiratory alkalosis.

Table: Characteristics of the Most Commonly Used Forms of Mechanical Ventilation

Ventilatory Mode	Variables Monitored By User (Dependent)	Advantages	Disadvantages
ACMV (assist-control ventilation)	• Peak, mean, and plateau airway pressures • VE • ABG • I/E ratio	• Patient control • Guaranteed ventilation	• Potential hyperventilation • Barotrauma and volume trauma • Every effective breath generates a ventilator volume
IMV (intermittent mandatory ventilation)	• Peak, mean, and plateau airway pressures • VE • ABG • I/E ratio	• Patient control • Comfort from spontaneous breaths • Guaranteed ventilation	• Potential dysnchrony • Potential hypoventilation
PSV (pressure-support ventilation)	• Tidal volume • Respiratory rate • VE • ABG	• Patient control • Comfort • Assures synchrony	• No timer backup • Potential hypoventilation
NIV (noninvasive ventilation)	• Tidal volume • Respiratory rate • VE • ABG	• Patient control	• Mask interface may cause discomfort and facial bruising • Leaks are common • Hypoventilation

12. Ans. (b) Pelizaeus-merzbacher disease

(Ref: Harrison 20th edition, page 3149)
- The tigroid pattern occurs on MRI head is seen in Pelizaeus-merzbacher disease, *due to creation of islands of perivascular myelin due patchy myelin deficiency*. It is a rare hypomyelination syndrome caused by mutation in proteolipid protein, PLP 1 gene at chromosome Xq22. The disease has autosomal or X-linked inheritance leading to equal incidence in both genders. Child will show slow psychomotor development with nystagmus, hypotonia, extrapyramidal symptoms and spasticity.

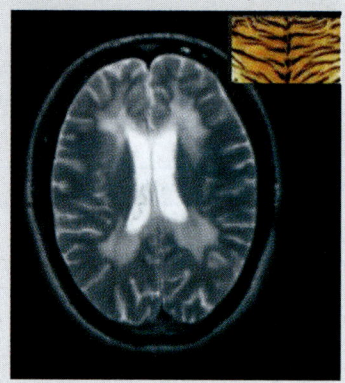

13. Ans. (c) Polycythemia vera

(Ref: Harrison 20th edition, page 734)
- The clinical diagnosis is based on presence of JAK 2 mutation with elevated cell counts and *characteristic aquagenic pruritus*. The elevated basophils produce histamine which leads to intense pruritus, post water exposure.

14. Ans. (a) Leucocyte depletion

(Ref: Wintrobe' clinical Hematology: 13th edition, page 554)
- In setting of recurrent of transfusions the donor leucocytes increase the risk of development of febrile non hemolytic transfusions as well as graft versus host disease.
- Of the methods available to reduce the number of WBC in blood products washing of Red cells, freezing and deglycerolization are effective and yield a product with short shelf life. Modern generation of leukoreduction filters and apheresis machines can provide greater than 4 log reduction of WBC.
- *Leukoreduction of blood products should produce blood products with residual WBC < 5 X 10^6 WBC per unit (99.9 percent or log 3 reduction).*

15. Ans. (b) Transfusion related circulatory overload (TACO)

(Ref: Harrison 20th edition, page 814)
- This C.K.D patient has developed severe anemia which is a compensated heart failure state. The patient was given first unit of blood in two hours instead of standard four hours and he is already in compensated heart failure.
- The acute decompensation due to volume overloading that has subsequently occurred will result in pulmonary edema and shortness of breath. This presentation is called as transfusion associated circulatory overload.
- Ideally patients of CKD should be given erythropoietin injections to reduce the incidence of having severe anemia.

16. Ans. (c) Insulinoma

(Ref: Harrison 20th edition, page 597, 608)
- The incidence of Insulinoma is 1-2% whereas the incidence of ZES is given as 0.5-1.5%.

Table: Gastrointestinal Neuroendocrine Tumor Syndromes

Name	Biologically active peptide(s) secreted	Incidence (new cases/10^6 population/year)	Tumor location
Well-established functional pNET syndromes			
Zollinger-Ellison syndrome	Gastrin	0.5-1.5	• Duodenum (70%) • Pancreas (25%)
Insulinoma	Insulin	1-2	Pancreas (>99%)
VIPoma (Verner-Morrison syndrome, pancreatic cholera, WDHA)	Vasoactive intestinal peptide	0.05-0.2	• Pancreas (99%, adult) Other (10%, neural, adrenal, periganglionic)
Glucagonoma	Glucagon	0.01-0.1	Pancreas (100%)
Somatostatinoma	Somatostatin	Rare	• Pancreas (55%) • Duodenum/jejunum (44%)

17. Ans. (d) Needle insert in in 2nd intercostal space

(Ref: Harrison 20th edition, page 2009)
- The clinical diagnosis based on history of rib fractures, respiratory distress and hypotension is pneumothorax. There can be concomitant hemothorax but treatment of obstructive shock caused by pneumothorax will take is the immediate step. This would be done with inserting a wide bore needle in second intercostal space to reduce the impact of obstructive shock and increase systolic blood pressure.

18. Ans. (b) Prevent transfusion related reactions

(Ref: Harrison 20th edition, page 814)
- The image shows a filter in blood transfusion set that will generate leuco-depleted blood. The second generation filters of size 40um can remove microaggregates of fibrin, platelets and leucocytes and reduce the number of leucocytes by magnitude of 5×10^8 per unit. The main immediate advantage is reduced incidence of febrile non hemolytic transfusions.

Potential benefits
- Reduced risk of platelet refractoriness,
- Reduced risk of febrile non-haemolytic transfusion reactions (FNHTR),
- Reduced risk of CMV transmission,
- Reduction in storage lesion effect,
- Reduction in the incidence of bacterial contamination of blood components,
- Possible reduced risk of transfusion-associated graft vs host disease (TA-GVHD)
- Possible reduction in transfusion related immuno-modulatory (TRIM) effects, including cancer recurrence, mortality, non-transfusion transmitted infection,
- Possible reduced risk of transmitting variant Creutzfeldt-Jakob Disease,

19. Ans. (c) Acute Respiratory failure

(Ref: Clinical intensive medicine, 2015 edition, page 533)
- The postoperative period following cardiac surgery is characterized by high incidence of respiratory complications with atelectasis being more prominent when Cardiopulmonary bypass is used. Post op pain and prolonged hospital stay of this patient can both explain the presentation of these patients.

Complications after CABG

- Death (3%)
- Respiratory failure
  - Atelectasis (70%)
  - Pleural effusion (~10%)
  - ARDS (rare as hen's teeth)
- Pulmonary hypertension
- Myocardial dysfunction
  - Cardiac tamponade (1.5%)
  - CABG graft ischaemia (4-5%)
- Vasoplegia
- Neurological complications:
  - Focal neurological deficit (3%)
  - Impairment of memory or cognition (3%)
- Renal failure (7%)
  - Renal failure requiring dialysis (1.25%)
- **Hyperglycaemia**

Sample Video Questions

1. **The following procedure was performed in a patient of spontaneous pneumothorax. It is called as?**

   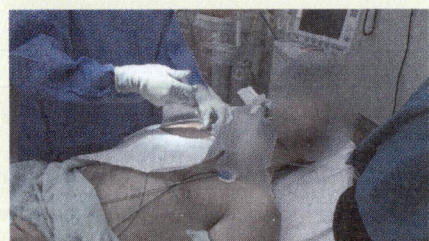

   a. Thoracentesis   b. Thoracic venting
   c. Wide bore needle aspiration
   d. V.A.T.S

2. **What is the abnormality shown in the ECG?**

   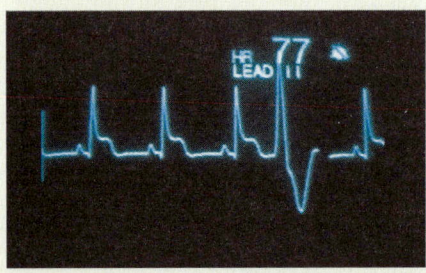

   a. Premature ventricular contractions
   b. Sine wave pattern
   c. ST segment depression
   d. Electrical alternans

3. **What is the treatment of this cardiac arrythmia?**

   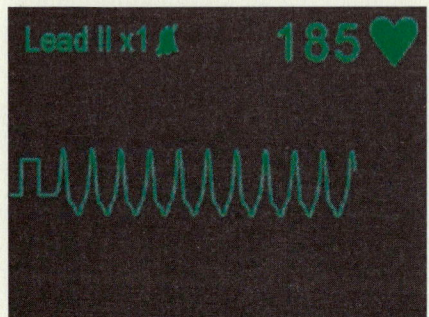

   a. Ibtilide   b. Adenosine
   c. Digoxin   d. Amiodarone

4. **Comment on the possible diagnosis in the patient?**

   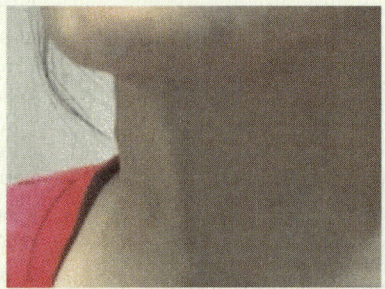

   a. Tricuspid regurgitation   b. Aortic regurgitation
   c. Mitral regurgitation   d. Cor-triatrium

5. **What is the ECG abnormality shown in the picture?**

   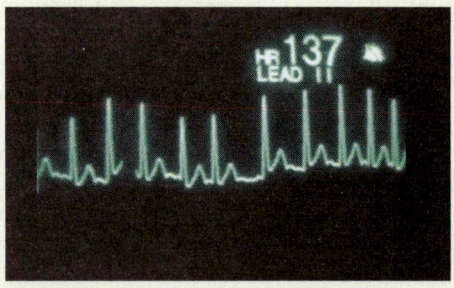

   a. Atrial fibrillation   b. Atrial flutter
   c. AVNRT   d. AVRT

6. **What is the ECG rhythm shown in the video?**

   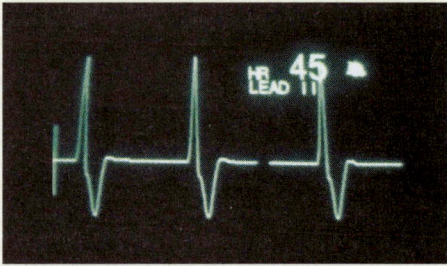

   a. Accelerated idioventricular rhythm
   b. Agonal rhythm
   c. Sine wave pattern
   d. Complete heart block

7. Comment on the character of apex beat shown in the video?

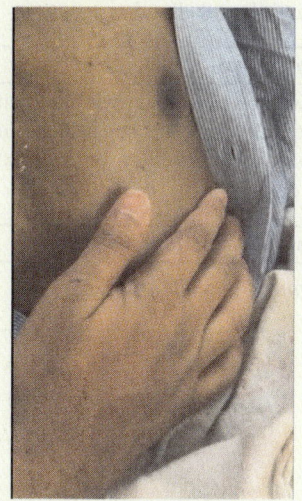

   a. Heaving   b. Hyperdynamic
   c. Tapping   d. Hypokinetic

8. The patient is having?

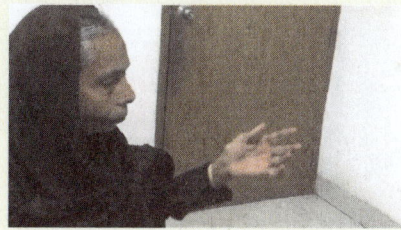

   a. Resting tremor   b. Past pointing
   c. Startle Myoclonus d. Asterixis

9. What is the gait abnormality shown in the video?

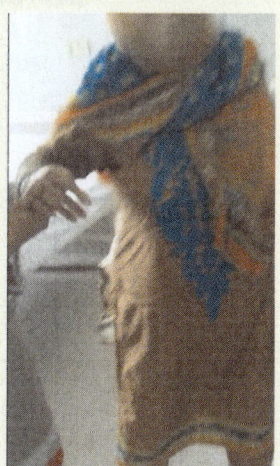

   a. Festinating gait   b. Stamping gait
   c. Magnetic gait   d. Equine gait

10. Which EEG pattern is shown here?

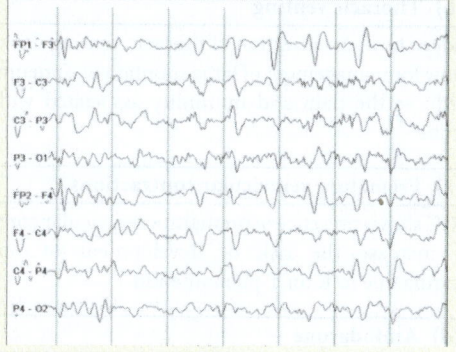

   a. Hepatic encephalopathy
   b. Creutzfeldt-Jakob Disease
   c. GTCS
   d. Herpes simplex encephalitis

11. Comment on the diagnosis?

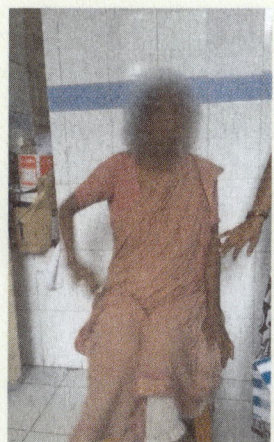

   a. Athetosis   b. Hemiballismus
   c. Gegenhalten   d. Asterixis

12. What clinical sign is shown in the video?

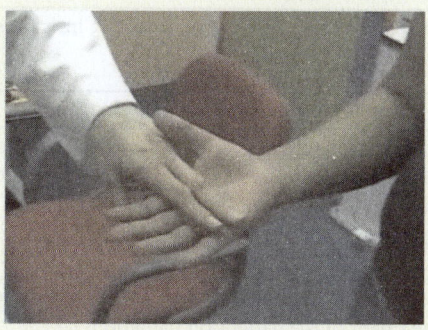

   a. Myoclonus   b. Paratonia
   c. Myotonia   d. Hoffman reflex

For video, scan this QR Code

ANSWERS FOR VIDEO QUESTIONS

1. Ans. (b) Thoracic venting
The video shows an insertion of thoracic venting device that is used now for management of large spontaneous pneumothorax and reduces the pain and morbidity associated with use of chest tube.

2. Ans. (a) Premature ventricular contractions
The ECG shows presence of premature ventricular contractions which increase the risk of development of ventricular tachycardia due to R on T phenomenon.

3. Ans. (d) Amiodarone
The rhythm show is monomorphic Ventricular tachycardia and is treated with iv amiodarone.

4. Ans. (a) Tricuspid regurgitation
- Notice the visible neck pulsations indicating elevated JVP. Choice C and D are ruled out as they are left sided lesions and usually do not lead to changes in JVP.
- The confusion can be with dancing carotids of aortic regurgitation versus giant CV waves of Tricuspid JVP.
- The dancing carotid produces an outward displacement and does not start from base of neck unlike the video shown in the image.

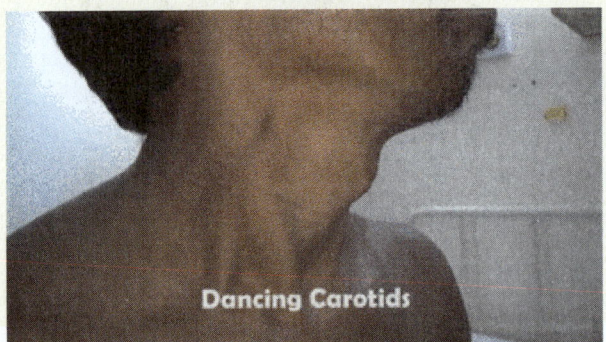

For video scan QR-Code given on page XXXIX

5. Ans. (a) Atrial fibrillation
The video shows presence of irregular RR interval suggestive of diagnosis of atrial fibrillation.

6. Ans. (a) Accelerated idioventricular rhythm
The video shows a heart rate of 45/min with broad complex QRS complexes suggestive of diagnosis of slow VT which is also called as AIVR. It happens to be a reperfusion arrythmia.

7. Ans. (a) Heaving
The video shows presence of heaving apex beat which has lifted the finger of the patient on palpation.

8. Ans. (b) Past pointing
Notice as the patient's finger is approaching the examiner's finger, the patient shows past pointing and intentional tremor. This is suggestive of cerebellar damage.

9. Ans. (c) Magnetic gait
The video shows a classical magnetic gait/ gait apraxia. Notice how she walked as if feet are stuck to ground and froze in between as she lost her concentration to walk. This is a feature of frontal lobe damage

10. Ans. (a) Hepatic encephalopathy
(Ref: Harrison 20th edition page 3059)

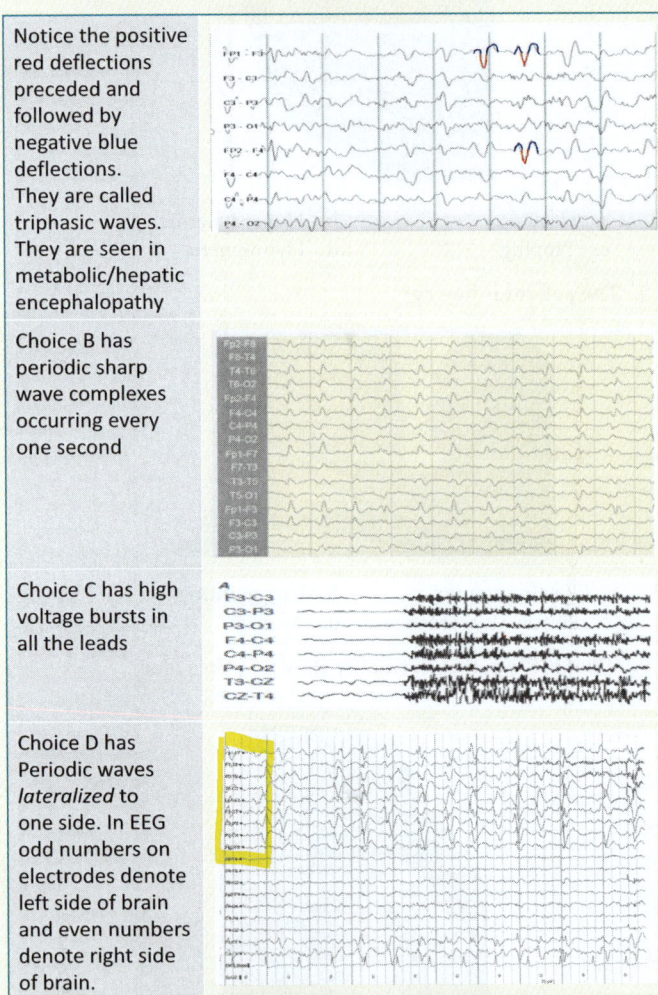

Notice the positive red deflections preceded and followed by negative blue deflections. They are called triphasic waves. They are seen in metabolic/hepatic encephalopathy

Choice B has periodic sharp wave complexes occurring every one second

Choice C has high voltage bursts in all the leads

Choice D has Periodic waves *lateralized* to one side. In EEG odd numbers on electrodes denote left side of brain and even numbers denote right side of brain.

11. Ans. (b) Hemiballismus
The patient is having involuntary movement at both proximal and distal part of right arm and leg indicating a movement disorder which is called hemiballismus.

12. Ans. (c) Myotonia
The video shows myotonia which is continuous contraction of muscle cells that persists after stimulation of muscle cells that persists after the stimulation or voluntary effort has stopped. You an notice the contracted adductor muscles of thumb at the end of the video.

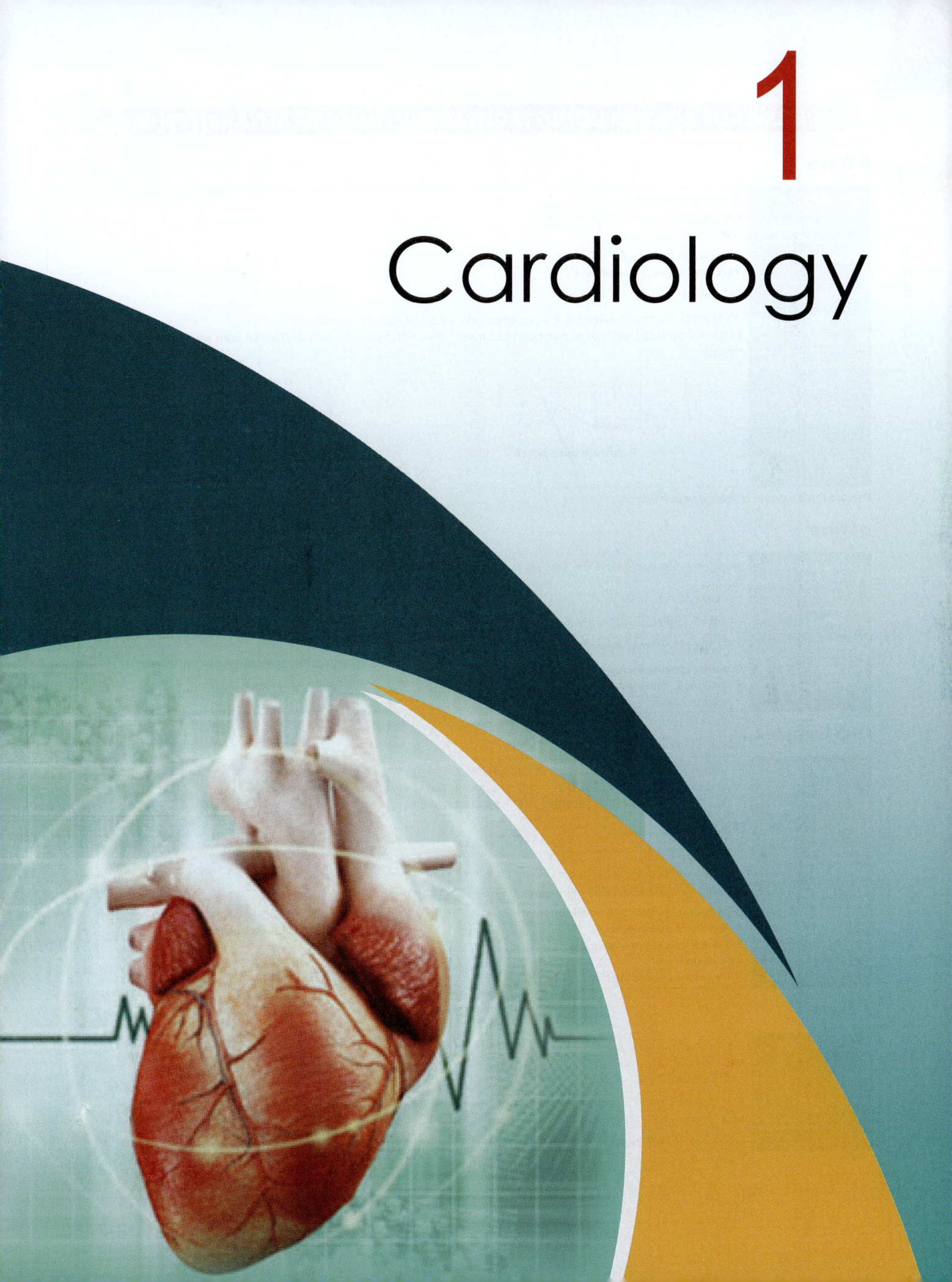

1 Cardiology

BASICS OF ECG INCLUDING TACHYARRHYTHMIA/BRADYARRHYTHMIA

P Wave

Configuration	Rounded and upright Positive in lead II and negative in aVR Biphasic in lead V_1
Amplitude	<2.5 mm in limb leads[Q] <1.5 mm in precordial leads
Duration	<120 msec
Remarks	Right atrial overload can lead to P wave amplitude > 2.5 mm called p-pulmonale Left atrial overload will lead to duration >120 msec with a notch called P mitrale (Can be seen with left atrial conduction delays)

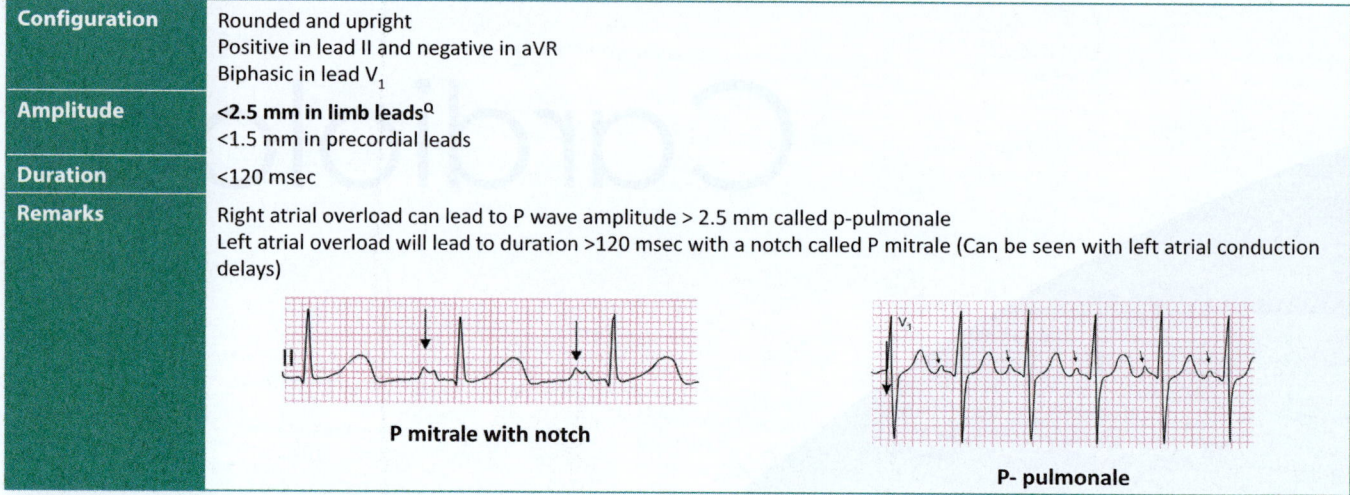

P mitrale with notch

P- pulmonale

Pseudo P-pulmonale is seen in hypokalemia.

q Wave

Configuration	Negative deflection before the R wave, due to septal activation Seen in I, aVL, V_5 and V_6 Usually not seen in V_1-V_3
Amplitude	< 25% of amplitude of R wave in same lead
Duration	< 40 msec (one small square)
Remarks	**Q waves are considered pathological if:**[Q] • > 40 ms (1 mm) wide • > 25% of depth of QRS complex • > 2 mm deep • Seen in leads V_{1-3}

QRS Complex

Configuration	• In leads I, II, III, aV_L, aV_F and V_4 to V_6, the deflection of the QRS complex is characteristically positive or upright. • In leads aV_R, V_1 and V_3, the QRS complex is usually negative or inverted. • R and S wave amplitude becomes equal in transition zone (V_3 and V_4).
Axis	-30° to 100°
Duration	80 – 100 msec
Remarks	Low QRS voltage= peak to trough QRS amplitude of <5 mm in six limb leads or < 10 mm in chest leads. Electrical Alternans= beat to variation in amplitude in cardiac tamponade
	Broad complex QRS (> 3 small squares)[Q] • Bundle branch blocks • Pre-excitation syndrome • Hyperkalemia • Ventricular paced rhythm	**Narrow complex QRS (< 2 small squares)** • All supraventricular tachycardia

T Wave

Configuration	Vector oriented concordant with mean QRS vector Upright in all except aVR and V_1 Indicates ventricular repolarization
Amplitude[Q]	Less than 5 mm in the limb leads Less than 10 mm in the precordial leads
Duration	Dependent on QT interval

Contd...

Remarks	• Tall-tented T waves in Hyperkalemia • Hyperacute T waves in Myocardial infarction • T wave inversion in Myocardial ischemia

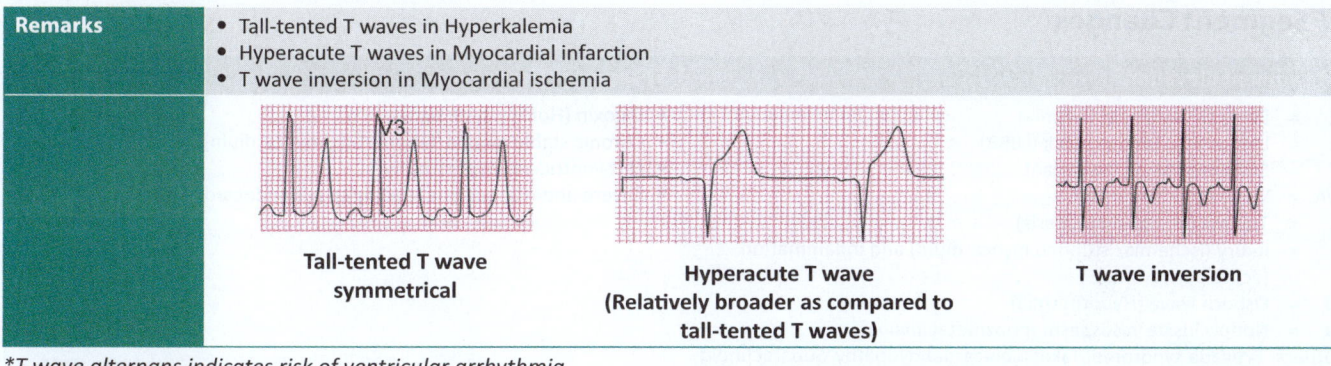

Tall-tented T wave symmetrical

Hyperacute T wave (Relatively broader as compared to tall-tented T waves)

T wave inversion

*T wave alternans indicates risk of ventricular arrhythmia

U Wave

Configuration	Small rounded deflection after T wave
Amplitude	< 1 mm
Remarks	• Prominent U waves in hypokalemia predispose to development of Torsades de pointes[Q] • Inverted U waves indicate myocardial ischemia

PR Interval

Duration	120–200 msec
Remarks	• PR interval duration is inversely related to heart rate • Short PR interval= WPW syndrome, Lown Ganong Levine syndrome • Prolonged PR interval= First degree heart block, Rheumatic fever

QT interval

Duration	360–440 msec (9–10 small squares) • Measured in lead II or V_5-V_6 • The maximum slope intercept method is used to measure T wave ending

Remarks	**QT prolongation[Q]**
	• Hypocalcemia
	• Hypomagnesemia
	• Hypokalemia (prolonged QU interval)
	• Class IA and III drugs
	• Subarachnoid hemorrhage
	• Long QT syndrome
	• Romano ward syndrome **QT shortening**
	    • Hypercalcemia
	    • Digoxin
	    • Congenital Short QT syndrome

	QTc (Bazzet Formula) = QT/ √ R-R interval • QTc is prolonged if > 440 ms in men or > 460 ms in women • QTc >500 is associated with increased risk of torsades de pointes • QTc is abnormally short if <350 ms • A useful rule of thumb is that a normal QT is less than half the preceding RR interval

ST Segment Changes

ST segment elevation[Q]	ST segment Depression
E = Electrolytes (Hyperkalemia) L = Left bundle branch block (LBBB) E = Early repolarization variant VA = Ventricular aneurysm T = Trauma (pericardiocentesis) I = Injury (ischemia/ stunned myocardium) and inflammation (acute pericarditis) O = Osborn wave (Hypothermia) N = Nonocclusive vasospasm (prinzmetal angina) Others- Brugada syndrome, Takotsubo cardiomyopathy, Subarachnoid hemorrhage.	• Digoxin (Hockey stick sign) • Chronic stable angina/hibernating myocardium) • Left ventricular hypertrophy • Severe anemia, cocaine leading to subendocardial ischemia

Electrolytes and ECG Abnormalities

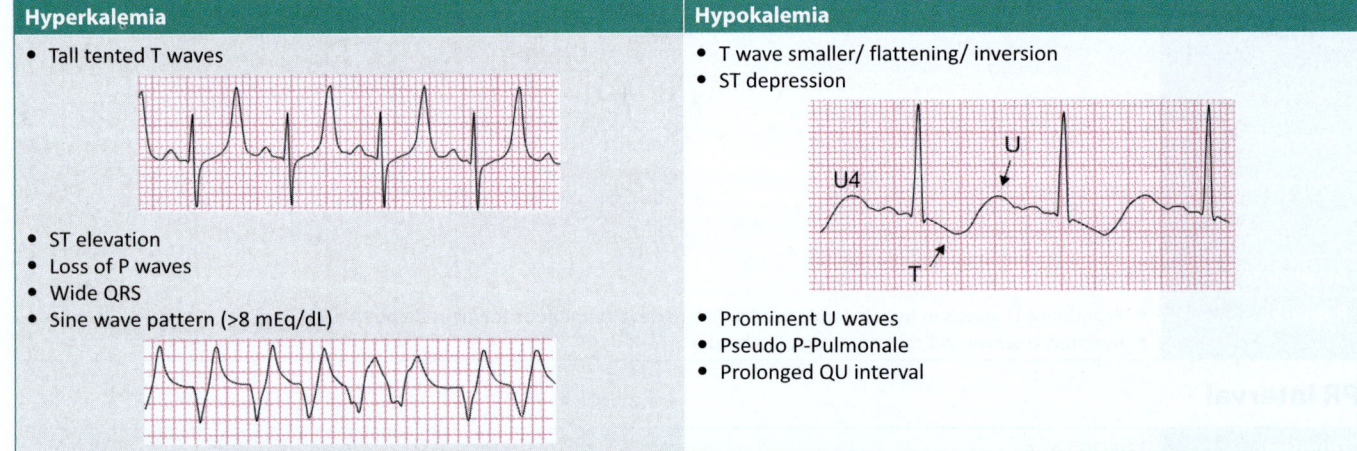

Hyperkalemia	Hypokalemia
• Tall tented T waves • ST elevation • Loss of P waves • Wide QRS • Sine wave pattern (>8 mEq/dL)	• T wave smaller/ flattening/ inversion • ST depression • Prominent U waves • Pseudo P-Pulmonale • Prolonged QU interval

Hypercalcemia	Hypocalcemia
• J waves (The same is seen in hypothermia!!) • QT shortening	QT prolongation

Hypermagnesemia	Hypomagnesemia
• Prolongation of PR, QRS, and QT intervals heart block (Value >10 mmol/L) asystole	• Prolonged PR • Prolonged QT intervals and QT_c (leads to Torsades de pointes) • T-wave flattening or inversion

*QT prolongation is seen with both hypermagnesemia and hypomagnesemia

Miscellaneous Aberrations

Abnormality	Cause	ECG appearance
Osborn wave/ J waves[Q]	• Hypothermia • Hypercalcemia • Subarachnoid hemorrhage	Osborn wave Notice the wave at J point

Contd...

Abnormality	Cause	ECG appearance
Epsilon wave[Q]	Arrhythmogenic right ventricular dysplasia	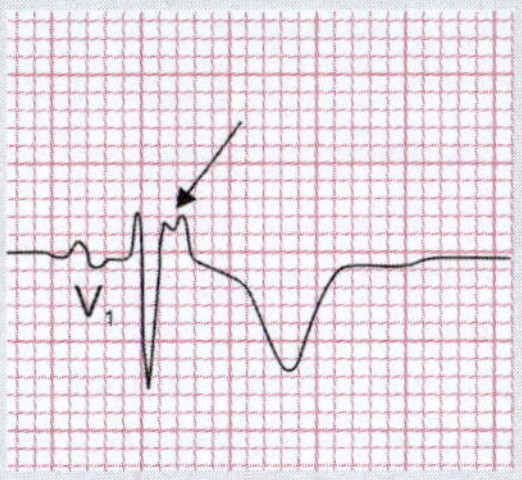 Notice the *notched* wave at the J point
Brugada pattern[Q] (not Brugada sign which is seen in VT)	Brugada syndrome (SCN5A- sodium channel defect)	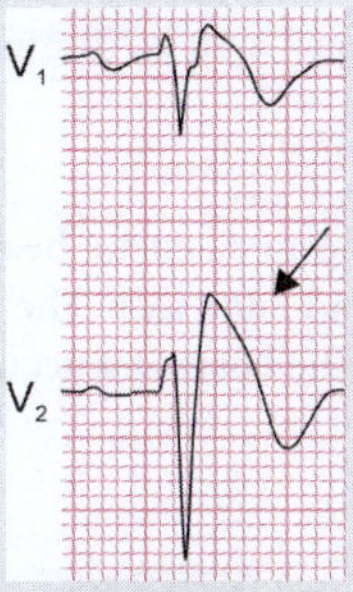
Hockey stick sign[Q]	Digoxin	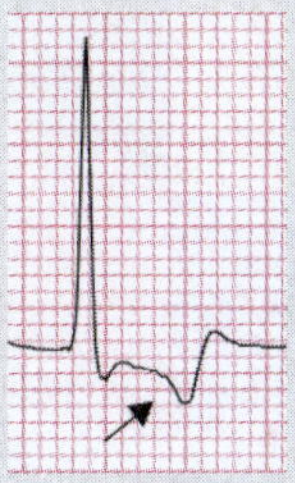 Scooped ST segment / reverse tick sign
$S_1Q_3T_3$ pattern[Q]	Massive pulmonary embolism	• Deep S wave in lead I • Deep Q waves in lead III • Inverted T waves in lead III

*Hockey stick sign on echocardiography is seen in mitral stenosis.

Heart Rate Calculation

Method 1: Count the number of large squares separating R-R interval

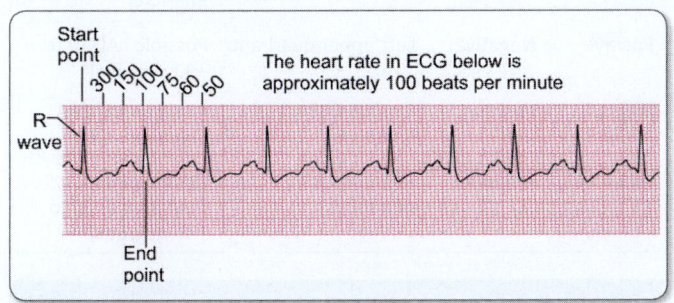

No of large squares between R-R waves	Heart rate
1	300
2	150
3	100

No of large squares between R-R waves	Heart rate
4	75
5	60
6	50
7	40

Method 2: Divide 1500/number of small squares counted between R-R interval

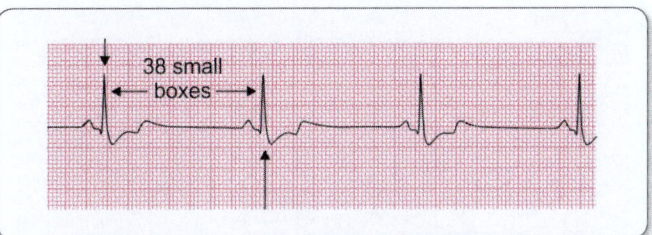

Contd...

Method 3: Heart rate calculation, if rhythm is abnormal

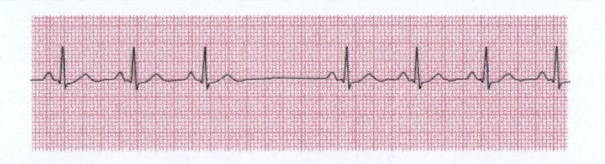

- Since the R-R interval of the patient is variable, count the number of R waves in a 6 second strip and multiply the same by 10.
- This would give 7 R waves in 6 second interval of this strip and hence the heart rate is 7 × 10 = 70/min.

Axis Calculation

The most efficient method to calculate heart axis is to calculate the mean QRS vector from lead I and aVF. The vectors can be plotted on the diagram below to get the heart axis accurately.

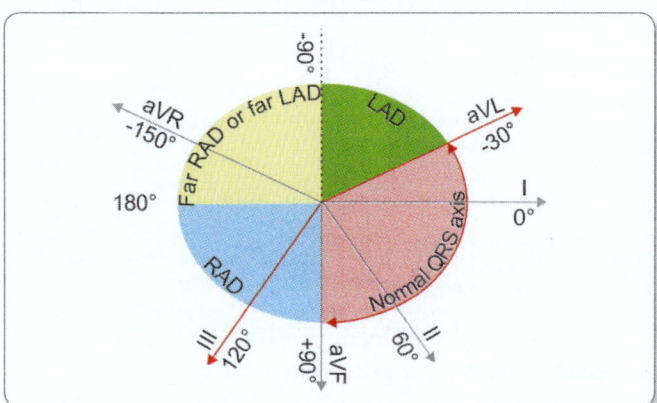

Interpretation

Lead I	Lead AVF	Quadrant	Axis
Positive	Positive	Left lower quadrant	Normal (0 to +90 degrees)
Positive	Negative	Left upper quadrant	Possible LAD (0 to −90 degrees)
Negative	Positive	Right lower quadrant	RAD (+90 to 180 degrees)
Negative	Negative	Right upper quadrant	Extreme Axis Deviation (−90 to 180 degrees)

Right Axis Deviation

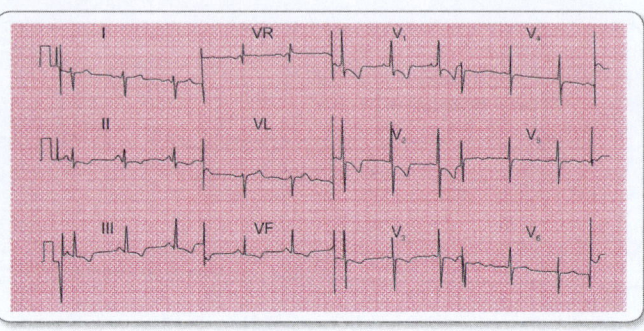

- The mean QRS vector in lead I is negative
- The mean QRS vector in lead aVF is positive
- Hence, the axis shows right axis deviation

Causes of Right Axis Deviation[Q]

1. Normal (children and young adults)
2. Left posterior fascicular block
3. Reversal of right and left arm electrodes
4. Pulmonary embolism
5. Pulmonary arterial hypertension (PAH)
6. Chronic obstructive pulmonary disease (COPD)
7. Lateral wall MI
8. Dextrocardia
9. Left pneumothorax
10. Wolff–parkinson–white (WPW) type A

Left Axis Deviation

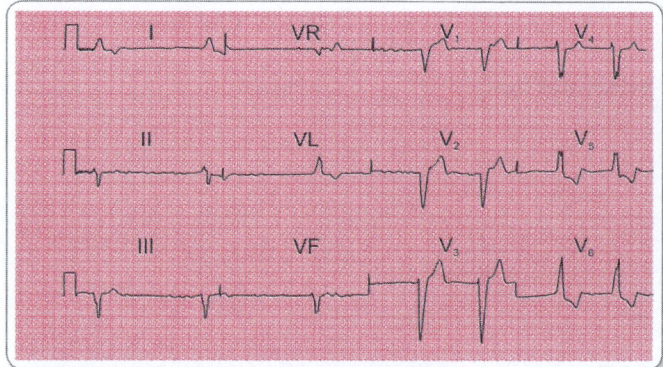

- The mean qRS vector in lead I is positive.
- The mean qRS vector in lead III is negative.
- Hence, the axis shows left axis deviation.

The most efficient way to estimate axis is to look at leads I + aVF.

Lead I	Lead AVF	Quadrant	Axis
Positive	Positive	Left lower quadrant	Normal (0 to +90 degrees)
Positive	Negative	Left upper quadrant	Possible LAD (0 to −90 degrees)
Negative	Positive	Right lower quadrant	RAD (+90 to 180 degrees)
Negative	Negative	Right upper quadrant	Extreme Axis Deviation (−90 to 180 degrees)

Causes of left axis deviation[Q]	Causes of extreme axis[Q] deviation
• Left anterior fascicular block • Left bundle branch block • Left ventricular hypertrophy • Inferior wall MI • Ventricular ectopy • Ventricular pacing	• Hyperkalemia • Right ventricular hypertrophy • Ventricular tachycardia • Accelerated idioventricular rhythm

Bundle Branch Block

Left bundle branch block (LBBB)

Mnemonic: WILLIAM
The slurring (arrow) is due to sequential rather than simultaneous activation of ventricles

Criteria
- QRS duration >120 msec
- Dominant S wave in Lead V_1
- Broad monophasic R wave in lateral leads (I, aVL and V_5-V_6)
- Absence of Q waves in lateral leads V_5-V_6
- Prolonged R wave peak time >60 msec in precordial leads

Causes of LBBB[Q]
1. Aortic stenosis
2. Ischemic heart disease (IHD)
3. Hypertension
4. Dilated cardiomyopathy
5. Anterior wall MI
6. Hyperkalemia
7. Digoxin toxicity
8. Lenegre's disease (degenerative fibrosis of conducting system)

Right bundle branch block (RBBB)

Mnemonic: MARROW

Criteria
- Broad QRS > 120 msec
- RSR' pattern in V_1-V_3
- Wide slurred S wave in lateral leads (I, aVL, V_5-V_6)

Causes of RBBB
1. Physiological
2. RVH/ Cor-pulmonale
3. Pulmonary embolism
4. Rheumatic heart disease
5. Myocarditis
6. Cardiomyopathy
7. Atrial septal defect

LBBB

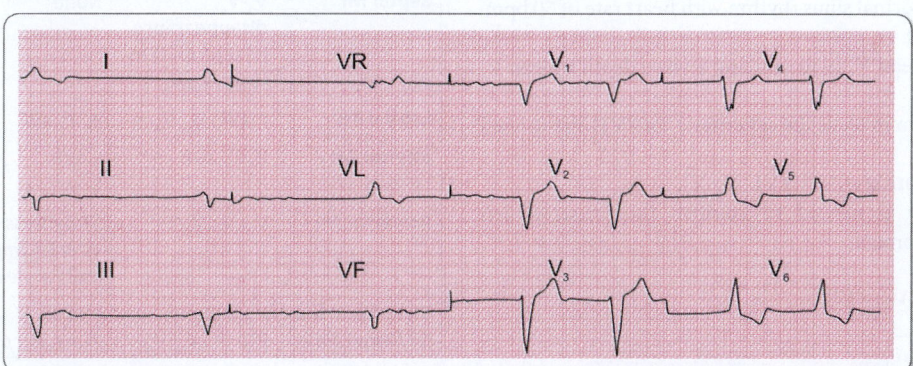

- Dominant S wave in Lead V_1
- Broad monophasic R wave in lateral leads (I, aVL and V_5-V_6)
- Absence of Q waves in lateral leads V_5-V_6
- Slurring of peak of R wave in V_5-V_6

RBBB

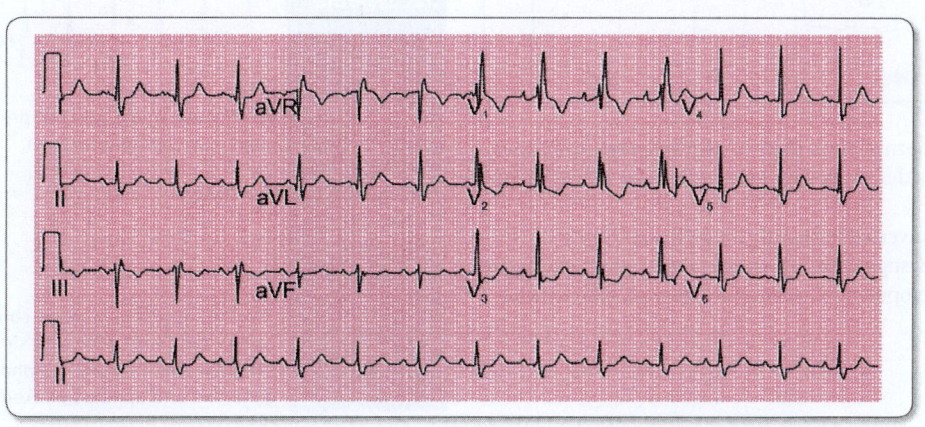

- Notice the RSR' pattern in V_1-V_3
- Wide slurred S wave in lateral leads (I, aVL, V_5-V_6)

Chamber Enlargement

Left Ventricular Hypertrophy	Right Ventricular Hypertrophy
• Precordial leads = SV_1 + RV5 or RV_6 > 35 mm • Limb leads= RaVL + SV_3 > 20 mm in women and >28 mm in men • Not very accurate in obese, persons and athletes	• Tall R in V1 with R amplitude> S amplitude • Right axis deviation • ST depression and T wave inversion in right to mid-precordial leads

Left Ventricular Enlargement

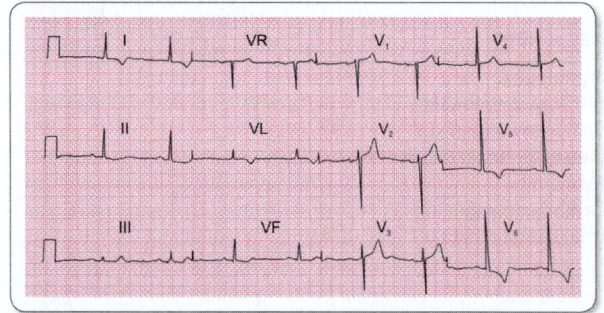

- The ECG shows normal sinus rhythm with heart rate of 50 bpm.
- The axis is normal
- R wave height in lead V_5 is 30 mm and S wave depth in lead V_1 is 20 mm
- The sum of the two exceeds the set criteria for LVH mentioned above
- Inverted T waves are seen in I, aVL, V_5-V_6.
- Echocardiography is needed to confirm the cause of left ventricular enlargement.

Right Chamber Enlargement

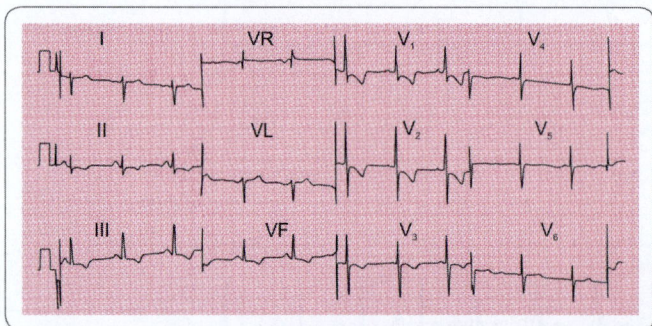

- The ECG shows normal sinus rhythm with heart rate of 75 bpm. There is right axis deviation with Peaked P waves in lead II and III.
- The T waves are inverted in lead II, III, aVF and V_1-V_2.
- The findings are suggestive of presence of right ventricular strain due to development of pulmonary artery hypertension.

ECG Findings of Myocardial Ischemia/Infarction Findings[Q]

Ischemia	T wave inversion and/ or ST segment depression
Injury	ST segment elevation
Infarction	Pathological Q wave (definition given in Q wave section)

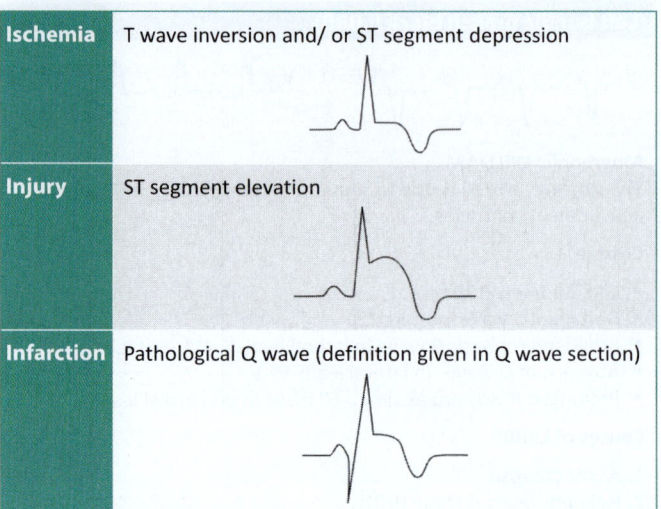

Infarct Localization[Q]

Localization of a myocardial infarct			
Localization	ST elevation	Reciprocal ST depression	Coronary artery
Anterior MI	V_1-V_6	None	LAD
Septal MI	V_1-V_4, disappearance of septum Q in leads V_5, V_6	None	LAD-septal branches
Lateral MI	I, aVL, V_5, V_6	II, III, aVF	LCX or MO
Inferior MI	II, III, aVF	I, aVL	RCA (80%) or RCX (20%)
Posterior MI	V_7, V_8, V_9	ST depression V1-V3 >2mm (mirror view)	RCX (Ramus circumflex)
Right Ventricle MI/Atrial MI	V_1, V_4R PTa in I,V_5, V_6	I, aVL PTa in I, II or III	RCA RCA

LAD = left anterior descending artery   MO = marginal obtuse branch
LCX = left circumflex artery   RCX= ramus circumflex

Quick Overview of Rhythm Abnormalities

Sinus Tachycardia	The P wave and T wave or preceding complex are close and rhythm is regular.
Atrial Premature Complexes	The PAC occurs as a single complex occurring earlier than next expected sinus complex leading to irregular rhythm. The morphology of P wave is also distorted and appears peaked.

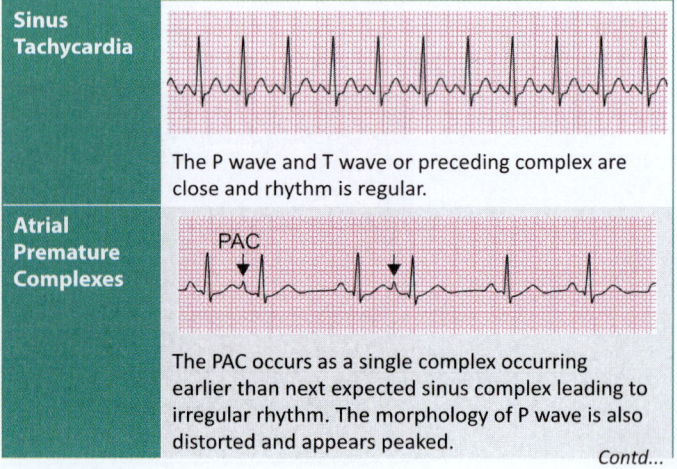

Contd...

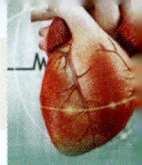

Paroxysmal supraventricular tachycardia (PSVT)	P waves are buried in T wave with narrow complex tachycardia which is due to atrioventricular re-entrant tachycardia.	Mobitz II heart Block	P-R interval before and subsequent to missed beat is of equal duration
Atrial flutter	The macro-entrant re-entry causes saw tooth waves with AV node limiting the number of waves conducting to the ventricles.	2:1 heart block	P-R interval is 200 msec (5 small squares) and is constant in the entire strip and every second P wave is not conducted to the ventricles resulting in dropped beats. This is a feature of 2:1 conduction block. It is highly likely to be misdiagnosed as Mobitz II heart block
Atrial fibrillation	Absence of P waves with normal QRS complex and irregularly irregular rhythm.	Third degree heart block	P-P interval is >> R-R interval. QRS complexes occurring independent of P waves
Multi-focal atrial tachycardia	Characterised by rhythm having at least three distinct P-wave morphologies with a rate of 100–150/min.	First degree heart block	Prolonged P-R interval of >200 msec but there are no dropped beats.
WPW	The change in slope of R wave is called Delta wave. P-R interval is short and P-J interval is normal		
Ventricular tachycardia (VT)	Broad complex QRS leading to spindle appearance		
Torsades de pointes	Broad complex QRS with variable amplitude is called torsades de pointes		
Ventricular fibrillation	Twitching of ventricles		
Mobitz I heart block	Serial PR prolongation followed by missed beat PR before and after missed beat are of different durations with the subsequent PR always having less duration than the previous PR interval.		

Contd...

Tachyarrhythmias

- Most common arrhythmia mechanism is re-entry (Ref: Chapter 273e: Harrison 19th edition).
- Most common sustained arrhythmia is atrial fibrillation.
- Most common benign rhythm identified is atrial premature contraction.
- Most common arrhythmia in COPD patient is multifocal atrial tachycardia (MAT).
- Postoperative atrial fibrillation is managed with landiolol hydrochloride.
- Atrial fibrillation getting converted to ventricular fibrillation is seen with accessory pathway conducting antegradely like bundle of Kent in WPW.
- Most common form of PSVT is AVNRT (AV nodal re-entrant tachycardia) and not AVRT (AV re-entry tachycardia).
- VT storm or electrical storm is >3 or more separate episodes of VT within 24 hours.
- Most commonly identified arrhythmia in cardiac arrest patients is ventricular fibrillation.
- Most common genetic cardiovascular disorder is hypertrophic obstructive cardiomyopathy.
- Most common reason of sudden death in hypertrophic cardiomyopathy (HCM) is polymorphic VT and Ventricular fibrillation (VF).

Mechanism of Arrhythmia

Type of arrhythmias	Mechanism of arrhythmia
Sinus bradycardia Sinus tachycardia	Suppression/acceleration of phase 4
Digitalis toxicity Reperfusion VT	Delayed after depolarization
Torsades des pointes	Early after depolarization
Ischemic VF AV block	Suppression of phase 0
Polymorphic VT Atrial fibrillation	AP prolongation, early after depolarization (EADs), delayed after depolarization (DADs) AP shortening
Monomorphic VT, atrial fibrillation	Excitable gap and functional re-entry

Comparison of Characteristics of Atrial Fibrillation and Atrial Flutter

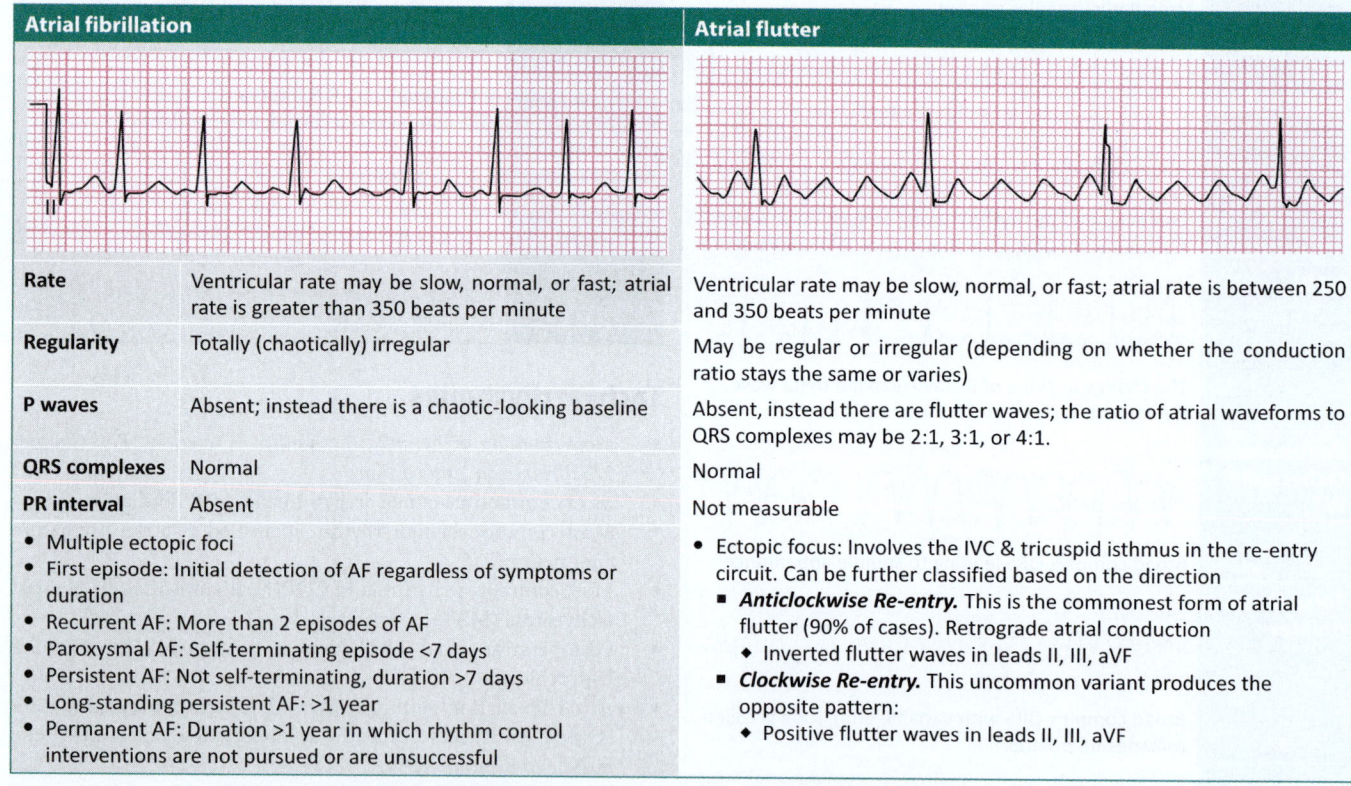

	Atrial fibrillation	Atrial flutter
Rate	Ventricular rate may be slow, normal, or fast; atrial rate is greater than 350 beats per minute	Ventricular rate may be slow, normal, or fast; atrial rate is between 250 and 350 beats per minute
Regularity	Totally (chaotically) irregular	May be regular or irregular (depending on whether the conduction ratio stays the same or varies)
P waves	Absent; instead there is a chaotic-looking baseline	Absent, instead there are flutter waves; the ratio of atrial waveforms to QRS complexes may be 2:1, 3:1, or 4:1.
QRS complexes	Normal	Normal
PR interval	Absent	Not measurable

- Multiple ectopic foci
- First episode: Initial detection of AF regardless of symptoms or duration
- Recurrent AF: More than 2 episodes of AF
- Paroxysmal AF: Self-terminating episode <7 days
- Persistent AF: Not self-terminating, duration >7 days
- Long-standing persistent AF: >1 year
- Permanent AF: Duration >1 year in which rhythm control interventions are not pursued or are unsuccessful

- Ectopic focus: Involves the IVC & tricuspid isthmus in the re-entry circuit. Can be further classified based on the direction
  - **Anticlockwise Re-entry.** This is the commonest form of atrial flutter (90% of cases). Retrograde atrial conduction
    - Inverted flutter waves in leads II, III, aVF
  - **Clockwise Re-entry.** This uncommon variant produces the opposite pattern:
    - Positive flutter waves in leads II, III, aVF

Comparison of Treatment Protocol for Atrial Fibrillation and Atrial Flutter

Atrial fibrillation	Atrial flutter
• *Acute rate control* with beta blocker and or **verapamil/diltiazem**[Q] • *Acute rate control with acute CHF* = digoxin **(beta blockers are contraindicated in acute CHF)**[Q] • Chronic rate control is done with beta blocker having calcium channel blocker (CCB) and digoxin. If it fails, go for catheter ablation • *Amiodarone is used for maintaining rhythm control in majority of patients in India.* • If duration of AF is > 48 hours then due to risk of thromboembolism, anti-coagulant with rivaroxaban or dabigatran. Then give DC shock. • On recurrence, give IBUTILIDE and repeat cardioversion • New onset AF producing hypotension, pulmonary edema should be managed with **synchronous DC shock of 200 J**[Q]	• For hemodynamic instability DC shock is warranted. **Cardioversion can be accomplished with synchronous DC, which often requires relatively low energies (approximately 50 J)**[Q] • The short-acting antiarrhythmic medication ibutilide can also be given IV • Anti-coagulation is advised for episodes lasting for > 48 hours • Recurrent episodes managed with sotalol, dofetilide, disopyramide • Catheter ablation of cavo-tricuspid isthmus is successful in 90% of cases • For risk of embolic stroke, CHA_2DS_2–VASc score is calculated and rivaroxaban is started

Multi-focal Atrial Tachycardia

- Characterised by rhythm having at least three distinct P-wave morphologies with a rate of 100–150/min.
- Clear isoelectric interval between P waves
- Occurs due to triggered automaticity and seen in COPD patients.

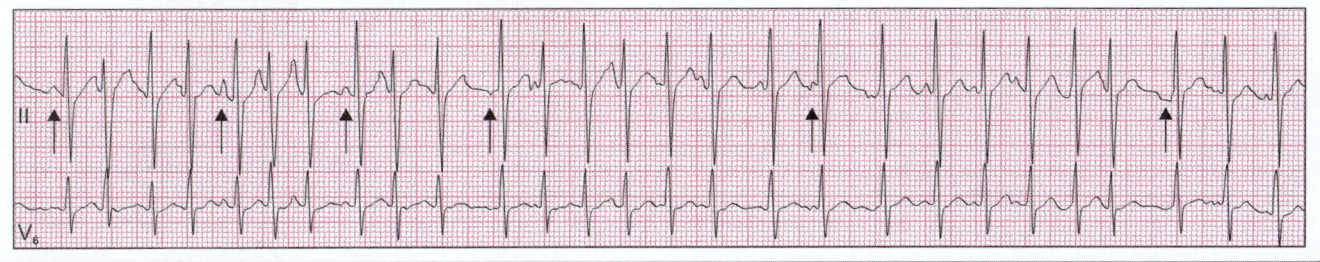

Treatment

1. DC shock is contraindicated
2. Treat the cause
3. Calcium channel blockers like verapamil or diltiazem may slow down atrial and ventricular rates

Risk Assessment in Atrial Fibrillation (CHA$_2$DS$_2$–VASc) and Need for Anticoagulants

Risk factors	Points	Estimated Annual Stroke Rate
C – Congestive heart failure	1	0
H – hypertension	1	1.3%
A – age ≥75 year	2	2.2%
D – diabetes mellitus	1	3.2%
S – stroke or TIA, embolus	2	4.0%
V – vascular disease	1	6.7%
A – age 65-75 y	1	>9%
Sex – female	1	

Treatment of AF with WPW

- Treatment with AV nodal blocking drugs e.g. adenosine, calcium-channel blockers, beta-blockers **may increase conduction** via the accessory pathway with a resultant increase in ventricular rate and **possible degeneration into VT or VF**
- In a hemodynamically unstable patient, urgent synchronized DC cardioversion is required.

Comparison of AVNRT (AV nodal re-entrant tachycardia) from AVRT (AV re-entry tachycardia)

AVNRT	AVRT
Typically paroxysmal and may occur upon provocation with exertion, coffee, tea or alcohol. It is more common in women than men (~75% of cases occur in women)	Incidence varies from 0.1 to 3/1000 in healthy subjects. The majority of AVRT occurs via accessory pathways, which are *located between the left ventricle and left atrium or in the posteroseptal area*, while right sided accessory pathway is seen with Ebstein's anomaly.
Re-entry is via the AV node and the current in circus movement leads to simultaneous activation of both the atria and ventricles. Hence P wave is inscribed during or slightly before or slightly after the QRS leading to difficulty in discerning the P wave	*Orthodromic AV entry:* Wave-front travels via the AV node to the HIS bundle and ventricles but travels retrograde via the accessory pathway *Antidromic AV entry:* Wave front travels via the accessory pathway to the ventricle and then retrogradely via the AV node back to the atria
ECG will typically show a tachycardia of 140–280 bpm with normal and regular QRS complexes. There will be either 1. No visible P-waves (hidden within the QRS complex) *or* 2. P-waves immediately after the QRS complex 3. Narrow QRS complex 4. Reduced RR interval, regular 5. ST depression	*ECG findings of orthodromic AVRT* 1. Rate usually 200 – 300 bpm 2. P waves may be buried in QRS complex or retrograde 3. QRS complex usually <120 ms 4. T wave inversion common

Contd...

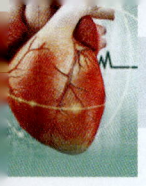

AVNRT	AVRT
NORMAL (ECG trace showing P, Q, R, S, T waves with 200 ms interval)	Diagrams showing Sinus node, AV node, Bundle branch, Normal conduction vs Accessory pathway, Pre-excitation; Delta wave, Secondary ST-T change, Short PR, Wide QRS
AVNRT (ECG trace)	**ECG findings of antidromic AVRT (WPW)** 1. PR interval: <120 ms 2. Delta wave: slurring slow rise of initial portion of the QRS 3. QRS prolongation: >110 ms 4. ST Segment and T wave discordant changes i.e. in the opposite direction to the major component of the QRS complex 5. PJ interval is normal
For management: • Vagal maneuvers like carotid sinus massage or Valsalva maneuver and face ice pack (preferred for pediatric AVNRT) • Adenosine, beta-blockers or calcium channel blockers can suppress an AVNRT event by blocking or slowing the AV node. Other second-line therapies may include amiodarone or flecainide • Cardioversion when the tachycardia is refractory to other medical therapies or the tachycardia is causing hemodynamic instability (falling blood pressure, development of heart failure etc.) • Radiofrequency catheter ablation can be offered to patients with frequent attacks for whom medical therapy isn't appropriate in the long term and can be curative	**For management:** • In presentation of hypotension with respiratory distress or hypotension, QRS synchronous DC shock is warranted • *Hemodynamically stable regular, narrow complex qRS tachycardia: vagal stimulation, intravenous adenosine and intravenous verapamil/diltiazem* • If arrhythmia persists, add ibutilide + AV node blocking agent • *Adenosine precipitates atrial fibrillation* (page 1484, Harrison 19th edition), so should be used cautiously in patients with WPW in whom AF may precipitate VF

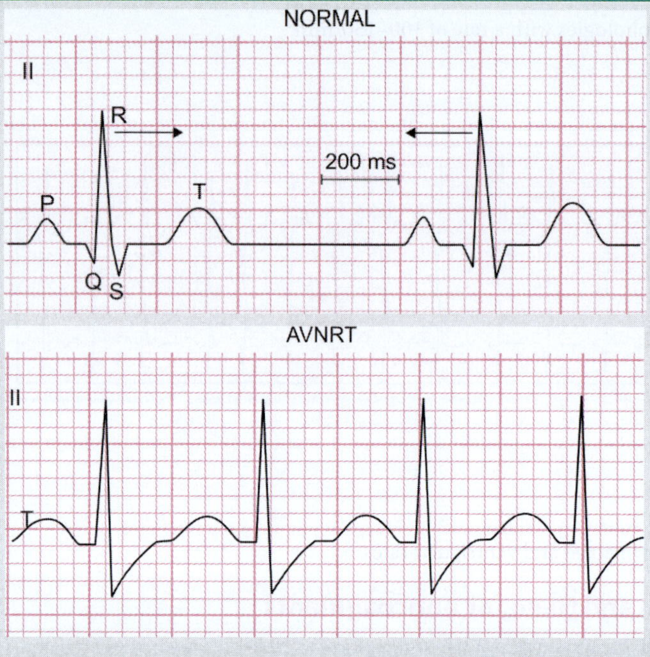

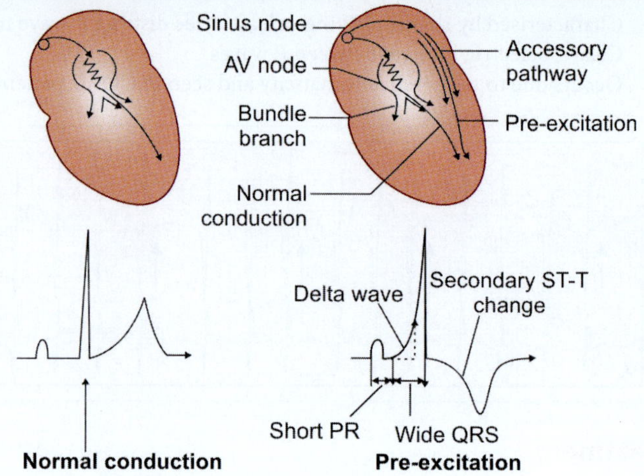

Wolff-Parkinson White Syndrome

- Bundle of kent leads to early excitation of partially filled ventricles. Thus cardiac output is lower and syncopal episodes are seen
- It can conduct both antegradely and retrogradely. The antegrade conduction via bundle of kent is called as orthodromic conduction. In contrast retrograde conduction to atria via His-Purkinje system is called as antidromic AV re-entry.
- Delta wave in ECG is change in slope in the upswing of R wave
- Doc for rapid pre-excited tachycardia is procainamide or ibutilide
- AV nodal blocking agents like verapamil, diltiazem, adenosine will increase conduction via bundle of kent leading to them being contraindicated in W.P.W.
- Invasive electrophysiological studies are done to evaluate whether the pathway can support dangerously rapid heart rates and simultaneous cathether ablation can be done
- For low risk patients showing orthodromic re-entry, vagal maneuvers, β-blockers, verapamil diltiazem or flecainide can reduce frequency of episodes

Major Features Differentiating Wide QRS Complex Tachycardia from Narrow Complex Tachycardia

Narrow QRS Complex Tachycardia	Wide QRS Complex Tachycardia
SVT	VT and SVT with aberrancy
Slowing or termination by vagal tone	Fusion beats
Onset with premature P wave	Capture beats
RP interval ≤100 msec	AV dissociation

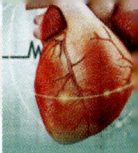

Monomorphic Ventricular Tachycardia

Duration	• Sustained = Duration > 30 seconds or requiring intervention due to hemodynamic compromise • Nonsustained = Three or more consecutive ventricular complexes terminating spontaneously in < 30 seconds
Clinical significance	• Ventricular tachycardia may impair cardiac output with consequent hypotension, collapse, and acute cardiac failure. This is due to extreme heart rates and lack of coordinated atrial contraction (loss of "atrial kick"). • The presence of pre-existing poor ventricular function is strongly associated with cardiovascular compromise
Mechanism	Most common mechanism is re-entry (due to different gradient between damaged tissue due to ischemia) > triggered activity > abnormal automaticity
ECG	• Classic monomorphic VT with uniform QRS complexes • Indeterminate axis • Very broad QRS (~200 ms) • Notching near the nadir of the S wave in lead III = Josephson's sign • VT storm or electrical storm is > 3 or more separate episodes of VT within 24 hours
	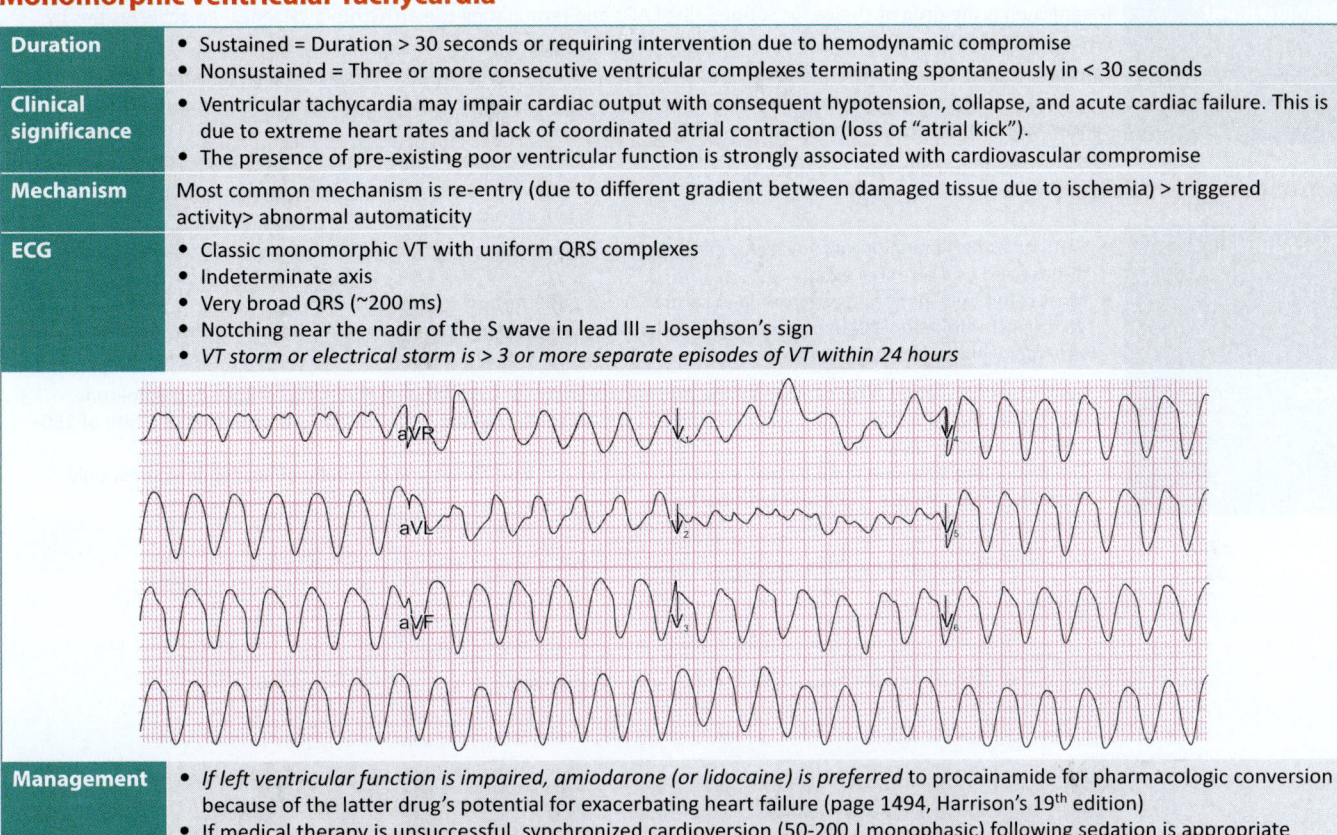
Management	• *If left ventricular function is impaired, amiodarone (or lidocaine) is preferred* to procainamide for pharmacologic conversion because of the latter drug's potential for exacerbating heart failure (page 1494, Harrison's 19th edition) • If medical therapy is unsuccessful, synchronized cardioversion (50-200 J monophasic) following sedation is appropriate • *Pulseless VT*, in contrast to other unstable VT rhythms, is treated with immediate defibrillation. High-dose unsynchronized energy should be used. The initial shock dose on a *biphasic defibrillator is 150–200 J,* followed by an equal or higher shock dose for subsequent shocks.

Polymorphic Ventricular Tachycardia

Causes[Q]	1. Prolongation of the QT interval 2. Jervell and Lange-Nielsen syndrome (congenitally long QT associated with congenital deafness) 3. Romano Ward syndrome (i.e., isolated prolongation of QT interval). Both of these syndromes are associated with sudden death due to either primary ventricular fibrillation or torsades de pointes 4. Brugada syndrome 5. Takotsubo cardiomyopathy 6. Hypokalemia and Hypomagnesemia 7. Class IA agents (e.g. quinidine, procainamide, disopyramide), class IC agents (e.g., encainide, flecainide), and class III agents (e.g., sotalol, amiodarone). 8. Drug interactions with the antihistamines astemizole (recalled from US market) and terfenadine (recalled from US market) can precipitate torsades; these drugs should never be used with class IA, IC, or III agents.
Features	The definition requires that the QT interval be increased markedly (usually to 600 msec or greater)
ECG	The morphology of the QRS complexes varies from beat to beat. The ventricular rate can range from 150 beats per minute (bpm) to 250 bpm
	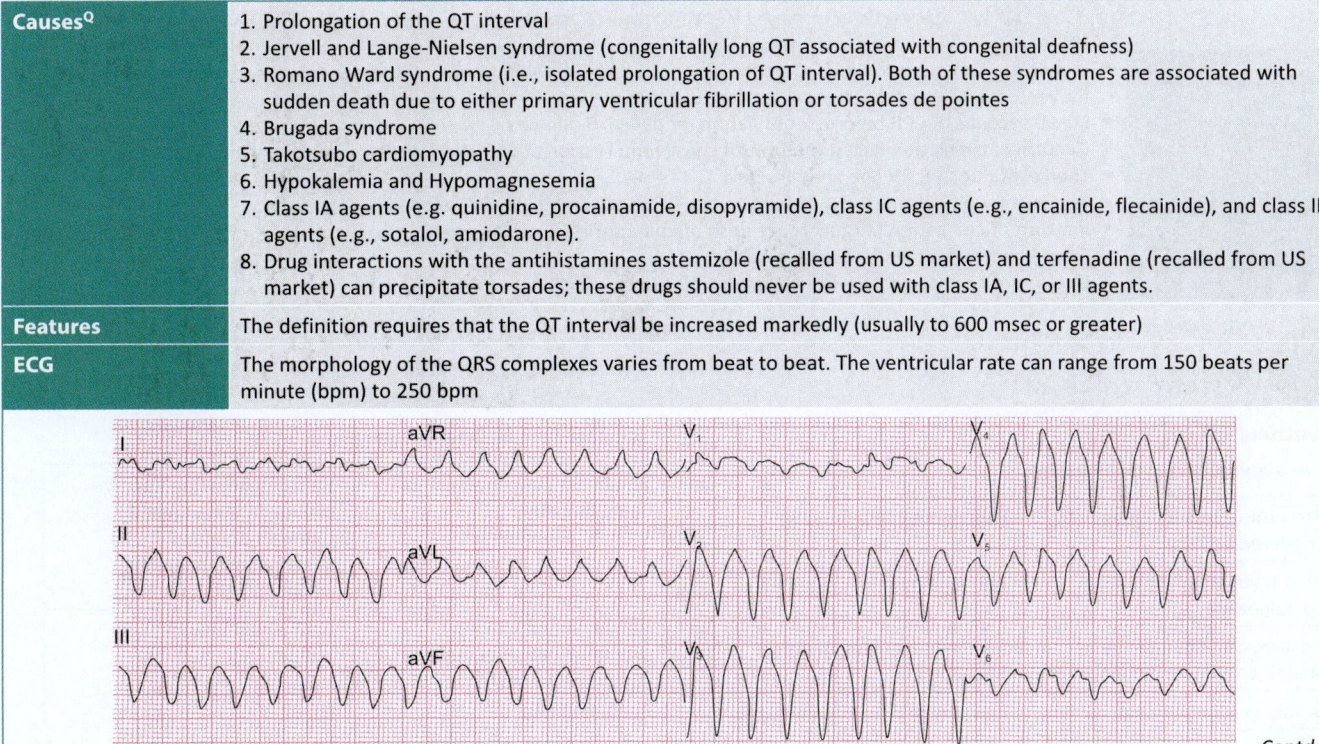

Contd...

Management	Magnesium is the drug of choice for suppressing EADs and terminating the arrhythmia. Magnesium achieves this by decreasing the influx of calcium, thus lowering the amplitude of EADs
	Isoproterenol accelerates AV conduction and decreases the QT interval by increasing the heart rate and reducing temporal dispersion of repolarization. *Beta-adrenergic agonists such as isoproterenol are contraindicated in the congenital form of long QT syndrome*

Ventricular Fibrillation

Mechanism	• Ventricular fibrillation occurs in various clinical situations but is most commonly associated with coronary artery disease and as a terminal event • Most commonly identified arrhythmia in cardiac arrest patients and commotio cordis • Ventricular fibrillation can occur during antiarrhythmic drug administration, hypoxia, ischemia, atrial fibrillation, and very rapid ventricular rates in the pre-excitation syndrome, after electrical shock administered during cardioversion
ECG	• Ventricular fibrillation is recognized by the presence of irregular undulations of varying contour and amplitude • Ventricular flutter is manifested as a sine wave in appearance—regular large oscillations occurring at a rate of 150–300/min (usually about 200). • The distinction between rapid VT and ventricular flutter can be difficult and is usually of academic interest only. Hemodynamic collapse is present with both.

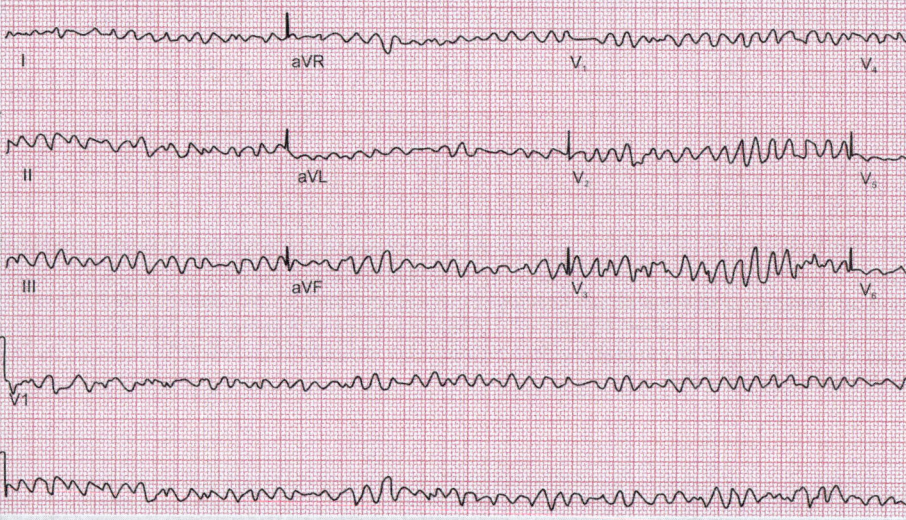

Management	• Immediate *non-synchronized DC electrical shock* using 200 – 400 J is mandatory therapy for ventricular fibrillation and for ventricular flutter that has caused loss of consciousness (within 5 minutes of onset) • 60–90 seconds of CPR before defibrillation for delay >5 minutes • If return of circulation fails, 2 minutes of chest compression at >100/min and repeat shock. Can repeat this step twice • Then continue CPR, IV line and intubate • Administer epinephrine 1 mg IV followed by DC shock within 30–60 seconds • If return of circulation fails, increase dose of epinephrine and use anti-arrhythmics (LAMP = lignocaine, amiodarone, magnesium sulfate and procainamide) • If return of circulation fails: Defibrillate—CPR—Drug—Shock

Recent advances

Ventricular Tachycardia

• Acute ventricular tachycardia

Structurally normal heart and triggered activity	Short acting beta blocker
Post-myocardial infarction sustained VT	Lignocaine
Post-myocardial infarction sustained VT with hypotension	Synchronized cardioversion 100–200 J
Stable ventricular tachycardia	Amiodarone^Q > Procainamide

• Chronic recurrent ventricular tachycardia

Sustained VT with structural heart disease	Beta blocker (*Don't answer anti-arrhythmic drugs*) Catheter ablation internal cardioverter defibrillator (ICD)
Nonsustained VT (> 3 premature ventricular beats for <30 seconds) with structural heart disease	Beta blockers with amiodarone ICD

*Lignocaine is never to be used prophylactically to prevent VT

Cardiac Arrest Score

The cardiac arrest score, can be used for patients with witnessed out-of-hospital cardiac arrest. The score uses 3 criteria:

1. Emergency department (ED) systolic blood pressure
2. Time to return of spontaneous circulation (ROSC) after loss of consciousness
3. Neurologic responsiveness. The score is calculated as follows
   - ED SBP: >90 mm Hg = 1 point; < 90 mm Hg = 0 points
   - Time to ROSC: < 25 minutes = 1 point; >25 minutes = 0 points
   - Neurologically responsive = 1 point; comatose = 0 points

Bradyarrhythmias

1st Degree Heart Block

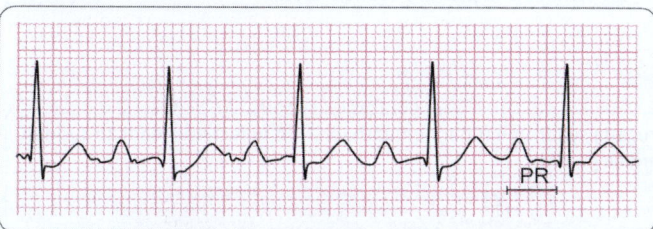

Normal PR interval is 120–200 msec (3–5 small squares)

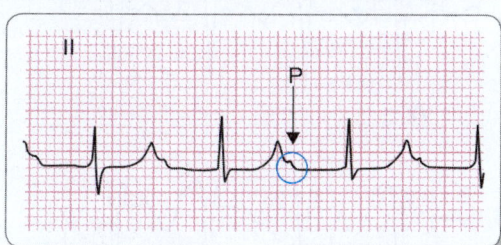

*Notice the prolonged PR interval with P wave buried in previous T wave

Causes of first degree heart block

1. Increased vagal tone
2. Athletic training
3. Inferior MI
4. Mitral valve surgery
5. Myocarditis (e.g. Lyme disease)
6. Electrolyte disturbances (e.g. hyperkalemia)
7. AV nodal blocking drugs (beta-blockers, calcium channel blockers, digoxin and amiodarone)

Mobitz I Heart Block/ Wenckebach Phenomenon

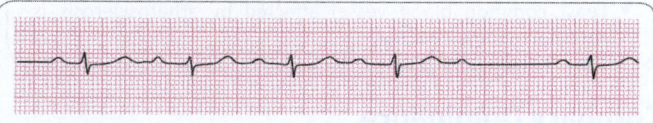

- Progressive prolongation of the PR interval culminating in a non-conducted P wave
- The P-R interval is the longest immediate before the dropped beat
- The P-R interval is the shortest immediately after the dropped beat

Causes

1. Drugs: Beta-blockers, calcium channel blockers, digoxin, amiodarone
2. Increased vagal tone (e.g. athletes)
3. Inferior MI
4. Myocarditis
5. Following cardiac surgery (mitral valve repair, tetralogy of Fallot repair)

It does not require pacing.

Mobitz II Heart Block

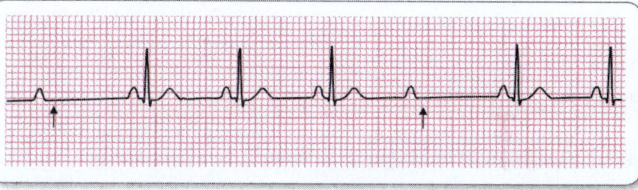

Notice the PR interval to be normal followed by sudden drop in conduction

- Mobitz II is usually due to the failure of conduction at the level of the bundle of His-Purkinje system (i.e. below the AV node).
- While Mobitz I is usually due to a functional suppression of AV conduction (e.g. due to drugs, reversible ischemia), Mobitz II is more likely due to *structural* damage to the conducting system (e.g. infarction, fibrosis, necrosis).

Causes

1. Septal infarction with necrosis of the bundle branches
2. Idiopathic fibrosis of the conducting system (Lenegre's or Lev's disease)
3. Cardiac surgery (especially surgery occurring close to the septum, e.g. mitral valve repair)
4. Inflammatory conditions (rheumatic fever, myocarditis, Lyme disease)
5. Autoimmune systemic lupus erythematosus [(SLE), systemic sclerosis]
6. Infiltrative myocardial disease (amyloidosis, hemochromatosis, sarcoidosis)
7. Hyperkalemia.

Third Degree Heart Block/ Complete Heart Block

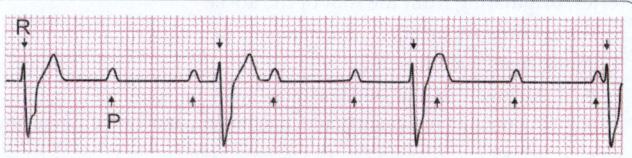

- The atrial rate is approximately 100 bpm.
- The ventricular rate is approximately 40 bpm.
- The two rates are independent; there is no evidence that any of the atrial impulses are conducted to the ventricles.

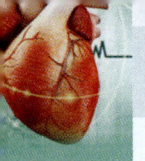

Causes

1. Inferior myocardial infarction
2. AV-nodal blocking drugs (e.g. calcium-channel blockers, beta-blockers, digoxin)
3. Idiopathic degeneration of the conducting system (Lenegre's or Lev's disease).
4. Metabolic/endocrine causes: **Hypothyroidism^Q**, adrenal insufficiency, hyperkalemia and sarcoidosis

These patients need urgent temporary pacing followed by permanent pacing.

BRUGADA Syndrome

- It is an autosomal dominant disorder with defect in SCN5A (Sodium channel).
- The defect leads to *reduced inward current in the region of RV outflow tract epicardium*.
- The large potential difference between the normal endocardium and RV outflow tract epicardium leads to *re-entry phenomenon* leading to development of life threatening tachyarrhythmias.
- It happens to be the *most common cause of sudden and unexpected death* in South Asian men
- It may present with history of palpitations and syncope. Family history of sudden death may be present.
- Characteristic ECG finding is *coved ST segment changes with T wave inversion*.
- Treatment of choice is **ICD^Q** to manage recurrent Ventricular arrhythmia and prevent sudden death.

Brugada Sign versus Brugada Syndrome

Brugada sign (used for diagnosis of Ventricular tachycardia)	Brugada syndrome (Channelopathy:SCN5A defect and leads to sudden cardiac death)
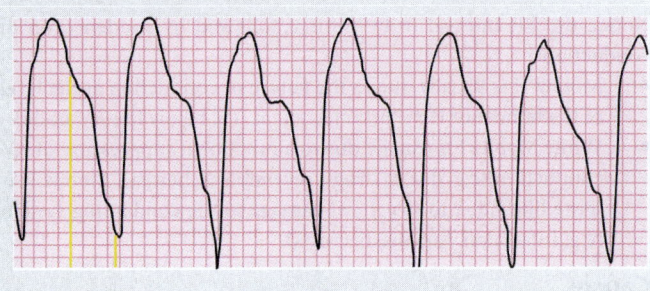	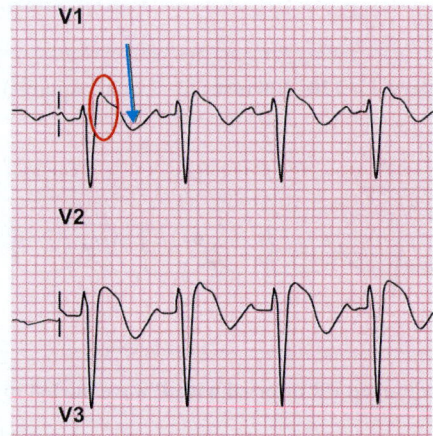
Normally the entire qRS complex is 80-10 mmsec. *In brugada sign, the interval from R wave to the bottom of S wave is >100 msec. The feature is seen in VT.*	Notice the Coved ST segment in V1 and V2 (*red marking*) and T wave inversion (*blue markings*)

CORONARY CIRCULATION

Arterial supply to the heart arises from the right and left coronary arteries, originating from the root of the aorta.
1. Right coronary artery
2. Acute marginal branches
   - Atrioventricular nodal artery
   - Posterior interventricular artery/posterior descending artery
3. Left main coronary artery
4. Left anterior descending artery
   - Septal branches
   - Diagonal branches
   - Left circumflex artery
   - Obtuse marginal branches

Extra Mile

- Coronary dominance is determined by Post-descending artery
- MC blood vessel in heart affected by atherosclerosis is LAD
- MC blood vessel overall affected by atherosclerosis is abdominal aorta
- Least common blood vessel affected by atherosclerosis is internal mammary artery

Coronary Dominance

- Right-dominant circulation: PIV and at least one posterolateral branch arise from RCA (80%)
- Left-dominant circulation: PIV and at least one posterolateral branch arise from LCX (15%)

- Balanced circulation: dual supply of posteroinferior LV from RCA and LCX (5%)
- The sinoatrial node is supplied by the SA nodal artery, which may arise from the RCA (60%) or LCA (40%)
- Most venous blood from the heart drains into the RA through the coronary sinus, although a small amount drains through the thebesian veins into all four chambers, contributing to the physiologic R-L shunt

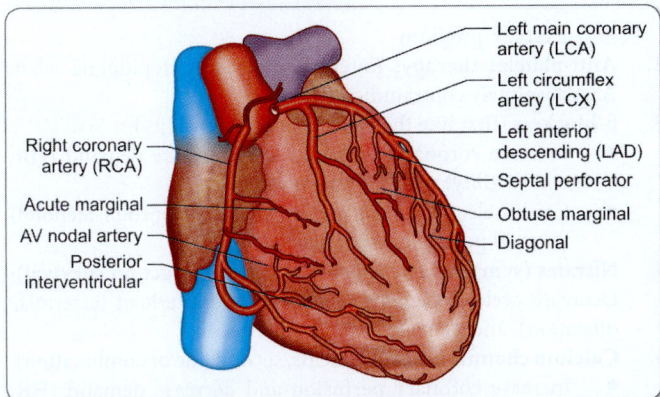

Coronary circulation

Significance of learning this anatomy is to be able to select the correct blood vessel blocked in Acute myocardial infarction

Blood vessel blocked	Type of MI	ST segment ELEVATION in corresponding ECG leads
LAD	Anterior wall MI	V_1-V_4, I, aVL
LAD (septal branch)	Septal MI	V_{1-2}, I, aVL
LCX/Diagonal	Lateral wall MI	V_5-V_6, I, aVL
Main left coronary artery	Extensive anterior wall MI	V_1-V_6, I, aVL
LCX or Post descending artery	Posterior wall MI	V_7-V_9 STE, V_1-V_2 STD
RCA	Inferior wall MI	Lead II, III, aVF

Ischemic Heart Disease (IHD)

Parameters of Framingham risk calculator for determining atherosclerotic cardiovascular heart disease

A.B.C.D. S2
- Age
- BP
- Cholesterol
- HDL
- Smoking
- SBP

The calculator gives a 10 year prediction for chance of developing a heart attack.

Epidemiology

- Peak incidence of symptomatic IHD is age 50–60 years (men) and 60–70 years (women).

Risks Factors for Atherosclerotic Heart Disease (Framingham Data)

Major Risks Factors	Minor Risks Factors

• Smoking
• Diabetes mellitus
• Hypertension
• Family history of MI
  ▪ First degree male relative <55 years
  ▪ Or first degree female relative <60 years
• Hyperlipidemia
	• Male, postmenopausal female
	• Obesity
	• Sedentary lifestyle
	• Homocysteinemia

MC lipid profile defect is Familial Combined Hyperlipidemia with incidence of 1 per 100–200 individuals (page 2439: Harrison 19th ed)

Markers for atherosclerosis:
- High sensitivity – CRP (Predictor for future coronary events)
- Total cholesterol/HDL ratio: >3.5
- Lipoprotein A/apolipoprotein B
- Homocystine levels elevation leads to premature atherosclerosis
- LDL
- HDL

Chronic Stable Angina/Reversible Ischemia

It develops when >70% luminal diameter is reduced due to atherosclerosis affecting any coronary artery.

Signs and Symptoms

1. Retrosternal chest pain, tightness or discomfort radiating to left (± right) shoulder/arm/neck/jaw, associated with diaphoresis, nausea, anxiety.
2. *Predictably precipitated by the "3E's": Exertion, Emotion and Eating.*
3. Brief duration, lasting <10–15 minutes and typically relieved by rest and nitrates.
4. **Levine's sign: Clutching fist over sternum when describing chest pain**.
5. Angina equivalents: Dyspnea, acute left ventricular failure, flash pulmonary edema.

Clinical Assessment

- Labs: Hemoglobin, fasting glucose, fasting lipid profile
- ECG (at rest and during episode of chest pain if possible)
- CXR (suspected heart failure, valvular disease, pericardial disease, aortic dissection/aneurysm, or signs or symptoms of pulmonary disease)
- **Stress Testing**
  A. **Treadmill Test:** The exercise time is based on using the standard Bruce protocol. The ischemic ST segment response is defined as flat or *downsloping ST depression of >0.1 mV below baseline and lasts for duration >80 msec.*

Contraindications to Exercise Testing

Absolute	Relative
• Acute myocardial infarction (within two days) • Uncontrolled cardiac arrhythmias causing symptoms or hemodynamic compromise • Symptomatic severe aortic stenosis • Acute aortic dissection • Acute myocarditis or pericarditis • Acute pulmonary embolus or pulmonary infarction • Unstable angina not previously stabilized by medical therapy • Uncontrolled symptomatic heart failure	• Left main coronary stenosis • Hemodynamically significant aortic stenosis • High – degree atrioventricular block • Electrolyte abnormalities • Tachyarrhythmias or brady-arrhythmias • Hypertrophic cardiomyopathy and other forms of outflow tract obstruction • Severe uncontrolled Hypertension • Mental or physical impairment leading to inability to exercise adequately

B. Dobutamine stress echocardiography
  ◆ Performed post-ACS and used to decide on potential efficacy of revascularization
  ◆ In patients unable to exercise and have contraindications to T.M.T.
C. Exercise myocardial perfusion imaging (MPI) using Thallium-201 or technetium-99.
D. PET scan (Rubidium-82). (Best test for Hibernating myocardium.)^Q

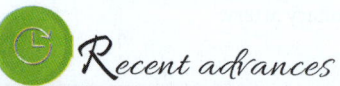 Recent advances

Role of Cardiac Imaging
- Stress cardiac MRI is *best initial noninvasive* test in symptomatic patient with suspected coronary artery disease.
- PET scan with high accuracy can distinguish between stunned myocardium and scar tissue.
- Electron beam CT scan can quantify coronary artery calcification.
- Gadolinium enhanced MRI is the most sensitive test to detect and quantify the extent of infarction.

Treatment of Chronic Stable Angina

1. **General Measures:**
   - Lifestyle modification
   - *Statins*

Guidelines for Statins use

	Old guidelines	New guidelines
Initiation of treatment	Start treatment to achieve Target LDL defined as <130 : normal population < 100: with Peripheral vascular disease (PVD) < 70 : diabetes mellitus	Start treatment in patients with • Atherosclerotic cardiovascular heart disease • >21 yrs with LDL >190 mg/dL • Diabetes mellitus, 40–75 years with LDL 70–189 mg/dL • Diabetes mellitus, 40-75 years with LDL 70–189 mg/dL and >7.5% mortality risk
Strategy	Dose was not specified, Neither the level to which LDL should fall was specified	• Low intensity statin to cause up to 30% reduction in LDL using Atorvastatin 10–20mg • Moderate intensity statin to cause 30–50% reduction in LDL • High intensity Statin to cause > 50% reduction in LDL using atorvastatin 80 mg

   - Exercise program
2. **Anti-platelet therapy:** Enteric-coated ASA/clopidogrel when ASA absolutely contraindicated.
3. **β-blockers** (first line therapy - decrease mortality):
   - Increase coronary perfusion and decrease demand (HR, contractility) and BP (afterload).
   - Cardioselective agents preferred (e.g. metoprolol, atenolol) to avoid peripheral effects.
4. **Nitrates (symptomatic control, no clear impact on survival):** Decrease preload (venous dilatation) and afterload (arteriolar dilatation), and increase coronary perfusion.
5. **Calcium channel blockers** (CCBs, second line or combination):
   - Increase coronary perfusion and decrease demand (HR, contractility) and BP (afterload)
   - Remember: Verapamil/diltiazem combined with beta-blockers may cause symptomatic sinus bradycardia or AV block
6. **ACE inhibitors**
   - Angina patients tend to have risk factors for cardiovascular disease which warrant use of an ACEI (e.g. hypertension, diabetes, proteinuric renal disease, previous MI with LV dysfunction). Angiotensin II receptor blockers (ARBs) when ACEIs contraindicated.
7. **Ranolazine:** Ranolazine is believed to have its effects via altering the transcellular late sodium current. It affects the sodium-dependent calcium channels during myocardial ischemia in rabbits by altering the intracellular sodium level. It also shifts ATP production from fatty acid to more oxygen-efficient carbohydrate oxidation

- Drug of choice in chronic stable angina is Beta blockers.
- Drug of choice for acute chest pain in chronic stable angina is SL nitrates.
- Major mortality reducing drug in chronic stable angina is Beta blockers > Statins > Aspirin

8. **Invasive Strategies:** Revascularization with percutaneous coronary intervention (PCI) and stenting

Protocol for invasive strategies

Single vessel disease	PCI with stenting
Double vessel disease	PCI with stenting
Triple vessel disease	CABG

Contd...

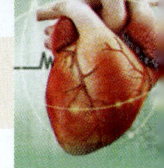

Stenting is usually done with drug eluting stents that are coated with products like Paclitaxel, Everolimus and Sirolimus that prevent redevelopment of atherosclerosis.

Percutaneous Coronary Intervention (PCI)

- Interventional technique aimed at relieving significant coronary stenosis
- Main techniques: Balloon angioplasty and stenting.

Indications

1. Medically refractory angina with hibernating myocardium
2. Non-ST-elevation myocardial infarction (NSTEMI), Unstable angina (UA) with high thrombolysis in myocardial infarction (TIMI) risk score within 90 min of presentation
3. Primary/rescue PCI for ST-elevation myocardial infarction (STEMI).

Coronary Artery Bypass Graft (CABG) Surgery

Indications

1. Significant left main artery disease
2. Triple vessel disease, survival benefit greatest in patients with abnormal LV function (EF <50%)
3. Two-vessel disease with significant proximal left anterior descending (LAD) disease and with abnormal LV function (EF <50%)
4. One or two vessel disease without significant LAD disease who have survived sudden cardiac death or sustained VT
5. Patients with one or two vessel disease without significant LAD disease but with a large **area** of viable myocardium and high risk criteria on noninvasive testing
6. Recurrent stenosis associated with a large area of viable myocardium or high risk criteria on noninvasive testing.

Conduits for CABG

Graft	Occlusion / Patency Rate
Saphenous vein grafts (SVG)	At 10 years, 50% occluded, 25% stenotic, 25% angiographically normal
Left internal thoracic / mammary artery (LITA/LIMA) (LIMA to LAD)	90–95% patent at 15 years

Variant Angina (Prinzmetal's Angina)

- Myocardial ischemia secondary to coronary artery *vasospasm*, with or without atherosclerosis.
- Typically occurs between midnight and 8 AM, unrelated to exercise, relieved by nitrates.
- Higher incidence in women with history of migraine or Raynaud's phenomenon.
- Typically ST elevation on ECG. **Only angina to have an ST segment elevation.**
- Many patients also exhibit multiple episodes of asymptomatic ST-segment elevation (silent ischemia).
- **Spasm seen usually in right coronary artery.**
- Spasm defined as >75% blockage in any of the coronary artery.
- Diagnose by provocative testing with Ergot vasoconstrictors (rarely done).
- Treat with nitrates and CCBs.
- On admission however first line treatment is NTG drip, followed by long acting nitrates and CCB on discharge.

Acute Coronary Syndrome (ACS)

Causes

1. Coronary atherosclerosis with superimposed thrombus on ruptured plaque
2. Coronary thromboembolism (e.g. infective endocarditis, intracavitary thrombus, paradoxical embolism) or cholesterol embolism
3. Severe coronary vasospasm
4. Coronary dissection
5. Increased demand can also contribute (e.g. tachycardia, anemia).

Spectrum of ACS

- UA/NSTEMI
- STEMI
- Sudden cardiac death

Unstable Angina (UA)/Non-ST Elevation MI (NSTEMI)

Unstable angina is clinically defined by any of the following:
- Accelerating pattern of pain: increased frequency, increased duration, with decreased exertion, decreased response to treatment.
- Angina at rest
- New onset angina
- Angina post-MI or post-procedure (e.g. PCI, CABG)

NSTEMI is clinically defined by the presence of 2 of the following 3 criteria:
- Symptoms of angina/ischemia
- Rise and fall of serum markers of myocardial necrosis
- Evolution of ischemic ECG changes (without ST elevation or new LBBB)

ST Elevation Myocardial Infarction (STEMI)

Acute plaque rupture and thrombosis with total coronary occlusion resulting in myocardial necrosis.

Diffuse chest pain lasting for > 20 minutes with any one of following
1. ECG criteria: ST elevation in 2 contiguous leads (>1 mm in limb leads or >2 mm in precordial leads) or new LBBB
2. Troponin I showing doubling/tripling above the 99th percentile upper reference limit
3. Intraoperative MI diagnosed by transesophageal echo showing stunned myocardium.
4. Identification of intracoronary thrombus by angiography.

ECG Changes with Infarction

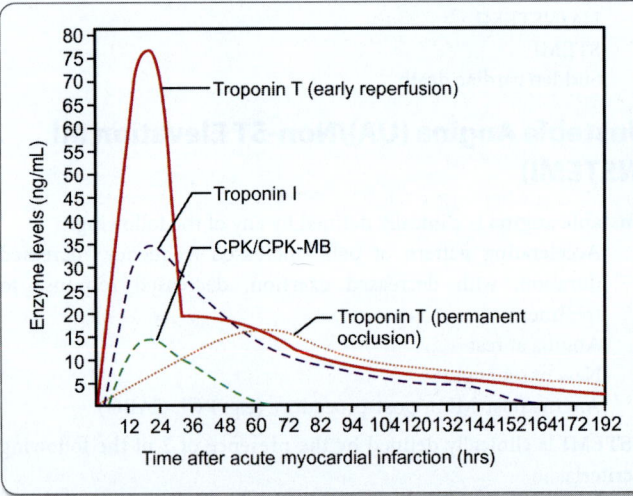

- Hyperacute T waves in the leads facing the infarcted area/T wave inversion
- ST elevation (Pardee sign) in the leads facing the infarcted area, usually in the first hour post infarct
- Significant Q waves (hours to days post-infarct)

Cardiac Biomarkers

They provide diagnostic and prognostic information and identify increased risk of mortality in acute coronary syndromes.

Cardiac biomarkers

- First to rise after MI is heart fatty acid binding protein > myoglobin
- New CK-MB elevation can be used to diagnose re-infarction after 72 hours.
- Reinfarction is best diagnosed by 20% increase over baseline Troponin T values
- **Copeptin and heart fatty acid binding protein are new biomarkers in acute coronary syndrome, and rise in the first hour**
- Normally LDH is predominant form in serum and LDH 1 is in heart. In case of MI, LDH 1 > LDH 2 due to myocardial necrosis. This is called as *flipped pattern*.

Enzyme	Peak	Duration Elevated	DDx of Elevation
Troponin I, Troponin T	1–2 days	Up to 2 weeks	MI, CHF, AF, acute pulmonary embolism, myocarditis, chronic renal insufficiency, sepsis, hypovolemia
CK-MB (Creatine phosphokinase-Myocardial Band)	1 day	3 day	Myocardial infarction, myocarditis, pericarditis, muscular dystrophy, cardiac defibrillation

Universal Definition of MI

- **Type 1**: Spontaneous MI is related to ischemia due to a primary coronary event such as plaque rupture, fissuring, or dissection
- **Type 2**: MI secondary to ischemia is due to either increased oxygen demand or decreased supply, e.g. coronary artery spasm, coronary embolism, anemia, arrhythmias, hypertension, or hypotension
- **Type 3**: Sudden unexpected cardiac death, including cardiac arrest, often with symptoms suggestive of myocardial ischemia, but death occurring before blood samples could be obtained, or at a time before the rise of cardiac biomarkers in the blood
- **Type 4**: Associated with coronary angioplasty or stents:
  - Type 4a:^{Q} MI associated with PCI (associated with 5 times elevation of troponin I)
  - Type 4b: MI associated with stent thrombosis as documented by angiography or at autopsy
- **Type 5**:^{Q} MI associated with CABG (associated with 10 times elevation of Troponin-I).

Acute Management STEMI

- Goal is to reperfuse artery: thrombolysis (EMS-to-needle) within 30 minutes^Q or primary PCI (EMS-to-balloon) within 90 minutes^Q.

Management of NSTEMI and STEMI

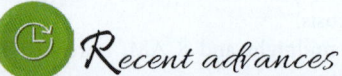

Role of Dual Antiplatelet Therapy in ACS
- Guidelines call for P2Y12 inhibitor to be added to aspirin for all patients of STEMI irrespective of reperfusion strategy.
- It should be continued for 14 days and subsequently up to 1 year.

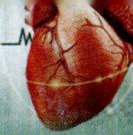

1. **General measures:**
   - ABCs: assess and correct hemodynamic status first
   - Bed rest, cardiac monitoring, oxygen
   - Nitroglycerin SL
   - Morphine IV.
2. **Anti-platelet and anticoagulation therapy:**
   - Acetyl salicylic acid (ASA) 162-325 mg chewed/clopidogrel 300 mg loading dose, then 75 mg OD in addition to ASA
   - Subcutaneous low molecular weight heparin (LMWH) or IV unfractionated heparin (UFH) (LMWH preferable, except in renal failure or if CABG is planned within 24 hour)
   - If PCI is planned: Clopidogrel 300 mg loading dose and IV GP IIb/IIIa inhibitor
   - Continue LMWH or UFH followed by oral anticoagulation at discharge if at high risk for thromboembolic event (large anterior MI, atrial fibrillation, severe LV dysfunction, CHF, previous DVT or PE, or echo evidence of mural thrombus).
3. **Beta-blockers**
   - First dose IV followed by oral administration
   - CCB in absence of severe LV dysfunction in patients with continuing or frequently recurring ischemia when beta-blockers are contraindicated (evidence suggests that CCBs do not prevent MI or decrease mortality)
4. **Invasive strategies and re-perfusion options:**

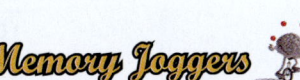

NSTEMI
- **A**bciximab, **β**-blocker, **E**noxapdrin, **M**orphine, **O**$_2$, **A**spirin and **N**itrates
  (Mnemonic: ABE-MOAN)
- If patient does not improve go for *delayed PCI*^{Q}.

- **STEMI**: Treatment of choice is PCI
  - Primary PCI (<12 hours after symptom onset and <90 minutes after presentation) improves mortality.
  - If patient reaches Non PCI capable hospital, transfer for primary PCI if first medical contact to device time is ≤ 120 minutes.
  - Thrombolysis: Preferred if patient presents in <12 hours of symptom onset, and <30 min after presentation to hospital.

- Thrombolysis is NOT administered for UA/NSTEMI
- Most common complication seen after thrombolysis is bleeding.
- First medical contact to device time should be < 90 minutes, if PCI is to be performed.

Contraindications for Thrombolysis in STEMI

Absolute	Relative
• Prior intracranial hemorrhage • Known structural cerebral vascular lesion • Known malignant intracranial neoplasm • Significant closed –head or facial trauma (< 3 months) • Ischemic stroke (< 3 months) • Active bleeding • Suspected aortic dissection	• Chronic, severe, poorly controlled hypertension • Uncontrolled hypertension (SBP> 180 mm Hg, DBP > 110 mm Hg) • Current anticoagulation • Noncompressible vascular punctures • Ischemic stroke (>3 months) • Recent internal bleeding (< 2–4 weeks) • Prolonged CPR or major surgery (<3 weeks) • Pregnancy • Active peptic ulcer

Complications of Myocardial Infarction

Complications	Etiology	Presentation	Therapy
Arrhythmia			
• Tachycardia	Ventricular fibrillation	Sudden death	DC shock
	Ventricular tachycardia	6-12 hours	Lignocaine
• Bradycardia	Mobitz 2 heart block	First 48 hrs	Temporary pacing
Myocardial Rupture			
• LV free wall	Transmural infarction	1–7 days	Surgery
• Papillary muscle rupture	Inferior infarction	1–7 days	Surgery
• Ventricular septum	Septal infarction	1–7 days	Surgery
Shock / CHF	Infarction or aneurysm	Within 48 hours	Ionotropes, intra-aortic balloon pump
Post-infarct angina	Persistent coronary stenosis multi-vessel disease	Anytime	Aggressive medical therapy PCI or CABG
Recurrent MI Thrombo-embolism	Reocclusion Mural/apical thrombus DVT	Anytime 7–10 days up to 6 months	

HEART FAILURE

Congestive Heart Failure (CHF)

Systolic Dysfunction (Impaired Ventricular Ejection)

- Impaired myocardial contractile function leading to decreased ejection fraction (LVEF) and stroke volume.

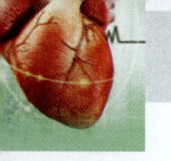

- Findings: apex beat displaced, S3, increased heart size on CXR. 50% patients with CHF have sleep disturbances, including Cheyne-Stokes breathing and sleep apnea (central or obstructive).

Causes
1. Hypertension
2. Diabetes mellitus
3. Alcohol
4. Myocarditis
5. Dilated cardiomyopathy

Diastolic Dysfunction (Impaired Ventricular Filling)

- At least 1/3 of all HF patients have normal systolic function (i.e. normal ejection fraction).
- Increased LV filling pressures produce venous congestion upstream (i.e. pulmonary and systemic venous congestion).
- **Findings:** HTN, apex beat sustained, S4, normal-sized heart on CXR, LVH on ECG/echo, normal LVEF.

Causes of Decreased Compliance
1. Severe hypertrophy (HTN, AS, HCM)
2. Restrictive cardiomyopathy (RCM)
3. MI

High-Output Heart Failure

- Caused by demand for increased cardiac output
- Often exacerbates existing heart failure or decompensates a patient with other cardiac pathology, but is infrequently a primary cause of heart failure
- Differential diagnosis: anemia, thiamine deficiency (Beri-Beri), hyperthyroidism, A-V fistula or L-R shunting, Paget's disease, renal disease and hepatic disease.

Framingham Criteria for Heart Failure

Major	Minor
Acute pulmonary oedema	Ankle edema
Cardiomegaly	Hepatomegaly
Hepatojugular reflux	Dyspnea on exertion
Neck vein distention	Nocturnal cough
Paroxysmal nocturnal dyspnea or orthopnea	Pleural effusion
S₃/Ventricular group	Tachycardia
Weight loss > 4.5 kg in 5 days in response to treatment	

Killip stage of heart failure
I: No clinical signs of heart failure
II: Rales/crackles in lung, S₃, elevated JVP
III: Frank acute pulmonary edema
IV: Cardiogenic shock or hypotension

- Heart failure is diagnosed when 2 major criteria or one major and two minor criteria are met

Investigations

1. N-Terminal ProB-type Natriuretic peptide: elevated
2. Uric acid
3. BUN
4. ECG - look for chamber enlargement, arrhythmia, ischemia/infarction
5. CXR - cardiomegaly, pleural effusion, redistribution, Kerley B-lines, bronchiolar alveolar cuffing
6. Electrocardiography - LVEF, cardiac dimensions, flow or wall motion abnormalities, valvular disease, pericardial effusion
7. Radionuclide angiography (MUGA) - LVEF
8. Myocardial perfusion scintigraphy (thallium or sestamibi SPECT).

Diagnostic Evaluation

Cardiac output and perfusion of extremities	Pulmonary edema (elevated PCWP)	What to be done?	Initial treatment
Warm to touch	Present (wet lungs)	Decrease pulmonary edema	Diuretics
Cold to touch	Present (wet lungs)	Increase the cardiac output	Dobutamine/dopamine
		Decrease pulmonary edema	Inodilators to unload the lungs
Warm to touch	Absent (dry lungs)	Pulmonary or hepatic disease	Treat lung disease
Cold to touch	Absent (dry lungs)	RV dysfunction	Fluid bolus

Management

Management of heart failure with preserved ejection fraction	
Drugs providing benefit and early promise are 1. Aldosterone antagonists 2. ARNI 3. ACEI play a role in prevention.	Sacubitril and valsartan—The most recently approved combination to improve clinical outcome in patients with heart failure with preserved as well as reduced LVEF, called as an angiotensin receptor-neprilysin inhibitor (ARNI). Compared to the ACE inhibitor enalapril, the ARNI was shown to reduce cardiovascular death and hospitalization for heart failure by 20% for patients with heart failure and reduced LVEF in a large randomized trial

Management of heart failure with reduced ejection fraction
1. ARNI 2. ACEI 3. β blockers: Metoprolol, bisoprolol, carvedilol

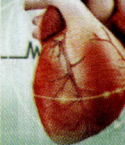

Acute Pulmonary Edema

- Treat acute precipitating factors (e.g. ischemia, arrhythmias)

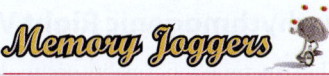

- L – **L**asix 40–500 mg IV
- M – **M**orphine 2–4 mg IV - decreases anxiety and preload
- N – **N**itroglycerine - topical/IV/SL
- O – **O**xygen
- P – **P**ositive airway pressure (CPAP/BiPAP) - decreases preload and need for ventilation
- P – **P**osition - sit patient up with legs hanging down unless patient is hypotensive

Cardiogenic Shock

- Norepinephrine/Dobutamine/Dopamine infusion
- Rarely used, but potentially life-saving measures:
  - Intra-aortic balloon pump (IABP)
  - L or R ventricular assist device (LVAD/RVAD)
  - Cardiac transplant

Procedural Interventions

- Resynchronization therapy: Symptomatic improvement with biventricular pacemaker
- Consider if QRS > 120 msec, LVEF <35%, and severe symptoms despite optimal therapy
- ICD: Mortality benefit in 1° and 2° prevention of sudden cardiac death
- Valve repair if patient is surgical candidate and has significant valve disease contributing to CHF.

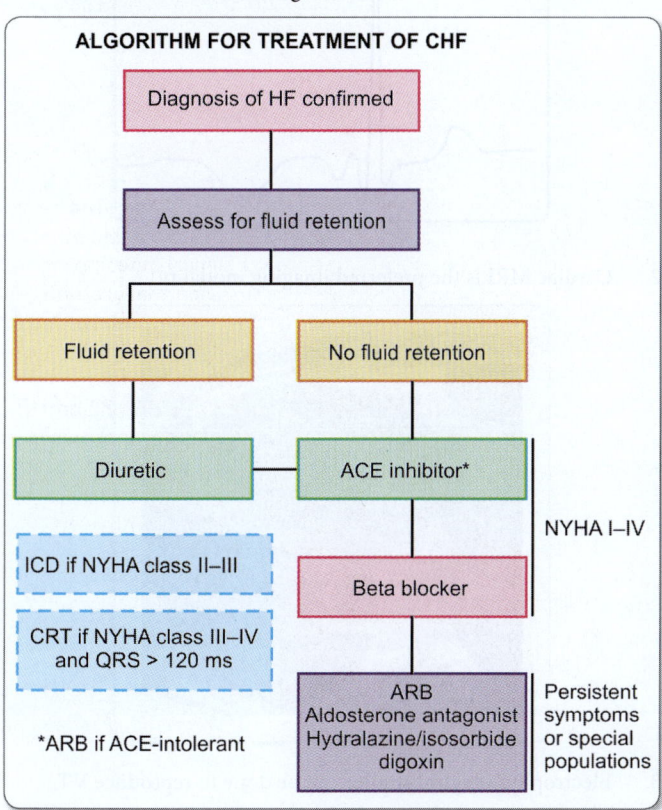

> Patients on ACEΘ exhibit increase in serum creatinine or potassium but do not require discontinuation. Even at serum creatinine values as high as 3 mg/dL, ACEΘ can be given. (page 413, CMDT 2018)
>
> However spirinolactone should be discontinued at high serum creatinine levels.

MYOCARDIAL DISEASE

Myocarditis

Definition

Inflammatory process involving the myocardium ranging from acute to chronic; an important cause of dilated cardiomyopathy

Etiology

1. Viral (most common): **Coxsackie B**^{Q}, echovirus, poliovirus, HIV, mumps
2. Bacterial: *S. aureus, C. perfringens, C. diphtheriae, Mycoplasma*
3. Fungi
4. Spirochaete (Lyme disease - *Borrelia burgdorferi*)
5. Chagas disease (*Trypanosoma cruzi*), toxoplasmosis
6. Toxic: Catecholamines, chemotherapy, cocaine
7. Hypersensitivity, eosinophilic: Drugs (antibiotics, diuretics, lithium, clozapine), insect /snake bites
8. **Systemic diseases:**^{Q} Collagen vascular diseases (SLE, RA, others), sarcoidosis, autoimmune
9. Other: Giant cell myocarditis, acute rheumatic fever.

Signs and Symptoms

- Constitutional illness
- Acute CHF
- Chest pain - Due to pericarditis or cardiac ischemia
- Arrhythmias
- Systemic or pulmonary emboli
- Sudden death.

Investigations

1. ECG: Non-specific ST-T changes ± conduction defects
2. Increased CK, troponin, LDH and AST with acute myocardial necrosis ± increased WBC, ESR, ANA, rheumatoid factor, complement levels
3. Blood culture, viral titers and cold agglutinins for Mycoplasma
4. CXR - Enlarged cardiac silhouette
5. Echo: Dilated, hypokinetic chambers, segmental wall motion abnormalities
6. Myocardial biopsy (in limited cases).

Management

- Supportive care
- Restrict physical activity
- Treat CHF
- Treat arrhythmias
- Anticoagulation
- Treat underlying cause, if possible.

CARDIOMYOPATHY (TAKOTSUBO CARDIOMYOPATHY, ARRHYTHMOGENIC RV DYSPLASIA)

Takotsubo Cardiomyopathy/Broken Heart Syndrome

Etiology

The *most common mechanism* is stress induced massive catecholamine release and toxicity. This leads to subsequent *stunning of myocardium*. Biopsy of myocardium reveals focal myocytolysis with mononuclear infiltrates and contraction band necrosis.

Modified Mayo criteria for Takotsubo Cardiomyopathy (T.C.M)/ Broken heart syndrome

1. Transient hypokinesia/ akinesia of Left ventricle
2. Absence of any coronary artery occlusion by a thrombus
3. ST segment elevation/T wave inversion or modest cardiac troponin elevation
4. Absence of pheochromocytoma or myocarditis

*Needs all four for diagnosis

Clinical Features

- Emotionally or physically stressful event like being stuck in a lift in middle of a massive earthquake
- The most common presenting symptoms are chest pain and dyspnea through palpitations, nausea, vomiting, syncope and cardiogenic shock
- Hypotension due to reduction in stroke volume with murmurs and rales on auscultation.
- ECG findings of ST segment with elevated Cardiac troponins will mimic STEMI.
- However when patient is taken up for PCI and Angiography is being done, the coronary vasculature is normal.
- Bed side echo may shows hypokinesia of LV with ballooning like a jar used to trap octopus.

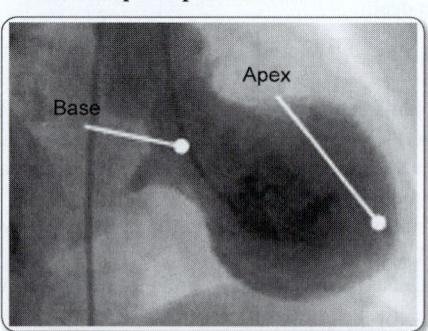

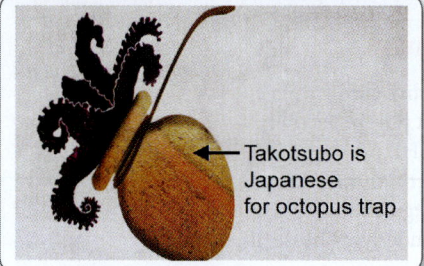
Takotsubo is Japanese for octopus trap

Management is with intra-aortic balloon pump to counter cardiogenic shock and *is the only cardiomyopathy where recovery will occur over* next few weeks.

Arrhythmogenic Right Ventricular Dysplasia

The structural abnormality occurs due to fatty infiltration and fibrosis of RV myocardium. This results in progressive RV dilatation and dysfunction. LV can also be involved but septum is spared. Electron microscopy shows defects in desmosomes which are responsible for cell to cell binding.

The most common pattern of inheritance is *autosomal dominant*.

Clinical Features

- *Most common symptoms* are palpitations and syncope. Family history of sudden cardiac death can be present.
- Most common ECG abnormalities are-ventricular ectopics, VT and ventricular fibrillation.
- RV malfunction leads to dyspnea and leg swelling.
- Important differenital diagnosis is UHL's Anomaly which has thin walled RV. The thin walled RV occurs due to lack of RV myocardium. In contrast ARVD, RV muscle is replaced by fibrofatty degeneration.

Investigations

1. ECG shows *epsilon wave*.

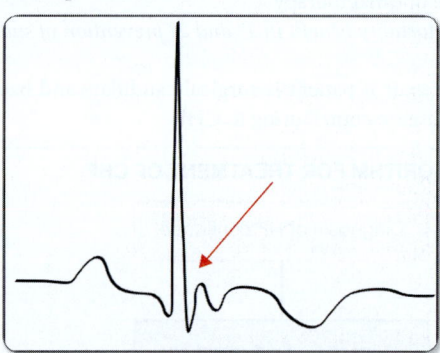

2. Cardiac MRI is the preferred imaging modality.

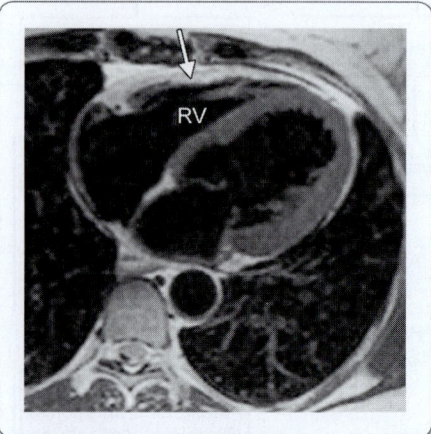

3. Electrophysiological studies can be done to reproduce VT.

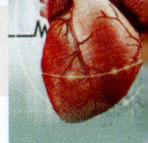

4. Histopathological finding of fibrosis is NOT pathognomonic because the fatty infiltration of myocardium can be seen in geriatric patients as well.

Treatment

- For secondary prevention of sudden cardiac death in patients with sustained VT or ventricular fibrillation, an *implantable cardioverter defibrillator* is required.
- Beta blockers are generally considered as first line drug therapy and sotalol is used.
  Sotalol is the most effective drug for inducible or non-inducible ventricular tachycardia.

Hypertrophic Cardiomyopathy (HCM)

- Most causes involve asymmetric septal hypertrophy with left ventricular outflow tract obstruction.
- It's an example of diastolic dysfunction and therefore, a secondary systolic dysfunction.
- The shape of left ventricle is referred to as banana-shaped.
- Prevalence of 1/500–1/1,000 in general population.
- It is autosomal dominant with defect of beta myosin gene with defect on chromosome 14.

Signs and Symptoms

- Due to elevated filling pressures, pulmonary edema develops with dyspnea as initial symptom. In lots of cases, it may not be recognized initially and patient may complain only of effort intolerance.
- Angina, pre-syncope/syncope (due to LV outflow obstruction or arrhythmia), CHF, arrhythmias, sudden cardiac death.
- Sudden death can occur during athletic activity like playing football due to ischemic ventricular fibrillation.
- *Pulses:* Rapid upstroke, bifid carotid pulse (Pulsus Bisfiriens).
- *Precordial palpation:* Well sustained double apical impulse, **'triple ripple' (triple apical impulse in HCM)**[Q], LV lift.
- *Precordial auscultation:* Normal or paradoxically split S2, S4, harsh systolic diamond-shaped murmur at LLSB or apex, enhanced by squat to standing or Valsalva (murmur secondary to LVOT obstruction as compared to aortic stenosis); often with pan-systolic murmur due to mitral regurgitation.

Investigations

1. ECG: LVH, high voltages across precordium, prominent Q waves or tall R wave in V_1, P wave abnormalities.
2. Echo: Asymmetric septal hypertrophy (less commonly apical), systolic anterior motion of Mitral valve and Mitral regurgitation.

Management

- Avoid factors which increase obstruction, including volume depletion and strenuous exertion.
- Treatment of HOCM (with LVOT obstruction)
  - Medical agents: DOC is Propranolol as it will decrease heart rate and reduce oxygen consumption. The comparative increase in duration of diastole will enhance the filling of the heart with corresponding increase in cardiac output. Verapamil may also be used.
  - NTG, digoxin, ACEI, diuretics are *contraindicated* in patients of HOCM.
- Management of patients with drug-refractory symptoms:
  - Surgical myomectomy
  - Septal ethanol ablation
  - Dual-chamber pacing
  - Treatment of ventricular arrhythmias: Amiodarone or ICD[Q]

Restrictive Cardiomyopathy (RCM)

- Impaired ventricular filling in a non-dilated, non-hypertrophied ventricle secondary to myocardial abnormality (stiffening, fibrosis and/or decreased compliance)
- Usually with intact systolic function
- Rarest *cardiomyopathy.*[Q]

Etiology

1. Infiltrative: Amyloidosis (most common cause),[Q] sarcoidosis
2. Non-infiltrative: Scleroderma, idiopathic myocardial fibrosis
3. Storage diseases: Hemochromatosis, Fabry's disease, glycogen storage diseases
4. Endomyocardial fibrosis, Loeffler's endocarditis or eosinophilic endomyocardial disease
5. Radiation heart disease (radiation can lead to mixed restrictive and constrictive pericarditis)
6. Carcinoid syndrome (may have associated TV or PV dysfunction).

Clinical Manifestations

- CHF (usually with preserved LV systolic function), arrhythmias.
- Elevated JVP with *prominent x and y descents*, Kussmaul's sign[Q].
- Patients may have distention of the abdomen secondary to ascites, but they frequently have profound bilateral peripheral edema. Abdominal discomfort or liver tenderness may be reported.
- Chest pain secondary to angina or chest pain mimicking myocardial ischemia can be observed, primarily in patients with amyloidosis, possibly due to myocardial compression of small vessels. Patients may complain of palpitations, frequently due to atrial fibrillation, which is common in idiopathic RCM.
- As many as one-third of patients with idiopathic RCM may present with thromboembolic complications, especially pulmonary emboli secondary to blood clots in the legs. If atrial fibrillation is present, a high risk of left atrial clots and systemic emboli is present.
- Heart sounds S_1 and S_2 are normal, with a normal S_2 split. A loud early diastolic filling sound (S_3) may be present but is uncommon in amyloidosis. *A fourth heart sound (S_4) is never present, possibly secondary to amyloid infiltration of the atria.* Murmurs due to mitral and tricuspid valve regurgitation may be heard, but they are secondary to the myocardial disease and usually not hemodynamically significant.

Clinical Features	Constrictive Pericarditis	Restrictive Cardiomyopathy
History	Prior history of pericarditis or condition that causes pericardial disease	History of systemic disease (e.g. Amyloidosis, hemochromatosis)

Contd...

Clinical Features	Constrictive Pericarditis	Restrictive Cardiomyopathy
General examination	—	Peripheral stigmata of systemic disease
Systemic examination-Heart sounds	**Pericardial knock^Q**, high-frequency sound	Presence of loud diastolic filling sound S_3, Low- frequency sound
Murmurs	No murmurs	Murmurs of mitral and tricuspid insufficiency
Prior chest radiograph	Pericardial calcification	Normal results of prior chest radiograph

Investigations

1. *ECG:* Low voltage, non-specific, diffuse ST-T wave changes ± non-ischemic Q waves
2. *CXR:* Mild cardiac enlargement
3. *Echo:* LVH, RVH, LAE, RAE, valve thickening
4. *Cardiac catheterization:* Increase end-diastolic ventricular pressures
5. *Endomyocardial biopsy:* To determine etiology (especially for infiltrative RCM and is investigation of choice)
6. Cardiac MRI

Management

- Exclude constrictive pericarditis
- *Treat underlying disease:* Control heart rate, anticoagulate if atrial fibrillation
- Supportive care and treatment for CHF, arrhythmias
- *Heart transplant:* might be considered for CHF refractory to medical therapy.

Dilated Cardiomyopathy (DCM)

Definition

Unexplained dilation and impaired systolic function of one or both ventricles.

Etiology

1. Idiopathic (presumed viral or genetic): 50% of DCM
2. Alcohol (MC Toxin leading to DCM)
3. Familial
4. Uncontrolled tachycardia (e.g. persistent atrial fibrillation)
5. *Collagen vascular disease:* SLE, PAN, dermatomyositis, progressive systemic sclerosis
6. *Infectious:* viral (Coxsackie B, HIV), Chagas disease, Lyme disease, Rickettsial diseases, acute rheumatic fever
7. *Neuromuscular disease:* Duchenne muscular dystrophy, Myotonic dystrophy, Friedreich's ataxia
8. *Metabolic:* Uremia, nutritional deficiency (thiamine, selenium, carnitine)
9. *Endocrine:* Hyper/ hypothyroidism, DM, pheochromocytoma
10. Peripartum cardiomyopathy
11. *Toxic:* Cocaine, heroin, organic solvents
12. *Drugs:* Chemotherapies (doxorubicin, cyclophosphamide), anti-retrovirals, chloroquine, clozapine.

Signs and Symptoms

- Systemic or pulmonary emboli
- CHF
- Arrhythmias
- Sudden death (major cause of mortality due to fatal arrhythmia).

Investigations

1. CBC, electrolytes, creatinine, bicarbonate, BNP, CK, troponin, LFTs
2. *ECG:* Variable ST-T wave abnormalities, poor R wave progression, conduction defects, arrhythmias (non-sustained VT)
3. *CXR:* Global cardiomegaly (globular heart), signs of CHF
4. *Echocardiography:* 4-chamber enlargement, global hypokinesia with depressed LVEF, MR and TR, mural thrombus
5. *Endomyocardial biopsy:* Not routine, used to rule out a treatable cause
6. *Angiography:* In selected patients to exclude ischemic heart disease.

Management

- Careful titration of diuretics as they can decrease cardiac ouput.
- *Thromboembolism prophylaxis:* anticoagulation with warfarin
- Treat symptomatic or serious arrhythmias
- Immunize against influenza and S. pneumonia
- Consider surgical options (e.g. LVAD, transplant, volume reduction surgery, AICDs) in appropriate candidates with severe, refractory disease.

Quick Comparison of Histopathological Features of Subtypes of Cardiomyopathies

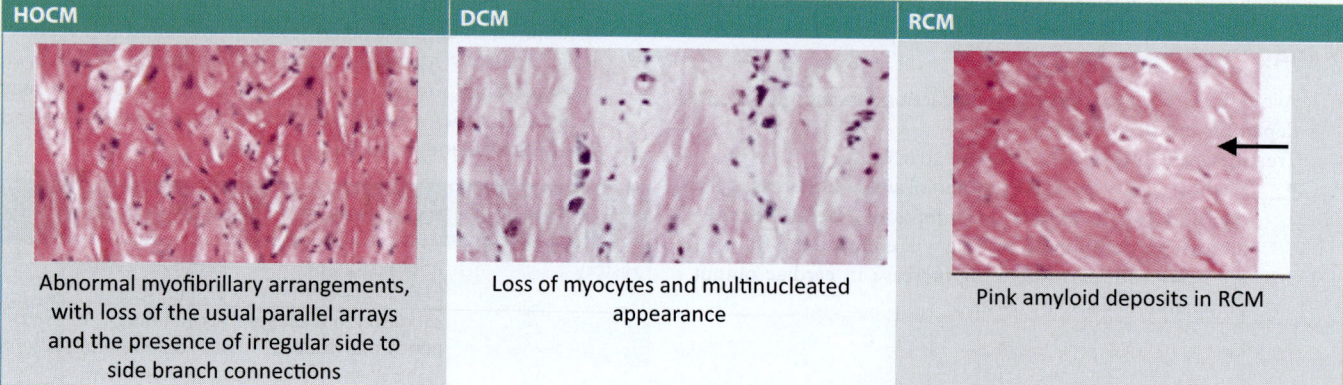

HOCM	DCM	RCM
Abnormal myofibrillary arrangements, with loss of the usual parallel arrays and the presence of irregular side to side branch connections	Loss of myocytes and multinucleated appearance	Pink amyloid deposits in RCM

INFECTIVE ENDOCARDITIS

Causative Organisms Associated with Infective Endocarditis

Sub-acute bacterial endocarditis	*Streptococcus viridans/enterococci*
IV drug abuser/Right sided endocarditis	*Staphylococcus aureus*
Left sided endocarditis	*S. aureus* > Enterococci
Prosthetic valve endocarditis	< 2 months: C.O.N.S (coagulase negative endocarditis) 2–12 months: C.O.N.S (coagulase negative endocarditis) > 1 year: *S. viridans*
Native valve endocarditis community acquired	*Streptococcus*
Health care associated	*S. aureus*
Culture negative endocarditis	*Granulicatella abiotrophia/Tropheryma whipplei/Coxiella/Bartonella*
Libman sacks endocarditis	SLE (Inferior surface of valves show fibrin deposits)
Non-bacterial thrombotic endocarditis	Endothelium damage leads to platelet fibrin thrombus

Manifestations of Infective Endocarditis

System involved	Manifestation
Cardiac involvement	Perivalvular abscess, CHF, pericarditis, bundle branch block, MI, new onset murmur due to fistula in the valve; The organisms in the deep layers are difficult to kill and are metabolically inactive
Peripheral manifestations (J.O.S.H)	**J**aneway lesions, **O**sler nodes, **S**plinter **H**emorrhage
CNS	Mycotic aneurysms
Kidney	Post infectious glomerulonephritis with low C3
Immunological manifestations	Roth spots, Osler nodes, glomerulonephritis

Causes of Roth Spots

1. Infective endocarditis
2. SLE
3. Polyarteritis nodosa
4. Severe anemia
5. Leukemia
6. Hypertension
7. Diabetes mellitus

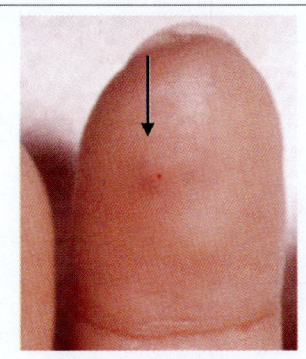
Osler nodes

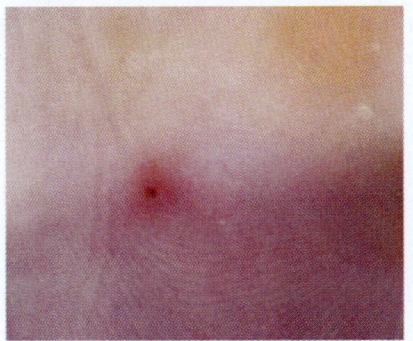
Janeway lesions

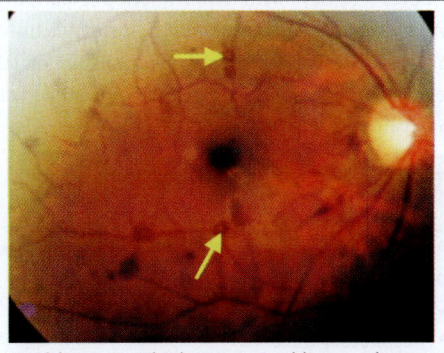
Roth's spots which are retinal hemorrhages with a white center

Major Blood Culture Criteria for IE

- Two blood cultures positive for organisms typically found in patients with IE
- Blood cultures persistently positive for one of these organisms, from cultures drawn more than 12 hours apart
- Three or more separate blood cultures drawn at least 1 hour apart.

Major Echocardiographic Criteria for IE

- Echocardiogram positive for IE, documented by an oscillating intracardiac mass on a valve or on supporting structures, in the path of regurgitant jets, or on implanted material, in the absence of an alternative anatomic explanation
- Myocardial abscess
- Development of partial dehiscence of a prosthetic valve
- New-onset valvular regurgitation.

Minor Criteria for IE

- Predisposing heart condition or intravenous drug use
- Fever of 38°C (100.4°F) or higher
- Vascular phenomenon, including major arterial emboli, septic pulmonary infarcts, mycotic aneurysm, intracranial hemorrhage, conjunctival hemorrhage, or Janeway lesions
- Immunologic phenomenon such as glomerulonephritis, Osler nodes, Roth's spots and rheumatoid factor
- Positive blood culture results not meeting major criteria or serologic evidence of active infection with an organism consistent with IE
- Echocardiogram results are consistent with IE but not meeting major echocardiographic criteria.

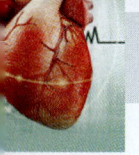

A definitive clinical diagnosis can be made based on the following:
- 2 major criteria
- 1 major criterion and 3 minor criteria
- 5 minor criteria

Treatment

Patient should be afebrile in < 7 days. Fever persisting for >7 days is suggestive of paravalvular abscess.

S. aureus	Naficillin + gentamycin and rifampicin x 8 weeks *rifampicin kills staphylococcus adherent to foreign material MRSA= add vancomycin
HACEK	Ceftriaxone X 4 weeks
Enterococci	Penicillin G + gentamycin X 4 weeks
Penicillin sensitive *S. bovis*	Penicillin G + ceftriaxone X 2 weeks
Penicillin resistant *S. bovis*	Same as above for 4 weeks

Indications for Surgery
- Aortic regurgitation leads to CHF
- Sinus of Valsalva rupture
- Perivalvular abscess
- Fever >10 days with hypermobile vegetations.

AHA guidelines recommend IE prophylaxis–only for patients with prosthetic valve material, past history of IE, certain types of unrepaired congenital heart disease or cardiac transplant recipients who develop valvulopathy.

Antibiotic prophylaxis is only for the following procedures:
- Dental
- Respiratory tract
- Procedures on infected skin/skin structures.

Not for gastrointestinal/genitourinary procedures specifically.

HEART SOUNDS AND MURMURS

Heart Sounds

1. Atrial Systole

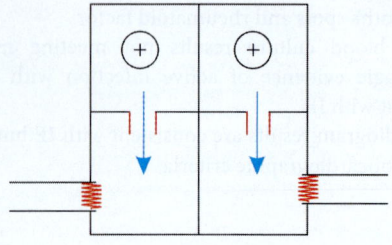

2. Isovolumetric Contraction (S_1 occurs)

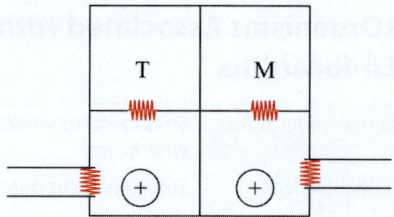

3. Ventricular Systole (ejection click)

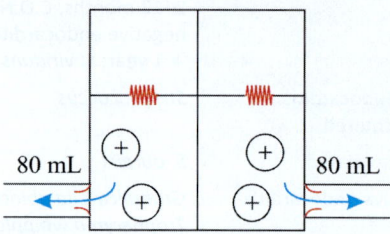

4. Isovolumetric Relaxation (S_2 occurs)

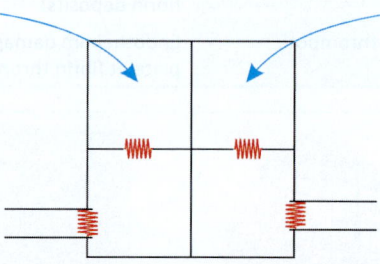

5. Ventricular Diastole (opening snap)

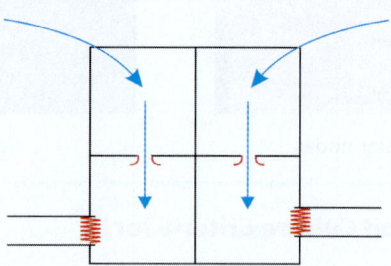

First Heart Sound S1 (25 –45Hz)

This is produced during the closure of MITRAL VALVE and TRICUSPID VALVE. It is heard with diaphragm of the stethoscope.

S_1 Loud	Tachycardia / MS / physiological in pregnancy, children
S_1 soft	Calcification of leaflet of MS / bradycardia / obesity, emphysema

* S_1 is lower frequency than S_2

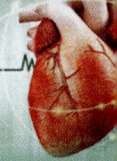

Second Heart Sound S2 (50 Hz)

This is due to closure of AORTIC VALVE and PULMONIC VALVE. It is heard with diaphragm of the stethoscope

Narrow split	Pulmonary atresia, TOF (single S2)
Wide variable split	MR, VSD, RBBB
Wide fixed split	ASD, PAH, pulmonary embolism
Loud S_2	PAH
Reversed Split	HTN, IHD, AS, LBBB, aortic pulmonary shunt

Ejection Sound/Click

Loud	Congenital bicuspid valve, aortic or pulmonary root dilatation
Soft	Calcified bicuspid aortic valve
Non ejection mid systolic	Clicks: Mitral valve prolapse

*Pulmonary ejection click is the only right sided acoustic event that decreases in intensity with inspiration

Third Heart Sound S3 [Early Diastolic]

Diastolic heart sound produced during ventricular filling. It's a low frequency diastolic heart sound. This is heard with the help of bell of stethoscope.
- Children
- MR
- AR
- DCM/CHF
- Constrictive pericarditis.

Fourth Heart Sound S4 [Late Diastolic]

Produced during atrial filling, heard with bell.
- HTN
- IHD
- HCM
- AS/PS.

* Low frequency heart sounds are: Tumor plop sound, S_3 and S_4.
* S_4 is absent in atrial fibrillation

Murmurs

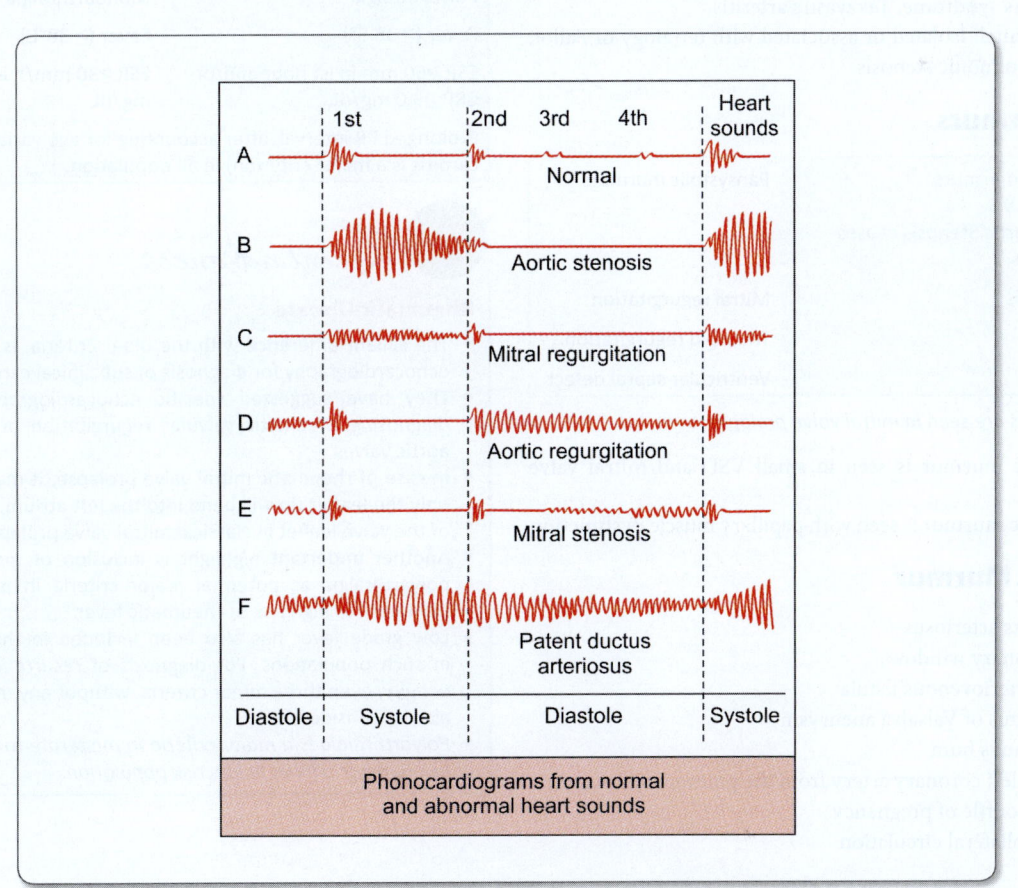

Phonocardiograms from normal and abnormal heart sounds

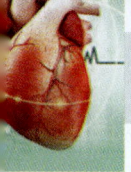

Diastolic Murmurs

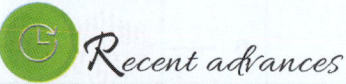

Early Diastolic Murmurs Mn: GAP	Mid Diastolic Murmurs
Graham steele murmur	**C**arey coombs murmur
Aortic regurgitation (mild)	**A**ustin flint murmur
Pulmonic regurgitation (mild)	**M**itral stenosis

- Flow murmurs are also mid-diastolic murmurs.
- *Carey Coombs: Mid diastolic murmur*
- Causes of Aortic regurgitation that have been asked in previous year questions are:
    - Valvular: Congenital (bicuspid valve), rheumatic endocarditis, prolapse, trauma, postvalvulotomy
    - Dilatation of the valve annulus: Aortic dissection, annulo-aortic ectasia, cystic medial degeneration, hypertension, ankylosing spondylitis, syphilis, Takayasu's arteritis.
- Causes of Pulmonary regurgitation that have been asked in previous years:
    - Valvular: Postvalvulotomy, endocarditis, rheumatic fever, carcinoid
    - Dilatation of the valve annulus: Pulmonary hypertension, Marfan's syndrome, Takayasu's arteritis
    - Congenital: Isolated or associated with tetralogy of Fallot, VSD, pulmonic stenosis.

Systolic Murmurs

Ejection systolic murmurs Mnemonic = P.A.S.S Pulmonic and Aortic Stenosis causes Systolic Murmurs	Pansystolic murmurs
Pulmonic stenosis	Mitral regurgitation
Aortic stenosis	Tricuspid regurgitation
HOCM	Ventricular septal defect

*Mid systolic clicks are seen in mitral valve prolapse

- Late systolic murmur is seen in small VSD and mitral valve prolapse.
- Early systolic murmur is seen with papillary muscle dysfunction

Continuous Murmur

1. Patent ductus arteriosus
2. Aortopulmonary window
3. Coronary arteriovenous fistula
4. Ruptured sinus of Valsalva aneurysm
5. Cervical venous hum
6. Anomalous left coronary artery from the pulmonary artery
7. Mammary souffle of pregnancy
8. Bronchial collateral circulation
9. Intercostal or pulmonary arteriovenous fistula.
10. Peripheral pulmonic stenosis

RHEUMATIC FEVER

(2015, Revised Jones criteria)

Major Criteria

Low-risk populations	Moderate- and high-risk populations
Carditis • Clinical and/or subclinical carditis	**Carditis** • Clinical and/or subclinical carditis
Arthritis • Polyarthritis only	**Arthritis** • Monoarthritis or polyarthritis • Polyarthralgia
Chorea	Chorea
Erythema marginatum	Erythema marginatum
Subcutaneous nodules	Subcutaneous nodules

Minor Criteria

Low-risk populations	Moderate- and high-risk populations
Polyarthralgia	Monoarthralgia
Fever ($\geq$ 38.5°)	Fever ($\geq$ 38°C)
ESR $\geq$60 mm in Ist hour and/or CRP $\geq$3.0 mg/dL	ESR $\geq$30 mm/h and/or CRP $\geq$3.0 mg/dL
Prolonged PR interval, after accounting for age variability (unless carditis is a major criterion) in all population.	

Recent advances

Rheumatic Update
- The salient difference with the older criteria, is the inclusion of echocardiography for diagnosis of subclinical carditis.
- They have suggested specific echocardiographic criteria for diagnosing rheumatic valvular regurgitation of the mitral and aortic valves.
- In case of rheumatic mitral valve prolapse, it may be noted that only the leaflet tip will bend into the left atrium, unlike the body of the valve leaflet in classical mitral valve prolapse.
- Another important highlight is inclusion of monoarthritis and polyarthralgia as potential major criteria in populations with moderate to high risk of rheumatic fever.
- Low grade fever has also been included in the minor criteria in such populations. For diagnosis of *recurrence of rheumatic activity*, even three minor criteria, without any major criteria can also be considered.
- *Polyarthralgia is a major criteria in moderate to high risk groups but is minor criteria in low risk population.*

Rheumatic Carditis

	Rheumatic pericarditis	Rheumatic myocarditis	Rheumatic endocarditis
Symptoms and findings	Chest pain at rest; Pericardial friction RUB	CHF with pulmonary edema; S3; Carey coombs murmur (characteristic murmur of rheumatic etiology)	Most common valvular lesion in ACTIVE CARDITIS is **Mitral regurgitation**[Q] Most common valvular lesion in rheumatic carditis is **mitral stenosis**[Q] Rarest involvement: **pulmonic valve**[Q]
ECG	ST segment elevation	Non-specific ST segment changes	P mitrale and P pulmonale in setting of pulmonary artery hypertension.
Treatment	Steroids	Diuretics	Valvuloplasty will relieve features of **acute CHF**[Q]

Medical Therapy for Acute Rheumatic Fever

- Treat group A streptococcal infection regardless of organism detection.
- Steroids and salicylates are useful in the control of pain and inflammation.
- Heart failure may require digitalis, fluid and sodium restriction, diuretics, and oxygen.
- Management of chorea

Mild cases	Provide calm environment
Moderate cases	Carbamazepine or valproate is preferred to haloperidol
Severe/Refractory	Steroids

- Administer prophylaxis against GABHS infections to patients who have developed ARF. Most authorities suggest that prophylaxis be given for 5 years. For those who have rheumatic carditis, some authorities suggest lifelong prophylaxis.

AHA Guidelines for Duration of Secondary Prophylaxis[Q]	
Rheumatic fever without carditis	For 5 years after last attack or up to 21 years of age
Rheumatic fever with Carditis but no residual valvular disease	For 10 years after last attack or up to 21 years of age
Rheumatic fever with Echo proven valvular damage	For 10 years after last attack or up to 40 years of age

VALVULAR HEART DISEASE

Comparison of Diseases of Aortic Valves

Aortic Stenosis

Etiology
1. Congenital (bicuspid, unicuspid valve)
2. Calcification, rheumatic disease
3. AVA:N 3–4 cm^2
4. Severe AS ≤1.0 cm^2
5. Critical AS <0.5 cm^2

Symptoms
Exertional angina, syncope, dyspnea, PND, orthopnea, peripheral edema

Physical Examination
Narrow pulse pressure, brachioradial delay, pulse parvus et tardus

Auscultation: Crescendo-decrescendo SEM radiating to R clavicle with musical quality at apex (Gallavardin phenomenon), S4, soft S2 with paradoxical splitting, S3 (late)

Aortic Regurgitation

Etiology
1. **Supravalvular:** Aortic root disease like Marfan's atherosclerosis and dissecting aneurysm, connective tissue disease
2. **Valvular:** Congenital (bicuspid AV, large VSD), infective endocarditis
3. **Acute onset:** IE, aortic dissection, trauma, failed prosthetic valve

Symptoms
- Usually only becomes symptomatic late in disease when LV failure develops
- Dyspnea, orthopnea, PND, syncope, angina

Aortic insufficiency

Auscultation: Early decrescendo diastolic murmur at LLSB (cusp) or RLSB (aortic root), best heard sitting, leaning forward, on full expiration, soft S1, absent S2, S3 (late)

Contd...

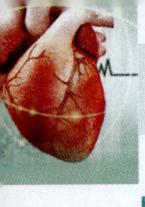

Aortic Stenosis	Aortic Regurgitation
Investigations 1. ECG: LVH and strain, LBBB, LAE, AF 2. CXR: Post-stenotic aortic root dilatation, calcified valve, LVH, LAE, CHF 3. ECHO: Reduced valve area, pressure gradient, LVH, reduced LV function	**Investigations** 1. ECG: LVH, LAE 2. CXR: LVH, LAE aortic root dilatation 3. Echo/TTE: Quantify AR, leaflet or aortic root anomalies 4. Cath: If > 40 yrs and surgical candidate – to assess for ischemic heart disease
Treatment Asymptomatic: Serial Echo monitoring and avoid exertion	**Treatment** Asymptomatic: Serial Echo monitoring and afterload reduction (ACEIs) e.g. nifedipine, hydralazine
Symptomatic: Avoid nitrates/arterial dilators and ACEIs in severe AS	**Symptomatic**: Avoid exertion, treat CHF
Surgery if: Symptomatic or LV dysfunction	**Surgery if**: NYHA class III-IV CHF, LVEF <50% with/without symptoms, increasing LV size
Surgical Options • **Valve replacement:** aortic rheumatic valve disease & trileaflet valve • Pregnancy • **Balloon valvuloplasty** (in very young patients)	**Surgical Options** • **Valve replacement:** Most patients • **Valve repair:** Limited role, repair of valves to improve coarctation • **Bentall procedure:** A Bentall procedure is a cardiac surgery operation involving composite graft replacement of the aortic valve, aortic root and ascending aorta, with re-implantation of the coronary arteries into the graft.

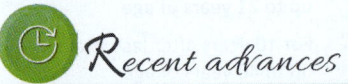

Aortic Stenosis

Severe aortic stenosis is defined as surface area < 1 cm^2 or 0.6cm^2/m^2 with low stroke volume <35 mL/m^2.

High gradient severe aortic stenosis	> 4 m/sec Doppler jet velocity > 40 mm Hg mean gradient
Super severe aortic stenosis	> 5 m/sec Doppler jet velocity > 55 mm Hg mean gradient

Asymptomatic patients with severe aortic stenosis with increased transvalvular gradient > 55 mm Hg need aortic valve replacement.

Aortic Regurgitation Management Update

- Aortic regurgitation will cause an increase in preload as well as afterload. Hence for AR with hypertension, ARB are to be given in place of beta blockers.
- Surgery is indicated in symptomatic patients and in asymptomatic patients with LV end diastolic pressure of > 65 mm Hg

Comparison of Diseases of Mitral Valve

Mitral Stenosis	Mitral Regurgitation
Etiology 1. Rheumatic disease (most common cause): 2. Congenital (rare) 3. Severe MS is MVA <1.2 cm^2	**Etiology** 1. Mitral valve prolapse 2. Congenital cleft leaflets 3. LV aneurysm 4. LV dilatation: CHF, DCM, myocarditis 5. IE abscess 6. Marfan's syndrome 7. HOCM, acute MI 8. Myxoma, MV annulus calcification, chordae /papillary muscle trauma/ischemia/rupture 9. Rheumatic disease
Symptoms Dysnea, orthopnea, fatigue, palpitations, peripheral edema, malar flush, pinched and blue facies (severe MS)	**Symptoms** Dyspnea, PND, orthopnea, palpitations, peripheral edema

The murmur of mitral regurgitation

Contd...

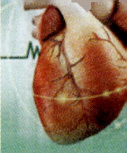

Mitral Stenosis	Mitral Regurgitation
Physical Examination • AF=no "a" wave on JVP • Left parasternal lift • Palpable diastolic thrill at apex	**Physical Examination** Displaced, hyperdynamic apex, left parasternal lift, apical thrill
Auscultation: Mid-diastolic rumble at apex, best with bell in LLD position following exertion, loud S1, OS following loud P2 (heard best during expiration), long murmur & **short A2-OS interval correlate with worse MS**^{Q}	**Auscultation:** Holosystolic murmur at apex, radiating to axilla ± mid-diastolic rumble, loud S2 (if pulmonary HTN), S3
Investigations 1. ECG: NSR/AF, LAE (P mitrale), RVH, RAD 2. CXR: LAE, CHF, MV calcification 3. Echo/TTE: Restricted opening of MV 4. Cath Lab: Concurrent CAD if > 40 yrs (male) or > 50 yrs (female)	**Investigations** 1. ECG: LAE, left atrial delay (bifid P waves), ±LVH 2. CXR: LVH, LAE, pulmonary venous HTN 3. Echo: Severity of MR, LV function, leaflets 4. Swan-Ganz cath: Prominent LA "v" wave
Treatment Avoid exertion, fever (increased LA pressure), treat AF and CHF, increase diastolic filling time (beta-blockers, digitalis)	**Treatment** • **Asymptomatic:** Serial echo monitoring • **Symptomatic:** Decrease preload (diuretics), decrease afterload (ACEIs) for severe MR and poor surgical candidate; stabilize acute MR with vasodilators before surgery

Hemodynamics of Mitral Stenosis

- The left atrial pressure exceeds the left ventricular pressure during diastole due to mitral stenosis and the consequent generation of a pressure gradient across the left atrium and left ventricle. This transvalvular gradient leads to faster opening of the mitral valve and a faster recoil which leads to a loud S_1.
- In future, in case of calcification of the valve, the elastic recoil will reduce, leading to soft S_1.
- In diastole, the stenotic mitral valve opens, which corresponds to the opening snap (OS) and the passage of blood across the mitral stenosis results in an audible decrescendo murmur. Left atrial contraction prior to S_1 increases the pressure gradient resulting in accentuation of the murmur before S_1 is audible.
- Severity of MS is decided by length of murmur or inversely related to A2—opening snap gap.
- Severity of MS is not decided by loud murmur or loud S_1 or loud P2.
- **The murmur of MS is mid diastolic murmur with a pre-systolic accentuation.**
- **Carey Coombs murmur is a mid diastolic murmur suggestive of rheumatic *myocarditis*.**^{Q}

PERICARDIAL DISEASE

Acute Pericarditis

Etiology of Pericarditis/Pericardial Effusion

1. Idiopathic is most common: Usually presumed to be viral
2. Infectious
    - Viral: Coxsackie virus A, B (most common), echovirus
    - Bacterial: *S. pneumoniae, S. aureus*
    - TB
    - Fungal: Histoplasmosis, Blastomycosis
3. Post-MI: Acute (direct extension of myocardial inflammation, 1-7 days), Dressler's syndrome (autoimmune, 2-8 weeks) post-cardiac surgery (e.g. CABG)
4. Metabolic: uremia (common), hypothyroidism
5. Neoplasm: Hodgkin's, breast Ca, lung Ca, renal cell Ca, melanoma
6. Collagen vascular disease: SLE, polyarteritis nodosa, RA, scleroderma
7. Vascular: Dissecting aneurysm
8. Others: drugs (e.g. hydralazine), radiation, infiltrative disease (sarcoidosis)

Signs and Symptoms

- **Diagnostic triad:** Chest pain, friction rub, and ECG changes
- **Pleuritic chest pain:** Alleviated by sitting up and leaning forward
- **Pericardial friction rub** - may be uni-, bi- or triphasic
- ± Fever, malaise.

Investigations

1. ECG:
    - Initially diffuse elevated ST segment in all leads except aVR ± depressed PR segment
    - The elevation in the ST segment is concave upwards
    - After 2–5 days, ST isoelectric with T wave flattening and inversion
2. CXR: Normal heart size, pulmonary infiltrates
3. Echo: Assess pericardial effusion

Treatment

- Treat the underlying disease
- Anti-inflammatory agents (high dose NSAIDs/ASA, steroids if severe or recurrent); analgesics

Prognosis

- Complications: recurrence, atrial arrhythmia, pericardial effusion, tamponade, constrictive pericarditis (uncommon)

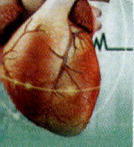

Pericardial Effusion

Etiology

1. Transudative (serous) = CHF, hypoalbuminemia
2. Exudative (serosanguinous or bloody)
   - Causes similar to the causes of acute pericarditis
   - May develop acute effusion secondary to hemopericardium (trauma, post MI myocardial rupture, aortic dissection)
3. Physiological consequences depend on type and volume of effusion, rate of effusion development, and underlying cardiac disease.

Signs and Symptoms

- May be asymptomatic or similar to acute pericarditis
- Dyspnea, cough due to extracardiac involvement like recurrent laryngeal nerve/tracheobronchial/phrenic nerve irritation
- JVP increased with dominant "x" descent
- Arterial pulse normal to decreased volume, decreased pulse pressure
- Auscultation: Distant heart sounds ± rub.

Investigations

1. ECG: Low voltage, flat T waves and **ELECTRICAL ALTERNANS**[Q]

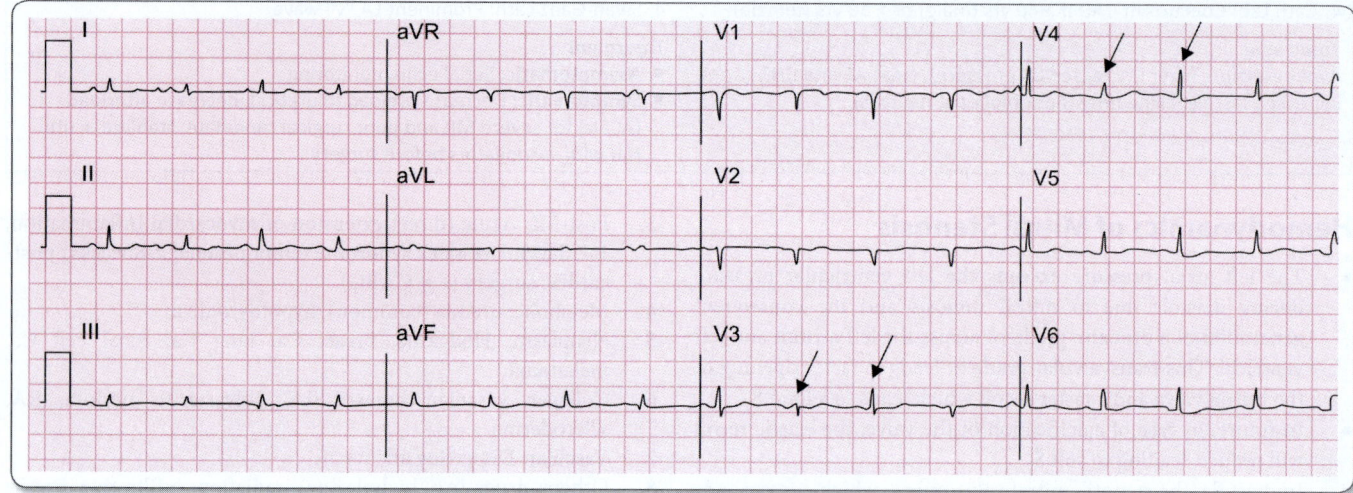

2. CXR: Cardiomegaly, rounded cardiac contour
3. Echo (procedure of choice)[Q]: Fluid in pericardial sac
4. Pericardiocentesis: Definitive method of determining transudate vs. exudate, identify infectious agents, neoplastic involvement.

Treatment

- Mild: Frequent observation with serial echocardiograms, treat the cause, anti-inflammatory agents for inflammation
- Severe: May develop cardiac tamponade.

Cardiac Tamponade

Etiology

1. Major complication of rapidly accumulating pericardial effusion; cardiac tamponade is a clinical diagnosis.
2. Any cause of pericarditis especially trauma, malignancy, uremia, idiopathic, proximal aortic dissection with rupture.
3. Not every massive pericardial effusion leads to cardiac tamponade as it is dependent on time over which it develops.
4. In hypothyroidism, serous cavity effusion like a massive pericardial effusion takes a long time to develop and therefore, pulsus paradoxus might not be present.

Signs and Symptoms

- Tachypnea, dyspnea, shock
- Pulsus paradoxus
- JVP "x" descent only, *absent "y" descent*[Q]
- Hepatic congestion/peripheral edema.

Investigations

1. ECG: Electrical alternans (pathognomonic variation in R wave amplitude), low voltage
2. Echo: Pericardial effusion, compression of cardiac chambers (RA and RV) in diastole
3. Cardiac catheterization.

Treatment

- Pericardiocentesis: Echo- or ECG-guided
- Pericardiotomy
- Avoid diuretics and vasodilators (these decrease venous return to already under-filled heart)
- Fluid administration i.e. saline load may temporarily increase CO.

Constrictive Pericarditis

Etiology

1. Chronic pericarditis resulting in fibrosed, thickened, adherent, and /or calcified pericardium

2. Any cause of acute pericarditis may result in chronic pericarditis
3. Major causes are idiopathic, post-infectious (viral, TB), radiation, post-cardiac surgery, uremia, MI.

Signs and Symptoms

- Dyspnea, fatigue, palpitations
- Abdominal pain
- May mimic CHF (especially right-sided HF)
- Ascites, hepatosplenomegaly, pedal edema
- Increased JVP, Kussmaul's sign (paradoxical increase in JVP with inspiration), Friedreich's sign (prominent "y" descent)
- BP usually normal (and usually no pulsus paradoxus)
- Pericardial knock (early diastolic sound)^Q

Investigations

1. ECG: Non-specific: low voltage, flat T wave, ± AF
2. CXR: Pericardial calcification, effusions
3. Echo/CT/MRI: Pericardial thickening. CT chest is the best test to demonstrate calcification of constrictive pericarditis.
4. Cardiac catheterization: Equalization of end-diastolic chamber pressures (diagnostic).

Treatment

- Medical: Diuretics, salt restriction
- Surgical: Pericardiectomy (only if refractory to medical therapy)
- Prognosis best with idiopathic or infectious cause and worst in post-radiation with death resulting from heart failure

Differentiation between Constrictive Pericarditis and Cardiac Tamponade

Characteristics	Constrictive Pericarditis	Cardiac Tamponade
JVP	"Y" > "X"	Prominent X with absent Y
Kussmaul's sign	Present	Absent
Pulsus paradoxus	Uncommon	Always
Pericardial Knock	Present	Absent
Hypotension	Variable	Severe

AORTIC DISSECTION

Tear in aortic intima allowing blood to dissect into the media; acute <2 weeks, chronic >2 weeks.

Classification

- De Bakey classification
  - Type I: Involves ascending and descending aorta
  - Type II: Ascending aorta only (stops at the innominate artery)
  - Type IIIA: Descending thoracic aorta only (distal to left subclavian artery and proximal to diaphragm)
  - Type IIIB: Type IIIA plus abdominal aorta
- Stanford
  - Type A: Involves ascending aorta ± aortic arch; requires emergency surgery
  - Type B: Only involves aorta distal to subclavian artery; emergency surgery only if complications of dissection (requires long-term follow-up to assess aneurysm size)

Etiology

1. Most common: Damage to aortic media (smooth muscle and elastic tissue), leading to degenerative/cystic changes due to hypertension^Q
2. Other: Cystic medial necrosis, atherosclerosis, connective tissue disease (Marfan's, Ehlers-Danlos), congenital conditions (coarctation of aorta, bicuspid aortic valves, patent ductus arteriosus), infection, trauma, arteritis (Takayasu's)

Clinical Features

Sudden onset tearing chest pain that radiates to back with:
- Hypertension (75–85% of patients)
- Asymmetric blood pressure and pulses between arms^Q
- Ischemic syndromes due to occlusion of aortic branches: coronary (MI), carotids (ischemic stroke), Horner's yndrome 1, splanchnic (ischemic gut)
- "Unseating" of aortic valve cusps (new diastolic murmur in 20–30%)
- Rupture into pleura (dyspnea, hemoptysis) or peritoneum (hypotension, shock) or pericardium (cardiac tamponade)
- Renal insufficiency
- Lower limb ischemia.

Investigations

1. CXR findings
2. Pleural cap (pleural effusion in lung apices)
3. Widened mediastinum
4. Left pleural effusion with extravasation of blood
5. TEE; can visualize aortic valve and thoracic aorta but not abdominal aorta (preferred bed side investigation)
6. ECG: LVH, pericarditis, heart block
7. Cardiac MRI is preferred in stable patients (Tennis ball appearance)

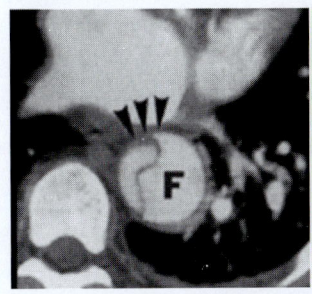 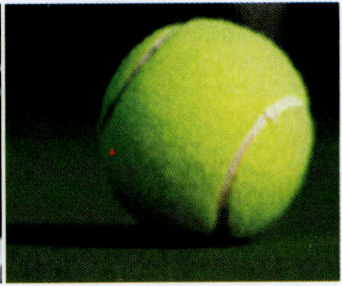

8. Troponin I to rule out MI.

Treatment

- Medical treatment
  - Esmolol/Labetalol to lower BP and decrease cardiac contractility
  - Target SBP of 110 mm Hg and HR 60 bpm

- Surgical treatment
    - Resection of intimal tear, re-constitution of flow through true lumen, replacement of the affected aorta with prosthetic graft, correction of any predisposing factors (e.g. bicuspid aortic valve, PDA, etc.)
    - **Type A:** Requires emergent surgery with cardiopulmonary bypass, may require hypothermic circulation for transverse arch dissections, valve replacement and coronary reimplantation for aortic root involvement, initial mortality rate without surgery is 1–2% per hour for first 48 hours
    - **Type B:** Initially managed medically; 10–20% require urgent operation for complications (expansion, rupture, compromise of branch arteries, refractory HTN).

SYNCOPE

- It is defined as sudden transient loss of consciousness due to global cerebral hypoperfusion.
- In case the patient requires CPR or cardioversion, then it is definitely not syncope.
- Most common cause is neurocardiogenic (vasovagal) followed by cardiovascular causes

Etiology

- *Neurocardiogenic:* The increased sympathetic tone leads to increased LV contraction. This activates the mechanoreceptors in LV and leads to increased vagal tone (Hyperactive Bezold Jarisch reflex). Cough, deglutition, defecation and micturition increase vagal tone.
- *Orthostatic Hypotension*
    - Hypovolemia or diuretics
    - Autonomic neuropathy

Primary autonomic neuropathy	Secondary autonomic neuropathy
• Parkinsonism • Multiple system atrophy • Lewy body dementia • Postural orthostatic tachycardia syndrome (Dysautonomia)	• Diabetes mellitus • CKD • Amyloidosis

- *Cardiovascular*
    - Bradyarrhythmias: Sick sinus syndrome, complete heart block
    - Tachyarrhythmias: VT, SVT, Wolff Parkinson White syndrome
    - Valvular disease: Aortic stenosis, Atrial Myxoma
    - Others: Cardiac tamponade, Hypertrophic Obstructive Cardiomyopathy
- *Neurological*
    - Vertebrobasilar insufficiency
    - SAH
    - TIA/ Stroke
    - Migraine
- *Miscellaneous* like hypoglycemia, narcolepsy and psychogenic causes

Transient convulsive activity may occur with cerebral hypoxia and can mimic seizure.
Patients with vasovagal syncope DONOT have increased risk of death, MI or stroke

HYPERTENSION

Classification	Systolic mm Hg	Diastolic mm Hg
Normal	<120	and < 80
Pre hypertension	120–139	or 80–89
Stage I hypertension	140–159	or 90–99
Stage II hypertension	> 160	or > 100
Isolated systolic	≥ 140	and < 90

- 24 hr blood pressure monitoring, showing an average of > 135/85 mm Hg and asleep BP > 120/75 mm Hg approximate clinic BP value of 140/90 mm Hg
- MC congenital cardiovascular cause of hypertension is coarctation of aorta
- Heart disease is the most common cause of death in hypertensive patients

Hypertension update 2017 *(only to be answered if specified)*

Categories of BP in Adults

BP category	SBP		DBP
Normal	<120 mm Hg	and	<80 mm Hg
Elevated	120–129 mm Hg	and	<80 mm Hg
Hypertension			
Stage 1	130–139 mm Hg	or	80–89 mm Hg
Stage 2	>140 mm Hg	or	>90 mm Hg

Based on average of ≥2 careful readings obtained on >2 occasions.

Causes of Secondary Hypertension

Cause	Clinical pointers	Screening tests
Obstructive sleep apnea	• Resistant hypertension • Obesity • Fitful sleep	Epworth sleepiness score Overnight oximetry
Renovascular disease	• **Flash pulmonary edema**[Q] • Early onset in women with fibromuscular dysplasia	Renal doppler
Primary aldosteronism	Hypertension with hypokalemia	Plasma aldosterone: renin ratio
Drug abuse cocaine, ephedrine amphetamines, smoking (nicotine)	Tremors (fine), Tachycardia, Chest pain	Urinary drug screen
Renal parenchymal disease	• UTI, analgesic abuse • Family history of polycystic kidneys	Renal ultrasound

BP Goals of Pharmacological Therapy in Patients with Hypertension

Clinical conditions	BP Goal (mmHg)
Clinical CVD or 10 yr ASCVD risk > 10%	<130/80
Diabetes mellitus	<130/80
Chronic kidney disease/Post transplantation	<130/80
Heart failure/Stable ischemic heart disease	<130/80
Secondary stroke prevention	<130/80

Management of Hypertensive Crisis

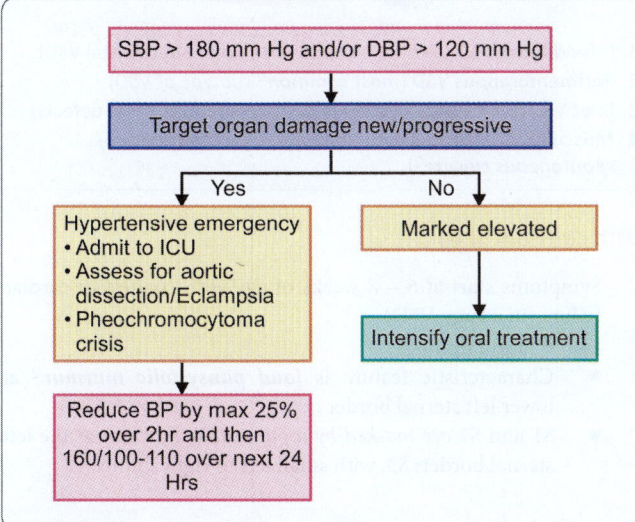

Unequal BP between Left and Right Arm

1. Takayasu's arteritis
2. Coarctation of aorta
3. Supravalvular aortic stenosis
4. Aortic dissection
5. Obstructive aortoarteritis

Coanda effect, is a tendency of jet stream to adhere to the right aortic wall causing disproportionately higher BP in right arm. This is seen in supravalvular aortic stenosis. Murmur of S.V.A.S is ejection systolic murmur.

- SBP in upper limbs > SBP in lower limb is seen in postductal coarctation of aorta
- SBP in lower limbs > SBP in upper limbs by a magnitude of >20 mmHg is seen in valvular aortic regurgitation

Hypertension with Metabolic Alkalosis (Liddle Syndrome)

- Autosomal dominant
- Gain of function of epithelial sodium channel (ENac)
- Expansion of plasma volume and gain of salt leads to HTN
- The corresponding urinary loss of potassium and H^+ leads to hypokalemic alkalosis
- To block ENac: Amiloride is the drug of choice.

Hypertension with Metabolic Acidosis (Pseudohypoaldosteronism)

- Renal tubular *unresponsiveness or resistance* to *action of aldosterone*
- Further subclassified as PHA Type 1 called as classic form and PHA Type 2/Gordon syndrome/Chloride shunt syndrome
- PHA Type 2/Gordon syndrome is an autosomal dominant disorder leading to mutation in genes encoding WNK kinases
- Sustained volume depletion, triggers hyperreninism and hyperaldosteronism leading to hypertension
- Avidity of distal nephron for chloride is increased and in turn limits the sodium and mineralocorticoid dependent voltage. This limited voltage gradient further limits driving force for potassium and hydrogen.

Preferred Parenteral Drugs for Selected Hypertensive Emergencies

Stroke	Nicardipine
Malignant hypertension	Labetalol
Myocardial infarction	Nitroglycerin
Acute LVF	Nitroglycerin
Aortic dissection	Nitroprusside, esmolol
Adrenergic crisis	Phentolamine
Hypertensive encephalopathy	Nitroprusside

Management of Hypertension

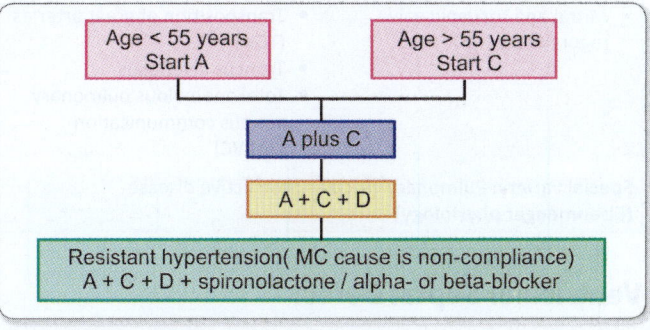

*Where A- ACE/ARB Inhibitor; C-Calcium channel blocker; D-Diuretic

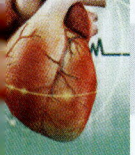

CONGENITAL HEART DEFECTS (CHD)

- Prevalence is 6 – 8 / 1000 live births
- Inheritance is multifactorial^Q

NADAS' Criteria for Diagnosis of Congenital Heart Disease

Major	Minor
Systolic murmur grade 3 or more with thrill	Systolic murmur less than 3
Diastolic murmur	Abnormal S2
Cyanosis	Abnormal ECG
Congestive heart failure	Abnormal X-ray
	Abnormal BP

Presence of 1 major or 2 minor criteria are essential for indicating the presence of heart disease.

Prenatal Risk Factors for CHD

- Intrauterine infections: (especially Rubella^Q associated with PDA, pulmonary stenosis and VSD)
- Gestational diabetes^Q (associated with VSD, PDA and cardiomyopathy)
- Maternal lupus (complete heart block)
- Teratogenic drugs^Q in first trimester like anticonvulsants, thalidomide and retinoic acid
- Phenylketonuria^Q (associated with VSD, TOF, PDA)

Classification of CHD

Acyanotic heart defects	Cyanotic heart defects
Left to right shunt: • ASD • VSD • PDA • AVSD (or Endocardial cushion defects) **Obstructive lesions:** • Aortic stenosis • Coarctation of aorta • Mitral and tricuspid valve regurgitation	**Decreased pulmonary blood flow:** • Pulmonary atresia/ critical pulmonary stenosis • Tetralogy of Fallot (TOF) • Ebstein's anomaly • Tricuspid atresia **Increased pulmonary blood flow:** • Transposition of great arteries (TGA) • Truncus arteriosus • Total anomalous pulmonary venous communication (TAPVC)

Special variety: Pulmonary vascular obstructive disease (Eisenmenger physiology)

Ventricular Septal Defect

- Most common form of CHD^Q

Types

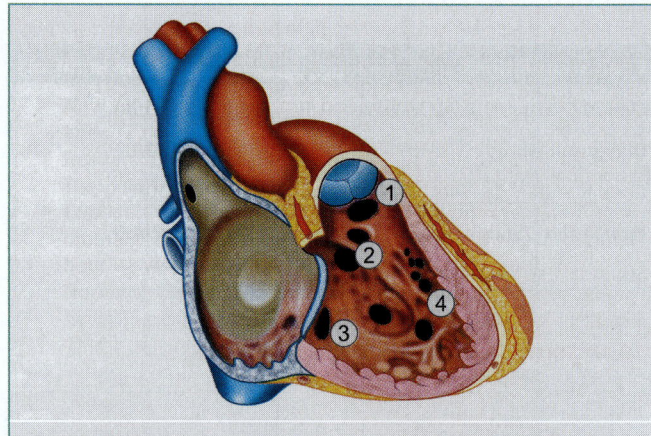

1. **Infundibular VSD** (also called as subarterial or supracristal VSD)
2. **Perimembranous VSD** (*most common^Q subtype of VSD*)
3. **Inlet** VSD (typically associated with endocardial cushion defects)
4. **Muscular** VSD (second common type; *has high chance of spontaneous closure^Q*)

Clinical Features

- Symptoms start at 6 – 8 weeks of age with congestive cardiac failure (in a large VSD)
- Examination findings:
  - Characteristic feature is **loud pansystolic murmur^Q** at lower left sternal border
  - S1 and S2 *are masked by a pansystolic murmur* at the left sternal border; S3: with small left to right shunts

X-ray Chest

- Cardiomegaly (depending on the magnitude of shunt)
- Small VSD have a normal sized heart shadow

ECG Findings

- Left axis deviation indicating left atrial and ventricular hypertrophy.

Complications

- *Congestive cardiac failure^Q*
- *Recurrent chest infections^Q*
- *Infective endocarditis^Q* (VSD is the *commonest congenital lesion complicated by infective endocarditis*)
- *Eisenmenger syndrome^Q* (development of pulmonary arterial hypertension and reversal of shunt – *explained below*)

Management

- *Assess the possibility of spontaneous closure (explained later)*
- Treatment of anemia and other complications
- **Surgical treatment:**
  - *Patch closure (treatment of choice)* or *catheter closure* (in children > 8 years of age with muscular VSD)

- Indications:
  - Early onset of CCF^Q (in infancy)
  - $Qp: Qs > 2:1^Q$ (i.e., pulmonary flow more than twice the systemic flow, indicating a large shunt)
  - Presence of *associated lesions like pulmonary stenosis*

Atrial Septal Defect

- Most common CHD *encountered in adults*^{Q}

Anatomical Types

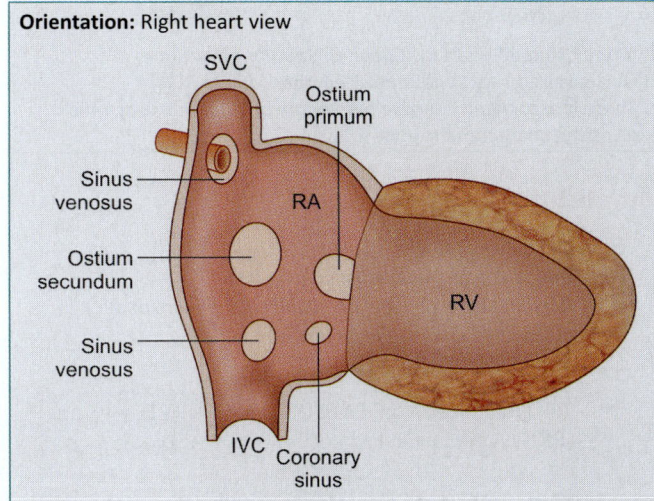

1. **Ostium secundum** (fossa ovalis) defect – **Most common**^{Q} type; (located in the central portion of atrial septum)
2. **Ostium primum** ASD (lower part of the atrial septum – *associated with endocardial cushion defects*^{Q})
3. **Sinus venosus** ASD (at the junction of superior vena cava and right atrium)
4. **Coronary sinus** ASD

- A **widely split and fixed S2**^{Q} is the characteristic auscultatory finding
- Unlike VSD, there is **no shunt murmur**^{Q} across the defect (*since there is no much pressure difference between left atrium and right atrium*)
- ECG usually shows right axis deviation – characteristic **rsR' pattern** is seen in >90% of patients (*Exception: ostium primum ASD is associated with left axis deviation*)
- Right atrium and right ventricle are enlarged
- Complications similar to VSD can occur but they are very rare and usually occur in adulthood
- ASD closure is recommended to prevent complications of atrial arrhythmias and heart failure in late adulthood.
- *Transcatheter closure using occluder device*^{Q} is usually recommended

Patent Ductus Arteriosus (PDA)

- Refers to unusual persistence of ductus arteriosus (which is a communication between the pulmonary artery and the aorta)
- **Female**^{Q} **predominance** (2:1); associated with **congenital rubella**^{Q} infection
- A significant PDA presents with CCF at 6 – 8 weeks of age

- Characteristic auscultatory findings are:
  - **Continuous "machinery" murmur**^{Q} – heard best in 2nd left intercostal space close to sternal border and below left clavicle (*reason for continuous murmur is due to flow across the ductus during both systole and diastole*)
  - *Large volume pulse and wide pulse pressure*^{Q}
  - S1: Accentuated
  - S2: Paradoxical splitting of S2 in large PDA
  - S3: Large shunt
- Complications are similar to VSD

Treatment

- **Preterm babies:** *Prostaglandin inhibitors*^{Q} like *Indomethacin or ibuprofen* is useful (*started before the age of 2 weeks*)
- **Term babies:** Surgical **ligation**^{Q} or catheter-based coil closure

Causes of continuous murmur in childhood
- Patent ductus arteriosus (PDA)^Q – Heard in 2nd left Intercostal space
- Rupture of sinus of Valsalva - RSOV^Q.
- Aortopulmonary window (AP Window)^Q.
- Anomalous origin of left coronary artery from pulmonary artery (ALCAPA).
- Surgical shunts - Blalock – Taussig shunt^Q in TOF.
- Bronchopulmonary collaterals seen in TOF (Tetralogy of Fallot) tricuspid atresia, truncus arteriosus.
- Peripheral pulmonary artery stenosis.
- Pulmonary and coronary AV fistula.
- Intercostal AV fistula.
- Collaterals in coarctation of aorta^Q. – heard over thoracic spine in the back
- Venous hum^Q and mammary souffle^Q

Assessing the Probability of Spontaneous Closure of Heart Defects

Variable	Likelihood of spontaneous closure
Age	- **PDA** in a term baby is **unlikely** to close; PDA in preterm has high chance of spontaneous closure - **ASD or VSD** persisting **beyond age of 3 years** is **unlikely** to close
Location	**VSD:** - **Muscular** VSD has high likelihood of **spontaneous closure**; - Inlet VSD and malaligned VSD (as in Tetralogy of Fallot) never close spontaneously **ASD:** - **Ostium secundum** ASD has high likelihood of **spontaneous closure**
Size	- **ASD > 8 mm** in size and large unrestrictive VSDs are **unlikely** to close spontaneously

Eisenmenger Syndrome

Physiology	Clinical features
Left to right shunt ↓ Increased pulmonary blood flow ↓ Vascular remodelling and endothelial dysfunction ↓ Increase in pulmonary vascular resistance and RVH ↓ (Inversion) Right to left shunt ↓ Cyanosis	• Paradoxical improvement in congestive symptoms followed by appearance of *cyanosis*^{Q} • *Clubbing*^{Q} • Parasternal heave^Q, **palpable S2**^{Q} **Chest X ray:** • Normal heart size • Plethora of hilar regions with oligemia in peripheral lung fields **Treatment** • **Heart – lung transplantation**^{Q} • Primary surgical correction of VSD/ASD/PDA is contraindicated^Q

Tetralogy of Fallot (TOF)

- *Cyanotic heart disease capable of survival (without surgery) beyond infancy is TOF*^{Q}
- Classic **tetrad**^{Q}:
  1. VSD^Q
  2. Over-riding aorta^Q
  3. Subpulmonic infundibular stenosis^Q (Most important determinant of cyanosis)
  4. Right ventricular hypertrophy^Q (concentric type).
- Usually symptom is slowly progressive cyanosis after birth
- *The severity of cyanosis is directly proportional to the severity of pulmonic stenosis, but the intensity of the systolic murmur is inversely related to the severity of pulmonic stenosis*^{Q}.

$$\text{pulmonary stenosis (severity)} \propto \frac{\text{cyanosis}}{\text{intensity of the systolic murmur}}$$

- **CCF is never seen**^{Q} [except if anemia/infective endocarditis/hypertension/aortic regurgitation or pulmonary regurgitation supervenes]
- **Examination findings:**
  - Loud, single S2^Q (**Reason**: It is the A2 since the pulmonic component is delayed and so soft that it is inaudible)
  - **No shunt (VSD) murmur** is heard^Q [**Reason**: i) VSD is large and allows free flow of blood; ii) As the systolic pressures between the two ventricles are identical there is little or no left to right shunt and the VSD is silent.]

- Chest X ray:

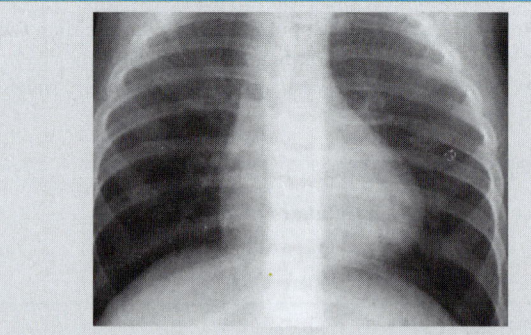

- '**Boot**^{Q}' shaped heart or '*Coeur en Sabot*' appearance
- Normal sized heart with **upturned apex** (due to RVH)
- There is associated *concave pulmonary arterial segment* which gives the characteristic boot shape

Complications

- Infective endocarditis^Q
- **Neurological complications:**
  - Cerebral thrombosis^Q (in children < 2 years of age)
  - Brain abscess^Q (> 2 years of age)
- Cyanotic spells^Q

  - TETRALOGY ^{Q} OF FALLOT – ASD + RVH + PS
  - PENTALOGY OF FALLOT – TOF + ASD

Cyanotic Spells (also called as "Tet" spells, Anoxic, Hypoxic or Hypercyanotic Spells)

- Age group: **2 months – 2 years**^{Q}
- *Precipitating factors*: vigorous crying^Q, exertion^Q
- Decrease in systemic vascular resistance (SVR) and spasm of infundibulum are two important events which occur during initiation of spell

Mechanism of Cyanotic Spell

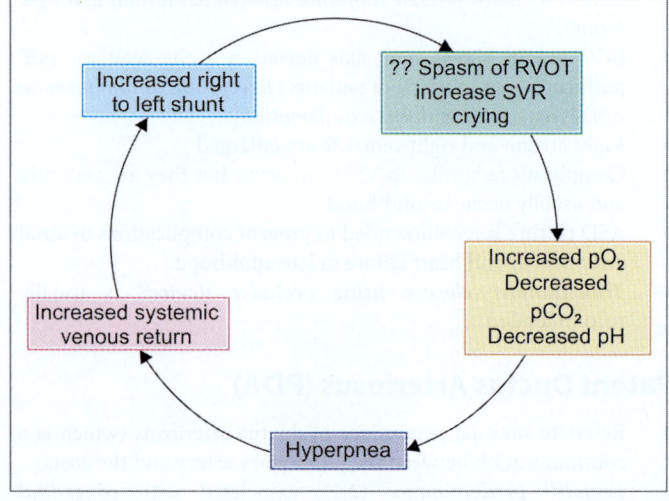

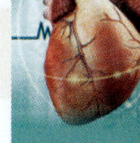

- During a spell, *increasing cyanosis*[Q], and *decreased intensity of the heart murmur*[Q] are observed
- If cyanotic spell is not treated promptly, *limpness, convulsion, cerebrovascular accident, or even death* may occur

Treatment of Cyanotic Spell

- *Knee-chest*[Q] *position*
- *Morphine*[Q] (*suppresses the respiratory center and abolishes hyperpnea*)
- *Sodium bicarbonate*[Q] (*to correct acidosis*)

- O₂ inhalation[Q]
- Beta blockers[Q] (to treat infundibular spasm)
- Alpha agonists[Q] (to increase systemic vascular resistance)

Prevention

- Correction of associated anemia
- *Palliative surgical (shunt) procedures*[Q] (Aim is to increase pulmonary blood flow in infants with uncontrollable hypoxic spells on whom the corrective surgery cannot safely be performed)

Shunt Procedures Performed in TOF

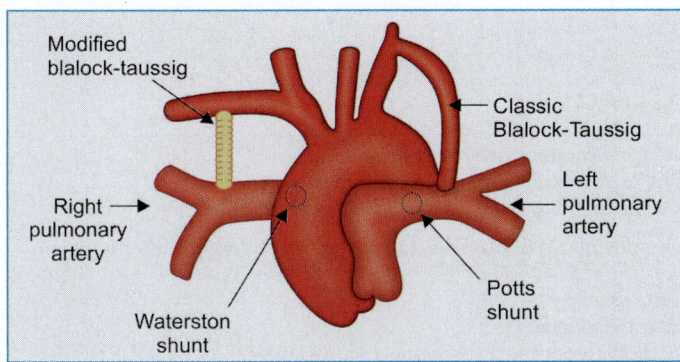

1. *Blalock-Taussig (B-T) shunt* – anastomosis between the subclavian artery and the ipsilateral PA (Pulmonary artery)
2. *Gore-Tex* interposition shunt (*modifed B-T shunt*) – between the subclavian artery and the ipsilateral PA
3. *Waterston* shunt – anastomosis between the ascending aorta and the right PA
4. *Potts* shunt – anastomosis between the descending aorta and the left PA

Transposition of Great Arteries (TGA)

Following are the types of TGA.

- **Complete Type:** The aorta arises from right ventricle and pulmonary artery from the left ventricle
- **Physiologically Corrected Type**[Q]: Here, the right atrium is corrected to morphologically inverted left ventricle, which is connected to the pulmonary artery while the left atrium is connected to the morphologically inverted right ventricle, which is connected to the aorta. *Since the route of blood flow is normal, it is called as TGA.*

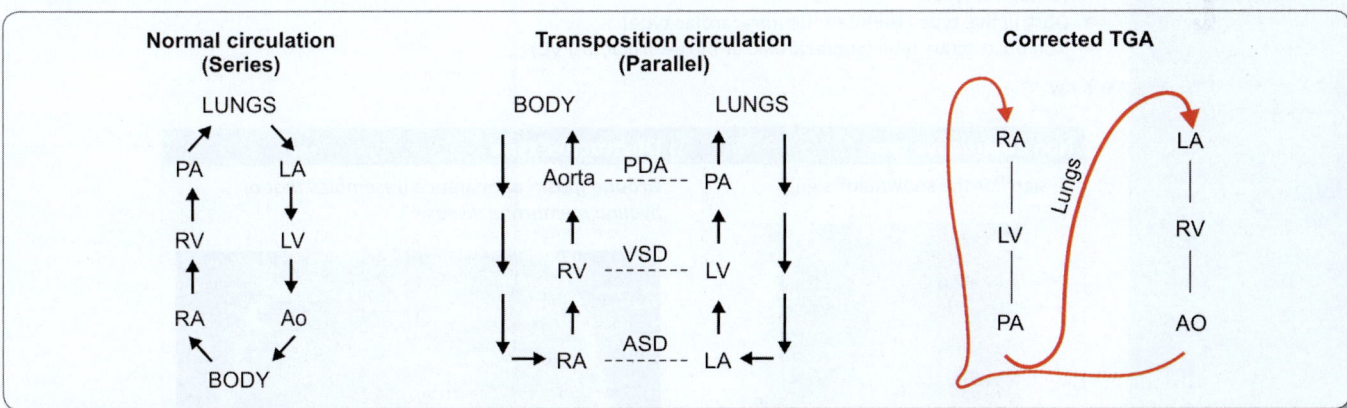

- *Complete* type is also called as *D – TGA*[Q] since aorta lies anterior and to the right of the pulmonary artery
- Survival depends on the presence of communication like VSD, ASD or PDA (*since the systemic and pulmonary circulations are separate*)

Clinical Features

- TGA with *intact ventricular septum*: *cyanosis at birth*[Q] *and CCF in first week*[Q] of life
- TGA *with VSD*: mild *cyanosis and CCF*[Q] at 6 – 8 weeks after birth; *single S2 is a characteristic*[Q] auscultatory finding
- **Chest X ray:** " **Egg on side (or) Egg on string** appearance" (*cardiomegaly with a narrow base and plethoric lung fields as depicted in the picture below*)

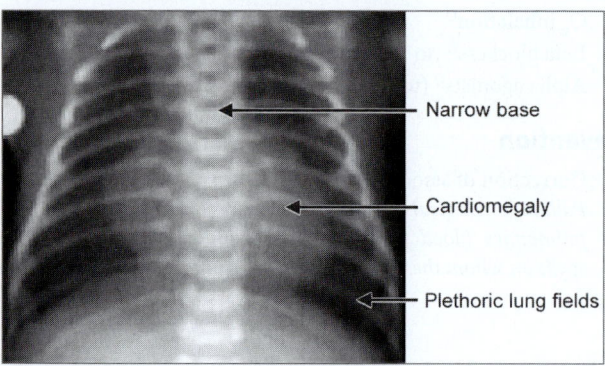

"EGG on side" appearance

Treatment

- **Arterial switch** operation – treatment of choice[Q]
- Temporary measures: Alprostadil (PGE1 – Keeps ductus open) and Balloon atrial septostomy

Salient Points About Other Cyanotic Congenital Heart Defects

Tricuspid atresia	• Congenital absence of the tricuspid valve resulting in **hypoplastic right ventricle** • Clinical features are *almost identical to TOF*[Q] (due to decreased outflow from right ventricle) • Presence of **left axis deviation in ECG**[Q] and **left ventricular hypertrophy**[Q] are characteristic distinguishing features
Ebstein's anomaly	• Characteristic abnormality of the tricuspid valve – downward displacement of **posterior and septal leaflet** causing **atrialization**[Q] *of a part of right ventricle* • Associated with maternal **lithium**[Q] intake during pregnancy • Clinically present with cyanosis, effort intolerance and fatigue • Characteristic auscultatory finding: **Mid systolic click**[Q] (produced by abnormal tricuspid valve) • X ray: **Box**[Q] **shaped heart**
TAPVC (Total anomalous partial venous connection)	• Anomaly of pulmonary veins wherein they don't drain into left atrium • Anatomical types (according to site of drainage of pulmonary veins):

Supracardiac	Drain into SVC or left innominate vein
Intra – cardiac	Enter into coronary sinus or right atrium
Infracardiac	Drain into IVC or portal vein

- Physiological types
  - Obstructive type (TAPVC of the infracardiac type)
  - Non obstructive type (Supracardiac or intra-cardiac TAPVC)
- X ray

Non obstructive type	Obstructive type
'8' sign[Q] or the snowman[Q] sign	**Ground glass**[Q] appearance (*resembles that of hyaline membrane disease*[Q])

Contd...

| Truncus arteriosus | • Presence of **single arterial trunk**^Q from which aorta, pulmonary arteries and coronary artery arises 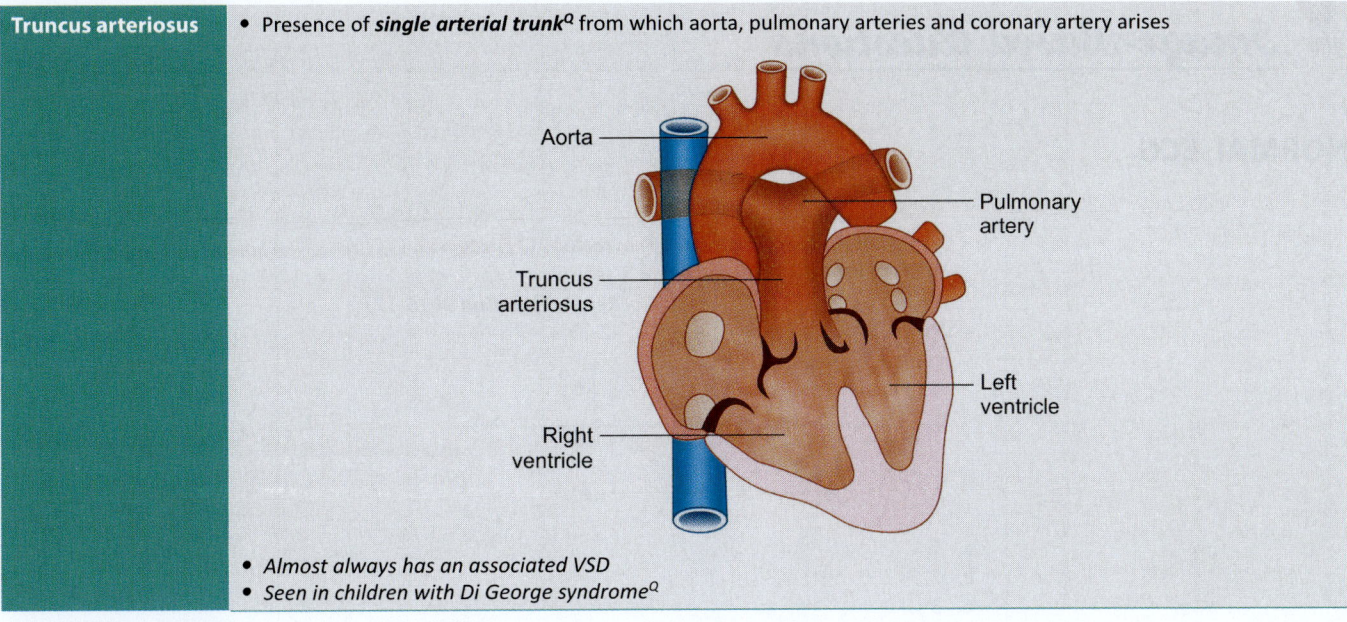 • Almost always has an associated VSD • Seen in children with Di George syndrome^Q |

Coarctation of Aorta

- Located at junction of arch with descending aorta. Otherwise it may be distal or proximal to the ductus or ligamentum arteriosum or left subclavian artery.
- Medial wall of aorta is spared in narrowing.
- **Preductal coarctation:** No collaterals formed in fetal life as there is **no obstruction to blood** flowing from ductus arteriosus into aorta before birth.
- **Postductal coarctation:** Collaterals seen as **obstruction to blood** flowing from ductus arteriosus into aorta before birth.

Clinical Features

Postductal coarctation presents with LVF in few weeks after birth.
- Pain, claudication in lower limbs
- Radio-femoral delay
- BP more in the upper limbs than in lower limbs
- Differential cyanosis
- S1 normal
- S2 normal split with loud A2
- Ejection systolic murmur with maximum intensity over the back
- Collaterals, pulsatile vessels seen in the back and inferior surfaces of ribs.

Investigations

- **Barium swallow:** E sign.
- Inferior rib notching

Complications

LVF/rupture berry aneurysm, aortic dissection.

Management

- Operate/balloon angioplasty after age of 1 yr
- Recurs and treated by balloon angioplasty.
- HTN can persist even after treatment.

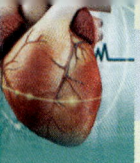

Image-Based Questions

NORMAL ECG

1. For calculation of rate related (corrected) QT interval, QT interval is divided by $\sqrt{X}$; where X is?
   (Recent Question 2016-17)

   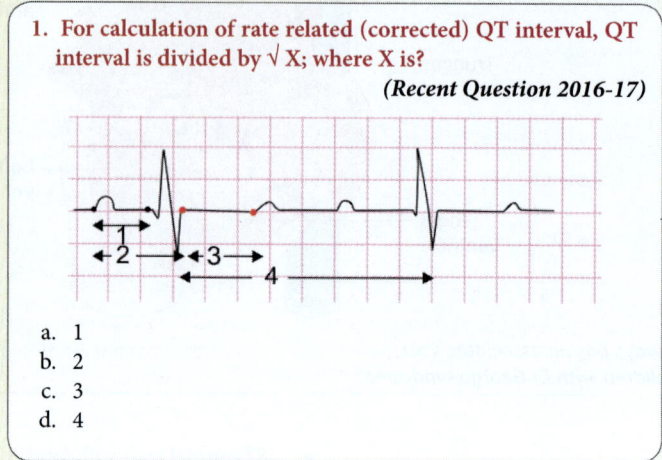

   a. 1
   b. 2
   c. 3
   d. 4

2. The marked part of the ECG called as 'X' points to which phase of cardiac action potential? *(Recent Question 2016-17)*

   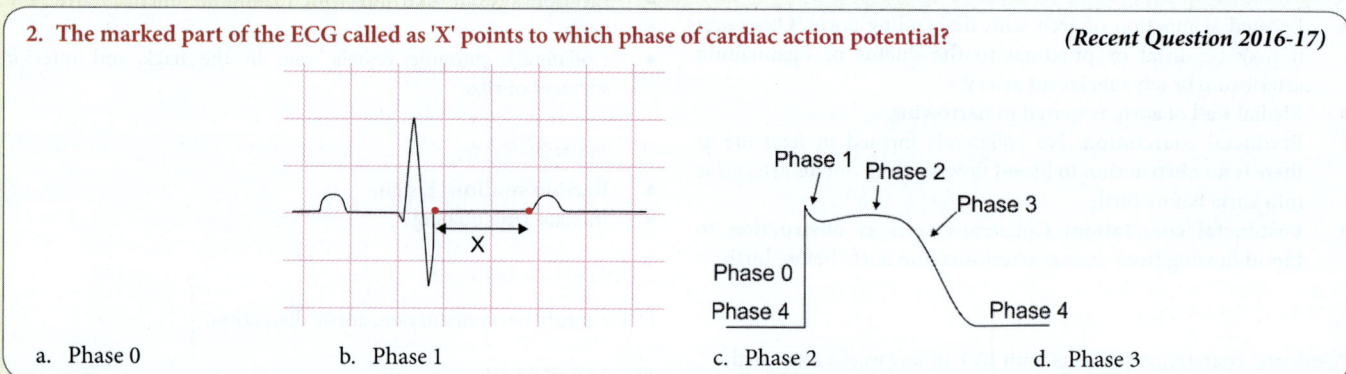

   a. Phase 0   b. Phase 1   c. Phase 2   d. Phase 3

TACHYARRHYTHMIAS

3. A 35 year old lady has been diagnosed as having anxiety neurosis by her psychiatrist. She came to you for second opinion. Comment on the diagnosis based on ECG?
   (Recent Question 2016-17)

   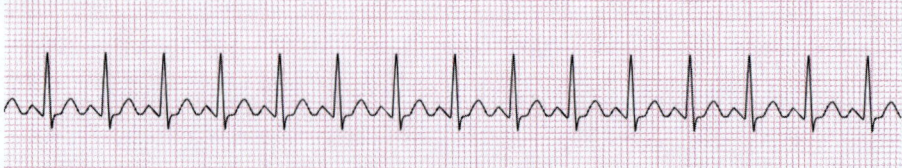

   a. Sinus tachycardia   b. WPW syndrome   c. Multifocal atrial tachycardia   d. Atrial fibrillation

4. Comment on the ECG findings *(Recent Question 2016-17)*

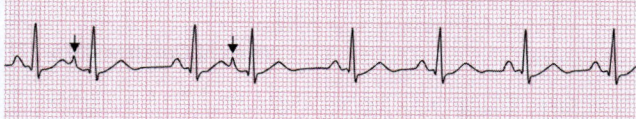

a. Atrial fibrillation
b. Atrial premature complexes
c. PSVT
d. WPW

5. A 25 year old woman presents with complaints of recurrent episodes of sudden onset palpitations. What does her ECG tracings shows? *(Recent Question 2016-17)*

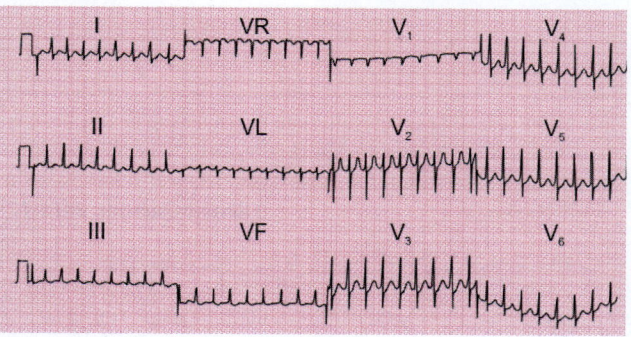

a. Atrial flutter
b. Atrial bigeminy
c. PSVT
d. Sinus tachycardia

6. A 52 year old male diabetic patient presents with palpitations to the AIIMS emergency. Urgent ECG was performed. What is the immediate next step in the management? *(AIIMS MAY 2016)*

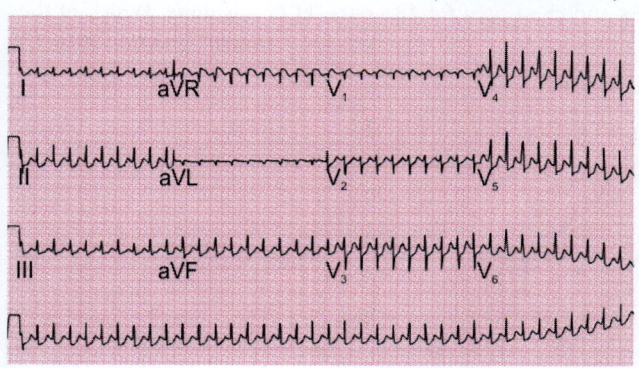

a. Electrical cardioversion
b. Amiodarone
c. Adenosine
d. Primary PCI

7. A 15 year old child of Valvular heart disease on heart failure treatment, has the following ECG tracing. What is the diagnosis? *(Recent Question 2016-17)*

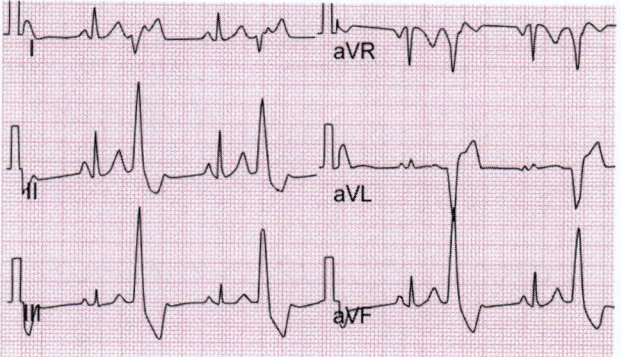

a. Tall tented T wave
b. Ventricular bigeminy
c. Non paroxysmal atrial tachycardia with irregular AV block
d. Non paroxysmal atrial tachycardia with regular AV block

8. A 1-year old child with CHD is on heart failure treatment. The ECG shows all except? *(Recent Question 2016-17)*

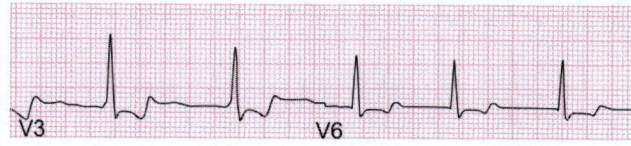

a. Ventricular bigeminy
b. Heart Rate of 60 bpm approximately
c. ST depression
d. U wave

9. What does the following ECG show? *(Recent Question 2016-17)*

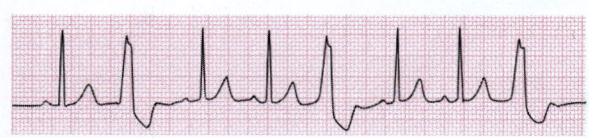

a. Ventricular bigeminy
b. Ventricular trigeminy
c. Atrial premature contraction
d. Atrial bigeminy

ISCHEMIC HEART DISEASE

10. A 75-year old male patient presents to the AIIMS emergency with retrosternal chest pain for 6 hours. The following ECG was done. What will be the primary management of the patient? *(AIIMS May 2016)*

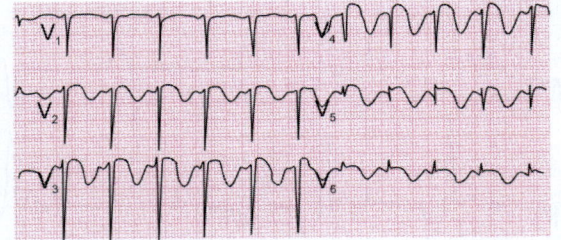

a. Primary PCI
b. Thrombolysis
c. Abciximab
d. Low molecular weight heparin

12. What ECG finding is shown here? *(Recent Question 2016-17)*

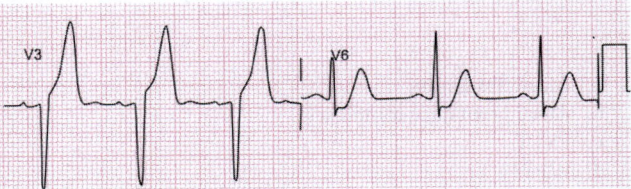

a. Hyperacute T wave
b. T wave Alternans
c. T wave inversion
d. Artefact

11. Which of the following finding is shown in the chest leads? *(Recent Question 2016-17)*

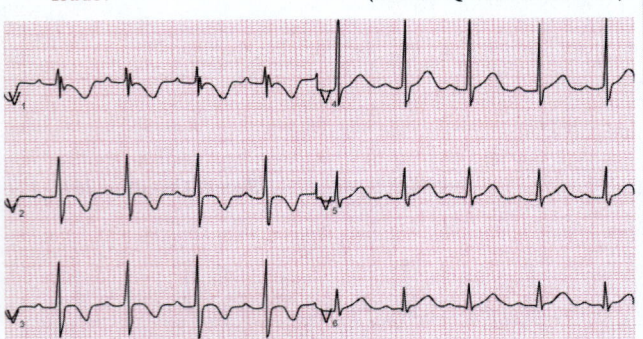

a. Myocardial ischemia
b. Myocardial injury
c. Digoxin
d. Digoxin toxicity

13. A 50-year old man develops an excruciating headache. On examination he has nuchal rigidity. NCCT performed after 4 hours shows blood in the Sylvian fissure. What does the ECG shows? *(Recent Question 2016-17)*

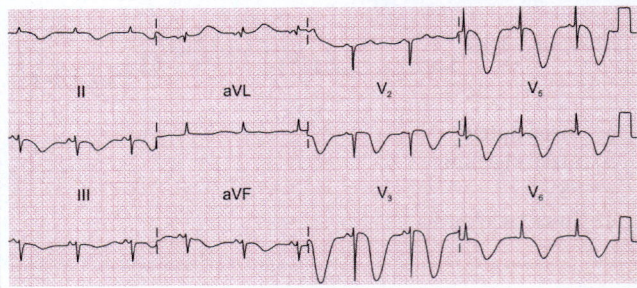

a. T wave inversion
b. Artifact
c. Premature ventricular complexes
d. Positive U waves

14. A 65 year old man is brought with complaints of breathlessness and chest pain for 18 hours. ECG was done. Which of the following is incorrect? *(Recent Question 2016-17)*

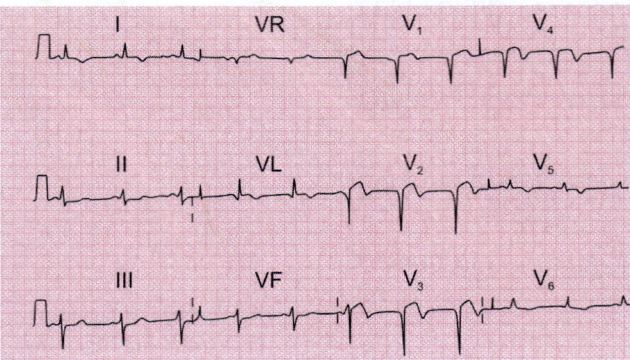

a. Normal sinus rhythm
c. ST elevation in V2-V4
b. Normal axis
d. Premature ventricular contractions

BRADYARRHYTHMIAS

15. Comment on the diagnosis from the ECG shown below?

(AIIMS Nov 2016)

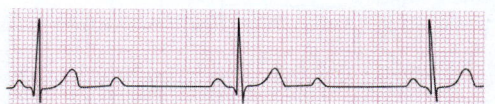

a. 2:1 heart block
b. Trifascicular block
c. First degree heart block
d. Atrial fibrillation

17. A 65 year old patient of STEMI underwent thrombolysis with STK. The ECG tracing performed after thrombolysis is shown below. What does it exhibits?

(Recent Question 2016-17)

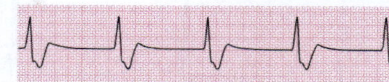

a. Ventricular bigeminy
b. Accelerated idioventricular rhythm
c. Ventricular tachycardia
d. Wenckebach phenomenon

16. Comment on the diagnosis. *(Recent Question 2016-17)*

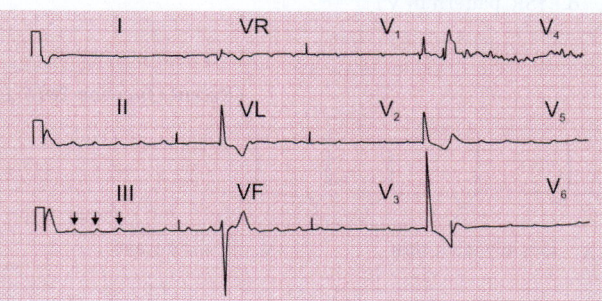

a. Left bundle branch block
b. Right bundle branch block
c. Complete heart block
d. Accelerated idioventricular rhythm

18. A 60-year old patient is having recurrent syncopal attacks post myocardial infarction. The ECG shows?

(Recent Question 2016-17)

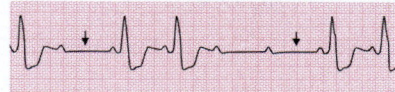

a. Accelerated idioventricular rhythm
b. Ventricular bigeminy
c. Mobitz II heart block
d. Wenckebach phenomenon

EFFECTS OF DRUGS ON ECG

19. A 35-year old female patient on amitriptyline is brought in the casualty with suspected intentional over-dosage. On admission BP was 80/60 mm Hg and GCS was 5/15. She was intubated and ECG was performed. Which of the following is the correct ECG interpretation and management?

(Recent Question 2016-17)

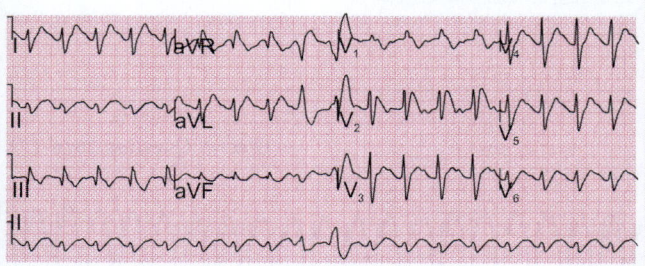

a. Broad complex qRS: Sodabicarbonate
b. Broad complex qRS : Amiodarone
c. Himalayan P waves: Ammonium chloride
d. Himalayan P waves: Procainamide

20. A 50 year old woman with rheumatic heart disease is on medication for heart disease. She feels unwell for most part of the day. Which of the following medicine should be prescribed for the condition shown below?

(Recent Question 2016-17)

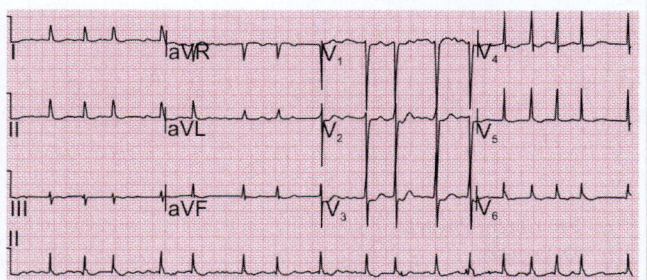

a. ACE inhibitor
b. Diuretics
c. Ivabradine
d. Digoxin

21. A 25-year old soldier is trapped in an avalanche in Siachen glacier. He is airlifted to the base hospital. On admission the pulse is thready and BP is unrecordable. ECG strip is shown below. All findings are seen *except*?
    (Recent Question 2016-17)

    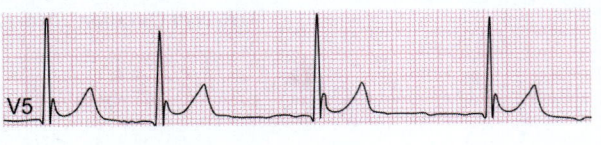

    a. Bradycardia
    b. Osborn wave
    c. ST segment elevation
    d. Atrial bigeminy

22. A 30-year old lady with scleroderma presents with progressive dyspnea on exertion. What does the ECG shows?
    (Recent Question 2016-17)

    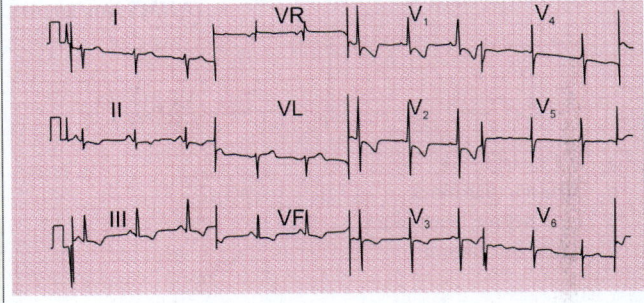

    a. Peaked P waves
    b. Right axis deviation
    c. T wave inversion in V1-V3
    d. rSR' pattern in V1

23. What does the following ECG shows? *(Recent Question 2016-17)*

    a. Osborn wave
    b. Delta wave
    c. Hockey stick sign
    d. Epsilon wave

MISCELLANEOUS

24. A 20 year old student collapsed while running after a bus to college. Which of the following waves is shown in the ECG?
    (Recent Question 2016-17)

    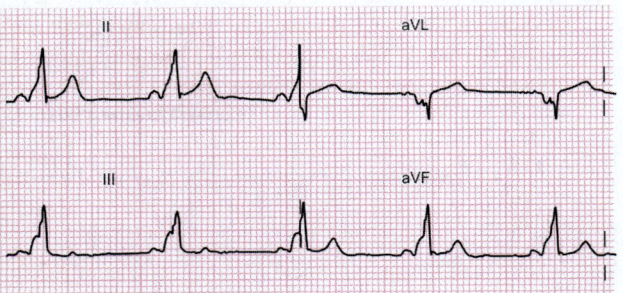

    a. Prominent P waves
    b. Delta wave
    c. Epsilon wave
    d. Prominent T waves

25. The below ECG shows *(Recent Question 2016-17)*

    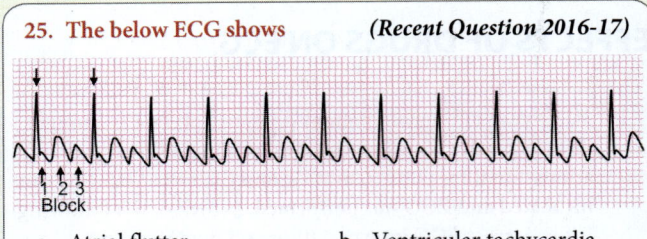

    a. Atrial flutter
    b. Ventricular tachycardia
    c. Atrial fibrillation
    d. PSVT

26. Which of the following abnormalities is shown in the ECG given below?
    (Recent Question 2016-17)

    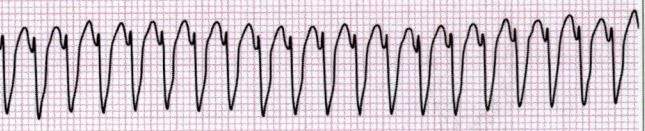

    a. Ventricular fibrillation
    b. Ventricular tachycardia
    c. Ventricular bigeminy
    d. Artifacts

27. A lady with no past history related to heart disease presents with history of palpitations off and on. She is feeling unwell since morning and says that after an episode of vomiting, the palpitations had subsided. ECG shows:
   (Recent Question 2016-17)

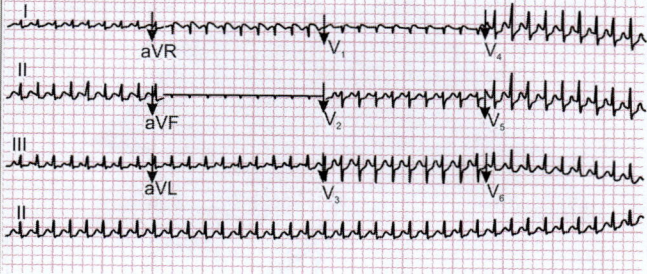

   a. PSVT
   b. VT
   c. V. fibrillation
   d. A. fibrillation

30. A 60-year old smoker lady developed severe chest pain since 6 am in the morning. On admission at 7 am, the cardiac enzymes were normal and ECG was as shown. Which coronary artery of the patient is involved?
   (Recent Question 2016-17)

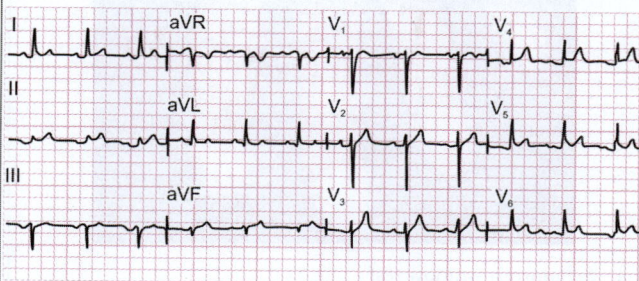

   a. Left anterior descending
   b. Left circumflex artery
   c. Right coronary artery
   d. Posterior descending artery

28. Which of the following is seen in the ECG shown below?
   (Recent Question 2016-17)

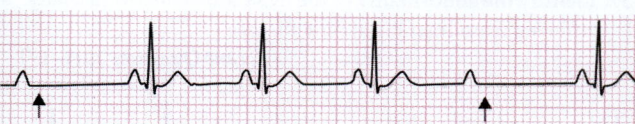

   a. 1st degree heart block
   b. Mobitz 1 heart block
   c. Mobitz II heart block
   d. 3rd degree heart block

31. A patient with MI has dyspnea grade 4. The pulse rate is 120 bpm and BP is 220/120 mm Hg. The CXR of patient is shown below. All are indicated for this patient except?

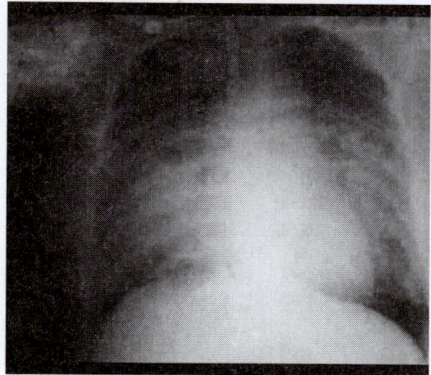

   a. Thrombolysis
   b. Morphine
   c. Aspirin
   d. Furosemide

29. Comment on the diagnosis in the ECG?
   (Recent Question 2016-17)

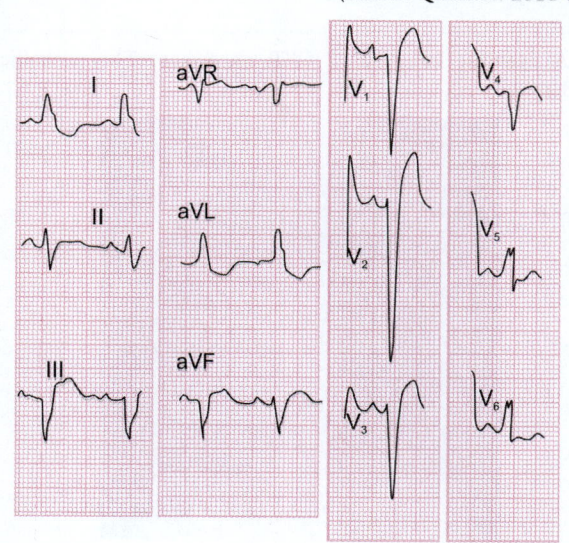

   a. RBBB
   b. LBBB
   c. Trifascicular block
   d. Mobitz II heart block

32. The CXR below shows:

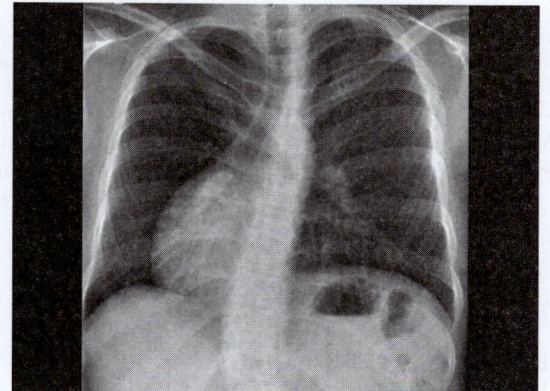

   a. Dextrocardia
   b. Pneumothorax
   c. Pneumomediastinum
   d. Pulmonary hamartoma

33. What is incorrect about the image shown below?

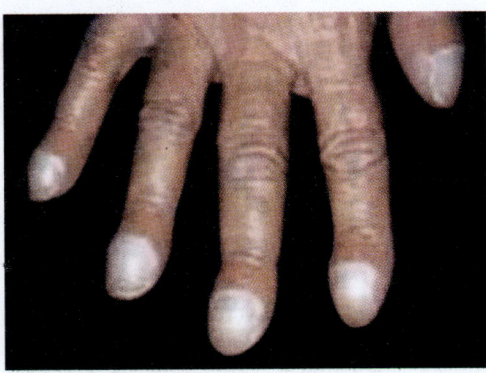

a. Schamroth window test
b. Seen with suppurative lung disease
c. Left to right shunts
d. Loss of Lovibond angle

34. The child shown below has which heart disease?

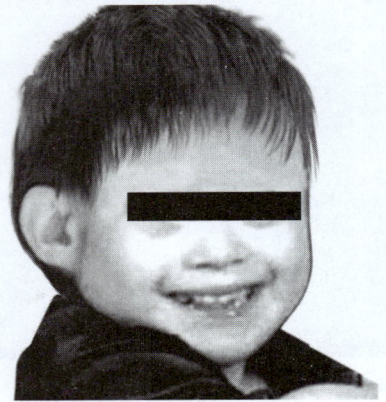

a. Endocardial cushion defect
b. Partial anomalous pulmonary venous connection
c. PDA
d. Tetralogy of Fallot

35. A martial arts exponent complains of dizziness and syncope. The ECG tracing is given below. The diagnosis is:
(Recent Question 2016-17)

a. First degree heart block
b. Mobitz 1 heart block
c. Mobitz 2 heart block
d. Third degree heart block

36. A child adopts this knee chest position many times and has dusky discoloration of tongue and extremities since birth. Which is not indicated in management of this child?

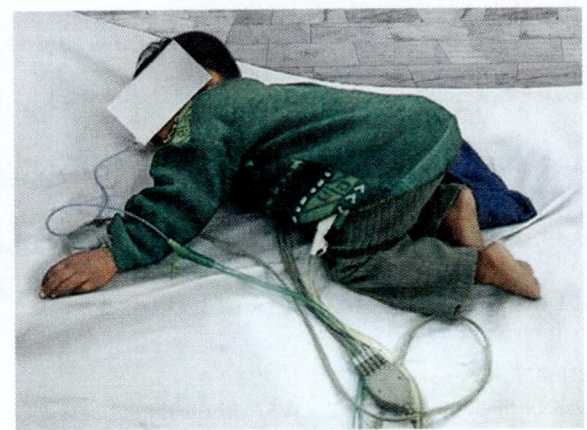

a. Morphine
b. Propranolol
c. Phenoxybenzamine
d. Phenylephrine

37. Identify the abnormality in the ECG shown below in a lady suffering from interstitial lung disease.
(Recent Question 2016-17)

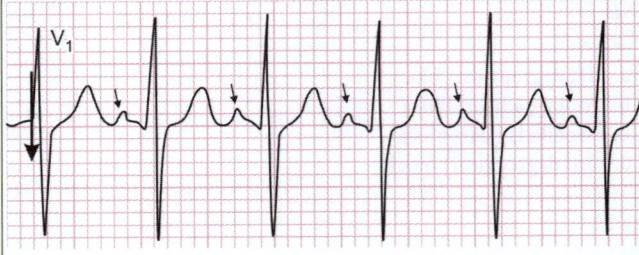

a. P pulmonale
b. P mitrale
c. PSVT
d. S1Q3T3

38. A cyanotic baby has a CXR as shown. The probable diagnosis is?

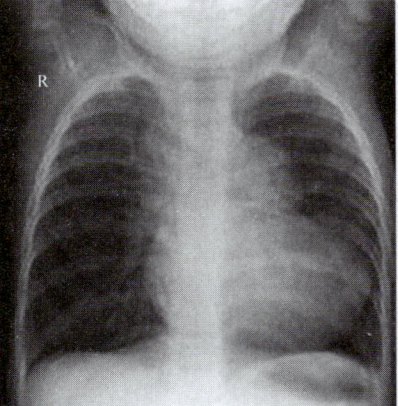

a. Boot-shaped heart
b. Snowman heart
c. Box-shaped heart
d. Normal heart

39. Which of the following conditions can be a probable diagnosis for the JVP recording mentioned below?

(Recent Question 2016-17)

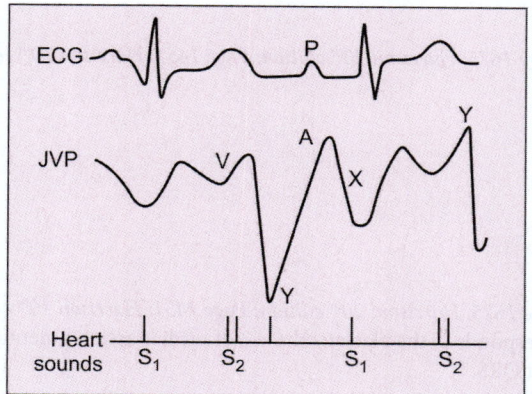

a. Constrictive pericarditis
b. Cardiac tamponade
c. Cor pulmonale
d. Cor Triatriatum

40. A hypertension patient is having severe chest pain after which he developed unilateral ptosis and hemiparesis. The CXR of patient is shown below. The clinical diagnosis is?

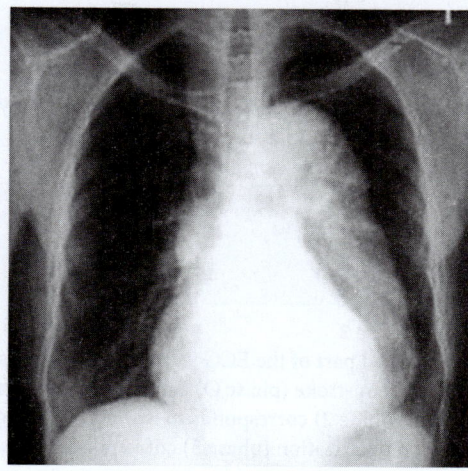

a. Aortic dissection
b. Acute myocardial infarction
c. Cardiac rupture
d. Atrial fibrillation with embolic stroke

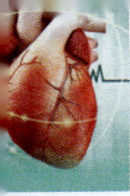

Answers of Image-Based Questions

NORMAL ECG

1. **Ans. (d) 4**   *(Ref: Page 1675: Harrison 20th edition; Page 1451: Harrison 19th edition)*
   - Corrected QT is defined as QT interval divided by √R-R interval
   - R-R interval in ECG is 4.

   Markings in the ECG given:-

   1. Is PR interval
   2. Is PJ interval
   3. Is ST segment
   4. Is RR interval

2. **Ans. (c) Phase 2**   *(Ref: page 1675: Harrison: 20th edition; Page 1451: Harrison 19th edition)*
   - The marked part of the ECG is the isoelectric ST segment which corresponds to the plateau, phase 2 of cardiac action potential
   - The rapid upstroke (phase O) action potential corresponds to onset of QRS.
   - Plateau (phase 2) corresponds to isoelectric ST segment.
   - Active repolarization (phase 3) corresponds to inscription of T wave

TACHYARRHYTHMIAS

3. **Ans. (a) Sinus Tachycardia**   *(Ref: Page 1733: Harrison 20th edition; Page 1477: Harrison 19th edition)*
   - The ECG shows normal sinus rhythm with heart rate of >100 bpm.
   - P waves are normal height and duration. PR interval is 120 msec and QRS duration is 80 msec.
   - The findings are diagnostic of sinus tachycardia
   - Sinus tachycardia is subdivided into physiological and non-physiological.
   - *Inappropriate sinus tachycardia* causes the sinus rate to increase spontaneously at rest or out of proportion to physiological stress or exertion. Affected patients are usually females. Misdiagnosis with anxiety disorder is common.

4. **Ans. (b) Atrial premature complexes**   *(Ref: page 1733: Harrison: 20th edition; Page 1477: Harrison 19th edition)*
   - The ECG shows variable RR interval. Atrial fibrillation and PSVT are both ruled out as P waves can be seen.
   - After the occurrence of Premature atrial contraction (second beat in rhythm strip) normal sinus rhythm was obtained.
   - The PAC reoccurs again after the end of T wave in the fourth beat followed by restoration of normal sinus rhythm.
   - WPW has delta wave with short PR and broad QRS complex.

5. **Ans. (c) PSVT**   *(Ref: Page 1739: Harrison 20th edition; Page 1480-81: Harrison 19th edition)*
   - The findings of the ECG are heart rate of 200 bpm. P waves are not visible.
   - The axis is normal with narrow qRS complexes.
   - This could either be junctional tachycardia or atrioventricular nodal re-entrant tachycardia.
   - Taking into consideration the age of the patient the incidence of junctional tachycardia can explain the patient experiencing multiple episodes in the past.

6. **Ans. (c) Adenosine**   *(Ref: Page 1739: Harrison: 20th edition; Page 1479: Harrison 19th edition)*
   - The ECG shows a heart rate of 200/min.
   - Axis is normal.
   - Rhythm is regular with absence of P waves.
   - Narrow complex QRS (<0.08 sec) is present. P waves buried in the preceding T wave.
   - This is seen in Paroxysmal supraventricular tachycardia.
   - The first line management is adenosine 6 mg intravenously.
   - In case the patient is having hemodynamic compromise, electrical cardioversion needs to be done.

7. **Ans. (b) Ventricular bigeminy**   *(Ref: page 214: Practical Cardiology 2nd edition)*

   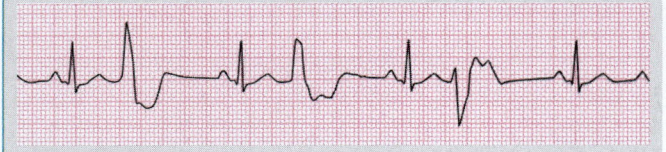

   Heart rate of the patient is 50 BPM
   The tracing shows normal sinus rhythm alternating with premature ventricular contraction. This is diagnostic of ventricular bigeminy which is the most common arrhythmia seen with digoxin toxicity.

8. **Ans. (a) Ventricular Bigeminy**   *(Ref: chapter 269e- Harrison 19th edition)*
   The ECG strip shows heart rate of approximately 60 bpm. ST segment depression (hockey stick sign) is seen followed by positive deflection of U waves

Abnormalities of U wave

Prominent U waves	Inverted U waves
• Bradycardia • Hypokalemia • Hypocalcemia • Hypomagnesemia • Hypothermia • Raised ICP • HOCM • LVH	• Myocardial Ischemia • HTN • Cardiomyopathy

9. **Ans. (b) Ventricular trigeminy** (Ref: page 214-15: Practical Cardiology: 2nd edition)

The image shows a pattern of two normal sinus rhythm beats followed by premature ventricular beats. This is seen in ventricular trigeminy.

ISCHEMIC HEART DISEASE

10. **Ans. (a) Primary PCI** (Ref: Figure 295-4, page 1604: Harrison: 19th edition)
    - The ECG shows heart rate of about 120/min.
    - T wave inversion is present from V2- V6
    - ST segment elevation > 2 mm is noted from V4-V6 exhibiting the traditional Pardee sign
    - *STEMI is best managed with primary PCI with first medical contact to device time to be kept <90 minutes*
    - If the patient is seen in non PCI capable hospital DIDO time should be less than 30 minutes for thrombolysis.

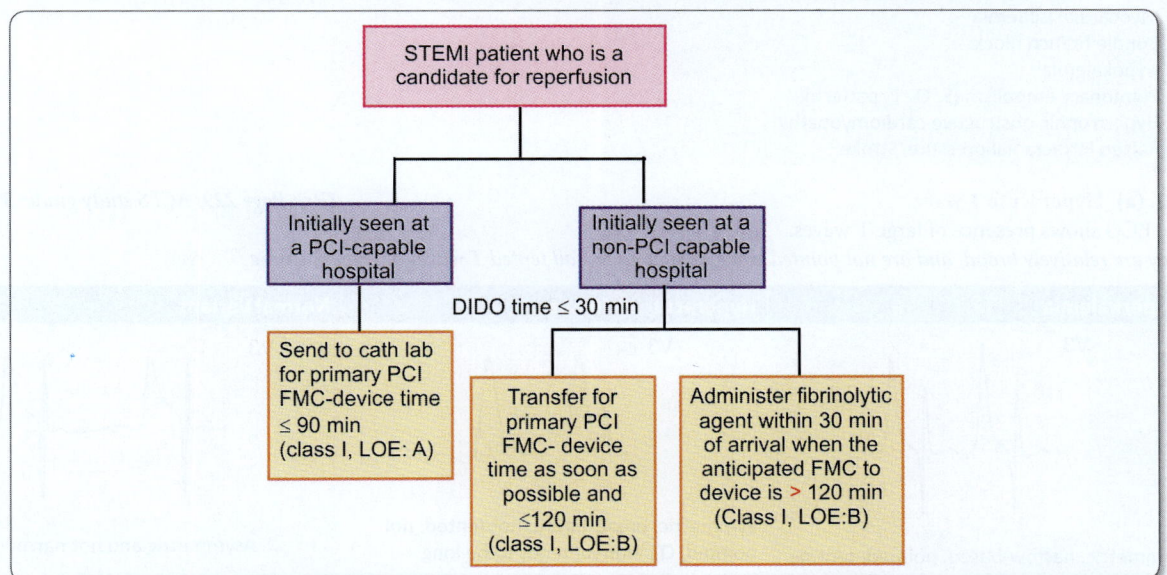

- The patient can be transferred from non PCI capable hospital to PCI capable hospital in case the First medical contact to device time is less than 120 minutes.
- In the question there is no mention of any PCI/ non PCI capable hospital.
- Due to paucity of transport facilities in India, the concept of transfer from non PCI to PCI capable centre with performance of PCI within 120 minutes looks impossible.

11. **Ans. (a) Myocardial Ischemia** (Ref: Page 1681: Harrison 20th edition; Page 1455-56: Harrison 19th edition)
    - The T wave is upright in all leads except aVR and V_1. In the strip provided, notice the predominant T wave inversion in V1-V4. This is seen in myocardial ischemia.

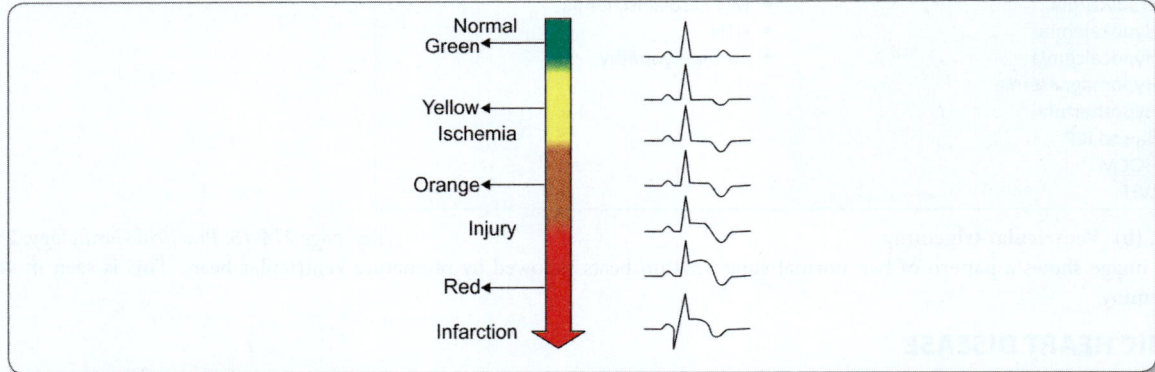

- Diagnosis of myocardial injury needs elevated cardiac biomarkers.
- Digoxin leads to ST segment depression
- Digoxin toxicity leads to Ventricular Bigeminy.

Causes of T Wave Inversion

- Normal in children
- Myocardial ischemia
- Bundle branch block
- Hypokalemia[Q]
- Pulmonary embolism ($S_1 Q_3 T_3$ pattern)
- Hypertrophic obstructive cardiomyopathy
- Raised intracranial pressure/Stroke[Q]

12. **Ans. (a) Hyperacute T wave** (Ref: Page 229; ACLS study guide: 5th edition)
    The ECG shows presence of large T waves.
    They are relatively broad, and are not pointed when compared to Tall tented T waves of Hyperkalemia.

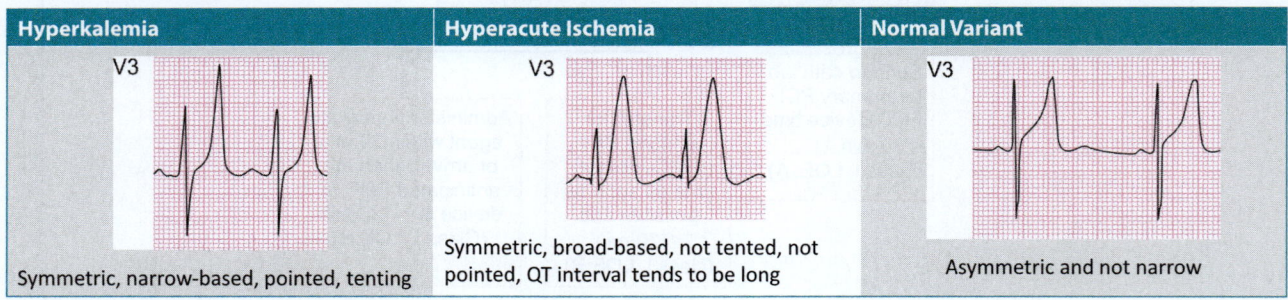

Hyperkalemia	Hyperacute Ischemia	Normal Variant
V3	V3	V3
Symmetric, narrow-based, pointed, tenting	Symmetric, broad-based, not tented, not pointed, QT interval tends to be long	Asymmetric and not narrow

13. **Ans. (a) T wave inversion** (Ref: Page 146: Braunwald: 10th edition and page 1457:Harrison 19th edition)
    - Hypothalamic stimulation as well as autonomic dysregulations have been implicated as causative for the ECG changes in SAH.
    - Heart rate is 60 bpm with left axis deviation. Deep symmetrical T wave inversion is noted in the chest leads.
    - The morphological ECG changes most frequently encountered in a subject with SAH are U waves, T-wave abnormalities, R-wave abnormalities and non-specific ST-T changes.
    - The predominant rhythm abnormalities seem to be relatively benign sinus tachycardias and bradycardias.

14. **Ans. (d) Premature ventricular contractions** (Ref: Page 1750: Harrison 20th edition; Page 1457: Harrison 19th edition)
    - The ECG shows normal sinus rhythm with heart rate of 75 bpm with normal axis.
    - Raised ST segment in lead V_2-V_4 and inverted T waves in lead I, aVL, V_2-V_4 are seen.

BRADYARRHYTHMIAS

15. **Ans. (a) 2:1 block** (Ref: page 1729: Harrison: 20th edition; Page 1473: Harrison 19th edition)
    - The heart rate is 30/min and normal P waves are present. This effectively rules out atrial fibrillation.(Choice D)
    - Missed beats are seen in the rhythm strip but are not a feature of 1st degree heart block. Hence Choice C is ruled out.
    - Tri-fascicular block is RBBB plus left anterior hemi-block plus left anterior posterior hemi-block. It will behave like 3rd degree heart block where Atrial rate (P-P) interval >>ventricular rate (R-R interval).

- Since in this question Atrial rate (P-P) interval = ventricular rate (R-R interval) tri-fascicular block is ruled out. Also the rSR' pattern typical of RBBB is not seen in the strip provided.
- PR interval is 200 msec (5 small squares) and is constant in the entire strip and every second P wave is not conducted to the ventricles resulting in dropped beats. This is a feature of 2:1 conduction block.

16. Ans. (c) **Complete heart block** (Ref: page 1729: Harrison: 20th edition); Page 1473: Harrison 19th edition
    - The image shows multiple nonconducted P waves with wide complex qRS escape rhythm. There is no relationship between the P waves and qRS complexes.
    - The atrial rate is faster than ventricular rate. This is seen in complete heart block.

17. Ans. (b) **Accelerated idioventricular rhythm** (Ref: Page 1882: Harrison: 20th edition; Page 1609: Harrison 19th edition)
    - The heart rate is 40 BPM with regular rhythm. Wide complex QRS is seen indicating origin from distal pacemakers. P waves are absent.
    - This bizarre appearance is called slow ventricular tachycardia. It is the most common arrhythmia seen post thrombolysis and is technically known as accelerated idio-ventricular rhythm. It is less commonly seen now days as most patients are managed with percutaneous coronary intervention.

18. Ans. (c) **Mobitz II heart block** (Ref: Page 1729: Harrison 20th edition; Page 1472: Harrison 19th edition)
    - The ECG shows more P waves than QRS complexes. This suggests a heart block.
    - P wave is upright and has a normal morphology. PR interval is 200 msec
    - *Dropped beats are present with PR interval remaining the same before the dropped beats.*

Comparison of Heart Blocks

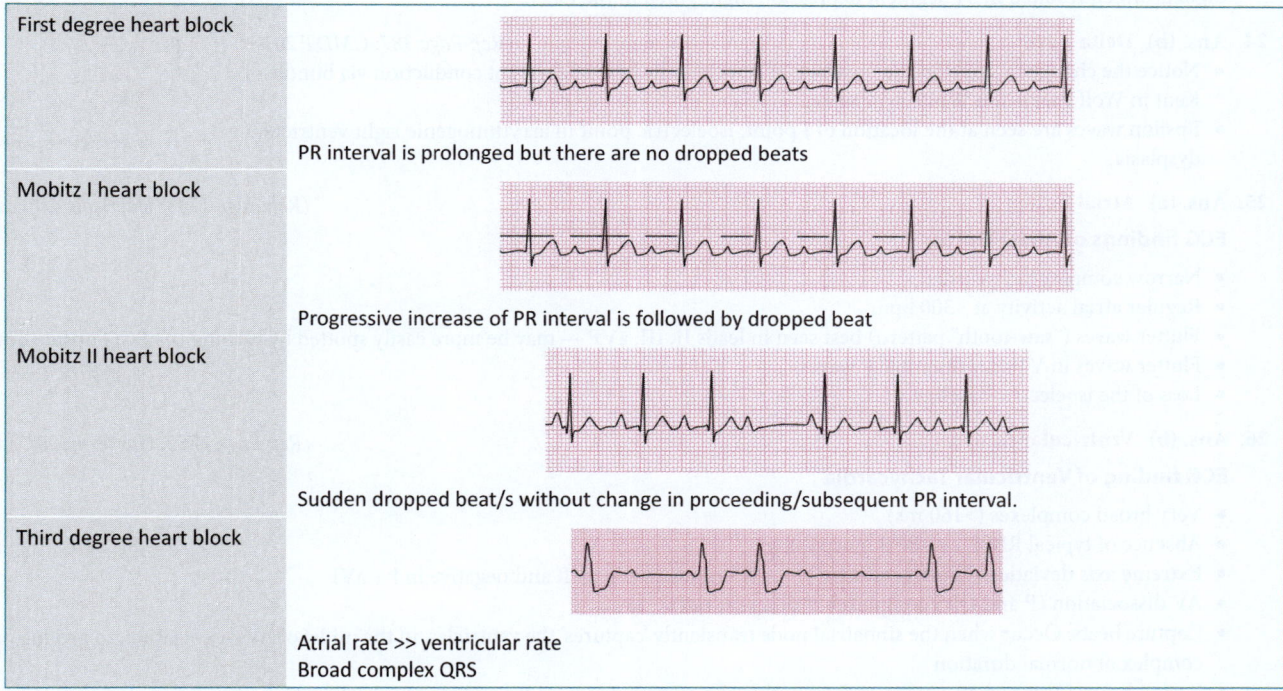

First degree heart block	PR interval is prolonged but there are no dropped beats
Mobitz I heart block	Progressive increase of PR interval is followed by dropped beat
Mobitz II heart block	Sudden dropped beat/s without change in proceeding/subsequent PR interval.
Third degree heart block	Atrial rate >> ventricular rate; Broad complex QRS

EFFECTS OF DRUGS ON ECG

19. Ans. (a) **Broad complex qRS: Soda-bicarbonate** (Ref: Page 1582: CMDT 2019)
    - The patient has presented with TCA toxicity. The ECG shows broad complex qRS with duration of 160 msec. ST segment elevation is seen in V_1 and V_2.
    - The correction of acidosis promotes protein binding of TCA and improves myocardial contractility.
    - Sodium bicarbonate is indicated for qRS intervals greater than 100 milliseconds, seizures, acidosis (pH level < 7), hypotension, cardiac arrest, or dysrhythmia.
    - Avoid drugs that exacerbate the cardiac effects of CAs, such as quinidine and procainamide (class IA), flecainide (class IC), and bretylium and amiodarone (class III).

20. Ans. (d) **Digoxin** (Ref: Page 1746: Harrison 20th edition; Page 1457: Harrison 19th edition)
    - The ECG shows irregularly irregular heart rhythm with absent P waves. This is diagnostic of atrial fibrillation.
    - Also seen is down-sloping ST segment depression pronounced in V_2-V_3 and in the rhythm strip.

- This patient of rheumatic heart disease is in atrial fibrillation for which she would have been put on digoxin by her physician.
- The combination of extracardiac side effects of digoxin and atrial fibrillation hemodynamic effects would explain the general unwell being of the patient.
- ACE inhibitor can lead to hyperkalemia and diuretics can lead to hypokalemia. However ECG changes of potassium deficit/excess are not seen.

21. **Ans. (d)   Atrial Bigeminy** (Ref: page 1681: Harrison 20th edition; Page 1457: Harrison 19th edition)

The V5 lead recording shows heart rate of 50 bpm with *absence of P waves and presence of Osborn wave at the J point*.

Concomitant ST Elevation is noted. The patient is suffering from hypothermia which explains the ECG changes. Atrial bigeminy should have discernible P waves.

22. **Ans. (d)   rSR' pattern in V1** (Ref: Page 1678-79: Harrison: 20th edition; Page 1453: Harrison 19th edition)
    - The ECG shows normal sinus rhythm with heart rate of 60bpm.
    - Right axis deviation is present.
    - Peaked P waves (>2.5 mm) are seen in Lead II, III
    - R>S in lead V1 (Normally its vice versa)
    - T wave inversion in lead II, III, aVF and V_1-V_3
    - rSR' pattern is seen in Right bundle branch block.

23. **Ans. (c)   Hockey stick sign** (Ref: page 125: Practical Cardiology: 2nd edition)

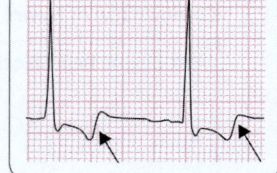

The image shows rhythm strip exhibiting a variable heart rate with ST segment depression. P wave is absent with narrow complex. The patient was probably having atrial fibrillation and was started on digoxin which resulted in ST segment depression highlighted in the ECG.

24. **Ans. (b)   Delta wave** (Ref: Page 387: CMDT 2017)
    - Notice the change in slope on the upstroke of R wave indicative of aberrant conduction via bundle of Kent in Wolf Parkinson White syndrome.
    - Epsilon waves are seen at the location of J point, isoelectric point in arrythmogenic right ventricular dysplasia.

25. **Ans. (a)   Atrial flutter** (Ref: Page 1743: Harrison: 20th edition)

ECG findings of Atrial Flutter
- Narrow complex tachycardia
- Regular atrial activity at ~300 bpm
- Flutter waves ("saw-tooth" pattern) best seen in leads II, III, aVF — may be more easily spotted by turning the ECG upside down!
- Flutter waves in V1 may resemble P waves
- Loss of the isoelectric baseline.

26. **Ans. (b)   Ventricular tachycardia** (Ref: Page 1752: Harrison: 20th edition)

ECG finding of Ventricular Tachycardia
- Very broad complexes (>160 ms)
- Absence of typical RBBB or LBBB morphology
- Extreme axis deviation ("northwest axis") — QRS is positive in aVR and negative in I + aVF
- AV dissociation (P and QRS complexes at different rates)
- Capture beats: Occur when the sinoatrial node transiently 'captures' the ventricles, in the midst of AV dissociation, to produce a QRS complex of normal duration
- Fusion beats: Occur when a sinus and ventricular beat coincide to produce a hybrid complex of intermediate morphology
- Positive or negative concordance throughout the chest leads, i.e. leads V1-6 show entirely positive (R) or entirely negative (QS) complexes, with no RS complexes seen
- Brugada's sign: The distance from the onset of the QRS complex to the nadir of the S-wave is > 100ms
- Josephson's sign: Notching near the nadir of the S-wave
- RSR' complexes with a taller "left rabbit ear". This is the most specific finding in favour of VT. This is in contrast to RBBB, where the right rabbit ear is taller.

27. **Ans. (a)   PSVT** (Ref: Page 1739: Harrison: 20th edition)
    - The most common arrhythmia in a setting of a structurally normal heart is PSVT. Vomiting is reverse peristalsis and is caused by vagal action. This explains the sudden termination of the arrhythmia and patient feeling better.
    - The ECG shows a heart rate of about 200 bpm or more with narrow complex QRS.
    - RR interval is constant in long lead II.
    - The apparent ST segment depression disappears with the arrhythmia treatment.
    - First line management of this patient is carotid sinus massage.

Also Know
- DOC for SVT: Verapamil
- DOC for PSVT: Adenosine
- Digitalis-induced arrhythmia: Lignocaine

28. **Ans. (c) Mobitz II heart block** *(Ref: Page 1728: Harrison: 20th edition)*
    - Notice the dropped beats marked by arrows which indicate 2nd degree heart block.
    - Now calculate PR interval prior to and following the dropped beat
    - The PR interval prior to the dropped beat and subsequent to the heart block is same 0.12 seconds, which is diagnostic of Mobitz II heart block.
    - In Mobitz I heart block, PR interval prior to dropped beat is the longest and subsequent to the dropped beat is the shortest.

29. **Ans. (b) LBBB** *(Ref: Page 1679: Harrison: 20th edition; Page 1455: Harrison 19th edition)*
    - The image shows heart rate of 75 bpm with Left axis deviation
    - P wave is 3 small squares and PR interval is about 5 small squares (normal)
    - QRS morphology shows broad complex QRS.
    - QS Complex is seen in Lead I
    - Lead V6 shows RR'
    - Wide R wave in Lead I, aVL, V_5 and V_6 is seen suggestive of delayed activation of left ventricle.
    - These findings are diagnostic of LBBB

Differentiating QRS pattern of BBB

Leads	RBBB	LBBB
V1	rSR'	QS
V6	qRS	Slurred R or RR' or RSR

30. **Ans. (b) Left circumflex artery** *(Ref: Page 263: ECG made easy 5th edition)*

The patient is having early morning attack of chest pain, which points to either Prinzmetal's or acute MI as ECG shows ST segment elevation in leads I, V_5 and V_6 which points to lateral wall MI. The main supply to lateral wall of heart is left circumflex artery.

Localization of a myocardial infarct			
Localization	ST elevation	Reciprocal ST depression	Coronary artery
Anterior MI	V_1-V_6	None	LAD
Septal MI	V_1-V_4, disappearance of septum Q in leads V_5, V_6	None	LAD-septal branches
Lateral MI	I, aVL, V_5, V_6	II, III, aVF	LCX or MO
Inferior MI	II, III, aVF	I, aVL	RCA (80%) or RCX (20%)
Posterior MI	V_7, V_8, V_9	ST depression V1-V3 >2mm (mirror view)	RCX (Ramus circumflex)
Right Ventricle MI/Atrial MI	V_1, V_4R PTa in I,V_5,V_6	I, aVL PTa in I, II or III	RCA RCA

LAD = left anterior descending artery
LCX = left circumflex artery
MO = marginalis obtunalis
RCX = ramus circumflex

31. **Ans. (a) Thrombolysis** *(Ref: Q.34 Page 261: ECG made easy 5th edition)*
    - Thrombolysis is contraindicated in patient with SBP > 180 mm Hg as it can lead to hemorrhagic stroke.
    - Morphine reduces pulmonary edema and will be useful in this patient as CXR shows bat wing pulmonary edema.
    - Chewable aspirin reduces clot propagation.
    - Furosemide will reduce this cardiogenic pulmonary edema.

32. **Ans. (a) Dextrocardia**
    - Situs solitus is the normal position, and situs inversus is the mirror image of situs solitus. Cardiac situs is determined by the atrial location.

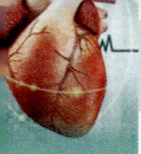

- In situs inversus, the morphologic right atrium is on the left, and the morphologic left atrium is on the right. The normal pulmonary anatomy is also reversed so that the left lung has 3 lobes and the right lung has 2 lobes.
- In addition, the liver and gallbladder are located on the left, whereas the spleen and stomach are located on the right. The remaining internal structures are also a mirror image of the normal.

33. **Ans. (c)** Left to right shunts (Ref: Page 169: CMDT 2019)

   Clubbing may be present in one of five stages
   - Fluctuation and softening of the nail bed.
   - Loss of the normal <165° angle (Lovibond angle) between the nailbed and the fold (cuticula)
   - Increased convexity of the nail fold
   - Thickening of the whole distal (end part of the) finger (resembling a drumstick)
   - Shiny aspect and striation of the nail and skin.

   Schamroth's test or Schamroth's window test is a popular test for clubbing. When the distal phalanges (bones nearest the fingertips) of corresponding fingers of opposite hands are directly opposed (place fingernails of same finger on opposite hands against each other, nail to nail), a small diamond-shaped "window" is normally apparent between the nailbeds. If this window is obliterated, the test is positive and clubbing is present.

34. **Ans. (a)** Endocardial cushion defect (Ref: OP Ghai, 7th ed, pg 613)

   The mongoloid slant of eyes with a saddle nose and a happy posing baby points to DOWN's syndrome which is associated with ASD ostium primum/ endocardial cushion defect.

35. **Ans. (b)** Mobitz 1 heart block (Ref: Page 1728: Harrison: 20th edition)
   - Due to intense training in martial arts etc these athletes are at the risk of developing first degree heart block or Mobitz 1 heart block.
   - In the tracing given you will notice a gradual onset progression of PR interval in the first four cardiac cycles counting from the left followed by a dropped beat.
   - In exam, since you will have 30–40 seconds for evaluation, you should locate the dropped beat in any ECG of bradycardia, then note the PR interval in beat preceding the dropped beat as well as subsequent beat
   - You will notice that in the beat preceding the dropped beat the PR interval will be much more than PR interval in the beat following the PR interval.

36. **Ans. (c)** Phenoxybenzamine (Ref: Page 422: OP Ghai 8th edition)
   - The child is in knee chest position and you can notice the cyanotic hue of the extremities. This child has tetralogy of Fallot and is probably having a Tet spell.
   - *Depending on the frequency and severity of hypercyanotic attacks, one or more of the following procedures should be instituted in sequence:*
     - Placement of the infant on the abdomen in the knee-chest position while ascertaining that the infant's clothing is not constrictive. Calming and holding the infant in a knee-chest position may abort progression of an early spell. Premature attempts to obtain blood samples may cause further agitation and be counterproductive.
     - Administration of oxygen (although increasing inspired oxygen will not reverse cyanosis caused by intracardiac shunting).
     - Injection of morphine subcutaneously in a dose not in excess of 0.2 mg/kg.
     - Vasopressors like phenylephrine to reduce right to left shunting.

37. **Ans. (a)** P pulmonale (Ref: Page 269: ECG made easy 5th edition)
   - The patient has tall P waves in ECG in setting of ILD which indicates pulmonary artery hypertension.
   - P wave should be > 1.5 mm in V_1-V_2, in chest leads or P wave >2.5 mm in limb leads for diagnosis of p- pulmonale.
   - Causes of P pulmonale are:

   1. PAH
   2. TOF and pulmonic stenosis in right to left sided shunts
   3. Tricuspid stenosis
   4. Cor pulmonale

38. **Ans. (a)** Boot-shaped heart (Ref: Page 422: OP Ghai, 8th edition)
   - "Boot-shaped" heart with an upturned cardiac apex due to right ventricular hypertrophy and concave pulmonary arterial segment, seen in patients with TOF
   - Most infants with TOF however may not show this finding.
   - Pulmonary oligemia due to decreased pulmonary arterial flow.
   - Right sided aortic arch is seen in 25% of patients.

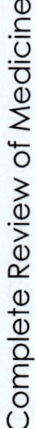

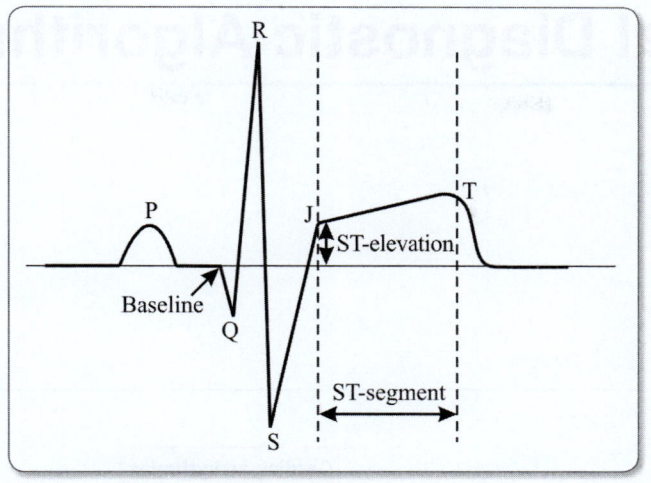

39. **Ans. (a) Constrictive pericarditis** *(Ref: Page 99: Braunwald, 10th edition)*

The JVP tracing shows a prominent × and prominent y descent.

Disease	X descent in JVP	Y descent in JVP
Cardiac tamponade	Absent	Absent
Constrictive pericarditis	Prominent	Prominent
Restrictive cardiomyopathy	Present	Rare

*The y descent, which follows the peak of the v wave, can become prolonged or blunted with obstruction to right ventricular inflow, as may occur with tricuspid stenosis (TS) or pericardial tamponade.

40. **Ans. (a) Aortic dissection** *(Ref: Page 1921: Harrison: 20th edition)*
    - The main point in diagnosis is CXR finding of widening of anterior mediastinum in patient of chest pain at rest with double aortic shadow. The lung fields are clear, thus rule out pulmonary edema due to acute MI.
    - Clinical indicators are chest pain at rest with development of Horner syndrome and stroke.
    - The closest choice in the question is atrial fibrillation due to embolic stroke. Due to hypertension structural damage to heart, atrial fibrillation can ensue. However, the acute chest pain presentation negates this possibility.

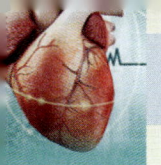

Conceptual Diagnostic Algorithm

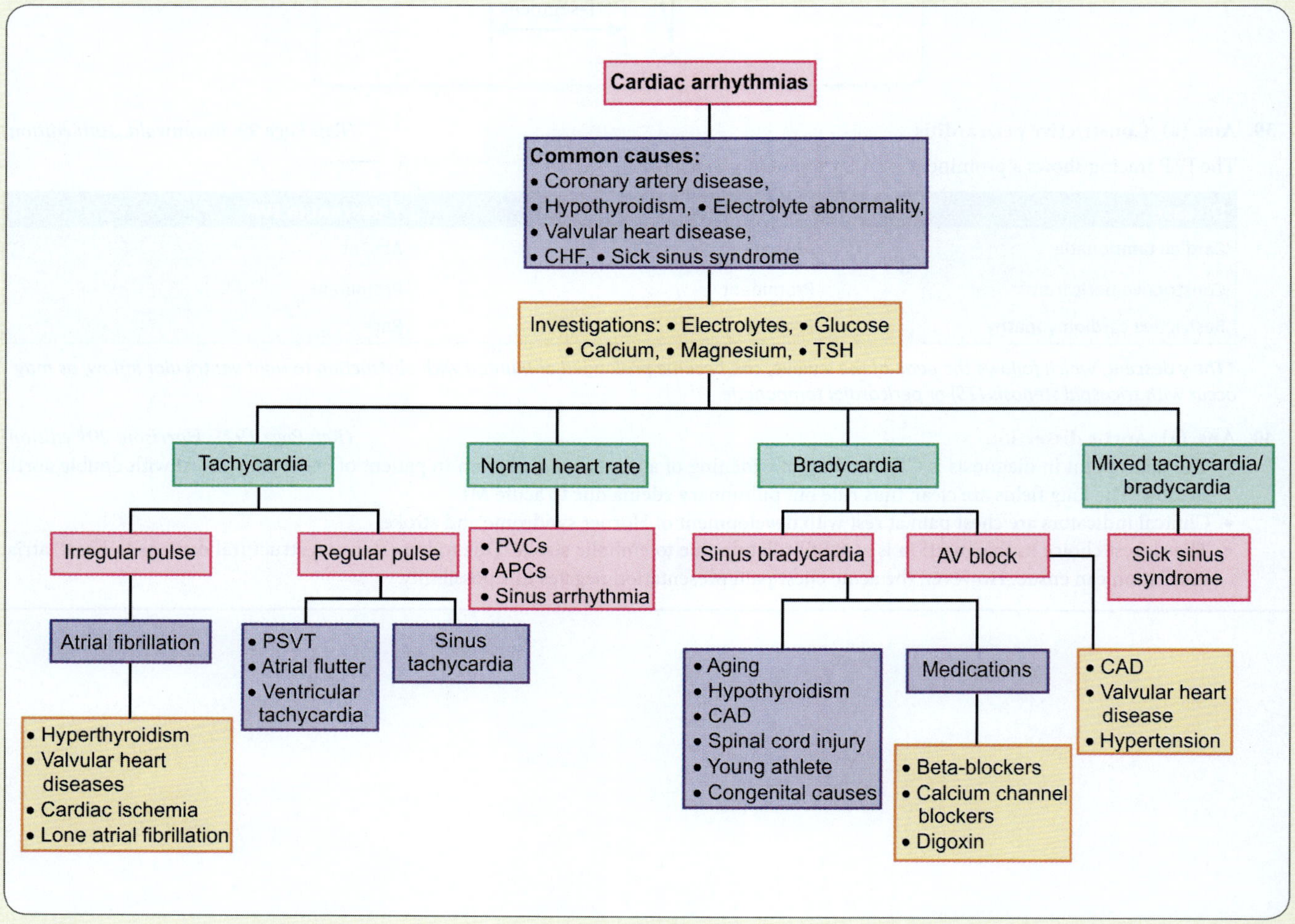

Cardiac arrhythmias

Common causes:
- Coronary artery disease,
- Hypothyroidism, • Electrolyte abnormality,
- Valvular heart disease,
- CHF, • Sick sinus syndrome

Investigations: • Electrolytes, • Glucose • Calcium, • Magnesium, • TSH

Tachycardia

Irregular pulse
Atrial fibrillation
- Hyperthyroidism
- Valvular heart diseases
- Cardiac ischemia
- Lone atrial fibrillation

Regular pulse
- PSVT
- Atrial flutter
- Ventricular tachycardia

Sinus tachycardia

Normal heart rate
- PVCs
- APCs
- Sinus arrhythmia

Bradycardia

Sinus bradycardia
- Aging
- Hypothyroidism
- CAD
- Spinal cord injury
- Young athlete
- Congenital causes

AV block
Medications
- Beta-blockers
- Calcium channel blockers
- Digoxin

Mixed tachycardia/bradycardia

Sick sinus syndrome
- CAD
- Valvular heart disease
- Hypertension

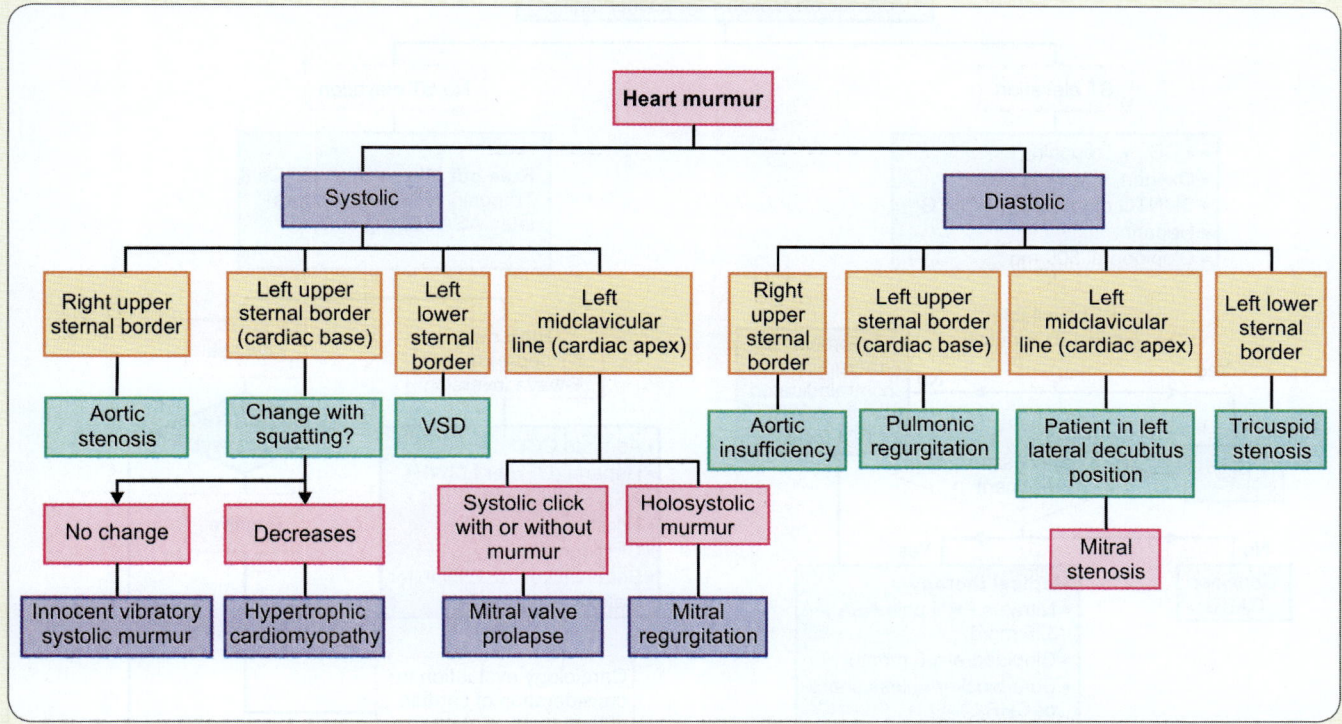

* MC murmur in children is a functional murmur. Best position to hear functional murmur is left lower sternal border
* Functional murmur is a systolic murmur
* All murmur decreases with valsava, standing and amylnitrate inhalation except HOCM murmur which becomes louder, MVP murmur which becomes longer.

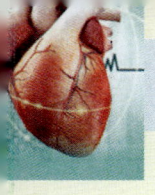

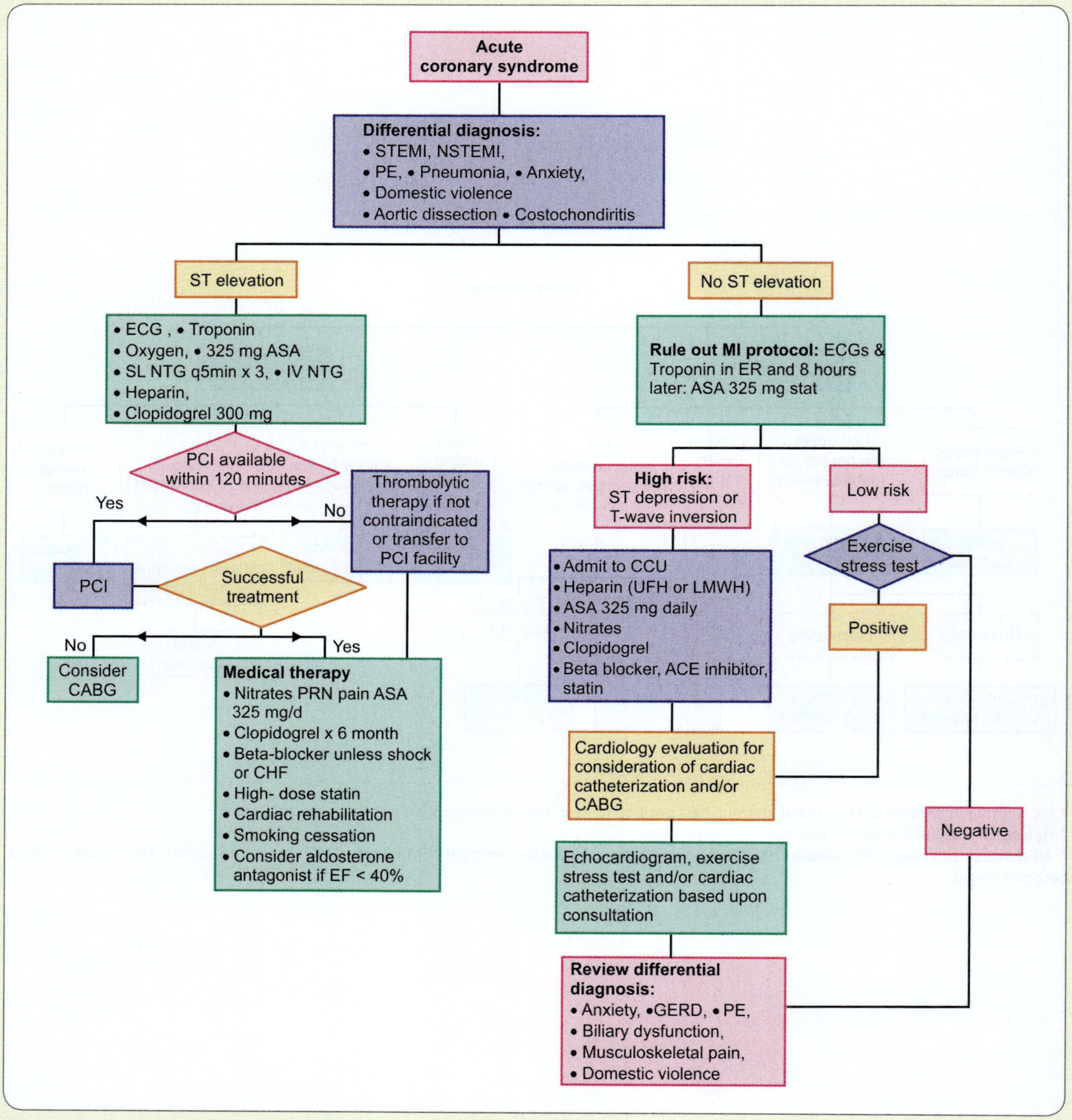

ALGORITHM

Acute coronary syndrome

Differential diagnosis:
- STEMI, NSTEMI,
- PE, • Pneumonia, • Anxiety,
- Domestic violence
- Aortic dissection • Costochondiritis

ST elevation
- ECG, • Troponin
- Oxygen, • 325 mg ASA
- SL NTG q5min x 3, • IV NTG
- Heparin,
- Clopidogrel 300 mg

PCI available within 120 minutes?
- Yes → PCI
- No → Thrombolytic therapy if not contraindicated or transfer to PCI facility

Successful treatment?
- No → Consider CABG
- Yes → **Medical therapy**
  - Nitrates PRN pain ASA 325 mg/d
  - Clopidogrel x 6 month
  - Beta-blocker unless shock or CHF
  - High-dose statin
  - Cardiac rehabilitation
  - Smoking cessation
  - Consider aldosterone antagonist if EF < 40%

No ST elevation
Rule out MI protocol: ECGs & Troponin in ER and 8 hours later: ASA 325 mg stat

High risk: ST depression or T-wave inversion
- Admit to CCU
- Heparin (UFH or LMWH)
- ASA 325 mg daily
- Nitrates
- Clopidogrel
- Beta blocker, ACE inhibitor, statin

Cardiology evaluation for consideration of cardiac catheterization and/or CABG

Echocardiogram, exercise stress test and/or cardiac catheterization based upon consultation

Review differential diagnosis:
- Anxiety, •GERD, • PE,
- Biliary dysfunction,
- Musculoskeletal pain,
- Domestic violence

Low risk → Exercise stress test
- Positive
- Negative

* FMC-device time should be < 90 minutes to perform P.C.I (first medical contact)

Multiple Choice Questions

Arrhythmias and Emergency Medicine

1. A patient presents with recent onset breathlessness and ECG was done. The diagnosis is? *(AIIMS May 2019, Nov 2018)*

   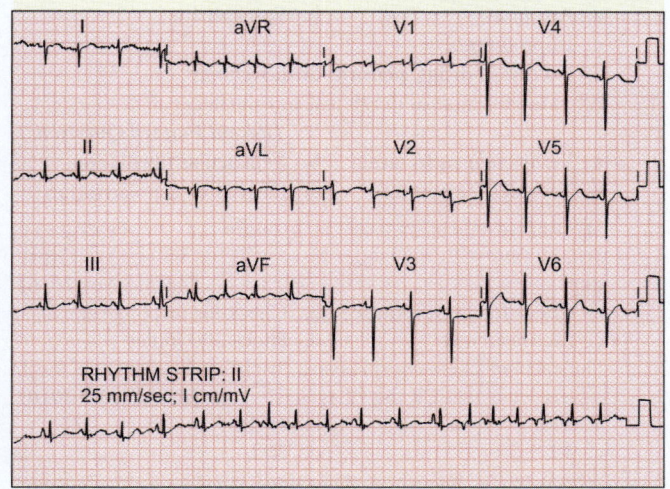

   a. Atrial fibrillation
   b. Paroxysmal supraventricular tachycardia
   c. Acute myocardial infarction
   d. Multi-focal atrial tachycardia

2. A 25-year-old female presented to ER unconscious. Her mother tells you about her having recurrent episodes of syncopal episodes. Her BP is 80/60 mm Hg and you order an ECG. Treatment is? *(Recent Question 2019)*

   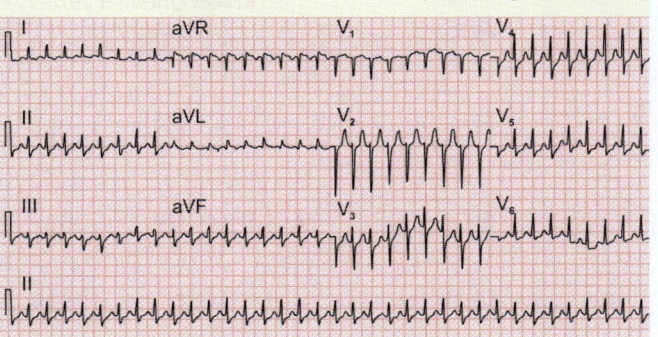

   a. Carotid sinus massage   b. Cardioversion
   c. Adenosine push   d. Verapamil

3. Comment on the diagnosis of the patient?
   (Recent Question 2019)

   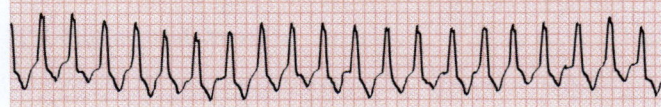

   a. Ventricular tachycardia
   b. Ventricular flutter.
   c. Ventricular fibrillation
   d. Electromechanical dissociation

4. Which of the following is associated with AV block?
   (Recent Pattern 2018)
   a. Hypothyroidism   b. Hyperthyroidism
   c. Cushing disease   d. Pheochromocytoma

5. Implantable cardioverter defibrillator is useful in?
   a. Brugada syndrome   *(Recent Pattern 2018)*
   b. Arrythmogenic RV dysplasia
   c. Post MI with structural damage
   d. All of the above

6. Which of the following drugs is an alternative to epinephrine in ACLS algorithm for a pulseless patient?
   a. Vasopressin   *(Recent Pattern 2018)*
   b. Low dose dopamine
   c. Atropine
   d. Desmopressin

7. Heart block is seen with all except? *(Recent Pattern 2018)*
   a. Coronary artery disease   b. Sarcoidosis
   c. Hypothyroidism   d. Cushing syndrome

8. You are posted in a high dependency ward where during the morning round a patient complains of palpitations with ECG showing narrow QRS tachycardia with heart rate around 150/ min and systolic BP of 96 mm Hg. What is the next best step to be done? *(AIIMS Nov 2017)*
   a. DC cardio version
   b. Carotid sinus massage
   c. IV adenosine
   d. Wait and watch

9. Identify the ECG pattern. *(AIIMS Nov 2017)*

   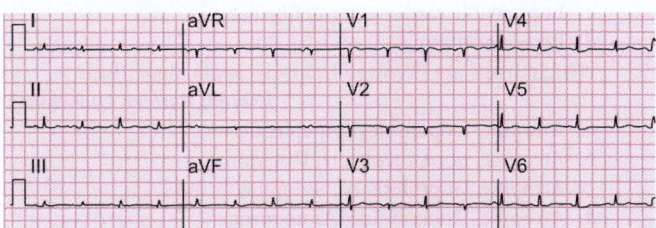

   a. P-Pulmonale
   b. Electrical Alternans
   c. Ventricular Bigeminy
   d. Wrong calibration

10. What is the correct sequence of events according to BLS?
    (AIIMS Nov 2017)
    a. Start CPR, give rescue breath, asses Pulse
    b. Give rescue breath, See pulse, start CPR
    c. Assess patient, activate emergency response team, call for defibrillator and start CPR
    d. Assess pulse, defibrillate, Start CPR

11. A patient has presented with complaints of amblyopia, episodes of palpitations and occasional exertional chest pain. ECG shows ventricular extra systoles. Which of the following is the probable cause? *(AIIMS May 2017)*
    a. Cocaine poisoning
    b. Nicotine poisoning
    c. Arsenic poisoning
    d. Cannabis ingestion

12. This 50-year-old patient developed syncope after having a coffee. ECG was done. Which is the most appropriate therapy for a patient suffering from the condition shown below? *(AIIMS May 2017)*

    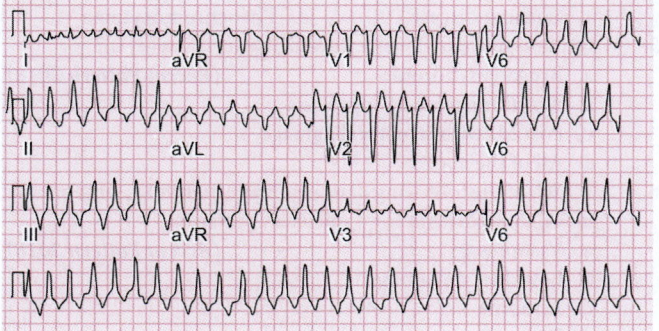

    a. Lignocaine b. DC shock
    c. Amiodarone d. Esmolol

13. Which of the following is recommended for management of symptomatic bradycardia non responsive to 0.5mg iv atropine? *(Recent Pattern Questions)*
    a. Atropine (higher dose) b. Vasopressin
    c. Epinephrine d. Isoproterenol

14. A 50-year-old patient presents with features of poor perfusion following MI. On examination heart rate is 40/min with BP of 60mmHg systolic. Atropine was given twice over 5 minutes, but the condition of patient is not improving. What is the next best step? *(Recent Pattern Questions)*
    a. Trans-venous Pacing b. Transcutaneous Pacing
    c. Implantable cardioverter defibrillator
    d. Repeat atropine

15. Which drugs are involved in bradycardia algorithm? *(Recent Pattern Questions)*
    a. Atropine, Dopamine, Epinephrine
    b. Atropine, norepinephrine, Dopamine
    c. Atropine, Isoproterenol, Norepinephrine
    d. Atropine, Dobutamine, Amiodarone

16. The primary decision point in bradycardia algorithm is determination of? *(Recent Pattern Questions)*
    a. Heart rate b. Rhythm
    c. Perfusion of organs d. Blood pressure

17. After determination of inadequate perfusion of organs in a patient with bradycardia, which of the following is the first step?
    a. Observation and monitoring *(Recent Pattern Questions)*
    b. Transcutaneous pacing
    c. Give intravenous atropine and monitor
    d. Use defibrillator at 200J

18. Comment on the diagnosis. *(Recent Pattern Questions)*

    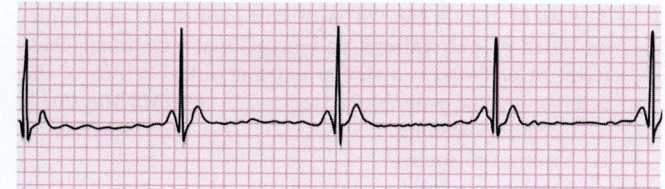

    a. Sinus bradycardia
    b. Mobitz type II heart block
    c. Wenckebach phenomenon
    d. Third degree/ complete heart block

19. Which of the following is not a cause of PEA? *(Recent Pattern Questions)*
    a. Low pO2 < 60mm Hg b. Hydrogen ion depletion
    c. Hypokalemia d. Hypovolemia

20. Which of the following drugs is used first line in management of PEA? *(Recent Pattern Questions)*
    a. Atropine b. Epinephrine
    c. Isoproterenol
    d. No role of drugs, perform cardioversion

21. What is the cause of death in Commotio cordis? *(Recent Pattern Questions)*
    a. Ventricular tachycardia b. Ventricular fibrillation
    c. Torsades De pointes d. Early after depolarization

22. An unresponsive patient is brought to the emergency department with no proper history. What will be your next step? *(AIIMS Nov 2016)*
    a. Check for carotid pulse b. Check for responsiveness
    c. Secure airway d. Shock 300 Joules

23. The ratio of chest compression to rescue breath ratio for a lone rescuer in CPR for all ages is? *(AIIMS Nov 2016)*
    a. 30:2 b. 15:2
    c. 3:1 d. 30:1

24. Which of the following statements is true about atropine and its role in cardiac arrest protocol? *(Recent Question 2016-17)*
    a. Atropine is not a part of the protocol
    b. Atropine is used only for bradycardia
    c. Atropine is used after failure of repeat epinephrine
    d. Atropine is used after failure of ROSC with defibrillation

25. A 30-year-old man presents with recurrent attacks of feeling dizzy. ECG was done. What is the diagnosis? *(Recent Question 2016-17)*

    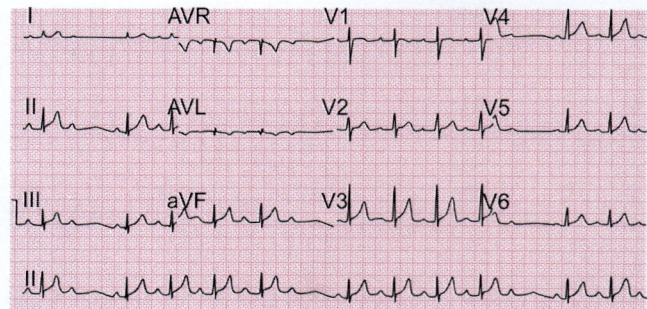

    a. Atrial fibrillation b. PSVT
    c. Mobitz I heart block d. Complete heart block

26. A 60-year-old retired banker complains of feeling dizzy with palpitations and breathlessness. His BP becomes unrecordable while ECG is being recorded. What should be done as first step in management of this patient? *(Recent Question 2016-17)*

    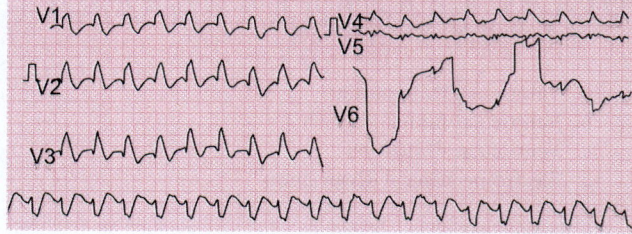

    a. IV Amiodarone 150mg b. IV Lasix 40mg
    c. Cardioversion d. IV lignocaine

27. Most common paroxysmal regular SVT is?
    (Recent Question 2016-17)
    a. Inappropriate sinus tachycardia
    b. Atrioventricular nodal re-entrant tachycardia
    c. Atrioventricular re-entrant tachycardia
    d. Paroxysmal atrial tachycardia

28. A 55-year-old diabetic hypertensive male smoker came with chest pain for last one day. His ECG is shown. Which of the following is the correct diagnosis? *(APPG 2016)*

    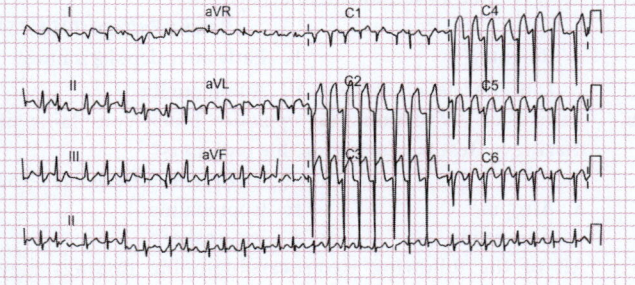

    a. Anterior STEMI with VT
    b. Inferior STEMI with VT
    c. Inferior STEMI with SVT
    d. Anterior STEMI with atrial fibrillation

29. Identify the ECG given in the figure below?
    (AIIMS Nov 15)

    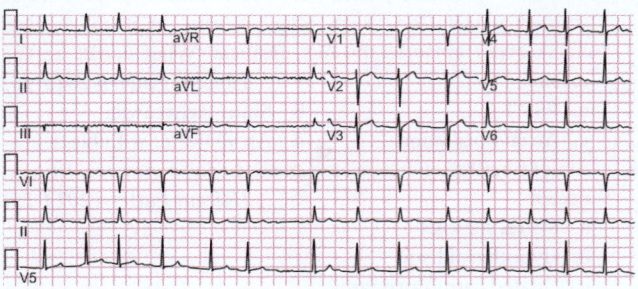

    a. Sinus rhythm   b. PSVT
    c. Atrial fibrillation   d. Ventricular fibrillation

30. In the ECG shown which drug is not to be given?
    (AIIMS Nov 15)

    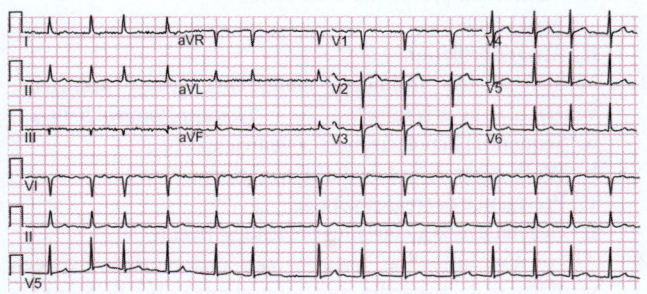

    a. Amiodarone   b. Adenosine
    c. Diltiazem   d. Beta blocker

31. Match List I with List II and select the correct answer using the code given below the lists: *(UPSC 2015)*

    List I (Emergency drugs)   List II (Clinical condition)
    A. Amiodarone   1. 1st degree heart Block
    B. Adenosine   2. Atrial fibrillation
    C. Digoxin   3. Ventricular tachycardia
    D. Atropine   4. Paroxysmal supraventricular tachycardia

    Code:
	A	B	C	D
a.	1	2	4	3
b.	1	4	2	3
c.	3	2	4	1
d.	3	4	2	1

32. Which of the auscultatory sign is absent in mitral stenosis in the presence of atrial fibrillation? *(UPSC 2015)*
    a. Mid diastolic murmur
    b. Pre-systolic accentuation
    c. Variable first heart sound
    d. Loud P_2

33. What is the drug of choice to control sudden onset supraventricular tachycardia? *(Bihar PG 15)*
    a. Adenosine   b. Propranolol
    c. Verapamil   d. Digoxin

34. Unconscious child, CPR was started and ECG shows normal QRS but peripheral pulse was absent inspite of chest compressions. What should be done next?
    (JIPMER Nov 2015)
    a. Epinephrine   b. Atropine
    c. Defibrillator   d. Synchronised cardioversion

35. New onset atrial flutter. Best treatment is?
    (JIPMER Nov 2015)
    a. Cardioversion   b. Procainamide
    c. Bretylium   d. Amiodarone

36. A 75-year-old patient clutches chest and falls down. A Physician arrives on the scene. What is the first thing to be done by the physician? *(JIPMER Nov 2015)*
    a. Call for help
    b. Clear patient airway
    c. Check peripheral pulse
    d. Chest compressions

37. In ECG lead II, III, and aVF are abnormal. Which of the following vessel is blocked? *(JIPMER May 2015)*
    a. Left coronary artery
    b. Left anterior descending
    c. Right coronary artery
    d. Right circumflex artery

38. A 55-year-old hypertensive patient has a standing BP 190/10 and sitting BP-180/100. He also has irregularly irregular rhythm, double apical impulse and bilateral basal crepitations. But no murmurs could be auscultated and heart rate could not be determined. What is the likely cause? *(JIPMER Nov 2014)*
    a. Left atrial Myxoma
    b. Mitral regurgitation
    c. Cor Pulmonale
    d. Left ventricular hypertrophy

39. If a person is having ventricular tachycardia, extra systoles appears in: *(Recent Question 2015-16)*
    a. P wave
    b. QRS complex
    c. T wave
    d. R wave

40. The image shows presence of: *(Recent Question 2015-16)*

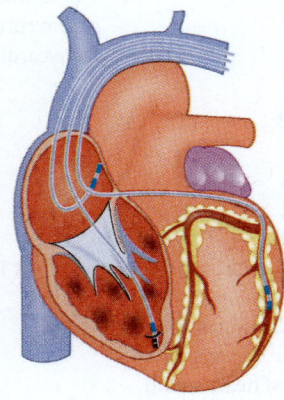

a. Implantable cardioverter defibrillator
b. Cardiac resynchronization therapy
c. Dual pacing
d. Transvenous pacemaker

41. A 70-year old hypertensive patient with complaint of palpitations and pre-syncope. On examination, his heart rate is 72 BPM and BP was 150/100. ECG done shows *(Recent Question 2015-16)*

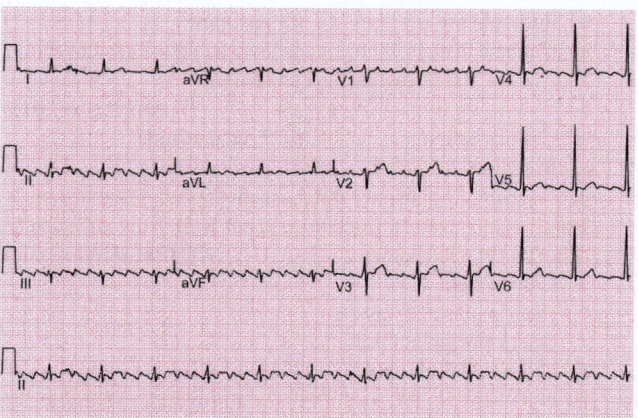

a. Atrial flutter
b. Atrial fibrillation
c. Multifocal atrial tachycardia
d. PSVT

42. A 62-year-old male with underlying COPD develops a viral upper respiratory infection and begins taking an over-the-counter decongestant. Shortly thereafter he experiences palpitations and presents to the emergency room, where the given rhythm strip is obtained, demonstrating: *(Recent Question 2015-16)*

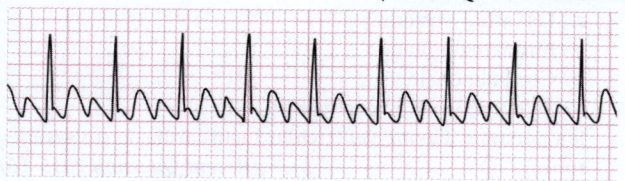

a. Junctional tachycardia
b. Atrial flutter
c. Paroxysmal atrial tachycardia
d. Complete heart block

43. A 40-year-old Lady intraoperatively develops HR = 220 bpm and Blood pressure of 70/40, ECG shows qRS complex = 110 milliseconds. Best management is? *(JIPMER 2014)*
a. Adenosine 6 mg/12 mg   b. Amiodarone
c. DC cardioversion   d. Esmolol

44. Most common arrhythmia in ICU patients: *(Recent Pattern 2015-16)*
a. Atrial flutter   b. Atrial fibrillation
c. PSVT   d. NPAT

45. Most common mechanism of arrhythmia? *(Recent Pattern 2014-15)*
a. Re-entry   b. Early after depolarization
c. Late after depolarization   d. Automaticity

46. Patient of AV conduction episodes block complains of dizziness. Best treatment for this patient is? *(Recent Pattern 2014-15)*
a. Atropine   b. Isoprenaline
c. Adrenaline   d. Pacemaker

47. All of the following electrocardiographic findings may represent manifestations of digitalis intoxication, except: *(Recent Pattern 2014-15)*
a. Ventricular Bigeminy
b. Junctional tachycardia
c. Bidirectional tachycardia
d. Multifocal Atrial tachycardia

48. 40-year-old female patient develops recurrent episodes of sudden palpitations with HR=150/min, rhythm regular. After every episode she has diuresis. What could be the cause? *(Recent Pattern 2014-15)*
a. PSVT   b. Sinus tachycardia
c. Atrial fibrillation   d. Atrial flutter with block

49. Atrial fibrillation may occur in all the following conditions, except- *(Recent Pattern 2014-15)*
a. Mitral stenosis
b. Hypothyroidism
c. Dilated cardiomyopathy
d. Mitral regurgitation

50. Which of the following arrhythmia is most commonly associated with alcohol binge in alcoholics? *(Recent Pattern 2014-15)*
a. Ventricular fibrillation
b. Ventricular premature contractions
c. Atrial flutter
d. Atrial fibrillation

51. Which of the following statements about premature ventricular beat is false? *(Recent Pattern 2014-15)*
a. Sequential depolarization of ventricles
b. Wide, Bizarre, Notched qRS complexes
c. Prevalence decreases with age
d. Palpitations is a common presenting feature

52. All of the following features can differentiate between ventricular tachycardia and supraventricular tachycardia except: *(Recent Pattern 2014-15)*
a. qRS < 0.12 seconds
b. Ventricular rate > 160/min
c. Variable first heart sound
d. Relieved by carotid sinus massage

53. Feature of Torsades de pointes is: *(Recent Pattern 2014-15)*
a. Hypermagnesemia   b. Short qRS complex
c. Prolonged QT_c interval   d. PQ segment

54. **Which of the following is the most common heart block in neonatal lupus.** *(Recent Pattern 2014-15)*
    a. 1st degree heart block
    b. Mobitz 2A heart block
    c. Mobitz 2B heart block
    d. 3rd degree heart block
55. **True about Torsades de pointes?** *(Recent Pattern 2014-15)*
    a. ST segment depression   b. QTc prolongation
    c. Narrow qRS Complex   d. PQ segment elevation
56. **A 40-year-old male presents to the office with a history of palpitations that last for a few seconds and occur two or three times a week. There are no other symptoms. ECG shows a single unifocal premature ventricular contraction. The most likely cause of this finding is:**
    (Recent Pattern 2014-15)
    a. Underlying coronary artery disease
    b. Valvular heart disease
    c. Hypertension
    d. Idiopathic
57. **A 78-year-old male with hypertension (controlled on anti-hypertensive drugs) presents with new onset of mild left hemiparesis and ECG finding of atrial fibrillation. Which of the following must be done?** *(Recent Pattern 2014-15)*
    a. Close observation   b. Permanent pacemaker
    c. Aspirin   d. Warfarin
58. **While at the ward round, you see an elderly lady attendant slump to the floor. Going to her aid, you notice her to be unresponsive and apneic. Your first step in Adult Basic Life Support(CPR) should be the following?**
    a. Cardioversion   *(Recent Pattern 2014-15)*
    b. Assess breathing
    c. Determine responsiveness
    d. Institute chest compression
59. **In the ICU, a patient suddenly becomes unresponsive, pulseless, and hypotensive, with cardiac monitor indicating ventricular tachycardia. The first therapeutic step among the following should be:** *(Recent Pattern 2014-15)*
    a. Amiodarone 300 mg IV push
    b. Lidocaine 1.5 mg / kg IV push
    c. Defibrillation at 200 joules biphasic
    d. Defibrillation at 360 joules uniphasic
60. **A 12-year-old wheel chair bound boy with scoliosis has presented with Dyspnea. ECG shows deep QS waves in V2, V3 with tall R waves in V5, V6. Probable diagnosis:**
    a. Amyotrophic lateral sclerosis *(Recent Pattern 2014-15)*
    b. Duchenne muscular dystrophy
    c. Pott's paraplegia
    d. Myotonic dystrophy
61. **Treatment of asymptomatic bradycardia is:**
    (Recent Pattern 2014-15)
    a. No treatment is required   b. Give atropine
    c. Isoprenaline   d. Cardiac pacing
62. **Which is incorrect about a pacemaker:**
    (Recent Pattern 2014-15)
    a. Deployed below skin of the chest
    b. Pacing leads lie in the right atrium and right ventricle
    c. Treatment of choice in Mobitz 1 heart Block
    d. Biventricular pacing is useful for dilated cardiomyopathy
63. **Frog sign is seen in:** *(Recent Pattern 2014-15)*
    a. AVNRT   b. Diabetic nephropathy
    c. Medullary sponge kidney   d. Budd Chiari syndrome
64. **Sinus Bradycardia is defined as heart rate of?**
    (Recent Pattern 2014-15)
    a. Less than 40/min   b. Less than 50/min
    c. Less than 60/min   d. Less than 70/min
65. **A person with mitral regurgitation and atrial fibrillation presents with syncope. On examination the person has a heart rate of 55. What is the most probable cause?**
    (Recent Pattern 2014-15)
    a. Digitalis toxicity   b. Junctional Tachycardia
    c. Stroke   d. Subarachnoid Hemorrhage
66. **All of the following are true about Atrial fibrillation, except:**
    a. Risk of thromboembolism   *(Recent Pattern 2014-15)*
    b. Digoxin for treatment
    c. Cardioversion followed by anticoagulation
    d. Ectopic originating in pulmonary vein
67. **Congenital long QT syndrome causes death due to?**
    a. Complete heart block   *(Recent Pattern 2014-15)*
    b. Polymorphic ventricular tachycardia
    c. Acute myocardial infarction
    d. Recurrent supraventricular tachycardia
68. **All are true about WPW syndrome except?**
    a. More common in females   *(Recent Pattern 2014-15)*
    b. Delta wave in ECG
    c. HIS bundle study is done for diagnosis
    d. Can occur in a normal heart
69. **Broad complex tachycardia, due to ventricular tachycardia is suggested by all except?** *(Recent Pattern 2014-15)*
    a. Fusion Beats
    b. A V dissociation
    c. Capture Beats
    d. Termination of tachycardia by carotid Sinus massage
70. **Drug of choice in maintenance therapy in P.S.V.T is:**
    (Recent Pattern 2014-15)
    a. Amiodarone   b. Lignocaine
    c. Verapamil   d. Adenosine
71. **In a patient with wide-complex tachycardia, the presence of all of the following in the ECG indicates ventricular tachycardia except?** *(Recent Pattern 2014-15)*
    a. Atrioventricular dissociation
    b. Fusion beats
    c. Typical right bundle branch block
    d. Capture beats
72. **A chronic alcoholic develops palpitations suddenly after alcohol binge. Which of the following arrhythmia is most commonly associated with alcohol binge in the alcoholics?**
    a. Ventricular fibrillations *(AIIMS Nov 01)*
    b. Ventricular premature contractions
    c. Atrial flutter
    d. Atrial fibrillation
73. **All of the following are features of Premature Ventricular Complexes, except:** *(AI 2003)*
    a. Wide qRS complex
    b. Absent P wave
    c. Complete compensatory pause
    d. Prolonged PR interval

74. **The drug of choice in patients with Wolff-Parkinson-White syndrome with atrial fibrillation is:** *(AIIMS Nov 2003)*
    a. Digitalis
    b. Procainamide
    c. Verapamil
    d. Adenosine
75. **Radiofrequency ablation is done for:** *(AIIMS June 1998)*
    a. Ventricular tachycardia
    b. PSVT
    c. WPW
    d. Atrial tachycardia
76. **All of the following are features of Mobitz Type I block, except:** *(AI-1992)*
    a. Constant PR interval
    b. Normal qRS morphology
    c. Regular Atrial Rhythm
    d. Atrial rate > ventricular rate

Atherosclerotic CVD and Myocardial Infarction

77. **"Flipping effect" is best explained by?** *(Recent Pattern 2018)*
    a. LDH 1 > LDH 2
    b. LDH 2> LDH 1
    c. LDH 2 > LDH 3
    d. LDH 3> LDH 2
78. **A post MI patient came for follow-up after 1 month. His lipid profile shows HDL of 32mg/dl, LDL of 126mg/dl and Triglycerides of 276mg/dl. What is the best management of this patient?** *(AIIMS May 2017)*
    a. Atorvastatin 80mg
    b. Rosuvastatin 20mg
    c. Fenofibrate
    d. Rosuvastatin + Fenofibrate
79. **A 60-year-old male is on aspirin, ACE inhibitor, nitrates and beta blocker for chronic stable angina. Since new-year party he is having long lasting angina pain every day for past 3 days at rest. ECG was normal and Troponin I levels are normal. Which is the best management of this patient?**
    a. Admit and start heparin *(Recent Pattern Questions)*
    b. Admit and start thrombolysis
    c. Admit and observe for rise of cardiac biomarkers
    d. Increase dose of long acting nitrates and manage as out patient
80. **A 55-year-old female presents with Levine sign, hiccups and vomiting episodes. On examination HR=50/min with BP =100/60 mm Hg with elevated JVP. ECG technician is yet to arrive. Which coronary artery is likely to be involved?**
    a. RCA *(Recent Pattern Questions)*
    b. LAD
    c. LCX
    d. Left main coronary artery
81. **A 45-year-old female tourist to India, presents with diffuse chest pain. She is admitted for observation and next morning she has recurrence of chest pain and ECG shows ST elevation in V1 to V4. Troponin is normal and pain is promptly relieved by SL NTG. Which of the following is the best management plan for this patient?** *(Recent Pattern Questions)*
    a. Echocardiography and anti-inflammatory therapy
    b. Exercise stress testing and long acting nitrates
    c. Coronary angiography with long acting nitrates and CCB
    d. Thallium scan and long acting nitrates
82. **A 67 year man with history of hypertension, hyperlipidemia and tobacco use has been diagnosed with infra-renal aortic aneurysm of size 3 X 3.5 cm. Which is best suited for this patient?** *(Recent Pattern Questions)*
    a. Endovascular stenting of aneurysm
    b. Serial follow up with MRI, major determinant of surgery being renal artery involvement
    c. Serial follow up with MRI, major determinant of surgery being size greater than 5-6cm
    d. Serial follow up with MRI, initiate Statins and operate in case of acute abdominal pain
83. **Which amongst the following endothelin is involved in MI?** *(Recent Question 2016-17)*
    a. Endothelin 1
    b. Endothelin 2
    c. Endothelin 3
    d. Endothelin 4
84. **VLDL is?** *(Recent Question 2016-17)*
    a. Triglyceride value/3
    b. Triglyceride value/5
    c. LDL- HDL
    d. LDL- IDL-HDL
85. **Friedewald's formula is used to calculate?**
    a. LDL cholesterol *(Recent Question 2016-17)*
    b. 10 year Mortality due to ASCVD
    c. Risk of death due to stroke
    d. Progression of ESRD
86. **High HDL cholesterol is seen in?** *(Recent Question 2016-17)*
    a. Abetalipoproteinemia
    b. Hyperalphalipoproteinemia
    c. Sitosterolemia
    d. Dysbetalipoproteinemia
87. **Choose the TRUE statement regarding the disease depicted in the given images?** *(APPG 2016)*

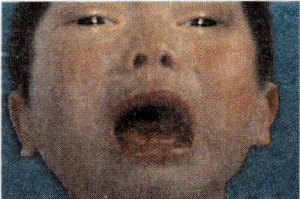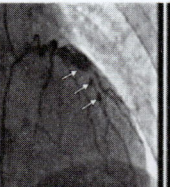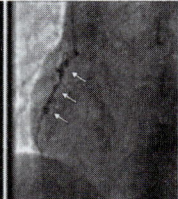

   a. Aspirin is contraindicated
   b. Bilateral purulent conjunctivitis
   c. IV immunoglobulin is used in treatment
   d. Lymphadenopathy is rare
88. **A 65-year-old elderly male has history of sweating and chest pain for last 24 hr with the following ECG. Which of the following is not given in managing the patient?** *(AIIMS Nov 15)*

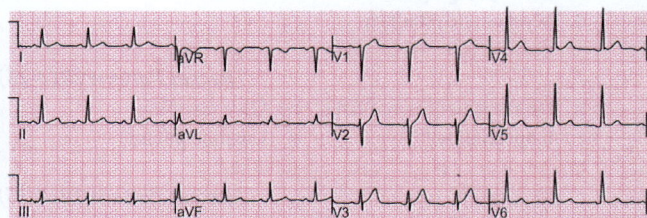

   a. Aspirin
   b. Statin
   c. Thrombolytic therapy
   d. Morphine

89. A 7-year-old boy presents with severe abdominal pain. On examination he has xanthomas. Blood drawn for work up has milky appearance of plasma. Which lipoprotein is increased? *(AIIMS May 2015)*
    a. Chylomicron
    b. Chylomicron remnants
    c. LDL
    d. HDL

90. The following statements in relation to right ventricular myocardial infarction are correct except: *(UPSC 2015)*
    a. It may occur along with inferior wall myocardial infarction
    b. The ECG shows segment elevation in right precordial leads
    c. Prognosis in right ventricular involvement in inferior wall MI is bad
    d. The treatment includes intravenous diltiazem

91. Match List-I with List-II and select the correct answer using the code given below the lists: *(UPSC 2015)*

List-I (Types of hyperlipidemia)	List-II (feature)
a. Hyper-Chylomicronaemia	1. Palmar plantar xanthoma
b. Familial hypercholesterolemia	2. Tendon xanthoma
c. Type III Hyper-lipoproteinaemia	3. Eruptive xanthoma over buttocks
d. Familial LPL deficiency	4. Triglyceride level above 1000 mg%

    Code:

	A	B	C	D
a.	3	1	2	4
b.	3	2	1	4
c.	4	1	2	3
d.	4	2	1	3

92. Which one of the following is not an early complication of acute myocardial infarction? *(Recent Question 2015-16)*
    a. Papillary muscle dysfunction
    b. Ventricular septal defect
    c. Pericarditis
    d. Dressler's syndrome

93. This 60-year-old male-diabetic and smoker-came with 3 hours of substernal pain. Which of the following statements is true regarding his ECG? *(APPG 2015)*

    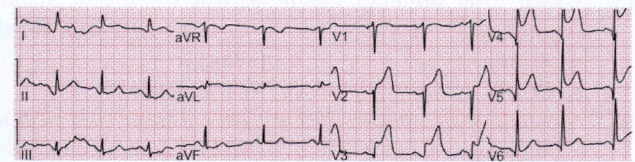

    a. Heart rate is 45/min
    b. ECG shows acute anterior myocardial infarction
    c. Patient should be given IV lidocaine
    d. ECG is suggestive of subendocardial, ischemia

94. Elevated triglycerides and decreased HDL is seen in? *(JIPMER Nov 2015)*
    a. Smoker
    b. Alcoholics
    c. Athlete
    d. Diabetes

95. Treatment of choice for STEMI? *(JIPMER Nov 2014)*
    a. Thrombolysis with altepase
    b. t-PA with streptokinase
    c. Primary percutaneous coronary intervention
    d. Low molecular weight heparin

96. Reversible myocardial ischemia is best diagnosed by: *(JIPMER Nov 2014)*
    a. MUGA scan
    b. Thallium scan
    c. PET scan
    d. Coronary angiogram

97. In an established case of coronary artery disease Post MI which of the following drug will not prolong life expectancy?
    a. ACE inhibitors
    b. Statin *(JIPMER Nov 2014)*
    c. Aspirin
    d. Nitrate

98. Feature of unstable angina: *(PGI Chandigarh May 2015)*
    a. ↑ Troponin
    b. Elevation of ST segment
    c. Depression of ST segment
    d. Q wave
    e. T wave inversion

99. Digitalis is used in mitral stenosis when patient develops? *(Recent Question 2015-16)*
    a. Atrial fibrillation
    b. Right ventricular failure
    c. Acute pulmonary edema
    d. Myocarditis

100. Which of the following is given to decrease Serum Triglycerides? *(Recent Question 2015-16)*
    a. Fibrates
    b. Statins
    c. Ezetimibe
    d. Niacin

101. Which is the best way to differentiate between stable angina and NSTEMI? *(Recent Question 2015-16)*
    a. ECG
    b. Cardiac-biomarker
    c. Trans thoracic Echocardiography
    d. Multi uptake gated Acquisition scan

102. Aetiology of Dressler Syndrome is? *(Recent Question 2015-16)*
    a. Viral
    b. Autoimmune
    c. Idiopathic
    d. Toxin mediated

103. A 65-year-old male had MI one year ago. Now the same patient presents with hypertension. Which of the following drug is best suited for this patient? *(Recent Question 2015-16)*
    a. Clonidine
    b. Thiazide
    c. Metoprolol
    d. Lisinopril

104. All are used for secondary prevention of MI except: *(Recent Question 2015-16)*
    a. Aspirin
    b. Statins
    c. Beta blockers
    d. Warfarin

105. Coronary artery disease is associated with all EXCEPT: *(Recent Question 2015-16)*
    a. Chlamydia
    b. Poor dental hygiene
    c. Smoking
    d. Alcohol

106. A 50-year old man who had recently joined a gym collapsed on the treadmill. He was rushed to the hospital where an ECG shows presence of: *(Recent Question 2015-16)*

    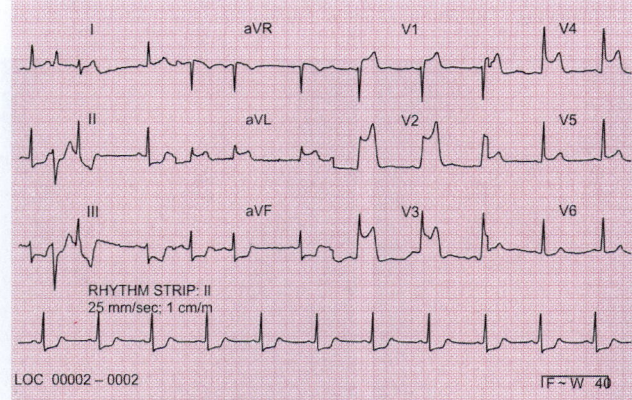

    a. Acute extensive anterior wall MI
    b. Brugada syndrome
    c. Catecholamine sensitive ventricular tachycardia
    d. Arrhythmogenic right ventricular dysplasia

107. A 65-year old man presents with crushing chest pain for 2 hours. On examination BP = 80/60 mm Hg and JVP is elevated 4 cm above the sternal angle. All are true about the condition shown except: *(Recent Question 2016-17)*

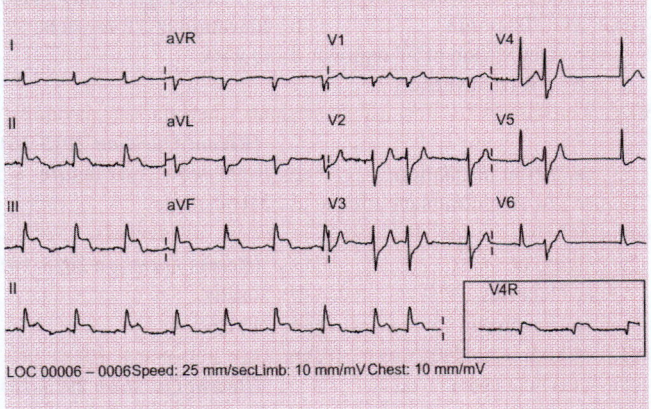

   a. ST elevation in V4R
   b. ST segment depression in lead II, III, aVF
   c. Right ventricular infarction
   d. Cardiogenic shock

108. A 65-year-old diabetic with extensive sweating and dizziness. ECG shows presence of: *(Recent Question 2016-17)*

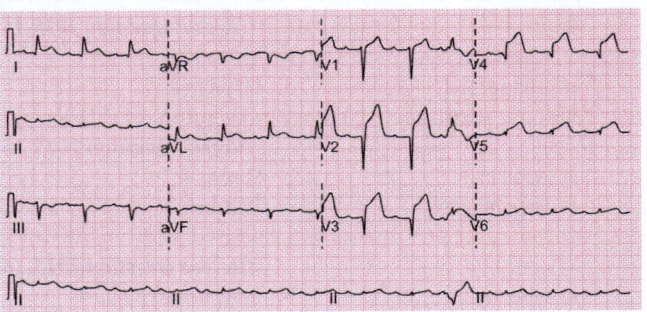

   a. Hypoglycemia
   b. Hypoglycemic unawareness
   c. Anterior wall MI
   d. Inferior wall MI

109. A 15-year old obese teenager presents with lesions on elbows and knees. He has positive family history of coronary artery disease. The images below show:

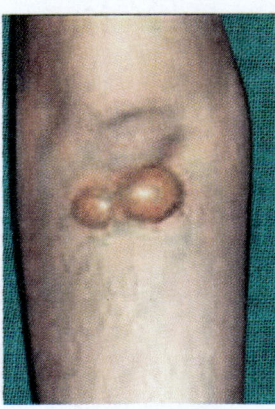
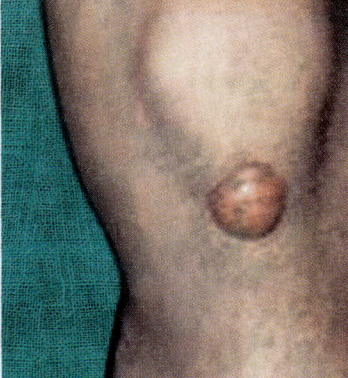

   a. Bursitis
   b. Eruptive xanthoma
   c. Tendon xanthoma
   d. Xanthoma disseminatum

110. A 25-year old patient with history of recent respiratory tract infection complains of severe chest pain at rest. The ECG of the patient is given. The most probable diagnosis of the patient is:

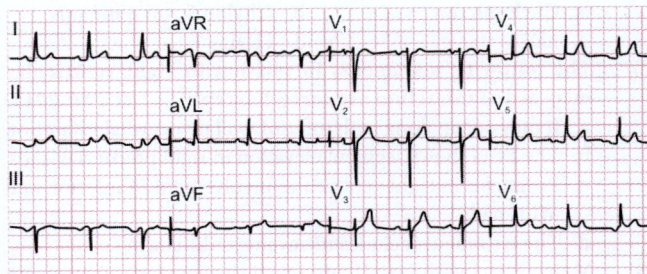

   a. Acute MI
   b. Prinzmetal angina
   c. Takotsubo cardiomyopathy
   d. Acute pericarditis

111. A patient undergoes a cardiac stress test the results of which are given below:

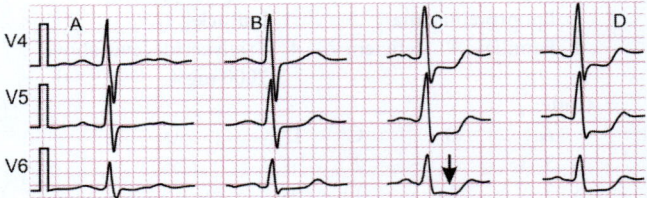

   What is incorrect about this patient?
   a. Patient has fixed stenotic lesion in left circulation
   b. ST depression of > 2 mm in chest leads is present
   c. Nitrates are mortality reducing drugs
   d. Chest pain lasts for duration less than 5 minutes

112. Which of the following is the best test for viable myocardium after MI? *(JIPMER 2014)*
   a. Thallium scan
   b. MUGA scan
   c. MDCT
   d. Stress Echocardiography

113. Which drug prolongs life in patient of chronic stable angina? *(JIPMER 2014)*
   a. Aspirin
   b. β Blocker
   c. CCB
   d. ACE inhibitor

114. A patient with anterior wall MI was thrombolysed within 6 hours with STK. On day 3 he had fever with chills and platelet count of 60,000. Which of the following is responsible for this presentation? *(Recent Pattern 2015-16)*
   a. Aspirin
   b. Ranolazine
   c. STK
   d. Clopidogrel

115. ROSE questionnaire is used for? *(Recent Pattern 2015-16)*
   a. Alcohol addiction
   b. Sex addiction
   c. Angina assessment
   d. Deep Vein thrombosis Assessment

116. Which is best for plaque morphology?
   a. CCTA *(Recent Pattern 2015-16)*
   b. MRI
   c. Optical Coherence Tomography
   d. IVUS

117. All are true regarding universal definition of MI except?
    a. Sudden death is seen in MI (AIIMS May 2012)
    b. New regional wall motion with increased biochemical marker is MI
    c. 3 x Troponin elevation is required for CABG related MI
    d. Re-infarction can be diagnosed if elevation in troponin level by 20% on serial sampling

118. A patient suffered a transmural myocardial infarction. He was started on streptokinase and warfarin. Which of the following finding on further examination is an indication for stopping thrombolytics? (AIIMS May 2013)
    a. Mobitz type II block
    b. Pericardial fluid collection on Echocardiography
    c. Deep vein thrombosis in the leg
    d. Pericardial friction rub

119. A young male patient presents with LDL 600 mg/dl, triglycerides 140 mg/dl. What would be the most likely finding on physical examination? (AIIMS May 2012)
    a. Tendon xanthoma   b. Lipemia retinalis
    c. Palmar xanthoma   d. Tuberous xanthoma

120. Thrombolytics can be given in treatment of acute myocardial infarction, if patient comes within:
    a. 3 hrs   b. 6 hrs   (AIIMS May 2013)
    c. 12 hrs   d. 24 hrs

121. Which of the following is not a contraindication to thrombolysis? (Recent Pattern 2014-15)
    a. BP>180/110 mm Hg
    b. Diabetic retinal flame shaped hemorrhage
    c. History of previous cerebral bleed
    d. Aortic dissection

122. Dose of streptokinase to be used in MI is? (Recent Pattern 2014-15)
    a. 0.15 Million units   b. 1.5 Million units
    c. 15 Million units   d. 150 Million units

123. Dose of reteplase for management of MI is? (Recent Pattern 2014-15)
    a. 5 IU   b. 10 IU
    c. 15 IU   d. 50 IU

124. Most common cause of sudden death (< 24 hours) in MI is? (Recent Pattern 2014-15)
    a. Cardiogenic shock   b. Ventricular fibrillation
    c. Mobitz 1 heart block d. Cardiac rupture

125. A patient of acute Myocardial infarction with ECG showing ST segment elevation has severe hypotension. Immediate management of the patient is: (Recent Pattern 2014-15)
    a. Intra-aortic balloon pump b. PCI with angioplasty
    c. Thrombolysis   d. Intravenous fluids

126. Wellen's syndrome is seen with: (Recent Pattern 2014-15)
    a. Stable angina   b. Unstable angina
    c. Prinzmetal angina   d. Ludwig angina

127. Half- life of alteplase? (Recent Pattern 2014-15)
    a. 3 min   b. 6 min
    c. 9 min   d. 12 min

128. Persistent ST segment elevation 24 hours after treatment for MI with P.C.I is due to (Recent Pattern 2014-15)
    a. Left ventricular aneurysm
    b. Impending cardiac rupture
    c. Dressler syndrome
    d. Coronary artery dissection

129. Most common arrhythmia seen after reperfusion strategy in MI? (Recent Pattern 2014-15)
    a. A.I.V.R   b. V.T
    c. V.fibrillation d. P.S.V.T

130. Correct sequence of ECG changes in acute Ml is? (Recent Pattern 2014-15)
    a. T inversion, ST elevation, Q wave
    b. ST elevation, T inversion, Q wave
    c. ST elevation, Q wave, T inversion
    d. Q wave, ST elevation, T inversion

131. False positive troponin I can be seen in all except?
    a. Blunt trauma chest (Recent Pattern 2014-15)
    b. Pulmonary embolism
    c. Chronic liver failure
    d. Renal failure

132. A hypertensive patient is brought with a BP of 220/130 mmHg to the casuality. CT scan shows an infarct. What should be the primary BP of the patient to start thrombolysis? (Recent Pattern 2014-15)
    a. <200/150   b. <180/110
    c. <165/120   d. <140/90

133. CAD is related to decreased levels of which HDL: (Recent Pattern 2014-15)
    a. HDL1   b. HDL 2
    c. HDL 3   d. HDL 4

134. Pulsus alternans is seen in? (Recent Pattern 2014-15)
    a. Anterior wall MI   b. Bronchial asthma
    c. Critical aortic stenosis d. Constrictive pericarditis

135. All are associated with increased risk of coronary events except: (Recent Pattern 2014-15)
    a. High sensitivity CRP
    b. High Agatson score
    c. Intravascular IVUS showing lumen reduction
    d. Ability to complete stage 3 of Bruce protocol treadmill

136. In myocardial infarction, the correct sequence of increase in enzyme levels is: (Recent Pattern 2014-15)
    a. CPK, AST, LDH   b. CPK, LDH, AST
    c. AST, CPK, LDH   d. LDH, CPK, AST

137. An athlete presents with chest pain, which of the following tests would be most sensitive and specific for diagnosis of myocardial infarction? (AIPG Jan 2012)
    a. Troponin I and T   b. Creatine kinase-MB
    c. Leukocytosis   d. C-reactive protein

138. All are true regarding Prinzmetal's Variant Angina (PVA) except? (Bihar PG 2014)
    a. Detection of transient elevation of ST segment with rest pain
    b. Silent ischemia
    c. Focal spasm is most common in left coronary artery
    d. Coronary angiography which demonstrates transient coronary spasm is the diagnostic hallmark

139. Which of the following is associated with atherosclerosis? (Recent Pattern 2014-15)
    a. Chlamydia trachomatis   b. Chlamydia pneumoniae
    c. Chlamydia psittaci   d. Chlamydia gingivalis

140. Usual duration of chest pain in chronic stable Angina is? (Recent Pattern 2014-15)
    a. 1–3 minutes   b. 5–10 minutes
    c. 15–30 minutes   d. >30 minutes

141. **Unstable angina is characterized by?** *(Recent Pattern 2014-15)*
    a. Decrescendo pattern of symptoms
    b. Crescendo pain with ECG findings
    c. ST segment elevation
    d. Normal cardiac biomarkers

142. **Which is incorrect about Dressler syndrome?**
    a. Post MI pericarditis *(Recent Pattern 2014-15)*
    b. Post MI pleuritis
    c. Autoimmune
    d. Treatment with steroids is necessary

143. **A 50-year-old lady presents with cold intolerance, constipation, hoarseness of voice. On Chest X-Ray cardiomegaly is present. Investigation to diagnose the condition:** *(AIIMS May 2013)*
    a. Coronary angiography   b. Lt ventriculography
    c. Rt.ventriculography   d. Echocardiography

144. **Dressler's syndrome is characterized by?**
    a. Onset within 72 hours *(Recent Pattern 2014-15)*
    b. Treatment of choice is steroids
    c. Pericardial effusion   d. Angina

145. **What is diagnostic of fresh myocardial infarction in ECG:**
    a. QT interval prolongation b. P mitrale *(AIIMS May 95)*
    c. ST segment elevation   d. ST segment depression

146. **Exercise testing is absolutely contraindicated in which one of the following:** *(AI 2003)*
    a. One week following myocardial infarction
    b. Unstable angina
    c. Symptomatic severe aortic stenosis
    d. Peripheral vascular disease

147. **All of the following are risk factors for atherosclerosis except:**
    a. Increased waist - hip ratio *(AI 2006)*
    b. Hyperhomocysteinemia
    c. Decreased fibrinogen levels
    d. Decreased HDL levels

148. **Which of the following is the best marker to predict future cardiac events** *(DNB June 2012)*
    a. hs CRP   b. Homocystine
    c. Interleuken-6   d. LDL

149. **Most important predictor of coronary artery disease is:**
    a. VLDL   b. LDL *(AIIMS May 2009)*
    c. Chylomicron   d. LDL/HDL

150. **Which of the following dietary interventions has shown to reduce mortality in patients with coronary heart disease.-**
    a. High Fibre diet   *(AIIMS May 2007)*
    b. Steral Esters
    c. Potassium supplements
    d. Omega 3 polysaturated fatty acids

151. **Most common site of myocardial infarction is:** *(AI 2007)*
    a. Anterior wall of left ventricle
    b. Posterior wall of left ventricle
    c. Posterior wall of right ventricle
    d. Inferior wall of left ventricle

152. **All of the following arteries are common sites of occlusion except:** *(AIIMS May 2005)*
    a. Left anterior descending
    b. Right coronary artery
    c. Circumflex coronary artery
    d. Marginal artery

153. **In stable angina:** *(AIIMS Nov 2003)*
    a. CK-MB is elevated
    b. Troponin I is elevated
    c. Myoglobin is elevated
    d. The levels of cardiac markers remain unchanged

154. **A patient presents 12 hours following a Myocardial infarction. Test of choice:** *(AIIMS June 1998)*
    a. Lactate dehydrogenase
    b. Cardiac troponins
    c. Creatinine phosphokinase
    d. Myoglobin

155. **Which of the following is the preferred marker for detecting Acute STEMI in Atheletes:** *(AI 2012)*
    a. CK-MB   b. Troponin T/I
    c. C-Reactive Protein   d. LDH

156. **Agent of first choice in an acute attack of Prinzmetal's angina is:** *(AI 1995)*
    a. Diltiazem   b. Nitrates
    c. Propranolol d. Verapamil

157. **A patient presents with acute anterior wall infarction and hyotension. Which will be the immediate treatment modality for this patient:** *(AI 2007)*
    a. Intra-aortic balloon counter pulsation
    b. Anticoagulation
    c. Thrombolytic therapy
    d. Primary angioplasty

158. **All of the following drugs are used in the management of acute myocardial infarction, except:** *(AIIMS May 2004)*
    a. Tissue Plasminogen activator
    b. Intravenous beta blockers
    c. Acetylsalicylic acid
    d. Calcium channel blockers

159. **Streptokinase and Urokinase are contraindicated in:**
    a. Intracranial malignancy *(AI 2010)*
    b. Massive pulmonary embolism
    c. AV fistula
    d. Thrombophlebitis

160. **A patient with acute inferior wall myocardial infarction has developed hypotension with kussmaul sign. Which of the following is the most likely cause of?** *(AIIMS May 2004)*
    a. Cardiac rupture
    b. Interventricular septal perforation
    c. Papillary muscle rupture
    d. Right ventricular infarction

161. **In a patient with myocardial infarction the valvular lesion is commonly seen in:** *(AIIMS May 2002)*
    a. Aortic stenosis   b. Mitral regurgitation
    c. Aortic regurgitation d. Septal defect

162. **A new systolic murmur after Acute myocardial infarction may be due to all of the following except:**
    a. Complete heart block *(AIIMS May 2002)*
    b. Rupture of Interventricular septum
    c. Papillary muscle dysfunction
    d. Ischemic cardiomyopathy

163. **Which test is performed to detect reversible myocardial ischemia?** *(AIIMS May 2003)*
    a. Coronary angiography   b. MUGA scan
    c. Thallium scan   d. Resting echocardiography

164. A young patient sustains cardiac arrest, in the medical ward. Immediate defibrillation is advised when the ECG shows: *(AI 2004)*
    a. Ventricular Tachycardia
    b. Asystole
    c. Electromechanical dissociation
    d. Persistant Bradyarrhythmia

165. All of the following statements regarding subendocardial infarction are true, except: *(AI 2006)*
    a. These are multifocal in nature
    b. These often result from hypotension or shock
    c. Epicarditis is not seen
    d. These may result in aneurysm

Valvular Lesions of Heart

166. Absence of loud first heart sound in mitral stenosis indicates all except? *(AIIMS Nov 2017)*
    a. Mild MS
    b. Calcified mitral valve
    c. Presence of aortic regurgitation
    d. 1st degree heart block

167. Which of the following is true about mitral valve prolapse? *(Recent Pattern Questions)*
    a. Displacement of one or both mitral valve leaflets posteriorly into left atrium during systole
    b. Migration of systolic click and systolic murmur towards S1 during squatting
    c. Prophylactic beta blockers
    d. Restriction of vigorous exercise to mitigate risk of sudden cardiac death

168. Which is the most common arrhythmia in patients with Mitral valve Prolapse? *(Recent Pattern Questions)*
    a. Premature ventricular contraction
    b. Atrial fibrillation
    c. Atrial flutter
    d. Ventricular tachycardia

169. Which of the following is not seen in MVP?
    a. Transient ischemic attack *(Recent Pattern Questions)*
    b. Infective endocarditis
    c. Premature ventricular contractions
    d. Defect in type IV collagen

170. All of the following clinical findings are seen in a patient with isolated aortic stenosis except? *(AIIMS May 2016)*
    a. Left ventricular impulse is displaced laterally
    b. Pulsus bisferiens is hallmark finding
    c. Systemic BP is normal in early stages of disease
    d. Carotid thrill

171. A 18-year-old boy is brought to your hospital with loss of consciousness. He regains consciousness in the ER, and GCS on admission is 12/15. CNS examination is normal and auscultation reveals a narrow split S2 and clear lungs. ECG was done. Diagnosis is? *(Recent Question 2016-17)*

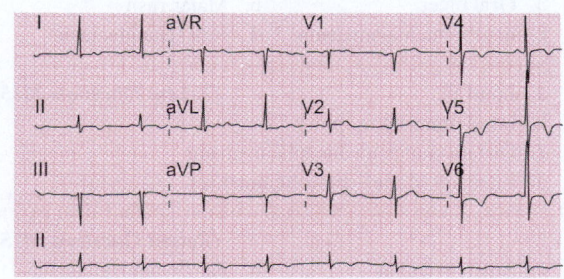

a. Left outflow tract obstruction
b. Right outflow tract obstruction
c. Atrial fibrillation with cerebral embolism
d. Subarachnoid haemorrhage with T wave inversion

172. Which is the valvular lesion being repaired in this 20-year-old man with malar flush? *(Recent Question 2016-17)*

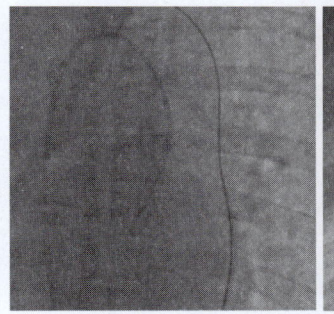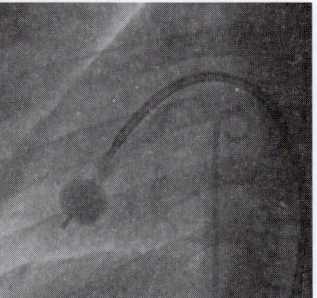

a. Mitral stenosis   b. Mitral regurgitation
c. Aortic stenosis   d. Aortic regurgitation

173. Hockey-stick appearance in echocardiography is a feature of? *(UPSC 2015)*
    a. Mitral stenosis   b. Mitral incompetence
    c. Aortic stenosis   d. Aortic regurgitation

174. Hepatomegaly with liver pulsation indicates?
    a. TR   b. MR
    c. Pulmonary hypertension d. MS

175. Murmur heard in aortic stenosis? *(Recent Question 2015-16)*
    a. Right 2nd intercostal, low pitch murmur
    b. Apex, low pitch murmur
    c. Left Sternal area, low pitch murmur
    d. Pan-systolic murmur, high pitch murmur

176. In a patient there is dyspnea in upright position which is relieved in supine position. Diagnosis?
    a. Tachypnea *(Recent Question 2015-16)*
    b. Orthopnea
    c. Paroxysmal nocturnal dyspnea
    d. Platypnea

177. Duroziez's sign is seen in? *(Recent Question 2015-16)*
    a. Aortic Regurgitation
    b. Aortic Stenosis
    c. Mitral Stenosis
    d. Mitral Regurgitation

178. Rheumatic Heart disease diagnostic criteria includes:
 (Recent Question 2015-16)
    a. Oral ulcer
    b. Malar rash
    c. Erythema Marginatum
    d. Nail telangiectasia
179. Severity of mitral stenosis is best identified by:
    a. Loud S1 (Recent Question 2015-16)
    b. Loud opening snap
    c. Duration of mid-diastolic murmur
    d. Intensity of mid-diastolic murmur
180. Which of the following is a cause of wide pulse pressure:
 (Recent Question 2015-16)
    a. Aortic stenosis
    b. Aortic regurgitation
    c. Mitral stenosis
    d. Tricuspid stenosis
181. All are associated with pulse being checked in the picture except:

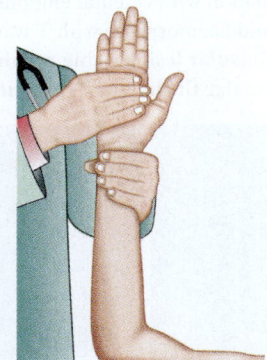

    a. Duroziez sign
    b. Early diastolic murmur
    c. Decreased LV end diastolic pressure
    d. Pulsus bisferiens
182. Which procedure is being done in the image shown?

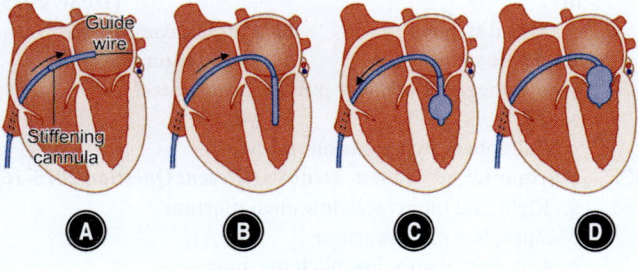

    a. Percutaneous mitral balloon valvotomy
    b. Percutaneous mitral valvuloplasty
    c. Percutaneous mitral valve repair
    d. Percutanous coronary intervention
183. Which of the following is not seen in mitral stenosis
 (AIIMS Nov 14)
    a. Loud S1
    b. Opening snap
    c. Mid diastolic murmur
    d. S3
184. In Mitral Stenosis double atrial shadow is due to enlargement of? (Recent Pattern 2015-16)
    a. Right atrium
    b. Left atrium
    c. Both atria
    d. Left auricle
185. In pregnancy which valvular disease is most dangerous?
 (Recent Pattern 2015-16)
    a. MR
    b. TS
    c. AS
    d. AR
186. A person with aortic stenosis could perform an exercise for 11 minutes in Bruce protocol. Exercise had to be stopped due to fatigue. He had a peak systolic gradient of 60 mm Hg across the aortic valve at rest. The best management for him would be (AIIMS May 2012)
    a. Medical management
    b. Aortic valve balloon dilation to prevent worsening
    c. Aortic valve replacement
    d. Coronary angiography
187. A lady presents with grade-III dyspnea. She has severe mitral stenosis with atrial fibrillation. Along with increased ventricular rate, clots in the left atrium are seen. Which of the following should not be done? (AIIMS Nov. 2012)
    a. Diltiazem to reduce the heart rate
    b. Warfarin therapy
    c. Open mitral commissurotomy and removal of clot
    d. Cardioversion with percutaneous balloon valvotomy
188. Criteria for mitral Valvotomy includes all except?
    a. Significant symptoms (Recent Pattern 2014-15)
    b. Isolated mitral stenosis
    c. Mobile non calcified valve
    d. Left atrial thrombus
189. Pulsatile liver is seen with (Recent Pattern 2014-15)
    a. Tricuspid regurgitation
    b. Tricuspid stenosis
    c. Dilated cardiomyopathy
    d. Pulmonic stenosis
190. A patient with angina, exertional syncope and Left ventricular hypertrophy is diagnosed as aortic stenosis. What is the predicted life span of this patient?
 (Recent Pattern 2014-15)
    a. 1 year
    b. 2 years
    c. 3 years
    d. 4 years
191. Displacement of cardiac apex to left and downwards indicates? (Recent Pattern 2014-15)
    a. Right ventricular hypertrophy
    b. Left ventricular hypertrophy
    c. Right atrial hypertrophy
    d. Left atrial hypertrophy
192. Incorrect about chronic aortic regurgitation is
 (Recent Pattern 2014-15)
    a. Chest pain
    b. Wide pulse pressure
    c. Quincke's sign
    d. Late systolic murmur
193. Dyspnea, syncope and angina pectoris occur most commonly in? (Recent Pattern 2014-15)
    a. MS
    b. AS
    c. MR
    d. AR
194. A patient recovered from right hemiparesis. On examination patient was found to have aortic valve lesion and is in sinus rhythm. What will you do to prevent further stroke?
    a. Anti-platelet only (AIIMS Nov. 2013)
    b. Anti-coagulant only
    c. Both anti-platelet and anticoagulant
    d. Low molecular weight heparin subcutaneously.
195. Most common valvular lesion seen with carcinoid syndrome is? (Recent Pattern 2014-15)
    a. Tricuspid stenosis and pulmonic stenosis
    b. Tricuspid insufficiency and pulmonic stenosis
    c. Mitral stenosis and aortic stenosis
    d. Mitral insufficiency and aortic stenosis

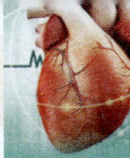

196. Area of mitral orifice in adults is: (AIIMS Dec 94)
    a. 6-8 cm²   b. 2-5 cm²
    c. 4-6 cm²   d. 1-4 cm²
197. All of the following statements about mitral valve prolapse are true except: (AIIMS Nov 93)
    a. It is more common in females
    b. Most patients are symptomatic
    c. It has a benign clinical course
    d. Transient cerebral ischemia is a known complication
198. A 26 yr old asymptomatic woman is found to have arrythmias and a systolic murmur associated with midsystolic clicks; which investigation would you use: (AI 2001)
    a. Electrophysiological testing
    b. Tc scan
    c. Echocardiography
    d. Angiography
199. Angina pectoris and Syncope are most likely to be associated with: (AI 1994)
    a. Mitral stenosis   b. Aortic stenosis
    c. Mitral regurgitation d. Tricuspid stenosis
200. Calcification of the aortic valve is seen in: (AI 95)
    a. Aortic stenosis   b. Aortic regurgitation
    c. Marfan's syndrome   d. Hurler's syndrome
201. Aortic regurgitation does NOT occur in: (AIIMS Sept 96)
    a. Acute MI   b. Marfan's syndrome
    c. Rheumatic heart disease d. Infective endocarditis
202. LVH is commonly seen with: (AI 1999)
    a. Pure mitral stenosis b. ASD with fossa-ovalis
    c. Aortic incompetence   d. Carcinoid syndrome
203. Obstruction in pulmonary stenosis may occur at the following sites: (AI 97)
    a. Supravalvular   b. Valvular
    c. Subvalvular   d. All of the above

Rheumatic Heart Disease

204. Which of the following drugs is recommended for refractory Sydenham's chorea? (Recent Pattern 2018)
    a. Steroids   b. Haloperidol
    c. Carbamazepine   d. Valproate
205. A patient presented with mitral valve stenosis, identify the diagnosis from the mitral valve histopathology depicted below? (AIIMS Nov 2017)

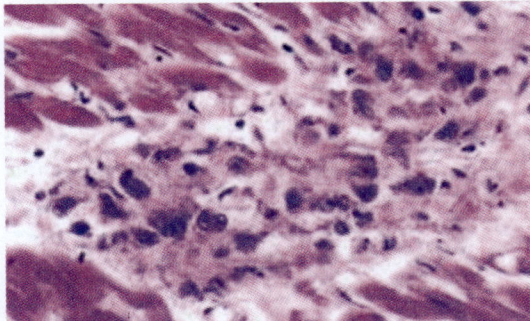

    a. Tuberculosis
    b. Rheumatic heart disease
    c. Myxomatous degeneration
    d. Viral myocarditis

206. The mechanism of autoimmunity in rheumatic fever is?
    a. Defective tolerance or regulation (APPG 2016)
    b. Molecular mimicry
    c. Break down of T cell anergy
    d. Abnormal display of self-antigen
207. A girl comes with Sydenhams chorea and acute rheumatic fever is suspected. Other major criteria of Rheumatic fever are absent. No evidence of sore throat. Best investigation to prove rheumatic etiology is? (AIIMS May 15)
    a. ASLS   b. ASLO
    c. Throat culture   d. Blood culture
208. Carey comb murmur is seen in? (Bihar PG 15)
    a. Severe mitral stenosis
    b. Acute rheumatic carditis
    c. Pure aortic regurgitation
    d. Severe pulmonary HT
209. Aschoff's nodules are seen in? (Bihar PG 15)
    a. Subacute bacterial endocarditis
    b. Libman-sacks endocarditis
    c. Rheumatic carditis
    d. Nonbacterial thrombotic endocarditis
210. In cases of streptococcal pharyngitis how early should the treatment be initiated to effectively prevent rheumatic fever? (JIPMER Nov 2014)
    a. 7 days   b. 8 days
    c. 9 days   d. 10 days
211. Not common in RHD? (AIIMS Nov. 14)
    a. MS   b. AS
    c. PS   d. TS
212. A patient presents with syncope, dyspnea & angina, what is the possible diagnosis? (AIIMS Nov. 14)
    a. Mitral stenosis   b. Aortic stenosis
    c. Pulmonic stenosis   d. Tricuspid stenosis
213. A girl presents with Syndenham's chorea. Which is the best test to prove recent infection? (AIIMS Nov. 14)
    a. ASO titer   b. Brain biopsy
    c. Anti-hyaluronidase   d. Throat swab
214. Sequel of rheumatic heart disease in a 5-year-old child is? (Recent Pattern 2014-15)
    a. Mitral regurgitation b. Mitral stenosis
    c. Tricuspid stenosis   d. Tricuspid regurgitation
215. A patient has got a history of hypersensitivity to penicillin. What is the drug that can be used for rheumatic fever prophylaxis in such a patient. (AIIMS May 2013)
    a. Sulfisoxazole   b. Sulfasalazine
    c. Streptomycin   d. Sulfadiazine
216. Which of the following is a minor criteria for diagnosis of Rheumatic Fever (RF) according to modified Jones criteria?
    a. ASO titre   (AI 2007)
    b. Past History of Rheumatic Fever
    c. Fever
    d. Subcutaneous nodules
217. Characteristic feature of Rheumatic carditis is: (AI 99)
    a. Pericarditis   b. Endocarditis
    c. Myocarditis   d. Pancarditis
218. Diagnostic feature in rheumatic heart disease is: (AI 97)
    a. Aschoff's nodule   b. Mc Callman patch
    c. Pancarditis   d. Fibrinoid Necrosis

219. True about Erythema Marginatum in Acute Rheumatic fever is: *(PGI Dec 01)*
    a. Pruritic
    b. Commonly involves face
    c. Common manifestation of Acute Rheumatic fever
    d. Usually associated with carditis

220. Earliest valvular lesion in the case of acute rheumatic fever is: *(AIIMS May 94)*
    a. Mitral regurgitation (MR)
    b. Aortic Regurgitation (AR)
    c. Mitral stenosis (MS)
    d. Aortic Stenosis (AS)

221. Site of lesion in endocarditis of RHD is: *(PGI Dec-97)*
    a. Along line of closure of valves
    b. Both sides of valves
    c. Valve cusps
    d. Free margin of valves

Murmurs and Heart Sounds

222. Which of the following murmur increases on standing? *(Recent Question 2019)*
    a. HOCM
    b. MR
    c. MS
    d. Ventricular septal defect

223. Phonocardiogram tracing is shown below with corresponding ECG. Identify the phase corresponding with S2 in phonocardiogram. *(AIIMS May 2017)*

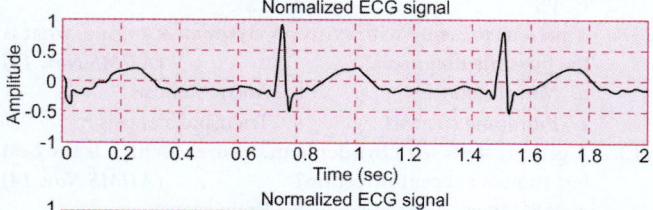
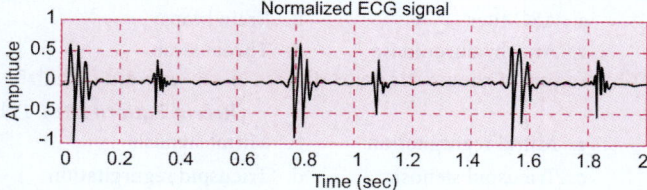

    a. A
    b. B
    c. C
    d. Data insufficient

224. A 75-year-old man is brought to the casualty with sudden syncopal episode while playing with his grandchildren. He is currently alert and describes occasional substernal heaviness and shortness of breath. His lungs have bibasilar rales and BP is 120/80mmHg. Which is the classical finding expected in this patient? *(Recent Pattern Questions)*
    a. Harsh ejection systolic murmur with Soft S2
    b. Harsh ejection systolic murmur with wide split S2
    c. Harsh Holosystolic murmur with soft 2
    d. Harsh pansystolic murmur with loud S2

225. Which is correct about Graham Steell murmur? *(Recent Pattern Questions)*
    a. High pitched, diastolic, decrescendo murmur
    b. Low pitched, diastolic, crescendo murmur
    c. High pitched, systolic, crescendo –decrescendo murmur
    d. High pitched, systolic, late systolic murmur

226. Which is correct about Austin Flint murmur? *(Recent Pattern Questions)*
    a. Soft low pitched, mid diastolic murmur
    b. Soft low pitched, mid systolic murmur
    c. Harsh high pitched, mid diastolic murmur
    d. Harsh high pitched, mid systolic murmur

227. Continuous murmur is seen in all of the following conditions except? *(AIIMS Nov 2016)*
    a. PDA
    b. Coronary AV fistula
    c. Pulmonary AV fistula
    d. VSD with aortic regurgitation

228. Match List I with List II and select the correct answer using the code given below the lists: *(UPSC 2015)*
    List I (Auscultatory findings)   List II (Cardiac condition)
    a. Wide fixed split in the second heart sound   1. Pulmonary hypertension
    b. Continuous/Machinery murmur   2. Atrial septal defect
    c. Muffled heart sounds   3. Patent ductus arteriosus
    d. Narrow split S_2 4. Pericardial effusion
    Code:
	A	B	C	D
a.	2	4	3	1
b.	2	3	4	1
c.	1	4	3	2
d.	1	3	4	2

229. Ross procedure involves: *(APPG 2015)*
    a. Replacement of aortic valve with pulmonic homograft
    b. Replacement of aortic valve with autologous pulmonic valve and implantation of pulmonic valve homograft
    c. Replacement of mitral valve with tissue prosthesis and repair of tricuspid valve
    d. Replacement of aortic valve with porcine valve and repair of pulmonary valve

230. Mid systolic click is classically heard in? *(APPG 2015)*
    a. Mitral valve prolapse
    b. Hamman- rich syndrome
    c. Rheumatic aortic regurgitation
    d. Congenital Mitral stenosis

231. Early diastolic murmur is/are seen in: *(PGI 2012)*
    a. VSD
    b. ASD
    c. Mitral stenosis
    d. AR
    e. PR

232. Reverse split S2 is seen in *(Recent Question 2015-16)*
    a. Aortic stenosis
    b. Mitral stenosis
    c. Pulmonary artery hypertension
    d. Pulmonic stenosis

233. Which is the location of Erb's point during auscultation?

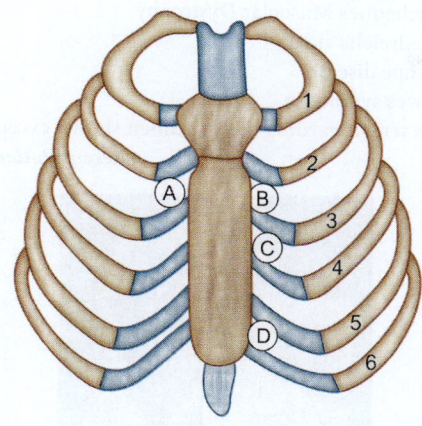

   a. A = 2nd intercostal space right parasternal line
   b. B = 2nd intercostal space left parasternal line
   c. C = 3rd intercostal space left parasternal line
   d. D = 5th intercostal space left parasternal line
234. Right murmur that decreases in intensity with inspiration *(JIPMER 2014)*
   a. Pulmonary ejection click in pulmonic stenosis
   b. Tricuspid stenosis
   c. Tricuspid regurgitation
   d. Pulmonic regurgitation
235. All form boundaries of triangle of auscultation except? *(Recent Pattern 2014-15)*
   a. Trapezius   b. Latissmus dorsi
   c. Scapula   d. Rhomboid major
236. Wrong about continuous murmur:
   a. Seen with coarctation of aorta *(Recent Pattern 2014-15)*
   b. Peaks at S2
   c. Heard both in systole and diastole
   d. Increase on squatting
237. Which is not a high pitched heart sound: *(Recent Pattern 2014-15)*
   a. Mid systolic click   b. Pericardial shudder
   c. Opening snap   d. Tumor plop sound
238. Narrow split S2 is seen in: *(Recent Pattern 2014-15)*
   a. Aortic stenosis
   b. Mitral stenosis
   c. Pulmonary artery hypertension
   d. Pulmonic stenosis
239. All are true about Physiological murmur except:
   a. Only Diastolic murmur *(Recent Pattern 2014-15)*
   b. Midsystolic murmur
   c. Present in child with anemia
   d. Not audible without stethoscope
240. Loud P2 is found in? *(Recent Pattern 2014-15)*
   a. Pulmonary HTN
   b. MS
   c. MR
   d. Aortic incompetence
241. Systolic murmur is associated with?
   a. Ejection click   *(Recent Pattern 2014-15)*
   b. Opening snap
   c. S4
   d. Pericardial knock

242. All of the following are true about S1, except:
   a. Lower frequency than S2 *(Recent Pattern 2015-16)*
   b. Caused by closure of mitral valve
   c. Heard at the end of ventricular systole
   d. Better heard with diaphragm of stethoscope
243. First heart sound is soft in all, except: *(AIIMS Dec 95)*
   a. Short PR interval   b. Ventricular septal defect
   c. Mitral regurgitation d. Calcified valve
244. Wide split S2 occurs in: *(AIIMS May 93)*
   a. VSD (ventricular septal defect)
   b. Mitral stenosis
   c. ASD (Atrial septal defect)
   d. Coarctation of aorta
245. Fixed splitting of S2 may be seen in all except: *(PGI June 95)*
   a. Pulmonary embolism   b. PS
   c. ASD   d. LBBB
246. Third heart sound is seen in all except: *(AIIMS Nov 2014)*
   a. Athletes   b. Mitral stenosis
   c. Constrictive pericarditis d. LVF
247. True about third heart sound is: *(PGI Dec-98)*
   a. Absent in chronic constrictive pericarditis
   b. Absent in aortic aneurysm
   c. Absent in MS
   d. Normal physiologically in athletes
248. S4 is seen in all of the following, except: *(AIIMS May 94)*
   a. Thyrotoxicosis
   b. Acute MI
   c. Atrial fibrillation
   d. Hypertrophic cardiomyopathy
249. All of the following heart sounds occur shortly after S2 except: *(AI 2003)*
   a. Opening snap   b. Pericardial knock
   c. Ejection click   d. Tumor plop
250. All of the following are diastolic sounds, except:
   a. S3   *(PGI- Dec-06)*
   b. S4
   c. Opening snap
   d. Ejection click
251. Which of the following murmurs increase with Valsalva maneuver? *(AIIMS Nov 2010)*
   a. MR   b. VSD
   c. AS   d. HOCM
252. Continuous murmur is found in all, EXCEPT:
   a. Mitral stenosis with mitral regurgitation *(AIIMS May 93)*
   b. Patent ductus arteriosus
   c. Rupture of sinus of Valsalva
   d. Systemic Arterio Venous (AV) fistula
253. Continuous murmur is present in (select two options)
   a. PDA   *(PGI June 06)*
   b. AS with AR
   c. Shunt between pulmonary & subclavian artery
   d. VSD with AR
254. During the cardiac cycle the opening of the aortic valve takes place at the: *(AI 04)*
   a. Beginning of systole
   b. End of isovolumetric contraction
   c. End of diastole
   d. End of diastasis

Cardiomyopathy

255. A healthy middle – aged man was arguing with his brother and got so emotionally upset due to the arguments, that he suddenly developed chest pain and collapsed. When brought to the hospital, he was declared dead. What is the diagnosis? **(AIIMS May 2018)**
    a. Takotsubo cardiomyopathy
    b. Dilated cardiomyopathy
    c. Arrhythmogenic right ventricle dysplasia
    d. Chronic ischemic cardiomyopathy

256. "Myocardial stunning" is seen in? **(Recent Pattern 2018)**
    a. Restrictive cardiomyopathy
    b. Cardiac tamponade
    c. Takotsubo cardiomyopathy
    d. Pericardial shudder

257. A multi parous P3 L3 young lady who delivered normally 3 weeks ago suddenly developed dyspnea with cardiac failure. She has no H/O cardiac disease before /during pregnancy. She had tachycardia and peripheral oedema. Her haemoglobin was 9 gm/dl. Her Echocardiogram has revealed an EF of 35%. Which one of the following is the Most Likely Diagnosis? **(APPG 2016)**
    a. Acute MI
    b. Deep vein thrombosis with pulmonary embolism
    c. Amniotic fluid embolism
    d. Peripartum cardiomyopathy

258. Which disorder of carbohydrate metabolism typically has Cardiac involvement? **(APPG 2016)**
    a. Glycogen Storage Disease Type II (Pompe)
    b. Galactosemia
    c. Glycogen Storage Disease Type I (von Gierke)
    d. Hereditary fructose intolerance

259. An athlete collapsed suddenly and died on field. Post-mortem heart is shown in the figure. There is family history of heart disease. What is your diagnosis? **(AIIMS Nov 15)**

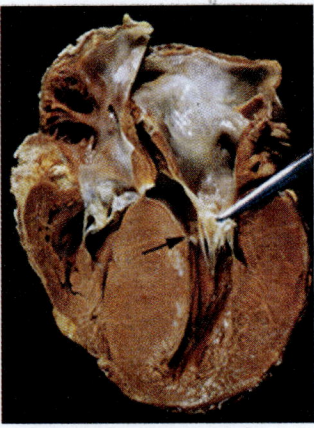

    a. Hypertrophic cardiomyopathy
    b. Mitral regurgitation
    c. Mitral stenosis
    d. Aortic stenosis with left ventricular hypertrophy

260. Which of the following drugs is not given in dilated cardiomyopathy? **(UPSC 2015)**
    a. Beta blocker
    b. Calcium channel blocker
    c. Spironolactone
    d. ACE inhibitors

261. Cardiomyopathy is not a feature of? **(Bihar PG 15)**
    a. Duchenne's Muscular Dystrophy
    b. Friedreich's ataxia
    c. Pompe disease
    d. Lowe's syndrome

262. All are true regarding the specimen shown except: **(Recent Pattern 2015-16)**

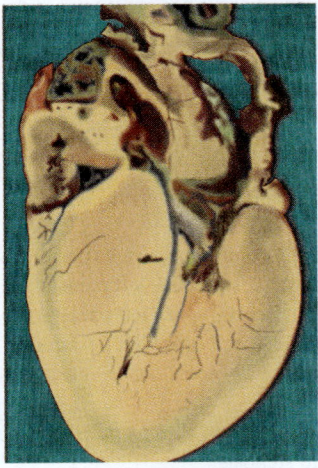

    a. Asymmetrical septal hypertrophy
    b. Left ventricular outflow tract obstruction
    c. Diamond-shaped cavity of left ventricle
    d. Diastolic dysfunction

263. Not a Single gene disorder? **(JIMPER-2014)**
    a. Mitral Valve Prolapse
    b. Hypertrophic obstructive Cardiomyopathy
    c. Dilated Cardiomyopathy
    d. Arrhythmogenic Right Ventricular Cardiomyopathy

264. 25-year-old footballer is elbowed in the chest by the rival defender during ball possession. Following the chest trauma the player collapses and dies. The most probable cause of death is: **(Recent Pattern 2014-15)**
    a. HOCM
    b. Commotio cordis
    c. Hemothorax
    d. Aortic transection

265. Cardiomyopathy does not occur in?
    a. Duchenne muscular dystrophy **(Recent Pattern 2014-15)**
    b. Alkaptonuria
    c. Pompe disease
    d. Fabry's disease

266. RCM is caused by all except: **(Recent Pattern 2014-15)**
    a. Fatty infiltration of myocardium
    b. Amyloidosis
    c. Daunorubicin
    d. Carcinoid syndrome

267. Incorrect about Broken heart syndrome?
    a. Catecholamine toxicity **(Recent Pattern 2014-15)**
    b. ST elevation
    c. Apical ballooning
    d. Dobutamine for cardiogenic dysfunction

268. Banana shaped left ventricle is seen in?
    a. HOCM **(Recent Pattern 2014-15)**
    b. DCM
    c. RCM
    d. Takotsubo cardiomyopathy

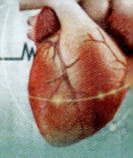

269. Which of following is a treatable cause of RCM?
    a. Fabry's disease   (Recent Pattern 2014-15)
    b. Amyloidosis
    c. Endomyocardial fibroelastosis
    d. Hypereosinophilic syndrome
270. Incorrect about restrictive cardiomyopathy:
    a. Kussmaul's sign   (Recent Pattern 2014-15)
    b. Pulsatile liver
    c. Pedal edema
    d. Dip and spike configuration in ventricular systolic pressure.
271. In case of sudden death in a young football player, the first clinical suspicion would rest on which of the following differentials?   (Recent Pattern 2014-15)
    a. Arrthymogenic right ventricular dysplasia
    b. Takotsubo cardiomyopathy
    c. Atrial septal defect
    d. Eisenmenger complex
272. Drug contraindicated in HOCM is?
    (Recent Pattern 2014-15)
    a. Verapamil   b. Propranolol
    c. Digoxin   d. None of the above
273. Dicrotic pulse is seen in?   (Recent Pattern 2014-15)
    a. HOCM   b. DCM
    c. RCM   d. Left ventricular failure
274. Which Cardiomyopathy is caused by chronic alcoholism?
    (Recent Pattern 2014-15)
    a. Dilated   b. Hypertrophic
    c. Atrophy   d. Restrictive
275. All are true about hypertrophic cardiomyopathy, except:
    a. Systolic dysfunction   (AIIMS 1996)
    b. Concentric hypertrophy
    c. Diastolic dysfunction
    d. Double apical impulse

Pericardial Diseases

276. A male patient is brought to ER after a car crash. He had dyspnea with chest pain and ecchymosis on the anterior chest wall. On examination pulse rate is 120/min with BP= 80/50 mm Hg, elevated JVP and reduced breath sounds on left side of chest. Pelvis and extremities are normal. Diagnosis is?   (AIIMS May 2018)
    a. Tension pneumothorax   b. Cardiac tamponade
    c. Neurogenic shock   d. Distributive shock
277. Which parameter is the best to differentiate cardiac tamponade from tension pneumothorax?
    a. Raised JVP   (AIIMS Nov 2018)
    b. Breath sounds
    c. Raised Heart rate
    d. Not improving after initial fluid resuscitation
278. While measuring blood pressure of cardiac tamponade patient what advise will you give him?   (AIIMS Nov 2018)
    a. Hold breath
    b. Breath normally
    c. Long and deep breathing
    d. Short and shallow breaths

279. A patient with suspected cardiac tamponade is admitted to your ward. Which of the following is correct about examination of the patient?   (AIIMS May 2016)
    a. BP cuff is inflated 20 mmHg above the systemic pressure
    b. Pulsus paradoxus is absent in patients with low pressure cardiac tamponade
    c. Patient is asked to take deep breaths during BP measurements
    d. BP is measured when the first korotkoff sound is heard only during expiration
280. Which of the following can differentiate between Cardiac tamponade and Tension pneumothorax?   (AIIMS Nov 15)
    a. JVP   b. Pulse volume
    c. Breath Sounds   d. Pulse rate
281. This patient, previously healthy, came with dyspnea and low grade fever since 4 months. His lungs are clear. JVP is normal. ECG showed low voltage complexes. What is the possible diagnosis?   (APPG 2015)

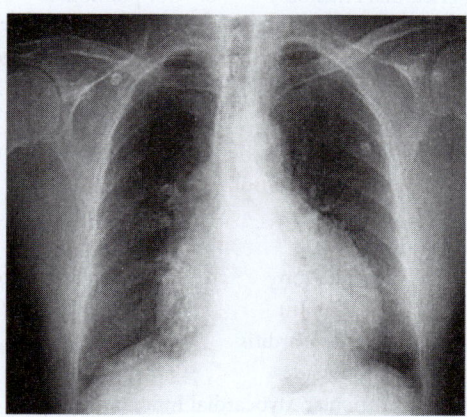

    a. Syphilitic aortic aneurysm
    b. Hypertrophic cardiomyopathy
    c. Rheumatic mitral stenosis
    d. Tuberculous pericardial effusion
282. Beck's triad of cardiac tamponade includes all, except?
    a. Hypotension   b. Increased JVP
    c. Muffled Heart sounds   d. Tachycardia
283. Features of Constrictive pericarditis which differentiate from restrictive cardiomyopathy:
    (PGI Chandigarh May 2015)
    a. Prominent X descent   b. Pericardial knock
    c. Fourth heart sound   d. Thickened pericardium
    e. Right ventricular hypertrophy
284. Hypotension with muffled sounds and congested neck veins is seen in?   (Recent Question 2015-16)
    a. Cardiac tamponade
    b. Pericardial effusion
    c. Constrictive pericarditis
    d. Acute congestive heart failure
285. Incorrect about Dressler syndrome is?
    a. Post MI pericarditis   (Recent Question 2015-16)
    b. Post MI pleuritis
    c. Autoimmune
    d. Treatment with steroids is necessary

286. A 60-year-old smoker presents with breathlessness for 2 weeks. On examination: heart rate is 100/min, BP = 90/60 mm Hg and neck veins are distended with a palpable liver. CXR is shown. Probable diagnosis is?

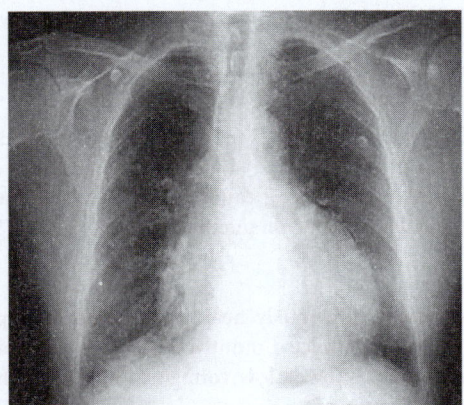

   a. Pericardial effusion   b. Cor pulmonale
   c. Broken heart syndrome   d. Brugada syndrome

287. Restrictive and constrictive pericarditis occurs together in: *(Recent Pattern 2014-15)*
   a. Radiation   b. Adriamycin
   c. Amyloidosis   d. Post cardiotomy syndrome

288. Most common presentation of cardiac lupus? *(Recent Pattern 2014-15)*
   a. Myocarditis   b. Pericarditis
   c. Aortic regurgitation d. Libman Sacks endocarditis

289. Beck's Triad is seen in: *(AI 2010)*
   a. Constrictive Pericarditis
   b. Cardiac tamponade
   c. Right Ventricular Myocardial Infarction (RVMI)
   d. Restrictive Cardiomyopathy

290. All of the following statements about chronic constrictive pericarditis are true except *(PGI Dec 99)*
   a. Commonest cause in India is 'Idiopathic'
   b. Kussmaul's sign is present
   c. Ascites
   d. Right ventricular End Diastolic pressure is raised

Congestive Heart Failure

291. Which of the following is not successful in measuring cardiac output? *(AIIMS Nov 2018)*
   a. Transthoracic Echocardiography
   b. Central Venous Pressure
   c. Thermodilution method
   d. Pulmonary artery catheterization

292. A 40-year-old lady presents with features of NYHA class III heart failure. Her serum potassium is 4.5mg% and Serum Creatinine is 2.5mg%. Which of the following drugs is best avoided? *(AIIMS May 2017)*
   a. Spirinolactone
   b. Carvedilol
   c. Enalapril
   d. Digoxin

293. A 60-year-old diabetic woman presents with breathlessness after discontinuing her medication for hypertension. CXR was performed. Identify the Kerley B lines *(Recent Question 2016-17)*

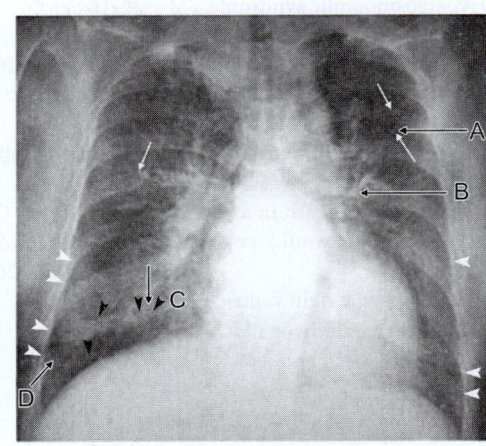

   a. Location A   b. Location B
   c. Location C   d. Location D

294. Which of the following drug is not used for management of acute pulmonary oedema? *(Recent Question 2016-17)*
   a. Norepinephrine   b. Dopamine
   c. Dobutamine   d. Phenylephrine

295. A patient came with dyspnoea, elevated JVP and oedema in the feet. Lungs are clear. There is a parasternal heave and S2 is palpable in the pulmonary area. Which one of the following is LEAST helpful in determining aetiology. *(APPG 2016)*
   a. Echo for mitral stenosis
   b. Anti-endomysial antibody estimation
   c. ELISA for HIV
   d. Urine / stool examination for Schistosoma ova

296. All are Hyperdynamic state except? *(AIIMS May 15)*
   a. Anemia   b. Beriberi
   c. Corpulmonale   d. Arterio-venous fistula

297. Treatment of digoxin over dose includes administration of all of the following except? *(Bihar PG 15)*
   a. Potassium   b. Lignocaine
   c. Phenytoin   d. Haemofiltration

298. A 26-year-old laborer presents with decreased urine output, swelling in both feet and tender hepatomegaly. CXR was done. All are true about findings of this patient except:

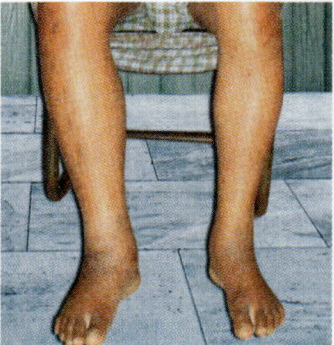 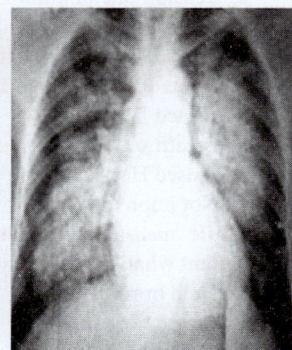

   a. Bat wing edema   b. Low urinary sodium
   c. High serum potassium d. Wide variable split S2

299. Not a marker of heart failure? (AIIMS Nov 14)
    a. CRP   b. Sirtuin
    c. BNP   d. Troponin
300. Inability to carry out any physical activity without discomfort comes under? (AIIMS Nov 14)
    a. NYHA1   b. NYHA2
    c. NYHA3   d. NYHA4
301. A patient with CHF with LVEF<40% should be given? (Recent Pattern 2015-16))
    a. ACEI + beta blocker   b. ACEI + furosemide
    c. ACEI + CCB   d. ACEI +ARB
302. Cheyne stokes breathing is seen in: (Recent Pattern 2014-15)
    a. Intracranial hypotension   b. Congestive heart failure
    c. Left atrial myoxma   d. Pickwinian syndrome
303. The treatment of acute pulmonary oedema includes all of the following except? (AIPG Jan. 2012)
    a. Morphine   b. Digoxin
    c. Frusemide   d. Positive ventilation
304. In a patient with chronic congestive cardiac failure, all of the following drugs prolong survival except:
    a. Metoprolol   b. Carvedilol (AIIMS May 04)
    c. Enalapril   d. Digoxin
305. All of the following statements about digoxin are true except: (AI 1997)
    a. Negative chronotropic effect
    b. Oral absorption is good
    c. Actively metabolized in liver
    d. Lipid soluble

Congenital Heart Disease

306. Lithium use in pregnancy leads to which effect on the baby? (AIIMS Nov 2018)
    a. CVS defect   b. Urogenital defect
    c. Neural tube defect d. Facial defect
307. Epstein syndrome is characterised by presence of?
    a. Tricuspid valve abnormality (Recent Question 2019)
    b. Large platelets
    c. Skeletal defects
    d. Joint laxity
308. Which of the following is compatible with tet spells in a 4 month old child with TOF? (AIIMS May 2016)
    a. O₂ saturation less than 75% in room air?
    b. Inability to hear a murmur
    c. Hepatomegaly   d. S3 Rhythm
309. Congenital heart disease associated with pre-excitation is? (UPSC 2015)
    a. Atrial septal defect   b. Bicuspid aorta valve
    c. Ebstein's anomaly   d. Patent ductus arteriosus
310. When should a very large ventricular septal defect be operated? (UPSC 2015)
    a. In school going age   b. Only if CHF is uncontrolled
    c. Before six months of age d. Soon after birth
311. Pulmonary blood flow increases in all except?
    a. ASD   (PGI Chandigarh May 2015)
    b. VSD
    c. TOF
    d. Transposition of great Artery
    e. PDA

312. In coarctation of aorta, site of rib notching is? (Recent Question 2015-16)
    a. Upper border   b. Lower border
    c. Costal surface   d. Vertebral end
313. Snow man appearance or figure of 8 appearance is seen in? (Recent Question 2015-16)
    a. Total anomalous pulmonary venous connection
    b. Transposition of great arteries
    c. Tetralogy of fallot   d. Tricuspid atresia
314. A neonate presents with anoxic spells and single S2. CXR shows all except:

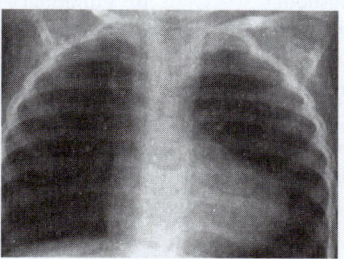

    a. Boot-shaped heart   b. Pulmonary plethora
    c. Right sided aortic arch
    d. Right ventricular hypertrophy
315. A 6-hour old child with cyanosis. On examination, S2 is loud and single. CXR was done. All are true about this condition except?

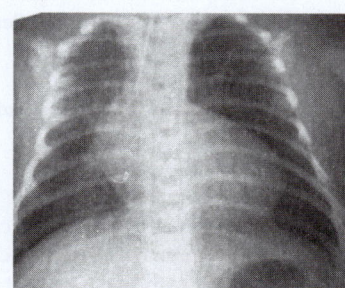

    a. Ductal dependent systemic circulation
    b. Alprostadil infusion
    c. Balloon atrial septostomy
    d. Associated with diabetes in the mother
316. A 5-year old child with episodes of recurrent pneumonia was found to have a mid-diastolic murmur. CXR was performed. All are correct about the image shown except?

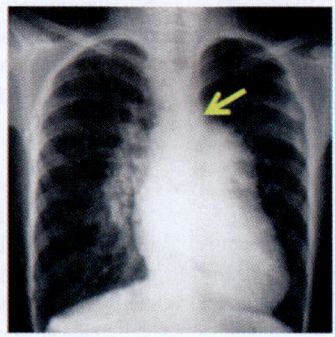

    a. Increased pulmonary plethora
    b. Enlarged left ventricle
    c. Dilated pulmonary artery trunk
    d. Increased CT ratio

317. Turner's syndrome is associated with?
    (Recent Pattern 2015-16)
    a. Coarctation of aorta   b. Aortic dissection
    c. Aortic regurgitation   d. Pulmonic stenosis
318. Most common cause of heart block in infants is?
    a. SLE   *(Recent Pattern 2015-16)*
    b. Surgery for congenital heart disease
    c. Viral myocarditis
    d. Rheumatic fever
319. A Preterm baby with PDA will have all except:
    (AIIMS Nov. 2012)
    a. CO_2 washout   b. Pulmonary hemorrhage
    c. Necrotising Enterocolitis d. Bounding pulses
320. All are causes of sudden death in infant except:
    a. Romano ward syndrome   *(Recent Pattern 2014-15)*
    b. Aortic stenosis
    c. Hypoplastic left heart syndrome
    d. Kawasaki disease
321. Neonate with cyanosis, heart failure and systolic murmur is suffering from: *(Recent Pattern 2014-15)*
    a. TOF   b. VSD
    c. TGA   d. Rheumatic fever
322. Which of the following is not given in treatment of cyanotic spell?   *(AIIMS Nov. 2013)*
    a. Phenylephrine   b. Propranolol
    c. Calcium chloride   d. Soda bicarbonate
323. Ductus arteriosus complete closure occurs at how many weeks in a term baby?   *(Recent Pattern 2014-15)*
    a. 1 week   b. 2 week
    c. 3 week   d. 4 week
324. Alprostadil is contraindicated in: *(Recent Pattern 2014-15)*
    a. Tricuspid atresia
    b. Transposition of great arteries
    c. Tetralogy of Fallot
    d. Total anomalous pulmonary venous connection (TAPVC)
325. Partial anomalous pulmonary venous connection is associated with which of the following defects?
    a. Sinus venosus ASD   *(Recent Pattern 2014-15)*
    b. Ostium primum ASD
    c. Endocardial cushion defect
    d. Tricuspid atresia.
326. Which of the following conditions causes both superior as well as inferior notching of the ribs?
    (Recent Pattern 2014-15)
    a. Coarctation of aorta   b. Hyperparathyroidism
    c. Interrupted aortic arch   d. Blalock Taussig shunt
327. Reversal of shunt is not possible in natural history of:
    (AIIMS Nov. 2012)
    a. ASD   b. VSD
    c. TOF   d. PDA
328. A preterm baby with Patent Ductus Arteriosus. All are true except: *(AIIMS May 2013)*
    a. Narrow pulse pressure   b. Necrotizing enterocolitis
    c. Continuous murmur   d. Congestive heart failure
329. Extremely bad prognosis is seen in which heart disease in pregnancy?   *(Recent Pattern 2014-15)*
    a. Repaired TOF
    b. Bicuspid aortic valve
    c. ASD
    d. Pulmonary artery hypertension
330. The commonest mode of inheritance of congenital heart disease is   *(AI 2002)*
    a. Autosomal dominant   b. Autosomal recessive
    c. Sex linked dominant   d. Multifactorial
331. All can cause recurrent pulmonary infection except:
    (AIIMS Sep 96)
    a. VSD   b. Recurrent LVF
    c. TOF   d. ASD
332. Essential criteria for TOF includes all except:
    (AIIMS Nov 07)
    a. Valvular stenosis   b. Infundibular stenosis
    c. Over riding of aorta   d. RVH
333. Which of the following is a component of Pentalogy of Fallot: *(AI 2007)*
    a. Atrial Septal Defect (ASD)
    b. Patent Ductus Arteriosus (PDA)
    c. Coarctation of Aorta (COA)
    d. Left Venticular Hypertrophy (LVH)
334. In which of the following a 'Coeur en Sabot' shape of the heart is seen: *(AI 2004)*
    a. Tricuspid atresia
    b. Ventricular septal defect
    c. Transposition of great arteries
    d. Tetralogy of Fallot
335. Potts shunt is: *(AI 2001)*
    a. Right subclavian artery to right pulmonary artery
    b. Descending aorta to left pulmonary artery
    c. Left subclavian to left pulmonary artery
    d. Ascending aorta to right pulmonary artery
336. All of the following are true about ASD except: *(AI 2001)*
    a. Right atrial hypertrophy
    b. Left atrial hypertrophy
    c. Right ventricular hypertrophy
    d. Pulmonary hypertension
337. MC cause of death in adult with PDA is: *(PGI Dec 99)*
    a. CCF   b. Infective endarteritis
    c. Rupture   d. Embolism
338. All of the following are characteristic features of Tricuspid Atresia Except: *(AIIMS Dec 98)*
    a. Left Axis deviation
    b. Right ventricular hypoplasia
    c. Pulmonary vascularity is diminished
    d. Splitting of S2
339. A 1-month-old boy is referred for failure to thrive. On examination, he shows feature of congestive failure. The femoral pulses are feeble as compared to branchial pulses. The most likely clinical diagnosis is: *(AI 2006)*
    a. Congenital aortic stenosis
    b. Coarctation of aorta
    c. Patent ductus arteriosus
    d. Congenital aortoiliac disease
340. The most common type of total anomalous pulmonary venous connection is: *(AI 2005)*
    a. Supracardiac   b. Infracardiac
    c. Mixed   d. Cardiac
341. The heart lesion not found in Congenital Rubella infection is: *(AI 1995)*
    a. ASD   b. VSD
    c. PDA   d. PS

Pulmonary Artery Hypertension

342. Which is the best anti-hypertensive drug in pulmonary hypertension? *(AIIMS May 15)*
    a. Bosentan b. Amlodipine
    c. Frusemide d. Digoxin

343. All are causes of pulmonary hypertension, except? *(Bihar PG 15)*
    a. Hyperventilation b. Morbid obesity
    c. High altitude d. Fenfluramine

344. A lady presents with complaints of dysnea. Pulse rate is 70/min while BP=110/70 mm Hg. On examination there is an early-diastolic murmur. CXR is given here. Diagnosis of the patient is?

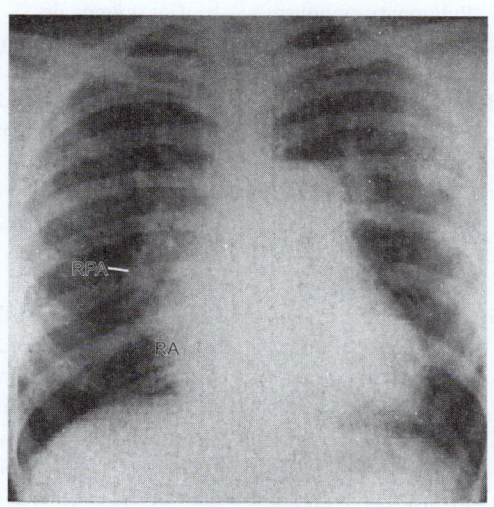

    a. Pulmonary artery hypertension
    b. Pulmonary venous hypertension
    c. Valvular lesion of left side of heart
    d. Congestive heart failure

345. All of the following pulmonary symptoms and non-pulmonary causes are correctly matched except
    a. Tachypnea : Acidosis *(AIIMS Nov. 14)*
    b. Wheezing : Congestive heart failure
    c. Cyanosis : Anxiety
    d. Chest pain : Pericarditis

346. A 35-year-old lady with Idiopathic pulmonary artery hypertension. Which findings best describe this patient *(Recent Pattern 2014-15)*
    a. Elevated JVP, normal S1 S2, diastolic murmur
    b. Elevated JVP, singular loud S2, systolic murmur
    c. Elevated JVP, wide fixed split S2, systolic murmur
    d. Elevated JVP, barrel chest reverse split S2

347. Precapillary Pulmonary hypertension is caused by all except: *(PGI June 03)*
    a. Mitral stenosis
    b. Pulmonary vasculitis
    c. Primary pulmonary hypertension
    d. Thromboembolism

348. Pulmonary hypertension in COPD is due to all, except:
    a. Hypoxia *(PGI Dec 97)*
    b. Pulmonary vasoconstriction
    c. High lung volume
    d. Bronchoconstriction

ECG

349. ECG shows a mean axis of 90 degrees. In which of the following would be present the maximum voltage of R wave? *(AIIMS Nov 2018)*
    a. III b. I
    c. aVF d. aVL

350. Pseudo-p-Pulmonale is seen in? *(Recent Pattern 2018)*
    a. Hypokalemia b. Hyperkalemia
    c. Hypomagnesemia d. Hypercalcemia

351. A 45-year-old lady presents with 1 year history of episodic leg edema and difficulty in breathing on exertion. ECG was performed. What is the most likely diagnosis?
    (Recent Pattern Questions 2018)

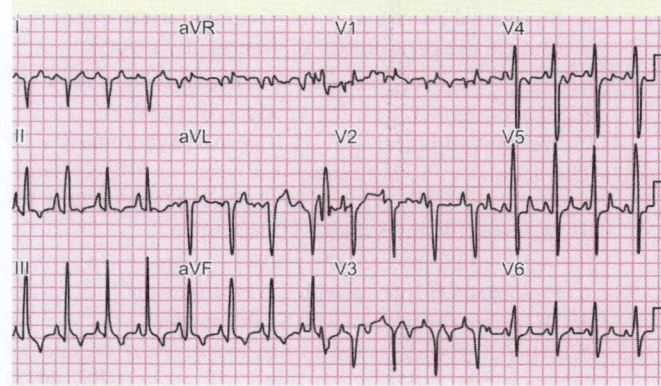

    a. Right bundle branch block
    b. Cor-pulmonale
    c. TakoTsubo cardiomyopathy
    d. Aortic stenosis

352. Which of the following is wrong about the ECG findings?
    (Recent Pattern Questions 2018)

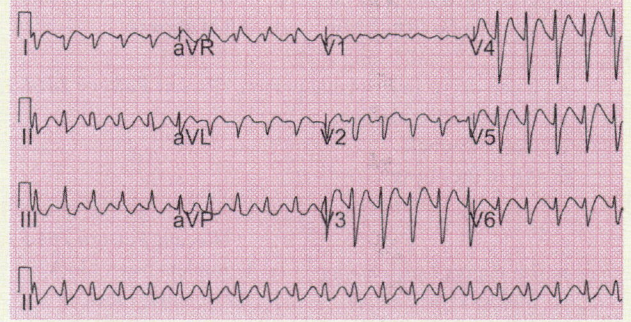

    a. Right axis deviation b. Heart rate of 150/min
    c. Broad QRS
    d. Electromechanical dissociation

353. Standard ECG leads are unable to detect?
    a. LVH b. RBBB *(JIPMER May 2015)*
    c. Right ventricular infarct d. Arrhythmia

354. LBBB is seen with all except: *(AIIMS May 2013)*
    a. Acute MI b. Ashmann syndrome
    c. Hypokalemia d. Hyperkalemia

355. What is not correct about LBBB? *(Recent Pattern 2014-15)*
    a. Can occur after MI
    b. ST segment elevation is seen
    c. A-V dissociation
    d. Cardiomyopathy is associated

356. **Epsilon waves in ECG are seen in:** *(Recent Pattern 2014-15)*
    a. Arrythmogenic right ventricular dysplasia
    b. Takotsubo cardiomyopathy
    c. Hyperthermia
    d. Restrictive cardiomyopathy

357. **QT prolongation is seen in all, except:**
    (Recent Pattern 2014-15)
    a. Hypothermia   b. Digitalis toxicity
    c. Hypocalcemia   d. Romano –ward syndrome

358. **QT interval is shortened in:** *(Recent Pattern 2014-15)*
    a. Hypocalcemia   b. Hypokalemia
    c. Hypercalcemia d. Digoxin

359. **ST elevation is seen in all of the following conditions except:**
    (Recent Pattern 2014-15)
    a. Myocardial infarction   b. Coronary artery spasm
    c. Constrictive pericarditis d. Ventricular aneurysm

360. **Inverted T waves are seen in?** *(Recent Pattern 2014-15)*
    a. Hyperkalemia   b. Hyperthermia
    c. Wellen syndrome d. Coronary syndrome X

361. **The following ECG findings are seen in Hypokalemia:**
    (Recent Pattern 2014-15)
    a. Increased PR interval with ST depression
    b. Increased PR interval with peaked T wave
    c. Prolonged QT interval with T wave inversion
    d. Decreased QT interval with ST depression

362. **Which ECG finding is most likely to be seen at the time of cardiac arrest** *(UPSC 2013)*
    a. Ventricular fibrillation
    b. Ventricular tachycardia
    c. Atrial fibrillation
    d. Paroxysmal atrial tachycardia

363. **Which of the following may occur due to hyper-kalemia:**
    (Recent Pattern 2014-15)
    a. Prolonged PR interval b. Prolonged qRS interval
    c. Ventricular fibrillation d. All of above

364. **Which of the following is cause of RBBB?**
    a. It can occur in a normal person *(Recent Pattern 2014-15)*
    b. Pulmonary embolism
    c. Corpulmonale
    d. All of the above

365. **Alternating RBBB with Left anterior hemiblock is seen in?**
    (Recent Pattern 2014-15)
    a. 1st degree heart block   b. Complete heart block
    c. Mobitz type II block   d. Bifascicular block

366. **Which is the following is the commonest ECG finding in pulmonary embolism?** *(Recent Pattern 2014-15)*
    a. Sinus Tachycardia   b. Inverted T wave in Lead III
    c. $S_1Q_3T_3$ d. Pathological Q

367. **Left axis deviation is seen in all except?**
    (Recent Pattern 2014-15)
    a. Left anterior hemi block b. Inferior wall MI
    c. ASD (Septum secundum)   d. Right pneumothorax

368. **Electrical alternans is seen in?** *(Recent Pattern 2014-15)*
    a. Cardiac tamponade   b. Constrictive pericarditis
    c. Severe LVF   d. Severe RVF

369. **Osborn wave is seen in?** *(Recent Pattern 2014-15)*
    a. WPW syndrome type I   b. Hypercalcemia
    c. Cardiac tamponade   d. Athlete

370. **All are ECG changes in hypokalemia, except:**
    a. U wave   *(Recent Pattern 2014-15)*
    b. ST segment sagging
    c. T-wave flattening or inversion
    d. QT interval shortening

371. **Low voltage ECG is seen in?** *(Recent Pattern 2014-15)*
    a. Hypothyroidism   b. Hyperthyroidism
    c. Diabetes   d. Addison's disease

372. **PR interval is reduced in?** *(Recent Pattern 2014-15)*
    a. Wenckebach phenomenon
    b. WPW syndrome
    c. Hypothyroidism
    d. Complete heart block

373. **Low voltage in ECG indicates?** *(Recent Pattern 2014-15)*
    a. Pulmonary embolism   b. Cor pulmonale
    c. Infective endocarditis d. Pericardial effusion

374. **All of the following are the electrocardiographic features of Hyperkalemia, except:** *(Recent Pattern 2014-15)*
    a. Prolonged PR interval   b. Prolonged QT interval
    c. Sine wave patterns   d. Loss of P waves

375. **In LVH, SV1 + RV6 is more than ……… mm?**
    (Recent Pattern 2014-15)
    a. 25   b. 30
    c. 35   d. 40

376. **In left sided massive pneumothorax, ECG shows all, except:**
    (Recent Pattern 2014-15)
    a. Left axis deviation   b. Absent R wave
    c. Pathological Q waves   d. Precordial T wave inversion

377. **ST elevation is seen in all of the following conditions except:**
    (AIIMS 2002)
    a. Myocardial infarction   b. Coronary artery spasm
    c. Constrictive pericarditis d. Ventricular aneurysm

378. **QT interval is shortened in:** *(AI 95)*
    a. Hypocalcemia   b. Hypophosphatemia
    c. Hypercalcemia   d. Hypernatremia

379. **All of the following may occur due to hyperkalemia, except:**
    (AI 06)
    a. Prolonged PR interval   b. Prolonged qRS interval
    c. Prolonged QT interval   d. Ventricular asystole

380. **Feature of Torsade de pointes is:** *(AIIMS Dec 97)*
    a. Wide qRS complex   b. Short qRS complex
    c. Prolonged QTc interval d. Short QTc interval

381. **Congenital long QT syndrome can lead to:**
    a. Complete heart block   *(AIIMS May 2003)*
    b. Polymorphic ventricular tachycardia
    c. Acute myocardial infarction
    d. Recurrent supraventricular tachycardia

382. **Constant PR interval is seen in:** *(PGI-1997)*
    a. First degree block
    b. Second degree – Mobitz type I block
    c. Second degree – Mobitz type II block
    d. Third degree block

383. **Electric alternans is seen in:** *(AI 1995)*
    a. Cardiac tamponade
    b. Restrictive cardiomyopathy
    c. Constructive pericarditis
    d. Right Ventricular MI (RVMI)

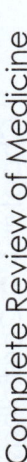

WPW and Brugada Syndrome

384. Digoxin is not used in the management of?
 (Recent Question 2016-17)
    a. Atrial fibrillation   b. Atrial flutter
    c. Low output CCF   d. W.P.W

385. A 16-year old boy has history of recurrent episodes of fainting in-school assembly. ECG was done. What is incorrect about the condition?

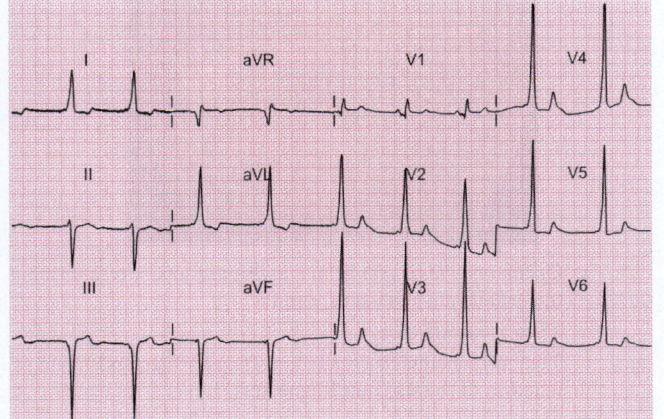

    a. Pre-excitation syndrome
    b. Wide QRS
    c. Delta wave
    d. Pacemaker is treatment of choice

386. An 18-year-old boy is asymptomatic. On ECG he has a short PR interval with delta waves. Which of the following is not required for these patients? (AIIMS May 2013)
    a. Electrophysiological studies
    b. Treadmill test
    c. Procainamide
    d. Beta blockers

387. What is incorrect about Brugada syndrome?
    a. SCN5A defect   (Recent Pattern 2014-15)
    b. Asymptomatic ST segment elevation
    c. Sudden death
    d. Pacemaker is treatment of choice

388. Brugada Syndrome is associated with: (AIIMS 2013)
    a. Left Bundle Branch Block
    b. Left Anterior Fascicular block
    c. Left Posterior Fascicular block
    d. Right Bundle Branch Block

JVP

389. 'a' wave in JVP indicates: (AIIMS May 2018)
    a. Right atrial contraction
    b. Closure of tricuspid valve
    c. Onset of ventricular systole
    d. Maximal atrial filling

390. C wave in JVP is due to? (Recent Pattern 2018)
    a. Atrial contraction   b. Atrial relaxation
    c. Tricuspid bulge   d. Early ventricular filling

391. 'a' wave in JVP represents. (AIIMS May 2017)
    a. Passive atrial filling   b. Right atrial contraction
    c. Ventricular filling   d. Ventricular relaxation

392. In a patient of lung cancer with full neck veins and low BP, which of the following is incorrect?
 (Recent Pattern Questions)
    a. Electrical alternans   b. Low voltage ECG
    c. Prominent Y descent   d. Absence of Kussmaul sign

393. In JVP y descent is absent and X wave is prominent? This suggests: (Recent Question 2015-16)
    a. Restrictive cardiomyopathy
    b. Cardiac tamponade
    c. Constrictive pericarditis
    d. Right Ventricular Failure

394. Internal jugular vein pressure determines pressure of:
 (Recent Question 2015-16)
    a. RA   b. RV
    c. LA   d. LV

395. Canon A wave is seen in:
    a. Atrial fibrillation   b. Complete heart block
    c. Ventricular fibrillation d. Mobitz 1 heart block

396. A wave in JVP is absent in: (Recent Question 2015-16)
    a. Atrial fibrillation   b. Heart block
    c. Tricuspid regurgitation   d. Complete heart block

397. Canon a waves are seen in: (Recent Question 2015-16)
    a. Atrial fibrillation   b. Junctional tachycardia
    c. Constrictive pericarditis d. Cardiac tamponade

398. Giant 'a' waves in JVP occur in all except: (AI 1996)
    a. Junctional rhythm   b. Pulmonary hypertension
    c. Tricuspid regurgitation d. Complete heart block

399. C wave in JVP indicates: (AI 2009)
    a. Atrial contraction   b. Bulging of tricuspid valve
    c. Ventricle systole   d. Rapid ventricular filling

Aortic Dissection

400. A 50-year male presented with high BP of 160/100 mm Hg and heart rate of 120/min. CECT is shown below. Which is best management of this condition? (AIIMS May 2018)

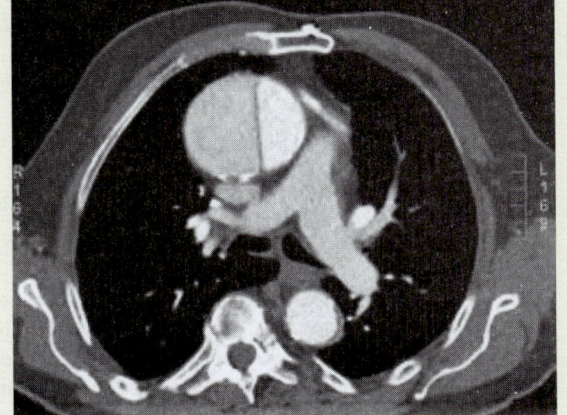

    a. Surgical repair   b. LMW heparin
    c. Beta blocker   d. Vitamin K inhibitors

401. A 70-year-old man with Hypertension wakes up with severe chest pain and diaphoresis. On examination he has bounding pulses with wide pulse pressure. A diastolic murmur is heard along the right sternal border. Which of the following is the possible aetiology?
    a. Aortic dissection   (Recent Question 2019)
    b. STEMI with papillary muscle dysfunction
    c. Myocarditis with functional regurgitation
    d. Flash pulmonary oedema

402. A 65-year old hypertension patient presents with Chest pain, difficulty in breathing for 1 hour. Chest X-ray done shows presence of:

    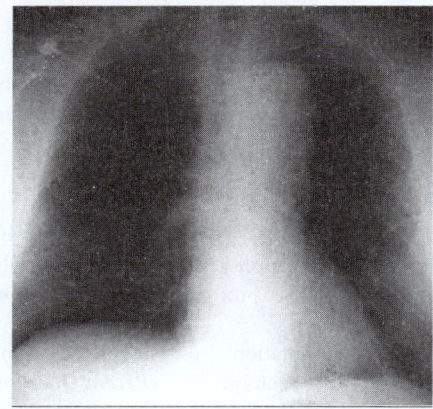

    a. Kerley B Lines   b. Aortic Dissection
    c. Hilar lymphadenopathy   d. Pneumomediastinum

403. Investigation of choice for aortic dissection with hypotension is ?   (Recent Pattern 2014-15)
    a. CT scan   b. Technetium99 scan
    c. MRI   d. T.E.E.

404. All of the following factors predispose to Aortic dissection, except: (PGI June 02)
    a. Systemic hypertension   b. Coarctation of aorta
    c. Ist trimester pregnancy d. Takayasu's arteritis

Infective Endocarditis

405. Treatment of choice for late cardiovascular syphilis is?   (AIIMS May 2018)
    a. Benzathine penicillin 2.4 million units in single dose i.m
    b. Benzathine penicillin 7.2 million units in three divided doses i.m
    c. Benzyl penicillin 12-24 million units for 21 days i.m
    d. Tetracycline 2g daily

406. Roth spots are seen in?   (Recent Pattern 2018)
    a. Leukemia   b. Uveal melanoma
    c. Starvation   d. Aortic dissection

407. A 40-year-old patient came with complaints of spikes of fever and difficulty in breathing. T.E.E shows multiple vegetations on surface of heart valves. Blood culture showed growth of Burkholderia Cepacia. Which of the following is first line management for this patient?   (AIIMS May 2017)
    a. Levofloxacin and Cefotaxime
    b. Aminoglycosides and Colistin
    c. Cefepime and Tigecycline
    d. Cotrimoxazole with Meropenem

408. A 50 year man came with a 'grey spot' in his vision. He had recurrent fevers and weight loss for the past 3 months. He had a history of mitral valve infection. Vision is 6/6. This is the picture of his fundus. Choose the FALSE statement?   (APPG 2016)

    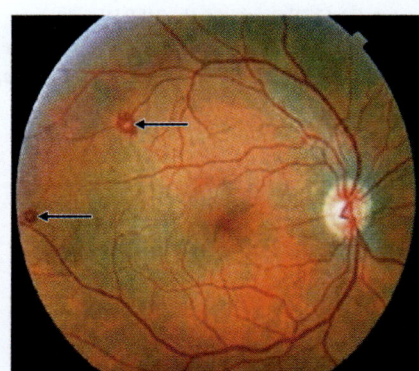

    a. Occur in several conditions including less severe virulent infections of a metastatic nature
    b. They are Roth spots
    c. They are characteristically associated with severe general reaction of the surrounding retina
    d. These findings can also occur in anemia, leukemia

409. Which of the following is not a part of Duke Criteria for infective endocarditis?   (AIIMS May 15)
    a. Splenomegaly   b. Fever > 100.4 Celsius
    c. IV drug user   d. Blood culture positive

410. Infective endocarditis is most commonly seen in?   (Bihar PG 15)
    a. ASD   b. VSD
    c. PDA   d. Pulmonary atresia

411. Osler's nodes are seen in?   (Recent Pattern 2014-15)
    a. Rheumatoid arthritis
    b. Rheumatic heart disease
    c. Subacute bacterial endocarditis
    d. Typhoid

412. What is not true about infective endocarditis?
    a. Hematuria   (Recent Pattern 2014-15)
    b. Rose spots seen
    c. Splinter hemorrhages seen
    d. Hemiplegia

413. Most common cause of infective endocarditis is?   (Recent Pattern 2014-15)
    a. Staphylococcus aureus   b. Streptococcus viridans
    c. Streptococcus pyogenes d. Streptococcus mutilan

414. Infective endocarditis where lifelong treatment is required: (Recent Pattern 2014-15)
    a. Aspergillus endocarditis b. Libman sacks endocarditis
    c. Fusarium solani   d. Enterococci

415. Infective endocarditis is least common in: (AIIMS Nov 93)
    a. Mitral stenosis   b. Aortic stenosis
    c. VSD   d. ASD

416. Least common site for vegetation is: (AIIMS May 94)
    a. Aortic Stenosis (AS)
    b. Mitral Stenosis (MS)
    c. Mitral Regurgitation (MR)
    d. Atrial Septal Defect (ASD)

417. Mitral valve vegetations do not usually embolise to: *(AIIMS Nov 2001)*
   a. Lung
   b. Liver
   c. Spleen
   d. Brain

418. Most common heart valve involved in IV drug user is: *(AIIMS Feb 97)*
   a. Mitral valve
   b. Aortic valve
   c. Pulmonary valve
   d. Tricuspid valve

419. A patient with a prosthetic heart valve develops endocarditis eight months after valve replacement. Most likely organism responsible is: *(AIIMS Nov 2010)*
   a. Staphylococcus Aureus
   b. Staphylococcus Epidermidis
   c. Streptococcus Viridans
   d. HACEK group

Hypertension

420. A patient of Hypertension on metoprolol, Verapamil was given. This is will result in? *(AIIMS Nov 2018)*
   a. Atrial fibrillation
   b. Bradycardia with AV Block
   c. Torsades De pointes
   d. Tachycardia

421. Which of the following leads to hypokalemic metabolic alkalosis with hypertension? *(Recent Pattern 2018)*
   a. Bartter Syndrome
   b. Gitelman Syndrome
   c. Renal tubular acidosis
   d. Liddle Syndrome

422. A patient came with early diastolic murmur in the second intercostal space and had differential BP recording in the upper limb with one arm showing measurement of 150/110 mm Hg and the other showing 90/60. All of the following can be a cause except? *(AIIMS Nov 2017)*
   a. Aortic dissection
   b. Takayasu Arteritis
   c. Coarctation of Aorta
   d. Supravalvular Aortic Stenosis

423. A 50-year-old construction worker continues to have elevated BP of 160/100 mmHg after a third agent (thiazide) is added to his anti-hypertensive regimen. Physical examination is normal, electrolytes are normal and he is not taking any over the counter medications. Which is the next helpful step in diagnosis of this patient? *(Recent Pattern Questions)*
   a. Check pill count
   b. Perform renal Doppler
   c. MRI aorta
   d. Adrenal CT scan

424. Osler manoeuvre is used for diagnosis of? *(Recent Question 2016-17)*
   a. Pseudo-hypertension
   b. Infective endocarditis
   c. Auscultation of murmur of mild AR
   d. Cutis Laxa

425. All are true about renal artery stenosis except? *(PGI Chandigarh May 2015)*
   a. ACE inhibitors can be used in bilateral renal artery stenosis
   b. ACE inhibitors can be used in unilateral renal artery stenosis
   c. ACE inhibitors are best drug to control DM associated hypertension
   d. Excision & Grafting is treatment of choice
   e. Angioplasty with or without stenting, and surgical bypass used only in refractory cases

426. A 40 year-old female has a SBP = 130 mm Hg and DBP = 100 mm Hg on two consecutive occasions. Her father is alos hypertensive and is on medication. Blood work up is normal. Best treatment is? *(Recent Question 2015-16)*
   a. D.A.S.H
   b. Sedative
   c. Anti –hypertensive drugs
   d. Error in BP Machine

427. Most common cause of aortic dissection: *(Recent Question 2015-16)*
   a. Syphilis
   b. Hypertension
   c. Marfan syndrome
   d. Cystic medial necrosis

428. Hypertension patient has presented with BP of 220/130 mm Hg in the emergency with headache but no CNS deficit. What is the goal BP for this patient? *(Recent Pattern 2014-15)*
   a. 200/150
   b. 180/110
   c. 160/90
   d. 140/90

429. Most common cause of Resistant hypertension is? *(Recent Pattern 2014-15)*
   a. Non-compliance of patient
   b. Obstructive sleep apnea
   c. Pheochromocytoma
   d. Renovascular disease

430. Most common cause of Secondary hypertension is? *(Recent Pattern 2014-15)*
   a. Renovascular disease
   b. Pheochromocytoma
   c. Renal parenchymal disease
   d. Hyperthyroidism

431. A lady on anti hypertensive medication comes with hemiparesis and speech difficulty for 2.5 hours. BP is 180/100. What is the best treatment for this patient? *(AIIMS Nov. 2013)*
   a. Aggressive Reduction of BP
   b. Modest Lowering of BP
   c. Thrombolysis with tissue plasminogen activator
   d. Aspirin and Clopidogrel loading dose.

432. Blood pressure is difficult to measure in a patient with: *(Recent Pattern 2014-15)*
   a. Mitral stenosis
   b. Aortic stenosis
   c. Complete heart block
   d. Atrial fibrillation

433. Pregnant lady with Hypertension with diabetes mellitus requires which drug to control her BP? *(Recent Pattern 2014-15)*
   a. ACE inhibitors
   b. Beta blocker
   c. ARB
   d. Diuretics

434. Most common cause of hypertension is? *(Recent Pattern 2014-15)*
   a. Renal artery stenosis
   b. Essential HTN
   c. Pheochromocytoma
   d. Chronic Glomerulonephritis

435. A hypertensive diabetic is having proteinuria, antihypertensive of choice is: *(AIIMS May 95)*
   a. Propanolol
   b. Clonidine
   c. Enalaprilat
   d. Alpha methyldopa

436. In Accelerated HTN what is metabolic defect: *(PGI June 2000)*
   a. Normal non-ionic metabolic acidosis
   b. Ionic gap met acidosis
   c. Hypomagnesemia
   d. Metabolic alkalosis

437. Most common cause of renal artery stenosis in young adults in India is: *(AIIMS Dec 97)*
    a. Atherosclerosis
    b. Non specific aorto-arteritis
    c. Fibro muscular dysplasia
    d. None of the above

438. A 10-year-old boy presents to the pediatric emergency unit with seizures. Blood pressure in the upper extremity is measured as 200/140 mm Hg. Femoral pulses were not palpable. The most likely diagnosis amongst the following is: *(AI 2010)*
    a. Takayasu Aortoarteritis
    b. Renal parenchymal disease
    c. Grandmal seizures
    d. Coarctation of Aorta

439. Which condition is most commonly associated with coarctation of aorta? *(AI 2008)*
    a. PDA
    b. Bicuspid aortic valve
    c. Aortic stenosis
    d. VSD

440. Coarctation of aorta is associated with all, except: *(AIIMS June 98)*
    a. Turner's syndrome
    b. Bicuspid aortic valve
    c. Pulmonary stenosis
    d. Atresia of aortic arch

Miscellaneous

441. In a patient with autonomic dysreflexia after a spinal cord injury, supine BP of the patient is 200/100 mm Hg with Heart rate of 58/min. Which of the following is required for initial management of these patients? *(Recent Question 2019)*
    a. Nicardipine
    b. Sodium nitroprusside
    c. Nitro-glycerine
    d. Labetalol

442. What is the treatment of anaphylactic shock?
    a. 1 ml i.v adrenaline 1 in 100000 *(AIIMS Nov 2017)*
    b. 0.5 ml i.m epinephrine 1 in 1000
    c. 0.5 ml i.m epinephrine 1 in 10000
    d. 1 ml i.v adrenaline 1 in 10000

443. Which of the following indicates modified shock index? *(AIIMS Nov 2017)*
    a. HR/MAP
    b. CO/MAP
    c. MAP/HR
    d. CO x MAP

444. What does balanced resuscitation mean?
    a. ABC management *(AIIMS Nov 2017)*
    b. Electrolyte imbalance management
    c. Fluid management
    d. Maintenance of acid base balance

445. Which of the following is the best guide for fluid administration? *(AIIMS Nov 2017)*
    a. Urine output
    b. CVP
    c. HR
    d. Blood pressure

446. Which of these factors is *not* used to assess the reliability of the relative while taking history? *(AIIMS Nov 2017)*
    a. Blood relation
    b. Time of cohabitation
    c. Education status
    d. Observational ability

447. A.C.L.S stands for? *(Recent Question 2016-17)*
    a. Advanced cardiac life support
    b. Acute cardiac life support
    c. Adult cardiac life support
    d. Adjunctive cardiac life support

448. A 25-year-old patient with abdominal trauma presents with Hypovolemic shock, and is unresponsive to crystalloids. What is the next step? *(Recent Question 2016-17)*
    a. Albumin
    b. Colloids
    c. Blood transfusion
    d. Immediate laparoscopy

449. This picture depicts the pressure recordings from _____ *(APPG 2016)*

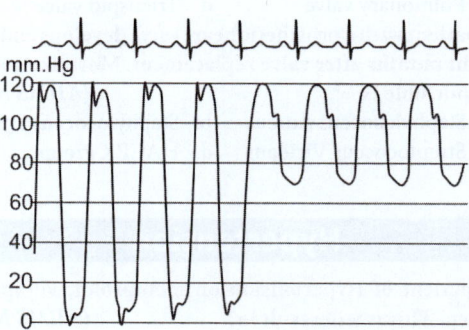

    a. LV & aorta in aortic regurgitation
    b. LV & aorta in a normal person
    c. RV & pulmonary artery in a normal person
    d. LV & aorta in aortic stenosis

450. Match the following drugs with their timing of administration *(APPG 2016)*

A.	At night	i	Alendronate
B.	Eccentric dose (8AM and 2 PM)	ii	Simvastatin
C	Before exercise	iii	Regular dose of isosorbide mononitrate
D	Once in the morning, before breakfast, sitting upright	iv	Cromolyn sodium

    a. ABCD = ii, i, iiii, iv
    b. ABCD = ii, iii, iv, i
    c. ABCD = i, ii, iv, iii
    d. ABCD = ii, i, iv, iii

451. Clinical markers in the revised Cardiac Risk Index (in preop evaluation) include the following EXCEPT.
    a. S3 gallop *(APPG 2016)*
    b. Serum creatinine > 2 mg%
    c. Diabetic on OHA with HbA1C of 7%
    d. Major intraperitoneal surgery

452. Match the following fundus findings and choose the best combination *(APPG 2016)*

P.	Cotton wool spots	X.	Cholesterol emboli
Q.	Cherry red spot	Y.	Hypertensive retinopathy
R.	Hollenhorst plaque	Z.	Central retinal artery occlusion

    a. PQR = YZX
    b. PQR = YXZ
    c. PQR = ZYX
    d. PQR = XZY

453. Atrial Myxoma is associated with the following except?
    a. Fever *(UPSC 2015)*
    b. Weight loss
    c. Systolic murmur at apex
    d. Subungual splinter hemorrhage

454. All of the following diseases affect the heart muscle except?
 (JIPMER May 2015)
 a. Scleroderma b. Fabry's
 c. Sarcoidosis d. Von gierke disease

455. A young woman present to the emergency departments with central cyanosis because her friends told her she looks bluish she is asymptomatic what could be the cause of bluish discolorations of tongue? *(JIPMER Nov 2014)*
 a. CO poisoning
 b. Severe anemia
 c. Drinking water contaminated with nitrates
 d. Lead poisoning

456. Energy selection in CPR according to AHA 2010 guideline is/are: *(PGI Chandigarh May 2015)*
 a. Monophasic 120-200 J, Biphasic 360 J
 b. Monophasic 200 J, Biphasic 360 J
 c. Monophasic 120 J, Biphasic 200 J
 d. Monophasic 360 J, Biphasic 120-200 J
 e. Monophasic 360 J, Biphasic 220 J

457. Which of the following are correct:
 (PGI Chandigarh May 2015)
 a. Pulsus paradoxus-Aortic regurgitation
 b. Pulsus bisferiens-Pulmonic stenosis
 c. Water-Hammer pulse-Aortic regurgitation
 d. Pulsus parvus et tardus-Aortic stenosis
 e. Collapsing pulse-Aortic regurgitation

458. What would you do immediately after a cardiac arrest?
 (Recent Question 2015-16)
 a. Give epinephrine b. Check for breathing,
 c. Check for pulse d. Chest Compressions

459. Initial ECG change in Hyperkalemia is?
 (Recent Question 2015-16)
 a. Tall tented T waves b. PR prolongation
 c. qRS widening d. ST segment depression

460. ECG finding of Hyperkalemia: *(Recent Question 2015-16)*
 a. T wave inversion b. ST depression
 c. P pulmonale d. Wide QRS complex

461. Pericardical cyst is seen at: *(Recent Question 2015-16)*
 a. Cardiophrenic angle b. Middle mediastinum
 c. Posterior mediastinum d. Lingula

462. Most common cause of unilateral pedal edema?
 (Recent Question 2015-16)
 a. Pregnancy b. Lymphedema
 c. Venous insufficiency d. Milroy disease

463. According to revised guidelines of American heart association, which of the following drugs is not recommended in Cardiac arrest? *(Recent Question 2015-16)*
 a. Adrenaline b. Atropine
 c. Amiodarone d. Vasopressin

464. A Patient presented with deficiency of thiamine. What could be possible outcome: *(Recent Question 2015-16)*
 a. Delayed wound healing b. Cardiac abnormality
 c. Memory loss d. Gingival bleeding

465. A 1-year-old male child is having a Heart Rate 40/min, BP 90/60. His serum Potassium = 6.5. What is the next best management? *(Recent Question 2015-16)*
 a. Ipratropium b. Adrenaline
 c. Sodium bicarbonate d. Calcium chloride

466. The structure marked by red arrow is:

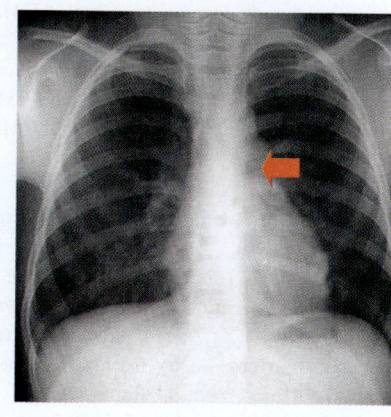

 a. Aortic knuckle b. Left atrial appendage
 c. Pulmonary artery trunk d. Left pulmonary artery

467. This patient can die due to which disease?

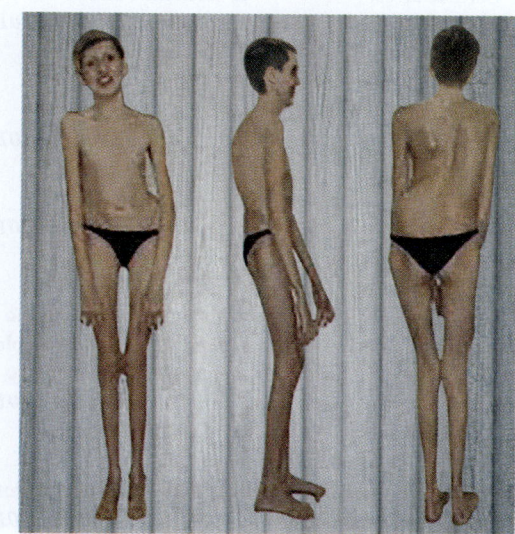

 a. Aortic dissection b. Mitral valve prolapse
 c. Ectopial entis d. Embolic stroke

468. Wrongly matched pair is? *(AIIMS May 2012)*
 a. NF 1 -renal artery stenosis
 b. Moyamoya-aortic aneurysm
 c. Marfans syndrome –dural ectasia
 d. Mulibrey nanism-constrictive pericarditis

469. Patient with ICD collapses, which ICD imaging modality is best suited for this patient? *(AIIMS Nov. 2012)*
 a. Chest X-ray b. MRI
 c. CT d. USG

470. DRESS syndrome is associated with all except:
 (Recent Pattern 2014-15)
 a. Eosinophilia b. Myocarditis
 c. Endocarditis d. Encephalitis

471. P.S.T is: *(Recent Pattern 2014-15)*
 a. Phenol sulfotransferase deficiency
 b. Post-traumatic stress disorder
 c. Protein S deficiency
 d. Paroxysmal supraventricular tachycardia

472. According to AHA 2010, drug not used in CPR is? *(AIIMS Nov. 2013)*
    a. Adrenaline
    b. Vasopressin
    c. Atropine
    d. Amiodarone

473. Beyond which critical value Shock Index [Heart rate/BP] in pregnancy is considered abnormal? *(AIIMS Nov. 2012)*
    a. 0.9-1.1
    b. 0.5 0-.7
    c. 0.3-05
    d. 0.7-0.9

474. Kerley B lines are seen at: *(Recent Pattern 2014-15)*
    a. Apex
    b. Cardiophrenic angle
    c. Lung fissure
    d. Pleural surface

475. Most common aortic branch involved in Takayasu Arteritis is? *(Recent Pattern 2014-15)*
    a. Left subclavian artery
    b. Common carotid artery
    c. Abdominal aorta
    d. Renal artery

476. Therapeutic hypothermia is of benefit in preventing neurological complications in *(Recent Pattern 2014-15)*
    a. Sepsis
    b. Poly-trauma
    c. Cardiac arrest
    d. Ischemic stroke

477. Who invented the stethoscope: *(Recent Pattern 2014-15)*
    a. Rene Laennec
    b. Leeuwenhoek
    c. Joseph Littmann
    d. William Osler

478. Cafe coronary term was coined by: *(Recent Pattern 2014-15)*
    a. Roger Hausen
    b. William Osler
    c. Christian Bernard
    d. Jean Marie Charcot

479. Dissecting aneurysm is seen in? *(Recent Pattern 2014-15)*
    a. Takayasu disease
    b. Atherosclerosis
    c. Syphilis aortitis
    d. Marfan syndrome

480. 60-year-old female patient with cardiac prosthetic valve has serum creatinine of 3 mg % with pyonephrosis. Investigation of choice for determining prosthetic valve damage is? *(Recent Pattern 2014-15)*
    a. Blood culture
    b. Cinefluorography
    c. Over penentrated CXR
    d. T.E.E.

481. Raised Intra-abdominal pressure to consider abdominal compartment syndrome is? *(Recent Pattern 2014-15)*
    a. 0-12 mm Hg
    b. >12 mm Hg
    c. >20 mm Hg
    d. >30 mm Hg

482. Pulsus paradoxus is seen in all except: *(AIIMS June 98)*
    a. IPPV
    b. COPD
    c. Cardiac Temponade
    d. Constrictive pericarditis

483. Pulsus alternans occurs in: *(PGI-June 98)*
    a. Constrictive pericarditis
    b. Viral myocarditis
    c. Hypokalemia
    d. MI

484. Water Hammer pulse is seen in: *(AIIMS May 07)*
    a. Aortic stenosis
    b. Aortic regurgitation
    c. Aortic stenosis and Aortic regurgitation
    d. Mitral regurgitation

485. Left atrial filling pressure closely approximates-
    a. Pulmonary capillary wedge pressure *(AIIMS May 93)*
    b. Central venous pressure
    c. Intrapleural pressure
    d. Intracranial pressure

486. Pulmonary edema associated with normal PCWP is observed. Which of these is not a cause: *(AI 01)*
    a. High altitude
    b. Cocaine overdose
    c. Post cardiopulmonary bypass
    d. Bilateral renal artery stenosis

487. All the following are radiological features of Chronic Cor pulmonale except: *(AI 1996)*
    a. Kerley B lines
    b. Prominent lower lobe vessels
    c. Pleural effusion
    d. Cardiomegaly

488. Pulsus paradoxus is a characteristic feature of:
    a. Constrictive pericarditis *(AIIMS Dec 92)*
    b. Cardiac Tamponade
    c. Hypertrophic obstructive cardiomyopathy
    d. Restrictive cardiomyopathy

489. The commonest tumor of the myocardium is: *(AI 94)*
    a. Myxoma
    b. Rhabdomyoma
    c. Sarcoma
    d. Fibroma

490. Vegetations on undersurface of A.V. valves are found in:
    a. Acute Rheumatic corditis *(AI 2001)*
    b. Libman Sack's endocarditis
    c. Non thrombotic bacterial endocarditis
    d. Chronic rheumatic carditis

491. Least conduction velocity is seen in: *(PGI Dec 98)*
    a. AV node
    b. Purkinje fibres
    c. Bundle of HIS
    d. Ventricular myocardial fibres

492. At the end of isometric relaxation phase *(AI 2000)*
    a. Atrioventricular valves open
    b. Atrioventricular valves close
    c. Corresponds to peak of "C" wave in JVP
    d. Corresponds to T wave in ECG

493. Mean arterial pressure is calculated as: *(AIIMS Nov 06)*
    a. (SBP + 2DBP)/3
    b. (DBP + 2SBP)/3
    c. (SBP + 3DBP)/2
    d. (DBP + 3SBP)/2

494. Most common cause of aortic aneurysm is: *(AI 98)*
    a. Syphilis
    b. Marfan's syndrome
    c. Atherosclerosis
    d. Congenital

495. During cardiac imaging the phase of minimum motion of heart is: *(Bihar PG 2016)*
    a. Late systole
    b. Mid systole
    c. Late diastole
    d. Mid diastole

496. Ideal site for checking core temperature? *(AIIMS Nov 2015)*
    a. Rectum
    b. Distal oesophagus
    c. Pulmonary artery
    d. Tympanic membrane

497. The term evidence based medicine was coined by? *(Bihar PG 2015)*
    a. Rutherford
    b. Stache
    c. Sackett
    d. Minstrel

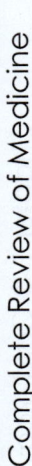

Answers with Explanations

Arrhythmia

1. Ans. (d) Multi-focal atrial tachycardia

(Ref: Harrison 20th edition, page 1547)

- The heart rate is irregular. Notice the horizontal rhythm strip markings.

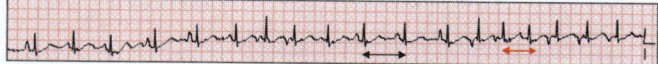

- Right axis deviation is present.

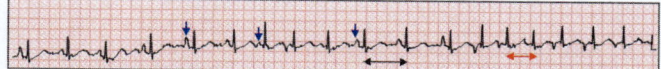

P wave is present and is showing different morphologies. The vertical markings highlight the different shapes of P waves.
- The presence of P waves automatically rules out atrial fibrillation and Paroxysmal supraventricular tachycardia.
- qRS complexes are of normal duration. ST segment is normal.
- Progression of R wave as we move to lateral chest leads is abnormal. Deep S waves in lateral leads point to a possible RV enlargement.
- The given findings point to diagnosis of multifocal atrial tachycardia.

2. Ans. (b) Cardioversion

(Ref: Harrison 20th edition, page 1743)

The heart rate is 200/min with normal axis. Narrow complex tachycardia is seen with Hidden P waves. There is wide spread ST segment depression seen in limb leads and chest leads. The patient is having an AV nodal re-entrant tachycardia/ Paroxysmal Supraventricular tachycardia. Since patient is unconscious and has hypotension, cardioversion should be done to restore normal sinus rhythm.

3. Ans. (a) Ventricular tachycardia

(Ref: Harrison 20th edition Page 1758)

- The ECG shows a heart rate of 200/min with broad complex tachycardia. Notching at nadir of S wave called as Josephson sign (arrow) is noted. Rabbit ear appearance (circle) is noted at peak of R wave. These findings are seen in Ventricular tachycardia.

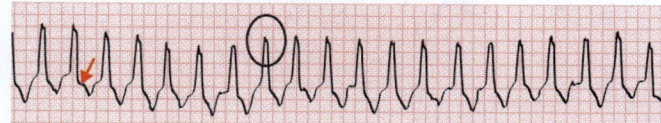

- Choice B should produce a sinusoidal pattern. Choice C should produce Twitching ventricles. Choice D produces Electrical Alternans.

4. Ans. (a) Hypothyroidism

(Ref: Harrison 20th edition, page 1728; Harrison 19th edition, page 1471)

Metabolic /endocrine causes of Atrioventricular Block

1. Hyperkalemia
2. Hypermagnesemia
3. Adrenal insufficiency
4. Hypothyroidism

5. Ans. (d) All of the above

(Ref: Harrison 20th edition, page 2066, 1756)

- Arrhythmogenic right ventricular dysplasia can affect either of the two ventricles and is a defect of desmosomal proteins. It leads to epsilon waves on ECG and can trigger VT. Hence ICD is indicated to prevent sudden death.
- Brugada syndrome is characterised by >0.2mv of ST segment elevation with coved ST segment and negative T waves in more than one anterior precordial leads. These patients can develop polymorphic VT in absence of structural heart disease and hence need an ICD.
- After 40 days or more of actual episode of MI, the patients with EF<35% and having inducible VT in electrophysiological lab are candidates for ICD.

Indications for ICD

Class I indications	Class IIA indications
• Structural heart disease with sustained VT	• ARVD with 1 or more risk factor
• Syncope due to inducible VT (documented by electrophysiological study)	• Brugada syndrome with syncope or VT
	• Catecholaminergic polymorphic VT
	• Cardiac sarcoidosis
• Post MI, LVEF<35% NYHA class II/ III	• Giant cell myocarditis
	• HOCM with 1 or more risk factor
• Post MI, LVEF<40% inducible VT or VF	• Long QT syndrome, syncope while on beta blockers
	• Non hospitalised patients awaiting a heart transplant

6. Ans. (a) Vasopressin

(Ref: Harrison 20th edition, page 2064; Harrison: 19th edition, page 1769)

This question was asked as per the 19th edition of Harrison.
- According to the current edition if there is no return of spontaneous circulation inspite of CPR adrenaline shock, then amiodarone 300 mg is given

The activities performed in ACLS are:
1. Defibrillation/ Cardioversion and pacing if required
2. Intubation with endotracheal tune
3. Insertion of iv line to administer life-saving drugs
   - After 2-3 unsuccessful defibrillation attempts epinephrine 1mg is given iv and attempts to defibrillate are repeated.
   - The dose of epinephrine may be repeated after intervals of 3-5 minutes
   - *Vasopressin* (Single dose 40 units intravenously) was suggested as an alternative to epinephrine, but has been removed in the current edition.

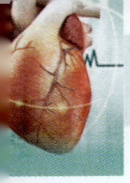

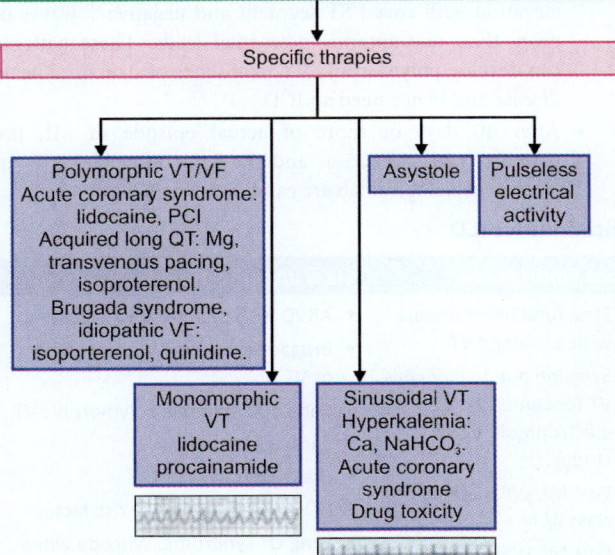

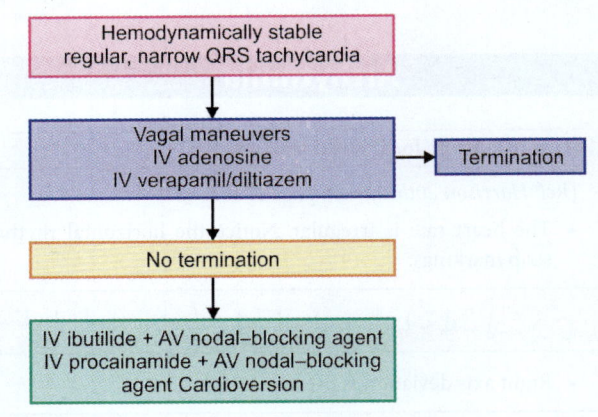

7. Ans. (d) Cushing syndrome

(Ref: Harrison 20th edition; table 275-1, page 1728; Harrison 19th edition, page 1491)

- Coronary heart disease can lead to ischemic damage to conduction system.
- Presence of non-caseating granulomas in sarcoidosis leads to damage to conduction system.
- Myxedema cardiomyopathy is associated with a reversible form of heart block that responds to thyroxine replacement
- Hence by exclusion, the answer is Cushing syndrome.

8. Ans. (b) Carotid sinus massage

(Ref: Harrison 20th edition, page 1742; Harrison 19th edition, page 1483)

- HDUs are wards for people who need more intensive observation, treatment and nursing care than is possible in a general ward but slightly less than that given in intensive care. The ratio of nurses to patients may be slightly lower than in intensive care but higher than in most general wards.
- The patient has developed narrow complex QRS tachycardia and since the BP is recordable, carotid sinus massage should be initiated.

9. Ans. (b) Electrical Alternans

(Ref: Harrison 20th edition, page 1682; Harrison, 19th Edition, page 1459)

- Notice the low voltage ECG which is defined as amplitude of all qRS complexes in limb leads less than 5 mm
- Also notice that *amplitude of qRS complexes is variable* in all the arrow marked leads.

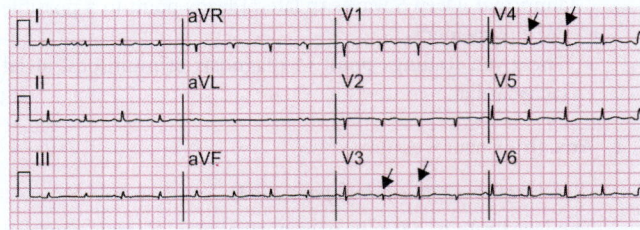

- Hence, the ECG is diagnostic of electrical alternans.
- The triad of sinus tachycardia with low voltage ECG and electrical alternans is highly suggestive of pericardial effusion

Variation in amplitude of qRS complexes

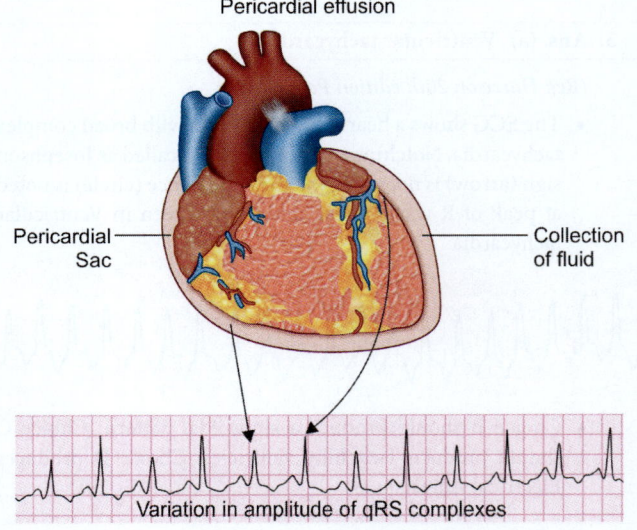

10. Ans. (c) Assess patient, activate emergency response team, call for defibrillator and start CPR

(Ref: AHA 2015 guidelines)

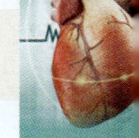

The first box of BLS algorithm is asked in the question (Highlighted Text)

BLS Healthcare provider
Adult cardiac arrest algorithm–2015 update

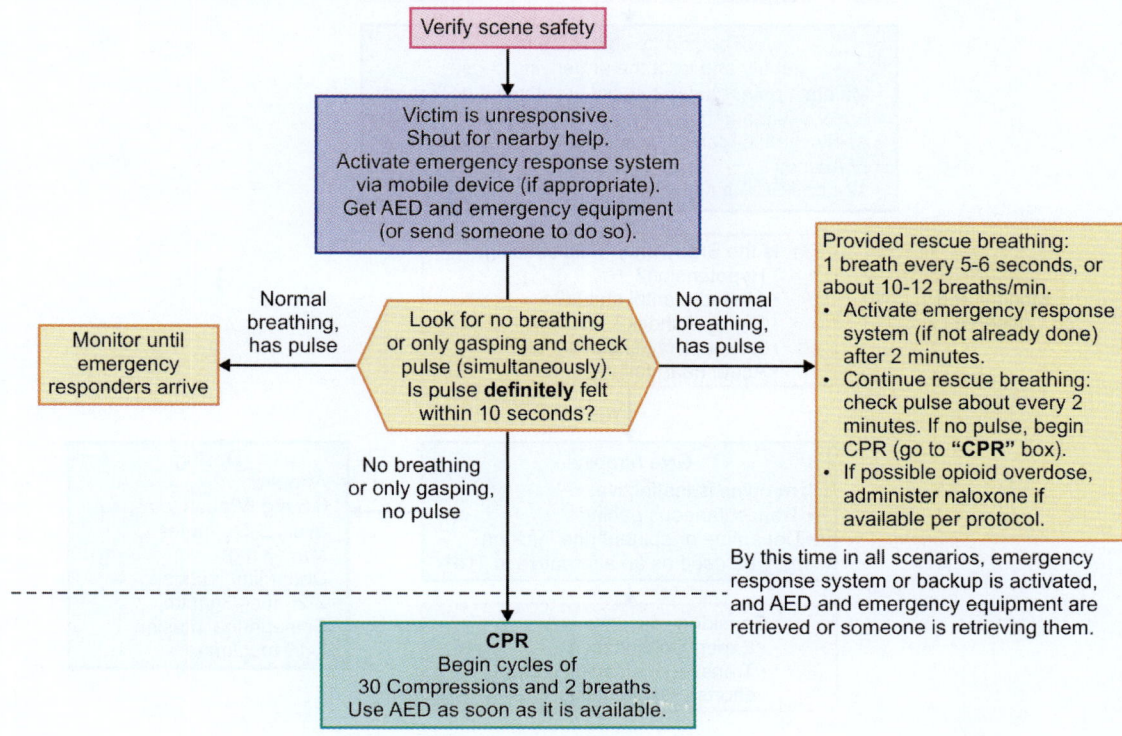

---

11. **Ans. (b) Nicotine poisoning**

    (Ref: APC Essentials of Forensic medicine and toxicology, page 585)

    Amblyopia is the key point which is ruling out choice A, C and D.

    Cardiovsacular symptoms and amblyopia indicate nicotine poisoning.

    Features of chronic nicotine poisoning:

    1. Respiratory system: Asthma like symptoms with coughing
    2. GIT: Diarrhea, PUD, nausea with vomiting
    3. CVS: Angina, arrhythmias, CAD, extrasystoles, Hypertension
    4. Eyes: Amblyopia and Blindness
    5. Women: Osteoporosis, PIH, Preterm labour and congenital malformations

    Poisoning from nicotine can occur from:
    1. Nicotine sulfate in insecticides
    2. Green tobacco sickness (tobacco harvesters who pick and brush up against wet tobacco leaves)
    3. Improper use of nicotine patches
    4. Ingestion of nicotine chewing gum

12. **Ans. (b) DC shock**

    (Ref: Harrison 20th edition, page 2064; Harrison 19th edition, page 1494)

    - The ECG shows heart rate of 200/min with normal axis.
    - *Broad qRS complex of 160msec is seen.*
    - Also notice the rabbit ear appearance of the peak of R wave seen in Ventricular tachycardia.
    - ACLS guidelines state qRS synchronous electrical cardioversion in case of Ventricular tachycardia in following conditions:

    1. Setting of hypotension
    2. Impaired consciousness
    3. Pulmonary oedema

    - Amiodarone is preferred DOC in case of stable VT.

13. **Ans. (c) Epinephrine**

    (Ref: AHA ACLS 2015 Manual, page 125)

    For management of symptomatic bradycardia following drugs are recommended

    Atropine 0.5 mg (Maximum 3mg)
    Epinephrine 2–10 µg/kg/min
    Dopamine 2–10 µg/ kg/min

14. **Ans. (b) Transcutaneous Pacing**

    Ref: ACLS 2015 guidelines

    In case of symptomatic bradycardia with signs of poor perfusion, transcutaneous pacing is recommended as per ACLS 2015 guidelines

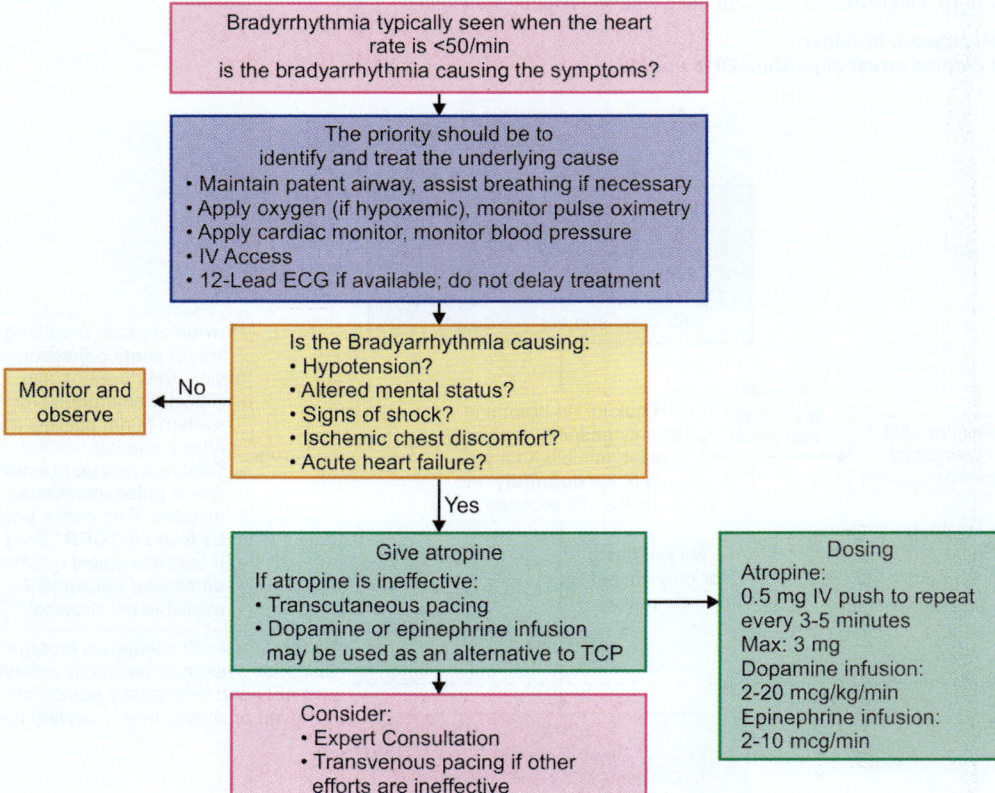

15. Ans. (a) Atropine, Dopamine, Epinephrine

(Ref: AHA ACLS provider manual 2015, page 125-126)

- First line drug for management of symptomatic bradycardia is atropine. It is given up to maximum dose of 3mg.
- If patient is still unstable, TCP (Transcutaneous pacing) is recommended.
- In case it is not available, two drugs dopamine and epinephrine are recommended.
- If patient is still unstable, trans-venous pacing is done.

16. Ans. (c) Perfusion of organs

(Ref: AHA ACLS manual, 2015, page 123)

The adequacy of perfusion of organ is the primary decision point to initiate bradycardia management algorithm.

17. Ans. (c) Give intravenous atropine and monitor

(Ref: AHA ACLS Manual, 2015, page 123)

The first and foremost step in management of symptomatic bradycardia is administration of atropine.

18. Ans. (a) Sinus bradycardia

(Ref: ECG interpretation made incredibly easy: 3rd edition, page 6)

- The ECG shows heart rate of 40/min with P wave of normal duration before every normal qRS complex.

- PR interval is constant and there are no dropped beats in the rhythm shown.
- The patient is having sinus bradycardia.

19. Ans. (b) Hydrogen ion depletion

(Ref: AHA ACLS 2015 guidelines)

- The 5 H and 5 T of pulseless electrical activity are mentioned below. PEA implies that electrical activity is seen on ECG but pulse is absent.
- The leading cause of PEA is hypoxia secondary to respiratory failure (40-50% cases) and hypovolemia.
- Hydrogen ion depletion implies alkalosis whereas PEA occurs with acidosis.

H	Hypovolemia	Hypoxia	Hydrogen ion (acidosis)	Hypo/Hyperkalemia	Hypothermia
T	Toxins	Tamponade	Tension Pneumothorax	Thrombosis (heart: acute, massive MI)	Thrombosis (lungs: massive PE)

20. Ans. (b) Epinephrine

(Ref: AHA ACLS 2015 guidelines)

In PEA the treatment algorithm to be followed is for asystole. Always push epinephrine and evaluate for reversible causes

Adult cardiac arrest circular algorithm—2015 update

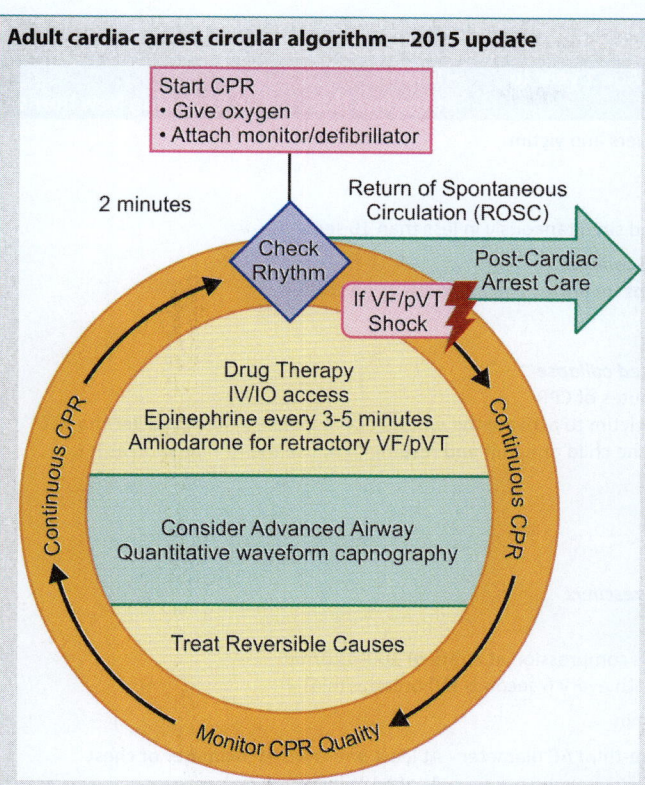

CPR quality

- Push hard (at least 2 inches (5cm) and fast (100-120/min) and allow complete chest recoil
- Minimize interruptions in compressions
- Avoid excessive ventilation
- Rotate compressor every 2 minutes, or sooner if fatigued
- If no advanced airway, 30:2 compression-ventilation ratio
- Quantitative waveform capnography
  - If $PETCO_2$ <10 mm Hg, attempt to improve CPR quality
- Intra-arterial pressure
  - If relaxation phase (diastolic) pressure <20 mm Hg, attempt to improve CPR quality

Shock energy for defibrillation

- **Biphasic:** Manufacturer recommendation (e.g. initial dose of 120-200 J); if unknown, use maximum available. Second and subsequent doses should be equivalent, and higher doses may be considered.
- **Monophasic:** 360 J

Drug therapy

- **Epinephrine IV/IO dose:** 1 mg every 3-5 minutes
- **Amiodarone IV/IO dose:** First dose: 300 mg bolus. Second dose: 150 mg

Advanced airway

- Endotracheal intubation or supraglottic advanced airway
- Waveform capnography or capnometry to confirm and monitor ET tube placement
- Once advanced airway in place, give 1 breath every 6 seconds (10 breaths/min) with continuous chest compressions

Return of spontaneous circulation (ROSC)

- Pulse and blood pressure
- Abrupt sustained increase in $PETCO_2$ (typically ≥40 mm Hg)
- Spontaneous arterial pressure waves wth intra-arterial monitoring

Reversible causes

- Hypovolemia
- Hypoxia
- Hydrogen ion (acidosis)
- Hypo-/hyperkalemia
- Hypothermia
- Tension pneumothorax
- Tamponade, cardiac
- Toxins
- Thrombosis, pulmonary
- Thrombosis coronary

---

21. Ans. (b) Ventricular fibrillation

(Ref: Harrison 20th edition, page 58; Harrison 19th edition, page 289e)

Non penetrating blunt trauma to chest can trigger *ventricular fibrillation* and lead to sudden cardiac death. This is called commotio cordis and occurs in sporting injuries. Trauma to chest at peak of T wave, often called as vulnerable period of heart triggers ventricular fibrillation.

22. Ans. (a) Check for carotid pulse

(Ref: Harrison 20th edition, page 2063)

- According to the AHA 2015 BLS guidelines, *since the patient is already mentioned as unresponsive*, the rescuer should quickly assess the carotid pulse and breathing of the patient for no more than 10 second period. Call for help to activate emergency response system.
- If the unresponsive patient is having no breathing and no carotid pulse, sequence C-A-B is applied and chest compressions are started at a rate of 30:2 across all age groups.
- If the unresponsive patient is having no breathing but carotid impulse is present, provide only rescue breaths once every 6 seconds to achieve a target of minimum 10 breaths per minute.
- Refer to guidelines in Question 2.

23. Ans. (a) 30:2

(Ref: AHA 2015 guidelines)

- The chest compression to ventilation ratio is 30:2 for all age groups except neonatal resuscitation where the ratio is 3:1. Even in infants and children the ratio is 30:2.
- For adults irrespective of number of rescuers the ratio of chest compression to ventilation ratio is 30:2
- For children if 1 rescuer is present the chest compression to ventilation ratio is 30:2
- For children if 2 or more rescuers are present the chest compression to ventilation ratio is 15:2

TABLE: Summary of High-Quality CPR Components for BLS Providers

Component	Adults and Adolescents	Children (Age 1 year to puberty)	Infants (Age less than 1 year, Excluding New borns)
Scene safety	Make sure the environment is safe for rescuers and victim		
Recognition of cardiac arrest	Check for responsiveness No definite pulse felt within 10 seconds Breathing and pulse check can be performed simultaneously in less than 10 seconds		
Activation of emergency response system	If you are alone with no mobile phone, leave the victim to activate the emergency response system and get the AED before beginning CPR Otherwise, send someone and begin CPR immediately; use the AED as soon as it is available	*Witnessed collapse* Follow steps for adults and adolescents on the left *Unwitnessed collapse* Give 2 minutes of CPR Leave the victim to activate the emergency response system and get the AED Return to the child or infant and resume CPR; use the AED as soon as it is available	
Compression ventilation ratio without advanced airway	1 or 2 rescuers 30:2	1 rescuer 30:2 2 or more rescuers 15:2	
Compression ventilation ratio with advanced airway	Continuous compression at a rate of 100–120/min Give 1 breath every 6 seconds (10 breaths/min)		
Compression rate	100–120/min		
Compression depth	At least 2 inches (5 cm)*	At least one-third AP diameter of chest About 2 inches (5 cm)	At least one-third AP diameter of chest About 1 ½ inches (4 cm)
Hand placement	2 hands on the lower half of the breastbone (sternum)	2 hands or 1 hand (optional for very small child) on the lower half of the breastbone (sternum)	1 rescuer 2 fingers in the center of the chest, just below the nipple line 2 or more rescuers 2 thumb-encircling hands in the center of the chest, just below the nipple line
Chest recoil	Allow full recoil of chest after each compression; do not lean on the chest after each compression		
Minimizing interruptions	Limit interruptions in chest compressions to less than 10 seconds		

24. Ans. (b) Atropine is used only for bradycardia

(Ref: Harrison 20th edition, page 2064; Harrison 19th edition, page 1769)

Atropine is used only for management of bradycardia and routine use during resuscitation is not recommended.

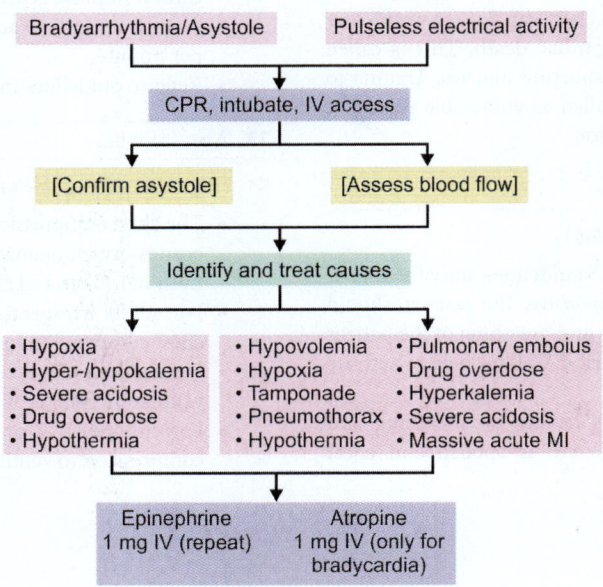

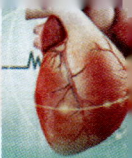

25. Ans. (c) Mobitz I heart Block

(Ref: Harrison 20th edition, page 1728; Harrison 19th edition, page 1473)

- The heart rate is regularly irregular due to change in rhythm.
- Approximate heart rate is 60/min (6 QRS complexes in 6 seconds in lead II [30 large squares]).
- Axis is normal.
- Progressive lengthening of PR interval followed by dropped beat is seen.
- PR interval before the dropped beat is more than PR interval in subsequent beats.
- The diagnosis is Mobitz I heart block.

26. Ans. (c) Cardioversion

(Ref: Harrison 20th edition, page 2064; Harrison: 19th edition, page 1491)

The ECG shows broad complex QRS tachycardia diagnostic of Ventricular tachycardia. Since the BP of the patient is crashing, a DC Shock should be given immediately.

27. Ans. (b) Atrio-ventricular nodal re-entrant tachycardia

(Ref: Harrison 20th edition, page 1739; Harrison: 19th edition, page 1479)

- Atrioventricular nodal reentrant tachycardia is the most common paroxysmal regular SVT.
- AVNRT occurs in the absence of structural heart disease and is usually well tolerated.
- Neck pulsations are usually felt because of the simultaneous atrial and ventricular contraction, and a "frog sign" can be identified on physical examination during the arrhythmia.
- It *develops because of the presence of two electro-physiologically distinct pathways* for conduction in the complex syncytium of muscle fibers that make up the AV node.
- The fast pathway in the more superior part of the node has a longer refractory period, whereas the pathway lower in the AV node region conducts more slowly but has a shorter refractory period.

28. Ans. (d) Anterior STEMI with atrial fibrillation

(Ref: Harrison 20th edition, page 1680, 1747; Harrison 19th edn, page 1456)

- The ECG shows variable heart rate with RR interval in lead II (see the inferior most lead) varying between 150-300 bpm. The axis is normal.
- P wave is absent with reduced RR interval and narrow complex qRS.
- Hyper-acute T waves are seen in V2 – V5 implying anterior wall MI.
- Hypertension is a risk factor for development of both sub-endocardial ischemia and atrial fibrillation
- Ventricular tachycardia has wide complex qRS and hence choice A and B are ruled out.

29. Ans. (c) Atrial fibrillation

(Ref: Harrison 20th edition, page 1747; Harrison 19th edn. page 1485)

The ECG shows presence of variable heart rate due to presence of irregularly irregular RR interval. The P waves in the ECG are not seen and QRS complex is normal duration. These point to presence of atrial fibrillation.

Arrhythmia	ECG pointers	ECG appearance
Choice A Sinus rhythm	P wave followed by normal duration qRS and concordant T wave.	
Choice B PSVT	Absent P waves Narrow qRS Regular RR interval ST depression	
Choice C Atrial fibrillation	Absent P waves Narrow qRS **irregular RR interval**	

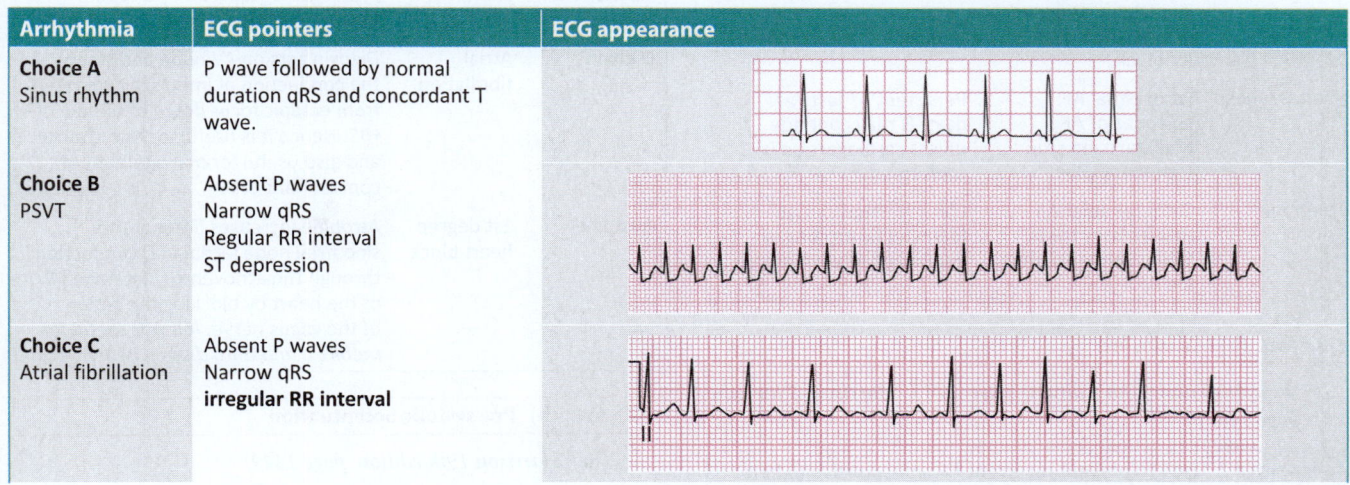

Contd...

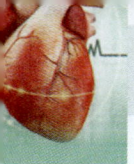

Arrhythmia	ECG pointers	ECG appearance
Choice D Ventricular fibrillation	Twitching with undulations seen on baseline ECG	(12-lead ECG showing leads I, aVR, V1, II, aVL, V2, III, aVF, V3, V1 with ventricular fibrillation pattern)

Atrial Fibrillation (AF)

Epidemiology	• It is the most common sustained arrhythmia • Prevalence increases with age, and more than 95% of AF patients are older than 60 years.		
Risk factors for developing AF 1. Age 2. Hypertension 3. Diabetes mellitus 4. Cardiac disease 5. Sleep apnea 6. Hyperthyroidism 7. acute alcohol intoxication 8. Myocardial infarction or pulmonary embolism, post cardiac surgery			
Clinical features	1. Rapid rates may cause hemodynamic collapse or heart failure exacerbations particularly in patients with impaired cardiac function 2. Exercise intolerance and easy fatigability 3. Dizziness or syncope 4. Asymptomatic in patients with high degree of AV block		
Clinical types	Paroxysmal AF: episodes of AF that start and stop spontaneously.	Persistent AF lasts >7 days, & may continue unless cardioversion is performed.	
Treatment	Catheter ablation that isolates these foci usually abolishes the AF.	Cardioversion can be followed by prolonged periods of sinus rhythm.	

30. Ans. (b) Adenosine

(Ref: Harrison 20th edition, page 1743; Harrison 19th edn. page 1487)

Amiodarone	Used to prevent recurrent AF unresponsive to beta blockade.
Adenosine	Adenosine blocks antegrade conduction through the AV node but doesn't affect accessory or bypass tracts like those seen in WPW syndrome. Because of this, adenosine can be dangerous when given to patients with atrial fibrillation, with bypass tract as atrial fibrillation will degenerate into ventricular fibrillation.
Diltiazem	Useful because it will prevent a rapid ventricular rate from developing if AF is converted to "slow" AFL with the drug therapy.
Beta blocker	Used for rate control in atrial fibrillation leading to hypotension and syncope.

31. Ans. (d) 3 4 2 1

(Ref: Harrison 19th edition, page 1489, 1479, 1485)

Amiodarone	Ventricular tachycardia	Prolongs the APD of the current generated due to re-entry or automaticity. This results in decrease in firing frequency of the ectopic focus and helps in termination of arrhythmia.
Adenosine	P.S.V.T	Prolongs AV nodal delay and re-establishes the superiority of SA node.
Digoxin	Atrial fibrillation	Digoxin acts on AV node and slows the conduction of impulses generated from ectopic focus down to bundle of HIS. Hence it is useful for rate control and also useful for management of concomitant CHF
Atropine	1st degree heart block	Atropine increases firing of the sinoatrial node (atria) and conduction through the atrioventricular node (AV) of the heart by blocking the action of the vagus nerve. *It is not useful for mobitz II and third degree heart block.*

32. Ans. (b) Pre-systolic accentuation

(Ref: Harrison 19th edition, page 1449)

The presystolic accentuation of mid-diastolic murmur of atrial fibrillation is due to atrial contraction against a closed mitral valve. With the onset of atrial fibrillation, since atria will be twitching, pre-systolic accentuation will disappear.

Other changes in findings of mitral stenosis with onset of atrial fibrillation are:

1. The first heart sound becomes variable in Intensity as heart rhythm is irregularly irregular

2. Opening snap continues to occur as long as the valves are pliable and non-calcified.
3. A2-O. Snap interval is usually less influenced by AF as it is primarily determined by mean LA pressure at the onset of diastole which has little variation beat to beat.
4. Length of the diastolic murmur varies.

33. Ans. (a) Adenosine

(Ref: Harrison 19th edition, page 1479-80)

- Treatment is directed at altering conduction within the AV node. Vagal stimulation, such as that which occurs with the Valsalva maneuver or carotid sinus massage, can slow conduction in the AV node sufficiently to terminate AVNRT.
- In patients in whom physical maneuvers do not terminate the tachyarrhythmia, the administration of adenosine, 6–12 mg IV, frequently does so. Intravenous beta blockade or calcium channel therapy should be considered as second-line treatment.
- If hemodynamic compromise is present, R-wave synchronous DC cardioversion using 100–200 J can terminate the tachyarrhythmia.

34. Ans. (a) Epinephrine

(Ref: APLS, 4th edition, page 133)

- Since the ECG is showing normal qRS and pulse is absent, the child is suffering from Pulseless electrical activity (PEA)
- It is a clinical condition characterized by unresponsiveness and lack of palpable pulse in the presence of organized cardiac electrical activity.
- Children with PEA are likely to have respiratory aetiology or shock unlike adults where arrhythmia like VT or ventricular fibrillation is more common.
- *Epinephrine should be administered in 1 mg doses IV/IO every 3-5 minutes during pulseless electrical activity (PEA) arrest.*

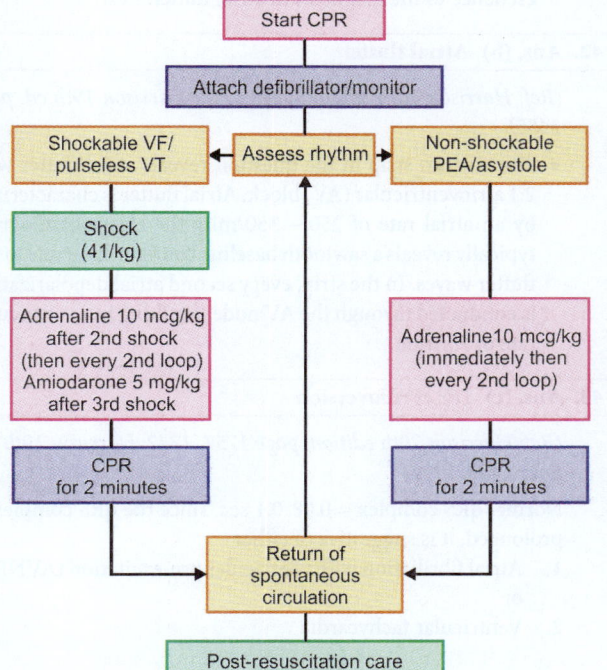

Etiology of PEA 5Hs and 5 Ts
- Hypoxia
- Hypovolemia
- Hydrogen ion (acidosis)
- Hyperkalemia/hypokalemia
- Hypothermia
- Tension pneumothorax
- Tarnponade (cardiac)
- Thrombosis (Coronary)
- Thrombosis (Pulmonary)
- Tablets (drug overdose)

35. Ans. (a) Cardioversion

(Ref: Harrison 20th edition, page 1743)

- In atrial flutter if class I agents are used it will lead to slowing of atrial flutter to a point where 1:1 conduction will occur and heart rate can jump up to 200bpm leading to hemodynamic compromise.
- Hence Ibutilide is recommended and 1 mg infusion over 60 minutes will work in 50-70% of patients reverting them back to normal sinus rhythm. However it is not in the choices
- *Electrical cardioversion of low intensity 25-50J can convert 90% of patients into normal sinus rhythm and is most effective therapy in recent onset atrial flutter*
- For recurrent atrial flutter, anti-arrhythmic drugs like sotalol, amiodarone can be used but 70% will experience recurrence. In this situation catheter ablation at cavo-tricuspid isthmus is more effective.

36. Ans. (a) Call for help

(Ref: AHA Basic life support 2015 guidelines)

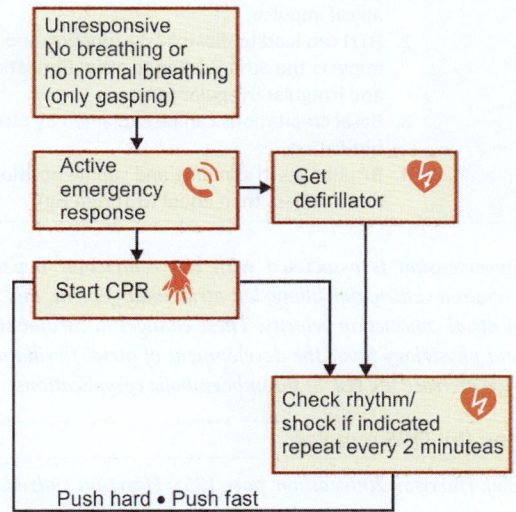

CPR Quality
- Push hard (≥2 inches [5 cm]) and fast ((≥100 /min) and allow complete chest recoil
- Minimize interruptions in compressions
- Avoid excessive ventilation
- Rotate compressor every 2 minutes
- If no advanced airway, 30:2 compression-ventilation ratio

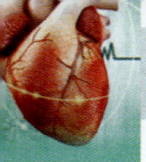

- Quantitative waveform capnography
  - If ET$_{CO_2}$ < 10 mm Hg, attempt to improve CPR quality
- Intra-arterial pressure
  - If relaxation phase (diastolic) pressure < 20 mm Hg, attempt to improve CPR quality

Return of Spontaneous Circulation (ROSC)
- Pulse and blood pressure
- Abrupt sustained increase in ET$_{CO_2}$ (typically ≥40 mm Hg)
- Spontaneous arterial pressure waves with intra-arterial monitoring

37. Ans. (c) Right coronary artery

(Ref: Harrison 20th edition, page 1680; Harrison 19th edition, page 1452)

Leads II, III, and aVF detect inferior wall ischemia, which is mainly supplied by right coronary artery.

38. Ans. (d) Left ventricular hypertrophy

(Ref: Harrison 20th edition, page 1894; Harrison 19th edition, page 289e-2, 1543, 1505)

Left atrial myxoma	More common in young female with symptoms of platypnea and low cardiac output since the tumor limits the blood flow into the left ventricle.
Mitral regurgitation	Ruled out as no murmur was auscultated in the patient
Cor pulmonale	Ruled out as primary lung disease or findings of RVF are absent
LVH	*Points in favour of diagnosis* 1. Hypertension can lead to LVH causing double apical impulse. 2. HTN can lead to diastolic dysfunction and impacts the atria leading to atrial fibrillation and irregular irregular pulse 3. Basal crepitations can be explained by atrial fibrillation. 4. BP changes in standing and supine position are normal (less than equal to 10mm Hg)

Hypertension is associated with left ventricular hypertrophy, impaired ventricular filling, left atrial enlargement, and slowing of atrial conduction velocity. These changes in cardiac structure and physiology favor the development of atrial fibrillation, and they increase the risk of thromboembolic complications.

39. Ans. (b) QRS complex

(Ref: Harrison 20th edition, page 1755; Harrison 19th ed. / 1489)

- The origin of premature beats/ ventricular extra systoles in the ventricle at sites remote from the Purkinje network produces slow ventricular activation and a wide QRS complex that is typically >140 ms in duration.
- Ventricular premature complexes are common and increase with age and the presence of structural heart disease.

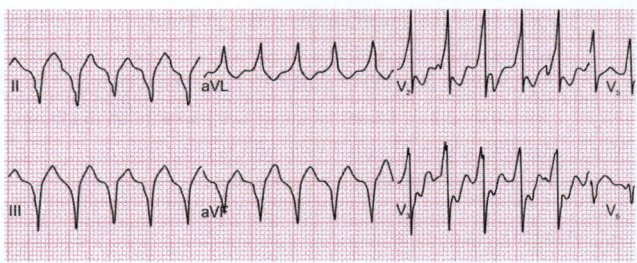

40. Ans. (b) Cardiac resynchronization therapy

(Ref: Harrison 20th edition, page 1777; Harrison 19th ed. page 1514)

- The image shows presence of Cardiac resynchronization therapy (CRT) device with three leads seen in color blue.
- The leads are touching right atrium and right ventricular endocardial surface.
- The third lead is seen on the left side inside a vein and is stimulating the left side of the heart.
- This startegy is useful for patients of dilated cardiomyopathy and congestive heart failure where the right and left ventricles donot contract simultaneously but asynchronously.

41. Ans. (a) Atrial flutter

(Ref: Harrison 20th edition, page 1743; Harrison 19th ed. page 1485)

- The ECG in lead II and other inferior leads shows presence of flutter waves.
- You can count 3 – 4 flutter waves before every narrow QRS complex.
- Since the ventricular rate is about 75 bpm (RR interval), atrial rate shall be obtained by multiplying the atrial rate by 4 which is 300 bpm
- The presence of risk factor of hypertension also lends credence to the diagnosis of atrial flutter.

42. Ans. (b) Atrial flutter

(Ref: Harrison 20th edition, page 1743; Harrison 19th ed. page 1485)

- The rhythm strip in the question reveals atrial flutter with 2:1 atrioventricular (AV) block. Atrial flutter is characterized by an atrial rate of 250 – 350/min; the electrocardiogram typically reveals a sawtooth baseline configuration due to the flutter waves. In the strip, every second atrial depolarization is conducted through the AV node, resulting in a ventricular rate of 75/min.

43. Ans. (c) DC cardioversion

(Ref: Harrison 20th edition, page 1757, 1742; Harrison 19th ed. Page 1482, 1494)

Normal qRS complex = 0.08-0.1 sec. since the qRS complex is prolonged, it is suggestive of either
1. Atrial fibrillation with ventricular pre-excitation (AVNRT) or
2. Ventricular tachycardia

Diagnostic criteria for ventricular tachycardia are:

- Presence of a qRS duration >140 ms in the absence of drug therapy,
- Superior and rightward qRS frontal plane axis,
- Bizarre qRS complex that does not mimic the characteristic qRS pattern associated with left or right bundle branch block,
- Slurring of the initial portion of the qRS
- qRS complex is usually >0.14 seconds but in the question this is 0.11 seconds

- *Hence The Patient Is Not Having Ventricular Tachycardia. In patients who manifest pre-excitation and AF, therapy should be aimed at preventing a rapid ventricular response. In life-threatening situations, DC cardioversion should be used to terminate the AF.*
- Acute treatment of AP-mediated macro-entrant orthodromic tachycardia is similar to that for AV nodal reentry and is directed at altering conduction in the AV node. Vagal stimulation with the Valsalva maneuver and carotid sinus pressure may create sufficient AV nodal slowing to terminate the AVRT. Intravenous administration of adenosine, 6–12 mg, is first-line pharmacologic therapy; the calcium channel blockers verapamil and diltiazem or beta blockers may also be effective.

44. Ans. (b) Atrial fibrillation

(Ref: Harrison 20th edition, page 1746; Cardiovascular Critical Care 3rd edition, Harrison 19th p 1486)

- Atrial arrhythmias are the most common among the CHF, post-op surgical patients admitted to ICU, and hypertensive patients.

45. Ans. (a) Re-entry

(Ref: Harrison 20th edition, page 1718; Harrison 19th ed. page 1466)

- The most common arrhythmia mechanism is re-entry. Fundamentally, re-entry is defined as circulation of an activation wave around an inexitable obstacle.
- Re-entry is due to in-homogeneities in myocardial conduction and/or recovery properties. The presence of a unidirectional block with slow conduction to allow for retrograde recovery of the blocked myocardium allows the formation of a circuit that, if perpetuated, can sustain a tachycardia.
- Re-entry appears to be the basis for most abnormal sustained Supra Ventricular Tachycardias (SVTs) and VTs.
- Two classic examples of re-entry that is primarily functional are VF due to acute myocardial ischemia and polymorphic VT in patients with a genetically determined ion channel abnormality such as the Brugada syndrome, LQTS, or catecholaminergic polymorphic VT.

46. Ans. (d) Pacemaker

(Ref: Harrison 20th edition, page 1730; Harrison 19th p 1474, page 1874)

- Temporary or permanent artificial pacing is the most reliable treatment for patients with symptomatic AV conduction system disease.

47. Ans. (d) Multifocal Atrial tachycardia

(Ref: Harrison 20th edition, page 1738; Harrison 19th p 1485; Page 218-219, Ketzung 19th edn)

Ectopic rhythms seen in digoxin toxicity are due to enhanced automaticity, reentry, or both, and may include the following:

1. Ventricular bigeminy
2. Premature ventricular contractions
3. Bidirectional ventricular tachycardia: Results from alterations in intraventricular conduction, junctional tachycardia with aberrant intraventricular conduction.
4. AV block
5. Non-paroxysmal atrial tachycardia with block

Digoxin causes a ST depression in V5-6 (Hockey stick sign). In digoxin toxicity, any arrhythmia or block may occur. Ventricular ectopics bigeminy is most common. Non-paroxysmal atrial tachycardia with variable block is characteristic.

48. Ans. (a) PSVT

(Ref: Harrison 19th p 1479)

- Choices C and D are ruled out as they would result in irregular rythm.
- Choice A is common in females in 2nd 4th decade and occurs in absence of structured heart disease. Simultaneous activation of atria and ventricles against a closed tricuspid valve can result in perception of fluttering sensation in neck. Elevated venous pressures result in release of natriures is leading to post tachycarida diuresis.
- Choice B can be a physiological response to stress and hence a less likely diagnosis.

49. Ans. (b) Hypothyroidism

(Ref: Harrison 20th p 1746; Harrison 19th p 1486)

Atrial fibrillation occurs in a structurally damaged heart like dilated cardiomyopathy, left atrial enlargement secondary to mitral valvular defects. It is also seen in thyrotoxicosis due to sympathetic overdrive caused by thyroid hormones can cause micro- voltage gradients to develop between the pulmonary vein musculature and atrial muscle.

50. Ans. (d) Atrial fibrillation

(Ref: Harrison 20th p 1746; Harrison 19th p 1486)

Alcoholic patients have a structurally damaged heart secondary to atrial fibrillation. Binge drinking can provoke an atrial fibrillation which can cause palpitations followed by syncope and crashing of BP. This sudden deterioration after binge drinking is referred to as holiday heart syndrome.
Remember Atrial fibrillation is the most common sustained arrythmia.

51. Ans. (c) Prevalence decreases with age

(Ref: Harrison 20th p 1756; Harrison 19th p 1492)

- P.V.C is a relatively common event where the heartbeat is initiated by Purkinje fibers in the ventricles rather than by

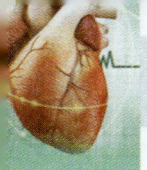

the SA node. The electrical events of the heart detected by the electrocardiogram allow a P.V.C to be easily distinguished from a normal heart beat and present as a broad complex qRS.
- Although a P.V. C can be a sign of decreased oxygenation to the myocardium often PVCs are benign and may even be found in otherwise healthy hearts but *prevalance increases with age.*
- A P.V.C may be perceived as a "skipped beat" or felt as palpitations in the chest.
- In a P.V. C, the ventricles contract first and before the atria have optimally filled the ventricles with blood, which means that circulation is inefficient. However, single beat PVC arrhythmias do not usually pose a danger and can be asymptomatic in healthy individuals.

52. Ans. (b) Ventricular rate> 160/min

(Ref: Harrison 20th p 1757; Harrison 19th p 1484, 1494)

PSVT	VT
ECG shows narrow complex qRS	ECG shows wide complex qRS
Heart rate usually 125-250 bpm	Heart rate 100-200 bpm
Patients who have limited hemodynamic reserve may be tachypneic and hypotensive. Crackles may be auscultated secondary to heart failure. An S3 may be present, and large jugular venous pulsations may also be visualized	The first heart sound may vary in intensity as a result of loss of atrioventricular (AV) synchrony. Episodes of VT are often associated with hypotension and tachypnea. Signs of diminished perfusion may be present, including diminished level of consciousness, pallor, and diaphoresis. Jugular venous pressure may be high, and Cannon a waves may be observed if the atria are in sinus rhythm.
Responsive to vagal maneuvers	Non responsive to vagal maneuvers

Electrocardiographic characteristics of the various SVTs are as follows:
- Sinus tachycardia - Heart rate greater than 100 bpm; P waves similar to sinus rhythm
- Inappropriate sinus tachycardia (IST) - Findings similar to sinus tachycardia; P waves similar to sinus rhythm
- Sinus nodal reentrant tachycardia (SNRT) - P waves similar to sinus rhythm; abrupt onset and offset
- Atrial tachycardia - Heart rate 120-250 bpm; P-wave morphology different from sinus rhythm; long RP interval (in general); AV block does not terminate tachycardia
- Multifocal atrial tachycardia - Heart rate 100-200 bpm; 3 or more different P-wave morphologies
- Atrial flutter- Atrial rate of 200-300 bpm; flutter waves; AV conduction of 2:1 or 4:1
- Atrial fibrillation - Irregularly irregular rhythm; lack of discernible P waves
- AV Nodal Reentrant Tachycardia (AVNRT) - Heart rate of 150-200 bpm; P wave located either within the QRS complex or shortly after the QRS complex; short RP interval in typical AVNRT and long RP interval in atypical AVNRT

- AV reentrant tachycardia (AVRT) - Heart rate of 150-250 bpm; narrow QRS complex in orthodromic conduction and wide QRS in antidromic conduction; diagnosis excluded by AV block during SVT; P wave after QRS complex.

53. Ans. (c) Prolonged QT$_c$ interval

(Ref: Harrison 20th p 1760; Harrison 19th p 1497)

Torsade de pointes: Looks like VF but is VT with varying axis. It is due to Prolonged QT interval.
Treatment: A. Correct electrolyte imbalance b. Mg sulfate c. Overdrive pacing

54. Ans. (d) 3rd degree heart block

(Ref: Harrison 20th p 2522; Harrison 19th p 2133)

- In patient of SLE, R_O antibody can be transferred via placenta to the fetus with resultant damage to AV node of the fetus. This results in baby being born with complete heart block /3rd degree heart block.
- The neonate is born with bradycardia and AV dissociation and requires pacing in first few days of life.

55. Ans. (b) QTc prolongation

(Ref: Harrison 20th p 1760; Harrison 19th p 1497)

Torsades de pointes ("Twisting of the Points"; polymorphic VT associated with long QT intervals)
- It refers to VT characterized by polymorphic qRS complexes that change in amplitude and cycle length, giving the appearance of oscillations around the baseline. This rhythm is, by definition, associated with QT prolongation.

Causes of Torsades de pointes
- Electrolyte disturbances (particularly hypokalemia and hypomagnesemia)
- Use of a variety of antiarrhythmic drugs (especially quinidine)
- Phenothiazine
- Tricyclic antidepressants
- Liquid protein diets
- Intracranial events
- Bradyarrhythmias, particularly third-degree AV block
- May occur as a congenital anomaly that most often presents with Torsades de Pointes (syncope or sudden death) at a young age

- The electrocardiographic hallmark is polymorphic VT preceded by marked QT prolongation, often in excess of 0.60s.
- These patients often have multiple episodes of nonsustained polymorphic VT associated with recurrent syncope, but they may also develop VF and sudden cardiac death.

56. Ans. (d) Idiopathic

(Ref: Harrison 20th p 1756; Harrison 19th p 1492)

PVCs are common in patients with and without heart disease, and are detected in 60% of adult males on Holter monitoring. Occasional unifocal PVCs do not suggest any of the underlying diseases described.

57. Ans. (d) Warfarin

(Ref: Harrison 20th p 1748; 1882, Harrison 19th p 1488)

- This patient has CHADS2 score of 5 (stroke=2 points, age=2 points and 1 point for hypertension)
- Aspirin alone might be sufficient for a stroke patient without the complicating factor of atrial fibrillation. However, in patients with atrial fibrillation, in whom the risk of stroke approaches 30%, therapeutic anticoagulation with warfarin reduces the incidence of future stroke to a greater extent than the use of aspirin.
- This particular patient may be a candidate for medical or electrical cardioversion, which requires pretreatment with Coumadin for 3 weeks (if the atrial fibrillation has been present for over 48 h or is of unknown onset).
- Alternatively, a transesophageal echocardiogram (TEE) could be performed to exclude the presence of left atrial thrombus, followed by cardioversion and then maintenance warfarin anticoagulation for 4 weeks. Lidocaine is useful in ventricular, not supraventricular, arrhythmias.

58. Ans. (d) Institute chest compression

(Ref: Harrison 20th p 2064; Harrison 19th p 1768)

- The BLS algorithm has been simplified, and "Look, Listen and Feel" has been removed from the algorithm. Performance of these steps is inconsistent and time consuming. For this reason the 2015 AHA Guidelines for CPR advocate immediate activation of the emergency response system and starting chest compressions for any unresponsive adult victim with no breathing or no normal breathing (i.e., only gasps).
- Encourage **Hands-Only (compression only) CPR** for the untrained rescuer.
- Initiate chest compressions before giving rescue breaths (**CA-B rather than A-B-C**). Chest compressions can be started immediately, whereas positioning the head, attaining a seal for mouth-to-mouth rescue breathing, or obtaining or assembling a bag-mask device for rescue breathing all take time. Beginning CPR with 30 compressions rather than 2 ventilations leads to a shorter delay to first compression.
- The recommended depth of compression for adult victims has increased from a depth of 1½ inches to a depth of at least 2 inches.

59. Ans. (c) Defibrillation at 200 joules biphasic

(Ref: Harrison 20th p 2063; Harrison 19th p 1769)

- The standard approach to ventricular fibrillation or pulseless ventricular tachycardia involves defibrillation with 200 joules followed if needed by epinephrine 1 mg IV push every 3 to 5 min AND/OR vasopressin for maintaining brain perfusion.
- Persistent ventricular fibrillation or pulseless ventricular tachycardia leads to consideration of amiodarone 300 mg IV push or lidocaine 1.0 to 1.5 mg/kg IV push. In addition, magnesium sulfate 1 to 2 g IV may be given in Torsade de Pointes or when arrhythmia due to hypo-magnesemia is suspected.

60. Ans. (b) Duchenne muscular dystrophy

(Ref: Harrison 20th p 3244, 1680 Harrison 19th p 1558, 462 e-5)

- All patient of DMD are boys who become wheel chair bound by the age of 12-15 years and then die of pneumonia. The heart is also involved in these patients and dilated cardiomyopathy can result in worsening of dyspnea due to concomitant pulmonary edema.
- ECG findings mentioned are suggestive of muscle hypertrophy of the heart with global dysfunction worsening the cardiovascular status of these patients.
- ALS is ruled out as it presents at 30-40 years and does not have cardiac involvement

61. Ans. (a) No treatment is required

(Ref: AHA ACLS 2015 guidelines)

Asymptomatic bradycardia requires no treatment. But patient having bradycardia with symptoms (fatigue, dizziness) should be treated by injection atrophine, or injection isoprenaline or pacemaker.

62. Ans. (c) Treatment of choice in Mobitz I heart Block

(Ref: Harrison 20th p 1732; Harrison 19th p 1475)

Indications for a permanent pacemaker
1. Complete AV block (Stokes-Adams attacks, congenital)
2. Mobitz type II block
3. Persistent AV block after anterior MI
4. Symptomatic bradycardia (e.g. sick sinus syndrome)

63. Ans. (a) AVNRT

(Ref: Harrison 19th p 1479)

- Atrioventricular Nodal Reentrant Tachycardia is the most common paroxysmal regular SVT.
- Neck pulsations due to simultaneous atrial and ventricular contraction, against a closed tricuspid valve produces can on a wave. They may be perceived as fluttering sensation in neck and is referred as frog sign.

64. Ans. (c) Less than 60/min

(Ref: Harrison 20th p 1722; Harrison 19th p 1470)

- By definition sinus bradycardia is a rhythm driven by the SA node with a rate of <60 beats/min

65. Ans. (a) Digitalis toxicity

(Ref: Harrison 20th p 1738; Harrison 19th p 309-310)

- All patients of mitral regurgitation have an increase in size of left atrium which predisposes to chronic atrial fibrillation. In these patients digoxin is initiated for rate control. Since it causes prolongation of AV nodal block, bradycardia can occur in this case, leading to syncope.
- Atrial fibrillation leads to embolic stroke that can present as stupor or coma with neurological deficit. In case of raised ICT due to stroke, bradycardia can be seen as a part of cushing reflex. However in question, presentation of patient

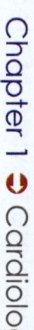

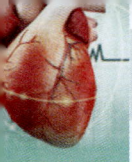

is of syncope with no neurological deficit. This rules out stroke.
- SAH presents with headache, nuchal rigidity and features of increased sympathetic activity

66. Ans. (c) Cardioversion followed by anticoagulation

(Ref: Harrison 20th p 1747-48; Harrison 19th p 1486-87)

In chronic atrial fibrillation, clots develop in the left atrial appendage and they can embolise to systemic circulation leading to embolic stroke. The protocol used for atrial fibrillation is

RACE Protocol

1. **R**ate control with esmolol
2. **A**nticoagulation with warfarin
3. **C**hemical cardioversion with amiodarone
4. **E**lectrical cardioversion in case chemical cardioversion fails

The decision to anticoagulate is made on basis of C.H.A.D.S2- VASc score

Condition	Points
CHF	1
HTN	1
Age >75yrs	2
Diabetes mellitus	1
Stroke/ T.I.A	2
Vascular disease like P.A.D	1
Age 65-74 yrs	1
Sex of patient- female	1

*The max score possible is 9

- Anticoagulation is of particular importance in patients who has known risk factors for stroke with AF.

Score	Risk	Anticoagulation Therapy	Considerations
0	Low	No anti-thrombotic therapy	No anti-thrombotic therapy (or Aspirin 75-325 mg/daily) (or Aspirin)
1	Moderate	Oral anticoagulant (or Aspirin)	Oral anticoagulant, either new oral anticoagulant drug e.g. Dabigatran or well controlled warfarin at INR 2.0-3.0 (or Aspirin 75-325 mg daily, depending on factors such as patient preference)
2 or greater	High	Oral anticoagulant	Oral anticoagulant, using either a new oral anticoagulant drug (Apixaban, Rivaroxaban) or well controlled warfarin at INR 2.0-3.0

Contd...

67. Ans. (b) Polymorphic ventricular tachycardia

(Ref: Harrison 20th p 1760; Harrison 19th p 1497)

- All forms of the long QT syndrome involve an abnormal repolarization of the heart. The abnormal repolarization causes differences in the refractory period of the heart muscle cells.
- After-depolarizations can be propagated to neighbouring cells due to the differences in the refractory periods, leading to re-entrant ventricular arrhythmias like torsades de pointes/ polymorphic VT.
- Early After-Depolarizations (EADs) that are seen in LQTS are due to re-opening of L-type calcium channels during the plateau phase of the cardiac action potential.
- Since adrenergic stimulation can increase the activity of these channels, this is an explanation for why the risk of sudden death in individuals with LQTS is increased during increased adrenergic states (i.e., exercise, excitement) — especially since repolarization is impaired. Normally during adrenergic states, repolarizing currents will also be enhanced to shorten the action potential. In the absence of this shortening and the presence of increased L-type calcium current, EADs may arise.
- The Jervell and Lange-Nielsen syndrome (JLNS) is an autosomal recessive form of LQTS with associated congenital deafness. It is caused specifically by mutation of the KCNE1 and KCNQ1 genes
- In untreated individuals with JLNS, about 50 percent die by the age of 15 years due to ventricular arrhythmias
- Romano-Ward syndrome is an autosomal dominant form of LQTS that is not associated with deafness.

68. Ans. (a) More common in female

(Ref: Harrison 20th p 1739; Harrison 19th p 1481; page 931, Ferri's clinical adviser 2018)

ECG findings in WPW syndrome

1. Short PR interval
2. Delta Wave with wide QRS
3. Secondary ST, T wave changes.
   - WPW syndrome is more common in males.
   - It can occur in a normal heart, it is seen in MVP, cardiomyopathy and Ebstein anomaly.

69. Ans. (d) Termination of tachycardia by carotid Sinus massage

(Ref: Harrison 20th p 1752, 1734; Harrison 19th p 1492, 1494)

Broad complex tachycardia

- ECG shows rate of > 100 and qRS complexes> 120ms

Differential diagnosis
1. VT
2. PSVT with aberrant conduction, e.g. AF, atrial flutter.

- Concordance means qRS complexes are all positive or all negative
- A fusion beat is when a 'normal beat fuses with a VT complex to create an unusual complex,
- Capture beat is a normal qRS between abnormal beats.

70. **Ans. (c)** Verapamil

(Ref: Harrison 20th p 1739; Harrison 19th p 1484)

a. PSVT. Narrow complex tachycardia (rate> 100 bpm, qRS width <120ms),
b. Acute management: Vagotonic maneuvers followed by IV adenosine, esmolol or verapamil (if not on B-blocker); DC shock if hemodynamically compromised.
c. Maintenance therapy: β-blockers or verapamil.

71. **Ans. (c)** Typical right bundle branch block

(Ref: Harrison 20th p 1756-58; Harrison 19th p 1494)

72. **Ans. (d)** Atrial fibrillation

(Ref: Harrison 20th p 3280; Harrison 19th p 1486)

73. **Ans. (d)** Prolonged PR interval

(Ref: Harrison 20th p 1756; Braunwald 8th/893-898, Harrison 19th p 1489)

74. **Ans. (b)** Procainamide

(Ref: Harrison 20th p 1741; Hurst 12th/981, Harrison 19th p 1483)

Choices A,C,D will prolong AV nodal delay and will lead to increased conduction via the aberrant pathway.

75. **Ans. (c)** WPW

(Ref: Harrison 20th p 1741; Harrison 19th p 1483)

76. **Ans. (a)** Constant PR interval

(Ref: Harrison 20th p 1728; Harrison 19th p 1472)

Mobitz I heart block has progressive increase of P-R interval.

Atherosclerotic CVD and Myocardial Infarction

77. **Ans. (a)** LDH 1 > LDH 2

(Ref: Ferri's Clinical Advisor: 2018, page 1470)

- LDH 2 is the predominant form in the serum whereas LDH1 is mainly in heart and Red blood cells. Hence in normal situation LDH2> LDH1

- In case of MI, the damaged myocytes will result in release of LDH1 in the blood stream resulting in LDH1 value in serum being more than LDH2 values. This LDH1 > LDH2 is called the *Flipped pattern*.
- However now, troponins levels are measured, post MI instead of the LDH1 and LDH2 values.

Role of LDH currently as tumour marker in:

1. Lymphoma
2. Ewing Sarcoma
3. Hepatitis
4. Haemolytic Anaemia

Isoenzymes

- Isoenzymes are multiple enzyme, isomers of enzyme
- There are five isoenzymes of LDH
- LDH-1 found in heart and in RBC as well as in brain
- LDH-2 found in the reticuloendothelial system
- LDH-3 found in the lungs
- LDH-4 found in the kidneys, placenta and pancreas
- LDH-5 found in the liver and striated muscle

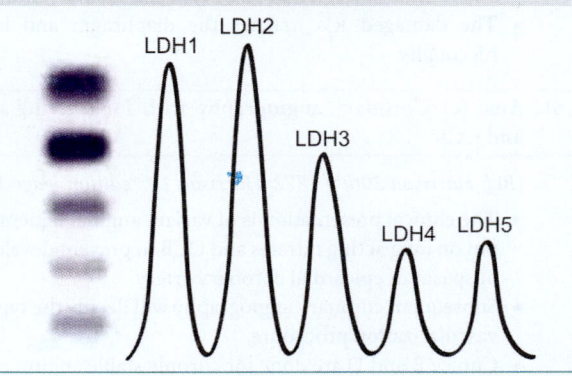

78. **Ans. (a)** Atorvastatin 80mg

(Ref: Harrison 20th p 2901; Harrison 19th edition, page 2439 and 2447)

- The lipid profile report of the patient shows *elevated LDL and triglycerides*. It points to the diagnosis of *Type IIB hyperlipoproteinemia*.
- The patient has already developed Atherosclerotic cardiovascular disease. Hence high dose statins must be started to reduce the future progression of atherosclerotic plaques in his coronary circulation.
- High intensity statins: Atorvastatin 40-80mg or Rosuvastatin 20-40mg.
- Fenofibrates are used in case of Triglyceride values shooting beyond 500mg%.

Guidelines for use of high dose statins

1. ASCVD (MI/ unstable angina/ Chronic stable angina/ Stroke/ TIA episodes/ PVD)
2. Asymptomatic with age > 21years and LDL>190mg/dl
3. LDL> 70 with DM
4. LDL >70 with age >40 years
5. 10 year CV risk by Framingham score of >7.5%

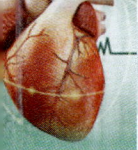

79. Ans. (a) Admit and start heparin

(Ref: Harrison 20th p 1866; Harrison 19th edition, page 1594)

- The patient is a known case of chronic stable angina and has presented with development of *unstable angina since angina episodes have become more pronounced, frequent and is occurring at rest.*
- Anti-thrombotic therapy with heparin, abciximab and intravenous beta blocker is recommended.
- TIMI score is calculated subsequently to decide the need for revascularization procedure.
- Thrombolysis is contraindicated in unstable angina.

80. Ans. (a) RCA

(Ref: Harrison 20th p 1680; Harrison 19th edition page 1608; Braunwald 9/e, page 1957)

- The RCA supplies the circulation to most of inferior myocardium. The proximal end in 60% of patients supplies the SAN and distal end in 90% patients supplies the AV node. Thus occlusion of RCA can lead to bradycardia.
- The damaged RV irritates the diaphragm and leads to hiccoughs.

81. Ans. (c) Coronary angiography with long acting nitrates and CCB

(Ref: Harrison 20th p 1872; Harrison 19th edition, page 1598)

- The clinical presentation is of variant angina. Patient will be put on long acting nitrates and CCB to prevent development of spasm of epicardial coronary artery.
- Subsequent coronary angiography will decide the type of revascularization procedure.
- Choice B and D are done for chronic stable angina
- Choice A will offer no diagnostic help.

82. Ans. (c) Serial follow up with MRI, major determinant of surgery being size greater than 5-6cm

(Ref: Harrison 20th p 1919; Harrison 19th edition, page 1693)

- The patient is having all important risk factors for development of abdominal aorta aneurysm.
- If size of AAA exceeds 5.5cm operative repair is recommended. Other indications for surgery are rapid expansion and onset of symptoms.
- Endovascular stent grafts for infra-renal AAA are achieving success in selected patients.

Risk of rupture of abdominal aorta aneurysm

AAA diameter (cm)	Rupture risk (%/y)
<4	0
4-5	0.5-5
5-6	3-15
6-7	10-20
7-8	20-40
>8	30-50

AAA = abdominal aortic aneurysm

83. Ans. (a) Endothelin1

(Ref: Harrison: 19th edition, page 265e-4)

- Plasma ET-1 levels are raised after acute myocardial infarction and it is due to coronary vasoconstriction which is responsible for myocardial ischemia and ventricular dysfunction.
- Endothelin (ET)-1 is a potent coronary vasoconstrictor.

84. Ans. (b) Triglyceride value/5

(Ref: Harrison 20th p 2900; Harrison 19th edition, page 2446)

The VLDL cholesterol is estimated by dividing the plasma concentration of triglcerides by 5. This reflects the ratio of TG to cholesterol in VLDL particles

85. Ans. (a) LDL cholesterol

(Ref: Harrison 20th p 2900; Harrison 19th edition, page 2446)

Friedewald formula is used to calculate the value of LDL-Cholesterol.

> LDL= Total cholesterol- TG/5- HDL

- The sample for lipids and lipoprotein levels should be collected after 12 hours of fasting. The Friedewald formula will calculate LDL accurately if Triglyceride value is less than 200 mg/dl. By convention the formula is not used if the value of triglycerides is more than 200 mg/dl.
- 10 year mortality due to atherosclerotic cardiovascular disease is calculated by Framingham risk calculator.

86. Ans. (b) Hyperalphalipoproteinemia

(Ref: Clinical Lipidology by Braunwald, page 73: 2014 edition, page 73)

- US National Cholesterol Education Program Adult Treatment Panel III guidelines state *an HDL cholesterol level (HDL-C) of 60 mg/dL or greater is a negative (protective) risk factor.*
- Hyperalphalipoproteinemia leads to elevated concentration of Apo-A-I and Apo-A-II and leads to elevated HDL.
- Persons with Hyperalpha-Lipoproteinemia do not have any unusual clinical features, and the *condition should not be considered a disease entity but rather a fortuitous condition that can increase longevity* because of the associated decreased incidence of CHD.
- Abetalipoproteinemia presents with low cholesterol and triglycerides. They present in infancy with diarrhea and fat malabosrbtion. Neurological features develop with loss of DTR, reduced vibration and proprioception. Spastic gait develops with pigmentary retinopathy leading to decreased night and colour vision.
- Sitosterolemia is due to inability to metabolise plant phytosterols. These patients have multiple tendon xanthomas with normal cholesterol.
- Dysbetaliporoteinemia presents with equal elevations of cholesterol and triglycerides and is a type III hyperlipidemia leading to premature atherosclerosis.

87. Ans. (c) IV immunoglobulin is used in treatment

(Ref: Harrison 20th p 2588; Harrison 19th edition, page 130t, 2192-93)

- The image shows a child with erythema over cheeks with evidence of stomatitis.
- The angiography reports shows multiple aneurysms in course of left main coronary artery
- Hence the diagnosis is Kawasaki disease.
- Choice A is wrong as aspirin prevents development of Myocardial infarction in patient of Kawasaki disease.
- Choice B is wrong as patients have bulbar congestion but absence of any discharge.
- Choice D is wrong as patients develop a unilateral cervical lymphadenopathy with fever in initial part of illness.

88. Ans. (c) Thrombolytic therapy

(Ref: Harrison 20th p 1878; Harrison 19th edn. page 1605)

- The ECG shows heart rate of 80 BPM with normal axis. P wave is normal with normal duration QRS seen after each P wave. T waves are hyper-acute in leads V2-V5 with simultaneous presence of ST segment elevation in chest leads V2-V5.
- This is diagnostic of STEMI involving anterior wall and the vessel blocked in left anterior descending artery.
- The symptoms of chest pain and diaphoresis are explained by the ECG findings of the pain.
- Ideal treatment of STEMI is PCI or thrombolysis
- Since PCI is not in choices we need to consider thrombolysis for the patient but it is *indicated only within 12 hours of onset of MI.*
- As per this question the patient presented late and hence *we will treat with aspirin to prevent future MI episode, Statin to stabilize the vulnerable plaques and morphine to calm the patient and reduce pulmonary edema.*
- E.C.G changes in acute infarction

ECG findings of ischemia	ECG finding of injury	ECG findings of cell death
• Tall wide (peaked) T wave • T wave inversion	• ST elevation (Pardee sign)	• Pathological Q wave

ST Elevation MI Management:
1. Nitrates
2. Morphine
3. Oxygen
4. Aspirin + Ticagrelor/Prasugrel
5. Start adjunctive Treatment
6. Beta Blockers (IV)
7. Nitroglycerine (IV)
8. Heparin (IV)
9. Reperfusion Therapy is the definitive treatment of choice if patient presents <12 hours.
   - Thrombolysis (Streptokinase) Door to needle time< 30 minutes
   - Early Primary PCI (Cath lab equipped hospital) Door to balloon time< 90 minutes

89. Ans. (a) Chylomicron

(Ref: Harrison's 20th, page 2893-94 and Harper's illustrated Biochemistry 28/e Pg 231-233)

- The milky plasma and abdominal pain in the child point to elevated triglycerides which can cause acute pancreatitis.
- **Milky plasma is seen in type I and type V Hyperlipoproteinemia.**
- Xanthomas are seen in type I, IIa, III and type V Hyperlipoproteinemia.
- Combination of milky plasma and xanthoma is seen in type 1 and type 5 hyper-lipoproteinemia
- In both chylomicrons are elevated, though in type V both chylomicrons and VLDL are elevated.

TABLE: Fredrickson Classification of Hyperlipoproteinemias

Phenotype	I	IIa	IIb	III	IV	V
Lipoprotein, elevate	Chylomicrons	LDL	LDL and VLDL	Chylomicron and VLDL remnants	VLDL	Chylomicrons and VLDL
Triglycerides	↑↑↑	N	↑	↑↑	↑	↑↑↑
Cholesterol (total)	↑	↑↑↑	↑↑	↑↑	N/↑	↑↑
LDL -cholesterol	↓	↑↑↑	↑↑	↓	↓	↓
HDL- cholesterol	↓↓↓	N/↓	↓	N	↓↓	↓↓↓
Plasma appearance	Lactescent	Clear	Clear	Turbid	Turbid	Lactescent
Xanthomas	Eruptive	Tendon, tuberous	None	Palmar, tuberoeruptive	None	Eruptive
Pancreatitis	+++	0	0	0	0	+++
Coronary atherosclerosis	0	+++	+++	+++	+/−	+/−
Peripheral atherosclerosis	0	+	+	++	+/−	+/−

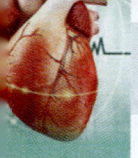

90. **Ans. (d)** The treatment includes intravenous diltiazem

(Ref: Harrison 20th p 1882; Harrison's 19th edition, page 1762, 269e-8f)

- Right ventricular (RV) infarction rarely occurs in isolation, with approximately between one-third and half of the patients with inferior-wall myocardial infarction (IWMI) having some RV involvement **(Choice A)**
- In clinical practice, RV infarction is frequently diagnosed electrocardiographically. An ST-segment elevation of >1 mm in lead V4R is considered significant and correlates closely with other noninvasive evidences of RV dysfunction. **(Choice B)**
- Patients with acute IWMI have a substantially increased risk of death during hospitalization if RV involvement is present.
- In a meta-analysis from patients undergoing thrombolysis, the mortality rate was noted to be higher in the presence of RV infarction. **(Choice C)**
- The clinical triad of hypotension, clear lung fields, and elevated jugular venous pressure has been traditionally considered as a marker of RV infarction in patients with IWMI.
- Diltiazem will *worsen the hypotension of right ventricular infarction*

91. **Ans. (d)** 4 2 1 3

(Ref: Harrison 20th p 2893; Harrison 19th, page 2439, 2441, 2443)

CHOICE	Plasma characteristics	Special feature	Alternative name
Hyperchylomicronemia	Turbid plasma with creamy supernatant	Triglycerides > 1000mg% And eruptive xanthoma	Type 1 Hyperlipoproteinemia
Familial hypercholestrolemia	Clear plasma	Tendon xanthoma	Type 2A hyperlipoproteinemia
Type III Hyperlipoproteinaemia	Turbid	Palmar and tubero-eruptive xanthoma	Familial Dysbetalipoproteinemia
Familial LPL deficiency	Turbid	Eruptive xanthoma	Primary lipid defect with single gene mutation

Types of Xanthoma

Type	Seen in	Alternative name
Eruptive	Type 1 Hyperlipoproteinaemia	Familial hyperchylomicronemia
Tendon	Type 2A Hyperlipoproteinaemia	Familial hypercholesterolemia
Palmar	Type 3 Hyperlipoproteinaemia	Familial dysbetalipoproteinemia

92. **Ans. (d)** Dressler's syndrome

(Ref: Braunwald 8th edition, Table 70-1)

Early Pericarditis	Late Pericarditis (Dressler's Syndrome)
• Occurs in 10% of patients with acute MI. • Risk factors: transmural MI. • Timing: Usually occurs 1-4 days after MI. • Symptoms: worsening of pain while supine, radiation of pain to the trapezius ridge • Physical exam: Pericardial friction rub. • Diagnosis: ECG may show evidence of pericarditis; echo may show pericardial effusion. • Treatment: aspirin. Avoid NSAIDs and corticosteroids (may interfere with healing of infarcted myocardium)	• Occurs in 1-3% of patients with acute MI. secondary to immune-medicated injury • Timing: Usually occurs 1-8 weeks after MI • Physical exam: Pericardial rub, fever • Diagnosis: ECG may show evidence of pericarditis; echocardiography may show pericardial effusion • Treatment: aspirin. If > 4 weeks since MI, can use NSAIDs and /or corticosteroids

93. **Ans. (b)** ECG shows acute anterior myocardial infarction

(Ref: Harrison 20th p 1680; Harrison 19th edition, page 1602t)

- Heart rate of the patient is about 75BPM.
- The current ECG shows presence of ST elevation in lead I, aVL and the precordial leads V2-V5 suggestive of anterior wall MI

Heart rate is 45/min	Wrong statement
Patient should be given lidocaine	It is given in case of post MI ventricular tachycardia
ECG is suggestive of hyperkalemia	ST elevation and Tall tented T waves should be present in all leads. P wave should disappear. qRS should be wide complex.

Regular rhythms can be quickly determined by counting the number of large graph boxes between two R waves. That number is divided into 300 to calculate bpm. The rates for the first one to six large boxes can be easily memorized.

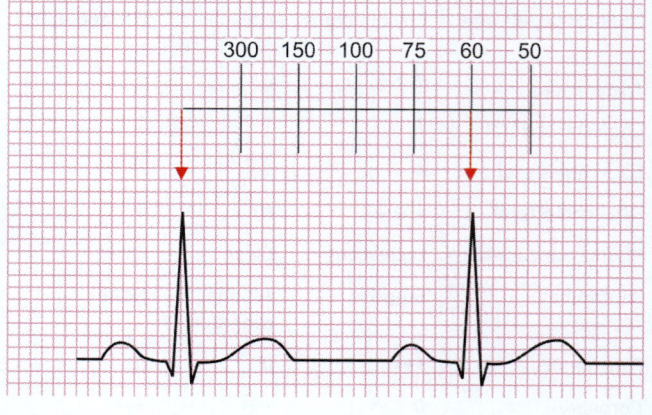

94. **Ans. (d)** Diabetes

(Ref: Harrison 20th p 2905; Harrison 19th edition, page 2428)

The most common pattern of dyslipidemia in diabetes mellitus is hypertriglyceridemia and reduced HDL levels.

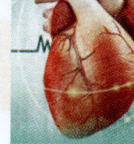

95. Ans. (c) Primary percutaneous coronary intervention

(Ref: Harrison 20th p 1878; page 1599, Harrison 19th edition)

Primary percutaneous coronary intervention PCI is the preferred therapy for ST segment elevation myocardial infarction with the objective of keeping *door to device time to be less than 90 minutes.*

96. Ans. (c) PET scan

(Ref: Harrison 20th p 1686, Table 236-1; Harrison19th, page 1582)

	SPECT	PET
Tracers used	Thallium-201 Technetium 99m 99Mtc	Rubidium 82 13N ammonia
Sensitivity	87%	90%
Specificity	73%	89%
Features	Myocardium perfusion imaging	Myocardial viability and inflammation imaging

MUGA scan: Multi-gated blood pool acquisition radionuclide angiography is used to assess LV function and volume.

For the diagnosis of angiographically significant CAD
1. SPECT using thallium 201
2. Technetium 99 m either exercise or pharmacologic stress
3. PET Myocardial perfusion imaging

The FDA approved PET tracers are-
1. Rubidium 82
2. 13-N ammonia
3. Fluro-deoxy-glucose FDG-18 assesses myocardial glucose metabolism which is an indicator of viability.

97. Ans. (d) Nitrate

(Ref: CMDT 2019, page 372 and Braunwald cardiology 8th edition, Chapter 54)

- After STEMII post MI the LV undergoes riches of changes in size shape and thickness called ventricular remodeling.
- This is reduced by ACE inhibitors ARBs
- Statins administered at dose of atorvastation 80 mg provides long term mortality benefits
- Aspirin used daily reduces the incidences of clinical events and improve survival
- Other oral antiplatelet agents like clopidogreal abciximab tirofiban and eptifibatide also improves survival
- There is no evidence that nitrates improves survival in myocardial infarction

Trials Showing Improvement in Mortality in Post MI

ACE inhibitors	SMILE, GISSI and ISIS4 trial
ARB	VALIANT
Spironolactone	RALES

98. Ans. (a, c, e) (a) ↑Troponin (c) Depression of ST segment, (e) T wave inversion

(Ref: Harrison 20th p 1868)

- Unstable angina is characterized by athero-embolism and blockage of perforators from clot fragments originating from epicardial coronary artery. The cardiac biomarkers become elevated though the doubling, tripling of Troponin levels like in myocardial infarction is not seen.
- ECG shows no ST segment change in 50% cases, ST depression in 25% cases and symmetrical T wave inversion in 25% cases.
- Rarely peaked T waves may be seen in all leads indicating disease process in Left main coronary artery called Wellen's syndrome.
- ST elevation is seen in Prinzmetal angina and hence it is called variant angina

99. Ans. (a) Atrial fibrillation

(Ref: Harrison 20th p 1747; Harrison 19th ed. / 1487-88)

- Beta blockers, nondihydropyridine calcium channel blockers (e.g., verapamil or diltiazem), and digitalis glycosides are useful in slowing the ventricular rate of patients with AF.
- Since left ventricular muscle function usually is normal in mitral stenosis, the use of digitalis is of little benefit to patients in sinus rhythm. In patients in atrial fibrillation, however, digitalis is used to slow ventricular rate. A rapid ventricular rate in mitral stenosis shortens diastole, thereby reducing left ventricular filling, which, in turn, further increases left atrial pressure and reduces cardiac output. β-Blockers and diltiazem or verapamil may be added to digoxin if further heart rate control is necessary.

100. Ans. (a) Fibrates

(Ref: Harrison 20th p 2899; Harrison 19th ed. / 2449)

- The fibrates, or fibric acid derivatives, act in part to stimulate the activity of peroxisome proliferator-activated receptors (PPARs), which are involved in fatty acid breakdown. *The main action of fibrates is to lower triglyceride levels (by 35 to 50 percent). Fibrates also raise serum high density lipoprotein (HDL) by 15 to 25 percent. Fibrates are the drugs of choice when treating isolated elevated triglycerides.*
- Niacin, fibrates, and prescription omega-3 fatty acids are approved for the treatment of patients with hypertriglyceridemia.
- Statins (or HMG-CoA reductase inhibitors) are a class of cholesterol lowering drugs that inhibit the enzyme HMG-CoA reductase which plays a central role in the production of cholesterol.
- Ezetimibe inhibits the absorption of cholesterol from the small intestine and decreases the amount of cholesterol normally available to liver cells, leading them to absorb more from circulation and thus lowering levels of circulating cholesterol

101. Ans. (b) Cardiac Biomarkers

(Ref: Harrison 20th p 1868; Harrison 19th ed. / 1580)

- Cardiac markers are used in the diagnosis and risk stratification of patients with chest pain and suspected acute coronary syndrome (ACS).

- The cardiac troponins, in particular, have become the cardiac markers of choice for patients with acute coronary syndrome which includes NSTEMI.
- Indeed, cardiac troponin is central to the definition of acute myocardial infarction (MI) in the consensus guidelines from the European Society of Cardiology (ESC) and the American College of Cardiology (ACC).
- *However in chronic Stable angina the symptoms arise on exertion/emotion or post-prandially and have characteristic ST segment depression on exercise testing. Cardiac biomarkers are normal as no cell death occurs in this case.*

102. Ans. (b) Autoimmune

(*Ref: Braunwald 8th edition, Table 70-1*)

- Post-pericardiotomy syndrome following myocardial infarction is called Dressler syndrome and is an autoimmune process.
- It also seen as an unusual complication after percutaneous procedures such as coronary stent implantation, after implantation of epicardial pacemaker leads and trans-venous pacemaker leads, and following blunt trauma, stab wounds, and heart puncture.
- It involves the pleura and pericardium and is also seen in patients who have undergone surgery that involves opening the pericardium.

103. Ans. (d) Lisinopril

(*Ref: Harrison 20th p 1871; Harrison 19th ed. / 1623*)

- ACEIs attenuate the development of left ventricular hypertrophy, improve symptomatology and risk of death from CHF, and reduce morbidity and mortality rates in post-myocardial infarction patients.
- Similar benefits in cardiovascular morbidity and mortality rates in patients with CHF have been observed with the use of ARBs.
- ACEIs provide better coronary protection than do calcium channel blockers, whereas calcium channel blockers provide more stroke protection than do either ACEIs or beta blockers.

104. Ans. (d) Warfarin

(*Ref: Harrison 20th p 1871*)

Aspirin and clopidogrel have been shown to reduce mortality due to MI.
- Statins regress atherosclerosis and β blockers due to oxygen conserving action will prevent future episode of MI.
- Warfarin is not routinely used in post MI Patients.

105. Ans. (d) Alcohol

(*Ref: Harrison 19th ed. / 95e-5*)

- Alcohol in mild amounts has been shown to have beneficial effect on heart.
- Studies have shown chylamydia as incriminating factor for atherosclerosis and so does poor dental hygiene.

106. Ans. (a) Acute extensive anterior wall MI

(*Ref: Harrison 20th p 1680; Harrison 19th ed. pg 1605*)

- The ECG shows patient in sinus Rhythm, normal QRS axis
- Upsloping ST segment elevation is seen in V2-V5 and aVL
- In extreme left premature ventricular beats can be noticed in Lead II and Lead III
- Rhythm strip lead II shows ST depression (right at the bottom)
- Brugada syndrome has ST elevation in V1-V3 and can present with sudden collapse during physical exertion but the collapse occurs due to ventricular tachycardia. ECG strip however does not show any tachyarrhythmia.
- Arrythmogenic right ventrcular dysplasia shows presence of epsilon waves.

107. Ans. (b) ST segment depression in lead II, III, aVF

(*Ref: Harrison 20th p 1680; Harrison 19th ed. page 1605*)

The ECG shows
- Sinus rhythm is present with normal QRS axis and tall T waves.
- ST elevation >1 mm in V4R and leads II, III, aVF.
- ST depression (reciprocal) is present in anterior leads.
- Hence the diagnosis is right ventricular MI.
- Right ventricular infarction leads to hypotension with clear lung fields and presence of elevated JVP (Kussmaul sign +).

108. Ans. (c) Anterior wall MI

(*Ref: Harrison 20th p 1680; Page 1605, Harrison 19th ed.*)

- ECG shows presence of ST elevation from V2-V5 which is diagnostic of anterior wall MI.

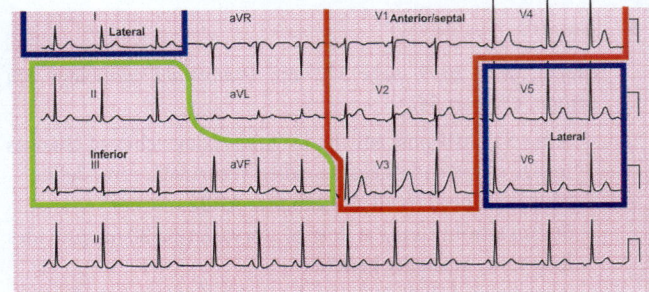

109. Ans. (c) Tendon xanthoma

(*Ref: Harrison 20th p 2893; Harrison 19th ed. page 2441, 2443*)

- Tendon xanthoma develops in pressure areas, such as the extensor surfaces of the knees, the elbows, and the buttocks.
- They appear as slowly enlarging subcutaneous nodules related to the tendons or the ligaments. Sometimes they might mimic gout-like lesions.
- Eruptive xanthomas erupt as crops of small, red-yellow papules on an erythematous base
- Xanthoma disseminatum presents in adults as red-yellow papules and nodules with a predilection for the flexures. Sometimes, they may have extensive eyelid involvement.

110. Ans. (d) Acute pericarditis

(Ref: Harrison 20th p 1841)

The history points to recent viral infection that could contribute to development of pericarditis. Most common cause of pericarditis is idiopathic or viral.

ECG findings:
- Heart rate= 75 bpm
- Axis= normal
- PR interval= 0.16 sec
- QRS= 0.08 sec
- QT= 400 msec
- Uniform ST segment elevation in all the leads but ST segment depression in aVR seals the diagnosis of pericarditis.

111. Ans. (c) Nitrates are mortality reducing drugs

(Ref: Harrison 19th ed. page 1582 & 1583; CMDT 2019, page 372)

- The tracing shows ST segment DOWNSLOPING depression >2 mm and is persisting for >80 msec, which is the necessary criteria for stable angina.
- The fixed stenotic lesion > 70% leads to symptoms of unstable angina.
- The chest pain develops on exertion/emotion and is relieved over 3–5 minutes by rest.
- The major mortality reduction with chronic stable angina is seen > beta blockers.

112. Ans. (a) Thallium scan

(Ref: Braunwald 8th edn, Table 16-1)

Thallium scan is a class I indication for Risk assessment, prognosis, and assessment of therapy after STE acute myocardial infarction and can be used to determine
1. Rest RV/LV function
2. Presence/extent of stress-induced ischemia
3. Detection of infarct size and residual viable myocardium

Thallium scan is also a class I indication for:
1. Diagnosis, prognosis, and assessment of therapy in patients with unstable angina/NSTEMI.
2. Diagnosis of symptomatic and selected patients with asymptomatic myocardial ischemia
3. Assessment of ventricular performance (rest or exercise)

113. Ans. (b) β Blocker

(Ref: CMDT 2019 p 372)

114. Ans. (d) Clopidogrel

(Ref: Harrison 20th p 846; Harrison 19th p 745)

Thrombocytopenia is a rare but dangerous adverse effect of clopidogrel, encompassing Thrombotic Thrombocytopenic Purpura (TTP), isolated thrombocytopenia and autoimmune thrombocytopenia.

115. Ans. (c) Angina assessment

(Ref: Braunwald 8th edn Ch 57)

- In ROSE assessment we ask the patient to point to chest pain with his hand. We ask for radiation of chest pain, how did it come at rest or exertion and how did it go away.
- The Rose Questionnaire was developed initially to diagnose both angina and intermittent claudication in epidemiological surveys. It questions whether the patient develops pain in either calf with walking and whether the pain occurs at rest, while walking at an ordinary or hurried pace, or when walking uphill.

116. Ans. (d) IVUS

(Ref: Evidence based cardiology consult, page 217, 2014 edition)

- Coronary lesions prone to rupture have a distinct morphology compared with stable plaques, and can be detected by noninvasive imaging to identify vulnerable plaques before they lead to clinical events.

(Intravascular ultrasound) ⟶ IVUS is the gold standard for evaluating coronary plaque, lumen and vessel characteristics

117. Ans. (c) 3 × Troponin elevation is required for CABG related MI

(Ref: Braunwalds 9th ed. page 1241 Harrison 20th p 1877; Harrison 19th p 1602 Table 295.2)

- Elevation of the troponin I level more than ten times the upper limit of normal is commonly considered diagnostic of MI in CABG related MI (Type 5 MI)
- Elevation of troponin I level five times the normal limit is associated with type 4A MI which is seen during the performance of percutaneous coronary intervention
- New regional wall motion in MI is suggestive of MI and/or expansion of the existing damage in the heart. It is also useful for diagnosis of intra-operative MI
- Sudden death is seen in MI and is seen with Type III MI. Usual cause is a ventricular fibrillation.
- In case of re-infarction the values of TROPONIN I will show an increasing trend over the admission values with significant cut off being >5%.

118. Ans. (b) Pericardial fluid collection on Echocardiography

(Ref: Harrison 20th p 1884; Harrison 19th p 1610)

- The diagnosis of this patient is transmural MI with extensive necrosis causing a hemorrhagic pericardial effusion.
- The patient was put on thrombolytic and anticoagulant which will cause the hemorrhagic effusion to increase in size.
- In fact some of these patients can develop cardiac tamponade. This will produce cardiogenic shock and drastic reduction in cardiac output.

- So thrombolytic agent and anticoagulant need to be stopped.
- Following thrombolysis, the most frequent and potentially the most serious complication is hemorrhage

119. Ans. (a) Tendon xanthoma

(Ref: Harrison 20th p 2893; Harrison 19th p 2440)

- Increased LDL cholesterol and triglycerides in the normal range suggests the diagnosis of hypercholesterolemia.
- The diagnosis of this patient is type IIA hyper-lipoproteinemia
- These disorders are characterized by mutation in the L.D.L. receptors.
- Tendon xanthoma are seen in type IIA hyper-lipoproteinemia

- ERUPTIVE xanthomas are seen in type I, III and Type V hyperlipoproteinemia.
- The most common hyperlipoproteinemia is type IIB and does not have any xanthoma
- Touton cells are found in xanthoma.

120. Ans. (c) 12 hrs

(Ref: CMDT 2019, page 386)

Fibrinolysis
- Since myocardium can be salvaged only before it has been irreversibly injured, the timing of reperfusion therapy, is of extreme importance.
- It is clear that every minute counts and that patients treated within 1–3 h of the onset of symptoms generally benefit most.
- *Although reduction of the mortality rate is more modest, the therapy remains of benefit for many patients seen 3–6 h after the onset of infarction, and some benefit appears to be possible up to 12 h, especially if chest discomfort is still present and ST segments remain elevated.*
- If no contraindications are present, fibrinolytic therapy should ideally be initiated within 30 min of presentation (i.e., door-to-needle time <30 min). The principal goal of fibrinolysis is prompt restoration of full coronary arterial patency.

121. Ans. (b) Diabetic retinal flame shaped hemorrhage

(Ref: Harrison 20th p 1879; Harrison 19th p 1605)

Fundus finding in Diabetic retinopathy of flame shaped hemorrhages is not an active bleeding and thrombolysis may be done. (Simply put, man can live without an eye but not without a heart.)

Contraindications and Cautions for Thrombolysis

Absolute	Relative
- Prior intracranial hemorrhage	- Pregnancy
- Known structure cerebral vascular lesion	
- Known malignant intracranial neoplasm	- Recent invasive surgical procedures

Absolute	Relative
- Significant closed–head or facial trauma (< 3 months)	- Prolonged CPR
- Ischemic Stroke (< 3 months) Active bleeding	- Active peptic ulcer
- Suspected aortic dissection - Uncontrolled hypertension (SBP> 180, DBP > 110)	- Hemorrhagic diabetic retinopathy

122. Ans. (b) 1.5 million units

(Ref: Harrison 20th p 856; Harrison 19th p 1605)

The adult dose of streptokinase for AMI is 1.5 million U in 50 mL of 5% dextrose in water (D5W) given IV over 60 minutes. Allergic reactions force the termination of many infusions before a therapeutic dose can be administered.

123. Ans. (b) 10 IU

(Ref: Harrison 20th p 857; Harrison 19th p 759)

Thrombolytics drugs used in acute MI	
Drug	**Dose**
1. Reteplase is a second-generation recombinant tissue-type plasminogen activator that seems to work more rapidly and has a lower bleeding risk than the first-generation agent alteplase. The drug is produced in Escherichia coli by means of recombinant DNA techniques.	Reteplase is FDA-approved for AMI and is administered as 2 boluses of 10 U given 30 minutes apart, with each bolus administered over 2 minutes.
2. Tenecteplase, the latest thrombolytic agent approved for use in clinical practice. It is produced by recombinant DNA technology using Chinese hamster ovary cells.	Tenecteplase is administered in a 30-50 mg IV bolus over 5 seconds.
3. Streptokinase is produced by beta-hemolytic streptococci **(Streptococcus equisimilus)**. Because streptokinase is produced from streptococcal bacteria, it often causes febrile reactions and other allergic problems. It can also cause hypotension that appears to be dose-related. Streptokinase usually cannot be administered safely a second time within 6 months, because it is highly antigenic and results in high levels of antistreptococcal antibodies.	The adult dose of streptokinase for AMI is 1.5 million U in 50 mL of 5% dextrose in water (D5W) given IV over 60 minutes.
4. Alteplase was the first recombinant tissue-type plasminogen activator and is identical to native tPA. Alteplase is fibrin-specific and has a plasma half-life of 4-6 minutes. It is the lytic agent most often used for treatment of coronary artery thrombosis, PE, and AIS.	Alteplase can be administered in an accelerated infusion (1.5 h) using 50-mg and 100-mg vials and reconstituted with sterile water to 1 mg/mL. *AIS = Acute Ischemic Stroke

Contd...

124. Ans. (b) Ventricular fibrillation

(Ref: Harrison 19th p 1602)

- Tachyarrythmia contributing to sudden death after MI is ventricular fibrillation or ventricular tachycardia
- Bradyarrythmia leading to sudden death after MI is Mobitz II heart block
- Prompt reperfusion, efforts to reduce infarct size and treatment of ongoing ischemia and other complications of MI appear to have reduced the incidence of cardiogenic shock from 20% to about 7%. Only 10% of patients with this condition present with it on admission, while 90% develop it during hospitalization.
- Rupture of the free wall of the left or right ventricles, as this is associated with immediate hemodynamic collapse and death secondary to acute pericardial tamponade. *Cardiac rupture is rare in this scenario of PCI facilities.*

125. Ans. (b) PCI with angioplasty

(Ref: Harrison 20th p 2054; Harrison 19th p 1762)

According to newer guidelines, PCI with angioplasty will be preferred over intra-aortic balloon pump for management of cardiogenic shock in AMI.

126. Ans. (b) Unstable angina

(Ref: Emergency of cardiolog by Amel Mettu: p 14 2018 edition)

Severe anterior wall ischemia (with or without infarction) may cause prominent T-wave inversions in the precordial leads. This pattern (sometimes referred to as Wellens T waves) is usually associated with a high-grade stenosis of the left anterior descending coronary artery and presents as unstable angina. Wellens syndrome is also referred to as LAD coronary T-wave syndrome.

Criteria include the following:
1. Characteristic T-wave changes
2. History of anginal chest pain
3. Normal or minimally elevated cardiac enzyme levels.
4. ECG without Q waves, without significant ST-segment elevation, and with normal precordial R-wave progression.
    - Recognition of this ECG abnormality is of paramount importance because this syndrome represents a preinfarction stage of coronary artery disease (CAD) that often progresses to a devastating anterior wall MI.

127. Ans. (b) 6 minutes

(Ref: Harrison 20th p 857; Harrison 19th p 759)

- Alteplase was the first recombinant tissue-type plasminogen activator and is identical to native tPA. In vivo, tissue-type plasminogen activator is synthesized and made available by cells of the vascular endothelium. It is the physiologic thrombolytic agent responsible for most of the body's natural efforts to prevent excessive thrombus propagation.
- *Alteplase is fibrin-specific and has a plasma half-life of 4-6 minutes.*

128. Ans. (a) Left ventricular aneurysm

(Ref: Harrison 20th p 1884; Harrison 19th p 1610)

- Persistent ST segment elevation after treatment for MI can be due to LV aneurysm or Re-thrombosis in infarct related artery.
- To differentiate between the two serial CPKMB levels matter. CPK levels showing an increasing trend point to diagnosis of re-thromobosis while when CPK MB levels plateau off is suggestive of LV aneurysm.
- Imaging like bed side Echo can also help in diagnosing a LV aneurysm where as a new motion wall abnormality points to arethrombosis of infarct related artery.
- Ischemic complication of MI can include infarct extension, recurrent infarction, and recurrent angina.
- The diagnosis of infarct expansion, re-infarction, or post-infarction ischemia can be made with echocardiography or nuclear imaging. A new wall motion abnormality, larger infarct size, new area of infarction, or persistent reversible ischemic changes help substantiate the diagnosis. CK-MB is a more useful marker for tracking ongoing infarction than troponin, given its shorter half-life. Re-elevation and subsequent decline in CK-MB levels suggest infarct expansion or recurrent infarction. Elevations in the CK-MB level of more than 50% over a previous nadir are diagnostic for reinfarction.

129. Ans. (a) A.I.V.R

(Ref: Harrison 20th p 1882)

- AIVR refers to a ventricular rhythm that is characterized by three or more complexes at a rate >40 beats/min and < 120 beats/min. Mechanism is due to abnormal automaticity originating distal to bundle of His
- AIVR has a characteristic gradual onset and offset and more variability in cycle length. It is typically a brief, self-limiting arrhythmia.
- AIVR can be seen in
    a. Acute myocardial infarction
    b. Cocaine intoxication
    c. Acute myocarditis
    d. Digoxin intoxication
    e. Postoperative cardiac surgery.
- In the setting of sustained AIVR, hemodynamic compromise can occur because of the loss of AV synchrony

130. Ans. (b) ST elevation, T inversion, Q wave

(Ref: Harrison 20th p 1680; Harrison 19th p 1456)

- The earliest presentation of acute myocardial infarction is the hyperacute T wave, which is treated the same as ST segment elevation.
- In practice this is rarely seen, because it only exists for 2–30 minutes after the onset of infarction. Hyper-acute T waves need to be distinguished from the peaked T waves associated with hyperkalemia.
- In the first few hours the ST segments usually begin to rise. Pathological Q waves may appear within hours or may take greater than 24 hr.
- The T wave will generally become inverted in the first 24 hours, as the ST elevation begins to resolve.
- Long term changes of ECG include persistent Q waves (in 90% of cases) and persistent inverted T waves.
- Persistent ST elevation is rare except in the presence of a ventricular aneurysm

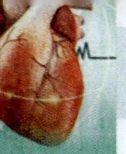

131. Ans. (c) Chronic liver failure

(Ref: Cardiac intensive care 2nd edition, pg. 199)

The best test for diagnosis of MI is troponin I which can be quantified as value more than 0.04ng/dl after 3 hours of onset of myocardial infarction. TROPONIN -I can be false positive in the following cases

System	Causes of Troponin Elevation
Cardiovascular	Acute aortic dissection Arrhythmia Medical ICU patients Hypotension Heart failure Apical ballooning syndrome Cardiac inflammation Endocarditis, myocarditis, pericarditis Hypertension Infiltrative disease Amyloidosis, sarcoidosis, hemochromatosis, Scleroderma Left ventricular hypertrophy
Myocardial Injury	Blunt chest trauma Cardiac surgeries Cardiac procedures Ablation, cardioversion, percutaneous intervention
Respiratory	Acute PE ARDS
Infectious/ Immune	Sepsis/SIRS Viral illness Thrombotic thrombocytopenic purpura
Gastrointestinal	Severe GI bleeding
Nervous system	Acute stroke • Ischemic stroke • Hemorrhagic stroke Head trauma
Renal	Chronic kidney disease
Endocrine	Diabetes Hypothyroidism
Musculoskeletal Inherited	Rhabdomyolysis Neurofibromatosis Duchenne muscular dystrophy

132. Ans. (b) <180/110

(Ref: Harrison 20th p 1879; Chapter 245, page 2028, Harrison 19th p 2562)

Thrombolysis is contraindicated with SBP > 180 and DBP >110 mm Hg

133. Ans. (b) HDL 2

(Ref: Clinical Lipidology: Braunwald, pg 97)

- The risk of development of acute myocardial infarction is inversely related to total HDL and HDL2.
- HDL is the smallest and densest lipoprotein. It has 2 major subfractions HDL2 and HDL3. HDL2 has higher lipid content then HDL 3.
- HDL 2 plays a role in reverse cholesterol transport from tissues to be excreted via bile.

134. Ans. (a) Anterior wall MI (See Table below)

(Ref: Harrison 20th p 1670; Harrison 19th p 1446)

Pulsus alternans is a pattern in which there is regular alteration of the pressure pulse amplitude, despite a regular rhythm. It is due to alternating left ventricular contractile force, which usually indicates severe impairment of left ventricular function/ and commonly occurs in patients who also have a loud third heart sound.

Type	Character	Disease
Pulsus paradoxus	Decrease in Systolic pressure > 12 mm Hg during inspiration	1. Cardiac tamponade 2. Chronic constrictive pericarditis 3. Inferior wall MI 4. Emphysema 5. Bronchial asthma (Severe) 6. SVC obstruction 7. Pulmonary embolism
Hypokinetic pulse	Small weak pulse, a narrow pulse pressure, and increased peripheral vascular resistance	Hypovolemia, Left ventricular failure, Restrictive pericardial disease, Aortic stenosis
Pulsus tardus (Pulsus parvus-et-tardus)	Slow rising pulse with delayed systolic peak	Severe aortic valve stenosis
Reversed pulsus paradoxus	Increase in systolic pressure during inspiration	HOCM, IPPV
Pulsus Bisfriens	2 systolic peaks Normal beat followed by premature beat followed by compensatory pause occurring in rapid succession resulting in alteration in strength of pulse(like pulsus alternans however in pulsus alternans there is no compensatory pause)	1. Severe Aortic regurgitation 2. Combined aortic stenosis & severe aortic regurgitation 3. H.O.C.M 4. Digitalis toxicity
Dicrotic pulse	1 systolic & 1 diastolic peak	1. Dilated cardiomyopathy 2. Cardiac tamponade 3. Typhoid 4. Dehydration
Pulsus alternans (Radial artery)	Alternate strong & weak beat with regular rhythm	1. Severe Left ventricular functional impairment (e.g Acute M.I) 2. May occur in paroxysmal tachycardia 3. Toxic myocarditis 4. For several beats following a premature beat
Water Hammer Pulse/ Collapsing/ Corrigan's Pulse	Large bounding pulse associated with increased stroke volume & decreased peripheral vascular resistance	Aortic regurgitation

135. Ans. (d) Ability to complete stage 3 of Bruce protocol treadmill

(Ref: Harrison 20th p 1858; Harrison 19th p 1582)

- Relative risk of future cardiovascular events based on hs-CRP testing is estimated as follows:
  1. Low risk: CRP < 1.0 mg/L
  2. Intermediate risk: CRP 1.0-3.0 mg/L
  3. High risk: CRP > 3.0 mg/L
- Agatson score is used to evaluate coronary artery calcification which is directly related to atherosclerosis severity.
- Intravascular USG showing lumen reduction of coronary artery is indicative of atherosclerosis.

136. Ans. (a) CPK, AST, LDH

(Ref: Pubmed)

137. Ans. (a) Troponin I and T

(Ref: Harrison 20th p 1876; Harrison 19th p 1600)

- Troponin is released during MI from the cytosolic pool of the myocytes.
- Its subsequent release is prolonged with degradation of actin and myosin filaments.
- Differential diagnosis of troponin elevation includes acute infarction, severe pulmonary embolism causing acute right heart overload, heart failure and myocarditis.
- Troponins can also help to calculate infarct size but the peak must be measured in the 3rd day.
- They are released in 2-4 hours and persist for up to 7 days.
- **This is the most sensitive and specific test for myocardial damage.**
- CK-MB resides in the cytosol and facilitates high energy phosphates into and out of mitochondria.
- It is distributed in a large number of tissues even in the skeletal muscle.
- It is relatively specific when skeletal muscle damage is not present.
- **REASON WHY AN ATHLETE DEVELOPS MI?**—Coronary anomalies of left coronary artery originating from the right aortic sinus along with an intramural course, which gets KINKED during high performance sports.

138. Ans. (c) Focal spasm is most common in left coronary artery

(Ref: Harrison 20th p 1871-72; Harrison 19th p 1598)

- Patients with Prinzmetal's Variant Angina are generally younger and have fewer coronary risk factors (with the exception of cigarette smoking) than patients with UA secondary to coronary atherosclerosis.
- The clinical diagnosis of variant angina is made with the detection of transient ST-segment elevation with rest pain. Many patients also exhibit multiple episodes of asymptomatic ST-segment elevation (silent ischemia). Small elevations of troponin may occur in patients with prolonged attacks of variant angina.
- Coronary angiography demonstrates transient coronary spasm as the diagnostic hallmark of PVA. Atherosclerotic plaques, which do not usually cause critical obstruction, in at least one proximal coronary artery occur in the majority of patients, and in them spasm usually occurs within 1 cm of the plaque.
- Focal spasm is most common in the right coronary artery, and it may occur at one or more sites in one artery or in multiple arteries simultaneously. Ergonovine, acetylcholine, other vasoconstrictor medications, and hyperventilation have been used to provoke focal coronary stenosis on angiography to establish the diagnosis. Hyperventilation has also been used to provoke rest angina, ST-segment elevation, and spasm on coronary arteriography.

139. Ans. (b) Chlamydia pneumoniae

(Ref: Harrison 20th p 1324; Harrison 19th p 1173)

Epidemiologic studies have demonstrated an association between serologic evidence of C. pneumoniae infection and atherosclerotic disease of the coronary and other arteries.

140. Ans. (b) 5-10 minutes

(Ref: Harrison 20th p 1853; Harrison 19th p 1580)

- **Duration:** More than 2 and less than 10 min
- Patient presents with Levine sign.
- **Quality:** Pressure, tightness, squeezing, heaviness, burning
- **Location:** Retrosternal, often with radiation to or isolated discomfort in neck, jaw, shoulders, or arms—frequently on left Precipitated by exertion, exposure to cold, psychological stress
- Associated Features: S4 gallop or mitral regurgitation murmur during pain

141. Ans. (b) Crescendo pain with ECG findings

(Ref: Harrison 20th p 1868; Harrison 19th 1594)

UA is defined as angina pectoris or equivalent ischemic discomfort with at least one of three features:
1. It occurs at rest (or with minimal exertion), usually lasting > 10 min
2. It is severe and of new onset (i.e., within the prior 4-6 weeks); and/or
3. It occurs with a crescendo pattern (i.e., distinctly more severe, prolonged, or frequent than previously)
4. In UA, ST-segment depression, transient ST-segment elevation, and/or T-wave inversion occur in 30-50% of patients, depending on the severity of the clinical presentation. In patients with the clinical features of UA, the presence of new ST-segment deviation, even of only 0.05 mV, is an important predictor of adverse outcome. T-wave changes are sensitive for ischemia but less specific, unless they are new, deep T-wave inversions (0.3 mV).

142. Ans. (d) Treatment with steroids is necessary

(Ref: Harrison 19th p 1610; CMDT 2019 pg 391-92)

Dressler syndrome is post MI pericarditis/Pleuritis and is characterized by autoimmunity causing damage to the heart. The resultant inflammation causes chest pain in these patients up to 6 weeks of a preceding myocardial inflammation. The investigations show ECG evidence of pericarditis with ST elevation with concavity in upwards direction.

The CPK-MB levels are normal. The treatment of these patients shall be aspirin 650mg TID for 3-5 days. Braunwald 10th edition states that glucocorticoids may impair helaing process and me best avoided.

143. Ans. (d) Echocardiography

(Ref: Harrison 19th p 270e, 2291)

The diagnosis of patient is **Hypothyroidism and the presentation of MYXEDEMA HEART is characterized by a massive pericardial effusion without any findings of hypotension or pulsus paradoxsus.**

Main cause of enlarged cardiac silhouette in hypothyroidism is pericardial effusion. Pericardial effusions occur in up to 30% of patients but rarely compromise cardiac function. Out of the choices mentioned, echocardiogram is the investigation of choice for diagnosis. Other Cardiopulmonary manifestations of hypothyroidism are as follows:

- Myocardial contractility and pulse rate are reduced
- Increased peripheral resistance- diastolic hypertension. Blood flow is diverted from the skin- cool extremities.
- Alterations in myosin heavy chain isoform expression -cardiomyopathy is unusual.
- Pulmonary function is generally normal, but dyspnea may be caused by pleural effusion, impaired respiratory muscle function, diminished ventilatory drive, or sleep apnea.

144. Ans. (c) Pericardial effusion

(Ref: Harrison 19th p 1610; Braunwald 10th edition pg 1136)

- Dressler's syndrome is also known as post-myocardial infarction syndrome and the term is sometimes used to also refer to post-pericardiotomy pericarditis which is a secondary form of pericarditis that occurs in the setting of injury to the heart or the pericardium.
- *It consists of a triad of features, fever, pleuritic pain and pericardial friction rub/pericardial effusion.*
- It is believed to result from an autoimmune inflammatory reaction to myocardial neo-antigens formed as a result of the MI.
- A similar pericarditis can be associated with any pericardiotomy or trauma to the pericardium or heart surgery.

145. Ans. (c) ST segment elevation

(Ref: Harrison 20th p 1680; Harrison 19th p 1456)

146. Ans. (c) Symptomatic severe aortic stenosis

(Ref: Harrison 19th p 1532, Braunwald 10th edition pg 168)

147. Ans. (c) Decreased fibrinogen levels

(Ref: Harrison 19th p 1587-88)

148. Ans. (a) hs CRP

(Ref: Braunwald's 8th/1013, 1014, Harrison 19th p 1582)

(Hypertension, pg 148: Companion to Braunwald 2nd/e)

149. Ans. (d) LDL/HDL

(Ref: Braunwald 8th/1008; Essential Cardiology 2nd/ 6;)

150. Ans. (d) Omega 3 polyunsaturated fatty acids

(Ref: Harrison 20th p 2901)

151. Ans. (a) Anterior wall of left ventricle

(Ref: Robbins 8th/557)

152. Ans. (d) Marginal artery

(Ref: Robbin's 8th/577-578; Snell's 7th/117-119)

153. Ans. (d) The levels of cardiac markers remain unchanged

(Ref: Harrison 20th p 1854; Harrison 19th p 1582)

154. Ans. (b) Cardiac troponins

(Ref: Harrison 20th p 1876; Harrison 19th p 1600)

155. Ans. (b) Troponin T/I

(Ref: Harrison 20th p 1876; Harrison 19th p 1600)

156. Ans. (b) Nitrates

(Ref: Harrison 20th p 1872; Harrison 19th p 1598)

157. Ans. (d) Primary angioplasty

(Ref: Harrison 20th p 2054; Harrison 19th p 1762)

158. Ans. (d) Calcium channel blockers

(Ref: Harrison 20th p 1877; Harrison 19th p 1603-4)

159. Ans. (a) Intracranial malignancy

(Ref: Harrison 20th p 1879; Braunwald's 8th/1237, Harrison 19th p 1605)

160. Ans. (d) Right ventricular infarction

(Ref: Harrison 20th p 1882; Harrison 19th p 1608)

- RVMI leads to decreased pulmonary flow and hypotension on presentation. RVF explains then kussmaul sign

161. Ans. (b) Mitral regurgitation

(Ref: Harrison 20th p 1874; Harrison 19th p 1543)

162. Ans. (a) Complete heart block

(Ref: Harrison 20th p 1874)

163. Ans. (c) **Thallium scan**

(Ref: Harrison 20th p 1686; Harrison 19th p 1585)

164. Ans. (a) **Ventricular tachycardia**

(Ref: Harrison 20th p 2064; Harrison 19th p 1769)

165. Ans. (d) **These may result in aneurysm**

(Ref: Robbins 8th/575)

For aneurysm formation, full thickness infarction is required.

Valvular Lesions of Heart

166. Ans. (a) **Mild MS**

(Ref: Harrison 20th p 1815; Harrison 19th edition pg. 1447)

- Calcified mitral valve will reduce the mobility of valve leaflets and produce soft S1.
- Aortic regurgitation leads to increase of LVEDP, which *decreases the gradient* between left atrium and left ventricle. The explains the soft S1
- Heart block will lead to bradycardia and produce soft S1.
- The intensity of S1 is determined by distance over which the anterior valve leaflet must travel to return to its annular plane. Mitral stenosis of any grade will lead to increase in LA minus LV gradient and resultant loud S1.

167. Ans. (a) **Displacement of one or both mitral valve leaflets posteriorly into left atrium during systole**

(Ref: Harrison 20th p 1822; Harrison 19th edition page 1546)

- In MVP, the mitral valve leaflets have systolic displacement of >2mm above plane of mitral annulus into left atrium. Hence choice A is correct
- During squatting the LV volume increases which pushes the mid-systolic click farther away from S1
- During standing venous return reduces, leading to reduced LV volume and mid-systolic click comes closer to S1. Hence choice B is wrong.

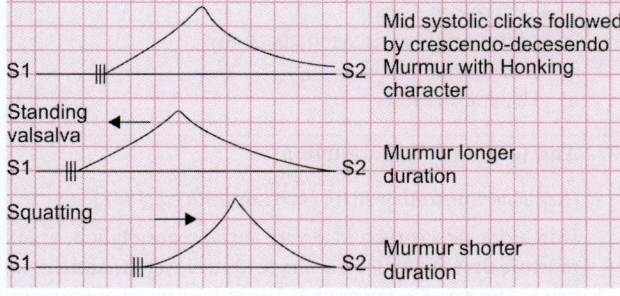

- Beta blockers are given only in select cases as most patients of MVP are asymptomatic. Hence Choice C is wrong.
- Sudden cardiac death is rare and occurs in patients with severe MR. Hence choice D is wrong.

168. Ans. (a) **Premature ventricular contraction**

(Ref: Harrison 20th p 1822; Harrison 19th p 1546)

MVP may lead to excessive stress on papillary muscles which will lead to dysfunction and ischemia of papillary muscles. The subjacent myocardium will suffer from ischemia leading to premature ventricular contractions recorded in ECG.

Arrhythmias seen in MVP

1. Premature ventricular contractions
2. PSVT
3. VT
4. Atrial fibrillation

169. Ans. (d) **Defect in type IV collagen**

(Ref: Harrison 20th p 1822; Harrison 19th p 1546)

- Transient ischemic attacks occur in MVP due to endothelial disruption which leads to cerebral emboli.
- Infective endocarditis occurs in MVP in patients with Mitral regurgitation
- Due to stress on papillary muscles and subjacent myocardium, PVC and PSVT can occur.
- A Defect in *type III collagen* has been incriminated in MVP with electron microscopy showing fragmentation of collagen fibrils.
- The pattern of inheritance of MVP is autosomal dominant with incomplete penetrance.

170. Ans. (b) **Pulsus bisferiens is a hallmark finding**

(Ref: Harrison 20th p 1805; Harrison 19th p 1530)

- Aortic stenosis results in left ventricular hypertrophy which will result in double apical impulse and shift of apex beat laterally.
- The characteristic pulse of aortic stenosis is Pulsus parvus et tardus. *Pulsus bisferiens is seen in HOCM, severe AR and concomitant AS and AR.*
- In early stages the BP is normal. In later stages as stroke volume reduces, it results in low SBP and reduced pulse pressure.
- The murmur in aortic stenosis is an ejection systolic murmur and the transvalvular gradient results in development of carotid thrill. It is not to be confused with dancing carotids seen in aortic regurgitation.

171. Ans. (a) **Left outflow tract obstruction**

(Ref: Harrison 20th p 1677, 1805; Harrison 19th p 1454)

- The ECG shows a heart rate of 55/min with left axis deviation
- SV1+RV5> 35 mm is suggestive of left ventricular hypertrophy
- Narrow split S2 indicates outflow tract obstruction
- Taking into consideration the age, the patient either suffers from HOCM or valvular aortic stenosis. The low cardiac output can lead to exertional syncope.

172. Ans. (a) **Mitral Stenosis**

(Ref: Harrison 20th p 1817; Harrison 19th p 1542)

- The image shows a balloon valvotomy procedure being performed which rules out regurgitant lesions.
- Aortic stenosis is ruled out since percutaneous aortic balloon valvuloplasty is preferred in children with aortic

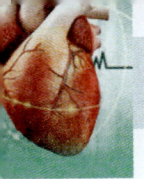

stenosis. It is not used in adults with severe calcific aortic stenosis because of high stenosis rates and procedural complications like embolic stroke.
- Mitral stenosis with surface area less than 1square cm/m² or <1.5 square cm/m² in adults is treated with percutaneous mitral balloon valvotomy. Successful valvotomy is defined as 50% percent reduction in mean mitral valve gradient and doubling of mitral valve area.

173. Ans. (a) Mitral stenosis

(Ref: Harrison 20th p 1699; Braunwald 8th edition, Chapter 62)

Hockey stick sign is seen in:

ECG	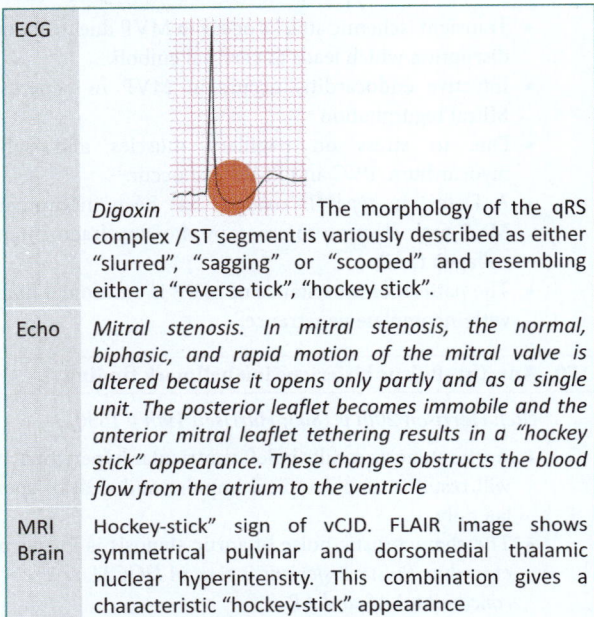 *Digoxin* The morphology of the qRS complex / ST segment is variously described as either "slurred", "sagging" or "scooped" and resembling either a "reverse tick", "hockey stick".
Echo	*Mitral stenosis. In mitral stenosis, the normal, biphasic, and rapid motion of the mitral valve is altered because it opens only partly and as a single unit. The posterior leaflet becomes immobile and the anterior mitral leaflet tethering results in a "hockey stick" appearance. These changes obstructs the blood flow from the atrium to the ventricle*
MRI Brain	Hockey-stick" sign of vCJD. FLAIR image shows symmetrical pulvinar and dorsomedial thalamic nuclear hyperintensity. This combination gives a characteristic "hockey-stick" appearance

174. Ans. (a) TR (Tricuspid regurgitation)

(Ref: Harrison 20th p 244, 1768; Harrison 19th p 1548)

With the onset of TR in patients with PA hypertension, symptoms of pulmonary congestion diminish, but the clinical manifestations of right-sided heart failure become intensified. The neck veins are distended with prominent *v* waves and rapid *y* descents, marked hepatomegaly, ascites, pleural effusions, edema, systolic pulsations of the liver, and a positive hepatojugular reflex.

175. Ans. (a) Right 2nd intercostal, low pitch murmur

(Ref: Harrison 20th p 1805; Harrison 19th ed. / 144B)

Aortic stenosis is the most common cause of a mid- systolic murmur in an adult.
- *The murmur of AS is low to medium pitch and rasping or harsh in character.*
- It is usually loudest to the right of the sternum in the second intercostal space (aortic area) and radiates into the carotids.
- Mid-systolic murmurs begin at a short interval after S1, end before S2, and are usually crescendo-decrescendo in configuration.

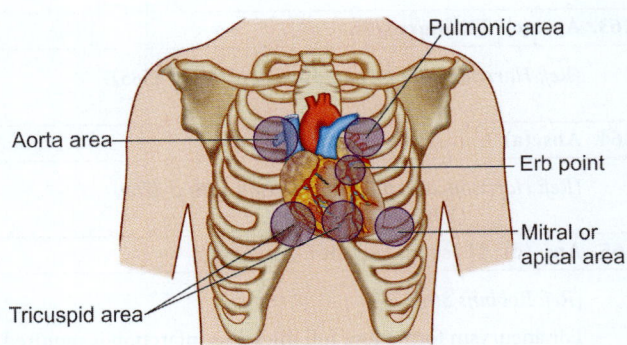

Transmission of the mid-systolic murmur to the apex, where it becomes higher-pitched, is common (Gallavardin effect).

176. Ans. (d) Platypnea

(Ref: Harrison 20th p 228, 2235; Harrison 19th ed./1992)

- Platypnea-orthodeoxia syndrome is a relatively uncommon but striking clinical syndrome characterized by dyspnea and deoxygenation accompanying a change to a sitting or standing from a recumbent position.
- In orthopnea (reverse findings are seen) the dysnea is seen in supine position and reduces in sitting position. It is usually due to acute CHF and bilateral diaphragmatic hernia.

Causes of Platypnea
1. ASD or PFO with position-dependent shunting
2. Other Cardiac conditions
   - Pericardial effusion
   - Constrictive pericarditis
   - Aortic aneurysm
3. Pulmonary
   - Multiple pulmonary emboli
   - Pulmonary emphysema
   - Radiation-induced bronchial stenosis
   - Hepatopulmonary syndrome
   - Amiodarone toxicity of the lungs
   - Pulmonary A-V communications
   - PCP pnuemonia
   - Fat embolism syndrome
4. Autonomic
   - Parkinson disease
   - Bilateral thoracic sympathectomy
5. Abdominal
6. Hepatic cirrhosis

177. Ans. (a) Aortic Regurgitation

(Ref: Harrison 20th p 1810; Harrison 19th ed. / 411)

Duroziez's sign is seen in severe aortic regurgitation, gradual pressure over the femoral artery leads to a systolic and diastolic bruit. The systolic murmur is heard best when the proximal femoral artery is compressed and the diastolic when the distal femoral artery is compressed.

178. Ans. (c) Erythema Marginatum

(Ref: Harrison 20th p 2544; Harrison 19th ed./2149)

Revised Jones Criteria (2015 Guidelines)	
A. Diagnosis	
For all patient populations with evidence of preceding gas infection Initial ARF – 2 Major or 1 major plus 2 minor Recurrent ARF- 2 Major or 1 major and 2 minor or 3 minor	
B. What are major criteria?	
Low-risk populations	Moderate-and high-risk population

• Carditis
  Clinical and/or subclinical carditis
	• Carditis
	  ▪ Clinical and/or subclinical carditis

• Arthritis
  ▪ Polyarthritis only
	• Arthritis
	  ▪ Monoarthritis or polyarthritis
	  ▪ Polyarthralgia

• Chorea	• Chorea
• Erythema marginatum	• Erythema marginatum
• Subcutaneous nodules	• Subcutaneous nodules
C. What are the minor criteria	
Low-risk populations	Moderate-and high-risk population
• Polyarthraigia	• Monoarthralgia
• Fever (>38.5°)	• Fever (>38°C)
• ESR>60 mm in 1st hour and/or CRP >3.0 mg/d	• ESR>30 mm/h and /or CRP >3.0
• Prolonged PR interval, after accounting for age variability (unless carditis is a major criterion) in all population	

179. Ans. (c) Duration of mid-diastolic murmur

(Ref: Harrison 20th p 1815; Harrison 19th ed. / 1539)

- Severity of mitral Stenosis implies that the mitral valve orifice has become smaller in size. This implies that the blood will take longer time to go from left atrium to left ventricle. This implies the LENGTH Of murmur will increase.

180. Ans. (b) Aortic regurgitation

(Ref: Harrison 20th p 1896; Harrison 19th ed. / 1534)

Pulse pressure is SBP – DBP. In aortic stenosis or mitral stenosis SBP is low leading to reduction of pulse pressure. In tricuspid stenosis since the blood flow into right side of heart is reduced, so is left side inflow and therefore reduction in SBP.

Other Changes in Pulse Pressure Include
- **Increased pulse pressure:** Aortic regurgitation, Aortic sclerosis
- **Decreased pulse pressure:** Aortic stenosis, Mitral stenosis
- **Increased diastolic pressure:** Mitral stenosis
- **Decreased diastolic pressure:** Aortic regurgitation, Patent ductus arteriosus

Causes of Wide Pulse Pressure
- Atherosclerosis
- Arteriovenous fistula
- Chronic aortic regurgitation
- Thyrotoxicosis
- Fever
- Anemia
- Pregnancy
- Anxiety

- Heart block
- Aortic dissection
- Endocarditis
- Raised intracranial pressure

181. Ans. (c) Decreased LV end diastolic pressure

(Ref: Harrison 20th p 1810-11)

- The image shows collapsing pulse being checked by the examiner which is seen in aortic regurgitation.
- Aortic regurgitation leads to early diastolic murmur while severe aortic regurgitation leads to mid diastolic murmur.
- Due to *rapid run off from the aorta back into left ventricle* the LV pressure keeps on rising, leading to *increased LV end diastolic Pressure*.
- Pulsus bisferiens can be seen in:
  1. HOCM
  2. Aortic regurgitation
  3. Aortic stenosis with aortic regurgitation

182. Ans. (a) Percutaneous mitral baloon valvotomy

(Ref: Harrison 20th p 1817; Harrison 19th p 1539-40)

- The image shows a deflated Baloon cathrether being advanced across the interatrial septum and then being inflated at the mitral valve to improve the symptoms in severe mitral stenosis. The procedure is referred to as PMBV (percutaneous mitral baloon valvotomy).

183. Ans. (d) S3

(Ref: Harrison 20th p 1815; Harrison 19th p 1540)

- The first heart sound (S1) is usually accentuated and slightly delayed.
- The pulmonic component of the second heart sound (P2) also is often accentuated, and the two components of the second heart sound (S2) are closely split.
- The opening snap (OS) of the mitral valve is most readily audible in expiration at, or just medial to, the cardiac apex. This sound generally follows the sound of aortic valve closure (A2) by 0.05–0.12 s. The time interval between A2 and OS varies inversely with the severity of the MS.
- The OS is followed by a low-pitched, rumbling, diastolic murmur, heard best at the apex with the patient in the left lateral recumbent position
- In general, the duration of this murmur correlates with the severity of the stenosis in patients with preserved CO

184. Ans. (b) Left atrium

(Ref: Harrison 20th p 1815; Grainger Radiology, 4th edition, page 684, Harrison 19th p 1540)

Double-density sign is seen on frontal chest radiograph in the presence of left atrial enlargement, and occurs when the right side of the left atrium pushes behind the right cardiac shadow, indenting the adjacent lung and forming its own distinct silhouette

185. Ans. (c) AS (Aortic Stenosis)

(Ref: Harrison 20th p 1831; Current medical diagnosis and Treatment, 2018, pg. 344)

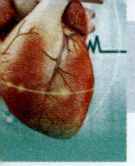

- Amongst all the mentioned options, AS is associated with mortality rate of 17% and fetal mortality rate of 32% and maternal mortality after MTP of a huge 40%.

> **Pregnancy is contraindicated in**
> 1. Pulmonary artery hypertension
> 2. Severe ventricular dysfunction (Liver < 30%)
> 3. Peripartum cardiomyopathy (Previous)
> 4. Severe mitral stenosis and severe symptomatic aortic stenosis
> 5. Morton syndrome with aorta dilated > 45 mm

186. Ans. (c) Aortic valve replacement

(Ref: Harrison 20th p 1807; Harrison 19th p 1533; Braunwald 9th ed., pg 1474)

- The diagnosis of the patient is severe aortic stenosis based on transvalvular peak gradient of 60 mm Hg.
- However since patient managed to perform on the Treadmill for up to stage 3 (beyond 9 minutes) of Bruce protocol without any ECG changes we will label him as ASYMPTOMATIC SEVERE AORTIC STENOSIS patient.
- In Modified Bruce protocol on a treadmill there are 7 stages of 3 minutes each for which the patient walks on the treadmill at a gradually increasing speed.
- According to 20th edition of Harrison, there is a change in guidelines with surgery being indicated for asymptomatic severe aortic stenosis due to progressive nature of disease.
- Other indications for which surgery can be considered include:
  1. An abnormal response to treadmill exercise
  2. Rapid progression of AS, especially when urgent access to medical care might be compromised
  3. Very severe AS defined by a valve area <0.6 cm^2/m^2 of body surface area.
  4. Severe LV hypertrophy suggested by a wall thickness of >15 mm. Exercise testing can be safely performed in the asymptomatic patient, as many as one-third of whom will show signs of functional impairment.

187. Ans. (d) Cardioversion with percutaneous balloon valvotomy

(Ref: Harrison 20th p 1816; Harrison 19th p 1542)

- In atrial fibrillation the clots that are formed are kept RETAINED in the left atria due to twitching activity of the atria.
- Moreover the mitral stenosis also reduces the chances of clot embolization.
- Hence in case cardioversion is done, the normal sinus rhythm ensues and the proper contraction of atria allows dislodgement of clots from the atria.
- The PMV procedure dilates the mitral annulus, relieves the annulus and the chances of clots embolizing via a bigger orifice increase.
- Usually, cardioversion should be undertaken after the patient has had at least 3 consecutive weeks of anticoagulant treatment to a therapeutic INR.
- If cardioversion is indicated more urgently, then intravenous heparin should be provided and TEE performed to exclude the presence of left atrial thrombus before the procedure. In the presence of left atrial thrombus, if cardioversion is performed it can dislodge the thrombus and can lead to thromboembolism.
- Cardioversion to sinus rhythm is rarely successful or sustained in patients with severe MS, particularly those in whom the LA is especially enlarged or in whom AF has been present for more than 1 year.

188. Ans. (d) Left atrial thrombus

(Ref: Harrison 20th p 1816; Harrison's, ch. 237, Valvular Heart Disease: page 1932, Harrison 19th p 1542)

- Mitral valvuloplasty will lead to dilatation of mitral annulus and will enhance the possibility of left atrial thrombus to embolise to systemic circulation.
- For critical mitral stenosis balloon valvotomy is recommended to reduce PCWP and symptoms. In case of mitral stenosis with significant mitral regurgitation balloon dilatation is not recommended as MS will improve whereas Mitral regurgitation can worsen.
- In case of calcification of valve the pliability of valves is reduced and balloon Valvotomy would not be recommended.
- For left atrial thrombus anti-coagulation using Warfarin is recommended.

189. Ans. (a) Tricuspid regurgitation

(Ref: Harrison 20th p 244, 1768; Harrison 19th p 1548)

- Pulsatile liver is seen with tricuspid regurgitation due to back flow of blood from RV to RA during systole and this pressure is transmitted to liver during systole.
- In tricuspid stenosis, pre-systolic pulsations of the liver can be seen

190. Ans. (c) 3 years

(Ref: Harrison 20th p 1806; Harrison 19th p 1532)

Predicted life span based on symptoms in patients of aortic stenosis
- Angina and exertional syncope 3 years
- Dyspnea 2 years
- CHF 1.5 years

191. Ans. (b) Left ventricular hypertrophy

(Ref: Harrison 20th p 1851; Harrison 19th p 1531)

- The normal left ventricular apex impulse is located at or medial to the left midclavicular line in the fourth or fifth intercostal space.
- Left ventricular hypertrophy results in exaggeration of the amplitude, duration, and often size of the normal left ventricular thrust. The impulse may be displaced laterally and downward into the sixth or seventh intercostal space, particularly in patients with a left ventricular volume load such as the one which occurs in cases of aortic regurgitation or lesions like aortic stenosis/HOCM.
- Right ventricular hypertrophy often results in a sustained systolic lift at the lower left parasternal area, which starts in early systole and is synchronous with the left ventricular apical impulse.

192. Ans. (d) Late systolic murmur

(Ref: Harrison 20th p 1811; Harrison 19th p 1536)

- In chronic aortic regurgitation due to back flow of blood, coronary artery pressure will reduce leading to coronary insufficiency leading to chest pain.
- Diastolic pressures are often lower than 60 mm Hg, with pulse pressures often exceeding 100 mm Hg, although younger patients with more compliant vessels may have a less widened pulse pressure. Associated physical examination findings include the following:
  - Becker sign - Visible systolic pulsations of the retinal arterioles
  - Corrigan pulse ("Water-hammer" pulse) - Abrupt distention and quick collapse on palpation of the peripheral arterial pulse
  - de Musset sign - Bobbing motion of the patient's head with each heartbeat
  - Hill sign - Popliteal cuff systolic blood pressure 40 mm Hg higher than brachial cuff systolic blood pressure
  - Duroziez sign - Systolic murmur over the femoral artery with proximal compression of the artery, and diastolic murmur over the femoral artery with distal compression of the artery
  - Müller sign - Visible systolic pulsations of the uvula
  - Quincke sign - Visible pulsations of the fingernail bed with light compression of the fingernail
  - Traube sign ("pistol-shot" pulse) - Booming systolic and diastolic sounds auscultated over the femoral artery

193. Ans. (b) AS (Aortic stenosis)

(Ref: Harrison 20th p 1804; Harrison 19th p 1531)

The valvular obstruction will cause concentric left ventricular hypertrophy which will lead to subendocardial ischemia and resultant angina. Thus CABG might be required in patients with aortic stenosis who undergo an aortic valve replacement.
- Crescendo decrescendo murmur
- Mid systolic murmur
- Ejection systolic murmur
- Pulsus anacrotic

194. Ans. (a) Anti-platelet only

(Ref: American stroke association 2010, guidelines and Harrison, Table 370-3, Harrison 19th p 2566, Table 446-3)

- Because of the calcific nature of the emboli, anticoagulation is not recommended, and antiplatelet therapy remains an empirical approach
- According to ASA 2010 guidelines for cardio-embolic stroke in Aortic Valve Disease

Recommendations are:
1. Antiplatelet therapy may be reasonable for patients with ischemic stroke or TIA and native aortic or nonrheumatic mitral valve disease who do not have AF.

Condition	Recommendation
Nonvalvular atrial fibrillation	Calculate CHADS2a score
CHADS2 score 0	Aspirin or no antithrombotic

Contd...

Condition	Recommendation
CHADS2 score 1	Aspirin or VKA
CHADS2 score >1	VKA (Vitamin K antagonist)
Rheumatic mitral valve disease	
With atrial fibrillation, previous embolization, or atrial appendage thrombus, or left atrial diameter >55 mm	VKA
Embolization or appendage clot despite INR 2–3	VKA plus aspirin
Aortic valve calcification	
Asymptomatic	No therapy
Otherwise cryptogenic stroke or TIA	Aspirin

195. Ans. (b) Tricuspid insufficiency and pulmonic stenosis

(Ref: Harrison 19th p 564)

- In carcinoid syndrome the serotonin based products cause fibrosis in the right side of the heart leading to Tricuspid Insufficiency and Pulmonic Stenosis (MNEMONIC: T.I.P.S)
- Carcinoid heart disease results from neoplasms of enterochromaffin cells. Patients who have carcinoid disease can survive up to 10 years after diagnosis, because the tumors, although malignant, are slow growing. These tumors are associated with the production of biologically active substances, depending on the tumor's site of origin. Serotonin is a common product of carcinoid tumors. Most such tumors contain tryptophan hydroxylase, which enables them to produce serotonin after hydroxylation and subsequent decarboxylation of the tryptophan. In turn, 5-hydroxyindole acetaldehyde, the oxidation product of serotonin, produces 5-HIAA, which is excreted in urine. Elevated levels of circulating serotonin have been associated with cardiac failure, due to fibrous deposits on the endocardium. These deposits are thought to be responsible for the fibrous degeneration of the valve apparatus.

196. Ans. (c) 4-6 cm^2

(Ref: Braunwald 6th/378, 1643, 1673, Harrison 19th p 1539)

197. Ans. (b) Most patients are symptomatic

(Ref: Harrison 19th p 1546)

198. Ans. (c) Echocardiography

(Ref: Harrison 19th p 1546)

199. Ans. (b) Aortic stenosis

(Ref: Harrison 19th p 1531)

200. Ans. (a) Aortic stenosis

(Ref: Harrison 19th p 1531)

201. Ans. (a) Acute myocardial infarction

(Ref: Harrison 19th p 1535)

202. Ans. (c) Aortic incompetence

(Ref: Harrison 19th p 1535)

203. Ans. (d) All of the above

(Ref: Ghai 5th/315, Harrison 19th p 1549)

Rheumatic Heart Disease

204. Ans. (a) Steroids

(Ref: Harrison 19th edition, page 2153)

Milder cases of Sydenham's chorea are managed by providing a calm environment.

In severe chorea carbamazepine or sodium valproate is preferred to haloperidol. Response takes 1–2 weeks to develop.

However for *severe and refractory cases of chorea, corticosteroids are effective* and lead to rapid symptom reduction. *If all of these fail, IVIG is used.*

205. Ans. (b) Rheumatic heart disease

(Ref: Robbins and Cotran pathologic basis of disease 9th edition page 558)

- The image shows cardiac myocytes in the periphery and *Aschoff bodies* in the middle of the slide. They are composed of mixed mononuclear inflammatory cells with associated necrosis.
- These inflammatory cells are activated macrophages showing prominent nucleoli and caterpillar like nuclear chromatin and are called Anitschkow cells. (These features are not visible in the image given in the question).
- Valvular lesion of mitral stenosis also helps in selecting the answer as rheumatic heart disease.
- Myxomatous degeneration leads to MVP and hence is clinically ruled out.
- TB of myocardium is extremely rare and hence ruled out.
- Viral myocarditis is diagnosed on basis of Dallas criteria and shows extensive myocyte disarray

Rheumatic heart disease

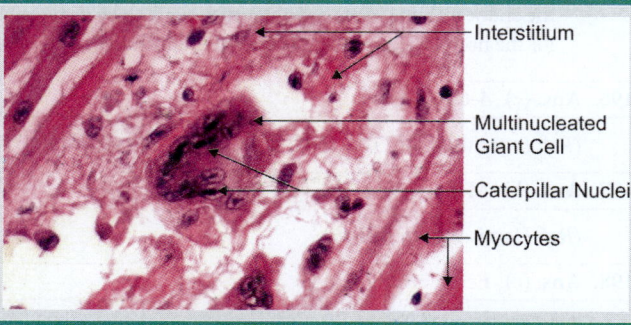

Viral myocarditis

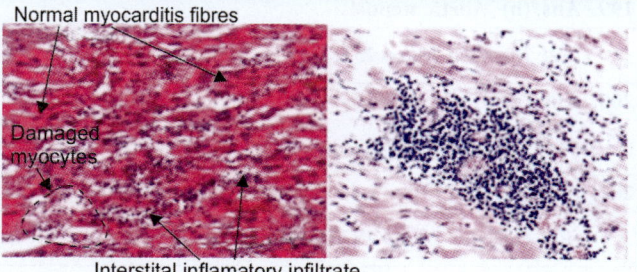

*N.B. established histological Dallas criteria defined as follows: histological evidence of inflammatory infiltrates within the myocardium associated with myocyte degeneration and necrosis of nonischemic origin

206. Ans. (b) Molecular mimicry

(Ref: Harrison 19th edition, page 372e, 2149)

The hallmark of the pathogenesis of rheumatic fever is Molecular mimicry where the streptococcal group A carbohydrate epitope, N-acetyl glucosamine, and the α-helical coiled-coil streptococcal M protein structurally mimic cardiac myosin in the human disease

207. Ans. (b) ASLO

(Ref: Harrison 20th p 2542; Harrison 19th edition, page 2149, 2151)

Revised Jones Criteria

Major Criteria

Low-risk populations	Moderate- and high-risk populations
1. Carditis ■ Clinical and/or subclinical carditis	Carditis ■ Clinical and/or subclinical carditis.
2. Arthritis ■ Polyarthritis only	Arthritis ■ Monoarthritis or polyarthritis ■ Polyarthralgia
3. Chorea	Chorea
4. Erythema marginatum	Arythema marginatum
5. Subcutaneous nodules	Subcutaneous nodules

Minor Criteria

Low-risk populations	Moderate and high-risk populations
1. Polyarthralgia	Monoarthralgia
2. Fever (≥38.5°)	Fever (>38°C)
3. ESR >60 mm in 1st hour	ESR ≥30 mm/h and/or CRP ≥3.0
4. Prolonged PR interval, after accounting for age variability (unless carditis is a major criterion) in all population.	

Supporting evidence of a preceding streptococcal infection within the last 45 days	• Elevated or rising anti-streptolysin 0 or other streptococcal antibody, or • A positive throat culture, or • Rapid antigen test for group A streptococcus, or • Recent scarlet fever

- Since chorea is a late feature of rheumatic fever and occurs about 3-6 months after a sore throat, the history of preceding sore throat may not be recalled and ASO Titers can fall back to normal.

208. Ans. (b) Acute rheumatic carditis

(Ref: Harrison 20th p 2542)

A short, mid-diastolic murmur is rarely heard during an episode of acute rheumatic fever (Carey-Coombs murmur) and probably is due to flow through an edematous mitral valve. An opening snap is not present in the acute phase, and the murmur dissipates with resolution of the acute attack

209. Ans. (c) Rheumatic carditis

(Ref: Harrison 20th p 2542; Robbins 8th edition, chapter 11)

- During acute RF, Aschoff bodies and are pathognomonic for RF
- Aschoff bodies consist of a central zone of degenerating, hyper-eosinophilic extracellular matrix infiltrated by lymphocytes (primarily T cells), occasional plasma cells, and plump activated macrophages called **Anitschkow cells.**
- The Anitschkow cells have abundant cytoplasm and central nuclei with chromatin arrayed in a slender, wavy ribbon (Caterpillar cells)
- Valve involvement results in fibrinoid necrosis along the lines of closure forming 1- to 2-mm vegetations (verrucae) that have little effect on cardiac function. These irregular, warty projections probably arise from the precipitation of fibrin at sites of erosion caused by underlying inflammation and collagen degeneration.

210. Ans. (c) 9 days

(Ref: Harrison 19th edition, page 2152-53)

- In case a course of penicillin is commenced within 9 days of sore throat onset, it will prevent almost all cases of ARF.
- Primary prevention for ARF remains primary prophylaxis (i.e, the timely and complete treatment of group A streptococcal sore throat with antibiotics).

211. Ans. (c) PS (Pulmonic stenosis)

(Ref: Harrison 20th p 2542; OP Ghai 8th edn p 436)

The functional consequence of RHD is valvular stenosis and regurgitation (stenosis tends to predominate). RHD is overwhelmingly the most frequent cause of mitral stenosis accounting for 99% of cases. The mitral valve alone is involved in 70% of cases of RHD, with combined mitral and aortic disease in another 25%; the tricuspid valve is usually less frequently and less severely involved, and the *pulmonic valve almost always escapes injury.*

212. Ans. (b) Aortic stenosis

(Ref: CMDT 2019 pg 353)

Aortic stenosis presents with
- Insidious progression of fatigue and dyspnea associated with gradual curtailment of activities.
- Dyspnea results primarily from elevation of the pulmonary capillary pressure caused by elevations of LV diastolic pressures secondary to reduced left ventricular compliance and impaired relaxation.
- Angina pectoris usually develops somewhat later and reflects an imbalance between the augmented myocardial oxygen requirements and reduced oxygen availability.
- Exertional syncope may result from a decline in arterial pressure caused by vasodilation in the exercising muscles and inadequate vasoconstriction in non-exercising muscles in the face of a fixed CO, or from a sudden fall in CO produced by an arrhythmia.
- Because the CO at rest is usually well maintained until late in the course, marked fatigability, weakness, peripheral cyanosis, cachexia, and other clinical manifestations of a low CO are usually not prominent until this stage is reached. Orthopnea, paroxysmal nocturnal dyspnea, and pulmonary edema, i.e., symptoms of LV failure, also occur only in the advanced stages of the disease.
- Severe pulmonary hypertension leading to RV failure and systemic venous hypertension, hepatomegaly, AF, and TR are usually late findings in patients with isolated severe AS.

213. Ans. (a) ASO titer

(Ref: Harrison 20th p 2543)

Supporting evidence of a receding streptococcal infection within the last 45 days (essential criteria)	Elevated or rising anti-streptolysin O or other streptococcal antibody, or A positive throat culture, or Rapid antigen test for group A streptococcus, or Recent scarlet fever

214. Ans. (a) Mitral regurgitation

(Ref: Harrison 20th p 2542; Harrison 19th p 2150-51)

- *In rheumatic heart disease, the damage to chordate tendinae by inflammatory Aschoff nodules results in development of mitral regurgitation in pediatric presentation.*
- The most common valve involvement >18years of age is mitral stenosis
- *Remember that pulmonic valve is not involved in rheumatic etiology.*

215. Ans. (d) Sulfadiazine

(Ref: AHA Guidelines 2010 and Nelson ch. 438)

Secondary Prophylaxis for Rheumatic Fever
Macrolide or azalide antibiotic (for patients allergic to penicillin and Sulfadiazine)
- *In a patient allergic to penicillin, sulfadiazine is the next consideration for prophylaxis.*
  - In a pt weighing 27 kg or less - 0.5 g PO/day
  - In a pt weighing 27 kg or less - 1 g PO/day
- Macrolide (Erythromycin/clarithromycin) is considered in a patient allergic to both Penicillin and sulfadiazine.

Bacterial Endocarditis
The AHA no longer recommends prophylaxis for infective endocarditis in most patients with rheumatic heart disease. The exceptions are:
1. Patients with prosthetic valves or valves repaired with prosthetic material,
2. Patients with previous endocarditis or specific forms of congenital heart disease, and
3. Cardiac transplant recipients who develop cardiac valvulopathy.

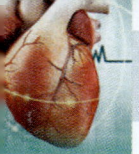

216. Ans. (c) Fever

(Ref: Harrison 20th p 2542; Harrison 19th p 2150)

217. Ans. (d) Pancarditis

(Ref: Harrison 20th p 2542; Harrison 19th p 2151)

218. Ans. (a) Aschoff's nodule

(Ref: Harrison 20th p 2542; Harrison 19th p 2151)

219. Ans. (d) Usually associated with carditis

(Ref: Harrison 20th p 2542; Harrison 19th p 2151)

220. Ans. (a) Mitral Regurgitation (MR)

(Ref: Harrison 20th p 2542; Harrison 19th p 2151)

221. Ans. (a) Along line of closure of valves

(Ref: Robbins 7th/597)

Murmurs and Heart Sounds

222. Ans. (a) HOCM

(Ref: Harrison 20th edition, page 247)

- HOCM has asymmetrical septal hypertrophy which leads to development of LV outflow tract obstruction. Due to peculiar banana shaped cavity of left ventricle, the volume of blood in chamber of LV decides the magnitude of LV outflow obstruction.
- The hypertrophied septum narrows the outflow tract of blood into aorta.

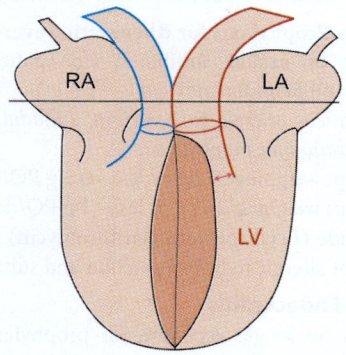

- More volume of blood in LV reduces the outlet obstruction. Due to less obstruction murmur will be softer.
- On standing the venous return will reduce leading to less blood in chamber of LV. Less blood in LV chamber increases the LV outlet obstruction leading to the murmur becoming louder

	Aortic stenosis	HCM	MVP
Standing or Valsalva (↓ venous return)	↓	↑	↑
Hand grip (↑ vascular resistance)	↓	↓	↓

Contd...

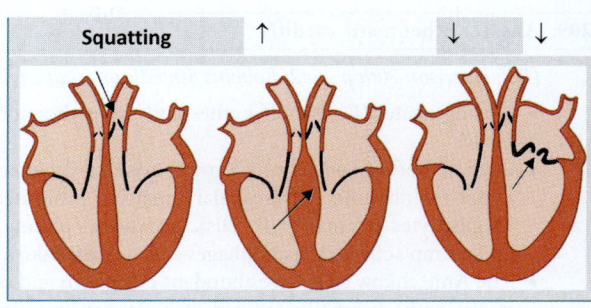

223. Ans. (b) B

(Ref: Harrison 20th p 1668; Harrison 19th edition, page 1448)

- S2 on Phonocardiogram corresponds to end of T wave where Aortic and pulmonic valves will snap shut.
- Marking A in diagram corresponds to qRS complex and represents starting of ventricular systole. At this time aortic and pulmonic valves are opening. It is known as ejection click.
- Marking B in diagram corresponds to end of T wave and represents end of ventricular systole. At this time aortic and pulmonic valves are closing. It is known as S2.
- Marking C in diagram corresponds to P wave when atrial systole is occurring and contributing to 30% filling of the ventricle.

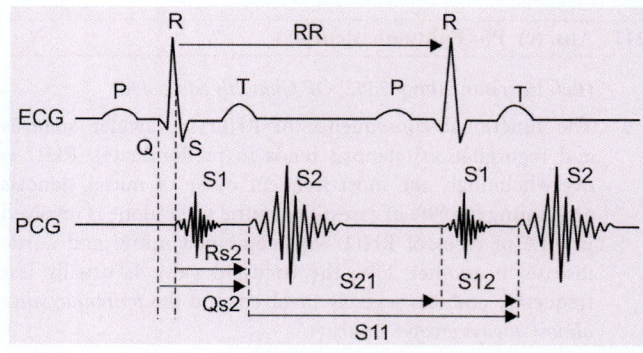

224. Ans. (a) Harsh ejection systolic murmur with Soft S2

(Ref: Harrison 19th edition, page 1531; CMDT 2019 pg 353)

- The clinical presentation of exertional syncope, angina equivalent and dyspnea in geriatric age group points to diagnosis of valvular Aortic stenosis.
- The auscultatory finding is of harsh ejection systolic murmur radiating to the carotids.
- Soft S2 is due to poor mobility of a stenosed valve.
- Choice B is wrong because in aortic stenosis, narrow split S2 or paradoxical split S2 is heard.
- Choice C and D are wrong due to presence of Ejection systolic murmur in aortic stenosis.

225. Ans. (a) High pitched, diastolic, decrescendo murmur

(Ref: Harrison 19th edition, page 1540; CMDT 2019 pg 362)

Graham Steell murmur occurs due to dilatation of pulmonic valve ring, and occurs in patients with mitral valve disease and severe pulmonary artery hypertension.

It is a high pitched, diastolic, decrescendo blowing murmur along the left sternal border.

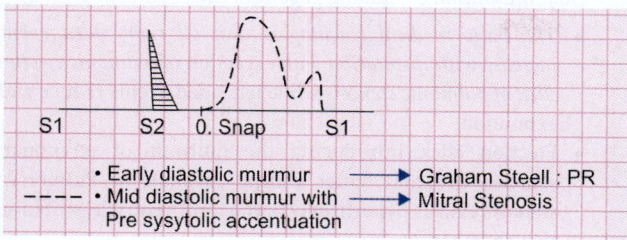

- Early diastolic murmur → Graham Steell ; PR
- Mid diastolic murmur with Pre sysytolic accentuation → Mitral Stenosis

226. Ans. (a) Soft low pitched, mid diastolic murmur

(Ref: Harrison 19th edition, page 1536; CMDT 2019 pg 358)

- Austin flint murmur is due to severe aortic regurgitation. It is produced by diastolic displacement of anterior leaflet of mitral valve by AR stream.
- It produces a soft low pitched, rumbling mid to late diastolic murmur.

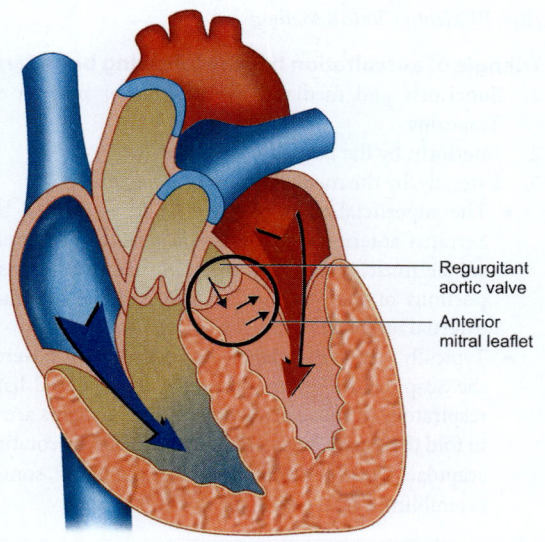

- Regurgitant aortic valve
- Anterior mitral leaflet

227. Ans. (d) VSD with aortic regurgitation

(Ref: Harrison 20th p 1674; Harrison: 19th edition, page 1449)

Continuous murmur is heard both in systole and diastole and peaks at S2. Both of these criteria should be satisfied to call it a continuous murmur. Causes-

1. PDA
2. AV fistula (Coronary, Pulmonary, Systemic)
3. Aorto-pulmonary window
4. Coarctation of aorta
5. Venous hum
6. Rupture of sinus of Valsava
7. Pregnancy(Mammary soufflé)
8. Peripheral pulmonary artery stenosis associated with William syndrome.

228. Ans. (b) 2 3 4 1

(Ref: Harrison 20th p 1672, 1674; 1447, Harrison 19th, 51-e-1f)

Wide fixed split S2	ASD	ASD being a low pressure shunt operates only during expiration when pressure in right atrium falls. Thus the amount of blood in right ventricle is same in both phases of respiration leading to fixed split S2.
Continuous machinery murmur	PDA	Aorta to pulmonary artery shunt operates in both phases of respiration leading to continuous murmur.
Muffled heart sounds	Pericardial effusion	Massive accumulation of fluid outside the heart will lead to muffling of heart sounds.
Narrow split S_2	PAH	Mean pressure>25mm Hg at rest is defined as PAH and this increased pressure affects the gradient between RV and pulmonary artery. This leads to early closure of P_2 and development of narrow split S_2.

229. Ans. (b) Replacement of aortic valve with autologous pulmonic valve and implantation of pulmonic valve homograft

(Ref: Nelson 18th edition, chapter 427; CMDT 2019 pg 334)

- The Ross Procedure is a type of specialized aortic valve surgery where the patient's diseased aortic valve is replaced with his or her own pulmonary valve.
- The pulmonary valve is then replaced with cryopreserved cadaveric pulmonary valve.
- In children and young adults, or older particularly active patients, this procedure offers several advantages over traditional aortic valve replacement with manufactured prostheses.

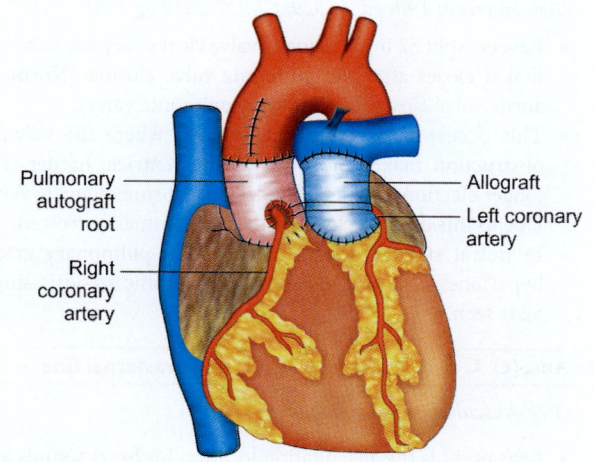

- Pulmonary autograft root
- Right coronary artery
- Allograft
- Left coronary artery

230. Ans. (a) Mitral valve prolapse

(Ref: Harrison 20th p 1821; Harrison 19th edition, page 1546)

- The words "midsystolic click" are virtually synonymous with prolapse of the mitral valve toward the left atrium during systole.
- It is most commonly the result of myxomatous degeneration of the valve with prolongation of the valve and/or chordae tendinae.

- The central problem lies in an abnormal ratio between the length of the mitral apparatus and the volume of the left ventricular chamber. The mitral valve is "too long" for the size of the ventricular chamber.
- Therefore, as ventricular systole proceeds and ventricular volume declines, the valve cannot be held in place.
- The valve then slips and as it is caught again to be held in place by subvalvular tissue, the sudden cessation in motion creates a high frequency sound, the midsystolic click.
- The midsystolic click may actually occur at almost any time during systole depending upon the length of the mitral apparatus and the volume of the left ventricle.

Hamman Rich syndrome	Idiopathic interstitial lung disease
Rheumatic aortic regurgitation	Can lead to early diastolic murmur In severe AR, mid diastolic murmur will be heard and is called Austin flint murmur.
Congenital mitral stenosis	Leads to mid diastolic murmur with presystolic accentuation.

231. Ans. (d) AR, (e) PR

(Ref: Harrison 20th p 1673; Harrison 19th/ Chap 51e-1449, 1550, 1156)

VSD	Pan-systolic murmur
ASD	No shunt murmur with mid-diastolic shunt murmur
Mitral stenosis	Mid diastolic murmur with pre-systolic accentuation
AR	Early diastolic murmur
PR	Early diastolic murmur

232. Ans. (a) Aortic stenosis

(Ref: Harrison 19th ed. / 1529; CMDT 2019 pg 353)

- Reverse split S2 implies aortic valve closes very late to a level that it closes after the pulmonic valve closure (Normally aortic valve closes first and then pulmonic valve).
- This occurs in severe aortic stenosis where the valvular obstruction makes the work of left ventricle harder. The longer ejection time leads to delayed closure of aortic valve. Due to this delayed closure the split becomes narrowed
- In mitral stenosis loud S1 is seen. In pulmonary artery hypertension loud P2 is seen. In pulmonic stenosis single S2 is seen.

233. Ans. (c) C = 3rd intercostal space left parasternal line

(Ref: Auscultation skills: Lippincott p 201)

- Erb's point is the auscultation location for heart sounds and heart murmurs located at the third intercostal space and the left lower sternal border

Aortic area	2nd right interspace close to the sternum
Pulmonic area	2nd left interspace close to the sternum
ERB's point	3rd left interspace close to the sternum
Tricuspid area	5th left interspace close to the sternum
Mitral area (apical)	5th left interspace medial to the MCL

234. Ans. (a) Pulmonary ejection click in pulmonic stenosis

(Ref: Braunwald 8th edition, page 106; Harrison 20th p 1671)

- *The basic medical teaching is that all right sided events increase with inspiration with exception of pulmonic ejection click of pulmonic stenosis while left sided events reduce with expiration.*
- Ejection click introducing the murmur of pulmonary stenosis becomes softer during inspiration. Pulmonary stenosis evokes hypertrophy of the right ventricle, stiffening that chamber.
- When blood is drawn into the right ventricle during inspiration, the thickened right ventricle does not distend normally, so pressure in the chamber rises, and the pulmonary valve is partially opened.
- Because the pulmonary valve is partially open when the right ventricle contracts, its excursion is less, and the ejection click associated with its maximal opening is softer and earlier

235. Ans. (d) Rhomboid major

(Ref: PJ Mehta Clinical Methods)

Triangle of auscultation has the following boundaries:
1. Superiorly and medially, by the inferior portion of the Trapezius
2. Inferiorly, by the Latissimus Dorsi
3. Laterally, by the medial border of the scapula
   - The superficial floor of the triangle is formed by the Serratus anterior and the lateral portion of the erector spinae muscles. Deep to these muscles are the osseous portions of the 6th and 7th ribs and the internal and external intercostal muscles.
   - Typically, the Triangle of Auscultation is covered by the Scapula. To better expose the triangle and listen to respiratory sounds with a stethoscope, patients are asked to fold their arms across their chest, medially rotating the scapulae, while bending forward at the trunk, somewhat resembling a fetal position.

236. Ans. (d) Increase on squatting

(Ref: Harrison 20th p 1674; Harrison 19th p 1449)

- A continuous murmur is predicated on a pressure gradient that persists between two cardiac chambers or blood vessels across systole and diastole.
- The murmurs typically begin in systole, envelop the second heart sound (S2), and continue through some portion of diastole.
- **Continuous murmurs are not affected by dynamic auscultation maneuvers like squatting etc. as it is the pressure gradient that decides this murmur.**
- They can often be difficult to distinguish from individual systolic and diastolic murmurs in patients with mixed valvular heart disease.
- The classic example of a continuous murmur is that associated with a patent ductus arteriosus, which usually is heard in the second or third interspace at a slight distance from the sternal border.

- Other causes of a continuous murmur include:
    1. Ruptured sinus of Valsalva aneurysm with creation of an aortic–right atrial or right ventricular fistula
    2. Coronary or great vessel arteriovenous fistula
    3. Arteriovenous fistula constructed to provide dialysis access.
    4. The cervical venous hum is heard in children or adolescents in the supraclavicular fossa. It can be obliterated with firm pressure applied to the diaphragm of the stethoscope, especially when the subject turns his or her head toward the examiner.
    5. The mammary souffle of pregnancy relates to enhanced arterial blood flow through engorged breasts. The diastolic component of the murmur can be obliterated with firm pressure over the stethoscope

2. Often position-dependent: Murmurs heard while supine and may disappear when upright or sitting.
3. Otherwise healthy individual, no concerns about growth, no symptoms of heart failure such as dyspnea on exertion. (In infants, ask if the baby tires during feeding, becomes diaphoretic, or develops a rapid respiratory rate. In older children, this can be elucidated by asking whether or not the child can keep up with peers during play.)
4. Occurs during systole or continuously during both systole and diastole. (Murmurs occurring only during diastole are always pathological)
5. Physiologic splitting of S2 (A2 and P2 components should only be resolvable during inspiration and should merge during expiration.)
6. No palpable thrill (A thrill is a vibration caused by turbulent blood flow.)

237. Ans. (d) Tumour plop sound

(Ref: Harrison 20th p 1848; Harrison 19th p 1447)

> **Low pitch heart sounds are:**
> 1. S3
> 2. S4
> 3. Tumor plop sound (atrial myxoma)

- Mid systolic clicks are heard in mitral valve prolapse during systole and are high pitch sounds.
- The pericardial knock (PK) is also high-pitched and occurs slightly later than the opening snap, corresponding in timing to the abrupt cessation of ventricular expansion after tricuspid valve opening and to an exaggerated y descent seen in the jugular venous waveform in patients with constrictive pericarditis.
- *A tumor plop is a lower-pitched sound that can be heard in patients with atrial myxoma. It may be appreciated only in certain positions and arises from the diastolic prolapse of the tumor across the mitral valve.*

238. Ans. (a) Aortic stenosis

(Ref: Harrison 19th p 1531; CMDT 2019 p 353)

- Reverse split S2 implies aortic valve closes very late, to a level that it closes after the pulmonic valve closure (Normally aortic valve closes first and then pulmonic valve).
- This occurs in severe aortic stenosis where the valvular obstruction makes the work of left ventricle harder. The longer ejection time leads to delayed closure of aortic valve. Due to this delayed closure the split becomes narrowed
- In mitral stenosis loud S1 is seen. In pulmonary artery hypertension loud P2 is seen. In pulmonic stenosis single S2 is seen.

239. Ans. (a) Only Diastolic murmur

(Ref: Nelson 20th/e p 322)

A functional murmur (innocent murmur, physiological murmur) is a heart murmur that is primarily due to physiological conditions outside the heart, as opposed to structural defects in the heart itself.

Characteristics of functional murmur:
1. Soft, less than 3/6 in intensity (although note that even when structural heart disease is present, intensity does not predict severity.)

240. Ans. (a) Pulmonary HTN

(Ref: Harrison 19th p 1655; CMDT 2019 p 24)

Causes of Loud P2
1. Pulmonary hypertension unless proved otherwise
2. Eisenmenger's syndrome due to ASD, VSD, PDA
3. Multiple pulmonary thrombi

241. Ans. (a) Ejection click

(Ref: Harrison 20th p 1671-72; Harrison 19th p 1448)

During a systolic murmur seen in stenotic lesion like aortic stenosis, the left ventricle shall generate more force to open the stenosed valve. Hence the forceful opening of these valves will cause loud ejection click.

Do not confuse with mid systolic clicks which are seen with mitral valve prolapse.

Heart sounds	Significance
• Loud EJECTION CLICK	Aortic or pulmonic stenosis
• Mid systolic click	Mitral valve prolapse
• Loud OPENING SNAP	Mitral or tricuspid stenosis
• Tumour plop sound	Atrial myxoma
• Pericardial shudder	Constrictive pericarditis

242. Ans. (c) Heard at the end of ventricular systole

(Ref: Harrison 20th p 1671; Harrison 19th p 1447)

S1 is heard at the start of ventricular systole and not at the end.

243. Ans. (a) Short PR interval

(Ref: Harrison 20th p 1671; Harrison 19th p 1447)

244. Ans. (c) >(a) (ASD > VSD)

(Ref: Harrison 20th p 1671; Harrison 19th p 1447)

245. Ans. (d) LBBB

(Ref: Hurst 12th /268; 'Cardiology' 3rd/ed, Harrison 19th p 1447)

246. Ans. (b) Mitral stenosis

(Ref: Harrison 20th p 1671-72; Harrison 19th p 1448)

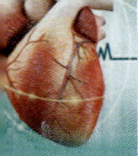

247. Ans. (c) Absent in MS

(Ref: Harrison 20th p 1671-72; Harrison 19th p 1448)

248. Ans. (c) Atrial fibrillation

(Ref: Harrison 20th p 1671-72; Harrison 19th p 1448)

249. Ans. (c) Ejection click

(Ref: Harrison 20th p 1671-72; Harrison 19th p 1447)

250. Ans. (d) Ejection click

(Ref: Harrison 20th p 1671-72)

251. Ans. (d) HOCM

(Ref: Harrison 20th p 1674; Harrison 19th p 1450)

All murmurs decrease with Valsalva, standing and amylnitrate inhalation except HOCM which becomes louder and MVP which becomes longer.

252. Ans. (a) Mitral stenosis with mitral regurgitation

(Ref: Harrison 20th p 1674; Hurst's 12th/290)

253. Ans. (a) PDA; **(c)** Shunt between pulmonary & subclavian artery

(Ref: Harrison 20th p 1674; Harrison 19th p 1449)

254. Ans. (b) End of isovolumetric contraction

(Ref: Harrison 20th p 1668; Guyton 10th/99)

Cardiomyopathy

255. Ans. (a) Takotsubo cardiomyopathy

(Ref: Harrison 20th edition, page 1790-91)

- The clinical history points to intense emotional trauma and catecholamine toxicity. The catecholamine toxicity leads to development of Takotsubo cardiomyopathy. It is also known as Broken heart syndrome. All the other options have a chronic presentation.
- The closest choice is ARVD which can present as sudden cardiac death but usually in setting of physical exertion and not emotional trauma.

256. Ans. (c) Takotsubo cardiomyopathy

(Ref: Harrison 20th p 1791; Harrison: 19th edition, page 1565)

- Takotsubo cardiomyopathy occurs due to catecholamine toxicity.
- It results in *intense sympathomimetic innervation* with *diffuse microvascular spasm* resulting in *myocardial stunning*.
- Hence the clinical presentation of *TTCM mimics myocardial infarction*.
- The ventricles show global ventricular dilatation with contraction at base resulting in a shape of narrow necked jar.

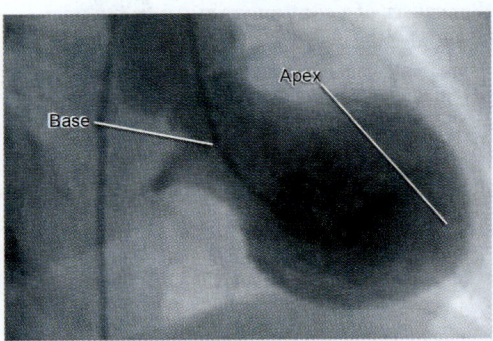

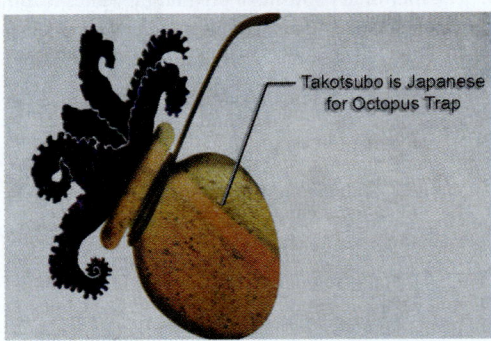

Pericardial shudder is the auscultatory finding of constrictive pericarditis.

257. Ans. (d) Peri partum cardiomyopathy

(Ref: Harrison 20th p 1788; Harrison 19th p 1562)

Acute MI	Ruled out as chest pain at rest, elevated cardio-markers or ECG changes are not present.
DVT with PE	Develops suddenly and is a close answer but point against is Echo finding of only low ejection fraction. In PE, Echo shows RV dyskinesia with or without tricuspid regurgitation. The interventricular septal deviation is also seen.
Amniotic fluid embolism	Ruled out as it occurs immediately during active labour.
Peri-partum cardiomyopathy	PPCM is diagnosed when the following 3 criteria are met: 1. Heart failure develops in the last month of pregnancy or within 5 months of delivery. 2. Heart pumping function is reduced, with an ejection fraction (EF) less than 45% 3. No other cause for heart failure with reduced EF can be found. In this question hemoglobin, MI and Pulmonary embolism have been ruled out.

258. Ans. (a) Glycogen Storage Disease Type II (Pompe)

(Ref: Nelson 20th p 2186)

Classic infantile form of Pompe disease presents with
1. Cardiomyopathy and conduction disorders,
2. Muscular hypotonia /floppy baby

3. Macroglossia
4. Organomegaly

- Cardiomyopathy is of hypertrophic type, showing a severe thickening of the septum, or of both the septum and free walls of the left and right heart.
- Glycogen storage involves not only cardiac myocytes, but also the special cells of the conduction system (particularly, the A-V node and the His-bundle cells), representing the histological background of classical electrocardiographic abnormalities in Pompe disease: pre-excitation patterns (short PR, delta waves), atrio-ventricular blocks and bundle branch abnormalities.

259. Ans. (a) Hypertrophic cardiomyopathy

(Ref: Harrison 20th p 1794; Harrison 19th p 1569)

- The image shows presence of a symmetrical septal hypertrophy and free wall hypertrophy of left ventricle.
- This is leads to small left ventricle reflecting low cardiac output and thereby limited coronary reserve.
- This also points to presence of sub-endocardial ischemia. During physical exertion, there is worsening of sub-endocardial ischemia leading to ventricular tachycardia or ventricular fibrillation.
- The pointer in the image points to left ventricular outflow tract obstruction
- Rigorous athletic training (athlete's heart) may cause intermediate degrees of physiologic hypertrophy difficult to differentiate from mild hypertrophic cardiomyopathy.
- Unlike hypertrophic cardiomyopathy, hypertrophy in the athlete's heart regresses with cessation of training, and is accompanied by supernormal exercise capacity, mild ventricular dilation & normal diastolic function

260. Ans. (b) Calcium channel blockers

(Ref: Harrison 20th p 1775; Harrison 19th p 1513)

Dilated cardiomyopathy presents with heart failure with low ejection fraction due to low ejection fraction.

Beta blockers	Beta blockers like carvedilol, bisoprolol and metoprolol have been shown to reduce improve survival in clinical trials
CCB	CCB like amlodipine, felodipine reduce BP but do not affect morbidity and mortality. First generation agents like verapamil, diltiazem may exert negative inotropic effects and destabilize previously asymptomatic patients. Hence there use should be discouraged.
ACE inhibitors	ACE inhibitors lead to 35% reduction in end point mortality in heart failure patients
Spironolactone	Aldosterone antagonism is associated with reduction in mortality in all stages of symptomatic NYHA class II to IV.

261. Ans. (d) Lowe's Syndrome

(Ref: Harrison 20th p 1784, 1792; Harrison 19th p 1565-66)

Causes of cardiomyopathy
Glycogen Storage Diseases
II – Pompe's (alpha 1,4 glucosidase)
III- Forbes:(amylo 1, 6 glucosidase)
Miscellaneous
Hemochromatosis
Familial amyloidosis – abnormal transthyretin
Friedreich's ataxia- frataxin
Dystrophin-related dystrophy (Duchenne's Becker's)
Mitochondrial myopathies (e.g, Kearns-Sayre syndrome)
Arrhythmogenic ventricular dysplasia
Hemochromatosis
Sphingolipidoses
Fabry's disease (alpha galactosidase A)
Gaucher disease (beta-glucocerebroside)

262. Ans. (c) Diamond-shaped cavity of left ventricle

(Ref: Harrison 20th p 1794)

- The image shows specimen of enlarged heart with interventricular septal hypertrophy that is reducing the cavity size of left ventricle. Thus it is an example of diastolic dysfunction as it reduces the end diastolic volume significantly.
- Morever the presence of *dynamic* left ventricular hypertrophy results in low cardiac output.
- *Banana-shaped cavity of left ventricle is seen with of HOCM.*

263. Ans. (b) Hypertrophic obstructive cardiomyopathy

(Ref: Harrison 20th p 1794; Harrison 19th p 1553)

- Familial HCM occurs as an autosomal dominant Mendelian-inherited disease in approximately 50% of cases.
- Greater than 100 mutations have been identified in at least 12 sarcomeric genes with the β-myosin heavy chain being most frequently affected, followed by myosin-binding protein C and troponin T. These three genes account for 70% to 80% of all cases of HCM.
- In Arrthymogenic right ventricular dysplasia the ventricular wall is severely thinned as a result of myocyte replacement by massive fatty infiltration and lesser amounts of fibrosis. Most cases are sporadic, but familial forms do occur with gene defects localized to chromosome 14 (autosomal dominant inheritance with variable penetrance). Most of the mutations seem to involve desmosomal junctional proteins.

264. Ans. (b) Commotio cordis

(Ref: Harrison 20th p 58)

- Blunt, nonpenetrating, often innocent-appearing injuries to the chest may trigger ventricular fibrillation even in absence of overt signs of injury.

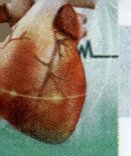

- This syndrome, referred to as commotiocordis, occurs most often in adolescents during sporting events (e.g., baseball, hockey, football) and probably results from an impact to the chest wall overlying the heart during the susceptible phase of repolarization just before the peak of the T wave. Survival depends on prompt defibrillation.

265. Ans. (b) Alkaptonuria

(Ref: Harrison 20th p 1784, 1792; Harrison 19th p 1558)

Cardiomyopathy of restrictive and pseudohypertrophic type:

Glycogen Storage Diseases
II–Pompe's (alpha 1,4 glucosidase)
III–Forbes: de-branching enzyme (amylo 1,6 glucosidase)
Glucose Metabolism (Defective PRKAG2a)
Fatty acid metabolism
Carnitine transport defect
Medium chain Acyl-CoA dehydrogenase
Long chain Acyl-CoA dehydrogenase
Sphingolipidoses
Fabry's disease (alpha galactosidase A)
Gaucher disease (beta-glucocerebroside)
Disorders of lysosomal function
Danon's disease–(lysosome-associated membrane protein, LAMP2)
Miscellaneous
Hemochromatosis–Fe metabolism
Familial amyloidosis–abnormal transthyretin
Friedreich's ataxia–frataxin

266. Ans. (a) Fatty infiltration of myocardium

(Ref: Harrison 20th p 1784, 1792; Harrison 19th p 1565)

Causes of Restrictive Cardiomyopathy

1. Amyloidosis
   Primary (light chain amyloid)
   Familial (abnormal transthyretin)
   Senile (normal transthyretin or atrial peptides)

2. Hemochromatosis (Iron)
3. Fabry's disease
4. Glycogen storage disease (II, III)
5. Radiation
6. Scleroderma
7. Tropical endomyocardial fibrosis
8. Hypereosinophilic syndrome (Löffler's endocarditis)
9. Carcinoid syndrome
10. Radiation
11. Drugs: e.g., serotonin, ergotamine

267. Ans. (d) Dobutamine for cardiogenic dysfunction

(Ref: Harrison 19th p 1565)

- Broken heart syndrome / Tako-tsubo-cardiomyopathy occurs due to catecholamine toxicity. This causes ballooning of the apex and loss of shape of heart contributes to myocardial dysfunction.
- Dobutamine should not be used as catecholamines are already increased in this patient. Hence intra-aortic balloon counter pulsation is used for the management of cardiogenic shock of these patients
- Broken heart syndrome has ST segment elevation and its presentation mimics myocardial infarction
- Causes of ST segment elevation are ELEVATION
  - E- electrolytes imbalance like hyperkalemia
  - L- LBBB
  - E- Early repolarization varaint
  - VA- Ventricular Aneurysm
  - T- Trauma (pericardiocentesis)
  - I- Injury like AMI
  - O- Osbourne waves (Hypothermia)
  - N- Non occlusive spasm (Prinzmetal angina)

268. Ans. (a) HOCM

(Ref: Harrison 20th p 1782, 1794; Harrison's, ch. 238; Cardiomyopathy page 1952, Harrison 19th p 1568)

Spherical Ventricle	Dilated cardiomyopathy
Apical ballooning	Stress cardiomyopathy/Tako-Tsubo
Spade-shaped Ventricle	Apical hypertrophic cardiomyopathy
Distortion of Ventricle	Myocardial infarctions/ aneurysms/ remodeling
Banana-shaped Ventricle	Hypertrophic cardiomyopathy

269. Ans. (a) Fabry's disease

(Ref: Harrison 20th p 1791; Harrison's, ch. 238 page 1965, Harrison 19th p 1565)

- Enzyme replacement therapy in form of beta-agalactisidase is used in Fabry's disease. It is manufactured using DNA recombinant technology and can prevent disease progression and reverse some symptoms.

Fabry's disease is a X linked disease and presents in childhood with:

1. Acroparasthesia
2. Kidney damage presenting with foamy urine due to proteinuria and renal failure
3. Cardiac involvement in form of restrictive cardiomyopathy
4. Skin involvement in form of angiokeratoma.

- Investigation of choice is leucocyte alpha galactosidase assay.
- Usual causes of Restrictive cardiomyopathy are untreatable and therefore cardiac transplantation is the only viable option left for all other causes.
- The most common cause of RCM is amyloidosis.

270. Ans. (d) Dip and spike configuration in ventricular...

(Ref: Harrison 20th p 1846)

- Restrictive cardiomyopathy has fibrosis in the muscle layer of the heart leading to reduced compliance of the ventricles. The right ventricle has less muscle mass and is first affected.
- The reduced compliance of right ventricle affects the rapid ventricular filling of the heart leading to paradoxical rise of JVP on inspiration which is called as Kussmaul sign
- The backward congestion will result in pulsatile liver (also seen with TR)
- The backward congestion leads to ascites which leads to a lots of these patients initially being wrongly diagnosed as those with liver dysfunction.

- This disease has diastolic dysfunction and hence the dip and spike configuration seen on cardiac catheterization is seen during diastole and not as wrongly mentioned in the question as systolic.

271. Ans. (a) Arrythmogenic RV dysplasia

(Ref: Harrison 20th p 1759; ch. 233 page 1897, Harrison 19th p 1564)

- The most important cause of sudden death in professional footballer in setting of beta myosin testing being available is not HOCM but arrythmogenic right ventricular dysplasia.
- The Desmin gene is responsible for a defect in muscle of right ventricle leading to fibrofatty replacement of the muscle. These patients in setting of adrenergic stimulation can develop a VT or Torsades de Pointes leading to death on the football field.
- Takotsubo cardiomyopathy presents in setting of catecholamine surge like an emotional break-up or getting stuck in an elevator during an earthquake.
- ASD presents with exercise intolerance due to secondary pulmonary artery hypertension
- *Eisenmenger patient will be so sick that he cannot be expected to be a football player!!*

272. Ans. (c) Digoxin

(Ref: Harrison 20th p 1796; Harrison 19th p 1569)

- Digoxin is contraindicated in hypertrophic cardiomyopathy and in patients with AV conduction blocks.
- Also drugs that reduce preload and afterload like nitrates, Frusemide, ACE inhibitors are contra-indicated in HOCM as they decrease the amount of inflow into the right side of the heart. Subsequently the flow of blood in to the left side of heart is also reduced and since in these patients the flow is already reduced, subendocardial ischemia in these patients will worsen.

273. Ans. (b) Dilated Cardiomyopathy (DCM)

(Ref: Harrison 20th p 1669-70)

Types of pulse seen are:
1. Anacrotic pulse / Pulsus parvus et tardus: Severe valvular AS
2. Bisferiens pulse : AR, AR with AS, HOCM
3. Water hammer/collapsing pulse/Corrigan pulse: aortic regurgitation/Wet beri-beri, patent ductus arteriosus.
4. Dicrotic pulse: Dilated cardiomyopathy
5. Pulsus alternans: Severe LVF / anterior wall MI
6. Pulsus bigeminus: Digoxin toxicity with ventricular bigeminy.
7. Pulsus paradoxus: the paradox is that the pulse disappears during inspiration, though the heart is beating
    i. Pericardial tamponade
    ii. Inferior wall MI
    iii. Constrictive pericarditis
    iv. Severe COPD / cor pulmonale
    v. Severe acute Bronchial Asthma
    vi. Pulmonary embolism/acute cor pulmonale
    vii. Superior vena cava obstruction (commonly caused by oat cell cancer of lung)

- Heart rate and pulse rate readings show disparity in people with tachy-arrhythmias like Ventricular tachycardia/ventricular bigeminy. Such a discrepancy is known as pulse deficit.
- RADIO-FEMORAL delay is seen in coarctation of aorta

274. Ans. (a) Dilated

(Ref: Harrison 20th p 1784; Harrison 19th p 1558)

- Long term alcohol intake causes damage to the myocytes and hence results in development of Dilated Cardiomyopathy.
- Hypertrophied obstructive cardiomyopathy is autosomal dominant condition due to defect of beta-myosin gene on chromosome 14.
- Restrictive cardiomyopathy occurs due to amyloidosis. Hemochromatosis, radiation to chest, scleroderma and POMPE's disease.

275. Ans. (a) Systolic dysfunction

(Ref: Harrison 20th p 1794)

In HOCM, the banana shaped cavity of left ventricle leads to decreased end diastolic volume which leads to low cardiac output.

Pericardial Diseases

276. Ans. (a) Tension pneumothorax

(Ref: Harrison 20th edition, page 2009)

- The findings of hypotension with elevated JVP and reduced breath sounds points to diagnosis of Tension pneumothorax.
- In cardiac tamponade same finding would be seen but breath sounds would not be affected.
- A large bore needle should be inserted into the pleural space through second intercostal space to allow escape of air and improvement in hemodynamic status of the patient. The needle should be left in place until a thoracostomy tube can be placed.

277. Ans. (b) Breath sounds

(Ref: Harrison 20th edition, page 1843, 2009)

Put explanation of Q 275: CROM 4e page 126

278. Ans. (b) Breath normally

(Ref: Harrison 20th edition, page 1670)

For demonstration of pulsus paradoxsus which is a feature of cardiac tamponade, the patient has to breath normally.
Procedure for measurement of Pulsus paradoxsus

- The patient is placed in a semi-recumbent position
- Respirations should be normal
- The blood pressure cuff is inflated to at least 20 mm Hg above the systolic pressure and slowly deflated until the first Korotkoff sounds are heard only during expiration.
- At this pressure reading, if the cuff is not further deflated and if pulsus paradoxus is present, the first Korotkoff sound is not audible during inspiration.

Contd...

- As the cuff is further deflated, the point at which the first Korotkoff sound is audible during both inspiration and expiration is recorded.
- If the difference between the first and second measurement is greater than 12 mm Hg, an abnormal pulsus paradoxus is present.
- The paradox is that while listening to the heart sounds during inspiration, the pulse weakens or may not be palpated with certain heartbeats.

279. Ans. (b) Pulsus paradoxus is absent in patients with low-pressure cardiac tamponade

(Ref: Harrison 20th p 1843; Braunwald: 9th edition, Chapter 75)

- BP cuff is inflated 20 mm Hg above systemic pressure in case of eliciting trousseau sign and not pulsus paradoxus. *Hence choice A is wrong.* Pulsus paradoxus is a >10 mm Hg fall in systolic pressure with inspiration and is considered pathological and a sign of pulmonary or pericardial disease.
- Cardiac tamponade is characterised by intra-pericardial pressure exceeding LVEDP leading to diastolic collapse of ventricles. This results in crashing of BP and appearance of pulsus paradoxus.
- In contrast the low pressure cardiac tamponade is characterized by intra-pericardial pressure exceeding *only the intra-atrial pressure* leading to under-filling of ventricles and results in *only hypotension*. Since it is a *milder* condition pulsus paradoxus will be absent. **Hence choice B is correct.**
- If patient is asked to take deep breaths in will result in possible syncope as pulse is disappearing on inspiration. *Hence choice C is wrong.*
- Pulsus paradoxus is measured by noting the difference between the systolic pressure at which the Korotkoff sounds are first heard (during expiration), and the systolic pressure at which the Korotkoff sounds are heard with each beat, independent of respiratory phase. *Hence choice D is wrong as it says only expiration.*
- Causes of Pulsus paradoxus-
  1. Pericardial tamponade
  2. Massive pulmonary embolus
  3. Hemorrhagic shock
  4. Severe obstructive lung disease
  5. Tension pneumothorax
  6. Obesity and pregnancy

280. Ans. (c) Breath sounds

(Ref: Harrison 20th p 1843, 2009)

	Cardiac Tamponade	Tension Pneumothorax
Disease Process	Beck's Triad • Hypotension • Muffled heart sounds • Elevated JVP (non- pulsatile)	The diagnosis is made by physical examination showing. • Enlarged hemithorax • No breath sounds • Hyper-resonance to percussion • Shift of the mediastinum to the contralateral side.
JVP	Elevated (compression of heart)	Elevated (due to kinking of SVC and IVC)
Pulse volume	Low volume/Pulsus paradoxus (decreased Venous return)	Low volume/Pulsus paradoxus (decreased Venous return)
Breath sounds	*Dullness to percussion egophony, and bronchial breath sounds may be appreciated at the inferior angle of the left scapula when the effusion is large enough to compress the left lower lobe of the lung, causing consolidation or atelectasis. Trachea will be central.*	*In a tension pneumo-thorax, the affected side will have diminished/absent breath sounds and will likely be hyper-resonant to percussion. Trachea will be deviated contralateral side.*
Pulse rate	Normal to increased	Normal to increased

281. Ans. (d) Tuberculous pericardial effusion

(Ref: Harrison 20th p 1844; Harrison 19th p 1577)

The presence of low grade fever and dyspnea indicates an infective pathology. The CXR shows an increased CT Ratio which could be a tuberculous pericardial effusion. The diagnosis is given more credence due to ECG showing Low voltage ECG which is seen with an effusion.

Syphilitic Aortic aneurysm	In Syphilitic aortitis, the vasa vasorum undergo hyperplastic thickening of their walls thereby restricting blood flow and causing ischemia of the outer two-thirds of the aortic wall. 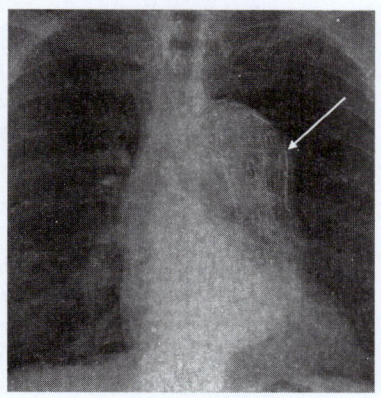 Sixty percent of thoracic aortic aneurysms involve the aortic root and/or ascending aorta, 40% involve the descending aorta, 10% involve the arch, and 10% involve the thoraco-abdominal aorta (with some involving >1 segment)
Hypertrophic cardiomyopathy	Presents with enlarged heart and T wave inversion due to sub-endocardial ischemia and deep Q waves in lateral and inferior leads to septal hypertrophy
Rheumatic Mitral Stenosis	Ruled out as the following features are not present History of gradual progression of DOE, orthopnea. Pulmonary edema is seen on CXR Straightening of left heart border ECG showing P- mitrale or P pulmonale

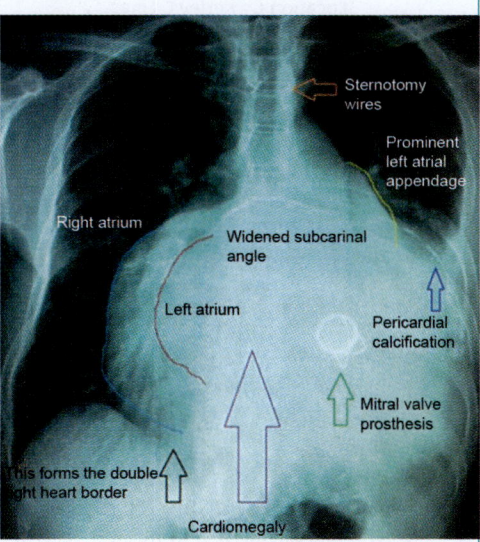

282. Ans. (d) Tachycardia

(Ref: Harrison 19th edition, page 1573)

- The three principal features of tamponade (*Beck's triad*) are hypotension, soft or absent heart sounds, and jugular venous distention with a prominent *x* descent but an absent *y* descent.
- There are both limitation of ventricular filling and reduction of cardiac output. The quantity of fluid necessary to produce this critical state may be as small as 200 mL when the fluid develops rapidly or >2000 mL in slowly developing effusions when the pericardium has had the opportunity to stretch and adapt to an increasing volume.
- Tamponade may also develop more slowly, and in these circumstances the clinical manifestations may resemble those of heart failure, including dyspnea, orthopnea, and hepatic engorgement.
- There may be reduction in amplitude of the QRS complexes, and *electrical alternans* of the P, QRS, or T waves should raise the suspicion of cardiac tamponade.

283. Ans. (b) Pericardial knock, (d) Thickened pericardium

(Ref: Harrison 20th p 1844; Harrison 19th/1573)

	Constrictive pericarditis	Restrictive cardiomyopathy
Pathology	Calcification around the heart	Fibrosis in cardiac muscle
Kussmaul sign	Present due to reduced RV compliance	Present due to Reduced RV compliance
JVP x and y descent	Prominent X Prominent Y	Prominent X Prominent Y (rare)
Auscultation	Pericardial knock/ shudder (mimics S3)	S3 (rare)
Chest X ray	Calcification around heart	Normal size heart minus calcification
Rightheart catheterization	Square root wave sign	Absent
RV and LV pressure	Disconcordance with respiratory cycle With equalization of diastolic pressures	Concordance with respiratory cycle.
BNP levels	Normal or mild elevation	Gross elevations

284. Ans. (a) Cardiac tamponade

(Ref: Harrison 20th p 1843)

Beck's triad is a collection of three medical signs associated with acute cardiac tamponade, an emergency condition wherein fluid accumulates around the heart and impairs its ability to pump blood. The signs are:
- Low arterial blood pressure
- Distended neck veins
- Distant, muffled heart sounds.

Constrictive pericarditis can present with hypotension and congested neck veins but muffled heart sounds are not present.

285. Ans. (d) Treatment with steroids is necessary

(Ref: CMDT 2019 p 439)

- Dressler syndrome is post MI pericarditis/Pleuritis and is characterized by autoimmunity causing damage to the heart. The resultant inflammation causes chest pain in these patients upto 6 weeks of a preceding myocardial inflammation. The investigations show ECG evidence of pericarditis with ST elevation with concavity in upwards direction. The CPKMM levels are normal. The treatment of these patients shall be aspirin 650 mg TID.

286. Ans. (a) Pericardial effusion

(Ref: CMDT 2019 p 439)

- Since in the CXR, the cardiac borders look bulging and CT ratio is increased, the finding is that of a water bottle heart/money bag appearance. In clinical setting of hypotension with distended neck veins, this patient is having a massive pericardial effusion and developing findings of a tamponade.
- The point against cor pulmonale is that it is characterized by right ventricular failure with pulmonary artery hypertension. But in this CXR, pulmonary artery segment is not bulging.

287. Ans. (a) Radiation

(Ref: Harrison 19th p 1577)

- Constrictive pericarditis and restrictive cardiomyopathy are clinical entities, which possess similar diagnostic signatures.
- However, constrictive pericarditis requires surgical treatment and is usually curable, while restrictive cardiomyopathy, needs cardiac transplantation.
- Therefore, the differentiation of constriction and restriction is important.
- Mixed physiology of constriction and restriction has been also reported in cases with prior radiation exposure to the chest
- *Progressive fibrosis can cause restrictive myocardial disease without dilation. Thoracic radiation, common for breast and lung cancer or mediastinal lymphoma, can produce early or late restrictive cardiomyopathy. Patients with radiation cardiomyopathy may present with a possible diagnosis of constrictive pericarditis, as the two conditions often coexist.*

288. Ans. (b) Pericarditis

(Ref: Harrison 20th p 2520; Harrison 19th p 2129)

- Pericarditis is the most common cardiac abnormality in Systemic Lupus Erythematosus (SLE) patients, but lesions of the valves, myocardium and coronary vessels may all occur. In the past, cardiac manifestations were severe and life threatening, often leading to death.
- Vascular occlusion, including coronary arteries, may develop due to vasculitis, premature atherosclerosis or anti-phospholipid antibodies associated with SLE. Premature atherosclerosis is the most frequent cause of coronary artery disease (CAD) in SLE patients.

289. Ans. (b) Cardiac tamponade

(Ref: Harrison 20th p 1843; Harrison 19th p 1573)

290. Ans. (a) Commonest cause in India is 'Idiopathic'

(Ref: Harrison 20th p 1846; Harrison 19th p 1575-76)

Congestive Heart Failure

291. Ans. (b) Central Venous Pressure

(Ref: Harrison 20th edition, page 1711-12)

CVP is used to asses filling of the right heart with low values seen in hypovolemic shock and elevated in cardiogenic shock. It cannot calculate cardiac output.

Thermodilution technique uses temperature deviation in pulmonary artery after injection of 10ml room temperature normal saline into the right atrium to calculate Cardiac output. Choices A and D are ruled out easily by English wording itself.

292. Ans. (a) Spirinolactone

(Ref: CMDT 2019 p 419)

- The given patient with findings of heart failure has *normal serum potassium* and *elevated creatinine*.
- Spironolactone has been documented to reduce mortality in heart failure by 30% but is **not** to be given if eGFR is <30ml/min, serum Creatinine is >2.5mg% and K+ is >5.0meq/dl.
- For ACE inhibitors, CMDT 2018 on page 413 has clearly mentioned "*Some patients may exhibit rise of serum creatinine and potassium but do not require discontinuation*".
- Beta blockers are preferred agents from management of chronic compensated CHF.
- Digoxin has not been shown to reduce mortality in CHF but is not contraindicated in case of elevated Serum creatinine.

293. Ans. (d) Location D

(Ref: Harrison 20th p 1829; Harrison: 19th edition, page 476e-3 and page 1552)

Location A= Kerley A Lines
Location B= Dilated Pulmonary Veins
Location C= Kerley C Lines
Location D= Kerley B Lines

- Kerley A lines are linear opacities extending from the periphery to the hila. They are caused by distention of anastomotic channels between peripheral and central lymphatics.
- Kerley B lines are *short horizontal lines situated perpendicular to the pleural surface at lung bases* and represent oedema of the interlobular septa
- Kerley C lines are reticular opacities at lung base.

294. Ans. (d) Phenylephrine

(Ref: Harrison 20th p 2057-58; Harrison Page 1761)

First Line of action In Management of Acute Pulmonary Oedema
1. Furosemide
2. Morphine
3. Oxygen
4. Nitroglycerin IV if SBP>100 mm Hg
5. Norepinephrine 0.5-30 μg/min IV if if SBP< 100 mm Hg and signs of shock are present.

6. Dopamine 5-15 µg/kg per minute if SBP< 100 mm Hg and signs of shock are present.
7. Dobutamine 2-20 µg/kg/minute IV if SBP 70-100 mm Hg and **no** Signs of shock are present

295. Ans. (b) Anti-endomysial antibody estimation

(Ref: Harrison 20th p 1939)

- The findings of dyspnea, elevated JVP and pedal oedema are suggestive of right sided CHF
- Parasternal heave and palpable S2 indicates pulmonary artery hypertension
- This also explains why lungs are clear since pulmonary oedema is absent in PAH
- Reduced RV compliance in RVH leads to elevated JVP and oedema in feet
- The reason for dyspnea is less pulmonary flow due to PAH.

Echo for mitral stenosis	Useful for diagnosis as PAH is seen in long standing MS
ELISA For HIV	Useful for diagnosis of Group 1 PAH
Urine and stool for Schistosoma	Useful for diagnosis of Group 1 PAH

WHO classification of PAH

Group 1	Idiopathic PAH HIV **Portal Hypertension (Schistosomiasis)** Drugs Connective tissue disorders Pulmonary veno-occlusive disease
Group 2	Pulmonary artery hypertension due to left heart disease
Group 3	PAH due to lung disease like COPD, interstitial lung disease.
Group 4	PAH due to secondary thromboembolism with occlusion of proximal or distal pulmonary arteries
Group 5	PAH due to Haematologicaldisorders: Myeloproliferative disorders Systemic disorders: Sarcoidosis, Langhans cell histiocytosis Metabolic disorders: glycogen storage disorders Miscellaneous: Tumour embolization

296. Ans. (c) Corpulmonale

(Ref: Harrison 20th p 1763;Harrison 19th edition, page 1505 and 96e-2)

Etiologies of Heart Failure

Depressed Ejection Fraction (<40%)	
• Coronary artery disease	• Nonischemic dilated cardio-myopathy
• Myocardial infarction	• Familial/genetic disorders
• Myocardial ischemia	• Infiltrative disorders
• Chronic pressure overload	• Toxic/drug-induced damage
• Hypertension	• Viral
• Obstructive valvular disease	• Chagas disease
• Chronic volume overload	• Disorders of rate and rhythm
• Regurgitant valvular disease	• Chronic bradyarrhythmias
• Intracardiac (left-to-right) shunting	• Chronic tachyarrhythmias
• Extracardiac shunting	

Contd...

Preserved Ejection Fraction (> 40 – 50%)	
• Pathologic hypertrophy	• Restrictive cardiomyopathy
• Primary (hypertrophic cardio-myopathies)	• Infiltrative disorders (amyloidosis, sarcoidosis)
• Secondary (hypertension)	• Storage diseases (hemochromatosis)
• Aging	• Fibrosis
	• Endomyocardial disorders
Pulmonary Heart Disease	
• Cor pulmonale	
• Pulmonary vascular disorders	
High output States	
• Metabolic disorders	• Excessive blood-flow requirements
• Thyrotoxicosis	• Systemic arteriovenous shunting
• Nutritional disorders: beriberi	• Chronic anemia

297. Ans. (d) Haemofiltration

(Ref: Harrison 18th edition, e-50)

For management of digoxin toxicity the following protocol is used:
1. Digoxin-specific antibody fragments for hemodynamically compromising dysrhythmias, Mobitz II or third-degree atrioventricular block, hyperkalemia (>5.5 meq/L; in acute poisoning only).
2. Temporizing measures include atropine, dopamine, epinephrine
3. External cardiac pacing for bradydysrhythmias
4. *Magnesium, lidocaine, or phenytoin, for ventricular tachydysrhythmias.*
5. Internal cardiac pacing and cardioversion can increase ventricular irritability

298. Ans. (d) Wide variable split S2

- The image shows presence of *bat wing pulmonary edema*.
- Due to forward failure low perfusion of kidneys leads to low urine output. Hence RAAS in stimulated to result in increased aldosterone levels. This leads to increased salt and water retention and explains low urinary sodium. The increase in potassium is due to kidney getting involved.
- Left ventricular failure leads to narrow split S2

299. Ans. (b) Sirtuin

(Ref: Harrison 20th p 1767; Braunwald heart disease, chapter 23)

- Both B-type natriuretic peptide (BNP) and N-terminal pro-BNP, which are released from the failing heart, are relatively sensitive markers for the presence of HF with depressed EF; they also are elevated in HF patients with a preserved EF, albeit to a lesser degree. Levels can be falsely low in obese patients and may normalize in some patients after appropriate treatment. At present, serial measurements of BNP are not recommended as a guide to HF therapy.
- Other biomarkers, such as troponin T and I, C-reactive protein, TNF receptors, and uric acid, may be elevated in HF and provide important prognostic information.
- A family of histone deacetylases known as sirtuins. An important member of this family is SIRT1, homologues of which enhance the lifespans of model organisms. SIRT1 is

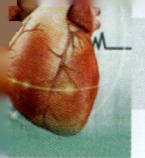

a putative target of resveratrol, which is thought to activate the enzyme and, therefore, might enhance lifespan and, presumably health span as well.

300. Ans. (d) NYHA4

(Ref: Harrison 20th p 1650; Harrison 19th p 1440)

Class	Patient Symptoms
Class I	No limitation of physical activity. Ordinary physical activity does not cause undue fatigue, palpitation (feeling heart beats), or dyspnea (shortness of breath).
Class II (Mild)	Slight limitation of physical activity. Comfortable at rest, but ordinary physical activity results in fatigue, palpitation, or dyspnea.
Class III (Moderate)	Marked limitation of physical activity. Comfortable at rest, but less than ordinary activity causes fatigue, palpitation, or dyspnea.
Class IV (Severe)	Unable to carry out any physical activity without discomfort. Symptoms of cardiac insufficiency at rest. If any physical activity is undertaken, discomfort is increased.

301. Ans. (a) ACEI + Beta blocker

(Ref: Harrison 20th p 1774-75; Harrison 19th p 1511)

- Beta-blocker therapy represents a major advance in the treatment of patients with a depressed Beta-blocker therapy represents a major advance in the treatment of patients with a depressed EF.
- These drugs interfere with the harmful effects of sustained activation of the adrenergic nervous system by competitively antagonizing one or more adrenergic receptors. Although there are a number of potential benefits to blocking all three receptors, most of the deleterious effects of adrenergic activation are mediated by the beta1 receptor.
- Therefore, beta blockers are indicated for patients with symptomatic or asymptomatic HF and a depressed EF <40%. Drugs that interfere with excessive activation of the RAA system and the adrenergic nervous system can relieve the symptoms of HF with a depressed EF by stabilizing and/or reversing cardiac remodeling.
- In this regard, ACE inhibitors and beta blockers have emerged as the cornerstones of modern therapy for HF with a depressed EF.

302. Ans. (b) Congestive heart failure

(Ref: Harrison 20th p 1766; Harrison 19th p 1504)

This abnormal pattern of breathing, in which breathing is absent for a period and then rapid for a period, can be seen in patients with:
1. Heart failure
2. Stroke [Bihemispheric damage]
3. Traumatic brain injuries and brain tumors.
4. Healthy people during sleep at high altitudes
5. Toxic metabolic encephalopathy like carbon monoxide poisoning.

303. Ans. (b) Digoxin

(Ref: Harrison 20th p 2057-58; Harrison, ch. 272 page 2236-37, Harrison 19th p 1761)

- Morphine acts as a venodilator and anxiolytic.
- Frusemide reduces fluid overload and possible vasodilator.
- Positive pressure ventilation reduces alveolar, interstitial edema thus reducing venous return. CPAP or BiPAP can be used.
- Digoxin is used when pulmonary edema is associated with AF and fast ventricular rate; otherwise the use is limited.

Acute Pulmonary Edema
Administer
• Furosemide IV 0.5 to 1.0 mg/kg
• Morphine IV 2 to 4 mg
• Oxygen/intubation as needed
• Nitroglycerin SL, then 10 to 20 mcg/min IV if SBP greater than 100 mm Hg
• Norepinephrine, 0.5 to 30 mcg/min IV or Dopamine, 5 to 15 mcg/kg per minute IV if SBP < 100 mm Hg and signs/symptoms of shock present
• Dobutamine 2 to 20 mcg/kg per minute IV if SBP 70 to 100 mm Hg and no signs/symptoms of shock

304. Ans. (d) Digoxin

(Ref: Harrison 19th p 1512)

305. Ans. (c) Actively metabolized in liver

(Ref: KDT 5th/ 461, 462, KDT 5th/ 461, 462)

Congenital Heart Disease

306. Ans. (a) CVS defect

(Ref: Harrison, page 1832)

Lithium is a teratogenic drug leading to Ebstein anomaly. It results in deformed tricuspid valve leading to regurgitation and sometimes stenosis. Some patients may also have WPW.

307. Ans. (b) Large platelets

(Ref: Harrison 20th edition, page 826)

Epstein syndrome (EPTS) is an autosomal dominant disease characterized by nephritis, mild hearing loss, and thrombocytopenia with giant platelets

308. Ans. (b) Inability to hear a murmur

(Ref: O.P Ghai: 8th edition, page 421)

- Tetralogy of fallot has sub-pulmonic stenosis and R to L shunting leading to cyanosis.
- The murmur due to RV outflow tract obstruction is ejection systolic murmur.
- In a tet spell the shunting from R to L increases. Now since RV contains a fixed amount of blood and most of the blood is going from R to left, the blood flow across the pulmonic valve reduces. This explains the worsening of cyanosis in a tet spell. Less blood across subpulmonic stenosis will lead to reduction in intensity of murmur and it may not be heard.
- Choice C and D are features of heart failure and are ruled out.

- Tet spells are common on waking up and following exertion. The child becomes dysneic and more blue. Subsequently he loses consciousness and convulsions may occur.

309. Ans. (c) Ebstein anomaly

(Ref: Harrison 20th p 1832; Harrison 19th edition, page 1527)

- Ebstein's anomaly is the most commonly occurring congenital abnormality associated with the Wolff-Parkinson-White (WPW) syndrome.
- Ebstein's anomaly of the tricuspid valve does not usually cause symptoms unless it is severe with cyanosis or associated with paroxysmal tachycardia due to pre-excitation.
- Ebstein's anomaly can often be suspected from the ECG, which may show sinus rhythm with right bundle branch block, often with rather low voltage secondary R-waves in V1 or right –sided pre-excitation with a short PR interval and complexes which resemble left bundle branch block. Occasionally the ECG may alternate between these two patterns.
- Patients with Ebstein's anomaly who suffer from atrioventricular re-entry tachycardia usually have more frequent attacks during pregnancy.

Congenital conditions with pre-excitation are:
1. Ebstein anomaly
2. Tricuspid atresia
3. Dextrocardia
4. Familial cardiomyopathy
5. Fibro-elastosis

310. Ans. (b) Only if CHF is uncontrolled

(Ref: Braunwald 8th edition, chapter 61 and Nelson 20th edition, page 2196)

Indications for surgical closure of a VSD include patients at any age with large defects in whom:
1. Clinical symptoms and failure to thrive cannot be controlled medically
2. Infants between 6 and 12 mouths of age with large defects associated with pulmonary hypertension, even if the symptoms are controlled by medication; and patients older than 24 months with a Qp : Qs ratio greater than 2 :1.
3. Patients with supra-cristal VSD of any size are usually referred for surgery because of the high risk for aortic valve regurgitation.
4. Severe pulmonary vascular disease is a contraindication to closure of a VSD.

The natural course of a VSD depends to a large degree on the size of the defect. A significant number (30–50%) of small defects close spontaneously, most frequently during the 1st 2 yr of life. Small muscular VSDs are more likely to close (up to 80%) than membranous VSDs are (up to 35%). The vast majority of defects that close do so before the age of 4 yr.

311. Ans. (c) TOF

(Ref: Nelson 20th p 2188; Harrison 19th/1521-22, 1526; O.P. Ghai 8th/415)

- ASD, VSD and PDA are Left to right sided shunts that increase pulmonary blood flow.
- In transposition of great arteries the reason for cyanosis is mixing of blood of two circuits. The malformation consists of the origin of the aorta from the morphological right ventricle and that of the pulmonary artery from the morphological left ventricle. Consequently, the pulmonary and systemic circulations are connected in parallel rather than the normal in-series connection.
- In TOF the pulmonary oligaemia is due to sub-pulmonic stenosis.

312. Ans. (b) Lower border

(Ref: Chest X Ray solutions, H. Singh 1st ed. pg 218)

- **Causes of inferior rib notching**
  - **Arterial:** aortic coarctation, aortic thrombosis, pulmonary-oligemia/AV malformation, Blalock Taussig shunt, Tetralogy of fallot, absent pulmonary artery and pulmonary stenosis.
  - **Venous:** AV Malfomations of chest wall, superior vena cava or other central venous obstruction.
  - **Neurogenic:** Intercostal neuroma, Neurofibromatosis type 1, poliomyelitis.
  - **Osseous:** Hyperparathyroidism, Thalassemia
- **Causes of superior rib notching**
  - Poliomyelitis
  - Osteogenesis Imperfecta
  - Neurofibromatosis
  - Marfan's Syndrome
  - Collagen vascular disease
  - Hyperparathyroidism.

313. Ans. (a) Total anomalous pulmonary venous connection

(Ref: Nelson 20th p 2227)

Total anomalous pulmonary venous connection	Figure of 8 or snowman heart
Transposition of great arteries	Egg on side appearance
T.O.F	Boot shaped heart
Ebstein anomaly	Box shaped heart

314. Ans. (b) Pulmonary plethora

(Ref: Harrison 19th ed, pg 1526-27. Nelson 20th p 2213)

- The CXR shows an heart with boot-shaped configuration and reduced vascularity of lungs. The clinical diagnosis is tetralogy of Fallot, which due to subpulmonic stenosis presents with pulmonic oligemia.

315. Ans. (a) Ductal dependent systemic circulation

(Ref: Harrison 19th ed, pg 1526-27. Nelson 20th p 2223)

The image shows presence of egg-shaped heart with presence of cyanosis since birth and loud S2.

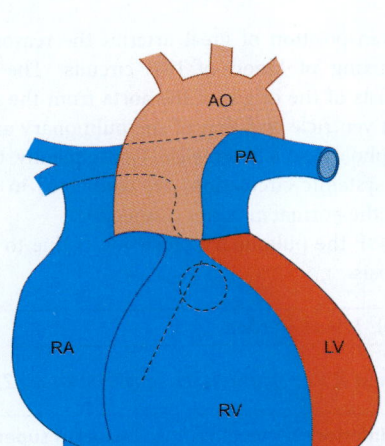

- This *indicates transposition of great arteries which is a ductal dependent pulmonary circulation.*
- Choice B is correct as PGE1 infusion will keep ductus patent and ensure survival. Balloon atrial septostomy will ensure reduction of cyanosis.
- Infant of diabetic mother is at risk for development of:
  1. VSD
  2. TGA
  3. Asymmetrical septal hypertrophy

316. Ans. (b) Enlarged left ventricle

(Ref: Harrison 19th ed, pg 1520. Nelson 20th p 2189-90)

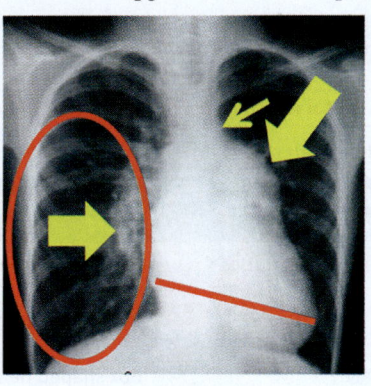

- The clinical age of presentation of 5 years with recurrent pneumonia point to L to R shunt. The presence of flow murmur (mid diastolic murmur) points to diagnosis of atrial septal defect.
- Large yellow arrow on right side points to pulmonary plethora
- Large yellow arrow on left side points to dilatation of pulmonary trunk
- Small yellow arrow on left side indicates site of aortic knuckle.
- Red line indicates enlarged heart.

317. Ans. (a) Coarctation of aorta

(Ref: Harrison 20th p 1837; Nelson 18th edn Ch 587: Harrison 19th p 1524)

- Turner syndrome is associated with isolated non-stenotic bicuspid aortic valves in one third to one half of patients. In later life, bicuspid aortic valve disease can progress to dilatation of the aortic root.
- Less frequent defects include aortic coarctation (20%), aortic stenosis, mitral valve prolapse, and anomalous pulmonary venous drainage

318. Ans. (b) Surgery for congenital heart disease

(Ref: O.P. Ghai 8th edn, Net source p 458)

In children, the most common cause of permanent acquired complete AV block is *surgery for congenital heart disease*. Postsurgical complete atrioventricular block (AVB) is the most common cause for acquired AV block in children, resulting from trauma to the AV node at the time of surgery (i.e., hemorrhage, ischemia, necrosis, inflammation, traumatic disruption).

The second most common cause is congenital heart disease associated with complete AV block. Other etiologies of acquired AV block are often reversible and include digitalis and other drug intoxications, viral myocarditis, acute rheumatic fever, Lyme disease, and infectious mononucleosis.

319. Ans. (a) Carbon dioxide washout

(Ref: Nelson Pediatrics ch. 101.4 Harrison 20th p 1834)

Manifestations of PDA may include:
1. Apnea for unexplained reasons in an infant recovering from RDS
2. A hyperdynamic precordium, bounding peripheral pulses, wide pulse pressure, and a continuous or systolic murmur with or without extension into diastole or an apical diastolic murmur, multiple clicks resembling the shaking of dice.
3. Carbon dioxide retention
4. Increasing oxygen dependence
5. X-ray evidence of cardiomegaly and increased pulmonary vascular markings;
6. Hepatomegaly.
7. Pulmonary hemorrhage can occur due to increased pressure in pulmonary circulation.
   The diagnosis is confirmed by echocardiographic visualization of a PDA with Doppler flow demonstrating.

320. Ans. (d) Kawasaki Disease

(Ref: Nelson 20th p 1209; Harrison 20th p 2588)

Romano Ward syndrome	Romano Ward syndrome is a variant of long Q-T syndrome, a group of channelo-pathies that affect ventricular repolarization, is also associated with sudden death and can mimic Sudden Infant Death Syndrome • The mechanism of sudden death is polymorphic VT (Torsades de pointes) • An initial presentation of sudden cardiac death is found in 9% of patients. • LQT 3 can present with death in sleep as well in children

Contd...

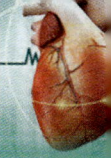

Aortic stenosis	Mortality is higher in patients presenting with severe or critical aortic valve stenosis during the first year of life, specifically in the neonatal period, although this risk has decreased significantly over the past 20 years. Undetected, severe aortic valve stenosis is a known cause of sudden death and accounts for approximately 1% of all causes of sudden death in young people.
Hypoplastic left heart syndrome	The hypoplastic LV cannot maintain system perfusion and presents with shock after death. Prostaglandin infusions in these patients shall help in survival
Kawasaki disease	It is also a cause of sudden death in children but is the best answer because of relatively better prognosis. Nelson states "Recovery is complete and without apparent long-term effects for patients who do not develop coronary disease. Recurrent acute illness occurs in only 1-3% of cases. The prognosis for patients with coronary abnormalities depends on the severity of coronary disease. Overall, 50% of coronary artery aneurysms resolve as assessed by echo-cardiogram 1-2 yr after the illness. Giant aneurysms are unlikely to resolve and are most likely to lead to thrombosis or stenosis."

Also note that amongst coronary artery causes of sudden death in children it is anomalous origin of coronary artery from Sinus of Valsava which is given as more common than Kawasaki. Nelson states "Coronary artery anomalies are also commonly associated with sudden death in children and adolescents. The most common abnormality associated with sudden death is the origin of the left main coronary artery from the right sinus of Valsava. The coronary artery therefore courses between the aorta and pulmonary artery. Exercise results in a rise in pulmonary and aortic pressure, which compresses the left main coronary artery and results in ischemia."

321. Ans. (c) TGA

(Ref: Harrison's, ch. 236: Congenital Heart page 1927, Harrison 19th p 1527; Nelson 20th p 2223)

- TGA is the most common cyanotic heart disease presenting in first few hour of life (it is a very shocking but true statement). TOF presents after one week of life
- Infants with transposition of the great arteries (TGA) are usually born at term, with cyanosis apparent within hours of birth. The clinical course and manifestations depend on the extent of inter-circulatory mixing and the presence of associated anatomic lesions.
- Transposition of the great arteries with large ventricular septal defect: Infants may not initially manifest symptoms of heart disease, although mild cyanosis (particularly when crying) is often noted. Signs of congestive heart failure (tachypnea, tachycardia, diaphoresis, and failure to gain weight) may become evident over the first 3-6 weeks as pulmonary blood flow increases
- *The points against diagnosis of TOF is heart failure, though cyanosis and murmur are present*
- *Rheumatic fever presents in 5-15 yr age group and does not have cyanosis.*
- *VSD presents at 6 weeks with CHF*

322. Ans. (c) Calcium chloride

(Ref: Nelson Textbook of Pediatrics, ch. 430; Nelson 20th p 2212)

Depending on the frequency and severity of hyper-cyanotic attacks, one or more of the following procedures should be instituted in sequence:
1. Placement of the infant on the abdomen in the knee-chest position
2. Administration of oxygen (although increasing inspired oxygen will not reverse cyanosis caused by intracardiac shunting)
3. Injection of morphine subcutaneously in a dose not in excess of 0.2 mg/kg. Calming and holding the infant in a knee-chest position may abort progression of an early spell.
4. Because metabolic acidosis develops when arterial pO_2 is <40 mm Hg, rapid correction (within several minutes) with intravenous **administration of sodium bicarbonate** is necessary if the spell is unusually severe and the child shows a lack of response to the foregoing therapy.
5. For spells that are resistant to this therapy, drugs that increase systemic vascular resistance, such as **intravenous phenylephrine,** can improve right ventricular outflow, decrease the right-to-left shunt, and improve the symptoms.
6. β-Adrenergic blockade by the intravenous administration of propranolol (0.1 mg/kg given slowly to a maximum of 0.2 mg/kg) is also useful.

Clinical presentation of TET SPELL
1. Usually are seen during the 1st and 2nd year of life. The infant becomes hyperpneic and restless, cyanosis increases, gasping respirations ensue, and syncope may follow.
2. The spells occur most frequently in the morning on initially awakening or after episodes of vigorous crying. Temporary disappearance or a decrease in intensity of the systolic murmur is usual as flow across the right ventricular outflow tract diminishes.
3. The spells may last from a few minutes to a few hours but are rarely fatal. Short episodes are followed by generalized weakness and sleep. Severe spells may progress to unconsciousness and, occasionally, to convulsions or hemiparesis.

323. Ans. (d) 4 weeks

(Ref: O.P. Ghai, 7th ed., pg. 395)

Functional closure of Ductus Arteriosus occurs by 7 days of life:
- O.P Ghai states complete closure occurs by upper limit of 28 days i.e 4 weeks.
- Prostaglandin E2 (PGE2), produced by both the placenta and the DA itself, is by far the most potent of the E prostaglandins, but prostaglandin E1 (PGE1) also has a role in keeping the ductus arteriosus open.
- PGE1 and PGE2 keep the ductus open by increasing the concentration of intracellular cAMP, and by using specific receptors such as EP2 or EP4 which are sensitive to PGE2.

- Throughout pregnancy the DA of the fetus remains open, due to prostaglandins, but immediately after birth the levels of both PGE2 and the EP4 receptors will reduce significantly.
- This allows the ductus arteriosus to close, so that the normal post-natal circulation of the heart can commence.

324. Ans. (d) Total anomalous pulmonary venous connection (TAPVC)

(Ref: Cloherty Manual of Neonatal Care: 7th ed., ch. 41)

- In TAPVC, alprostadil infusion will keep the ductus patent and will cause more blood to flow into the lungs. This blood will now rush into the abnormal pulmonary veins which again drain this blood back to right atrium instead of left atrium.
- This will lead to volume based overloading of the right side of the heart as it receives the normal venous return as well the blood from the abnormal veins which has increased due to our wrong decision to keep the ductus patent
- Ductus dependant pulmonary circulation = TOF/TGA/ tricuspid atresia
- Ductus Dependant systemic circulation= mitral atresia/ hypoplastic left heart syndrome/aortic atresia/ interrupted aortic arch
- Ductus INDEPENDENT circulation= TAPVC/ A. L. C. A. P. A/ Truncus arteriosus

325. Ans. (a) Sinus venosus ASD

(Ref: Harrison 20th p 2191; Nelson, 18th ed., ch. 256)

- PAPVC is similar to Total Anomalous Pulmonary Venous Connection (TAPVC); however, TAPVC differs in that all or most pulmonary venous vessels connect to the right side of the heart in TAPVC
- The most common type of ASD is sinus venosus type associated with PAPVC. The anomalous pulmonary vein, usually the right upper or middle pulmonary vein can either override the intra-atrial septum (anomalous drainage) or can drain separately into the superior vena cava (true anomalous connection). Usually, the connection is unobstructed.
- It is also associated with Scimitar sign-where the anomalous venous return on CXR looks like a curved sword.

326. Ans. (b) Hyperparathyroidism

(Ref: Principles of cardiovascular radiology, pg. 86, ch. 7)

- PTH hormone will cause bone resorbtion irrespective of the surface of the bone.
- In Coarctation and interrupted aortic arch the collaterals will cause inferior surface of rib erosion
- In blalock taussig shunt the vascular graft pulsations can cause the same (involves only upper 2 rib spaces)

327. Ans. (c) TOF

(Ref: Harrison 20th p 1834-35; TOF: OP Ghai, 7th ed. pg 408, Harrison 19th p 1526)

- In all L-R shunts, increased pulmonary blood flow causes pulmonary artery hypertension. Subsequently the increased pressure in Pulmonary artery causes shunt reversal, referred to as Eisenmenger complex

- As the systolic pressures between the two ventricles are identical, there is little or no left to right shunt and the ventricular septal defect is silent. The right to left shunt is also silent since it occurs at insignificant difference in pressure between the right ventricle and the aorta. The flow from the right ventricle into the pulmonary artery occurs across the pulmonary valve producing an ejection systolic murmur. The more severe the pulmonic stenosis, the less the flow into the pulmonary artery and the bigger the right to left shunt. In definitive repair, undertaken at 6 months- 1 year of age, VSD needs to be closed . Defective closure can therefore technically result in shunt reversal.

328. Ans. (a) Narrow pulse pressure

(Ref: Harrison 20th p 1834; Nelson Textbook of Pediatrics 18th ed./ch. 426 and 102.2, Harrison 19th p 1523)

- A large PDA will result in striking physical signs attributable to the wide pulse pressure, most prominently, bounding peripheral arterial pulses. The apical impulse is prominent and, with cardiac enlargement, is heaving. A thrill, maximal in the 2nd left interspace, is often present and may radiate toward the left clavicle, down the left sternal border, or toward the apex. It is usually systolic but may also be palpated throughout the cardiac cycle. The classic continuous murmur is described as being like machinery or rolling thunder in quality.
- The greatest risk factor for NEC is prematurity. NEC probably results from an interaction between loss of mucosal integrity due to a variety of factors (ischemia, infection, inflammation) and the host's response to that injury (circulatory, immunologic, inflammatory) resulting in necrosis of the affected area.

329. Ans. (d) Pulmonary artery hypertension

(Ref: Table 31-3, current diagnosis and treatment in cardiology 2nd edition and Harrison 20th p 1831)

High maternal risk conditions are as follows:
1. Poor functional class before pregnancy (NYHA functional classification II or more) or cyanosis
2. Pulmonary hypertension
3. Eisenmenger syndrome
4. Impaired systemic ventricular function (ejection fraction < 40%)
5. Mitral valve stenosis (area < 2 cm^2), aortic valve stenosis (area < 1.5 cm^2), left ventricular outflow tract peak pressure gradient greater than 30 mm Hg before pregnancy
6. Preconception history of adverse cardiac events such as symptomatic arrhythmia, stroke, transient ischemic attack, and pulmonary edema
7. Marfan syndrome

330. Ans. (d) Multifactorial

(Ref: Nelson 20th page 2183)

331. Ans. (c) TOF

(Ref: Harrison 20th p 1835; Ghai 6th/406 – 409, Harrison 19th p 1526)

332. **Ans. (a) Valvular stenosis**

(Ref: Harrison 20th p 1835; Harrison 19th p 1526)

333. **Ans. (a) Atrial septal defect (ASD)**

(Ref: Dorland's Medical Dictionary 28th/1253, 1746; Stedman's Medical Dictionary 28th/1452)

334. **Ans. (d) Tetralogy of Fallot**

(Ref: Harrison 20th p 1837; Ghai 5th /303, Harrison 19th p 1527)

335. **Ans. (b) Descending aorta to left pulmonary artery**

(Ref: Sabiston 15th/2023-4, O.P. Ghai p 422 8th edn)

336. **Ans. (b) Left arterial hypertrophy**

(Ref: Harrison 20th p 1832; Harrison 19th p 1521)

ASD is associated with RA and RV hypertrophy but not LA hypertrophy.

337. **Ans. (a) CCF; (b) Infective Endarteritis**

(Ref: Nelson 20th p 2198; Harrison 19th p 1523)

338. **Ans. (d) Splitting of S2**

(Ref: Nelson 20th p 2218; Ghai 6th/408, 410, 414-415, Harrison 19th p 1527)

339. **Ans. (b) Coarctation of aorta**

(Ref: Harrison 20th p 1837; Ghai 6th/419, Harrison 19th p 1525)

340. **Ans. (a) Supracardiac**

(Ref: Harrison 20th p 2227 Schwartz 8th/ 622, O. P Ghai 8th edn p 427)

341. **Ans. (a) ASD**

(Ref: O. P Ghai 8th edn p 401)

Pulmonary Artery Hypertension

342. **Ans. (a) Bosentan**

(Ref: Harrison 20th p 1941; Harrison's 19th edition, page 1659)

Endothelin receptor antagonist	Bosentan is approved by US FDA and improves exercise tolerance in 6-minutes-walk test.
Amlodipine	Not approved by US FDA and only 20% respond to CCB in the long term.
Diuretics	Will worsen PAH
Digoxin	Used in CHF and no role in PAH

343. **Ans. (a) Hyperventilation**

(Ref: Harrison 20th p 1939; Harrison 19th edition, page 1658)

- Hypoxia leads to constriction of pulmonary artery and development of pulmonary artery hypertension.
- Morbid obesity leads to obstructive sleep apnea and can lead to PAH
- High altitude will also lead to hypoxia and development of PAH.
- A causal relationship has been established between exposure to several anorexigens, including aminorex and the fenfluramines, and the development of PAH.

344. **Ans. (a) Pulmonary artery hypertension**

(Ref: Harrison 20th p 1936-37)

- In view of prominent pulmonary artery segment with early diastolic murmur the clinical diagnosis is pulmonary artery hypertension causing a mild pulmonary regurgitation. The gender female is suggestive of a connective tissue disorder that can lead to pulmonary artery hypertension.
- The striking feature in this chest X-ray is the remarkably prominent main pulmonary artery segment (MPA), which appears to be aneurysmally dilated. Right pulmonary artery (RPA) is also enlarged. Enlargement of right pulmonary artery differentiates it from the post-stenotic dilatation of main pulmonary artery in pulmonary stenosis. In post-stenotic dilatation, even though the left pulmonary artery, which is in line with the main pulmonary artery may be dilated, the right pulmonary artery, which does not have the effect of the jet and eddy currents is not dilated.
- This X-ray also shows a prominent right atrial contour, indicating right atrial dilatation as a consequence of pulmonary hypertension and right ventricular hypertrophy.
- The end on views of blood vessels seen through the right pulmonary artery shadow are tiny, indicating that the RPA dilatation is unlikely to be due to increased pulmonary blood flow. Large end on vessels are a feature of pulmonary hypertension due to excessive left to right shunt causing increased pulmonary blood flow.

345. **Ans. (c) Cyanosis: anxiety**

(Ref: Harrison 19th p 1442)

346. **Ans. (b) Elevated JVP with singular loud S2, systolic murmur**

(Ref: Harrison 20th p 1937)

- PAH is characterized by presence of large 'a' waves leading to elevated JVP. S2 is loud and hides S1. Hence S2 is singular. Loud P2 is a finding of PAH. Wide fixed split S2 is seen with ASD.
- The systolic murmur in these patients is explained by the presence of tricuspid regurgitation developing due to severe PAH
- Barrel shaped chest is seen with COPD.

347. **Ans. (a) Mitral stenosis**

(Ref: Harrison 20th p 1939; Internal Medicine 5th/293)

348. **Ans. (d) Bronchoconstriction**

(Ref: Harrison 20th p 1939; Harrison 19th p 1505)

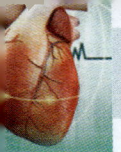

ECG

349. Ans. (c) aVF

(Ref: Harrison 20th edition, page 1676)

90 degrees cardiac axis corresponds to lead aVF in ECG and therefore the maximum R wave amplitude would be seen in that lead only.

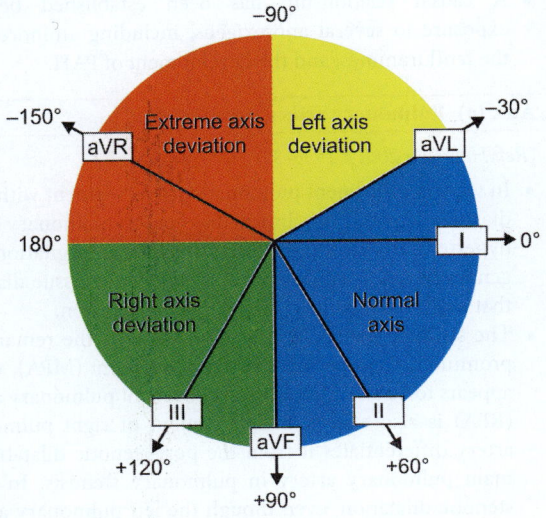

350. Ans. (a) Hypokalemia

Ref: Oxford Handbook of Clinical Medicine, 10th edition, Page 96

- P- pulmonale (tall P wave in leads II, III, aVF) in absence of right atrial enlargement is termed as Pseudo- P- Pulmonale.
- Hypokalemia leads to gradient change across the cell membrane and leads to more sodium entry into the cell. This causes the P wave amplitude to increase which is called pseudo P-pulmonale.
- Conversely the gradient change in hyperkalaemia ensures less entry of sodium into cells and leads to reduction in amplitude of P waves.

351. Ans. (b) Cor-pulmonale

(Ref: Harrison 20th p 1769, Harrison 19th edition, page 1454)

- The ECG shows heart rate of 100/min with right axis deviation.
- Peaked P waves are seen in lead II, III and aVF
- S>R in lead V6.
- T wave inversion is noted in V2-V3 with non-specific ST segment changes.
- These changes and clinical feature of pedal edema point to right ventricular etiology. Hence the diagnosis is choice B.
- Choice A is ruled out as RSR' pattern in V1 is not seen.
- Choice C is ruled out as it presents as acute coronary syndrome.
- Choice D is ruled out as it presents with left axis deviation and left ventricular enlargement.

352. Ans. (d) Electromechanical dissociation

(Ref: Harrison 20th p 1682; Harrison 19th edition, page 1453)

The ECG shows a heart rate of 150 bpm with right axis deviation. P waves are not seen with broad QRS complex. Since clinical history is not given, the ECG shows broad complex tachycardia. Electrolytes and cardiac biomarkers of the patient should be checked.

Electromechanical dissociation is seen in cardiac rupture seen post MI.

353. Ans. (c) Right Ventricular Infarct

(Ref: Harrison 20th p 1676-77; page 1452: Harrison 19th edition)

The standard precordial chest leads and limb leads can study the heart in the following fashion.

1. One or more of the precordial leads (V1 through V6) and in leads I and aVL with acute transmural anterior or anterolateral wall ischemia
2. Leads V1 to V3 with anteroseptal or apical ischemia
3. Leads V4 to V6 with apical or lateral ischemia;
4. Leads II, III, and aVF with inferior wall ischemia
5. However to study *right ventricular ischemia right-sided precordial leads V3R, V4R* need to be deployed
6. Posterior wall infarction, which induces ST elevation in leads placed over the back of the heart such as leads V7 to V9, can be induced by lesions in the right coronary artery or left circumflex artery

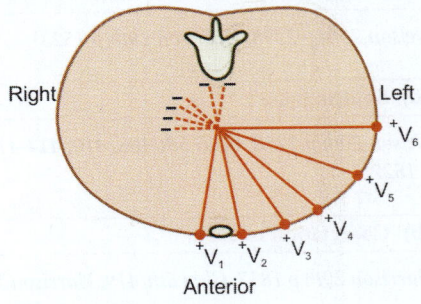

354. Ans. (c) Hypokalemia

(Ref: Harrison 20th p 1678-79; Current Diagnosis and Management in Cardiology, Ch. 19: Supraventricular Tachycardia, Harrison 19th p 1455)

Causes of LBBB
- Aortic stenosis
- Ischaemic heart disease
- Hypertension
- Dilated cardiomyopathy
- **Anterior MI**
- Primary degenerative disease (fibrosis) of the conducting system (Lenegre disease)
- **Hyperkalaemia**
- Digoxin toxicity
- **Ashmann phenomenon (has both LBBB and RBBB)**

1. In acute MI, ischemia can damage the left bundle leading to LBBB.
2. Hyperkalemia can cause defective repolarization and hence cause Bundle branch block pattern in ECG that culminates in sine wave pattern.
3. Atrial fibrillation has a narrow complex qRS but Ashmann phenomenon seen in atrial fibrillation is characterized by broad complex qRS with usually a RBBB morphology. Thus if an impulse lands on the bundle of HIS and finds the right

bundle refractory then RBBB will occur. Also remember that the refractory period of right fascicle is more than that of the left fascicle resulting in RBBB mostly in these patients.

355. Ans. (c)   A-V dissociation

(Ref: Harrison 20th p 1678-79; Harrison's, ch. 228 page 1835, Harrison 19th p 1454)

- Left bundle branch block alters both early and later phases of ventricular depolarization.
- The major qRS vector is directed to the left and posteriorly. In addition, the normal early left-to-right pattern of septal activation is disrupted such that septal depolarization proceeds from right to left as well.
- As a result, left bundle branch block generates wide, predominantly negative (QS) complexes in lead V1 and entirely positive (R) complexes in lead V6.
- A pattern identical to that of left bundle branch block, preceded by a sharp spike, is seen in most cases of electronic right ventricular pacing because of the relative delay in left ventricular activation.
- ST segment changes and T waves are opposite to direction of major waves in each leads

Causes of LBBB
- **Ischemia**- aortic stenosis and MI
- **Structural damage** – Hypertension, dilated cardiomyopathy
- **Electrolytes** – hyperkalemia

356. Ans. (a)   Arrythmogenic right ventricular dysplasia

(Ref: Harrison 20th p 1759; Harrison 19th p 1564)

- Arrythmogenic right ventricular dysplasia is a non-ischemic cardiomyopathy that involves the right ventricle. It is characterized by hypokinetic areas involving the free wall of the right ventricle, with fibrofatty replacement of the right ventricular myocardium, with associated arrhythmias originating in the right ventricle.
- The epsilon wave is found in about 50% of those with ARVD. This is described as a terminal notch in the QRS complex. It is due to slowed intra-ventricular conduction.

357. Ans. (b)   Digitalis toxicity

(Ref: Harrison 20th p 1681; Harrison 19th p 1457)

QT Interval
1. Normal QT= 0.36-0.44sec
2. QT interval: It varies with rate. Calculate corrected QT interval (QTc) (By using BAZZETT'S Formula)
3. Prolonged QT interval: Congenital like in Romano-Ward syndrome Electrolyte imbalance (Hypokalemia, Hypocalcemia, Hypomagnesemia), Class 1A anti arrhythmic drugs (quinidine), head injury, hypothermia, sotalol. Macrolides (e.g. erythromycin), amiodarone, Tricyclic, Torsades De Pointes, cerebrovascular accident.
4. Short QT interval: Hypercalcemia, Hypermagnesemia, Class 1 B anti arrhythmic drugs Acute MI

358. Ans. (c)   Hypercalcemia

(Ref: Harrison 20th p 1681; Harrison 19th p 1457)

Remember that QT interval shows a inverse relation with values of potassium, calcium and magnesium.

Comparison of ECG findings of hypocalcemia versus hypercalcemia

Hypocalcemia	Hypercalcemia
• Narrowing of the qRS complex • Reduced PR interval • T wave flattening and inversion • Prolongation of the QT-interval • Prominent U-wave • Prolonged ST and ST-depression	• Mild: broad based tall peaking T waves • Severe: extremely wide qRS, low R wave, disappearance of P waves, tall peaking T waves • QT shortening

ECG finding with digoxin administration are
- PR interval prolongation
- ST segment depression
- QT shortening

359. Ans. (c)   Constrictive pericarditis

(Ref: Harrison 20th p 1680; Harrison 19th p 1456)

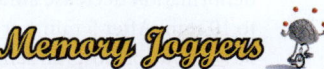

Mnemonic for ST segment elevation is E.L.E.V.A.T.I.O.N
E = electrolytes like hyperkalemia
L = LBBB
E = early repolarization variant
VA = ventricular aneurysm
T = trauma like pericardiocentesis
I = injury eg AMI
O = osbourne waves
N = non occlusive (Prinzmetal) spasm

360. Ans. (c)   Wellen's syndrome

(Ref: Harrison 20th p 1680; Harrison's Ch-45 Harrison 19th p 1457 and p 310)

- Severe anterior wall Ischemia (with or without infarction) may cause prominent T-wave inversions in the precordial leads. This pattern (sometimes referred to as Wellens T waves) is usually associated with a high-grade stenosis of the left anterior descending coronary artery.
- Hyperkalemia has tall Tented T waves
- Coronary syndrome X is characterised by blockage of perforators while the epicardial coronary artery is normal. In these patients stenting of coronaries is not useful. Nitrates are mainstay of therapy.

361. Ans. (a)   Increased PR interval with ST depression

(Ref: Harrison 20th p 1681; Harrison 19th p 1457 and p 310)

The question is very smartly worded as on first look choice C also looks correct. But QT interval in hypokalemia is an apparent prolongation due to merging of T and U waves. This also predisposes the patient to develop torsades de pointes.

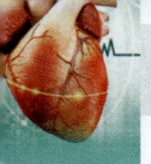

- ST depression is due to concordance with T wave which becomes inverted in hypokalemia.
- Due to slow repolariztion, PR interval is prolonged.

362. Ans. (a) Ventricular fibrillation

(Ref: Harrison 20th p 2061; Harrison 19th p 1768)

- When the onset is instantaneous or abrupt, the probability that the arrest is cardiac in origin is >95%.
- Continuous electrocardiographic (ECG) recordings fortuitously obtained at the onset of a cardiac arrest commonly demonstrate changes in cardiac electrical activity during the minutes or hours before the event.
- There is a tendency for the heart rate to increase and for advanced grades of PVCs to evolve. Most cardiac arrests that are caused by VF begin with a run of nonsustained or sustained VT, which then degenerates into VF.
- The probability of achieving successful resuscitation from cardiac arrest is related to the interval from onset of loss of circulation to institution of resuscitative efforts, the setting in which the event occurs, the mechanism (VF, VT, PEA, asystole), and the clinical status of the patient before the cardiac arrest.
- Return of circulation and survival rates as a result of defibrillation decrease almost linearly from the first minute to 10 min. After 5 min, survival rates are no better than 25–30% in out-of-hospital settings.

363. Ans. (d) All of above

(Ref: Harrison 20th p 310; Harrison 19th p 1457)

364. Ans. (d) All of the above

(Ref: Harrison 20th p 1678; Harrison 19th p 1454-55)

Causes of RBBB
1. Normal physiological
2. Pulmonary embolism/ corpulmonale
3. Pulmonary artery hypertension
4. ASD
5. Rheumatic heart disease

365. Ans. (d) Bifascicular block

(Ref: Harrison 20th p 1678-79; Harrison 19th p 1455)

1. Bifascicular block is combination of RBBB with either Left anterior hemiblock or left posterior hemiblock
2. Tri fascicular block is RBBB plus either LAHB/LPHB+ first degree AV block
3. Complete heart block is destruction of AV node leading to AV dissociation

366. Ans. (a) Sinus Tachycardia

(Ref: Harrison 20th p 1912; Harrison 19th p 1633)

- Most common ECG finding of pulmonary embolism is sinus tachycardia
- Most characteristic ECG finding of pulmonary embolism is S1 Q3 T3
- The S1Q3T3 is the ECG manifestation of acute pressure and volume overload of the right ventricle

- An S wave in lead I signifies a complete or more often incomplete RBBB
- In lead III, look for a Q wave, slight ST elevation, and an inverted T wave. These findings are due to the pressure and volume overload over the right ventricle which causes repolarization abnormalities.

367. Ans. (c) ASD (Septum secundum)

(Ref: Harrison 20th p 1676-77; Harrison 19th p 1453)

Causes of right axis deviation are:	Causes of left axis deviation
1. Left posterior fascicular block	1. Left ventricular hypertrophy
2. Lateral myocardial infarction	2. Left anterior fascicular block
3. ASD septum secondum	3. Inferior wall MI
4. Right ventricular hypertrophy	4. Ostium primum ASD
5. Acute lung disease (e.g. PE)	5. Left bundle branch block
6. Chronic lung disease (e.g. COPD)	6. WPW type A
7. Ventricular ectopy	
8. Hyperkalaemia	
9. Sodium-channel blocker toxicity	
10. WPW syndrome	
11. Normal in children or thin adults with a horizontally positioned heart	

*Ostium primum is associated with cleft mitral valve that leads to left atrial enlargement and left axis deviation.

368. Ans. (a) Cardiac tamponade

(Ref: Harrison 20th p 1682; Harrison 19th p 1459)

Electrical alternans occurs due to the to and fro swinging activity of the heart while it is encased in a pericardial sac filled with lots of fluid.

369. Ans. (b) Hypercalcemia

(Ref: Harrison 20th p 3340, 1681; Harrison 19th p 1457)

- Characteristically seen in hypothermia (typically T<30°C), but they are not pathognomonic.
- J waves may be seen in a number of other conditions:
  1. Normal variant
  2. Hypercalcaemia
  3. Medications
  4. Neurological insults such as intracranial hypertension, severe head injury and subarachnoid haemorrhage

370. Ans. (d) QT interval shortening

(Ref: Harrison 20th p 1681; Harrison's 19th p 307)

Remember that QT interval shows an inverse relation with values of potassium, calcium and magnesium.

Comparison of ECG findings of hypokalemia and hyperkalemia

Hypokalemia	Hyperkalemia
• Increased amplitude and width of the P wave • Prolongation of the PR interval • T wave flattening and inversion • ST depression • Prominent U waves (best seen in the precordial leads) • Apparent long QT interval due to fusion of the T and U waves (= long QU interval)	• Tall tented T waves • Prolongation of PR interval • Loss of P waves • Widening of qRS • Sine wave pattern

371. Ans. (a) Hypothyroidism

(Ref: Harrison 20th p 1681; Harrison 19th p 1457)

The qRS is said to be low voltage when:
- The amplitudes of all the qRS complexes in limb leads are less than 5 mm; or
- The amplitudes of all the qRS complexes in precordial leads are less than 10 mm

There are several etiologies of low voltage ECG:
1. Obesity
2. Emphysema
3. Pericardial effusion, Pleural Effusion
4. Severe hypothyroidism (myxedema)
5. Subcutaneous emphysema
6. Pneumothorax or Pneumopericardium
7. Old large MI
8. End-stage dilated cardiomyopathy
9. Infiltrative/restrictive diseases such as amyloidosis or hemochromatosis.

372. Ans. (b) WPW Syndrome

(Ref: Harrison 20th p 1740-41; Harrison 19th p 1481)

- PR interval in ECG shows an inverse relation with heart rate
- Choice a and d mention heart block which implies that bradycardia ensues leading to PR interval prolongation.
- Hypothyroidism patients also have bradycardia, leading to P-R prolongation.
- In WPW, the bundle of Kent is an accessory pathway which allows fast conduction to the ventricles and consequently leads to complaints of palpitations and reduction of PR interval.

373. Ans. (d) Pericardial effusion

(Ref: Harrison 20th p 1681; Harrison 19th p 1457)

Low voltage is indicative of conditions where the electrical signal from the heart is attenuated either because of a heart condition in itself or because of conditions outside the heart. Possible reasons include:
- Pericardial effusion
- Constrictive pericarditis
- Severe ischemic heart disease
- Infiltrative disease, e.g. amyloidosis
- Hypothyroidism
- Pulmonary emphysema
- Pleural effusion
- Pneumothorax
- Generalized edema

374. Ans. (b) Prolonged QT interval

(Ref: Harrison 20th p 310; Harrison 19th p 310)

375. Ans. (c) 35

(Ref: EGG problem 3rd edition John R. Hampton, Harrison 19th p 1454)

Left Ventricular hypertrophy criteria is = Sum of S wave in V1 and R wave in V6 is >35mm (SV1 + RV6 > 35) or R wave in aVL> 11mm.

376. Ans. (a) Left axis deviation

(Ref: Harrison 20th p 1676; Harrison 19th p 1453)

- The ECG manifestations of a left tension pneumothorax
  1. Rightward shift of the mean frontal qRS axis
  2. Reduced precordial R-wave voltage
  3. Decreased and/or alternating qRS amplitude (electrical alternans)
  4. Precordial T-wave inversions.

Commonly, two or three of the above are present, and less often, all four are present.
- Non infarction Q waves
  1. Normal variant Q waves in V_1-V_2, III, aV_F
  2. Left pneumothorax or dextrocardia
  3. Myocarditis
  4. LBBB
  5. WPW

377. Ans. (c) Constrictive pericarditis

(Ref: Harrison 20th p 1681; Harrison 19th p 1456)

378. Ans. (c) Hypercalcemia

(Ref: Harrison 20th p 1681; Harrison 19th p 1457)

379. Ans. (c) Prolonged QT interval

(Ref: Harrison 20th p 310; Harrison 19th p 310)

380. Ans. (c) Prolonged QTc interval

(Ref: Harrison 20th p 1760)

381. Ans. (b) Polymorphic ventricular tachycardia

(Ref: Harrison 20th p 1760; Harrison 19th p 1491)

382. Ans. (a) First –degree block; (c) Second degree Mobitz type II

(Ref: Harrison 20th p 1728)

383. Ans. (a) Cardiac tamponade

(Ref: Harrison 20th p 1682; Harrison 19th p 1573)

WPW and Brugada Syndrome

384. Ans. (d) WPW

(Ref: Harrison 20th p 1740-41; Harrison 19th edition, page 1484)

Patients with symptomatic Wolff-Parkinson-White (WPW) syndrome should not be treated with calcium channel blockers or digoxin because of the potential for rapid ventricular rates and development of atrial fibrillation or atrial flutter which can result in dramatic hemodynamic collapse.

385. Ans. (d) Pacemaker is treatment of choice

(Ref: Harrison 20th p 1740-41; Harrison 19th ed. pg. 1481)

- The ECG shows normal sinus rhythm with left axis deviation
- Short PR interval with wide QRS showing *prolonged upstroke of QRS (delta wave). The prolonged upstroke with slight change of slope in seen in this ECG in lead V3 and V4.*

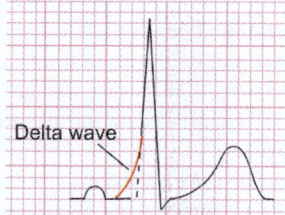

- The accessory pathway, Bundle of Kent can explain these abnormalities and the boy suffers from Wolf Parkinson White syndrome.
- *The treatment of choice in case of positive family history of sudden death, recurrent episodes of syncope is implantable cardioverter defibrillator. This can deliver a DC shock and can terminate a life threatening arrhythmia.*

386. Ans. (b) Treadmill test

(Ref: Harrison 20th p 1741-42; Harrison 19th p 1483)

- **The clinical diagnosis of the patient is Wolf Parkinson white syndrome.** These patients have a bypass tract that allows conduction of impulses from atria to ventricles without having to be subjected to the decremental property of AV node.
- Invasive electro physiology study is recommended to assses if pathway leads to rapid ventricular rates and in same setting curative catheter ablation can be done.
- β-blockers and vagal maneuvers can be done at onset of episode.
- *Walking on Treadmill will lead to sympathetic stimulation and precipitate arrhythmia and thus would not be recommended for patient of W.P.W.*
- Rapid pre excited tachycardia should be treated with electrical cadioversion or intravenous procainamide or ibutilide.

387. Ans. (d) Pacemaker is treatment of choice

(Ref: Harrison 20th p 1756; Harrison 19th p 1497-98)

- The major clinical features of Brugada syndrome include manifest, transient, or concealed ST segment elevation in V1 to V3 that typically can be provoked with the sodium channel-blocking drugs ajmaline, flecainide, and procainamide and a risk of polymorphic ventricular arrhythmias.
- **Defect:** *It occurs due to a diminished inward sodium current in the region of the RV outflow tract epicardium.*
- A loss of the action potential dome in the RV epicardium due to unopposed ITo potassium outward current results in dramatic shortening of the action potential.
- The large potential difference between the normal endocardium and rapidly depolarized RV outflow epicardium gives rise to ST-segment elevation in V1–V3 in sinus rhythm and predisposes to local ventricular reentry.
- The majority of genetic abnormalities responsible for the syndrome have not been described; however, in ~20% of patients, mutations of SCN5A genes have been identified.
- Although identified in both genders and all races with an autosomal dominant inheritance pattern, the arrhythmia syndrome is most common in young male patients (~75%) and is thought to be responsible for the Sudden and Unexpected nocturnal Death Syndrome (SUDS) described in Southeast Asian men.
- The ventricular arrhythmia characteristically occurs with rest or during sleep. Fever and other sodium channel-blocking drugs also precipitate ventricular arrhythmias.
- For patients who have had syncopal attacks, I.C.D. implantable cardioverter defibrillator is used and not the pacemaker which cannot deliver a DC shock to terminate the arrhythmia developing in these patients.

388. Ans. (d) Right Bundle Branch Block

(Ref: Harrison 20th p 1761; Harrison 19th p 1497)

- Brugada syndrome is a genetically determined channelopathy and has autosomal dominant pattern. The defect lies in Transmembrane sodium current that affects right ventricular endocardium differently from epicardium. This could lead to block pattern in ECG.

JVP

389. Ans. (a) Right atrial contraction

(Ref: Harrison 20th edition, page 1668)

'a' wave in JVP indicates Atrial contraction.

390. Ans. (c) Tricuspid bulge

(Ref: Harrison 20th p 1668; Harrison 19th edition, page 1444)

Waveform component	Phase of cardiac cycle	Mechanical event
a wave	End diastole	Atrial contraction
c wave	Early systole	Tricuspid bulging (IVC)
v wave	Late systole	Systolic filling of the atrium
x descent	Mid systole	Atrial relaxation
y descent	Early diastole	Early ventricular filling

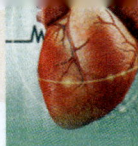

Abnormality		Causes	What it represents
Loss of 'a' wave	(waveform showing v, y)	Atrial fibrillation	Loss of effective atrial contraction
Systolic V wave	(waveform showing cV)	Tricuspid regurgitation	• 'x' descent lost and replaced by very prominent upright systolic wave representing blood shooting back up into the neck as right ventricle contracts • Synchronous with carotid pulse and called systolic 'V' wave (not to be confused with 'v' wave) • Sometimes called 'cV' wave • Frequently seen rising to the earlobes; 'y' descent steep as a result
Prominent 'a' wave	(waveform showing a, v, x, y)	• Tricuspid stenosis • Pulmonary hypertension of any cause resulting in right ventricular overload • Pulmonary stenosis	Atrium contracting against resistance; 'y' descent also slowed because ventricular filling impeded

391. Ans. (b) Right atrial contraction

(Ref: Harrison 20th p 1668; Harrison 19th edition, page 1443-1444)

The *a* wave reflects right atrial pre-systolic contraction and occurs just after the electrocardiographic P wave preceding the first heart sound.

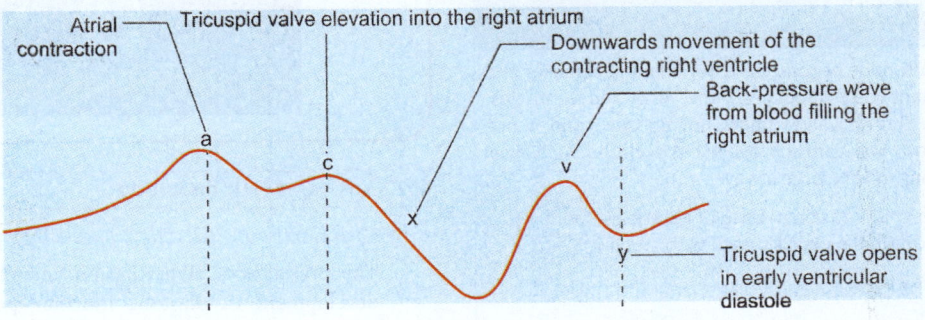

392. Ans. (c) Prominent Y descent

(Ref: Harrison 20th p 1669; Harrison 19th edition, page 1543)
- Lung cancer can exhibit metastasis to heart leading to development of pericardial effusion.
- As more fluid would have accumulated, patient developed cardiac tamponade leading to hypotension and full neck veins.
- Y descent is absent in cardiac tamponade.
- Due to swinging motion of heart in a sac of fluid, Electrical alternans is seen.
- Kussmaul sign is a paradoxical rise of JVP on inspiration. But in tamponade, due to extreme magnitude of pressure in pericardial space, Kussmaul sign becomes absent.

393. Ans. (b) Cardiac tamponade

(Ref: Harrison 20th p 1669; Harrison 19th ed. / 1573)

JVP Findings

JVP Waves	Findings Constrictive pericarditis	Findings Cardiac tamponade
X wave	Prominent	Prominent
Y wave	Prominent	Absent

394. Ans. (a) Right atrium (RA)

(Ref: Harrison 20th p 1668)

Normal JVP = 5-8 cm of water
- Elevated JVP is indicative of right sided CHF
- Kussmaul sign is seen in constrictive pericarditis
- *Kussmaul sign is not seen in cardiac tamponade*
- **Canon a waves are seen AV dissociation/ ventricular tachycardia/ junctional tachycardia**

395. Ans. (b) Complete heart block

(Ref: Harrison 20th p 1668)

- The *a* wave reflects right atrial presystolic contraction and occurs just after the electrocardiographic P wave, preceding the first heart sound (S1).
- The *a* wave is not present with atrial fibrillation.
- Canon *a* wave occurs with
  - Atrioventricular (AV) dissociation/ complete heart block due to right atrial contraction against a closed tricuspid valve.
  - Wide complex tachycardia like ventricular tachycardia
- A prominent *a* wave is seen in patients with reduced right ventricular compliance like Right ventricular failure.

396. Ans. (a) Atrial fibrillation

(Ref: Harrison 20th p 1668; Harrison 19th ed. / 1443-1444)

- A wave in JVP is due to atrial contraction. In atrial fibrillation, since the atria are twitching, the power of atria is reduced to a level that a wave would be absent.
- Heart block will have large a waves.
- Tricuspid Regurgitation has absent x and large v waves.
- Constrictive Pericarditis has a large y descent.

397. Ans. (b) Junctional tachycardia

(Ref: Harrison 20th p 1668; Harrison 19th ed. / 1480)

	Absent 'a' waves
Atrial fibrillation	
Junctional tachycardia	The AVN node becomes the dominant pacemaker and simultaneously depolarizes the Atria and ventricles. Hence the AV valves might not be open and hence the atria will contract against the closed AV valves resulting in very large a waves
Constricitive pericarditis	Due to impaired compliance of ventricles, rapid ventricular filling occurs leading to steep y
Cardiac tamponade	Absent y waves

398. Ans. (c) Tricuspid regurgitation

(Ref: Harrison 20th p 1669; Harrison 19th p 1444)

399. Ans. (b) Bulging of tricuspid valve

(Ref: Harrison 20th p 1668; Harrison 19th p 1444)

Aortic Dissection

400. Ans. (a) Surgical repair

(Ref: Harrison 20th edition, page 1921)

- The image shows CT chest with an ascending aorta dissection (tennis ball appearance). Posterior to it is the pulmonary artery bifurcation which is normal and does not exhibit any embolus.
- Emergent or urgent surgical correction is preferred treatment for acute ascending aortic dissections and intramural hematomas.
- Type B aortic dissections involve transverse and/or descending aorta.
  - For uncomplicated/stable distal lesions and intramural type B hematomas medical therapy is preferred.
  - For complicated type B surgical correction is indicated.

Type A aortic dissection

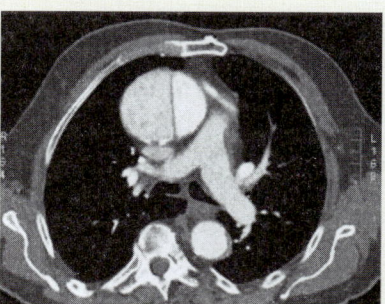

Type B Aortic dissection

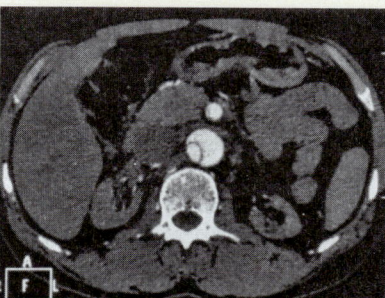

401. Ans. (a) Aortic dissection

(Ref: Harrison 20th edition, page 1921)

The presence of Hypertension and chest pain followed by development of diastolic murmur points to development of aortic regurgitation. Acute onset Aortic regurgitation is a complication of retrograde spread of aortic dissection.

Choice B: Papillary muscle dysfunction would lead to systolic murmur.

Choice C: Regurgitation leads to Systolic murmur

Choice D: Seen with renal artery stenosis and presents with heart failure.

402. Ans. (b) Aortic dissection

(Ref: Harrison 20th p 1921; Harrison 19th ed. page 1640)

- The X ray of hypertension patient shows presence of mediastinal widening which is the most common plain radiographic finding in aortic dissection.

403. Ans. (d) T.E.E.

(Ref: Harrison 20th p 1921; Harrison 19th p 1641)

- The diagnosis of aortic dissection can be established by noninvasive techniques such as echocardiography, CT, and MRI. Aortography is used less commonly because of the accuracy of these noninvasive techniques.
- Transthoracic echocardiography can be performed simply and rapidly and has an overall sensitivity of 60–85% for aortic dissection. For diagnosing proximal ascending aortic dissections, its sensitivity exceeds 80%; it is less useful for detecting dissection of the arch and descending thoracic aorta.
- Transesophageal echocardiography requires greater skill and patient cooperation but is very accurate in identifying dissections of the ascending and descending thoracic aorta but not the arch, achieving 98% sensitivity and approximately 90% specificity. Echocardiography also provides important information regarding the presence and severity of aortic regurgitation and pericardial effusion.
- CT and MRI are both highly accurate in identifying the intimal flap and the extent of the dissection and involvement of major arteries; each has a sensitivity and specificity >90%. They are useful in recognizing intramural hemorrhage and penetrating ulcers. MRI can also detect blood flow, which may be useful in characterizing antegrade versus retrograde dissection.
- The relative utility of transesophageal echocardio-graphy, CT, and MRI depends on the availability and expertise in individual institutions as well as on the hemodynamic stability of the patient, with CT and MRI obviously less suitable for unstable patients.

404. Ans. (c) Ist trimester pregnancy

(Ref: Harrison 20th p 1920; Harrison 19th p 1641)

Infective Endocarditis

405. Ans. (b) Benzathine penicillin 7.2 million units in three divided doses i.m

(Ref: Harrison 20th edition, page 1285)

For management of late latent syphilis, cardiovascular syphilis Penicillin G Benzathine is given 2.4MU i.m. weekly for 3 weeks.

Type of syphilis	Treatment
Primary, secondary and early latent	CSF normal or not examined Benzathine single dose 2.4mU IM
Late latent or cardiovascular	CSF normal or not examined Benzathine single dose 2.4mU IM x 3 weeks
Neurosyphilis (Asymptomatic or Symptomatic)	Aqueous Crystalline penicillin G IV for 14 days Aqueous procaine penicillin G + oral probenecid for 14 days

406. Ans. (a) Leukemia

(Ref: Harrison 19th edition, 40e-2)

Roth spots are white centered haemorrhage.

Cause of Roth spots

1. Bacteria endocarditis and sepsis
2. Lymphoproliferative disorders
3. Diabetes mellitus
4. Hypertension
5. Anaemia
6. Connective tissue disorders

407. Ans. (d) Cotrimoxazole with Meropenem

(Ref: Harrison 20th p 1169, 1172; Harrison 19th edition, page 1048)

- Burkholderia cepacia is resistant to most antibiotics.
- Hence due to intrinsic resistance TMP-SMX, meropenem and Doxycycline are most effective agents
- Fluoroquinolones and third generation cephalosporins should be used only after susceptibility against these agents is known.
- Burkholderia cepacia leads to cepacia syndrome. It is characterised by rapidly progressive distress and sepsis. It causes
  1. Recurrent pneumonia in cystic fibrosis
  2. Ventilator associated pneumonia
  3. Catheter associated infection
  4. Wound infections

408. Ans. (c) They are characteristically associated with severe general reaction of the surrounding retina

(Ref: Harrison 20th p 923; Harrison 19th edition and Chapter 40e-2, page 816:)

- The fundus examination in patient of mitral valve infection shows Roth spots. Choice B is true.
- The presence of recurrent fevers in a patient of pre-existing heart disease predisposes to development of infective endocarditis.
- Acute bacterial endocarditis is seen with staphylococcus and Subacute variety with Streptococcus iridians> Enterococci. It can occur with less virulent infections and hence choice A is true.

Causes of Roth's spots
1. Infective endocarditis
2. SLE
3. PolyarteritisNodosa
4. Severe anaemia
5. Leukaemia
6. Diabetes mellitus
7. Hypertension

409. Ans. (a) Splenomegaly

(Ref: Harrison 20th p 925; Harrison 19th edition, page 819-820)

The Duke Criteria for the Clinical Diagnosis of Infective Endocarditis

Major Criteria

Positive blood culture:

- Typical microorganism **for infective endocarditis from** two separate blood cultures

- *Viridans streptococci*, Streptococcus gallolyticus, *HACEK group*, Staphylococcus aureus, *or*
- Community-acquired enterococci in the absence of a primary focus, or
- Persistently positive blood culture, **defined as recovery of a** microorganism consistent with infective endocarditis from:
- Blood cultures drawn >12 h apart; or
- All of 3 or a majority of greater then or equal to 4 separate blood cultures, with first and last drawn at least 1 h apart
- Single positive blood culture for Coxiella burnetii or phase I IgG antibody titer of > 1: 800
- Evidence of endocardial involvement

Minor Criteria
- Predisposition: predisposing **heart condition** or **injection drug use**
- Fever >38.0°C (>100.4°F)
- **Vascular phenomena**: major arterial emboli, septic pulmonary infarcts, mycotic aneurysm, intracranial hemorrhage, conjunctival hemorrhages, Janeway lesions
- **Immunologic phenomena**: glomerulonephritis, Osier's nodes, Roth's spots, rheumatoid factor
- **Microbiologic evidence**: positive blood culture but not meeting major criterion as noted previously or serologic evidence of active infection with organism consistent with infective endocarditis

Definite endocarditis is **defined by documentation** of *two major criteria, of one major criterion and three minor criteria, or of five minor criteria.*

Transesophageal echocardiography **is recommended for assessing possible prosthetic valve endocarditis or complicated endocarditis.**

Excluding single positive cultures for coagulase-negative staphylococci and diphtheroids, which are common culture contaminants, and organisms that do not cause endocarditis frequently, such as gram-negative bacilli.

410. Ans. (b) VSD

(Ref: Nelson 20th/e 2264; CMDT 2019 pg 1466)

- Infective endocarditis lesions are seen based on pressure gradient. In adults the highest incidence is with mitral regurgitation while in children it is with VSD.
- Infective endocarditis is least common in ASD. Highest risk of adverse outcome after infective endocarditis for which prophylaxis
  1. Prosthetic cardiac valves
  2. Unrepaired cyanotic congenital heart disease
  3. Completely repaired defects with prosthetic material
  4. Rheumatic fever (Mitral stenosis aortic regurgitation)
  5. VSD, congenital aortic stenosis

411. Ans. (c) Subacute bacterial endocarditis

(Ref: Harrison 20th p 925)

Peripheral manifestations of injective endocardites
1. Osler nodes
2. Subungual hemorrheages
3. Janeway lesions
4. Roth spots
5. Petechiae

412. Ans. (b) Rose spots seen

(Ref: Harrison 20th p 923; Harrison 19th p 817)

- With dental procedures is recommended
- Rose spots are bacterial emboli to the skin and occur in approximately 1/3 of cases of typhoid fever.
- They are one of the classic signs of untreated disease, but can also be seen in other illnesses as well, including Shigellosis and non-typhoidal salmonellosis.
- They appear as a rash between the seventh and twelfth day from the onset of symptoms. They occur in groups of five to ten lesions on the lower chest and upper abdomen, and they are more numerous following paratyphoid infection.
- Rose spots typically last three to four days.
- Hematuria can occur as a manifestation of post infectious glomerulonephritis in IE
- Hemiplegia can occur after brain abscess formation in IE

413. Ans. (a) Staphylococcus aureus (See Table below)

(Ref: Harrison 20th p 927; Harrison 19th p 816)

ORGANISMS CAUSING MAJOR CLINICAL FORMS OF ENDOCARDITIS								
	Native Valve Endocarditis		Prosthetic Valve Endocarditis at Indicated times of Onset (months) after Valve Surgery			Endocarditis in Injection Drug users		
	Community – Acquired	Health care-Associated	<2	2-12	>12	Right Sided	Left Sided	Total
MC organism	Staphylococcus aureus	Staphylococcus aureus	Coagulase negative staphylococci	Coagulase negative staphylococci	Streptococci	Staphylococcus aureus	Enterococci	Staphylococcus aureus

414. Ans. (a) Aspergillus endocarditis

(Ref: Current diagnosis and treatment in Cardiology 2nd edition, chapter 29)

- Fungal endocarditis is a very rare disease accounting for only 2–4% of all cases of endocarditis
- Aspergillus was the etiologic agent in 24% of cases of fungal endocarditis

- The most important aspect regarding the treatment of Aspergillus endocarditis is early recognition followed by rapid surgical resection or debridement in combination with antifungal therapy because of the high risk of embolic complications and cardiac decompensation.
- The Infectious Diseases Society of America recommends Voriconazole as the preferred agent.
- In case of candida endocarditis liposomal amphotericin B or caspofungin for 6-8 weeks with or without flucytosine and then lifelong management with fluconazole
- Because of the risk of recurrent infections, especially following surgical treatment of infected prosthetic valves, consider lifelong prophylactic treatment with oral triazoles.

415. Ans. (d) ASD

(Ref: API 9th/500)

416. Ans. (d) Atrial septal defect (ASD)

(Ref: API 9th/500)

417. Ans. (a) Lung

(Ref: Harrison 20th p 924; Harrison 19th p 816)

Mitral valve vegetation would obviously not go to the lung, as that would involve a 'backward flow'.

418. Ans. (d) Tricuspid valve

(Ref: Harrison 20th p 922; Harrison 19th p 816)

419. Ans. (b) Staphylococcus Epidermidis

(Ref: Harrison 20th p 922; Harrison 19th p 817)

Hypertension

420. Ans. (b) Bradycardia with AV Block

(Ref: Goodman Gilman 13th edition, page 214)

Verapamil acts on AV node and slows the heart rate. The combination with beta blocker will further slow the heart.

421. Ans. (d) Liddle Syndrome

(Ref: Harrison 20th p 1899; Harrison 19th edition, page 306)

- **Liddle syndrome** exhibits gain of function of epithelial sodium channel at plasma membrane of principal cells.
- This results in net gain of salt and water leading to hypertension
- The corresponding urinary loss of potassium and hydrogen explains hypokalemic alkalosis.
- Bartter syndrome (defect at TAL) and Gitelman syndrome (defect at DCT) both have hypokalemic alkalosis but hypertension in not present
- RTA is easiest to rule out on account of acidosis.

422. Ans. (d) Supravalvular Aortic Stenosis

(Ref: Harrison 20th p 1669; Harrison 19th edition, page 1445 and 51e-2:)

- Supravalvular aortic stenosis is characterized by an external hourglass deformity of the aorta with a corresponding luminal narrowing at a level just distal to the coronary artery ostia.
- Discrepancies between carotid pulsations and upper extremity pulses and blood pressure are the characteristic clinical findings in SVAS (Supravalvular aortic stenosis).
- The discrepancies occur because the jet of blood flow from SVAS has a preferential trajectory into the brachiocephalic (innominate) artery (i.e. Coanda effect).
- However in SVAS, the characteristic systolic murmur is crescendo-decrescendo in shape, low pitched, and best heard at the base of the heart, sited higher than in valvular aortic stenosis. (Chapter 51e-2, Harrison 19th).
- The patient had early diastolic murmur. This makes SVAS the answer to the question.
- For unequal BP between Left and right arm, the defect should be present between the right brachiocephalic trunk and left common carotid artery.
- In Takayasu's arteritis, the ostial narrowing of left and right subclavian arteries can lead to differential BP.
- Coarctation of aorta of pre-ductal variety involves the arch of aorta and lead to unequal BP between left and right arm.
- Similarly in aortic dissection unequal BP between two arms and dusky appearance of toes is useful for early diagnosis.

EXTRA MILE

BP difference between both arms should be less than 10mmHg
BP value differential exceeding this threshold may be associated with:-
1. Atherosclerosis or inflammatory subclavian artery disease
2. Supravalvular aortic stenosis
3. Coarctation of aorta
4. Aortic dissection

423. Ans. (a) Check pill count

(Ref: Harrison 20th p 477, 479)

- The patient is suffering from resistant hypertension and the leading cause of resistant hypertension is non- compliance on the part of patient.
- Resistant hypertension is defined as blood pressure that remains above goal in spite of the concurrent use of 3 antihypertensive agents of different classes. Ideally, one of the 3 agents should be a diuretic and all agents should be prescribed at optimal dose amounts.

424. Ans. (a) Pseudo-hypertension

(Ref: Harrison 20th p 1905; Page 1626: Harrison 19th edition)

- Blood pressure may be falsely elevated in geriatric patients due to severely sclerotic arteries. This leads to over diagnosis of hypertension in these patients. Hence it is called pseudo-hypertension. The clinical sign used to diagnose it is called Osler manoeuvre.
- Osler manoeuvre is characterised by palpable radial artery impulse in spite of occlusion of brachial artery by BP cuff.

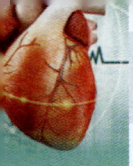

425. Ans. (a) ACE inhibitors can be used in bilateral renal artery stenosis; (d) Excision & Grafting is treatment of choice

(Ref: Harrison 19th/1628- 29)

- ACE inhibitors are contraindicated in bilateral renal artery stenosis. The drug for management of HTN in bilateral R.A.S is Calcium channel blocker.
- In case of poor response, bilateral renal artery stenosis is managed with percutaneous trans-renal angioplasty with stenting.
- ACE inhibitors are the DOC for management of unilateral renal artery stenosis and also preferred agents in diabetes patients for slowing nephropathy progression and BP control.

426. Ans. (a) D.A.S.H

(Ref: World Journal of hypertension guidelines)

Reduction of diastolic blood pressure to less than 60–80 mm Hg does not improve mortality and may lead to adverse cardiovascular events.

This is called as J-curve phenomenon. Consindering her positive family history, dietary approaches to stop hypertension is the best possible intervention.

Causes of Isolated Diastolic Hypertension are

1. Essential hypertension
2. Hypothyroidism
3. Conn syndrome
4. Cushing syndrome

427. Ans. (b) Hypertension

(Ref: Harrison 20th p 1920; Harrison 19th ed. / 1640)

- 70% cases of aortic dissection occur due to hypertension. The tear occurs in tunica media and causes a tearing pain in the chest with maximum intensity in inter-scapular area. The IOC for aortic dissection is trans-esophageal echocardiography.
- Marfan syndrome also can present with aortic dissection, which in fact is the leading cause of death in these patients. Syphilis involves the arch of aorta and causes an aneurysm that can rupture anyday.

428. Ans. (c) 160/90

(Ref: European Society of Cardiology Guidelines 2015)

Hypertensive encephalopathy presents with nausea vomiting and unconsciousness.	Reduce MAP by 25% over 8 hours using sodium nitroprusside
Acute ischemic stroke	Since thrombolysis is indicated keep SBP <185 and DBP <110 using labetalol/nicardipine
Intracranial hemorrhage with raised ICP	Keep MAP< 130 and SBP <180
No features of Raised ICT SAH	Keep MAP <110 and SBP <160 Keep DBP <90

In this question since no neurological deficit was mentioned, it implies patient did not have any CNS event and BP should be gradually reduced to SBP <160/90.

429. Ans. (a) Non-compliance of patient

(Ref: The Cleveland Clinic Foundation Intensive Review of Internal Medicine,edited by James K. Stoller, Harrison 19th p 1626; CMDT 2019 pg 479)

- Refractory hypertension was defined as uncontrolled blood pressure (systolic/diastolic > 140/90 mm Hg) on > 5 antihypertensive drug.
- *Resistant hypertension (RHTN) is defined as a blood pressure remaining above goal despite the concurrent use of 3 antihypertensive medications of different classes, including, ideally a diuretic.*

	Resistant hypertension	Refractory hypertension
Definition	Resistant hypertension (RHTN) is defined as blood pressure remaining above goal despite the concurrent use of 3 antihypertensive medications of different classes, including, ideally a diuretic	3.6% of all cases of resistant hypertension is refractory. Refractory hypertension was defined as uncontrolled blood pressure (systolic/diastolic, >140/90 mm Hg) on ≥ 5 antihypertensive drug.
MC cause	Inadequate treatment has been mentioned in several published series.	No case based data mentioned
Other causes	Causes of resistant hypertension include improper BP measurement, volume overload, drug-induced or other causes, and associated conditions such as obesity or excessive alcohol intake.	Treat secondary causes of HTN
Treatment	Catheter-based renal sympathetic denervation is a novel investigational treatment for resistant hypertension (defined here as a SBP >160 mm Hg taking > 3 antihypertensive drugs, including a diuretic). This treatment is based on the importance of renal sympathetic and somatic nerves in modulating blood pressure Baroreceptor Activation Treatment (BAT) by an implantable stimulator can potentially safely reduce SBP over the long term in patients with resistant hypertension	Treatment like CPAP for OSA

430. Ans. (c) Renal parenchymal disease

(Ref: Harrison 20th p 1895; Harrison 19th p 1617)

- Secondary hypertension is much less common accounting to only 5-10 % of all causes of hypertension. Renal disease is the most common cause of secondary hypertension. Both renal parenchymal and reno-vascular diseases can cause secondary hypertension. Accounting for up to 2-5% of all cases of hypertension, renal parenchymal damage is the most common cause of secondary hypertension. As chronic glomerulonephritis has become less common, hypertensive nephrosclerosis and, to an even greater degree, diabetic nephropathy have become the most common causes of chronic renal disease
- Reno-vascular disease is the most common cause of secondary hypertension in the elderly.
- Atherosclerosis is the most common renovascular cause of secondary hypertension in elderly while Fibromuscular dysplasia is the most common renovascular cause of secondary hypertension in young.

431. Ans. (b) Modest Lowering of BP

(Ref: American stroke association 2015 guidelines)

In this case the mean arterial pressure is
SBP+ 2(DBP)/3 = 127 mm Hg approximately.
The AHA/ASA recommendations for treating elevated BP are as follows:
1. If systolic BP is over 200 mm Hg or Mean Arterial Pressure (MAP) is over 150 mm Hg, then consider aggressive reduction of BP with continuous IV infusion; check BP every 5 minutes
2. If systolic BP is over 180 mm Hg or MAP is over 130 mm Hg and intracranial pressure is elevated, then consider monitoring intracranial pressure and reducing BP using intermittent or continuous intravenous medications, while maintaining a cerebral perfusion pressure of 60 mm Hg or higher
3. *If systolic BP is over 180 or MAP is less than 130 mm Hg and there is no evidence of elevated intracranial pressure, then consider modest reduction of BP (target MAP of 110 mm Hg or target BP of 160/90 mm Hg) using intermittent or continuous intravenous medications to control it, and perform clinical reexamination of the patient every 15 minutes*

A simpler way to solve this question is that sudden/aggressive lowering of blood pressure leads to reduction in cerebral perfusion and CNS ischemia. Permissive hypertension is recommended to maintain perfusion in case of CNS events.

432. Ans. d. Atrial fibrillation

(Ref: Harrison 20th p 1746; Harrison 19th p 1486)

- Since patients of atrial fibrillation have an irregularly irregular pulse the routine oscillo-metric devices would falter on BP measurement and hence the N.I.C.E (British HTN guidelines) advise the auscultatory method only.
- Complete heart block has bradycardia but the rhythm is regular and hence BP can still be measured by both oscillometric and auscultatory method.

433. Ans. (b) Beta blockers

(Ref: CMDT 2019 pg 480)

- Evidence-based guidelines from the American Association of Clinical Endocrinologists single out methyldopa or Labetalol as preferable anti-hypertensive medications in pregnancy, with magnesium sulfate for women with preeclampsia who are at high risk for seizures.
- ACE inhibitors should be avoided during pregnancy, as they are associated with fetal renal dysgenesis or death when used in the second and third trimesters, as well as with increased risk of cardiovascular and central nervous system malformations when used in the first trimester.

434. Ans. (b) Essential HTN

(Ref: CMDT 2019 pg 453; Harrison 19th p 1616)

ADULT : Essential hypertension
CHILDREN : Chronic glomerulonephritis

Depending on methods of patient ascertainment, 80-95% of hypertensive patients are diagnosed as having "essential" hypertension (also referred to as primary or idiopathic hypertension). In the remaining 5-20% of hypertensive patients, a specific underlying disorder causing the elevation of blood pressure can be identified

435. Ans. (c) Enalaprilat

(Ref: CMDT 2019 pg 465; Harrison 19th p 1623)

436. Ans. (d) Metabolic alkalosis

(Ref: Harrison 20th p 321; Harrison 19th p 322)

437. Ans. (b) Non specific aorto-arteritis

(Ref: Disease of kidney and urinary tract 8th/1279)

438. Ans. (d) Coarctation of Aorta

(Ref: Harrison 20th p 1899; Hurst 11th/ed 1809, Harrison 19th p 1525)

439. Ans. (b) Bicuspid aortic valve

(Ref: Harrison 20th p 1917; Harrison 19th p 1525)

440. Ans. (c) Pulmonary stenosis

(Ref: Harrison 20th p 1917; Harrison 19th p 1525)

Miscellaneous

441. Ans. (c) Nitro-glycerine

(Ref: Harrison 20th edition, page 3163)

- The patient due to spinal cord injury above T6 developed massive sympathomimetic surge leading to splanchnic vasoconstriction and development of hypertension. This triggered reflex bradycardia. Choice D is ruled out in setting of bradycardia.

- Since the patient is not having target organ damage currently in form of papilledema or any CNS event Choice A and B are ruled out. Choice A is used in Hemorrhagic stroke with Hypertensive crisis and Choice B in Hypertensive encephalopathy.
- The patient with supine hypertension will be managed by placing him in sitting position and giving him a buccal spay of NTG followed by NTG Drip if required.
- The usual trigger for Autonomic Dysreflexia in patients of spinal cord injury is blocked or kinked Foley's catheter or stool impaction. Hence taking care of these two eventualities would also help.

442. Ans. (b) 0.5 ml i.m epinephrine 1 in 1000

(Ref: Harrison 20th p 2507; Harrison 19th edition pg. 2117)

Management of anaphylaxis:

1. 0.3-0.5mL of 1:1000 (1mg/ml) Epinephrine SC or IM with repeated doses as required at gap of 5 to 20 minutes.
2. If antigenic material was injected into an extremity, apply tourniquet and give 0.2ml of 1:1000 epinephrine into the site.
3. Volume expanders like normal saline
4. Vasopressors like dopamine
5. Diphenhydramine
6. Aminophylline
7. Prednisolone is not useful for acute event but reduces later recurrence of bronchospasm.

443. Ans. (a) HR/MAP

(Ref: ncbi.nlm.nih.gov)

Modified Shock index is used to predict the development of shock.

$$\text{MSI} = \frac{\text{HR}}{\text{MBP}} = \frac{\text{HR}}{\text{CO} \times \text{SVR}} = \frac{1}{\text{SV} \times \text{SVR}}$$

- A *high* MSI denotes a low Systemic vascular resistance, a sign of hypodynamic circulation.
- A *low* MSI indicates that Systemic Vascular resistance is high, a sign of hyperdynamic circulation.
- Meta-analysis shows that MSI of >1.3 indicates increased probability of ICU admission and death.
- Conversely low MSI is indicator of increased mortality as well and is seen in CVA and arrhythmias.
- It is a better predictor of mortality than blood pressure and heart rate.

444. Ans. (c) Fluid management

(Ref: ATLS students manual 10th edition page 53, 56, 59)

Balanced resuscitation is the goal of perfusion with the risks of re-bleeding by accepting a lower than normal blood pressure. The objective is to strike a balance and not cause hypotension as it can jeopardize the tissue perfusion.

It called permissive hypotension/ balanced resuscitation/ hypotensive resuscitation.

445. Ans. (a) Urine output

(Ref: Bailey and Love: 26th edition, page 18)

- Urine output is an accurate guide that represents end organ perfusion.
- CVP can be influenced by intra-thoracic pressures (PEEP from ventilation, obstructive lung disease), valvular heart disease and pericardial disease (Cardiac Tamponade) and hence it is not reliable.
- HR can be influenced by drugs and can be low in neurogenic shock.
- Blood pressure falls only when physiological countermeasures are getting exhausted.

446. Ans. (d) Observational ability

(Ref: None)

- The question is based on common sense. Time of cohabitation will determine how accurately a relative can describe the symptoms of the patient. For example son is staying abroad and is now describing progression of symptoms of Huntington's disease in his father to you. This will not be a reliable history.
- Especially for diseases that have a genetic basis, blood relations are important.
- Educated family members can better verbalize and empathize with the patient

447. Ans. (a) Advanced Cardiac life support

(Ref: AHA 2015 Guidelines)

448. Ans. (c) Blood transfusion

(Ref: Bailey 26th edition, page 17)

Choice A and B	This statement is direct quote from Bailey page 17, 26th edition "*On balance, there is little evidence to support the administration of colloids, which are more expensive and have worse side-effect profiles.*" Most importantly, the oxygen carrying capacity of crystalloids and colloids is zero.
Choice C	If blood is being lost, the ideal replacement fluid is blood, although crystalloid therapy may be required while awaiting blood products.
Choice D	Fluid resuscitation must be done before General anesthesia can be given and surgeon can proceed with immediate laparoscopy.

449. Ans. (b) LV and aorta in normal person

(Ref: Braunwald cardiology, 8th edition figure 19.14 and Valvular heart disease, companion to Braunwald's Cardiology, 4th edition, page 102)

- Notice the red line (in the diagram shown here) drawn from the peak of R wave to LV waveform indicating LV end diastolic pressure which appears close to normal value of 6-12 mm Hg. An elevated LVEDP indicates LVF or diastolic dysfunction and low LVEDP indicates hypovolemia.
- Now if you compare the systolic pressure of LV waveform with systolic pressure of aorta waveform, both show same value of about 120mmHg.

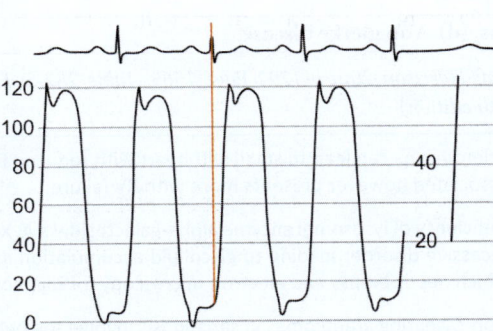

- Conclusion is that LV and aorta systolic and diastolic values given in the recording are normal.

Normal LV pressure = 120/6-12 mm Hg
Normal Aorta pressure = 120/80 mm Hg

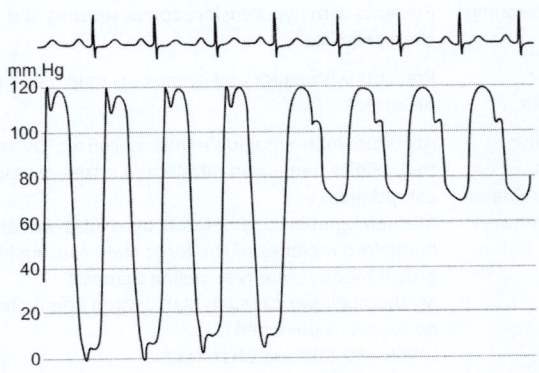

Aortic stenosis	In aortic stenosis, LV systolic pressure will be more than aortic pressure. This is because the calcified stenotic valve will increase the work load of LV. 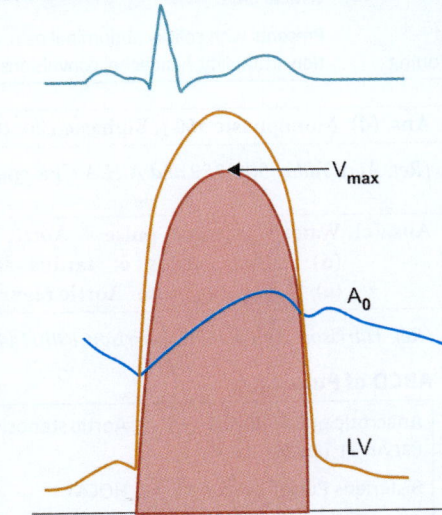
Aortic regurgitation	The LVEDP will increase due to regurgitation of blood. Notice the red line drawn from peak of R wave to DBP on the curve shown on right side of this tracing.

Contd...

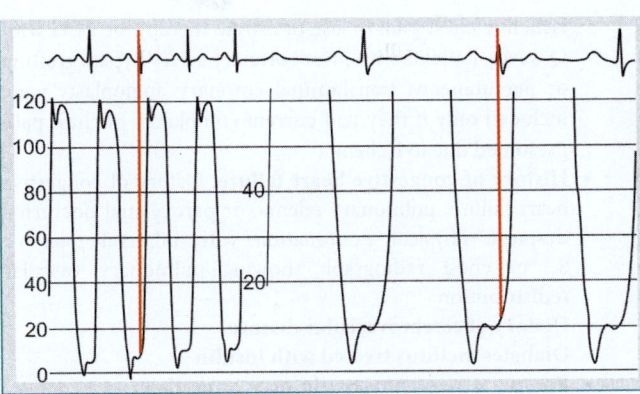

450. Ans. (b) ABCD = ii, iii, iv, i

(Ref: Chapter 102e-1: Harrison 19th edition, Chapter 39, Page 524: Essentials of Pharmacology 7th edition; Harrison 20th p 2955)

At night: Simvastatin	For atorvastatin which is long acting, the timing of the day does not matter, but since simvastatin has shorter action, a bed time dose is recommended. The logic is that *HMG CoA reductase is most active at night when dietary intake is low, simvastatin is recommended to be taken at night.*
Eccentric dose: isosorbide mononitrate	Tolerance to anti-anginal effect of nitrates develops if given spaced evenly and dose escalation does not help in overcoming resistance. According to 19th edition of Harrison since there is development of tolerance to nitrates, a nocturnal drug free interval should be present to reduce tolerance. *For achieving this eccentric drug dosing schedule should be racticed like 30 mg at 7am, 12 am and 5 pm and avoid nocturnal blood levels.*
Before exercise: Sodium Cromoglycate	For exercise induced asthma following strategies are used in decreasing order of efficacy. 1. Inhaled Steroids 2. Inhaled Ipratropium 3. Inhaled Sodium Cromoglycate
One in morning, before breakfast in sitting upright: Alendronate	Bisphosphonates lead to development of reflux esophagitis.

451. Ans. (c) Diabetic on OHA with HbA1C of 7%

(Ref: The Cleveland intensive review of Clinical medicine 5th edition, page 67)

Revised Goldman Cardiac Risk Index (LEE RISK INDEX)
- **High-risk type of surgery:** Intraperitoneal, Intrathoracic, or suprainguinal vascular procedure
- **History of ischemic heart disease:** history of myocardial infarction, positive exercise stress test, current complaint of

ischemic chest pain or use of nitrate therapy, or ECG with Q waves. Patients with prior coronary artery bypass grafting or percutaneous transluminal coronary angioplasty were included only if they had current complaints of chest pain presumed due to ischemia
- **History of congestive heart failure:** history of congestive heart failure, pulmonary edema, or paroxysmal nocturnal dyspnea, physical examination with bilateral rales or S_3, or chest radiograph showing pulmonary vascular redistribution
- **History of cerebrovascular disease**
- **Diabetes mellitus treated with insulin**
- **Preoperative serum creatinine > 2 mg/dL**

452. Ans. (a) PQR = YZX

(Ref: Harrison 20th p 3082; Harrison 19th edition, page 201, 1443, 40e-4)

Cotton wool spots are seen in hypertensive retinopathy	Earliest finding in hypertensive retinopathy is focal attenuation of arterioles. Later AV nipping, cotton wool spots and flame shaped haemorrhages are seen. These are evidence of target organ damage and necessitate strict BP control
Cherry red spot is seen in CRAO	Mnemonic: "Cherry Trees Never Grow Tall in Sand" **C**entral retinal artery occlusion **T**ay-Sachs disease **N**iemann-Pick disease **G**aucher's disease **T**rauma (Berlin's edema) **S**andhoff disease
Hollenhorst plaques are seen due to cholesterol embolization	75% of patients with Hollenhorst plaques are asymptomatic but due to association with carotid artery stenosis, Doppler study of carotid artery is recommended.

453. Ans. (d) Subungual splinter hemorrhage

(Ref: 289e-1: Harrison's 19th edition; Braunwald page 1865; Harrison 20th p 1848)

Myxomas present with constitutional signs and symptoms like:
1. Fever,
2. Weight loss
3. Cachexia, malaise, Arthralgias, rash
4. Digital clubbing,
5. Raynaud's phenomenon
6. Hypergammaglobulinemia.

- Atrial myxoma *can lead to damage to mitral valve leading to systolic murmur of mitral regurgitation.* The obstructive effects of tumor can lead to mitral stenosis but incidence is lower.
- A characteristic low-pitched sound, a *"tumor plop,"* may be appreciated on auscultation during early or mid-diastole and is thought to result from the impact of the tumor against the mitral valve or ventricular wall in case of ventricular myxoma. *Both in atrial and ventricular myxoma, the sound produced is diastolic.*

454. Ans. (d) Von gierke disease

(Ref: Harrison 20th p 1792 Page 1565, Table 287-5: Harrison 19th edition)

Scleroderma can lead to small stiff heart with reduced EF. PAH associated however presents more with RV failure.
Deficiency of lysosomal enzyme alpha-galactosidase A, X-linked recessive disorder leading to glycolipid accumulation in heart which needs biopsy and electron microscopy for diagnosis.
Non-caseating granulomas in sarcoidosis involve the heart leading to restrictive cardiomyopathy.

455. Ans. (c) Drinking water contaminated with nitrates

(Ref: Harrison 20th p 695; Harrison 19th edition p 636)

CO poisoning	Presents with hypotension, coma, seizures and cherry red lips
Severe anemia	Presents with pallor and cyanosis is milder and can be absent.
Drinking water contaminated with nitrates	Acquired methemoglobinemia is caused by toxins that oxidize heme iron nitrate and nitrite containing compounds. Methemoglobin is generated by oxidations of the heme iron moieties of the ferric state causing bluish brown muddy color resembling cyanosis Methemoglobin has such high oxygen affinity hence no oxygen is delivered Levels >50-60% are often fatal Methemoglobin should be suspected in patients with hypoxic symptoms who appear cyanotic but PaO2 and oxygen saturation are normal. Muddy appearance of freshly drawn blood can be a critical clue.
Lead poisoning	Presents with colicky abdominal pain, anemia, constipation, irritability, headache, convulsions and Coma

456. Ans. (d) Monophasic 360 J, Biphasic 120-200 J

(Ref: Ajay Yadav 5th/ 259 and A.H.A CPR guidelines 2015)

457. Ans. (c) Water-Hammer pulse- Aortic regurgitation:
(d) Pulsus parvus et tardus -Aortic stenosis:
(e) Collapsing pulse- Aortic regurgitation

(Ref: Harrison 20th p 1670; Harrison 19th/1445-46)

ABCD of Pulse

Anacrotic pulse/ Pulsus Parvus et Tardus	Aortic stenosis
Bisferiens Pulse	HOCM
Collapsing Pulse/ Water Hammer/ Corrigan pulse	Aortic regurgitation
Dicrotic pulse	Dilated cardiomyopathy
Pulsus paradoxus	Cardiac tamponade Shock of any etiology Status asthmaticus Acute corpulmonale
Irregularly irregular pulse	Atrial fibrillation

458. Ans. (d) Chest Compressions

(Ref: Harrison 20th p 2064; Harrison 19th ed. / 1768)

- According to AHA 2010 guidelines, the basic life support entails C_A_B and a shift from ABC protocol. Therefore the first thing to be done is chest compressions@100 times per minute. The depth of sternal depression should be 2 inches (5 cm)
- ALSO remember that in Advance cardiac life support the drugs used are epinephrine, and amiodarone. ATROPINE has been withdrawn and this is a change from 2005 guidelines.

459. Ans. (a) Tall tented T waves

(Ref: Harrison 20th p 310; Harrison 19th ed. / 310)

Serum potassium > 5.5 mEq/L is associated with repolarization abnormalities:
- Peaked T waves (usually the earliest sign of hyperkalemia) Serum potassium > 6.5 mEq/L is associated with progressive paralysis of the atria:
- P wave widens and flattens
- PR segment lengthens
- P waves eventually disappear

Serum potassium >7.0 mEq/L is associated with conduction abnormalities and bradycardia:
- Prolonged QRS interval with bizarre QRS morphology
- High-grade AV block with slow junctional and ventricular escape rhythms
- Any kind of conduction block (bundle branch blocks, fascicular blocks)
- Sinus bradycardia or slow AF
- Development of a sine wave appearance (a pre-terminal rhythm)

Serum potassium level of > 9.0 mEq/L causes cardiac arrest due to:
- Asystole
- Ventricular fibrillation

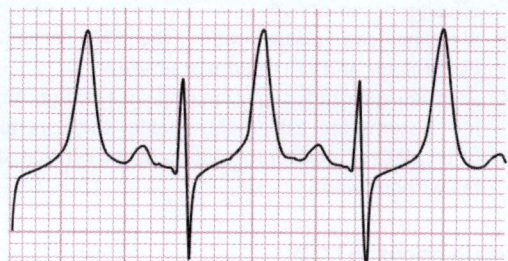

460. Ans. (d) Wide QRS complex

(Ref: Harrison 20th p 310; Harrison 19th ed. / 310)

ECG Findings of Hyperkalemia
- The first ECG finding in hyperkalemia is tall tented T waves followed by slowing of depolarization of heart.
- This results in prolonged PR interval with QRS widening.
- Subsequently the P waves start becoming smaller.
- Sine wave pattern leading to ventricular fibrillation/ diastolic arrest of heart.

461. Ans. (a) Cardiophrenic angle

(Ref: Harrison 20th p 2010; Harrison 19th ed./1719)

- Pericardial cyst is most commonly located at right costophrenic angle and identified incidentally on chest X-Ray.

462. Ans. (c) Venous insufficiency

(Ref: Harrison 20th p 1934; Harrison 19th ed. / 253)

- Edema is defined as a palpable swelling caused by an increase in interstitial fluid volume. The most likely cause of leg edema in patients over age 50 is venous insufficiency.
- The most important cause of unilateral pedal edema is venous insufficiency which must be evaluated using a Doppler exam.

463. Ans. (b) Atropine

(Ref: AHA 2015 guidelines; Management of Cardiac Arrest)

464. Ans. (b) Cardiac abnormality

(Ref: Harrison 20th p 1789; Harrison 19th ed. / 96e-1t)

- Vitamin B1 deficiency causes Beri-Beri which is of two types- WET BERI-BERI having cardiac failure and DRY BERI-BERI causing CNS problems like Wernicke encephalopathy and Korsakoff psychosis.
- Gingival bleeding and delayed wound healing (choice A) is seen with scurvy. Memory loss is seen with niacin deficiency.

465. Ans. (d) Calcium chloride

(Ref: Harrison 20th p 310; Harrison 19th ed. / 312)

- In a clinical setting of hyperkalemia in 1-year-old child, cardiac arrhythmias associated with hyperkalemia include sinus bradycardia, sinus arrest, slow idioventricular rhythms, ventricular tachycardia, ventricular fibrillation, and asystole
- Intravenous calcium serves to protect the heart while measures are taken to correct hyperkalemia.
- Calcium raises the action potential threshold and reduces excitability without changing the resting membrane potential. By restoring the difference between the resting and threshold potentials, calcium reverses the depolarization blockade caused by hyperkalemia.
- *The recommended dose of treatment of hyperkalemia is 10 mL of 10% calcium gluconate (3–4 mL of calcium chloride), infused intravenously over 2 to 3 min with cardiac monitoring.*
- The effect of the infusion starts in 1–3 min and lasts 30–60 min; the dose should be repeated if there is no change in ECG findings or if they recur after initial improvement.

466. Ans. (c) Pulmonary artery trunk

The structures forming left heart border are:

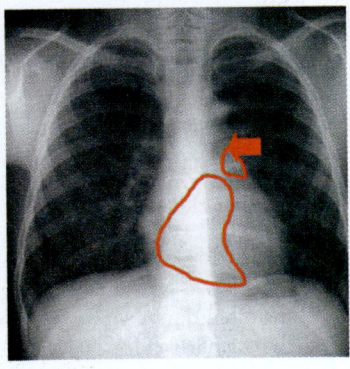

1. Aortic knuckle
2. Pulmonary artery trunk
3. Left ventricle

The left atrium does not form the left heart border. Enlargement of left atrium is picked up by widened carinal angle.

EXTRA MILE

- *Straightening of left heart border occurs in mitral stenosis.*

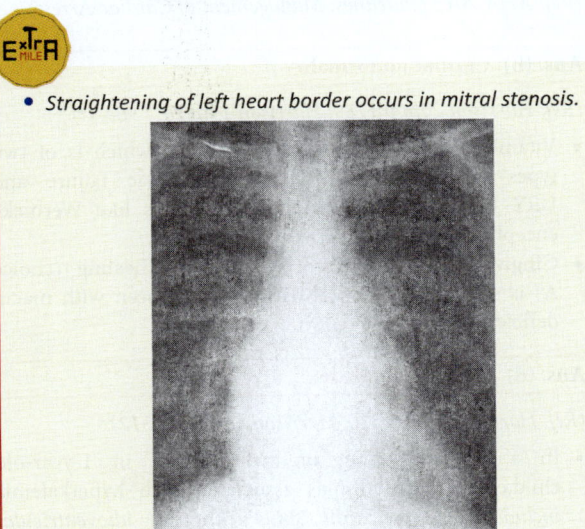

It is due to 4 factors.
1. Hypoplastic aorta
2. LAA
3. PA
4. Under filled LV

467. Ans. (a) Aortic dissection

(Ref: Harrison 20th p 1920)

- The patient is very tall with long arms with pectus excavatum with exaggerated lumbar lordosis.
- This leads to suspicion of Marfan syndrome with defect in protein fibrillin on chromosome 15.
- The most common cause of death in these patients is due to aortic dissection

468. Ans. (b) Moya Moya disease-aortic aneurysm

(Ref: Harrison 20th p 3086; Harrison; 18 ed, ch. 310, pg. 3297)

- **Moya-Moya disease** is a progressive, occlusive disease of the cerebral vasculature with particular involvement of the circle of Willis and the arteries that feed it. The term moyamoya (Japanese for **"puff of smoke"**) refers to the appearance on angiography of abnormal vascular collateral networks that develop adjacent to the Stenotic vessels.
- Associations are vascular diseases like - Atherosclerotic disease, coarctation of the aorta and fibromuscular dysplasia and hypertension.

Neurofibromatosis is associated with
Pheochromocytomas and
Vascular stenosis (i.e., renal artery stenosis secondary to Fibromuscular dysplasia)
Marfan's Syndrome: Dural ectasia occurs in approximately 90% of Marfan patients, and its severity increases with ageing.
Mulibrey Nanism Syndrome: A very rare inherited malformation characterized by dwarfism, pericardial constriction and yellow dots in fundus of the eye.

469. Ans. (a) Chest X-ray

(Ref: Harrison 20th p 1754; Harrison 19th p 1499)

Complications of implantable cardioverter defibrillator
1. Lead dislodgment generally occurs within few days of device implantation pacer and may be seen on chest radiography as the leads are radio-opaque.
2. Free-floating ventricular leads may trigger malignant arrhythmias.
3. Device-associated venous thrombosis is rare but generally presents as unilateral arm edema. Treatment includes extremity elevation and anticoagulation.
4. Collapse of the lung (pneumothorax) occurs in about 1 percent of cases and can usually be treated by inserting a chest tube.
5. Perforation of the heart, causing a collection of blood to develop within the sac around the heart (pericardial effusion or tamponade).
6. Bleeding can occur under the skin around the defibrillator and can require drainage.
7. Premature battery depletion or device failure. Although ICD systems are extremely reliable, they are like any other piece of electronic equipment and can occasionally fail without warning.

Details about an I.C.D
An ICD is approximately the size of a pager. The main parts include:
- The ICD — The ICD is powered by a battery and generates an electrical shock. It is also called the battery, device, or pulse generator. It is a single unit that is usually inserted into a "pocket" created under the skin (or muscle) in the chest below the collarbone (in the pectoral region). The longevity of the ICD is defined by the length of life of the battery (usually three to five years).
- The leads — Flexible, insulated wires, or leads, monitor the electrical impulses and report the heart's electrical activity back to the ICD. These leads deliver electrical charges from the generator to the heart muscle when needed. During

implantation, the ICD leads are passed through a vein into the heart.
- The leads are connected to the ICD. When the ICD reaches the end of battery life and is replaced, the original leads are usually left in place and connected to the new device. The leads may last for 20 years or more.

470. Ans. (c) Endocarditis

(Ref: CMDT 2019 p 711; Harrison 19th p 382)

- The life-threatening DRESS (Drug Rash with Eosinophilia and Systemic Symptoms) syndrome is characterized by the presence of at least three of the following findings: fever, exanthema, eosinophilia, atypical circulating lymphocytes, lymphadenopathy, and hepatitis
- The DRESS syndrome is most frequently caused by aromatic anticonvulsants (phenytoin, phenobarbital, and carbamazepine); however, other drugs such as sulfonamides, metronidazole, minocycline, sulfasalazine, allopurinol, and antiretrovirals such as nevirapine and abacavir have been implicated
- Due to association with HHV 6, encephalitis has been reported
- The organ involvement in DRESS syndrome in decreasing order of prevalence is:
  1. Liver–hepatitis ranging from enzyme derangement to fulminant course causing ENCEPHALOPATHY.
  2. Kidney –Hematuria due to interstitial nephritis
  3. Colitis
  4. Pneumonitis
  5. Myocarditis
  6. Encephalitis
  7. Arthritis
  8. Myositis

Treatment: Most important steps in managing patients with DRESS are recognizing the presence of this syndrome and immediately stopping the offending drug. Management is essentially supportive. The role of corticosteroids and intravenous immunoglobulins in the treatment of DRESS syndrome are controversial.

471. Ans. (a) Phenol sulfotransferase deficiency

(Ref: Net Source: Pubmed)

- P.S.T- Phenolsulfotransferase activity.
- Patients with dietary migraine were found to have significantly lower levels of platelet phenolsulpho-transferase activity than either migrainous patients without a history of dietary provocation or normal controls.
- Of the two known human variants of this enzyme, the phenol-inactivating P form, for which no endogenous substrate has so far been identified, was more severely involved than the M enzyme, which inactivates monoamines (including tyramine). Such commonly implicated dietary triggering agents as chocolate and cheese may contain as-yet-unidentified phenolic substrates of phenolsulphotransferase P; if the platelet enzyme deficiency were mirrored by low gut activity, abnormally large amounts of potentially toxic substances might gain access to the circulation in consequence.

472. Ans. (c) Atropine

(Ref: AHA 2015 guidelines; Harrison 19th p 1770)

Every 5 years the American Heart Association has a meeting where they hammer out new CPR and ACLS guidelines based upon the data collected from the previous 5 years.

ACLS: De-emphasis of Devices, Drugs and other Distracters

1. Atropine is no longer recommended for routine use in management of PEA/asystole. Atropine: deleted from pulse less arrest algorithm
2. Chronotropic drug infusions are now recommended as alternative to pacing in symptomatic and unstable bradycardia.
3. Adenosine is recommended as safe and potentially effective for treatment and diagnosis in initial management of undifferentiated regular monomorphic wide-complex tachycardia.
4. Sodium Bicarbonate: Routine use not recommended (Class III, LOE B).
5. Calcium: Routine administration for treatment of cardiac arrest not recommended (Class III, LOE B).

> - Adrenaline 1 mg iv/IO, 3-5 minutes every 10 minute. It increases coronary perfusion.
> - Vasopressin 40 Units iv/IO can replace 2nd or 3rd dose of epinephrine. It increases cerebral perfusion.
> - Amiodarone for refractory VT/VF: 300mg i.v. bolus first dose/ repeat 150 mg iv repeat.
> - 8-10 breaths per minute with continuous chest compressions
> - Compression rate at least 100 per minute.
> - Compress at least 2 inches (2005 recommendation was 1½ to 2 inches).
> - Why change to C-A-B: To reduce delay to CPR, sequence begins with skill that everyone can perform. Emphasize primary importance of chest compressions for professional rescuers
> - Supplementary oxygen is not needed for patients without evidence of respiratory distress if the oxy-hemoglobin saturation is <94%.

473. Ans. (a) 0.9-1.1

(Ref: Net source: Pubmed)

Any patient presenting with shock must have an early working diagnosis, an approach to urgent resuscitation, and then confirmation of the working diagnosis. The following points should be considered for early diagnosis of sepsis:

- Patients with sepsis may present in a myriad of ways, and high clinical suspicion is necessary to identify subtle presentations.
- Septic patients should be screened for evidence of tissue hypo-perfusion.
- Cool or clammy skin, mottling, and elevated shock index (heart rate/systolic blood pressure > 0.9) may be signs of tissue hypoperfusion.
- A lactic acid level higher than 4 mmol/dL has been used as an entry criterion for early goal-directed therapy and an indicator of severe tissue hypoperfusion.

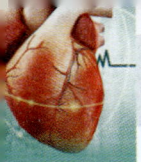

474. Ans. (d) Pleural surface

(Ref: Sutton Textbook of Radiology, 7th ed., page 131,145)

Kerley B lines
- These are short parallel lines at the lung periphery.
- These lines represent interlobular septa, which are usually less than 1 cm in length and parallel to one another at right angles to the pleura.
- They are located peripherally in contact with the pleura, but are generally absent along fissural surfaces.
- They may be seen in any zone but are most frequently observed at the lung bases at the costophrenic angles on the PA radiograph, and in the substernal region on lateral radiographs. Kerley B lines are seen in Congestive Heart Failure (CHF) and Interstitial Lung Diseases (ILD).
- Kerley A lines are longer (at least 2 cm and up to 6cm) unbranching lines coursing diagonally from the hila out to the periphery of the lungs. They are caused by distension of anastomotic channels between peripheral and central lymphatics of the lungs. Kerley A lines are less commonly seen than Kerley B lines. Kerley A lines are never seen without Kerley B or C lines.
- Kerley C lines are the least commonly seen of the Kerley lines. They are short, fine lines throughout the lungs, with a reticular appearance. They may represent thickening of anastomotic lymphatics or superimposition of many Kerley B lines.

475. Ans. (a) Left subclavian artery

(Ref: Harrison 20th p 2585; Harrison's, ch. 326: Vasculitis Syndrome page 2796, Harrison 19th p 2189)

Artery	Percent of Arteriographic Abnormalities	Potential Clinical Manifestations
Subclavian	93	Arm claudication, Raynaud's phenomenon
Common carotid	58	Visual changes, syncope, transient ischemic attacks, stroke
Abdominal aorta	47	Abdominal pain, nausea, vomiting
Renal	38	Hypertension, renal failure

476. Ans. (c) Cardiac arrest

(Ref: Harrison 20th p 2063, 2065)

- Inducing mild therapeutic hypothermia in selected patients surviving out-of-hospital sudden cardiac arrest can significantly improve rates of long-term neurologically intact survival and may prove to be one of the most important clinical advancements in the science of resuscitation.
- Patients who have been shown to benefit from induced hypothermia include the following:
  - Intubated patients with treatment initiated within 6 hours after cardiac arrest (nonperfusing ventricular tachycardia [VT] or VF)
  - Patients able to maintain a systolic blood pressure >90 mm Hg, with or without pressors, after CPR.
- The types of medical events that hypothermic therapies may effectively treat fall into four primary categories:
  1. Cardiac arrest- validated by clinical studies
  2. *Ischemic stroke- Harrison and internet data mention clinical trial on animals only*
  3. Traumatic brain or spinal cord injury without fever –validated by clinical studies
  4. Neurogenic fever following brain trauma- validated by clinical studies

477. Ans. (a) Rene Laennec

(Ref: Medical Encyclopedia)

- The stethoscope was invented in France in 1816 by René Laennec at the Necker-Enfants Malades Hospital in Paris
- Joseph Littman- Dummy choice!
- William Osler- Founder of John Hopkin university and famed osler residency

- Father of Neurology- Jean Mary Charcot
- Father of Medicine – Hippocrates

478. Ans. (a) Roger Hausen

(Ref: Medical Encyclopedia)

- It's a misnomer coined café coronary but not related to coronary blockage.
- Early recognition of airway obstruction is imperative, because hypoxia of only four to six minutes' duration may result in irreversible brain damage. Fortunately, the foreign body preventing adequate air exchange can often be dislodged and expelled once the correct emergency procedures are implemented.
- The Heimlich maneuver or external subdia-phragmatic abdominal thrust is recognized as the basic procedure for relief of complete larynx/trachea obstruction. This technique, by elevating the diaphragm, can force a sufficient quantity of air from the lungs to create an artificial cough that is often of adequate force and duration to expel the obstructing foreign body from the airway. If noninvasive procedures prove to be ineffective, a cricothyrotomy should be performed by trained rescuers. Many of the victims of foreign body airway obstruction are either children or elderly with alcohol consumption.

479. Ans. (d) Marfan syndrome

(Ref: Harrison 20th p 1920; Harrison 19th p 1641)

- Syphilitic aneurysms result in marked aortic root dilatation with ascending aneurysms but are extremely rare.
- Dissections are common in Marfan syndrome, idiopathic T.A.A (thoracic aorta aneurysm), and TAA associated with bicuspid aortic valve, because the medial degeneration is devoid of significant scarring and results in laminar weakness of the wall.
- Inflammatory aortitides are associated with aneurysm, but the significant adventitial fibrosis that accompanies Takayasu aortitis inhibits dissections, despite the medial inflammation, whereas the aortitis of giant cell aortitis

is more frequently associated with aneurysms, because fibrosis is less prominent.

480. Ans. (d) T.E.E

(Ref: Harrison 20th p 1683-84; Harrison 19th ed. p 820)

- Trans-Esophageal Echocardiography has emerged as the imaging study of choice in patients with a suspected prosthetic valve complication. This applies especially to prosthetic mitral valves, where transthoracic Doppler is often insensitive. Adequately excluding prosthetic valve regurgitation with a transthoracic echocardiogram is difficult.
- TEE provides a unique window for High resolution imaging of posterior structure of heart, particularly left atrium, mitral valve and aorta.
- Cinefluorography may detect impaired occluder movement but often cannot readily determine the etiology.
- An Over penetrated antero-posterior chest radio-graph helps to delineate the valvular morphology and whether or not the valve and occluder are intact. In more stable patients, a lateral chest film helps identify the valve position and type.

481. Ans. (b) >12 mm Hg

(Ref: Schwartz textbook of surgery 9th ed., page 316)

- Intra-abdominal hypertension is defined as a pressure over 12 mm Hg in adults. However, if the pressure continues to rise over 20 mm Hg and organs begin to fail, the syndrome has now progressed to the end stage of the highly fatal process termed abdominal compartment syndrome. These pressure measurements are relative. Small children get into trouble and develop compartment syndromes at much lower pressures while young previously healthy athletic individuals may tolerate an abdominal pressure of 20 mm Hg very well.

IAP can be easily monitored by measuring bladder pressure. Measurement of intraluminal bladder pressure consists of instilling about 50 mL of saline into the urinary bladder through the Foley catheter.

The following grading system has become accepted if IAH is present:

- Grade I: 10-15 mm Hg
- Grade II: 15-25 mm Hg
- Grade III: 25-35 mm Hg
- Grade IV, greater than 35 mm Hg

- End-organ damage has been observed with IAH at values ranging from 20-40 mm Hg.

482. Ans. (a) IPPV

(Ref: Harrison 20th p 1843; Harrison 19th p 1446)

483. Ans. (d) MI

(Ref: Harrison 20th p 1670; Harrison 19th p 1446)

484. Ans. (b) Aortic regurgitation

(Ref: Harrison 20th p 1670; Harrison 19th p 1445)

485. Ans. (a) Pulmonary capillary wedge pressure

(Ref: Harrison 20th p 1711; Hurst 12th/494, Harrison 19th p 1461)

486. Ans. (d) Bilateral renal artery stenosis

(Ref: Harrison 19th p 1617; CMDT 2019 p 390)

487. Ans. (b) Prominent lower lobe vessels

(Ref: Harrison 20th p 1768)

488. Ans. (b) Cardiac Tamponade

(Ref: Harrison 20th p 1843)

489. Ans. (a) Myxoma

(Ref: Harrison 20th p 1847)

490. Ans. (b) Libman Sack's Endocarditis

(Ref: Harrison 20th p 2520; Harrison 19th p 817)

491. Ans. (a) AV node

(Ref: Ganong 22nd/547-549)

492. Ans. (a) Atrios-ventricular valves open

(Ref: Guyton 10th/99)

493. Ans. (a) (SBP + 2DBP)/3

(Ref: Chaudhary 5th/244)

494. Ans. (c) Atherosclerosis

(Ref: Harrison 20th p 1917; Harrison 19th p 1639)

495. Ans. (d) Mid diastole

(Ref: Advances in Cardiology by Braunwald p 227)

496. Ans. (c) Pulmonary Artery

(Ref: Miller's Anaesthesia 8th edition, page 1643, Chapter 54)

Measurement of Core Temperature

- Core temperature refers to the deep body temperature that is carefully regulated by the hypothalamus to be independent of transient small changes in ambient temperature.
- Ideal sites of temperature measurement would be protected from heat loss, painless, and convenient to use.
- Core temperature is *best measured* from the pulmonary artery, distal esophagus, tympanic membrane, or nasopharynx.
- Oral, axillary, rectal, and bladder temperatures approximate core temperature in most clinical circumstances, except during rapid changes in temperature.
- If the question is framed as preferred site for checking core temperature, the answer is lower esophagus.

497. Ans. (c) Sackett

(Ref: http://www.ncbi.nlm.nih.gov/pmc/articles/PMC3263217)

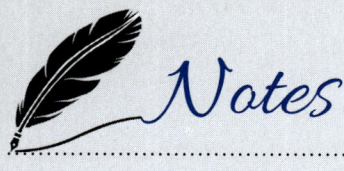

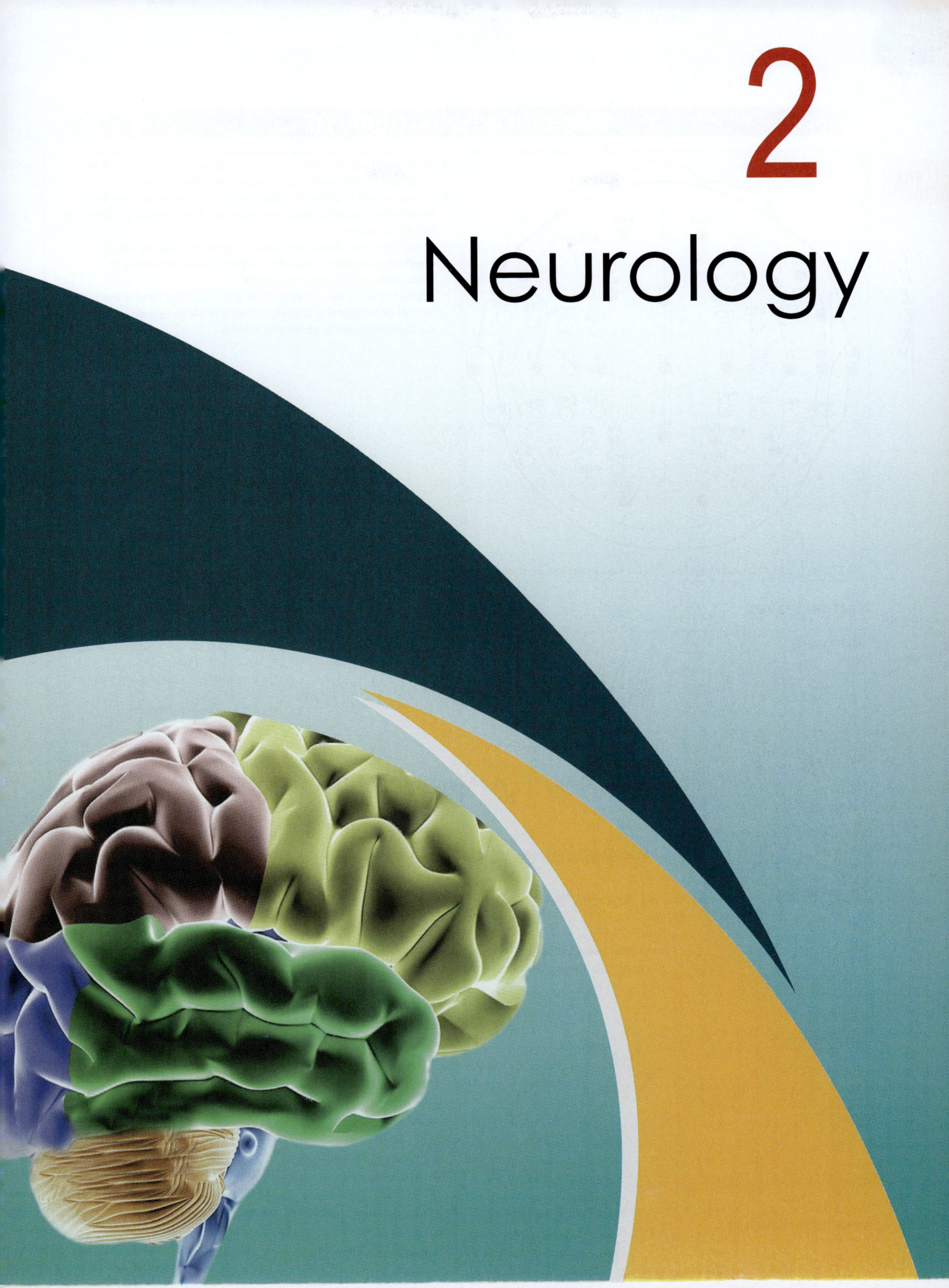

2 Neurology

ELECTROENCEPHALOGRAPHY

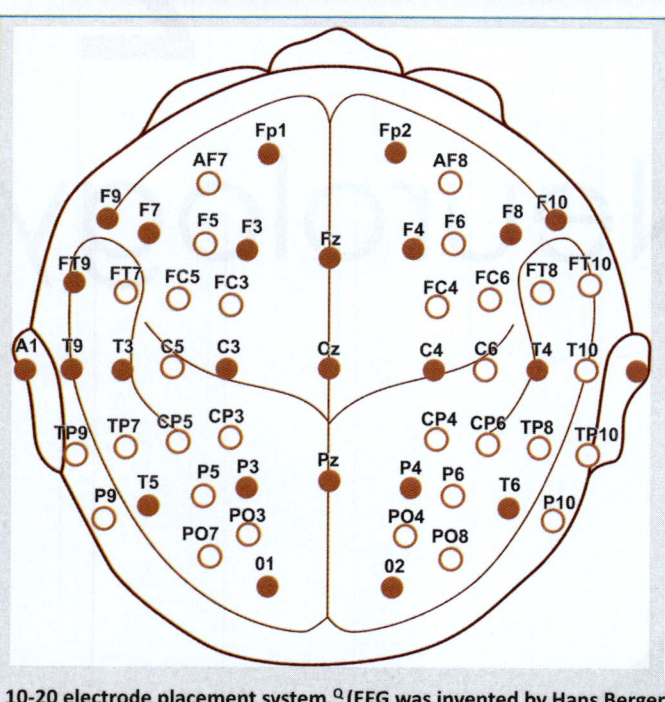

- Right sided placements are indicated by even numbers and left sided placements with odd numbers and midline by Z
- The recording is called *montage* with x axis showing time and vertical axis showing electrical discharge from frontal or central or temporal regions
- Maneuvers like photic stimulation, hyperventilation, sleep deprivation or sleep induction help in certain situations to precipitate an abnormal discharge
- Artifacts due to eye movement or jaw clenching can be seen in frontal or temporal leads respectively, while in epilepsy all or multiple leads show abnormal activity

10-20 electrode placement system.^{Q} (EEG was invented by Hans Berger)

Normal Waves

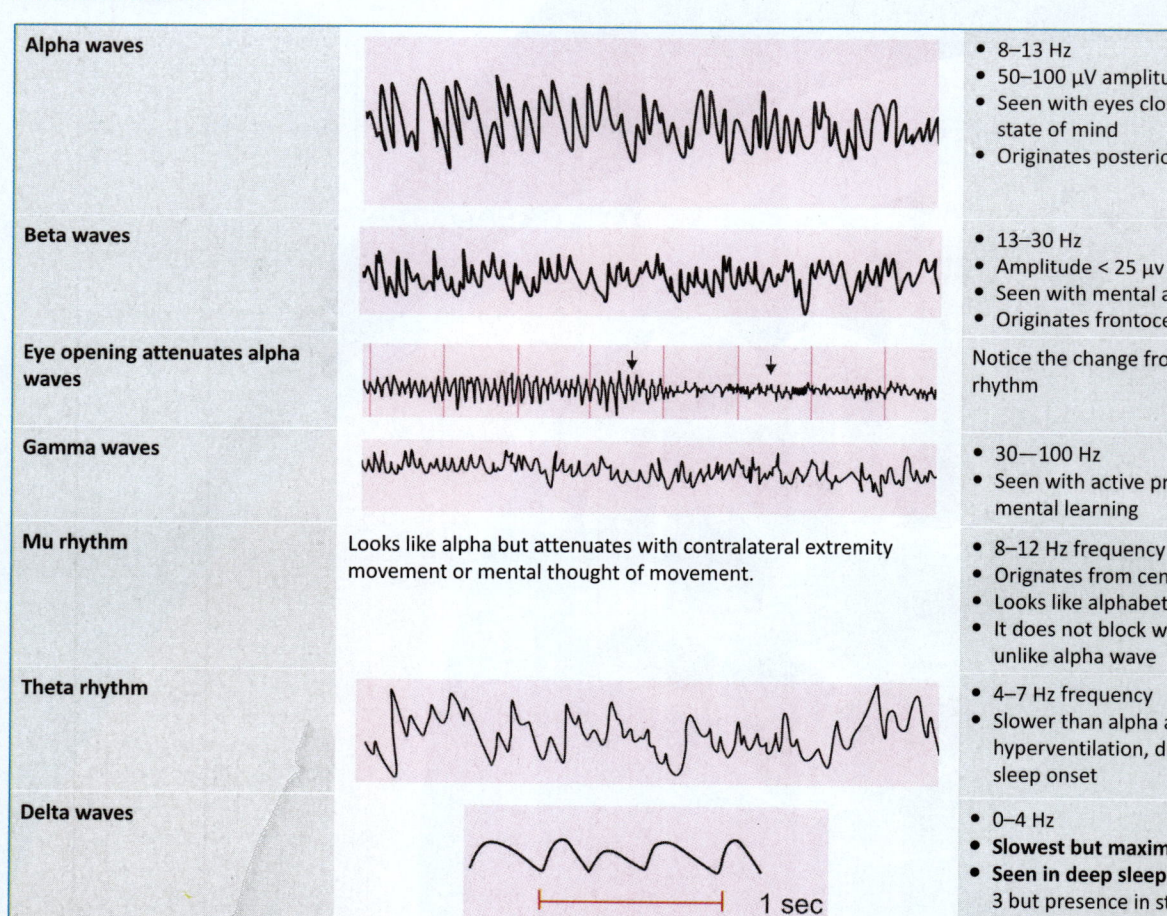

Alpha waves		• 8–13 Hz • 50–100 μV amplitude • Seen with eyes closed and relaxed state of mind • Originates posteriorly
Beta waves		• 13–30 Hz • Amplitude < 25 μv • Seen with mental alertness • Originates frontocentral
Eye opening attenuates alpha waves		Notice the change from alpha to beta rhythm
Gamma waves		• 30—100 Hz • Seen with active problem solving, mental learning
Mu rhythm	Looks like alpha but attenuates with contralateral extremity movement or mental thought of movement.	• 8–12 Hz frequency • Orignates from centroparietal area • Looks like alphabet small "m" • It does not block with eye opening unlike alpha wave
Theta rhythm		• 4–7 Hz frequency • Slower than alpha and seen with hyperventilation, drowsiness and sleep onset
Delta waves	1 sec	• 0–4 Hz • **Slowest but maximum amplitude**^{Q} • **Seen in deep sleep like NREM stage**^{Q} 3 but presence in stuporose patient indicates hepatic encephalopahty

*Alpha coma is seen in hypoxic ischemic encephalopathy, pontine or diffuse cortical damage. It is not altered rhythm by environmental stimuli, unlike normal alpha.

Contd...

SLEEP EEG

NREM stage 2	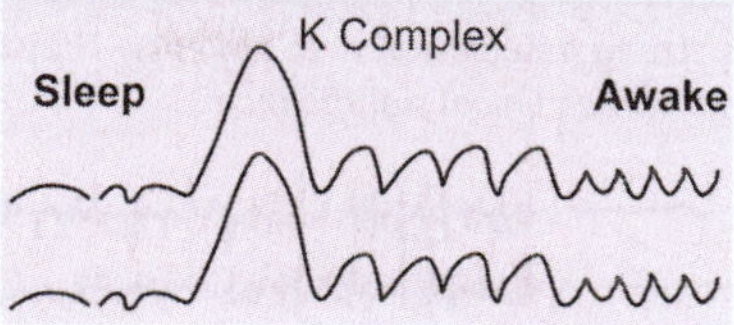 K Complex diagram (Sleep — K Complex — Awake)	K complexes are high amplitude (>100 µV), broad (>200 ms), diphasic and transient
Lambda waves/Positive occipital sharp transients of sleep (POSTS)	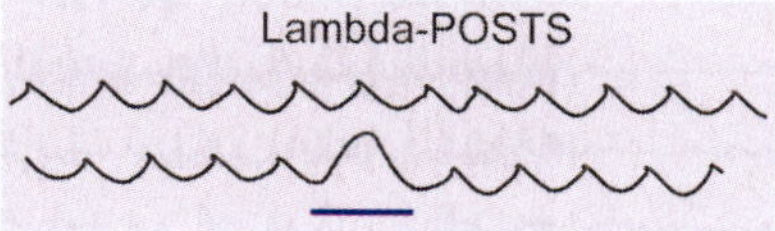 Lambda-POSTS diagram	They have a positive maximum at the occiput, are contoured sharply and occur in early sleep (stages I and II). Their morphology is classically described as "reverse check mark," and their amplitude is 50–100 µV
NREM stage 3 and 4 (called as slow wave sleep)	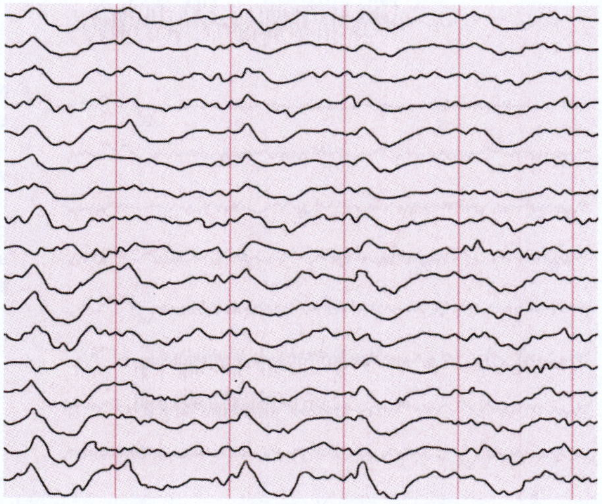 EEG tracing	Notice the slow delta waves
Comparison of EEG in sleep stages	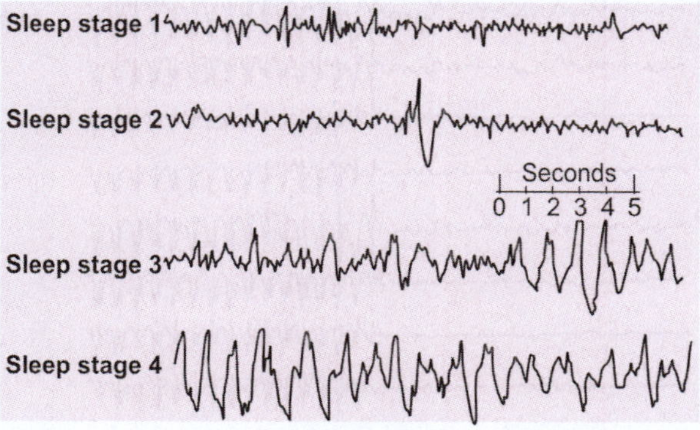 Sleep stages 1–4 tracings (Seconds 0 1 2 3 4 5)	Notice the K complex in stage 2 and slowing to delta rhythm in stage 3 and 4
Saw tooth waves[Q]	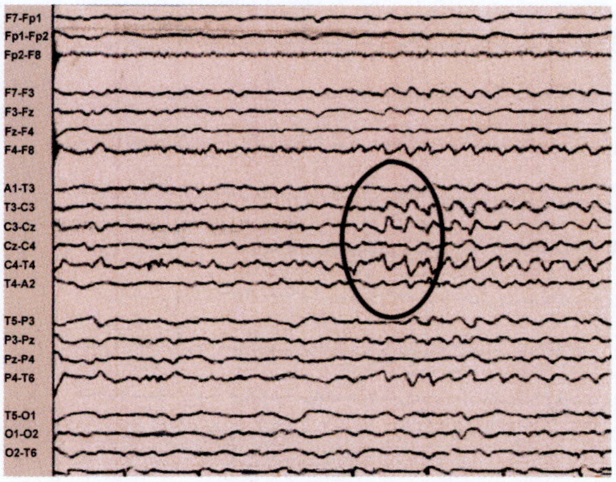 EEG tracing	Train of vertex waves in REM Sleep

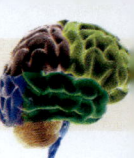

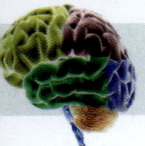

Abnormal Waveforms in EEG

Spikes and sharp waves are sharp transients that have a strong association with epilepsy. They can be distinguished by their duration (spikes, <70 ms; sharp waves, 70–200 ms) but have essentially the same clinical significance

GTCS	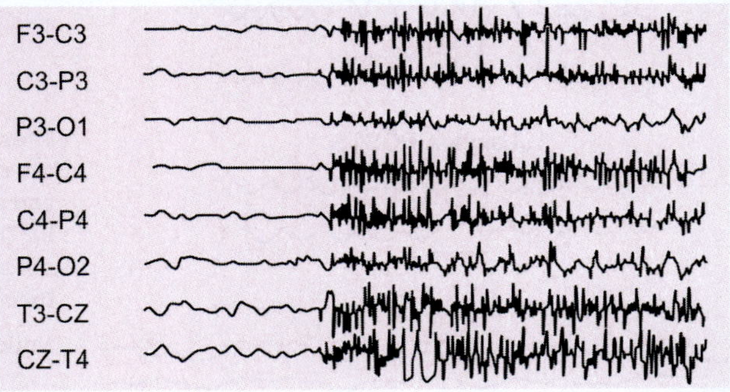 (EEG tracing: F3-C3, C3-P3, P3-O1, F4-C4, C4-P4, P4-O2, T3-CZ, CZ-T4)	Generalized repetitive sharp activity with synchronicity in all leads
Periodic lateralized epileptiform discharge[Q]	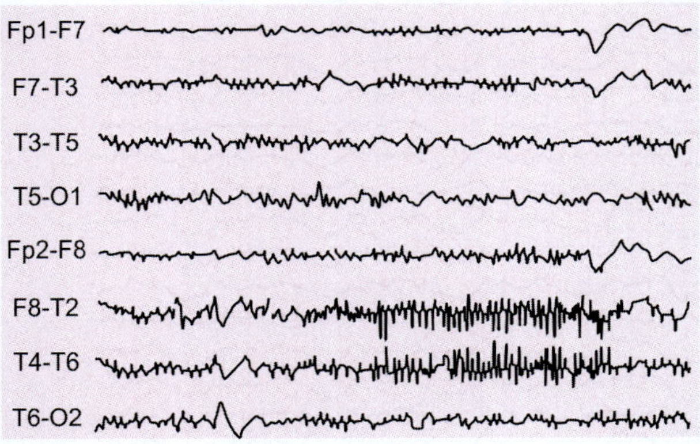 (EEG tracing: Fp1-F7, F7-T3, T3-T5, T5-O1, Fp2-F8, F8-T2, T4-T6, T6-O2)	• Notice the repetitive burst of activity over temporal area • In herpes simplex encephalitis, which mainly affects the temporal lobe, EEG shows periodic discharges over the temporal lobe, which are called *periodic lateralized epileptiform discharge*[Q]
3/sec spike and slow wave pattern of absence seizures	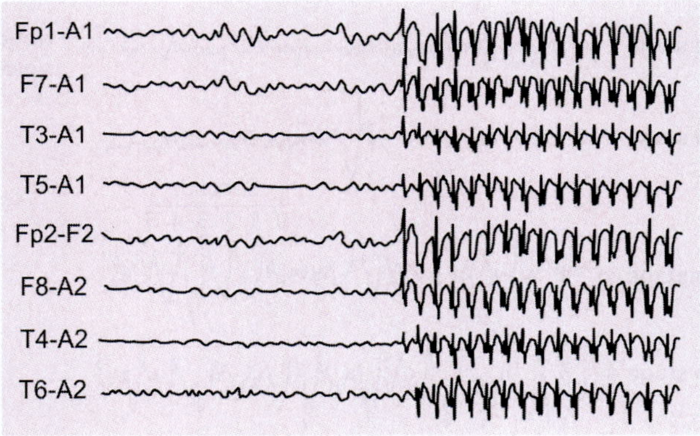 (EEG tracing: Fp1-A1, F7-A1, T3-A1, T5-A1, Fp2-F2, F8-A2, T4-A2, T6-A2)	The pattern can be **precipitated by hyperventilation or photic stimulation**
Periodic sharp wave complexes[Q]	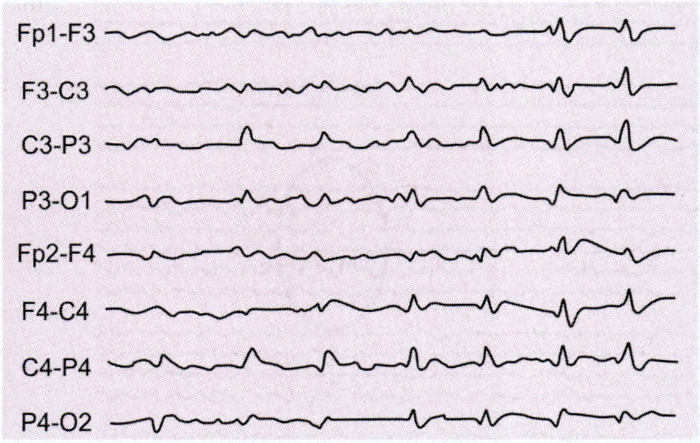 (EEG tracing: Fp1-F3, F3-C3, C3-P3, P3-O1, Fp2-F4, F4-C4, C4-P4, P4-O2)	The high voltage bursts occur periodically every 1 second and are seen in variant Creutzfeldt Jakob disease

Contd...

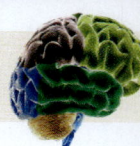

Hypsarrhythmia[Q]	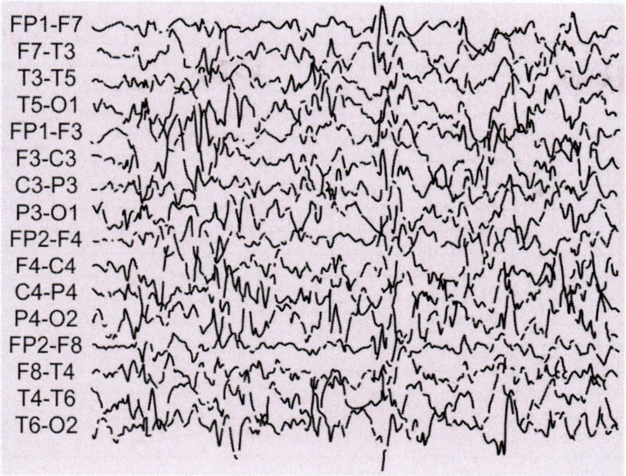 [EEG tracing]	• Characterstic pattern of infantile spasm where gross chaos is seen • It is defined as continuous (during wakefulness), high-amplitude (>200 Hz), generalized polymorphic slowing with no organized background and multifocal spikes
Polyspike and wave pattern in juvenile myoclonic epilepsy[Q]	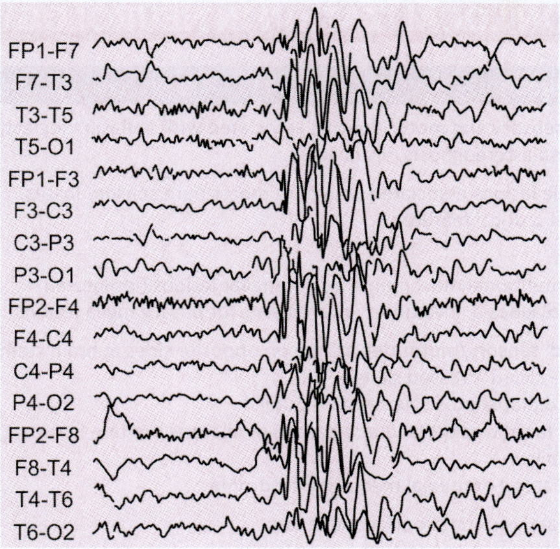 [EEG tracing]	These spikes are seen at 4–6Hz
Triphasic waves[Q]	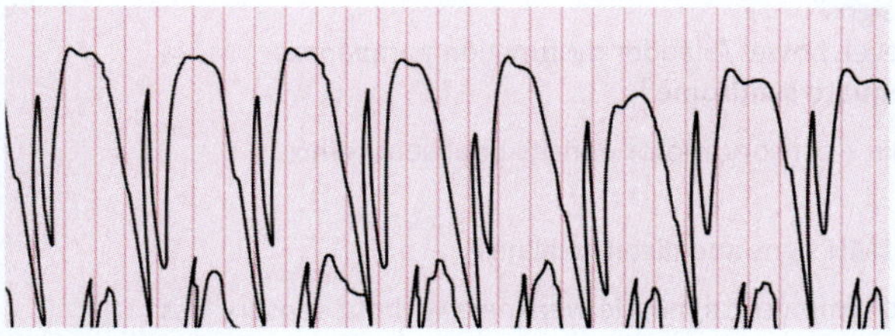 [EEG tracing] *Notice the pattern* 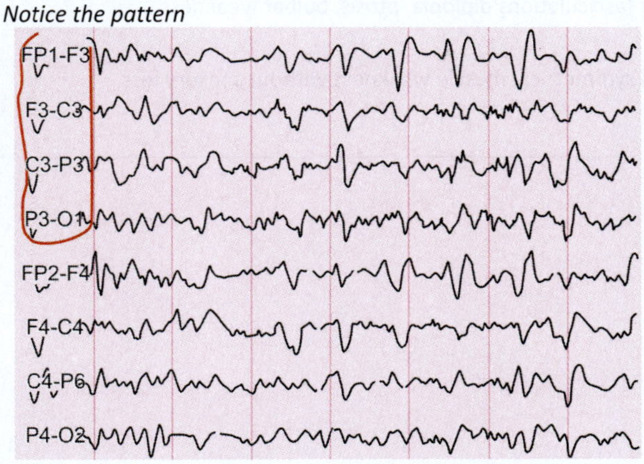 [EEG tracing]	Hepatic encephalopathy

Contd...

Burst suppression pattern[Q]

Causes-
1. Coma
2. Hypothermia
3. Drug intoxication
4. Childhood encephalopathies
5. Prolonged anesthesia

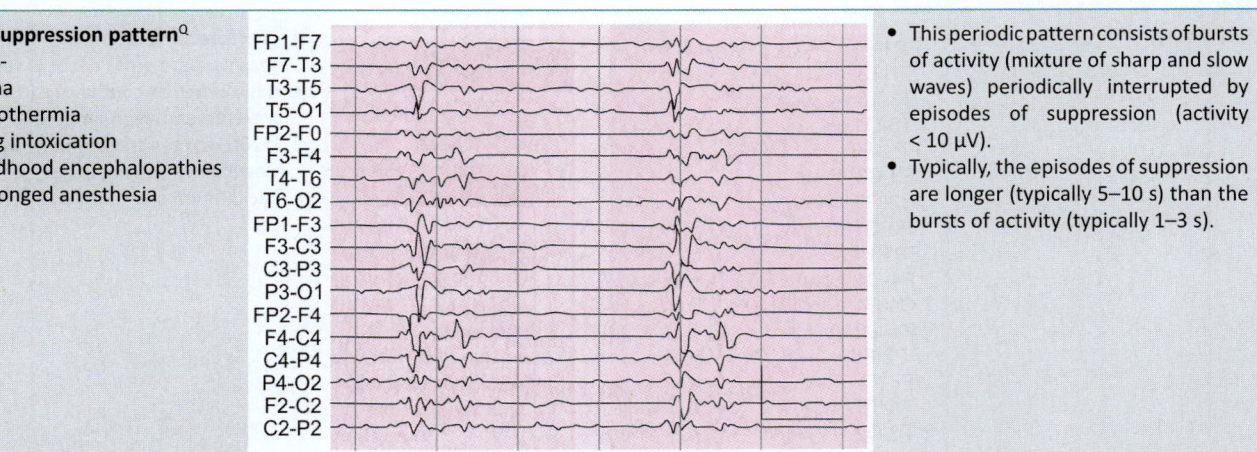

- This periodic pattern consists of bursts of activity (mixture of sharp and slow waves) periodically interrupted by episodes of suppression (activity < 10 μV).
- Typically, the episodes of suppression are longer (typically 5–10 s) than the bursts of activity (typically 1–3 s).

LESION LOCALIZATION IN NEUROLOGY

Location of the lesion	General symptoms	Remarks
Cortex and internal capsule	Contralateral sensory and motor deficits, associated with aphasia, neglect, agraphaestheisa astereognosia, visual loss Internal capsule lesions associated with pure motor pure sensory losses, and absence of cortical features	Seizure disorder (cortex only) Coma Stroke
Cerebellum and Basal ganglia	Incoordination • Abnormal intentional movements for cerebellar lesions (ipsilateral) • Tremor, bradykinesia, involuntary movements for basal ganglia lesions	Cerebellar degeneration Parkinson's disease stroke
Brainstem (unilateral) Mid brain CN 3-4; Pons CN 6-7; Medulla CN 8-10	CN defects and sensory/motor deficits are on opposite sides in brain stem lesions and are called "crossed signs" • MIDBRAIN: diplopia ptosis, unreactive pupil. • PONS: LMN facial weakness, quadriparesis in bilateral pontine lesions, pinpoint pupils. • MEDULLA: Lateral or medial medullary syndrome.	Cranial nerve palsies
Spinal cord (unilateral)	• Ipsilateral paralysis and proprioceptive loss • Contralateral pain – temperature loss below the level of the lesion- "Crossed signs" • Sensory level, bowel /bladder dysfunction paraparesis **Brown-Sequard syndrome**[Q]	Spinal cord syndromes
Nerve root	Radicular pain + sensory/motor deficits or absent reflex	Nerve root compression Disk herniation
Peripheral nerve	Presence of LMN signs and distal weakness	Neuropathies
Neuromuscular junction	Proximal and symmetrical muscle weakness without sensory loss fatigability or fasciculations diplopia, ptosis, bulbar weakness	Myasthenia gravis Lambert–Eaton syndrome Botulism
Muscle	Proximal and symmetrical muscle weakness without sensory loss	Muscular dystrophies Myopathies including polymyositis Dermatomyositis

CN = Cranial nerve

HEADACHE

Common Causes of Headache

Primary headache	Secondary headache
Tension-type	Systemic infection
Migraine	Head injury
Idiopathic	Vascular disorders
Exertional	Subarachnoid hemorrhage
Cluster	Brain tumor

- Most common type of headache is **tension headache**.
- Most common type of 2° headache is due to infection.

Migraine

Migraine, the second most common cause of primary headache is usually an episodic headache associated with certain features such as sensitivity to light, **sound or movement**[Q] nausea and vomiting often accompany the headache. Migraine can often be recognized by its activators, referred to as *triggers*.

Classical Migraine with Aura

- It is more common in female patients.
- Aura comprises visual complaints like Photopsia and Scotomas.
- One of the mediators behind migraine is serotonin, which leads to vasoconstriction of intracranial blood vessels. This vasoconstriction leads to reflex vasodilatation of extracranial blood vessels.
- Dura mater is the pain sensitive structure in the brain and reflex vasodilatation of vessels cause stretching of dura, which manifests as pain.

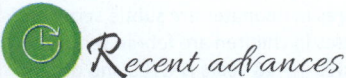

New Theory for Migraine
- Calcitonin gene related peptide acting on vascular terminations of Vth nerve
- Cortical spreading depression

Clinical Features

1. Recurrent attacks (defined as >5 episodes per year)
2. Headache can be unilateral or bilateral and it is pulsating and throbbing in nature
3. Nausea/vomiting
4. Photophobia/Phonophobia
5. Aggravation by physical movements like walking, climbing, etc.

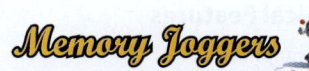

For diagnosis of migraine POUND Mnemonic is used:
P – Pulsating headache
O – One day duration (4–72 hours)
U – Unilateral
N – Nausea
D – Disabling in character

Repeated attacks of headache lasting 4–72 hours in patients with a normal physical examination, no other reasonable cause for the headache and:

At least 2 of the following features:	Plus at least 1 of the following features:
• Unilateral pain • Throbbing pain • Aggravation by movement • Moderate or severe intensity	• Nausea/vomiting • Photophobia and phonophobia

Abortive Treatment for Migraine

- First line treatment for mild to moderate attacks is NSAIDS.
- Triptans are migraine-specific drugs that bind to serotonergic receptors. They are considered first-line therapy for moderate to severe migraine, or mild to moderate attacks unresponsive to nonspecific analgesics.

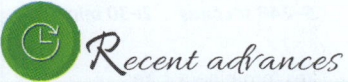

- Rizatriptan has a faster/quicker onset of action than sumatriptan.
- Rizatriptan and eletriptan are most efficacious.
- For severe migraine, prochlorperazine and dihydroergotamine are used intravenously.

Prophylaxis of Migraine

- Propranolol
- Flunarizine
- Gabapentin
- Pregabalin
- Amitriptyline.

Migraine Variants

Cluster Headache

Cluster headache is a rare form of primary headache.
- The pain is deep, usually retro-orbital, often excruciating in intensity, non-fluctuating and explosive in quality.
- A core feature of cluster headache is periodicity. At least one of the daily attacks of pain recurs at about the same hour each day for the duration of a cluster bout.
- The typical cluster headache patient has daily bouts of 1–2 attacks of relatively short-duration unilateral pain for 8–10 weeks in a year. This is usually followed by a pain-free interval that averages a little less than a year.

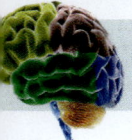

Clinical Features
1. Epiphora
2. Nasal stuffiness
3. Red eye (Bulbar congestion)
4. Attack duration: < 3 hours

Treatment
- Acute cluster headache:
    - *High flow oxygen at 12 L/min (First Line Treatment)*
    - Sumatriptan injection
    - Gabapentin/pregabalin
- Prophylaxis
    - Verapamil
    - Greater occipital nerve block.

Clinical features of the trigeminal autonomic cephalalgias

	Cluster Headache	SUNCT	Paroxysmal Hemicrania
Pain excruciating			
Type	Stabbing, boring	Burning/stabbing	Throbbing/boring, stabbing
Site	Orbit, temple	Periorbital	Orbit, temple
Attack frequency	1/alternate day–8/day	3–200/day Diagnosis requires ≥ 20 attacks	1–40/day (>5/day for more than half the time)
Duration of attack	15–180 min	5–240 seconds	2–30 min
Autonomic features	Yes	Yes (prominent conjunctival injection and lacrimation)	Yes
Active treatment	Sumatriptan *Oxygen inhalation*	Lidocaine (IV)	No effective treatment
Prophylactic treatment	*Short term prevention:* Prednisolone *Long term prevention:* Verapamil, Lithium	Lamotrigine Topiramate Gabapentin	Indomethacin

SUNCT = Short-lasting unilateral neuralgiform headache attack with Conjunctival injection and lacrimation

- Retro-orbital pain with nausea and vomiting for more than 6 hrs and vertically fixed, poorly reacting pupil indicates acute angle closure glaucoma
- Thunderclap headache indicates subarachnoid hemorrhage.

Basilar Migraine

Patients with basilar migraine (also known as **migraine with brainstem aura**) usually present with symptoms of vertebrobasilar insufficiency, which may precede a headache. The most common symptoms are dizziness and vertigo.

Ophthalmoplegic Migraine

This condition presents with pulsating headache *followed by* ipsilateral 3rd nerve palsy with rare involvement of 4th and 5th nerve. It presents with ipsilateral ptosis and squint. Diplopia is masked by presence of ptosis.

Familial Hemiplegic Migraine

It is a calcium channel defect. Family history of migraine is present with development of hemiparesis, lasting for days.

EPILEPSY

It is due to paroxysmal hypersynchronous discharge of cerebral neurons, which causes release of excitatory neurotransmitters like aspartate and glutamate. **Epilepsy** is a chronic condition characterized by *two or more unprovoked seizures*.
- Safest anti-epileptic drug in pregnancy: Lamotrigine > carbamazepine = topiramate > valproate > phenobarbitone (Reference: William Obstetrics Table 14.5).
- Best treatment for medically refractory seizures is surgery.
- **Status epilepticus:** Seizure lasting >30 minutes without spontaneous cessation or recurrent seizures without full return to consciousness interictally.
- **Generalized convulsive status epilepticus (GCSE)** is defined as convulsion lasting for *>5 minutes*.

Treatment of GCSE
- Start lorazepam/clonazepam.
- If it fails, then phenytoin/valproate levetiracetam are given.
- If the above steps fail, then the diagnosis is refractory SE and give IV midazolam and/or propofol.

- Most common type of seizures in neonates are subtle seizures.
- Most common type of seizures in children are febrile seizures.
- Most common type of seizures in <18 years is GTCS and occurs due to drug abuse.
- Most common cause of seizure in adults (>35 years) is cerebrovascular accident.
- Juvenile myoclonic epilepsy (Janz Syndrome) presents in adolescents, who in future years will develop GTCS.
- Most common epilepsy in children is benign rolandic epilepsy with DOC as carbamazepine.
- Serum prolactin levels are increased in post ictal state

AES Guidelines for Status Epilepticus

- **Stabilization phase** (0–5 minutes of seizure activity): During this phase, standard initial first aid for seizures (e.g., airway, breathing, circulation) should be initiated, after initial assessments and monitoring.
- **Initial therapy phase** (5–20 minutes of seizure activity): When it's clear the seizure requires medical intervention, a benzodiazepine that (specifically IM midazolam, IV lorazepam, or IV diazepam) is recommended as initial therapy.

- **Second therapy phase** (20–40 minutes of seizure activity): If seizures continue, reasonable options include IV fosphenytoin, valproic acid, or levetiracetam. If none of these is available, IV phenobarbital is a reasonable alternative.
- **Third therapy phase** (40+ minutes of seizure activity): There is no clear evidence to guide therapy in this phase. If the second therapy fails to stop the seizures, treatment considerations should include repeating second-line therapy or anesthetic doses of thiopental, midazolam, pentobarbital, or propofol (all with continuous EEG monitoring).

Difference between Seizures and Syncope

Characteristics	Seizures	Syncope
Time of onset	Day or night	Day
Position	Any	Upright, not recumbent
Onset	Sudden or brief	Gradual
Aura	Possible specific aura	Dizzy, blurring, lightheaded
Color of lips	Normal or cyanotic	Pallor
Autonomic features	Uncommon outside of ictus	Common; diaphoresis
Duration of tonus/clonus	30–60 seconds	<15 seconds
Incontinence	Common	Possible sometimes
Post-ictal	Occurs in tonic-clonic or complex partial	Rare
Motor activity	Common	Occasional brief jerks
Injury	(Common) tongue biting	Rare, unless from fall
Automatisms	Common in absence or complex partial	None
EEG	Normal or Abnormal	Normal
Duration of unconsciousness^Q	Minutes	Seconds

Generalized Tonic Clonic Seizures

- The patient is uneasy and irritable, hours before the attack (premonitory symptoms).
- **Tonus**: 10–30 secs.
- **Clonus**: 1–5 minutes, Violent jerking of limbs, tongue bite, incontinence.
- **Post-ictal deficit**: Unconsciousness, flaccid limbs, corneal reflexes, extensor plantars for a few hours.

Absence Seizures/Petit Mal Epilepsy

- Usual age of presentation is at 5 yrs.
- Patient presents with vacant staring spells and become unresponsive for few seconds. During the attack muscle tone is normal.
- Tonus and clonus are absent, consciousness is preserved and post-ictal deficit is absent.
- **EEG finding: 3/sec spike and slow wave pattern^Q**.
- Attack can be precipitated by hyperventilation and photic stimulation.

Myoclonic Seizures/Janz Syndrome

- Involuntary movements involve few muscles or a group of muscles, and is called myoclonus.
- Usual age of presentation is around 10–19 years, and occur as early morning attacks.
- EEG-findings: 4–6 Hz **poly-spike activity^Q**.

Focal Seizures

- **Motor**: Activity arises in precentral gyrus causing partial seizures affecting contralateral arm and trunk. Sometimes, the attack begins in one part like mouth, thumb, great toe, followed by gradual spread of neurons called **Jacksonian epilepsy**. Prolonged episodes are associated with paresis of involved limbs called **TODD's palsy**.
- **Sensory**: Activity arises in postcentral gyrus causing electrical tingling sensation.
- **Versive**: Frontal epileptic focus with conjugate deviation of eyes.
- **Visual**: Characterized by visual hallucinations of faces, images, etc.
- **Psychomotor**:
    - Alterations of mood, memory, perception (called temporal lobe epilepsy).
    - Associated with:
        - Déjà vu [undue familiarity]
        - Jamai vu [being unfamiliar with a person or situation]
        - Complex hallucinations of sound, smell and taste
        - Automatic movements like lip smacking.

Aura is *not* seen in G.T.C.S. It is a feature of focal seizures.

Drugs of Choice for Epilepsy

Seizure type	Drug of choice
Atonic/Myoclonic/Absence seizures	Valproate
Febrile seizures (episode)	Intranasal midazolam/ rectal diazepam
Prophylaxis of febrile seizures	Oral clobazam
Infantile spasm	ACTH
Infantile spasm in Tuberous sclerosis	Vigabatrin
Status epilepticus	Lorazepam
Refractory status epilepticus	Midazolam
GTCS	Lamotrigine, valproate and levetiracetam
Female patient with epilepsy	Levetiracetam lamotrigine

Source: Harrison 20th edition, pg 3064

Rare Epilepsy Syndromes

Mesial Temporal Lobe Epilepsy (MTLE)
- It is the most common syndrome associated with focal dyscognitive features and is an example of an epilepsy syndrome with distinctive clinical, electroencephalographic and pathologic features.
- These patients have a past history of febrile seizures in childhood (atypical variety usually) with family history of epilepsy. Subsequently, these patients present with focal seizures with complex automatisms.
- EEG shows unilateral or bilateral anterior temporal spikes on EEG.
- High-resolution MRI can detect the characteristic hippocampal sclerosis that appears to be essential in the pathophysiology of MTLE for many patients. Recognition of this syndrome is especially important *because it tends to be refractory to treatment with anticonvulsants but responds extremely well to surgical intervention.*[Q]

Lennox-Gastaut Syndrome
- It occurs in children and is defined by the following triad:
  1. Multiple types (usually including generalized tonic-clonic, atonic, and atypical absence seizure)
  2. *EEG showing slow (2.5 Hz) spike-and-wave discharges*[Q] and a variety of other abnormalities
  3. Impaired cognitive function in most but not all cases.
- Lennox-Gastaut syndrome is associated with CNS disease or dysfunction from a variety of causes, including developmental abnormalities, perinatal hypoxia/ischemia, trauma, infection, and other acquired lesions.
- The multifactorial nature of this syndrome suggests that it is a nonspecific response of the brain to diffuse neural injury.

Juvenile Myoclonic Epilepsy (JME)
- It is a generalized seizure disorder of unknown cause that appears in early adolescence and is usually characterized by bilateral myoclonic jerks that may be single or repetitive.
- Myoclonus is most frequent in the morning after awakening and can be provoked by sleep deprivation.
- Consciousness is preserved unless the myoclonus is especially severe. Many patients also experience generalized tonic-clonic seizures, and up to one-third have absence of seizures. Although complete remission is relatively uncommon, they respond well to appropriate anticonvulsant medication.

Lafora Disease/ Progressive Myoclonic Epilepsy
- Fragmentary, symmetric, or generalized myoclonus and/or generalized tonic-clonic seizures.
- Visual hallucinations (occipital seizures).
- Progressive neurologic degeneration including cognitive and/or behavioral deterioration, dysarthria, ataxia and at later stages, spasticity and dementia.
- Slowing of background activity, loss of α-rhythm and sleep features, and photosensitivity on early EEGs
- Periodic acid Schiff-positive intracellular inclusion bodies (Lafora bodies) on skin biopsy.
- Normal MRI of the brain at onset

Unverricht-Lundborg Disease
- It is a neurodegenerative disorder characterized by onset from the age of 6 – 15 years, stimulus-sensitive myoclonus, and tonic-clonic epileptic seizures.

PARKINSONISM

- Parkinson's disease (PD) is the second most common neurodegenerative disease, exceeded only by Alzheimer's disease (AD).
- Pathologically, the hallmark features of PD are degeneration of dopaminergic neurons in the substantia nigra pars compacta (SNc), reduced striatal dopamine and intracytoplasmic proteinaceous inclusions known as Lewy bodies.
- Among the different forms of Parkinsonism, PD is the most common (approximately 75% of cases). Historically, PD was diagnosed based on the presence of two of three parkinsonian features (tremor, rigidity and bradykinesia).
- Clinicopathologic correlation studies subsequently determined that Parkinsonism associated with rest tremor, asymmetry and a good response to levodopa was more likely to predict the correct pathologic diagnosis. With these revised criteria (known as **the UK Brain Bank Criteria**), the clinical diagnosis of PD is confirmed pathologically in 99% of cases.

Causes of Parkinsonism
1. Parkinson's disease is caused due to genetic or sporadic reasons (Most common cause of parkinsonism)
2. **Secondary Parkinsonism**
   - Drugs (Anti-psychotics)
   - Tumors
   - Infections
   - Toxins: Manganese, carbon monoxide and carbon disulfide
   - Liver failure
   - **Normal pressure hydrocephalus**[Q]
3. **Atypical Parkinsonism**
   - Multiple system atrophy (Shy Dragger syndrome)
   - Progressive supranuclear gaze palsy
   - Corticobasilar degeneration.

Other diseases having Parkinsonism-like features
- Wilson's disease
- Huntington's chorea
- Neurodegeneration with brain iron accumulation.

> - Progressive supranuclear gaze palsy has damage at superior colliculus leading to impaired downward gaze. This explains repeated falls and spilling of food while eating. EOG reveals involuntary movements called "square wave Jerks".
> - Multiple system atrophy presents with autonomic symptoms or cerebellar symptoms.

Clinical Features

Cardinal features	Other motor features (Non-dopaminergic features)	Non-motor features
Bradykinesia	Micrographia	Anosmia
Resting tremor (Most common)	Masked facies	Sensory disturbances (like pain)
Rigidity	Reduced eye blink	Mood disorders (like depression)
Festinating Gait/ postural instability	Soft voice	Sleep disturbances
	Dysphagia	Autonomic disturbances
	Freezing	Orthostatic hypotension
		Gastrointestinal disturbances
		Genitourinary disturbances
		Sexual dysfunction
		Cognitive impairment

(Anosmia precedes development of motor symptoms by 4 years).

Investigations

Imaging of the brain dopamine system in PD with positron emission tomography (PET) or single-photon emission computed tomography shows reduced uptake of striatal dopaminergic markers, particularly in the posterior putamen.

Imaging can be useful in difficult cases or research studies but is rarely necessary in routine practice, as the diagnosis can usually be established on clinical criteria alone.

- Freezing phenomenon in Parkinsonism is seen with degeneration of noradrenergic locus coeruleus.
- Levodopa is absolutely contraindicated in melanoma

Management

- **Levodopa** is routinely administered in combination with a **peripheral decarboxylase inhibitor** to prevent its peripheral metabolism to dopamine and the development of nausea and vomiting due to activation of dopamine receptors in the area postrema that are not protected by the BBB.

  Acute dopaminergic side effects include nausea, vomiting, and orthostatic hypotension. These are usually transient and can generally be avoided by gradual titration
- Initial **dopamine agonists** were ergot derivatives (e.g., bromocriptine, pergolide, cabergoline) and were associated with ergot-related side effects, including cardiac valvular damage. *They have largely been replaced by a second generation of non-ergot dopamine agonists (e.g., pramipexole, ropinirole, rotigotine)*
- *Rotigotine* is administered as a once-daily transdermal patch.
- **Apomorphine** is a dopamine agonist with efficacy comparable to levodopa, but it must be administered parenterally and has a very short half-life and duration of activity (45 min). It is generally administered SC as a rescue agent for the treatment of severe "off" episodes
- **Inhibitors of monoamine oxidase type B (MAO-B)** block central dopamine metabolism and increase synaptic concentrations of the neurotransmitter. Selegiline and rasagiline are relatively selective suicide inhibitors of the MAO-B enzyme
- When levodopa is administered with a decarboxylase inhibitor, it is primarily metabolized by **catechol-O-methyltransferase (COMT)**. Inhibitors of COMT increase the elimination half-life of levodopa and enhance its brain availability. Combining levodopa with a COMT inhibitor reduces "off" time and prolongs "on" time in fluctuating patients, while enhancing motor scores
- Most surgical procedures for PD performed today utilize **deep brain stimulation (DBS).** Here, an electrode is placed into the target area and connected to a stimulator inserted SC over the chest wall. DBS simulates the effects of a lesion without necessitating a brain lesion.
- **DBS for PD primarily targets the STN or the GPi.** It provides dramatic results, particularly with respect to "off" time and dyskinesias, but *does not improve features that fail to respond to levodopa and does not prevent the development or progression of nondopaminergic features such as freezing, falling, and dementia*

MRI Brain Findings
- Tigroid appearance on MRS: Pelizaeus merzbacher
- Face of panda appearance: Wilson's disease
- Eye of tiger sign: Pantothenate kinase associated neuro-degenerative/neurodegeneration in brain with iron accumulation
- Hot cross bun sign: Multiple system atrophy
- Humming bird sign: Progressive supranuclear gaze palsy

Clinical Features of Localized Cerebral Lesions

Parietal lobe lesions	**Dominant Parietal Lobe** 1. Acalculia 2. Alexia 3. Finger agnosia 4. Right-left confusion 5. Agraphia 6. Aphasia 7. Dyslexia 8. Homonymous hemianopia **Nondominant parietal lobe** 1. Neglect 2. Apraxia [constructional and dressing apraxia]
Temporal lobe lesions	**Nondominant temporal lobe lesion** 1. Prosopagnosia 2. Disturbed memory 3. Disturbed sense of smell 4. Complex hallucinations 5. Homonymous hemianopia **Dominant temporal lobe lesion** 1. Wernicke's aphasia 2. Dyslexia 3. Word deafness

Contd...

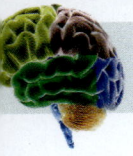

Frontal lobe lesions	1. Disinhibition 2. Lack of initiative 3. **Antisocial behavior** 4. Impaired memory 5. **Incontinence** 6. Grasp reflex 7. Anosmia 8. **Abulia/ Broca's aphasia** 9. **Gait apraxia/ magnetic gait**
Occipital lobe lesions	1. Visual hallucinations 2. Palinopsia 3. Asimultagnosia 4. Visual agnosia 5. Homonymous hemianopia 6. Prosopagnosia

* *Prosopagnosia is due to interruption of fibers from occipital cortex to centers where memory of faces is stored (pg 125, Bradley Neurology 2015 ed)*

Blood supply to brain

Area of brain	Blood supply
Thalamus	Branches of post communicating and basilar artery
Midbrain	Postcerebral artery P1 segment
Pons	Basilar artery
Medulla	Vertebral artery
Cerebellum	Superior cerebellar, and inferior cerebellar, post. inferior cerebellar artery
Internal capsule	Anterior limb: Lenticulostriate branch of MCA (superior half) + Recurrent artery of Hebneur (inferior half) Posterior limb: Lenticulostriate branch of MCA (superior half) + Anterior choroidal A (inferior half) Genu: Lenticulostriate branch of middle cerebral artery

STROKE

- It is defined as sudden onset of neurological deficits of vascular basis lasting longer than 24 hours.
- **Transient Ischemic Attack (TIA):** Sudden onset of neurological deficits of a vascular basis that resolves after a brief period within 24 hours.
- **Reversible Ischemic Neurological Deficit (RIND or minor stroke):** Sudden onset of neurological deficits of vascular basis lasting >24 hours that resolve completely or near completely within 72 hours.

Risk of Stroke following TIA: The ABCD2 Score

Clinical Factor	Score
Age ≥ 60 years	1
SBP > 140 mm Hg or DBP > 90 mm Hg	1
Clinical symptoms Unilateral weakness Speech disturbance without weakness	2 1
TIA duration > 60 minutes 10-59	2 1
Diabetes (oral medications or insulin)	1
Total score	7
More the ABCD2 score more is the likelihood of 3-month rate of stroke (%)	

Stroke Syndromes According to Vascular Territory

- **ACA:** Contralateral paresis and sensory loss, loss of bladder control (hypertonic detrusor)
- **MCA:** Proximal occlusion involves all of the below findings:
  - *Superior division:* Contralateral face and arm paresis and sensory loss, Broca's (expressive) aphasia
  - *Inferior division:* Contralateral homonymous hemianopsia (esp. inferiorly), contralateral graphesthesia and astereognosis, anisognosia, contralateral neglect, Wernicke's (receptive) aphasia
- **Internal carotid:** Transient monocular blindness (amaurosis fugax)
- **PCA:**
  - *Parinaud syndrome:*[Q] Difficulty in looking upward with pseudo-Argyl Robertson pupils.
  - *Claude's syndrome:*[Q] Ipsilateral 3rd nerve palsy, contralateral resting tremors and contralateral ataxia.
  - *Weber's syndrome:*[Q] Ipsilateral 3rd nerve palsy and contralateral hemiplegia
  - Cortical blindness or prosopagnosia (occlusion of P_2 segment of PCA)
- Cortical blindness is blindness with preserved pupillary light reflex. The patient is unaware of blindness and deny it (Anton syndrome). Some islands of central vision are preserved with loss of peripheral vision. This is called as "**gun barrel vision**".
- **Basilar artery:**
  - *Millard Gubler syndrome:* Ipsilateral 6th, 7th nerve palsy with contralateral hemiplegia

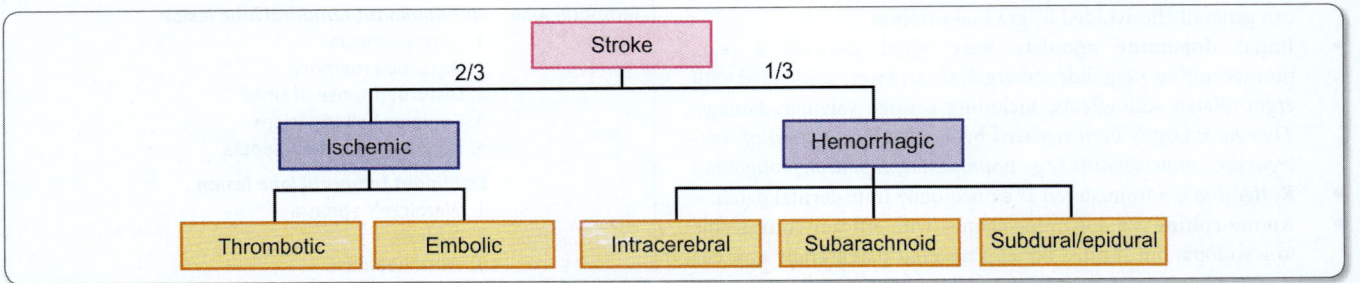

Types of stroke

- **PICA (Lateral Medullary syndrome or Wallenburg Syndrome):**^{Q}
  - Ipsilateral ataxia
  - Ipsilateral Horner's syndrome
  - Ipsilateral facial sensory loss
  - Contralateral limb impairment of pain and temperature
  - Nystagmus, vertigo, N/V
  - Dysphagia, dysarthria, hiccup

Distinct Clinical Syndromes Associated with Lacunar Infarcts

- **Pure motor hemiparesis**
  - Most common **lacunar syndrome.**^{Q}
  - Results from infarction of contralateral internal capsule (may also be seen with infarcts in corona radiata and pons)
  - The face, arms and legs are equally affected.
  - There is no sensory loss, homonymous hemianopia, aphasia or hemineglect.
- **Pure sensory stroke**
  - **Infarction almost always involves the thalamus.**^{Q}
  - Sensory loss is present throughout the contralateral side.
  - Sensation is usually decreased for all sensory modalities, and no other neurologic deficits are present.
  - Patient often complains of abnormal spontaneous sensation, such as "pins-and-needles" or skin tightness.
- **Anterior choroidal artery stroke**^{Q}
  - This artery arises from the internal carotid artery.
  - It supplies the posterior limb of the internal capsule and the white matter posterolateral to it, through which pass some of the geniculocalcarine fibers.
  - The complete syndrome of anterior choroidal artery occlusion consists of:

    > 1. Contralateral hemiplegia
    > 2. Hemianesthesia (hypesthesia)
    > 3. Homonymous hemianopia

  - However, because this territory is also supplied by penetrating vessels of the proximal MCA and posterior communication and posterior choroidal arteries, *minimal deficits may occur*, and patients frequently recover substantially.
- **Balint syndrome:**^{Q} Seen in patients who recovered after CPR due to damage in parieto-occipital area.
  - Inability to perceive the visual field as a whole **(asimultagnosia)**^{Q}
  - Difficulty in fixating the eyes (oculomotor apraxia)
  - Inability to move the hand to a specific object by using vision **(optic ataxia).**^{Q}

- Ocular bobbing has fast downward and slow upward movement of eyes. It is seen in bilateral pontine lesion.
- Ocular dipping has slow downward and fast upward movement of eyes. It is seen in diffused critical anoxic damage.

Etiology of Ischemic Stroke

1. **Thrombosis:** Stepwise deficits, preceded by TIAs
2. **Embolic Stroke:** Abrupt onset, no warning TIA; maximal at onset; multifocal if it is of cardiac origin; seizure more likely.

Conditions Associated with Increased Risk of Cerebral Ischemia

- **Vascular disorders:** Atherosclerosis, vasculitis, SLE, syphilis, AIDS, carotid or vertebral dissection, drug abuse (cocaine, amphetamines, heroin), migraines, venous or sinus thrombosis, lacunar infarcts (due to chronic HTN)
- **Cardiac disorders:** Mural thrombus, rheumatic heart disease, arrhythmia, endocarditis, mitral valve prolapse, prosthetic heart valves
- **Hematologic disorders:** Thrombocytosis, polycythemia, sickle cell disease, leukocytosis, hypercoagulable states.

Hemorrhagic Stroke

Etiology

1. **Intracerebral (ICH):** Hypertension, amyloid angiopathy
2. **Subarachnoid (SAH):** Aneurysm, AVM
3. **Epidural/Subdural Hematoma**

Investigations

1. Blood investigations: CBC, ESR, VDRL, serum glucose, cholesterol and lipids
2. ECG
3. NCCT Head
4. Lumbar puncture (rule out subarachnoid hemorrhage)
5. Intra-arterial angiography or MRA (anterior circulation TIAs or dissection)
6. Carotid doppler or transcranial doppler
7. Echocardiography

Treatment for Stroke

1. **Surgical:** Decompression to prevent herniation if cerebellar hematoma or superficial hemorrhage of cerebral white matter
2. Antihypertensive to lower BP with Nicardipine up to 160/90 mm Hg
3. Corticosteroids for vasogenic edema
4. **Blood sugar:** Avoid hyperglycemia which will increase the infarct size
5. *Thrombolysis with reteplase (recombinant tissue plasminogen activator) within 4.5 hours of acute ischemic stroke onset (NINDS trial). The 4.5 hours window period is taken from onset of symptoms. Ideally thrombolysis done within 3 hrs produces better neurological outcomes.*
6. Carotid artery stenosis is managed with endarterectomy
7. Anti-platelet therapy is indicated for primary prevention
8. Hypercholesterolemia: Statins reduce the risk of stroke in patients with CAD or at high risk for cardiovascular events, even with normal cholesterol.
9. Mechanical thrombectomy can be done upto 8 hours of symptom onset. (Page 2562 : Harrison 19th)
10. **Malignant cerebral edema**^{Q} leading to midline shift requires hemicraniectomy.

Guidelines for Blood Pressure Control in Stroke
- Do not lower the blood pressure unless the hypertension is severe i.e. > 220/130 and lower to < 185/110, if thrombolysis is indicated.
- Antihypertensive therapy is withheld for at least 5 days after thromboembolic stroke unless there is acute MI, renal failure, aortic dissection, SBP above 220 mmHg or DBP above 120 mmHg.
- Most patients with an acute cerebral infarct are initially hypertensive and their BP will fall spontaneously within 1–2 days
- IV Nicardipine/Clevidipine or labetalol is usually first line, if needed.

Major syndromes

Name of syndrome	Site of lesions	Clinical features
Weber's	Anterior cerebral peduncle mid brain	• Ipsilateral 3rd palsy • Contralateral hemiplegia
Nothnagel	Superior cerebellar peduncle	• Ipsilateral 3rd nerve palsy • Contralateral cerebellar signs
Parinaud's	Dorsal mid brain tectum	• Vertical gaze palsy • Convergence disorders • Convergence retraction nystagmus • Pupillary and lid disorders
Millard Gubler's	Basilar artery involvement leading to lesion of the ventrocaudal pons	• Ipsilateral lateral rectus weakness due to cranial nerve VI fasicle and nucleus of 6th nerve is spared. • Ipsilateral peripheral facial paresis, due to cranial nerve VII involvement • Contralateral hemiplegia (sparing the face) due to pyramidal tract involvement
Wallenberg's	Lateral medulla	• Ipsilateral 5th, 8th, 9th, 10th, 11th nerve palsy • Ipsilateral Horner's syndrome • Ipsilateral cerebellar signs • Contralateral spinothalamic sensory loss • Vestibular disturbance

*Foville syndrome has same features as Millard Gubler syndrome except eye findings of lateral gaze palsy. Millard Gubler has lateral rectus weakness because abducens fasicle is damaged rather than the nucleus.

- Patient looks toward the side of lesion in cortical stroke.
- Patient looks away from lesion in Brain stem stroke.

SUBARACHNOID HEMORRHAGE (SAH)

- **Saccular (Berry) aneurysms** occur at the bifurcations of the large to medium-sized intracranial arteries. Rupture is into the subarachnoid space in the basal cisterns and often into the parenchyma of the adjacent brain.
- Approximately, 85% of aneurysms occur in the anterior circulation, mostly on the adjacent brain.
- As an aneurysm develops, it typically forms a neck with a dome. The length of the neck and the size of the dome vary greatly and are factors that are important in planning neurosurgical obliteration or endovascular embolization.
- The arterial internal elastic lamina disappears at the base of the neck.
- The media thins and connective tissue replaces smooth-muscle cells. At the site of rupture (most often the dome) the wall is thin, and the tear that allows bleeding is often <0.5 mm long.
- **Most common cranial nerve affected in *unruptured* berry aneurysm is 3rd nerve**
- Most common cause of death in SAH patients is **Vasospasm**.
- *Those >7 mm in diameter and those at the top of the basilar artery and at the origin of the posterior communicating artery are at the greatest risk of rupture.*

Grading Scales for Subarachnoid Hemorrhage

Grade	Hunt-Hess Scale^Q	World Federation of Neurosurgical Societies (WFNS) Scale
1	Mild headache, normal mental status, no cranial nerve or motor findings	GCS score 15, no motor deficits
2	Severe headache, normal mental status, may have cranial nerve deficit	GCS score 13–14, no motor deficits
3	Somnolent, confused, may have cranial nerve or mild motor deficit	GCS score 13–14, with motor deficits
4	Stupor, moderate to severe motor deficit, may have intermittent reflex posturing	GCS score 7–12, with or without motor deficits
5	Coma, reflex posturing or flaccid	GCS score 3–6, with or without motor deficits

Investigations in Subarachnoid Hemorrhage

1. **Noncontrast CT scan**: Investigation of choice (LP is not indicated prior to imaging procedure). Blood is seen in the Sylvian fissure. (Source: middle cerebral artery)
2. **CSF examination:**
   - Hallmark is bloody CSF
   - **Xanthochromic CSF**: Lysis of RBCs and Subsequent conversion of Hb to bilirubin stains the spinal fluid yellow within 6-12 hours. Peaks at 48 hours and lasts for 1–4 weeks.
   - MR angiography: For unruptured aneurysm.
3. ECG shows prolonged QT interval and can exhibit findings of MI (due to catecholamine surge).
4. **Serum sodium:** Reduced due to natriuresis caused by release of B-type natriureteric peptide.

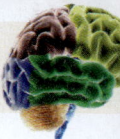

Treatment

1. Airway protection and BP control.
2. Prevent vasospasm: Nimodipine, (drug of choice). It can cause hypotension. Hence, fluids should be given to mantain CPP of 60–80 mm Hg.
3. Judicious use of vasopressors like phenylephrine and norepinephrine. Treatment with hypertension and hypervolemia requires monitoring of arterial and central venous pressure.
4. Vasodilation by direct angioplasty. Verapamil, nicardipine and papaverine are also used.
5. Endovascular coiling *(Treatment of choice for unruptured Berry aneurysm).*

CADASIL (**C**erebral **A**utosomal **D**ominant **A**rteriopathy with **S**ubcortical **I**nfarcts and **L**eucoencephelopathy) occurs due to defect in Notch-3 gene.

COMA AND BRAIN DEATH

GCS-P Score

Eye opening	Scores	Verbal response	Scores	Motor activity	Scores
Spontaneous	4	Orientation	5	Obeys commands	6
To speech	3	Confused	4	Localizes pain	5
To pain	2	Inappropriate words	3	Normal flexion	4
Nil	1	Incomprehensible sounds	2	Abnormal flexion	3
		Nil	1	Extensor response	2
				Nil	1

Pupil Reactivity Score

Pupil unreactive to light	Pupil reactivity score
Both pupil	2
One pupil	1
Neither pupil	0

*Higher score is assigned to non reactive score
*No longer recommended to assigned 1 point to non testable elements. Any element that is non testable should be marked as NT.

Tests for Confirming Brain Death

Presence of irreversible coma with
1. **All brain stem reflexes are absent.**
2. Pupils are fixed, unreactive to light.
3. Corneal reflexes are absent.
4. Vestibulocochlear reflexes are absent.
5. No motor response to cranial nerve distribution.
6. No gag or suction reflex.
7. No respiratory movement after patient disconnected from ventilator long enough to allow carbon dioxide to rise above threshold for $pCO_2 > 50$ mm Hg.
(Spinal reflexes can be elicited in brain dead patients. Spontaneous twitching movements of fingers and toes may be seen)

LMNL	UMNL/ pyramidal tract lesion/ corticospinal lesion
Superficial reflexes absent	Superficial reflexes are absent
Deep tendon reflexes absent/areflexia	Deep tendon reflexes brisk

Clinical Features of Extrapyramidal Lesions

Features	Lesion
Rigidity	Substantia nigra
Resting Tremors	Substantia nigra
Hypokinesia	Substantia nigra
Chorea	Caudate nucleus
Hemiballismus	Subthalamic nuclei
Dystonia, atheotosis	Globus pallidus

BASIC NEUROLOGY

Differences between LMNL and UMNL

LMNL	UMNL/ pyramidal tract lesion/ corticospinal lesion
Weakness of muscles	Loss of voluntary movements and fine movements
Hypotonia	Spasticity
Flexor plantars	Extensor plantar reflexes
Wasting/ fasciculations	No wasting

Cerebellar Lesions

Lesions like tumors, trauma, and infections can have multitude of presentations of cerebellar lesions
- Intentional tremors/ head tilt/head tremors
- Dysmetria /past pointing
- Dysdiadochokinesia (breaking up of complex movements)
- Ataxia with leaning towards sign of lesion
- Dysarthria (staccato speech)

Contd...

- Nystagmus
- Hypotonia
- *Pendular knee jerk*[Q].

- Gait ataxia occurs due to damage of **palaeocerebellum**
- Do not confuse with Gait APRAXIA which is seen with Frontal lobe damage (MAGNETIC GAIT)
- Trucal ataxia occurs due to damage of **archicerebellum**.
- Limb ataxia occurs due to damage of **neocerebellum**.

Segmental Supply of Tendon Reflexes

Deep tendon reflex	Lesion at
Trapezius	Spinal accessory nerve and $C_{1,2}$
Biceps	$C_{5,6}$ **(Musculocutaneous nerve)**[Q]
Brachioradialis	$C_{5,6}$ (Radial nerve)
Triceps	C_7 (Radial nerve)
Finger flexors	$C_{6,7,8}$ and T_1
Knee jerk	$L_{2,3,4}$ (Femoral nerve)
Ankle	S_1 **(Medial popliteal nerve)**[Q]

Monosynaptic Reflexes

Stapedial reflex[Q]	VIII, VII
Jaw jerk	V, V
Corneal reflex	V, VII
Plantar [extension of great toe, abduction of toes]	S_1
Abdominal reflexes	T_6–T_{12}
Cremasteric reflex	L_1
Bulbocavernous	S_{2-3}
Anal reflex[Q]	S_4–S_5

*Beevor sign is displacement of umbilicus on elicitation of abdominal reflexes in spinal cord lesions

Cranial Nerve Lesions

Lesions of III, IV and VI Cranial Nerves

3, 4, 6 cranial nerves lesions lead to pupillary abnormalities
Various disorders of cranial nerves

Disorder	Defect	Light reflex	Consensual light reflex	Accommodation/ light reflex
Optic neuritis	Afferent defect	Light reflex is impaired	Consensual light reflex is impaired	Near reflex absent
Argyl Robertson pupil	Neurosyphilis	Light reflex is impaired	Consensual light reflex normal	Near reflex present
Horner's syndrome	Cervical sympathetic chain	Light reflex is impaired	Consensual light reflex normal	Normal

- Argyl Robertson pupil is ALSO seen in (apart from neurosyphilis):
  - Diabetes mellitus
  - Multiple sclerosis
  - Sarcoidosis
  - Syringobulbia.
- Reversed Argyl Robertson pupil is seen in **encephalitis lethargica**.[Q]
- Site of lesion in Argyl Robertson pupil is pretectum of midbrain.
- Marcus Gunn Pupil is seen in multiple sclerosis and optic nerve meningioma.

Fifth Nerve Lesion: Trigeminal Neuralgia

- Paroxysms of sharp lancinating pain in region of trigeminal sensory divisions.
- Pain sets off by washing, shaving, tooth cleaning, eating, talking, and exposure to cold.
- The paroxysms of pain may last a few seconds; repetitive, dull ache; spontaneous remissions. No motor or sensory signs.
- DOC is carbamazepine

Remember
- Mobius syndrome has presentation of congenital bilateral seventh nerve palsy with sometimes third and sixth nerve palsy too. It is associated with periconceptional intake of misoprostol.
- Bitemporal inferior quadrantopia is seen with craniopharyngioma.

Seventh Nerve Lesion: Bell's Palsy

The nerve is damaged in facial canal and constitutes lower motor neuron type of lesion.

Etiology
Idiopathic/ viral/ trauma/ cold exposure/ vascular damage

Clinical Features
- Subacute onset in a few hours.
- It is associated with pain in face/around ear followed by loss of movement on one side of face. *The mouth deviates to the healthy side.*
- Taste in anterior 2/3rd of tongue is diminished.
- Hyperacusis.
- Drooling of saliva/ failure to close eyes as it is attempted. Instead there may be upward deviation of eyes when the patient tries to close it (Bell's sign).

Occipitofrontalis muscle of face, responsible for wrinkling on forehead has bilateral innervations from facial nerve of both sides. Hence wrinkling on the forehead is preserved in UMN lesion of the 7th nerve.

- Clonus is grade 4 DTR
- Root value of stapedial reflex is (8, 7)
- Wartenberg reflex is equivalent of Balbinski sign in case of amputation of both lower limbs.

Bulbar Palsy and Pseudobulbar Palsy

Bulbar palsy is caused by lower motor neuron lesions of cranial nerves: IX, X, XII
- Palatal and pharyngeal muscle weakness
- Tongue weakness, which leads to tongue deviation on protrusion to same side of lesion
- Dysarthria
- Absent gag reflex.

Pseudobulbar palsy occurs due to damage to corticobulbar fibers supplying the cranial nerves. V, VII, IX, X, XII
- The gag reflex is brisk.
- Tongue is spastic causing spastic dysarthria.
- The tongue deviates to opposite side of lesion on tongue protrusion.
- Brisk jaw jerk.
- **Donald duck voice**[Q] (As if patient is trying to sequence out words from tight lips).
- Emotional lability

INFECTIONS OF THE CNS

Most Common Causes of Bacterial Meningitis

Age group	Predominant causative organism
Neonate (global)	Group B streptococci
Neonate (India)	*Klebsiella> S.aureus> E. coli*
Child	Pneumococcus
Adult	Pneumococcus
Adults (Epidemic situations)	N. meningitidis

CSF Parameters of Common CNS Infections

Manifestation in	Pressure	Color	Cells	Sugar	Protein
Normal	10–20 mm Hg	Clear	0–4 lymphocytes/mm^3	2/3 blood sugar	15–45 mg%
Pyogenic meningitis	Increased	Turbid	Increased >1000 cells polymorphs/mm^3	Decreased	Increased
TBM	Increased	Straw coloured	Increased cells 100 – 1,000 cells /mm^3 (predominantly lymphocytes)	Decreased	Increased up to 100 mg%
Viral meningitis	Normal	Clear	Increased cells >25 lymphocytes/cu.mm	Normal	Normal

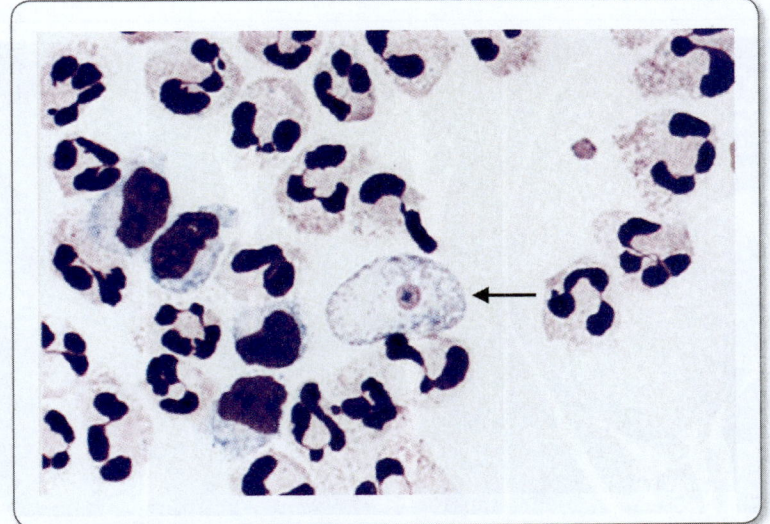

Slide showing neutrophils, monocytes and Trophozoites of Naegleria in CSF preparation

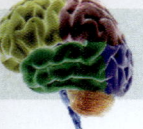

- Mollaret meningitis (recurrent meningitis): It is an aseptic meningitis called benign recurrent lymphocytic meningitis. CSF shows large endothelial cells and PMN.
- Most common cause of meningitis in AIDS patients is *Cryptococcus neoformans*.
- CSF electrophoresis is done in multiple sclerosis showing presence of oligoclonal IgG bands.
- Most common cause of viral encephalitis is Herpes simplex.
- Most common cause of viral encephalitis in India is Japanese B encephalitis.

Herpes Virus Encephalitis

- HSE results from primary HSV-1 infection, predominantly occurring under the age of 18; or over 50 years of age.
- HSE is thought to be caused by the retrograde transmission of virus from a peripheral site on the face following HSV-1 reactivation, along a nerve axon, to the brain.
- The virus lies dormant in the ganglion of the trigeminal cranial nerve. *The olfactory nerve may also be involved in HSE, which may explain its predilection for the temporal lobes of the brain, as olfactory nerve sends branches there.*
- Without treatment, HSE results in rapid death in approximately 70% of cases.
- Lumbar puncture shows bloody CSF
- MRI shows frontal and temporal lobe enhancement.
- EEG shows *periodic lateralized epileptiform discharge known as PLED*

- Empirical acyclovir treatment should be started on admission.

- Whenever MCQ mentions fever with irrelevant talking or altered sensorium without meningeal signs, Acyclovir should be the first line of treatment pending a PCR CSF for herpes.

Neurocysticercosis

- Most common central nervous system parasitic infection; occurs due to larval stage (cysticercosis cellulosae) lodging in the brain.
- **Most common presentation of Neurocysticercosis is Seizures.**
- Parenchymal brain calcifications are the most common findings on NCCT.
- These cysts are located in the following order of frequency in:
  - CNS (neurological manifestations are the most common)
  - Subcutaneous tissue (Rice grain calcification)
  - Striated muscle
  - Globe of the eye.
- **Most common sites of Neurocysticercosis :** Parenchymatous> interventricular> subarachnoid> spinal> orbital.
- MC presentation is focal seizures

Stages of NCC
- **Vesicular:** Cyst with eccentric scolex.
- **Colloidal:** Cyst contracts, walls have focal lymphoid nodules and scolex converted to mineralized granules.
- **Granular nodular:** Granulation tissue laid down
- **Nodular calcified:** Calcification and subsides edema

Investigation

1. On MRI, scolex is hyperintense of isointense relative to white matter.
2. Mostly it is described as SSECTL (single, small contrast enhancing CT lesion).
3. Calcified lesion appear hypointense on all MRI gradient echo acquisitions.

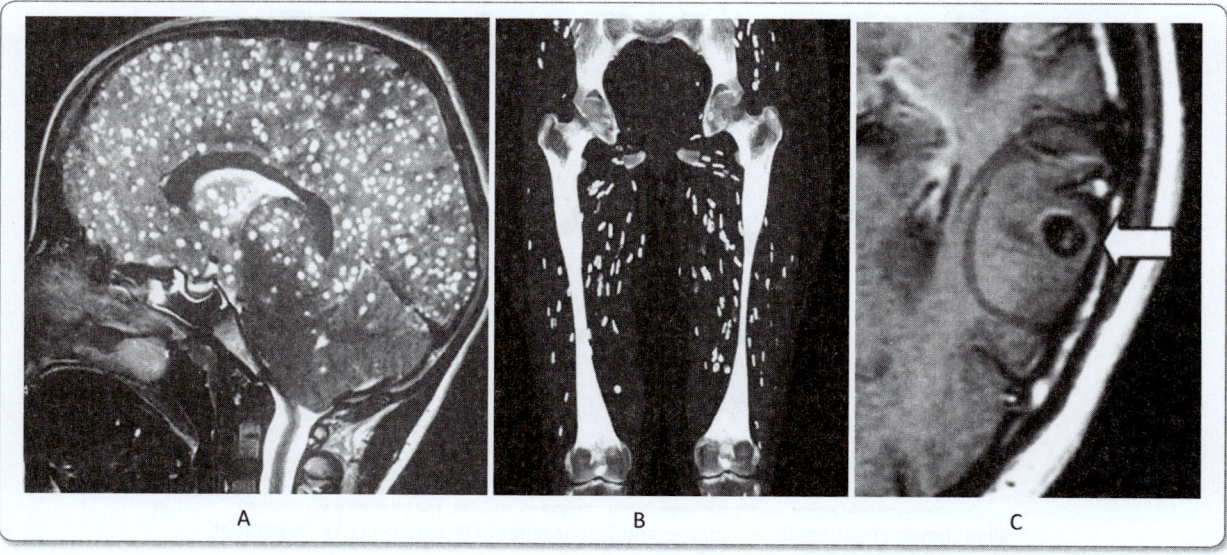

A-Starry sky appearance on MRI head seen in NCC
B- Rice grain calcification seen due to dead larva in cysticercosis
C- Vesicular lesion with central white dot in NCC

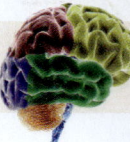

Treatment

- Niclosamide is ineffective for neurocysticercosis.
- Albendazole and praziquantel are both effective in treatment.
- **DOC is albendazole (8–28 days)**.
- Anticonvulsants (antiepileptics) should be given during drug treatment and probably for an indefinite time afterwards.
- Corticosteroids are used during the acute phase of cysticercotic encephalitis, if intracranial hypertension is present. (It is used for the prevention of development of hydrocephalus, and does not have much role once hydrocephalus is already present.)

TUMORS OF BRAIN

- Most common brain tumor is secondaries (oat cell Ca lung, Ca breast, malignant melanoma).
- Most common malignant brain tumor is glioma.
- Most common benign brain tumor is meningioma.
- Most common cause of leptomeningeal metastasis is Ca breast.
- **From question perspective, remember:**
  Incidence of metastasis: Meningioma>>Astrocytoma.

Pediatric Brain Tumors

- Most common malignant brain tumor in children is medulloblastoma.
- Brain tumor with worst prognosis in children is brain stem glioma.
- Most common benign brain tumor in children is craniopharyngioma.
- Brain tumor that can be visualized on X-ray skull is Cranio-pharyngioma (due to calcification).

Hereditary Syndromes Associated with Brain Tumors

Syndrome	Nervous system neoplasms
Neurofibromatosis type 1 (von Recklinghausen's disease)	Optic glioma
Neurofibromatosis type 2	Schwannoma
Tuberous sclerosis	Astrocytoma
Von Hippel-Lindau	Hemangioblastoma of retina, cerebellum and spinal cord; pheochromocytoma
Li-Fraumeni	Malignant glioma
Retinoblastoma	Pineoblastoma, malignant glioma
Turcot	Medulloblastoma, malignant glioma
Gorlin (basal cell nevus syndrome)	Medulloblastoma

Clinical Features

Increased intracranial tension
- Headache
- Nausea, vomiting
- Papilledema/ seizures/ cranial nerve palsies/ epilepsy.

Examination

1. Bradycardia. hypertension (Cushing reflex)
2. Pupillary signs like ipsilateral pupillary dilatation.
3. **Kernohan Woltman sign**^{Q} (Ipsilateral Hemiparesis) due to pressure on crus cerebri and is a false localizing sign.

Investigations

1. IOC is Gadolinium-enhanced MRI
2. Cerebral angiography.
3. Stereotactic surgery: Best suited for isolated lesions in the brain

Management

- Dexamethasone: For cerebral edema
- Chemotherapy: Temozolomide
- Radiation: Best suited for metastasis of brain

Normal Pressure Hydrocephalus

Characterized by Intermittent increase in pressure at night
- *Dementia, ataxia, incontinence (Triad)* and gait apraxia is seen
  Management: Acetazolamide and VP shunting
- Fisher test is done in NPH where 25-40 cc of CSF is withdrawn. The gait of the patient before and after withdrawl of CSF is compared. The benefit in gait improvement persists for several weeks.

Pseudotumor Cerebri

- Idiopathic in young obese females
- Seen in children with hypervitaminosis A
- The pressure in ventricles is increased but the ventricular size is normal unlike hydrocephalus where both ventricular size and pressure are increased

DEMYELINATING DISORDERS

Affecting brain mainly with some component affecting PNS	Affecting peripheral nervous system exclusively
• Multiple sclerosis • Acute disseminated encephalomyelitis • Tabes dorsalis • Vitamin B12 deficiency • Central pontine myelinosis • Leukodystrophies	• Guillain-Barré syndrome • Chronic inflammatory demyelinating polyneuropathy (CIDP) • Charcot Marie tooth disease • Copper deficiency

Multiple Sclerosis

Immune-mediated inflammatory disease that attacks myelinated axons in the central nervous system, *destroying the myelin and the axon in variable degrees* and producing significant physical disability within 20–25 years in more than 30% of patients. The hallmark of MS is symptomatic episodes that occur months or years apart and affect different anatomic locations.

Clinical Patterns of MS

1. Relapsing remitting (RRMS): 85% (most common type)
2. Primary progressive (PPMS): rare, most severe, no therapy available
3. Progressive relapsing (PRMS)
4. Secondary progressive (SPMS)

* RRMS can become SPMS

MS Variants

- **Devic's disease/neuromyelitis optica (NMO):** Severe optic neuritis and extensive transverse myelitis extending >3 vertebral segments
- **Clinically isolated syndrome (CIS):** Single MS-like episode
- **Fulminant MS (Marburg):** Rapidly progressive and fatal MS associated with severe axonal damage, inflammation and necrosis.

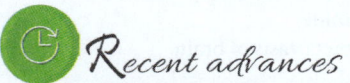

Diagnostic Criteria for Neuromyelitis Optica
- Must required: Optic neuritis and transverse myelitis
  with
- MRI spine showing >3 vertebral segments or anti-aquaporin-4 antibody positivity
  with
- Anti aquaporin-4 antibody

Etiology

1. Genetic
2. Polygenetic: The HLA-DR2 gene has been demonstrated to be a genetically susceptible area. 30% concordance for monozygotic twins
3. Environmental MS is more common in regions with less sun exposure and thus, lower stores of vitamin D
4. MS has also been linked to certain viruses, particularly with EBV.

Symptoms of MS

1. **Sensory loss: MC symptom (37%).**^{Q}
2. **Optic neuritis (ON) (36%) can be the first demyelinating event**. ON is characterized by loss of vision (or loss of color vision) in the affected eye and pain on movement of the eye. Much less commonly, patients with ON may describe phosphenes (transient flashes of light or black squares) lasting from hours to months. Phosphenes may occur before or during an ON event or even several months following recovery.
3. Spasticity occurs most frequently in muscles that function to maintain upright posture.
4. Cognitive dysfunction: The estimated prevalence of cognitive dysfunction in MS ranges from 40 to 70%.
5. Pain: Primary pain is related to the demyelinating process itself. This neuropathic pain is often characterized as having a burning, gnawing, or shooting quality. Secondary pain in MS is primarily musculoskeletal in nature and possibly results from poor posture, poor balance, or abnormal use of muscles or joints as a result of spasticity.
6. Urinary symptoms are common in MS with most patients experiencing problems at some point in their disease. Patients with impaired storage have a small, spastic bladder with hypercontractility of the detrusor muscle. Symptoms experienced may include urgency, frequency, incontinence and nocturia.
7. Constipation may be the result of a neurogenic bowel or due to immobility.
8. Persons with MS often experience an increase in symptoms of **fatigue or weakness** when exposed to high temperatures due to weather (especially hot, humid weather), exercise, hot showers or baths, or fever. Overheating, may result in blurring of vision (**Uhthoff sign**), usually in an eye previously affected by ON. These symptoms result from elevation of core body temperature, which further impairs conduction by demyelinated nerves, and they typically reverse rapidly when exposure to high temperature ends.
9. **Acute transverse myelitis**: Loss of motor, sensory, autonomic, reflex, and sphincter function below the level of the lesion indicates acute transverse myelitis. It is usually seen in MS variant called as **Devic's disease**^{Q}.
10. **Lhermitte's sign**: *Flexion of neck causes electric shock sensation down back into legs.*

- Most common presentation of multiple sclerosis is sensory loss > optic neuritis

Investigations

1. **MRI:** Demyelinating plaques appear as hyperintense lesions on T2 weighted MRI, with active lesions showing enhancement with gadolinium
2. **Typical locations:** Periventricular, corpus callosum, cerebellar peduncles, brainstem, juxtacortical region and dorsolateral spinal cord
3. **Dawson's fingers:** Periventricular lesions extending superiorly into corpus callosum
4. **CSF:** Oligoclonal bands in 90%, increased IgG concentration
5. **Evoked potentials (visual/auditory/somatosensory):** Delayed but well-preserved wave forms.

Diagnosis

Dissemination in space and in time as based on the *Revised McDonald criteria*

- **Dissemination in Time**: 2 or more attacks, new gadolinium enhancing lesion 3 months later, or new T2 lesions >1 month after first attack.
- **Dissemination in Space**: Clinical evidence of 2 or more lesions; or three of (1 gadolinium enhancing or 9 T2 lesions), (infratentorial lesion), (1 juxtacortical lesion), (3 periventricular lesions).

Treatment

- **Acute exacerbation and first episode treatment:** Methylprednisolone 500–1000 mg IV daily X 3–7 days ± taper for optic neuritis

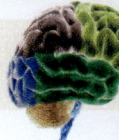

Disease modifying therapy (DMT):
1. IFN-beta-1a
2. IFN-beta-1b
3. Glatiramer acetate
4. Natalizumab
5. Fingolimod
6. Mitoxantrone
7. Dimethyl fumarate
8. Teriflunomide and
9. Alemtuzumab.

- **IFN-beta** is a class I interferon originally identified by its antiviral properties *(Drug of choice)*[Q]
    - Efficacy in MS probably results from immune-modulatory properties, including downregulating expression of MHC molecules on antigen-presenting cells and limiting the trafficking of inflammatory cells in the CNS.
    - IFN-beta reduces the attack rate and improves disease severity measures such as EDSS progression and MRI-documented disease burden.
- **Glatiramer acetate** is a synthetic, random polypeptide composed of four amino acids (l-glutamic acid, l-lysine, l-alanine and l-tyrosine).
    - Glatiramer acetate reduces the attack rate (whether measured clinically or by MRI) in RRMS.
    - Glatiramer acetate should be considered in RRMS patients. Its usefulness in progressive disease is entirely unknown.
    - *Clinical trials suggest that glatiramer acetate has about equal efficacy to high IFN beta doses.*
- **Natalizumab** is a monoclonal antibody against the alpha 4 subunit of alpha-4 beta 1 integrin, a cellular adhesion molecule expressed on the surface of lymphocytes.
    - It prevents lymphocytes from binding to endothelial cells, thereby preventing lymphocytes from entering the CNS.
    - Natalizumab greatly reduces the attack rate and significantly improves all measures of disease severity[Q] in MS. This is the drug causing **maximum reduction in EDSS** (expanded disability severity score)
    - However, because of the development of progressive multifocal leukoencephalopathy (PML) in approximately 0.2% of patients treated with natalizumab for more than 2 years, natalizumab is currently recommended for JC antibody negative patients.
- **Fingolimod** is a sphingosine-1-phosphate (S1P) inhibitor.
    - Its mechanism of action is probably due, in part, to the trapping of lymphocytes in the periphery and the prevention, thereby, of lymphocytes reaching the brain.
- **Mitoxantrone** is indicated for use in SPMS, in PRMS, and in patients with worsening RRMS (defined as patients whose neurologic status remains significantly abnormal between MS attacks). *Page 2670, Harrison 19/e, mentions it being rarely used now a days.*
    - It can be cardiotoxic and hence at currently approved doses the maximum duration of therapy can be only 2–3 years.

Drug causing maximum change in EDSS score in multiple sclerosis is Natalizumab (page 2669, Harrison 19/e) (Please donot go by facebook posts)

Acute Disseminated Encephalomyelitis

- Immune-mediated disease of the brain that occurs following a viral infection but may appear following vaccination, bacterial or parasitic infection, or even appear spontaneously.
- As it involves autoimmune demyelination, it is similar to multiple sclerosis, and is considered part of the multiple sclerosis borderline diseases.
- Although it occurs in all ages, most reported cases are in children and adolescents, with the average age around 5–8 years, with mortality rate as high as 5%; however, full recovery is seen in 50 – 75% of cases.
- ADEM produces multiple inflammatory lesions in the brain and spinal cord, particularly in the white matter.
- Usually these are found in the subcortical and central white matter and cortical gray-white junction of both cerebral hemispheres, cerebellum, brainstem, and spinal cord, but periventricular white matter and gray matter of the cortex, thalami and basal ganglia may also be involved.
- The widely accepted first-line treatment is high doses of intravenous corticosteroids, such as methylprednisolone or dexamethasone, followed by 3–6 weeks of gradually lower oral doses of prednisolone.

Central Pontine Myelinosis

- Central pontine myelinosis presents most commonly as a complication of treatment of patients with profound, life-threatening hyponatremia.
- It occurs as a consequence of a rapid rise in serum tonicity following treatment in individuals with chronic, severe hyponatremia who have made intracellular adaptations to the prevailing hypotonicity.
- Hyponatremia should be corrected at a rate of no more than 4–6 mmol/L of sodium per day to prevent central pontine[Q] myelinosis.
- Brain cells adjust their osmolarities by changing levels of certain osmolytes like inositol, betaine, and glutamine. In hyponatremia, the levels of these osmolytes fall, causing the cells to absorb free-water. The reverse is true for hypernatremia, in which cells will shrink to dilute the hypernatremic fluid. Therefore, rapid correction of sodium in hyponatremia would cause the extracellular fluid to be relatively hypertonic. Free water would then move out of the cells to decrease this relative hypertonicity. This leads to a central pontine myelinosis, manifesting as the paralysis. The brain appears to shrink.
- Clinical features are–acute para-or quadraparesis, dysphagia, dysarthria, diplopia, loss of consciousness, and other neurological symptoms associated with brainstem damage.

- The patient may experience locked-in syndrome where cognitive function is intact, but all muscles are paralyzed with the exception of eye blinking. These result from a rapid myelinosis of the corticobulbar and corticospinal tracts in the brainstem.

Central pontine myelinosis is more common with fast correction of chronic hyponatremia.

LEUKODYSTROPHIES

It is a group of disorders characterized by degeneration of the white matter in the brain. Myelin in the CNS is produced by oligodendrocytes. When damage occurs to the white matter tissue, immune responses can lead to inflammation in the CNS, along with loss of myelin.

1. **Adrenoleukodystrophy**
   - X-linked disorder of peroxisomal fatty acid metabolism
   - **ABCD1 gene**^{Q}
   - Treated by: Mixture of unsaturated fatty acids (glycerol trioleate and glyceryl trierucate in a 4:1 ratio), known as Lorenzo's oil that inhibits elongation of saturated fatty acids in the body
2. **Adrenomyeloneuropathy**: Variant of above disorder with adult presentation
3. **Metachromatic leukodystrophy**:
   - **Arylsulfatase B deficiency**^{Q}
   - Affected children begin to have difficulty in walking after the first year of life, usually at 15–24 months. Symptoms include muscle wasting and weakness, muscle rigidity, developmental delays, progressive loss of vision leading to blindness, convulsions, impaired swallowing, paralysis, and dementia. Children may become comatose. If left untreated, most children with this form of MLD die by the age of 5 years.
4. **Krabbe's disease:**
   - Mutations in the GALC gene located on chromosome 14 (14q31), which causes a deficiency of an enzyme called galactocerebrosidase.
   - Symptoms begin between the ages of 3 and 6 months with irritability, fever, limb stiffness, seizures, feeding difficulties, vomiting, and slowing of mental and motor development. In the initial stages, the disease can be misdiagnosed as cerebral palsy. Other symptoms include muscle weakness, spasticity, deafness, optic atrophy, optic nerve enlargement, blindness, paralysis, and difficulty while swallowing.
5. **Pelizaeus-Merzbacher disease** is generally caused by a recessive mutation of the gene on the long arm of the X-chromosome (Xq21-22) that codes for a myelin protein *called* proteolipid protein 1 *or* PLP1
6. **Canavan's disease**
   - Canavan's disease is caused by a defective ASPA gene, which is responsible for the production of the enzyme aspartoacylase.
   - Decreased aspartoacylase activity prevents the normal breakdown of N-acetyl aspartate, wherein the accumulation of N-acetylaspartate, or lack of its further metabolism interferes with growth of the myelin sheath of the nerve fibers in the brain.
7. **Alexander's disease** is caused by mutations in the gene for glial fibrillary acidic protein *(GFAP)* that maps to chromosome 17q21. It is inherited in an autosomal dominant manner
8. **Refsum's disease**
   - Adult Refsum's disease may be divided into the adult Refsum's disease 1 and adult Refsum's disease 2 subtypes. The former stems from mutations in the phytanoyl-CoA hydroxylase (*PAHX* aka *PHYH*) gene, while the latter stems from mutations in the peroxin-7 (*PEX7*) gene.
   - Adult Refsum's disease should not be confused *with infantile Refsum's disease, a* peroxisome biogenesis disorder resulting from *deficiencies in the catabolism of very long chain fatty acids* and branched chain fatty acids (such as phytanic acid) and plasmalogen biosynthesis.

Progressive Multifocal Leukoencephalopathy

Progressive multifocal leukoencephalopathy (PML) is a demyelinating disease of the CNS characterized by widespread lesions due to infection of oligodendrocytes by a human papovavirus.

About JC virus

- The virus is thought to enter the body via the respiratory or oral route. After its entry, it becomes latent in the kidneys, lymphoreticular tissues, and brain.
- As many as 90% of healthy individuals have serum antibodies to this virus, but less than 10% show any evidence of ongoing viral replication. In cases associated with the initiation of highly active antiretroviral therapy (HAART), immune recovery may uncover pre-existing subclinical PML.

Prognosis

In the pre-HAART era, the prognosis in patients with PML was dismal, with death occurring in approximately 95% of patients within 4–6 months after diagnosis in most cases. Approximately, 8% of patients experience spontaneous recovery. *With the widespread adoption of highly active antiretroviral therapy (HAART), the incidence of PML has decreased substantially*

Clinical Features

1. Patients with progressive multifocal leukoencephalopathy (PML) typically experience *insidious onset* and steady progression of focal symptoms that include behavioral, speech, cognitive and motor symptoms (eg, head tremor and visual impairment).
2. *Focal neurological signs include aphasia, hemiparesis, ataxia, cortical blindness, limb apraxia, brainstem symptoms and less frequently, head tremor.* **Focal signs tend to be related to posterior brain (occipital lobes).**
3. Gait abnormalities occur in up to 65% patients and cognitive dysfunction is seen at the time of presentation in up to 30% people.
4. Conjugate gaze abnormalities are common.

Investigations

1. MRI of the brain shows single or multiple confluent lesions most frequently in the parieto-occipital white matter. Occasional infratentorial lesions are usually asymmetrical. The demyelinating plaques involve subcortical U fibers but tend to spare the cortical ribbons and deep gray matter structures. Subcortical gray matter or the spinal cord may be involved, but rarely. *Gray matter involvement has a scalloped appearance.*
2. Polymerase chain reaction (PCR) of the CSF has been shown to be highly specific (92–99%) and sensitive (74–93%) for the detection of JC virus in patients with PML.
3. Brain biopsy has a sensitivity of 74–92% and a specificity of 92–100% in progressive multifocal leukoencephalopathy.

Treatment

No definitive treatment is available till yet.

VARIANT CREUTZFELDT JAKOB DISEASE

It is the progressive neuropsychiatric illness for 6 months with psychiatric symptoms usually preceding the neurological symptoms. It is seen due to consumption of tainted beef.

- **EEG shows periodic sharp wave complexes**^{Q}
- Brain MRI shows bilateral symmetrical pulvinar high-signal intensity (relative to the signal intensity of the other deep gray matter nuclei and cortical gray matter). MRI findings are:
  1. Pulvinar sign
  2. **Hockey stick sign**^{Q}
  3. **Cortical ribboning**^{Q}
- Positive findings on tonsil biopsy (biopsy not routinely recommended).
- CSF study
  - Tau protein has the best sensitivity (80%) and specificity (94%) of *any of the proteins investigated in variant CJD*
  - The detection of CSF 14-3-3 is nonspecific
- Postmortem brain biopsy showing multiple florid plaques with severe spongiform change and neuronal loss.

HUNTINGTON'S CHOREA

- Autosomal dominant
- Polyglutamine (CAG) repeats >40 located on huntingtin gene located on short arm of chromosome 4.
- Intraneuronal inclusions containing aggregates of ubiquitin and mutant protein huntingtin are seen in nuclei of affected neurons.
- MRI head shows atrophy of caudate nucleus with concomitant enlargement of frontal horns of lateral ventricles called as "Box car" ventricles.
- PET study shows reduced metabolic activity of caudate nucleus and putamen.

  The clinical features of Huntington's disease (HD) include
  1. **Movement disorder:** Chorea
  2. **Cognitive disorder:** The dementia syndrome associated with HD includes early onset behavioral changes, such as irritability, untidiness, and loss of interest
  3. **Behavioral problems.**

4. In advanced disease, patients develop an akinetic-rigid syndrome, with minimal or no chorea. Other late features are spasticity, clonus, and extensor plantar responses
5. **Juvenile HD (Westphal variant),** defined as having an age of onset of younger than 20 years, is characterized by parkinsonian features, dystonia, long-tract signs, dementia, epilepsy, and mild or even absent chorea.

Management is done with a presynaptic dopamine depleter, **tetrabenazine.**^{Q} Overuse can cause secondary parkinsonism. For management of psychosis, clozapine is used.

FRIEDREICH'S ATAXIA

- Most common form of **inherited ataxia**^{Q}
- Frataxin gene on chromosome 9q13 with **GAA**^{Q} triplet repeats
- Patients have 200–900 GAA repeats
- Genetic defect leads to mitochondrial iron accumulation leading to irreversible neuronal injury

Clinical Features

1. The disease presents in individual below 25 years of age with staggering gait and recurrent falls and titubation
2. Dysarthria is presenting symptom
3. MRI shows spinal cord atrophy.

Lesions in Friedreich ataxia	Clinical correlation
Involvement of corticospinal pathway	Extensor plantars
Involvement of peripheral nerves	Absence of deep tendon reflux
Involvement of dorsal column	Sensory ataxia due to loss of proprioception
Cardiac involvement	Symmetrical hypertrophy with conduction defects
Pancreatic beta cell dysfunction	Diabetes mellitus
Musculoskeletal abnormalities	Pes cavus, scoliosis
Degeneration of glossopharyngeal, vagus, hypoglossal and deep cerebellar nuclei	• Cannot eat • Cannot drink • Cannot speak

MOTOR NEURON DISEASE

Impaired neuronal viability due to
- Superoxide dismustase 1 transgenes
- **Hexanucleotide repeats**^{Q}
- ALS gene leading to defective axonal cytoskeleton

Site of lesion	Nomenclature
Death of anterior horn cells in spinal cord and cranial nerve nuclei innervating bulbar muscles	Progressive muscular atrophy/ Spinomuscular atrophy
Death of motor neurons in layer five of motor cortex or corticospinal pathways	Primary lateral sclerosis
Combination of above two	Amyotrophic lateral sclerosis

Amyotrophic lateral sclerosis is most common type of motor neuron disease.

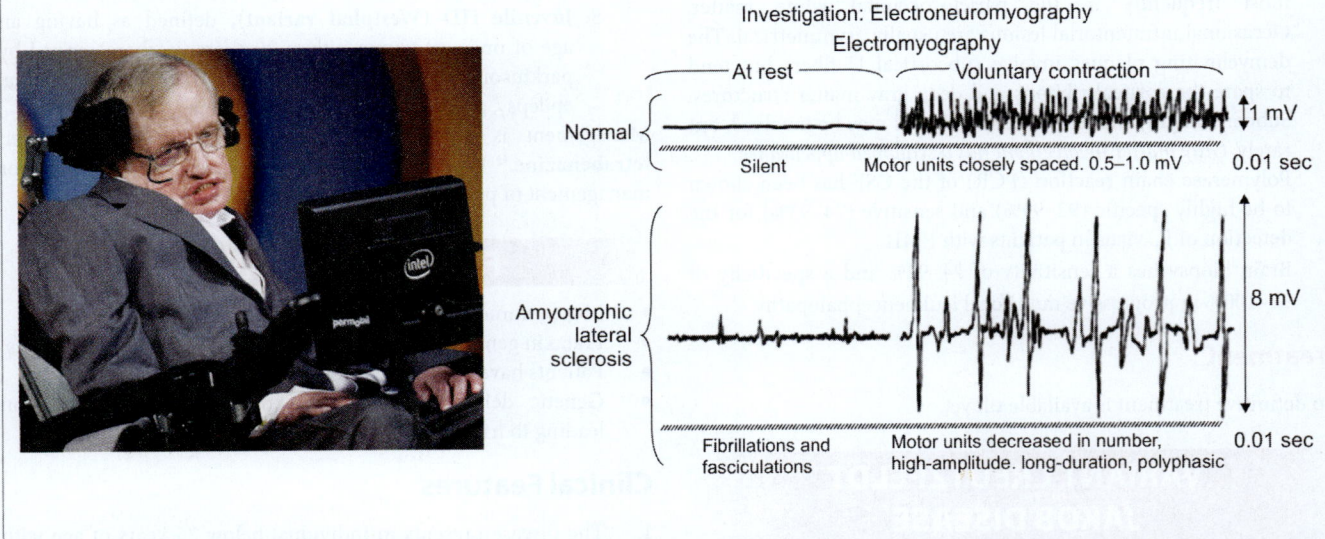

Stephen Hawking (Astrophysicist) who died of pneumonia, secondary to Motor neuron disease

Clinical Features

1. Asymmetrical muscle weakness present distally. So walking on slippery surface shall be difficult.
2. Bulbar palsy can lead to difficulty in chewing, swallowing and tongue movements. Tongue fasciculations are noted.
3. Spasticity and brisk reflexes occur due to corticospinal involvement.
4. Pseudobulbar palsy results in dysarthria and exaggeration of emotion-like involuntary crying or laughing.
5. Death occurs due to respiratory paralysis.
6. Diagnosis is considered definitive if three out of four areas are involved- bulbar, cervical, thoracic and lumbosacral motor neurons.

Treatment

Riluzole produces survival benefit by reducing glutamate production and reducing excitotoxicity. New drug used is edavarone.

DISEASES OF SPINAL CORD

Syringomyelia

Etiology

1. **Associated with Chiari type 1 malformation**[Q]. (Arnold Chiari type 2 malformation is associated with myelomeningocele)
2. Congenital malformation presenting as dilatation of central canal and exerts pressure on adjoining tracts

Clinical Features

1. Occurs mostly in third and fourth decade; insidious onset of illness with pain in shoulder and wasting of small muscles of hand.
2. *It is associated with dissociated sensory loss (patchy loss of pain temperature with sparing of proprioception).* Painless burn in hand and neglect of injury is seen.
3. Wasting of muscles of hand, as syrinx expands spasticity of legs, bladder and bowel dysfunction ensues.
4. Patient has trophic ulcers and parlayzed painless joints called **Charcot's joints.**
5. Syringobulbia leading to palatal and vocal cord paralysis, dysarthria, nystagmus, vertigo and tongue weakness.

Investigations

MRI shows a syrinx compressing spinal cord tracts

Management

- Surgical decompression

Barber chair sign/Lhermitte sign is positive in
1. Tabes dorsalis
2. Multiple sclerosis
3. Cervical spondylosis
4. Syringomyelia
5. Subacute combined demyelination of spinal cord (SACD)
6. Tumor of spinal cord

Brown-Séquard Syndrome (Hemi-section of Spinal Cord)

If one-half of spinal cord is damaged transversely, the manifestations are:
1. *Ipsilateral weakness with ipsilateral loss of proprioception*

2. Opposite side loss of pain and temperature sensation, one or two levels below lesion
3. Lower motor neuron lesion at the level of lesion
4. Corticospinal lesion leading to *ipsilateral spastic weakness*.

Subacute Combined Demyelination of Spinal Cord (SACD)

The posterior column is demyelinated in patches causing the following symptoms.

Clinical Features

- Parasthesia of hands and feet along with loss of proprioceptive stimuli.
- Presence of sensory ataxia. It is associated with optic atrophy and irritability.
- Spasticity due to demyelination of corticospinal tract.
- Brisk DTR.
- Loss of reflexes due to peripheral neuropathy and concomitant presence of Babinski sign is an important clue.

Investigations

1. Low serum vitamin B_{12} levels
2. Schilling test (not done now a days)
3. Increased homocysteine
4. Methylmalonic acid.

Management

Vitamin B_{12} mega-dosages

NEUROPATHY

Peripheral Neuropathies

Anatomic classification of peripheral neuropathies

Mononeuropathy	Distribution of a single peripheral nerve
Mononeuritis multiplex	Motor, sensory and reflex deficits affecting multiple nerves Stepwise progression asymmetrical Can eventually summate to a symmetric stocking glove pattern
Polyneuropathy	Diffuse, symmetric distal stocking glove pattern distal hyporeflexia

Mononeuritis Multiplex

Causes

1. PAN (most common cause in world)
2. Rheumatoid arthritis
3. Diabetes mellitus
4. Leprosy (most common cause in India)
5. Sarcoidosis

Differential diagnosis of Mononeuritis Multiplex and Investigations to be Performed

	Etiology	Key Investigations
Vascular	1. Polyarteritis nodosa	1. LP (lymphocytosis and increased protein) 2. Nerve biopsy 3. Hepatitis B serology 4. p-ANCA
	2. SLE	5. ANA, anti-ds DNA 6. Nerve biopsy
	3. RA	7. ANA, Rheumatoid factor 8. Nerve biopsy
Infectious	4. HIV	9. HIV serology
	5. Lyme disease	10. Lyme serology
	6. Syphilis	11. VDRL
Endocrine	7. Diabetes mellitus	12. HbA1C
Immune	8. Chronic inflammatory demyelinating Polyneuropathy 9. Sarcoidosis	13. EMG 14. LP (Oligoclonal banding on electrophoresis) 15. Serum ACE 16. Nerve biopsy

Causes of Peripheral Neuropathy

1. Deficiency of vitamins: B_6, B_{12}, E, folate
2. **Drugs**: Vincristine, amiodarone, hydralazine, phenytoin, alcohol.
3. **Hereditary**: MC type is Charcot Marie tooth disease. Most subtypes are autosomal dominant. The most common subtype is CMT1 with patients presenting with distal weakness foot drop in first to third decade. Atrophy of muscles below knee result in inverted champagne bottle legs. Nerve biopsy reveals a *onion bulb* appearance.
4. **Metabolic**: Diabetes mellitus, rheumatoid arthritis, liver failure, acute intermittent porphyria, hypothyroidism
5. **Connective tissue**:
   - PAN
   - RA
   - SLE
   - Sarcoidosis: MC cranial nerve involved in 7th nerve
6. Overall MC cause of peripheral neuropathy is diabetes mellitus. Distal sensory and sensorimotor polyneuropathy (DSPN) is most common form of diabetic neuropathy. Nerve biopsy will show axonal degeneration and not demyelination. In diabetics, MC cranial nerve involved is 3rd nerve palsy with pupillary sparing.

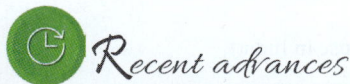 Recent advances

Axonal Degeneration versus Segmental Demyelination		
	Axonal degeneration	Segmental demyelination
CMAP amplitude	Decreased	Normal^Q
Conduction velocity	Normal	Slow
F wave	Normal^Q	Prolonged
H reflex	Normal^Q	Prolonged
Needle EMG fibrillations	Present	Absent

Clinical Features

- Distal paresthesia of feet and hands
- Loss of superficial touch called glove and stocking sensation
- Depressed deep tendon reflexes.

Investigations

1. NCV
2. Metabolic screen.

Management

- Multivitamins and cause specific treatment

Mononeuropathy

Carpal tunnel syndrome	Median nerve
Tarsal tunnel syndrome	Post tibial nerve
Meralgia paresthetica	Lateral cutaneous nerve of thigh
Foot drop	Peroneal nerve in leprosy
Supracondylar fracture of humerus	Ulnar nerve in trauma

Causes of Carpal Tunnel Syndrome

1. Idiopathic
2. Occupational (I.T. Professionals)
3. Pregnancy
4. Diabetes mellitus
5. Hypothyroidism.

The H-reflex on stimulation of the tibial nerve in the popliteal fossa is routinely used in the diagnosis of first sacral (S1) nerve-root radiculopathy.

Clinical Features

- Pain; paresthesia on palmar aspect, arm and shoulders; paralysis of abductor pollicis brevis

Management

- Rest to joint
- Splinting
- Surgical decompression.

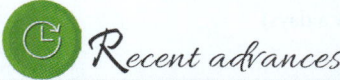 Recent advances

- MC cause of ICU admission is acute kidney injury
- MC cause of acute generalized weakness leading to ICU admission are
  - GBS
  - Myasthenia gravis/crisis
  - Critical illness polyneuropathy
  - Critical illness myopathy
- CIP and CIM are a complication of sepsis and multiorgan failure and present with inability to wean a patient from ventilator.
- Toxins due to sepsis or MODS lead to axonal degeneration.

DISORDERS OF MUSCLES

Myopathies

Clinical Approach to Muscle Diseases

	Etiology	Key clinical features	Key investigations
Inflammatory	Polymyositis	Myalgias Ptosis is not seen Pharyngeal involvement	Increased CK Biopsy: endomysial infiltrates: necrosis
	Dermatomyositis	Myalgias similar to polymyositis Heliotrope rash can be paraneoplastic	Increased CK Biopsy perifascicular atrophy
	Sarcoidosis	Hilar lymphadenopathy	ACE level Biopsy granulomas
	Inclusion body myositis	Weak quadriceps and deep finger flexors	Increased CK Biopsy: Inclusion bodies.
Endocrine	Thyroid derangement Cushing's syndrome Parathyroid derangements	(Read endocrinology chapter)	TSH, Serum cortisol, calcium panel

Contd...

	Etiology	Key clinical features	Key investigations
Toxic	Medication Critical illness myopathy	Medication or toxin history ICU patient Steroids Nondepolarizing paralyzing agents Failure to wean from ventilation	Toxicology screen Biopsy: selective loss of thick myosin filaments
Infectious	Parasitic, bacterial or viral	Myalgias Inflammatory myopathy	Elevated Myoglobin
Hereditary dystrophy	Duchenne Becker Myotonic dystrophy	Early onset (Duchenne and Becker) Progressive proximal muscle weakness Calf pseudohypertrophy Distal myopathy Myotonia Genetic anticipation	Biopsy: abnormal dystrophin staining Genetic testing
Hereditary metabolic	McArdle's	Exercise related myalgias, cramping, and Myoglobinuria	↑lactate ↑ serum/ urinary myoglobin Post – exercise
Hereditary periodic paralysis	Periodic paralysis	Episodic weakness Normal between attacks	↑ or ⁻K
Hereditary mitochondrial	MERRF MELAS Kearns Sayre	Ptosis, opthalmoparesis common Proximal >distal myopathy Exercise intolerance Rhabdomyolysis	Increased lactate Biopsy: ragged red fibers

Duchenne's Muscular Dystrophy: X-linked Recessive Condition

- Duchenne's dystrophy is present at birth, but the disorder usually becomes apparent between ages 3 and 5 years.
- The boy falls frequently and has difficulty keeping up with friends when playing. Running, jumping, and hopping are invariably abnormal. By the age of 5 years, muscle weakness is obvious by muscle testing.
- On getting up from the floor, the patient uses his hands to climb up himself (**Gowers' sign**).
- **Pseudohypertrophy of calf muscles**^{Q}
- Contractures of the heel cords and iliotibial bands become apparent by age of 6 years, when toe walking is associated with a lordotic posture.
- Loss of muscle strength is progressive, with predilection for proximal limb muscles and the neck flexors; leg involvement is more severe than arm involvement.
- By the age of 12 years, most patients are dependent on wheelchairs. Contractures become fixed, and a progressive scoliosis often develops that may be associated with pain.
- The chest deformity with scoliosis impairs pulmonary function, which is already diminished by muscle weakness.
- By the age of 16–18 years, patients are predisposed to serious, sometimes *fatal pulmonary infections (Most common cause of death)*.
- Other causes of death include aspiration of food and acute gastric dilation.
- CPKMM is a screening test. Values can be falsely normal due to significant muscle wasting.

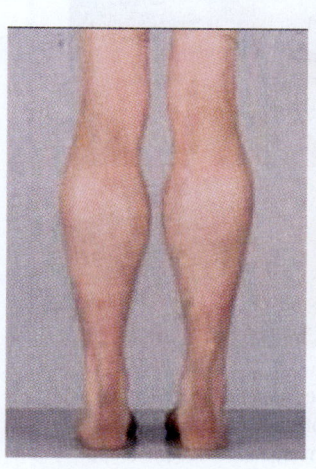

Pseudo-hypertrophy of calf muscles in Duchenne' muscular dystrophy

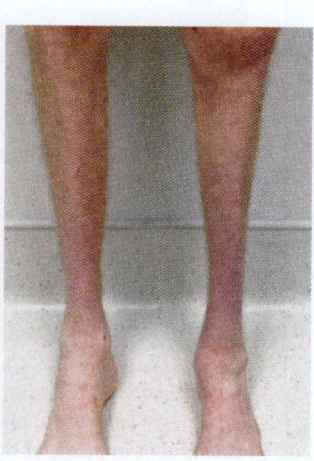

Stork leg appearance in Charcot-Marie tooth disease

Neuromuscular Junction Abnormalities

Myasthenia Gravis

Pathology

- Receptors for acetycholine in post functional membrane are blocked by antibodies. Thus, the muscle after a little work is fatigued.
- **65% patients have thymus hyperplasia and 10% have a thymoma.**^{Q}
- HLA B8/ HLA DR W3
- Antibodies associated with thyroiditis/Grave's disease/ rheumatoid arthritis/ SLE.

Clinical Features

1. Overall, women are affected more frequently than men, in a ratio of 3:2.
2. The cardinal features are *weakness* and *fatigability* of muscles. The weakness increases during repeated use (fatigue) and shows a diurnal variation of symptoms.
3. Exacerbations and remissions may occur, particularly during the first few years after the onset of the disease.
4. Unrelated infections or systemic disorders can lead to increased myasthenic weakness and may precipitate "crisis.
5. *Asymmetrical ptosis.*
6. *Diplopia.*
7. *Weakness while chewing, swallowing and speaking.*

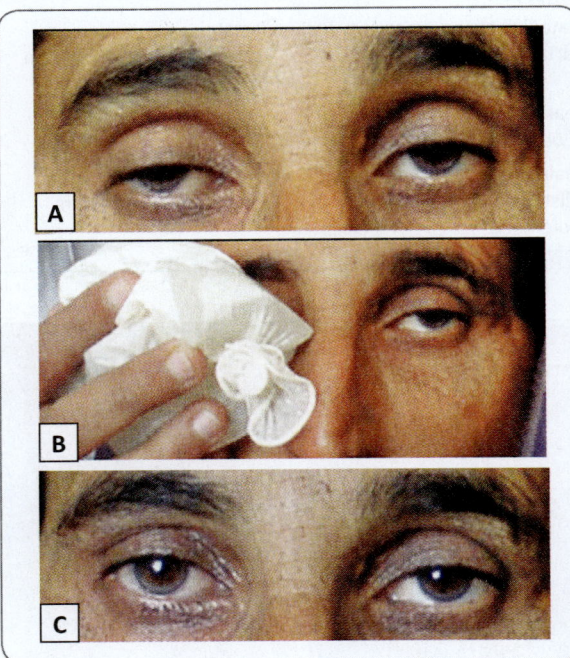

(A) Bilateral ptosis (more marked in right eye);
(B) Ice pack application on right eye;
(C) Improvement in ptosis of right eye after ice pack application

Ice pack test in Myasthenia Gravis.

8. Shoulder girdle weakness.
9. Respiratory muscle weakness.
10. Antibodies transferred by placenta to baby who may fail to establish respiration after birth. Later on problems with breast feeding due to weak sucking capacity.
11. *Deep tendon reflexes are normal.*

Relapse
- Emotional/physical effort
- Pregnancy
- Infections.

Investigations

1. **Anti-AcH receptor blocking antibodies**: 85% positive in generalized MG and 50% positive in ocular MG. A negative test does not rule out possibility of M. gravis. *(Most specific test)*

2. **Repetitive nerve stimulation**: Electric shocks are delivered at a rate of two or three per second to the appropriate nerves, and action potentials are recorded from the muscles. In normal individuals, the amplitude of the evoked muscle action potentials does not change at these rates of stimulation. **However, in myasthenic patients, there is a rapid reduction of >10–15% in the amplitude of the evoked responses. (DECREMENTAL RESPONSE)**

3. **Single nerve fiber EMG**: Confirmatory test/Investigation of choice

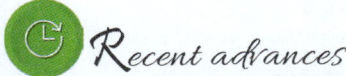

- SFEMG is more sensitive than RNS in assessing MG.
- **Most accurate test for diagnosis of M.Gravis is single fiber EMG**

4. **Tensilon test**:
   - Edrophonium is used most commonly for diagnostic testing because of the rapid onset (30 s) and short duration (5 min) of its effect. An objective end-point must be selected to evaluate the effect of edrophonium, such as weakness of extraocular muscles, impairment of speech, or the length of time that the patient can maintain the arms in forward abduction.
   - An initial IV dose of 2 mg of edrophonium is given. If definite improvement occurs, the test is considered positive and is terminated. If there is no change, the patient is given an additional 8 mg IV.
   - The dose is administered in two parts because some patients react to edrophonium with side effects such as nausea, diarrhea, salivation, fasciculations, and rarely with severe symptoms of syncope or bradycardia. Atropine (0.6 mg) should be drawn up in a syringe, ready for IV administration if cholinergic crisis develops.

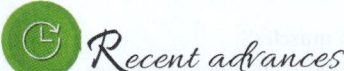

- **The edrophonium test is now reserved for patients with clinical findings that are suggestive of MG but who have negative antibody and electrodiagnostic test results.**
- False-positive tests occur in occasional patients with other neurologic disorders, such as amyotrophic lateral sclerosis, and in placebo-reactors.
- False-negative or equivocal tests may also occur.

5. Thyroid function test
6. CT chest to evaluate the presence of Thymoma
7. Ice pack Test
8. **Anti-musk A/b:** Muscle specific kinase antibody in ocular M. gravis.

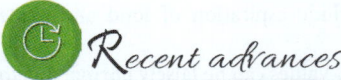

- The ice pack test (i.e., placing ice over the lid) is done for assessing improvement in ptosis and diplopia in ocular MG. The rationale behind this test is that cooling of muscle may improve neuromuscular transmission.

Management

- **Anticholinesterase drugs**
  - Anticholinesterase medication produces at least partial improvement in most myasthenic patients, although improvement is complete in only a few.
  - Pyridostigmine is the most widely used anticholinesterase drug. The beneficial action of oral pyridostigmine begins within 15–30 min and lasts for 3–4 h, but individual responses vary. Treatment begins with a moderate dose, e.g., 30–60 mg three to four times daily.
- **Myasthenic crisis** is best managed with IVIG/ Plasmapheresis.
- **Azathioprine/steroids**: For the intermediate term, glucocorticoids and cyclosporine or tacrolimus generally produce clinical improvement within a period of 1–3 months. The beneficial effects of azathioprine and mycophenolate mofetil usually begins after many months (as long as a year), but these drugs have advantages for the long-term treatment of patients with MG.
- **Thymectomy** must be done once disease spreads to extraocular muscles. It should be carried out in all patients with generalized MG who are between the ages of puberty and at least 55 years. (**Treatment of choice for generalized M. gravis.**) Treatment of choice for ocular M. gravis is steroids.

Comparison of pathophysiology of Myasthenia Gravis and Lambert Eaton Syndrome

	Myasthenia gravis	Lambert Eaton syndrome
Defect	Post junctional defect	Pre-junctional defect
Associated with	Thymoma	Oat cell Cancer of lung
Antibody seen	Anti- ACH receptor Blocking antibody Anti- MUSK antibody	Anti- P/Q antibody
Clinical features	Asymmetrical ptosis with diurnal variation; Chewing weakness	Ptosis without diurnal variation
Investigation of choice	Single fiber; EMG showing a decremental response	Single fiber EMG showing an incremental response
Drug of choice	Neostigmine/ pyridostigmine	3,4 diaminopyridine

Chronic Progressive External Ophthalmoplegia

- It is the most frequent manifestation of mitochondrial myopathies.
- Bilateral, symmetrical, progressive ptosis, followed by ophthalmoparesis, months or years later. Ciliary and iris muscles are not involved. Diplopia is not seen due to symmetrical ptosis. When ptosis progresses, the patient may use the frontalis muscle to elevate the eyelids, adopt a chin-up head position, and eventually resort to manual elevation of the eyelids.
- It may be presentation in Kearns-Sayre syndrome, which is a mitochondrial myopathy.
  - Presents before the age of 20 years
  - Pigmentary retinopathy
  - Cardiac conduction defects
  - Cerebrospinal fluid (CSF), proteins greater than 100 mg/dL.

CHANNELOPATHIES

	Calcium Channel	Sodium Channel		Potassium Channel
Feature	Hypokalemic PP	Hyperkalemic PP	Paramyotonia congenita	Anderson's syndrome
Mode of inheritance	AD	AD	AD	AD
Age of onset	Adolescence	Early childhood	Early childhood	Early childhood
Myotonia	No	Yes	Yes	No
Frequency of attacks of weakness	Daily to yearly	May be 2–3/day	With cold	Daily to yearly
Duration of attacks of weakness	2 – 12 h	From 1 – 2 h to > 1 day	2 – 24 hours	2 – 24 h
Serum K⁺ level during attacks of weakness	Decreased	Increased or normal	Usually normal	Variable

*PP: periodic paralysis

Comparison of clinical presentation of Neuromuscular junction diseases with Botulism

	Myasthenia gravis	Lambert– Eaton	Botulism
Ocular/bulbar paresis	+	-	++ (early)
Limb weakness	+	+	+
Fatigability	+	+	+
Post- exercise enhancement	-	+	+
Reflexes	N	↓	↓
Autonomic anticholinergic S&S	-	-	++
Sensory S&S	-	-	-
Associated conditions	Thymoma	Small cell carcinoma	GI signs and symptoms
EMG Response to repetitive stimulation	Reduced	↓ (rapid stimu-lation) – (slow stimu-lation)	↓ (rapid stimu-lation) – (slow stimula-tion)

CSF Parameters in Various Neurological Disorders

Condition	Color	Protein	Glucose	Cells	Other
Normal	Clear	<0.45 g/L	60% of serum Glucose >3 mmol/L	0-4 WBC 0 RBC 0 Neutrophils	
Guillain–Barré syndrome	Clear of cloudy	Markedly increased	Normal	Normal	Albumino-cytological dissociation
Multiple Sclerosis	Clear	Normal or increased	Normal	0-20 x 10⁶/L Lymphocytes	Oligoclonal banding on protein electrophoresis
Pseudo-tumor Cerebri	Clear	Normal	Normal	Normal	Elevated opening pressure
Neoplasm (Neoplastic meningitis)	Clear of Xanthochromia	Normal or increased	Normal or deceased	Normal or increased lymphocytes	Cytology positive
Traumatic tap	Bloody, no xanthochromia	Normal	Slightly increased	RBCs = peripheral blood less RBCs in tube 4 than tube 1	
Subarachnoid hemorrhage	Bloody or xanthochromia after 2-8 h	Increased	Normal	WBC/RBC ratio same as blood same number of RBCs in tubes 1 & 4	

- The LP needle is introduced *cephalad* (aiming for the umbilicus of the patient). At the time of manometric pressure recording the legs of the patient should be extended to reduce the chances of false elevation of pressure of CSF due to hyperflexion of spine.
- Persistent excruciating headache >24 hours after LP can be managed with bed rest, caffeine oral/ intravenous. Low volume blood patch can be used in still in distress patients. The blood of the patient is used to seal the tear/rent in the dura mater which is leading to persistent CSF leakage.

Comparison of quincke versus sprotte (atraumatic needle for LP).

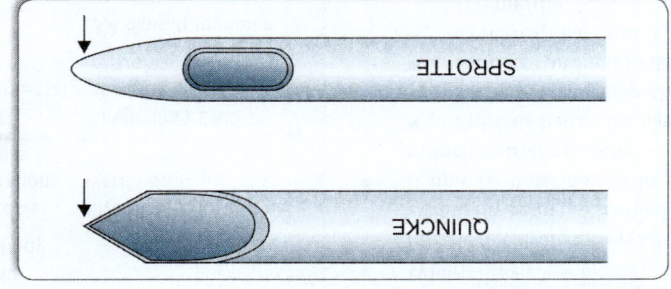

- 20-30 ml CSF can be safely removed in single Tap.

Measures to lower post-LP headache

Effective strategies
- Use of small-diameter needle (22-gauge or smaller)
- Use of atraumatic needle (sprotte and others)
- Replacement of stylet prior to removal of needle
- Insertion of needle with bevel oriented in a cephalad to caudad direction (when using standard needle)

Ineffective strategies
- Bed rest (up to 4 h) following LP
- Supplemental fluids
- Minimizing the volume of spinal fluid removed
- Immediate mobilization following LP

Image-Based Questions

1. A 35-year-old man presented with progressive myoclonus and apathy. MRI was done. Diagnosis is?

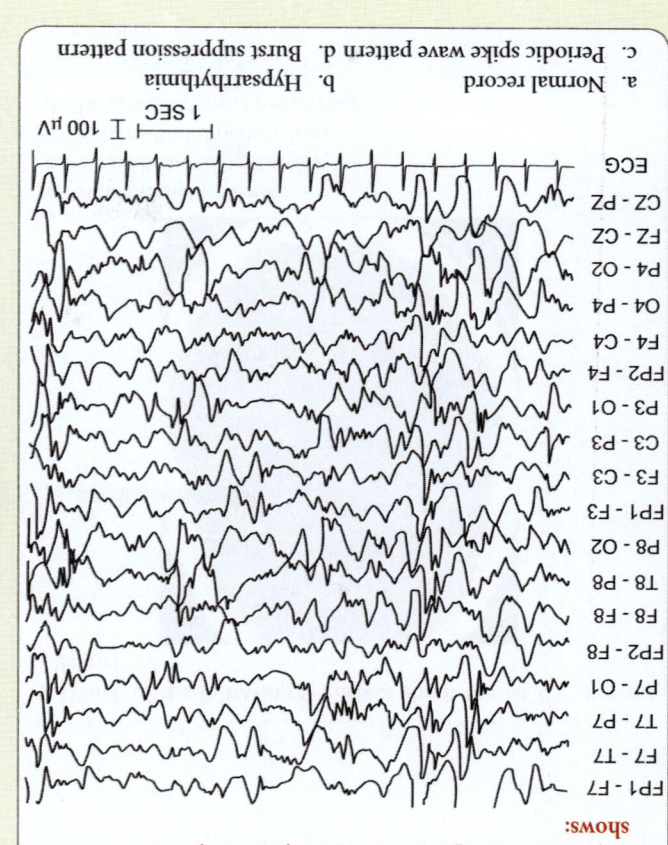

a. Herpes simplex encephalitis
b. SSPE
c. Variant Creutzfeldt Jakob disease
d. Mesial temporal sclerosis

2. 1-year old child presented with myoclonic jerks. EEG done shows:

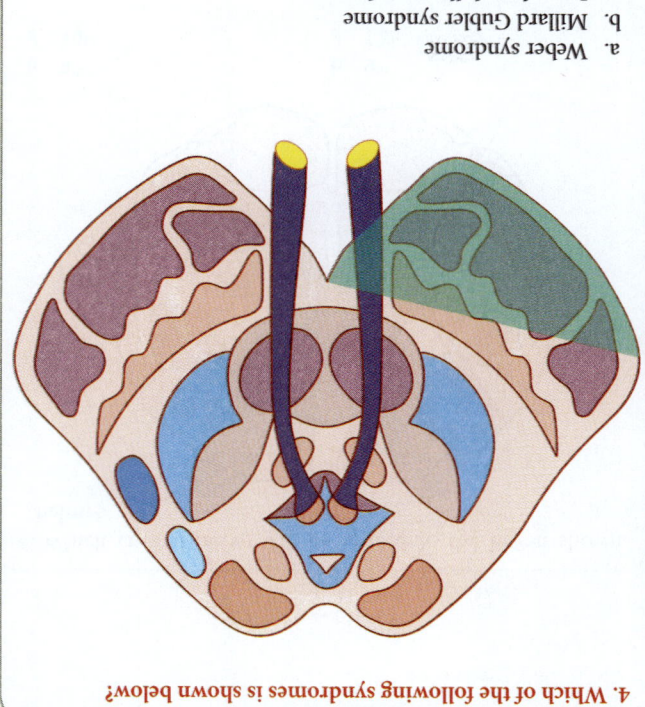

a. Normal record
b. Hypsarrythmia
c. Periodic spike wave pattern
d. Burst suppression pattern

3. A 60-year-old man presented with history of memory loss and fatigue. On examination, he has bradykinesia with axial rigidity. Resting tremor is absent and patient has broad based gait with tendency to fall. MRI was done. All are true about the condition except:

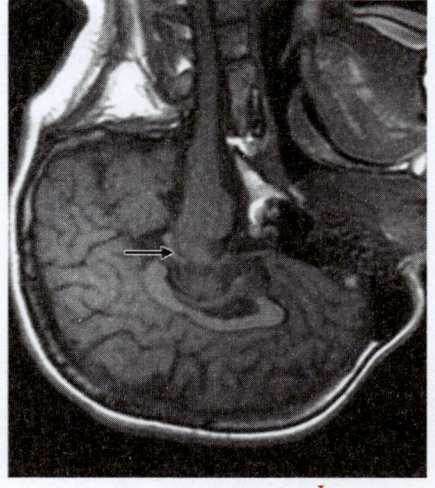

a. Poor response to levodopa
b. Gaze palsy
c. Pseudobulbar palsy
d. Intracranial hypotension

4. Which of the following syndromes is shown below?

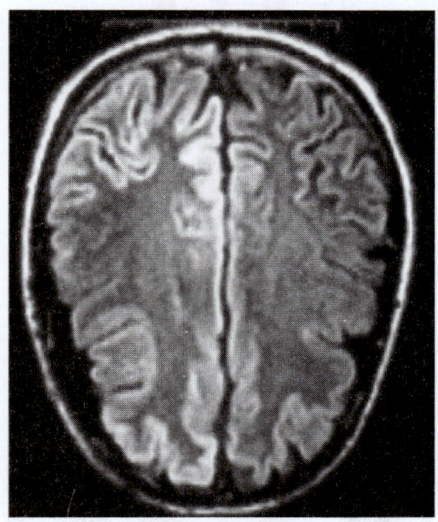

a. Weber syndrome
b. Millard Gubler syndrome
c. Lateral medullary syndrome
d. Anton syndrome

Complete Review of Medicine

5. Which of the following will not be seen in the lesion at this level?

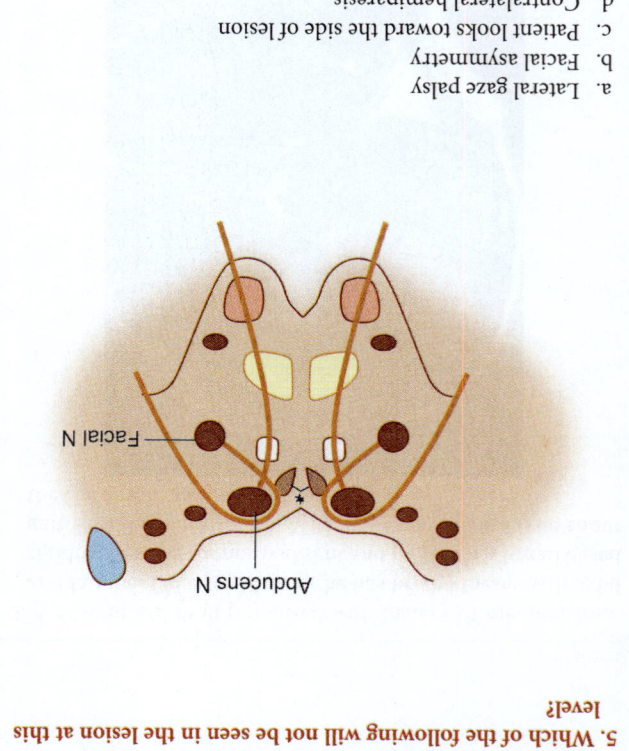

a. Lateral gaze palsy
b. Facial asymmetry
c. Patient looks toward the side of lesion
d. Contralateral hemiparesis

6. Which cranial nerve will be spared in the lesion shown below?

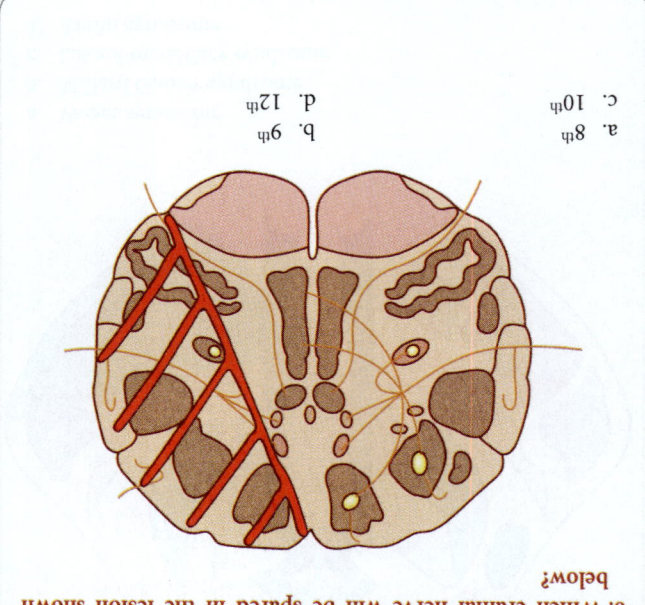

a. 8th   b. 9th
c. 10th   d. 12th

7. Medial medullary syndrome leads to blockage of which of the following blood vessel?

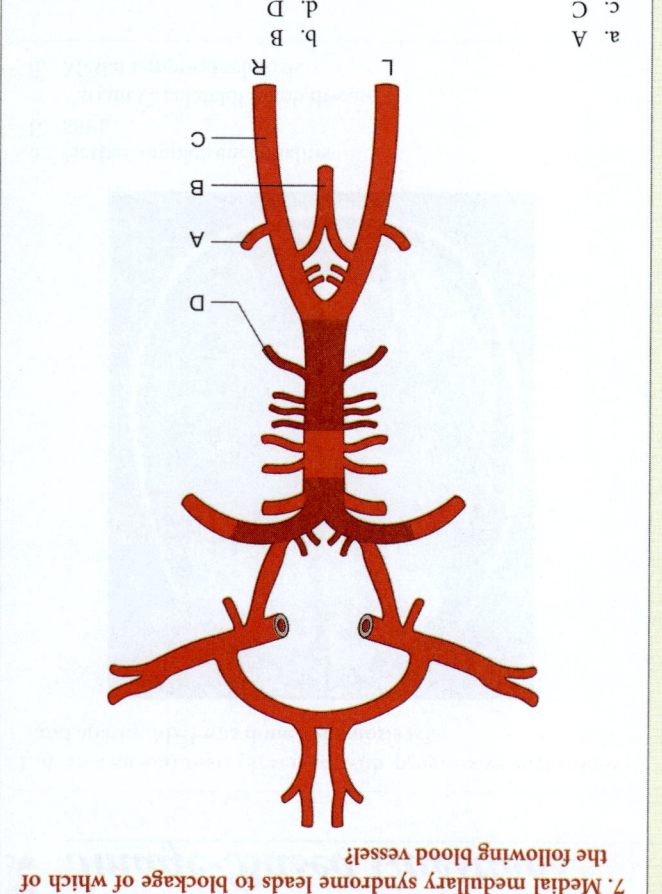

a. A   b. B
c. C   d. D

8. Which of the following is correct about the NCCT shown below?

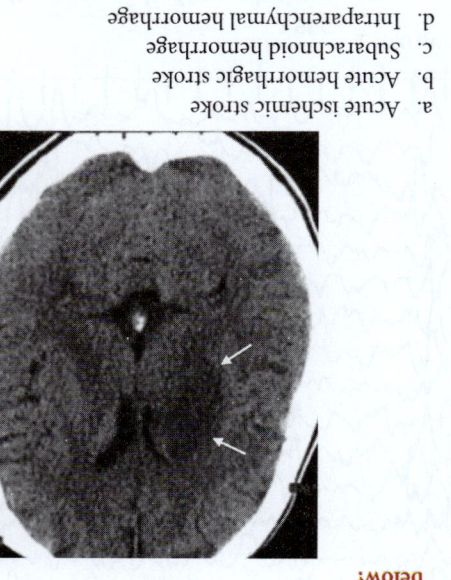

a. Acute ischemic stroke
b. Acute hemorrhagic stroke
c. Subarachnoid hemorrhage
d. Intraparenchymal hemorrhage

9. The NCCT shows presence of:

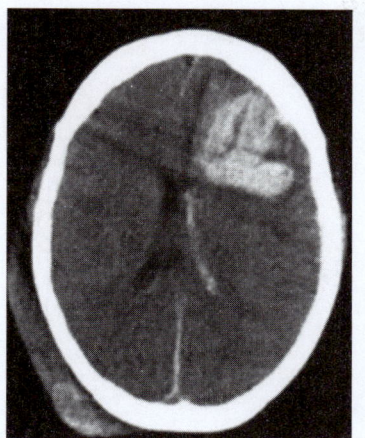

a. Left intraventricular hemorrhage
b. Right intraventricular hemorrhage
c. Left intraparenchymal hemorrhage
d. Right intraparenchymal hemorrhage

10. Patient presents with worst headache of his life. NCCT was done. All are true about the condition except:

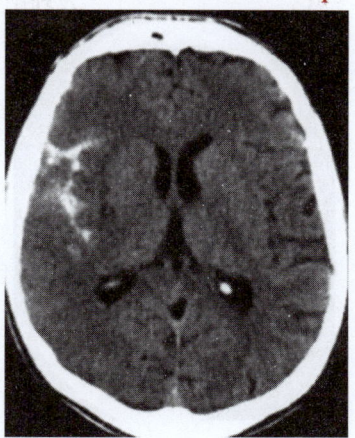

a. Xanthochromic CSF
b. Prolonged QT interval
c. Most common cause of death is rebleeding
d. Nimodipine is drug of choice

11. 45-year-old woman presents with one-sided ptosis, severe headache for last 4 hours. Patient was non-cooperative during physical examination due to severe headache. CT scan and ECG were done and shows presence of ?

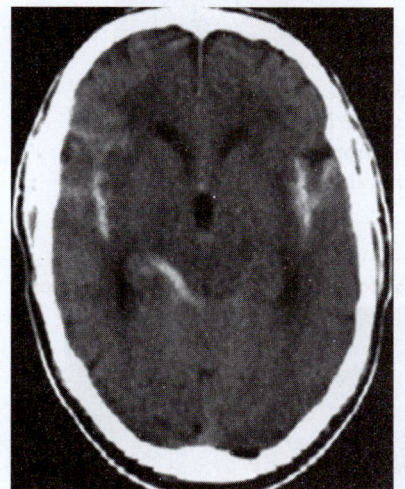
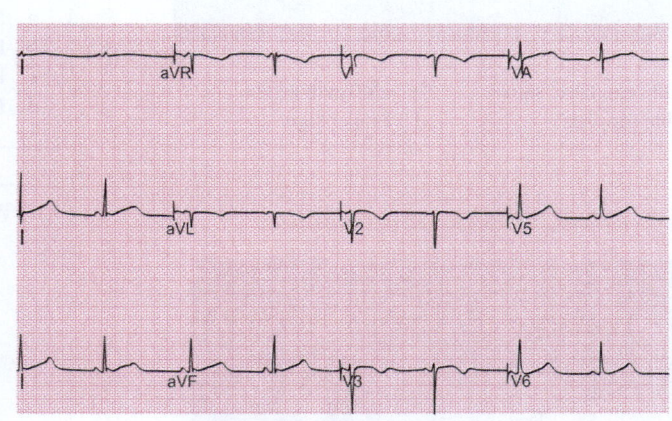

a. SAH and prolonged QT interval
b. SAH and shortened QT interval
c. SAH and ST segment depression
d. SAH and ST segment elevation

12. NCCT was performed on a 40-year old head injury patient. The finding shown is:

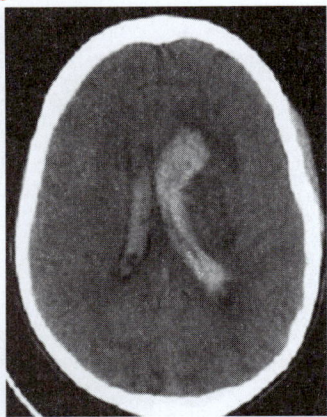

a. Intraparenchymal bleed b. Intraventricular bleed
c. Subarachnoid bleed d. All of the above

15. Which reflex is being tested here?

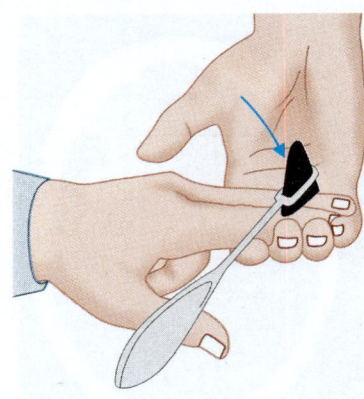

a. Brachioradialis Reflex b. Hoffman Reflex
c. Finger flexor Reflex d. Supinator reflex

13. Which clinical sign is being elicited?

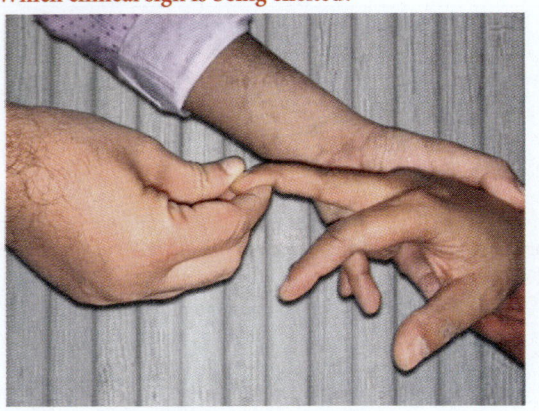

a. Hoffman-Tinel sign b. Hoffman reflex
c. Table top sign d. Prayer sign

16. All are true about the reflex being tested except?

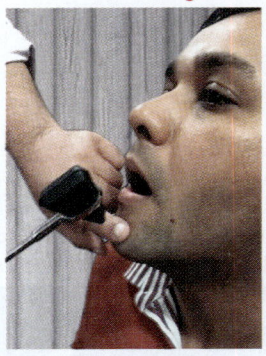

a. Mediated via mesencephalic nucleus
b. Efferent is via V3 branch of trigeminal
c. Brisk in amyotrophic lateral sclerosis
d. Brisk in cervical myelopathy at C5 level

14. Which test is being performed in the patient?

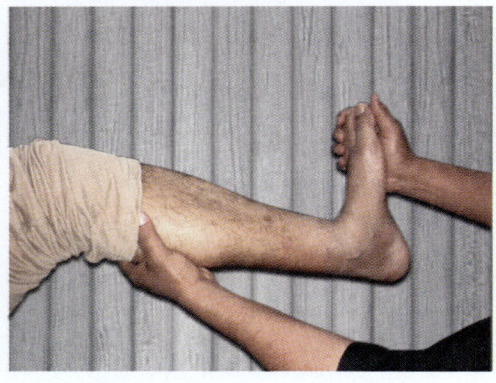

a. Gordon sign b. Hoffman sign
c. Ankle clonus d. Oppenheimer sign

17. Which of the following is correct about the lesion?

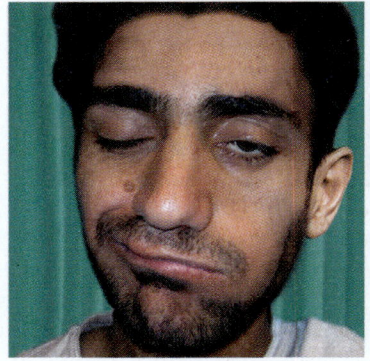

a. Right infranuclear seventh nerve palsy
b. Left supranuclear seventh nerve palsy
c. Left infranuclear seventh nerve palsy
d. Right supranuclear seventh nerve palsy

18. All of the following layers are pierced by this needle except:

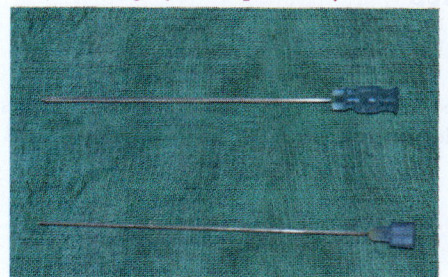

   a. Supraspinous ligament
   b. Interspinous ligament
   c. Ligamentum flavum
   d. Ligmanetum denticulatum

19. A 35-year old patient complains of daily headaches for a month and has suffered from multiple episodes of GTCS since last one week and speech deficit. MRI shows a solitary lesion with perilesional edema. All are true about the condition except?

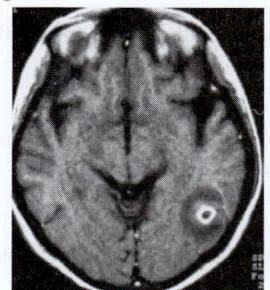

   a. Steroids must be given in the racemose form
   b. MRI shows colloidal stage of NCC
   c. CSF eosinophilia
   d. Enzyme linked immune-electrotransfer blot assay is more sensitive than CSF ELISA

20. 25-year-old lady presented with complaint of night time bedwetting for last 3 consecutive nights and stiffness in legs for last few months. She reported her symptoms are worsened by physical exertion. MRI head was performed. Which is correct?

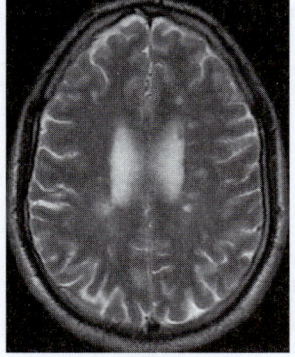

   a. Presence of periventricular lesions
   b. Raised intracranial pressure
   c. Cortical atrophy
   d. Loss of corticomedullary differentiation

21. A child with mental retardation and skin rash on cheeks was subjected to CT scan. The diagnosis of the child is:

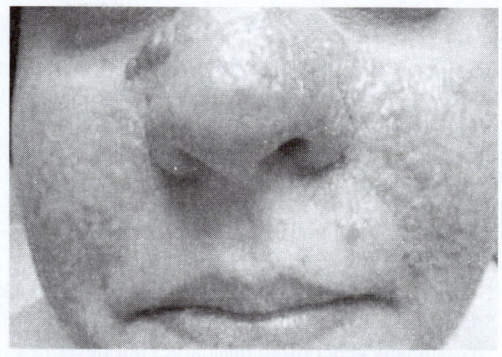

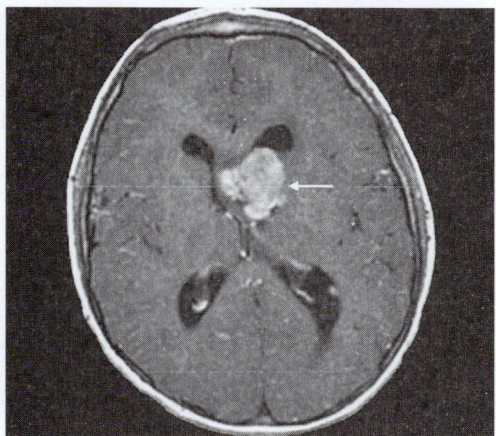

   a. Tuberous sclerosis
   b. Von Hippel Lindau
   c. Sturge Weber syndrome
   d. Ataxia telangiectasia

22. 14-year-old boy presents with bilateral foot deformity. On examination, thickened peripheral nerves and sensory gait ataxia is noted. On biopsy of the nerve, a typical onion bulb appearance is noted. The probable diagnosis is?

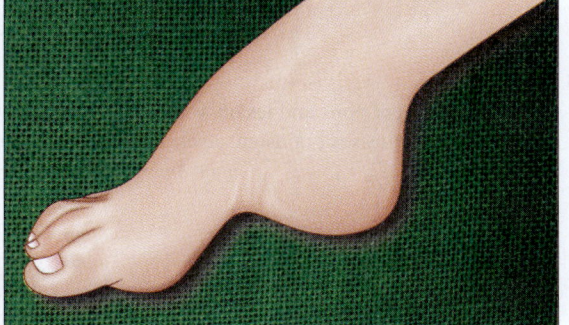

   a. Friedreich ataxia
   b. Ataxia telangiectasia
   c. Charcot Marie tooth disease
   d. Leprosy

Answers of Image-Based Questions

1. **Ans. (c) Variant Creutzfeldt Jakob disease**
   - The image shows MRI head showing cortical ribboning with clinical feature of myoclonus and apathy which favors diagnosis as vCJD.
   - Choice A involves mainly temporal lobes. Choice B is seen in children. Medial temporal sclerosis leads to focal seizures and needs surgery.

2. **Ans. (b) Hypsarrhythmia**
   Criteria for hypsarrhythmia:
   - Essentially continuous electrical discharge
   - Present in both wakefulness and sleep
   - Consist of random high voltage slow waves and spikes
   - Spikes vary in location and duration: focal or multifocal
   - Occasionally generalized discharges but never in a rhythmic or highly organized pattern

   Choice C is seen with prion disease while choice D is seen with cerebral anoxia or birth asphyxia.

3. **Ans. (d) Intracranial hypotension**
   - The clinical information of poor response to levodopa with bradykinesia and rigidity indicates atypical parkinsonism. Moreover resting tremor is absent and tendency to recurrent falls points to diagnosis of progressive supranuclear gaze palsy.
   - MRI head shows a *humming bird* appearance.
     - Atrophy of the midbrain, which looks like head of a bird with beak anteriorly towards optic chiasma (notice the black arrow)
     - Perservered pons forms the body of the bird.

4. **Ans. (a) Weber's syndrome**
   - The lesion shown in the image is of midbrain stroke involving the crus cerebri (corticospinal pathway) and oculomotor nerve. This results in ipsilateral 3rd nerve palsy with contralateral hemiplegia and is called Weber's syndrome.
   - Choice B leads to ipsilateral 6th and 7th cranial nerve palsy with contralateral hemiplegia.
   - Choice C leads to 5th, 7th, 8th, 9th, 10th and 11th cranial nerve palsy with crossed hemi-anesthesia.
   - Choice D leads to bilateral occipital cortex lesions leading to gun barrel vision and subsequent cortical blindness.

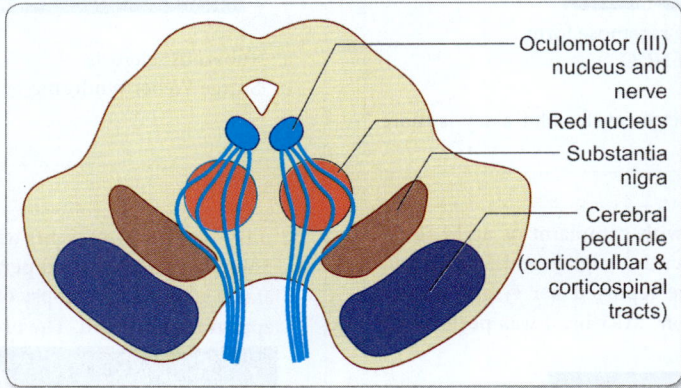

5. **Ans. (c) Patient looks toward the side of lesion**
   - The image is of pons and lesion at this level can involve the sixth nerve and seventh nerve as it arches across the 6th nerve nucleus. Clinical diagnosis is brainstem stroke, Foville syndrome.

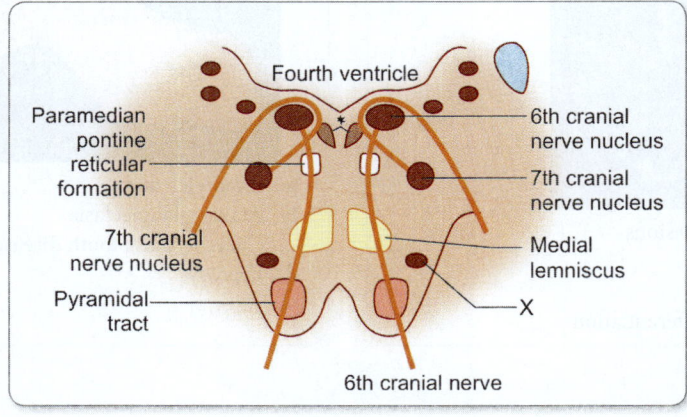

- Choice A is correct as manifestation of 6th nerve involvement.
- Choice B is correct as manifestation of 7th nerve involvement.
- Choice D is correct due to involvement of pyramidal pathway.
- In cortical stroke, patient looks towards the lesion.
- *In brainstem stroke, patient looks away from the lesion.*
- The brainstem centers for lateral conjugate gaze are in the pons, very close to the sixth nerve nuclei.
- The right frontal center connects with the left pontine center, and the left frontal center with the right pontine center.
- The left pontine center controls lateral conjugate eye movement to the left, and the right pontine center controls lateral conjugate eye movement to the right.
- *Thus, a patient who has a destruction of one pontine center will look away from the lesion and towards the paralyzed side because of the unopposed action of the opposite pontine center.*

6. Ans. (d) 12th
   - The image shows presence of lateral medullary syndrome with involvement of nucleus of tractus solitarius and nucleus ambiguus but spares the 12th nerve, which originates medially.

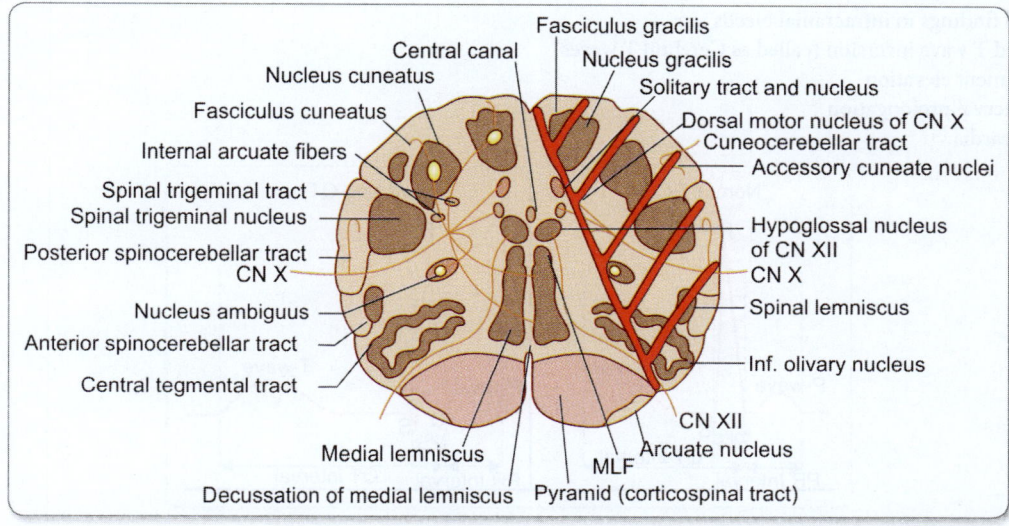

7. Ans. (b) **Anterior spinal artery**
   The following diagram and its branches should be remembered.

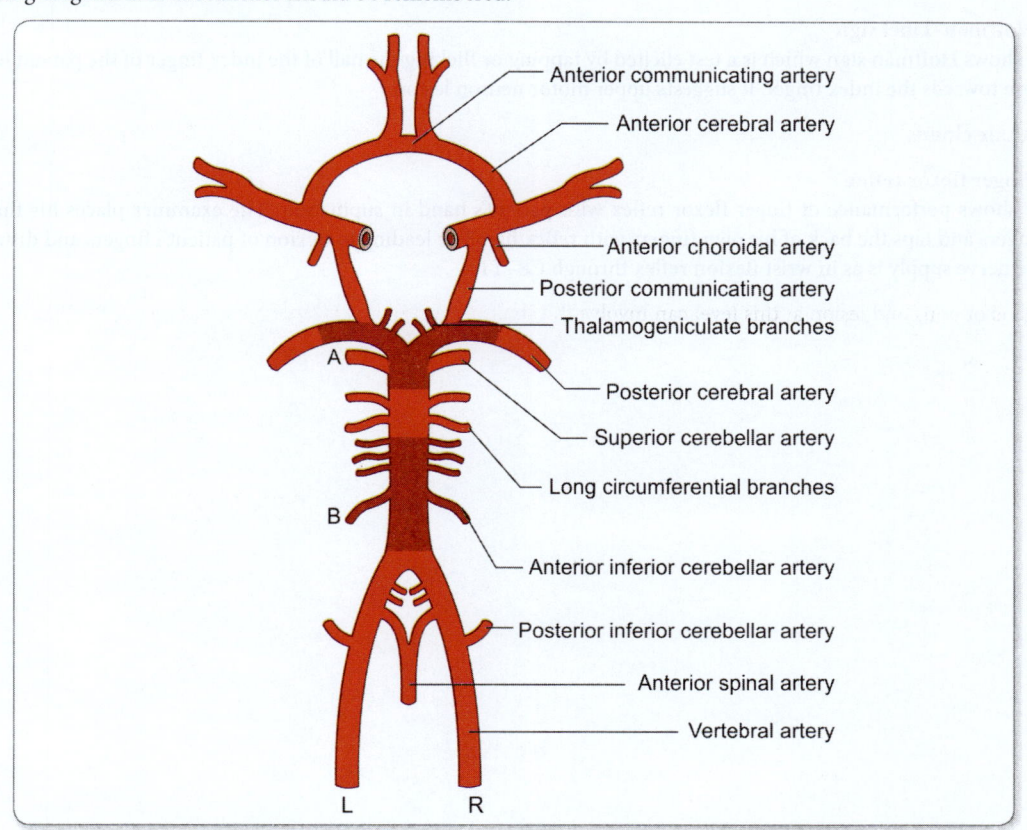

8. **Ans. (a) Acute ischemic stroke**
   The image shows NCCT with hypodensity diagnostic of right ischemic stroke.

9. **Ans. (c) Left intraparenchymal hemorrhage**
   The image shows NCCT showing a hyperdensity in left frontoparietal area suggestive of intraparenchymal hemorrhage.

10. **Ans. (c) Most common cause of death is rebleeding**
    The image shows NCCT showing presence of blood in Sylvian fissure suggestive of diagnosis of subarachnoid hemorrhage.
    - Choice A is correct because in delayed presentation of SAH, RBC will lyse and lead to yellow CSF called xanthochromic CSF.
    - Choice B is correct with catecholamines released due to stress of SAH leading to QT prolongation.
    - Choice C is *wrong* as most common cause of death is vasospasm.
    - Choice D is correct as Nimodipine reduces the vasospasm in surrounding area and reduces mortality.

11. **Ans. (a) SAH and prolonged QT interval**
    - The presence of severe headache and CT scan showing hyperdensity in Slyvian fissure is diagnostic of subarachnoid hemorrhage. The most common cranial nerve involved in ruptured berry aneurysm is oculomotor nerve.
    - The ECG findings in intracranial bleeds are:
      - Marked T wave inversion (called as Cerebral T waves)
      - ST segment elevation
      - QT interval prolongation
      - Bradycardia.

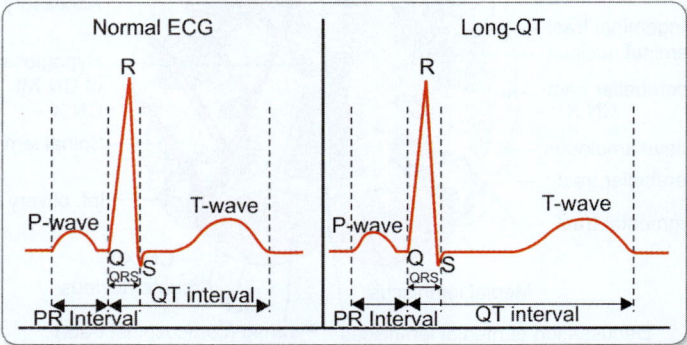

12. **Ans. (b) Intraventricular bleed**
    The NCCT shows hyperdensity in the ventricles indicating intraventricular bleed and periventricular edema.

13. **Ans. (b) Hoffman-Tinel sign**
    The image shows Hoffman sign which is a test elicited by tapping or flicking the nail of the index finger of the patient leading to flexion of the thumb towards the index finger. It suggests upper motor neuron lesion.

14. **Ans. (c) Ankle clonus**

15. **Ans. (c) Finger flexor reflex**
    The image shows performance of finger flexor reflex with patient's hand in supination. The examiner places his fingers against the patient's fingers and taps the back of his own fingers with reflex hammer leading to flexion of patient's fingers and distal phalanx of the thumb. The nerve supply is as in wrist flexion reflex through C8–T1.

16. Ans. (d) Brisk in cervical myelopathy at C5 level

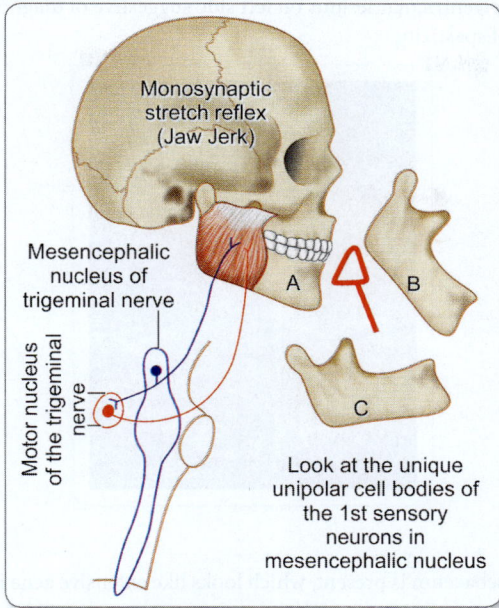

To elicit the jaw reflex, the examiner places his index finger or thumb over the middle of the patient's chin, holding the mouth open about midway with the jaw relaxed. The response is an upward jerk of the mandible.

Afferent impulse of this reflex is carried through the sensory portion of the trigeminal nerve, possibly through the mesencephalic root. *Efferent impulse* is carried through its motor portion. The reflex center is in the pons.

Interpretation:
- In normal individuals, the jaw jerk is minimally active or absent.
- Its greatest use is in distinguishing limb hyperreflexia due to a cervical spine lesion (where the jaw jerk is normal) from a state of generalized hyperreflexia (where the jaw jerk is increased along with all the other reflexes).
- Exaggerated with lesions affecting the corticobulbar pathways above the motor nucleus, especially if bilateral, as in pseudobulbar palsy or amyotrophic lateral sclerosis (ALS).

17. Ans. (c) Left infranuclear seventh nerve palsy
The patient is able to close his eyes on the right side and shows face deviation to right side (normal side). On left side, there is inability to close eye with slight up-rolling of eye on forcible closure. No lines on forehead indicate inability to produce wrinkles on forehead.

18. Ans. (d) Ligamentum denticulatum
The layers pierced when the lumbar puncture needle is advanced are:
- Skin
- Subcutaneous tissue
- Supraspinous ligament
- Interspinous ligament
- Ligamentum flavum
- Dura mater

The pia mater is a vascular membrane that closely covers the spinal cord. It is thickened on either side between the nerve roots to form the **ligamentum denticulatum**, which passes laterally to adhere to the arachnoid and the dura mater.

19. Ans. (a) Steroids must be given in the racemose form

Choice A	In cases of multiple cysts in the subarachnoid space (i.e., the racemose form), urgent *surgical extirpation* is recommended. If the obstruction is due to arachnoiditis, placement of a ventricular shunt should be done.
Choice B	The image shows presence of perilesional edema with cyst wall enhancement, which indicates colloidal stage of NCC. In vesicular stage hyperintense lesion in T2 is seen but perilesional edema and cyst wall enhancement are not seen In nodular granular stage, calcification is seen around the lesion with absence of edema.
Choice C	CSF eosinophilia is seen in • NCC • Neuro-syphilis • TB meningitis
Choice D	Enzyme-linked immunosorbent assay (ELISA) is the most widely used test of cerebrospinal fluid (CSF); it has a sensitivity of 50% and a specificity of 65% for neurocysticercosis. Enzyme-linked immunoelectrotransfer blot (EITB) assay in serum using lentil lectin glycoprotein antigens of *T. solium* cysts is also highly sensitive and specific, initially described as 98% and 100%, respectively for detection of antibodies in serum and cerebrospinal fluid.

20. **Ans. (a) Presence of Periventricular Lesions**
    The image shows presence of small periventricular lesions on left side suggestive of diagnosis of multiple sclerosis. The lesions explain nocturnal enuresis and development of spasticity.

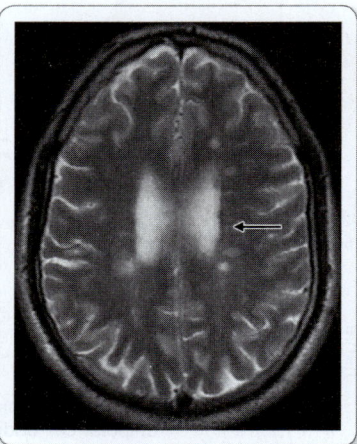

21. **Ans. (a) Tuberous sclerosis** (Ref: Nelson 18th ed. ch. 596.2)
    - In the picture, on the left adenoma sebaceum is present, which looks like extensive acne in a butterfly distribution. The CT scan head shows a big lesion obliterating the ventricular system. These are subependymal nodules seen in tuberous sclerosis.
    - Point against Sturge Weber is the absence of cutaneous lesion of port wine stain.
    - VHL is associated with cerebellar hemangioblastoma.

22. **Ans. (c) Charcot Marie tooth disease**
    The image shows presence of pes cavus which indicates distal muscle weakness. Concomitant sensory deficit is leading to gait ataxia. Classical onion bulb appearance on nerve biopsy nails the diagnosis as Charcot Marie tooth disease.

Conceptual Diagnostic Algorithm

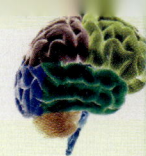

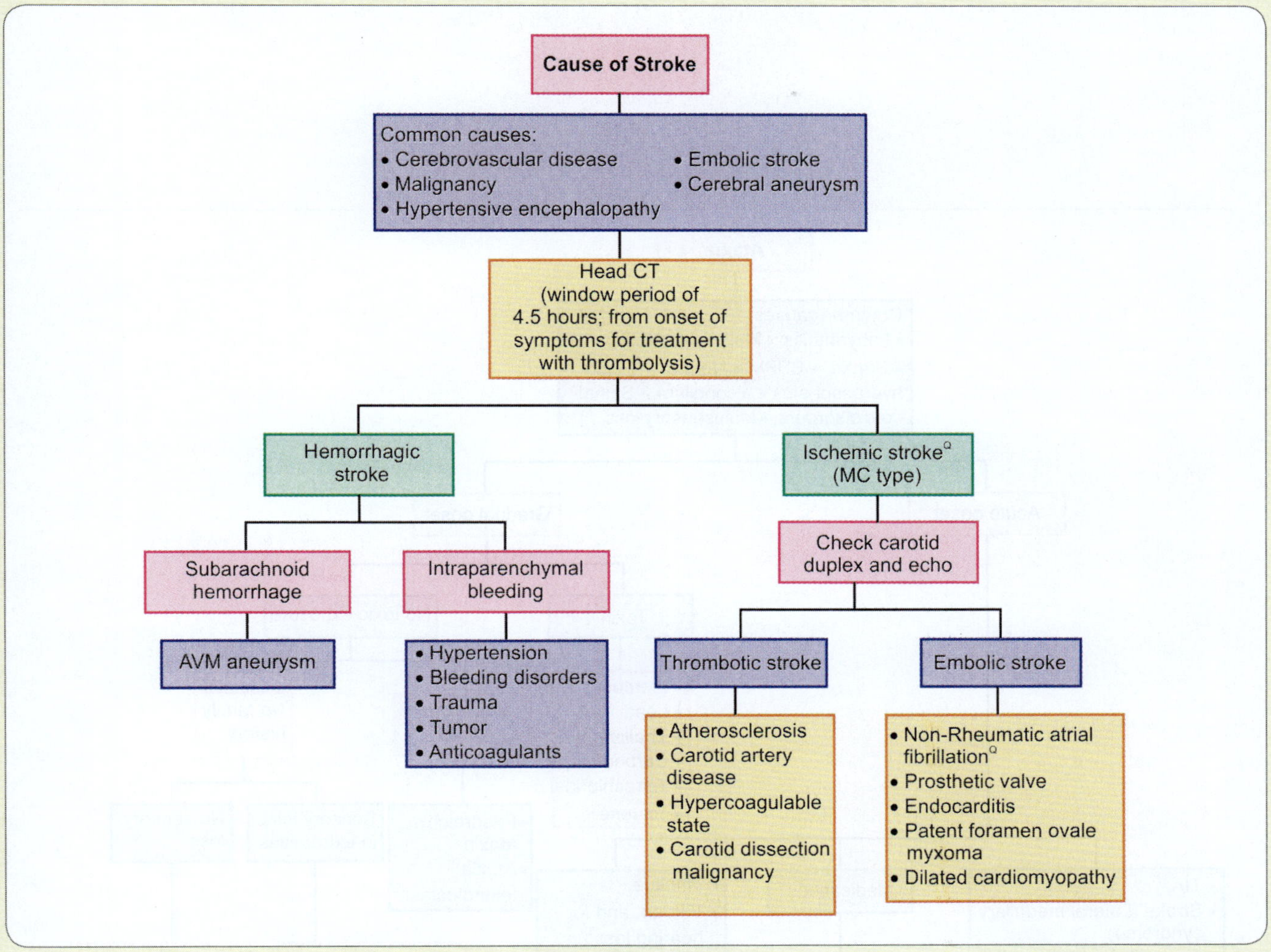

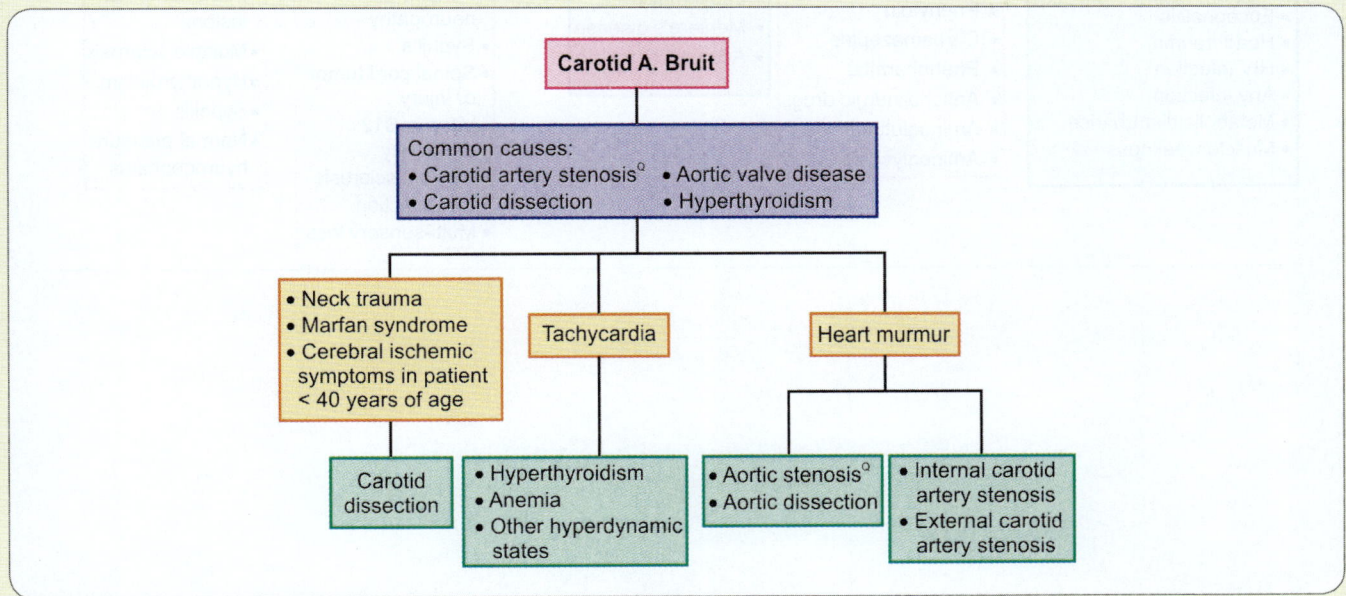

* Ejection systolic murmur of aortic stenosis radiates to neck and felt as Carotid Thrill.
* Donot mix with dancing carotids, seen in Aortic Regurgitation
* Cartid sinus message is contraindicated in patient with Carotid Artery Bruit

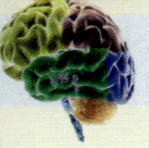

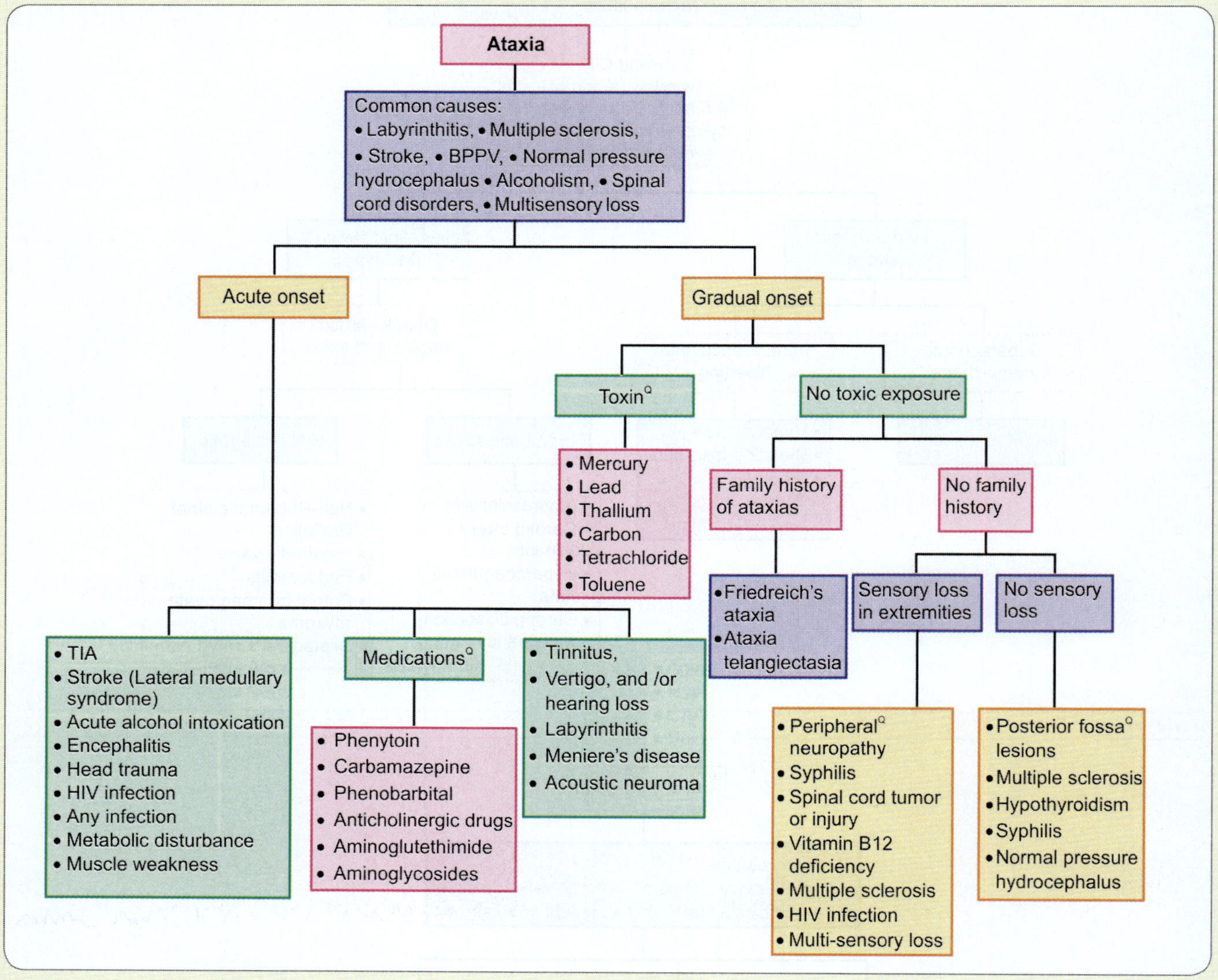

Ataxia

Common causes:
- Labyrinthitis, • Multiple sclerosis,
- Stroke, • BPPV, • Normal pressure hydrocephalus • Alcoholism, • Spinal cord disorders, • Multisensory loss

Acute onset
- TIA
- Stroke (Lateral medullary syndrome)
- Acute alcohol intoxication
- Encephalitis
- Head trauma
- HIV infection
- Any infection
- Metabolic disturbance
- Muscle weakness

Medications^Q
- Phenytoin
- Carbamazepine
- Phenobarbital
- Anticholinergic drugs
- Aminoglutethimide
- Aminoglycosides

- Tinnitus, Vertigo, and/or hearing loss
- Labyrinthitis
- Meniere's disease
- Acoustic neuroma

Gradual onset

Toxin^Q
- Mercury
- Lead
- Thallium
- Carbon Tetrachloride
- Toluene

No toxic exposure

Family history of ataxias
- Friedreich's ataxia
- Ataxia telangiectasia

No family history

Sensory loss in extremities
- Peripheral^Q neuropathy
- Syphilis
- Spinal cord tumor or injury
- Vitamin B12 deficiency
- Multiple sclerosis
- HIV infection
- Multi-sensory loss

No sensory loss
- Posterior fossa^Q lesions
- Multiple sclerosis
- Hypothyroidism
- Syphilis
- Normal pressure hydrocephalus

Multiple Choice Questions

Epilepsy

1. A 16-year-old girl was on anti-epileptic for treatment of focal seizure episodes while asleep. She has had no seizure for last 6 months. NCCT and EEG is normal. What is the further management? *(AIIMS Nov 2018)*
   a. Stop treatment
   b. Continue for 2 years
   c. Lifelong treatment
   d. Stop treatment and follow up with 6 monthly EEG

2. A man falls in front of a liquor shop and becomes unconscious. On admission he has fast pulse, feeble respiratory events and slurring of speech. He is kept in observation overnight and when he wakes up he is normal but could not recall the events of the previous night. What is the likely explanation? *(AIIMS May 2017)*
   a. Epilepsy
   b. Drunkenness
   c. Concussion
   d. Diffuse axonal injury

3. A 25 year old epileptic patient is on levetiracetam 1000mg twice daily for last 2 years. He started to develop anger and aggressive behaviour as an intolerable side effect which is affecting his quality of life. What is the next step in management of the patient? *(AIIMS May 2017)*
   a. Gradually taper levetiracetam over 6 months
   b. Stop levetiracetam immediately
   c. Continue the same dose for the next 5 years
   d. Stop the drug and initiate alternative anti-epileptic drug.

4. Negative myoclonus is seen in? *(Recent Pattern Questions)*
   a. Hepatic encephalopathy
   b. Variant CJD
   c. Janz Syndrome
   d. Salaam Seizures

5. Which of the following is associated with mesial temporal sclerosis? *(Recent Pattern Questions)*
   a. History of febrile seizures
   b. Hypothyroidism
   c. Neurofibromatosis
   d. Recurring Oral aphthous ulceration

6. Which is the most efficacious treatment of mesial temporal lobe epilepsy syndrome? *(Recent Pattern Questions)*
   a. Amygdalohippocampectomy
   b. Levetiracetam
   c. Primidone
   d. Vagus nerve stimulation

7. A known case of GTCS is on Valproate for last 1 year. He has been seizure free for last 1 year. Recent EEG is normal. Anti-epileptics withdrawl should be initiated ____ years of initiation? *(Recent Pattern Questions)*
   a. 1
   b. 2
   c. 3
   d. 4

8. A 35 year patient recalls episodes where he smells pungent odour, becomes sweaty and loses consciousness. His family member says while unconscious he was having facial twitching with lip smacking movements. What is the diagnosis? *(Recent Pattern Questions)*
   a. Focal seizures
   b. Hysteria
   c. Atonic seizures
   d. Myoclonic seizures

9. Lennox Gastaut Syndrome is characterized by?
   a. Single seizure type *(Recent Question 2016-17)*
   b. Atyical febrile seizures
   c. Good prognosis with adequate control
   d. EEG showing less than 3 Hz Spike and Wave discharge

10. Which drug is suitable for epilepsy related to brain tumour? *(Recent Question 2016-17)*
    a. Levetiracetam
    b. Phenytoin
    c. Carbamazepine
    d. Phenobarbitone

11. Gender specific side effect of Valproate? *(AIIMS Nov 2015)*
    a. Alopecia
    b. Weight loss
    c. PCOD
    d. Tremor

12. The following statement are true regarding epilepsy except: *(AP PG 2015)*
    a. Jacksonian epilepsy is a spreading seizure activity
    b. Serum level of prolactin increases dramatically after tonic clonic convulsions
    c. Changes in memory/perception and "blackouts" are not features of complex partial seizures
    d. Absence seizures are briefer and more frequent without postictal confusion

13. Patient presents with history of lip smacking and staring for 3minutes. Past history of Headache for 6 months. He was unaware of event. MRI shows a mass in temporal lobe showing hyper-intensity on T2 weighted image Diagnosis is?
    a. Meningioma *(JIPMER Nov 2015)*
    b. Astrocytoma
    c. Craniopharyngioma
    d. Glioblastoma multiforme

14. All are used in early generalised convulsive status epilepticus treatment except? *(JIPMER Nov 2015)*
    a. Phenobarbitone
    b. Fosphyenytoin
    c. Lorazepam
    d. Valproate

15. The below EEG of a 1 year old infant shows: *(APPG 2015)*

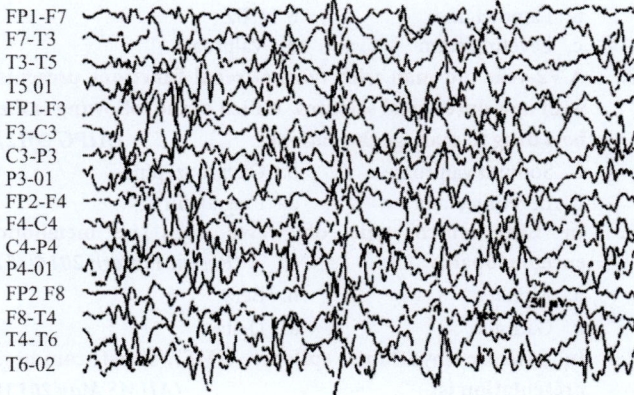

   a. Hypsarrhythmia
   b. Burst suppression pattern
   c. Spike and slow wave
   d. Periodic lateralized epileptiform discharge

16. 7-year old girl is easily distracted in class and exhibits poor scholastic performance. Seizures are precipitated by hyperventilation. Diagnosis is? *(AIIMS May 2014)*

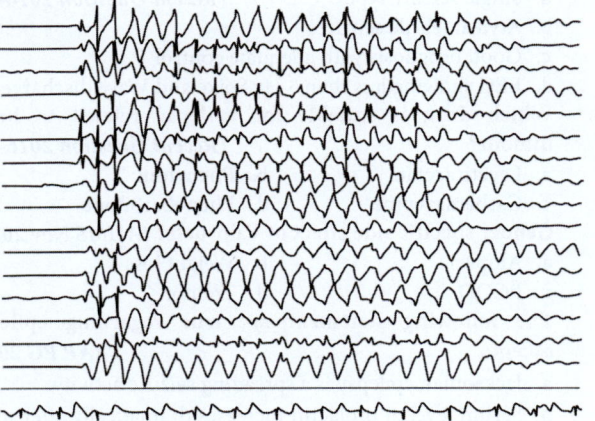

   a. Myoclonic seizures b. Absence seizures
   c. Atonic seizures d. Myotonia

17. Lafora's disease presents with
   (Recent Question 2015-2016)
   a. G.T.C.S b. Myoclonic epilepsy
   c. Petit mal epilepsy d. Partial seizures

18. Person suffers seizure on platform while waiting for train. He has a band showing him to be epileptic and the medicines he takes are in his pocket. So what should you do? *(AIIMS Nov 14)*
   a. Take person away from train make sure he does not fall on tracks, meanwhile call for medical help and transfer to hospital
   b. Take person away from train stuff handkerchief in his mouth hold his hands and feet till seizure subsides then transfer to hospital
   c. Take person away from train make him lie down hold his leg up give the meds and water then transfer to hospital
   d. Take person away from train give meds and water then transfer to hospital

19. DOC of GTCS in pregnancy? *(Recent Pattern 2015-16)*
   a. Lamotrigine b. CBZ
   c. Levetiracetam d. Valproate

20. A 72-year old man with normal renal functions presents with new onset focal seizures. Which of the following is the best drug to manage the patient? *(AIPG 2012)*
   a. Sodium valproate b. Oxcarbazepine
   c. Levetiracetam d. Pregabalin

21. In EEG which type of waves seen in metabolic encephalopathy: *(Recent Pattern 2014/15)*
   a. Alpha b. Beta
   c. Gamma d. Delta

22. In Juvenile myoclonic epilepsy (JME), most common presentation is? *(AIIMS May 2013)*
   a. GTCS during sleep b. GTCS on awake state
   c. Myoclonus d. Absence seizures

23. New anti-epileptic drug for Lennox Gastaut syndrome is: *(AIIMS Nov 2012)*
   a. Lacosamide b. Vigabatrin
   c. Rufinamide d. Zonisamide

24. A pregnant lady is a known case of juvenile myoclonic epilepsy and is receiving sodium valproate. Which of the following drugs is best suited after valproate for management of this patient. *(AIIMS May 2013)*
   a. Phenytoin b. Carbamazepine
   c. Lamotrigine d. Lacosamide

25. Which can differentiate between seizures and syncope?
   a. Recovery from unconsciousness *(AIIMS May 2013)*
   b. Injury due to fall
   c. Urinary incontinence
   d. Tongue bite

26. Most effective management in medically intractable seizures? *(AIIMS May 2013)*
   a. Ketotic diet b. Vagus nerve stimulation
   c. Deep brain stimulation d. Surgery

27. A neurosurgeon in parent teacher meeting saw a child with precocious puberty and uncontrollable laughing. He suggested the parent of child to get a MRI done to evaluate for the possibility of: *(AIIMS Nov 2012)*
   a. Hypothalamic Hamartoma
   b. Pineo-germinoma
   c. Pituitary adenoma
   d. Craniopharyngioma

28. Most common electrolyte abnormality causing seizures in hospitalized patients is: *(Recent Pattern 2014/15)*
   a. Hyponatremia b. Hypernatremia
   c. Hypokalemia d. Hyperkalemia

29. Incorrect about Lafora's disease is: *(Recent Pattern 2014/15)*
   a. Myoclonus
   b. Autosomal recessive
   c. Diagnosis by DNA sequencing
   d. Treatment with glucocerebrosidase infusions

30. EEG showing < 3Hz polyspike activity is seen in:
   a. Lennox Gastaut syndrome *(Recent Pattern 2014/15)*
   b. Absence seizures
   c. Juvenile myoclonic epilepsy
   d. GTCS

31. Hypsarrythmia on EEG is seen in: *(Recent Pattern 2014/15)*
   a. Infantile tremor syndrome
   b. Petit mal epilepsy
   c. Rolandic epilepsy
   d. Infantile spasm

32. Periodic lateralized slowing on EEG is seen in:
   a. Herpes simplex encephalitis *(Recent Pattern 2014/15)*
   b. Mesial temporal sclerosis
   c. SSPE
   d. Variant Creutzfelt Jakob disease

33. Drug of choice in neonatal seizures:
   (Recent Pattern 2014/15)
   a. Phenobarbitone b. Phenytoin
   c. Pentobarbital d. Topiramate

34. Atypical febrile seizures are associated with:
   (Recent Pattern 2014/15)
   a. Complex partial seizures b. No post ictal deficit
   c. Neuro-degeneration d. Raised ICT

35. Pyknolepsy is seen in: *(Recent Pattern 2014/15)*
   a. Lennox Gastaut syndrome
   b. Absence seizure
   c. Narcolepsy
   d. Adrenoleukodystrophy

36. **Best drug for photosensitive epilepsy:**
    (Recent Pattern 2014/15)
    a. Valproate b. Topiramate
    c. Ethosuximide d. Zonisamide
37. **Periodic epileptiform discharges in EEG are seen in:**
    a. S.S.P.E *(Recent Pattern 2014/15)*
    b. Herpes simplex encephalitis
    c. Subdural effusion
    d. Status epilepticus
38. **6 year old child with abnormal twitching of the face during sleep noticed by mother. EEG shows spikes over centro-temporal area. Diagnosis:** *(Recent Pattern 2014/15)*
    a. GTCS b. Rolandic epilepsy
    c. Absence seizure d. Subtle seizure
39. **A 29-year old, 4-month pregnant primigravida has history of juvenile myoclonic epilepsy. She has been regularly taking sodium valproate and now seeking an opinion for her antiepileptic regimen. What would you suggest her?**
    (AIIMS May 2012)
    a. Immediately taper valproate and start lamotrigine
    b. Continue valproate with monitoring of drug level
    c. Switch to carbamazepine
    d. Add lamotrigine to valproate
40. **Absence seizures are seen in:** *(AIIMS Dec 98)*
    a. Grand mal epilepsy b. Myoclonic epilepsy
    c. Petitmal epilepsy d. Hyperkinetic child
41. **Absence seizures are characterized on EEG by:** *(AI 2003)*
    a. 3 Hz spike & wave b. 1-2 Hz spike & wave
    c. Generalized poly spikes d. Hypsarrythmia
42. **All of the following are features of juvenile Myoclonic epilepsy, except** *(AIIMS May 04)*
    a. Myoclonus on awakening
    b. Generalized tonic-clonic seizures
    c. Automatism
    d. Absence seizures
43. **Myoclonic seizure is typically seen in:** *(PGI Dec 98)*
    a. SSPE b. Cerebellar lesion
    c. Pontine lesion d. Thalamic lesion
44. **Commonest type of seizure in newborn:** *(AI 08)*
    a. Clonic b. Tonic
    c. Subtle d. Myoclonic
45. **The drug of choice for absence seizure** *(AIIMS Nov 06)*
    a. Valproate b. Gabapentin
    c. Carbamezepine d. Phenytoin
46. **Which of the following is the most common location of intracranial neurocysticercosis :** *(AIIMS Nov 05)*
    a. Brain parenchyma b. Subarachnoid space
    c. Spinal cord d. Orbit

Raised ICP

47. **An intubated patient exhibits eye opening to pressure and abnormal flexion. What is the GCS score?**
    (AIIMS May 2018)
    a. E2 VT M3 b. E2 VT M4
    c. E2 V1 M3 d. E2 V1 M3
48. **In a patient of head injury, the following sign is noted on his handkerchief. Which is the next test to confirm the diagnosis?** *(Recent Question 2019)*

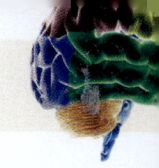

    a. Beta 2 micro-globulin b. Beta trace protein
    c. Beta amyloid d. Beta glucuronidase
49. **Patient had a RTA and was put on mechanical ventilation. He is opening his eyes on verbal command. He moves all his limbs spontaneously. What will be his GCS score?**
    a. 9T b. 10T *(AIIMS Nov 2018)*
    c. 11T d. 12T
50. **Calculate the GCS of a patient with spontaneous eye opening, who moves away his limb on painful stimulus and speaks inappropriate words?** *(AIIMS Nov 2017)*
    a. 10
    b. 11
    c. 12
    d. 13
51. **A lady had a normal vaginal delivery and was discharged. On 3rd day she came back with fever, tachycardia and seizures. Fundus examination shows papilledema with no focal deficits. What is the diagnosis?** *(AIIMS May 2017)*
    a. Meningitis
    b. Acute migraine
    c. Cortical vein thrombosis
    d. Subarachnoid haemorrhage
52. **A 30 year old female was admitted to casualty with a history of head trauma. On examination she is lying with both legs in extended posture. She opens her eyes to pain, moans and localises pain on left hand. Calculate her GCS?**
    a. 7 b. 8 *(AIIMS May 2017)*
    c. 9 d. 11
53. **Which is not a sign of raised ICP?**
    a. Blurring of disc margins *(AIIMS May 2017)*
    b. Positive Kernig Sign
    c. Ipsilateral pupil dilatation
    d. Ipsilateral hemiplegia
54. **CT scan Head should be done before Lumbar puncture in all of the following except?** *(Recent Pattern Questions)*
    a. Hypertension
    b. Immunocompromised state
    c. Kernohan Woltman sign
    d. Low GCS score

55. **All of the following are seen in brain death except?**
    (Recent Pattern Questions)
    a. Elicitation of Deep Tendon reflexes
    b. Dorsiflexion of great toe bilaterally
    c. Constricted pupil
    d. Absent gag reflex

56. **Foraminal brain herniation leads to?**
    a. Ipsilateral pupillary dilatation *(Recent Pattern Questions)*
    b. Locked in state
    c. Respiratory arrest
    d. Ipsilateral hemiplegia

57. **A 40 year old patient is brought with head injury. Which of the following will help in decreasing the value of Raised ICP?** *(AIIMS May 2016)*
    a. Administer Nimodipine
    b. Increase oxygen content of blood
    c. Prevent the fall of CO_2 levels in the blood
    d. Administer sedative

58. **How much ml CSF can be safely removed in a routine lumbar puncture?** *(Recent Question 2016-17)*
    a. 10-20 ml   b. 20-30 ml
    c. 30-40 ml   d. 40-50 ml

59. **How much CSF can be tapped in case of Normal pressure hydrocephalus to determine the likelihood of response to CSF shunting?** *(Recent Question 2016-17)*
    a. 10-20 ml   b. 20-40 ml
    c. 40-60 ml   d. 60-80 ml

60. **A 75 year old woman presents with progressive memory impairment. Her son says that she behaves like a child with uncontrollable laughing or crying and he found her sitting in a puddle of her urine. Gait abnormality is present. CT head was performed. Diagnosis is?**
    (Recent Question 2016-17)

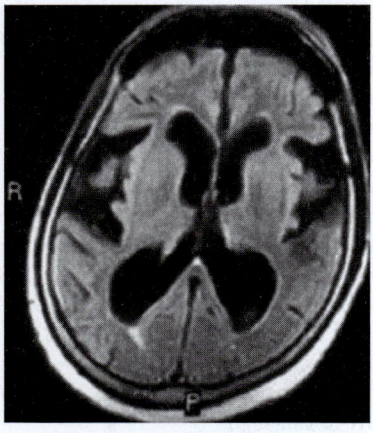

    a. Normal pressure hydrocephalus
    b. Parkinsonism
    c. Dementia with Lewy bodies
    d. Binswanger disease

61. **Decorticate posturing is due to?**
    (Recent Question 2016-17)
    a. Bilateral damage to rostral midbrain
    b. Bilateral damage to caudal diencephalon
    c. Bilateral lesion in ventral pons
    d. Bilateral lesion in medulla

62. **Ocular bobbing is seen in?** *(Recent Question 2016-17)*
    a. Mid brain damage
    b. Pontine damage
    c. Medulla damage
    d. Cerebellum damage

63. **Alpha Coma is seen in?** *(Recent Question 2016-17)*
    a. Diffuse Cortical Damage
    b. Hyperthermia
    c. Central pontine Myelinosis
    d. Critical illness polyneuropathy

64. **Horizontal displacement of pineal calcification > ____ mm is associated with coma.** *(Recent Question 2016-17)*
    a. 1-3 mm
    b. 3-5 mm
    c. 6-8 mm
    d. 9 mm

65. **All are used for management in head injury patient except?** *(Recent Question 2016-17)*
    a. Neuromuscular paralysis
    b. Nor epinephrine
    c. Sedation
    d. Glucocorticoids

66. **Most common form of brain herniation is?**
    a. Transtentorial herniation *(Recent Question 2016-17)*
    b. Transfacial herniation
    c. Foraminal herniation
    d. Transcalvarial herniation

67. **Which of the following is a foraminal herniation of brain?**
    (Recent Question 2016-17)

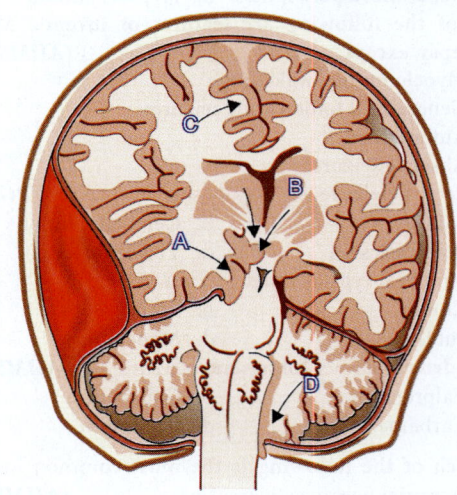

    a. A
    b. B
    c. C
    d. D

68. **This is the plain CT scan of a male who sustained an injury with a baseball bat. Which of the following statements are TRUE regarding this condition?** *(AP PG 2016)*
    P. Middle meningeal artery is the vessel commonly injured
    Q. Usually occurs several weeks after a trivial injury, often forgotten
    R. Lucid interval is classical but seen only in 1/5th to 1/3rd patients
    S. May be associated with a Hutchinson pupil

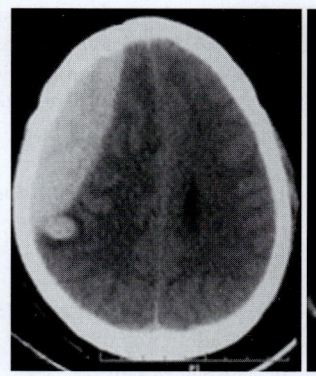 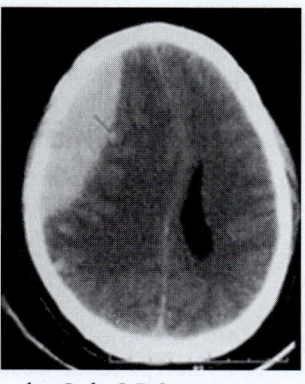

    a. Only P, R, S are correct   b. Only Q,R,S are correct
    c. P,Q,R,S all are correct   d. Only P, R are correct

69. All are seen in Benign Intracranial Hypertension except? *(AIIMS Nov 2015)*
    a. Normal ventricles   b. Papilledema
    c. Proptosis   d. Lateral rectus palsy

70. In Glasgow coma scale maximum and minimum scores are? *(AIIMS Nov 2015)*
    a. 18 and 3   b. 18 and 0
    c. 15 and 3   d. 15 and 0

71. Commonly used shunt in hydrocephalus management? *(AIIMS May 2015)*
    a. Ventriculo atrial   b. Ventriculo peritoneal
    c. Ventriculo pericardial   d. Ventriculo pleural

72. A 10 year old child "blanks out" in class (e.g. stops talking midsentence and then continues as if nothing had happened). During spells there is slight quivering of lips. What is the most probable diagnosis? *(UPSC 2015)*
    a. Brain tumor   b. Autism
    c. Adjustment disorder   d. Absence seizure

73. Which of the following is not a component of Glasgow Coma Scale? *(Bihar PG 2015)*
    a. Eye opening   b. Motor response
    c. Pupil size   d. Verbal response

74. Patient has space occupying lesion in temporal and occipital lobe. What will occur? *(JIPMER Nov 2015)*
    a. Trans-tentorial herniation
    b. Cerebellar tonsil herniation
    c. Cingulate herniation
    d. Trans-falcial herniation

75. A-22 year old obese female experience right eye diplopia. She had increased weight gain in last year and her current BMI is 35. Her fundus examinationa reveals papilledema on the right side. The most likely cause for her symptoms is? *(JIPMER Nov 2014)*
    a. Craniopharyngioma
    b. Idiopathic intracranial hypertension
    c. Optic neuritis
    d. Sagittal sinus thrombosis

76. Which of the following is/are the feature(s) of headache due to increase in intracranial pressure: *(PGI May 2015)*
    a. Increase on coughing/sneezing
    b. Most commonly presents as focal severe acute headache
    c. Pulsatile in nature
    d. Throbbing character
    e. Analgesics are not very helpful

77. Glasgow coma scale motor 4 represents? *(Recent Question 2015-16)*
    a. Withdrawal on flexion   b. Decorticate posturing
    c. Decerebrate posturing   d. Localise pain

78. Increased intra-cranial tension is related to: *(Recent Question 2015-16)*
    a. Hyotension and tachycardia
    b. Hypertension and tachycardia
    c. Hypertension and bradycardia
    d. Hypotension and bradycardia

79. A road traffic accident patient in the casualty is comatose with unilaterally dilated pupil. The NCCT of the patient shows a Lesion peripherally present with concavo – convex border. What is the probable diagnosis? *(Recent Question 2015-16)*
    a. Sub-dural hematoma
    b. Epi-dural hematoma,
    c. Sub-arachnoid hemorrhage
    d. Intra-parenchymal bleeding

80. Extradural hemorrhage on NCCT Head is seen as: *(Recent Question 2015-16)*
    a. Hyperdense biconvex   b. Hypodense biconcave
    c. Hyperdense biconcave   d. Hypodense biconvex

81. A patient after an accident was unconscious. On physical examination there was unilateral papillary dilatation. Possible reason for the same is? *(Recent Question 2015-16)*
    a. Uncal herniation   b. Tonsillar herniation
    c. Cingulate herniation   d. Transcalvarial herniation

82. Stenosis of aqueduct of sylvius results in? *(Recent Question 2015-16)*
    a. Enlargement of lateral ventricles
    b. Enlargement of fourth ventricle
    c. Enlargement of lateral and third ventricle
    d. Enlargement of lateral and fourth ventricle

83. The following fundus finding is seen in?

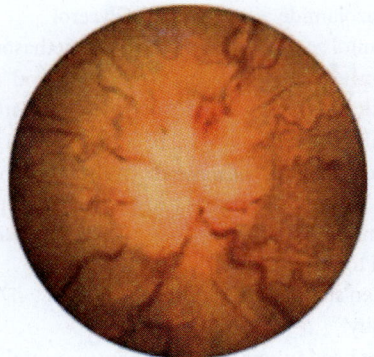

    a. Retinitis pigmentosa   b. Multiple sclerosis
    c. Hysterical blindness   d. ICSOL

84. Cushing's triad has all except? *(AIIMS Nov 14)*
    a. Bradycardia   b. Hypertension
    c. Abnormal breathing   d. Posturing

85. Increased ICT is shown by? *(Recent Pattern 2015-16)*
    a. Miosis   b. Systemic hypotension
    c. Tachycardia   d. Reduction in GCS

86. Not essential for brain death: *(Recent Pattern 2015-16)*
    a. Negative Apnea test   b. Loss of brain stem function
    c. Loss of pupillary reflex   d. Loss of deep tendon reflexes

87. **All are true about CNS leukemia except:**
    a. CNS irradiation is given *(Recent Pattern 2014/15)*
    b. Intrathecal methotrexate is given
    c. Seen with chronic myeloid leukemia
    d. Single blast in CSF is sufficient for diagnosis

88. **Which of the following is a sign of brainstem death?**
    a. Doll's eye reflex absent *(AIIMS Nov 2012)*
    b. Fixed non-reactive pupil
    c. Horner's pupil
    d. Positive vestibulo cochlear reflex

89. **Pseudotumor Cerebri is seen in?** *(AIIMS May 2013)*
    a. Obese women in the age group 20–40 yrs
    b. Obese males 20-40 yrs
    c. Thin females 50-60 yrs
    d. Thin males 50-60 yrs

90. **A 65 yr old male fainted in the bathroom. His relatives informed that his stool was black in colour. He is hypertensive and has got history of coronary artery disease. He was on long term treatment with atenolol, aspirin and sorbitrate. His BP=80/50 and HR 150/min. Most probable diagnosis:** *(AIIMS May 2011)*
    a. Myocardial infarction with cardiogenic shock
    b. Cerebrovascular accident
    c. Gastric ulcer and bleed
    d. Septic shock

91. **In Glasgow coma scale, withdrawal to pain comes under which score?** *(AIIMS Nov 2012)*
    a. M2
    b. M3
    c. M4
    d. M5

92. **Cerebral perfusion pressure to be maintained in road traffic accident case is:** *(Recent Pattern 2014/15)*
    a. 10-30 mm Hg
    b. 30-50 mm Hg
    c. 50-70 mm Hg
    d. >90 mm Hg

93. **DOC for idiopathic intra-cranial hypertension: (I.I.H)** *(Recent Pattern 2014/15)*
    a. Acetazolamide
    b. Glycerol
    c. Mannitol
    d. Dexamethasone

94. **Ipsilateral 3rd nerve palsy with ipsilateral hemiplegia is seen with:** *(Recent Pattern 2014/15)*
    a. Uncal herniation
    b. Cingulate herniation
    c. Millard Gubler syndrome
    d. Weber syndrome

95. **Pseudo-Tumour Cerebri is caused by all except:**
    a. Vitamin A toxicity *(Recent Pattern 2014/15)*
    b. PCM toxicity
    c. Sudden stoppage of steroids
    d. Obesity

96. **In case of head injury in children intracranial pressure to be maintained below:** *(Recent Pattern 2014/15)*
    a. 5 mm Hg
    b. 10 mm Hg
    c. 20 mm Hg
    d. 30 mm Hg

97. **Transtentorial uncal herniation causes all except:**
    a. Ipsilateral dilated pupils *(Recent Pattern 2014/15)*
    b. Ipsilateral hemiplegia
    c. Cheyne stokes respiration
    d. Withdrawal reflex

98. **A waves in ICP monitoring is due to:** *(Recent Pattern 2014/15)*
    a. Atrial contraction
    b. Cheyne stokes breathing
    c. BP fluctuations
    d. Brain herniation

99. **You are a doctor in C.H.C. when a patient of acute head injury comes with worsening of GCS leading to coma. Patient has unilateral dilatation of pupil and hemiplegia. You decide to do burr hole at?** *(AIIMS Nov 2014)*
    a. Refer to higher centre if not known which side bleed is present
    b. If no localizing signs, hole in left temporal (dominant lobe)
    c. Burr hole in middle
    d. Burr hole contralateral to the dilated pupil

100. **Dilated ventricles with normal CSF pressure is seen in:** *(Recent Pattern 2014/15)*
    a. Hydrocephalus
    b. Pseudotumour cerebri
    c. Hydrocephalus ex-vacuo
    d. Normal variant

101. **Incorrect about Mannitol:** *(Recent Pattern 2014/15)*
    a. Increases cerebral oxygen delivery
    b. Prolonged use leads to damage to blood brain barrier
    c. Exacerbates cerebral edema
    d. Osmotic properties take 3 hours to develop

102. **Therapeutic hypothermia is of benefit in preventing neurological complications in:** *(Recent Pattern 2014/15)*
    a. Sepsis
    b. Poly-trauma
    c. Cardiac arrest
    d. Ischemic stroke

103. **'Duret Hemorrhages' are seen in :** *(AIIMS May 08)*
    a. Brain
    b. Kidney
    c. Heart
    d. Lung

104. **Triad of normal-pressure hydrocephalus includes:**
    a. Tremor, aphasia dementia *(AI 1999)*
    b. Ataxia, aphasia, gait disorder
    c. Gait disorder, urinary incontinence, dementia
    d. Gait disorder, urinary incontinence, lower cranial nerve palsy

105. **All the following are features of Pseudotumor Cerebri except :** *(AI 1996)*
    a. Normal-sized ventricles on CT scan
    b. Increased protein in CSF
    c. Papilledema
    d. Absence of focal neurological deficit

106. **A head injured patient, who opens eyes to painful stimulus, is confused and localizes to pain. What is the Glasgow coma score:**
    a. 7
    b. 9 *(AIIMS Nov 05)*
    c. 11
    d. 13

107. **In a patient with head injury, damage in the brain is aggravated by** *(AI 2010)*
    a. Hyperglycemia
    b. Hypothermia
    c. Hypocapnia
    d. Serum osmolality

108. **An elderly female presented with history of progressive right-sided weakness and speech difficulty. She gives a history of a fall in her bathroom two months back. The most likely clinical diagnosis is :** *(AI 91)*
    a. Progressive supranuclear palsy
    b. Left cerebral tumor
    c. Left sided stroke
    d. Left chronic subdural haematoma

109. **The earliest manifestations of increased intracranial pressure following head injury is :** *(AI 2005)*
    a. Ipsilateral papillary dilatation
    b. Contralateral papillary dilatation
    c. Altered mental status
    d. Hemiparesis

Headache

110. True statement regarding migraine in pregnancy?
    a. Ketorolac is preferred   (JIPMER May 2018)
    b. NSAIDs are first line drugs
    c. Improved symptoms with pregnancy
    d. Sumatriptan preferred over chlorpromazine

111. Which of the following best describes a patient with classical migraine?   (Recent Pattern Questions)
    a. Unilateral headache with unilateral visual loss and muscle aches
    b. Left retro-orbital headache with rhinorrhoea and red eye
    c. Visual deficit that persists cessation of unilateral headache
    d. Pulsating unilateral headache worsened with movements of head

112. A patient with past history of recurrent headache, presents with irregular, dazzling, enlarging visual phenomena that obstructs vision in the affected region and remains for several minutes. The symptoms are indicative of:
    a. Acute angle closure glaucoma   (UPSC 2015)
    b. Retinal detachment
    c. Migraine
    d. Intumescent cataract

113. A patient presents with sudden onset occipital headache, ataxia, vomiting and drowsiness and down beating nystagmus. What is the diagnosis?   (JIPMER Nov 2014)
    a. Acute cerebellar hemorrhage
    b. Subarachnoid hemorrhage
    c. Transient ischemic attack
    d. Herpes simplex encephalitis

114. A 22-yrs old man present with history of headache for 6 months which is mainly on frontal region occasionally associated with nausea He has been taking paracetamol 3g per day hydroxycodeine 50 mg 3 times a day and aspirin 300 mg 3 times a day for headache but only with temporary relief from symptoms no focal signs on neurological examinations he also has history of depression and is on treatment for 2 year with paroxetine now What is the diagnosis?   (JIPMER Nov 2014)
    a. Cluster headache
    b. Migraine
    c. Depression associated headache
    d. Analgesic abuse headache

115. All of the following are causes of primary headache EXCEPT: (Recent Question 2015-16)
    a. Migraine   b. Tension headache
    c. Cluster headache   d. Sinusitis

116. A 65yr old lady underwent mastectomy. 6 months later she developed headache with pain at temple region with ESR= 55mm fall in 1 st hour. Diagnosis?   (JIPMER 2014)
    a. Giant cell arteritis
    b. Meningeal metastasis
    c. Tension headache
    d. P.A.N

117. Sumatriptan is contraindicated in all except:
    a. Basilar migraine   (Recent Pattern 2014/15)
    b. Ischemic heart disease
    c. Pregnancy
    d. Ergot alkaloids in last one week

118. A 70 year old retired Military person with good previous medical record complains of bi-temporal headache which is decreased in lying down position. He states that he gets relief by giving pressure over bilateral temples. The patient also complains of loss of appetite with feeling feverish. The most probable diagnosis is: (AIIMS Nov 2012)
    a. Chronic tension headache
    b. Temporal arteritis
    c. Migraine
    d. Fibromyalgia

119. Cluster headache is characterized by all, except: (AI 2005)
    a. Affects predominantly females
    b. Unilateral headache
    c. Onset typically in 20-50 years of life
    d. Associated with conjunctival congestion

120. A female has episodic, recurrent headache in left hemicranium with nausea and parasthesia on right upper and lower limbs is most probably suffering from:
    a. Migraine   (AIIMS June 2000)
    b. Glossopharyngeal neuralgia
    c. Herpes zoster infection of trigeminal Nerve
    d. Brain tumour

121. A female aged 30, presents with episodic throbbing headache for past 4 yrs. It usually involves one half of the face and is associated with nausea and vomiting. There is no aura. Most likely diagnosis is: (AI 2001)
    a. Migraine
    b. Cluster headache
    c. Angle closure glaucoma
    d. Temporal arteritis

122. A 35 year old Lady has unilateral headache, nausea, vomiting and visual blurring. The diagnosis is:
    a. Cluster headache   (AIIMS June 99)
    b. Glaucoma
    c. Subarachnoid haemorrhage
    d. Migraine

123. What is drug of choice for acute attack of migraine-
    a. Methysergide   (AIIMS May 95)
    b. Caffeine
    c. Amitryptiline
    d. Sumatriptan

Neurocutaneous Disorders

124. All are criteria for NF-1 except?   (Recent Pattern 2018)
    a. Acoustic neuroma   b. Café-Au-Lait macules
    c. Pseudoarthrosis   d. Scoliosis

125. Schwannoma of spinal nerve roots is seen in?
    a. Neurofibromatosis 1   (Recent Question 2016-17)
    b. Neurofibromatosis 2
    c. Turcot syndrome
    d. Li-Fraumeni Syndrome

126. Lisch nodules are seen in which of the following conditions?
    a. Von Recklinghausen's disease   (UPSC 2015)
    b. Louis-bar syndrome
    c. Tuberous sclerosis
    d. Von Hippel-Lindau syndrome

127. A 6-year old child with port wine stain, mental retardation and recurrent focal seizures. All are true about the condition except?

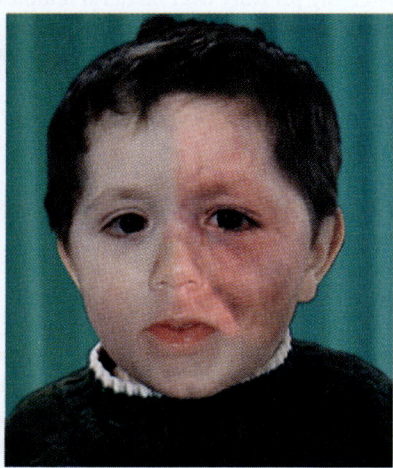

   a. Optic nerve cupping
   b. Tram track appearance on X ray skull
   c. Vagal nerve stimulation
   d. Hemangioma

128. Not seen in tuberous sclerosis (AIIMS Nov 14)
   a. Giant cell Astrocytoma
   b. White matter migration lines
   c. Sub-ependymal nodules
   d. Ependymoma

129. All of the following are true about von Hippel Lindau syndrome except? (Recent Pattern 2014/15)
   a. Multiple tumours are uncommon
   b. Hemangio-pericytomas are seen in the cranio-spinal axis
   c. Supra-tentorial lesions are seen
   d. Tumors of Schwann cells are seen

130. 48 year old woman with history of seizures has presented with gross haematuria and left flank pain. Abdominal CT scan reveals left perinephric hematoma with 3 cm angiomyolipoma along with multiple right renal angiomyolipomas measuring from 1.5 to 6.5 cm. The most likely diagnosis is:
   a. Tuberous sclerosis (AIIMS Nov 2012)
   b. Von Hippel Landau syndrome
   c. Familial angiolipomatosis
   d. ADPKD

131. Tuberculosis sclerosis is associated with all except:
   a. Ash leaf macule (APPG 2014)
   b. Shagreen patch
   c. Schwannoma
   d. Adenoma sebaceum

132. A child presented to the casualty with seizures. On examination an oval hypo-pigmented macules were noted on the trunk, along with sub-normal IQ. Probable diagnosis of the child is: (AIIMS Nov 2012)
   a. Neurofibromatosis
   b. Sturge Weber
   c. Tuberous sclerosis
   d. Incontinentia Pigmenti

133. An 8 year old boy has mental retardation. On examination he is found to have a well defined kidney lump. CT scan shows a well-defined hypo-echoic lesion in the kidney and multiple lesions in the liver showing density of -50 to -80 Hounsfield units. Probable diagnosis is: (AIIMS Nov 2012)
   a. Autosomal recessive polycystic kidney
   b. Tuberous sclerosis
   c. Von Hippel Landau
   d. Paraganglioma

134. The diagnosis of a patient presenting with Seizures, Mental retardation and Sebaceous adenoma is: (AI 1995)
   a. Hypothyroidism   b. Tuberous sclerosis
   c. Toxoplasmosis   d. Down's syndrome

135. Brain tumor is associated with A/E: (PGI Dec 99)
   a. Tuberous sclerosis
   b. Von Hippel Landau syndrome
   c. Neurofibromatosis
   d. Sturge Weber syndrome

Stroke and SAH

136. A 60-year-old male diabetic and hypertensive patient was found unconscious in the morning. On examination pulse rate is 120/min, BP=160/100 mm Hg and bilateral extensor plantars are elicited. What is the next step to be done for management? (AIIMS May 2018)
   a. Order CT scan
   b. Check blood glucose
   c. Give intravenous mannitol
   d. Immediately reduce BP with antihypertensives

137. A patient of RTA presents in emergency. On examination, the patient was moaning with inability to speak but was able to understand what he wanted to speak. Which of the following marked area of brain is involved in this? (AIIMS May 2018)

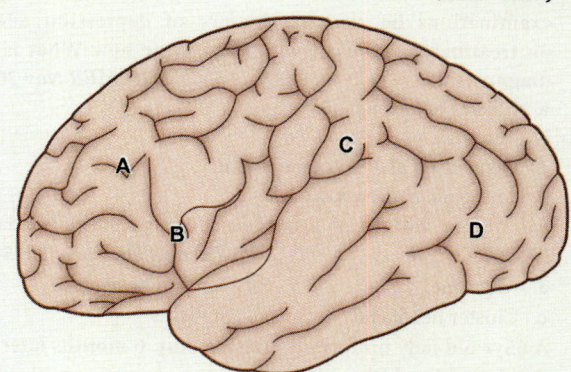

   a. A   b. B
   c. C   d. D

138. A 60-year-old female presents with left sided weakness for more than one hour and left sided facial weakness with BP of 160/100 mm Hg. CT is normal. What is the next best step? (AIIMS Nov 2018)
   a. Start thrombolysis
   b. Give loading dose of aspirin and clopidogrel
   c. Manage BP Alone
   d. No intervention required

139. Occlusion of blood supply of the area marked in red will lead to all of the following except? *(AIIMS Nov 2018)*

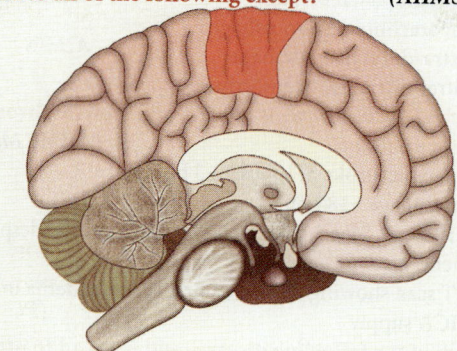

 a. Urinary incontinence b. Rectal incontinence
 c. Apraxia (Constructional) d. Peri-anal anaesthesia

140. A 70-year-old patient presents with dizziness and headache followed by left sided hemiparesis with right pupillary dilatation and ptosis. Most probable blood vessel damaged is? *(JIPMER May 2018)*
 a. Middle cerebral artery b. Anterior cerebral artery
 c. Posterior cerebral artery d. Basilar artery

141. What is the site of lesion in a patient with Alexia without agraphia? *(JIPMER May 2018)*
 a. Fusiform gyrus b. Cingulate gyrus
 c. Paracentral lobule d. Splenium

142. All are differential diagnosis for 'Thunderclap headache' except? *(JIPMER May 2018)*
 a. Encephalitis b. Ischemic stroke
 c. Subarachnoid hemorrhage d. Meningitis

143. All are true about Weber syndrome except? *(Recent Pattern 2018)*
 a. Dorsal Mid brain lesion
 b. Cerebral peduncle is involved
 c. Ipsilateral 3rd nerve palsy
 d. Contralateral hemiplegia

144. A middle aged patient presents with the worst headache of his life. What is the investigation of choice?
 a. NCCT b. CECT *(AIIMS Nov 2017)*
 c. MRI d. Lumbar puncture

145. A middle aged patient presents with history of left sided weakness for 2 days. Currently the patient is extremely drowsy and underwent a NCCT brain. Which of the following is the best treatment for this patient? *(AIIMS Nov 2017)*

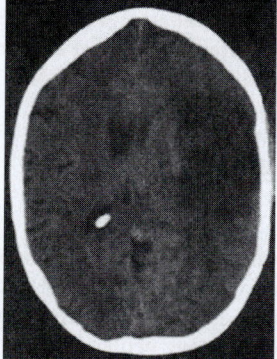

 a. Aspirin/Clopidogrel b. Mechanical Thrombectomy
 c. Mannitol d. Decompressive surgery

146. The digital subtraction angiography given below shows? *(AIIMS Nov 2017)*

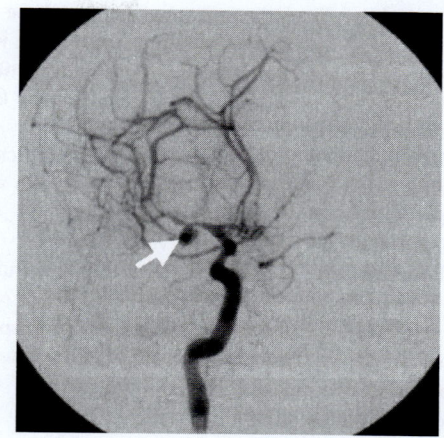

 a. Intracranial pseudoaneurysm
 b. Carotid-cavernous fistula
 c. Angiofibroma tumor blush
 d. Vein of Galen malformation

147. What is the window period of thrombolysis in a stroke patient? *(AIIMS May 2017)*
 a. 1.5 hours b. 2.5 hours
 c. 3.5 hours d. 4.5 hours

148. Which of the following complications of stroke need not be treated? *(AIIMS May 2017)*
 a. Fever b. Spasticity
 c. Neglect d. Dysphagia

149. A 65 year old diabetic woman develops weakness in the left side of face, right arm and right leg. She also has diplopia on left lateral gaze. What is the site of lesion? *(Recent Pattern Questions)*
 a. Right pons b. Left pons
 c. Right midbrain d. Left midbrain

150. A 25 year old is admitted with loss of consciousness after cocaine over-dosage. On examination BP= 200/100 with GCS of 7/15. Right sided pupil is dilated and shows sluggish reaction to light. Which is not recommended for this patient? *(Recent Pattern Questions)*
 a. Administer mannitol at 1g/kg body weight
 b. Administer hypertonic fluids to maintain sodium of 145mEq/dl
 c. Initiate sodium nitroprusside to achieve MAP below 130 mmHg
 d. Neuromuscular paralysis

151. An 80 year old lady develops CVA. She describes unrelenting pain on right side of body as if somebody poured acid on her. Where is the lesion located?
 a. Habenular commissure *(Recent Pattern Questions)*
 b. Internal capsule
 c. Pulvinar
 d. Ventro-posterolateral nucleus

152. Paradoxical embolism is detected by? *(Recent Pattern Questions)*
 a. MRI Chest
 b. Bubble contrast Echocardiography
 c. CT scan Chest
 d. Impedance plethysmography

153. An 80 year old chronic alcoholic was diagnosed with atrial fibrillation five years ago. His son describes stepwise decline in his father's overall memory over these years. On examination he is having pseudobulbar affect with brisk DTR in left upper extremity and up-going plantars. What is the diagnosis? (Recent Pattern Questions)
    a. Binswanger's disease
    b. Alzheimer's
    c. Multi infarct dementia
    d. Vitamin B_{12} deficiency

154. Which of the following is preserved in locked in state? (Recent Pattern Questions)
    a. Horizontal gaze
    b. Vertical gaze
    c. Phonation
    d. Diaphragmatic function

155. A 65 year old patient of CAD develops sudden onset right side face and arm weakness and expressive dysphasia. On admission BP= 160/100 mm Hg. NCCT was done. Which is the best step in management of this patient?
    (Recent Pattern Questions)

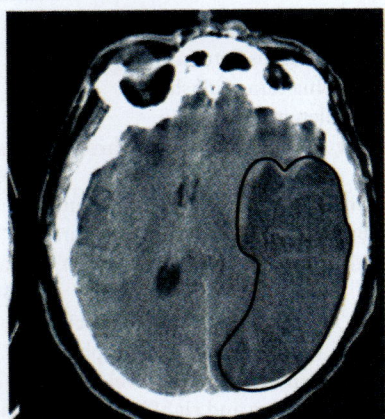

    a. Intravenous Nicardipine
    b. Intravenous Labetalol
    c. Intravenous Reteplase
    d. Intravenous Mannitol

156. All of the following reduce the risk of atherothrombotic stroke except? (Recent Pattern Questions)
    a. Aspirin
    b. BP control
    c. Statin
    d. Rivaroxaban

157. A 25 year old unconscious patient is brought to the ER. On examination his BP = 140/90 mm Hg, pulse rate is 88/minute, respiratory rate is 10/min, body temperature is 96 degrees F and pin point pupils. What is the diagnosis of the patient? (AIIMS Nov 2016)
    a. Pontine haemorrhage
    b. Opium poisoning
    c. Metabolic encephalopathy
    d. Sepsis

158. A 50 year old patient presents with complaints of weakness on right side and left sided loss of sensation. On examination both upper limb and lower limb of right side has decreased tone and on right side horner syndrome is present. He is having dysarthria and difficulty in swallowing. He has hemi-sensory loss on left side of the body with loss of touch, pain and temperature. Which is the cause of symptoms in these patients? (AIIMS Nov 2016)
    a. Right posterior inferior cerebellar artery occlusion
    b. Left posterior inferior cerebellar artery occlusion
    c. Right middle cerebral artery occlusion
    d. Basilar artery occlusion

159. Nimodipine is used in the management of? (AIIMS May 2016)
    a. Subdural haemorrhage
    b. Subarachnoid haemorrhage
    c. Extra-dural haemorrhage
    d. Intraventricular haemorrhage

160. Which of the following is not an indication for thrombolysis in stroke patient? (AIIMS May 2016)
    a. Ischemic stroke of less than 3 hours
    b. Patient age >18 hours
    c. Sustained Blood pressure>185/110 mm Hg despite treatment
    d. CT scan showing non-haemorrhage or oedema in >1/3rd of MCA supply

161. Which of the following diseases will not lead to ptosis? (Recent Question 2016-17)
    a. Miller Fisher Syndrome
    b. Guillain Barre syndrome
    c. Lambert Eaton syndrome
    d. Parinaud Syndrome

162. Which is not a feature of MCA blockage? (Recent Question 2016-17)
    a. Anosognosia
    b. Apraxia
    c. Dysarthria
    d. Abulia

163. Which is not a feature of Gerstmann syndrome? (Recent Question 2016-17)
    a. Jargon speech
    b. Acalculia
    c. Alexia
    d. Finger Agnosia

164. A patient of un-ruptured berry aneurysm has 6th nerve palsy and visual deficit. This indicates presence of berry at which of the following site? (Recent Question 2016-17)
    a. Cavernous sinus
    b. Posterior communicating artery
    c. Posterior inferior cerebellar artery
    d. Anterior communicating artery

165. Which of the following Berry Aneurysm will have the highest chances of rupture? (Recent Question 2016-17)
    a. > 7 mm and top of basilar artery
    b. >7 mm and anterior communicating artery
    c. >7 mm and middle cerebral artery
    d. >7 mm and posterior inferior cerebellar artery

166. Which type of amyloid is deposited in cerebral amyloid angiopathy? (Recent Question 2016-17)
    a. A-beta
    b. A- beta 2
    c. ATTR
    d. Apo E

167. A man comes with aphasia. He is unable to name things and repetition is poor. However comprehension, fluency and understanding of written words is unaffected. He is probably suffering from? (AIIMS Nov 2015)
    a. Conduction aphasia
    b. Anomic aphasia
    c. Transcortical sensory aphasia
    d. Broca's aphasia

168. Hypertensive hemorrhage is most commonly seen in?
    a. Basal ganglia
    b. Thalamus (AIIMS May 2015)
    c. Brain stem
    d. Cerebrum

169. Which of the following ocular findings is a component of Foville syndrome? (UPSC 2015)
    a. Lateral gaze palsy
    b. Medial gaze palsy
    c. 3rd Nerve Palsy
    d. Nystagmus

170. This hypertensive patient was admitted with right hemiplegia. Plain CT scan shows: *(AP PG 2015)*

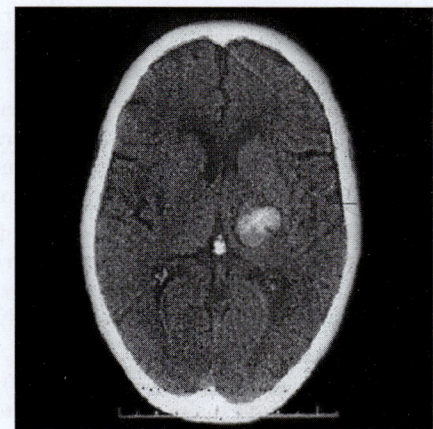

   a. Ischemic infarct in left parietal lobe
   b. Hemorrhage in left thalamus and internal capsule
   c. Hemorrhage in left frontal lobe
   d. Ischemic infarct in right internal capsule

171. A 67 years old male patient presents with sudden onset diplopia right sided facial nerve palsy involving both upper and lower part of the face and left sided hemiparesis. Most probable site of the lesion? *(JIPMER Nov 2014)*
   a. Right midbrain   b. Right pons
   c. Left mid brain   d. Left medulla

172. Right internal carotid artery stenosis leads to all except?
   a. Dysphasia   *(JIPMER Nov 2014)*
   b. Contralateral hemiparesis
   c. Contralateral hemi-sensory loss
   d. Drop attacks

173. Most common site of brain Hemorrhage is?
                                    (Recent Question 2015-16)
   a. Putamen   b. Internal capsule
   c. Ventral pons   d. Cerebellum

174. Commonest cause of cerebrovascular accident:
                                    (Recent Question 2015-16)
   a. Infarction   b. Hemorrhage
   c. Embolism   d. Aortic dissection

175. Which of the following nerve is first affected in berry aneurysm: *(Recent Question 2015-16)*
   a. 3rd nerve   b. 4th nerve
   c. 5th nerve   d. 6th nerve

176. Duration of TIA is less than? *(Recent Question 2015-16)*
   a. 12 hours   b. 24 hours
   c. 48 hours   d. 36 hours

177. In Balint syndrome all are seen except?
                                    (Recent Pattern 2015-16)
   a. Opsoclonus   b. Optic ataxia
   c. Simultagnosia   d. Ocular apraxia

178. A patient presents with subarachnoid haemorrhage. NCCT reveals blood in the fourth ventricle. The bleeding is most likely to occur from an aneurysm of which of the following arteries?   *(AI 2012)*
   a. Anterior communicating artery
   b. Basilar top region
   c. AICA
   d. PICA

179. A hypertensive patient with severe headache and vomiting. He has got neck stiffness but no Focal Neurological Deficit. What is the most probable diagnosis?
   a. Intra-cerebral bleed   *(Recent Pattern 2014/15)*
   b. Subarachnoid haemorrhage
   c. Meningitis
   d. Meningo-encephalitis

180. Aneurysm of Posterior communicating artery will compress which cranial nerve?   *(Recent Pattern 2014/15)*
   a. Trochlear   b. Trigeminal
   c. Optic   d. Oculomotor

181. Gait apraxia is seen in: *(AIIMS Nov 2011)*
   a. ACA   b. MCA
   c. PCA   d. Posterior choroidal artery

182. A 26 year old healthy female got pregnant for the first time and a LSCS was done for fetal distress. Mild hypertension was present during pregnancy. 2 days after delivery she had headache and seizures. CT shows 2X3 cm Para-sagittal Lesion. Urinalysis shows no proteinuria. Diagnosis is:
   a. Eclampsia   *(AIIMS Nov 2013)*
   b. Hypertensive I.C.H.
   c. Sagittal sinus thrombosis
   d. Pituitary apoplexy

183. A patient developed sudden severe headache 2 hours ago and became unconscious. On regaining consciousness he developed photophobia and neck rigidity. What is the next line of management?   *(AIIMS Nov 2013)*
   a. NCCT   b. IV antibiotics
   c. CSF   d. MRI

184. A patient has developed confusion and keeps bumping into objects. He can speak fluently and on examination patient has inability to differentiate between fingers, cannot write. On MRI T2 images show cortical and sub cortical lesions: Diagnosis is: *(AIIMS May 2013)*
   a. Gerstmann syndrome   b. Anton syndrome
   c. Millard Gubler syndrome d. Locked in syndrome

185. Pure word blindness is seen due to lesion at?
   a. Superior temporal gyrus
   b. Inferior temporal gyrus
   c. Angular gyrus
   d. Arcuate fasciculus

186. A middle aged hypertensive male develops sudden onset unconsciousness, with nuchal rigidity. Rest of the neurological examination is within normal limits. Diagnosis is?   *(AIIMS May 2013)*
   a. SAH   b. Intra-parenchymal bleed
   c. Extra-dural hemorrhage d. Sub dural haemorrhage

187. A third cranial nerve palsy associated with pupillary dilation, loss of ipsilateral light reflex, focal pain behind the eye may occur with?   *(APPG 2014)*
   a. Aneurysm in the cavernous sinus
   b. Expanding supraclinoid carotid aneurysm
   c. Expanding aneurysm at the junction of posterior communicating and internal carotid artery
   d. Expanding anterior cerebral artery aneurysm

188. Ocular bobbing is seen in: *(Recent Pattern 2014/15)*
   a. Damage to M.L.F   b. Severe refractive error
   c. Pontine lesions   d. Cerebellum damage

189. **Cranial nerves involved in Millard Gubler syndrome are:**
    (Recent Pattern 2014/15)
    a. 3rd and 4th nerve
    b. 4th and 5th nerve
    c. 6th and 7th nerve
    d. 7th and 8th nerve

190. **A diabetes mellitus patient with BP of 220/130 mm Hg is brought to the casualty in coma. CT scan shows a large infarct. What is the target BP of this patient to initiate thrombolysis?** *(Recent Pattern 2014/15)*
    a. Less than 200/130
    b. Less than 180/110
    c. Less than 160/100
    d. Less than 140/90

191. **Hypertensive Patient presents with one day history of headache, Nausea, vomiting and difficulty in walking. Diagnosis is?** *(Recent Pattern 2014/15)*
    a. Extradural hemorrhage
    b. Intraparenchymal haemorrhage
    c. Sub-dural haemorrhage
    d. Sub-arachnoid haemorrhage

192. **Cerebral infarct is earliest detected by:**
    a. Diffusion weighted MRI *(Recent Pattern 2014/15)*
    b. P.E.T scan
    c. MRI scan
    d. CT scan

193. **All are true about Broca's aphasia except:**
    a. Non fluent aphasia *(Recent Pattern 2014/15)*
    b. Damage to posterior part of inferior frontal Gyrus
    c. Repetition is preserved
    d. Syntax is preserved

194. **Death after Rupture of Berry Aneurysm is due to:**
    a. Re-bleeding *(Recent Pattern 2014/15)*
    b. Cerebral ischemia
    c. Intraventricular hemorrhage
    d. Myocardial infarction

195. **Duret haemorrhage is seen in:** *(Recent Pattern 2014/15)*
    a. Brain
    b. Adrenal gland
    c. Lungs
    d. Liver

196. **The most common cause of embolic stroke:**
    (Recent Pattern 2014/15)
    a. Non rheumatic atrial fibrillation
    b. Carotid artery atherosclerosis
    c. Paradoxical embolism
    d. LV aneurysm

197. **What is true about Lacunar stroke:**
    a. Female on OCP *(Recent Pattern 2014/15)*
    b. Male with hypertension
    c. Young male with AV malformation
    d. Young male with mycotic aneurysm

198. **Thrombosis of the Superior branch of middle cerebral artery leads to:** *(Recent Pattern 2014/15)*
    a. Motor aphasia
    b. Urinary retention
    c. Bitemporal hemianopia
    d. Grasp reflex

199. **Presence of hemiplegia with homonymous hemianopia with gaze to same side is seen with occlusion of which brain vessel?** *(Recent Pattern 2014/15)*
    a. Middle cerebral artery
    b. Basilar artery
    c. Anterior cerebral artery
    d. Internal cartoid artery

200. **Hemianopia, cortical blindness, amnesia and thalamic pain are associated with the occlusion of:**
    (Recent Pattern 2014/15)
    a. Anterior cerebral artery
    b. Middle cerebral artery
    c. Posterior cerebral artery
    d. Basilar artery

201. **Ipsilateral 3rd nerve palsy with Contralateral hemiplegia is known as:** *(Recent Pattern 2014/15)*
    a. Millard Gubler syndrome
    b. Weber's syndrome
    c. Foville syndrome
    d. Benedicts syndrome

202. **Characteristic features of a lesion in the lateral part of the medulla include all except:** *(Recent Pattern 2014/15)*
    a. Ipsilateral Horner's syndrome
    b. Contralateral loss of proprioception to the body and limbs
    c. Nystagmus
    d. Dysphagia

203. **Most common site of cerebral infarction is in the territory of:**
    a. Anterior cerebral artery *(Recent Pattern 2014/15)*
    b. Middle cerebral artery
    c. Posterior cerebral artery
    d. Posterior inferior cerebellar artery

204. **Pyrexia, pin point pupils and unconsciousness is characteristic of:** *(Recent Pattern 2014/15)*
    a. Brain stem lesion
    b. Cerebellar lesion
    c. Thalamic lesions
    d. Internal capsule lesions

205. **Lateral medullary syndrome is due to thrombosis of:**
    (Recent Pattern 2014/15)
    a. Posterior inferior cerebellar artery
    b. Anterior inferior cerebellar artery
    c. Superior cerebellar artery
    d. Posterior communicating branch of middle cerebral artery

206. **Lateral medullary syndrome is associated with:**
    a. Dissociative anesthesia *(Recent Pattern 2014/15)*
    b. Dense hemianesthesia
    c. Crossed hemianesthesia
    d. No sensory deficit is seen

207. **Hemiplegia is most often caused by thrombosis of:**
    a. Anterior cerebral artery *(Recent Pattern 2014/15)*
    b. Middle cerebral artery
    c. Posterior cerebral artery
    d. Basilar artery

208. **Which of the following is not a usual feature of right middle cerebral artery territory infarct?** *(Recent Pattern 2014/15)*
    a. Aphasia
    b. Hemiparesis
    c. Facial weakness
    d. Dysarthria

209. **Cranial nerve most commonly compressed by intracranial aneurysm:** *(Recent Pattern 2014/15)*
    a. Oculomotor
    b. Facial
    c. Optic
    d. Trigeminal

210. **Thrombosis of Anterior cerebral Artery, distal to the communicating branch leads to:** *(Recent Pattern 2014/15)*
    a. Contralateral Hemiparesis
    b. Ipsilateral hemiparesis
    c. Incontinence
    d. Seizures

211. **Anterior inferior cerebellar arterial occlusion can cause:**
 (Recent Pattern 2014/15)
    a. Contralateral lower leg weakness
    b. Urinary retention
    c. Hemianopia
    d. Hemianaesthesia of same side of the face

212. **Which of the following is not involved in lateral medullary syndrome?** *(Recent Pattern 2014/15)*
    a. Sympathetic tract
    b. IX, X, XI cranial nerves
    c. XIIth cranial nerve
    d. Spinothalamic tract

213. **Least common site for Berry Aneurysm:**
    a. Vertebral artery *(Recent Pattern 2014/15)*
    b. Basilar artery
    c. Junction of anterior cerebral artery and internal cartoid artery
    d. Posterior cerebral artery

214. **Hemiparesis is *not* seen with:** *(Recent Pattern 2014/15)*
    a. Posterior inferior cerebellar artery stroke
    b. Middle cerebral artery stroke
    c. Posterior cerebral artery stroke
    d. Anterior spinal artery stroke

215. **In a patient with ruptured cerebral aneurysm, cause of delayed neurological symptoms are, all except:**
    a. Enlargement of aneurysm *(Recent Pattern 2014/15)*
    b. Rebleed
    c. Spasm
    d. Hydrocephalus

216. **The most common cause of Intraparenchymal bleed is:**
 (Recent Pattern 2014/15)
    a. Thrombocytopenia
    b. Diabetes
    c. Hypertension
    d. Berry aneurysm

217. **Elderly man complains of three episodes of visual loss in right eye over 20 minutes. Blood vessel involved is:**
    a. Anterior cerebral artery *(Recent Pattern 2014/15)*
    b. Middle cerebral artery
    c. Internal carotid artery
    d. Basiliar artery

218. **Which is true about CADASIL?** *(Recent Pattern 2014/15)*
    a. Monogenic stroke syndrome
    b. White matter changes
    c. Onset is usually in the fourth or fifth decade of life
    d. All of the above

219. **The investigation to be performed in patient of SAH with normal CT scan?** *(Recent Pattern 2014/15)*
    a. Contrast enhanced CT
    b. Three tube test
    c. MRI
    d. Gadolinium enhanced MRI

220. **Following are features of ischemia in anterior choroidal artery territory except:** *(Recent Pattern 2014/15)*
    a. Hemiparesis
    b. Hemisensory loss
    c. Homonymous hemianopia
    d. Predominant involvement of the anterior limb of internal capsule

221. **Pontine Stroke is associated with all except:**
    a. Bilateral pin point pupil *(Recent Pattern 2014/15)*
    b. Pyrexia
    c. Vagal palsy
    d. Quadriparesis

222. **Which cranial nerve is involved in Locked in syndrome?**
    a. 7
    b. 9 *(PGI May 2012)*
    c. 10
    d. 12
    e. All of the above

223. **Posterior cerebral artery occlusion leads to loss of memory due to involvement of:** *(Recent Pattern 2014/15)*
    a. Superior temporal gyrus
    b. Supra marginal gyrus
    c. Angular gyrus
    d. Hippocampus

224. **History of transient ischemic attack, excludes:**
    a. Amaurosis fugax *(Recent Pattern 2014/15)*
    b. Weak shoulder shrugging
    c. Asymmetrical mouth retraction
    d. Seizures

225. **Features of posterior inferior cerebellar artery thrombosis include all of the following except:** *(Recent Pattern 2014/15)*
    a. Sudden onset of severe vertigo
    b. Acute cerebellar S/S with Nystagmus to the side of lesion the involvement
    c. Palsy of 10,11,12 nerves
    d. Horner's syndrome

226. **80 year diabetic presents with right sided face, arm and leg weakness. Sensation, speech and comprehension are intact. Blood vessel involved is:** *(Recent Pattern 2014/15)*
    a. Anterior cerebral artery
    b. Lenticulostriate artery
    c. Internal carotid artery
    d. Basilar artery

227. **Pin point pupils are due to damage to:**
    a. Edinger Westphal nucleus *(Recent Pattern 2014/15)*
    b. Superior colliculus
    c. Lateral geniculate body
    d. Descending sympathetic pathways

228. **Lesion in inferior frontal gyrus causes:**
    a. Defect in articulation *(AIIMS Dec 97)*
    b. Incomprehension of written language
    c. Incomprehension of spoken language
    d. Motor aphasia

229. **Most common cause of intracranial haemorrhage is:**
    a. Sub arachnoid haemorrhage *(AIIMS Nov 98)*
    b. Intracerebral hemorrhage
    c. Subdural haemorrhage
    d. Extradural haemorrhage

230. **Which of the following is the most common location of hypertensive hemorrhage?** *(AI 2003)*
    a. Pons
    b. Thalamus
    c. Putamen/external capsule
    d. Subcortical white matter

231. **Commonest cause of subarachnoid haemorrhage is:**
    a. Rupture of circle of Willis aneurysm *(AI 1998)*
    b. Rupture or vertebral artery aneurysm
    c. Rupture of venecomitants of corpus striatum
    d. Rupture of dural sinuses

232. **Berry aneurysm is caused by:** *(AIIMS May 2011)*
    a. Degeneration of internal elastic lamina
    b. Degeneration of tunica media
    c. Degeneration of muscular layer
    d. Degeneration of external elastic lamina

233. Which is least common site of berry aneurysm:
    a. Basilar artery *(AIIMS Dec 95)*
    b. Vertebral artery
    c. Anterior cerebral artery
    d. Posterior cerebral artery
234. Which of the following is the most common cause of late neurological deterioration in a case of cerebrovascular accident : *(AIIMS Nov 2000)*
    a. Rebleeding
    b. Vasospasm
    c. Embolism
    d. Hydrocephalus
235. "Prosopagnosia" is characterised by : *(AI 2005)*
    a. Inability to read
    b. Inability to identify faces
    c. Inability to write
    d. Inability to speak

Parkinsonism and Dementia

236. A medical student presented to the ED with protracted vomiting. For this he was given an anti-emetic drug following which he developed abnormal posturing. Which of the following is the most likely drug to be given to the patient? *(AIIMS May 2018)*
    a. Metoclopramide
    b. Ondansetron
    c. Domperidone
    d. Dexamethasone
237. What is correct about Parkinsonism?
      (Recent Pattern Questions)
    a. Early initiation of therapy with levodopa predisposes to higher incidence of dyskinesia
    b. Early therapy with deep brain stimulation slows progression of disease
    c. Initial therapy with dopamine agonists controls symptoms in most patients
    d. Initial therapy with levodopa prevents development of recurrent falls
238. An 18 year old boy is admitted with psychotic behaviour. On examination he is having dystonia and incoordination. Liver enzymes are elevated. Which of the following is a possible diagnosis? *(Recent Pattern Questions)*
    a. Rheumatic Chorea
    b. Westphal variant of Huntington disease
    c. Wilson disease
    d. Hallervorden Spatz disease
239. A 40 year old man is brought to the doctor by his family for rapid intellectual decline. Examination shows fast semi-purposive movements in hands. His father and grandfather had a similar illness. What is the diagnosis?
    a. Pre-senile Dementia *(Recent Pattern Questions)*
    b. Lewy body dementia
    c. Corticobasilar degeneration
    d. Huntington chorea
240. A 79-year-old male with Parkinson's disease presented to the emergency department after a sudden fall. The patient was on treatment with aspirin for AF. The image shows?
      (Recent Question 2016-17)

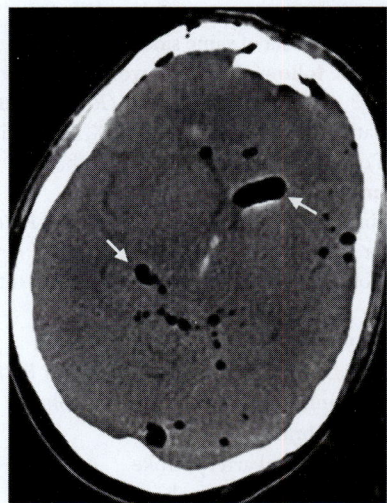

    a. Hydrocephalus
    b. Pneumocephalus
    c. Intra-ventricular bleed
    d. Subarachnoid haemorrhage
241. Which one of the following cerebral blood flow patterns is likely in a patient with huntington's disease: *(AP PG 2015)*
    a. Hyperemia to basal ganglia with reduced flow to other areas in brain
    b. Bilateral reduction in blood flow to caudate nucleus
    c. Bilateral reduction in blood flow starting from occipital cortex and spreading anteriorly
    d. Decreased blood flow to temporal Lobes
242. Hippocampal formation includes all, except?
    a. Dentate gyrus *(Bihar PG 2015)*
    b. Subiculum complex
    c. Amygdaloid nucleus
    d. Entorhinal cortex
243. All of the following are known predisposing factors for Alzheimer's disease except? *(Bihar PG 2015)*
    a. Down syndrome
    b. Low education level
    c. Smoking
    d. Female sex
244. Features of Parkinsonism include all except:
    a. Mask like facies
    b. Rigidity
    c. Intention tremor
    d. Resting tremor
    e. Flaccidity
245. Which is the earliest symptom of Parkinsonism?
    a. Tremors *(Recent Question 2015-16)*
    b. Rigidity
    c. Bradykinesia
    d. Chorea

246. Two patients in neurology department were asked to draw concentric circles inside the red reference line. Which of the two patients is likely to be suffering from essential tremors

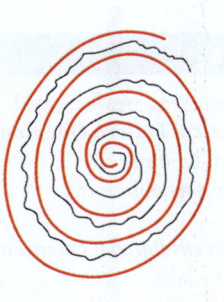
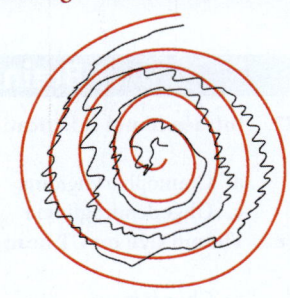

A   B

   a. Patient A has essential tremors
   b. Patient B has essential tremors
   c. Both   d. None
247. The patient B has lesion at which of the following sites?

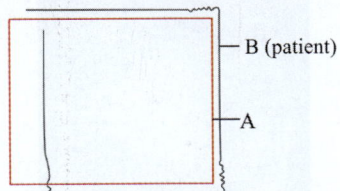

   a. Cerebellum   b. Basal ganglia
   c. Thalamus   d. Putamen
248. Element causing Parkinsonism? *(Recent Pattern 2015-16)*
   a. Manganese   b. Copper
   c. Iron   d. Lead
249. Not seen in Alzheimer's Disease? *(Recent Pattern 2015-16)*
   a. Cerebral atrophy
   b. Ventricular shrinkage
   c. Sun downing
   d. Apraxia
250. Anosmia is early clinical feature of? *(Recent Pattern 2015-16)*
   a. Alzheimer   b. Parkinson's disease
   c. Huntington's chorea d. All of the above
251. All are seen in Alzheimer's disease except:
   a. Aphasia   *(AIIMS Nov 2011)*
   b. Acalculia
   c. Apraxia
   d. Agnosia
252. Which of the following disease causes loss of cortical neurons? *(AIIMS May 2012)*
   a. Spinocerebellar ataxia
   b. Progressive Supranuclear gaze palsy
   c. Corticobasilar degeneration
   d. Multiple system atrophy
253. In a patient of Parkinson's disease with intractable tremors, the most preferred site of DBS (Deep Brain Stimulation) is: *(AIIMS Nov 2012)*
   a. Globus Pallidus externa
   b. Putamen
   c. Subthalamic nucleus
   d. Substantia nigra

254. Neurofibrillary tangles are seen in case of Alzheimer's disease. Which of the following areas of brain is resistant to neurofibrillary tangle formation? *(AIIMS Nov 2012)*
   a. Area of visual association
   b. Cuneal gyrus of area VI
   c. Entorhinal cortex
   d. Lateral geniculate nucleus
255. All of the following are true about Alzheimer's disease except: *(AIIMS May 2012)*
   a. Number of Senile plaques correlate with age
   b. Underlying tau proteins suggest neurodegeneration.
   c. Number of neurofibrillary tangles is associated with the severity of dementia
   d. Extracellular inclusions can be found in the absence of intracellular inclusions
256. Regarding Alzheimers disease(AD), Small vessel disease (SVD) and Cerebral amyloid angiopathy (CAA) which of the following is false? *(AIIMS Nov 2011)*
   a. SVD is not related to AD
   b. CAA can be seen in patients with AD
   c. SVD is related to AD
   d. CAA is associated with SVD
257. A 50 year old lady presents with slowness of movement for 2 years, rigidity and vertical square wave jerks. What is the most probable diagnosis? *(AIIMS Nov 2012)*
   a. Parkinson's disease
   b. Lewy body dementia
   c. Progressive supranuclear paralysis
   d. Multiple system atrophy
258. With ageing, a slight decrease in cognitive impairment is seen due to increase in level of: *(AIIMS May 2010)*
   a. Homocysteine   b. Taurine
   c. Methionine   d. Cysteine
259. Coarse tremors in tongue are seen in all except:
   a. Parkinsonism   b. Alcohol *(AIIMS Nov 2013)*
   c. Thyrotoxicosis   d. General paresis
260. Lobes affected in Alzheimer's: *(AIIMS May 2013)*
   a. Frontal and temporal lobe b. Temporal and parietal lobe
   c. Parietal and occipital lobe d. Parietal and frontal lobe
261. Cases of fatal hepatic toxicity have been reported requiring periodic monitoring of liver function tests with:
   a. Tolcapone   *(Bihar PG 2014)*
   b. Entacapone
   c. Rasagiline
   d. Ropinirole
262. In Huntington's Chorea the causative mutation in the protein Huntington is a: *(APPG 2014)*
   a. Point mutation
   b. Gene deletion
   c. Frame shift mutation
   d. Trinucleotide repeat expansion
263. Reversible dementia is seen in *(Recent Pattern 2014/15)*
   a. Wilson
   b. Huntington disease
   c. Alzheimer's
   d. Myxedema

264. **Wheel chair sign is seen in:** *(Recent Question 2016/17)*
    a. Parkinsonism
    b. Duchenne muscular dystrophy
    c. Becker's dystrophy
    d. Thomsen disease
265. **Pick's body in Pick's disease is:** *(Recent Pattern 2014/15)*
    a. Tau protein
    b. Alpha synuclein
    c. Beta synuclein
    d. A β amyloid
266. **Levo-dopa is contraindicated in:** *(Recent Pattern 2014/15)*
    a. Malignant melanoma
    b. Multiple system atrophy
    c. Shy dragger syndrome
    d. Olivopontocerebellar atrophy
267. **Which of the following is predominantly involved in Alzheimer's dementia:** *(AIIMS May 08)*
    a. Frontal cortex
    b. Temporo-Parietal cortex
    c. Fronto-Parietal cortex
    d. Fronto-Temporal cortex
268. **A chromosomal anomaly associated with Alzheimer's dementia is:** *(AI 2001)*
    a. Trisomy 18
    b. Patau syndrome.
    c. Trisomy 21
    d. Turner's syndrome
269. **Which of the following is not seen in early onset Alzheimer's Disease:** *(AIIMS Nov 2011)*
    a. Aphasia
    b. Apraxia
    c. Acalculia
    d. Agnosia
270. **The following is not a feature of Alzheimer's disease:** *(AI 2004)*
    a. Neurofibrillary tangles
    b. Senile (neuritic) plaques
    c. Amyloid Angiopathy
    d. Lewy bodies
271. **In Parkinsonism what is not present:** *(AIIMS May 94)*
    a. Tremors at rest
    b. Past pointing
    c. Akinesia
    d. Rigidity
272. **Deep brain Stimulation of which part of the brain has been shown to reduce frequency of symptoms in Parkinsonism:** *(AI 2012)*
    a. Striatus
    b. Globus Pallidus Externus
    c. Subthalamic nucleus
    d. Putamen
273. **All are true about Huntington's disease except:** *(AI 2001)*
    a. Chorea
    b. Behavioral disturbance
    c. Dopamine depletion
    d. Cog-wheel rigidity.
274. **An elderly man presents with features of dementia, ataxia, difficulty in downward gaze and a history of frequent falls. Likely diagnosis is:** *(AI 2001) (AIIMS May 01)*
    a. Parkinson's disease
    b. Progressive supranuclear gaze palsy
    c. Alzheimers disease
    d. None of the above
275. **A 45-year-old man presents with history of frequent falls. He has difficulty in looking down also. What is the most probable diagnosis :** *(AIIMS Nov 2000)*
    a. Normal pressure hydrocephalus
    b. Parkinson's disease
    c. Alzheimer's disease
    d. Progressive supranuclear palsy

276. **Pick's body in Pick's disease is:** *(AI 2008)*
    a. Tau protein
    b. Alpha synuclein
    c. Beta synuclein
    d. Aamyloid beta

Brain Tumors

277. **Intra-tumoral calcification in brain is seen in all except?** *(Recent Pattern Questions)*
    a. Craniopharyngioma
    b. Meningioma
    c. Oligodendroglioma
    d. Hemangioblastoma
278. **Thumb sign on CT head is seen in?** *(Recent Pattern Questions)*
    a. Chordoma
    b. Metastasis
    c. Glioblastoma multiforme
    d. Astrocytoma
279. **A 50 year old woman presents with complaints of headache and feeling low for last one year. She is being treated for depression. Last night she had an episode of GTCS. NCCT scan shows?** *(Recent Question 2016-17)*

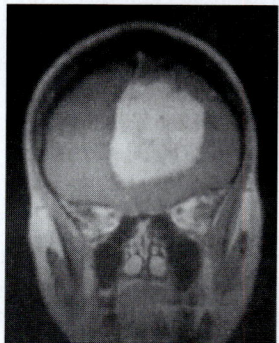

    a. Brain abscess
    b. Brain infarction
    c. Meningioma
    d. Hydatid cyst
280. **Meningioma is composed of?** *(Recent Question 2016-17)*
    a. Arachnoid cap cells
    b. Protoplasmic astrocytes
    c. Pia matter cells
    d. Ependymal cells
281. **Which is the most common type of primary CNS lymphoma in AIDS Positive patients?** *(Recent Question 2016-17)*
    a. Centroblastic large cell lymphoma
    b. Immunoblastic Large cell lymphoma
    c. Anaplastic B- Cell Lymphoma
    d. Lympho-plasmacytic Lymphoma
282. **A 45 year old man presents with diminished vision in right eye. On examination Marcus Gunn pupil is noted. MRI head was performed. Diagnosis is?** *(Recent Question 2016-17)*

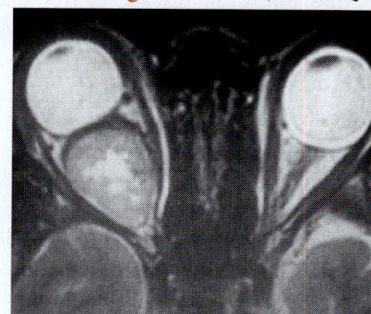

    a. Neuromyelitis optica
    b. Rhabdomyosarcoma
    c. Retinoblastoma
    d. Optic nerve Glioma

283. A patient with a mass in brain is managed by chemo and radiation. After 2 months, she develops vomiting and headache again. What is the investigation of choice to detect the mass?
   a. Contrast enhanced MRI   b. PET Scan   *(JIPMER 2014)*
   c. MRI   d. CT scan

284. Brain tumour with worst prognosis in children:
   (Recent Pattern 2014/15)
   a. Cerebellar astrocytoma   b. Brainstem glioma
   c. Craniopharyngioma   d. Pineal body tumour

285. Most common intracranial tumour is:
   (Recent Pattern 2014-15)
   a. Meningioma   b. Astrocytoma
   c. Craniopharyngioma   d. Oligodendroglioma

286. Which of the following is the most common type of Glial tumors?
   a. Astrocytomas   b. Medulloblastomas   *(AI 06)*
   c. Neurofibromas   d. Ependymomas

287. Most common site of sub ependymal astrocytoma (giant cell)
   a. Trigone of lateral ventricle   *(AIIMS Nov 07)*
   b. Foramen of Munro
   c. Temporal horn of lateral ventricle
   d. 4th ventricle

288. All of the following tumors may be malignant except:
   a. Glioma   b. Astrocytoma   *(AI 1997)*
   c. Hemangioblastoma   d. Ependymoma

289. Which of the following brain tumors does not spread via CSF?   *(AI 2004)*
   a. Germ cell tumors   b. Medulloblastoma
   c. CNS Lymphoma   d. Craniopharyngioma

290. All the following are true of Craniopharyngioma except:
   a. Derived from Rathke's pouch   *(AI 1994)*
   b. Contains epithelial cells
   c. Present in sellar or infra-sellar location
   d. Causes visual disturbances

291. Neurofibromatosis I is most commonly associated with:
   a. Brain stem gliomas   *(AIIMS Nov 07)*
   b. Optic nerve glioma
   c. Sub ependymal pilocytic astrocytoma
   d. Glioblastoma multiforme

292. CNS tumor seen in Von Hippel Lindau syndrome is:
   a. Meningioma   *(PGI Dec 99)*
   b. Cerebellar hemangioblastoma
   c. CNS lymphoma   d. Glioma

293. A patient presents with unilateral painful ophthalmoplegia. Imaging revealed an enlargement of cavernous sinus on the affected side. The likely diagnosis is: *(AIIMS May 08)*
   a. Gradenigo syndrome
   b. Cavernous sinus thrombosis
   c. Tolosa-Hunt Syndrome   d. Orbital Pseudotumor

CNS Infection and Prion Disease

294. A patient presented with headache and fever for 7 days. While doing a lumbar puncture, it was noticed that the opening CSF pressure increased on jugular vein compression and became normal on relieving the pressure on jugular vein. What is the interpretation of this?
   a. Subdural blockage   *(AIIMS May 2018)*
   b. Subarachnoid blockage
   c. Arachnoid villi blockage
   d. Patent subarachnoid space

295. A patient with undulating fever presents with features of encephalitis. He is treated successfully with doxycycline and rifampicin. Probable diagnosis is?   *(JIPMER May 2018)*
   a. Brucellosis
   b. Bordetella pertussis
   c. Francisella tularensis
   d. Mycoplasma pneumoniae

296. A patient presented with history of fever for 3 days with head ache and photophobia. On examination Kernig's sign is positive. CSF findings report mentions lymphocyte count of 36/ml with normal glucose levels, increased protein level with increased opening pressure. Identify the etiological agent.   *(AIIMS Nov 2017)*
   a. Coxsackie virus   b. Mycobacterium tuberculosis
   c. Neisseria   d. Cryptococcus Neoformans

297. A patient presents with fever and altered sensorium. You suspect meningococcal sepsis. Which of the following antibiotic is recommended as the first line for empirical therapy?   *(AIIMS May 2017)*
   a. Ceftriaxone   b. Penicillin –G
   c. Piperacillin- Tazobactum   d. Co-trimoxazole

298. What is the correct sequence to be followed in suspected bacterial meningitis?   *(Recent Pattern Questions)*
   a. Draw blood culture sample, empirical antibiotics, neuroimaging followed by LP
   b. Empirical antibiotics, neuroimaging, blood culture sample followed by LP
   c. LP, Empirical antibiotics and CSF culture
   d. Empirical antibiotics, mannitol, LP followed by neuroimaging

299. Variant Creutzfeldt Jakob disease occurs in which of the following population groups?   *(Recent Pattern Questions)*
   a. Patients accidently inoculated during surgery
   b. Sporadic cases worldwide in fifth or sixth decades
   c. Young adults exposed to tainted beef products
   d. Well defined germ line mutation in Autosomal dominant inheritance

300. An AIDS positive truck driver develops seizures. NCCT head is shown below. What is the diagnosis?
   (Recent Pattern Questions)

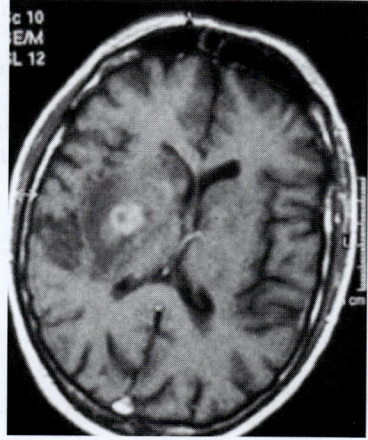

   a. Neurocysticercosis
   b. Cerebral Toxoplasmosis
   c. Primary CNS Lymphoma
   d. Tubercular meningitis

301. **Startle myoclonus in a 60 year old man with rapidly progressive deficits in cortical dysfunction is seen in which of the following?** *(Recent Pattern Questions)*
    a. Myoclonic epilepsy
    b. Lewy body dementia
    c. Prion disease
    d. Multiple system atrophy

302. **Which of the following is incriminated in causing non-infectious chronic meningitis?** *(Recent Pattern Questions)*
    a. Ibuprofen
    b. Acyclovir
    c. Beta-lactam antibiotics
    d. Phenobarbital

303. **A 50 year old woman is on immunosuppressive therapy with steroids post kidney transplantation. She presents with 3 day history of fever, headache and confusion. LP reveals 200 PMN cells /cu.mm with elevated CSF protein. India ink preparation slide is shown. What is the diagnosis?**
    (Recent Pattern Questions)

    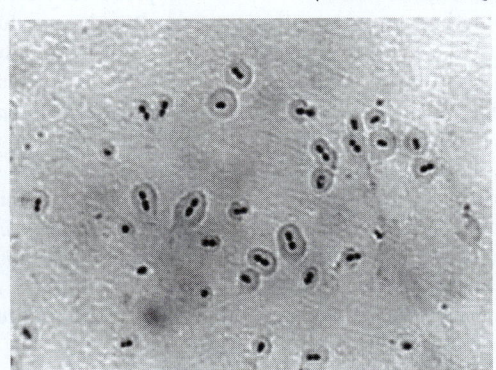

    a. Pneumococcal meningitis
    b. Cryptococcal meningitis
    c. Aseptic meningitis
    d. Cerebral toxoplasmosis

304. **All are true about lumbar puncture except?**
    a. Needle inserted in cephalad direction *(AIIMS May 2016)*
    b. Lateral recumbent position, the bevel of needle should face up
    c. Legs should be straightened during measurement of opening pressure
    d. Needle inserted at L1-L2 space.

305. **All are absolute criteria for diagnosis of NCC except?**
    (Recent Question 2016-17)
    a. Neuro-radiological demonstration of lesions showing Scolex
    b. Visualization of parasite in eye by Fundoscopy
    c. Demonstration of antibodies to cysticerci in serum by enzyme linked immune-electroblot
    d. Demonstration of cysticerci by histological examination of biopsy material

306. **Identify the instrument shown in the figure below?**
    (AIIMS Nov 2015)

    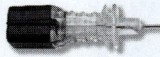

    a. LP needle
    b. Pleural tap
    c. Liver biopsy
    d. Bone marrow aspiration needle

307. **Tropical spastic Para paresis is caused by?**
    a. Hepatitis B virus *(AIIMS May 2015)*
    b. Human T-cell Lymphotropic virus
    c. HIV
    d. Ebstein Barr Virus

308. **Less in CSF when compared to plasma is all except?**
    (JIPMER May 2015)
    a. Glucose
    b. Chloride
    c. Protein
    d. Calcium

309. **32 years old AIDS positive female presented with headaches and nuchal stiffness. On lumbar puncture examination clear CSF was obtained with leucocytes >100/cu.mm. India ink staining was positive. The most probable diagnosis is?**
    a. Candida Meningitis *(Recent Question 2015-16)*
    b. Tubercular Meningitis
    c. Cryptosporidium
    d. Cryptococcus meningitis

310. **DOC for listeria meningitis:** *(Recent Question 2015-16)*
    a. Ampicillin
    b. Cefotaxime
    c. Ceftriaxone
    d. Ciprofloxacin

311. **A Patient presents with headache and Nuchal rigidity. Lumbar Puncture was performed and CSF shows normal protein and normal glucose with clear CSF. Microscopic examination of CSF showed 50 lymphocytes/cu.mm with lymphocytic pleocytosis. What is the diagnosis?**
    (Recent Question 2015-16)
    a. Bacterial meningitis
    b. Viral meningitis
    c. Neoplastic meningitis
    d. Fungal meningitis

312. **Which of the following is not seen in tubercular meningitis:**
    (Recent Question 2015-16)
    a. Evidence of old pulmonary lesions or a miliary pattern is found on chest radiography
    b. Culture of CSF is diagnostic in majority of cases and remains the gold standard.
    c. It is seen most often in young children but also develops in adults.
    d. Cerebrospinal fluid reveals a low leukocyte count.

313. **Incorrect about the image provided in the question?**

    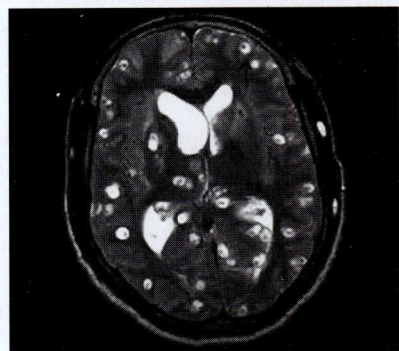

    a. Starry sky appearance
    b. Dexamethasone is given
    c. CSF eosinophilia
    d. ELISA CSF for NCC is the investigation of choice

314. **Aseptic meningitis is caused by?** *(Recent Pattern 2015-16)*
    a. Indomethacin
    b. Ibuprofen
    c. Aspirin
    d. Icatibant

315. **Herpes zoster infection can lead to?** *(Recent Pattern 2015-16)*
    a. Frontal lobe infarction
    b. Parietal lobe infarction
    c. Temporal lobe infarction
    d. Occipital neuralgia

316. **All are true about Ramsay hunt syndrome except?**
    (Recent Pattern 2015-16)
    a. Facial palsy
    b. Vesicles in meatus
    c. Vertigo
    d. Palatal myoclonus

317. Fever blisters can occur due to: *(Recent Pattern 2014/15)*
    a. HHV6
    b. Varicella
    c. Primary HSV 1 infection
    d. Reactivation of HSV-1

318. A patient presented with headache, vomiting. CT scan showed presence of brain abscess. Culture and antibiotic sensitivity result is awaited. Which antibiotic can be given empirically in this patient till getting the report?
    a. Penicillin G *(Recent Pattern 2014/15)*
    b. Ceftriaxone + Metronidazole
    c. Amikacin
    d. Gentamicin

319. A patient with Tubercular meningitis was taking ATT regularly. At end of 1 month of regular intake of drugs deterioration in sensorium is noted in condition of the patient. Which of the following investigations is not required on emergency evaluation? *(AIIMS Nov 2012)*
    a. MRI
    b. NCCT
    c. CSF examination
    d. Liver function tests

320. Which of following is correct about prions?
    a. Long incubation period *(AIIMS Nov 2010)*
    b. Destroyed by autoclaving at 121°C
    c. Nucleic acid present
    d. Immunogenic

321. A Bengali woman had fever for 2 days and has irrelevant talking. She is complaining of weakness in arms. Which of the following drugs can be given in ER to her, pending investigations? *(AIIMS May 2013)*
    a. Mannitol
    b. Acyclovir
    c. Penicillin
    d. Amphotericin B

322. In HIV infection all are affected except: *(AIIMS Nov 2012)*
    a. Cingulate gyrus
    b. Caudate nucleus
    c. Globus pallidus
    d. Cerebral white matter

323. Locomotor ataxia, a late manifestation of syphilis due to parenchymatous involvement of the spinal cord is called:
    a. General paralysis of insanity *(APPG 2014)*
    b. Tabes dorsalis
    c. Meningovascular syphilis
    d. Syphilitic amyotrophy

324. Which of the following does not require a lumbar puncture in children? *(AIIMS Nov 2012)*
    a. ALL
    b. HL
    c. NHL
    d. AML

325. A 30 year old patient is having high grade fever with altered sensorium. On third day the patient develops seizures and has Nuchal rigidity. The CSF examination of the patient shows presence of 300 cells/cu.mm, protein 70 mg%, glucose 54 mg% (BLOOD GLUCOSE= 95 mg%) with polymorph 65% and the rest being lymphocytes. The most probable diagnosis of the patient is : *(AIIMS Nov 2012)*
    a. Viral meningitis
    b. Tubercular meningitis
    c. Pyogenic meningitis
    d. Cerebral malaria.

326. Which of the following enzymes can be detected in CSF:
    a. GGT and ALT *(AIIMS Nov 2012)*
    b. CK-MB and ALP
    c. LDH and CK
    d. Deaminase and superoxide dismutase

327. Eosinophilic meningitis is seen with all except:
    a. Coccidiomycosis *(Recent Pattern 2014/15)*
    b. Cryptococcal meningitis
    c. Lepto-meningeal metastasis
    d. Helminthic infections

328. Steroids are contraindicated in all except? *(Recent Pattern 2014/15)*
    a. DM
    b. TB
    c. Peptic ulcer
    d. Brain tumor

329. Treatment for Neurocysticerosis in children: *(Recent Pattern 2014/15)*
    a. Albendazole 15 mg/kg /day for 8 days
    b. Albendazole 15 mg/kg /day for 2 week
    c. Albendazole 15 mg/kg /day for 3 week
    d. Albendazole 15 mg/kg /day for 6 week

330. Disease spread by cannibalism: *(Recent Pattern 2014/15)*
    a. Nipah virus
    b. Nocardiosis
    c. Kuru
    d. Madras motor neurone disease

331. CSF glucose level is: *(Recent Pattern 2014/15)*
    a. Half the plasma glucose
    b. 2/3 plasma glucose
    c. 1/3 plasma glucose
    d. Same as plasma glucose

332. A person whose CSF grows Streptococcus pneumoniae on culture is most likely to show? *(AIPG 2011)*
    a. Pleocytosis, high protein, reduced sugar
    b. Pleocytosis, high protein, high sugar
    c. Lymphocytosis, high protein, normal sugar
    d. Lymphocytosis, low protein, normal sugar

333. In Pneumococcal meningitis the empirical treatment given is: *(Recent Pattern 2014/15)*
    a. Penicillin G
    b. Doxycycline
    c. Tetracycline
    d. Vancomycin+ceftriaxone

334. Limb girdle muscle dystrophy includes all of the following groups of disorder except: *(AIPG 2011)*
    a. Sarcoglycanopathy
    b. Dystrophinopathy
    c. Dysferlinopathy
    d. Calpainopathy

335. The CSF findings in TB meningitis are all the following except: *(AI 1995)*
    a. Raised protein
    b. Low sugar
    c. Raised chloride
    d. High RBC count

336. Which of the following is the classical CSF finding seen in TBM? *(AI 2007)*
    a. Increased protein, decreased sugar, increased lymphocytes
    b. Increased protein, sugar and lymphocytes
    c. Decreased protein, increased sugar and lymphocytes
    d. Increased sugar, protein and neutrophils

337. Characteristic finding in CT in a TB case is :
    a. Exudate seen in basal cistern *(AI 2001)*
    b. Hydrocephalus is non communicating
    c. Calcification commonly seen in cerebellum
    d. Ventriculitis is a common finding

338. Pneumococcal meningitis is associated with the following CSF findings: *(AI 2012)*
    a. Pleocytosis with low protein and low sugar
    b. Pleocytosis with high protein and low sugar
    c. Lymphocytosis with low protein and low sugar
    d. Lymphocytosis with high protein and low sugar

339. The drug of choice in Cryptococcal Meningitis is: *(AI 1995)*
    a. Pentostatin
    b. Amphotericin B
    c. Clotrimazole
    d. Zidovudine

340. Subdural empyema is most commonly caused by:
    a. H influenza   (AI 2000)
    b. Staphylococcus aureus
    c. Streptococcus pneumoniae
    d. E. Coli

341. Which of the following viruses is not a common cause of viral encephalitis?   (AI 2004)
    a. Herpes simplex virus type 2
    b. Japanese encephalitis virus
    c. Nipah virus
    d. Cytomegalovirus

342. Which of the following is the most common cause of meningoencephalitis in children: (AI 2010)
    a. Mumps   b. Arbovirus
    c. HSV   d. Enterovirus

343. A young male develops fever, followed by headache, confusional state, focal seizures and right hemiparesis. The MRI performed shows bilateral frontotemporal hyper intense lesion. The most likely diagnosis is: (AI 2004)
    a. Acute pyogenic meningitis
    b. Herpes simplex encephalitis
    c. Neurocysticercosis
    d. Carcinomatous meningitis

344. The drug of choice in Herpes Simplex Encephalitis is:
    a. Acyclovir   b. Zidovudine   (AI 1994)
    c. Amantadine   d. Vidarabine

345. Which of the following statements about Prions is true:
    a. They are infectious proteins   (AI 2008)
    b. They are made up of bacteria and virus
    c. They have rich nuclear material
    d. They can be cultured in cell free media

346. Which one of the following is not a Prion associated disease:
    a. Scrapie   b. Kuru   (AI 2005)
    c. Creutzfeldt-Jakob disease   d. Alzheimer's disease

347. All of the following statements about Creutzfeldt-Jakob disease are true, except :   (AIIMS May 04)
    a. It is a neurodegenerative disease
    b. It is caused by infectious proteins
    c. Myoclonus is rarely seen
    d. Brain biopsy is specific for diagnosis

Guillain Barre Syndrome, Neuropathy and Myopathy

348. A patient wakes up with development of ascending paralysis, areflexia and sphincter sparing. Diagnosis is?
          (Recent Question 2019)
    a. Botulinism   b. G.B.S
    c. Snake bite   d. Polio

349. A patient presents with ascending muscle weakness for 2 days. On examination, limb is flaccid. What investigation should be done first?   (AIIMS May 2017)
    a. Serum calcium
    b. Serum magnesium
    c. Serum potassium
    d. Serum sodium

350. A 12 year old girl presented with on and off colicky abdominal pain for last 1 year. She exhibits aggressive behaviour and developed paraparesis of last 2 days. What is the likely diagnosis?   (AIIMS May 2017)
    a. Conversion disorder
    b. Acute inflammatory demyelinating polyneuropathy
    c. Acute intermittent porphyria
    d. Chronic inflammatory demyelinating polyneuropathy

351. A patient with dermatomyositis reports improvement of symptoms on steroids for last 6 months. Labs done today show Creatine kinase of 1300 Units/L. What is the next step in management?   (Recent Pattern Questions)
    a. Continue same dose of steroids
    b. Raise dose of steroids
    c. Start mycophenolate
    d. Perform muscle biopsy

352. A 35 year old lady presents with progressive weakness of both legs and sensory loss below the belly button. She gives history of low grade fever in last week. DTR are normal. All investigations should be done except?
          (Recent Pattern Questions)
    a. ANA   b. EMG
    c. LP   d. MRI Spine

353. Which of the following is not transmitted from the female parent?   (Recent Pattern Questions)
    a. Duchenne muscular dystrophy
    b. Kearns Sayre syndrome
    c. Myoclonic Epilepsy with Ragged Red fibres
    d. Limb girdle muscular Dystrophy

354. Post herpetic neuralgia is seen after?   (AIIMS Nov 2016)
    a. 1 weeks   b. 2 weeks
    c. 3 weeks   d. 4 weeks

355. What is the diagnosis of this patient?   (AIIMS Nov 2016)

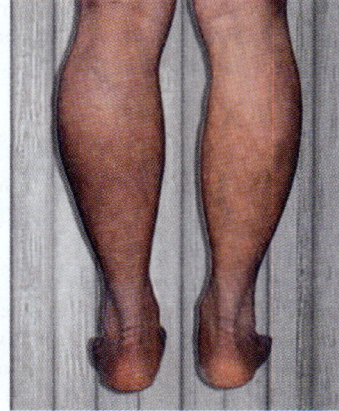

    a. Myasthenia gravis   b. Congenital myopathy
    c. Inclusion body myositis d. Muscular dystrophy

356. A factory worker employed to polish glass comes with complaints of tingling sensation in limbs, constipation and frequent episodes of abdominal pain. X-Ray of limbs shows increased shadows in the femur. Which of the following tests will be useful to diagnose the etiology of symptoms?
    a. Mercury levels in blood   (AIIMS May 2016)
    b. ALA levels in the urine
    c. RBC cholinesterase
    d. Cyanmeth-hemoglobin levels in the blood

357. Keyboard operators and typists are especially susceptible to injury of the? (UPSC 2015)
   a. Axillary nerve   b. Median nerve
   c. Ulnar nerve   d. Radial nerve

358. Charcot's joint include all of the following except?
   a. Syringomyelia   (Bihar PG 2015)
   b. Leprosy
   c. Diabetes
   d. Arthrogryposis Multiplex congenita

359. Gower's manoeuvre is classically seen in? (AP PG 2016)
   a. Parkinsonism
   b. Cerebral palsy
   c. Duchenne muscular dystrophy
   d. Friedreich's ataxia

360. All are true about Miller fisher syndrome except?
   (JIPMER Nov 2015)
   a. Arreflexia   b. Muscle weakness
   c. Pupillary paralysis d. Opthalmoplegia

361. A man has acute onset of paraplegia with symmetrical bilateral areflexia. Diagnosis is:
   (Recent Question 2015-16)
   a. Acute transverse myelitis
   b. Subacute combined degenerative disorder
   c. Guillian Barre syndrome
   d. Poliomyelitis

362. CSF finding in Guillain Barre syndrome is?
   (Recent Question 2015-16)
   a. Normal cells with increased protein
   b. Increased protein with normal cells
   c. Normal cells and normal protein
   d. Increased cells with low sugar

363. Which of the following is correct for the gait abnormalities shown?

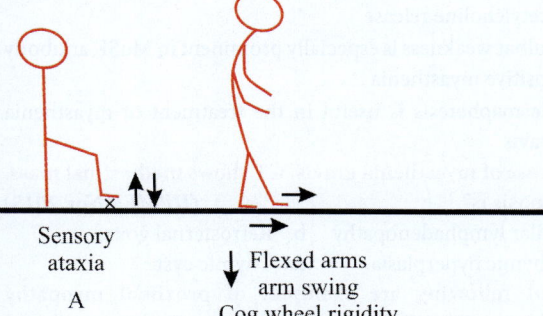

Sensory ataxia
A

Flexed arms
arm swing
Cog wheel rigidity
B

   a. A: Normal pressure hydrocephalus, B: Parkinsonism
   b. A: Tabes dorsalis, B: Parkinsonism
   c. A: Frontal lobe damage, B: Parkinsonism
   d. A: Astasia abasia, B: Parkinsonism

364. Arsenic poisoning causes? (Recent Pattern 2015-16)
   a. Polyneuritis
   b. Mononeuritis multiplex
   c. Radiculopathy
   d. Myelopathy

365. Protein defective in congenital muscular dystrophy:
   (Recent Pattern 2014/15)
   a. Merosin   b. Dystrophin
   c. Laminin   d. Sarcoglycan

366. A 14-year-old girl presents with quadriparesis, facial palsy, winging of scapula and ptosis. There is h/o similar illness in father and brother but less severe. Her CPK level is also raised (500IU/L). She is probably suffering from?
   a. Emery-Dreifuss muscular dystrophy (AIPG 2011)
   b. Becker muscular dystrophy
   c. Limb girdle dystrophy
   d. Scapulofaciohumeral dystrophy

367. Conduction velocity of nerve is NOT affected in which of the following? (Recent Pattern 2014/15)
   a. Leprosy   b. Motor neuron disease
   c. Hereditary neuropathy d. A.I.D.P

368. Small fibre neuropathy is seen in? (AIPG 2010)
   a. HIV   b. Vitamin B_{12} deficiency
   c. AIP   d. Cisplatin toxicity

369. Which of the following is Not true about polymyositis?
   a. Limb girdle weakness (AIIMS Nov 2012)
   b. Ophthalmoplegia
   c. Para-neoplastic syndrome
   d. Spontaneous discharge in EMG

370. A 10 year old child with large leg muscles and low levels of CPK-MM is suggestive of diagnosis: (AIIMS Nov 2012)
   a. Duchenne's muscular dystrophy
   b. Beckers muscular dystrophy
   c. Congenital myopathy
   d. Hereditary sensori-motor neuropathy

371. Which is not seen in Miller Fisher syndrome:
   (Recent Pattern 2014/15)
   a. Anti-GQ1 antibodies b. Ataxia
   c. Cranial nerve palsy d. Postural hypotension

372. A 60 year old female is having proximal muscle weakness with increased serum creatinine kinase. The probable diagnosis is:
   a. Polymyositis   (Recent Pattern 2014/15)
   b. Dermatomyositis
   c. Inclusion body myositis
   d. Limb girdle muscle dystrophy

373. Palpable nerves are seen in: (Recent Pattern 2014/15)
   a. Charcot Marie Tooth disease
   b. Diabetes mellitus
   c. Neurosyphilis   d. Myotonic dystrophy

374. Which of the following shows predominant motor involvement? (Recent Pattern 2014/15)
   a. Lead poisoning   b. Arsenic poisoning
   c. Thallium poisoning d. Mercury poisoning

375. All are true about peripheral-neuropathy except:
   a. Glove and stocking anaesthesia (AI 1999)
   b. Proximal muscle weakness
   c. Nerve-conduction deficit d. Decreased reflexes

376. All of the following are feature of autonomic neuropathy, Except:
   a. Resting Tachycardia (AIIMS May 08)
   b. Silent Myocardial Infarction
   c. Orthostatic Hypotension d. Bradycardia

377. All of the following are predominant motor neuropathy except: (AIIMS May' 06)
   a. Acute inflammatory demyelinating polyradiculoneuropathy
   b. Porphyric neuropathy
   c. Lead intoxication
   d. Arsenic intoxication

378. Pure motor paralysis is seen in : **(AI 2000)**
   a. Polio
   b. Guillain Barre syndrome
   c. Diabetes mellitus
   d. Sub-Acute Combined Degeneration

379. All of the following are true about Guillain Barre Syndrome(GBS), Except: **(AI 2010)**
   a. Ascending paralysis
   b. Flaccid paralysis
   c. Sensory level
   d. Albumino-Cytological Dissociation

380. Dystrophin gene mutation leads to : **(AIIMS May 03)**
   a. Myasthenia gravis
   b. Motor neuron disease
   c. Poliomyelitis
   d. Duchenne's muscular dystrophy

381. In Duchenne's muscular dystrophy, which muscle is not involved : **(AIIMS Feb 97)**
   a. Gastrocnemius
   b. Vastus medialis
   c. Brachioradialis
   d. Infraspinatus

382. All are Congenital Myopathies, except:
   a. Central-core Myopathy **(AIIMS Nov 01)**
   b. Nemaline Myopathy **(AIIMS May 2011)**
   c. Z band Myopathy
   d. Centro-nuclear Myopathy

383. Which of the following antibodies is specific for myositis: **(AIIMS Nov 08)**
   a. Anti–Jo-1
   b. Anti–Scl-70
   c. Anti-Sm
   d. Anti-ku

384. Which is NOT a feature of polymyositis?
   a. Pharyngeal muscle involvement **(AIIMS-97)**
   b. Gottron's rash
   c. Proximal muscle involvement
   d. Pain in limbs

385. All of the following are feature of dermatomyositis, Except: **(AIIMS Nov 09)**
   a. Salmon Patch
   b. Gottron's patch
   c. Mechanic finger
   d. Periungual telengiectasias

Myaesthenia Gravis and Channelopathies

386. A patient is having ptosis and hypotropia. After administration of an intravenous drug to the patient, in 6 minutes his symptoms have resolved. The diagnosis of the patient is. **(AIIMS Nov 2018)**

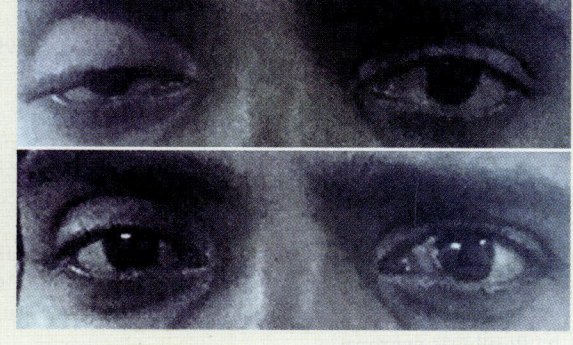

   a. Sixth nerve palsy
   b. Myasthenia gravis
   c. Third nerve palsy
   d. Tolosa-Hunt syndrome

387. A patient had ptosis and diplopia, which was relieved within 5 mins of administering an IV drug. What is the diagnosis? **(AIIMS Nov 2017)**
   a. Myasthenia gravis
   b. 3rd nerve palsy
   c. Grave's ophthalmopathy
   d. 6th nerve palsy

388. All are seen in Myasthenia Gravis except? **(AIIMS May 2017)**
   a. Ptosis
   b. Muscle fatigability
   c. Absent DTR
   d. Normal pupillary reflexes

389. What is not useful for diagnosis of myasthenia gravis?
   a. AChR antibodies **(Recent Pattern Questions)**
   b. Voltage gated calcium channel antibodies
   c. Muscle specific kinase antibodies
   d. Edrophonium test

390. All of the following tests must be done before initiating treatment of M. Gravis? **(Recent Pattern Questions)**
   a. CT Chest
   b. Pulmonary function test
   c. CRP
   d. TSH

391. What is incorrect about M. Gravis?
   a. Symmetrical ptosis **(Recent Pattern Questions)**
   b. Dysphagia
   c. Normal DTR
   d. Thymectomy for generalised M. Gravis

392. Which of the following is not a sodium channel defect? **(Recent Question 2016-17)**
   a. Hyperkalemic periodic paralysis
   b. Brugada Syndrome
   c. Paramyotonia congenita
   d. Anderson Tawi syndrome

393. The following are true regarding myasthenia gravis except: **(AP PG 2015)**
   a. Thymoma or thymic hyperplasia is common
   b. Antibodies to presynaptic voltage gated channels impair acetylcholine release
   c. Bulbar weakness is especially prominent in MuSK antibody positive myasthenia
   d. Plasmapheresis is useful in the treatment of myasthenia gravis

394. In a case of myasthenia gravis, CT shows mediastinal mass. Diagnosis is? **(JIPMER Nov 2015)**
   a. Hilar lymphadenopathy
   b. Retrosternal goiter
   c. Thymic hyperplasia
   d. Thymic cyst

395. All of following are examples of proximal myopathy (weakness) EXCEPT? **(Recent Question 2015-16)**
   a. Myasthenia gravis
   b. Thyroid myopathy
   c. Drug induced myopathy
   d. Duchenne's muscular dystrophy

396. Which of the following is a Channelopathy?
   a. Ataxia Telangiectasia **(Recent Pattern 2015-16)**
   b. Friedreich Ataxia
   c. Amyotrophic lateral sclerosis
   d. Andersen Tawi Syndrome

397. Good syndrome is? **(Recent Pattern 2015-16)**
   a. Thymoma with immunodeficiency
   b. Thymoma with M. Gravis
   c. Thymoma with serum sickness
   d. Thymoma with pure red cell aplasia

398. Episodic muscle weakness can be caused by all of the following except: *(AIPG 2011)*
    a. Hypercalcemia
    b. Channelopathies
    c. Lambert-Eaton syndrome
    d. Hyper-phosphatemia

399. Ice pack test is done for: *(Recent Pattern 2014/15)*
    a. M. Gravis
    b. Multiple system atrophy
    c. Hyperparathyroidism
    d. Hypokalemic periodic paralysis

400. SCN4A defect is seen in: *(Recent Pattern 2014/15)*
    a. Brugada syndrome
    b. Hyper-kalemic periodic paralysis
    c. Lambert Eaton syndrome
    d. Para-myotonia congenital

401. A 35 year old man presents with complaints of ptosis, with difficulty in chewing and occasionally swallowing. On examination there is a asymmetrical ptosis, lateral arm abduction time of 60 seconds. Repetitive nerve stimulation test shows decremental response. EMG shows myopathic response. Anti–Ach receptor antibodies are negative. Probable diagnosis is: *(AIIMS May 2013)*
    a. Ocular M. Gravis
    b. Generalised M. Gravis
    c. Since Anti-Ach receptor antibodies are negative consider other diagnosis
    d. Chronic Progressive external opthalmoplegia

402. Which one of the following is correct regarding Eaton-Lambert syndrome- *(AIIMS Nov 04)*
    a. It commonly affects the ocular muscle
    b. Neostigmine is the drug of choice for this syndrome
    c. Repeated electrical stimulation enhances muscle power in it
    d. It is commonly associated with adenocarcinoma of lung

403. All of the following are neurologic channelopathies, except
    a. Hypokalemic periodic paralysis *(AIIMS May 04)*
    b. Episodic ataxias
    c. Familial hemiplegic migraine
    d. Huntington's disease

Basic Neurology

404. What is the diagnosis? *(AIIMS Nov 2018)*

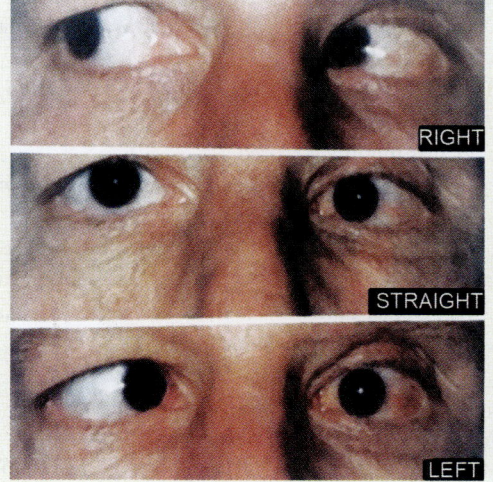

    a. 2nd nerve palsy
    b. 3rd nerve palsy
    c. 4th nerve palsy
    d. 6th nerve palsy

405. Deep tendon reflex requires all of the following structures to be functional except? *(Recent Pattern Questions)*
    a. α-motor neurons
    b. ϒ-motor neurons
    c. Pyramidal neurons
    d. Spindle afferent neurons

406. Which of the following is the correct method for testing the corresponding cranial nerves? *(Recent Pattern Questions)*
    a. Olfactory nerve: sniff alcohol or ammonia
    b. Optic nerve: check ocular Saccades
    c. Trigeminal nerve: Test eyebrow elevation and forehead wrinkling
    d. Accessory nerve: Check Shoulder Shrug

407. Which nerve is *not* involved in control of speech? *(Recent Pattern Questions)*
    a. Vagus
    b. Phrenic
    c. Trigeminal
    d. Hypoglossal

408. "Donald Duck" voice is heard in?
    a. Devic's disease *(Recent Pattern Questions)*
    b. Pseudobulbar palsy
    c. Progressive supra-nuclear gaze palsy
    d. Palatal myoclonus

409. The picture below is of a doctor performing a deep tendon reflex. Which of the following is correct about the picture shown in the image? *(AIIMS May 2016)*

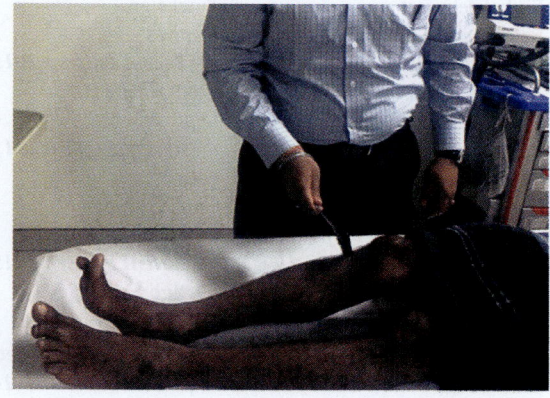

    a. Reflex is always brisk in case of motor neuron disease
    b. Examiner is doing the test wrongly
    c. Reflex is always absent in case of peripheral nerve disease
    d. Root value is L1, L2, L3

410. The inability to perceive the texture & shape an object occurs in lesion of ? *(AIIMS Nov 2015)*
    a. Lateral Spinothalamic tract
    b. Nucleus Gracilis
    c. Spino reticular tract
    d. Nucleus cuneatus

411. Right 12th nerve damage leads to ? *(Recent Question 2015-16)*
    a. Tongue deviation to left on protrusion
    b. Tongue deviation to right on protrusion
    c. Nasal twang to voice
    d. Scanning speech defects

412. Which of the following is not a test for integrity of 7th and 9th nerve: *(Recent Question 2015-16)*
    a. Position of uvula
    b. Palate symmetry
    c. Taste
    d. Tongue protrusion

413. Cranial Nerve 8 palsy causes all EXCEPT:
 (Recent Question 2015-16)
 a. Gag reflex   b. Vertigo
 c. Motion sickness   d. Tinnitus

414. A patient is unable to solve mathematical calculations, which part of his brain is damaged?
 (Recent Question 2015-16)
 a. Temporal lobe   b. Frontal lobe
 c. Parietal lobe   d. Occipital lobe

415. The test being performed is?

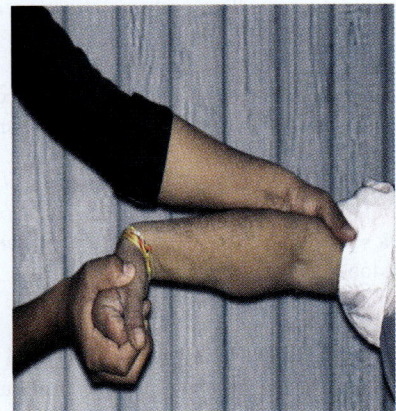

 a. Finkelstein test   b. Tinel sign
 c. Fromment sign   d. Jeanne's sign

416. High Steppage Gait is seen in? (Recent Pattern 2015-16)
 a. Foot drop   b. Frontal lobe stroke
 c. Tabes dorsalis   d. Leprosy

417. Hung- up reflexes are seen in? (Recent Pattern 2015-16)
 a. Chorea   b. Atheotosis
 c. Cerebral palsy   d. Cerebellar palsy

418. Cranial Nerve 8 palsy causes all except?
 (Recent Pattern 2015-16)
 a. Gag reflex   b. Vertigo
 c. Motion sickness   d. Tinnitus

419. The triad of strabismus, diplopia and ptosis are caused due to damage of which nerves: (Recent Pattern 2014/15)
 a. Oculomotor   b. Trochlear
 c. Abducent   d. Cervical sympathetic truk

420. Anterior Corticospinal injury is associated with all except:
 a. Loss of superficial abdominal reflexes (AIIMS May 2012)
 b. Loss of fine movements of fingers and hands
 c. Babinski sign positive
 d. Clasp knife rigidity

421. Blink reflex is used for diagnosis of: (AIIMS Nov 2012)
 a. Mid pontine lesions
 b. Neuromuscular transmission defect
 c. Axonal neuropathy
 d. Motor neuron disease

422. Inability to perform rapid alternating movements is called:
 a. Dysdiadochokinesia   b. Dysarthria (APPG 2014)
 c. Dyssynergia   d. Dystonia

423. Inverse stretch reflex: (Bihar PG 2014)
 a. Is a monosynaptic reflex
 b. Is a bi-synaptic reflex
 c. Is a polysynaptic reflex
 d. Has lower threshold than stretch reflex

424. What is incorrect about Charcot neurological triad:
 a. Scanning speech (Recent Pattern 2014/15)
 b. Intentional tremor
 c. Nystagmus
 d. Rigidity

425. Pendular knee jerks are due to defect of:
 (Recent Pattern 2014/15)
 a. Ischemic stroke   b. Neocerebellum
 c. Paleocerebellum   d. Archicerebellum

426. Micturition reflex Centre is seen in:
 a. Barrington nucleus (Recent Pattern 2014/15)
 b. Para-median pontine reticular pathway
 c. Pulvinar
 d. Peri-ventricular nucleus

427. Dorello's canal carries: (Recent Pattern 2014/15)
 a. 3rd nerve   b. 4th nerve
 c. 5th nerve   d. 6th nerve

428. Muscle tone increasing on patient trying to relax the muscles is seen in: (Recent Pattern 2014/15)
 a. Paratonia   b. Myotonia
 c. Spasticity   d. Rigidity

429. Urine urge occurs at what bladder capacity?
 a. 50 ml (Recent Pattern 2014/15)
 b. 150 ml
 c. 250 ml
 d. 400 ml

430. Argyl robertson pupil is seen in all except:
 (Recent Pattern 2014/15)
 a. Chronic alcoholism   b. Encephalitis
 c. Diabetes mellitus   d. Hypertension

431. All of the following are features of Pseudobulbar palsy, except: (AI 1991)
 a. Dysarthria   b. Dysphagia
 c. Emotional lability   d. Hypoactive jaw jerk

432. Which is pathgnomonic for motor neuron disease
 a. Fasciculation (AIIMS Dec 95)
 b. Bladder, bowel involvement
 c. Pseudohypertrophy
 d. Sensory loss in patchy manner

433. Amyotrophic lateral sclerosis involve: (PGI June 03)
 a. Anterior horn cell   b. Posterior horn cell
 c. Dorsal root ganglia   d. Ventral root ganglia
 e. Myoneural junction

434. Motor neuron disease, TRUE is: (AIIMS May 94)
 a. Sensory involvement
 b. Ocular motility is spared
 c. Involvement of anterior and lateral columns of spinal cord
 d. Intellectual improvement

435. A ventrolateral cordotomy is performed to produce relief of pain from the right leg. It is effective because it interrupts the:
 a. Left Dorsal Column (AI 2012)
 b. Left Lateral Spinothalamic tract
 c. Right Lateral Spinothalamic tract
 d. Right Corticospinal tract

436. Type of sensation lost on same side in Brown sequard syndrome is: (AIIMS Nov 93)
 a. Pain   b. Touch
 c. Proprioception   d. Temperature

437. The following are components of Brown Sequard syndrome except : *(AI 2007)*
    a. Ipsilateral extensor plantar response
    b. Ipsilateral pyramidal tract involvement
    c. Contralateral spinothalamic tract involvement
    d. Contralateral posterior column involvement
438. Beevor's Sign is seen in: *(AIIMS May 09)*
    a. Abdominal muscle   b. Facial muscle
    c. Respiratory muscle   d. Hand muscle
439. Most common drug used in spasticity in patients with spinal cord injury is: *(Recent Pattern)*
    a. Diazepam   b. Tinazidine
    c. Salicylates   d. Baclofen
440. After a minor head injury a young patient was unable to close his left eye and had drooling of saliva from left angle of mouth. He is suffering from:
    a. VIIth nerve injury   *(AIIMS May 03)*
    b. Vth nerve injury
    c. IIIrd nerve injury
    d. Combined VIIth and IIIrd nerve injury
441. TRUE regarding upper motor neuron VIIth nerve paralysis is: *(AIIMS Dec 95)*
    a. Ipsilateral upper face paresis
    b. Ipsilateral lower face paresis
    c. Contralateral upper face paresis
    d. Contralateral lower face paresis

Pediatric Neurology

442. A neonate presented with periventricular calcification on CT brain. What is the best method of diagnosis of etiological agent? *(AIIMS Nov 2017)*
    a. Liver biopsy   b. CSF
    c. Blood   d. Urine
443. Myotonic dystrophy 1 is due to defect on which chromosome? *(Recent Pattern Questions)*
    a. 9   b. 11
    c. 14   d. 19
444. Which of the following is incorrect about myotonic dystrophy type 1? *(Recent Pattern Questions)*
    a. Trinucleotide Repeats
    b. Cardiac conduction defect
    c. Distal muscle weakness
    d. Hatchet face appearance
445. A 7 year old boy presents with progressive gait difficulty with twisting of ankles, and foot deformities. On examination stork leg appearance of legs was seen. The first probable diagnosis is? *(Recent Question 2016-17)*
    a. Becker's muscular dystrophy
    b. Charcot marie Tooth disease
    c. Chronic inflammatory demyelination polyneuropathy
    d. Inclusion body myositis
446. Which type of Arnold Chiari malformation is associated with congenital hydrocephalus? *(JIPMER Nov 2015)*
    a. Type 1   b. Type 2
    c. Type 3   d. Type 4
447. Which type of Meningocele is associated with cerebellar herniation? *(JIPMER Nov 2015)*
    a. Dandy walker syndrome
    b. Arnold chiari I malformation
    c. Arnold chiari II malformation
    d. Hydromelia
448. Small posterior fossa is seen in? *(Recent Pattern 2015-16)*
    a. Arnold chiari malformation
    b. Dandy walker
    c. Medulloblastoma
    d. Schizencephaly
449. SSPE is diagnosed by all except? *(Recent Pattern 2015-16)*
    a. EEG
    b. Antibodies to measles in CSF
    c. Antibodies to measles in blood
    d. Antigen in brain biopsy
450. A 5 year old child presents with loss of vision and axial proptosis. Pupillary examination shows relative afferent pupillary defect. Probable diagnosis is? *(APPG 2014)*
    a. Optic nerve glioma
    b. Optic nerve sheath meningioma
    c. Retinoblastoma
    d. Optic disc melanocytoma
451. Bilateral proptosis in children is seen in:
    a. Neurofibromatosis   *(AIIMS Nov 2012)*
    b. Leukemia
    c. Cavernous hemangioma
    d. Malignant fibrous Histiocytoma
452. During antenatal ultrasonography if the shape of cerebellum shows "banana sign" it suggests: *(Recent Pattern 2014/15)*
    a. Anencephaly   b. Hydrocephaly
    c. Spina bifida   d. Neoplasm
453. Which is true about hydrancephaly:
    a. Sun setting sign   *(Recent Pattern 2014/15)*
    b. Normal size ventricles
    c. Mental retardation
    d. Absent cerebral hemispheres
454. Which of the following is a neuronal migration defect? *(Recent Pattern 2014/15)*
    a. Gaucher disease   b. Schizencephaly
    c. SSPE   d. Sphingolipidosis

Multiple Sclerosis

455. Latest drug approved for Amyotrophic Lateral Sclerosis is? *(AIIMS May 2018)*
    a. Piracetam   b. Edavarone
    c. Ocrelizumab   d. Nitisinone
456. A patient has had recurrent optic neuritis bilaterally with transverse myelitis. Visual acuity in right eye is 6/60 and left eye is 6/18. Patient showed a 50% response to steroids. Diagnosis is? *(AIIMS Nov 2018)*
    a. Neuromyelitis Optica
    b. Subacute combined degeneration of spinal cord
    c. Post cerebral artery stroke
    d. Neurosyphilis

457. **Which of the following is used in acute exacerbation of multiple sclerosis?** *(Recent Question 2019)*
    a. Methylprednisolone b. Fingolimod
    c. Beta interferon d. Natalizumab

458. **Which of the following is the least likely presentation of multiple sclerosis?** *(Recent Pattern Questions)*
    a. Inter-nuclear ophthalmoplegia
    b. Colour blindness
    c. Nocturnal Enuresis
    d. Transverse myelitis

459. **Which of the following tests is not required for diagnosis of multiple sclerosis?** *(Recent Pattern Questions)*
    a. Lumbar puncture
    b. Gadolinium enhanced MRI
    c. Visual evoked potential
    d. Electronystagmogram

460. **A 30-year old female presents with complaints of gradual onset weakness of legs for one month with reduction in visual acuity and urinary incontinence for past few days. Contrast MRI shows periventricular lesions. Which of the following drugs is not used in these patients?**

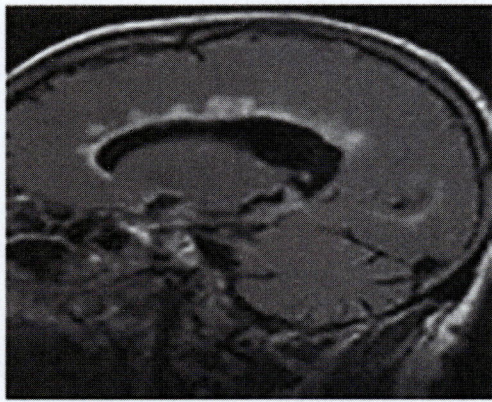

    a. Fingolimod b. Beta interferon
    c. Glatiramer acetate d. Mitotane

461. **Which of the following clinical features of demyelinating myelopathy is least likely to suggest a progression to multiple sclerosis?** *(AIIMS May 2012)*
    a. Complete cord transection
    b. Bilateral visual loss
    c. Absence of oligoclonal bands
    d. Poor prognosis

462. **Drug that causes maximum reduction in appearance of new lesions and change in disease severity in relapsing remitting multiple sclerosis is:** *(Recent Pattern 2014/15)*
    a. Natalizumab b. Glatiramer
    c. Interferon beta 1a d. Interferon beta 1b

463. **A 30 year old female presents with complaints of gradual onset weakness of legs for one month with reduction in visual acuity and urinary incontinence for past few days. Contrast MRI shows periventricular lesions. Which of the following drugs is not used in these patients?**
    (Recent Pattern 2014/15)
    a. Fingolimod b. Beta interferon
    c. Glatiramer acetate d. Mitotane

464. **Which of the following condition improves with pregnancy?** *(Recent Pattern 2014/15)*
    a. Multiple sclerosis b. SLE
    c. Myasthenia gravis d. Rheumatoid arthritis

465. **Pulfrich effect is seen in:** *(Recent Pattern 2014/15)*
    a. Multiple sclerosis b. C.I.D.P
    c. C.R.P.S d. Red green color blindness

466. **Which of the following is used in the treatment of Multiple Sclerosis:** *(AIIMS Nov 2006)*
    a. Interferon Alpha b. Interferon Beta
    c. Infliximab d. Interferon gamma

Diseases of Spinal Cord

467. **Which is the most common presentation of cervical degenerative disc disease?** *(Recent Pattern Questions)*
    a. Biceps weakness
    b. Loss of sensation over nape of neck
    c. Loss of sensation in axilla and medial arm
    d. Wasting of intrinsic hand muscles

468. **A 35 year old patient presents with numbness over neck. On examination decreased pain and temperature sensation in found in distribution of C4, C5. Scalp sensation, cranial nerve function and limb examination is normal. Bladder and bowel sphincter control is normal. What is the diagnosis?** *(Recent Pattern Questions)*
    a. Amyotrophic lateral sclerosis
    b. Intramedullary tumour
    c. Neuro-syphilis
    d. A.I.D.P

469. **A 28 year old smoker construction worker presents with low back pain. The pain is worse on standing and improves with sitting. Reflexes are diminished in right lower limb with absence of sensation in both lower limbs. What is the likely diagnosis?** *(Recent Pattern Questions)*
    a. Lumbar canal stenosis
    b. Occlusive Aortoiliac disease
    c. Tethered cord syndrome
    d. Vertebral metastasis

470. **What is correct about Syringomyelia?** *(Recent Pattern Questions)*
    a. Vibration and position sense is usually diminished
    b. Best treated by neurosurgical excision of syrinx
    c. Developmental defect associated with Chiari malformation
    d. Crossed hemi-anaesthesia

471. **Which of the following is an indication for surgery in a patient with intervertebral disk herniation at L5-S1?** *(Recent Pattern Questions)*
    a. Root pains and Night time symptoms
    b. Absent ankle jerks
    c. Pain killer requirement for more than 2 weeks/ month
    d. Progressive weakness on serial examinations

472. **Which of the following tests is abnormal in patients of ALS (Amyotrophic Lateral Sclerosis)?** *(Recent Pattern Questions)*
    a. V.E.P b. MRI whole spine
    c. CT whole Spine d. Electromyography

473. A Patient after trauma has developed priapism. The lesion is at? *(Recent Question 2016-17)*
    a. Medullary damage
    b. Mid brain damage
    c. Cortical damage
    d. Spinal cord damage
474. Patient was treated for mantle cell Hodgkin lymphoma with radiation therapy. After 6 months he develops an electric shock like pain along the spine on flexing his neck. What is the diagnosis? *(JIPMER Nov 2014)*
    a. Cervical arthritis
    b. Lhermitte sign
    c. Uthoff sign
    d. Spinal cord compression
475. Cauda equina is differentiated from conus medullaris by presence of: *(PGI May 2015)*
    a. Both Ankle jerk and knee jerks may be lost
    b. Asymmetric areflexic paraplegia
    c. Motor changes
    d. Bladder & bowel involvement as initial presentation
    e. Root pain
476. All of the following features are seen in myelopathies except?
    a. Facial sensory impairment *(AIIMS May 2012)*
    b. Brisk jaw jerks
    c. Brisk pectoral jerks
    d. Urgency and incontinence of micturition
477. Most common cranial nerve involvement causing opthalmoparesis in Guillain Barre syndrome is due to: *(Recent Pattern 2014/15)*
    a. 6th nerve
    b. 7th nerve
    c. 8th nerve
    d. 9th nerve
478. In cervical syringomyelia all are seen except:
    a. Burning sensation in hands *(AIIMS Nov 2012)*
    b. Hypertrophy of abductor pollicis brevis
    c. Plantar extensor
    d. Absent biceps reflex.
479. Most common slowly growing vascular tumor of spinal cord, cerebellum and brain is: *(AIIMS Nov 2012)*
    a. Hemangioblastoma
    b. Pilocytic astrocytoma
    c. Meningioma
    d. Medulloblastoma
480. What is true about critical illness myoneuropathy? *(AIIMS Nov 2013)*
    a. Diaphragm atrophy due to mechanical ventilation
    b. Cranial nerves are more commonly involved than peripheral nerves
    c. Peripheral nerves histology shows demyelination
    d. Injury is completely irreversible.
481. In Wernicke's encephalopathy amnestic defect is correlated most closely with inflammation and necrosis of:
    a. Mamillary bodies *(APPG 2014)*
    b. Midline cerebellum
    c. Peri-acqueductal gray matter
    d. Dorso-medial thalamus
482. Most common extra-dural tumour of the spine is: *(Bihar PG 2014)*
    a. Neurofibroma
    b. Glioma
    c. Meningioma
    d. Metastasis
483. Most common cancer showing leptomeningeal metastasis to brain: *(Bihar PG 2014)*
    a. Lung cancer
    b. Malignant melanoma
    c. Breast cancer
    d. Prostate cancer
484. Onion skin pattern of sensory loss in face is seen:
    a. Syringomyelia *(Recent Pattern 2014/15)*
    b. Diabetes mellitus
    c. Amyloidotic polyneuropathy
    d. Leprosy
485. Dissociative sensory loss is seen in all except:
    a. Anterior spinal artery occlusion *(Recent Pattern 2014/15)*
    b. Leprosy
    c. Multiple system atrophy
    d. Hydromyelia
486. All of the following metastatic tumours cause spinal cord compression except: *(Recent Pattern 2014/15)*
    a. Lung cancer
    b. Breast cancer
    c. Lymphoma
    d. Meningioma
487. Dissociative sensory loss is not seen in:
    a. Syringomyelia *(Recent Pattern 2014/15)*
    b. Cauda equina syndrome
    c. Diabetes mellitus
    d. Damage to spino-thalamic pathways
488. All the following are complications of subarachnoid block except: *(Recent Pattern 2014/15)*
    a. Post dural puncture headache
    b. Backache
    c. Hypertension
    d. Bloody tap
489. Sub-acute combined degeneration of spinal cord is seen in:
    a. Thiamin deficiency *(Recent Pattern 2014/15)*
    b. Tuberculosis of spine
    c. Addisonian pernicious anemia
    d. Industrial toxin damage to spinal cord
490. Dose of methylprednisolone following spine injury:
    a. 30 mg/kg within 3 hrs of injury *(Recent Pattern 2014/15)*
    b. 45 mg/kg within 6 hrs of injury
    c. 50 mg/kg within 9 hrs of injury
    d. 60 mg/kg within 12 hrs of injury
491. Hypotension in Acute Spinal Cord injury is due to:
    a. Loss of Sympathetic tone *(Recent Pattern 2014/15)*
    b. Loss of Parasympathetic tone
    c. Vasovagal Attack
    d. Orthostatic Hypotension
492. Which of the following is not a feature of extramedullary tumour: *(AI 2008)*
    a. Early Corticospinal signs and paralysis
    b. Root pain or midline Back –pain
    c. Abnormal CSF
    d. Sacral sparing
493. Clinical features of Conus Medullaris syndrome include all of the following Except:
    a. Plantar Extensor *(AI 2008)*
    b. Absent knee & ankle jerks
    c. Sacral anesthesia
    d. Lower sacral & coccygeal involvement
494. Hypotension in Acute Spinal Cord Injury is due to :
    a. Loss of Sympathetic tone *(AIIMS Nov 06)*
    b. Loss of Parasympathetic tone
    c. Vasovagal Attack
    d. Orthostatic Hypotension

495. Which of the following signs is not suggestive of a cervical spinal cord injury : *(AIIMS Nov 05)*
    a. Flaccidity
    b. Increased rectal sphincter tone
    c. Diaphragmatic breathing
    d. Priapism

496. Spastic paraplegia is caused by all, except: *(AI 2009)*
    a. Vitamin B_{12} deficiency
    b. Cervical spondylosis
    c. Lead poisoning
    d. Motor neuron disease

497. Anterior spinal Artery thrombosis is characterized by all, except: *(PGI Dec 2000)*
    a. Loss of pain & touch
    b. Loss of vibration sense
    c. Loss of power in lower limb
    d. Sphincter dysfunction

498. A 65 year old man presents with anaemia and posterior column dysfunction, the likely cause is: *(AIIMS May 95)*
    a. B_1-deficit
    b. B_{12}-deficit
    c. SSPE
    d. Multiple sclerosis

499. Features of syringomyelia include all of the following, except: *(PGI 09)*
    a. Dissociative sensory loss
    b. Bilateral involvement
    c. Segmental sensory loss
    d. Wasting of small muscles of hand
    e. Ascending weakness

Miscellaneous

500. The given image shows which of the following condition? *(AIIMS Nov 2018)*

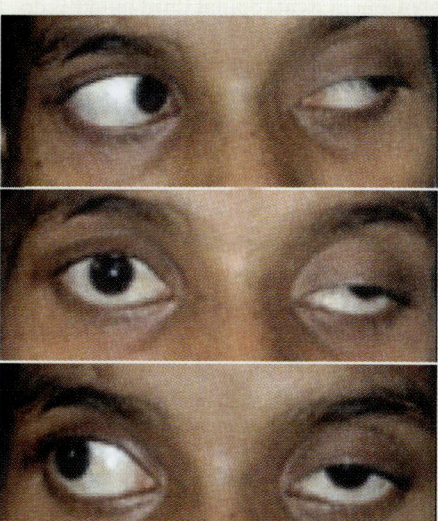

    a. Inter-nuclear ophthalmoplegia
    b. Oculomotor nerve palsy
    c. Lateral rectus palsy
    d. Trochlear nerve palsy

501. A 55 year old man presents with gait ataxia. MRI head was done. Which of the following best describes this patient? *(Recent Pattern Questions)*

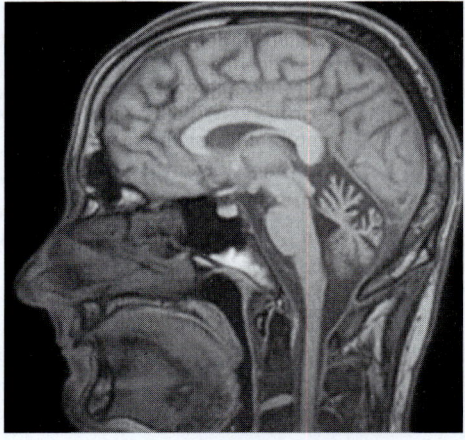

    a. Dementia, gait ataxia, urinary incontinence
    b. Dementia, Chorea, Myoclonus
    c. Vertical gaze palsy, recurrent falls, Axial Rigidity
    d. Scanning speech, oscillatory tremor of head and nystagmus

502. What is the Muscle biopsy finding in fibromyalgia? *(Recent Pattern Questions)*
    a. Endomysial deposits of amyloid
    b. Normal Myocytes
    c. Intense inflammatory infiltrate in proximal muscle groups
    d. Ragged Red fibres in distal muscle groups

503. A patient complains of repeated episodes of excruciating pain in gums and lips after brushing teeth. What is the diagnosis? *(Recent Pattern Questions)*
    a. Dental caries
    b. Tic Douloureux
    c. Root abscess
    d. Glossopharyngeal neuralgia

504. A 70 year old man complains of recurrent episodes of syncope. He believes that episodes occur when he turns his head too quickly. The last episode occurred when he was shaving. Which of the following is not helpful in diagnosis of this patient? *(Recent Pattern Questions)*
    a. Holter
    b. Dix Hallpike's manoeuvre
    c. Carotid sinus massage with ECG monitoring
    d. CT spine and base of brain

505. Which of the following is not useful in a patient of trigeminal neuralgia? *(Recent Pattern Questions)*
    a. Glucocorticoids   b. Carbamazepine
    c. Phenytoin   d. Oxcarbazepine

506. A confused 25 year old girl is brought to your casualty. Her relatives tell that she is on some psychiatric medication but cannot offer more details. Her general physical examination is normal except for tremors in hands, gait ataxia and moderate sized diffuse goitre. Which of the following is most beneficial for the patient? *(Recent Pattern Questions)*
    a. IV saline and observation
    b. Gastric lavage and charcoal
    c. Fluamazenil
    d. Parenteral haloperidol

507. What is the most frequently used drug for restless legs syndrome? *(Recent Pattern Questions)*
    a. Zolpidem
    b. Trazodone
    c. Multivitamins and stretching exercises
    d. Pramipexole

508. All are associated with decreased sense of smell except? *(Recent Pattern Questions)*
    a. Parkinsonism   b. Kallmann Syndrome
    c. Influenza B   d. HIV infection

509. Which of the following patient has the highest chances of developing delirium? *(Recent Pattern Questions)*
    a. 25 year old lady admitted with deep vein thrombosis after delivery
    b. 55 year old man post –op day 2 after colectomy
    c. 65 year old man admitted in ICU post hip joint surgery
    d. 85 year old man living alone in old age home

510. All are true about Wernicke's disease except? *(Recent Question 2016-17)*
    a. Amnestic defect is due to lesion in dorsal medial nuclei of thalamus
    b. Glucose infusions followed by mega dosages of thiamine
    c. Gait ataxia occurs due to polyneuropathy and vestibular paresis
    d. Horizontal nystagmus

511. These images depict a disease that may present with seizures. Select the correct statement. *(AP PG 2016)*

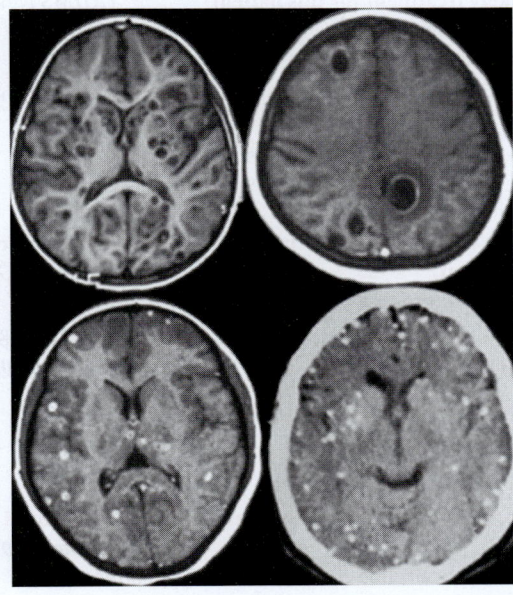

    a. IV contrast enhancement of MRI is the preferred imaging mode
    b. Viable cysts appear as thin walled cysts with minimal inflammation
    c. X-ray of the legs may show multifocal rice grain like calcification
    d. All these statements are true

512. Which one is not used in Alcohol detoxification? *(AIIMS Nov 2015)*
    a. Flumazenil   b. Disulfiram
    c. Acamprosate   d. Naltrexone

513. Most specific sign of metabolic encephalopathy? *(AIIMS Nov 2015)*
    a. Apraxia   b. Asterixis
    c. Anosmia   d. Abulia

514. Features of Friedreich's Ataxia include all of the following, except? *(Bihar PG 2015)*
    a. Progressive weakness
    b. Absent lower limb reflexes
    c. Increased tone in lower limbs
    d. Extensor plantar Response

515. Which of the following is the correct diagnosis? *(AIIMS Nov 2015)*

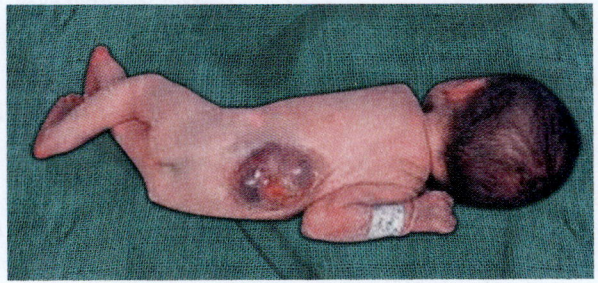

    a. Myelomeningocele
    b. Cystic Hygroma
    c. Sacrococcygeal Teratoma
    d. Spina bifida

516. A previously well 2 year old boy presents with a brief single episode of generalized seizure. There is no past or family history of seizures. On examination, child is alert, active, with axillary temperature of 40°C. Except for bilateral tonsillar enlargement and congestion, systemic examination is normal. Management at this time may include: *(UPSC 2015)*
    a. Immediate reduction of body temperature
    b. Intravenous diazepam and phenytoin, followed by a lumbar puncture
    c. Institution of phenytoin for maintenance therapy for at least one year
    d. Rectal diazepam every 8 hourly for 2-3 days to reduce the risk of recurrence

517. For cancer pain, ladder 2 step in WHO's pain step ladder includes: *(PGI May 2015)*
    a. Oral morphine
    b. Injectable morphine
    c. Codeine
    d. Fentanyl
    e. Tramadol

518. A lady can't speak but can tell by writing. Which of the following brain areas is affected? *(Recent Question 2015-16)*
    a. Broca's area   b. Wernicke's area
    c. Paracentral lobule d. Insula

519. A patient after alcoholic drink fell asleep in chair overnight with hanging arm and develops Saturday Night Palsy. Which of the following best describes the clinical manifestations? *(Recent Question 2015-16)*
    a. Neuropraxia
    b. Axonotmesis
    c. Neurotmesis
    d. Necroptosis

520. **The submerged part of cerebral cortex is?**
    (Recent Question 2015-16)
    a. Insula
    b. Broadman area
    c. Corpus callosum
    d. Piriform sulcus
521. **Unilateral ptosis is NOT seen In?**
    (Recent Question 2015-16)
    a. Myasthenia Gravis
    b. Thyroid Opthalmopathy
    c. Marfan syndrome
    d. Pancoast tumor
522. **CSF is absorbed by :-**   (Recent Question 2015-16)
    a. Choroid plexus
    b. Sub-arachnoid granulations
    c. Dura matter
    d. Pia matter
523. **Incorrect about Dementia pugilistica:**
    (Recent Question 2015-16)
    a. Seen in boxers
    b. Difficulty in gait
    c. Decreased cognition
    d. Nystagmus
524. **Two point discrimination test exhibits maximum sensitivity in?**   (Recent Question 2015-16)
    a. Shin
    b. Toes
    c. Finger pads
    d. Soles
525. **Hemiballismus is due to lesion in?**
    a. Ipsilateral Caudate nucleus   (Recent Question 2015-16)
    b. Contralateral sub-thalamic lesion
    c. Contralateral Putamen
    d. Ipsilateral sub-thalamic lesion
526. **Which vessel DOESN'T form circle of willis:**
    a. Middle cerebral artery   (Recent Question 2015-16)
    b. Anterior cerebral artery
    c. Posterior cerebral artery
    d. Internal carotid artery
527. **Duret haemorrhage is?**   (Recent Question 2015-16)
    a. Traumatic brain haemorrhage in contre-coup injury
    b. Adrenal haemorrhage in water house friderichsen
    c. Brain hemorrhage due to tear of basiliar artery branches
    d. Petechial hemorrhages in fat embolism
528. **What are nitrergic neurons:**   (Recent Question 2015-16)
    a. Post ganglionic neurons releasing nitric oxide
    b. 1st order neurons releasing nitric oxide
    c. Post ganglionic neurons releasing substance P
    d. 1st order neurons releasing calcitonin Gene related peptide
529. **H reflex is used for?**   (AIIMS Nov 14)
    a. S1 radiculopathy
    b. L5 radiculopathy
    c. L4 radiculopathy
    d. L3 radiculopathy
530. **Wernicke's encephalopathy does not involve** (JIPMER 2014)
    a. Thalamus
    b. Mammillary body
    c. Hippocampus
    d. Periventricular white matter
531. **DOC for Tourette syndrome?**   (Recent Pattern 2015-16)
    a. Haloperidol
    b. Valproate
    c. B complex
    d. Clonidine
532. **A patient presents with ataxia. On examination ankle and knee jerks are absent. Plantars are extensor. The diagnosis would be:**   (AIPG 2010)
    a. Friedreich's ataxia
    b. Neuromyelitis optica
    c. Vitamin B_{12} deficiency
    d. Tabes Dorsalis
533. **A 30-year old man complains of falling asleep at work frequently, which he attributes to disturbed sleep at night. He also gives h/o falls while partying with friends. Which of the following problems he might be facing?**
    a. Paralysis during sleep-wake transition with hallucinations
    b. Snoring and witnessed apneas   (AIIMS Nov 2012)
    c. Leg problems while going off to sleep
    d. Generalized seizures in the wake state
534. **Most common type of spinocerebellar ataxia in India**
    (AIIMS Nov 2012)
    a. SCA1
    b. SCA2
    c. SCA3
    d. SCA4
535. **Left lobe of the brain is responsible for:**
    (Recent Pattern 2014/15)
    a. Enjoying music
    b. Spatial orientation
    c. Fine motor movement
    d. Processing of speech
536. **A 16 year old girl has recurrent abdominal pain. On work up USG abdomen and LFT was normal. She has now developed sudden onset bilateral loss of vision, pupils were bilaterally responding to light, with CT head and MRI head being normal. Diagnosis of the patient is:**
    (AIIMS Nov 2013)
    a. Bilateral optic neuritis
    b. PCA infarct
    c. Malingering
    d. Devic's disease
537. **A chronic alcoholic for 15 years stopped consuming alcohol for religious reasons. On the first day he developed nausea and vomiting and on second day seizures. What is the most likely treatment for this patient**   (AIIMS Nov 2013)
    a. Diazepam
    b. Sodium valproate
    c. Phenytoin
    d. Carbamazepine
538. **Which is not correct about Bell's Palsy?**   (AIIMS Nov 2012)
    a. Steroid is mandatory
    b. Unilateral facial weakness
    c. Urgent surgical decompression
    d. HSV 2 is not the cause
539. **The aqueous pressure is higher than intracranial pressure by about:**   (Bihar PG 2014)
    a. 1 to 5 mm Hg
    b. 6 to 10 mm Hg
    c. 15 to 18 mm Hg
    d. More than 20 mm Hg
540. **Steroids are used in:**   (Recent Pattern 2014/15)
    a. Severe typhoid
    b. Cerebral malaria
    c. E. coli septicemia
    d. H. influenzae meningitis
541. **In which of the following vomiting is not associated?**
    (Recent Pattern 2014/15)
    a. Hypocalcemia
    b. Hyponatremia
    c. Diabetes Mellitus
    d. Hypercapnia
542. **Candle wax dripping sign is seen in:**
    a. Sarcoidosis   (Recent Pattern 2014/15)
    b. SLE
    c. HIV
    d. Rheumatoid arthritis
543. **Cause of death in Rett syndrome is:**
    a. Arrhythmia   (Recent Pattern 2014/15)
    b. Pneumonia
    c. Hypoglycaemia
    d. Birth asphyxia

544. Which is not correct regarding chronic fatigue syndrome?
    a. Non tender lymph nodes   (Recent Pattern 2014/15)
    b. Fatigue>6 months
    c. Impairment of recent memory and intelligence
    d. Myalgia/arthralgia
545. Werner syndrome is characterized by all except:
    a. Premature ageing   (Recent Pattern 2014/15)
    b. Bird like facies
    c. Premature atherosclerosis
    d. Pituitary adenoma
546. Drug of choice for Hyper-ammonemia in urea cycle disorders is: (Recent Pattern 2014/15)
    a. Benzoic acid   b. Sodium phenylbutyrate
    c. Cysteamine   d. lactulose
547. Iron deposition in basal ganglia is seen in:
    a. Halloverden Spatz disease   (Recent Pattern 2014/15)
    b. Hemochromatosis
    c. Hemosiderosis
    d. All of above
548. Miller Fisher test is used for: (Recent Pattern 2014/15)
    a. Evaluating gait and cognition in normal pressure hydrocephalus
    b. Severity of paralysis in Guillain Barre syndrome
    c. Grading muscle involvement in ALS
    d. Measuring disability in multiple sclerosis
549. Kluver Bucy Syndrome has?   (Recent Pattern 2014/15)
    a. Hypersomnia   b. Mood changes
    c. Hypersexuality   d. Aggression
550. All are true about Wolman Syndrome except:
    a. Autosomal recessive   (Recent Pattern 2014/15)
    b. Defect in cholestol ester transfer protein
    c. Adrenal calcification
    d. Failure to thrive
551. All of the following cause metabolic headache except: (Recent Pattern 2014/15)
    a. Hypoxia   b. Hypercapnia
    c. Hypokalemia   d. Hyponatremia
552. Severe Hyperphosphatemia is not found associated with?   (Recent Question 2016/17)
    a. Hypocalcemia   b. Hypercalcemia
    c. Tetany   d. QT prolongation
553. Christmas tree appearance of urinary bladder is seen in: (Recent Pattern 2014/15)
    a. Neurogenic bladder   b. Stress incontinence
    c. Autonomous bladder   d. Enuresis
554. Patient complains of dysphagia for solids and liquids. The level of lesion is at: (Recent Pattern 2014/15)
    a. Cortical level   b. Brainstem damage
    c. Cranial nerve palsy   d. Esophagus
555. Diencephalic pupils are due to damage to: (Recent Pattern 2014/15)
    a. Superior colliculus   b. Lateral geniculate body
    c. Optic pathway   d. Hypothalamus
556. Drug used in amyotrophic lateral sclerosis: (Recent Pattern 2014/15)
    a. Riluzole   b. Pramipexole
    c. Rotigotine   d. Ropirinole

557. Retrograde amnesia is seen with: (Recent Pattern 2014/15)
    a. Post traumatic head injury
    b. Temporal lobe epilepsy
    c. Drug addiction
    d. Lennox gastaut syndrome
558. A 25 year old man complains of syncope on shaving without any sweating palpitations. Diagnosis is:
    a. T.I.A   (Recent Pattern 2014/15)
    b. Carotid sinus hypersensitivity
    c. Trigeminal neuralgia
    d. Glossopharyngeal neuralgia
559. Which cranial nerve is involved in Tic Douloureux?
    a. V   (Recent Pattern 2014/15)
    b. VI
    c. VIII
    d. IX
560. Incorrect about Reye syndrome: (Recent Pattern 2014/15)
    a. Prothrombin time is increased
    b. Liver enzymes are elevated
    c. Neuroglucopenia
    d. Liver necrosis
561. The cause of systemic secondary insult to injured brain include all except: (Recent Pattern 2014/15)
    a. Hypocapnia
    b. Hypoxaemia
    c. Hypotension
    d. Hypothermia
562. Hexanucleotide repeats are seen in:
    a. Motor neuron disease   (Recent Pattern 2014/15)
    b. Spinocerebellar ataxia
    c. Huntington chorea
    d. Spinomuscular atrophy
563. Incorrect about cerebellar disease is:
    a. Rhomberg sign   (Recent Pattern 2014/15)
    b. Rebound phenomenon
    c. Dysaidokinesia
    d. Dysmetria
564. All of the following are features of Friedreich's Ataxia, Except: (AI 1992)
    a. Progressive Ataxia is the most common presentation
    b. Cardiomyopathy is a common association
    c. Diabetes mellitus may be associated
    d. Extensor plantar with brisk lower limb reflexes.
565. Pyramidal tract involvement with absent ankle jerk is seen in:
    a. Friedreich's ataxia   (AIIMS May 01)
    b. Subacute combined degeneration of the spinal cord
    c. Lathyrism
    d. Tabes dorsalis
566. Earliest presentation of Friedreich's ataxia is-
    a. Ataxia   (AIIMS Nov 93)
    b. Seizures
    c. Optic atrophy
    d. Stuttering
567. All are feature of Wernicke's encephalopathy, Except:
    a. Cogwheel rigidity   (AIIMS Feb 97)
    b. Alteration in mental function
    c. Ophthalmoplegia
    d. Ataxia

568. Which of the following is not involved in Wernicke's Korsakoff psychosis: (AI 2012)
   a. Mamillary body
   b. Thalamus
   c. Periventricular Grey matter
   d. Hippocampus

569. Memory impairment is most likely to occur in:
   a. Down's Syndrome (AIIMS Nov 99)
   b. Alkaptonuria
   c. Attention deficit disorder
   d. Conduct disorder

570. Non-noxious stimuli perceived as pain is termed as:
   a. Allodynia (AIIMS May 08)
   b. Hyperalgesia
   c. Hyperesthesia
   d. Hyperpathia

571. All of the following clinical findings are seen in Horner's syndrome, Except: (AIIMS May 2011)
   a. Miosis   b. Anhidrosis
   c. Heterochromia of Iris   d. Apparent Exophthalmos

572. A symmetric high-voltage, triphasic slow wave pattern is seen on EEG in the following :
   a. Hepatic encephalopathy (AIIMS May' 06)
   b. Uremic encephalopathy
   c. Hypoxic encephalopathy
   d. Hypercarbic encephalopathy

573. Metabolic encephalopathy presents with:
   a. Broca's aphasia (AIIMS June 99)
   b. Anomic aphasia
   c. Transcortical sensory aphasia
   d. Transcortical motor aphasia

574. Hand knee gait is seen in?
   a. Polio
   b. Avascular necrosis of hip
   c. Leprosy
   d. Spastic hemiplegia

Answers with Explanations

Epilepsy

1. Ans. (b) Continue for 2 years

(Ref: Harrison 20th edition, page 3065)

The clinical details provided in the question are:
- Single seizure type with adequate control
- No family history mentioned
- Normal EEG
  - In this clinical setting it is reasonable to withdraw therapy after 2 years.
  - Juvenile myoclonic epilepsy also occurs in adolescent age group but the seizures *occurs after awakening* and are usually myoclonic jerks or GTCS. Some cases may have absence seizures but focal seizures are not seen in juvenile myoclonic seizures.

2. Ans. (b) Drunkenness

(Ref: Harrison 20th p 3055, 3186; Harrison 19th edition, page 2724)

Harrison quotes "approximately 35% of drinkers and much higher proportion of alcoholics experience a *blackout*". It is an episode of *temporary antegrade amnesia* in which the person forgets all or part of what occurred during a drinking evening. You would have seen many such cases in your casualty as well. Another consequence of alcohol intake is impaired judgement and coordination. Neuroimaging reveals cerebellar atrophy.

Concussion or mild traumatic brain injury is defined as blow to head which results in:

1. Loss of consciousness <30 minutes (Few seconds to minutes)
2. Altered consciousness for <24 hours (usually < 30 minutes)
3. Post traumatic amnesia< 24 hours (usually <30minutes)
4. Glasgow coma scale (13-15)
5. Focal neurological signs: none or transient
6. Neuroimaging is normal

Concussion is a close choice but *points against the diagnosis of concussion* are:
1. As per Harrison concussion is seen in military war veterans and not alcoholics.
2. Loss of consciousness is usually for seconds or minutes in concussion while in this case the person was sleeping under influence of alcohol intoxication.
3. Post traumatic amnesia is usually for < 30minutes.

3. Ans. (a) Gradually taper levetiracetam over 6 months

(Ref: Harrison 20th p 3061, 3065; Harrison 19th edition, page 2554 and 2556)

- Sudden stoppage of AED leads to development of *breakthrough seizures*. Hence the drug should be gradually tapered.
- While the dose of levetiracetam is being reduced over 2-3 months, second drug needs to be introduced gradually.
- Levetiracetam is used for focal onset seizures in a dose of 1000-300mg/day. Therapeutic levels are 5-45µg/dl.
- Side effects are sedation, fatigue, incoordination, mood changes, anaemia and leukopenia.

4. Ans. (a) Hepatic encephalopathy

(Ref: Harrison 20th p 3138; Harrison 19th edition, page 2623)

Myoclonus is a rapid, shock like jerky movement consisting of single or repetitive muscle discharges. Types of myoclonus:

1. Action myoclonus: Occurs with voluntary movement
2. Reflex/ startle myoclonus: Occurs with external stimulus like loud noise
3. Negative myoclonus: Other term for Asterixis/ Flapping tremors
4. Hypnogogic jerks : Occurs in normal people on going to sleep in NREM1

5. Ans. (a) History of febrile seizures

(Ref: Harrison 20th p 3053; Harrison 19th edition, page 2544 and 2546)

- Mesial temporal sclerosis is associated with lower seizure threshold and *history of febrile seizures since childhood*.
- It is the most common syndrome associated with focal seizures with dyscognitive features in adult age group.
- Aura is common with behavioural arrest like staring.
- Complex automatism with post ictal disorientation is noted.
- MRI shows hippocampal sclerosis.

6. Ans. (a) Amygdalohippocampectomy

(Ref: Harrison 20th p 3053; Harrison 19th edition, page 2546)

Mesial temporal lobe epilepsy is due to hippocampal sclerosis. These patients have epilepsy refractory to medical therapy and hence need devices like vagal nerve stimulation. However definitive treatment involves

1. Resection of Antero-medial temporal lobe or limited removal of hippocampus and amygdala (Amygdalohippocampectomy)
2. Focal seizures may be abolished by focal neocortical resection with precise removal of an identified lesion (Lesionectomy).

7. Ans. (b) 2

(Ref: Harrison 20th p 3065; Harrison 19th edition, page 2556)

It is *reasonable to withdraw AED after 2 years* of a patient who meets the following criteria:

1. Complete medical control for 1-5 years
2. Single seizure type like focal /GTCS
3. Normal neurological examination
4. Normal cognition
5. Normal EEG

8. Ans. (a) Focal seizures

(Ref: Harrison 20th p 3051; Harrison 19th edition, page 2542)

- The patient is exhibiting focal seizures which are accompanied by transient impairment of patient's ability to maintain normal contact with environment.
- *Chewing, lip smacking, swallowing or picking movements of hands are called automatisms.*

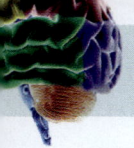

- The full recovery after the episode may range from seconds to an hour. Due to involvement of temporal lobe, patient was having abnormal olfactory sense before the episode.

9. Ans. (d) EEG showing less than 3 Hz Spike…

(Ref: Harrison 20th p 3052; O.P Ghai: 8th edition, page 557-561)

Lennox-Gastaut syndrome has the following triad:

1. Multiple seizure types (usually including generalized tonic-clonic, atonic, and atypical absence seizures)
2. EEG showing slow (<3 Hz) spike-and-wave discharges and a variety of other abnormalities
3. Impaired cognitive function in most but not all cases.

Lennox-Gastaut syndrome has a multifactorial nature and is associated with CNS disease or dysfunction, developmental abnormalities, and perinatal hypoxia/ischemia.

10. Ans. (a) Levetiracetam

(Ref: Harrison 20th p 3061; Harrison 19th edition, page 1793 and Epilepsy and brain tumour by Newton: 2015 edition, page 199)

- In epilepsy caused by brain tumour, agents of choice are those drugs that *do not* induce the hepatic microsomal enzyme system. These include levetiracetam, topiramate, lamotrigine, valproic acid, or lacosamide.
- *Other drugs such as phenytoin and carbamazepine are used less frequently because they are potent enzyme inducers that can interfere with both glucocorticoid metabolism and the metabolism of chemotherapeutic agents needed to treat the underlying cerebral oedema, systemic malignancy or the primary brain tumour.*

11. Ans. (c) P.C.O.D

(Ref: Goodman and Gilman, 12th edition, page 597; KD Tripathi 7th edition, page 405-09)

- Menstrual abnormalities and PCOD are side effects of valproate seen in females.
- Most common side effects are transient GIT side effects
- CNS side effects are sedation, ataxia and tremors
- Rare complication is fulminant hepatitis.

12. Ans. (c) Changes in memory/perception and "blackouts" are not features of complex partial seizures

(Ref: Harrison 20th p 3051; Harrison 19th edition, page 2543 and 2550)

Jacksonian epilepsy is a spreading seizure activity	Correct	In Jacksonian spread, motor movements may begin in a very restricted region such as the fingers and gradually progress (over seconds to minutes) to include a larger portion of the extremity.
Serum level of prolactin increases dramatically after tonic clonic convulsions	Correct	Measurement of serum prolactin levels may also help to distinguish between organic and psychogenic seizures, since most generalized seizures and some focal seizures are accompanied by rises in serum prolactin (during the immediate 30-minute postictal period), whereas psychogenic seizures are not
Absence seizures are briefer and more frequent without postictal confusion	Correct	Absence seizures are characterized by brief lapses of consciousness without loss of postural control. The seizure typically lasts for only seconds, consciousness returns as suddenly as it was lost, and there is *no postictal confusion*

13. Ans. (b) Astrocytoma

(Ref: Epilepsy and Brain tumour, edition, page 111, 2015)

The clinical features are those of focal seizures with dyscognitive features. Since MRI shows features of brain tumour the diagnosis is brain tumour related epilepsy. The brain tumour with 100% epilepsy association is dys-embryoblastic neuro-epithelial tumour followed by low grade astrocytoma.

Brain tumour related epilepsy

Tumor Histology	Seizure Frequency (%)
Dysembryoblastic neuroepithelial tumor	100
Ganglioglioma	80-90
Low-grade astrocytoma	75
Meningioma	29-60
Oligodendroglioma	53
Anaplastic astrocytoma	43
Glioblastoma multiforme	25
Ependymoma	25
Metastasis	20-35
Primary CNS lymphoma	10

MRI findings of Brain tumours

Meningioma	They appear as well-circumscribed, smoothly marginated extra-axial mass abutting the dura. Some can show calcification.
Astrocytoma	Low-grade astrocytomas are typically *hyperintense on T2-weighted images.* On T1-weighted images, most low-grade astrocytomas are hypointense relative to white matter. Contrast enhancement may be absent or, mild.
Craniopharyngioma	The lesion is seen in sellar or suprasellar area and has surrounding calcification.
Glioblastoma multiforme	MRI findings demonstrate a heterogeneous mass that is generally of low signal intensity on T1-weighted images and high signal intensity on T2-weighted images. *There are internal cystic areas, internal flow voids representing prominent vessels, internal areas of high signal intensity on T1 (hemorrhagic foci), neovascularity, necrotic foci, significant peritumoral vasogenic edema, and significant mass effect*

Contd...

14. Ans. (a) Phenobarbitone

(Ref: Harrison 20th p 3067; Harrison 19th edition, page 2258 and American epilepsy society 2016 guidelines)

In latest guidelines, Phenobarbitone is not used for GCSE.

Treatment for impending and early SE
Intravenous benzodiazepines: Lorazepam, midazolam, clonazepam
Intravenous anti-epileptics: phenytoin, valproate or levetiracetam
Treatment for established and early refractory SE (30minutes to 48 hours)
Intravenous midazolam or propofol
Late refractory Status Epilepticus
Pentobarbital or Thiopentone

15. Ans. (a) Hypsarrhythmia

(Ref: OP Ghai, 8th edition, page 559)

Hypsarrhythmia is an abnormal interictal pattern, consisting of high amplitude and irregular waves and spikes in a background of chaotic and disorganized activity seen on electroencephalogram and frequently encountered in an infant diagnosed with infantile spasms.

16. Ans. (b) Absence seizure

(Ref: Harrison 20th p 3051-52; Nelson, Pg 593.4)

- Simple (typical) absence (petitmal) seizures are characterized by a sudden cessation of motor activity or speech with a blank facial expression and flickering of the eyelids.
- These seizures, which are uncommon before the age of 5 years, are more prevalent in girls, are never associated with an aura, rarely persist longer than 30 sec and are not associated with a postictal state.
- These features tend to differentiate absence seizures from complex partial seizures.
- Children with absence seizures may experience countless seizures daily, whereas complex partial seizures are usually less frequent. Patients do not lose body tone, but their head may fall forward slightly.
- Immediately after the seizure, patients resume pre-seizure activity with no indication of postictal impairment.
- Automatic behavior frequently accompanies simple absence seizures. Hyperventilation for 3–4 min routinely produces an absence seizure.
- The EEG shows a typical 3/sec spike and generalized wave discharge. Complex (atypical) absence seizures have associated motor components consisting of myoclonic movement of the face, fingers, or extremities and occasionally loss of body tone.
- These seizures produce atypical EEG spike and wave discharges at 2–2.5/sec.

17. Ans. (b) Myoclonic epilepsy

(Ref: Harrison 20th p 3053; Harrison 19th edition, page 2545)

- Laforas disease is due to defect on chronosome 6
- Autosomal recessive with presentation between 6–19 years
- Brain degeneration with polyglucosan intracellular inclusion bodies
- Death by 10 years of disease onset
- Laforin is a protein involved in glycogen metabolism.

18. Ans. (a) Take person away from train make sure he does not fall on tracks, meanwhile call for medical help and transfer to hospital

(Ref: American epilepsy society guidelines 2015)

What NOT to do during a convulsion in an epileptic:

1. Do not try to put anything in the persons mouth;
   - There is no place for the "tongue blade" at the bedside or in the home. In fact, it is dangerous. Many sticks, teeth, and other things have been broken by persons attempting to prevent "swallowing of the tongue". The same applies to fingers - never place anything in the mouth of a person who is actively seizing/convulsing.
2. Do not try to restrain the convulsing limbs;
   - Soften the surface, remove obstacles/furnishings, get the person to a safe spot, cushion head with your hands.
   - Restraining the patient can lead to muscle tear or hematoma formation.
3. If a person known to have 'convulsive' epilepsy shows a color change toward blue in face, lips, nail-beds at the onset of a seizure- count to 60;
   - The cyanosis (bluing of lips, nails, skin) that may accompany what in essence is a brief "respiratory arrest" at the beginning of a convulsion is caused by contracted and 'stuck' respiratory muscles. It is not something that can be altered by any bystander/caregiver. It should pass relatively quickly, with improvement in color as the convulsion proceeds.
   - If the above state lasts beyond a minute, OR if it is followed by relaxation (instead of convulsive movements) with persistent bluish color, it would probably be wise to assume that this IS a respiratory arrest and NOT a seizure. [In which case the proper response would be Basic Life Support].
4. Do not attempt to give the person medication/fluids while they are non-interactive;
   - The person should be talking before any attempt is made to give anything by mouth.

Summary of Things Never to be done in seizure
Restrain the person's movements
Put anything in the person's mouth
Try to move them unless they are in danger
Give them anything to eat or drink until they are fully recovered
Attempt to bring them round.

19. Ans. (a) Lamotrigine

(Ref: Adam and Victor, principles of neurology, 8th edition, page 329-330)

- Risk of developing major congenital malformations is 4-5% with women on valproate while the risk of same in ordinary population is 2-3%.
- The risk with Lamotrigine is comparable to the risk of N.T.D with ordinary population.

20. Ans. (c) Levetiracetam

(Ref: Harrison 20th p 2556, 3064; Harrison 19th p 2552)

- Partial seizure are now called as Focal seizures.
- Levetiracetam has the advantage of having no known drug interactions. Therefore it is useful in eldery and patients who are taking multiple concurrent medications in geriatric age group.

21. Ans. (d) Delta

(Ref: Handbook of stroke, 2nd ed., pg 99)

- There is a good correlation between the severity of the EEG changes, the severity of the hepatic encephalopathy, and the clinical state of the patient.
- In mild encephalopathy associated with mild clouding of consciousness and confusion, there is at first slowing of the posterior dominant rhythm, which decreases from a higher to a lower alpha frequency and then into the theta frequency range.
- Severe encephalopathy is associated with deeper levels of coma, and the background *consists mainly of high-amplitude irregular delta activity.*
- With further deterioration in the encephalopathy, the amplitude of all activities drop below 20 μV and the EEG may consist of relatively low-amplitude, invariant delta activity.
- The most extreme type of abnormality in metabolic encephalopathy is lack of any cerebral activity (i.e., electro-cerebral inactivity).

Metabolic encephalopathy	EEG rhythm
Grade I (almost normal)	Dominant activity is alpha rhythm with minimal theta activity
Grade II (mildly abnormal)	Dominant theta background with some alpha and delta activities
Grade III (moderately abnormal)	Continuous delta activity predominates, little activity of faster frequencies
Grade IV (severely abnormal)	*Low-amplitude delta activity* or suppression-burst pattern
Grade V (extremely abnormal)	Nearly "flat" tracing or electrocerebral inactivity

Other important EEG patterns

- **Burst suppression pattern** seen in subacute sclerosing panencephalitis: high-voltage (300-1500 pV), repetitive, polyphasic sharp and slow wave complexes of 0.5- to 2-second duration that recur every 4-15 seconds.
- **Periodic sharp wave complexes** seen in Creutzfeldt-Jacob Disease: As the disease advances, the pattern becomes generalized and synchronous with continuous periodic stereotypic 200- to 400-millisecond sharp waves occurring at intervals of 0.5-1.0 seconds.

- **Lambda waves:** occur when reading and occasionally when watching TV. Amplitude <20 μV and duration 150-250 msec
- **Mu waves:** seen best when the cortex is exposed or if bone defects (e.g., postsurgical) are present in the skull.
- **3-Hz generalized spike and wave discharges** -Childhood Absence Epilepsy.
- **<3Hz (1.5-2.5 Hz) slow spike wave activity** is seen in lennox gastaut syndrome
- **Sleep spindles**-Spindles are groups of waves that occur during many sleep stages but especially in stage 2 NREM.
- **Saw tooth waves:** REM sleep

22. Ans. (c) Myoclonus

(Ref: Harrison 20th p 3052; Harrison 19th p 2544)

Juvenile Myoclonic Epilepsy
- Onset: Early adolescence
- Clinical features: Most common - Myoclonus bilaterally or single and prominent in morning after awakening. Consciousness is preserved unless very severe.
- In future life these patients develop GTCS
- Strong family history- polygenic inheritance
- Treatment - first line- Valproate, lamotrigine or topiramate
- Second line- clonazepam, felbamate

23. Ans. (c) Rufinamide

(Ref: Harrison 20th p 3063; Harrison 19th p 2555 t)

Drug	Role in LGS
Lacosamide	Lacosamide caused worsening of tonic seizures and electroencephalographic pattern.
Vigabatrin	Vigabatrin was approved by US Food and Drug Administration (FDA) in 2009 as monotherapy for patients with infantile spasms aged 1 month to 2 years and as adjunctive therapy for adults with refractory complex partial seizures
Rufinamide	• An antiepileptic agent that is structurally unrelated to current antiepileptics. • Rufinamide modulates sodium channel activity, particularly prolongation of the channel's inactive state. • It significantly slows sodium channel recovery and limits sustained repetitive firing of sodium-dependent action potentials. • In 2008, this drug was approved by the FDA for adjunctive therapy in children aged 4 years older with seizures associated with LGS
Zonisamide	Not recommended < 16 years of age

* Clobazam is the latest drug for L.G.S introduced in 2012

24. Ans. (c) Lamotrigine

(Ref: Harrison 20th p 3067; Harrison 19th p 2559)

- Juvenile myoclonic epilepsy is a frequent form of idiopathic generalized epilepsy that is usually and easily controlled by valproate monotherapy. However, juvenile myoclonic epilepsy is often misdiagnosed, and carbamazepine and phenytoin, have an aggravating effect. Hence choice a and b are ruled out.

Contd...

- Inutero valproate exposure continues to show the highest risk of congenital malformations and of adverse cognitive outcomes, including autism, compared to other AEDs.
- In utero exposure to *lamotrigine*, carbamazepine, phenytoin, and levetiracetam has been evaluated in large numbers of offspring, and all of these AEDs have a *low risk of major congenital malformations*, near 2.5%.

25. Ans. (a) Recovery from unconciousness

(Ref: Harrison 20th p 3060; Harrison 19th p 2551)

- Harrison's mentions clearly that urinary incontinence is present with both of these conditions. Injury due to fall can occur in both. *Unconsciousness will occur in both though the duration of unconsciousness varies and so does the recovery.*

Features	Seizure	Syncope
Immediate precipitating factors	Usually none	Emotional stress, Valsalva, orthostatic hypotension, cardiac etiologies
Premonitory symptoms	None or aura (e.g., odd odor)	Tiredness, nausea, diaphoresis, tunneling of vision
Posture at onset	Variable	Usually erect
Transition to unconsciousness	Often immediate	Gradual over seconds
Duration of unconsciousness	Minutes	Seconds
Incontinence	Sometimes	Sometimes
Tongue bite	Sometimes	Rarely
Facial appearance during event	Cyanosis, frothing at mouth	Pallor
Disorientation and sleepiness after event	Many minutes to hours	<5 min

26. Ans. (d) Surgery

(Ref: Harrison 20th p 3065; OP Ghai, pubmed.nl and Harrison 19th p 2557)

Ketotic diet	Useful in Pediatric seizures like Rett syndrome, Lennox Gastuat syndrome. It entails consumption of 3-4 grams of fat per gram of carbohydrates. This probably works by reducing the metabolism of the epileptogenic focus.
Vagus nerve stimulation	Vagal nerve stimulation (VNS) is a palliative device approved to treat medically refractory focal-onset epilepsy in adults. Some studies demonstrate its efficacy in focal-onset seizures and in a small number of patients with primary generalized epilepsy. Randomized studies showed modest efficacy at 3 months.
Deep brain stimulation (emedicine)	The NeuroPace RNS System, a device that is implanted into the cranium, senses and records electrocorticographic patterns and delivers short trains of current pulses to interrupt ictal discharges in the brain. The Neurological Devices panel of the US Food and Drug Administration (FDA) has concluded that this device is safe and effective in patients with partial-onset epilepsy in whom other antiepileptic treatment approaches have failed and that the benefits outweigh the risks

Contd...

Surgery (Harrison's)	About 70% of patients treated with temporal lobectomy will become seizure free, and another 15–25% will have at least a 90% reduction in seizure frequency. Marked improvement is also usually seen in patients treated with hemispherectomy for catastrophic seizure disorders due to large hemispheric abnormalities. Postoperatively, patients generally need to remain on antiepileptic drug therapy, but the marked reduction of seizures following resective surgery can have a very beneficial effect on quality of life.

- **The surgical approaches used for medically refractory epilepsy is :**
  1. Resection of the antero-medial temporal lobe (temporal lobectomy is the most commonly done procedure)^Q
  2. Removal of the underlying hippocampus and amygdala (amygdalohippocampectomy).
  3. Removal of an identified lesion (lesionectomy).
- Medically refractory epilepsy is defined as uncontrolled seizures or intolerable side effects of AED interfering with quality of life.
- MC cause of refractory epilepsy is temporal lobe epilepsy.^{Q}
- Uncontrolled seizures are defined as > 2 per month for 2 years in spite of supervised monotheraphy/polytherapy.

27. Ans. (a) Hypothalamic Hamartoma

(Ref: Nelson 20th 2838; Nelson 18th ed., ch. 563.2 /Precocious Puberty Resulting from Organic Brain Lesions)

Etiology

- Hypothalamic hamartomas are the most common brain lesion causing true precocious puberty by interrupting pubertal restraint pathways.

Clinical Manifestations

1. Rapidly progressive sexual precocity in very young children.
2. Hypothalamic signs or symptoms such as diabetes insipidus, adipsia, hyperthermia, *unnatural crying or laughing (Gelastic seizures)*, obesity, and cachexia should suggest the possibility of an intracranial lesion.

Treatment

1. In those patients with hypothalamic hamartoma and associated intractable gelastic or psycho-motor seizures, however, stereotactic radiation therapy (gamma knife surgery) is effective and less risky than neurosurgical intervention.
2. Therapy with GnRH agonists is as effective in children with organic brain lesions causing central precocious puberty as it is in children with idiopathic sexual precocity, and these analogs are the therapy of choice to halt premature sexual development.

28. Ans. (a) Hyponatremia

(Ref: Harrison 20th p 298; Harrison 19th p 298)

- Hyponatremia is the most common electrolyte abnormality in hospitalized patients and values less than 120 mEq/dl lead to cerebral edema and resultant seizures
- Hyponatremia is defined as a plasma Na+ concentration <135 mM, is a very common disorder, occurring in up to 22% of hospitalized patients.

- This disorder is almost always the result of an increase in circulating AVP and/or increased renal sensitivity to AVP, combined with any intake of free water; a notable exception is hyponatremia due to low solute intake

29. Ans. (d) Treatment with glucocerebrosidase infusions

(Ref: Harrison 20th p 3053; Harrison 19th p 2545t)

Lafora's disease
- It is a Progressive myoclonic epilepsy with autosomal recessive inheritance
- Onset age 6–19 years
- Death within 10 years
- Brain degeneration associated with poly-glucosan intracellular inclusion bodies in numerous organs.
- Investigation of choice is DNA sequencing which shows abnormality in EPM2A and EPM2B gene. Also demonstration of Lafora bodies within the apocrine sweat gland of the skin by an axillary skin biopsy examination.
- Management: Zonisamide has shown good results but as such textbook does not mention regarding the drug of choice.

30. Ans. (a) Lennox Gastaut syndrome

(Ref: Harrison 20th p 3052-53; Harrison 19th p 2544)

Lennox-Gastaut syndrome occurs in children and is defined by the following triad

1. Multiple seizure types (usually including generalized tonicclonic, atonic, and atypical absence seizures);
2. EEG showing slow (<3 Hz) spike-and-wave discharges and a variety of other abnormalities
3. Impaired cognitive function in most but not all cases.

- Lennox-Gastaut syndrome is associated with CNS disease or dysfunction from a variety of causes, including developmental abnormalities, perinatal hypoxia/ischemia, trauma, infection, and other acquired lesions.
- Latest drug for management is Rufinamide/Clobazam.

31. Ans. (d) Infantile spasm

(Ref: Nelson 20th p 2840; Nelson, 18th ed., Ch: 593.2)

High amplitude waves and spikes are present, randomly appearing and with no topographical distribution identified; also, there is no frequency nor amplitude gradient, indicating a highly disorganized brain activity and seen in INFANTILE SPASMS.

32. Ans. (a) Herpes simplex encephalitis

(Ref: Harrison 20th p 156, 1349; Harrison 19th p 895)

- **Periodic Lateralizing Epileptiform Discharges (PLEDs),** are strongly suggestive of Herpes simplex encephalitis
- In sporadic CJD (sCJD), the EEG exhibits characteristic changes depending on the stage of the disease, ranging from nonspecific findings such as diffuse slowing and frontal rhythmic delta activity (FIRDA) in early stages to disease-typical **periodic sharp wave complexes (PSWC)** in middle and late stages to a reactive coma traces or even alpha coma in pre-terminal EEG recordings. The periodic discharges take the form of diphasic or triphasic sharp waves, which repeat regularly at a frequency close to one per second. There is a fairly close relationship between the periodic complexes and myoclonic jerks; the latter may occur a few milliseconds before or after the electrical event.

33. Ans. (a) Phenobarbitone

(Ref: O.P. Ghai pg. 527, 7th ed.,..)

34. Ans. (a) Complex partial seizures

(Ref: Nelson 20th p 2829-30; Nelson, 18th ed., Ch. 593.1)

- Atypical febrile seizures are associated with post ictal deficit. There is also high incidence of positive family history and these patients in future go on to develop complex partial seizures.
- In this subset of patients some patients have mesial temporal sclerosis close to hippocampus which is amenable to surgery.

35. Ans. (b) Absence seizures

(Ref: Nelson 20th p 2831)

Pyknolepsy describes a patient with recurrent attacks of petit mal /absence seizures. It should be treated akin to status epilepticus in petit mal seizures.

36. Ans. (a) Valproate

(Ref: Epilepsy comprehensive textbook volume 3, 2nd edition page 2561)

- Majority of patients do not need anticonvulsant therapy, but, when needed, the drug of choice is valproate in monotherapy.
- Clobazam could be a helpful adjunct. Lamotrigine, topiramate, and levetiracetam have also been recommended as possible second choices.
- The most effective treatment is avoidance of the provoking stimulus. This can be difficult if the real trigger is not known. The parents of children with television-induced seizure should ensure that they are not closer than 2 meters from the set and do not approach it to switch or adjust the controls.

37. Ans. (a) S.S.P.E.

(Ref: Nelson 20th p 1545 Nelson, 18th ed., ch. 275;)

Disease	EEG findings
SSPE	Periodic epileptiform discharges occurring after every 4-15 seconds
Herpes encephalitis	Periodic LATERALISED slow waves with high voltage bursts due to temporal lobe involvement
Subdural effusion	Focal flattening with normal discharge in other areas
Status epilepticus	The seizures characteristically begin with a flattening of the normal background rhythms, followed by generalized low voltage fast activity or polyspikes that increase in amplitude and decrease in frequency until these patterns become obscured by muscle and movement artifact
CJD	PERIODIC SHARP WAVE COMPLEXES occur in about two-thirds of patients with sCJD, with a positive predictive value of 95%.

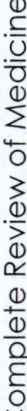

38. Ans. (b) Rolandic epilepsy

(Ref: Nelson 20th p 2828; Nelson, 18th ed., Ch. 593.2)

- Benign childhood epilepsy with centrotemporal spikes presents in children between 2-13 years.
- Seizures occur in sleep and focal seizures
- Self-limiting course by adolescence
- Inter-ictal EEG shows spike over centrotemporal or Rolandic area.

39. Ans. (b) Continue valproate with monitoring of drug level

(Ref: Harrison 20th p 3067; Harrison 19th p 2559)

- The patient is in second trimester of pregnancy.
- Organogenesis occurs in early pregnancy and damage may have already occurred.
- The fetus may already be having a NTD and hence there is no point in changing her treatment plan.
- If patient had presented when she was planning her pregnancy, the course of action would be to gradually reduce valproate dose and initiate lamotrigine.

40. Ans. (c) Petitmal epilepsy

(Ref: Harrison 20th p 3051; Harrison 19th p 2543)

41. Ans. (a) 3 Hz spike and wave

(Ref: Harrison 20th p 3051; Harrison 19th p 2543)

42. Ans. (c) Automatism

(Ref: Harrison 20th p 3051; Harrison 19th p 2543)

43. Ans. (a) SSPE

(Ref: Nelson 20th p 1545; Harrison 19th p 2543)

44. Ans. (c) Subtle

(Ref: Manual of Neonatal Care by Cloherty 6th/484)

45. Ans. (a) Valproate

(Ref: Harrison 20th p 3063; Harrison 19th p Table 445-8. 2552)

46. Ans. (a) Brain parenchyma

(Ref: Harrison 20th p 1015; Harrison 19th p 1431, Table 260-1)

Raised ICP

47. Ans. (a) E2 VT M3

(Ref: Harrison 20th edition and NCBI, page 3183)

Eye opening to pressure= 2 Intubated status= T Abnormal flexion/ Decorticate posturing= 3	Glasgow coma scale			
	Eye opening (E)		Verbal response (V)	
	Spontaneous	4	Oriented	5
	To speech	3	Confused	4
	To pressure	2	Words	3
	None	1		
	Best motor response (M)			
	Obeying commands	6		
	Localizing	5		
	Normal flexion	4		
	Abnormal flexion	3		
	Extension	2		
	None	1		

48. Ans. (b) Beta trace protein

(Ref: CSF in clinical neurology: 2ND edition, page 403)

- The image shows *halo sign/target sign* where a clear ring surrounds a central bloody spot after the bloody nasal discharge is dropped on a handkerchief or paper towel.
- *Beta trace protein* is found in CSF and is produced by the meninges and choroid plexus. It has a Prostaglandin D2 synthase activity and value is 1.5mg/L in ventricular CSF.
- Remember: Beta 2 micro-globulin levels are checked in urine for prognosis of patients of multiple myeloma.

49. Ans. (a) 9T

(Ref: Harrison 20th edition and NCBI Bookshelf, page 3183)

- Opening eyes on command = 3
- Moving limbs/obeying commands = 6
- Intubated = T
- The total score is 9T

The maximum score in intubated patient can be 10T and minimum as 2T.

Glasgow coma scale- P
The GCS-P is calculated by subtracting the Pupil Reactivity Score (PRS) from the glasgow come scale (GCS) total score:
- GCS-P = GCS-PRS

The pupil reactivity score is calculated as follows.
Pupils unreactive to light—Pupil reactivity score
- Both pupils-2
- One pupil-1
- Neither pupil-0

50. Ans. (c) 12

(Ref: Harrison 20th p 3183; Harrison: 19th ed., Table 457e-1:)

- Spontaneous eye opening is score of 4
- Patient can localize pain and hence is moving his arm away from painful stimulus is a score of 5.
- Inappropriate words are a score of 3.
- Hence the total score is 12.

TABLE: Glasgow coma scale for head injury

Eye opening (E)		Verbal Response (V)	
Spontaneous	4	Oriented	5
To loud voice	3	Confused, disoriented	4
To pain	2	Inappropriate words	3
Nil	1	Incomprehensible sounds	2
		Nil	1
Best Motor Response (M)			
Obey	6		
Localizes	5		
Withdraws (flexion)	4		
Abnormal flexion posturing	3		
Extension posturing	2		
Nil	1		

51. Ans. (c) Cortical vein thrombosis

(Ref: Harrison 20th p 3085; Harrison 19th edition, page 2566)

- The main risk factor for *cortical vein thrombosis* is a prothrombotic state like pregnancy and puerperium. Patients present with headache (gradual or thunderclap onset) with features of raised ICP. Patients may develop headache with/without focal deficits depending on the area involved.
- Cranial nerve palsies may occur. Magnetic resonance Venography is best imaging modality.
- Meningitis is ruled out due to absence of meningeal signs.
- Migraine is ruled out as it does not have raised ICP/papilledema.
- SAH presents with thunderclap headache with meningeal signs.

52. Ans. (c) 9

(Ref: Harrison 20th p 3183; Harrison 19th edition, page 457e-5)

- Opening eyes to pain is score of E2
- Moaning implies non comprehensible sounds and is a score of V2
- Localises pain is a score of M5
- Hence the total score of the patient is 9

53. Ans. (b) Positive Kernig Sign

(Ref: Harrison 20th p 999-1000; Harrison 19th edition, page 883 and 1779)

- Positive Kernig sign is a feature of meningeal irritation and not raised ICP.
- Ipsilateral hemiplegia occurs due to Kernohan Woltman sign seen in uncal herniation.
- The pupil of the same side of CNS bleed dilates and shows sluggish reaction to light. It is seen in uncal herniation and is called *Hutchinson's pupil*.
- Blurring of disc margins is an early finding in papilledema

54. Ans. (a) Hypertension

(Ref: Harrison 20th p 1000; Harrison 19th edition p 443e)

Neuroimaging should be done prior to LP in the following patients:

1. Altered level of consciousness
2. Focal neurological deficit
3. New onset seizure
4. Papilledema
5. Immunocompromised state

These patients are at increased risk of for potentially fatal cerebellar or tentorial herniation following lumbar puncture. Choices B, C and D satisfy the above mentioned requirements.

55. Ans. (c) Constricted pupil

(Ref: Harrison 20th p 2073; Harrison 19th edition, page 1735)

- In brain death, brain stem is dead but spinal cord is alive. Hence Deep Tendon reflexes are elicitable and Babinski sign can be seen bilaterally.
- Gag reflex is absent due to damage to medulla
- The *pupils are dilated and show no reaction to light due to damage to midbrain*.
- For diagnosis of brain death, sedative effect, hypothermia and neuromuscular paralysis must be ruled out.
- If in doubt the cerebral blood flow studies and EEG should be done.

56. Ans. (c) Respiratory arrest

(Ref: Harrison 20th p 2069; Harrison 19th edition, page 1772)

- Foraminal brain herniation leads to compression of medulla and respiratory arrest.
- Third nerve palsy causing ipsilateral pupillary dilatation and ipsilateral hemiplegia occurs in uncal (midbrain) herniation
- Locked in state occurs due to lesion of ventral pons.

57. Ans. (d) Administer sedative

(Ref: Harrison 20th p 2077; Harrison 19th edition, page 1780)

In patients with raised ICP: 20-25 mm Hg for > 5 minutes, the following *steps* are used for management of raised ICP-

1. Elevate head end
2. Drain CSF via ventriculostomy
3. Osmotherapy using mannitol
4. Glucocorticoids for vasogenic oedema (don't give in head injury and stroke)
5. **Sedation with morphine, propofol or midazolam and neuromuscular paralysis if necessary.**
6. Hyperventilation to maintain $PaCO_2$ 30-35 mm Hg. *SHORT TERM USE or skip the step*, due to limited efficacy.
7. Pressor therapy with phenylephrine, dopamine and norepinephrine to ensure CPP of >60 mm Hg.
8. Second tier therapy
   a. Decompressive craniectomy
   b. Pentobarbital coma
   c. Therapeutic Hypothermia to 33 degrees

This question is closely worded and is a typical AIIMS question.

Points against hyperventilation and keeping pCO$_2$=30-35mm Hg

1. In step wise management of Raised ICP as per Harrison, sedation is given before hyperventilation. Secondly hyperventilation is mentioned as a short term step or as skip the step.
2. In Bradley's textbook of neurology it is mentioned that elective hyperventilation does not cause reduction in CO$_2$.
3. In BTF 2016 guidelines "Hyperventilation should be avoided during the first 24 hours after injury when cerebral blood flow (CBF) is often critically reduced."

58. Ans. (b) 20-30 ml

(Ref: Harrison 19th edition, page 443 2e:)

In general 20-30 ml CSF can be safely removed from adults. It is used for cell counts with differential, CSF biochemistry, culture, smears, PCR, immune-electrophoresis, oligoclonal banding and cytology. CSF should be allowed to drip into collection tubes and never withdrawn with a syringe.

59. Ans. (b) 20-40 ml

(Ref: Meritt's neurology, page 359)

- For determining the efficacy of CSF shunting in NPH a tap test called Fisher test is done. *The best tolerated is a tap of 25-40ml through lumbar puncture with recording of opening and closing pressures.*
- Objective measurement is made by comparison of videotaped gait of the patient before and after the procedure. Gait usually improves several hours after the procedure with loss of benefit after few weeks.
- Other methods used are more invasive and might be refused by the patient. They are-
  1. Multiple LP over 3-5 days
  2. Insertion of continuous lumbar CSF drain
  3. Radionuclide Cisternogram

60. Ans. (a) Normal Pressure Hydrocephalus

(Ref: Harrison 20th p 3112; Harrison: 19th edition, page 2606-2607)

- The CT image shows dilated ventricles and favours the diagnosis of normal pressure hydrocephalus over Biswanger's disease.
- The presence of dementia, gait abnormalities and urinary incontinence favours diagnosis of normal pressure hydrocephalus.
- *Biswanger's disease* is associated with hypertension which is not present in this patient. It leads to development of vascular dementia. The concomitant white matter lesions lead to pyramidal signs. Parkinsonian rigidity can also be seen. CT shows bilateral leukoaraiosis (ischemic demyelination).
- *Dementia with lewy bodies* presents with visual hallucinations, REM sleep disorder and capgras syndrome. The lesion is mainly posterior parietal lobe atrophy. Gait abnormalities like in Parkinsonism are seen.

61. Ans. (a) Bilateral damage to rostral midbrain

(Ref: Harrison 20th p 2071; Harrison: 19th edition, page 1774)

Type of posturing	Lesion	Remarks
Decorticate	Bilateral damage to rostral midbrain	Flexion of elbows and wrists with supination of arms.
Decerebrate	Damage to motor tracts in the midbrain/ caudal diencephalon	Extension of elbows and wrists with pronation of arms.

The less frequent presentation of *arm extension with limb flexion* is seen in lesion in pons.

62. Ans. (b) Pontine damage

(Ref: Harrison 20th p 2072; Harrison 19th page 1775)

- Ocular bobbing is a brisk downward and slow upward movement of eyes associated with loss of horizontal eye movements.
- It indicates *bilateral pontine damage*. The cause is thrombosis of basiliar artery.
- In contrast ocular dipping is slower arrhythmic downward movement followed by faster upward movement in patients with normal reflex horizontal gaze. It *indicates diffuse cortical anoxic damage.*

63. Ans. (a) Diffuse cortical damage

(Ref: Harrison 20th p 2073; Harrison 19th page 1775)

- Alpha rhythm has discharge frequency of 8–13 Hz .On eye opening the pattern changes to beta rhythm.
- In pontine or diffuse cortical anoxia a special pattern of alpha coma is defined by widespread alpha rhythm that resembles the normal rhythm but does *not* alter on environmental stimuli.

64. Ans. (d) >9 mm

(Ref: Harrison 20th p 2070; Harrison: 19th edition, page 1772)

Drowsiness and stupor can occur with horizontal displacement of the diencephalon (Thalamus). The lateral shift can be quantified on a CT scan or MRI.
In case of acutely enlarging mass, horizontal displacement of pineal calcification is measured:
1. Displacement of 3-5 mm is associated with drowsiness.
2. Displacement of 6-8 mm is associated with stupor
3. Displacement > 9 mm is associated with coma

65. Ans. (d) Glucocorticoids

(Ref: Harrison 20th p 2077; Harrison: 19th edition, page 1780)

- Glucocorticoids are useful for management of vasogenic oedema from tumour or brain abscess.
- In contrast glucocorticoids are avoided in case of head trauma, ischemic and haemorrhagic stroke.
- Nor epinephrine or pressor therapy is used to maintain MAP to maintain CPP>60 mm Hg.
- Sedation is done with propofol or midazolam.
- Neuro-muscular paralysis will be necessary and patient will need ventilator support. This will ensure securing the airway and keeping pCO$_2$ between 30-35 mmHg.

66. Ans. (a) Transtentorial herniation

(Ref: Harrison 20th p 2069; Harrison 19th edition, page 1772)

The most common form of brain herniation is trans-tentorial herniation. The brain tissue is displaced from the supra-tentorial to the infra-tentorial compartment. This type of brain herniation is subdivided into-

1. Uncal trans-tentorial herniation: Impaction of medial temporal gyrus into tentorial opening just anterior to and adjacent to the midbrain. This results in ipsilateral third nerve palsy with ipsilateral hemiplegia which is called Kernohan Woltman sign.
2. Central trans-tentorial herniation: symmetric downward movement of thalamic structures through the tentorial opening with compression of midbrain. This results in miotic pupils and stupor.

Transfacial herniation occurs due to displacement of cingulate gyrus under the falx and across the midline. In contrast the downward forcing of cerebellar tonsils into foramen magnum is called *foraminal herniation*. This leads to compression of vital centres in the brain

67. Ans. (d) D

(Ref: Harrison 20th p 2069; Harrison 19th edition, page 1772)

- Pointer A: Uncal herniation
- Pointer B: Central herniation
- Pointer C: Transfacial herniation
- Pointer D: Foraminal herniation

68. Ans. (a) Only P, R, S are correct

(Ref: Bailey and Love, 26th edition, page 316)

The image shows presence of lenticular hyper-density in fronto-parietal area on left side. This is diagnostic of extradural bleeding. The artery involved in EDH is middle meningeal artery. Lucid interval which is consciousness between two periods of unconsciousness may not be seen in all cases. On side of the bleed the pressure on same oculomotor nerve will lead to ipsilateral mid dilated pupil. This is known as Hutchinson pupil. Choice B is false as presentation several weeks later after trivial head injury is seen in chronic subdural haemorrhage.

69. Ans. (c) Proptosis

(Ref: Harrison 20th p 186; Harrison 19th edition, page 203)

- Patients with Benign Intracranial Hypertension /Idiopathic intracranial hypertension (IIH) usually present with symptoms related to increased intracranial pressure (ICP) and papilledema,
- Symptoms include headache, transient visual obscurations, and diplopia due to unilateral or bilateral abducens nerve palsy.
- Hence choice B and D are ruled out

Diagnostic pointers to presence of pseudotumour cerebri/ idiopathic intracranial hypertension (by international society for headache)
1. *High rate of occurrence in obese women during the childbearing years.*
2. *Reduced conductance to CSF outflow.*
3. *Normal ventricular size; no hydrocephalus*
4. *No histologic evidence of cerebral edema*

Clinical features of pseudotumour cerebri
1. Elevated intracranial pressure (VIth CN palsy may be seen as a false localizing sign of raised intracranial tension)
2. Normal or Small sized Ventricular system^Q
3. No focal neurological signs^Q
4. Papilledema (enlarged blind spot in visual fluid)
5. Normal CSF findings^Q
6. Normal CT scan, MRI and isotope Scan
7. Excessive slow-wave activity on ECG

70. Ans. (c) 15 and 3

(Ref: Harrison 20th p 3183; Harrison 19th edition, page 260)

Glasgow Coma Scale

Eye opening (E)		Verbal response (V)	
Spontaneous	4	Oriented	5
To speech	3	Confused	4
To pressure	2	Words	3
None	1	Sounds	2
		None	1
Best motor response (M)			
Obeying commands	6		
Localizing	5		
Normal flexion	4		
Abnormal flexion	3		
Extension	2		
None	1		

Note: Revised GCS (2014)

Glasgow Coma Scale Update

- The GCS score is derived by assigning notation to the level in each of the three subcomponents of the GCS and summing the results of a patient's assessment. Further information on the GCS score can be accessed here. The **Pupil Reactivity Score** summarises information about of pupil reactivity to light and is calculated as follows:

Pupils unreactive light	Pupil reactivity score
Both pupils	2
One pupil	1
Neither pupil	0

The GCS-P is calculated by subtracting the pupil reactivity score (PRS) from the Glasgow Coma Scale

GCS-P = GCS-PRS

Minimum score 3, Max score 15

Intubation indicated when score less than 8

71. Ans. (b) Ventriculo peritoneal shunt

(Ref: Nelson 20th p 1296; Nelson 19th edition, page 2008-2011)

The preferred type of shunt is ventriculo-peritoneal shunt which has a one way valve that can regulate intra-cranial pressure and allows drainage of CSF to peritoneal cavity.

72. Ans. (d) Absence seizure

(Ref: Harrison 19th edition, page 2550)

- The history of repeated blanking out accompanied by subtle, motor activity like quivering of lips is diagnostic of presence of absence seizures.

Characteristics of Absence Seizures:
1. Sudden, brief lapses of consciousness without loss of postural control.
2. *Typically lasts for only seconds, consciousness returns as suddenly as it was lost, and there is no postictal confusion.*
3. Usually *accompanied by subtle, bilateral motor signs* such as rapid blinking of the eyelids, chewing movements, or small-amplitude, clonic movements of the hands.
4. As the clinical signs of the seizures are subtle, especially to parents, the first clue to absence epilepsy is often unexplained "daydreaming" and a decline in school performance recognized by a teacher.
5. The electro-physiologic hallmark of typical absence seizures is a generalized, symmetric, 3-Hz spike-and-wave discharge that begins and ends suddenly, superimposed on a normal EEG background and can be precipitated by hyperventilation and photic stimulation.

73. Ans. (c) Pupil size

(Ref: Harrison 19th edition, page 457 e-5)

Glasgow coma scale includes Eye opening, verbal response and motor activity.

74. Ans. (a) Trans-tentorial herniation

(Ref: Harrison 19th edition, page 1772)

Trans-tentorial herniation	Most common type of brain herniation
Uncal herniation	It refers to impaction of the anterior medial temporal gyrus (the uncus) into the tentorial opening just anterior to and adjacent to the midbrain
Cerebellar tonsil herniation/ foraminal herniation	Pressure on the posterior fossa contents from above or from within compresses the pons against the clivus and displaces the cerebellar tonsils into the foramen magnum. This causes compression of the medulla, respiratory arrest, and death
Cingulate herniation/ transfalcial herniation	Displacement of the cingulate gyrus under the falx and across the midline

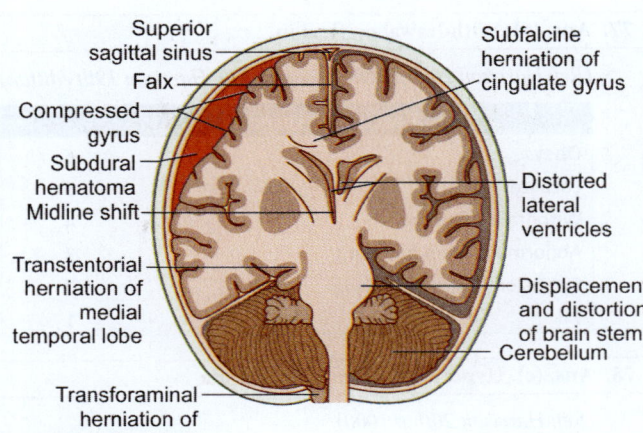

75. Ans. (b) Idiopathic intracranial hypertension

(Ref: Harrison 20th p 186; Harrison 19th edition, page no 202, 203)

Craniopharyngioma	Presents in children and adults after 55 years with features of raised ICT and visual field defects like bitemporal hemianopia
Idiopathic intracranial hypertension	Occurs in obese women and presents with headache and sixth nerve palsy
Optic neuritis	It is an acute inflammatory condition of the optic nerve. It cause painful eye movements and visual loss. Fundus looks normal due to retro-bulbar pathology
Sagittal sinus thrombosis	Occurs in setting of risk factors like OCP, pregnancy, post-partum period, Polycythemia and APLAS. Presents with headache vomiting, seizures and neurological deficits like paraparesis

76. Ans. (a) Increase on coughing/sneezing; (e) Analgesics are not very helpful

(Ref: Harrison 19th/110; Emergency Medicine by SN Chugh 4th/235-38)

Pulsatile/ throbbing nature of headache is seen with migraine and shows response to migraine.

Diagnostic criteria for headache due to raised ICP
- Diffuse non-pulsating headache with at least one of the following characteristics and fulfilling criteria mentioned below
  - Associated with nausea and/or vomiting
  - Worsened by physical activity and/or manoeuvres known to increase intracranial pressure (such as Valsalva manoeuvre, coughing or sneezing)
  - Occurring in attack-like episodes
  - Criteria
1. Space-occupying intracranial tumour demonstrated by CT or MRI and causing hydrocephalus
2. Headache develops and/or deteriorates in close temporal relation to the hydrocephalus
3. Headache improves within 7 days after surgical removal or volume-reduction of tumour

77. Ans. (a) Withdrawal on flexion

(Ref: Harrison 20th p 3183; Chapter 370: Harrison 19th edition)

Best motor response (M)	
Obeys	6
Localizes	5
Withdraws (flexion)	4
Abnormal flexion posturing	3
Extension flexion posturing	2
Nil	1

78. Ans. (c) Hypertension and bradycardia

(Ref: Harrison 20th p 1000)

- Cushing's reflex = a hypothalamic response to brain ischemia wherein the sympathetic nervous system is activated which causes increased peripheral vascular resistance with a subsequent increase in BP.
- The increased BP then activates the parasympathetic nervous system via carotid artery baroreceptors, resulting in vagal-induced bradycardia.
- The brain ischemia that leads to cushings reflex is usually due to the poor perfusion that results from increased ICP due to head bleeds or mass lesions.
- Cushing's reflex leads to the clinical manifestation of Cushing's triad.
- *Cushing's triad = hypertension, bradycardia, and irregular respirations (Cheyne-Stokes breathing).*
- *Cushing's triad signals impending danger of brain herniation*, and thus, the need for decompression. Consider administering mannitol, hyperventilation, and elevation of the head of bed as temporizing measures

79. Ans. (a) Sub-dural hematoma

(Ref: Harrison 20th p 3184; Harrison 19th edition, page 1772, 442e)

Sub dural hematoma	Concavo-convex bleed hyper-density
Extra dural hemorrhage	Biconvex /flame shaped hyper-density
Sub arachnoid hemorrhage	Intra-ventricular bleed/blood in slyvian fissure
Intra –parenchymal bleed	Mostly a lesion or hyper-density in basal ganglia secondary to hypertension.

80. Ans. (a) Hyperdense biconvex

(Ref: Harrison 20th p 3184)

- Extradural hemorrhage: Bleeding occurs between skull and duramatter. Bleeding occurs due to the rupture of Middle meningeal artery. Lucid Interval (Consciousness between two periods of unconsciousness) exists.
- **NCCT head shows hyperdensity which is bi-convex or flame shaped.**
- Subdural hemorrhage: Occurs due to rupture of Cortical bridging veins. *In NCCT it shows concavo-convex or sickle shaped bleed.*

81. Ans. (a) Uncal herniation

(Ref: Harrison 20th p 2069; Harrison 19th ed. / 1772)

- In uncal or mid brain herniation, the raised ICT compresses the same side third cranial nerve while it originates from Edinger -Westphal nucleus. This causes ptosis, diplopia and divergent squint. The reason for unconsciousness can be damage to reticular activating system in the midbrain.

82. Ans. (c) Enlargement of lateral and third ventricle

(Ref: Harrison 19th ed. / 174)

- Aqueduct of slyvius connects the third ventricle to the fourth one. Therefore the obstruction to this area will not only cause enlargement of third ventricle but will also dilate the lateral ventricles proximal to the obstruction.

83. Ans. (d) ICSOL

(Ref: Harrison 19th edition, page 457e-5)

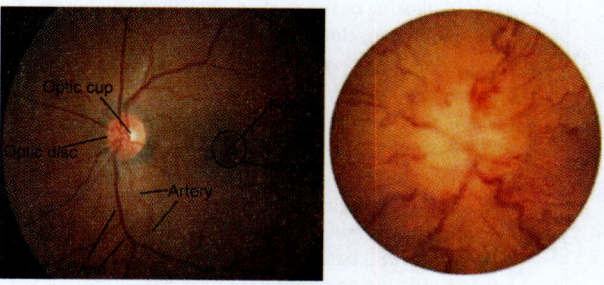

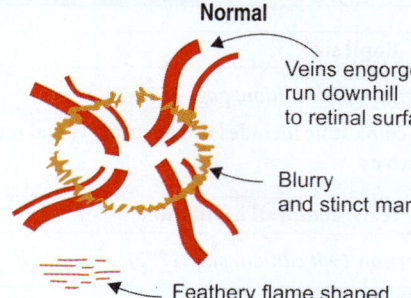

Papilledema: With blurring of margins of optic disc

84. Ans. (d) Posturing

(Ref: Greenburg Handbook of Neurosurgery, chapter 27, 7th edition, page 868)

- When CSF pressure and the pressure within the intra-cranial cerebral arteries start to equilibrate, the cerebral arteries become compressed and begin to collapse. This compromises cerebral blood flow. Cushing's reflex is activated, and the arterial pressure rises to a level higher than the CSF pressure, allowing cerebral blood flow to be reestablished and ischemia to relieved. The blood pressure is maintained at a new, higher level, and the brain is protected from further loss of adequate blood flow. Cushing's reflex causes the symptoms of Cushing's triad.

- The triad refers to three signs caused by Cushing's reflex:
  1. Bradycardia
  2. Hypertension (with widened pulse pressure)
  3. Bradypnea (often irregular)

It is indicative of an advanced increase in intracranial pressure, that is, the brain's "last gasp." The triad and the reflex are late findings, and irreversible neurologic damage may have already occurred by the time they are recognized.

85. Ans. (d) Reduction in GCS

(Ref: Harrison 20th p 2078; Harrison 19th p 1779)

Increased ICT leads to bradycardia with Hypertension. Uncal herniation of brain leads to ipsilateral pupillary dilatation. Reduction in GCS due to damage to reticular activating system leads to development of coma.

The proper functioning of R.A.S system, its ascending projections to the cortex, and the cortex itself are required to maintain alertness and coherence of thought. It follows that the principal causes of coma are:
1. Lesions that damage the RAS in the upper midbrain or its projections
2. Destruction of large portions of both cerebral hemispheres
3. Suppression of reticulo-cerebral function by drugs, toxins, or metabolic derangements such as hypoglycemia, anoxia, uraemia, and hepatic failure.

- Pupillary enlargement with loss of light reaction and loss of vertical and adduction movements of the eyes suggests that the lesion is in the upper brainstem.
- Conversely, preservation of pupillary light reactivity and of eye movements absolves the upper brainstem and indicates that widespread structural lesions or metabolic suppression of the cerebral hemispheres is responsible for coma.

86. Ans. (d) Loss of deep tendon reflexes

(Ref: Harrison 20th p 2073; Harrison 19th p 1775, 1776)

Brain death criteria include three essential elements:
1. Widespread cortical destruction that is reflected by deep coma and unresponsiveness to all forms of stimulation
2. Global brainstem damage demonstrated by absent pupillary light reaction and by the loss of oculovestibular and corneal reflexes
3. Destruction of the medulla, manifested by complete apnea. Apnea testing can be done safely by the use of diffusion oxygenation prior to removing the ventilator. This is accomplished by pre-oxygenation with 100% oxygen, which is then sustained during the test by oxygen administered through a tracheal cannula, CO_2 tension increases 0.3–0.4 kPa/min (2–3 mmHg/min) during apnea. At the end of a period of observation, typically several minutes, arterial pCO_2 should be at least >6.6–8.0 kPa (50–60 mmHg) for the test to be valid. Apnea is confirmed if no respiratory effort has been observed in the presence of a sufficiently elevated Pco_2

Loss of deep tendon reflexes is not required because the spinal cord remains functional.

87. Ans. (c) Seen with chronic myeloid leukemia

(Ref: OP. Ghai, 583, 7th ed, Ghai 8th 602-603)

- Lymphoblasts can cross the blood brain barrier. Acute lymphoblastic leukemia is associated with CNS leukemia.
- However, the control of central nervous system (CNS) leukemia remains a therapeutic challenge in childhood ALL, partly because of the late complications arising from cranial irradiation. In most current pediatric protocols, cranial irradiation (12 to 18 Gy) is given to 5% to 25% of patients—those with T-cell ALL, overt CNS disease (CNS3 status) or high-risk cytogenetics.
- Normally blasts are never seen in CSF and presence of a single blast in CSF is suggestive of CNS involvement.

88. Ans. (b) Fixed non-reactive pupil

(Ref: Harrison 20th p 2073; Harrison 19th p 1776)

- Enlarged and poorly reactive pupil signifies compression or stretching of the third nerve from the effects of a cerebral mass above.
- The most extreme pupillary sign, bilaterally dilated and unreactive pupils, indicates severe midbrain damage, usually from compression by a supratentorial mass.
- Reactive and round pupils of midsize (2.5-5mm) essentially exclude midbrain lesion.

Doll's eye reflex	Oculocephalic reflexes, are elicited by moving the head from side to side or vertically and observing eye movements in the direction opposite to head movement, depend on the integrity of the ocular motor nuclei and their interconnecting tracts that extend from the midbrain to the pons and medulla. The movements, somewhat inappropriately called 'doll's eyes', are normally suppressed in the awake patient. Absence of oculocephalic reflex is called as doll eye reflex present and indicates cerebral dysfunction
Horner pupil	The patient who has Horner's syndrome has a weak dilator muscle in one iris (due to reduced sympathetic activity) and, as a result, that pupil dilates more slowly than the normal pupil. If the sympathetic lesion is complete, the affected pupil dilates only by sphincter relaxation. The resultant asymmetry of pupil dilatation produces an anisocoria that is largest 4-5 seconds after the lights have been turned out-the process is much slower than is generally thought.
Positive vestibulo-cochlear reflexes	Thermal or caloric stimulation of the vestibular apparatus (oculo-vestibular response) is performed by irrigating the external auditory canal with cool water in order to induce convection currents in the labyrinths. After a brief latency, the result is tonic deviation of both eyes to the side of the cool water irrigation and nystagmus in the opposite direction. The loss of induced conjugate ocular movements indicates brainstem damage.

89. Ans. (a) Obese women in the age group 20-40 yrs

(Ref: Harrison 20th p 186; Harrison 19th p 203)

Pseudo tumor cerebri (Benign Intracranial hyper-tension). The majority of patients are young, female, and obese. It is a diagnosis of exclusion and diagnosis is made after Neuroimaging to rule out intracranial lesions.

Investigations
1. Fundus- Papilledema +
2. MR angiogram in selected cases to search dural venous sinus occlusion or AV shunt.
3. If neuroimaging is negative, subarachnoid opening pressure to be measured with LP.
4. An elevated pressure with normal CSF indicates Pseudo tumor cerebri (Idiopathic intracranial hypertension)

Risk Factors
Obesity
Obese women under the age of 44 are nearly 20 times more likely to develop the disorder.

Medications Causing Pseudotumour Cerebri
- Growth hormone
- Tetracycline- especially outdated ones
- Discontinuation of steroids
- Excess vitamin A
- Oral contraceptives

Treatment
1. Temporary relief by letting out 20-30 ml CSF by LP- (Diagnostic and therapeutic)
2. Acetozolamide- reduce CSF production
3. Weight reduction
4. Shunt - In case of failure to above measures and progressive visual loss
5. Emergency surgery- in case of sudden blindness by fulminant papilledema.

---

90. Ans. (c) Gastric ulcer and bleed

(Ref: Harrison 20th p 273; Harrison 19th p 1778, 1918)

- Patient has a history of GI bleed in the form of melena (likely precipitated by aspirin induced gastric ulcer). Hypotension and tachycardia support this diagnosis.
- CVA is associated with Bradycardia and hypertension on account of raised ICT and thereby to maintain the brain perfusion cushing's reflex comes into force.
- There is no setting for septic shock in the clinical profile mentioned.
- The closest choice to be ruled out is MI with cardiogenic shock but the history of fainting is only given with no mention of chest pain or ECG findings in the question.

91. Ans. (c) M4

(Ref: Harrison 20th p 3183; Harrison 19th p 1777)

Glasgow Coma Scale

Eye opening (E)		Verbal response (V)	
Spontaneous	4	Oriented	5
To speech	3	Confused	4
To pressure	2	Words	3
None	1	Sounds	2
		None	1

Eye opening (E)		Verbal response (V)	
Best motor response (M)			
Obeying commands	6		
Localizing	5		
Normal flexion	4		
Abnormal flexion	3		
Extension	2		
None	1		

Note: Revised GCS (2014)

Glasgow Coma Scale Update

- The GCS score is derived by assigning notation to the level in each of the three subcomponents of the GCS and summing the results of a patient's assessment. Further information on the GCS score can be accessed here. The **Pupil Reactivity Score** summarises information about of pupil reactivity to light and is calculated as follows:

Pupils unreactive light	Pupil reactivity score
Both pupils	2
One pupil	1
Neither pupil	0

The GCS-P is calculated by subtracting the pupil reactivity score (PRS) from the Glasgow Coma Scale
$$GCS\text{-}P = GCS\text{-}PRS$$

92. Ans. (c) 50-70 mm Hg

(Ref: Harrison 20th p 3094)

- After brain injury, and especially in the multiply injured patient, cerebral blood flow may be lowered to the ischaemic threshold.
- To prevent further neuronal death (the secondary brain injury), this flow of well oxygenated blood must be restored. Optimum level of CPP, is atleast 50-70 mm Hg.
- Mortality increases approximately 20% for each 10 mm Hg loss of CPP. In those studies where CPP is maintained above 70 mm Hg, the reduction in mortality is as much as 35% for those with severe head injury.

93. Ans. (a) Acetazolamide

(Ref: Walsh and Hoyt Clinical Neuro-ophthalmology Pg. 285-86)

- Acetazolamide appears to be the most effective agent for lowering ICP in idiopathic intracranial hypertension. Most patients experience adequate relief of symptoms (typically, headache) with this first-line agent
- In the event of intolerance to acetazolamide, furosemide may be used as a replacement diuretic in this group.
- Patients with I.I.H may experience headaches that have many of the features of migraine. These headaches can often be controlled with amitriptyline, propranolol, or other commonly prescribed migraine prophylaxis agents

- Patients experiencing a progressive loss of visual field in one or both of the eyes should immediately be placed on high-dose (60-100 mg/day) oral prednisone (or an equivalent corticosteroid regimen).
- Despite close follow-up care and maximum medical treatment, some patients experience deterioration of their visual function. In this situation, surgical intervention may be considered.
  1. Optic nerve sheath fenestration (decompression)
  2. Cerebrospinal fluid (CSF) diversion (i.e., via a lumboperitoneal or ventriculoperitoneal shunt)

94. Ans. (a) Uncal herniation

(Ref: Harrison 20th p 2069; Harrison 19th p 1772)

Uncal herniation	Ipsilateral 3rd nerve palsy with ipsilateral hemiplegia
Cingulate herniation	The innermost part of the frontal lobe is scraped under part of the falx cerebri
Millard Gubler syndrome	Ipsilateral 6,7th nerve palsy with contralateral hemiplegia
Weber syndrome	Ipsilateral 3rd nerve palsy with contralateral hemiplegia

Uncal Herniation Manifestations
1. Subtype of trans-tentorial herniation, the innermost part of the temporal lobe, the uncus, can be squeezed so much that it moves towards the tentorium and puts pressure on the midbrain.
2. The uncus can *squeeze the third cranial nerve*, which may affect the parasympathetic input to the eye on the side of the affected nerve, causing the pupil of the affected eye to dilate and fail to constrict in response to light as it should.
3. Pupillary dilation often precedes the somatic motor effects of cranial nerve III compression. The symptoms occur in this order because the parasympathetic fibers surround the motor fibers of CNIII and are hence compressed first.
4. False localizing sign, the so-called Kernohan's notch, which results from compression of the ipsilateral cerebral crus containing descending cortico-spinal and some corticobulbar tract fibers. This leads to ipsilateral hemiparesis (as these tracts are above their decussation where they are compressed
5. Distortion of the brainstem leading to Duret hemorrhages in the median and paramedian zones of the mesencephalon and pons.
6. The disrupted brainstem can lead to decorticate posture, respiratory center depression and death. Other possibilities resulting from brain stem distortion include lethargy, slow heart rate, and pupil dilation.
7. Compression of the ipsilateral posterior cerebral artery will result in ischemia of the ipsilateral primary visual cortex and contralateral visual field deficits in both eyes (contralateral homonymous hemianopsia).

95. Ans. (b) PCM toxicity

(Ref: Walsh and Hoyt Clinical Neuro-ophthalmology Pg. 280)

In pediatric age group vitamin A toxicity can present with pseudotumour cerebri. Steroids are used in management of this condition but sudden stoppage. will lead to these patients developing worsening of features.

Most cases of IIH occur in young women who are obese; a considerably smaller percentage occurs in men who are otherwise healthy. Patients with higher body mass indexes (BMIs) and recent weight gain are at increased risk.

96. Ans. (a) 5 mm Hg

(Ref: Nelson Table 602.1, 18th edition)

Normal ICP is 50-80 mm water and converted into mm Hg is 3.6 to 5.8 mm Hg. Hence the Ans: < 5 mm Hg.

If the question is asked regarding cerebral perfusion pressure for children it should be 45 mmHg, while it should be atleast 70mm Hg in adults.

97. Ans. (d) Withdrawl reflex

(Ref: Harrison 20th p 2069; Harrison 19th p 1772)

- In uncal herniation there is kinking of ipsilateral III rd nerve leading to ipsilateral mid-dilated pupils
- The uncal herniation compresses the opposite crus cerebri against the skull. This results in a finding of ipsilateral hemiplegia contrary to expectation of contralateral hemiplegia. This is known as Kernohan's Woltman sign.
- Raised ICT leads to Cheyne Stokes breathing
- Decerebrate rigidity is extensor posturing seen due to lesions rostral to midbrain herniation and is usually seen with Pontine stroke.

98. Ans. (d) Brain herniation

(Ref: Handbook of Neurosurgery, Greenberg, Pg: 653)

ICP Waveforms
- A waves or plateau waves—These comprise a steep rise in ICP from near normal values to 50 mm Hg or more, persisting for 5–20 minutes and then falling sharply. These waves are always pathological and indicate greatly reduced compliance. They are frequently accompanied by neurological deterioration and indicate early brain herniation.
- B waves—These rhythmic oscillations occur every 1–2 minutes. ICP rises in a crescendo manner to levels 20–30 mm Hg higher than baseline and then falls abruptly. These waves were originally always associated with Cheyne-Stokes respiration. However, they also occur in ventilated patients and are probably related to changes in cerebrovascular tone and cerebral blood volume. B waves are also indicative of failing intracranial compensation and indicate cerebral vasospasm.
- C waves—These oscillations occur with a frequency of 4–8 per minute and are of smaller amplitude than B waves. They are synchronous with spontaneous Traub-Hering-Meyer type variations in blood pressure and are probably of limited pathological significance.

99. Ans. (b) If no localizing signs, hole in left temporal (dominant lobe)

(Ref: Greenfield handbook of neurosurgery, chapter 27, page 864-65)

INDICATIONS in E/R for BURR HOLE
Clinical criteria based on deteriorating neurologic exam.
1. Patient dying of rapid trans-tentorial herniation
2. Brainstem compression that does not improve or stabilize with mannitol and hyperventilation.
   - Indicators of transtentorial herniation/brainstem compression:
     1. Sudden drop in Glasgow Coma Scale (GCS) score
     2. One pupil fixes and dilates
     3. Paralysis or decerebration (usually contralateral to blown pupil)
   - Recommended situations where criteria should be applied:
     1. Neurologically stable patient undergoes witnessed deterioration as described above
     2. Awake patient undergoes same process in transport, and changes are well documented by competent medical or paramedical personnel

Choice of Side for initial Burr Hole
Start with a temporal burr hole on the side:
1. Ipsilateral to a blown pupil. This will be on the correct side in > 85% of epidurals and other extra-axial mass lesions.
2. If both pupils are dilated, use the side of the first dilating pupil (if known)
3. If pupils are equal, or it is not known which side dilated first, place on side of obvious external trauma
4. *If no localizing clues, place hole on left side (to evaluate and decompress the dominant hemisphere)*

100. Ans. (c) Hydrocephalus ex-vacuo

(Ref: OP. Ghai, 549, 8th ed)

- Hydrocephalus ex vacuo also refers to an enlargement of cerebral ventricles and subarachnoid spaces, and is usually due to brain atrophy (as it occurs in dementias), post-traumatic brain injuries
- As opposed to hydrocephalus, this is a compensatory enlargement of the CSF-spaces in response to brain parenchyma loss - it is not the result of increased CSF pressure

101. Ans. (d) Osmotic properties takes 3 hours to develop

(Ref : Goodman gilman 12th ed., pg 748)

- Mannitol, a 6-carbon sugar and an osmotic diuretic and can have significant beneficial effects on ICP, cerebral blood flow and brain metabolism.
- *Mannitol has two main mechanisms of action. Immediately after bolus administration it expands circulating volume, decreases blood viscosity and therefore increases cerebral blood flow and cerebral oxygen delivery.*
- *Its osmotic properties take effect in 15-30 minutes when it sets up an osmotic gradient and draws water out of neurons.*
- *However after prolonged administration (continuous infusion), mannitol molecules move across into the cerebral interstitial space and may exacerbate cerebral oedema and raise ICP.*
- Mannitol itself directly contributes to this breakdown of the blood brain barrier.
- Mannitol is therefore best used by bolus administration where an acute reduction in ICP is necessary. For example the patient with signs of impending herniation (unilateral dilated pupil / extensor posturing) or with an expanding mass lesion may benfit from mannitol to acutely reduce ICP during the time necessary for CT scanning and/or operation.
- Mannitol is wholly excreted in the urine and causes a rise in serum and urine osmolality. Patients with poor renal perfusion (shock), sepsis, receiving nephrotoxic drugs or with a serum osmolality over 320mOsm are at risk of acute tubular necrosis. Hypovolemia should be avoided with the infusion of isotonic fluids as necessary.

102. Ans. (c) Cardiac arrest

(Ref: Harrison 20th p 2063; Harrison 19th p 1781)

- *Inducing mild therapeutic hypothermia in selected patients surviving out-of-hospital sudden cardiac arrest can significantly improve rates of long-term neurologically intact survival and may prove to be one of the most important clinical advancements in the science of resuscitation.*
- Patients who have been shown to benefit from induced hypothermia include the following:
- Intubated patients with treatment initiated within 6 hours after cardiac arrest (nonperfusing ventricular tachycardia [VT] or VF)
- Patients able to maintain a systolic blood pressure >90 mm Hg, with or without pressors, after CPR.
- The types of medical events that hypothermic therapies may effectively treat fall into four primary categories
  1. Cardiac arrest- validated by clinical studies
  2. Ischemic stroke- Harrison's and internet data mention clinical trial on animals only
  3. Traumatic brain or spinal cord injury without fever –validated by clinical studies
  4. Neurogenic fever following brain trauma- validated by clinical studies

103. Ans. (a) Brain

(Ref: 'Handbook of Clinical Neurology' by Young/85; 'Fundamentals of Diagnostic Radiology' by Brant & Helms 3rd/73)

104. Ans. (c) Gait disorder, urinary incontinence & dementia

(Ref: Harrison 20th p 3112; Harrison 19th p 2606-07)

105. Ans. (b) Increased protein in CSF

(Ref: Harrison 20th p 186; Harrison 19th p 203)

106. Ans. (c) 11

(Ref: Harrison 20th p 3186)

107. Ans. a > c. Hyperglycemia > Hypocapnia

(Ref: Harrison 19th p 1780)

108. Ans. (d) Left chronic subdural haematoma

(Ref: Harrison 20th p 3184)

109. Ans. (c) Altered mental status

(Ref: Harrison 20th p 2078; Harrison 19th p 457e-1)

Headache

110. Ans. (b) NSAIDs are first line drugs

(Ref: Adam and Victor, 10th edition, page 188)
- NSAIDS like acetaminophen and ibuprofen can be used in migraine. (Risk Category B)
- 60-70% of migraineurs improve spontaneously during pregnancy, usually in the third or fourth month.
- Ergotamines are contraindicated (risk category X), and triptans are not recommended (risk category C; risk cannot be ruled out).

Status of currently used drugs in migraine during pregnancy and breast feeding

Generic name	Level of risk in pregnancy	Breastfeeding
Acetaminophen	B	Caution
Dihydroergotamine	×	Contraindicated
Ergotamine	×	Contraindicated
5-HT1 agonists	C	Probably compatible
Aspirin	C (D in 3rd trimester)	Compatible
Caffeine	B	Compatible
Ibuprofen	B (D in 3rd trimester)	Compatible
Naproxen	B (D in 3rd trimester)	Compatible
Codeine	C (D at term or prolonged use)	Compatible

111. Ans. (d) Pulsating unilateral headache worsened with movements of head

(Ref: Harrison 20th p 3096; Harrison 19th edition, page 2590)
- Choice A is description of Giant cell arteritis
- Choice B is description of Cluster headache
- Choice C is description of ophthalmoplegic migraine

Simplified Diagnostic Criteria for Migraine

Repeated attacks of headache lasting 4-72 h in patients with a normal physical examination, no other reasonable cause for the headache, and:	
At least 2 of the following features:	Plus at least 1 of the following features:
Unilateral pain	Nausea/vomiting
Throbbing pain	Photophobia and phonophobia
Aggravation by movement	
Moderate or severe intensity	

112. Ans. (c) Migraine

(Ref: Harrison 20th p 3096; Harrison 19th p 2586)

Migraine	Dazzling and enlarging visual phenomenon and obstruction of vision occurs in scintillating scotoma. They are transient in nature and are associated with recurrent episodes of headache which makes this as the answer to the question.
Acute angle closure glaucoma	Will present with retro-orbital pain with nausea and vomiting. The eye will have ciliary congestion with shallow anterior chamber of eye. Corneal haze will be present with vertical oval dilated pupil. Hence it is ruled out.
Retinal detachment	Will cause blindness and hence is ruled out
Intumescent cataract	Cataract will cause visual blurring for whole day whereas in the question visual blurring is given for few minutes. Intumescent cataract will then lead to pupillary block and development of angle closure glaucoma that will called as phacomorphic glaucoma. Hence it is ruled out.

113. Ans. (a) Acute cerebellar hemorrhage

(Ref: Harrison 20th p 3154-55; Harrison 19th page 2579, 1785, 1179)

Acute cerebellar hemorrhage	Symptoms develop over few hours - Gait ataxia - Occipital headache - Repeated headache and vomiting Dizziness and vertigo - Gaze paresis and ipsilateral sixth nerve palsies - Down beating nystagmus - Dysarthria Dysphagia followed by stupor and coma due to obstructive hydrocephalus due to fourth ventricular compression - Nuchal pain
Subarachnoid hemorrhage	- Sudden onset of severe headache loss of hematoma and external neck stiffness and vomiting. - Anterior communicating artery of M.C.A bifurcation aneurysms cause hemiparesis, aphasia and abulia - Posterior communicating artery aneurysm cause retro-orbital pain 3rd cranial nerve palsy papillary dilation loss of light reflex. - Occipital pain indicate P.I.C.A or A.I.C.A aneurysm
Transient ischemic attack	- TIA is a transient focal neurological deficit which recovers within 24 hours. - Leads to development of Amaurosis fugax which is a transient monocular blindness due to emboli to central retinal artery due to carotid stenosis.
Herpes simplex encephalitis	Presents with Fever, Headache, psychiatric symptoms, seizures and focal weakness.

114. Ans. (d) Analgesic abuse headache

(Ref: Harrison 20th p 87, 3103; Harrison 19th edition, page 109)

Analgesic abuse headache	Points in favour of diagnosis are : • Presence of headaches which are refractory to analgesic and occurs daily • Headaches are accompanied by asthenia, nausea and other gastrointestinal symptoms, restlessness, anxiety, irritability, memory problems, and difficulty in intellectual concentration and depression • Evidence of tolerance to analgesics over time, with patients needing progressively larger doses and use for > 15 days per months • The slightest physical or intellectual effort may bring on headache. In these patients threshold for head pain appears to be low
Migraine	More common in women, presents with pulsating throbbing kind of headache with photophobia and responds to medication.
Depression associated headache	It is close choice but clinically speaking we should first rule out analgesic abuse headache by seeing response of the patient to withdrawal of NSAIDS.
Cluster headache	Presents with retro-orbital pain with epiphora and red eye.

115. Ans. (d) Sinusitis

(Ref: Harrison 20th p 85)

Primary Headache		Secondary Headache	
Type	%	Type	%
Tension –Type	69	Systemic infection	63
Migraine	16	Head injury	4
Idiopathic stabbing	2	Vascular disorders	1
Extertional	1	Subarachnoid hemorrhage	<1
Cluster	0.1	Brain tumor	0.1

116. Ans. (a) Giant cell arteritis

(Ref: Harrison 20th p 86)

	Giant cell arteritis	Meningeal metastasis
Symptoms	The headache of GCA has no pathognomonic features, but typically—and most importantly—**the headache is either new, in a patient without a history of headaches, or of a new type, in a patient with a history of chronic headache.** The headache is usually localized to the temporal or occipital area	• The symptoms are protean and can include the following: ▪ Headaches (usually associated with nausea, vomiting, lightheadedness) ▪ Gait difficulties from weakness or ataxia ▪ Memory problems ▪ Incontinence ▪ Sensory abnormalities There is a predilection for sites with slow CSF flow and gravity dependent areas allowing tumour cells to seed. Median survival in untreated cases is 4 to 6 weeks
Investigations	The laboratory hallmark of giant cell arteritis (GCA) is an elevation in the erythrocyte sedimentation rate (ESR) and C-reactive protein (CRP) level. The ESR usually exceeds 50 mm/h and may exceed 100 mm/h	• The diagnosis is made with positive CSF cytologic results (the most useful test), or identified on radiologic studies,

117. Ans. (d) Ergot alkaloids in last one week

(Ref: Harrison 19th p 2591; CMDT 2019 p 991)

- Sumatriptan causes vasoconstriction of blood vessels and this Vasoconstriction of Basiliar artery and its branches will worsen the cranial nerve deficits seen in these patients like diplopia, vertigo, difficulty in swallowing
- The vasoconstriction is the reason it will create trouble in patients with I.H.D
- It is categorized at pregnancy category C drug.

118. Ans. (b) Temporal arteritis

(Ref: Harrison 19th p 2188)

- Giant cell arteritis has a presentation at 72 years of age and accounts for 15% of all cases of fever of unknown origin in patients over the age of 65 yrs.
- Headache is the most common chief complaint and presents in over two thirds of patients with temporal arteritis. The *headache tends to be new or different in character than previous headaches and is typically sudden in onset, localizing to the temporal region.*
- However, pain with temporal arteritis can occur diffusely through the occipital, frontal, or parietal regions as well. Therefore, any new headache in patients older than 50 years warrants a consideration of temporal arteritis.
- Based on the 1990 American College of Rheumatology criteria for classification of temporal arteritis, at least 3 of the following 5 items must be present.

> 1. Age of onset older than 50 years
> 2. New-onset headache or localized head pain
> 3. Temporal artery tenderness to palpation or reduced pulsation
> 4. Erythrocyte sedimentation rate (ESR) greater than 50 mm/h
> 5. Abnormal arterial biopsy (necrotizing vasculitis with granulomatous proliferation and infiltration)

- Migraine is common in young females and presents with pulsating headache with photophobia, phono-phobia, nausea and vomiting and is ruled out
- Fibromyalgia presents as musculo-skeltal pain in women and is ruled out.

Read On For Why Answer Is Not Chronic Tension Headache:
In elderly patients, the practicing physician should never assume that headache onset is due to benign causes, such as tension-type head-aches, until pathologic etiologies are explored. Pain onset in tension-type headache can have a throbbing quality and is usually more gradual than onset in

Contd...

migraines. Compared with migraines, tension-type headaches are more variable in duration, more constant in quality, and less severe. IHS diagnostic criteria for tension-type head-aches states that 2 of the following characteristics must be present

1. Pressing or tightening (non-pulsatile quality)
2. Frontal-occipital location
3. Bilateral - Mild/moderate intensity
4. Not aggravated by physical activity

New headache onset in elderly patients should suggest etiologies other than tension headache.

119. Ans. (a)   Affects predominantly females

(Ref: CMDT 2019 pg 992-93; Harrison 19th p 2595)

120. Ans. (a)   Migraine

(Ref: CMDT 2019 pg 990; Harrison 19th p 2590)

121. Ans. (a)   Migraine

(Ref: CMDT 2019 pg 990; Harrison 19th p 2590)

122. Ans. (b)   Glaucoma

(Ref: Harrison 20th p 183; Harrison 19th p 205)

The clinching point in the question is a vertically dilated pupil with poor reaction to light pointing to diagnosis of glaucoma.

123. Ans. (d)   Sumatriptan

(Ref: CMDT 2019 pg 991; Harrison 19th p 2591)

Neurocutaneous Disorders

124. Ans. (a)   Acoustic neuroma

(Ref: Harrison 20th p 649; Harrison 19th edition, page 2331)

- Bilateral acoustic neuromas are the most distinctive feature of NF-2.
- Optic glioma is the most common CNS tumour seen in NF-1.
- 6 more C.A.L.M of size>5mm in pre-pubertal and >15mm in post-pubertal age group is hallmark feature of NF-1.
- Cortical thinning of bones with or without pseudoarthrosis is seen in NF-1
- Scoliosis happens to be most common orthopaedic manifestation of NF-1 though it is not specific enough to be included as diagnostic criterion.

125. Ans. (a)   Neurofibromatosis 1

(Ref: Harrison 20th p 649; Harrison: 19th edition, page 603)

- Schwannoma is a benign tumour arising from the Schwann cells of cranial and spinal nerve roots.

- The most common schwannoma is *vestibular schwannoma* or *acoustic neuroma* and arises from the vestibular portion of the eighth cranial nerve.
- Patients with neurofibromatosis type 2 have a high incidence of vestibular schwannomas that are frequently bilateral.
- *Neurofibromatosis type 1 is associated with an increased incidence of schwannomas of the spinal nerve roots.*

126. Ans. (a)   Von Recklinghausen's disease

(Ref: O.P Ghai 8th edition, page 586)

Von Reck-linghausen disease	Also called NF-1 or peripheral neurofibromatosis Deletion on chromosome 17 Diagnosis is made if 2 or more out of 6: 1. Café au lait spots 2. Two or more neurofibroma 3. Axillary freckling 4. Optic glioma 5. >2 Lisch nodules/ sphenoid bone dysplasia 6. First degree relative with NF1
Louis bar syndrome	1. Alternative name for Ataxia telangiectasia 2. Caused by breaks on chromosome 11q producing failure of DNA repair. 3. Autosomal recessive 4. Child 2-7 years with Ataxia, ocular apraxia with loss of proprioception. 5. Conjunctival telangiectasia 6. Recurrent pulmonary infections(low IgA)
Tuberous Sclerosis	Child with hypopigmented macules, adenoma sebaceum and seizures.
Von Hippel Landau syndrome	Child with nystagmus ataxia and raised ICT Cerebellar and retinal hemangioblastoma Spinal cord angiomas Cystic tumors of pancreas, kidneys and epididymis.

127. Ans. (d)   Hemangioma

(Ref: OP Ghai, 8th edition, page 586)

- The clinical diagnosis is *Sturge Weber syndrome*.
- Choice A is correct as due to presence of glaucoma, cupping of optic disc can be seen.
- Choice B is correct due to presence of intracranial calcification, which on X-Ray skull produces a tram-track appearance
- Choice C is correct as refractory focal seizures in the patient will require a vagal nerve stimulation to control recurrent seizures.
- Differential diagnosis of Sturge Weber syndrome:
  - Klippel-Trenaunay-Weber syndrome consists of port-wine stains of the extremities and face, as well as hemi-hypertrophy of soft and bony tissues.
  - Beckwith-Wiedemann syndrome consists of a facial port-wine stain (PWS), macroglossia, omphalocele, and visceral hyperplasia. Severe hypoglycemia resulting from pancreatic islet-cell hyperplasia may be life threatening.

128. Ans. (d)   Ependymoma

(Ref: Swaiman text book of pediatric neurology page no: 504, Harrison 20th p 649; Harrison 19th p 604)

> **Major features of TSC include the following:**
> - Facial angiofibromas or forehead plaque
> - Non-traumatic Ungual or periungual fibroma
> - Hypomelanotic macules (>3)
> - Shagreen patch
> - Multiple retinal nodular hamartoma
> - Cortical tuber
> - *Subependymal nodule*
> - *Subependymal giant cell astrocytoma*
> - Cardiac rhabdomyoma, single or multiple
> - Lymphangioleiomyomatosis
> - Renal angiomyolipomas
>
> **Minor features of TSC include the following:**
> - Multiple randomly distributed pits in dental enamel
> - Hamartomatous rectal polyps
> - Bone cysts
> - *Cerebral white matter radial migration lines*
> - Gingival fibromas
> - Retinal achromic patch
> - "Confetti" skin lesions
> - Multiple renal cysts

The following are the diagnostic criteria for TSC:
- Definite TSC - Two major features or one major feature plus two or more minor features
- Possible TSC - Either one major feature or two or more minor features

129. Ans. (a) Multiple tumors are uncommon

(Ref: Harrison 20th p 2155, 2745)

VHL is characterized by a predisposition to *bilateral and multi-centric* retinal angiomas, central nervous system (CNS) hemangioblastomas; renal cell carcinomas; pheochromocytomas; islet cell tumors of the pancreas; endolymphatic sac tumors; and renal, pancreatic, and epididymal cysts.

CNS hemangioblastoma is the most commonly recognized manifestation of VHL and occurs in 40% of patients.

Option B: Hemangiopericytomas are seen in the craniospinal axis
- Intracranial hemangiopericytomas are neoplasms of the pericytes that originate in the meninges.
- **An association with von Hippel Lindau disease is noted in 10% of patients.**
- The location of intracranial hemangiopericytomas is similar to that of meningiomas. Histologically, hemangiopericytomas are highly cellular, vascular tumors composed of angular pericytes surrounding often ill-defined capillaries in a branching pattern (staghorn vascularity).
- **Imaging of the cranio-spinal axis documents these lesions in patients with von Hippel Lindau disease.**

Option C: Supratentorial lesions are seen
- The vast majority of CNS tumours associated with the Von Hippel Lindau syndrome are cerebellar hemangioblastomas, which are mainly infratentorial.
- However, some Supratentorial lesions may also be seen in this condition.

Option D: Tumors of Schwann cells are common
- **Schwannoma near the sciatic nerve was identified in association with von Hippel Lindau syndrome.**

130. Ans. (a) Tuberous sclerosis

(Ref: Harrison 20th p 649; Nelson ch. 596.2, Harrison 19th p 604)

Tuberous sclerosis	Presents with Seizures and renal angiomylipomas which can bleed leading to the perinephric hematoma formation as mentioned in the question
Von Hippel Landau	Autosomal dominant. The most common tumours found in VHL are central nervous system and retinal hemangioblastomas, clear cell renal carcinomas, pheochromocytomas, pancreatic neuroendocrine tumours, pancreatic cysts, endolymphatic sac tumors and epididymal papillary cystadenomas. It results from a mutation in the von Hippel–Lindau tumor suppressor gene on chromosome 3p.
Familial angiolipomatosis	It's an important a differential diagnosis of Neurofibromatosis 1. The patients have seizures and lesion on skin which contain fat but may be wrongly ascribed to neurofibromas
Autosomal dominant polycystic kidney	Presents at 30-45 yrs of age with HTN, hematuria and bilaterally enlarged kidneys showing multiple large cysts. CNS manifestation is berry aneurysm and hence is ruled out.

More Details About Tuberous Sclerosis from Radiological Perspective

1. Angiomyolipomas are usually well-marginated, cortical heterogeneous tumors with predominantly fatty attenuation. The average attenuation depends on the relative proportions of fat and other soft tissue in the angiomyolipoma. **Attenuations of less than −20 Hounsfield units (HU) are widely accepted as confirming the presence of fat; this finding virtually confirms the diagnosis of angiomyolipoma.**
2. The most common neurological manifestations of Tuberous Sclerosis consist of seizures, cognitive impairment, and behavioral abnormalities including autism. The characteristic brain lesion is a cortical tuber. Tubers are located in the convolutions of the cerebral hemispheres and are also present in the subependymal region, where they undergo calcification and project into the ventricular cavity, producing a candle-dripping appearance.
3. TS may present during infancy with infantile spasms and a hypsarrhythmic EEG pattern.
4. Histopathology of angiomyolipoma
   - No true capsule
   - Commonly bleed
   - Tumor composed of fat, smooth muscle, aggregates of thick-walled blood vessels

131. Ans. (c) Schwannoma

(Ref: ch. 596.2 Nelson Textbook of Pediatrics, Harrison 19th p 604; Harrison 20th p 649)

Skin manifestations of tuberous sclerosis
1. More than 90% of cases show the typical hypomelanotic macules that have been likened to an ash leaf on the trunk and extremities. Visualization of the hypo-melanotic

macule is enhanced by the use of a Wood ultraviolet lamp, particularly in the infant. At least three hypo-melanotic macules must be present.

2. Sebaceous adenomas develop between 4 and 6 yrs of age; they appear as tiny red nodules over the nose and cheeks and are sometimes confused with acne. Later, they enlarge, coalesce, and assume a fleshy appearance.
3. A shagreen patch is also characteristic of TS and consists of a roughened, raised lesion with an orange-peel consistency located primarily in the lumbosacral region.
4. Subungual or periungual fibromas arise from the stratum lucidum of the finger and toe in many patients with TS during adolescence.

132. Ans. (c) Tuberous sclerosis

(Ref: Harrison 20th p 649; O.P. Ghai 7th Ed., Pg. No. 564, Harrison 19th p 604)

Tuberous Sclerosis Complex
- It inherited as an autosomal dominant trait. The presenting features vary with age.
- Cardinal features are skin lesions, convulsion and mental retardation. Early skin lesions are hypo-pigmented, ash-leaf shaped macules, red or pink papules (Angio-fibromas) called adenoma sebaceum on face.
- These appear and also enlarge with age. Other lesions are Shagreen patches, Subungual fibromas and oral fibromas.
- Retinal hamartoma may be present.
- In early life tumors in heart and kidneys may be detected on ultrasonography. In infancy, myoclonic jerks often lead to detection of this entity and are an important cause of West syndrome. Vigabatrine is a useful medication in these cases.

Incontinentia Pigmenti
- It's an X-linked dominant disorder IP is inherited in an X-linked dominant manner.
- Affected women have a 50% risk of transmitting the mutant IKBKG allele at conception; however, most affected male conceptuses miscarry.
- Skin lesions in IP evolve through characteristic stages:
  1. Blistering (from birth to about four months of age),
  2. Wart-like rash
  3. Swirling macular hyperpigmentation (from about six months of age into adulthood)
  4. Linear hypopigmentation
  5. Alopecia, hypodontia, abnormal tooth shape, and dystrophic nails.
  6. Some patients have retinal vascular abnormalities predisposing to retinal detachment in early childhood. Cognitive delays/mental retardation are occasionally seen.
  7. Discolored skin is caused by excessive deposits of melanin (normal skin pigment).
  8. Most newborns with IP will develop discolored skin within the first two weeks. The pigmentation involves the trunk and extremities, is slate-grey, blue or brown, and is distributed in irregular marbled or wavy lines. The discoloration sometimes fades with age.
  9. Neurological problems can include: cerebral atrophy, the formation of small cavities in the central white matter of the brain, and the loss of neurons in the cerebellar cortex.

133. Ans. (b) Tuberous sclerosis

(Ref: ch. 596.2 Nelson 18th edition, Harrison 20th p 649; Harrison 19th p 604)

This question tests your radiology as well as medicine skills. You should know that typical values in Hounsfield units are for different elements and tissues range from -1000 to more than +1000, air versus bone. Of importance is that fat is -100, muscle and blood around +40.

NOW WHY IS THE LESION MENTIONED IN THE QUESTION NOT A CYST?

Fluid filled spaces, for example cysts, could contain something close to water or have an attenuation corresponding to blood – which is positive 35-40 Hounsfield units.

Substance	HU
Air	-1000
Lung	-700
Fat	-84
Water	0
CSF	15
Blood	+30 to +45
Muscle	+40
Soft Tissue	+100 to +300
Cancellous Bone	+700
Dense Bone	+3000

Now let us evaluate the choices provided individually

ARPKD	• Mental retardation or seizures is not seen. • As mentioned above the cysts have positive hounsfield units where as in the question the units are negative which are indicative of fat / angiomylipoma. • Hence ARPKD is ruled out on basis of 2 points mentioned above • Patients in ARPKD present prenatally with massively enlarged kidneys and oligohydramnios. In infants, Potter facies with low-set, flattened ears; short, snubbed nose; deep eye creases; and micrognathia, all secondary to oligohydramnios, can be found.
Tuberous sclerosis	• Seizures or mental retardation is present dependant on number of tubers or subependymal nodules seen in these patients. • AMLs are benign mesenchymal tumors, composed of blood vessels, smooth muscle, and mature adipose tissue, that arise primarily in the kidneys.
VHL	• The primary cause of morbidity and mortality in von Hippel-Lindau disease, as well as the most serious sequela of the condition, involves the malignant degeneration of renal cysts. Renal cysts are seldom clinically significant; however, in von Hippel-Lindau disease they have an appreciable rate of malignant transformation. • Consequently, renal cell carcinoma is the leading cause of death in patients with von Hippel-Lindau disease. • LIVER INVOLVEMENT IN VHL IS HEMANGIOMA WHICH HAS POSITIVE HOUNSFIELD UNITS. • The kidneys are affected in three-quarters of patients, and half these patients develop clear cell carcinomas in the renal cysts. It is noteworthy that VHL mutations also account for 60% of spontaneous clear cell carcinomas of the kidney.

Contd...

Paraganglioma	• Paraganglioma is a rare neuroendocrine neoplasm that may develop at various body sites (including the head, neck, thorax and abdomen) • About 97% are benign and cured by surgical removal; the remaining 3% are malignant because they are able to produce distant metastases. "Paraganglioma" is now the most-widely accepted term for these lesions, that have been also described as: glomus tumor, chemodectoma, perithelioma, fibroangioma, and sympathetic nevi

134. Ans. (b) Tuberous Sclerosis

(Ref: Nelson 18th/2483, 2484, Harrison 20th p 649; Harrison 19th p 604)

135. Ans. (d) Sturge Weber Syndrome

(Ref: Nelson 20th p 2879)

Stroke and SAH

136. Ans. (b) Check blood glucose

Ref: Harrison 20th page 2072

- Choice C is ruled out since no features of raised ICP are given.
- Choice D is ruled out since BP lowering is done in case of CNS events if the BP> 185/110 mm Hg. Moreover, CT is required for diagnosis of a CNS event. At lower BP values reducing BP would be counterproductive and can lower Brain perfusion.
- Now we have to choose between the two choices CT scan and blood glucose.
- As per the algorithm of management of an unconscious patient, blood sugar levels should be checked first.
- In any unconscious patient of diabetes mellitus, status of blood sugar should be assessed immediately as hypoglycemia/hyperglycemia would change the line of management.
- Once these two possibilities are ruled out then CT head is to be performed to rule out a CNS event.
- Page 2072: 20th edition of Harrison quotes "the studies most useful in diagnosis of coma are chemical- toxicologic analysis of blood and urine followed by Cranial CT/MRI, EEG and CSF examination".

137. Ans. (b) B

Ref: Harrison 20th edition, page 3070

- The patient is having motor aphasia due to damage to Broca's area. Since he can understand commands/comprehension, Wernicke's area is normal.
- The markings in the question are as follows:

A = Contraversive eye center
B = Broca's area
C = Wernicke's area
D = Occipital cortex

138. Ans. (a) Start thrombolysis

Ref: Harrison 20th edition, page 3081, 3087

The patient has presented with features of right sided cortical stroke leading to focal deficits on the left side.
How to Interpret the normal CT head given in the question?

- Haemorrhagic stroke is ruled out
- Most importantly *CT scan showing no haemorrhage or oedema > 1/3 of MCA territory is an indication for thrombolysis* (Table 420-1 20th edition Harrison)

- In this scenario, the patient is treated as a case of ischemic stroke and managed with thrombolysis. The cut off for management of Thrombolysis is >4.5hours from symptom onset.
- The closest choice is choice B which is used for management of Transient ischemia attack. As per the definition of TIA symptoms resolve within 24 hours and most cases within one hour (Page 3087). TIA usually resolves before presenting to the physician.
- Choice C , BP should not be lowered in CNS events as it mantains brain perfusion. Only if BP is > 185/110 mm Hg that lowering of BP should be done before initiating thrombolysis.

139. Ans. (c) Apraxia (Constructional)

Ref: Neuroanatomical basis of clinical neurology, page 125

The image shows paracentral lobule which is a U-shaped convolution that loops below the medial part of the central sulcus on the medial side of the cortex and lies posterior to superior frontal gyrus and superior to cingulate gyrus.

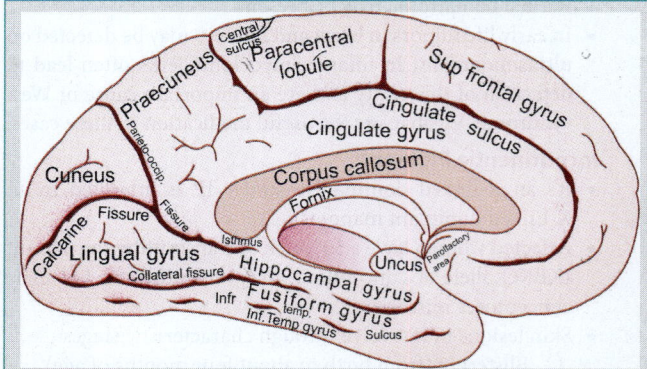

It is supplied by anterior cerebral artery. The control of leg, perineal and pelvic muscle floor lies in this area. Damage to this area leads to
- Spastic paralysis of contralateral leg
- Bowel incontinence (inability to control pelvic floor muscles)
- Urinary incontinence (inability to control pelvic floor muscles)
- Loss of perineal sensation

Apraxia is a disorder characterised by the inability to execute learned voluntary functions without any detectable motor, sensory or comprehen *sion deficits*. Kinetic apraxia is loss of ability to perform voluntary skilled movements in one extremity due to lesion of contralateral motor cortex (Broadman area 4).

140. Ans. (c) Posterior cerebral artery

Ref: Harrison 20th edition, page 3072

- The clinical information of headache followed by hemiparesis indicates development of stroke. Right pupillary dilatation and ptosis indicates the involvement of oculomotor nerve. Oculomotor nerve originates from the

141. Ans. (d) Splenium

Choice A: MCA territory stroke will lead to cortical stroke without any cranial nerve palsy
Choice B: ACA territory stroke will lead to abulia and bilateral pyramidal signs and paraparesis/quadriparesis.
Choice D: Basilar Artery stroke will lead to pontine stroke with cerebellar dysfunction.

midbrain and is supplied by posterior cerebral artery P1 segment.

Ref: Bradley neurology E-Book: 7th edition, page 138 and Harrison 20th edition, page 160

Alexia without agraphia (or pure alexia) means that the patient is unable to read, despite preservation of other aspects of language such as spelling and writing. It occurs due to lesions in left occipital cortex and posterior sector of corpus callosum known as splenium. It occurs due to interruption of visual input into language network. The blood vessel involved is posterior cerebral artery.

142. Ans. (b) Ischemic stroke

Ref: Bradley Neurology E-book:7th edition, page 1691

Thunderclap headache is a severe headache that peaks within 60 seconds of onset, and its causes are:

- Subarachnoid hemorrhage
- Intracranial hypotension
- Raised intracranial pressure
- Reversible cerebral vasoconstriction syndrome
- Cervical artery dissection, cerebral venous thrombosis
- Migraine
- Cluster headache
- Pituitary apoplexy

143. Ans. (a) Dorsal Mid brain lesion

(Ref: Harrison 20th p 3073; Harrison 19th edition, page 208 and 210)

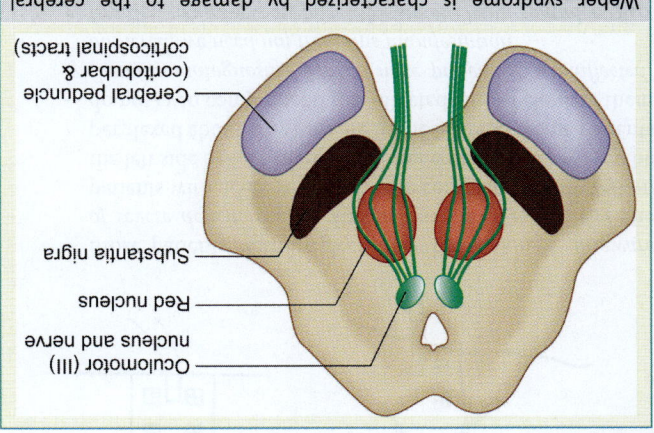

Weber syndrome is characterized by damage to the cerebral peduncle. This leads to damage to corticospinal pathway (purple) and oculomotor nerve (green). Hence the patient will develop ipsilateral third nerve palsy and contralateral hemiplegia. The blood vessel compromised is perforating branch of posterior cerebral artery.

Dorsal midbrain syndrome is Parinaud syndrome/ Supra-nuclear vertical gaze disorder caused by damage to posterior commissure.

1. Loss of up-gaze
2. Sun setting sign
3. Convergence retraction nystagmus
4. Lid retraction
5. Skew deviation
6. Pseudo-abducens palsy
7. Light near dissociation of pupils

144. Ans. (a) NCCT

(Ref: Harrison 20th p 2084; Harrison 19th edition, page 1785)

- The major complaint of SAH is severe headache associated with exertion. The patient often calls the headache as worst headache of his life. It is a generalized headache and associated with nuchal rigidity.
- The first investigation to evaluate this CNS bleed is NCCT Head.

ExTRA FILE

- Least common cause of primary headache is cluster headache.
- Least common cause of secondary headache is brain tumor.
- Most common secondary cause of new persistent daily headache is subarachnoid hemorrhage.

145. Ans. (d) Decompressive surgery

Ref: Schwartz 10th edition, page 1727-28 and Ultimate review for neurology boards, 3rd edition, page 147

NCCT scan shows a large hypo-density occupying more than 50% of MCA territory (marked red). It is also causing a significant midline shift (notice the obliterated lateral horn, color yellow).

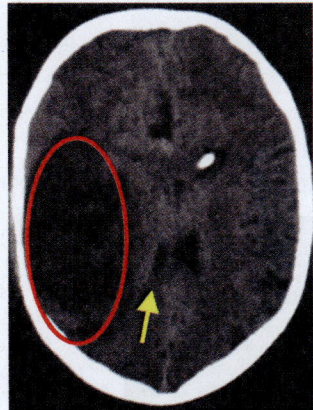

- Most ischemic infarcts evolve over a couple of days and lead to significant cerebral edema. This is also known as malignant cerebral edema due to large size infarction. It also explains the development of coma in this patient.
- The patient would require a decompressive craniectomy for definitive management. While the surgical measures are being planned, anti-edema measures should be instituted.

146. Ans. (a) Intracranial pseudoaneurysm

Ref: Harrison 19th edition, 440e

The image shows an outpouching at terminal intracranial part of internal carotid artery.

Hence the answer is A. Pseudo-aneurysm is a breach in vessel wall such that the blood leaks through the wall but is contained by adventitia or surrounding perivascular soft tissue.

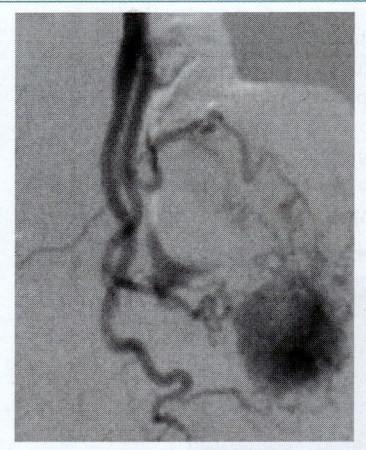

Vein of Galen malformation is an arteriovenous fistula resulting in dilatation of median prosencephalic vein which is the embryonic precursor to vein of Galen. The increased flow through MPV leads to neonatal presentation of non-cardiac CCF

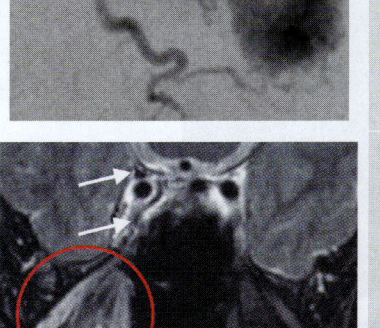

Carticocavernous fistula shows evidence of cavernous sinus thrombosis which is orbital proptosis, enlarged extraocular muscles (red) and enlarged draining veins especially superior ophthalmic veins.

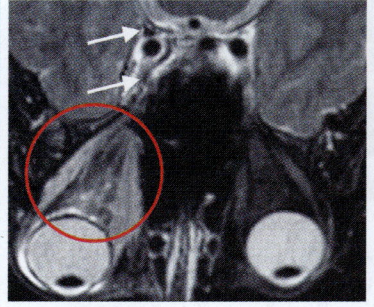

Angiofibroma tumor blush

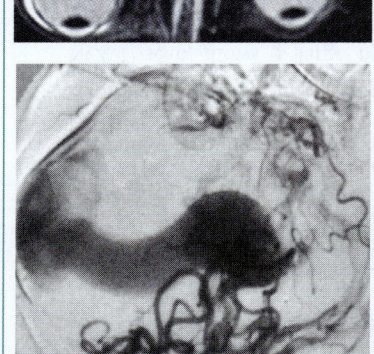
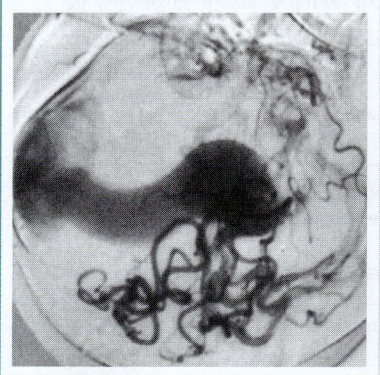

- Dual antiplatelet therapy will not manage the current episode and has role in prophylaxis.
- Mechanical thrombectomy is *not* an answer because it should be done within 8 hours of ischemic stroke symptoms (P: 2562: Harrison 19th edition). In the given question the patient presented on the second day of symptom onset.
- Endovascular Mechanical Thrombectomy is done for:
  1. Contraindications to Ischemic Stroke
  2. Failure to achieve vascular recanalization with iv thrombolysis

147. Ans. (d) 4.5 hours

Ref: Harrison 20th p 3081; Harrison 19th edition, page 2562

- Thrombolysis for AIS is ideally performed in a 3 hour window period. However due to favourable results now the usage has been extended upto 4.5 hours from onset of symptoms of stroke.
- Time of stroke onset is defined as time when the patient's symptoms were witnessed to begin or time when the patient was last seen as normal.

Indications for thrombolysis for acute ischemic stroke

Indication

- Clinical diagnosis of stroke
- Onset of symptoms to time of drug administration <4.5h
- CT scan showing no hemorrhage or edema of >1/3 of the MCA territory
- Age 18 > years
- Consent by patient or surrogate

148. Ans. (c) Neglect

Ref: Harrison 20th p 3070; Harrison 19th edition, page 2573

- Hemi-neglect or spatial agnosia implies blockage of inferior division of MCA and is seen more common in non-dominant parietal lobe lesion. Most patients will not be able to copy left side of the image. See the pic

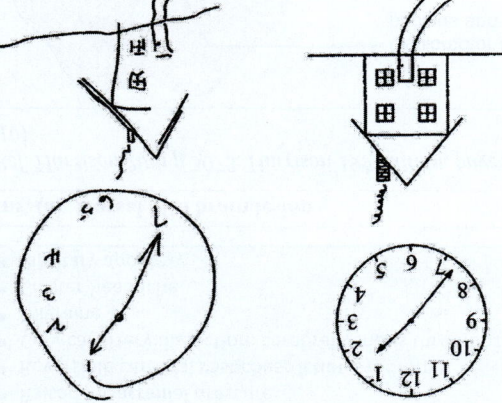

- Most patients with neglect may be strikingly *unaware of severe deficits* on the affected side. For example, some patients with acute stroke who are completely paralyzed on the left side believe there is nothing wrong and may even be perplexed about why they are in the hospital. Some patients do not even comprehend that affected limbs belong to them (hemiasomatognosia). Hence since patient is not affected/bothered, we need not treat this manifestation.
- Bradley neurology on page 399 states "hemi-spatial neglect can improve spontaneously over 3 weeks".
- *Fever* is always detrimental and contributes to worsening of neurological features. Stroke patients with fever are more likely to die in the next 10 days than those with normal body temperature.
- *Spasticity* causes disability and pain. The psychosocial impact of both necessitates treatment with Baclofen or Tizanidine.

- If not managed *dysphagia* will lead to aspiration and is a big time management issue in stroke patients.

149. Ans. (b) Left pons

(Ref: Harrison 20th p 190; Harrison 19th edition, page 209)

- The patient is having weakness in left side of face, and arm and leg weakness on right side. This is called *crossed hemiplegia* and is characteristically seen with pontine stroke.
- The damage to same side 6th and 7th cranial nerve can explain facial weakness and diplopia on looking to left.
- The corticospinal tract damage in pons will leads to contralateral spastic weakness in arms and legs.

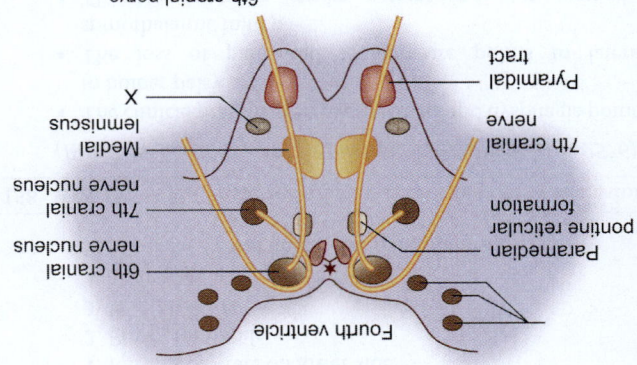

150. Ans. (c) Initiate sodium nitroprusside to achieve MAP below 130 mmHg

(Ref: CMDT 2019 Page 480, Table 11.13; CMDT 2018 Table 11-12)

- The patient is having CNS bleed due to cocaine overdose. The dilated right side pupil indicates evidence of uncal herniation.
- Sodium nitroprusside is not recommended to manage hypertensive crisis in CNS event. The current guidelines recommend use of nicardipine or labetalol.
- Mannitol or 3% saline can be used to lower raised ICP.
- NM paralysis is useful to reduce ICP. Airway compromise is always present in GCS less than 8. Hence NM paralysis and intubation is to be done.

Condition	First line drug	Drugs to avoid
Ischemic stroke (Systolic blood pressure > 180-200 mm Hg)	Nicardipine Clevidipine Labetalol	Nitroprusside, methyldopa, clonidine, nitroglycerin
Intracerebral haemorrhage (Systolic blood pressure > 140-160 mm Hg)	Nicardipine Clevidipine Labetalol	Nitroprusside, methyldopa, clonidine, nitroglycerin

151. Ans. (d) Ventro-posterolateral nucleus

(Ref: Harrison 20th p 3072; Harrison 19th edition, page 2575 and De Jong Neurological examination, page 554)

- The clinical presentation is of thalamic pain syndrome which can follow a lacunar infarct.

Contd...

- The pain is persistent on contralateral side of nucleus in facio brachio crural distribution. Also present is hemi-anesthesia, hemi-ataxia, choreoathetosis. It is also called Dejerine Roussy syndrome.
- The lesion in thalamus is in ventropostrolateral nucleus and adjacent white matter

152. Ans. (b) Bubble contrast Echocardiography

(Ref: Harrison 20th p 3083; Harrison 19th edition, page 2564)

Paradoxical embolism is a condition where a clot from venous return enters into left atrium and left ventricle. Here forth it can travel to brain leading to cryptogenic stroke.
These patients have a patent foramen ovale which allows transit of clot(s) in this fashion. For diagnosis, bubble contrast echocardiography is performed.

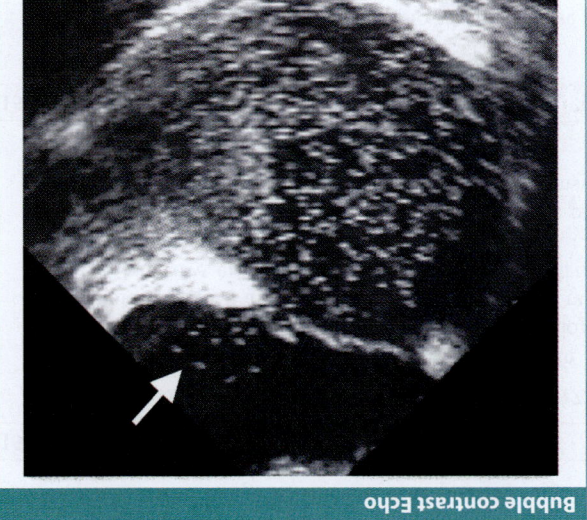

Bubble contrast Echo

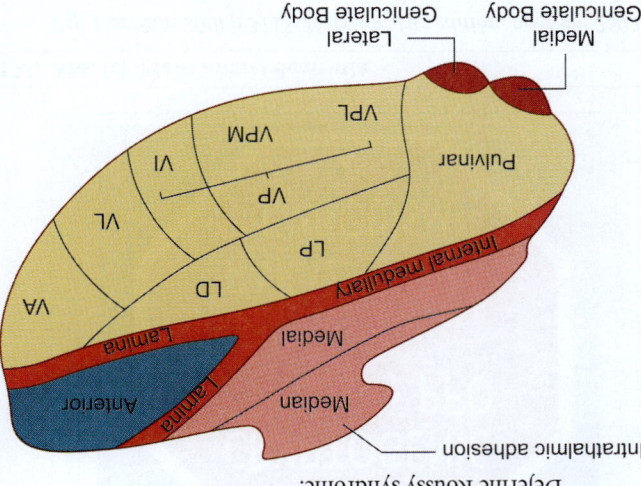

Intrathalamic adhesion

Lateral nuclei — LD - Lateral Dorsal nucleus
LP - Lateral Posterior nucleus
Medial nuclei
Anterior nuclei — VA - Ventral Anterior nucleus
VL - Ventral Lateral nucleus
VP - Ventral Posterior nucleus
VI - Ventral Intermediate nucleus
VPM - Ventral Posteromedial
VPL - Ventral Posterolateral

153. Ans. (c) Multi infarct dementia

Ref: Harrison 20th p 3118, Harrison 19th edition, page no: 2602

- Chronic alcoholism leads to development of dilated cardiomyopathy and atrial fibrillation. The emboli from heart can lead to multi small infarcts in brain. This leads to development of multi- infarct dementia.
- Binswanger's disease is seen in patients with long standing hypertension and atherosclerosis. It is associated with diffuse subcortical white matter damage.
- Vitamin B_{12} deficiency in setting of alcoholism will lead to development of myelopathy involving dorsal column. The dementia seen is subcortical.

154. Ans. (b) Vertical gaze

Ref: Harrison 20th p 2069, Harrison 19th edition, page no: 1771

- Locked in state is seen due to damage to ventral pons secondary to basilar artery damage.
- Bilateral Corticospinal damage leads Quadriplegia
- Bilateral Corticobulbar damage to 3rd, 4th, 6th and 7th nerves leads to loss of horizontal gaze, facial diplegia.
- Bilateral Corticobulbar damage to 9,10,12th nerves leads to aphonia and tongue paralysis
- Brain stem damage leads to loss of respiratory function.

155. Ans. (c) Intravenous Reteplase

Ref: Harrison 20th p 3081, Harrison 19th ed., page no: 1771

- The NCCT head shows large hypo-density in MCA distribution on left side diagnostic of acute ischemic stroke.
- Choice A and B are not required as BP is not in range of Hypertensive crisis. Lowering this BP Value will reduce cerebral perfusion and worsen the patient.
- Mannitol is given when features of raised ICP are present. Since the question is asking best step the answer is thrombolysis with Reteplase.

156. Ans. (d) Rivaroxaban

(Ref: Harrison 20th p 3080; Harrison 19th ed p 2585)

Atherothrombotic stroke occurs due to atherosclerotic plaque in intracerebral circulation. Hence aspirin and statins are recommended with strict BP control.

157. Ans. (b) Opium poisoning

(Ref: Harrison 20th p 3092, 3285; Harrison 19th edition, page 468e-3, 2593)

- The key word in the question is pin point pupils which narrows the choices to A and B. Pontine haemorrhage has pin point pupils but is associated with hyperthermia and is ruled out.
- Sepsis will have tachycardia and tachypnea. Metabolic encephalopathy will have pupils showing poor reaction to light.
- Clinical Pointers in the question for diagnosis of opioid Poisoning are:
  1. Respiratory rate on lower side
  2. Pin-point pupils
  3. Hypothermia
  4. Young age
  5. Absence of focal deficit like quadriparesis

158. Ans. (a) Right Posterior inferior cerebellar artery occlusion

(Ref: Harrison 20th p 3073; Harrison: 19th edition, page 2576)

- The clinical presentation of dysartharia and dysphagia points to bulbar palsy.
- The loss of pain and temperature points to lateral spinothalamic injury.
- The hypotonia in stroke patient indicates cerebellar involvement.
- The presence of these findings localise the lesion to the lateral part of medulla and patient is having lateral medullary syndrome.

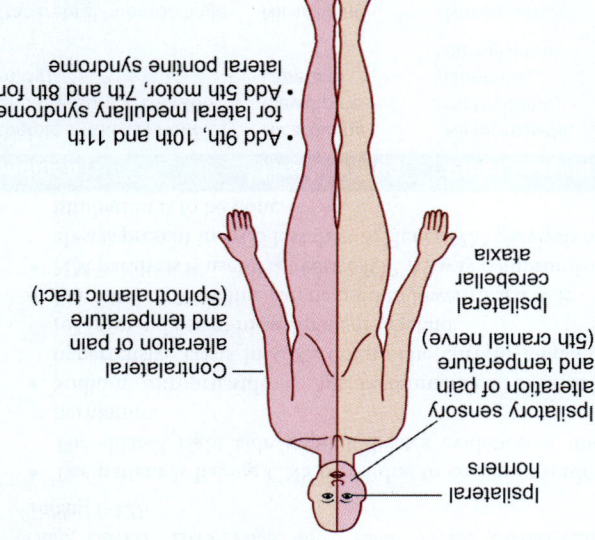

- Since the sensory involvement in lateral medullary involvement is crossed, it implies left sided hemi-sensory loss is due to lesion on right side.

Clinical pointers to the diagnosis in this question

1. The patient is having blockage of right posterior inferior cerebellar artery leading to Right sided horner syndrome
2. Right sided weakness in arm and leg
3. Right sided LMN paralysis of cranial nerve 10
4. Left sided loss of pain and temperature.

159. Ans. (b) Subarachnoid Haemorrhage

(Ref: Harrison 20th p 2085; Harrison: 19th edition, page 1787)

- The major cause of death in SAH is vasospasm of surrounding vessels. This can lead to brain infarction. Hence to prevent the development of vasospasm of these vessels, CCB nimodipine is used.
- This is however a double edged sword as the use of the drug can cause symptomatic hypotension.
- Hence judicious use of the drug plus volume expansion and vasopressors is used for treatment. Vasopressors used are phenylephrine or nor-epinephrine.

160. Ans. (c) Sustained Blood Pressure >185/110 mm Hg despite treatment

(Ref: Harrison 20th p 3081; Harrison: 19th edition, page 2562)

Indications for thrombolysis in stroke
1. Clinical diagnosis of stroke
2. Onset of symptoms to time of drug administration <4.5 hours
3. Age >18 years
4. Consent by parent/ surrogate
5. CT scan showing no haemorrhage or edema > 1/3rd of the MCA territory

Contraindications of thrombolysis
Sustained Blood pressure >185/110 mmHg despite treatment
Bleeding diathesis
Platelet count< 1 lac/cu.mm, haematocrit<25% and blood glucose <50 or >400mg%
Use of heparin within 48 hours and prolonged PTT or prolonged PT
Recent history of stroke (within previous 3 months)
Major surgery in last 2 weeks
GIT bleeding last 3 weeks
Recent MI
Coma or stupor
Rapidly improving symptoms

161. Ans. (d) Parinaud Syndrome

(Ref: Harrison 20th p 190, 192; Harrison 19th edition, page 46 2e-1)

Common neurological causes of Ptosis

Peripheral Neuropathy
Guillain-Barre syndrome
Miller Fisher Syndrome

Neuromuscular Junction
Botulism
Lambert-Eaton syndrome
Myasthenia gravis
Congenital myasthenia

Myopathy
Mitochondrial myopathies
Progressive external ophthalmoplegia
Oculopharyngeal and oculopharyngodistal muscular dystrophy
Myotonic dystrophy (ptosis only)
Congenital myopathy
Nemaline Rod myopathy (ptosis only)

162. Ans. (d) Abulia

(Ref: Harrison 20th p 3071; Harrison 19th edition, page 2572-73)

Abulia is a feature of ACA territory stroke.

Features of entire MCA blockage at the origin (Penetrating and cortical branches are blocked)

1. Contralateral hemiplegia
2. Hemi-anaesthesia
3. Homonymous hemianopia
4. Patient will look towards the lesion
5. Dysarthria due to facial weakness.
6. Due to involvement of dominant lobe global aphasia is present.
7. Due to involvement of non-dominant lobe anosoagnosia, constructional apraxia and neglect are found.

163. Ans. (a) Jargon speech

(Ref: Harrison 20th p 160; Harrison 19th edition, page 2573)

Features of Gerstmann syndrome

1. Acalculia
2. Dysgraphia
3. Finger anomia
4. Right left confusion

164. Ans. (a) Cavernous sinus

(Ref: Harrison 20th p 2084; Harrison 19th edition, page 1785)

The location of abducens nerve in the cavernous sinus makes it vulnerable to expanding supraclinoid carotid or anterior cerebral artery aneurysm.

Associated Cranial nerve palsy	Location of berry aneurysm
3rd nerve palsy with pupillary dilatation and loss of ipsilateral light reflex	At junction of Posterior communicating artery with internal carotid artery
6th nerve palsy	Cavernous sinus aneurysm of carotid artery or anterior cerebral artery
Occipital pain	P.I.C.A or A.I.C.A aneurysm
Pain behind eye or low temple	MCA aneurysm

165. Ans. (a) >7mm and top of basilar artery

(Ref: Harrison 20th p 2084; Harrison 19th edition, page 1785)

The size of aneurysm and site are important in predicting the risk of rupture. The size > 7mm in diameter and anatomical location of top of basilar artery are at greatest risk of rupture.

166. Ans. (a) A-β

(Ref: Harsh Mohan: 7th edition, page 70)

Types of amyloidosis	Biochemical type deposited	Organs involved
Senile cardiac	ATTR	Heart
Senile cerebral	Aβ (Cerebral amyloid angiopathy) APrP (Prion disease)	Cerebral vessels, plaques Neuro-Fibrillary Tangles

Contd...

Types of amyloidosis	Biochemical type deposited	Organs involved
Endocrine	Pro-calcitonin Pro-insulin	Thyroid Type 2DM
Tumour forming	AL	Respective anatomical location

167. Ans. (a) Conduction aphasia

(Ref: Harrison 20th p 159; Harrison 19th edition, page no 177, 178)

- Comprehension is a function of Wernicke's area and fluency is a function of Broca's area.
- Since in the question comprehension, fluency and understanding written words is not affected it implies damage is not in Wernicke or Broca's area
- The catch in the question is "unable to name things and repetition is poor" implying damage to arcus fasiculus and conduction aphasia.

Clinical Features of Aphasias and Related Conditions

Types of Aphasia	Compre-hension	Repetition of Spoken Language	Naming	Fluency
Conduction	Preserved	Impaired	Impaired	Preserved
Fluent (sensory) transcortical	Impaired	Preserved	Impaired	Preserve
Anomic	Preserved	Preserved	Impaired	Preserved except for word-finding pauses
Global	Impaired	Impaired	Impaired	Decreased
Wernicke's (Sensory)	Impaired	Impaired	Impaired	Preserved or increased
Broca's (motor)	Preserved (except grammar)	Impaired	Impaired	Decreased
Non-fluent (motor) Transcortical	Preserved	Preserved	Impaired	Impaired

168. Ans. (a) Basal ganglia

(Ref: Harrison 20th p 3092; Harrison's 19th edition, page 2582-83)

Causes of Intracranial Hemorrhage

Cause	Location	Comments
Head trauma	Intra-parenchymal: frontal lobes, anterior temporal lobes; subarachnoid	Coup and contre-coup injury during brain deceleration
Hypertensive hemorrhage	Putamen, globus pallidus, thalamus, cerebellar hemisphere, pons	Chronic hypertension produces hemorrhage from small vessels in these regions
Metastatic brain tumor	Lobar	Lung, choriocarcinoma, melanoma, renal cell carcinoma, thyroid, atrial myxoma
Drug	Lobar, subarachnoid	Cocaine, amphetamine, phenylpropanolamine
Arteriovenous Malformation	Lobar, intraventricular, subarachnoid	Risk is 2-4% per year for bleeding
Aneurysm	Subarachnoid, intra-parenchymal, rarely subdural	Mycotic and nonmycotic forms of aneurysms

Contd...

169. Ans. (a) Lateral gaze palsy

(Ref: Harrison 20th p 190; Harrison 19th edition, page 209)

Foville's syndrome after dorsal pontine injury includes
1. Lateral gaze palsy
2. Ipsilateral facial palsy
3. Contralateral hemiparesis incurred by damage to descending corticospinal fibers.

Anatomy:
Pons: Unilateral lesion in the dorsal pons

Blood vessel involved
- Basilar artery: Paramedian branches and short circumferential arteries

Signs & Symptoms

Side	Manifestation	Comments
Contralateral	Weakness – upper and lower extremity	Corticospinal tract
Ipsilateral	Weakness – face – entire side	VII nucleus / fascicle
Ipsilateral	Lateral gaze weakness	PPRF or CN VI nucleus

170. Ans. (b) Hemorrhage in left thalamus and internal capsule

(Ref: Harrison 20th p 3092; Harrison 19th edition, page 2582-83)

The N.C.C.T shows presence of left sided Hyper-intense lesion adjacent to third ventricle close to putamen, thalamus and internal capsule. With concurrent history of hypertension followed by right sided hemiplegia the diagnosis is left sided hemorrhage in left thalamus and internal capsule

171. Ans. (b) Right pons

(Ref: Harrison 20th p 190; Harrison 19th page 2577)

- Diplopia indicates 6th nerve palsy and facial weakness of half side involving both upper and lower part indicates involvement of corticobulbar fibers. Since 6th and 7th cranial nerves originate from the pons it is a pontine lesion.
- The left sided hemiparesis indicates lesion in right pons.

Name of syndrome	Site of lesions	Clinical features
Weber	Anterior cerebral peduncle mid brain[Q]	Ipsilateral 3rd palsy Contralateral hemiplegia
Claude	Cerebral peduncle involving red nucleus	Ipsilateral 3rd nerve palsy Contralateral cerebellar ataxia
Parinaud	Dorsal mid brain tectum	Vertical gaze palsy Convergence disorders Convergence retraction nystagmus Pupillary and lid disorders
Millard gubler	Basiliar artery involvement leading to lesion of *ventral pons* and the fascicles of cranial nerves VI and VII	Ipsilateral lateral rectus weakness with diplopia due to cranial nerve VI involvement. Ipsilateral peripheral facial paresis, due to cranial nerve VII involvement Contralateral hemiplegia (sparing the face) due to pyramidal tract involvement
Foville	Lesion of *dorsal pons* affecting nucleus of abducens, seventh nerve and corticospinal pathway	Lateral gaze palsy ipsilateral facial palsy Contralateral Hemiparesis
Wallenberg	Lateral medulla	Ipsilateral 5th, 8th, 9th, 10th, 11th nerve palsy Ipsilateral Horner's syndrome Ipsilateral cerebellar signs Contralateral spinothalamic sensory loss

172. Ans. (d) Drop attacks

(Ref: Harrison 20th p 146, 3072; Harrison 19th edition, page number 2574)

The clinical picture of internal carotid occlusion depends on site and etiology like low flow or clot propagation.
- In majority of cases, the cortex supplied by middle cerebral artery will suffer leading to features of proximal MCA occlusion. Since the right internal carotid artery is involved, left sided hemiplegia and hemi-anesthesia will be seen. *Choice B and C are correct.*
- When the origins of both the ACA and MCA are occluded at the top of the carotid artery Abulia or stupor occurs with the hemiplegia hemi-anesthesia and aphasia or anosognosia. *Choice A is correct.*
- Internal carotid artery also supplies the ipsilateral optic nerve and retina via the ophthalmic artery. The disease causes recurrent transient monocular blindness *amaurosis fugax*
- Drop attacks are sudden spontaneous falls while standing or walking, with complete recovery in seconds or minutes. There is usually no recognized loss of consciousness and the event is remembered.

Causes and types of falls /drops attacks
1. Transient ischemic attacks
2. Vertebrobasilar insufficiency
3. Third ventricular and posterior fossa tumors
4. Parkinson's disease
5. Progressive supranuclear palsy
6. Neuromuscular disorder (myopathy and neuropathy)
7. Myelopathy
8. Cataplexy
9. Vestibular disorder
10. Cyptogenic falls

173. Ans. (a) Putamen

(Ref: Harrison 20th p 3092; Harrison 19th ed. / 2582)
- Most common site of brain hemorrhage is Putamen.
- Intra-parenchymal hemorrhage is most lethal and has mortality rate of 40%.
- The IOC is NCCT.

174. Ans. (a) Infarction

(Ref: Bringham Intensive review of Internal Medicine 2nd ed./ 888)
- Most common type of stroke is ischemic stroke caused by extracranial and intracranial atherosclerosis.

175. Ans. (a) 3rd nerve

(Ref: Harrison 19th ed. / 1784-85)
- Most common cranial nerve affected in unruptured berry aneurysm is the 3rd cranial nerve which will present as ipsilateral ptosis, diplopia and strabismus.

176. Ans. (b) 24 hours

(Ref: Harrison 20th p 2084; Harrison 19th ed. / 2568)
- The standard definition of TIA requires that all neurologic signs and symptoms resolve within 24 hours regardless of whether there is imaging evidence of new permanent brain injury; stroke has occurred if the neurologic signs and symptoms last for >24 hours.

177. Ans. (a) Opsoclonus

(Ref: Harrison 20th p 3074; Harrison 19th p 2575)

Balint's Syndrome, results from infarctions secondary to low flow in the "watershed" between the distal PCA and MCA territories, as occurs after cardiac arrest.

It occurs due to lesion of bilateral visual association area.

Clinical manifestations: [S.O.P : Mnemonic]
1. Inability to synthesize whole of an image (**SIMULTANAGNOSIA**).
2. Disorder of the orderly visual scanning of the environment (**OPTIC ATAXIA/OCULAR APRAXIA**)
3. Patients may experience persistence of a visual image for several minutes despite gazing at another scene (**PALINOPSIA**)

The hallmark is the sudden onset of bilateral signs, including ptosis, pupillary asymmetry or lack of reaction to light, and somnoloscence.

178. Ans. (d) PICA

(Ref: Handbook of Neurosurgery, Greenberg, Pg. 2601)

- PICA originates from the intracranial portion of Vertebral Artery in 80-95% patients, approximately 8.6 mm above the foramen magnum and 1cm proximal to the vertebro-basilar junction.
- PICA aneurysms may present with only IVth ventricular blood without subarachnoid hemorrhage.

Clinical presentation	Aneurysm location
Intraventricular bleed in 3rd ventricle	Basiliar artery aneurysm
Intraventricular bleed in 4th ventricle	Post inferior cerebellar artery
Isolated occulomotor paralysis	Basiliar apex aneurysm
Isolated abducens paralysis	Vertebrobasiliar aneurysm
9,10,11th nerve paralysis	PICA

Most common site overall for intra-cranial aneurysms occur in the terminal portion of the internal carotid artery and the branching sites on the large cerebral arteries in the anterior portion of the circle of Willis.

179. Ans. (b) Subarachnoid haemorrhage (SAH)

(Ref: Harrison 20th p 2084; Harrison 19th p 1785)

In clinical setting of hypertension and sudden onset neck stiffness the most probable diagnosis is SAH. This patient does not have meningitis or meningo-encephalitis as there is no history of fever or seizures and altered sensorium.

Clinical Features
1. Most unruptured aneurysms are completely asymptomatic.
2. Ruptured aneurysm leads to sudden transient loss of consciousness.
3. Thunderclap headache. "Worst headache of a person's life"
4. Severe headache associated with exertion is the presenting complaint.
5. Vomiting, neck stiffness are seen due to meningeal irritation
6. Absence of focal neurological deficits.

Major causes of delayed neurological deficits:
1. Re-rupture
2. Hydrocephalus
3. Vasospasm
4. Hyponatremia

Lab evaluation and imaging-
1. Non-contrast CT scan is the initial investigation of choice. Hallmark of aneurysmal rupture is blood in CSF
2. Lumbar puncture; only if the scan fails to pick up the bleed.(xanthochromic CSF)
3. Four vessel conventional X-ray Angiography for confirmation.

Treatment options - Nimodipine to prevent vasospasm.
To prevent rupture: aneurysmal clip/Coiling of aneurysm.

180. Ans. (d) Oculomotor

(Ref: Harrison 20th p 2084; Harrison 19th p 1785)

- Progressively enlarging un-ruptured aneurysm most commonly involves the occulomotor nerve. This usually occurs from an expanding aneurysm at junction of posterior communicating artery and internal carotid artery.
- Posterior inferior cerebellar artery (PICA) aneurysm constitute 2% of all intracranial aneurysms and its proximity to 4th ventricle makes PICA aneurysms to present as isolated 4th ventricle bleed.
- Cavernous sinus aneurysm can produce 6th nerve palsy.
- Supra-clinoid carotid or anterior cerebral artery aneurysm can produce visual field defects.
- Posterior inferior cerebellar artery or anterior inferior cerebellar artery aneurysm may present as occipital and posterior cervical pain.
- An expanding middle cerebral artery aneurysm can produce pain in or behind the eye and in the low temple.
- Ophthalmic artery aneurysm can cause visual loss by compressing optic nerve.

181. Ans. (a) ACA

(Ref: Harrison 20th p 144; Harrison 19th p 163)

- Frontal gait disorder, sometimes known as gait apraxia is common in the elderly and has a variety of causes.
- Typical features include a wide base of support, short stride, shuffling along the floor, and difficulty with starts and turns. Many patients exhibit difficulty with gait initiation, descriptively characterized as the "slipping clutch" syndrome.
- The term lower body Parkinsonism is also used to describe such patients. Strength is generally preserved, and patients are able to make stepping movements when not standing and maintaining balance at the same time.
- The most common cause of frontal gait disorder is vascular disease, particularly subcortical small-vessel disease. Lesions are frequently found in the deep frontal white matter and centrum ovale.

182. Ans. (c) Sagittal sinus thrombosis

(Ref: William's 23rd ed. pg 1169)

Eclampsia	Most cases of eclampsia present in the third trimester of pregnancy, with about 80% of eclamptic seizures occurring intrapartum or within the first 48 hours following delivery.
Hypertensive ICH	The risk of stroke is generally thought to increase during pregnancy because of a hypercoagulable state; however, studies suggest that the period of risk occurs primarily in the postpartum period and that both ischemic and hemorrhagic strokes may occur at this time. This condition REQUIRES A HIGH BP whereas here mild hypertension is given.
Sagittal vein thrombosis	Pregnancy and puerperium are hyper-coagulable states in setting of clinical features of stroke due to Cerebral Venous thrombosis. It's a diagnosis of exclusion and requires MR venography for determination. Most common type is lateral or superior sagittal sinus thrombosis
Pituitary apoplexy	Present with visual deficit in form of bi-temporal superior quadrantopic effect with optic nerve involvement. It is best diagnosed with contrast based MRI.

183. Ans. (a) NCCT

(Ref: Harrison 20th p 2084; Harrison 19th p 1785)

The clinical picture is of a patient of a subarachnoid hemorrhage with a probable "warning leak".

- Subarachnoid hemorrhage has a characteristic clinical picture. Its onset is with sudden headache of a severity never experienced previously by the patient. This may be followed by nausea and vomiting and by a loss or impairment of consciousness that can either be transient or progress inexorably to deepening coma and death.
- If consciousness is regained, the patient is often confused and irritable and may show other symptoms of an altered mental status. Neurologic examination generally reveals nuchal rigidity and other signs of meningeal irritation, except in deeply comatose patients.
- *Occasional patients with aneurysms have headaches, sometimes accompanied by nausea and neck stiffness, a few hours or days before massive subarachnoid hemorrhage occurs. This has been attributed to "warning leaks" of a small amount of blood from the aneurysm.*
- A CT scan (preferably with CT angiography) should be performed immediately to confirm that hemorrhage has occurred and to search for clues regarding its source. CT findings sometimes are normal in patients with suspected hemorrhage, and the cerebrospinal fluid must then be examined for the presence of blood or xanthochromia before the possibility of subarachnoid hemorrhage is discounted.

184. Ans. (a) Gerstmann syndrome

(Ref: Harrison 20th p 160; Harrison 19th p 179, 2573)

GERSTMANN syndrome	Gerstmann syndrome is characterized by four primary symptoms: 1. Dysgraphia/agraphia: deficiency in the ability to write. 2. Acalculia: difficulty in learning or comprehending mathematics. 3. Finger agnosia: inability to distinguish the fingers on the hand. 4. Left-right disorientation.
Anton syndrome	• Anton–Babinski syndrome is a rare symptom of brain damage occurring in the occipital lobe. • Those who suffer from it are "cortically blind", but affirm, often quite adamantly and in the face of clear evidence of their blindness, that they are capable of seeing. Failing to accept being blind gets dismissed by the sufferer through confabulation
Millard Gubler syndrome	Symptoms result from the functional loss of several anatomical structures of the pons, **including the sixth and seventh cranial nerves and fibers of the cortico-spinal tract.** 1. Paralysis of the abducens (CN VI) leads to diplopia, internal strabismus. 2. Disruption of the facial nerves (CN VII) leads to symptoms including flaccid paralysis of the muscles of facial expression and loss of the corneal reflex. 3. Disruption of the cortico-spinal tract leads to contralateral hemiplegia of the extremities

Locked in syndrome	• Locked-in syndrome usually results in quadriplegia and the inability to speak in otherwise cognitively intact individuals.
	• The site of lesion is bilateral ventral pons/ brainstem leading to bilateral cortico- spinal pathway leading to quadriplegia.
	• The damage to cortico-bulbar fibers causes facial paralysis
	• The midbrain area of superior colliculus is preserved and hence vertical gaze is preserved
	• Clinical features of locked in syndrome
	  1. Sustained eyes opening and preserved vertical eye movement
	  2. Preserved higher cortical functions
	  3. Aphonia or severe hypophonia
	  4. Quadriplegia or quadriparesis
	  5. Primary mode of communication that uses vertical eye movements or blinking
	Individuals with the syndrome lack coordination between breathing and voice. This restricts them from producing voluntary sounds, though the vocal cords are not paralysed.

185. Ans. (c) Angular gyrus

(Ref: Localization in clinical Neurology, 6th edition, page 519)

Pure word blindness is referred to as alexia without agraphia. These patient cannot read but are able to write on dictation. It occurs due to damage to pathways converging visual input from both hemispheres to dominant angular gyrus. In contrast pure word deafness occurs due to lesion in left superior temporal gyrus.

186. Ans. (a) SAH

(Ref: Harrison 19th p 1785)

- At the moment of aneurysmal rupture with major SAH, the ICP suddenly rises. This may account for the sudden transient loss of consciousness that occurs in nearly half of patients. Sudden loss of consciousness may be preceded by a brief moment of excruciating headache, but most patients first complain of headache upon regaining consciousness. The patient often calls the headache "the worst headache of my life"; however, the most important characteristic is sudden onset. **The headache is usually generalized, often with neck stiffness, and vomiting is common**.
- Anterior communicating artery or MCA bifurcation aneurysms may produce deficits that can include hemiparesis, aphasia, and abulia.
- A third cranial nerve palsy, particularly when associated with pupillary dilation, loss of ipsilateral (but retained contralateral) light reflex, and focal pain above or behind the eye, may occur with an expanding aneurysm at the junction of the posterior communicating artery and the internal carotid artery.
- A sixth nerve palsy may indicate an aneurysm in the cavernous sinus, and visual field defects can occur with an expanding supraclinoid carotid or anterior cerebral artery aneurysm.
- Occipital and posterior cervical pain may signal a posterior inferior cerebellar artery or anterior inferior cerebellar artery aneurysm
- Pain in or behind the eye and in the low temple can occur with an expanding MCA aneurysm. Thunderclap headache if written in question again favours diagnosis of SAH.

187. Ans. (c) Expanding aneurysm at the junction of posterior communicating and internal carotid artery

(Ref: Localization of Neurological Lesion: 6th ed., by W. Brazin, Harrison 20th p 2084; Harrison 19th p 1785)

- **Choice A:** Cavernous sinus aneurysms causes painful opthalmoplegia with 3rd or multiple cranial nerve palsies with a SMALL pupil due to oculosympathetic dysfunction. Pain and numbness is seen in distribution of the fifth nerve.
- Choice B is ruled out as Expanding supra-clinoidal carotid aneurysm will have 3rd nerve palsy, optic atrophy will cause light reflex to be absent but eye pain is not present and patients have bi-temporal hemianopia.
- Logically speaking choice D is easiest to remove as it will cause mainly frontal lobe damage manifestations.

Aneurysm in cavernous sinus	**It presents with** 1. Isolated or combined ophthalmoplegia with involvement of 3rd, 4th, 6th cranial nerves 2. Painful ophthalmoplegia 3. Decreased pain sensation in the V1 ophthalmic division They represent 5–8% of all intracranial aneurysms with 60% arising from the internal carotid artery. Cavernous aneurysms do not carry a significant risk of subarachnoid haemorrhage; if they rupture they do so locally, resulting in the formation of a carotid cavernous fistula.
Expanding supraclinoid carotid aneurysm	• Supraclinoid aneurysms may cause ophthalmoplegia due to compression of cranial nerve (CN) III or variable visual defects and optic atrophy due to compression of the optic nerve. • Chiasmal compression may produce bilateral temporal hemianopsia. Hypopituitarism or anosmia may be seen with giant aneurysms. Cavernous-carotid aneurysms exert mass effects within the cavernous sinus, producing ophthalmoplegia and facial sensory loss. Rupture of these aneurysms typically produces a carotid-cavernous fistula, SAH, or epistaxis
Expanding aneurysm at junction of posterior communica- ting artery and internal carotid artery	Posterior communicating artery: Aneurysms present at the junction of the termination of the ICA and PCoA account for 23% of cerebral aneurysms; they are directed laterally, posteriorly, and inferiorly. Pupillary dilatation, ophthalmoplegia, ptosis, mydriasis, and hemiparesis may result.
Expanding aneurysm of anterior cerebral artery	Anterior cerebral artery: Aneurysms of this vessel, excluding ACoA, account for about 5% of all cerebral aneurysms. Most are asymptomatic until they rupture, although frontal lobe syndromes, anosmia, or motor deficits may be noted. Anterior communicating artery: This is the most common site of aneurysmal SAH (34%). Usually, ACoA aneurysms are silent until they rupture. Suprachiasmatic pressure may cause altitudinal visual field deficits, abulia or akinetic mutism, amnestic syndromes, or hypothalamic dysfunction. Neurological deficits in aneurysmal rupture may reflect intraventricular hemorrhage (79%), intraparenchymal hemorrhage (63%), acute hydrocephalus (25%), or frontal lobe strokes (20%).

188. Ans. (c) Pontine lesions

(Ref: Harrison 20th p 2072; Harrison 19th p 1775)

- *Ocular bobbing is a jerky downward deviation of the eyes with slow return, seen in comatose patients and believed to be due to a pontine lesion.*
- *Ocular dipping is inverse of ocular bobbing and slow downward deviation with fast upward movement and occurs due to diffuse cortical suppression in patients of cerebral anoxia like after CPR.*
- *Damage to medial longitudinal fasiculus leads to ataxic nystagmus*
- *Severe refractive errors or macular disease will lead to pendular nystagmus*
- *Downbeat nystagmus is seen with cerebellar lesions.*
- *Upbeat nystagmus with brainstem lesions.*

189. Ans. (c) 6th and 7th nerve

(Ref: Harrison 20th p 190; Harrison 19th p 209)

- Symptoms result from the functional loss of several anatomical structures of the pons, including the sixth and seventh cranial nerves and fibers of the corticospinal tract.
- Paralysis of the abducens (CN VI) leads to diplopia, internal strabismus, and loss of power to rotate the affected eye outward
- Disruption of the facial nerves (CN VII) leads to symptoms including flaccid paralysis of the muscles of facial expression and loss of the corneal reflex.
- Disruption of the corticospinal tract leads to contralateral hemiplegia of the extremities.

190. Ans. (b) Less than 180/110

(Ref: J.N.C 8 guidelines, Harrison 19th p 1627; Harrison 20th p 1905)

Hypertension complication	Target BP	Drugs to be used
Hypertensive encephalopathy	Reduce MAP by 25% maximum over 8 hours	Sodium nitroprusside/ labetalol/ clevidipine/ fenoldopam
Acute ischemic stroke	For thrombolysis to be initiated keep SBP< 185 and DBP < 110	Nicardipine/ labetalol
Intracranial hemorrhage with raised ICT	Keep MAP< 130 and SBP<180	Nicardipine/ labetalol*good BP control reduces hematoma growth
SAH	Keep SBP <160	Nimodipine
High BP without raised ICT	Keep SBP< 160	High dose ACE-

Remember in JNC 8 HYPERTENSION GUIDELINES vs JNC 7 guidelines

1. Goal BP in Patients age > 60 years: <150/90. Change from goal of < 140/90
2. Goal BP in patients age < 60 years: <140/90. Change from goal of < 130/80
3. Goal BP in Patients age 18-59 yrs with diabetes or renal disease: <140/90. Change from goal of <130/80 mm Hg
4. Begin treatment with either a thiazide-type diuretic, CCB, ACE inhibitor, or ARB. Most important change is that Beta blockers are not any more first line drugs for HTN!!
5. If a patient's goal BP is not achieved within 1 month of treatment, increase the dose of the initial agent or add an agent from another of the recommended drug classes; if 2-drug therapy is unsuccessful for reaching the target BP, add a third agent from the recommended drug classes

191. Ans. (b) Intraparenchymal hemorrhage

(Ref: Harrison 20th p 3092; Harrison 19th p 2582)

The bleed in this patient is a hyper-density in the area of basal ganglia and is an intraparenchymal bleed. The bleed is also causing a slight effacement of the ventricular system adjacent to which it is situated which explains the symptoms of raised ICT in these patients.

192. Ans. (a) Diffusion weighted MRI

(Ref: Imaging in stroke, Michael Hennerici Pg. 60; Harrison 19th p 2580)

- Cytotoxic edema, which is caused by the accumulation of intracellular water due to cell membrane damage minutes after onset of acute cerebral ischemia, causes a restriction of microscopic proton diffusion. In diffusion-weighted MRI, this decrease in water diffusion is presumably reflected in a decrease of the apparent diffusion coefficient, which is visualized as a hyper-intensity on the diffusion-weighted images (DWI). Ischemic changes were detected with DWI as early as 2 to 6 hours after onset of symptoms.
- In the ealy stage of ischemia, CT is the technique of choice to distinguish between hemorrhagic and nonhemorrhagic stroke. *However, with CT 30% to 60% of the ischemic lesions are still invisible in the acute stage.*
- During the first 24 hours after an ischemic stroke, proton density–weighted (PD-w) and T2-w MRI have 20% to 30% false-negative results. This percentage increases to 30% to 50% during the first 3 to 6 hours after stroke.
- As a consequence, CT or conventional MRI is not generally used to predict the presence and extent of ischemic damage in the acute stage after stroke.

193. Ans. (d) Syntax is preserved

(Ref: Harrison 20th p 159; Harrison 19th p 177t, 178)

- Syntax means logic in sentence. For example if a Broca's aphasia patient is asked to repeat: man is bitten by dog. He will respond by saying the dog—— bitten ——by man.
- So repetition is preserved in a sense but without retaining the original message of the sentence.
- Fluency, expression and syntax are functions of Broca's area and damage will cause loss of fluency.

194. Ans. (b) Cerebral ischemia

(Ref: Harrison 20th p 2085; Harrison 19th p 1785)

- Rebleeding of SAH occurs in 20% of patients in the first 2 weeks. The re-bleeds in the first days ("blow out" hemorrhages) are thought to be related to the unstable nature of the aneurysmal thrombus, as opposed to lysis of the clot sitting over the rupture site.
- *Delayed cerebral ischemia from arterial smooth muscle contraction is the most common cause of death and disability following aneurysmal SAH. Vasospasm can lead to impaired cerebral auto-regulation and may progress to cerebral ischemia and infarction. It typically has an onset by third day, maximal at 6-8th day and resolves around 12th day*

- Intra-ventricular bleed is associated with bad prognosis but occurs in a few % of patients.
- LV systolic dysfunction in humans with SAH is associated with normal myocardial perfusion and abnormal sympathetic innervation. These findings may be explained by excessive release of norepinephrine from myocardial sympathetic nerves, which could damage both myocytes and nerve terminals and result in MI.

195. Ans. (a) Brain

(Ref: Neuro-Imaging, Roy Riascos, 3rd edition, page 1032)

Duret hemorrhages are caused by *downward/trans-tentorial cerebral herniation* due to raised ICP. It has high incidence of death and persistent vegetative outcome.

196. Ans. (a) Non rheumatic atrial fibrillation

(Ref: Harrison 20th p 3082)

Non rheumatic atrial fibrillation leads to clot formation in left atrial appendage that can embolize to the brain leading to neurological deficits.

Since atrial fibrillation is the commonest sustained arrhythmia is clinical practice, the most common arrhythmia leads to the embolic stroke.

197. Ans. (b) Male with hypertension

(Ref: Harrison 20th p 3071; Harrison 19th p 2565)

In setting of HTN, Diabetes mellitus, mechanisms of lacunar stroke are microatheroma and lipohyalinosis. At the beginning, lipohyalinosis was thought to be the main small vessel pathology, but microatheroma now is thought to be the most common mechanism of arterial occlusion (or stenosis). Occasionally, atheroma in the parent artery blocks the orifice of the penetrating artery (luminal atheroma), or atheroma involves the origin of the penetrating artery (junctional atheroma).

198. Ans. (a) Motor aphasia

(Ref: Harrison 20th p 3070; Harrison 19th p 2573)

- In the Sylvian fissure, the MCA in most patients divides into superior and inferior divisions (M2 branches).
- Branches of the inferior division supply the inferior parietal and temporal cortex, and those from the superior division supply the frontal and superior parietal cortex.
- Hence due to damage of the blood supply of the Broca's area the main feature shall be motor aphasia.

199. Ans. (a) Middle cerebral artery

(Ref: Harrison 20th p 3070; Harrison 19th p 2573)

- If the entire MCA is occluded at its origin (blocking both its penetrating and cortical branches) and the distal collaterals are limited, the clinical findings are contralateral hemiplegia, hemi-anesthesia, homonymous hemianopia, and *a day or two of gaze preference to the ipsilateral side*.
- Dysarthria is common because of facial weakness. When the dominant hemisphere is involved, global aphasia is present also, and when the non-dominant hemisphere is affected, anosognosia, constructional apraxia, and neglect are found.

200. Ans. (c) Posterior cerebral artery

(Ref: Harrison 20th p 3072; Harrison 19th p 2575)

- Occlusion of the penetrating branches of thalamic and thalamogeniculate arteries of posterior cerebral artery produces less extensive thalamic and thalamocapsular lacunar syndromes. The thalamic Déjérine-Roussy syndrome consists of contralateral hemisensory loss followed later by an agonizing, searing or burning pain in the affected areas. It is persistent and responds poorly to analgesics.
- Bilateral infarction in the distal PCAs produces cortical blindness (blindness with preserved pupillary light reaction)
- Visual agnosia for faces, objects, mathematical symbols, and colors and anomia with paraphasic errors (amnestic aphasia) may also occur in this setting, even without callosal involvement. Occlusion of the posterior cerebral artery can produce peduncular hallucinosis (visual hallucinations of brightly colored scenes and objects).

201. Ans. (b) Weber's syndrome

(Ref: Harrison 20th p 3072; Harrison 19th p 2575)

Syndrome	Lesion	Clinical profile
Foville syndrome	Pons Damage to 6th and 7th along with P.P.R.F	I/L 6th and 7th nerve palsy with contralateral hemiplegia with internuclear opthalmoplegia
Weber syndrome	Mibrain damage to 3rd nerve and crus cerebri	I/L 3rd nerve palsy with contralateral hemiplegia
Claude syndrome	Dorsal tegmentum and dentato-rubral pathway	Combination of Nothnagel and Benedict syndrome
Nothnagel syndrome	Midbrain tectum involving quadragemial plate which is linked to superior cerebellar penduncle	I/L 3rd nerve palsy with C/L Ataxia
Benedicts syndrome	Damage to TEGMENTUM of midbrain	I/L 3rd nerve palsy + C/L Tremors>Chorea

202. Ans. (b) Contralateral loss of proprioception to the body and limbs

(Ref: Harrison 20th p 3073; Harrison 19th p 2576)

Lateral medullary syndrome results in contralateral loss of pain and temperature due to involvement of lateral spinothalamic pathway.

203. Ans. (b) Middle cerebral artery

(Ref: Harrison 20th p 3069; Harrison 19th p 2572)

The MCA is by far the largest cerebral artery and is the vessel most commonly affected by cerebrovascular accident. The MCA supplies most of the outer convex brain surface, nearly all the basal ganglia, and the posterior and anterior internal capsules. Infarcts that occur within the vast distribution of this vessel lead to diverse neurologic sequelae.

204. Ans. (a) Brain stem lesion

(Ref: Harrison 19th p 1774)

Pin point pupils are size of 1mm are seen due to damage to descending sympathetic pathways which are present in the brain stem.

205. Ans. (a) Posterior inferior cerebellar artery

(Ref: Harrison 20th p 3092; Harrison 19th p 2576)

The constellation of vertigo, numbness of the ipsilateral face and contralateral limbs, diplopia, hoarseness, dysarthria, dysphagia, and ipsilateral Horner's syndrome is called the lateral medullary (or Wallenberg's) syndrome.
Most cases result from ipsilateral vertebral artery occlusion; in the remainder, PICA occlusion is responsible. Occlusion of the medullary penetrating branches of the vertebral artery or PICA results in partial syndromes.

206. Ans. (c) Crossed hemianesthesia

(Ref: Harrison 20th p 3073; Harrison 19th p 2576)

- Due to damage to the sensory nucleus of the trigeminal nerve there is complete sensory loss on the same side of the face.
- Due to damage to lateral spinothalamic pathway which crosses over to the other side the manifestation is loss of pain and temperature in the body of the opposite side.
- This is known as crossed hemi-anaesthesia

EXTRA MILE

Dissociative anesthesia	Syringomyelia/anterior spinal artery occlusion
Crossed hemi anesthesia	Lateral medullary syndrome due to occlusion of vertebral artery
Dense hemi anesthesia	Internal capsule due to lenticulostriate artery occlusion.

207. Ans. (b) Middle cerebral artery

(Ref: Harrison 20th p 3069; Harrison 19th p 2572-73)

- Hemiplegia occurs most commonly due to occlusion of middle cerebral artery
- Paraplegia occurs due to occlusion of anterior cerebral artery
- Posterior cerebral artery occlusion (P_2 segment) leads to homonymous visual-field cut, usually a complete hemianopia, caused by a lesion in the contralateral occipital lobe. Macular or central field sparing can occur if the occipital pole remains intact through blood supply from a branch of the middle cerebral artery.

- Basilar artery stroke presents with Motor deficits such as hemiparesis or tetraparesis and facial paresis, dysarthria and speech impairment, vertigo, Vomitting and visual disturbances.

208. Ans. (a) Aphasia

(Ref: Harrison 20th p 3070; Harrison 19th p 2573)

- In right handed people the dominant parietal lobe is the left parietal lobe and it is supplied by left middle cerebral artery.
- It is the involvement of left parietal lobe that causes aphasia.
- *The question is however on right middle cerebral artery which if occluded will cause damage to right parietal lobe leading to apraxia and neglect as primary symptoms.*
- Occlusion of right middle cerebral artery will cause left sided face weakness and hemiplegia. Dysarthria can be explained by facial weakness.

209. Ans. (a) Oculomotor

(Ref: Harrison 20th p 2084; Harrison 19th p 1785)

The third cranial nerve is more susceptible to compression against the interclinoid ligaments above and the petroclinoid ligament below than the other cranial nerves in the cavernous sinus. For this reason, isolated third cranial nerve palsy may result from lateral extension of pituitary adenoma or other primary intrasellar mass

210. Ans. (c) Incontinence

(Ref: Harrison 20th p 3071; Harrison 19th p 2573)

- Occlusion of the proximal ACA is usually well tolerated because of collateral flow through the anterior communicating artery and collaterals through the MCA and PCA.
- Occlusion of distal ACA can lead to profound abulia (a delay in verbal and motor response) and bilateral pyramidal signs with paraparesis or quadriparesis and urinary incontinence

211. Ans. (d) Hemianesthesia of same side of face

(Ref: Harrison 20th p 3077; Harrison 19th p 2576)

Anterior inferior cerebellar artery produces variable degrees of infarction because the size of this artery and the territory it supplies vary inversely with those of the PICA. The principal symptoms include:
1. Ipsilateral deafness, facial weakness, vertigo, nausea and vomiting, nystagmus, tinnitus, cerebellar ataxia, Horner's syndrome, and paresis of conjugate lateral gaze; and
2. Contralateral loss of pain and temperature sensation

212. Ans. (c) XIIth cranial nerve

(Ref: Harrison 20th p 3073; Harrison 19th p 2576)

Lateral medullary syndrome aka Wallenburg is characterized by blockage of vertebral artery and results in damage to the cranial nerves originating from medulla with SPARING of the 12th cranial nerve which gets supply from the anterior spinal artery.

Features of lateral medullary syndrome	
Dysfunction	**Effects**
Vestibular nuclei	Vestibular system: vomiting, vertigo, nystagmus
Inferior cerebellar peduncle	Ipsilateral cerebellar signs including ataxia, dysmetria (past pointing), dysdiadochokinesia
Central tegmental tract	Palatal myoclonus
Lateral spinothalamic tract	Contralateral deficits in pain and temperature sensation from body (limbs and torso)
Spinal trigeminal nucleus and tract	Ipsilateral loss of pain, and temperature sensation from face
Nucleus ambigus- (which affects vagus nerve and glossopharyngeal nerve.)	Ipsilateral laryngeal, pharyngeal, and palatal hemiparalysis: dysphagia, hoarseness.
Descending sympathetic pathways	Ipsilateral Horner's syndrome (ptosis, miosis, and anhydrosis)

213. Ans. (a) Vertebral artery

(Ref: Neuro-Imaging, Roy Riascos, Pg 1061)

Approximately 85% of aneurysms develop in the anterior part of the circle of Willis, and involve the internal carotid arteries and their major branches that supply the anterior and middle sections of the brain.

The most common sites include the:
- Anterior Communicating artery (32 - 35%)
- Bifurcation of the Internal Carotid and Posterior Communicating artery (30 - 35%)
- Bifurcation of Middle cerebral (20%)
- Basilar artery bifurcation (5%)
- Remaining posterior circulation arteries (5%)

214. Ans. (a) Posterior inferior cerebellar artery stroke

(Ref: Harrison 20th p 3073; Harrison 19th p 2576-77)

- MCA occlusion will damage motor cortex leading to hemiplegia.
- PCA occlusion will damage corticospinal tract travelling through mid-brain leading to hemiplegia.
- Anterior spinal artery supplies medial part medulla and its occlusion damages corticospinal pathway.
- PICA supplies lateral part of medulla while corticospinal pathway travels via medial part of medulla. Hence hemiparesis will not be seen.

215. Ans. (a) Enlargement of aneurysm

(Ref: Harrison 20th p 2084; Harrison 19th p 1785)

Some complications of SAH include the following:
1. **Hydrocephalus:** It presents as a relatively abrupt mental status change, including lethargy, stupor, or coma. CT scan differentiates hydrocephalus from rebleeding.
2. **Rebleeding:** The incidence of the complication of rebleeding is greatest in the first 2 weeks. The peak is within 24-48 hours following initial SAH (approximately 6%), with a rate of 1.5% per day for the next 12-13 days. Clinical factors that increase the likelihood of rebleeding include Hypertension, Anxiety, Agitation, Seizure
3. **Vasospasm:** delayed ischemia from arterial smooth muscle contraction of the large capacitance vessels at the base of the brain is the *leading cause of death and disability* following aneurysmal SAH. Vasospasm is symptomatic in 36% of patients. The incidence of angiographic vasospasm is 30-70%;
4. **Seizures:** Generalized, partial, and complex-partial seizures are observed after SAH.
5. **Cardiac dysfunction:** Arrhythmias occur in as many as 90% of patients and most commonly include Premature ventricular complexes (PVCs), Bradyarrhythmias and Supraventricular tachycardia.

216. Ans. (c) Hypertension

(Ref: Harrison 20th p 3092; Harrison 19th p 2582)

- Intraparenchymal hemorrhage accounts for approx. 8-13% of all strokes and results from a wide spectrum of disorders.
- It is more likely to result in death or major disability than ischemic stroke or subarachnoid hemorrhage, and therefore constitutes an immediate medical emergency.
- Intracerebral hemorrhages and accompanying edema may disrupt or compress adjacent brain tissue, leading to neurological dysfunction
- Nontraumatic intraparenchymal hemorrhage most commonly results from hypertensive damage to blood vessel

217. Ans. (c) Internal carotid artery

(Ref: Harrison 20th p 3072; Harrison 19th edition, page 2568)

The clinical profile given is that of a transient ischemic attack in which an embolus via anterior circulation of brain i.e. internal carotid artery travels to cause transient blockage of ophthalmic artery supplying the retina.

Patient complains of a sweeping down-shade that affects the vision. The recurrent transient monocular vision is celled as amaurosis fugax.

218. Ans. (d) All of the above

(Ref: Harrison 20th p 3087; Harrison 19th p 2568)

- CADASIL (Cerebral Autosomal Dominant Arteriopathy with Subcortical Infarcts & Leukoencephalopathy)- This autosomal dominant condition is caused by one of several mutations in *Notch-3*, gene on *chromosome 19*. IT IS A HEREDITARY STROKE DISORDER.
- It is a monogenic disorder that presents as small-vessel strokes, progressive dementia, and extensive symmetric white matter changes visualized by MRI.
- Approximately 40% of patients have migraine with aura, often manifest as transient motor or sensory deficits,
- Onset is usually in the fourth or fifth decade of life
- The disease progresses to subcortical dementia associated with pseudobulbar palsy and urinary incontinence.

- It is different from Biswanger disease which has white matter atrophy due to hypertension.

219. Ans. (b) Three tube test

(Ref: Merritt's Neurology 2nd/ed p 84)

- LP is traditionally performed as a follow-up test when a CT scan has shown no SAH and has excluded possible contraindications to LP such as significant intracranial mass effect, elevated ICP, obstructive hydrocephalus, or obvious intracranial bleed.
- LP should not be performed if the CT scan demonstrates an SAH because of the (small) risk of further intracranial bleeding associated with a drop in ICP.
- An LP is performed to evaluate the cerebrospinal fluid for the presence of red blood cells (RBCs) and xanthochromia. Three tube test though redundant helps in differentiating a CSF bleed from a traumatic lumbar puncture.
- CSF samples taken within 24 hours of the ictus usually show a WBC-to-RBC ratio that is consistent with the normal circulating WBC-to-RBC ratio of approximately 1:1000.
- After 24 hours, CSF samples may demonstrate a polymorphonuclear and mononuclear polycytosis secondary to chemical meningitis caused by the degradation products of subarachnoid blood.

220. Ans. (d) Predominant involvement of the anterior limb of internal capsule

(Ref: Harrison 20th p 3071; Harrison 19th p 2573-74)

- **Anterior Choroidal Artery** arises from the internal carotid artery and supplies the **posterior** limb of the internal capsule and the matter posterolateral to it, through which pass some of the geniculocalcarine fibers.
- The complete syndrome of anterior choroidal artery occlusion consists of **contralateral hemiplegia, hemianesthesia (hypesthesia), homonymous hemianopia.**
- This territory is also supplied by penetrating vessels of proximal MCA and the posterior communicating and posterior choroidal arteries, minimal deficits may occur, patients frequently recover substantially.

Blood supply of internal capsule:

ANTERIOR LIMB	A.C.A (Medial striate A) + M.C.A (Lateral striate A)
GENU	I.C.A (Ant Choroidal A)
POSTERIOR LIMB	I.C.A (Ant Choroidal A) + M.C.A (lateral striate A)

221. Ans. (c) Vagal palsy

(Ref: Harrison 20th p 3074; Harrison 19th p 2579f)

- Features of pontine stroke develop due to involvement of the basilar artery.
- It is characterized by irritative disturbance of the descending sympathetic pathways from the hypothalamus via the brain stem.

Manifestations are:
1. Pinpoint pupil
2. Hyperpyrexia
3. Quadriparesis
4. Hypertension
5. Hyperhidrosis
6. Hyperventilation
7. Decerebrate rigidity
8. Coma

222. Ans. (e) All of the above

(Ref: Harrison 20th p 3076; Harrison 19th p 2578)

- The locked-in state is a pseudocoma in which an awake patient has no means of producing speech or volitional movement but retains voluntary vertical eye movements and lid elevation, thus allowing the patient to signal. The pupils are normally reactive.
- Cause is an infarction or hemorrhage of the ventral pons that transects all descending motor (corticospinal and corticobulbar) pathways.
- The patient is conscious, alert and awake as the tegmental ascending reticular activating system (ARAS) concerned with arousal is intact.
- Vertical movements are intact as it is controlled by the interstitial nucleus of cajal and the rostral part of the medial longitudinal fasciculus (MLF), which is situated in the tegmentum of the midbrain, which is spared in the locked in syndrome
- Horizontal movements of eyes are lost especially when the ventral part of the basalis pontis is involved, leading to involvement of the 6th cranial nerve fascicle
- **Patient may be aphonic because of the involvement of the corticobulbar fibers and motor nucleus of the lower cranial nerves especially the 7th, 9th, 10th, 12th cranial nerves.**
- Patient is quadriplegic due to involvement of pyramidal fibers in the lateral 2/3rd of cerebral peduncle of the midbrain or the basis pontis or the ventral aspect of the medulla.

223. Ans. (d) Hippocampus

(Ref: Harrison 20th p 3073; Harrison 19th p 2575)

- The superior temporal gyrus contains several important structures of the brain, including:
  1. Brodmann areas 41 and 42, marking the location of the primary auditory cortex, the cortical region responsible for the sensation of sound;
  2. Wernicke's area, Brodmann 22p, an important region for the processing of speech so that it can be understood as language.
- Supramarginal gyrus is a portion of the parietal lobe. It is probably involved with language perception and processing, and lesions in it may cause receptive aphasia
- Angular gyrus is involved in a number of processes related to language, number processing and spatial cognition, memory retrieval, attention, and theory of mind. It is Brodmann area 39 of the human brain.

Manifestations of posterior cerebral artery peripheral branches

Memory defect	Hippocampal lesion bilaterally or on the dominant side only.

Contd...

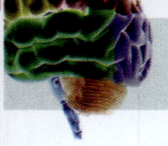

Homonymous hemianopia	Calcarine cortex or optic radiation
Bilateral homonymous hemianopia, cortical blindness, awareness or denial of blindness; tactile naming, achromatopia (color blindness), failure to see to-and-fro movements, inability to perceive objects not centrally located, apraxia of ocular movements, inability to count or enumerate objects, tendency to run into things that the patient sees and tries to avoid	Bilateral occipital lobe with possibly the parietal lobe involved.
Simultanagnosia, hemivisual neglect	Dominant visual cortex
Visual hallucinations, peduncular hallucinosis, metamorphopsia	Calacrine cortex

224. Ans. (d) Seizures

(Ref: Harrison 20th p 3068; Harrison 19th p 2568)

The following signs may be present in patients with T.I.A:
- Ocular dysmotility and Amaurosis fugax
- Forehead wrinkling asymmetry
- Incomplete eyelid closure
- Asymmetrical mouth retraction
- Loss of the naso-labial crease
- Swallowing difficulty
- Lateral tongue movement
- Weak shoulder shrugging
- Visual field deficits

The cerebellar system can be tested by assessing ocular movement, gait, and finger-to-nose and heel-to-knee movements, with an eye to signs of past-pointing and dystaxia, hypotonia, overshooting, gait dystaxia, and nystagmus

225. Ans. (c) Palsy of 10, 11, 12 nerves

(Ref: Harrison 20th p 3073; Harrison 19th p 2576)
- The 12th nerve involvement is a feature of medial medullary syndrome.

226. Ans. (b) Lenticulostriate artery

(Ref: Harrison 20th p 3071; Harrison 19th p 2572)

The patient has an embolic stroke due to athero-sclerosis secondary to diabetes. The anterior circulation damage causes *pure motor paralysis without sensory deficit*. The blood vessel causing such deficit is lenticulo-striate artery which is the branch of the largest blood vessel in the brain i.e. middle cerebral artery.

227. Ans. (d) Descending sympathetic pathways

(Ref: Harrison 20th p 3092; Harrison 19th p 1774)

Pin point pupils are size of 1mm and are seen due to damage to descending sympathetic pathways. Other structures mentioned in choice A,B,C are part of midbrain and hence can't be involved in pontine stroke.

228. Ans. (d) Motor aphasia

(Ref: Harrison 20th p 159; Harrison 19th p 177)

229. Ans. (b) Intracerebral hemorrhage

(Ref: Harrison 20th p 3092; Harrison 19th p 2582)

230. Ans. (c) Putamen / external capsule

(Ref: Harrison 20th p 3092; Harrison 19th p 2582)

231. Ans. (a) Rupture of circle of Willis aneurysm

(Ref: Harrison 20th p 2084; Harrison 19th p 1784)

232. Ans. (b) Degeneration of tunica media

(Ref: Harrison 20th p 2084; Harrison 19th p 1785)

233. Ans. (b) Vertebral artery

(Ref: Harrison 20th p 2084; Harrison 19th p 1784)

234. Ans. (b) Vasospasm

(Ref: Harrison 20th p 2084; Harrison 19th p 1785)

235. Ans. (b) Inability to identify faces

(Ref: Harrison 20th p 163; Harrison 19th p 182)

Parkinsonism and Dementia

236. Ans. (a) Metoclopramide

Ref: Katzung 13th edition, Page 1070

The presentation is of extrapyramidal side effects in the form of dystonia caused by metoclopramide. Dystonia can develop since this drug crosses the BBB and acts on D2 receptors. It responds to treatment with anti-cholinergic and anti-histaminic drugs.

237. Ans. (c) Initial therapy with dopamine agonists controls symptoms in most patients

(Ref: Harrison 20th p 3127; Harrison 19th edition, page 2615)

- Levodopa induced dyskinesia is *more common in advanced PD* as compared to early PD. Hence choice A is wrong.
- Deep brain stimulation is *used in medically refractory PD*. Hence choice B is wrong.
- Since dopamine agonists are long acting and have less dyskinesia they are used for initial treatment of Parkinson disease. Hence choice C is correct
- The *disease continues to progress* with features like falling, freezing and autonomic dysfunction in spite of levodopa. These non-dopaminergic features are primary source of disability. Levodopa *cannot* prevent development of non-dopaminergic features. Hence choice D is wrong.

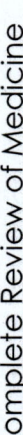

238. Ans. (c) Wilson disease

(Ref: Harrison 20th p 3140; Harrison 19th page 2625)

- Rheumatic chorea presents with emotional lability and poor handwriting, hung up reflexes, pronator sign and darting tongue. LFT is normal. Hence choice A is ruled out.
- Choice B presents with akinetic-rigid Parkinsonism like picture and LFT is normal
- Choice D presents with Parkinsonism like features with cognitive decline and retinal pigmentary changes. It occurs due to iron deposition in putamen.
- The features of Basal ganglia and deranged liver function point to diagnosis to Wilson disease. The disease shows astrogliosis mainly in corpus striatum.

239. Ans. (d) Huntington chorea

(Ref: Harrison 20th p 3137; Harrison 19th edition, page 2621)

- The fast semi-purposive movements are a description for Chorea. Huntington's disease has an autosomal dominant pattern of inheritance and hence presents in every generation. Intellectual decline is a common feature. With advancing age chorea reduces and dystonia, rigidity and myoclonus appear.
- Pre senile dementia is seen in Down's syndrome
- Lewy body dementia presents with hallucinations, delusions and dementia.
- Corticobasal ganglionic degeneration is manifest by asymmetric dystonia, apraxia (Loss of visuospatial skills), focal limb myoclonus or Alien hand syndrome. *Alien limb phenomenon* is characterised by position of the limb in space with the patient not being aware of it.

240. Ans. (b) Pneumocephalus

(Ref: Neuro-radiology imaging by Zasler: 2017 edition, page 274)

- The image shows a NCCT Head with multiple air pockets diagnostic of pneumocephalus. This can occur after a severe fall in Parkinsonism.
- Air on CT will have very low density (–1024 HU) but care needs to be taken in ensuring that it is not fat which is of higher density (–90 HU).

241. Ans. (b) Bilateral reduction in blood flow to caudate nucleus

(Ref: Harrison 20th p 3136-37; Harrison 19th edition, page 2621-22)

- The disease predominantly strikes the striatum.
- Single photon emission computerized tomography (SPECT), using Tc-99m-HMPAO shows significant reductions in tracer uptake in caudate nucleus and putamen
- Progressive atrophy of the caudate nuclei, which form the lateral margins of the lateral ventricles, can be visualized by MRI.
- More diffuse cortical atrophy is seen in the middle and late stages of the disease. Genetic testing can be used to confirm the diagnosis and to detect at-risk individuals in the family,
- The neuropathology of HD consists of prominent neuronal loss and gliosis in the caudate nucleus and putamen; similar changes are also widespread in the cerebral cortex.

Huntington chorea (must know facts)
- Autosomal dominant disorder with high penetrance.
- Intraneuronal inclusions containing aggregates of ubiquitin and the mutant protein huntingtin are found in the nuclei of affected neurons
- HD is caused by an increase in the number of polyglutamine (CAG) repeats (>40) in the coding sequence of the huntingtin gene located on the short arm of chromosome 4.

Clinical features
1. Onset is typically between the ages of 25 and 45 years
2. HD is characterized by semi-purposive, choreiform movements.
3. Dysarthria, gait disturbance, and oculomotor abnormalities are common features.
4. With advancing disease, there may be a reduction in chorea and emergence of dystonia, rigidity, bradykinesia, myoclonus, and spasticity.
5. HD can present as an akinetic-rigid or parkinsonian syndrome (Westphal variant). Depression with suicidal tendencies, aggressive behavior, and psychosis can be prominent features.
6. Associated findings: Non-insulin-dependent diabetes mellitus and neuroendocrine abnormalities, e.g., hypothalamic dysfunction.
7. Tetrabenazine has recently been approved for the treatment of chorea.

---

242. Ans. (c) Amygdaloid nucleus

(Ref: Ganong 25th edition, page 288; Atlas of neuroanatomy 2nd edition, page 203)

- The hippocampal formation is a compound structure in the medial temporal lobe of brain containing the dentate gyrus, the hippocampus proper and the subiculum and others including also the pre-subiculum, para-subiculum, and entorhinal cortex.
- Amygadala primary role in the processing of memory, decision-making, and emotional reactions, the amygdalae are considered part of the limbic system.

243. Ans. (c) Smoking

(Ref: Harrison 20th p 3108; Harrison 19th edition, page 2598)

The most important risk factors for AD are:
1. Old age
2. Positive family history.
3. Female sex may also be a risk factor independent of the greater longevity of women.
4. Past history of head trauma with concussion.
5. Low educational attainment but education influences test-taking ability, and it is clear that AD can affect persons of all intellectual levels.
6. Environmental factors, including aluminium, mercury, and viruses.
7. Diabetes increases the risk of AD threefold. Elevated homocysteine and cholesterol levels; hypertension; diminished serum levels of folic acid
8. Low dietary intake of fruits, vegetables, and red wine; and low levels of exercise are all being explored as potential risk factors for AD.

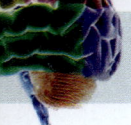

244. Ans. (c) Intention tremor & (e) Flaccidity

(Ref: Harrison 20th p 3121; Harrison 19th/2609-11)

Intentional tremor is a low frequency tremor of 5Hz and is seen in cerebellar lesions. Flaccidity is seen with lower motor neuron lesions.

245. Ans. (a) Tremors

(Ref: Harrison 19th ed. / 2609)

- In the early presentation, about 70 % patients experience a slight tremor in the hand or foot on one side of the body, or less commonly in the jaw or face. The tremor consists of a shaking or oscillating movement, and usually appears when a person's muscles are relaxed, or at rest, hence the term "resting tremor.
- The tremor of PD can be exacerbated by stress or excitement, sometimes attracting unwanted notice. The tremor often spreads to the other side of the body as the disease progresses, but usually remains most apparent on the initially affected side.

246. Ans. (b) Patient B has essential tremors

(Ref: Harrison 20th p 3121, 3123; Harrison 19th edition, page 2619, 2609)

- Patients with essential tremors have high frequency tremors, which significantly distorts fine movements.
- Parkinson patients have low frequency tremors 4-6 Hz and have micrographia, which though is not present in the pic above.

247. Ans. (a) Cerebellum

(Ref: Chapter 45/e-2, Harrison 19th edition)

Points in favour of cerebellar lesion
1. Notice the *low frequency tremors* at the turning point of line B. These tremors are coming at the terminal point where the line should end. More importantly, the patient overshoots the reference line and undershoots the reference line in the end.
2. The intentional tremor of cerebellar lesion does not begin at initiation of movement but in the terminal part of movement.
3. *The inability to finish the geometric figure points to dysmetria where orientation of geometric shapes and sizes is lost.*

248. Ans. (a) Manganese

(Ref: Harrison 20th p 3123; Harrison 19th p 2610)

Causes of Secondary Parkinsonism
1. Drug-induced
2. Tumor
3. Infection
4. Vascular
5. Normal-pressure hydrocephalus
6. Trauma
7. Liver failure
8. *Toxins (e.g., carbon monoxide, manganese, MPTP, cyanide, hexane, methanol, carbon disulfide)*

249. Ans. (b) Ventricular shrinkage

(Ref: Harrison 20th p 3108-09; Harrison 19th p 2598-99)

- MRI findings in patients of AD have hippocampal atrophy in addition to posterior-predominant cortical atrophy. The cortical atrophy leads to pseudo-appearance of dilated ventricles.
- Depression in these patients leads to development of aggressive behavior in evening hours which is referred to as sun downing phenomenon.
- 4 **A's** of Alzheimer's Disease are:
  1. Amnesia
  2. Apraxia
  3. Anosoagnosia
  4. Aphasia

250. Ans. (d) All of the above

(Ref: chapter 12, table 12.1, Adam and Victor Principles of neurology 9th edition)

CNS causes of Anosmia

1.	Head injury with tearing of olfactory filaments
2.	Cranial surgery
3.	Subarachnoid hemorrhage, meningitis
4.	Toxic (organic solvents, certain antibiotics-aminoglycosides, tetracyclines, corticosteroids, methotrexate, opiates, l-dopa)
5.	Metabolic (thiamine deficiency, adrenal and thyroid deficiency, cirrhosis, renal failure, menses)
6.	Wegener granulomatosis
7.	Compressive and infiltrative lesions (craniopharyngioma, meningioma, aneurysm, meningoencephalocele)
8.	Degenerative diseases (Parkinson, Alzheimer, Huntington)
9.	Temporal lobe epilepsy
10.	Malingering and hysteria

251. Ans. (b) Acalculia

(Ref: Harrison 20th p 3108; Harrison 19th p 2598-99)

The 4A of dementia are – AMNESIA/ APRAXIA/ APHASIA and ANOSOAGNOSIA

The DSM-IV criteria for dementia of the Alzheimer's type are:
- Memory impairment: impaired ability to learn new information as well as recall previously learned information.
- One or more of the following cognitive disturbances:
  - Language disturbance.
  - Apraxia (inability to carry out motor activities despite intact motor function).
  - Agnosia (failure to recognise or identify objects despite intact sensory function).
  - Disturbance of planning, organising, sequencing, abstracting and other higher functioning.
- Damage to the parietal and temporal cortex explains the features of aphasia and apraxia. Loss of cortical neurons explains dementia and agnosia

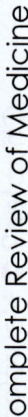

252. Ans. (c) Corticobasilar degeneration

(Ref: Harrison 19th p 2605)

Cortico-basal degeneration shows neuronal loss in cortex and basal ganglia

Disease	Clinical profile	Brain imaging/ biopsy findings
Cortico-basal degeneration	Asymmetric onset of rigidity, dystonie myoclonus, apraxia and alien limb syndrome. The affected limb performs unintended motor actions like grasping, groping.	Degeneration of peri-rolandic cortex and basal ganglia.
Progressive supranuclear gaze Palsy	Atypical parkinsonism with inability to look downwards leading to recurrent falls	Tau-positive cortical lesions found in highest concentration in the pre-central and angular gyrus, primarily affecting the deep cortical layers, and involved both small and large neurons. BUT NO ATROPHY OF CORTEX.
Spinocerebellar ataxia (The number of dominantly inherited SCAs that have been described has increased to 29)	Slowly progressive cerebellar syndrome with combinations of oculomotor disorders, dysarthria, dysmetria/kinetic tremor, and ataxic gait are key presenting features.	Patterns of atrophy are described on brain MRI: pure cerebellar atrophy, olivopontocerebellar atrophy.
Multiple system atrophy	One of three groups of symptoms predominates. These are: 1. Parkinsonism (slow, stiff movement, writing becomes small and spidery) 2. Cerebellar dysfunction 3. Autonomic nervous system dysfunction (impaired automatic body functions) including: postural or orthostatic hypotension, resulting in dizziness or fainting upon standing up urinary incontinence or urinary retention impotence	

253. Ans. (c) Subthalamic nucleus

(Ref: Harrison 20th p 3129; Harrison 19th p 2616)

- DBS for PD primarily targets the STN or the Globus pallidus interna
- It provides dramatic results, particularly with respect to "off" time and dyskinesias, but does not improve features that fail to respond to levodopa and does not prevent the development or progression of non-dopaminergic features such as freezing, falling, and dementia.
- *Recent studies indicate that benefits following DBS of the STN and GPi are comparable, but that GPi stimulation may be associated with a reduced frequency of depression*
- The procedure is thus primarily indicated for patients who suffer disability resulting from levodopa-induced motor complications that cannot be satisfactorily controlled with drug manipulation.

254. Ans. (d) Lateral geniculate nucleus

(Ref: Harrison 20th p 3109; Harrison 19th p 2598)

- In Alzheimer's disease, accumulation of amyloid in the blood vessels in cortex and leptomeninges is seen.
- Areas of visual association, cuneal gyrus and entorhinal cortex are cortical areas. Hence, accumulation of amyloid may be seen. The most severe degeneration is found in medial temporal lobe like entorhinal cortex.
- However, lateral geniculate nucleus is a part of thalamus, which is subcortical. Hence, amyloid deposition is not seen in this area.

Visual association area	Related to cortical visual cortex
Cuneal gyrus	The cuneus (Brodmann area 17) receives visual information from the contralateral superior retina representing the inferior visual field. *It is most known for its involvement in basic visual processing*
Entorhinal cortex	An area of the brain located in the medial temporal lobe and functioning as a hub in a widespread network for memory and navigation. *The EC is the main interface between the hippocampus and neocortex*
Lateral geniculate body	*The lateral geniculate nucleus (LGN) is a sensory relay nucleus in the thalamus of the brain which is a sub cortical area*

255. Ans. (d) Extracellular inclusions can be found in the absence of intracellular inclusions

(Ref: Adams & Victor Principles of Neurology 8th ed.Ch. 39)

- Neuritic plaques and neurofibrillary changes are found in all the association areas of the cerebral cortex, but it is the neurofibrillary tangles and neuronal alterations and loss, not the plaques, that correlate best with the severity of the dementia.
- It is not unusual to find a scattering of senile plaques in individuals who were thought-to be mentally normal during life. Neuritic plaques can be seen in normal aged brain also so they are non-pathogenic in all cases.
- TAU proteins are formed intra-cellularly leading to neuronal degeneration leading to Alzheimer disease.

256. Ans. (c) Small vessel disease is related to AD

(Ref: Adam's and Victor's Neurology 8th ed. P-738)

- Cerebral amyloid angiopathy (CAA) is an organ specific form of amyloid deposition in *small and medium sized arteries*, veins, of the cerebral cortex and meninges, in the elderly.
- It can be *associated with Alzheimer's disease*, Down's syndrome, cerebral vasculitis, cerebral irradiation and dementia pugilistica. Alzheimer's patients appear to be at an increased risk for amyloid angiopathy. Hence choice B and D are correct.

- Small Vessel Stroke refers to infarction following atherothrombotic or lipohyalinotic occlusion of a small artery (30-300 μm) in the brain. It results in development of multi infarct dementia and not Alziehemer's
- Irrespective of how so ever tricky this question looks, the bottom line is small vessel disease does not contribute to AD and choice C is the false statement.

257. Ans. (c) Progressive supranuclear paralysis

(Ref: Harrison 20th p 3116; Harrison 19th p 2612)

- *Square-Wave Jerks (SWJ) are inappropriate saccades that take the eye off the target, followed by a nearly normal inter-saccadic interval (approximately 200 msec), and then a corrective saccade that brings the eye back to the target.*
- It is a normal finding but occurs at an exaggerated frequency in patients of Progressive supra-nuclear gaze palsy.
- PSP is a Parkinsonism variant with concomitant damage at superior colliculus.
- Superior colliculus is one of the generators of Square wave jerks and this explains why textbook mentions the Square wave jerks on Electro-oculography as suggestive of diagnosis of PSP
- It also explains the recurrent falls in these patients and continuous snarling expression on the face.
- The development of early gait disturbance, falls, hyperextension of neck and characteristic abnormalities of vertical gaze suggest progressive supranuclear palsy (PSP)
- Early urinary incontinence, orthostatic hypotension, and dysarthria suggest multiple system atrophy (MSA).
- The early appearance of drug-induced hallucinations will suggest diagnosis of DLB.

258. Ans. (a) Homocysteine

(Ref: Harrison 20th p 3109; Harrison 19th p 434e)

Homocystiene is now referred to as a metabolic marker in Alzheimer and related to cognitive decline.
Increased homocysteine level is associated with a higher risk of strokes. Carotid stenosis appears to have a graded response to increased levels of homocysteine. Increased carotid plaque thickness has been associated with high homocysteine and low B-12 levels. Several mechanisms have been suggested as the possible cause of accelerated vascular disease, including the following:
- Endothelial cell damage
- Smooth muscle cell proliferation
- Lipid peroxidation
- Upregulation of prothrombotic factors (XII and V)
- Downregulation of antithrombotic factors or endothelial-derived nitric oxide

259. Ans. (c) Thyrotoxicosis

(Ref: DeJong's The Neurologic Examination, William W. Campbell, ch. 30, pg. 495)

- Tremor is the most common movement disorder. It is characterized by rhythmic, involuntary, oscillating movement of a body part. Abnormal functioning of the cerebellum can produce tremor. Positron emission tomography studies have shown cerebellar activation in almost all forms of tremors.
- Tremor can be classified on a clinical and etiologic basis. It can occur at rest (Parkinson's disease) or with posture and action (essential tremor) or classified on basis of frequency as coarse or fine tremors
- Differential diagnosis of tremor includes myoclonus, clonus, asterixis, and epilepsia partialis continua.
- **Coarse tremor is defined as slow <8 per second. The causes are:**

> 1. Pill rolling tremor of Parkinsonism
> 2. In Wilson and extra-pyramidal syndrome
> 3. Delirium tremens
> 4. **General paresis** (seen in neurosyphilis 10-30 years after primary syphilis)
> 5. **Cerebellar tremor** is a low-frequency (<5 Hz) intention tremor that usually occurs unilaterally.
> 6. **Holmes' tremor or rubral tremor** designates a combination of rest, postural, and action tremors due to midbrain lesions in the vicinity of the red nucleus. This type of tremor is irregular and low frequency (4.5 Hz). Signs of ataxia and weakness may be present. Common causes include cerebrovascular accident and multiple sclerosis, with a possible delay of 2 weeks to 2 years in tremor onset and occurrence of lesions.

In contrast physiological tremors have frequency of 8-12 Hz and are associated with anxiety/fright /physical exertion like after rock climbing. The enhanced physiological tremors are seen with thyrotoxicosis and are clearly visible or can be seen after making the patient stand with outstretched arms. We can place a paper sheet on outstretched fingers. The fine tremor of closed eyelids in thyrotoxicosis is called as ROSENBACH SIGN.

> For patients with severe, disabling, medication-refractory essential tremor, surgery is a reasonable treatment option. Surgical management includes ablative therapy through stereotactic thalamotomy or chronic thalamic deep brain stimulation. The ventral intermediate nucleus of the thalamus is the best target for both ablative and deep brain stimulation surgeries. Contraindications for surgical management of essential tremor include unstable medical illnesses, swallowing difficulty, and marked cognitive problems.

260. Ans. (b) Temporal and parietal lobe

(Ref: Harrison 20th p 3108-09; Harrison 19th p 2597-98)

- AD most often presents with an insidious onset of memory loss followed by a slowly progressive dementia over several years.
- **Pathologically, atrophy is distributed throughout the medial temporal lobes, as well as lateral and medial parietal lobes and lateral frontal cortex.**
- The main purpose of imaging is to exclude other disorders, such as primary and secondary neoplasms, vascular dementia, diffuse white matter disease, and NPH; it also helps to distinguish AD from other degenerative disorders with distinctive imaging patterns such as FTD or CJD.
- **Functional imaging studies in AD reveal hypoperfusion or hypometabolism in the posterior temporal-parietal cortex.**

261. Ans. (a) Tolcapone

(Ref: Harrison 20th p 3128; Harrison 19th p 2615)

- Tolcapone has demonstrated significant hepatotoxicity that limits the drug's utility.
- This hepatoxicity can be attributed to elevated levels of transminases, but studies have shown that minimal risk exists for those without preexisting liver conditions when their enzyme levels were being monitored. No clear mechanism is implicated in Tolcapone induced liver toxicity, but it has been hypothesized that it has something to do with abnormal mitochondrial respiration due to the uncoupling of oxidative phosphorylation.
- Entacapone, another COMT inhibitor, is an alternative selection for L-DOPA adjunct therapy in the treatment of Parkinson's disease, largely since it has a more favorable toxicity profile.

262. Ans. (d) Trinucleotide repeat expansion

(Ref: Harrison 20th p 3136; Harrison 19th p 2621)

- Huntington's disease (HD) is caused by a mutation in the huntingtin gene, where excessive (more than 36) CAG repeats result in formation of a protein that is unstable. These expanded repeats lead to production of a huntingtin protein that contains an abnormally long poly-glutamine tract at the N-terminus.
- This makes it part of a class of neurodegenerative disorders known as trinucleotide repeat disorders or polyglutamine disorders. The key sequence which is found in Huntington's disease is a tri-nucleotide repeat expansion of glutamine residues beginning at the 18th amino acid. In unaffected individuals, this contains between 9 and 35 glutamine residues with no adverse effects. However, 36 or more residues produce an erroneous form of Htt, mHtt (standing for mutant Htt). Reduced penetrance is found in counts 36-39.

Classification of the trinucleotide repeat, and resulting disease status, depends on the number of CAG repeats

Repeat count	Classification	Disease status
<28	Normal	Unaffected
28–35	Intermediate	Unaffected
36–40	Reduced penetrance	+/- Affected
>40	Full penetrance	Affected

263. Ans. (d) Myxedema

(Ref: Harrison 20th p 152; Harrison 19th p 171)

Causes of Reversible dementia
1. Hypothyroidism
2. Thiamine deficiency
3. Vitamin B12 deficiency
4. Normal pressure Hydrocephalus
5. Subdural hematoma
6. Chronic infection
7. Brain abscess

264. Ans. (a) Parkinsonism

(Ref: Harrison 20th p 3127)

- Usage of Levodopa leads to on and off phenomenon.
- When levodopa starts acting the rigid akinetic wheelchair bound Parkinsonism patient will be in a position to get out of a chair and start pushing the wheelchair.
- When the effect weans off the same patient will be restricted to a wheelchair. This is called as wheel chair sign.

265. Ans. (a) Tau protein

(Ref: Harrison 20th p 3116; Harrison 19th p 175)

Protein Aggregations in major dementias and related cognitive disorders:

Disease	Protein
Alzheimer's disease	A-beta, Tau
Fronto temporal dementia, Pick's disease	Tau
Progressive supranuclear palsy	Tau
Corticobasal degeneration	Tau
Parkinson's disease	Alpha-synuclein
Multiple system atrophy	Alpha-synuclein
Huntington's disease	Huntingtin
Prion disease	Prion protein
Spinocerebellar ataxia	Ataxin

Facts to Remember:
- Pick's bodies contain Tau protein
- Lewy bodies contain α (alpha) synuclein

266. Ans. (a) Malignant melanoma

(Ref: 250 Cases in Clinical Medicine, RR Baliga;)

Levodopa has a causal relationship with malignant melanoma due to their shared dopamine biochemical pathway and is not recommended.

267. Ans. (b) Temporo-Parietal cortex

(Ref: Robbins 7th/138, Harrison 20th p 3108; Harrison 19th p 2599)

268. Ans. (c) Trisomy 21

(Ref: Harrison 20th p 3109; Harrison 19th p 2600-01)

269. Ans. (c) Acalculia

(Ref: Kaplan and Sadock's Synopsis of Psychiatry 10th (2007)/342; Harrison 19th p 2598-99

270. Ans. (d) Lewy bodies

(Ref: Harrison 20th p 3109; Harrison 19th p 2600)

271. Ans. (b) Past pointing

(Ref: Harrison 20th p 3121; Harrison 19th p Table 449-1, p 2609)

272. Ans. (c) Subthalamic nucleus

(Ref: Harrison 20th p 3129; Harrison 19th p 2616)

273. Ans. (c) Dopamine depletion

(Ref: Harrison 20th p 3136; Harrison 19th p 2621)

Huntington's disease has dopamine excess and is rather treated by a dopamine depleter by name of tetrabenazine.

274. Ans. (b) Progressive Supranuclear gaze palsy

Ref: Harrison 20th/p 3117; Harrison 19th p 2612

275. Ans. (d) Progressive supranuclear palsy

(Ref: Harrison 20th/p 3117; Harrison 19th p 2612)

276. Ans. (a) Tau protein

(Ref: Harrison 20th/p 3116; Harrison 19th p 175)

Brain Tumors

277. Ans. (d) Hemangioblastoma

Ref: Walsh and Hoyt Neuro-Ophthalmology, page 1396

- Intra-tumoral calcification develops in slow growing tumours like Craniopharyngioma, meningioma and Oligodendroglioma.
- Hemangioblastoma is a highly vascular tumour.

278. Ans. (a) Chordoma

Ref: Neurology image based review page 160; Harrison 19th edition, page 2264

- Thumb sign on CT head is seen in Chordoma.
- Sella Chordoma usually presents with bony clival erosion and local invasion.
- Calcification also occurs and mucinous material may be obtained by FNAC.

279. Ans. (c) Meningioma

(Ref: Harrison 20th p 648; Harrison: 19th edition, page 602)

- The CT scan shows a calcified lesion originating from falx cerebri. Also notice the tail like appearance of the dura matter superior to the ICSOL. The clinical diagnosis is meningioma.
- The tumor is causing a midline shift and raised ICP explaining the long history of headaches in this patient.
- Meningioma is the most common primary brain tumour constituting 35% of total brain tumour.

280. Ans. (a) Arachnoid cap cells

(Ref: Harrison 20th p 648; Harrison: 19th edition, page 602)

Meningiomas arise from the dura matter and are composed of neoplastic meningothelial cells called *arachnoid cap cells*. Meningiomas are most commonly located over the cerebral convexities adjacent to saggital sinus.

281. Ans. (b) Immunoblastic large cell lymphoma

(Ref: Harrison 20th p 647; Harrison 19th edition, page 601)

- Primary CNS lymphoma in *immuno-competent* patients is diffuse large B cell Lymphoma.
- Primary CNS lymphoma in *immune-deficient* patients like HIV infected or organ transplant recipients on immune-suppression is large cell with immunoblastic and more aggressive features.
- Immunoblastic lymphoma is one of 3 morphologic variants of diffuse large B cell lymphoma (DLBCL). The other 2 variants are centroblastic lymphoma and anaplastic B-cell lymphoma.

282. Ans. (d) Optic nerve glioma

(Ref: Harrison 20th p 189; Harrison 19th edition, page 206-7)

- The image shows a large retro-bulbar lesion indenting the eyeball on right side. This is a feature of optic nerve glioma and this explains the Marcus gunn pupil (Relative afferent pupillary defect).
- Rhabdomyosarcoma presents in first decade of life with proptosis and is hence a less likely diagnosis.
- Neuromyelitis optica will present with transverse myelitis leading to ascending paralysis and optic neuritis.

283. Ans. (b) PET Scan

(Ref: Imaging in clinical oncology 5th edition, page 140)

- Radiation necrosis in the brain commonly occurs in three distinct clinical scenarios, namely, radiation therapy for head and neck malignancy or intracranial extraaxial tumor, stereotactic radiation therapy (including radiosurgery) for brain metastasis, and radiation therapy for primary brain tumors.
- Conventional magnetic resonance (MR) imaging findings of these two entities overlap considerably, and even at histopathologic analysis, tumor mixed with radiation necrosis is a common finding. Advanced imaging modalities such as diffusion tensor imaging and perfusion MR imaging (with calculation of certain specific parameters such as apparent diffusion coefficient ratios, relative peak height, and percentage of signal recovery), MR spectroscopy, and positron emission tomography can be useful in differentiating between recurrent tumor and radiation necrosis.
- *In everyday practice, the visual assessment of diffusion-weighted and perfusion images is helpful by favoring one diagnosis over the other.*
- PET has several uses in the diagnosis of brain tumors. *PET can help distinguish between recurrent tumor and radiation necrosis, may differentiate low-grade lesions from high-grade lesions, and may guide stereotactic biopsy to the site of active or high-grade tumor within an apparently low-grade lesion seen on MRI.* FDG is the most commonly used isotope for evaluating brain tumors. The differential accumulation of this metabolite in brain tumor tissue compared with normal brain can provide information about tumor grade.

284. Ans. (b) Brainstem glioma

(Ref: OP. Ghai, 545, 7th ed)

- Brainstem glioma is an aggressive and dangerous cancer. Without treatment, the life expectancy is typically a few months from the time of diagnosis. With appropriate treatment, 37% survive more than one year, 20% survive 2 years and 13% survive 3 years.

- Diffuse intrinsic Pontine Glioma has a 10 percent survival rate. The median overall survival of children diagnosed with DIPG is approximately 9 months.

285. Ans. (a) Meningioma

(Ref: Neurooncology by Bernstein 2nd/254; Textbook of Medical oncology 2nd/493, Harrison 19th p 598)

Remember: Metastasis > Meningioma > Astrocytoma
Investigation of choice for brain tumour: Gadolinium-enhanced MRI.

286. Ans. (a) Astrocytomas

(Ref: Harrison 20th p 644; Harrison 19th p 599)

287. Ans. (b) Foramen of Munro

(Ref: Neurology in clinical practice 4th/1428)

288. Ans. (c) Hemangioblastoma

(Ref: Chandrasoma Taylor 2nd / 933)

289. Ans. (d) Craniopharyngioma

(Ref: Text book on Clinical and radiation Oncology, Harrison 19th p 603)

290. Ans. (c) Present in sellar or infra-sellar location

(Ref: Harrison 20th p 649; Harrison 19th p 603)

291. Ans. (b) Optic nerve glioma

(Ref: Rudolph's Pediatrics 21st/2399)

292. Ans. (b) Cerebellar hemangioblastomas

(Ref: Harrison 20th p 2155)

293. Ans. (c) Tolosa-Hunt syndrome

(Ref: 'Imaging of the Globe and Orbit: A Guide to Differential Diagnosis' by Norbert Hosten 1998/128)

CNS Infection and Prion Diseases

294. Ans. (d) Patent subarachnoid space

Ref: AACN Procedure Manual for critical care: E-Book, page 883
- The description given in the question is of Queckenstedt's maneuver.
- The pressure on the internal jugular veins will cause increased venous congestion in the brain. This leads to increase of ICP which is transmitted to the spinal canal in 5-10 seconds. It indicates a patent subarachnoid space.
- In the setting of spinal block, the pressure to the manometer attached to LP needle would not be transmitted.
- In the current scenario, imaging in form of MRI spine is used to identify spinal block.

295. Ans. (a) Brucellosis

Ref: Harrison 20th edition, page 1194
- Choice B leads to pertussis and Choice C leads to ulceroglandular fever and presence of eschar. Choice D presents as atypical pneumonia. Hence the answer by exclusion is brucellosis.
- Neurological involvement can occur in brucella with development of meningo-encephalitis. The main clue to the answer is however response to combination of doxycycline with rifampicin.
- The gold standard treatment for brucella is injectable streptomycin and doxycycline for 3 weeks. However the WHO regimen recommends doxycycline and Rifampicin.

296. Ans. (a) Coxsackie virus

(Ref: Harrison 20th p 1003; Harrison 19th edition, page 891 and 1291)
- The presence of normal glucose concentration in CSF rules out options B and C and points to viral etiology of meningitis.
- Lymphocytes are the predominant cell type seen in viral meningitis with cell counts in range of 25-500/μL.
- Cryptococcus neoformans meningitis shows mononuclear cells with normal cell count. Moreover it is seen in AIDS patient and in this question no such clinical information is given.

297. Ans. (a) Ceftriaxone

(Ref: Harrison 20th p 1002; Harrison 19th edition, page 1000)
- For suspected meningococcal disease, empirical antibiotic therapy in the form of third generation cephalosporin is recommended. The most commonly used drug is ceftriaxone or cefotaxime. The total duration of treatment is 7 days.
- Cultures become sterile within 24 hours of initiation of therapy. Role of glucocorticoids remains controversial.

Antibiotics used in empirical therapy of bacterial meningitis and focal central nervous system infections

Indication	Antibiotics
Immunocompetent children >3 months and adults <55	Cefotaxime, ceftriaxone, or cefepime + vancomycin
Adults > 55 and adults of any age with alcoholism or other debilitating illnesses	Ampicillin + cefotaxime, ceftriaxone or cefepime + vancomycin
Hospital - acquired meningitis, post-traumatic or postneurosurgery meningitis, neutropenic patients with impaired cell-mediated immunity	Ampicillin + ceftazidime or meropenem + vancomycin

298. Ans. (a) Draw blood culture sample, empirical ...

(Ref: Harrison 20th p 1000; Harrison 19th edition, page 443e)

The following sequence has been mentioned in Harrison for suspected bacterial meningitis patient.

1. Blood culture sample
2. Give empirical antibiotic
3. Perform neuroimaging in case of findings of raised ICP and focal deficit
4. Perform diagnostic Lumbar puncture

Remember that Complement fixation tests and rapid antigen detection tests are not altered by empirical antibiotics.

299. Ans. (c) Young adults exposed to tainted beef products

(Ref: Harrison 20th p 3151; Harrison 19th edition, page 453e)

Disease	Host	Mechanism of pathogenesis
Human		
Kuru	Fore people	Infection through ritualistic cannibalism
ICJD	Humans	Infection from prion-contaminated hGH, dura mater grafts, etc.
vCJD	Humans	Infection from bovine prions
fCJD	Humans	Germline mutations in PRNP
GSS	Humans	Germline mutations in PRNP
FFI	Humans	Germline mutations in PRNP (D178N, M129)
sCJD	Humans	Somatic mutation or spontaneous conversion of PrP^c into PrP^{sc}?

300. Ans. (b) Cerebral Toxoplasmosis

(Ref: Harrison 20th p 1445; Harrison 19th edition, page 1265)

- The NCCT Scan shows a space occupying lesion in basal ganglia adjacent to third ventricle. The clinical history of AIDS positive patient with seizures and CT scan favours diagnosis of CNS toxoplasmosis.
- Choice A is ruled out as it has multiple lesions spread all over the brain.
- Choice D is ruled out as there is no hydrocephalus.

Points differentiating Cerebral Toxoplasmosis from PCNSL

Features that favour cerebral toxoplasmosis include:	Features that favour primary CNS lymphoma include:
Multiple lesions	Single lesion
Scattered though basal ganglia and corticomedullary junction	Subependymal spread
Ring or nodular enhancement	Solid enhancement
Haemorrhage occasionally occurs mostly in periphery of lesion	No haemorrhage before treatment
Thallium SPECT negative	Thallium SPECT positive

301. Ans. (c) Prion disease

(Ref: Harrison 20th p 3152; Harrison 19th edition, page 453 e-4)

- Prion disease leads to neurodegeneration and presents as myoclonus with cognitive decline. Startle myoclonus is triggered by loud sounds and bright lights.
- Choice A is seen in age group of 10-20 years with early morning myoclonic jerks and EEG finding of 4-6 Hz Poly-spikes.
- Choice B will present with hallucinations, delusions and dementia.
- Choice D presents with orthostatic hypotension with either Parkinsonism or cerebellar features.

302. Ans. (a) Ibuprofen

(Ref: Harrison 20th p 1010; Harrison 19th edition, page 909)

- Drug hypersensitivity is incriminated in causing chronic meningitis
- CSF shows mononuclear cells or eosinophils
- CBC shows eosinophilia

Drugs incriminated are:

• NSAIDS	• Penicillin
• Sulfonamides	• Lamotrigine
• INH	• OKT 3 antibodies
• Ciprofloxacin	• IV immunoglobulins

303. Ans. (a) Pneumococcal meningitis

(Ref: Harrison 20th p 1068; Harrison 19th edition, page 885, 888)

- Since the patient is on immunosuppressive regimen, the CMI of the patient is depressed. The altered sensorium of patient has necessitated performing a lumbar puncture.
- The presence of neutrophils indicates a bacterial infection. India ink preparation slide also shows capsulated diploccoci. Hence answer is A.
- Cryptococcal infection has CSF picture of lymphocytosis with capsulated organisms in India ink as budding yeast cells (red mark – refer table below).

India ink preparations

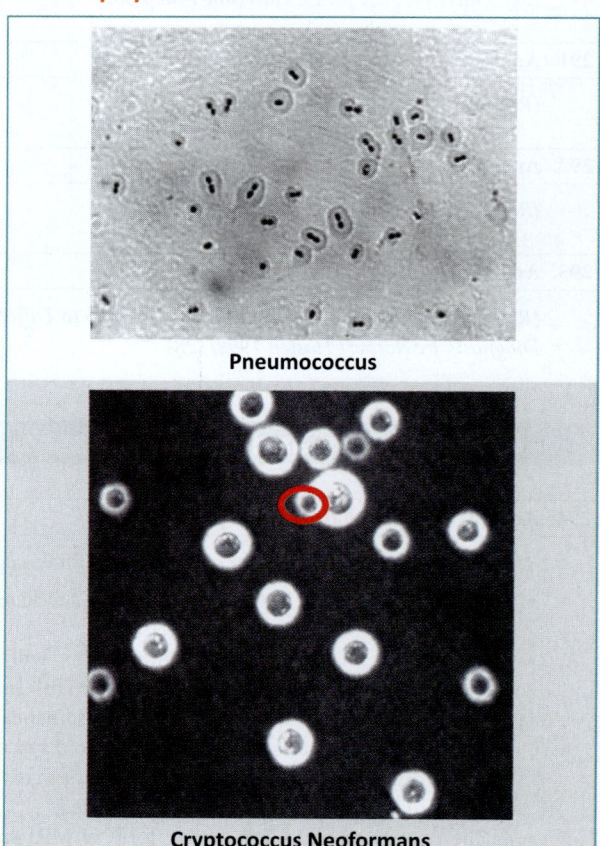

Pneumococcus

Cryptococcus Neoformans

304. Ans. (d) Needle inserted at L1-L2 space

(Ref: Harrison 20th p 59; Harrison 19th edition, page 443 e2)

- The position of the patient for lumbar puncture is essential. The patient is asked to lie on the edge of the bed and asked to roll up into a ball.
- The neck is gently anteflexed and thighs pulled up towards the abdomen. Shoulders and pelvis should be vertically aligned.
- The spinal cord ends at L1 in 94% of individuals and remaining 6%, conus medullaris extends to the L2-L3 interspace.
- *Hence LP is permitted at L3-L4 interspace or below.* The anatomical guide is a line joining the posterior superior iliac crests.
- The needle is inserted 10 degrees cephalad with bevel facing upwards. This way the cutting edge of the needle is parallel to the fibers of dura matter.
- The needle used is typically 20-22 gauge and should be inserted in midline with bevel facing pointed upward. This will minimise the injury to the fibres as the dura is penetrated. The pop sound on entry in subarachnoid space is felt and CSF is allowed to drip into the testing tubes.
- To record the pressure a manometer with 3 way stop cock is attached. The assistant can help the patient extend his legs and gently return the neck back to neutral position. The reading on manometer can be checked and variation of pressure with respiration noted.

305. Ans. (c) Demonstration of antibodies to cysticerci in serum by enzyme linked immune-electroblot

(Ref: Harrison 20th p 1643; Harrison: 19th edition, page 1431-32)

TABLE: Diagnostic criteria for Human Cysticercosis

1. Absolute criteria
   a. Demonstration of cysticerci by histologic or microscopic exmination of biopsy material
   b. Visualizationof the parasite in the eye by funduscopy
   c. Neuroradiologic demonstration of cystic lesions containing a charcteristic scolex

2. Major criteria
   a. Neuroradiologic lesions suggestive of neurocysticercosis
   b. Demonstration of antibodies to cysticerci in serum by enzyme-linked immunoelectrotransfer blot
   c. Resolution of intracranial cystic lesions spontaneously or after therapy with albendazole or praziquantel alone

3. Minor criteria
   a. Lesions compatible with neurocysticercosis detected by neuroimaging studies
   b. Clinical manifestations suggestive of neurocysticercosis
   c. Demonstration of antibodies to cysticerici or cysticercal antigen in cerebrospinal fluid by ELISA
   d. Evidence of cysticercosis outside the central nervous system (e.g., cigar-shaped soft-tissue calcifications)

306. Ans. (a) LP needle

The image shows presence of lumbar puncture needle with sharp cutting edge and hub at back which indicates the CSF.

The stylet is gradually withdrawn to collect CSF for cytology and biochemistry.

Pleural tap needle
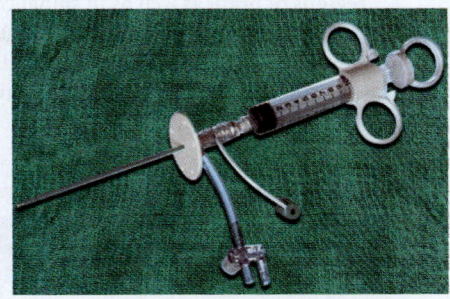

Liver biopsy needle
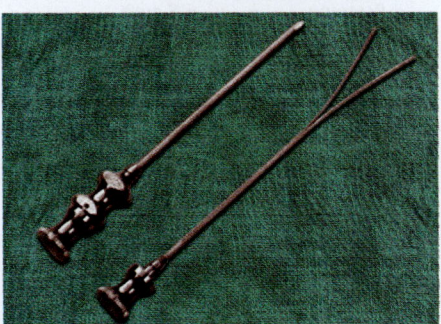

Bone marrow aspiration needle
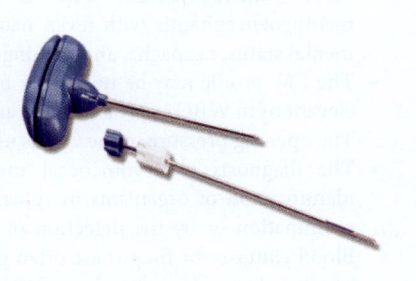

307. Ans. (b) Human T-cell Lymphotropic Virus

(Ref: Harrison 20th p 3179; 225e: section 14: Harrison 19th edition)

Tropical Spastic Paraparesis/HTLV-I-associated myelopathy (HAM)

- Caused by retro-virus HTLV-1
- Characterized by symmetric degeneration of lateral columns of spinal cord, including corticospinal tracts; an inflammatory infiltrate in the spinal meninges & cord parenchyma with myelin destruction.
- Occurs after a **shorter latency (1-3 years)** following HTLV infection and is most common in individuals who acquire the virus during adulthood from transfusion or sexual intercourse.
- **Clinical features:**
  1. Weakness or stiffness in one or both legs (spastic paraparesis or paraplegia with hyperreflexia, ankle clonus& extensor plantar responses)
  2. Back pain
  3. Urinary incontinence
  4. Mild sensory changes
  5. Peripheral neuropathy
  6. Cognitive function is usually spared

Investigations:
1. **MRI reveals lesions in white matter & paraventricular regions of brain as well as in spinal cord.**
2. **Antibodies to HTLV-I** are present in the serum and appear to be produced in the CSF of HAM patients, where titers are often higher than in the serum

308. Ans. (b) Chloride

(Ref: CSF in clinical practice 2nd edition page 149)

	Blood value	CSF value
Glucose	Fasting < 100mg%	2/3 (blood value)
Protein	6-8 gm%	15-45 mg%
Calcium	9-11mg%	2.3-3.2 mg%
Chloride	96 -106 meq/dl	120 meq/dl

309. Ans. (d) Cryptococcus meningitis

(Ref: Harrison 20th p 1443)

- *C. neoformans* is the leading infectious cause of meningitis in patients with AIDS
- It is the initial AIDS-defining illness in <2% of patients and generally occurs in patients with CD4+ T cell counts <100/μL
- Most patients present with a picture of subacute meningoencephalitis with fever, nausea, vomiting, altered mental status, headache, and meningeal signs.
- The CSF profile may be normal or may show only modest elevations in WBC or protein levels and decrease in glucose. The opening pressure in the CSF is usually elevated.
- The diagnosis of cryptococcal meningitis is made by identification of organisms in spinal fluid with India ink examination or by the detection of cryptococcal antigen. Blood cultures for fungus are often positive. A biopsy may be needed to make a diagnosis of CNS cryptococcoma.
- The prostate gland may serve as a reservoir for smoldering cryptococcal infection.
- Treatment is with IV amphotericin B 0.7 mg/kg daily, or liposomal amphotericin 4–6 mg/kg daily, with flucytosine 25 mg/kg qid for at least 2 weeks and, if possible, until the CSF culture turns negative. This is followed by fluconazole 400 mg/d PO for 8 weeks, and then fluconazole 200 mg/d until the CD4+ T cell count has increased to >200 cells/uL for 6 months in response to cART.

310. Ans. (a) Ampicillin

(Ref: Harrison 20th p 1102; Harrison 19th edition, page 983)

311. Ans. (b) Viral meningitis

(Ref: Harrison 20th p 1003; Harrison 19th ed. / 890)

- The key word in the diagnosis of patient is **lymphocytic pleocytosis**. Pleocytosis means a dimorphic cell population where first neutrophils and later lymphocytes are predominant".
- Harrison states clearly that "As a rule, a lymphocytic pleocytosis with a low glucose concentration should suggest fungal or tuberculous meningitis, or noninfectious disorders (e.g., sarcoid, neoplastic meningitis)". Where as in this question CSF sugar is normal. Hence the answer is viral meningitis.
- In contrast viral meningitis has the following features" The most important laboratory test in the diagnosis of viral meningitis is examination of the CSF. The typical profile is a lymphocytic pleocytosis (25–500 cells/L), a normal protein concentration (20–80 mg/dL), a normal glucose concentration, and a normal or mildly elevated opening pressure (100–350 mmH$_2$O).

CSF	Normal	Acute bacterial meningitis	Tubercular meningitis	Viral meningitis	Guillain–Barre syndrome	Fungal meningitis
Pressure	50 – 180 mmH$_2$O	Increased	Increased	Increased	Normal	Elevated
Color	Clear	**Turbid**	Straw	**Clear**	Normal	Clear
Cells	0-4 lymphocytes/ cu.mm	>1000 Neutrophils/ cu.mm	>100 Lymphocytes/ cu.mm	>25 Lymphocytes/ cu.mm	Normal	25-500 Lymphocytes/ cu.mm
Sugar	2/3rd of blood sugar	Decreased	Decreased	Normal	Normal	Low
Protein	15-45 mg %	Increased	Increased	Increased	Increased (albumin-cytological disassociation)	Normal/elevated

312. Ans. (d) Cerebrospinal fluid reveals a low leukocyte count.

(Ref: Harrison 20th p 1006; Harrison 19th ed. / 898-99)

Refer to above table
- Tubercular meningitis is seen most often in young children but also develops in adults, especially those infected with HIV.
- Tubercular meningitis results from the hematogenous spread of primary or post primary pulmonary TB.
- The disease often presents subtly as headache and slight mental changes after a prodrome of weeks of low-grade fever, malaise, anorexia, and irritability.

- *In general, examination of cerebrospinal fluid (CSF) reveals a high leukocyte count (up to 1000/µL), usually with a predominance of lymphocytes but sometimes with a predominance of neutrophils in the early stage; a protein content of 1–8 g/L (100–800 mg/dL); and a low glucose concentration.*
- Culture of CSF is diagnostic in up to 80% of cases and remains the gold standard. Polymerase chain reaction has a sensitivity of up to 80%, but rates of false-positivity reach 10%.
- Imaging studies (CT and MRI) may show hydrocephalus and abnormal enhancement of basal cisterns or ependyma.

313. Ans. (d) ELISA CSF for NCC is the investigation of choice

(Ref: Harrison 20th p 1643)

CSF findings include the following:
- Mononuclear pleocytosis
- Normal or low glucose levels
- Elevated protein levels
- High IgG index
- Oligoclonal bands, in some cases
- Eosinophilia (5-500 cells/µL); however, this also occurs in neurosyphilis and CNS tuberculosis
- *CSF ELISA for neurocysticercosis only has a sensitivity of 50% and a specificity of 65%.*
- MRI is the imaging modality of choice for neurocysticercosis, especially for evaluation of intraventricular and cisternal/subarachnoidal cysts. Findings on MRI include the following:

1. Vesicular stage: Cysts follow the CSF signal; T2 hyperintense scolex may be seen, with no edema and usually no enhancement.
2. Colloidal stage: Cysts are hyperintense to the CSF; there is surrounding edema, and the cyst wall enhances.
3. Nodular-granular stage: The cyst wall thickens and retracts, there is a decrease in edema, and nodular or ring enhancement is present.

314. Ans. (b) Ibuprofen

(Ref: Dubois hand book of Lupus, 7th edition, page 1150)

Ibuprofen is a common non-steroidal anti-inflammatory drug that is the most frequent cause of aseptic meningitis induced by drugs.

Medications Known to cause aseptic meningitis		
Medications	**Common**	**Uncommon**
NSAIDs	Ibuprofen	Sulindac Naproxen Diclofenac Rofecoxib
Antimicrobials	Trimethoprim/sulfamethoxazole	Sulfonamides
Immunomodulating agents	Monoclonal antibody OKT3 Intravenous IgG	Azathioprine

Causes of Acute Aseptic Meningitis	
Infectious cases	
Bacterial	Lyme disease Leptospirosis Mycobacterium tuberculosis infection Subacute bacterial endocarditis Parameningeal infection (epidural subdural abcess, sinus or ear infection) Partially treated bacterial meningitis
Viral	Echovirus infection Coxsackie virus infection Mumps Herpes simplex virus type 2 infection HIV infection Lymphocytic choriomeningitis Poliovirus infection

315. Ans. (d) Occipital neuralgia

(Ref: Essentials of Pain Medicine, 3rd edition, Page 290.)

- Occipital neuralgia is seen with:
  1. Temporal arteritis
  2. Neuro-syphilis
  3. Vascular compression
  4. Herpetic neuralgia(Varicella Zoster)
  5. Arthrosis of the C1-2 facet joint and scarring from previous surgeries in the area.

Herpes simplex virus causes viral encephalitis with predilection for temporal lobe.

316. Ans. (d) Palatal myoclonus

(Ref: Harrison 20th p 1355; Harrison 19th p 2648)

- *The symptoms and signs of Ramsay Hunt Syndrome include acute facial nerve paralysis, pain in the ear, taste loss in the front two-thirds of the tongue, dry mouth and eyes, and eruption of an erythematous vesicular rash in the ear canal, the tongue, and/or hard palate.*
- *Since the vestibulocochlear nerve is in proximity to the geniculate ganglion, it may also be affected, and patients may also suffer from tinnitus, hearing loss, and vertigo.*
- Patients lose their sense of taste in the anterior two-thirds of the tongue while developing ipsilateral facial palsy. The geniculate ganglion of the sensory branch of the facial nerve is involved.
- Possible involvement of the trigeminal nerve can cause anesthesia of the face.
- Palatal myoclonus is a rapid spasm of the palatal muscles, which results in clicking or popping in the ear. It is often due to lesions of the central tegmental tract (which connects the red nucleus to the ipsilateral inferior olivary nucleus) and the clicking noise does not subside when the patient sleeps.

317. Ans. (d) Reactivation of HSV-1

(Ref: Harrison 20th p 1345; Harrison 19th p 1177)

- Fever blisters are Grouped vesicles and erosions over the angle of the mouth -recurrent herpes labialis caused by HSV 1.
- HSV 1 is generally associated with orofacial infections.

- HSV 2 is associated with genital infections.
- Grouped umbilicated vesicles are hallmark of HSV infections.
- After the primary infection, the virus becomes established in a nerve ganglion (latent infection).
- The secondary phase is characterised by recurrent disease at the same site.

Recurrent HSV infections:
- Herpes facialis or labialis
- Herpes genitalis
- Kaposi's varicelliform eruption (eczema herpeticum)
- Herpetic whitlow
- Keratoconjuctivitis

318. Ans. (b) Ceftriaxone + Metronidazole

(Ref: Harrison 20th p 1015; Harrison 19th p 1097-98)

Brain Abscess
- Empirical therapy of community-acquired brain abscess in an immune-competent patient typically includes a third- or fourth-generation cephalosporin (e.g., cefotaxime, ceftriaxone, or cefepime) and metronidazole.
- In immune-competent individuals the most important pathogens are Streptococcus spp. [anaerobic, aerobic, and viridans (40%)], Enterobacteriaceae[Proteus spp., E. coli sp., Klebsiella spp. (25%)], anaerobes [e.g., Bacteroides, Fusobacterium(30%)], and staphylococci (10%).
- Optimal therapy of brain abscesses involves a combination of high-dose parenteral antibiotics and neurosurgical drainage.
- Aspiration and drainage of the abscess under stereotactic guidance are beneficial for both diagnosis and therapy. Complete excision of a bacterial abscess via craniotomy or craniectomy is generally reserved for multi-loculated abscesses or those in which stereotactic aspiration is unsuccessful.

319. Ans. (c) CSF examination

(Ref: OP Ghai 7th ed)

Clinically the reasons for patient deterioration can be:
1. Hyponatremia due to SIADH
2. Hydrocephalus → can be evaluated by CT
3. End arteritis/ brain infarction → can be evaluated by MRI
4. TB encephalopathy
5. Hemorrhagic -Leukencephalopathy
6. Ventriculitis/arachnoiditis
7. Iatrogenic drug induced hepatitis → can be evaluated with LFT
   - The CSF of patients with treated TB meningitis is commonly abnormal even at 12 months the rate of resolution of the abnormality bears no correlation with clinical progress or outcome, and is not an indication for extending or repeating treatment; repeated sampling of CSF by lumbar puncture to monitor treatment progress should therefore not be done.
   - In TBM, despite adequate treatment of hydrocephalus and various other complications, patients commonly fail to improve. This poor outcome is often associated with the extensive tuberculous exudate in the subarachnoid cisterns of the brain, which affects cerebral vessels and induces ischemia. Hence, treatment modalities should include optimizing physiological variables to preserve cerebral perfusion.

Therefore the following logical conclusion can be:
1. **ALTERED SENSORIUM** due to Hepatic encephalopathy secondary to hepatotoxicity of ATT. Hence LFT should be performed.
2. **ALTERED SENSORIUM** due to **Obstructive hydrocephalus** could lead to raised ICT leading to pressure on midbrain and resultant status. Therefore a MRI scan can identify the process and necessitate a neurosurgical consult.
3. **ALTERED SENSORIUM** due to **end-arteritis resulting in brain infarction** and hypo-dense lesions. **Tubercular encephalopathy** results in diffuse edema of brain simulating post -infective allergic encephalopathy. **Necrotizing or hemorrhagic leukoencephalopathy** may occur in TB meningitis. . In choice NCCT is given and it can identify infarction as well cerebral Edema.

320. Ans. (a) Long incubation period

(Ref: Harrison 20th p 3149; Harrison 19th p 453e-1)

- Patients who received injections of human growth hormone **developed CJD from injections of prion contaminated prepara-tions of human growth hormone, the possible incubation periods range from 4 to 30 years.**
- Prions are extremely resistant to common inactivation procedures. Autoclaving at 134°C for 5 h or treatment with 2 NNaOH for several hours is recommended for sterilization of prions. The term sterilization implies complete destruction of prions; any residual infectivity can be hazardous.
- *sCJD (sporadic CJD) prions bound to stainless steel surfaces are resistant to inactivation by autoclaving at 134°C for 2 h; exposure of bound prions to an acidic detergent solution prior to autoclaving rendered prions susceptible to inactivation.*
- *Prions are the only known infectious pathogens that are devoid of nucleic acid; all other infectious agents possess genomes composed of either RNA or DNA that direct the synthesis of their progeny.*
- Hallmark of all prion diseases, whether sporadic, dominantly inherited, or acquired by infection, is that they **involve the aberrant metabolism of PrP. This abnormal protein in cytoplasm of neuron hijacks the control centre of the neuron and results in dysfunction.**

321. Ans. (b) Acyclovir

(Ref: Harrison 20th p 1352; Harrison 19th p 896)

- Acyclovir is of benefit in the treatment of HSV and should be started empirically in patients with suspected viral encephalitis, especially if focal features are present, while awaiting viral diagnostic studies.
- Patients with encephalitis may have hallucinations, agitation, personality change, behavioral disorders, and, at times, a frankly psychotic state. Focal or generalized seizures occur in many patients with encephalitis.

- Acyclovir acts as an antiviral agent by inhibiting viral DNA polymerase and by causing premature termination of nascent viral DNA chains

Algorithm for patient with CNS infection

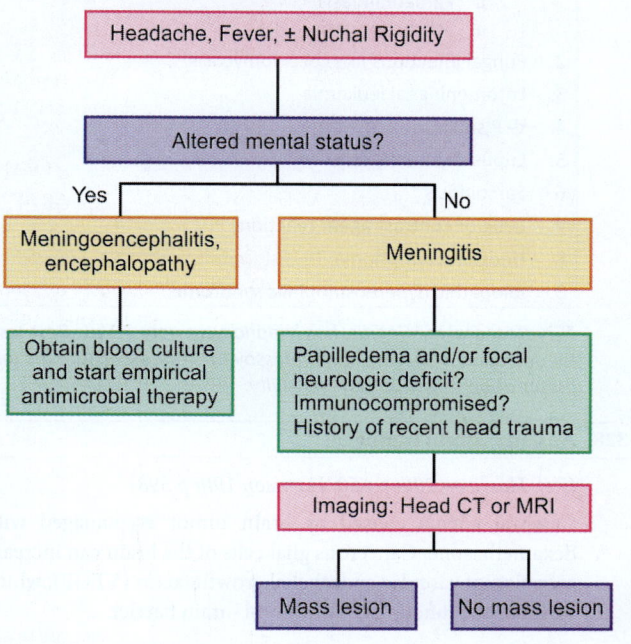

322. Ans. (a) Cingulate gyrus

(Ref: Harrison 20th p 1443; Harrison 19th p 1264-65)

- HIV causes subcortical dementia and basal ganglia involvement is seen. Cerebral white matter involvement is also mentioned in Harrison's. Hence by exclusion the Ans: A.
- AIDS related dementia causes psychomotor slowing, apathy, bradykinesia and altered posture and gait similar to those observed in advanced Parkinson's disease. The dementia has the hallmarks attributed to subcortical dementia. The exquisite sensitivity of many of these patients to dopamine receptor blockade suggested a profound and, perhaps, selective abnormality of striatal dopaminergic systems.
- Patients with HIV encephalopathy may also have motor and behavioral abnormalities. *The motor problems are unsteady gait, poor balance, tremor, and difficulty with rapid alternating movements. Increased tone and deep tendon reflexes may be found in patients with spinal cord involvement. Late stages may be complicated by bowel and/or bladder incontinence.*

323. Ans. (b) Tabes dorsalis

(Ref: Harrison 20th p 1283; ch. 169, Harrison 19th p 1136, 1138)

- Locomotor ataxia is the inability to precisely control one's own bodily movements. Persons afflicted with this disease may walk in a jerky, nonfluid manner. They will not know where their arms and legs are without looking, but can, for instance, feel and locate a hot object placed against their feet. It is often a symptom of tabes dorsalis, which is a key finding in tertiary syphilis.

- General paresis of insanity presents with delusions of grandeur etc. Symptoms of the disease first appear from 10 to 30 years after infection. Typical symptoms include loss of social inhibitions, asocial behavior, gradual impairment of judgment, concentration and short-term memory, euphoria, mania, depression, or apathy. Subtle shivering, minor defects in speech and Argyll Robertson pupil may become noticeable. Delusions, which are common, tend to be poorly systematized and absurd. They can be grandiose, melancholic, or paranoid.
- Meningovascular syphilis presents as a gumma causing bulbar or pseudo-bulbar palsy.
- Syphilitic amyotrophy presents with painless and progressive weakness.

324. Ans. (b) Hodgkins lymphoma (HL)

(Ref: 495.2 Nelson Acute leukemia and 496.2)

- CNS Leukaemia is a known manifestation of ALL. Thus intra-thecal methotrexate is given in ALL along with CNS radiation. Samples are also sent for CSF cytology to evaluate for CNS relapse while intra-thecal Methotrexate is being given.
- NHL spreads hematogenously to cause meningeal seeding and so does AML albeit the incidence for AML being less than 5%.
- Chloromas in AML involve the orbit and epidural space. CNS symptoms are more common in AML than ALL

325. Ans. (c) Pyogenic meningitis

(Ref: Harrison 20th p 1000; Harrison 19th p 888)

Data provided in question		Interpretation
CSF cytology	300 cells/cu mm	In bacterial meningitis counts are > 1000 cells/cu.mm.
CSF protein	70mg%	In favour of bacterial as well as viral encephalitis
CSF sugar	60 mg% against a blood glucose of 95mg%	Normally CSF sugar is 2/3 rd of blood sugar which means that a value of blood sugar of 95mg%, normal CSF sugar would be 63.3 mg%. Hence the value of 54% given in the question is less than the normal value
CSF / serum glucose ratio	60/95 = 0.63	In bacterial meningitis it should be less than 0.4.
CSF cells	65% polymorpho-nuclear cells	In favour of bacterial meningitis. Harrison states in viral encephalitis persisting CSF neutrophilia should prompt consideration of bacterial infection, leptospirosis, amebic infection, and noninfectious processes such as acute hemorrhagic leukoencephalitis

Contd...

Data provided in question		Interpretation
Clinical data	Short duration fever with subsequent development of seizures and nuchal rigidity satisfying the clinical triad for meningitis of bacterial etiology	Cerebral malaria –CSF is normal TBM- long duration with cob web coagulum with straw CSF, low sugar with protein upto 1-2 g% Viral encephalitis- due to irritation of brain parenchyma leading to patient with encephalitis commonly has an altered level of consciousness or a depressed level of consciousness to coma, and evidence of either focal or diffuse neurologic signs and symptoms. Patients with encephalitis may have hallucinations, agitation, personality change, behavioral disorders, and, at times, a frankly psychotic state. Focal or generalized seizures occur in many patients with encephalitis

* In lieu of low CSF sugar and predominant neutrophil population in CSF, Pyogenic meningitis is the diagnosis.

326. Ans. (c) LDH and CK

(Ref: Textbook of Medical Biochemistry by Chatter jee: 8th ed., pg. 730)

Various CSF enzymes have been investigated in CNS disorders

> (a) Creatine kinase
> - Normal <5 units/L
> - Increase up to ten times of normal are found due to release of the enzyme from damaged brain tissue when there has been an anoxic insult.
>
> (b) Lactate Dehydrogenase (LDH)
> - Normal CSF LDH is 5 to 40 U/L. Similar to AST, increase of CSF LDH observed in abscess, cerebral haemorrhage/ infarction and metastatic carcinoma.
> - LDH isoenzyme pattern is similar to serum. Increase of LDH4 isoenzyme of CSF has been reported in tubercular meningitis.

327. Ans. (b) Cryptococcal meningitis

(Ref: Nelson 20th p 2984)

CSF eosinophilia is defined as more than 10 eosinophils/cu.mm of CSF. The most common cause of CSF eosinophilia is parasitic infections enumerated below.

> 1. Helminthic infections
>   a. Nematode:
>   i. Angiostrongyliasis
>   ii. Gnathostomiasis
>   iii. Strongyloidiasis
>   iv. Toxocariasis
>   v. Trichinosis
>   b. Cestodes
>   i. Cysticercosis
>   ii. Echinococcosis
>   c. Trematodes
>   i. Paragonimiasis
>   ii. Schistosomiasis
> 2. Fungal infections like coccidomycosis
> 3. Letomeningeal leukemia
> 4. V- P shunts
> 5. Lupus erythematosis
> 6. Sarcoidosis
> 7. Drug or contrast agent reactions
> 8. Hodgkin's lymphoma
> 9. Idiopathic hypereosinophilic syndrome

*Cryptococcal meningitis, has lymphocytes upto 20/μL. Best test for detection is enzyme immunoassay for cryptococcus. India ink preparation shows 25-50% sensivity.

328. Ans. (d) Brain tumor

(Ref: Harrison 20th p 650; Harrison 19th p 598)

Cerebral edema caused by brain tumor is managed with dexamethasone. Cancerous glial cells of the brain can increase secretion of vascular endothelial growth factor (VEGF), which weakens the junctions of the blood–brain barrier.

329. Ans. (a) Albendazole 15 mg/kg/day for 8 days

(Ref: Harrison 20th p 1015)

- Albendazole is initially administered at doses of 15 mg/kg/d for 8 days. It can be taken with fatty meal to improve absorption. Use of steroids ameliorates the host response to dying parasite.
- An advantage of albendazole over praziquantel is that the former also destroys subarachnoid and ventricular cysts due to its better penetrance in the CSF.
- However, it seems that patients with subarachnoid cysts may need prolonged courses of albendazole (up to 1 month).
- Praziquantel is most often used at doses of 50 mg/kg/d for 15 days, but recommended dosages have ranged from 10 to 100 mg/kg for 3 to 21 days.

330. Ans. (c) Kuru

(Ref: Harrison 20th p 3044; Harrison 19th p 455e)

Kuru is an incurable degenerative neurological disorder endemic to tribal regions of Papua New Guinea. It is a type of transmissible spongiform encephalopathy, caused by a prion found in humans due to cannibalistic behavior.

331. Ans. (b) 2/3 plasma glucose

(Ref: Harrison 20th p 1000; Harrison 19th p 888)

332. Ans. (a) Pleocytosis, high protein, reduced sugar

(Ref: Harrison 20th p 1000; Harrison 19th p 888)

The classic CSF abnormalities in bacterial meningitis are:
- Elevated opening pressure (> 180 mm H2O in 90%)
- Polymorphonuclear leukocytosis (> 100 cells/μL in 90%)

Contd...

- Decreased glucose concentration (< 2.2 mmol/L or < 40 mg/dL and/or CSF/serum glucose ratio of < 0.4 in ~ 60%)
- Elevated protein concentration (> 45 mg/dL)

333. Ans. (d) Vancomycin+ceftriaxone

(Ref: Harrison 20th p 1000; Harrison's 19th ed. p 884)

- As a result of increased prevalence of resistant pneumococci, first line therapy for persons more than 1 month of age is a combination of Vancomycin and Cefotaxime/ ceftriaxome.
- If children are hypersensitive to beta lactam antibiotics, Rifampicin can be substituted for cefotaxime/ceftriaxone.
- A lumbar puncture must be considered after 48 hours if the organism is not susceptible to penicillin and information on cephalosporin sensitivity is not yet available, if the patient's clinical condition does not improve or deteriorates or if dexamethasone has been administered and may be compromising clinical evaluation.

334. Ans. (b) Dystrophinopathy

(Ref: Harrison 20th p 3247; Harrison 19th p 462e)

Caplain, Sarcoglycans (α, β and λ) and Dysferelin examples of defective gene/locus in Limb girdle dystrophies. Dystrophin is associated with Duchenne's and Becker type of muscular dystrophies and is not associated with Limb girdle dystrophies.

Limb -Girdle muscular dystrophy

- These are also called autosomal muscular dystrophies as these are caused due to defect in autosomes (the other muscular dystrophies i.e. duchenne and becker are x-linked).
- They are inherited in either an autosomal dominant (type I) or an autosomal recessive (type 2) pattern.
- Six subtypes of the dominant dystrophies (1A to 1F) and ten subtypes of the recessive limb girdle dystrophies (2A to 21) have been identified.
- They usually affect proximal musculature of the trunk and limbs.
- Mutation of the sarcoglycan complex of proteins have been identified in four of the limb girdle muscular dystrophies.

Disease	Clinical Features	LOCUS or Gene
LGMD1A	Onset 3rd to 4th decade Muscle weakness affects distal limb muscles, vocal cords, and pharyngeal muscles	Myotilin
LGMD1B	Onset 1st or 2nd decade Proximal lower limb weakness and cardiomyopathy with conduction defects.	Lamin A/C
LGMD1C	Onset in early childhood Proximal weakness Gowers' sign, calf hypertrophy	Caveolin-3
LGMD1D	Onset 3rd to 5th decade Proximal muscle weakness Cardiomyopathy and arrhythmias	Linked to chromosome 7q Gene unidentified
LGMD1E	Childhood onset Proximal muscle weakness EMG myopathic	Linked to chromosome 6q23 Gene unidentified

Contd...

Autosomal recessive Limb girdle muscular dystrophy		
LGMD2A	Onset 1st or 2nd decade Tight heel cords, Contractures at elbows, wrists, and fingers.	Calpain-3
LGMD2B	Onset 2d or 3d decade Proximal muscle weakness at onset, later distal (calf) muscles.	Dysferlin
LGMD2C-F	Onset in childhood to teenage years Clinical condition similar to Duchenne and Becker muscular dystrophies	Sarcoglycans γ, α, β,δ
LGMD2G	Onset age 10 to 15 Proximal and distal muscle weakness	Telethonin
LGMD2H	Onset 1st to 3d decade Proximal muscle weakness	TRIM32 gene
LGMD2I	Onset 1st to 3d decade Clinical condition similar to Duchenne or Becker dystrophies.	Fukutin-related protein
LGMD2J	Onset 1st to 3d decade Proximal lower limb weakness Mild distal weakness.	Titin

335. Ans. (c) Raised chloride

(Ref: Harrison's 19th p 904)

CSF chloride content is higher than blood chloride levels. In bacterial meningitis, CSF chloride is reduced.

336. Ans. (a) Increased protein, decreased sugar, increased Lymphocytes

(Ref: Harrison 20th p 1006; Harrison 19th p 888)

337. Ans. (a) Exudate seen in basal cisterns

(Ref: Cranial MRI & CT, Lee Rao & Zimmer Man – 4th/ 479)

338. Ans. (b) Pleocytosis with high protein and low sugar

(Ref: Harrison 20th p 1000; Harrison 19th p 888)

339. Ans. (b) Amphotericin B

(Ref: Harrison 20th p 1444; Harrison 19th p 899)

340. Ans. (c) Streptococcus pneumoniae

(Ref: Harrison 20th p 1016; Harrison 19th p 903)

Subdural empyema accounts for 15-25% of focal suppurative CNS infections. Sunusits is the most common predisposing condition. Aerobic and anaerobic streptococci are most common causative organism.

341. Ans. (a) Herpes simplex virus type 2

(Ref: Harrison 19th p 890)

342. Ans. (d) Enterovirus

(Ref: Harrison 20th p 2946; Nelson's 18th/2521)

343. Ans. (b) Herpes simplex encephalitis

(Ref: Harrison 20th p 993; Harrison 19th p 893, 895)

344. Ans. (a) Acyclovir

(Ref: Harrison 20th p 995; Harrison 19th p 896)

345. Ans. (a) They are infectious proteins

(Ref: Harrison 20th p 3149; Ananthnarayanan 7th/567; Jawetz 24th/581)

Prions are infectious proteins devoid of any nucleic acid.

346. Ans. (d) Alzheimer's disease

(Ref: Harrison 20th p 3149)

347. Ans. (c) Myoclonus is rarely seen

(Ref: Harrison 20th p 3152)

Guillain Barre Syndrome, Neuropathy and Myopathy

348. Ans. (b) G.B.S

(Ref: Harrison 20th edition, page 3225)

- Choice A is ruled out as it presents with descending paralysis.
- Ascending paralysis, areflexia and sphincter sparing is feature of GBS
- Snake bite will have autonomic features and is unlikely that patient does not feel the pain
- Polio is ruled out as it has descending paralysis.

349. Ans. (c) Serum potassium

(Ref: Harrison 20th p 138; Harrison 19th edition, page 307)

- Potassium deficit leads to hyperpolarization of skeletal muscle and thus impairs the capacity to depolarise and contract the skeletal muscle. This can present as weakness and lead to paralysis. Hypokalemia also leads to periodic paralysis.
- The first impression on reading the question is of GBS which presents with "rubbery legs" and ascending paralysis.
- Calcium and magnesium deficit lead to tetany and are easily ruled out.
- Sodium deficit will lead to altered sensorium and seizures.

Severe hyperphosphatemia can also mimic GBS presentation.

350. Ans. (c) Acute intermittent porphyria

Ref: (Harrison 20th p 2990; Harrison 19th edition, page 2526)

- Conversion disorder/ functional neurological symptom disorder is used to specify individuals whose somatic complaints involve one or more symptoms of altered voluntary or sensory functions that cannot be medically explained. However it cannot be taken as first diagnosis
- AIDP leads to ascending symmetrical flaccid paralysis (progression < 4weeks) but does not present with recurrent abdominal pain or personality change.
- CIDP presents like AIPD but progresses over >4 weeks. Hence by exclusion the diagnosis is acute intermittent porphyria

Acute intermittent porphyria
- Autosomal dominant disorder
- Reduced *HMB synthase* activity
- Attacks are triggered by drugs, steroid hormones and diet
- Presents with
  1. Recurrent episodes of abdominal pain
  2. Abdominal distention and decreased bowel sounds.
  3. Tachycardia, hypertension, restlessness and sweating due to sympathomimetic over-activity.
  4. Peripheral neuropathy occurs due to axonal degeneration.
  5. Motor neuropathy affects proximal muscles. Sensory changes and paraesthesias are common.
  6. Mental symptoms like depression, paranoia and hallucinations can occur.
- Treatment with intravenous hemin, carbohydrate loading, narcotic analgesia and phenothiazines.

351. Ans. (a) Continue same dose of steroids

(Ref: Harrison 20th p 2596; Harrison 19th edition, page 2200)

- The main objective of treatment in dermatomyositis is to improve muscle strength and reduce extra-muscular symptoms.
- Harrison states : "Unfortunately there is *tendency to chase CK levels* instead of muscle weakness which leads to prolonged and unnecessary use of immune-suppressive drugs"
- Hence in the case given above since symptomatic improvement has occurred though CK levels are highly elevated, oral prednisolone dose should remain the same.

352. Ans. (b) EMG

(Ref: Harrison 20th p 3175; Harrison 19th edition, page 2655)

The clinical history points towards etiology as myelopathy. Since the disease is in initial phase, reflexes can be normal. EMG is not indicated in these patients.

Causes of Non- compressive myelopathy and required investigations

1. Spinal cord infarction due to vasculitis: MRI Spine	3. Demyelination: MRI spine
2. Infections: Viral studies for HIV, HTLV-1	4. Systemic causes like SLE: ANA
	5. Idiopathic

353. Ans. (d) Limb girdle muscular dystrophy

(Ref: Harrison 20th p 3244; 462e-4: Harrison 19th edition)

- Choice A is XLR and mother will be a carrier for dystrophin gene.
- Choice B and C follow mitochondrial pattern of inheritance and hence come from the maternal side.
- Choice D has autosomal recessive as well as autosomal dominant forms. Hence it can be seen in either of the genders.

354. Ans. (d) 4 weeks

(Ref: Ferri's Clinical Advisor: 2015, page 569)

- The technical definition of post-herpetic neuralgia is neuropathic pain seen after 30 days of onset of rash.
- Immunocompromised hosts are more prone to neurological complications like encephalitis, myelitis, cranial and peripheral nerve palsies and more importantly acute retinal necrosis. The mortality rate is 10-20% in immunocompromised hosts with disseminated zoster.

Management
1. Wet compresses using burrow's solution applied 4-5 times/day are useful to break vesicles and remove serum and crust
2. Valcyclovir, Famcyclovir for 7-10 days

355. Ans. (d) Muscular dystrophy

(Ref: Bradley's Neurology in Clinical practice: 7th edition, page 283)

The image shows pseudo-hypertrophy of calf muscles seen in duchenne's muscular dystrophy. Causes of pseudo-hypertrophy of calf muscles-

1. Dystrophinopathy like Becker's and Duchenne's
2. Limb girdle muscular dystrophy
3. Spinal muscular atrophy
4. Glycogen storage disorders
5. Myxedema in Hypothyroidism
6. Sarcoidosis, Cysticercosis and amyloidosis
7. Focal myositis
8. Ruptured muscle tendon
9. Muscle tumour or muscle hernia

True Hypertrophy is seen in acquired neuro-myotonia and S1 radiculopathy

356. Ans. (b) ALA levels in the urine

(Ref: Harrison 20th p 3298; Harrison: 19th edition, page 2689)

- The clinical presentation is of an occupational exposure leading to neuropathy and GIT complaints like abdominal pain and constipation.
- The key-words in the question are the "radiological finding of increased shadows in the femur."
- These shadows are called lead lines but are not due to deposition of lead. Instead they are caused due to increased mineralization or calcification leading to increase in bone density in metaphyseal plate.
- Mercury poisoning has neurological features due to damage at dorsal root ganglia. Bone findings are not seen. GIT involvement will occur if button batteries are lodged in the gut and lead to liquefactive necrosis.
- Hence the test to be done is urine ALA levels to detect lead poisoning.

Lead poisoning	Mercury poisoning
Insidious onset motor neuropathy involving wrist and finger extensors Abdominal pain Burtonian line on gums	Metal fume fever leading to fatigue, weakness, dizziness and ejaculatory pain *Acrodynia*: pink disease with erythema of palms and soles with desquamation. Constipation or diarrhea and hair loss. *Erethism* is irritability and social withdrawal with insomnia.
Labs Microcytic hypochromic anaemia Basophilic stippling of RBC Elevated serum lead Elevated serum coproporphyrin> 150mg/L Urine amino- levulinic acid> 5mg/L	*Labs* Mercury levels are checked in hair and blood.

Lead poisoning does not involve ALA Synthetase

357. Ans. (b) Median nerve

(Ref: Harrison 20th p 101)

Keyboard operators and typists due to repetitive activity at the wrist joint are vulnerable to develop carpal tunnel syndrome involving development of median nerve compression.

Clinical Features

Manifestations include pain in the wrist that may radiate with paresthesia to the thumb, second and third fingers, and radial half of the fourth finger and, at times, atrophy of thenar musculature.

Examination findings
1. Positive Tinel's (Paresthesia in a median nerve distribution is induced or increased by either "thumping" the volar aspect of the wrist)
2. Phalen's sign. (Pressing the extensor surfaces of both flexed wrists against each other)

Causes of carpal tunnel syndrome is
1. Pregnancy
2. Edema due to repetitive activities at the wrist joint
3. Trauma
4. OA
5. Inflammatory arthritis
6. Infiltrative disorders (e.g., amyloidosis).

358. Ans. (d) Arthrogryposis multiplex congenita

(Ref: Harrison 20th p 2641-42; Harrison 19th edition p 2243-44)

359. Ans. (c) Duchenne muscular dystrophy

(Ref: Harrison 20th p 3244; Harrison's 19th edition, 462e-1)

Patients of Duchenne's muscular dystrophy have a proximal muscle weakness. These patients have difficulty in standing up from a sitting position due to weakness of muscles around the hip joint. This is called Gower sign.

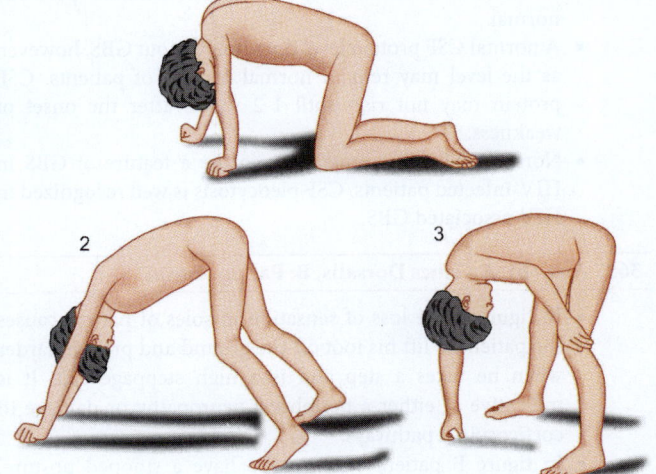

360. Ans. (b) Muscle weakness

(Ref: Harrison 20th p 3229; Harrison 19th edition, page number 2695)

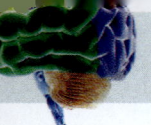

Miller Fisher Syndrome
• Rapidly evolving ataxia • Arreflexia of limbs *without weakness*[Q] • Opthalmoplegia with pupillary weakness • Anti GQ1b antibodies[Q] • Electro-diagnosis showing axonal or demyelinating disorder • IVIG is preferred over plasmapheresis in patients of MFS

361. Ans. (c) Guillain Barre syndrome

(Ref: Harrison 20th p 3229)

	Poliomyelitis	**Guillain-Barre syndrome**	**Transverse myelitis**	**Traumatic neuritis**
Fever	Present; may be biphasic	*May have a prodromal illness*	May have a prodromal illness	Absent
Symmetry Sensations	Asymmetric Intact; may have diffuse myalgias	*Symmetrical Variable*	Symmetrical Impaired below the level of the lesion	Asymmetric May be impaired in distribution of the affected nerve
Respiratory insufficiency	May be present	*May be present*	May be present	Absent
Cranial nerves	Affected in bulbar and bulbospinal variants	*Usually affected*	Absent	Absent
Radicular signs	May be present	*Present*	Absent	Absent
Bladder, bowel complaints	Absent	*Transient; due to autonomic dysfunction*	Present	Absent
Nerve conduction	May be abnormal	*Abnormal*	Normal	Abnormal
Cerebrospinal fluid	Lymphocytic pleocytosis; normal or increased protein	*Albumino-cytologic dissociation*	Variable	Normal
MRI spine	Usually normal	*Usually normal*	Characteristic	Normal

362. Ans. (a) Normal cells with increased protein

(Ref: Harrison 20th p 3229; Harrison 19th ed. / 2694)

Also refer to above table
- The characterized feature of GBS is albumin-cytological dissociation, characterized by elevated proteins due to autoimmunity while the cell count remains perfectly normal.
- A normal CSF protein level does not rule out GBS, however, as the level may remain normal in 10% of patients. CSF protein may not rise until 1-2 weeks after the onset of weakness.
- Normal CSF cell counts may not be a feature of GBS in HIV-infected patients. CSF pleocytosis is well recognized in HIV-associated GBS.

363. Ans. (b) A: Tabes Dorsalis, B: Parkinsonism

- In figure A the loss of sensation in soles of patient causes the patient to lift his foot off the ground and press it harder when he takes a step and is a high steppage gait. It is indicative of either a peripheral neuropathy or damage to corticospinal pathways.
- In figure B patient is shown to have a stooped posture, with semiflexed elbows and taking short shuffling steps indicative of festinating gait of Parkinsonism.

364. Ans. (a) Polyneuritis

(Ref: Harrison 20th p 3220; Harrison 19th p 2689)

Arsenic is another heavy metal that can cause a toxic sensorimotor polyneuropathy. The neuropathy manifests 5–10 days after ingestion of arsenic and progresses for several weeks, sometimes mimicking GBS.

365. Ans. (a) Merosin

(Ref: OP. Ghai, 566, 7th ed)

Classification of Congenital Muscular Dystrophy

- **Defects of structural proteins**
  - Merosin deficient CMD; Laminin α2
  - UCMD1; Collagen 6A1
  - UCMD2; Collagen 6A2
  - UCMD3; Collagen 6A3
  - Integrin α7-deficient CMD; Integrin α7
  - CMD with Epidermolysis bullosa;
- **Defects of glycosylation**
  - Walker-Walburg syndrome;
  - Muscle-eye brain disease,
  - Fukuyama CMD; Fukutin

366. Ans. (d) Scapulofaciohumeral dystrophy

(Ref: Nelson 20th p 2965; Harrison 19th p 462e, 2707)

- The question can be solved on logic that facial muscle involvement is not seen with Becker and Limb girdle muscular dystrophy
- Emery Dreifuss and Becker are XLR and hence present in boys while in question the patient is a girl child.

- Hence by exclusion the diagnosis is D: scapulo-faciohumeral dystrophy
- Facio-scapulo-humeral dystrophy is transmitted as autosomal dominant inheritance and has an onset in childhood or young adulthood.
- In most cases, facial weakness is the initial manifestation, appearing as an inability to smile, whistle or fully close the eyes.
- Weakness of the shoulder girdles, leading to loss of scapular stabilizing muscles makes arm elevation difficult.
- Scapular winging becomes apparent with attempts at abduction and forward movement of the arms.
- The serum CK level may be normal or mildly elevated.
- No specific treatment is available, ankle-foot orthoses are helpful for footdrop.

367. Ans. (b) Motor neuron disease

(Ref: Harrison 20th p 3142-43; Harrison 19th p 2632-33)

- *The site of lesion in motor neuron disease is anterior horn cell, pyramidal neurons and not the nerves. Thus the conduction velocity in the nerves is normal*
- Leprosy as a disease affects nerves and both Sensory nerve conduction /Motor nerve conduction studies may demonstrate reduced amplitude in affected nerves but occasionally may reveal demyelinating features.
- Charcot-Marie-Tooth disease (CMT) is the most common type of hereditary neuropathy, and has reduced motor nerve conduction velocity
- Acute Inflammatory Demyelinating polyneuropathy is the most common variant of GBS. The disease involves segmental demyelination in spinal cord and peripheral nerves. The earliest features are prolonged F-wave latencies, prolonged distal latencies and reduced amplitudes of compound muscle action potentials, probably owing to the predilection for involvements of nerve roots and distal motor nerve terminals early in the course.

368. Ans. (a) HIV

(Ref: Harrison 19th p 2684-85)

Causes of Small Fiber Neuropathy

1. Diabetes mellitus
2. Leprosy
3. Amyloidosis
4. Tangier's disease
5. Fabry's disease
6. HIV
7. Sarcoidosis/lupus vascaulitis/Sjogren syndrome

It occurs from damage to the small unmyelinated peripheral nerve fibers. These fibers, categorized as C fibers, are present in skin, peripheral nerves, and organs. The role of these nerves is to innervate the skin (somatic fibers) and help control autonomic function.

369. Ans. (b) Ophthalmoplegia

(Ref: Harrison 19th p 2194)

Polymyositis presents with symmetrical proximal muscle weakness. Pelvic girdle muscles are more involved than upper body muscles. *Ocular muscles are never involved in generalised polymyositis.* The actual onset of Poly-myositis is often not easily determined, and patients typically delay seeking medical advice for several months. This is in contrast to dermatomyositis, in which the rash facilitates early recognition.

Polymyositis mimics many other myopathies and is a diagnosis of exclusion. *It is a subacute inflammatory myopathy affecting adults, and rarely children, who do NOT have any of the following:*

1. Rash, involvement of the extraocular and facial muscles,
2. Family history of a neuromuscular disease,
3. History of exposure to myotoxic drugs or toxins,
4. Endocrinopathy, neurogenic disease, muscular dystrophy
5. Biochemical muscle disorder (deficiency of a muscle enzyme)

370. Ans. (a) Duchenne's muscular dystrophy

(Ref: Harrison 20th p 3244; Harrison 19th p 595)

- Duchenne's dystrophy is present at birth, but the disorder usually becomes apparent between ages 3 and 5 years. The usual history is a boy child falling frequently and have difficulty keeping up when playing.
- GOWER sign is seen with pseudohypertrophy of the calf muscles.
- Serum CK levels are invariably elevated to between 20 and 100 times normal. *The levels are abnormal at birth but decline late in the disease because of inactivity and loss of muscle mass.*
- Contractures of the heel cords and iliotibial bands become apparent by age 6 years, when toe walking is associated with a lordotic posture
- By age 12 years, most patients are wheelchair dependent.

371. Ans. (d) Postural hypotension

(Ref: Harrison 20th p 3229; Harrison 19th p 2698)

- Postural hypotension is usually an autonomic involvement seen with Guillain Barre syndrome in which ascending paralysis can cause involvement of T4-T8 sympathetic outflow to heart.
- Miller fisher syndrome consists of

1. Acute external ophthalmoplegia
2. Ataxia
3. Areflexia (Without weakness)

- More than 90% of MFS patients have serum antibodies to the gangliosides GQ1b and GT1a. These antibodies are most likely induced during antecedent infection by molecular mimicry.
- MFS patients with bulbar weakness or progression to GBS may benefit from treatment with intravenous immunoglobulin or plasma exchange

372. Ans. (a) Polymyositis

(Ref: Harrison 20th p 2592; Harrison 19th p 2194-96)

- It is a subacute inflammatory myopathy affecting adults, without Rash, involvement of eye, family history of neuromuscular disease
- Dermatomyositis is identified by a rash preceding muscle weakness.
- Inclusion body myositis has a asymmetrical muscle involvement.

373. Ans. (a) Charcot Marie Tooth disease

(Ref: Harrison 20th p 3208)

Causes of enlarged peripheral nerves are:

1. Leprosy
2. Hereditary sensory and motor neuropathy (charcot marie tooth disease)
3. Neurofibromatosis
4. Refsum disease
5. Perinuroma
6. Nerve tumor
7. Amyloidosis

In patients with Charcot-Marie-Tooth disease (CMT), distal muscle wasting may be noted in the legs, resulting in the characteristic stork leg or inverted champagne bottle appearance. Pes Cavus, thoracic scoliosis, claw hand are skeletal abnormalities

374. Ans. (a) Lead poisoning

(Ref: Harrison 20th p 3219; Harrison 19th p 2688)

- The most common presentation of lead poisoning is encephalopathy. However it also leads to primary motor neuropathy involving the radial nerve. Sensation is preserved.
- In contrast, arsenic leads to toxic sensori-motor neuropathy.
- Thallium poisoning leads to autonomic involvement with labile heart rate and BP.
- Mercury poisoning presents with parasthesias of hands and feet.

375. Ans. (b) Proximal muscle weakness

(Ref: Harrison 20th p 3206; Harrison 19th p 2675)

376. Ans. (d) Bradycardia

(Ref: Morgan's 4th/804, 805; Harrison 19th edtion, p 619)

Autonomic neuropathy with cholinergic or adrenergic dysfunction can occur at pre- or post ganglionic levels. It can lead to
1. Gastrointestinal paresis with pseudo-obstruction
2. Resting tachycardia
3. Cardiac arrhythmia
4. Orthostatic hypotension
5. Dry mouth
6. Anhidrosis
7. Erectile dysfunction
8. Problems in sphincter control.

377. Ans. (d) Arsenic intoxication

(Ref: Harrison 20th p 3220; Harrison 19th p 2688)

378. Ans. (a) Polio

(Ref: Harrison 20th p 1469; Harrison 19th p 1290-91)

379. Ans. (c) Sensory level

(Ref: Harrison 20th p 3229; Harrison 19th p 2694)

380. Ans. (d) Duchenne's muscular dystrophy

(Ref: Harrison 20th p 3244; Harrison 19th p 462e)

381. Ans. (b) Vastus medialis; (d) Infraspinatus

(Ref: Ghai 6th/548; Harrison 19th p 462e)

382. Ans. (c) Z band Myopathy

(Ref: Robbins 7th/1340)

383. Ans. (a) Anti-Jo-1

(Ref: The Washington Manual Rheumatology Subspecialty Consult (2003)/ 31, 32; Rheumatology: Diagnosis & Therapeutics 2nd/87; Harrison 19th p 2196)

384. Ans. (b) Gottron's rash

(Ref: Harrison 20th p 2592; Harrison 19th p 2195)

385. Ans. (a) Salmon Patch

(Ref: Harrison 20th p 2592; Harrison 19th p 2195)

Myasthenia Gravis and Channelopathies

386. Ans. (b) Myasthenia gravis

(Ref: Harrison 20th edition, page 3232)

The first image shows presence of asymmetrical ptosis. After administration of a drug (edrophonium: short acting anticholinesterase) there is resolution of neurological deficit. The clinical diagnosis of the patient is Myasthenia gravis.

387. Ans. (a) Myasthenia gravis

(Ref: Harrison 20th p 3244; : Harrison 19th edition, page 2701)

Ptosis with diplopia and relief of symptoms with edrophonium (Tensilon test) is diagnostic of M.Gravis.

388. Ans. (c) Absent DTR

(Ref: Harrison 20th p 3232-33; Harrison 19th edition, page 2702)

- Myasthenia Gravis presents with *fatigability and weakness* of muscles. It is worsened with repeated usage and improves following rest or sleeping.
- *Ptosis* is an early clinical feature along with diplopia. But light reflex is normal
- Facial weakness produces a snarling facies.
- Chewing muscle weakness and nasal timbre in speech contributes to dysarthria.
- Oro-pharyngeal muscle weakness is present and contributes to dysphagia.
- DTR reflexes are preserved in M. Gravis.

389. Ans. (b) Voltage gated calcium channel antibodies

(Ref: Harrison 20th p 3235; Harrison 19th edition, page 444 e-2)

Voltage gated calcium channel antibodies are used for diagnosis of Lambert Eaton syndrome.

Choices A, C and D are used for diagnosis of M. Gravis.

390. Ans. (c) CRP

Ref: Harrison 20th p 3233-34; Harrison 19th edition, page 2704

- Generalised M. Gravis is associated with Thymic hyperplasia or Thymoma. Hence CT chest is recommended.
- Baseline PFT will help in case of development of Myasthenia **Crisis** by the patient
- Since thyroid abnormalities like Hashimoto's thyroiditis is associated with M. Gravis, TSH is performed.

Recommended laboratory test or procedures
• CT or MRI of chest
• Test for lupus erythematosus, antinuclear antibody, rheumatoid factor, antithyroid antibodies
• Thyroid function test
• PPD skin tests
• Fasting blood glucose, hemoglobin A1c
• Pulmonary function test
• Bone densitometry

391. Ans. (a) Symmetrical ptosis

Ref: Harrison 20th p 3232; Harrison 19th edition, page 2701

- The ocular manifestations of M. Gravis result from dysfunction of myoneural junction.
- Common clinical signs are asymmetrical ptosis and diplopia.
- Snarling facies are present with nasal timbre in voice.
- Difficulty in swallowing may occur as a result of weakness of palate, tongue or pharynx giving rising to nasal regurgitation or aspiration of liquids. Bulbar weakness in seen in MuSK antibody positive MG.
- Treatment of choice for generalised M. Gravis is
- Characteristic features of M. Gravis are:

1. Eye muscle weakness that exacerbates during fatigue
2. Periodic remission
3. Responsiveness to Edrophonium
4. Normal DTR

392. Ans. (d) Anderson Tawi syndrome

(Ref: Harrison 20th p 3252; Harrison 19th edition, page 462-17)

Hyperkalemic periodic paralysis	Gain of function of sodium channel SCN4A
Brugada syndrome	Loss of function of Sodium Channel SCN5A
Paramyotoia congenital	Gain of function of sodium channel SCN4A
Anderson Tawi Syndrome	Defect in inward sending potassium channel

- Hyperkalemic periodic paralysis and paramyotonia congenita lead to development of myotonia.
- Brugada syndrome presents as ST elevation in lead V1-V2 and incomplete RBBB. It can lead to sudden death due to polymorphic ventricular tachycardia.
- Anderson Tawi syndrome leads to episodic weakness, arrhythmias and dysmorphic features. The prolongation of QT interval can lead to polymorphic Ventricular Tachycardia and possible sudden death. Incidence wise Brugada is more common than Anderson Tawi.

393. Ans. (b) Antibodies to presynaptic voltage gated channels impair acetylcholine release

(Ref: Harrison 20th p 3235; Harrison 19th edition, page 2702-2703)

Thymoma or thymic hyperplasia is common	1. The thymus is abnormal in 75% of patients with MG 2. In 65% the thymus is "hyperplastic," with the presence of active germinal centers detected histologically, though the hyperplastic thymus is not necessarily enlarged. 3. An additional 10% of patients have thymic tumors (thymomas)
Antibodies to presynaptic voltage gated channels impair acetylcholine release	The antibodies are directed against post synaptic antibodies. Pre-synaptic antibodies are seen in lambert Eaton syndrome.
Bulbar weakness is especially prominent in MuSK antibody positive myasthenia	Muscle-specific tyrosine kinase- (MuSK) antibodies-positive Myasthenia Gravis accounts for about one third of Seronegative Myasthenia Gravis and is clinically characterized by early onset of prominent bulbar, neck, shoulder girdle, and respiratory weakness. The response to medical therapy is generally poor
Plasmapharesis is useful in the treatment of myasthenia gravis	If immediate improvement is essential either because of the severity of weakness or because of the patient's need to return to activity as soon as possible, IVIg should be administered or plasmapheresis should be undertaken. Situation warranting IVIG usage is myaesthenic crisis.

394. Ans. (c) Thymic hyperplasia

(Ref: Harrison 20th p 3233; Table 461.3: Harrison 19th edition, Page number 2704)

- Thymus gland abnormalities are seen in 75% of anti Ach Receptor positive antibodies patients.
- CT chest can identify a Thymic Hyperplasia or a thymoma which though benign can produce mass effects.

395. Ans. (a) Myasthenia gravis

(Ref: Harrison 20th p 3232; Harrison 19th ed. / 2701)

- Myasthenia gravis is characterized by eye muscle weakness, ptosis and diplopia. In contrast all myopathies have proximal weakness (exception being Myotonic dystrophy).

396. Ans. (d) Anderson Tawi syndrome

(Ref: Harrison 20th p 3252; Harrison 19th p 462e-18)

Frederich ataxia	Chromosome 9 frataxin gene GAA Trinucleotide repeats
Ataxia telangiectasia	AT gene defective DNA Repair
Amyotrophic Lateral sclerosis	SOD 1 defect Hexanucleotide repeats

Clinical Features of Periodic Paralysis

Features	Calcium channel defect	Sodium channel defect		Potassium channel defect
	Hypokalemic PP	Hyper-kalemic PP	Paramyotonia Congenita	Andersen-Tawi
Syndrome	AD	AD	AD	AD
Age of onset	Adolescence	Early childhood	Early childhood	Early childhood
Myotonia	No	Yes	Yes	No
Episodic weakness	Yes	Yes	Yes	Yes
Frequency of attacks of weakness	Daily to yearly	May be 2-3/d	With cold, usually rare	Daily to yearly
Serum K+ level during attacks of weakness	Decreased	Increased or normal	Usually normal	Variable

397. Ans. (a) Thymoma with immunodeficiency

(Ref: Washington Manual of oncology, 2nd edition, page 172)

Good's syndrome (thymoma with immunodeficiency) is a rare cause of combined B and T cell immunodeficiency in adults. The clinical characteristics of Good's syndrome are increased susceptibility to bacterial infections with encapsulated organisms and opportunistic viral and fungal infections. The most consistent immunological abnormalities are hypogammaglobulinaemia and reduced or absent B cells. This disorder should be treated by resection of the thymoma and immunoglobulin replacement to maintain adequate trough IgG values.

398. Ans. (a) Hypercalcemia

(Ref: Harrison 20th p 3251, 3255; Harrison 19th p 444e, 2703)

Channelopathies	• The Sodium channels at Neuro-muscular junction like SCN4A may exhibit loss of function or gain of function. • Either way the depolarization of muscles is affected leading to muscle weakness • SCN4A gain of function results in hyperkalemic periodic paralysis • SCN4A loss of function will lead to hypokalemic periodic paralysis
Lambert Eaton syndrome	• Anti P/Q antibodies produced by Oat Syndrome Cell carcinoma will damage the neuromuscular junction leading less Ach production and thereby weakness. • It is a pre-junctional defect characterized by Ptosis and proximal muscle weakness
Hyperphosphatemia	• Features will develop due mainly to the formation of widespread calcium phosphate precipitates and resulting hypocalcemia.

Contd...

- Thus, tetany, seizures, accelerated nephrocalcinosis (with renal failure, hyperkalemia, hyperuricemia, and metabolic acidosis) will occur.
- Low calcium and increased potassium in these patients can lead to weakness as a symptom.

399. Ans. (a) M. Gravis

(Ref: Neurological signs by AJ Larner, 2013)

Ice pack test, is a simple test, safe, cheap, fast and reliable to be used routinely in patients suspec-ted of palpebral ptosis and/or ophthalmoparesis due to myasthenia gravis, and which has a high validity, safety, and reproducibility as a diagno-stic test.

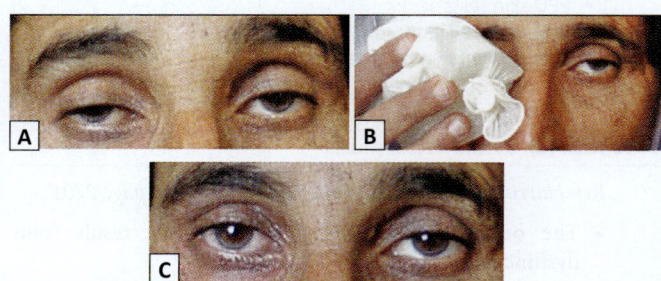

Figure: (A) Bilateral ptosis (more marked in right eye); (B) Ice pack application on right eye; (C) Improvement in ptosis of right eye after ice pack application

Investigations for the choices mentioned in the question

Multiple system atrophy	MRI showing hot cross buns sign and putaminal atrophy
Hyperparathyroidism	PTH assay and Technetium scan parathyroidism.
Hypokalemic periodic paralysis	C.M.A.P compound muscle action potential shows low amplitude and shows no improvement on exercise.

400. Ans. (b) Hyperkalemic periodic paralysis

(Ref: Harrison 20th p 3252; Harrison 19th p 444e)

Hyperkalemic periodic paralysis is a sodium channel defect seen in patients with mutations in SCN4A, therefore, the channel is unable to inactivate, sodium conductance is sustained and the muscle remains permanently tense. Since the motor end plate is depolarised, further signals to contract have no effect (paralysis). The condition is hyperkalemic because a high extracellular potassium ion concentration will make it even more unfavourable for potassium to leave the cell to repolarise it to the resting potential. This further prolongs the sodium conductance and keeps the muscle contracted.

401. Ans. (b) Generalised M. Gravis

(Ref: Harrison 20th p 3233; Harrison 19th p 2702)

- The main concept is that absence of Anti-Ach receptor blocking antibodies does not rule out M.gravis.
- Asymmetrical ptosis and swallowing difficulty are seen in M. gravis.

- Symmetrical ptosis and absence of swallowing complaints are seen in chronic progressive external opthalmoplegia.

MCQ choice	Clinical features	Investigations
Ocular M.Gravis	It affects individuals in all age groups, but peaks of incidence occur in women in their twenties and thirties and in men in their fifties and sixties. Overall, women are affected more frequently than men, in a ratio of 3:2. The cardinal features are weakness and fatigability of muscles. The weakness increases during repeated use (fatigue) or late in the day, and may improve following rest or sleep	Anti-AChR antibodies are detectable in the serum of 85% of all myasthenic patients but in only about 50% of patients with weakness confined to the ocular muscles. The presence of anti-AChR antibodies is virtually diagnostic of MG, but a negative test does not exclude the disease
C.P.E.O	CPEO tends to begin in young adulthood. Ptosis usually is the first clinical sign, and ophthalmoplegia may not become apparent for months to years. *The ptosis is usually bilateral and symmetrical.* As the ptosis progresses, the patient may use the frontalis muscle to elevate the eyelids, adopt a *chin-up head position*, and eventually resort to manual elevation of the eyelids, as ptosis often becomes complete. Because of the symmetric nature of this disorder, patients often *do not complain of diplopia*. The course of CPEO is characterized by *constant progression* without periods of remission or exacerbation.	A positive acetylcholine receptor antibody test may establish the diagnosis of myasthenia gravis. In contrast to myasthenia gravis, patients with CPEO usually report little to no variability in their ptosis.

Must Know
- Tensilon test is to be done for difficult to diagnose cases.
- Tensilon test is a provocative test and can precipitate cholinergic crisis. It can be false positive in A.L.S
- Thymectomy is done in all cases of generalized M. gravis between age of puberty to 55 yrs.
- Ocular M. gravis is managed with pyridostigmine and steroids/immunomodulators.
- Anti-M.U.S.K (muscle specific kinase antibody) is seen in 30% cases of ocular M. gravis.

402. Ans. (c) Repeated electrical stimulation enhances muscle power in it

(Ref: Harrison 20th p 3235; Harrison 19th p 2703)

Lambert Eaton syndrome has incremental response on EMG. Lower limbs with proximal muscle weakness is the most common clinical presentation in LEMS. It is associated with small cell lung cancer.

403. Ans. (d) Huntington's disease

(Ref: Harrison 20th p 3251-52; Harrison 19th p 2621)

Basic Neurology

404. Ans. (d) 6th nerve palsy

(Ref: Review of ophthalmology: 6th edition, page 5)

- The image shows left side 6th nerve palsy.
- On looking to right, both eyes are moving normally implying lateral rectus of right side and medial rectus of left side are working normally
  On looking to left, the right eye medial rectus is working normally leading to adduction but *left eye lateral rectus fails to abduct the eye*

405. Ans. (c) Pyramidal neurons

(Ref: Clinical neuroanatomy: 27th edition, page 58)

- The reflex arc operates independent of upper motor neurons (pyramidal neurons).
- A deep tendon reflex is elicited when a tap on a tendon stretches muscle spindles which are chronically activated by ϒ motor neurons.
- Spindle afferent neurons directly stimulate α motor neurons in the spinal cord causing a muscle contraction.

406. Ans. (d) Accessory nerve: Check Shoulder Shrug

(Ref: Harrison 20th p 3028; Harrison 19th edition, page 2537)

- Choice A is wrong because patient should be asked to sniff a mild agent like coffee or toothpaste. *Alcohol or ammonia stimulates trigeminal nerve which is involved in chemoreception.* Trigeminal nerve endings are typically activated by chemicals classified as irritants, including air pollutants (e.g. Sulphur dioxide), ammonia (smelling salts), ethanol (liquor), acetic acid (vinegar), carbon dioxide (in soft drinks), menthol (in various inhalants), and capsaicin (the compound in chili peppers that elicits the characteristic burning sensation).
- Choice B is wrong because ocular saccades utilize cranial nerve 3, 4 and 6 along with PPRF.
- Choice C is wrong as eyebrow elevation and forehead wrinkling is done to test the facial nerve.

407. Ans. (c) Trigeminal

(Ref: Harrison 20th p 3028; Harrison 19th edition, page 2537-38)

The speech is controlled by speech areas in dominant cortex. The corticobulbar fibers then descend down send signals to the following nerves
1. Vagus
2. Facial nerve
3. Hypoglossal nerve
4. Phrenic nerve

408. Ans. (b) Pseudobulbar palsy

(Ref: Macleod's clinical diagnosis E book page 109)

Comparison of signs in bulbar and pseudobulbar palsy

	Bulbar	Pseudobulbar
Speech	Nasal tone; difficulty forming consonants (especially "R"); may become slurred	'Donald duck' voice
Tongue	Weak, wasted with fasciculation	Small, stiff
Jaw jerk	Normal or absent	Brisk
Gag reflex	Absent	Present
Emotions	Normal	Labile (e.g. uncontrollable laughing/crying)

409. Ans. (b) Examiner is doing the test wrong

(Ref: Macleod's clinical examination e-Book 14th edition, page 140; Harrison 19th edition, page 2538, 2632, 2675)

A is wrong	Motor neuron disease can have features of both LMNL and UMNL in the same patient. Hence the statement of reflex is always brisk in motor neuron disease is technically wrong.
B is correct	The reflex should be done with the knees of the patient being partially flexed and rested on the examiner's forearm. The *anterior part of the thigh should be exposed* to check for visible contraction of the quadriceps femoris muscle. *Correct method 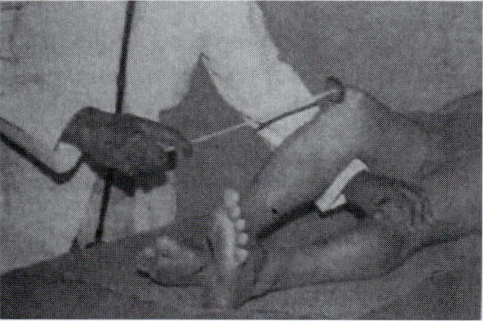
C is wrong	Peripheral neuropathy can have sensory, motor or autonomic features. If patient is having only dysautonomia like in case of diabetes then orthostatic hypotension will be a feature but DTR will be normal. In case of sensory neuropathy involving unmyelinated C fibers the patient will have dull poorly localised pain called protopathic pain. Due to involvement of A delta fibers, patients will have sharp and lancinating pain called epicritic pain. *In these situations motor nerves may not be involved and DTR will be normal.* Hence the statement that DTR is always absent in neuropathy is technically wrong.
D is wrong	The root value is L2,L3,L4

410. Ans. (d) Nucleus cuneatus

(Ref: Harrison 20th p 142; Harrison 19th edition, page 160 and Diagnostic Clinical Neuropsychology, 3rd edition, page 32)

- Astereognosis is impaired or lost ability to discriminate between various forms, as well as deficits in finger localization and in graphesthesia (ability to recognize palm writing). If a lesion occurs at or above the level of the thalamus, it commonly results in astereognosis,
- Now Since Nucleus cuneatus gets information from T5 upwards including the upper limb its lesion results in astereognosis.
- The onset of ataxia is somewhat later than in ataxia-telangiectasia but usually occurs before age 10 yr. The ataxia is slowly progressive and involves the lower extremities to a greater degree than the upper extremities.

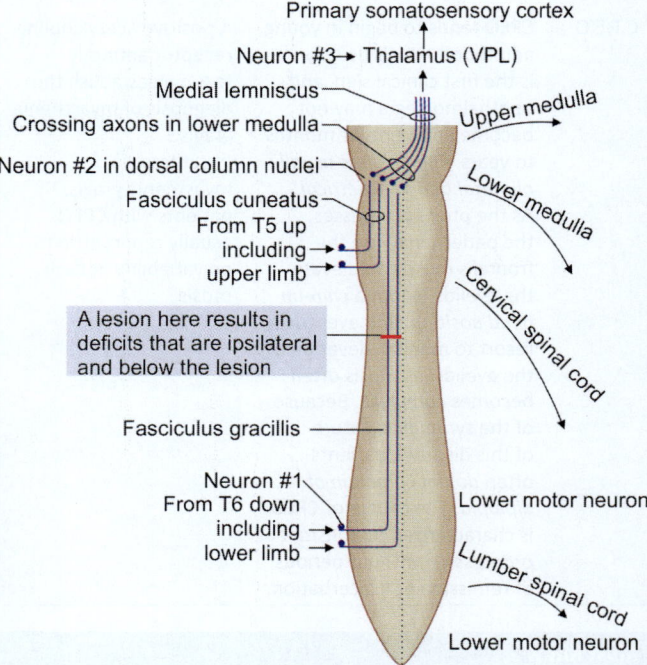

- The fasciculus gracilis (graceful, like a ballerina's legs) conveys information from the lower part of the body T6 and below.
- Together the fasciculus gracilis and cuneatus are referred to as the posterior columns, because they occupy a position at the posterior of the spinal cord.
- The posterior columns travel up the ipsilateral side of the spinal cord and synapse in the nucleus gracilis and nucleus cuneatus at the level of the medulla. From there, the fibers decussate (cross over) and continue on toward the thalamus in a pathway synapses in the thalamus, and from there the information is relayed to the postcentral gyrus, known as the somatosensory cortex.

411. Ans. (b) Tongue deviation to right on protrusion

(Ref: Harrison 20th p 3028; Harrison 19th ed. / Ch 367)

Following a lesion of the hypoglossal nucleus or nerve

1. ATROPHY of the muscles of the IPSILATERAL one-half of the tongue occurs.
2. FASCICULATIONS (tiny, spontaneous contractions) can be seen.
3. *Upon protrusion, the tongue will deviate TOWARD the side of the lesion (i.e., same side)*. This is due to the unopposed action of the genioglossus muscle on the normally innervated side of the tongue (the genioglossus pulls the tongue forward).

The corticobulbar input to the hypoglossal nucleus arises from motor cortex and is predominantly CROSSED. Thus, a lesion in motor cortex will result in deviation of the tongue toward the opposite side or CONTRALATERAL to the lesion. In contrast to the atrophy and fasciculations seen in lesions of the hypoglossal nucleus and nerve (lower motor neuron), NO such signs are present after lesions of the corticobulbar tract.

412. Ans. (d) Tongue protusion

(Ref: Harrison 20th p 3028; Harrison 19th ed. / 2537-38)

Functions of the Glossopharyngeal Nerve
- Receives general sensory fibers from the tonsils, the pharynx, the middle ear and the posterior 1/3 of the tongue.
- Receives visceral sensory fibers from the carotid bodies, carotid sinus.
- Receives special sensory fibers from the posterior one-third of the tongue
- Supplies parasympathetic fibers to the parotid gland via the otic ganglion.
- Supplies motor fibers to stylopharyngeus muscle, the only motor component of this cranial nerve.
- Contributes to the pharyngeal plexus.

Testing of 9th Nerve
- Testing the gag reflex using a wooden spatula
- Asking the patient to swallow or cough
- Evaluating for speech impediments.
- Test the posterior one-third of the tongue with bitter and sour substances to evaluate for impairment of taste.

413. Ans. (a) Gag reflex

(Ref: Harrison 20th p 3028; Harrison 19th ed. / 2537-38)

Damage to the vestibulocochlear nerve may cause the following symptoms:
- Hearing loss
- Vertigo
- False sense of motion
- Loss of equilibrium (in dark places)
- Nystagmus
- Motion sickness
- Gaze-evoked tinnitus

The gag reflex has the following pathway
- The sensory limb is mediated predominantly by CN IX (glossopharyngeal nerve)
- The motor limb by CN X (Vagus nerve).

The gag reflex involves a brisk and brief elevation of the soft palate and bilateral contraction of pharyngeal muscles evoked by touching the posterior pharyngeal wall

414. Ans. (c) Parietal lobe

(Ref: Harrison 20th p 160; Harrison 19th ed. / 209)

Performing Mathematical calculations is a function of parietal lobe. Damage to the left hemisphere of this lobe will result in problems in mathematics, long reading, writing, and understanding symbols. The parietal association cortex enables individuals to read, write, and solve mathematical problems.

415. Ans. (a) Finkelstein test

(Ref: Page 340, Essential Orthopedics 4e 5 Minute Sports Medicine Consult page 114)

- **Finkelstein test**: *Flex the thumb of the patient into the palm after stabilizing the forearm. Then force the wrist towards the ulna. Development of sudden severe pain is positive for De quervain tenosynovitis.*
- **Tinel Sign**: Percuss the median nerve, using the broad side of hammer while the hand of the patient is dorsiflexed. Paraesthesia percieved by the patient in thumb, index finger and middle finger is called as Tinel sign.
- **Fromment sign**: It is done to test ulnar nerve entrapment at the elbow.
- **Jeanne's sign**: It is similar to Fromment sign and seen in response to pinch forces. Instead of isolated thumb IP flexion, the IP flexion is accompanied by MP joint hyperextension.

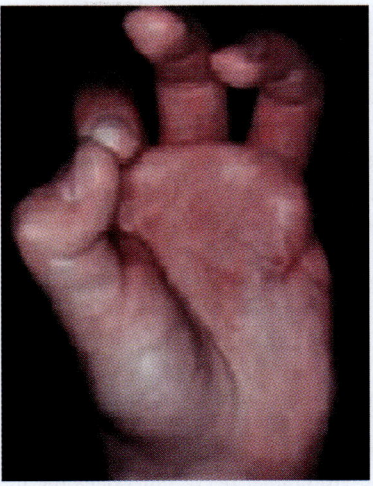

416. Ans. (c) Tabes Dorsalis

(Ref: Macleod's clinical examination e-Book 14th edition, page 44; Harrison 20th p 1283; Harrison 19th p 1136)

- The gait in foot drop is referred to as Equine Gait
- Frontal Lobe stroke leads to Magnetic Gait
- Leprosy can lead to foot drop and thereby equine gait due to involvement of peroneal nerve.
- In Tabes Dorsalis, due to peripheral neuritis the loss of sensation would lead to development of stamping gait/High Steppage Gait.

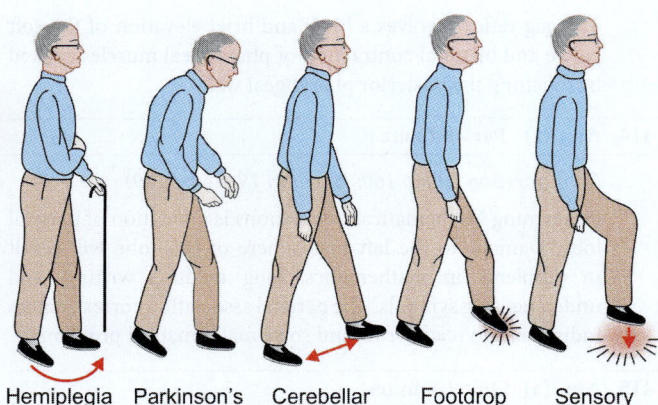
Types of gait abnormalities

417. Ans. (a) Chorea

(Ref: OP Ghai 8th edition p 579)

- It is called hung-up reflex in chorea due to superimposition of choreic (involuntary) movement on tendon reflex.

418. Ans. (a) Gag reflex

(Ref: Harrison 20th p 3082; chapter 367 and e42, Harrison 19th p 2538)

Damage to the vestibulocochlear nerve may cause the following symptoms:
1. Hearing loss
2. Vertigo
3. False sense of motion
4. Loss of equilibrium (in dark places)
5. Nystagmus
6. Motion sickness
7. Gaze-evoked tinnitus

The gag reflex has the following pathway
- The sensory limb is mediated predominantly by CN IX (glossopharyngeal nerve)
- The motor limb by CN X (Vagus nerve).

The gag reflex involves a brisk and brief elevation of the soft palate and bilateral contraction of pharyngeal muscles evoked by touching the posterior pharyngeal wall

419. Ans. (a) Oculomotor

(Ref: Harrison 20th p 3028; Harrison 19th p 2537)

- The 3rd cranial nerve innervates the medial, inferior and superior recti, inferior oblique, levator palpebrae superioris and the iris sphincter.
- *Total palsy of the oculomotor nerve causes ptosis, results in a dilated pupil (mydriasis), and leaves the eye 'down and out' because of the unopposed action of the lateral rectus and superior oblique.*
- Diplopia due to paralysis of these extra-ocular muscles, may not seen due to presence of ptosis.
- Cervical sympathetic trunk damage causes HORNER SYNDROME.
- Abducents and trochlear nerve palsy will cause diplopia and squint but ptosis will not be seen.

420. Ans. (b) Loss of fine movements of fingers and hands

(Ref: Physicon by Sanoop KS, 1st edition, page 106)

- Choice A and C are easily ruled out as they are features of UMNL. For the remaining two choices read the text given below.
- Corticospinal pathways are of 2 types
  1. Lateral corticospinal pathway which provides motor impulses to the spinal cord and is responsible for controlling fine and precise movements of the fingers and hands to control the skilled movement
  2. Anterior cortico-spinal pathway makes postural adjustment and helps in gross movements
- Extrapyramidal pathway is a tract functioning since birth and is responsible for co-ordination of large muscle groups leading to upright posture, locomotion, head and neck control and plays an important role like while turning to a special stimulus.
- Clasp knife rigidity/clasp knife spasticity are terms in literature used to describe UMNL.

421. Ans. (a) Mid pontine lesions

(Ref: Walsh and Hoyt's Clinical Neuro Opthalmology Vol. 1 pg 1254)

- *The motor arm of Blink reflex i.e. Motor nucleus is located at mid-pontine level medial to main sensory nucleus of Vth nerve, near the floor of fourth ventricle. Therefore it would be completely destroyed in mid pontine lesions.*
- In **Myasthenia gravis** in setting of ptosis induced on upward gaze it would be difficult to comment on blink reflex.
- In **Axonal Neuropathy** i.e. in early AIDP, distal demyelination occurs in parallel in many nerves. These abnormalities of blink reflexes most likely represent demyelination in either the facial and/or the trigeminal nerves, reflecting the multifocal nature of demyelination in AIDP. In unilateral facial palsy therefore only one eye will blink fully.
- In **Motor Neuron Disease** destruction of cranial nerve nuclei occurs, bulbar palsy ensues but eye movements, bladder and bowel are spared. Thus logically blink reflex would be unaffected and thus choice D is excluded.

Blink reflex pathway

1. Afferent: supra-orbital divison of Opthalmic division of fifth nerve sends impulses via the first order neurons synapsing in chief sensory nucleus in the tegmentum of pons.
2. Motor nucleus – mid-pontine level /Medial to main sensory nucleus of Vth nerve, near the floor of fourth ventricle.
3. The second order neurons project to bilateral VII nerve nuclei.
4. Supranuclear control – cortico-bulbar fibres from precentral gyrus.
5. Motor root: EXITS from motor nucleus, passes through substance of pons and emerges from anterolateral aspect of pons anterior and medial to the large sensory root. It then passes forward in posterior fossa, Pierces the dura mater beneath attachment of tentorium to tip of petrous part of temporal bone. It now enters the Meckel's cave leaves skull via Foramen Ovale. It joins the mandibular division of Vth N to form mandibular nerve – supplies masticatory muscles.

Midbrain lesions will not affect while mid pontine lesions will affect both afferent and efferent arms of blink reflex.

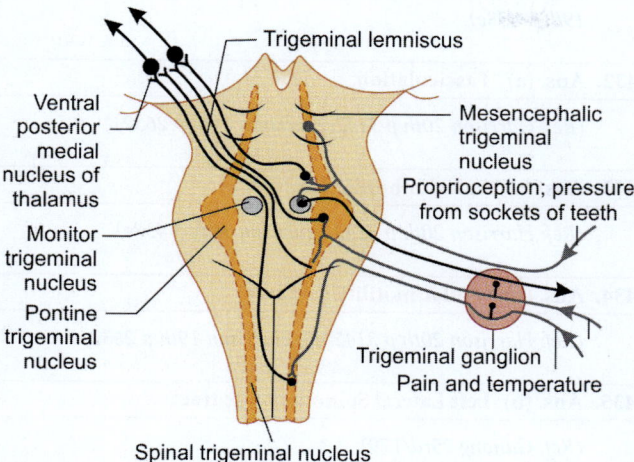

422. Ans. (a) Dysdiadochokinesia

(Ref: Macleod's clinical examination e-Book 14th edition, page 115; Harrison 19th p 2626)

Dysdiado-chokinesia	Breaking up of complex movements/ inability to perform rapid alternating movements like alternate pronation and supination of hands
Dysarthria	Difficulty in speaking due to cranial nerve palsy causing in poorly understood speech. The context of speech is fine as broca and Wernicke area are working fine.
Dyssynergia	A condition marked by generalized intention tremors associated with disturbance of muscle tone and of muscular coordination; due to disorder of cerebellar function.
Dystonia	Abnormal tone leading to abnormal posturing in the body in basal ganglia damage Positive Kernig's test is most likely in • Perichondritis • Normal individuals • Conductive deafness
Meningitis	KERNIG SIGN is positive when the thigh is bent at the hip and knee at 90 degree angles, and subsequent extension in the knee is painful (leading to resistance).This may indicate subarachnoid hemorrhage or meningitis. The pain felt on Kernig's sign is due to meningeal irritation caused by movement of the spinal cord within the meninges. BRUDZINSKI SIGN: a clinical sign in which forced flexion of the neck elicits a reflex flexion of the hips. It is found in patients with meningitis, subarachnoid haemorrhage and possibly encephalitis. In the Brudzinski's neck sign, this movement with neck flexion is cancelled out by the flexion of the hip; much like two persons pulling on either side of a single rope.

423. Ans. (b) Is a bi-synaptic reflex

(Ref: Ganong 25th edition, pg 232; ch. 367)

- The Golgi tendon reflex (also called negative or inverse stretch reflex) is a bi-synaptic reflex, initiated by the Golgi tendon organ located in muscle tendons.
- Like muscle spindles, Golgi tendon organs are also stretch receptors. However unlike the muscle spindle, which acts as a length-detector, the Golgi tendon organ acts as a tension-detector. This difference in sensory function occurs because muscle spindle is disposed in parallel to the extrafusal fibers while the Golgi tendon organ is disposed in series to the extrafusal fibers.
- *The Golgi tendon reflex is a protective reflex that prevents excessive rise in muscle tension. When the muscle contracts isometrically, the tendon gets stretched and the tension in the tendon rises markedly. This rise in tension is sensed by the Golgi tendon a which stimulates the I-b afferents. These afferents stimulate the inhibitory interneurons in the spinal cord and thereby, inhibit the á-motoneuron discharge to the muscle, which consequently relaxes. This reflex relaxation of the extrafusal muscle fibers response to rise in muscle tension is called the negative (inverse) stretch reflex.*

424. Ans. (d) Rigidity

(Ref: Oxford Illustrated companion to medicine, p 647)

Charcot's neurologic triad is the combination of nystagmus, intention tremor, and scanning or staccato speech and indicates cerebellar damage.

Rigidity is a feature of basal ganglia damage/extra-pyramidal damage

425. Ans. (b) Neocerebellum

(Ref: Sapira's Art and Science of Bedside Diagnosis, Page 559)

Choices in the question	Manifestation in case of lesions
Ischemic stroke	Brisk D.T.R with Balbinski sign
Neo-cerebellum	Lesions of this area cause hypotonia. This manifests as pendular knee jerk which freely swings back and forth. Also developing in these patients is dysmetria, dysaidokinesia, scanning speech.
Paleo-cerebellum	Gait ataxia, loss of tandem gait
Archi-cerebellum	Trucal ataxia, titubation

Hung up reflexes are seen in chorea. Hung up ankle reflex is seen in hypothyroidism.

426. Ans. (a) Barrington nucleus

(Ref: Autonomic Neurology, Wolfgang singes, 3rd edition, Pg 8)

- Barrington nucleus is a collection of cell bodies located in the rostral pons in the brainstem involved in the supra-spinal regulation of micturition.
- It makes connections with other brain centers to control micturition, including the medial frontal cortex, insular cortex, hypothalamus and periaqueductal gray (PAG).

- The PAG in particular acts a relay station for ascending bladder information from the spinal cord and incoming signals.

427. Ans. (d) 6th nerve

(Ref: Neuro-Oncology, ed, Pg 136, 2011)

- Dorello's canal is a fibrous ligament that extends from the petrous apex to the lateral dorsum sellae and creates a canal containing the abducent nerve.
- The close proximity explains why in conditions ranging from intracranial hypotension to middle ear infections the sixth nerve gets involved.

428. Ans. (a) Paratonia

(Ref: Harrison 20th p 135; Harrison 19th p 2574)

- Paratonia or Gegenhalten is defined as "a form of hypertonia with an involuntary variable resistance during passive movement."
- Attempting to move the limb of a person with paratonia will result in that person involuntarily resisting the movement. The amount of resistance is determined by the speed of the movement: faster, more forceful movements will result in greater amounts of resistance. It is also present regardless of the direction of the movement.
- Paratonia can be distinguished from spasticity by observing a lack of exaggerated deep tendon reflexes and a lack of a clasp-knife response.
- It can be distinguished from Parkinsonian (aka "lead-pipe") rigidity in that the amount of resistance in Parkinsonian rigidity does not vary with the velocity of the movement.
- Paratonia develops during a period of dementia and the degree of effect is dependent upon the disease's progress.

429. Ans. (b) 150 ml

(Ref Oxford hand book of Urology 3rd ed. pg 618; Harrison 19th p 1778)

Awareness of urine the bladder occurs at 50 ml while the urge to urinate occurs at 150 ml

430. Ans. (d) Hypertension

(Ref: 250 Cases in Clinical Medicine, pg. 38-39)

Argyl Robertson pupil is seen in: B.C.D.S3
1. Brainstem encephalitis
2. Chronic alcoholics
3. Diabetes mellitus
4. Sarcoidosis
5. Multiple sclerosis
6. Syringobulbia
    - The characteristics of A.R.P are small irregular pupils with absent light reflex and accommodation reflex is intact. Though alcohol is not a direct cause, chronic alcoholism can lead to promiscuous behavior and resultant develop-ment of syphilis and its complications.
    - Damage to light reflex requires damage to any of the following areas- superior colliculus, Decussation of Meynert and Edinger-westphal nucleus.
    - It is different from Holmes adie pupil in a sense that the pupil is large, irregular, oval or circular. This pupil is called as myotonic pupil as well.

431. Ans. (d) Hypoactive jaw jerk

(Ref: Harrison 20th p 136; Clinical Neurology 6th/40; Harrison 19th p 438e)

432. Ans. (a) Fasciculation

(Ref: Harrison 20th p 3142; Harrison 19th p 2632)

433. Ans. (a) Anterior horn cells

(Ref: Harrison 20th p 3142; Harrison 19th p 438e)

434. Ans. (b) Ocular motility is spared

(Ref: Harrison 20th p 3142-43; Harrison 19th p 2632)

435. Ans. (b) Left Lateral Spinothalamic tract

(Ref: Ganong 25rd/179)

436. Ans. (c) Proprioception

(Ref: Harrison 20th p 3173-74; Harrison 19th p 2652)

437. Ans. (d) Contralateral posterior column involvement

(Ref: Harrison 20th p 3173-74; Harrison 19th p 2652)

438. Ans. (a) Abdominal muscle

(Ref: Harrison 20th p 3173; Harrison 19th p 2651)

439. Ans. (d) Baclofen

(Ref: Practical Pharmacology in Rehabilitation (Human Kinetics) 2013/152; Harrison 19th p 2672)

440. Ans. (a) VII nerve injury

(Ref: API medicine 6th/ 730; Dhingra 3rd/ 123 (2nd/ 99)); Harrison 19th p 2647)

441. Ans. (d) Contralateral lower face paresis

(Ref: Fuller 2nd/ 85; Macleods 10th/ 206, Harrison 19th p 2647)

Pediatric Neurology

442. Ans. (d) Urine

Ref: Vople's Neurology of Newborn, 5th edition, Page 855

In neonates the usual cause of intracranial calcifications is CMV and Toxoplasmosis.

	CT head	Confirmatory test
Congenital CMV	Intracranial calcifications are classically *periventricular*	Confirmed by virus isolation from *urine*, saliva, bronchoalveolar washings, breast milk, cervical secretions, buffy coat, and tissues obtained by biopsy.

Contd...

	CT head	Confirmatory test
		Rapid identification within 24 hr is routinely available with the centrifugation-enhanced rapid culture system based on the detection of CMV early antigens using monoclonal antibodies
Congenital Toxoplasma	Intracranial calcifications are scattered diffusely.	Presence of *Toxoplasma*-specific IgM in *CSF* that is not contaminated with blood or confirmation of local antibody production of *Toxoplasma*-specific IgG antibody in CSF establishes the diagnosis of congenital *Toxoplasma* infection

443. Ans. (d) 19

(Ref: Harrison 20th p 3248; Harrison 19th edition, 462 e-9)

Myotonic dystrophy type 1: defect on chromosome 19
Myotonic dystrophy type 2: defect on chromosome 3

Important features of myotonic dystrophy

1. CTG repeats
2. Muscle weakness *distal*
3. Tenting of upper lips

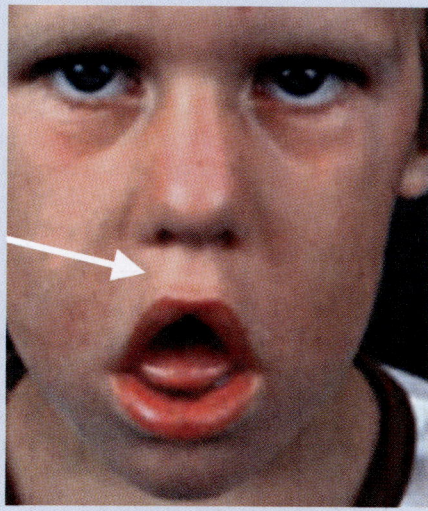

4. Wasting of temporalis, masseter leading to *hatchet facies*
5. Testis atrophy
6. Myotonia
7. Posterior sub capsular cataracts
8. First degree heart blocks

444. Ans. (c) Distal muscle weakness

(Ref: Harrison 20th p 3248; Harrison 19th edition, 462 e-9)

Myotonic Dystrophy has a proximal muscle weakness. The disease occurs due to trinucleotide repeats on chromosome 19.

445. Ans. (b) Charcot Marie Tooth Disease

(Ref: Harrison 20th p 3208; O.P. Ghai, 8th edition, page 591)

Becker's Dystrophy	Presents after 10 years with large calf muscles
Chronic inflammatory demyelination polyneuropathy	Will lead to progressive symmetric proximal and distal weakness in both upper and lower extremities with concomitant sensory loss.
Inclusion body myositis	Presents in adults with asymmetric distal weakness

Charcot-Marie-Tooth (CMT)

- Most common inherited neuromuscular disorder.
- The mutation results in abnormal myelin that is unstable and spontaneously breaks down. This process results in demyelination, leading to uniform slowing of conduction velocity
- Repeated cycles of demyelination and remyelination result in a thick layer of abnormal myelin around the peripheral axons. These changes cause what is referred to as an onion bulb appearance.

Clinical features

1. Frequent falling/tripping due to foot and distal leg weakness.
2. Frequent ankle sprains and falls are characteristic.
3. Parents may report that a child is clumsy
4. Intrinsic foot muscle weakness commonly results in the foot deformity (pes cavus)
5. Hand weakness results in complaints of poor finger control, poor handwriting, difficulty using zippers and buttons.

Investigation of Choice: DNA-based testing for the *PMP-22* duplication (CMT 1A) is widely available and detects more than 98% of patients with CMT 1A.

EMG shows same degree of marked slowing in all nerves tested, sensory and motor

446. Ans. (b) Type 2

(Ref: Rudolph Paediatrics 22nd edition, page 2343)

Congenital hydrocephalus is associated with Arnold Chiari type II malformation

Arnold chiari malformation type 1	Most common variety Least severe variety of the spectrum Often diagnosed in adulthood. Hallmark is caudal displacement of peg like cerebellar tonsils below the level of the foramen magnum
Arnold chiari malformation type 2	Chiari type II malformation is less common and more severe, almost invariably associated with myelomeningocele. Greater severity and hence it becomes symptomatic in infancy or early childhood. Hallmark is caudal displacement of lower brainstem (medulla, pons, 4th ventricle) through the foramen magnum. Symptoms arise from dysfunction of brainstem and lower cranial nerves.
Arnold chiari malformation type 3	Herniation of cerebellum into a high cervical myelomeningocele
Arnold chiari malformation type 4	Associated with cerebellar agenesis

447. Ans. (c) Arnold Chiari II malformation

(Ref: Rudolph Paediatrics 22nd edition, page 2343)

- The Chiari II malformation is a congenital malformation of the brain, nearly always associated with myelomeningocele
- It is the most common serious malformation of the posterior fossa.
- This condition has downward displacement of the medulla, fourth ventricle, and cerebellum into the cervical spinal canal, as well as elongation of the pons and fourth ventricle, probably due to a relatively small posterior fossa.
- Dandy-Walker malformation is characterized by agenesis or hypoplasia of the cerebellar vermis, cystic dilatation of the fourth ventricle, and enlargement of the posterior fossa.

448. Ans. (a) Arnold Chiari malformation

(Ref: Nelson 20th/e 2150)

- Small posterior fossa is a term used to describe Arnold chiari Malformation, type II. In contrast dandy walker syndrome, has a large posterior fossa.

449. Ans. (c) Antibodies to measles in blood

(Ref: chapter 243: Nelson 18th edition; Nelson 20th/e 2917)

The diagnosis of SSPE can be established through documentation of a compatible clinical course and at least 1 of the following supporting findings:

1. Measles antibody detected in CSF
2. Characteristic electroencephalographic findings called Rademecker complex.
3. Typical histologic findings and/or isolation of virus or viral antigen in brain tissue obtained by biopsy or postmortem examination.
4. CSF analysis reveals normal cells but elevated IgG and IgM antibody titers in dilutions of >1:8. Electroencephalographic patterns are normal in stage I, but in the myoclonic phase suppression-burst episodes are seen that are characteristic of but not Pathognomic for SSPE.

450. Ans. (a) Optic nerve glioma

(Ref: Nelson 20th/e 3059)

The key word in the question is Relative afferent pupillary defect. The causes are:

1. Optic neuritis/ ischemic optic disease or retinal disease
2. Severe glaucoma causing trauma to optic nerve
3. Direct optic nerve damage (trauma, radiation, tumor)
4. Retinal detachment
5. Very severe macular degeneration
6. Retinal infection (CMV, herpes)

451. Ans. (b) Leukemia

(Ref: Nelson ch. 632/Tumors of the Orbit)

- Cavernous hemangiomas are the most common intra-orbital tumors found in adults and hence ruled out.
- Neurofibromatosis presents with sphenoid dysplasia resulting in pulsating proptosis. It is unilateral. These benign, vascular lesions are slow growing and can manifest as a painless, progressively proptosis. The mass is usually located unilaterally. Bilateral is rare.
- **Malignant fibrous Histiocytoma:** It is a pleomorphic undifferentiated sarcoma. It occurs commonly in adults and is rare in children. It occurs mainly in extremities and retroperitoneum.

452. Ans. (b) Hydrocephaly

(Ref: Neural tube defects: Diego F. Wysyzinki, 2006 Pg 646; Nelson 20th/e 2150)

- The banana sign describes the posterior convexity of the cerebellum within the posterior cranial fossa. The cerebellar hemispheres were curved anteriorly with simultaneous obliteration of the cisterna magna. This is suggestive of ARNOLD CHIARI MALFORMATION and hence the Answer hydrocephaly. Which is an alternative term for hydrocephalus.
- The lemon sign describes a concave or flattened frontal contour of the fetal calvarium rather than a normal convex frontal contour and seen in Arnold–Chiari malformation.

453. Ans. (d) Absent cerebral hemispheres

(Ref Nelson 19th edn ch. 592.7)

The term hydrancephaly should *not be confused* with hydrocephalus.

Hydranencephaly is a condition in which the brain's cerebral hemispheres are absent to varying degrees and the remaining cranial cavity is filled with cerebrospinal fluid. Usually the cerebellum and brain stem are formed normally, although in some cases the cerebellum may also be absent

454. Ans. (b) Schizencephaly

(Ref: Nelson 20th/e 2807)

Neuronal migrational defects can have following possible manifestations:

Schizencephaly	Abnormal continuity of grey matter extending from the ependyma of the cerebral ventricles to the pia mater. *Type I schizencephaly* has a cord of grey matter tissue, either with no fluid cleft or with ventricular or cortical lips closing one end of an abnormal fluid cleft through the hemisphere. *Type II schizencephaly* shows a cerebrospinal fluid-filled cleft of varying size and shape extending through the hemisphere from the ependyma centrally to the pia peripherally
Lissencephaly	Lissencephaly, which literally means *smooth brain*, is a rare brain formation disorder caused by defective neuronal migration during the 12th to 24th weeks of gestation resulting in a lack of development of brain folds
Porencephaly	Characterized with *cysts or cavities* within the cerebral hemisphere. Patients with severe cases of porencephaly suffer epileptic seizures and developmental delays.

Multiple Sclerosis

455. Ans. (b) Edavarone

Ref: NCBI-NIH

- Edavarone is a free radical scavenger which has been recently approved for management of Amyotrophic Lateral Sclerosis.
- Ocrelizumab is the first drug for management of Primary progressive multiple sclerosis.
- Nitistinone is used for management of alkaptonuria.
- Piracetam is nootropic drug designed to enhance memory and boost cognitive function.

456. Ans. (a) Neuromyelitis Optica

Ref: Harrison 20th edition, Page 3202

- The combination of optic neuritis and transverse myelitis is a feature of Neuromyelitis optica which occurs due to aquaporin-4 antibodies.
- Choice B will present with loss of proprioception with macrocytic anaemia.
- Choice C will present with 3rd nerve palsy and features dependant on part of midbrain involved.
- Choice D presents with Argyl Robertson pupil and/or dorsal column involvement.

457. Ans. (a) Methylprednisolone

Ref: Harrison 20th edition, page 3194

- Glucocorticoids are used to manage first attacks or acute exacerbations of multiple sclerosis, which usually present as optic neuritis. They will provide short term clinical benefit by reducing the severity and shortening the duration of attacks.
- For treatment naïve patients who are JCV negative Interferon- beta and Glatiramer is initiated. The efficacy of both is rated as modest while natalizumab is rated as highly effective. It is however not recommended first line in treatment naïve patients.

458. Ans. (d) Transverse myelitis

(Ref: Harrison 20th p 3188; page 2663: Harrison 19th edition)

- Multiple sclerosis is a demyelinating disorder of brain and does not involve the spinal cord. Hence answer is D.
- Spinal cord involvement is rare in multiple sclerosis. If it is present, it is called Devic's Disease. It is characterised by presentation of Transverse myelitis and Optic neuritis.
- The most common presentation of multiple sclerosis is sensory loss followed by optic neuritis.

Symptom	% of cases
Sensory loss	37
Optic neuritis	36
Weakness	35
Paresthesias	24
Diplopia	15

Contd...

Symptom	% of cases
Ataxia	11
Vertigo	6
Paroxysmal attacks	4
Bladder	4

459. Ans. (d) Electronystagmogram

(Ref: Harrison 20th p 3191-92; Harrison 19th edition, page no: 2664-65)

According to revised McDonald criteria for diagnosis of multiple sclerosis following investigation should be done:

1. MRI (contrast enhanced): shows Plaques
2. Lumbar puncture to obtain CSF. CSF electrophoresis shows Oligo-clonal IgG bands
3. Visual evoked potential which shows reduced amplitude of voltage generated due to plaques in optic nerve.

460. Ans. (d) Mitotane

(Ref: Harrison 20th p 3196)

- Mitotane is used for treatment of inoperable adrenal carcinoma.
- The disease modifying therapy for multiple sclerosis is
  - IFN-beta 1a
  - IFN-beta -1a
  - IFN-beta-1b
  - Glatiramer acetate
  - Natalizumab
  - Fingolimod

461. Ans. (c) Absence of oligoclonal bands

(Ref: Harrison 20th p 3192; Harrison 19th p 2665)

- CSF studies suggest that patients with mono-symptomatic disease with positive oligo-clonal bands (OCB) have higher risk of evolution to MS than without OCBs.
- *OCBs are detected by agarose gel electrophoresis. Two or more OCBs are found in 75–90% of patients with MS.*

462. Ans. (a) Natalizumab

(Ref: Harrison 20th p 3196; Harrison 19th p 2669)

The following drugs are used as disease modifying therapy in multiple sclerosis:
(1) IFN-beta 1a, (2) IFN-beta -1a, (3) IFN-beta-1b, (4) Glatiramer acetate, (5) Natalizumab, (6) Fingolimod, and (7) Mitoxantrone

On comparison of results of each one of these drugs Natalizumab reduces the disease severity by 42% and reduces appearance of new lesions by 83%.

On facebook academic forums, mitoxantrone has been mentioned as best. Please check on page 3198, mitoxantrone is rarely used in multiple sclerosis.

463. Ans. (d) Mitotane

(Ref: Harrison 20th p 3196; Harrison 19th p 2669)

- Mitotane is used for treatment of inoperable adrenal carcinoma.

- The disease modifying therapy for multiple sclerosis is
    1. IFN-beta 1a
    2. IFN-beta -1a,
    3. IFN-beta-1b
    4. Glatiramer acetate
    5. Natalizumab
    6. Fingolimod, and
    7. Mitoxantrone

On comparison of results of each one of these drugs: Natalizumab reduces the disease severity by 42% and reduces appearance of new lesions by 83%, which is maximum in comparison of all the drugs tested in drug trials.

464. Ans. (d) Rheumatoid arthritis

(Ref: Harrison 20th p 2540; Harrison 19th ed p 2148)

Over 75% of rheumatoid arthritis patients report improvement of symptoms, during pregnancy.

465. Ans. (a) Multiple sclerosis

(Ref: Comprehensive Ophthalmology by Khurana: 2015 6th edition, page 63)

The Pulfrich effect is a psychophysical percept wherein lateral motion of an object in the field of view is interpreted by the visual cortex as having a depth component, due to a relative difference in signal timings between the two eyes.

Even if you neglect the physics associated with the term it seen in multiple sclerosis where optic nerve damage by the plaques leads to the effects mentioned above.

466. Ans. (b) Interferon Beta

(Ref: Harrison 20th p 3196; Harrison 19th p 2269)

Diseases of Spinal Cord

467. Ans. (a) Biceps weakness

Ref: Harrison 20th p 100; Harrison 19th edition page 2657 and page 577: PACES for MRCP)

- The most common site of cervical disk disease is C5, C6 and C6 and C7. Hence biceps and triceps weakness will occur.
- Sensory deficits with abnormal sensation in thumb and finger
- Sensation to axilla and medial arm is mediated by C8 and T1.

Cervical radiculopathy

Level	Reflex to be evaluated	Pain distribution
C5	Biceps	Lateral arm, medial scapula
C6	Biceps	Lateral forearm, thumb, index finger
C7	Triceps	Posterior arm
C8	Finger flexors	4th and 5th fingers, medial forearm
T1	Finger flexors	Medial arm, axilla

468. Ans. (b) Intramedullary tumor

(Ref: Harrison 20th p 3174; Harrison 19th edition, page 2652)

- Amyotrophic lateral sclerosis presents with asymmetric motor weakness with findings of LMNL and UMNL. Hence choice A is ruled out.
- Neurosyphilis can involve the spine and lead to tabes dorsalis. It presents as Lhermitte sign, sensory ataxia and urinary incontinence. Hence choice C is ruled out.
- AIDP (Subtype of GBS) presents as fast onset paraplegia/quadriplegia with/ without diaphragmatic paralysis. Hence choice D is ruled out.
- The patient is having features suggestive of central cord syndrome with involvement of lateral spinothalamic tract leading to decreased pain and temperature sensation.
- Urgent MRI spine is recommended.

469. Ans. (a) Lumbar canal stenosis

(Ref: Harrison 20th p 93; Harrison 19th edition, page 115)

- The history points to neurogenic claudication. Pain is worse on standing and improves with sitting. Focal deficit of diminished reflexes can be explained by same.
- Vascular claudication develops on walking and not on standing. Hence choice B is ruled out.
- In a construction worker, spinal cord trauma can occur while lifting bricks etc. which results in spinal canal stenosis.
- Tethered cord syndrome presents as cauda equine syndrome leading to urinary complaints and saddle anaesthesia.
- Vertebral metastasis is unlikely at this age.

470. Ans. (c) Developmental defect associated with Chiari malformation

(Ref: Harrison 20th p 3180; Harrison 19th edition, page 2658)

- Syringomyelia occurs due to Arnold Chiari malformation type 1. The syrinx leads to central cord syndrome with loss of pain and temperature sensation.
- The pain and temperature sensation loss is patchy and is called dissociative anaesthesia.
- Crossed hemi-anaesthesia is a feature of lateral medullary syndrome
- MRI is the investigation modality of choice for syringomyelia. For management decompression in posterior fossa is done. Direct decompression of syrinx is also performed with debatable results but *excision of syrinx is definitely not done.*

471. Ans. (d) Progressive weakness on serial examinations

(Ref: Manual of spine surgery, page 117-118)

Indications for surgical repair of intervertebral disc herniation:

1. Objective progressive motor weakness
2. Bladder and bowel incontinence
3. Incapacitating nerve root pains despite medical treatment

472. Ans. (d) Electromyography

(Ref: Harrison 20th p 3141; Harrison 19th edition, page 2634)

- ALS is a neurodegenerative disorder characterised by death of anterior horn cells in spinal cord and their brainstem homologues innervating bulbar muscles.
- Motor neurons originating in layer five of motor cortex are also destroyed.
- V.E.P is used for evaluation of optic nerve involvement in multiple sclerosis.
- CT/MRI spine cannot visualize loss of anterior horn cells or pyramidal cells in cortex.
- In patients suspected to have a motor neuron disease, clinicians should perform a thorough electro-diagnostic evaluation, including peripheral nerve conduction studies and needle electromyography to both exclude treatable disease and gather evidence toward a diagnosis of amyotrophic lateral sclerosis.
- Needle Electromyography is the most important component of electro-diagnostic evaluation of LMN involvement even before it becomes clinically evident. EMG should show evidence of chronic neurogenic change or acute denervation.
- Positive sharp waves, fibrillations and fasciculations are seen.

473. Ans. (d) Spinal cord damage

(Ref: Dejong neurological examination, 7th edition, page 661)

- Patients of spinal cord injury will develop non ischemic priapism.
- The mechanism of priapism in most patients with SCI is that *abrupt loss of sympathetic input to the pelvic vasculature leads to increased parasympathetic input and uncontrolled arterial inflow directly into the penile sinusoidal spaces.* The sympathetic outflow arises from the thoracolumbar spine, that is, the spinal cord from approximately T2 to the conus (L1-2).

Non ischemic priapism	Ischemic priapism
Increased arterial flow	Decreased venous outflow leading to increased inter-cavernosal pressure
1. Penile or perineal trauma 2. leading to fistula formation 3. Between cavernous artery and corpora 4. Acute spinal cord injury 5. Urological surgery	1. Idiopathic 2. Drugs 3. Pelvic vascular thrombosis 4. Sickle cell anaemia and trait 5. Leukemia 6. Hyperleucocytosis 7. TPN with fat infusions (Hyperviscosity) 8. Drugs like CPZ, cocaine 9. Tertiary syphilis

474. Ans. (b) Lhermitte sign

(Ref: Harrison 19th edition, page 121)

Cervical Arthritis	Presents with stiffness in neck muscles and reduced neck movements
Lhermite Sign	Seen is cervical spinal cord pathology when neck flexion produces an unpleasant electric shock sensation radiating down the extremities
Uthoff Sign	Seen in multiple sclerosis and characterized by worsening of symptoms like fatigue, optic neuritis with increase in body temperature.

Spinal cord compression	Presents with deficits like paraplegia, bladder and bowel involvement

Lhermittes sign/Barber chair syndrome

Etiology of Lhermite sign:
- Demyelination
- Head and neck radiotherapy
- Subacute combined degeneration of cord due to vitamin B12 deficiency
- Traumatic or compressive cervical myelopathy
- Epidural or subdural intraparencymal tumors
- Radiation myelitis
- Pyridoxine toxicity
- Inflammation SLE, Behcet disease herpes zoster myelitis
- Cavernous Angioma of cervical cord

475. Ans. (a) Both Ankle jerk and knee jerks may be lost; (b) Asymmetric areflexic paraplegia; (c) Motor changes & (e) Root pain

(Ref: Harrison 19th/115,1791,2651; Robbins 9th/; P.J.M 20th/336; L & B 26th/)

	Conus medullaris syndrome	Cauda equine syndrome
Presentation	Sudden and bilateral	Gradual and unilateral
Reflexes	Knee jerks preserved but ankle jerks affected	Both ankle and knee jerks affected
Radicular pain	Less severe	More
Low back pain	Moe	Less
Sensory symptoms and signs	Numbness tends to be more localized to perianal area; symmetrical and bilateral; sensory dissociation occurs	Numbness tends to be more localized to saddle area; asymmetrical, may be unilateral; no sensory dissociation; loss of sensation in specific dermatomes in lower extremities with numbness and paresthesia; possible numbness in pubic area, indluding glans penis or clitoris
Motor strength	Typically symmetric, hyperreflexic distal paresis of lower limbs that is less merked, fasciculations may be present	Asymmetric areflexic paraplegia that is more marked; fasciculations rare, atrophy more common
Impotence	Frequent	Less frequent; erectile dysfunction that includes inability to have erection, inability to maintain erectio, lack of sensation in pubic area (including glans penis or clitoris), and inability to ejaculate

Contd...

	Conus medullaris syndrome	Cauda equine syndrome
Sphincter dysfunction	Urinary retention and atonic anal sphincter cause overflow urinary incontinence and fecal incontinence; tend to present early in course of disease	Urinary retention; tends to present late in course of disease

476. Ans. (b) Brisk jaw jerks

(Ref. De Jong Neurological examination Ch. 15,. Pg No.194, 201 and. Ch. No.38 Pg no. 474.)

Facial sensory impairment	Trigeminal nerve has its nucleus in pons as well has a spinal nucleus which extends down through the lower pons and medulla into spinal cord as far as C3/C4. Through which sensory fiberswill pass thus carrying sensations of the face. Hence due to high cervical cord lesion till C3/ Facial sensory impairment will occur.
Brisk jaw jerk	*Afferent* impulse of this reflex are carried through sensory portion of the trigeminal nerve, the *efferent* impulse through trigeminal nerve with its reflex centre in PONS. *Hence this jerk like any other jerk will become brisk in a UMN lesion/supra-nuclear lesion OR a lesion above pons, never in a lesion with the spinal cord.*
Brisk pectoral reflex	With patients arm in mid-position between abduction and adduction, the examiner places her finger as nearly as possible on the tendon of pectoralis major muscle near its insertion on the greater tuberosity of the humerus. Tapping the finger causes adduction and slight internal rotation of the arm of the shoulder. The contraction of the muscle may be felt but usually not seen in normal individual. *In patients with cervical spondylotic myelopathy, a hyper- active/brisk pectoralis reflex indicates spinal cord compression at C2-3 and C3-4 levels. This reflex is mediated by the medial and lateral (anterior thoracic) nerves (C5-T1).*
Urgency and incontinence	Any spinal cord lesion will cause bladder lesions.

477. Ans. (a) 6th nerve

(Ref: Harrison 19th p 2697)

- The most common cranial nerve involved in GBS is the 7th cranial nerve involvement BUT the question was regarding cranial nerve involvement causing opthalmo-paresis in GBS.
- Hence the Ans: 6th nerve.
- Remember the number 7-6-3 as cranial nerves involved in GBS.
- Ophthalmoparesis may be observed in up to 25% of patients with GBS. Limitation of eye movement most commonly results from a symmetrical palsy associated with cranial nerve VI. Ptosis from cranial nerve III (oculomotor) palsy also is often associated with limited eye movements.

478. Ans. (b) Hypertrophy of abductor pollicis brevis

(Ref: Harrison 19th p 2658)

The Sensory Involvement in Syringomyelia

1. Dysesthetic pain, a common complaint in syringomyelia, usually involves the neck and shoulders, but may follow a radicular distribution in the arms or trunk. The discomfort, which is sometimes experienced early in the course of the disease, generally is deep, aching and can be severe.
2. The sensory deficit is recognizable by loss of pain and temperature sensation with sparing of touch and vibration in a distribution that is "suspended" over the nape of the neck, shoulders, and upper arms (cape distribution) or in the hands.

The Motor Involvement in Syringomyelia

1. Muscle wasting in the lower neck, shoulders, arms, and hands with asymmetric or absent reflexes in the arms reflects expansion of the cavity into the gray matter of the cord.
2. As the cavity enlarges and further compresses the long tracts, spasticity and weakness of the legs, bladder and bowel dysfunction, and Horner's syndrome appear.
3. Some patients develop facial numbness and sensory loss from damage to the descending tract of the trigeminal nerve (C2 level or above).
4. In cases with Chiari malformations, cough-induced headache and neck, arm, or facial pain are reported.
5. The extension of the syrinx into the medulla, syringebulbia, causes palatal or vocal cord paralysis, dysarthria, horizontal or vertical nystagmus, episodic dizziness, and tongue weakness.

479. Ans. (a) Hemangioblastoma

(Ref: Harrison 19th p 2654)

The clinical presentation of hemangioblastoma usually depends on the anatomical location and growth patterns.

1. Cerebellar lesions may present with signs of cerebellar dysfunction, such as ataxia and lack of coordination, or with symptoms of increased intracranial pressure due to associated hydrocephalus. In general, intracranial hemangioblastomas present with a long history of minor neurological symptoms that, in most cases, are followed by a sudden exacerbation, which may necessitate immediate neurosurgical intervention.
2. Patients with spinal cord lesions most frequently present with pain, followed by signs of segmental and long-track dysfunction due to progressive compression of the spinal cord.
3. Patients with VHL disease may present with ocular or systemic symptoms due to involvement of other organs and systems.
4. The polycythemia that may develop in some patients with hemangioblastomas usually is clinically asymptomatic

480. Ans. (c) Peripheral nerves histology shows demyelination

(Ref: Review Clinical review: Critical illness polyneuropathy and myopathy: Critical Care 2008, 12:238, Harrison 19th p 2684)

- Critical illness polyneuropathy is characterized by failure to wean off from ventilator (in absence of lung or heart disease) with reduction in spontaneous leg movements, symmetrical paresis with reduction in muscle tone and wasting.

- The failure to wean off ventilator is due to damage to phrenic nerve either due to cytokines released during SIRS when the patient required ventilation or neuromuscular blockers gaining access to peripheral nerves during the course of SIRS, where direct toxicity is incriminated.
- Critical illness myoneuropathy shares the major clinical sign of flaccid and usually symmetrical weakness. Other clinical signs include the reduction in or absence of deep tendon reflexes. Patients with CIP may show a distal loss of sensitivity to pain, temperature, and vibration.
- *Although facial muscles are relatively spared, ophthalmoplegia may occur.* Weaning problems are described to the involvement of the phrenic nerves and the diaphragm, and intercostal and other accessory respiratory muscles can be affected as well. It should be noted that CIP represents the response of the peripheral nervous system to critical illness, but the central nervous system also is frequently affected by critical illness, manifesting as a diffuse encephalopathy that occurs very early in the process. The cranial nerve involvement causing facial diplegia is documented but is very rare
- **Investigations**
    1. **Electrophysiological studies show-** *axonal degeneration*
    2. **Electromyography-** reduction in S.N.A.P and C.M.A.P
    3. **Phrenic Nerve conduction velocity** shows latency period increment
    4. **Muscle biopsy** of chest muscles and diaphragm shows denervation, neurogenic atrophy with spontaneous muscle fibrillations
- **Treatment:** intensive insulin therapy during ventilation duration has improved survival. Intravenous immunoglobulins have shown to improve survival. *50% of cases have been shown to have recovery*
- **Differential diagnosis** of critical illness myoneuropathy: Guillain Barre syndrome: differentiated by previous illness and recovery followed by ascending symmetrical paralysis with bilateral 7th nerve involvement. The lumbar puncture findings with NCV showing segmental de-myelination and antibodies demonstrated against myelin will aid in diagnosis.

481. Ans. (d) Dorso-medial thalamus

(Ref: Harrison 19th p 1783)

Amnestic defect is due to lesions in dorso medial thalamus. The appearance of acute Wernicke encephalopathy on MRI demonstrates abnormal hyperdensity of the dorso-medial thalamus and periaqueductal gray matter with associated abnormal enhancement on T1-weighted images. Depending on the location of the brain lesion different symptoms are seen.

1. **Brainstem tegmentum:** Ocular pupillary changes, Extraocular muscle palsy; gaze palsy and nystagmus.
2. **Hypothalamus, Medulla and dorsal nucleus of Vagus -** Autonomic dysfunction leading to cardio-circulatory and respiratory abnormalities.
3. **Cerebellum:** Ataxia.
4. **Diffuse cerebral dysfunction:** Altered cognition: global Confusional state.
5. **Brainstem periaqueductal gray matter:** Reduction of consciousness

482. Ans. (d) Metastasis

(Ref: Harrison's ch. 377: Tumours of Spinal Cord, Harrison 19th p 2654)

- Extradural tumors are mostly metastases from primary cancers elsewhere (commonly breast, prostate and lung cancer)
- The propensity of solid tumors to metastasize to the vertebral column probably reflects the high proportion of bone marrow located in the axial skeleton. Almost any malignant tumor can metastasize to the spinal column, with breast, lung, prostate, kidney, lymphoma, and plasma cell dyscrasia being particularly frequent. The thoracic spinal column is most commonly involved; exceptions are metastases from prostate and ovarian cancer, which occur disproportionately in the sacral and lumbar vertebrae, probably resulting from spread through Batson's plexus, a network of veins along the anterior epidural space.
- Most intradural mass lesions are slow-growing and benign. Meningiomas and neurofibromas account for most of these, with occasional cases caused by chordoma, lipoma, dermoid, or sarcoma.
- Primary intramedullary tumors of the spinal cord are uncommon. They present as central cord or hemicord syndromes, often in the cervical region; there may be poorly localized burning pain in the extremities and sparing of sacral sensation. In adults, these lesions are ependymomas, hemangioblastomas, or low-grade astrocytomas

483. Ans. (c) Breast cancer

(Ref: Harrison 19th p 605)

TABLE: Frequency of Nervous System Metastases by Common Primary Tumors

	LM %	Brain %
Lung	17	41
Breast	58	19
Melanoma	12	10
Prostate	1	1
GIT	–	7
Renal	2	3
Lymphoma	10	<1
Sarcoma	1	7
Other	–	11

LM stands for leptomeningeal metastasis

484. Ans. (a) Syringomyelia

(Ref: Harrison 19th p 2658)

The onion skin pattern of sensory loss is possible only if lesion involves the spinal nucleus of the trigeminal nerve which extends from pons to upper part of cervical cord.

In syringomyelia and its complication syringobulbia the expansion of central canal can lead to pressure over the sensory nucleus of trigeminal and resultant patchy loss of various sensory deficits will ensue.

485. Ans. (c) **Multiple system atrophy**

(Ref: 250 cases in clinical medicine pg. 70-71)

- Dissociative sensory loss implies loss of pain and temperature in a patchy fashion due to involvement of lateral spino-thalamic pathway.
- However conditions like diabetes, leprosy and amyloidotic polyneuropathy can affect peripheral nerves asymmetrically leading to manifestations of patchy loss of pain and temperature.
- Hydromelia is different from syringomyelia in a sense that it is expansion of ependymal lined central canal while syringomelia causes cleft like cavity in the inner portion of the cord. But hydromelia will also due to anatomic proximity affect lateral spino-thalamic pathway leading to dissociative sensory loss
- Multiple system atrophy has features of atypical parkinsonism with autonomic insufficiency and/or cerebellar signs.

486. Ans. (d) **Meningioma**

(Ref: Harrison 19th p 2653)

- Choice A, B, C are all tumors that metastasize to the brain while meningioma is a benign tumor of the spinal cord.
- Meningiomas are the second most common tumor in the intradural extramedullary location, second only to tumors of the nerve sheath.
- Meningiomas account for approximately 25% of all spinal tumors.
- Approximately 80% of spinal meningiomas are located in the thoracic spine, followed by cervical spine (15%), lumbar spine (3%), and the foramen magnum (2%). Most intradural spinal tumors are benign and potentially resectable.

487. Ans. (b) **Cauda equina syndrome**

(Ref: Harrison 19th p 2651)

- In cauda equina syndrome, the peripheral nerve fibers from the sacral segments of the cord, as well as various lumbar dorsal and ventral nerve roots, may also be involved.
- This results in an asymmetric and higher distribution of motor and sensory symptoms and signs in the lower extremities.
- The saddle anaesthesia seen has complete loss of all sensations like pin prick, temperature unlike dissociative anasesthesia
- Incontinence of bowel and bladder is not severe and develops late for the same reason.
- Symptoms of cauda equina syndrome include the following:
  1. Low back pain
  2. Unilateral or bilateral sciatica
  3. Saddle and perineal hypoesthesia or anesthesia
  4. Bowel and bladder disturbances
  5. Lower extremity motor weakness and sensory deficits
  6. Reduced or absent lower extremity reflexes

Urinary manifestations of cauda equina syndrome include the following:
- Retention
- Difficulty initiating micturition
- Decreased urethral sensation
- Typically, urinary manifestations begin with urinary retention and are later followed by an overflow urinary incontinence.

Bowel disturbances may include the following:
- Incontinence
- Constipation
- Loss of anal tone and sensation

488. Ans. (d) **Bloody tap**

(Ref: 1. Clinical Anesthesiology: Morgan's; 5th/e (2013); Pg : 9662. Lee's Synopsis of Anaesthesia, 12th/e; Pg : 684-689)

Although all the options mentioned may be observed during subarachnoid block, Bloody tap is a procedural finding & should not be considered as a complication of the block.

Complications of Neuraxial Anesthesia
1. Adverse or exaggerated physiological responses
   - Urinary retention
   - High block (Can lead to hypotension)
   - Total spinal anaesthesia
   - Cardiac arrest
   - Anterior spinal artery syndrome
   - Horner's syndrome
2. Complications related to needle/catheter placement
   - Backache
   - Dural puncture/leak
   - Postdural puncture headache
   - Diplopia
   - Tinnitus
   - Spinal cord damage
   - Cauda equina syndrome
   - Intraspinal/epidural hematoma
   - Subdural block
   - Inadvertent intravascular injection
   - Catheter shearing/retention
   - Inflammation
   - Arachnoiditis
   - Infection
   - Meningitis
   - Epidural abscess
3. Drug toxicity
   - Systemic local anesthetic toxicity
   - Transient neurological symptoms
   - Cauda equina syndrome

489. Ans. (c) **Addisonian pernicious anemia**

(Ref: Kumar & Clark: Clinical Medicine, 2012, Pg 816)

Subacute combined degeneration of spinal cord refers to degeneration of the posterior and lateral columns of the spinal cord as a result of

1. Vitamin B_{12} deficiency (most common)
2. Copper deficiency
3. Vitamin E deficiency
4. It is usually associated with pernicious anemia

Clinical Features
1. Early in the course, poor joint position and vibration sense predominate. Typically, the legs are affected before the arms. Rarely are all limbs affected simultaneously. A Romberg sign is commonly found. The gait may be wide based.
2. On presentation, 50% of patients have absent ankle reflexes with relative hyperreflexia at the knees. Plantars are initially flexor and later extensor. A Hoffman sign may be found.
3. As the disease progresses, ascending loss of pinprick, light touch, and temperature sensation occurs. Later, depending on the predominance of posterior column versus cortical spinal tract involvement, ataxia or spastic paraplegia predominates. Then, PNS involvement causes distal limb atrophy.
4. Cognitive testing may reveal mild impairment or frank dementia.
5. **Non-neurologic manifestations include the following:**
   - **General:** Lemon-yellow waxy pallor, premature whitening of hair, flabby bulky frame, mild icterus, and blotchy skin pigmentation in dark-skinned patients
   - **Cardiovascular:** Tachycardia, congestive heart failure
   - **Gastrointestinal:** Beefy, red, smooth, and sore tongue with loss of papillae that is more pronounced along edges
   - **Investigations:** Serum vitamin B12, methylmalonic acid levels with FLAIR MRI
   - **Treatment:** Parenteral im/sc vitamin B12. Cobalamin 1000 mcg IM/SC daily for 5 days followed by 1000 mcg/wk for 5 weeks, then 100-1000 mcg/month for life.

490. Ans. (a) 30 mg/kg within 3 hrs of injury

(Ref: CMDT 2013, Pg 1018)

491. Ans. (a) Loss of Sympathetic tone

(Ref: CMDT 2013, Pg 1018)

492. Ans. (d) Sacral sparing

(Ref: Harrison 19th p 2651-52)

493. Ans. (b) Absent knee and ankle jerks

(Ref: Principles of Surgical patient care 2nd /501, De Jong's Neurological examination 6th/578)

494. Ans. (a) Loss of sympathetic tone

(Ref: Harrison 19th p 2651)

495. Ans. (b) Increased rectal sphincter tone

(Ref: Harrison 19th p 438e)

496. Ans. (c) Lead poisoning

(Ref: Neurology by Anish Bahra/68; Oxford Handbook of tropical Medicine 2nd/436)

497. Ans. (b) Loss of vibration sense

(Ref: Current Diagnosis & Treatment in Neurology 1st/268, 270; Harrison 19th p 2652)

498. Ans. (b) B_{12} deficit

(Ref: Harrison 19th p 2659)

499. Ans. (e) Ascending weakness

(Ref: Harrison 19th p 2658)

Ascending weakness is not a typical feature of syringomyelia

Miscellaneous

500. Ans. (b) Oculomotor nerve palsy

(Ref: Kanski Clinical ophthalmology: 8th edition, page 821-30)

- The image shows presence of left sided ptosis with outgaze due to unopposed activity of lateral rectus muscle. There is an impaired adduction on the left side. The findings are characteristic of oculomotor nerve palsy.
- Lateral rectus palsy will lead to impaired abduction causing the patient to turn the face to the same side.
- Trochlear nerve palsy will lead to ipsilateral hypertropia due to limitation of depression.

Internuclear ophthalmoplegia is seen in multiple sclerosis. The lesion is at medial longitudinal fasciculus and is characterized by impaired adduction of the ipsilateral eye (marking C) with nystagmus of the abducting eye. Convergence is maintained.

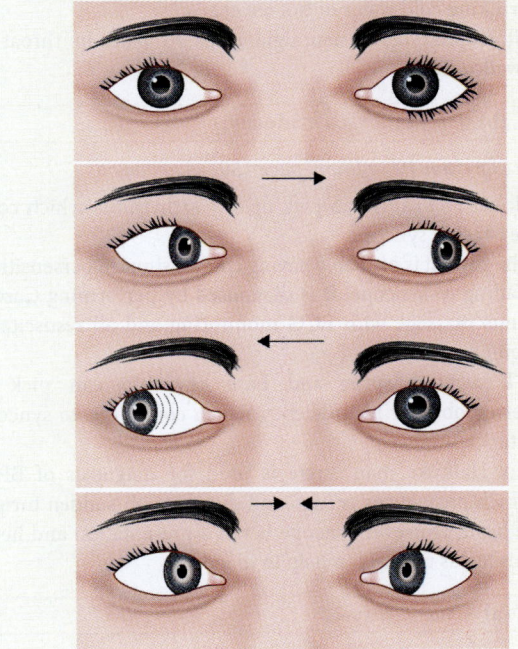

501. Ans. (d) Scanning speech, oscillatory tremor of head and nystagmus

(Ref: Harrison 19th edition, page 2628)

- The MRI head shows atrophy of cerebellum. Ventricles appear normal. Diagnosis is spinocerebellar ataxia.
- Choice A is feature of Normal pressure hydrocephalus.
- Choice B is seen in Huntington's chorea.
- Choice C is seen in Progressive Supra-nuclear gaze palsy

502. Ans. (b) Normal Myocytes

(Ref: Harrison 19th edition, page 2240)

- Fibromyalgia presents as chronic widespread musculoskeletal pain and tenderness. It occurs due to altered sensory afferent pain processing and impaired descending noxious inhibitory control leading to hyperalgesia and allodynia. Muscles and nerves are perfectly normal.
- Choice D is seen in MERRF (Myoclonic Epilepsy with Ragged Red Fibers).
- Choice C is seen in polymyositis.
- Choice A is dummy choice.

503. Ans. (b) Tic Douloureux

(Ref: Harrison 19th edition, page 2646)

- The clinical presentation is of trigeminal neuralgia also known as tic douloureux. It occurs due to ectopic generation of action potential in pain sensitive afferent of trigeminal nerve before it enters into pons.
- The pain may last for few seconds or minutes and may make the patient wince with pain.
- Triggers are washing face, brushing teeth and cold draft of air.
- Dental problems cause deep seated pain in tooth after drinking cold water or hot tea etc.
- Glossopharyngeal neuralgia leads to pain in throat on swallowing.

504. Ans. (b) Dix Hallpike's manoeuvre

(Ref: Harrison 19th edition, page 150)

- Holter recording can pick up any arrhythmia which could be causing syncope.
- The patient is probably having carotid sinus hypersensitivity leading to syncope. It is diagnosed by performing Carotid sinus massage with ECG monitoring and all resuscitative equipment.
- CT cervical spine and base of brain can pick up vertebrobasilar insufficiency which could lead to syncopal attacks.
- Dix Hallpike manoeuvre is used for diagnosis of BPPV which presents as vertigo and dizziness on sudden turning of head. However syncope is not a presentation and hence this test is unlikely to help in diagnosis.

505. Ans. (a) Glucocorticoids

(Ref: Harrison 19th edition, page 2646)

- The main drug used in trigeminal neuralgia is carbamazepine. It causes relief in 75% of patients.
- Alternative agent is oxcarbazepine which has less bone marrow toxicity.
- Lamotrigine and phenytoin are also used. However steroids have no role in management of trigeminal neuralgia.

Surgery is recommended in medically refractory cases

1. Microvascular decompression via sub-occipital craniotomy
2. Gamma knife radiosurgery of trigeminal roots
3. Radiofrequency thermal Rhizotomy

506. Ans. (a) IV saline and observation

(Ref: Harrison 19th edition, 47e-12)

The presence of a remarkable size goitre points to the drug being used as lithium. Lithium toxicity also leads to tremors and ataxia.

507. Ans. (d) Pramipexole

(Ref: Harrison 19th edition, page 192)

Restless legs syndrome is managed as:
1. Treat Iron deficiency anaemia if present
2. Dopamine agonists are most commonly used: Pramipexole/Ropinirole
3. Opioids, BZD and Gabapentin/ pregabalin

508. Ans. (c) Influenza B

(Ref: Harrison 19th edition, page 214)

- Non motor symptoms of Parkinsonism are constipation, anosmia and REM behaviour sleep disorder.
- Kallmann syndrome presents with anosmia due to olfactory bulb agenesis/ hypoplasia.
- HIV infection can also affect olfactory bulbs leading to anosmia
- Influenza B leads to Reye syndrome.

509. Ans. (c) 65 year old man admitted in ICU post hip joint surgery

(Ref: Harrison 19th edition, page 166-67)

- Delirium is commonly seen in hospitalized patients especially elderly and those undergoing hip surgery.
- It is a deficit of attention though cognitive domains like memory, executive function, visuospatial tasks and language are involved. There are two presentations.
  1. Hyperactive patients are easily identified by severe agitation, tremor and hallucinations.
  2. Hypoactive patients are often overlooked in the ward and ICU.

510. Ans. (b) Glucose infusion is followed by mega dose of thiamine

(Ref: Harrison: 19th edition, page 1783)

- Glucose infusions will worsen the neurological symptoms as metabolism of glucose utilizes thiamine. Thiamine is a cofactor in transketolase, pyruvate dehydrogenase and alpha ketoglutarate dehydrogenase. *Hence whatever residual thiamine is present will be consumed.*
- Wernicke's disease is a medical emergency and needs 100mg iv or im thiamine. Thiamine deficiency produces a

diffuse decrease in cerebral glucose utilization and results in mitochondrial damage.
- Site of lesions in Wernicke's disease-
  1. Periventricular third and fourth ventricle
  2. Aqueduct
  3. Atrophy of mammillary bodies
  4. Dorsal medial nucleus of thalamus(Amnestic effect)

511. Ans. (d) All these statements are true

(Ref: Harrison 19th edition, page 903, 1430-31)

Choice A	MRI is superior to CT in imaging the lesions of Neuro-cysticercosis
	• Detecting cystic lesions in the base of the brain, CSF spaces (Example, ventricular NCC, cisternal NCC), and intramedullary lesions.
	• Scolex may be more readily apparent on MRI than on CT.
	• Demonstrating inflammation around the cyst
Choice B	The image shows presence of Neuro-cysticercosis. The stages of disease progression are:
	• Vesicular stage: Viable cysticerci are associated with minimal inflammation
	• Colloid stage: Due to host's immune response, the cyst wall becomes infiltrated and is surrounded by predominantly mononuclear cells. Inflammatory cells enter the cyst fluid.
	• Granular-nodular stage: As the host's immune response progresses, fibrosis encompasses the cysticercus, with concomitant collapse of the cyst cavity.
	• Calcified nodule, which presumably forms as a result of dystrophic calcification of the necrotic larva.
Choice C	On radiographs, calcified cysticerci appear as multiple elongated lesions shaped like cigars or grains of rice. These lesions are arranged in the direction of the muscle fibers in affected skeletal muscle.

512. Ans. (a) Flumazenil

(Ref: Harrison 19th edition, page 2727)

Disulfiram	Induces vomiting and autonomic instability due to production of acetaldehyde.
Acamprosate	Inhibits NMDA receptors and decreases withdrawl symptoms
Naltrexone	Opioid antagonist which decreases the feeling of pleasure on taking alcohol by blocking the activity in dopamine rich ventral tegmental reward system

513. Ans. (b) Asterixis

(Ref: Harrison 19th edition, page 1782)

Apraxia	Constructional apraxia is seen with non-dominant parietal lobe damage. It can be an early sign in metabolic encephalopathy*but not specific as would be seen in a patient with stroke as well*
Asterixis	Flapping tremor of the extremities is also observed in patients with uremia, pulmonary insufficiency, and barbiturate toxicity and distinguishes this patient from a patient with stroke.

Asterixis can be elicited in lethargic but awake patients by having patients extend their arms and bend their wrists back. In this maneuver, patients who are encephalopathic have a "flap movement"—i.e., a sudden forward movement of the wrist like beating of wings of a bird.	
Anosmia	Can been even with URTI
Abulia	Abulia (a delay in verbal and motor response) is seen with anterior cerebral artery infarction.

Manifestations of Metabolic Encephalopathy
1. Lethargy, drowsiness and poor cognition
2. Constructional apraxia
3. Asterixis
4. Patients with hepatic encephalopathy show evidence of fetor hepaticus, a sweet musty aroma of the breath believed to be secondary to the exhalation of mercaptans.
5. Hyperventilation
6. Decreased body temperature.
7. Extrapyramidal symptoms—including tremor, bradykinesia, cog-wheel rigidity, and shuffling gait—have been described in patients with portosystemic shunting.

514. Ans. (c) Increased tone in lower limbs

(Ref: Harrison 19th edition, page 2629)

- Friedreich ataxia is inherited as an autosomal recessive disorder involving the spinocerebellar tracts, dorsal columns in the spinal cord, the pyramidal tracts, and the cerebellum and medulla.
- The majority of patients are homozygous for a GAA repeat
- Patients develop decreased tone in legs with extensor plantars and arreflexia.

> **Must Know**
>
> **Friedreich ataxia**
> - GAA Triplet repeats in FXN gene
> - Autosomal recessive
> - Defect on chromosome 9
> - Dying back phenomenon of axons
> - Loss of ambulation after 15 yr
> - Slow clumsy tabetocerebellar gait (combination of sensory and cerebellar gait)
> - Arreflexia with extensor plantars
> - Dysarthria
> - Associated with diabetes mellitus and cardiomyopathy

515. Ans. (a) Myelomeningocele

(Ref: CPDT 22nd edition 2015, page number 810)

- The image shows a baby with translucent sac at the back indicating a presence of myelomeningocele.
- Myelomeningocele results from failed closure of the caudal end of the neural tube, resulting in an open lesion or sac that contains dysplastic spinal cord, nerve roots, meninges, vertebral bodies, and skin
- Myelomeningocele is associated with Chiari type II malformation is characterized by cerebellar hypoplasia and varying degrees of caudal displacement of the lower

Contd...

brainstem into the upper cervical canal through the foramen magnum.
- This deformity impedes the flow and absorption of cerebrospinal fluid (CSF) and causes hydrocephalus, which occurs in more than 90% of infants with myelomeningocele.

516. Ans. (a) Immediate reduction of body temperature

(Ref: O.P.Ghai, 8th edition, page 556)

The description give is of a case of typical febrile seizure which occurs within 24 hours of fever and lasts less than 10 minutes and is usually a single episode per every febrile episode. There is no post ictal deficit. For management of this case
1. Prompt reduction of fever with hydrotherapy
2. Semi-prone position with adequate airway
3. Rule out meningitis
4. Avoid aspirin
5. Diazepam or Lorazepam for control of seizures.

517. Ans. (c) Codeine & (e) Tramadol

(Ref: L & B 26th/ 245; http://www.paincommunitycentre.org/article/who-analgesic-ladder; http://www.who.int/cancer/palliative/painladder/en/)

WHO PAIN RELIEF LADDER

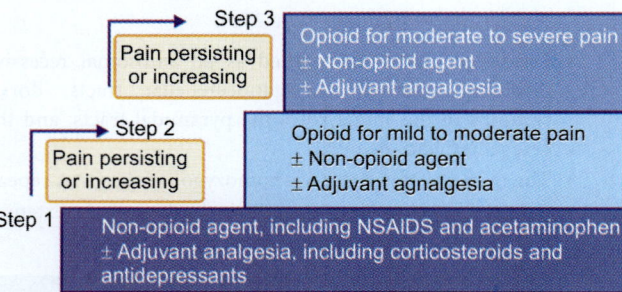

MODIFICATION OF WHO PAIN LADDER

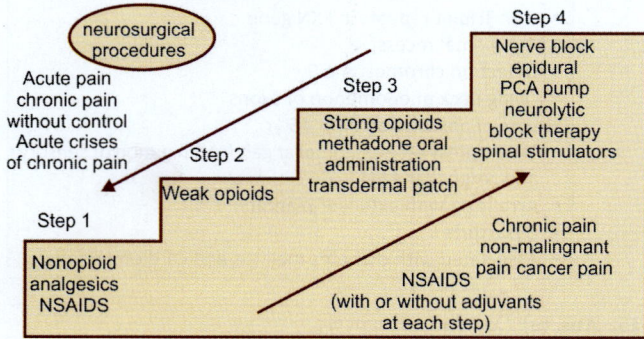

518. Ans. (a) Broca's area

(Ref: Harrison 19th ed. / 177)

- Broca's area damage is called expressive aphasia (non-fluent aphasia).
- Pattern has loss of the ability to produce language (spoken or written).
- Patient has insight to his problem and is frustrated.
- *Remember: Broca is broke. Speaks broken words.*
- Damage to paracentral lobule would lead to loss of control over urination and lead to urge incontinence.
- Damage to insula leads to loss of hand eye coordination and loss of social skills.

519. Ans. (a) Neuropraxia

(Ref: Maheshwari 5th ed. /69)

- In most cases of compressive radial neuropathy, the type of injury is a "neuropraxia" that does not involve damage to the axon.
- Neuropraxia is classified as a transient conduction block of motor or sensory function without neuronal degeneration. Therefore, despite decreased motor function, patients with neuropraxia are able to regain normal neurologic function within several weeks to months.
- Posture-induced radial neuropathy, known as *Saturday night palsy*, occurs because of compression of the radial nerve. The clinical symptoms of radial neuropathy are similar to stroke or a herniated cervical disk, which makes it difficult to diagnose.

	Neurotmesis	Axonotmesis	Neurapraxia
Pathological			
Anatomical continuity	May be lost	Preserved	Preserved
Essential damage	Complete disorganisation, Schwann sheaths preserved	Nerve fibres interrupted	Selective demyellnation of larger fibres, no degeneration of axons
Clinical			
Motor paralysis	Complete	Complete	Complete
Muscle atrophy	Progressive	Progressive	Very little
Sensory paralysis	Complete	Complete	Usually much sparing
Autonomic paralysis	Complete	Complete	Usually much sparing
Electrical phenomena			
Reaction of degeneration	Present	Present	Absent
Nerve conduction distal to the lesion	Absent	Absent	Absent
Motor-unit action potentials	Absent	Absent	Absent
Fibrillation	Present	Present	Occasionally detectable
Recovery			
Surgical repair	Essential	Not necessary	Not necessary

520. Ans. (a) Insula

(Ref: Textbook of Anatomy Vol.3 by Vishram singh, P 391)

- *Insula is also known as Island of Reil.*
- The word insula means hidden. *The insula is the submerged portion of cerebral cortex in the floor of lateral sulcus*.
- It is divided into 2 regions: Anterior and Posterior by a central sulcus. The anterior region represents 3 or 4 short gyri call *gyri brevia* and posterior region presents 1 or 2 long gyri called *gyri longa.*
- The insulae are believed to be involved in consciousness and *play a role in diverse functions usually linked to emotion or the regulation of the body's homeostasis*. These functions include perception, motor control, self-awareness, cognitive functioning, and interpersonal experience.

521. Ans. (b) Thyroid opthalmopathy

(Ref: Harrison 19th ed. / 2294-95)

The question is on unilateral ptosis whereas thyroid opthalmopathy has PROPTOSIS.

- In myasthenia gravis, due to anti-Ach-receptor blocking antibodies there is ptosis which can be unilateral or asymmetrical which will again appear unilateral.
- Marfan syndrome has congenital Ptosis.
  - Pancoast tumor causes Horner syndrome in which ipsilateral sympathetic chain is compressed leading to Ptosis, Miosis, Anhidrosis, Enopthalmos and loss of Cilio-spinal reflex.

522. Ans. (b) Sub-arachnoid granulations

(Ref: Harrison 19th ed. / 443e-4)

CSF is produced by the choroid villi in the lateral ventricles and third ventricles. The CSF flows via aqueduct of slyvius to the 3rd ventricle and then via foramen of Munro to the 4th ventricle. The CSF emerges out of Foramen of Luschka and Magendie and accumulates at the base of the skull in basal cisterns.

- This CSF is then reabsorbed via the arachnoid granulations back into the blood stream.
- The CSF is produced at a rate of 20ml per hour and reabsorbed at the same rate. The total amount of CSF at any point of time is 150 ml.

523. Ans. (d) Nystagmus

(Ref: Harrison 19th ed. / 2608)

- Dementia pugilistica is seen in athletes who participate in body contact sport like martial arts, boxing etc.
- Repeated blows to the head of the athlete over entire career span of the boxer can lead to cortical damage and Parkinson like features. *(Best example to remember this is Muhammad Ali, the greatest boxer of all times, suffered from dementia pugilistica).*
- It presents with personality and social disability changes.
- Nystagmus is not a clinical feature of this disease and is rather seen with vestibular diseases or cerebellar lesions.

524. Ans. (c) Finger pads

(Ref: De Jong neurological examination, 7th ed/542)

- Two-point discrimination is the ability to discern that two nearby objects touching the skin are truly two distinct points, not one. It is often tested with two sharp points during a neurological examination and is assumed to reflect how finely innervated an area of skin is.
- The maximum sensitivity for this test is in lips and finger tips which can be remembered as the most sensitive areas in the body.

525. Ans. (b) Contralateral sub-thalamic lesion

(Ref: Harrison 19th ed./2623)

Lesion	Manifestation
Caudate nucleus	Contralateral chorea
Globus pallidus	Contralateral atheotosis
Sub-thalamic nucleus	Contralateral hemiballismus
Cerebellum	Ipsilateral intentional tremors
Internal capsule	Contra-lateral hemiplegia with hemi-anesthesia
Ventral pons	Locked in syndrome

526. Ans. (a) Middle cerebral artery

(Ref: Gray's Anatomy 40th ed. / 246)

- The Circle of Willis is a part of the cerebral circulation and is composed of the following arteries:
  - Anterior cerebral artery (left and right)
  - Anterior communicating artery
  - Internal carotid artery (left and right)
  - Posterior cerebral artery (left and right)
  - Posterior communicating artery (left and right)
  The basilar artery and middle cerebral arteries, supplying the brain, are not considered part of the circle.

527. Ans. (c) Brain hemorrhage due to tear of basiliar artery branches

(Ref: Radiology review Manual 7th ed/234)

- The classical appearance of a Duret hemorrhage is located in the midline near the ponto-mesencephalic junction.
- Often however, these hemorrhages can be multiple or even extend into the cerebellar peduncles.
- Usually it is seen in patients with severe herniation for 12-24 hours prior to death

528. Ans. (b) 1st order neurons releasing nitric oxide

(Ref: Vascular medicine 3rd ed. / 84)

529. Ans. (a) S1 radiculopathy

(Ref: E 45: Harrison 18th edition)

- The H reflex is easily recorded only from the soleus muscle (S1) in normal adults. It is elicited by low-intensity stimulation of the tibial nerve and represents a monosynaptic reflex in which spindle (Ia) afferent fibers constitute the afferent arc and alpha motor axons the efferent pathway. *The H reflexes are often absent bilaterally in elderly patients or with polyneuropathies and may be lost unilaterally in S1 radiculopathies.*

- The H reflex is most commonly used to evaluate for an S1 radiculopathy or to distinguish from an L5 radiculopathy.
- Needle EMG is used to assess both nerve and muscle function. A small-diameter monopolar pin or coaxial needle is placed into a muscle to evaluate insertional activity, resting activity, voluntary recruitment, morphology, and size of motor units, as well as motor unit recruitment.

530. Ans. (c) Hippocampus

(Ref: Harrison 19th p 1783)

- Periventricular lesions in Wernicke's encephalopathy surround the third ventricle, aqueduct, and fourth ventricle, with petechial haemorrhages in occasional acute cases and atrophy of the mamillary bodies in most chronic cases.
- There is frequently endothelial proliferation, demyelination, and some neuronal loss. These changes may be detected by MRI scanning
- The amnestic defect is related to lesions in the dorsal medial nuclei of the thalamus.

531. Ans. (d) Clonidine

(Ref: Harrison 19th edition, page 2623)

Earlier Haloperidol was considered as DOC for Tourette syndrome. But according to recent changes in treatment modality, Clonidine is considered as DOC for Tourette syndrome.

532. Ans. (a) Friedreich's ataxia

(Ref: Harrison's 'Principles of Internal Medicine'; 18/e, pg 3343, Harrison 19th p 2629-2630)

- Friedreich's ataxia presents before 25 years of age with progressive staggering gait, frequent falling and titubation.
- The areas involved in these patients are spinocerebellar pathways, corticospinal pathway, dorsal column and peripheral nerves.
- Corticospinal pathway damage explains Extensor plantar responses, absence of deep tendon reflexes and weakness is explained by peripheral neuropathy.
- Rest of neurologic examination reveals nystagmus, loss of fast saccadic eye movements, truncal titubation, dysarthria, dysmetria and ataxia of trunk and limb movements.
- Loss of vibratory and proprioceptive sensation occurs due to dorsal column involvement.
- Dysarthria is occasionally the presenting symptom; rarely, progressive scoliosis, foot deformity, nystagmus or cardiomyopathy seen.

533. Ans. (a) Paralysis during sleep-wake transition with hallucinations

(Ref: Harrison 19th p 189)

- In obstructive sleep apnea patient usually falls asleep during day with no loss of postural tone. It mostly occurs in setting of obesity which is not mentioned here.
- Choice C points to restless legs syndrome but does not have history of falls.
- History of fall is highly suggestive of atonia/paralysis may be due to Narcolepsy. Narcolepsy is both a disorder of the ability to sustain wakefulness voluntarily and a disorder of REM sleep regulation.
- The classic "narcolepsy tetrad" consists of excessive daytime somnolence plus three specific symptoms related to an intrusion of REM sleep characteristics (e.g., muscle atonia, vivid dream imagery) into the transition between wakefulness and sleep.
    1. Sudden weakness or loss of muscle tone without loss of consciousness, often elicited by emotion (cataplexy)
    2. Hallucinations at sleep onset (hypnogogic hallucinations) or upon awakening (hypnopompic hallucinations)
    3. Muscle paralysis upon awakening (sleep paralysis).

534. Ans. (b) SCA2

(Ref: Harrison 19th p 2628)

- The most common type of SCA reported in India is SCA2.
- The age of onset ranges from 2–65 years, and there is considerable clinical variability within families. Although neuropathologic and clinical findings are compatible with a diagnosis of SCA1, including slow saccadic eye movements, ataxia, dysarthria, parkinsonian rigidity, optic disc pallor, mild spasticity, and retinal degeneration.
- Machado Joseph disease/SCA3 is the common type of SCA worldwide whereas the reported prevalence of MJD/SCA3 from India is very low.

535. Ans. (d) Processing of speech

(Ref: Harrison's 18th ed. P-202)

Assuming that the patient is a right handed individual, the left part of the parietal lobe will be his DOMINANT LOBE

Dominant parietal lobe functions (LEFT) functions	Non dominant Parietal Lobe (right)
Speech	Spatial orientation
Mathematical calculations	Musical awareness
Reading and understanding text and writing	Attending to contralateral side of body
L and R orientation	

- The language network shows a left hemisphere dominance pattern in the vast majority of the population.
- In approximately 90% of right-handers and 60% of left-handers, aphasia occurs only after lesions of the left hemisphere.
- A language disturbance that occurs after a right hemisphere lesion in a right hander is called crossed aphasia.

536. Ans. (c) Malingering

(Ref: Harrison 19th p 2656 and p 196, 202)

- PCA infarct presents with acute vision loss with new onset posterior cranium headache. The most common examination finding is homonymous visual field cut caused by lesion in opposite occipital lobe This is associated with limb weakness, memory loss and language problems in

setting of risk factors like HTN/family history/ trauma to neck. Macular sparing can occur if occipital lobe is spared. The deep branches of PCA supply the thalamus and mid brain and therefore hemiplegia may also be seen. CT shows hypo-density in occipital lobe and since none of this is present in the case, it is ruled out.
- Optic neuritis usually occurs due to compressive optic neuropathy due to mass lesions, toxic methanol poisoning and ischemic optic neuropathy which is ruled out since MRI imaging is normal.
- Devic's disease (Neuromyelitis optica) has sudden onset usually a unilateral blindness with features of transverse myelitis which is not seen in this case.
- Hence the diagnosis by exclusion is MALINGERING.

537. Ans. (a) Diazepam

(Ref: Harrison's ch. 392, Harrison 19th p 2727)

- If the patient agrees to stop drinking, sudden decreases in alcohol intake can produce withdrawal symptoms, many of which are the opposite of those produced by intoxication. Features include tremor of the hands (shakes); agitation and anxiety; autonomic nervous system overactivity including an increase in pulse, respiratory rate, and body temperature; and insomnia.
- These symptoms usually begin within 5–10 h of decreasing ethanol intake, peak on day 2 or 3, and improve by day 4 or 5, although mild levels of these problems may persist for 4–6 months as a protracted abstinence syndrome.
- **About 2–5% of alcoholics experience a withdrawal seizure, with the risk increasing in the context of concomitant medical problems,** misuse of additional drugs, and higher alcohol quantities. The same risk factors also contribute to a similar rate of delirium tremens (DTs), where the withdrawal includes delirium (mental confusion, agitation, and fluctuating levels of consciousness) associated with a tremor and autonomic overactivity (e.g., marked increases in pulse, blood pressure, and respirations). The risks for seizures and DTs can be diminished by identifying and treating any underlying medical conditions early in the course of withdrawal.
- *The next step is to recognize that because withdrawal symptoms reflect the rapid removal of a CNS depressant, alcohol, the symptoms can be controlled by administering any depressant in doses that decrease the agitation and then gradually tapering the dose over 3–5 days. While most CNS depressants are effective, benzodiazepines have the highest margin of safety and lowest cost and therefore, the preferred class of drugs.*

538. Ans. (c) Urgent surgical decompression

(Ref: Harrison's ch. 376, Harrison 19th p 2647)

- Herpes simplex virus (HSV) type 1 DNA was frequently detected in endo-neural fluid and posterior auricular muscle, suggesting that a reactivation of this virus in the geniculate ganglion may be responsible for most cases.

Clinical Manifestations:
1. Pain behind the ear may precede the paralysis for a day or two.
2. The onset of Bell's palsy is fairly abrupt, maximal weakness being attained by 48 h as a general rule.
3. Taste sensation may be lost unilaterally, and hyperacusis may be present. In some cases there is mild cerebrospinal fluid lymphocytosis.
4. MRI may reveal swelling and uniform enhancement of the geniculate ganglion and facial nerve and, in some cases, entrapment of the swollen nerve in the temporal bone. Approximately 80% of patients recover within a few weeks or months.

Differential Diagnosis
1. Lyme disease
2. The Ramsay Hunt syndrome, caused by reactivation of herpes zoster in the geniculate ganglion, consists of a severe facial palsy associated with a vesicular eruption in the external auditory canal.
3. Sarcoidosis
4. Leprosy frequently involves the facial nerve, and facial neuropathy may also occur in diabetes mellitus, connective tissue diseases including Sjögren's syndrome, and amyloidosis.
5. Melkersson-Rosenthal syndrome consists of recurrent facial paralysis; recurrent—and eventually permanent—facial (particularly labial) edema; and, less constantly, plication of the tongue.
6. Acoustic neuromas frequently involve the facial nerve by local compression. Infarcts, demyelinating lesions of multiple sclerosis, and tumors are the common pontine lesions that interrupt the facial nerve fibers;

Treatment:
1. Use of paper tape to depress the upper eyelid during sleep and prevent corneal drying, and massage of the weakened muscles.
2. A course of glucocorticoids, given as prednisone 60–80 mg daily during the first 5 days and then tapered over the next 5 days, modestly shortens the recovery period and improves the functional outcome.
3. Although two large recently published randomized trials found no added benefit of antiviral agents valacyclovir (1000 mg daily for 5–7 days) or acyclovir (400 mg five times daily for 10 days) compared to glucocorticoids alone, the overall weight of evidence suggests that the combination therapy with prednisone plus valacyclovir may be marginally better than prednisone alone, especially in patients with severe clinical presentations
4. Patients with a poor prognosis, identified by facial nerve testing or persistent paralysis, appear to benefit the most from surgical intervention. Surgery may be considered in patients with complete Bell palsy that has not responded to medical therapy and with greater than 90% axonal degeneration, as shown on facial nerve EMG within 3 weeks of the onset of paralysis. The problem must be localized with MRI. The surgeon can then decide if the

maxillary segment should be decompressed externally or if the labyrinthine segment and geniculate ganglion should be decompressed with a middle fossa craniotomy. The best surgical results were obtained when the procedure was done within 14 days after the onset of paralysis.

539. Ans. (a) 1 to 5 mm Hg

- In the healthy eye, flow of aqueous humor against resistance generates an average intraocular pressure of approximately 15 mm Hg. IOP is necessary to inflate the eye and maintain the proper shape and optical properties of the globe
- Normal ICP is 8-18 mm Hg, and values > 20 mmHg necessitate treatment to be initiated. Hence the difference between ICP and IOP can be best answered as the first choice

540. Ans. (d) H. influenzae meningitis

(Ref: ch. 602, Nelson Textbook of Pediatrics 18th ed.,)

- Rapid killing of bacteria in the CSF effectively sterilizes the meningeal infection but releases toxic cell products after cell lysis (cell wall endotoxin) that precipitates the cytokine-mediated inflammatory cascade. The resultant edema formation and neutrophilic infiltration may produce additional neurologic injury with worsening of CNS signs and symptoms. Therefore, agents that limit production of inflammatory mediators benefit patients with bacterial meningitis.
- *Infectious Diseases Society of America considers the use of dexamethasone in the treatment of HiB meningitis in infants and children to be an A-I recommendation.*
- The recommended dose is 0.15 mg/kg every 6 hours for the first 2 days after initial diagnosis and treatment. Administering the dexamethasone either before or concomitant with the first dose of antimicrobial therapy is likely of considerable importance if a positive effect is expected. No evidence indicates that this form of treatment with dexamethasone, administered during the first 2 days of illness, compromises the outcome of appropriate antimicrobial therapy.
- *Steroids reduce the chances of deafness by mitigating the gliosis that ensues in the eight nerve.*
- Septic shock steroids are not recommended as the toxins of bacteria have already caused endothelial damage.
- Corticosteroids do not constitute a recommended therapy for cerebral malaria, ARDS and massive hemolysis (Blackwater Fever).

541. Ans. (d) Hypercapnia

(Ref: Harrison 19th p 300, 2422, 2559)

Disease	Reason for association with vomiting
Hypocalcemia	Chronic vomiting will cause LOSS of ACID from the body. The resultant metabolic alkalosis will result in displacement of protons from proteins which act as a buffer base. The vacant space on proteins is now taken by ionized calcium. Hence the ionized calcium will decrease

Contd...

Disease	Reason for association with vomiting
Hyponatremia	Chronic vomiting leads to hyponatremia.
Diabetes mellitus	Vomiting can occur due to gastro-paresis secondary to diabetic neuropathy
Hypercapnia	Associated with carbon dioxide narcosis but vomiting is not mentioned

542. Ans. (a) Sarcoidosis

(Ref: Harrison 19th p 2207)

- Neuro-sarcoidosis causes posterior segment of eye involvement where Periphlebitis is seen and perivasculitis is limited to the retinal veins, tends to be segmental, and involves the small branch veins.
- En taches de bougie (candle-wax drippings) is the term used to describe the perivenous exudates. Periphlebitis tends to resolve dramatically on steroid therapy.

543. Ans. (b) Pneumonia

(Ref: Nelson 18th ed., ch. 29.4)

- Death in Rett syndrome may be sudden and often is secondary to pneumonia. Risk factors include seizures, loss of mobility, and difficulties with swallowing.
- Rett syndrome is a neurodevelopmental disorder that occurs almost exclusively in females and has a typically degenerative course. It is related to various mutations on the MECP2 gene, which codes for methyl-CpG binding protein-2 (MECP2).
- RS progresses through 4 stages, typically reached at the following ages:
  - Stage I - Developmental arrest (6-18 months)
  - Stage II - Rapid deterioration or regression (1-4 years)
  - Stage III - Pseudostationary (2-10 years)
  - Stage IV - Late motor deterioration (>10 years)

544. Ans. (a) Non tender lymph nodes

(Ref: Harrison 19th p 464e1)

According to the Centers for Disease Control and Prevention (CDC), in order to receive a diagnosis of CFS, a patient must
1. Have severe chronic fatigue of at least 6 months' duration, with other known medical conditions excluded by clinical diagnosis,
2. Concurrently have 4 or more of the following symptoms:
   - Substantial impairment in short-term memory or concentration
   - Sore throat
   - *Tender lymph nodes*
   - Muscle pain
   - *Multi-joint pain without swelling or redness*
   - Headaches of a new type, pattern or severity
   - *Unrefreshing sleep*
   - Post-exertional malaise lasting more than 24 hours

The symptoms must have persisted or recurred during 6 or more consecutive months of illness and must not have predated the fatigue.

545. Ans. (d) Pituitary adenoma

(Ref: Nelson 18th ed.,ch:90)

- Werner Syndrome is the most common of the premature aging disorders.
- It is an autosomal recessive disorder that affects connective tissue throughout the body. This segmental progeroid syndrome is caused by null mutations at the WRN locus
- The hallmark of this syndrome is a striking disproportion between the patient's real age and the patient's appearance.
- In general, this is an adult-onset disorder, with the earliest sign the lack of a growth spurt during adolescence.
- A prematurely aged appearance with gray hair and sclerodermatous cutaneous changes begins in the 20-30s in association with cataracts, diabetes mellitus, atherosclerosis, cancers, and osteoporosis.
- Pituitary adenoma is seen with WERMER Syndrome(M.E.N type 1) which is inherited as an autosomal dominant disorder. The combination of parathyroid tumors, pancreatic islet cell tumors, and anterior pituitary tumors is characteristic of MEN1.

546. Ans. (b) Sodium Phenylbutyrate

(Ref: Nelson 18th ed, Ch: 85.11: Urea cycle defects)

- In urea cycle disorders, the nitrogen accumulates in the form of ammonia, a highly toxic substance, and is not removed from the body.
- The baby may be irritable at first, followed by vomiting and increasing lethargy. Soon after, seizures, hypotonia, respiratory distress, and coma may occur. If untreated, the child will die. These symptoms are caused by rising ammonia levels in the blood.
- Acute neonatal symptoms are most frequently seen in, but not limited to, boys with OTC Deficiency
- Phenylbutyrate is a prodrug. In the human body it is metabolized by beta-oxidation, mainly in the liver and kidneys, to phenylacetate. Phenylacetate conjugates with glutamine to phenylacetylglutamine, which is eliminated with the urine. It contains the same amount of nitrogen as urea, which makes it an alternative to urea for excreting nitrogen.
- Cysteamine cleaves the disulfide bond with cystine to produce molecules that can escape the metabolic defect in cystinosis and cystinuria. It is also used for treatment of radiation sickness
- Lactulose is used for treatment of hepatic encephalopathy as it binds to ammonia produced by gut bacteria.

547. Ans. (a) Halloverden spatz disease

(Ref: Harrison 19th p 2611, 2626)

- The typical MRI findings of Halloverden Spatz disease include bilaterally symmetrical, hyperintense signal changes in the anterior medial globus pallidus, with surrounding hypointensity in the globus pallidus, on T2-weighted images. These imaging features, which are fairly diagnostic of HSD, have been termed the "eye-of-the-tiger sign."
- The hyperintensity represents pathologic changes, including gliosis, demyelination, neuronal loss, and axonal swelling.
- The surrounding hypointensity is due to loss of signal secondary to iron deposition

548. Ans. (a) Evaluating gait and cognition in normal pressure hydrocephalus

(Ref: Neurology Review, Andrew Tarulli, 2011, page 625)

Miller fisher test involves slow removal of approximately 30 ml of CSF in symptomatic patient of normal pressure hydrocephalus and re-evaluating the cognition of the patient.

549. Ans. (c) Hypersexuality

(Ref: Handbook of Clinical Neurology, Olivier dulac, Harvery B. Sarnat;) Ref: Olivier dulac, Harvery B. Sarnat, p 236

- Klüver–Bucy syndrome may present with Hyperphagia, Hypersexuality, Hyperorality, Visual agnosia, and docility.
- It results from bilateral lesions of the anterior temporal lobe (including amygdaloid nucleus).
- Sometimes Hypermetamorphosis may be seen which is an irresistible impulse to notice and react to everything within sight.

550. Ans. (b) Defect in cholestrol ester transfer protein

(Ref: Nelson 18th ed., ch: 86.4)

Wolman Disease
- It is an autosomal recessive disease.
- The Wolman disease phenotype is characterized by severe diarrhea and malnutrition in infancy. Nearly all patients with Wolman disease have adrenal-gland calcification.
- Lysosomal acid lipase (LAL) is the enzyme necessary for the hydrolysis of triglycerides and cholesteryl esters from endocytosed lipoproteins in lysosomes.
- Its deficiency produces 2 human phenotypes: Wolman disease and Cholesteryl Ester Storage Disease (CESD)
- Characteristic abdominal CT findings (enlarged liver with decreased density and calcified adrenal glands), elevated blood acid phosphatase levels, and histologic findings on liver tissue of microvesicular steatosis suggest a diagnosis of Wolman syndrome.

551. Ans. (c) Hypokalemia

(Ref: Harrison 19th p 118)

Hypoxia	Causes cerebral vasodilation and causes headache. Acute mountain sickness presents with headache due to same reason
Hypercapnia	Causes cerebral vasodilation and stretching of meninges which have nerve ending carrying pain.
Hyponatremia	Cerebral edema leads to headache and seizures

552. Ans. (b) Hypercalcemia

(Ref: Harrison 19th p 313, 2469)

Hyperphosphatemia can cause Hypocalcemia by following mechanisms
1. By precipitating calcium, the product of calcium and phosphate if exceeds 55, then they bind with each other and ectopic calcification occurs.
2. Decreasing vitamin D production
3. Interfering with PTH-mediated bone Resorption

For choice C and D: You can recall tumor lysis syndrome manifestations
1. Hyperphosphatemia
2. Hypocalcemia
3. Hyperuricemia
4. Hyperkalemia

Prolonged Hyperphosphatemia
1. Promotes soft-tissue calcification, in which an abnormal deposition of calcium phosphate occurs in previously healthy connective tissues, such as cardiac valves, and in solid organs, such as muscles.
2. Excess free serum phosphate is taken up into vascular smooth muscle via a type 3 sodium-phosphate co-transporter. The increased cellular phosphate activates a gene, CBFA1, that triggers a transformation in the vascular cell, causing smooth muscle cells to engage in Osteogenesis. Vascular walls become calcified and arteriosclerotic, leading to increased systolic blood pressure, widened pulse pressure, and subsequent left ventricular hypertrophy.

553. Ans. (a) Neurogenic bladder

(Ref: Clinical Pediatric Nephrology, 2nd ed., Pg 96)

Neurogenic bladder, typically occurs in those with sacral abnormalities at birth. The appearance has been described as a Christmas tree of pine cone bladder. The shape of the bladder is highly abnormality with an elongated appearance, with the dome like the top of a Christmas tree. The associated bladder wall hypertrophy gives an outline, which mimics the decorations that adorn a Christmas tree.

	Automatic bladder	Autonomous bladder
Lesion site	Above T5 or higher	Cauda equina damage lower motor neuron damage
Manifestations	Small spastic bladder	Large flaccid bladder
Why this name?	Urge comes again and again due to repeated contractions and hence empties repeatedly after some time.	Has no urge sensation and continuous DRIBBLING occurs. So it is like the bladder is working all the time but BRAIN HAS NO CONTROL OVER IT and hence called autonomous bladder.
Radiological data	Christmas tree appearance	No VUR but still bladder is large and holds lots of residual urine.

554. Ans. (d) Esophagus

(Ref: Harrison 19th p 257)

In dysphagia caused due to CNS the patient complains of Oro-pharyngeal dysphagia with nasal regurgitation of fluids and runs a risk of aspiration. but the patient in question has no such problems.

Areas of Brain Related to Swallowing

Step 1: Voluntary initiation of swallowing	Brain areas located in the precentral, posterior-inferior, and frontal- gyri
Step 2: Impulses travel via cortico-bulbar tract, to a swallowing center in the medulla	1. The nucleus ambiguous (of the vagus and glossopharyngeal 2. The dorsal motor nucleus (of the vagus nerve) 3. The hypoglossal nucleus (of the hypoglossal nerve)
Step 3: Cranial nerves helping with swallowing	Trigeminal (cranial nerve V) Facial (cranial nerve VII) Glossopharyngeal (cranial nerve IX) Vagus (cranial nerve X)

Contd...

Nerve signals originating in the mouth bring information to the brain about the food we are chewing. For instance they "tell" the brain about the size, temperature and texture of food. This information directs the efforts of the muscles of chewing which work together to generate a food bolus that is suitable for swallowing. As the swallowing reflex advances through its different phases, these nerves trigger the reflexive closing of the larynx and the epiglottis, which prevent food and liquid particles from entering the lungs.

555. Ans. (d) Hypothalamus

(Ref: Harrison's, 18th ed., ch: 370;)

Diencephalic pupils are a result of bilateral hemispherical dysfunction and are small. Damage occurs at and close to hypothalamus and will lead to damage to origin of sympathetic fibers which will lead to small but reactive pupils.

Midposition (4-7mm) Unreactive pupils are a result from direct midbrain (tectal region) damage.

556. Ans. (a) Riluzole

(Ref: Harrison 19th p 2635)

RILUZOLE delays the onset of ventilator-dependence or tracheostomy in selected patients and may increase survival by approximately two-to-three months.

For extending life or slowing disease progression in A.L.S, the evidence is best for use of noninvasive ventilation (NIV), percutaneous endoscopic gastrostomy (PEG), and riluzole.

557. Ans. (b) Temporal lobe epilepsy

(Ref: Harrison's 18th ed., ch. 28)

558. Ans. (b) Carotid sinus hypersensitivity

(Ref: CMDT 2013, Pg 977)

- Carotid sinus hypersensitivity (CSH) is an exaggerated response to carotid sinus baro-receptor stimulation. It occurs in older males and results in dizziness or syncope from transient diminished cerebral perfusion.
- Clinically and historically, 3 types of CSH have been described.
  1. The cardioinhibitory type comprises 70-75% of cases. The predominant manifestation is a decreased heart rate, which results in sinus bradycardia, atrioventricular block, or asystole due to vagal action on sinus and atrioventricular nodes. This response can be abolished with atropine.

2. The vasodepressor type comprises 5-10% of cases. The predominant manifestation is a vasomotor tone decrease without a change in heart rate. The significant resulting drop in blood pressure is due to a change in the balance of parasympathetic and sympathetic effects on peripheral blood vessels. This response is not abolished with atropine.
3. The mixed type comprises 20-25% of cases. A decrease in heart rate and vasomotor tone occurs.
- Permanent pacemaker implantation is generally considered an effective treatment for cardio-inhibitory CSH and mixed forms of CSH.

559. Ans. (a) V

(Ref: Harrison 19th p 2623)

560. Ans. (d) Liver necrosis

(Ref: OP. Ghai, 543, 7th ed)

- Reye syndrome is characterized by glycogen depletion and liver cell inflammation but not necrosis.
- Histologic changes include cytoplasmic fatty vacuolization in hepatocytes, astrocyte edema and loss of neurons in the brain, and edema and fatty degeneration of the proximal tubules in the kidneys
- The damage to liver causes increase in PT and hence vitamin K is given
- Blood sugar and CSF sugar are reduced and hence dextrose infusion should be given.
- The main feature of this disease is ANICTERIC hepatitis where liver enzymes are elevated but serum bilirubin is normal.

561. Ans. (d) Hypothermia

(Ref: Harrison 19th p 1781)

- Secondary insults promote excitotoxic secondary brain damage. Detection and correction of secondary insults appear to offer the best therapeutic strategy.
- *After brain trauma, systemic hypotension, compromised CPP, raised ICP, elevated temperature, hypoxemia, and jugular bulb venous desaturation are associated with poor prognosis.*
- Following adult brain trauma maintenance of CPP above at least 65 mmHg (probably > 40 mmHg in children below 8 years) seems important to improve outcome. Therapeutic hypothermia improves survival in Traumatic Brain injury.

562. Ans. (a) Motor neuron disease

(Ref: Harrison 19th p 2633)

- Motor neuron disease in associated with C9orf72 gene is located on the short (p) arm of chromosome 9.
- It consists of hexanucleotide repeat expansion of the six letter string of nucleotides GGGGCC.
- In a normal person, there are up to 30 repeats of this hexanucleotide, but in people with the mutation, the repeat can occur in the order of hundreds
- Thus the resultant accumulation of RNA in the nucleus and cytoplasm becomes toxic, and RNA binding protein sequestration occurs.
- *Two main CNS diseases showing hexa-nucleotide repeats are fronto-temporal dementia and motor neuron disease.*

563. Ans. (a) Rhomberg sign

(Ref: Harrison 19th p 2539)

- Rhomberg sign is a feature of dorsal column damage and indicates sensory ataxia
- Breaking up of complex movements and hypotonia is seen with cerebellar lesions. The hypotonia explains the rebound phenomenon due to lack of resistance.
- Dysmetria implies inability to judge distance between 2 points and is evaluated by finger nose test.

564. Ans. (d) Extensor plantar with brisk lower limb reflexes

(Ref: Harrison 19th p 2629)

565. Ans. (a) Friedreich's ataxia

(Ref: Harrison 19th p 2629)

566. Ans. (a) Ataxia

(Ref: Harrison 19th p 2629)

567. Ans. (a) Cogwheel rigidity

(Ref: Harrison 19th p 1782)

568. Ans. (d) Hippocampus

(Ref: Harrison 19th p 1783)

569. Ans. (a) Down's syndrome

(Ref: Harrison 19th p 2600)

570. Ans. (a) Allodynia

(Ref: Harrison 19th p 2643)

571. Ans. (d) Apparent exophthalmos

(Ref: Localization in Clinical Neurology (Lippincott Williams) 2011/208; Anatomic Basis of Neurological Diagnosis (Thieme) 2009/467)

Iris heterochromia is seen with Horner syndrome developing in child <2 years of age. Pigmentation of iris is under sympathetic control and is completed by age of 2 years.

572. Ans. (a) Hepatic encephalopathy

(Ref: Harrison 18th/p 2601)

573. Ans. (b) Anomic aphasia

(Ref: Harrison 19th p 178)

574. Ans. (a) Polio

Normally to transmit the weight of limb, midstance the knee is locked by quadriceps contraction. If it is weak, locking is hampered and buckling at knee will occur. Hence to stabilize the knee for weight bearing, patient places his hand in front of knee and lower thigh. This is called as hand knee gait.

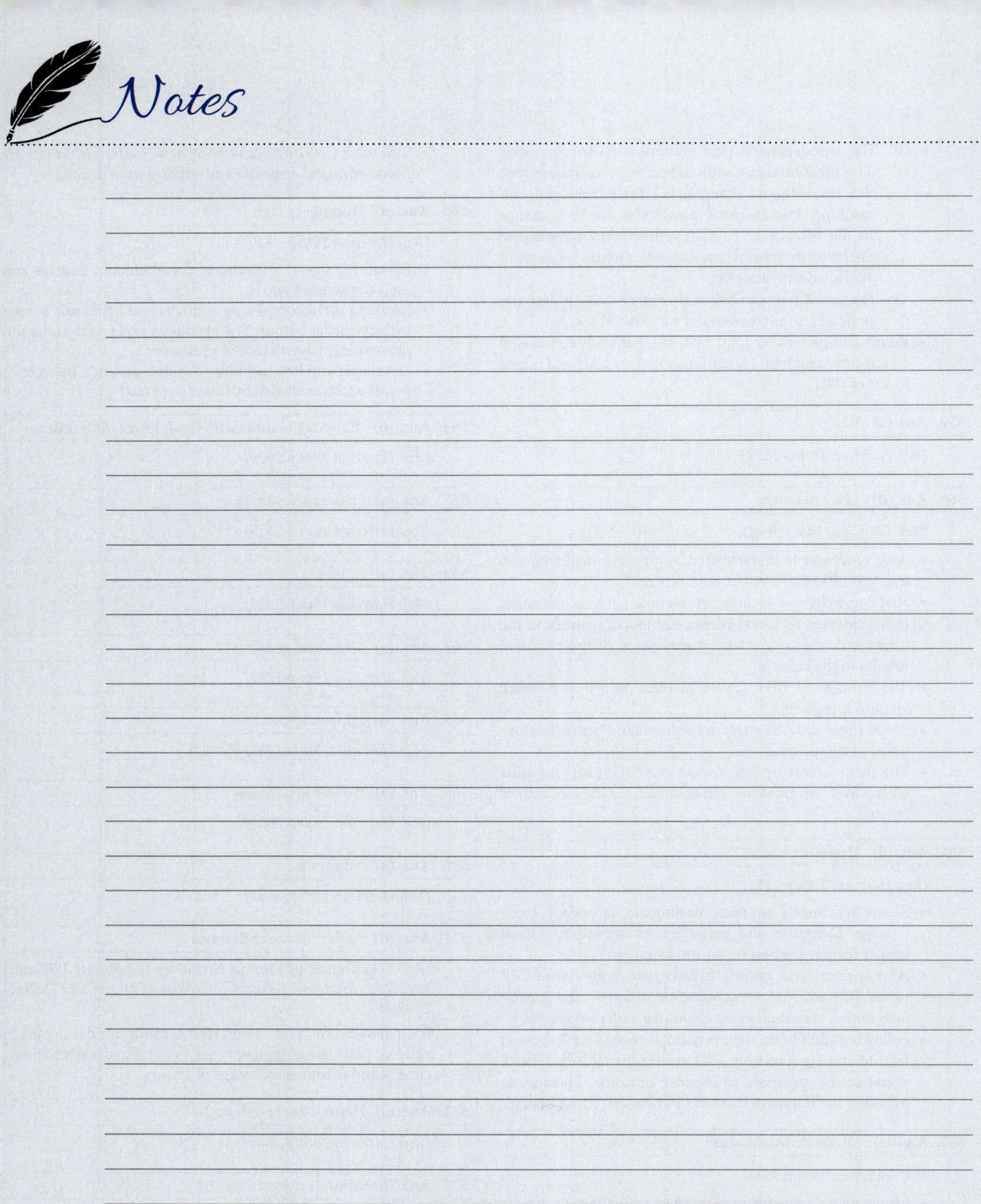

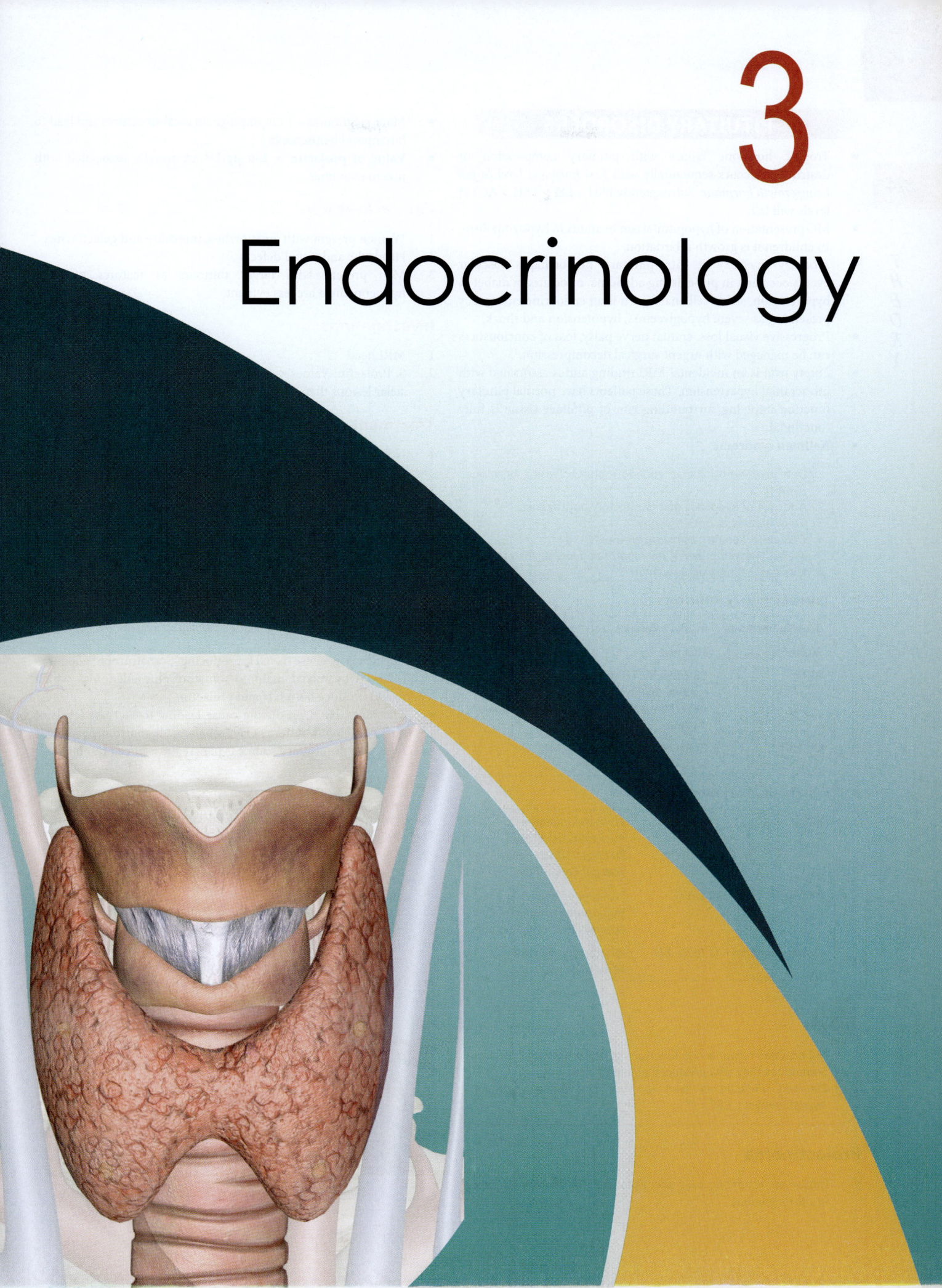

3 Endocrinology

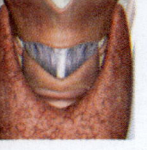

PITUITARY DISORDERS

- Trophic hormone failure with pituitary compression or destruction occurs sequentially with *first hormone level to fall being growth hormone*. Subsequently FSH > LH > TSH > ACTH levels will fall.
- MC presentation of hypopituitarism in adults in hypogonadism. In children it is growth retardation.
- *Pituitary apoplexy* is intra-pituitary hemorrhagic vascular events occuring in pre-existing adenoma, or occurs in diabetes, hypertension, sickle cell anaemia. It is an endocrine emergency presenting as severe hypoglycemia, hypotension and shock.
- Progressive visual loss, cranial nerve palsy, loss of conciousness can be managed with urgent surgical decompression.
- *Empty sella* is an incidental MRI finding and is associated with intracranial hypertension. These patients have normal pituitary function implying surrounding rim of pituitary tissue is fully functional.
- **Kallman syndrome**

  1. Defective hypothalamic gonadotrophia releasing hormone (GnRH)
  2. Anosmia or hyposmia due to olfactory bulb agenesis
  3. Color blindness, optic atrophy
  4. CNS abnormalities: Mirror movements
  5. Males: Delayed puberty, micropenis and low testosterone
  6. Females: Primary amenorrhea

- **Tests of pituitary sufficiency**

Growth hormone	Insulin tolerance test
Prolactin	TRH test
ACTH	CRH test, ACTH stimulation test (cosyntropin test) ACTH stimulation test for primary addison disease
LH, FSH	GnRH test with basal LH, FSH, testosterone, estrogen

- **Familial pituitary tumor syndromes**

MEN1	(11q13)	Pituitary adenoma Hyperparathyroidism Zollinger Ellison syndrome^Q Foregut carcinoids^Q
MEN4	(12p13)	Pituitary adenoma Hyperparathyroidism Reproductive organ tumors
Carney complex	(17q23–24)	Pituitary hyperplasia Atrial myxoma

> **EXTRA MILE**
> - MC pituitary tumor is non functioning/null cell tumor
> - Sometimes they may produced gonadotropins
> - Elevated prolactin is seen in post ictal period, primary hypothyroidism, CRF

Prolactinoma

- Tumor of lactotrope cells accounts for 50% of all *functioning pituitary tumours.*
- Macroadenomas > 1 cm impinge on local structures and lead to bitemporal hemianopia.
- Value of prolactin > 250 µg/L^Q are usually associated with macroadenomas.

Clinical Features

1. Women present with amenorrhea, infertility and galactorrhea
2. Headache and visual defects
3. Men present with larger tumours as features of male hypogonadism are less evident.

Investigations

1. MRI head
2. S. Prolactin: Values < 100 µg/L are caused by microadenomas, sellar lesions that decrease dopamine inhibition.

Treatment

1. No treatment is needed if patients are asymptomatic and fertility is not desired, since microadenomas rarely progress to macroadenomas.
2. Cabergoline is long acting dopamine agonist with high D_2 receptor affinity. The drug effectively supresses PRL for >14 days after single dose. It induces prolactinoma shrinkage in most patients.
3. Bromocriptine has short action and is used when pregnancy is desired. It has no teratogenic effects.

Acromegaly

- The leading cause is GH producing Somatotroph adenoma followed by mixed mammo-somatotrophic adenomas which would produce both GH and prolactin.
- The MC GHRH producing cause leading to increase levels of GH is carcinoid tumour > Hypothalamic hamartoma.
- Rarely extra-pituitary source is pancreatic islet cell tumour

Clinical Features

1. Frontal bossing with increase in size of hand and feet
2. Prognathism with widened space between lower incisors
3. Frequent change of shoe size, glove size, ring tightening and spade like hands
4. Increased heel pad thickness
5. Coarse facies wit hyperhidrosis and acanthosis nigricans
6. Hypertension leading to LVH and ischemic cardiomyopathy
7. Impaired glucose tolerance/ diabetes mellitus
8. Arthropathy and muscle weakness
9. Visual field defects due to optic chiasma compression
10. Increased risk of colonic polyps

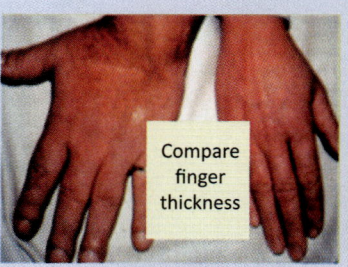

Spade like Hands

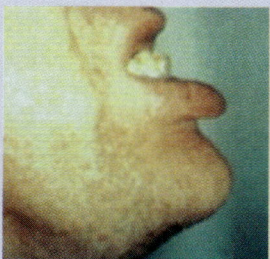

Prognathism

Work up
1. Screening test is IGF-1 levels
2. IOC is glucose challenge test which shows failure of GH level suppression to <0.4ug/L with oral glucose load
3. Increased prolactin level
4. Reduced TSH production due to the mass effect of tumour

Treatment
1. Trans sphenoidal surgery for resection of the macroadenoma
2. Earliest response to surgery is reduction of soft tissue swelling followed by reduction of GH hormone levels by 1 hour and IGF-1 levels by 3-4 hours.
3. Somatostatin analogues given subcutaneously to reduce the size of tumour and they act on SSTR2, SSRT5 receptors to reduce GH production.
   Lanreotide/Octreotide/Pasireotide
4. Pegvisomant antagonises the effect of GH at the receptor level but does not act on pituitary adenoma.

DIABETES MELLITUS

Causes of Type 1 Diabetes Mellitus

- **Autoimmunity** (HLA DQ-A1* 0301, DR-3 & DR-4)
- *Gene involved in T1DM is CTLA-4 gene.* This gene regulates insulin production.
- **Viral Damage:** Coxsackie–B, mumps, rubella (fulminant diabetes)
- **Bronze diabetes**
- **Latent autoimmune diabetes:** In adults, this condition is a variant of type–1 DM due to auto antibody anti GAD (glutamate acid decarboxylase). It destroys β-cell and is also called Type 1.5 diabetes mellitus.

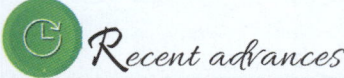

Type 1 Diabetes Mellitus has been reclassified
- Type 1A: Due to genetic or environmental factors
- Type 1B: Idiopathic

Diagnostic Sensitivity and specificity of Autoimmune Markers in Patients with Newly Diagnosed Type 1 Diabetes Mellitus.

Antibodies seen in type 1 Diabetes	Sensitivity
ICA antibody	44–100%
Glutamic acid decarboxylase (GAD65)	70–90%
Tyrosine phosphatase (IA-2)	50–70%
Zinc transporter 8 (ZnT8)	50–70%
Insulin (IAA)	40–70%

Causes of Type 2 Diabetes Mellitus

Type 2 DM has a strong genetic component. The concordance of type 2 DM in identical twins is between 70 and 90%. Individuals with a parent with type 2 DM have an increased risk and if both parents have type 2 DM, the risk approaches 40%. It occurs due to insulin resistance and defective insulin production. The levels of plasma insulin (fasting) is elevated in type 2 diabetes mellitus.

MODY: Maturity Onset Diabetes of Young

- *Maturity-onset diabetes of the young* (MODY) is a subtype of DM characterized by autosomal dominant inheritance, early onset of hyperglycemia (usually <25 years)
- MODY is of 6 types: 1, 2, 3, 4, 5 and 6
- Most Common type of MODY is 3.^{Q}

Genetic Defects of Pancreatic β Cell Function

MODY 1	HNF-4α; rare
MODY 2	Glucokinase; less rare
MODY 3	HNF-1α (accounts for two-thirds of all MODY), defect on chromosome 12
MODY 4	PDX1
MODY 5	HNF-1β
MODY 6	NeuroD1

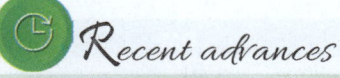

Type A Insulin Resistance Syndrome
- Autosomal dominant or recessive
- Mutations in INSR gene lead to defective insulin receptor
- Type 2 diabetes mellitus has insulin resistance due to polygenetic and receptor malfunction is due to factors like centripetal obesity.

Clinical features
- More common in females with primary amenorrhea or oligomenorrhea.
- Ovarian cysts
- Hirsutism
- Acanthosis nigricans
- *Obesity is not seen.*

Clinical Features of DM

Classic symptoms include polyuria, polydipsia and weight loss.
1. Polyuria : >3L/day
2. Polydipsia
3. Polyphagia
4. Weight loss and asthenia. Weight gain is a feature of Type 2 diabetes mellitus
5. Recurrent infections like UTI/vulvovaginitis
6. Postprandial blurring of vision.

Features of MODY
- No antibodies
- No obesity
- DKA uncommon
- No insulin resistance

Investigations

1. **HbA1c ≥ 6.5%**[Q]
   - Normal HbA1c < 5.6 %
   - HbA1c = 5.7–6.4 % - Impaired glucose tolerance

- HbA1c is indicative of sugar control for the previous 8–12 weeks.
- It is a retrospective test.
- It provides long term control of DM.
- It is the best test for determining the compliance of patient.
- Severity of DM is best determined by HbA1c.
- Investigation of choice for diagnosis of diabetes mellitus is HbA1c.

2. **Blood sugar**

Blood sugar	Normal	IGT	DM
Fasting	< 100 mg %	100–125 mg %	> 126 mg %
2 hour value	< 140 mg %	140–199 mg %	> 200 mg %

3. **Lipid profile**

	Normal	DM
S. cholesterol	< 200 mg	Normal
S. triglycerides	<150 mg	↑↑↑
LDL	<100	Normal
HDL	>30	↓

4. Urine for ketones/ proteins/sugar : Microalbuminuria indicates renal damage and ACE ⊖ should be initiated to slow the progression to ESRD.

- Best test for **short term control of diabetes is serum fructosamine.**
- Serum fructosamine is a retrospective test for previous 2 weeks.

Remember the Diagnostic Criteria for Diabetes Mellitus

Symptoms of diabetes plus random blood glucose concentration > 11.1 mmol/L (200 mg/dL)
Fasting plasma glucose >126 mg/dL
HbA1C > 6.5%
Two-hour plasma glucose >200 mg/dL, during an oral glucose tolerance test

Treatment of Type 2 Diabetes Mellitus

- Exercise has multiple positive benefits including cardiovascular risk reduction, reduced blood pressure, maintenance of muscle mass, reduction in body fat, and weight loss.
  - For individuals with type 1 or type 2 DM, exercise is also useful for lowering plasma glucose (during and following exercise) and increasing insulin sensitivity.
  - In patients with DM, the ADA recommends 150 min/week (distributed over at least 3 days) of moderate aerobic physical activity. The exercise regimen should also include resistance training.

Oral Hypoglycemic Drugs (see table below)

Drug category	Mechanism of action	Names	Lowering of HbA1c in %
Oral			
Biguanides	↓ Hepatic glucose production	Metformin	1–2
α-glucosidase inhibitors	↓ GI glucose absorption	Acarbose, miglitol	0.5–0.8
Dipeptidyl peptidase IV inhibitors	Prolong endogenous GLP-1 action	Saxagliptin, sitagliptin, vildagliptin	0.5–0.8
Insulin secretagogues: sulfonylureas	↑ Insulin secretion		1–2
Thiazolidinediones	↓ Insulin resistance, ↑ Glucose utilization	Rosiglitazone, Pioglitazone	0.5–1.4
Bile acid sequestrants	Bind bile acids; mechanism of glucose lowering not known	Colesevelam	0.5
Parenteral			
Insulin	↑ Glucose utilization, ↓ hepatic glucose production and other anabolic actions		Not limited
GLP-1 receptor agonists	↑Insulin, ↓glucagon, slow gastric emptying, satiety	Exenatide, liraglutide	0.5–1.0
Amylin agonists	Slow gastric emptying, ↓ glucagon	Pramlintide	0.25–0.5
Medical nutrition therapy and physical activity	↓Insulin resistance, ↑insulin secretion	Low-calorie, low-fat, diet, exercise	1–3

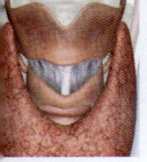

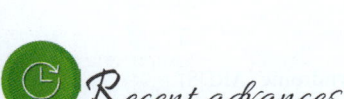

Recent advances

Algorithm for the Treatment of Type 2 Diabetes based on the Recommendations of the Consensus Panel of the American Diabetes Association

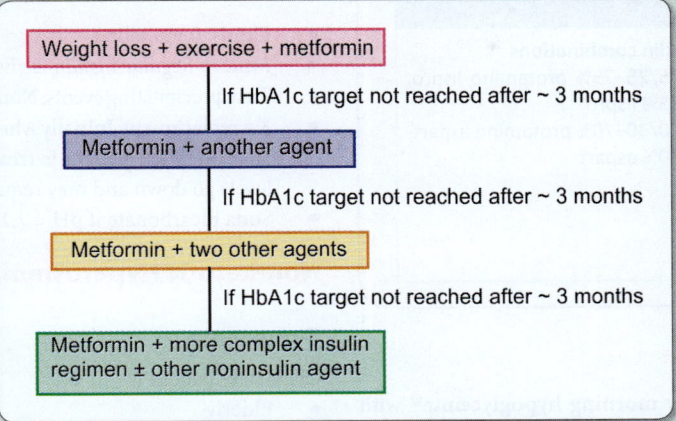

Effect on weight
- Metformin and DPP-4 inhibitors are weight neutral
- GLP-1 receptor agonists and SGLT2 inhibitors promote weight loss
- Sulfonylureas, insulins and pioglitazone are associated with weight gain.

Major side effects
- Metformin can cause lactic acidosis
- Pioglitazone is associated with fluid retention, fracture risk, and possibly bladder cancer
- GLP-1 receptor agonists are associated with nausea and vomiting and possibly pancreatitis
- DPP-4 inhibitors may be associated with pancreatitis risk.

Recently, bromocriptine has been approved as an antidiabetic drug
- It improves glycemic control and glucose tolerance in obese type 2 diabetic patients.
- Both reductions in fasting and postprandial plasma glucose levels appear to contribute to the improvement in glucose tolerance.

- **Insulin Therapy**
  - Current insulin preparations are generated by recombinant DNA technology and consist of the amino acid sequence of human insulin or variations thereof. In United States, most insulin is formulated as U-100 (100 units/mL).
  - Regular insulin formulated as U-500 (500 units/mL) is available and sometimes useful in patients with severe insulin resistance. Human insulin has been formulated with distinctive pharmacokinetics or genetically modified to more closely mimic physiologic insulin secretion. Insulins can be classified as short-acting or long-acting.
- **Uses of Insulin**
  1. Type-2 diabetes mellitus refractory to oral hypoglycemic drugs
  2. Type-1 diabetes mellitus
  3. Diabetic ketoacidosis
  4. Non-ketotic hyperosmolar coma
- **Insulin Delivery**
  - **Insulin pump**^{Q} **(Most effective delivery)**
  - Insulin pen
  - Inhaled insulin
  - Multi-dose vial
- **Sites of insulin administration**^{Q}
  1. Abdominal wall
  2. Thigh and arm
  3. Buttocks

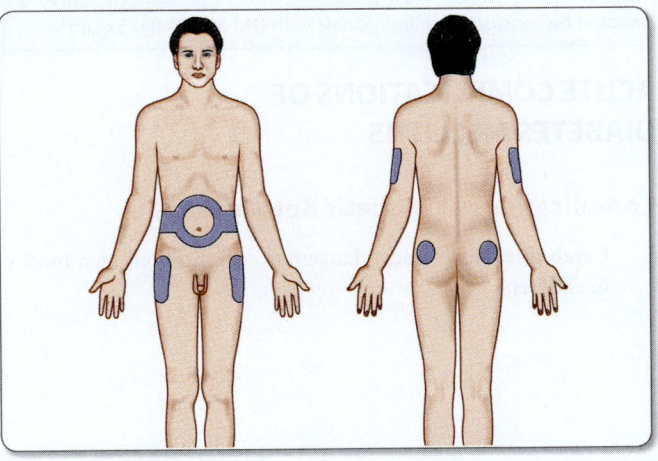

The *abdomen is preferred site* as it absorbs faster as compared to other sites.

Preparation of Insulin

Short-acting	Insulin combinations
• Aspart	• 75/25–75% protamine lispro, 25% lispro
• Glulisine	
• Lispro	• 70/30–70% protamine aspart, 30% aspart
• Regular	
Long-acting	
• Detemir	
• Glargine	
• NPH	

Side Effect of Insulin Usage

- **Somogyi phenomenon:** Early morning hypoglycemia[Q] with Prebreakfast hyperglycemia.
- **Dawn phenomenon:** Early morning hyperglycemia[Q] with Prebreakfast hyperglycemia.

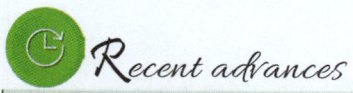 Recent advances

New Trends in Management of Diabetes Mellitus

Whole pancreas transplantation (performed concomitantly with a renal transplant) may normalize glucose tolerance. If it is not feasible then *the beta cell extract is infused in recipient's portal vein*.

After Successful pancreatic transplantation
- Complication that may be reversed/healed
  - Early diabetic nephropathy (microalbuminuria stage)
  - Diabetic neuropathy
- Complications that cannot be reversed/healed
  - Diabetic retinopathy
  - Peripheral vascular disease

Closed-loop pumps that infuse the appropriate amount of insulin in response to changing glucose levels.

Bariatric surgery for markedly obese individuals with type 2 diabetes. The ADA clinical guidelines state that bariatric surgery should be considered in individuals with DM and BMI>35kg/m².

ACUTE COMPLICATIONS OF DIABETES MELLITUS

Complications of Diabetic Ketoacidosis

1. **Cerebral edema**[Q] (most dangerous complication, seen mostly in children)
2. Venous thrombosis
3. Acute respiratory distress syndrome (ARDS)
4. Myocardial infarction (MI)
5. Acute gastric dilatation

Treatment of Diabetic Ketoacidosis

- Fluids: 0.9% saline
- *Insulin: Regular insulin is given IV in DKA*
- Treat precipitating events: Non-compliance, infection by antibiotics.
- K+ replacement: Initially when patient comes, he is hyperkalemic, later on when patient is treated with insulin, serum potassium levels go down and may require potassium replacement.
- Soda bicarbonate if pH < 7.15

Non-ketotic Hyperosmolar Coma

Symptoms

Classically patient is
- Elderly
- H/O polyuria of several weeks with weight loss and decrease oral intake
- Mentally confused.

Signs

- Tachycardia
- Hypotension
- Dehydration
- Altered sensorium, coma

Hyperglycemic Hyperosmolar State

- Hyperglycemia> 600 mg/dL
- Serum osmolality> 310 mosm
- No acidosis
- Bicarbonate > 15 mEq/L
- Normal anion gap

Treatment

- Fluid: Total fluid deficit (9–10 L) should be reversed over 1–2 day
- Initially give normal saline to stabilize the patients hemodynamically (to bring systolic BP above 90 mm Hg). After that give 0.45% saline
- Regular insulin to be given intravenously.
- Subcutaneous heparin should be given because these patients are prone to venous thrombosis.

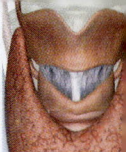

Laboratory Diagnosis of Coma in Diabetic Patients

Related to diabetes	Urine glucose	Acetone	Plasma glucose	Bicarbonate	Acetone
Hypoglycemia	0	0 or +	Low	Normal	0
Diabetic ketoacidosis	++++	++++	High	Low	++++
Hyperglycemic hyperosmolar state coma	++++	0	High	Normal or slightly low	0
Lactic acidosis	0 or +	0 or +	Normal or low or high	Low	0 or +

Lactic Acidosis

- Lactic acidosis is characterized by low pH in body tissues and blood.
- Elevated lactate is indicative of tissue hypoxia, hypoperfusion and state of acute circulatory failure.
- It is very common in type 2 diabetic patients who are on metformin therapy.

Lactic Acidosis
- Acidosis with hyperventilation
- Blood pH <7.3
- Serum bicarbonate < 15 mEq/L
- High anion gap
- Serum lactate >5 mmol/L
- Absent serum ketones.

Signs

- Deep and rapid breathing
- Vomiting
- Abdominal pain.

Treatment

- Lactic acidosis is typically associated with tissue hypoperfusion. Appropriate measures include treatment of shock, restoration of circulating fluid volume, improved cardiac function, identification of sepsis source and appropriate therapy, and resection of any potential ischemic regions.
- Sodium bicarbonate is given intravenously if pH < 7.2 inspite of adequate fluid resuscitation.
- Thiamine: Thiamine deficiency may be associated with cardiovascular compromise and lactic acidosis. The response to thiamine repletion may be dramatic and potentially life-saving.

Wolfram Syndrome/ DIDMOAD
- Due to WFS1 gene mutation
- Central diabetes insipidus
- Diabetes mellitus
- Optic atrophy
- Deafness

LONG-TERM COMPLICATIONS OF DIABETES

Duration of DM is the most important determinant for diabetes complications.

Diabetic Retinopathy

A diabetic patient has 25 times increased chances of blindness.

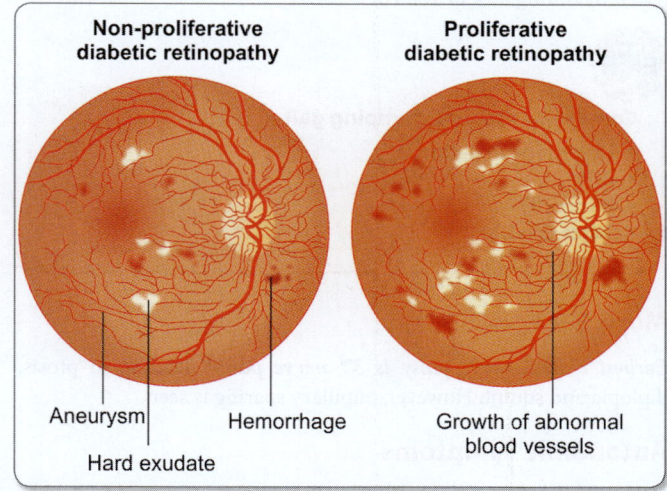

On Fundus Examination

- Earliest manifestation is formation of microaneurysms seen in *inner nuclear or outer plexiform layers*.
- Non-proliferative retinopathy leads to macular edema and progressive visual loss.
- *The appearance of neovascularization in response to retinal hypoxemia is the hallmark of proliferative diabetic retinopathy. These newly formed vessels appear near the optic nerve and/or macula and rupture easily, leading to vitreous hemorrhage, fibrosis, and ultimately retinal detachment.*
- Not all individuals with non-proliferative retinopathy develop proliferative retinopathy, but in the more severe or the non-proliferative disease, there are greater chances of evolution to **proliferative retinopathy within 5 years.**
- This creates an important opportunity for early detection and treatment of diabetic retinopathy

- S. homocysteine and S. creatinine elevations predict development of diabetic retinopathy
- **Treatment of neovascularization:** Pan-retinal photocoagulation with ND-YAG laser + inj. anti- VEGF (Bevacizumab)

Recent advances

Best measure to reduce microvascular and macrovascular complications In type 2 diabetes mellitus is blood pressure control rather than glycemic control.

Infections

- Rhinocerebral mucormycosis
- Invasive aspergilloma
- Malignant otitis externa
- Emphysematous pyelonephritis

Diabetic Neuropathy

First to be involved is sensory system characterized by distal sensory loss. Earliest sensation lost is vibration sense. Vibration sense is tested by tuning fork of 128 Hz.

Conditions causing stamping gait
- Diabetic neuropathy
- INH
- B6 toxicity
- Tabes dorsalis

Motor Symptoms

Earliest cranial nerve palsy is **3rd nerve palsy**^{Q} leading to ptosis, diplopia and squint. However, pupillary sparing is seen.

Autonomic Symptoms

- Silent myocardial infarction can lead to sudden death
- Postural hypotension
- Resting tachycardia
- Nocturnal diarrhea
- Constipation
- Gastroparesis.

Postural hypotension
- When SBP & DBP fall due to change in position from supine to standing in 3 minutes it is defined as postural hypotension.
- Systolic blood pressure fall > 20 mm Hg
- Diastolic blood pressure fall > 10 mm Hg
- Patient complains of dizziness, vertigo, pre-syncope
- Treatment: Elastic stocking & increase salt intake
- Drug of choice: Midodrine (oral)

Note:
- Most reliable symptom of hypoglycemia in DM is sweating.
- Non-selective β-blockers are contraindicated in DM.

Diabetic Nephropathy

Harrison 20th update
- American Diabetic Association *no longer uses* the term microalbuminuria or macroalbuminuria and instead uses the term albuminuria. (*It is still given below for you to be able to solve questions of previous years*)
- It is defined as spot urinary albumin to creatinine ratio > 30mg/g Cr
- Albuminuria is a risk factor for cardiovascular disease and progression of CKD

- During the first 5 years of DM, thickening of the glomerular basement membrane occurs.
- After 5–10 years of type 1 DM, 40% of individuals begin to excrete small amounts of albumin in the urine.
- *Microalbuminuria is defined as 30–299 mg/day in a 24-hour collection or 30–299 μg/mg creatinine in a spot collection (preferred method).*
- Although the appearance of microalbuminuria in type 1 DM is an important risk factor for progression to macroalbuminuria (>300 mg/day).
- Microalbuminuria is a risk factor for cardiovascular disease.
- Once macroalbuminuria is present, there is a steady decline in GFR, and 50% of individuals reach ESRD in 7–10 years.
- *Most common histopathological feature* of diabetic nephropathy is diffuse glomerulosclerosis.
- *Most characteristic finding in diabetic nephropathy* is nodular glomerulosclerosis.

Chronic kidney disease	GFR
Stage – I	90 mL / min / 1.73 m²
Stage – II	60–89 mL / min / 1.73 m²
Stage – III	30–59 mL / min / 1.73 m²
Stage – IV	15–29 mL / min / 1.73 m²
Stage – V	< 15 mL / min / 1.73 m²

- Stage – IV is hemodialysis dependent
- Stage – V is transplant dependent
- **Treatment:** ACE – inhibitors have been shown to slowdown the progression of the disease.

Diabetic Dermatopathy

- The most common skin manifestation in diabetics is *xerosis* and pruritis.
- Wound healing is always delayed.
- Pigmented pretibial papules begin as erythematous macule that develops into area of circular hyperpigmentation.
- Necrobiosis lipoidica diabeticorum presents as lesions with shallow central ulcerations or erosions in pre-tibial region in young women.

- Acanthosis nigricans has hyperpigmented velvety plaques on neck, axilla or extensor surfaces.

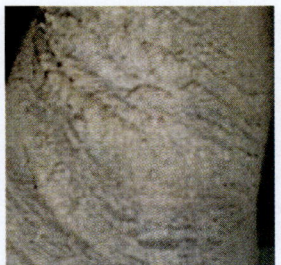

Acanthosis nigricans

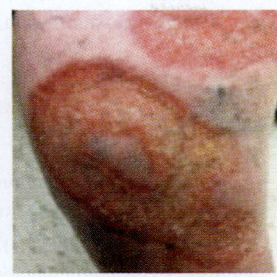

Necrobiosis lipoidica diabeticorum

Summary of Complications of Diabetes Mellitus

Microvascular
- Retinopathy (Non-proliferative/proliferative)
- Neuropathy
- Nephropathy
- Ischemic cardiomyopathy

Macrovascular
- Coronary heart disease (3–5 times higher than normal population)
- Peripheral arterial disease (100 times higher than normal population)
- Cerebrovascular disease

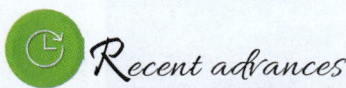

Treatment Goals for Adults with Diabetes

Index	Goal
Glycemic control	
• HbA1c	<7.0%
• Preprandial capillary plasma glucose peak	80–130 mg/dL
• Postprandial capillary plasma glucose	<180 mg/dL
Blood pressure	<140/90 mmHg
Lipids	
• Low-density lipoprotein	<100 mg/dL
• High-density lipoprotein	>40 mg/dL in men >50 mg/dL in women
• Triglycerides	<150 mg/dL

Landmark Trials in Diabetes Mellitus Whose Data is Asked and Is Highlighted

- The DCCT demonstrated that improvement of glycemic control
  - Reduced nonproliferative and proliferative retinopathy (47% reduction)
  - Microalbuminuria (39% reduction)
  - Clinical nephropathy (54% reduction)
  - Neuropathy (60% reduction)
  - Improved glycemic control also slowed the progression of early diabetic complication
  - *There was a nonsignificant trend in reduction of macrovascular events during the trial.*
- The UKPDS demonstrated that each percentage point reduction in A1C was associated with a 35% reduction in microvascular complications.
- One of the major findings of the UKPDS was that strict blood pressure control significantly reduced both macro and microvascular complications. In fact, the beneficial effects of blood pressure control were greater than the beneficial effects of glycemic control, lowering blood pressure to moderate goals (114/82 mmHg) reduced the risk of DM-related death, stroke, microvascular end-points, retinopathy and heart failure (risk reductions between 32 and 56%).

METABOLIC SYNDROME

Also known as syndrome X.
1. **Centripetal obesity:** Waist circumference >102 cm in males, >88 cm in females
2. **Hyperlipidemia:** Characterized by elevated triglycerides and low HDL.
3. **Hypertension:** ≥ 130 mm Hg systolic or ≥ 80 mm Hg diastolic
4. **Fasting plasma glucose** > 100 mg% or previously diagnosed type 2 diabetes.

It should not be confused with coronary syndrome X where the perforator vessels are blocked by atherosclerosis and not the major epicardial coronary artery. Hence, percutaneous coronary intervention would not work in coronary syndrome X. Drug of choice for coronary syndrome X is nitrates.

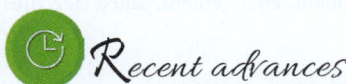

- Most common environmental factor affecting insulin resistance is obesity.
- Syndrome Z is a combination of metabolic syndrome and obstructive sleep apnea.

ADRENAL GLAND

- The right adrenal gland is triangular/pyramidal in shape, whereas the left adrenal gland is semilunar in shape. They weigh approximately 4–5 gram each.
- Each adrenal gland has two distinct structures, the outer adrenal cortex and the inner medulla, both of which produce hormones.
- The cortex mainly produces cortisol, aldosterone and androgens, while the medulla chiefly produces adrenaline and noradrenaline.
- In contrast to the direct innervation of the medulla, the cortex is regulated by neuroendocrine hormones secreted from the pituitary gland, which are under the control of the hypothalamus, as well as by the renin-angiotensin system.

Hormone	Abnormality
Aldosterone	↑: Conn's Syndrome (primary hyperaldosteronism) ↓: Addison's Disease
Cortisol	↑: Cushing syndrome
Sex-steroids	↑: Congenital adrenal hyperplasia ↓: Hypogonadism
Medulla	Pheochromocytoma

Congenital Adrenal Hyperplasia

- **Pattern of inheritance:** Autosomal recessive.
- **Enzyme deficiency:** 21-α-hydroxylase.
- Cholesterol is the substrate required for the synthesis of adrenal hormones.
- Out of the three hormones produced by adrenal cortex, aldosterone and cortisol require the enzyme 21-α-hydroxylase.
- Due to deficiency of 21-α-hydroxylase, aldosterone and cortisol production decreases and all the cholesterol is diverted to the synthesis of sex steroids leading to virilization of the girl child.
- The decrease in hormones trigger negative feedback mechanism increasing the production of ACTH hormone, which explains the hyperpigmentation around the genitals of girl child. (ACTH has a partial MSH like action)

Clinical Features of CAH

1. Salt wasting
2. Hypotension
3. Hypoglycemia
4. Virilization of the girl baby that leads to ambiguous genitalia
5. The genitals of the male baby at birth are normal. But later on, precocious puberty develops. This is presented as short stature, stocky muscular child with phallic enlargement, called **Hercules appearance**.

Investigations

1. **Screening:** Elevated 17-keto-steriod levels in mother's urine
2. **IOC:** Elevated 17-keto-steroids levels in baby (Cordocentesis)

Treatment

- Start dexamethasone in the mother.
- This is known as fetal therapy as it decreases severity of the disease in the fetus.

Other Defects in CAH

Enzyme defect	Clinical manifestation	Genitalia appearance
21-α-hydroxylase	MAP↓, Sugar↓	Girl baby with virilization
11-α-hydroxylase	HTN	Girl baby with virilization
17-α-hydroxylase	HTN	Male with ambiguous genitalia
3-α-hydroxylase	MAP↓	Male with ambiguous genitalia

Addison's Disease

It is characterized by decrease in aldosterone, cortisol and sex steroids, though the manifestations of aldosterone deficiency will manifest earlier.

Causes of Addison's Disease

- *MC infectious cause is HIV > TB (pg 309, 20th/e Harrison)*
- *Autoimmune (most common cause worldwide)*
- Addisonian Crisis (due to sudden stoppage of steroids)
- Waterhouse Friderichsen syndrome
- Secondary Addison's disease due to Sheehan's syndrome which has pituitary infarction.
- Non obstetric cause of pituitary damage is called as *Simmond's disease.*

Clinical Features

1. Salt wasting due to loss of salt and water
2. Polyuria: > 3L/24hrs
3. Mean blood pressure decreases, due to this the patient complains of dizziness, pre-syncope and syncope
4. Hyperkalemia
5. Metabolic acidosis
6. ACTH increase (since ACTH can behave like melanocyte stimulating hormone) leading to *hyperpigmentation* of oral mucosa, palmar and sole creases, previous surgical scars.
7. Hypoglycemia
8. Loss of pubic/axillary hair

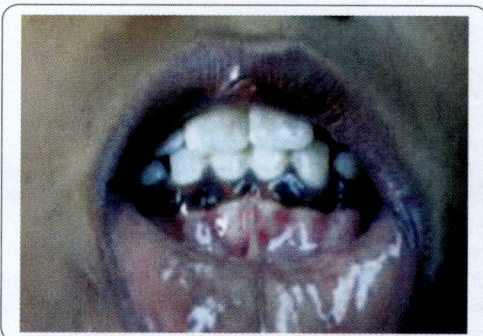

Hyperpigmentation of oral mucosa in Addison's disease

Investigations

1. Na⁺ decreases (normal value: 135–145 mEq)
   K⁺ increases (normal value: 3.5–5.5 mEq)
2. **Investigation of choice:** ACTH stimulation test/COSYNTROPIN test which fails to stimulate the gland.
3. **CT abdomen:** Evidence of damaged gland.
4. Gene XPERT for MTB.

Treatment

- Fludrocortisone: Promotes salt and water retention
- Dexamethasone: Cortisol like activity reduces hypoglycemic symptoms
- **DOC for Addison disease:** Hydrocortisone, replacement dose is 15–30 mg hydrocortisone daily in 2 or 3 divided dosages.

- **Drug of choice for Addisonian Crisis**: IV hydrocortisone + fluid resuscitation
- On administration of dextrose, **glucose fever** can develop.

Conn's Syndrome

Conn's syndrome is due to adrenal adenoma/adrenal carcinoma. [The incidence of Conn Syndrome and bilateral (micronodular) adrenal hyperplasia in causing hyperaldosteronism is given to be equal (pg 2728, 20th/e Harrison)]

Clinical Features of Conn's Syndrome

1. Hypertension.
2. Potassium (K+) decreases: Muscle cramps and fatigue
3. Hydrogen (H+) decreases: Metabolic alkalosis
4. *Pedal edema is absent*
5. Polyuria, Polydipsia

Investigations

1. Sodium (Na+) increased
2. Potassium (K+) decreased
3. **CT abdomen**: Presence of tumor in zona glomerulosa
4. **Screening test**: Plasma aldosterone : Renin ratio. Due to presence of hypertension, negative feedback ensues and leads to decreased renin levels.
5. **Investigation of choice**: Saline infusion test > Salt loading test

Treatment

- **Definitive treatment**: Surgical resection
- **DOC for Hyperaldosteronism**: Spirinolactone

Comparison of Primary Addison's and Conn's Syndrome

ADDISON's disease	CONN's syndrome
MC cause: autoimmunity	MC cause: Adrenal adenoma
Blood pressure ↓	Blood pressure ↑
K+ ↑	K+ ↓
H+ ↑	H+ ↓
Hyperpigmentation of palmar, sole creases	Pedal edema absent
IOC: ACTH stimulation test	IOC: Salt loading test
DOC: Hydrocortisone	DOC: Spironolactone

Conditions for Isolated Diastolic Hypertension

1. Essential hypertension
2. Myxedema
3. Cushing syndrome.

Cushing Syndrome

It is characterized by loss of diurnal variation and elevated levels of cortisol.

Causes

1. **Iatrogenic steroids**: This is the most common cause among all and ACTH levels are found to be low (Exogenous cause).
2. Ectopic ACTH production due to bronchial carcinoid is noticed and due to which, there is 24 hour stimulation of the adrenal gland resulting in increased production of cortisol.
3. **Pituitary adenoma**: This condition represents tumor in the pituitary gland resulting in increased cell production and their products, therefore increased level of ACTH and cortisol is seen. *It is called Cushing disease (endogenous cause).*
4. **Adrenal adenoma**: This condition represents tumor in the adrenal gland resulting in the increased production of cells and their products, as the tumor is in the adrenal gland, cortisol levels are increased but ACTH levels are decreased.

ACTH ↑	ACTH ↓
Oat cell cancer / ectopic ACTH	Iatrogenic steroids
Pituitary adenoma	Adrenal adenoma

Clinical Features of Cushing Syndrome

Earliest finding is loss of diurnal variation of cortisol production.

Body Compartment/ System	Signs and Symptoms
Body fat	Weight gain, central obesity, rounded face, fat pad on back of neck ("buffalo hump")
Skin	Facial plethora, thin and brittle skin, easy bruising, broad and purple stretch marks, acne, hirsutism
Bone	Osteopenia, osteoporosis (vertebral fractures), decreased linear growth in children
Muscle	Weakness, proximal myopathy (prominent atrophy of gluteal and upper leg muscles)
Cardiovascular^Q system	Diastolic hypertension, hypokalemia, edema, atherosclerosis
Metabolism	Glucose intolerance/diabetes, dyslipidemia
Reproductive system	Decreased libido, in women amenorrhea (due to cortisol-mediated inhibition of gonadotropin release)
Central nervous system	Irritability, emotional lability, depression, sometimes cognitive defects; in severe cases, paranoid psychosis
Blood and immune system	Increased susceptibility to infections, increased white blood cell count, eosinopenia, hypercoagulation with increased risk of deep vein thrombosis and pulmonary embolism

Investigation

1. **Screening test**: 24 hrs urinary cortisol levels (elevated up to twice the normal value) or salivary cortisol values

2. **Investigation of choice**: *Low-dose* dexamethasone suppression test (Plasma cortisol > 50 nmol/L after 0.5 mg dexamethasone q6h for 2 days)
3. **Imaging**: MRI head to evaluate pituitary adenoma
   - CT chest to rule out lung cancer
   - CT abdomen to evaluate adrenal adenoma
4. **ACTH levels**: Normal or high > 15 pg/mL : ACTH dependant cushing
   < 5 pg/mL : ACTH independent cushing

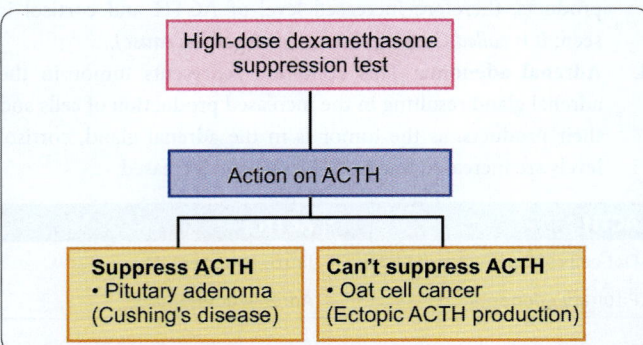

Lab Investigations in Common Etiologies of Cushing's Syndrome

	Adrenal	Pituitary adenoma	Ectopic ACTH
Diurnal variation of cortisol production	Absent	Present	Lost
ACTH levels	Reduced	Increased	Increased
High dose dexamethasone suppression test	Not suppressed	Suppressed	Not suppressed
Imaging	CT scan abdomen	MRI head and Inferior petrosal Sinus Sampling	Somatostatin receptor scinitigraphy and CT chest and abdomen.

Treatment

- Decrease the dose of the steroids in case the cause is iatrogenic steroids
- Chemotherapy (IV Etoposide + Cisplatin) in case of oat cell cancer of lung
- Trans-sphenoidal surgery for pituitary adenoma
- Medical adrenalectomy (Inhibits the production of cortisol)
  1. Ketoconazole (oral): Drug of choice
  2. IV aminogluthetimide
  3. Mitotane/Metyrapone.

Nelson syndrome: Hyperpigmentation postoperatively after bilateral surgical adrenalectomy due to increased ACTH

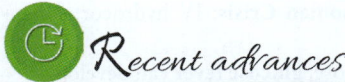

Polyglandular Autoimmune Syndrome

Type 1: Autoimmune Polyendocrinopathy Candidiasis (ectodermal dystrophy)
- Autosomal recessive with defect in T-cell function and presents in childhood
- Mucocutaneous candidiasis
- Hypoparathyroidism with dystrophy of nails and teeth
- Addison's disease.

Type 2
- Autoimmune adrenal insufficiency
- Type 1 diabetes mellitus
- Autoimmune thyroid disease
- Combination of Addison's disease and hypothyroidism is called Schmidt's syndrome
- Vitiligo, alopecia areata, Sjögren's syndrome.

Conditions with Hyperpigmentation (ACTH ↑)
- Ectopic ACTH (oat cell cancer)
- Pituitary adenoma (Cushing's syndrome)
- Addison's disease
- Nelson syndrome

Condition with No Hyperpigmentation (ACTH ↓)
- Addisonian crisis
- Pituitary damage (secondary Addison's disease): Alabaster coloured pale skin
- Tertiary Addison's disease.

PHEOCHROMOCYTOMA

Physiologically	Epinephrine > nor-epinephrine production
Pheochromocytoma secretes	Norepinephrine > epinephrine 80% 20%
Only if the question mentions	1. Size of tumor < 5 cm 2. Tumor associated with M.E.N 2A (sipple syndrome) Epinephrine >Nor-epinephrine production

- 10% are Malignant.
- 15% are Extraadrenal in location. (Organ of zuckerkandl)
- 10–15% are familial. (MEN2A: Sipple syndrome)
- 10% are Bilateral

- To distinguish between benign and malignant pheochromocytoma, MRI is performed.
- Imaging modality of choice for medullary pheochromocyte is MRI abdomen (pg 2330: Harrison 19th ed.) > MIBG scintigraphy
- Most common extramedullary site is organ of Zuckerkandl near inferior mesenteric artery.

Clinical Features

1. Headaches: MC symptom
2. Sweating attacks
3. Palpitations and tachycardia
4. **Hypertension (episodic or paroxysmal or sustained)**
5. Anxiety and panic attacks
6. Pallor
7. Abdominal pain
8. Weight loss
9. Paradoxical response to antihypertensive drugs
10. Polyuria and polydipsia
11. Constipation
12. **Orthostatic hypotension**^{Q}
13. Dilated cardiomyopathy
14. **Erythrocytosis**^{Q}
15. **Elevated blood sugar**^{Q}

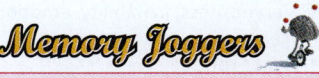

P.H.D: Palpitations, Hypertension and Diaphoresis: Triad for suspecting pheochromocytoma.

Investigations

1. **Screening test:** 24 hours urinary fractionated metanephrine levels > 24 hour urinary Vanillylmandelic acid levels
2. **Investigation of Choice:** Blood test – plasma fractionated metanephrine > plasma catecholamines
3. MRI abdomen for location, size and metastasis of tumor
4. MIBG scan, if MRI is normal.
5. PET scan for extra-adrenal pheochromocytoma

Treatment

- Definitive treatment is surgical resection but it is contraindicated in malignant pheochromocytoma.
- **Preoperative management of hypertension**: Oral phenoxybenzamine (non-selective α-blocker)
- **Intraoperative hypertension management**: IV phentolamine
- **Postoperative hypertension management**: IV Labetalol
- **Intraoperative hypertension crisis management**: IV Nitroprusside.

THYROID

Investigations in Thyroid Dysfunction

Assessment of Thyroid Function Test

↓ T4, and ↑ TSH	Primary hypothyroidism
Normal T4, ↑ TSH	Subclinical hypothyroidism (TSH being the main determinant in deciding)
↑ TSH ↑ T4	TSH secreting pituitary tumor or thyroid hormone resistance
↓ TSH, ↑ T4 or ↑ T3	Hyperthyroidism
↓ TSH, Normal T4 & T3	Subclinical hyperthyroidism
↓ TSH, ↓ T4 ↓ T3	Sick euthyroidism, Secondary hypothyroidism due to hypopituitarism

T3 Resin Uptake Test

This binding of the labeled T3 to the resin is increased in:
- TBG deficiency
- Hyperthyroidism
- The binding of the labelled T3 to the resin is decreased in hypothyroidism

Isotope Scan: (123, 125, 131 or 99 Technetium Pertechnetate)

- Useful for determining the cause of hyperthyroidism
- Detect retrosternal goiter
- Ectopic thyroid tissue
- Thyroid metastases (using whole body CT scan)
- 20% of 'cold' nodules are malignant
- Few neutral and almost no hot nodules are malignant.

Causes of Thyrotoxicosis with decreased RAIU

1. Thyrotoxicosis factitia
2. Hashi thyrotoxicosis
3. Struma ovary
4. Excess iodine ingestion
5. Functional metastatic follicular carcinoma
6. Amiodarone therapy
7. De-Quervain thyroiditis.

Causes of increased uptake in Radioactive iodine
- Hyperthyroidism
- Iodine deficiency
- Pregnancy
- Recovery phase of subacute, silent, or postpartum thyroiditis (Not illness phase of subacute thyroiditis)
- Rebound after withdrawal of antithyroid medication
- Lithium carbonate therapy
- Hashimoto thyroiditis

Endemic Cretinism

- If a pregnant female suffers from iodine deficiency, the baby born to this female will suffer from hypothyroidism and this condition is referred to as **endemic cretinism**.
- Blood profile of a baby suffering from hypothyroidism
  - Levels of T3 & T4 decreased
  - Levels of free T3 & T4 decreased
  - Thyroid stimulating hormone is elevated.

Clinical Features

1. Large baby (>4 kg), less cry, sleeps all the time and decreased activity.
2. Hypothermic state and coarse skin (Myxedema).
3. Reduced UDPGT activity, leads to prolongation of physiological jaundice >14 days.
4. Hypothyroidism causes delayed brain myelination, this leads to delayed social smile, decreased stranger anxiety and in future develops mental retardation.
5. Low levels of thyroid hormones causes delayed muscle development resulting in delayed onset of walking and delayed motor milestones.

Diagnostic Test

- **Screening**: Heel prick test is the best screening test for endemic cretinism. Heel prick test on day zero can be false positive because of birth asphyxia, and hence should always be performed after 72 hr of birth.
- **Thyroid function test:**
  - T3 & T4 ↓
  - Free T3 & T4 ↓
  - TSH ↑

Treatment

If there is no residual function, the daily replacement dose of levothyroxine is usually 1.6 µg/kg body weight (typically 100–150 µg).

SICK EUTHYROID SYNDROME

- In any systemic illness, TFT may become deranged.
- *The most common hormone pattern in sick euthyroid syndrome (SES) is a **decrease in total and unbound T3 levels (low T3 syndrome) with normal levels of T4 and TSH.***
- The magnitude of the fall in T3 correlates with the severity of the illness. T4 conversion to T3 via peripheral deiodination is impaired, leading to increased reverse T3 (rT3).
- Despite this effect, decreased clearance rather than increased production is the major basis for increased rT3. Also, T4 is alternately metabolized to the hormonally inactive T3 sulfate.
- This low T3 state is adaptive, because it can be induced in normal individuals by fasting.
- Very sick patients may exhibit a dramatic fall in total T4 and T3 levels (low T4 syndrome).
- In the vary advanced stage, the typical pattern is of 'everything to be low' (↓TSH, ↓T4 ↓T3)

Thyrotoxicosis

Primary	Secondary
Defect in the thyroid gland	Defect in the pituitary gland
Graves' disease: Autoimmune (LATS)	Pituitary adenoma
T4↑, T3↑ & TSH ↓↓	T4↑, T3↑ & TSH↑

Primary Thyrotoxicosis/GRAVE's Disease

- Grave's disease is an autoimmune condition affecting females. Antibody responsible for this condition is LATS (long acting thyroid stimulating antibody)
- **Thyroid profile**: T4↑, T3↑ &TSH ↓↓

Secondary Thyrotoxicosis

- It is characterized by the defect in the pituitary gland.
- Usual age of presentation is >60 years.
- Example of secondary thyrotoxicosis is by pituitary adenoma.
- Thyroid profile: T4↑, T3↑ & TSH↑

Common Features of Primary and Secondary Thyrotoxicosis

Clinical Features of Thyrotoxicosis
Goiter: There is diffuse thyroid enlargement ± bruit.
Gastrointestinal
• Weight loss despite normal or increased appetite
• Diarrhea, alimentary glycosuria can occur
Cardiorespiratory
• Palpitation, sinus tachycardia, atrial fibrillation, *dancing carotid*
• Increased pulse pressure, soft systolic murmur
• Angina, cardiomyopathy and cardiac failure
• "Means Lerman scratch" (the scratchy sound heard over the precordium)
• Some patients with thyrotoxicosis develop a reversible diastolic dysfunction and a low-output failure
Neuromuscular
• Nervousness, irritability, emotional liability, psychosis
• Tremor
• Hyper-reflexia
• Muscle weakness, hypokalemic periodic paralysis, bulbar myopathy
• *Common neurologic manifestations include hyper-reflexia, muscle wasting and proximal myopathy without fasciculation. Chorea is rare.*
Dermatological
• Finger clubbing (thyroid acropathy)
• Pretibial myxedema
Reproductive
• Amenorrhea/oligomenorrhea
• Infertility, spontaneous abortion
• Loss of libido, impotence
Ocular
Following Eye signs are seen in all cases of hyperthyroidism
• Wide staring appearance (**Kocher Sign**)
• Upper Lid retraction (**Dalrymple sign**)
• Lid lag with down gaze (**Von Graefe sign**)
• Decreased blinking (**Stellwag sign**)

Differences Between Primary and Secondary Thyrotoxicosis

Primary	Secondary
LATS present	LATS absent
Proptosis present	Proptosis absent
Myxedema present	Myxedema absent
Clubbing / acropathy present	Clubbing / acropathy absent
Atrial fibrillation absent	Atrial fibrillation present
TSH ↓	TSH ↑

LATS = Long Acting Thyroid Stimulating antibody

Investigations

1. **Thyroid function test:** Total T4 & T3 ↑
   Free T4 & T3 ↑
2. **Thyroid scan:** I-123 (half-life: 8 hrs)

Treatment

- **Patient <45 years**: Anti-thyroid drugs
  - Anti-thyroid drugs can lead to agranulocytosis, sub-total thyroidectomy can be done in this condition (6–8 g of the gland is left behind)
  - Anti-thyroid drugs propyl thiouracil and methimazole, inhibit coupling reaction
  - Propyl-thiouracil is safe in pregnancy and breast feeding
- **Patient >45 years**: Radio-iodine: I-131 (thyroid ablation).

Thyroid Storm

- During the surgery of toxic nodular goiter, massive release of T4 hormone occurs into the circulation. This T4 converts into T3 peripherally, which is the active form.
- This sudden elevated T3 triggers sympathetic activity in the body leading to various symptoms such as increased heart rate leading to high output congestive cardiac failure.
- *This intraoperative complication is referred to as thyroid storm.*

Treatment of Thyroid Storm

1. IV hydrocortisone
2. **Drug of choice**: Propylthiouracil via NG Tube/Rectum (pg 2707: Harrison 20th/e)
3. External cooling
4. Sodium bicarbonate
5. Lugol I_2/Potassium iodide

Prevention of Thyroid Storm

Lugol's-iodine to be administered for 10 days. It decreases the size of the gland and decreases iodine trapping (Wolff-Chaikoff effect)^Q

Conditions with Increased T4
1. Grave's disease
2. Pituitary adenoma
3. Thyrotoxicosis factitia consumption of tainted beef containing thyroid-gland of cattle
4. Struma ovary
5. Gestational trophoblastic neoplasia (hCG mimic TSH action)

Grave's Ophthalmopathy

1. Retraction of Müllers muscle leads to stare sign. It leads to decreased blink rate resulting in corneal xerosis.
2. External opthalmoplegia causes diplopia. Most common eye muscle involved is inferior rectus.^{Q}
3. Proptosis can be unilateral, bilateral or asymmetrical.
4. Retrobulbar neuritis leads to blindness.
5. Treatment is pulse methylprednisolone

Hypothyroidism

Diffrence between primary and secondary hypothroidism

Primary Hypothyroidism	Secondary Hypothyroidism
Defect in Thyroid gland	Defect in Pituitary gland
Thyroid profile: TSH↑, T3↓ & T4↓	Thyroid profile: TSH↓, T3↓ & T4↓
Causes:	Causes:

• Thyroiditis
• Endemic goiter
• Amiodarone
• Food goitrogens
  ▪ Cabbage
  ▪ Cassava beans
  ▪ Turnip
	• Sheehan syndrome (Anterior pituitary infarction due to PPH)
	• Pituitary apoplexy (bleeding in the pituitary gland)
	• Empty sella syndrome (Idiopathic CSF leakage leading to pituitary compression)

Symptoms of Hypothyroidism

Symptoms	Signs
• Dry skin • *Cold intolera*nce • Hair loss • Difficulty concentrating and poor memory • Constipation • Weight gain with poor appetite • Dyspnea • Hoarse voice • Menorrhagia (later oligomenorrhea or amenorrhea) • Paresthesia • Impaired hearing	• Dry coarse skin; cool peripheral extremities • Puffy face, hands, and feet (myxedema) • Diffuse alopecia • Bradycardia • Peripheral edema • *Delayed tendon reflex rela*xation • Carpal tunnel syndrome • Serous cavity effusions • **Diastolic hypertension**^{Q}

Complications of Hypothyroidism

- **Myxedema Heart**: Pericardial effusion/accelerated atherosclerosis
- **Myxedema Madness**: Psychosis
- **Myxedema Coma** presents with hypothermia (core temperature < 35° celsius). Treatment of myxedema coma is IV liothyronine (T3) and levothyroxine.

Thyroiditis

	Hashimoto's Thyroiditis	Riedel's Thyroiditis	De Quervain's Thyroiditis
Cause	Autoimmune	Idiopathic	Viral etiology
Antibody	Anti-TPO Anti-microsomal A/b Anti-thyro-globulin A/b	—	—

Contd...

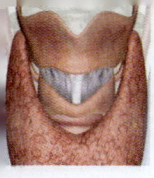

	Hashimoto's Thyroiditis	Riedel's Thyroiditis	De Quervain's Thyroiditis
Features	Autoantibodies destroy thyroid gland and leads to fibrosis of the gland	Stony hard consistency mimics anaplastic cancer of thyroid	Painful thyroiditis, can occur as a consequence of upper respiratory tract infection
Thyroid state	Initially hyperthyroid and after 5–20 years due to fibrosis it turns hypothyroid	Never hyperthyroid, presents with hypothyroidism	Self-limiting condition; initially hyperthyroid then turns hypothyroid and finally becomes euthyroid
Treatment	Thyroxine	Thyroxine	Steroids (prednisolone)

Insulinoma

- Insulinoma is an endocrine tumor of pancreas derived from β-cells of the pancreas.
- This increased insulin level in the body causes hypoglycemia.

WHIPPLE'S Triad[Q]
1. Presence of symptoms of Hypoglycemia
2. Documented low blood sugar at the time symptoms are present
3. Reversal of symptoms by glucose administration.

The average age of occurrence is 40–50 years old. The most common clinical symptoms are due to the effect of the hypoglycemia on the CNS (neuroglycemic symptoms) and include confusion, headache, disorientation, visual difficulties, irrational behavior, and even coma.

Diagnosis

Investigation of choice for Insulinoma: *72 hrs prolonged fasting test.*[Q]

Diagnostic Criteria for Insulinoma after a 72-Hour Fast

Laboratory Test	Result
Plasma glucose	< 45 mg/dL
Plasma insulin (RIA)	≥ 6 microunit/mL
Plasma C-peptide	≥ 200 pmol/L (0.2 nmol/L)
Plasma proinsulin	≥ 5 pmol/L
Beta-hydroxybutyrate	≤ 2.7 mmol/L
Sulfonylurea screen (including repaglinide and nateglinide)	Negative

For preoperative localization of insulinoma endoscopic ultrasound is the imaging modality of choice.[Q]

Treatment

DOC for insulinoma: *Octreotide.* Surgical treatment ranging from enucleation to distal pancreatectomy is curative.

Causes of Hypoglycemia
Fasting (Postabsorptive) Hypoglycemia
• Drugs: Insulin, sulfonylureas, ethanol, quinine, pentamidine, salicylates, sulfonamides
• Critical illnesses ■ Hepatic, renal, or cardiac failure ■ Sepsis ■ CRF
• Hormone deficiency: ■ Cortisol (Addison's) ■ Growth hormone (Hypopituitarism) ■ Glucagon deficiency ■ Epinephrine deficiency (in insulin-deficient diabetes)
• Non-beta-cell tumors: Hepatomas, adrenocortical carcinomas, carcinoids
• Endogenous hyperinsulinism: Insulinoma
• Autoimmune (autoantibodies to insulin or the insulin receptor)

Multiple Endocrine Neoplasia (MEN syndrome)

MEN - 1 (Wermer)	MEN-2A (Sipple Syndrome)	MEN-2B (also called MEN 3)
• Pituitary adenoma • Parathyroid adenoma • Pancreatic adenoma • Most common pancreatic adenoma in MEN-1 is gastrinoma[Q] • Most common skin manifestation is angiofibroma	• Parathyroid adenoma • Medullary carcinoma of thyroid • Pheochromocytoma • Hirschsprung's disease • Cutaneous lichen amyloidosis	• Medullary carcinoma of thyroid • Pheochromocytoma • Mucosal neuroma • Marfanoid features • Gastrointestinal neuromas

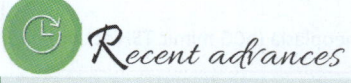

Multiple Endocrine Neoplasia

Men 3 (Men 2B)[Q]
- Autosomal dominant with ret proto-oncogene
- Infants with parent having MEN 3 and child having ret proto-oncogene must undergo prophylactic total thyroidectomy by the age of 6 months

MEN 4 (12 p 13)[Q]
- Gene involved CDKN1B
- Pituitary, parathyroid and pancreatic involvement like MEN1
- *Reproductive organ tumors (testicular cancer, neuroendocrine cervical carcinoma) and renal tumors*

PARATHYROID GLAND

Serum Alkaline Phosphatase

- In multiple myeloma there is no increased activity of osteoblasts. Therefore, serum alkaline phosphate (ALP) levels are normal in MM and bone scan is also normal.
- Other bone conditions with increased ALP
  - Paget's disease
  - Bone metastases
  - Rickets and osteomalacia.
- Low serum alkaline phosphatase levels are seen in hypophosphatasia.

Biochemical markers of Bone Metabolism in Clinical Use

Bone formation[Q]	Bone resorption
• Serum bone-specific alkaline phosphatase • Serum osteocalcin • Serum propeptide of type I procollagen	• Urine and serum cross-linked N-telopeptide • Urine and serum cross-linked C-telopeptide • Urine total free deoxypyridinoline

Manifestations of Hyperparathyroidism					
General	Renal	Bones	Abdomen	Cardiac	Calcification
• Anorexia • Nausea • Vomiting • Fatigue • Mental confusion • Psychic moans	• Polyuria • Nocturia • Renal colic	• Bone pain • Bone cysts • Brown tumor	• Peptic ulceration (abdominal groans) • Constipation	• Short QT interval in ECG (arrhythmias, hypertension)	• Ectopic calcification • Chondrocalcinosis

Serum abnormalities in Hyperparathyroidism				
	Serum Ca	Serum phosphate	Alkaline phosphatase	PTH
Primary hyperparathyroidism	↑	↓	↑	↑
Secondary hyperparathyroidism	↓	↑	↑	↑
Tertiary hyperparathyroidism	↑	↓	↑	↑

Hypercalcemia

Causes of Hypercalcemia

1. Lithium, thiazide, phenytoin
2. Ca of breast lung, kidney, MM, lymphoma
3. Vitamin D intoxication, vitamin A intoxication, aluminium intoxication
4. Hyperparathyroidism, hyperthyroid, pheochromocytoma
5. Sarcoidosis
6. Prolonged immobilization
7. Milk alkali syndrome
8. Familial hypercalciuric hypercalcemia
9. MC cause of asymptomatic hypercalcemia is primary hyperparathyroidism.

Management of Acute Hypercalcemia

1. It can be managed by hydration alone.
2. **Hydration with saline forced diuresis**: Loop diuretics (furosemide) promotes calcium excretion. Bolus furosemide will cause dehydration and increase calcium values, so it should be given as a drip.
3. **Bisphosphonates (Drug of choice)**: Bisphosphonates reduce calcium resorption
   - 1st generation : Etidronate
   - 2nd generation : Pamidronate
   - 3rd generation : Zoledronate
4. **Glucocorticoids**: Effective in particular situations such as Vitamin D intoxication, Sarcoidosis, Malignancy
5. **Inhaled Calcitonin**
6. **Dialysis**: Quick and effective and is likely to be needed in severe cases with renal failure

Hypoparathyroidism

Causes

1. Primary (due to gland failure)
   - *Idiopathic (Autoimmune)*: Most common cause
   - Infantile hypoparathyroidism: It is associated with thymic aplasia (Di George syndrome)
2. Secondary
   - **Postoperative**: Surgery (thyroidectomy).
   - Post radio-iodine therapy
   - Hypomagnesemia (Mg is required for PTH secretion)
3. *Pseudohypoparathyroidism (PHP)*
   - It is a group of disorders characterized by hypocalcemia due to renal resistance to PTH
   - PTH levels are high
   - Various phenotypic abnormalities in various tissues are associated. Classically, short stature, round face, obesity, short fourth metacarpals, ectopic bone formation, mental retardation and cataract.
4. *Pseudopseudohypoparathyroidism (PPHP- due to defect in Gs-alpha gene)*
   - Patients without hypocalcemia but sharing the phenotypic abnormalities (as of pseudohypoparathyroidism)
   - These patients have normal serum PO_4^- and normal serum PTH
   - In pseudohypoparathyroidism, defect lies at PTH receptor level, while in pseudopseudohypoparathyroidism deficiency lies at gene transcription level beyond the PTH receptors.

Condition	PTH levels	Calcium	Pattern of inheritance Imprinting
Hypoparathyroidism	Low	Low	Not applicable
Pseudohypoparathyroidism	Increased	Low	Genetic defect from mother
Pseudopseudohypopar-athyroidism	Increased	Normal	Genetic defect from father

Magnesium Metabolism

- Normal serum magnesium: 1.5 – 2.3 mg%
- Serum calcium and Serum magnesium levels always go parallel.
- The notable exceptions are CRF (hypocalcemia and hypermagnesemia), and Gitelman syndrome (normocalcemia and hypomagnesemia)
- Magnesium is required for PTH secretion and for PTH action

Causes of Hypermagnesemia
- ARF, CRF
- Addison disease
- Magnesium containing drugs.
- Hemolysis

Causes of hypomagnesemia
- Reduce intake especially common in alcoholic patient and TPN
- GI losses: chronic diarrhea
- Kidney loss: diuretics, Gitelman syndrome
- Acute pancreatitis
- Drugs: Foscarnet

Comparison of Findings in Magnesium Deficit and Excess

Hypermagnesemia	Hypomagnesemia
Inhibits PTH release Inhibits calcium reabsorbtion from TAL	Resistance to PTH Decreased production of vitamin D3
Vasodilation: Hypotension (earliest feature)	Tetany
Neuromuscular blockade: DTR inhibited	Vertigo/ataxia/nystagmus Depression/psychosis
Respiratory failure: decreased respiratory rate	
Bowel sounds reduced/ileus	
Pupils dilated	
ECG: PR, qRS and QT prolongation	ECG: PR and QT prolongation with T wave inversion

Note: QT prolongation is seen with both of them

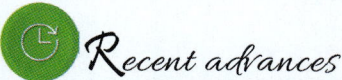

Gastroenteropancreatic Neuroendocrine Tumors (GEP-NTS)
- 50% Of GEP-NTS is non secretory. Hence most common presentation is incidental detection.
- Most common functional GEP-NTS is insulinoma.
- Functional GEP-NTS is associated with one the four mentioned
  - MEN1
  - Von Hippel Lindau syndrome
  - NF-1
  - Tuberous sclerosis complex

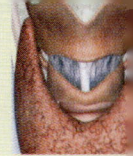

Image-Based Questions

1. A diabetic with HbA1c of 11% will require all for management except?

   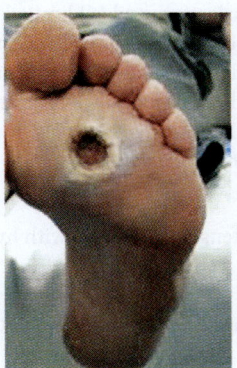

   a. Off loading
   b. Debridement
   c. Antiseptic agent dressings
   d. Antibiotics

2. A patient presents with hypertension and hypokalemia. CT abdomen was performed. Diagnosis is?

   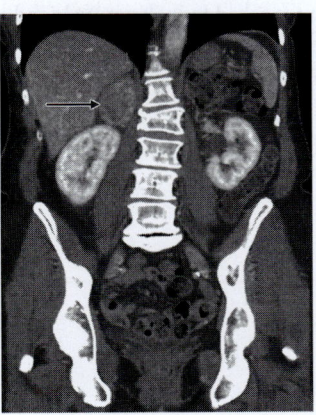

   a. Pheochromocytoma
   b. Conn's syndrome
   c. Liddle's syndrome
   d. Secondary hyperaldosteronism

3. All are true about the condition shown except?

   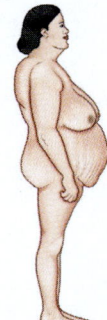

   a. Facial plethora
   b. Purplish striae
   c. Hyperkalemia
   d. Metabolic alkalosis

4. Probable diagnosis of this patient is

   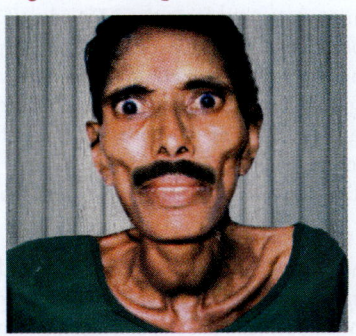

   a. Hashi thyrotoxicosis
   b. Hypothyroidism
   c. Retrosternal goiter
   d. Multinodular goiter

5. A 25-year old lady with constipation, kidney stones, hypertension and the following lesion on hand can be diagnosed of?

   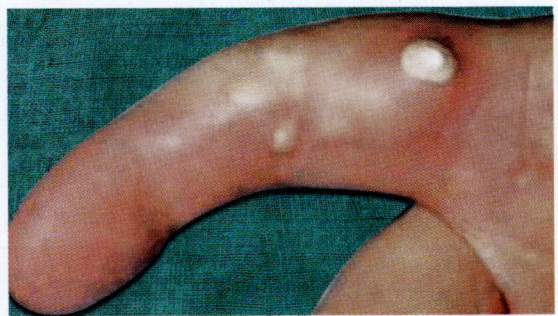

   a. Calcinosis cutis
   b. Cutaneous xanthoma
   c. Necrobiosis lipidoica
   d. Felon

6. The clinical sign below denotes:

   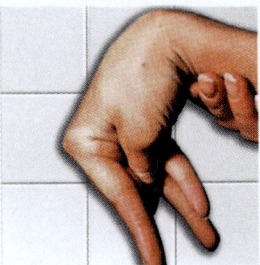

   a. Tetany
   b. Tetanus
   c. Median nerve palsy
   d. Radial nerve palsy

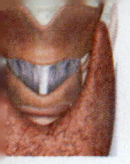

Answers of Image-Based Questions

1. **Ans. (c) Antiseptic agent dressings**
   - Consensus statement from the ADA identifies six interventions with demonstrated efficacy in diabetic foot wounds: (1) off-loading, (2) debridement, (3) wound dressings, (4) appropriate use of antibiotics, (5) revascularization, and (6) limited amputation.
   - Off-loading is the complete avoidance of weight bearing on the ulcer, which removes the mechanical trauma that retards wound healing. Bed rest and a variety of orthotic devices or contact casting limit weight bearing on wounds or pressure points.
   - Surgical debridement is important and effective, but clear efficacy of other modalities for wound cleaning (enzymes, soaking, whirlpools) are lacking. Dressings such as hydrocolloid dressings promote wound healing by creating a moist environment and protecting the wound. ***Antiseptic agents should be avoided. Topical antibiotics are of limited value***.

2. **Ans. (b) Conn's syndrome**
   - The image shows mass on top of kidney, indicative of adrenal pathology. Since hypertension is present with hypokalemia, increased aldosterone from adrenal adenoma is diagnostic of Conn's syndrome.
   - Pheochromocytoma has hypertension but hypokalemia is not seen.
   - Liddle syndrome is autosomal dominant disorder with over-activity of epithelial sodium channel, but does not present as an adrenal mass.

3. **Ans. (c) Hyperkalemia**
   The image shows a patient of Cushing's syndrome, which presents with hypokalemic alkalosis due to partial mineralocorticoid activity of cortisol.

4. **Ans. (d) Multinodular goiter**
   - The patient is a middle aged person, who has a prominent thyroid gland with presence of stare sign.
   - Substernal extension/ retrosternal extension cannot be made out unless the patient is asked to look upwards and suffusion of face is noted.
   - Hashi thyrotoxicosis may develop during pregnancy in patients of Hashimoto thyroiditis.

5. **Ans. (a) Calcinosis cutis**
   The findings of constipation and kidney stones point to presence of increased calcium and the image showing chalky-white compound deposited on the skin are suggestive of calcinosis cutis.

6. **Ans. (a) Tetany**
   The picture shows carpopedal spasm, which is diagnostic of tetany.

Conceptual Diagnostic Algorithm

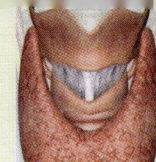

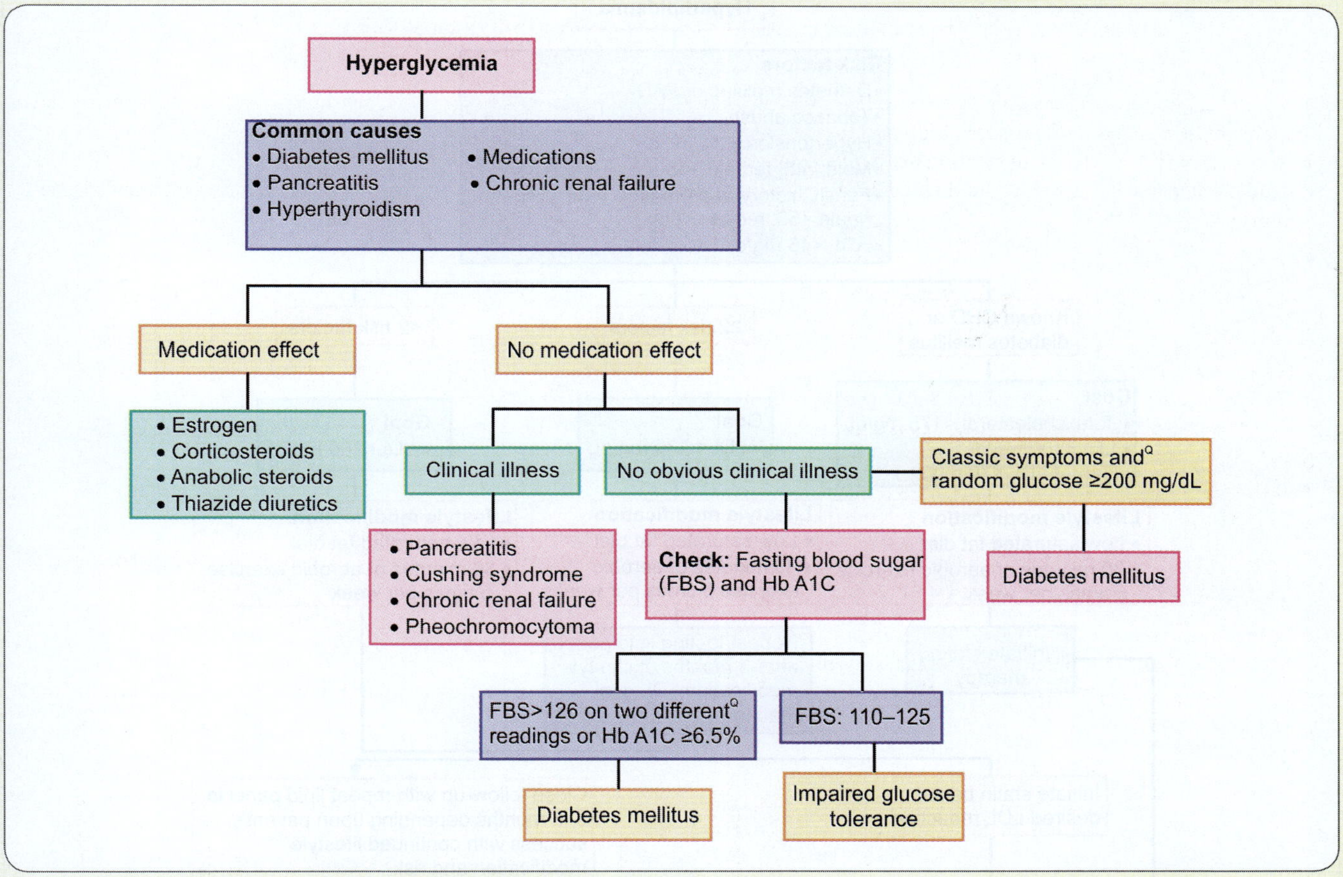

```
Hyperglycemia
    │
Common causes
• Diabetes mellitus      • Medications
• Pancreatitis           • Chronic renal failure
• Hyperthyroidism
    │
    ├─────────────────────────────┐
Medication effect            No medication effect
    │                             │
• Estrogen                        ├──────────────────────────────┐
• Corticosteroids            Clinical illness         No obvious clinical illness    Classic symptoms and
• Anabolic steroids               │                          │                       random glucose ≥200 mg/dL
• Thiazide diuretics              │                          │                              │
                          • Pancreatitis              Check: Fasting blood sugar       Diabetes mellitus
                          • Cushing syndrome          (FBS) and Hb A1C
                          • Chronic renal failure           │
                          • Pheochromocytoma                ├──────────────────┐
                                                  FBS>126 on two different    FBS: 110–125
                                                  readings or Hb A1C ≥6.5%         │
                                                            │                Impaired glucose
                                                     Diabetes mellitus           tolerance
```

* Classic symptoms are polyuria, polydipsia and weight loss
* 2° diabetes occurs in cushing syndrome, cystic fibrosis and chronic pancreatitis
* Neural tube defects are not seen in infant born to mother with gestational diabetes. Infant born to mother with pre-existing diabetes would develop congenital malformations.

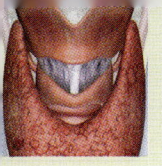

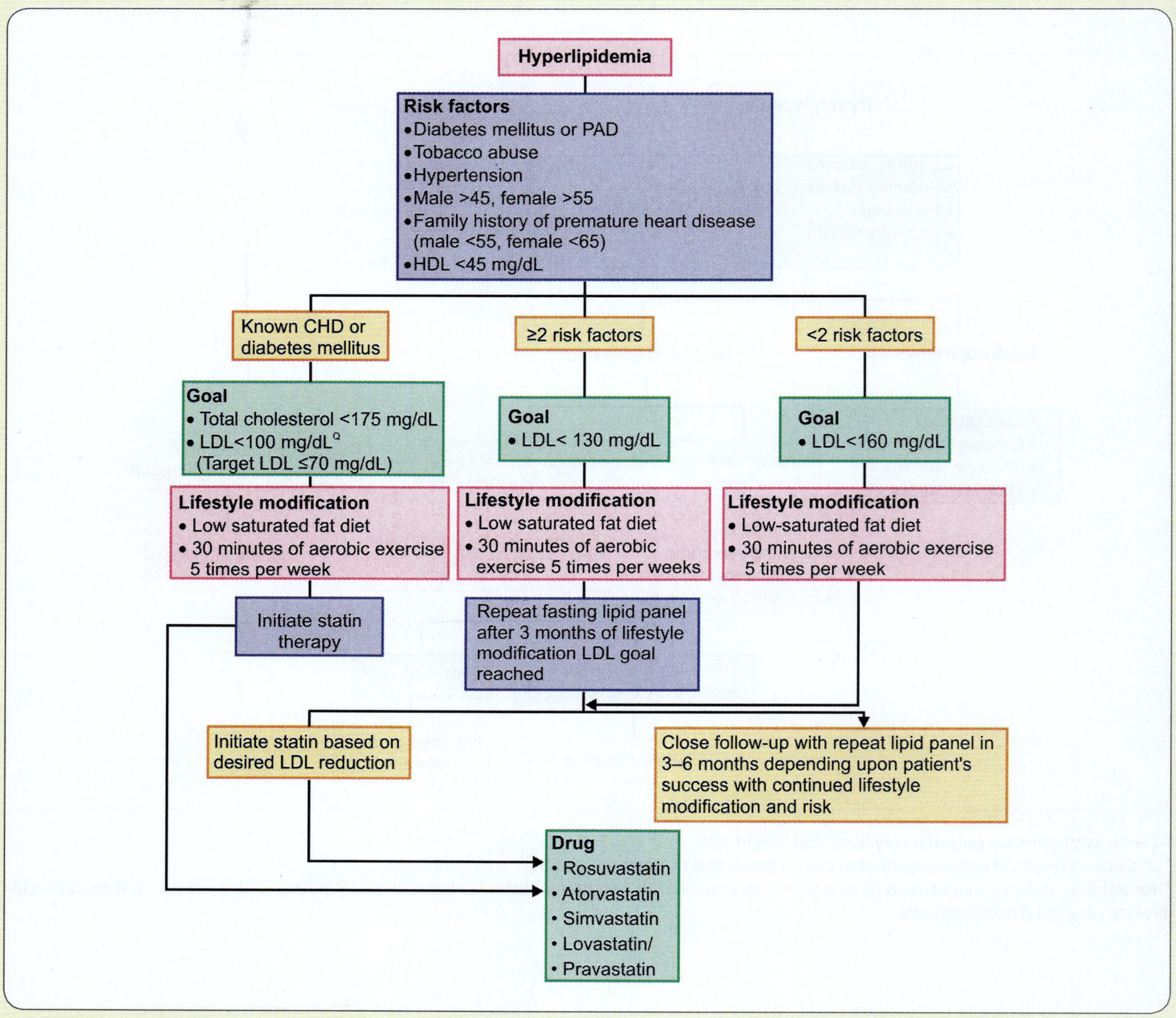

ALGORITHM

```
                    ┌─────────────────┐
                    │ Hyperlipidemia  │
                    └─────────────────┘
                             │
         ┌───────────────────────────────────────┐
         │ Risk factors                          │
         │ • Diabetes mellitus or PAD            │
         │ • Tobacco abuse                       │
         │ • Hypertension                        │
         │ • Male >45, female >55                │
         │ • Family history of premature heart   │
         │   disease (male <55, female <65)      │
         │ • HDL <45 mg/dL                       │
         └───────────────────────────────────────┘
```

Known CHD or diabetes mellitus

- **Goal**
  - Total cholesterol <175 mg/dL
  - LDL <100 mg/dL^Q
  - (Target LDL ≤70 mg/dL)

- **Lifestyle modification**
  - Low saturated fat diet
  - 30 minutes of aerobic exercise 5 times per week

- **Initiate statin therapy**

≥2 risk factors

- **Goal**
  - LDL <130 mg/dL

- **Lifestyle modification**
  - Low saturated fat diet
  - 30 minutes of aerobic exercise 5 times per weeks

- Repeat fasting lipid panel after 3 months of lifestyle modification LDL goal reached

- Initiate statin based on desired LDL reduction

<2 risk factors

- **Goal**
  - LDL <160 mg/dL

- **Lifestyle modification**
  - Low-saturated fat diet
  - 30 minutes of aerobic exercise 5 times per week

- Close follow-up with repeat lipid panel in 3–6 months depending upon patient's success with continued lifestyle modification and risk

Drug
- Rosuvastatin
- Atorvastatin
- Simvastatin
- Lovastatin/
- Pravastatin

Multiple Choice Questions

Diabetes Mellitus & Insulinoma

1. The following lesion was noticed in a patient with history of involuntary weight loss. What is the diagnosis?
   (Recent Question 2019)

   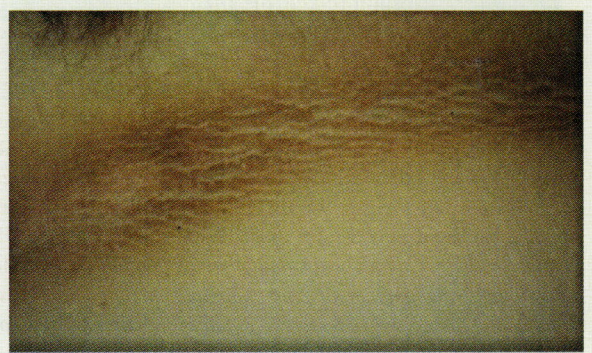

   a. Acanthosis nigricans
   b. Leser-Trelat sign
   c. Actinic keratosis
   d. Intertriginous candida

2. A morbidly obese diabetic patient on metformin presents with uncontrolled blood sugar level even after increasing dosage. He has a history of pancreatitis and a family history of bladder cancer. Patient does not want to take injections. What will you prescribe next? *(AIIMS Nov 2017)*
   a. Sitagliptin
   b. Liraglutide
   c. Canagliflozin
   d. Pioglitazone

3. Which of the following drugs is to be immediately stopped in a patient of diabetes with hypertension, severe septicemia and serum creatinine level of 5.7 mg? *(AIIMS Nov 2017)*
   a. Metoprolol
   b. Linagliptin
   c. Metformin
   d. Insulin

4. Which of the following is known as Type 1A diabetes mellitus? *(Recent Pattern Questions)*
   a. Immune mediated type 1
   b. Idiopathic type 1
   c. Latent autoimmune diabetes in adults
   d. Maturity onset diabetes in young

5. Zinc transporter 8 antibody is seen in?
   a. Hashimoto's thyroiditis *(Recent Pattern Questions)*
   b. Hypoparathyroidism
   c. Type 1 diabetes mellitus
   d. Type A insulin resistance

6. HNF- 1β gene defect is seen in? *(Recent Pattern Questions)*
   a. MODY2
   b. MODY3
   c. MODY4
   d. MODY5

7. Which type of diabetes has impaired glucose induced secretion of insulin with preserved β cell mass?
   a. MODY *(Recent Pattern Questions)*
   b. Wolfram syndrome
   c. Type 1 diabetes
   d. Latent autoimmune diabetes in adults

8. Hyperglycemia is seen in all except?
   (Recent Pattern Questions)
   a. Cirrhosis
   b. Myotonic dystrophy
   c. Lipodystrophy
   d. Sarcoma

9. Falsely elevated HbA1C is seen in?
   a. Thalassemia *(Recent Pattern Questions)*
   b. Recovery from acute blood loss
   c. Erythropoietin supplementation in CKD
   d. Splenectomy

10. Which is correct about syndrome X?
    (PGI Pattern)(Recent Pattern Questions)
    a. Elevated uric acid
    b. Dense LDL
    c. Reduced HDL
    d. Low plasminogen activator inhibitor
    e. Mutant insulin

11. Which is best for ascertaining glycemic control in a diabetic woman at the time of conception?
    (Recent Pattern Questions)
    a. Urine dipstick (DIASTIX)
    b. Serum fructosamine
    c. Glycosylated haemoglobin
    d. OGTT

12. Which is best for ascertaining glycemic control in bronze diabetes? *(Recent Pattern Questions)*
    a. Urine dipstick (DIASTIX)
    b. Serum fructosamine
    c. Glycosylated haemoglobin
    d. OGTT

13. False positive OGTT is seen in *all except*?
    (Recent Pattern Questions)
    a. Malnourished
    b. Infection
    c. Severe emotional stress
    d. Exercise

14. High Glycemic index is defined as value more than?
    (Recent Pattern Questions)
    a. 55
    b. 60
    c. 70
    d. 100

15. Which sulfonylurea drug has the highest insulinotropic potency? *(Recent Pattern Questions)*
    a. Glyburide
    b. Glipizide
    c. Glimepiride
    d. Gliclazide

16. Which of the following sulfonylureas cannot be used in patients with kidney failure? *(Recent Pattern Questions)*
    a. Glyburide
    b. Glipizide
    c. Gliclazide
    d. Glimepiride

17. Which is not a side effect of Thiazolidinediones?
    (Recent Pattern Questions)
    a. Hypoglycemia
    b. CHF
    c. Increase fracture risk
    d. Fatal liver damage

18. Hemorrhagic pancreatitis is a side effect of?
    (Recent Pattern Questions)
    a. Exenatide
    b. Canagliflozin
    c. Mitiglinide
    d. Pramlintide

19. Once a week preparation used in diabetes management is?
    (Recent Pattern Questions)
    a. Alogliptin
    b. Empagliflozin
    c. Albiglutide
    d. Glimepiride

20. An 11 year old type 1 diabetes mellitus patient was on CSII. While on holiday with her family she has become disoriented. On admission Na=126mEq/dl, potassium= 4.3mEq/dl, BUN= 100mg/dl, bicarbonate is 10mEq/dl and blood sugar is 600mg%. All are required for management except?
    a. ABG *(Recent Pattern Questions)*
    b. Potassium hydrogen phosphate
    c. Intravenous potassium
    d. 3% saline

21. Which of the following is known as peakless insulin?
    (Recent Pattern Questions)
    a. Isophane   b. Degludec
    c. Glulisine   d. Lispro

22. Weight loss is seen with all except?
    (Recent Pattern Questions)
    a. GLP-1 Agonists   b. SGLT-2 Inhibitors
    c. Pramlintide   d. DPP-4 inhibitors

23. Which long acting insulin can be mixed with rapid acting insulin? *(Recent Pattern Questions)*
    a. Glargine
    b. Degludec
    c. Detemir
    d. Can't be mixed due to difference in pH

24. All are complications due to use of the medical device shown here except? *(Recent Pattern Questions)*

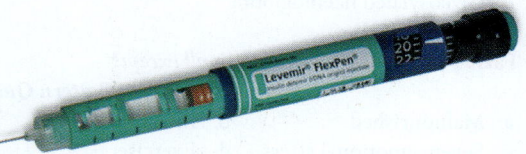

    a. Lipohypertrophy
    b. Neuroglucopenia
    c. Pre-breakfast hyperglycemia
    d. Molar ratio of insulin/C-peptide <1

25. Which is the most common cause of death in type 1 diabetes mellitus? *(Recent Pattern Questions)*
    a. Kidney disease   b. Myocardial disease
    c. Stroke   d. Infections

26. Which is the most common cause of death in type 2 diabetes mellitus? *(Recent Pattern Questions)*
    a. Kidney disease   b. Myocardial disease
    c. Stroke   d. Infections

27. The medical device shown below is used to deliver?
    (Recent Pattern Questions)

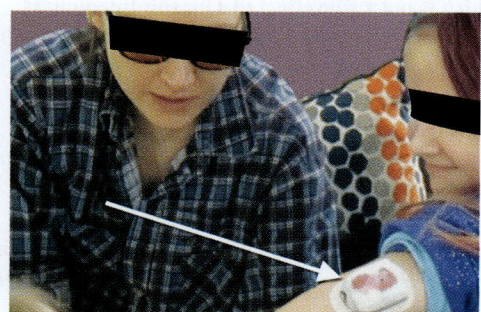

    a. Insulin   b. Ivacaftor
    c. Indacaterol   d. Vincristine

28. A type 1 DM patient on insulin is having consistent values of Pre-breakfast hyperglycemia. Hence the physician ordered self- monitoring of blood glucose including at night. The record of blood sugar of patient is given below. Which is the correct description for the recording shown?
    (Recent Pattern Questions)

Blood glucose in mg%		
10 PM	3AM	7AM
110mg%	40mg%	200mg%

    a. Dawn phenomenon   b. Somogyi phenomenon
    c. Waning of insulin effect   d. Factitious hypoglycaemia

29. A type 1 DM patient on insulin is having consistent values of Pre-breakfast hyperglycemia. Hence the physician ordered self- monitoring of blood glucose including at night. The following record of blood sugar of patient is given below. Which is the correct description for the recording shown below? *(Recent Pattern Questions)*

Blood glucose in mg%		
10 PM	3AM	7AM
110mg%	110mg%	200mg%

    a. Dawn phenomenon
    b. Somogyi phenomenon
    c. Waning of insulin effect
    d. Factitious hypoglycaemia

30. Which of the following is the best to reduce incidence of macrovascular complications in type 2 diabetes?
    a. Strict BP control   *(Recent Pattern Questions)*
    b. HbA1C< 6.5%
    c. Urine MICRAL
    d. Fasting Capillary blood glucose values of <180mg%

31. Which is the most common complication in type 2 diabetes mellitus?   *(Recent Pattern Questions)*
    a. Neuropathy   b. Nephropathy
    c. Retinopathy   d. Coronary artery disease

32. The following test is being performed on a patient of type 2 diabetes mellitus with HbA1c of 10.2%. Name the test.
    (Recent Pattern Questions)

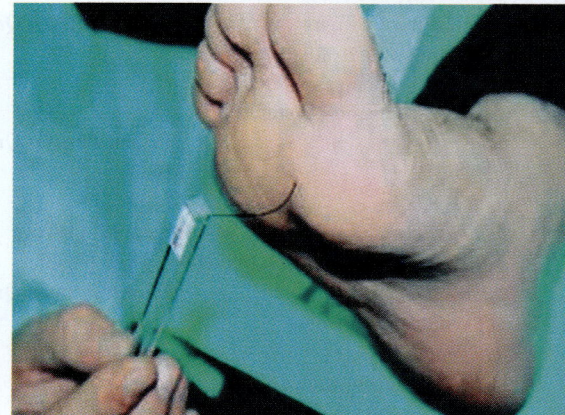

    a. Semmes Weinstein filament test
    b. Ipswich touch test
    c. Bio-Esthesiometry
    d. Two point discrimination test

33. Which of the following is correct about diabetic nephropathy? *(Recent Pattern Questions)*
    a. Urine dipsticks can easily detect microalbuminuria
    b. 24 hr urine albumin is more sensitive than spot sample urine albumin: urine creatinine
    c. Microalbuminuria correlates with nocturnal spike in Systolic blood pressure
    d. Most common cause of death in type 2 diabetes mellitus

34. Diabetic Amyotrophy presents with? *(Recent Pattern Questions)*
    a. Pain in front of thigh
    b. 3rd nerve palsy with pupillary sparing
    c. Distal areflexia
    d. Asymmetric motor weakness

35. All are sites of insulin administration except? *(Recent Pattern Questions)*
    a. Dorsum of hands
    b. Arms
    c. Lateral aspect of thigh
    d. Around umbilicus

36. Which of the following anti-diabetic drugs can be used safely in renal failure? *(Recent Pattern Questions)*
    a. Metformin
    b. Sitagliptin
    c. Linagliptin
    d. Canagliflozin

37. An unconscious diabetic is brought to the ER. His medical records show he is on warfarin for atrial fibrillation. Which of the following investigations will not be done in this patient for work up? *(AIIMS Nov 2016)*
    a. Lumbar puncture
    b. Random Blood sugar
    c. NCCT
    d. ECG monitoring

38. Which of the following anti-diabetic drugs can be used safely in renal failure? *(AIIMS Nov 2016)*
    a. Metformin
    b. Sitagliptin
    c. Linagliptin
    d. Canagliflozin

39. Gene involved in pathogenesis of Type 1 Diabetes mellitus is? *(Recent Question 2016-17)*
    a. CTLA-4
    b. ABCD1
    c. HNF-1 Alpha
    d. HNF-4 Alpha

40. Amyloid fibril deposition is seen in which type of diabetes? *(Recent Question 2016-17)*
    a. Type 1
    b. Type 2
    c. MODY
    d. Latent autoimmune diabetes of young

41. A diabetic normotensive patient of Enterococcus faecalis sepsis, on i.v. Linezolid developed high anion gap metabolic acidosis with increased serum lactate and negative ketone. The acid base abnormality is most probably? *(APPG 2016)*
    a. Type 'A' lactic acidosis due to sepsis
    b. Metabolic acidosis of uncertain etiology
    c. Diabetic ketoacidosis
    d. Type 'B' lactic acidosis due to Linezolid

42. Match the antidiabetic drug which is NOT to be used in the given situation. *(APPG 2016)*

    | P | Diabetes with recurrent UTI | W | Thiazolidinediones |
    | Q | Diabetic nephropathy with CKD | X | Glibenclamide |
    | R | Diabetes with heart failure | Y | Gliflozins |

    a. PQR = YXW
    b. PQR = XWY
    c. PQR = WYX
    d. PQR = XYW

43. A middle aged man comes with RTA and bleeding from the scalp. He is unconscious. A card in his pocket reveals that he is a known diabetic on Glimipiride + Metformin 2 tablets twice daily. What should be the next step? *(AIIMS May 2015)*
    a. Send blood for tests, start iv glucose and send to CT
    b. Start normal saline and send to CT
    c. Dextrose solution, CT scan
    d. Airway, CT scan, Blood Sugar if <70 start dextrose

44. A patient of hypoglycemia fails to regain consciousness after blood glucose is restored to normal. The complication to be suspected is? *(UPSC 2015)*
    a. Cerebral edema
    b. Lacunar infarct
    c. Post ictal state
    d. Cerebral hemorrhage

45. Consider the following conditions: *(UPSC 2015)*
    a. Thyrotoxicosis, pheochromocytoma and acromegaly
    b. Haemochromatosis
    c. Conn's syndrome (primary hyperaldosteronism)
    d. Pancreatic carcinoma
    Which of the above may result in secondary diabetes mellitus?
    a. B and C only
    b. A, B and D
    c. A, C and D
    d. A, B and C

46. Common site of injection of islet cells in islet cell transplant for diabetes mellitus: *(APPG 2015 Medicine)*
    a. Pelvis
    b. Portal vein
    c. Pancreas
    d. Forearm muscles

47. Whipple's triad is diagnostic of? *(APPG 2015 Medicine)*
    a. Gastrinoma
    b. Insulinoma
    c. somatostatinoma
    d. Glucogonoma

48. A 50 year old patient with signs of peripheral neuropathy is found to have diabetes mellitus. He has no ocular symptoms. When would you refer this patient for retina evaluation? *(UPSC 2015)*
    a. When he develops ocular symptoms
    b. Immediately
    c. If he needs insulin for blood sugar
    d. Five years after diagnosis

49. Which is related to MODY2? *(JIPMER Nov 2015)*
    a. HNF 1 alpha
    b. HNF 4 alpha
    c. Glucokinase
    d. PDX1

50. Initial imaging modality of choice for insulinoma?
    a. USG *(JIPMER May 2015)*
    b. CT abdomen
    c. Somatostatin receptor scan (SRS)
    d. E.U.S

51. All are true about diabetic ketoacidosis except?
    a. Glucose and ketones cause diuresis *(JIPMER May 2015)*
    b. It is an early presentation in type 1 DM
    c. Sodium Nitroprusside test is done to detect ketones
    d. Serum bicarbonate > 15mmol/L

52. Which of the following is true about glycosylated haemoglobin? *(JIPMER May 2015)*
    a. Increased in diabetic patients with sickle cell anaemia
    b. It is not a poor indicator of long term diabetic status in patient with renal disease
    c. Contain Haemoglobin with sugar moiety
    d. Half-life is 45 days in adults

53. **Hyperglycemic Hyperosmolar state (HHS) is characterized by:** *(PGI May 2015)*
    a. Hyperglycemia
    b. Acidosis
    c. Dehydration
    d. Coma

54. **Female with blood sugar of 600 mg% and sodium of 110 mEq. Insulin was given, what will happen to serum sodium levels?** *(Recent Questions 2015-16)*
    a. Sodium increase
    b. Sodium decrease
    c. Sodium unaffected
    d. Relative sodium deficiency

55. **Earliest finding in Diabetic nephropathy is:**
    a. Shrunken kidney is hallmark *(Recent Questions 2015-16)*
    b. Fibrin Caps
    c. Elevated Creatinine Clearance
    d. Urine albumin > 30 mg/dl

56. **Glucose fever is related with:** *(Recent Questions 2015-16)*
    a. Glucagon
    b. Parathyroid
    c. GH
    d. Aldosterone

57. **Glucose intolerance is caused by deficiency of?** *(JIPMER 2014)*
    a. Selenium
    b. Magnesium
    c. Chromium
    d. Zinc

58. **Not associated with diabetes mellitus:** *(Recent Pattern 2015-16)*
    a. Cushing syndrome
    b. Acromegaly
    c. Hypothyroidism
    d. Phaeochromocytoma

59. **Most common oral infection in diabetes mellitus?** *(Recent Pattern 2015-16)*
    a. Candida
    b. Aspergillus
    c. Mucormycosis
    d. Staphylococcus

60. **GTT post 1 hour sugar for gestational diabetes is > _____ mg %?** *(Recent Pattern 2015-16)*
    a. 140
    b. 150
    c. 180
    d. 200

61. **Aldose reductase inhibitor drugs are useful in?** *(Recent Pattern 2015-16)*
    a. Cataract
    b. Diabetes mellitus
    c. Hereditary fructose intolerance
    d. Essential fructosuria

62. **Foot Ulcers in diabetes are due to all except?** *(Recent Pattern 2015-16)*
    a. Decreased immunity
    b. Neuropathy
    c. Microangiopathy
    d. Macroangiopathy

63. **Cause of death in diabetic ketoacidosis in children?** *(Recent Pattern 2014-15)*
    a. Cerebral edema
    b. Hypokalemia
    c. Infection
    d. Acidosis

64. **According to ADA guidelines, the diagnosis of diabetes is made when the fasting blood glucose is more than:** *(Recent Pattern 2014-15)*
    a. 126 mg/dl
    b. 100 mg/dl
    c. 140 mg/dl
    d. 200 mg/dl

65. **Mauriac's syndrome is characterized by all except:** *(Recent Pattern 2014-15)*
    a. Diabetes
    b. Obesity
    c. Dwarfism
    d. Cardiomegaly

66. **Which of the following is used in management of diabetes?** *(Recent Pattern 2014-15)*
    a. Bromocriptine
    b. Octreotide
    c. Prednisolone
    d. Pegvisomant

67. **All are short acting insulin, except:** *(Recent Pattern 2014-15)*
    a. Lispro
    b. Aspart
    c. Glulisine
    d. Detemir

68. **Chances of blindness in diabetic patient as compared to non-diabetic patient is?** *(Recent Pattern 2014-15)*
    a. 5 times
    b. 10 times
    c. 15 times
    d. 25 times

69. **Diabetes is diagnosed when:** *(Recent Pattern 2014-15)*
    a. The level of fasting glucose is > 100 mg/dL and that of postprandial glucose is > 140 mg/dL
    b. The level of fasting glucose is > 126 mg/dL and that of postprandial glucose is > 199 mg/dL
    c. The level of plasma insulin is >6 lU/dL
    d. The HbA1c level is >5.5%

70. **The glucose lowering effect is least and delayed by several weeks with the following oral hypoglycaemic agents:**
    a. Insulin secretogogues *(Recent Pattern 2014-15)*
    b. DPP – IV inhibitors
    c. Biguanides
    d. Alpha-Glucosidase inhibitors

71. **A diabetes mellitus patient presents with fungal infection of sinuses and peri-orbital region with significant visual impairment. Best treatment among following is?**
    a. Amphotericin B *(AIIMS Nov 2012)*
    b. Itraconazole
    c. Ketoconazole
    d. Broad spectrum antibiotics

72. **Consider 2 patients with Atherosclerosis, one is diabetic and other is non-diabetic. When compared to non-diabetic, diabetic patient has 100 times increased risk of:**
    a. Myocardial infarction *(AIIMS Nov 2011)*
    b. Stroke
    c. Lower limb ischemia
    d. Vertebro basilar insufficiency

73. **Which is not seen in diabetic ketoacidosis:**
    a. Normal serum potassium *(Recent Pattern 2014-15)*
    b. Plasma osmolality 380 mOsm
    c. Urine Rothera test positive
    d. Urine Benedicts test positive

74. **Diabetes mellitus is present in all except:**
    a. Hemochromatosis *(Recent Pattern 2014-15)*
    b. Ataxia telengeictasia
    c. Friedreich ataxia
    d. Myotonic dystrophy

75. **Secondary diabetes may be noted in all except?**
    a. Acromegaly *(Recent Pattern 2014-15)*
    b. Addison's disease
    c. Haemosiderosis
    d. Glucagonoma

76. **Diabetic ketoacidosis is associated with all except:** *(Recent Pattern 2014-15)*
    a. ↑Utilization of glucose
    b. ↑In protein catabolism
    c. ↑ Anion gap
    d. Lipolysis

77. The following statements concerning diabetic keto-acidosis are correct except: *(Recent Pattern 2014-15)*
    a. Abdominal pain
    b. Low BUN
    c. Dehydration is out of proportion to the severity of vomiting
    d. Low-dose insulin therapy is the treatment of choice:

78. Which one of the following statements about diabetes is not correct? *(Recent Pattern 2014-15)*
    a. Insulin may be given subcutaneously in patient of diabetic ketoacidosis
    b. Insulin antibodies are a hallmark for diagnosis of insulin resistance
    c. During hypoglycaemic episodes patient may complain of difficulty in vision
    d. Positive test for ketone bodies in urine even after patients of diabetic ketosis are treated.

79. An obese patient presented in casualty with random blood sugar 400 mg%, urine sugar +++ and ketones 1+. Drug useful in management will be: *(Recent Pattern 2014-15)*
    a. Glibenclamide
    b. Troglitazsone
    c. Insulin
    d. Metformin

80. Retinopathy is most likely to be seen with:
    a. IDDM of 5 years duration *(Recent Pattern 2014-15)*
    b. NIDDM of 8 years duration
    c. Gestational diabetes
    d. Juvenile diabetes started before puberty

81. Insulin resistance is not seen in: *(Recent Pattern 2014-15)*
    a. Type 1.5 DM   b. Lipodystrophy
    c. Werner's syndrome d. Ataxic telangiectasia

82. Hypoglycemic unawareness is because of: *(Recent Pattern 2014-15)*
    a. Shifting of oral hypoglycemics to insulin
    b. Insulin resistance
    c. Autonomic neuropathy
    d. Necrobiosis lipoidica

83. Necrobiosis lipoidica diabeticorum is most marked on: *(Recent Pattern 2014-15)*
    a. Forearms   b. Face
    c. Pre-tibial   d. Sole of foot

84. An obese lady aged 45 years was brought to emergency in a semi-comatose condition. The laboratory investigation showed K+ (5.8 m mol/L); Na + (136 m mol/L); blood pH (7.1), HCO3 (12 m mol/L) Ketone bodies (350 mg/dl). Probable blood glucose is ? *(AIPG 2011)*
    a. < 45 mg/dl   b. < 120 mg/dl
    c. > 180 mg/dl   d. < 75 mg /dl

85. Oral anti-diabetic drug of choice in renal failure is: *(Recent Pattern 2014-15)*
    a. Glyburide   b. Chlorporamide
    c. Glipizide   d. Metformin

86. A patient with DM of 4 years duration presents with dizziness and HR 52/min, Probable cause is: *(Recent Pattern 2014-15)*
    a. Hypoglycaemia   b. Inferior wall MI
    c. Sick-sinus syndrome d. Autonomic dysunction

87. What is correct in diabetic ketoacidosis? *(Recent Pattern 2014-15)*
    a. Low serum potassium b. Increased anion gap
    c. Metabolic alkalosis d. Respiratory acidosis

88. Dose of insulin in diabetic nephropathy: *(Recent Pattern 2014-15)*
    a. Insulin dose should be increased in patient with ESRD
    b. Insulin dose should be decreased in patients with ESRD
    c. Insulin does not need change in ESRD
    d. Add inhaled insulin to conventional administration

89. The most effective correction of acidosis in diabetic ketoacidosis is by: *(Recent Pattern 2014-15)*
    a. I.V. bicarbonate   b. I.V. saline
    c. I.V. insulin   d. Oral bicarbonate

90. The complication of diabetes which cannot be prevented by strict control of blood sugar is: *(Recent Pattern 2014-15)*
    a. Amyotrophy
    b. Nerve conductivity
    c. Fluorescein dye leak
    d. Microalbuminuria

91. Incorrect about gestational diabetes mellitus?
    a. Congenital malformations *(Recent Pattern 2014-15)*
    b. Metformin used
    c. Prolonged labour
    d. Large for date baby

92. Microalbuminuria refers to urinary albumin excretion rate of: *(Recent Pattern 2014-15)*
    a. 30-300 mg/24 hour
    b. 400-600 mg/24 hour
    c. 700-900 mg/24 hour
    d. > 100 mg/24 hour

93. Diabetes mellitus patient presents with HbA1C of 9.6%. All improve with tight glycemic control except: *(Recent Pattern 2014-15)*
    a. Neuropathy   b. Nephropathy
    c. Retinopathy   d. Peripheral vascular disease

94. Necrobiosis lipoidica is seen in: *(Recent Pattern 2014-15)*
    a. Diabetes insipidus b. Lyme disease
    c. Diabetes mellitus   d. Simmonds disease

95. Which type diabetes is HLA associated: *(AI 2002)*
    a. Type I diabetes
    b. Type II diabetes
    c. Malnutrition related type disease
    d. Pregnancy related type diabetes

96. A 29 years old person is known diabetic on oral hypoglycemic agents since 3 years. He has lost weight and never had DKA. His grand father is diabetic but his father is nondiabetic. Which is the likely diagnosis: *(AI 2009)*
    a. MODY   b. DM type I
    c. DM type II   d. Pancreatic diabetes

97. All of the following are true about Type I DM, Except: *(Recent Question 2016-17)*
    a. Family history is present in 90% of cases
    b. Antibodies against β cells
    c. Prone to Diabetic Ketoacidosis (DKA)
    d. Insulin is required for management of DKA

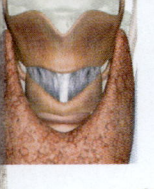

98. A 40 year old male patient is suffering from type II diabetes mellitus and hypertension. Which of the following antihypertensive drugs should not be used in such patients: (AIIMS Nov 03)
    a. Lisinopril
    b. Hydrochlorthiazide
    c. Losartan
    d. Trandolopril
99. Which of the following is not a test for diabetes mellitus (AIIMS Nov 2010)
    a. Fasting blood glucose
    b. Random blood glucose
    c. D-Xylose test
    d. Oral Glucose tolerance test
100. Which of the following findings can establish a diagnosis of Diabetes Mellitus: (AIIMS Nov 2011)
    a. Fasting plasma glucose 100mg/dl and 2 hour prandial glucose 140 mg/dl
    b. Fasting plasma glucose 125 mg/dl and 2 hour postprandial glucose 199 mg/dl
    c. Symptoms of Diabetes plus random blood glucose of 190 mg/dl
    d. Glycosylated Haemoglobin (HbA1C) > 6.5%
101. HbA1C level in blood explains: (AI 2004)
    a. Acute rise of sugar
    b. Long terms status of blood sugar
    c. Hepatorenal syndrome
    d. Chronic pancreatitis
102. The characteristic and common presentation of diabetic neuropathy is: (PGI Dec 98)
    a. Amyotrophy
    b. Mononeuropathy
    c. Distal sensory neuropathy
    d. Autonomic neuropathy
103. Recombinant human insulin is made by
    a. C-DNA from any eukaryote cell (AIIMS June 2000)
    b. Genome of any eukaryote
    c. C-DNA of pancreatic cell
    d. Genome of pancreatic cell
104. Which of the following tests is not used in the diagnosis of insulinoma: (AI 2011)
    a. Fasting blood glucose   b. D-Xylose test
    c. C- peptide levels   d. Insulin /Glucose Ratio
105. All cause weight gain, except: (AIIMS Sept 96)
    a. Diabetes mellitus   b. Cushing's syndrome
    c. Hypothyroidism   d. Insulin secreting tumour
106. Obesity is not a feature of : (AIIMS May 95)
    a. Hypothyroidism   b. Adrenal insufficiency
    c. Hypogonadism   d. Cushing's syndrome
107. Which is the best indicator for short term control (2-3 weeks) of blood glucose? (Recent Questions 2015-16)
    a. Serum fructosamine   b. HbA1c
    c. Blood sugar   d. Urine sugar
108. Which of the following drugs used for Diabetes Mellitus causes lactic acidosis: (Recent Questions 2015-16)
    a. Phenformin   b. Metformin
    c. Glipizide   d. Pioglitazone
109. Post Prandial capillary glucose should be_____ mg/dl for adequate diabetes control: (Recent Questions 2015-16)
    a. < 100 mg/dl   b. < 140 mg/dl
    c. < 180 mg/dl   d. < 200 mg/dl

Disorders of Adrenal Cortex

110. All are true about the condition shown except? (Recent Pattern Questions)

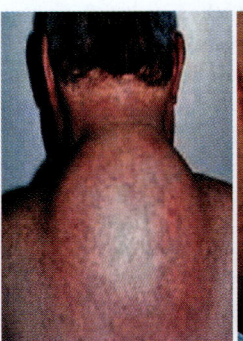 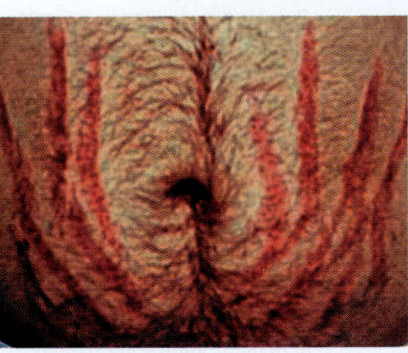

    a. Hyperpigmentation   b. Purplish striae
    c. Hyperkalemia   d. Metabolic alkalosis
111. All of the following investigations are needed for the following case except? (Recent Questions 2016-17)

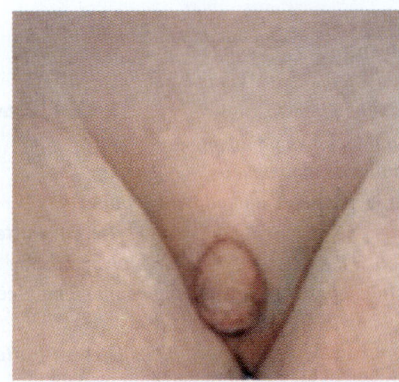

    a. X ray wrist and elbow   b. Karyotype
    c. Serum electrolytes   d. 24 hour urinary chloride
112. All are features of glucocorticoid deficiency except? (AIIMS Nov 2015)
    a. Weight loss   b. Fever
    c. Hyperkalemia   d. Postural hypotension
113. Following are the common features of Cushing's syndrome except? (UPSC 2015)
    a. Truncal obesity   b. Osteoporosis
    c. Distal myopathy   d. Glucose intolerance
114. Causes of diffuse hyperpigmentation include the following except: (APPG 2015 Medicine)
    a. Busulfan administration
    b. Nelson's syndrome
    c. Addison's disease
    d. Hermansky-pudlak syndrome
115. Addison's disease is characterized by all, except? (Bihar PG Medicine 2015)
    a. Hyperglycemia   b. Hypotension
    c. Hyperkalemia   d. Hyponatremia
116. The most common cause of Cushing's syndrome is? (Bihar PG Medicine 2015)
    a. Pituitary adenoma   b. Adrenal adenoma
    c. Ectopic ACTH   d. Iatrogenic steroids

117. Investigation to be performed in a patient with hypertension and hypokalemia? *(JIPMER May 2015)*
    a. Renin aldosterone ratio
    b. ACTH stimulation test
    c. 24 hour Urinary Catecholamine's
    d. Octreoscan

118. ACTH dependent Cushing syndrome is/are caused by:
    a. Pituitary adenoma *(PGI May 2015)*
    b. Adrenal adenoma
    c. Adrenocortical carcinoma
    d. Pheochromocytoma

119. Hyperpigmentation is seen with which hormone? *(Recent Questions 2015-16)*
    a. FSH   b. LH
    c. TSH   d. ACTH

120. All are seen in Addison's disease EXCEPT? *(Recent Questions 2015-16)*
    a. Hyponatremia   b. Hyperkalemia
    c. Hypotension   d. Metabolic alkalosis

121. Congenital adrenal hyperplasia due to 11 beta hydroxylase deficiency presents with all EXCEPT? *(Recent Questions 2015-16)*
    a. Metabolic acidosis   b. Hypokalemia
    c. Virilization   d. Hypertension

122. 40 year Male presents with primary infertility. Testis is present with azoospermia and absent vas deferens
    a. CFTR mutation   *(AIIMS Nov 14)*
    b. A.I.S
    c. Mullerian dysgenesis
    d. Congenital adrenal hyperplasia

123. Which of the following is not seen in Secondary Adrenal insufficiency? *(Recent Pattern 2015 -16)*
    a. Pigmentation   b. Hyponatremia
    c. Hypoglycemia   d. Lassitude

124. Obesity is seen in all except: *(Recent Pattern 2014-15)*
    a. Cushing syndrome   b. Pickwinian syndrome
    c. Prader willi syndrome d. Sipple syndrome

125. The most common cause of malignant adrenal mass is:
    a. Adrenocortical carcinoma   *(Recent Pattern 2014-15)*
    b. Malignant Phaeochromocytoma
    c. Lymphoma
    d. Metastasis from another solid tissue tumor

126. Primary hyperaldosteronism can be diagnosed by all of the following criteria except: *(Recent Pattern 2014-15)*
    a. Hypertension without edema
    b. Metabolic acidosis present
    c. Low plasma rennin activity that is not stimulated by volume depletion
    d. Hyperaldosteronism which is not suppressed by volume expansion.

127. Drug of choice for prenatal treatment of CAH due to 21 alpha hydroxylase deficiency: *(Recent Pattern 2014-15)*
    a. Dexamethasone   b. Betamethasone
    c. Prednisolone   d. Hydrocortisone

128. Cushing syndrome is commonly caused by:
    a. Adrenal adenoma   *(Recent Pattern 2014-15)*
    b. Adrenal hyperplasia
    c. Ectopic adrenal hormone production
    d. Adrenal carcinoma

129. Most common cause of Cushing's syndrome is:
    a. Pituitary adenoma   *(Recent Pattern 2014-15)*
    b. Adrenal adenoma
    c. Ectopic ACTH
    d. Iatrogenic steroids

130. Not seen in Cushing's syndrome: *(Recent Pattern 2014-15)*
    a. Hypoglycemia   b. Hypertension
    c. Frank psychosis   d. Hypokalemia

131. A 28-year-old lady has put on weight (10 kg over a period of 3 years) and has oligomenorrhoea followed by amenorrhoea for 8 months. The blood pressure is 160/100 mm of Hg. Which of the following is the most appropriate investigation? *(AIPG 2011)*
    a. Serum electrolytes
    b. Plasma cortisol
    c. Plasma testosterone and ultrasound
    d. T3, T4 and TSH

132. A patient presents with hemoptysis and cushingoid features with a lack of dexamethasone suppression, the likely reason could be: *(Recent Pattern 2014-15)*
    a. Adrenal hyperplasia   b. Adrenal adenoma
    c. CA lung   d. Ectopic ACTH production

133. Conn's syndrome is characterized by all except: *(Recent Pattern 2014-15)*
    a. Polyuria   b. Polydypsia
    c. Weakness   d. Anasarca

134. All are true about Cushing syndrome except? *(Recent Pattern 2014-15)*
    a. Association with MEN 2 syndrome
    b. Bronchial carcinoid causes cushing syndrome
    c. Hypokalemia
    d. Associated with coronary accidents

135. Best for management of hypoglycemia in a girl child with Congenital adrenal hyperplasia ? *(Recent Pattern 2014-15)*
    a. Betamethasone   b. Beclomethasone
    c. Budesonide   d. Hydrocortisone

136. Congenital 17-hydroxylase deficiency leads to hypertension due to accumulation of? *(Recent Pattern 2014-15)*
    a. Deoxycorticosterone   b. Cortisol
    c. 17 hydroxy pregnediol d. 17 hydroxy progesterone

137. Decreased plasma renin activity is seen in:
    a. Primary hyperaldosteronism *(Recent Pattern 2014-15)*
    b. Barter syndrome
    c. Pregnancy induced Hypertension
    d. Secondary aldosteronism

138. Salt losing type of adreno-genital syndromes is associated with: *(Recent Pattern 2014-15)*
    a. Hypoglycemia   b. Hypernatremia
    c. Hypertension   d. Hypokalemia

139. Patient with arthritis, skin hyperpigmentation and hypogonadism is diagnosed to have: *(Recent Pattern 2014-15)*
    a. Hemochromatosis
    b. SLE
    c. Ectopic ACTH secreting tumor of lung
    d. Wilson's disease

140. Pseudo-cushing syndrome is seen in: *(Recent Pattern 2014-15)*
    a. Chronic alcoholism   b. Incidentaloma
    c. Adrenal carcinoma   d. Nelson syndrome

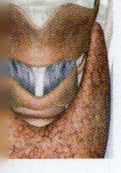

141. Incorrect about Addison's disease is?
    a. Hypoglycemia   (Recent Pattern 2014-15)
    b. Hypokalemia
    c. Loss of axillary and pubic hair
    d. Salt craving
142. A child presents with ambiguous genitalia without hyperpigmentation and normal blood pressure, 2.5 cm phallus with no opening at its tip, labia developed. Gonads are not seen in inguinal region and Mullerian structures are present on USG. The most probable diagnosis is:
    a. AIS   (Recent Pattern 2014-15)
    b. Maternal virilising tumor
    c. CAH
    d. 5-alpha-reductase deficiency
143. In Conn's syndrome, all the following are seen, except:
                             (Recent Pattern 2014-15)
    a. Hypokalemia   b. Hypernatremia
    c. Hypertension   d. Edema
144. Hypertension with hypokalemia is seen in following except:
    a. Cushing syndrome   (Recent Pattern 2014-15)
    b. Liddle syndrome
    c. End stage renal disease
    d. Primary hyperaldosteronism
145. Endogenous cause of Cushing's syndrome is: (AIIMS May 93)
    a. Cancer producing ectopic ACTH
    b. Pituitary adenoma
    c. Adrenal tuberculosis
    d. Bronchial Carcinoid
146. All of the following are true about Cushing's syndrome, except   (PGI 08)
    a. Violet striae
    b. Increased adrenaline
    c. Proximal muscle weakness
    d. Edema
147. A patient with cushinoid features presents with hemoptysis; he shows no response to dexamethasone suppression test; most likely diagnosis here is: (AI 2001)
    a. Adrenal hyperplasia
    b. Adrenal adenoma
    c. Ca lung with ectopic ACTH production.
    d. Pituitary microadenoma
148. A chronic smoker presented with mild haemoptysis. He also gave a history of hypertension and obesity. Lab data showed raised ACTH levels, which were not suppressed by high dose dexamethasone. The cause for the Cushing's syndrome in the patient is : (AIIMS May 02)
    a. MEN I
    b. Pituitary adenoma
    c. Adrenal cortical adenoma
    d. Ectopic ACTH secreting tumor
149. Which of the following is the earliest manifestation of Cushing 's syndrome?   (AI 2004)
    a. Loss of diurnal variation
    b. Increased ACTH
    c. Increased plasma Cortisol
    d. Increased urinary metabolites of Cortisol

Disorders of Adrenal Medulla

150. All are true about pheochromocytoma except?
    a. Urinary V.M.A is most specific   (JIPMER May 2018)
    b. Paraganglioma occurs at skull base
    c. 10% extra adrenal
    d. Organ of Zuckerkandl is most common extra adrenal site
151. VMA is elevated in which of the following conditions?
                             (Recent Pattern 2018)
    a. Primary micronodular adrenal hyperplasia
    b. Conn's Syndrome
    c. Neuroblastoma
    d. Tuberous Sclerosis
152. Which of the following is true about Pheochromocytoma:
    a. Sestabimi scan is done before surgery (PGI May 2015)
    b. Mostly are malignant
    c. Surgery is mainstay of treatment
    d. Prior α blocker is given
    e. Prior β blocker is given
153. Drug for management of hypertension in Phaeochromocytoma?   (Recent Pattern 2015-16)
    a. Phenoxybenzamine   b. Phentolamine
    c. Labetalol   d. Esmolol
154. In a case of Phaeochromocytoma, the diagnostic test best avoided is: (Bihar PG 2014)
    a. MRI scan   b. Urinary Metanephrines
    c. MIBG scan   d. FNAC
155. Which of the following is not found in pheochromocytoma?
                             (Recent Pattern 2014-15)
    a. Episodic hypertension   b. Postural hypotension
    c. Increased hematocrit   d. Hypocalcemia
156. A patient with pheochromocytoma would secrete which of the following in a higher concentration?
                             (Recent Pattern 2014-15)
    a. Norepinephrine   b. Epinephrine
    c. Dopamine   d. VMA
157. Pheochromocytoma is associated with:
    a. Vitiligo   (Recent Pattern 2014-15)
    b. Café-au-lait spots
    c. Ash leaf amelanotic macules
    d. Acanthosis Nigricans
158. In a patient with phenochromocytoma, all the following are seen except: (Recent Pattern 2014-15)
    a. Diarrhoea   b. Orthostatic hypotension
    c. Episodic hypertension d. Weight gain
159. The metastasis in phaeochromocytoma is treated by:
                             (Recent Pattern 2014-15)
    a. Strontium   b. Phosphorus
    c. Cobalt-60   d. MIBG
160. All the following drugs are used in pheochromocytoma except: (Recent Pattern 2014-15)
    a. Prazosin   b. Atenolol
    c. Nitroprusside   d. Metyrosine
161. Pheochromocytoma predominantly secretes: (AIIMS Nov 01)
    a. Epinephrine   b. Norepinephrine
    c. Dopamine   d. DOPA

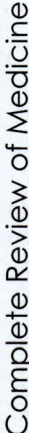

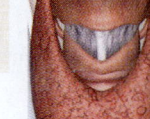

162. All of the following are features of phaeochromocytoma except: **(AI 2002)**
    a. Hypertensive paroxysm   b. Headache
    c. Orthostatic hypotension d. Wheezing

163. All are clinical features of pheochromocytoma, except: **(AIIMS Feb 97)**
    a. Increased hematocrit   b. Orthostatic hypotension
    c. Low cortisol level   d. Impaired glucose tolerance

Carcinoid Tumor and Syndrome

164. Best test for diagnosis of Carcinoid tumor:
    a. 24 hour urinary 5H.I.A.A **(Recent Questions 2015-16)**
    b. 24 hour catecholamines
    c. 24 hour vaniylmandelic acid levels
    d. 24 hour metanephrine levels

165. Which of the following is produced by Argentaffinoma of ileum? **(Recent Questions 2015-16)**
    a. G.A.B.A   b. Serotonin
    c. Epinephrine   d. Nor-epinephrine

166. Carcinoid Tumor of lung originates from? **(JIPMER 2014)**
    a. Type 2 Alveolar cell
    b. Clara cell
    c. Mucus (Goblet) cell
    d. Kulchitsky cell

167. Carcinoid syndrome produces valvular disease primarily of the: **(Recent Pattern 2014-15)**
    a. Venous valve   b. Tricuspid valve
    c. Mitral valve   d. Aortic valve

168. In carcinoid syndrome, the part of heart mostly affected is: **(Recent Pattern 2014-15)**
    a. Inflow tract of RV   b. Inflow tract of LV
    c. Mural endocardium   d. Pericardium

169. Carcinoid syndrome is associated with all except: **(Recent Pattern 2014-15)**
    a. Flushing of skin   b. Skin lesions like pellagra
    c. VMA in urine   d. Bronchospasm

Disorders of Thyroid Gland

170. A female patient was brought to the Emergency with altered sensorium. On examination BP was 80/60 mm with a pulse of 60/min. Rectal temperature was 34° Celsius. There was associated history of constipation, dry skin and menorrhagia. What is the diagnosis? **(AIIMS May 2018)**
    a. Myxedema coma
    b. Septic shock
    c. Hypothermia
    d. Cardiogenic shock

171. Which of the following is reason for thyroid storm after thyroid surgery? **(AIIMS Nov 2018)**
    a. Infection
    b. Inadequate preoperative preparation
    c. Thyroiditis
    d. Rough handling of thyroid at surgery

172. Comment on the diagnosis of the image shown below. **(AIIMS Nov 2017)**

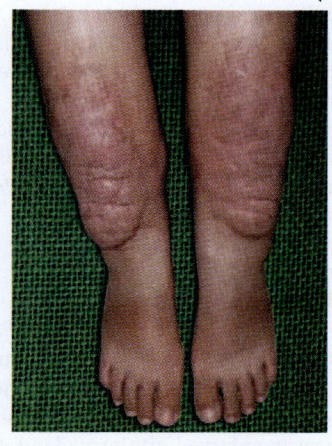

    a. Hypothyroidism   b. Hyperthyroidism
    c. Sarcoidosis   d. Diabetes

173. Thyroid function test of patient shows high TSH with a subnormal T4. What is the diagnosis? **(AIIMS May 2017)**
    a. Primary Hypothyroidism
    b. Hyperthyroidism
    c. Subclinical Hypothyroidism
    d. Secondary hypothyroidism

174. A young lady with tremors & diarrhea with elevated T4 and TSH levels were 8.5 mIU/L. Further examination reveals bi-temporal hemianopia. Next step of management: **(AIIMS May 2015)**
    a. Start anti-thyroid drugs, and do urgent MRI Brain
    b. Start beta blockers
    c. Conservative management
    d. Start anti-thyroid drugs and wait for symptoms to resolve

175. Patient present with thyrotoxicosis and both eyeballs protruded. Thyroid test done reveals? **(JIPMER May 2015)**
    a. T3 increased, T4 increased, TSH normal
    b. T3 decreased, T4 decreased, TSH increases
    c. T3 increased, T4 increased, TSH decreased
    d. T3 decreased, T4 normal, TSH decreased

176. Not a symptom of hyperthyroidism? **(JIPMER Nov 2014)**
    a. Hyperactivity   b. Palpitation
    c. Diarrhea   d. Hair loss

177. Which of the following present with hypothyroidism? **(Recent Questions 2015-16)**
    a. Struma ovarii
    b. Grave's disease
    c. Myasthenia gravis
    d. Toxic multinodular goiter

178. All are true about Hyperthyroidism EXCEPT: **(Recent Questions 2015-16)**
    a. Anxiety   b. Palpitations
    c. Tachycardia   d. Weight gain

179. Wolf Chaikoff effect is due to: **(Recent Questions 2015-16)**
    a. Iodine deficiency
    b. Excessive iodine
    c. Iodine metabolism defect
    d. TPO enzyme deficiency

180. Which of the following is NOT a feature of thyrotoxicosis?
    (Recent Questions 2015-16)
    a. Palpitation   b. Anxiety
    c. Weight loss   d. Menorrhagia
181. Proptosis not seen in?   (Recent Questions 2015-16)
    a. Primary thyrotoxicosis   b. Sarcoidosis
    c. Pituitary adenoma   d. Hypothyroidism
182. All are true about Hashimoto encephalopathy except:
    (Recent Pattern 2014-15)
    a. Myoclonus
    b. Seizures
    c. Steroid responsive encephalopathy
    d. EEG is normal
183. DOC for Hashimoto encephalopathy:
    (Recent Pattern 2014-15)
    a. Steroids   b. Prophythiouracil
    c. I-131   d. Liothyronine infusion
184. A 17-year old girl who was evaluated for short height was found to have an enlarged pituitary gland. Her T4 was low and TSH was increased. Which of the following is the most likely diagnosis?   (Recent Pattern 2014-15)
    a. Pituitary adenoma
    b. TSH-secreting pituitary tumour
    c. Thyroid target receptor insensivity
    d. Primary hypothyroidism
185. Extremely sensitive TSH detection tests can detect TSH at a minimum level of, less than?   (Recent Pattern 2014-15)
    a. 0.4 mU/L   b. 0.04 mU/L
    c. 0.004 mU/L   d. 0.0004 mU/L
186. The occurrence of hyperthyroidism following administration of supplemental iodine to subjects in endemic area of iodine deficiency is due to?   (Recent Pattern 2014-15)
    a. Wolf-Chaikoff effect   b. Jod-Basedow effect
    c. Pemberton effect   d. Graves' effect
187. All are true about Central hypothyroidism except?
    a. Craniopharyngioma is an etiology   (AIPG 2012)
    b. Treatment is done by monitoring TSH level in plasma
    c. TSH level may be normal
    d. Before starting treatment checkout for adrenal insufficiency
188. Thyroid storm is seen in: (Recent Pattern 2014-15)
    a. Thyroid surgery   b. Neonatal thyrotoxicosis
    c. Peri-operative infection   d. All of the above
189. Heel pad thickness is useful in: (Recent Pattern 2014-15)
    a. Hypothyroidism   b. Acromegaly
    c. PEM   d. All of the above
190. Hypothyroidism is associated with the following clinical problems, except: (Recent Pattern 2014-15)
    a. Menorrhagia   b. Early abortions
    c. Galactorrhoea   d. Thromboembolism
191. Pemberton sign is seen in?   (Recent Pattern 2014-15)
    a. Retrosternal goiter   b. Grave opthalmopathy
    c. Thyroid crisis   d. Addisonian crisis
192. Reversible Dementia is a feature of?
    (Recent Pattern 2014-15)
    a. Hyperparathyroidism   b. Hypothyroidism
    c. Hyperthyroidism   d. Cushing's disease
193. Which of the following are not related to Myxedema?
    a. Coronary atherosclerosis   (APPG 2014)
    b. Type III hyperlipoproteinaemia
    c. Massive Pericardial effusion
    d. Absence of pulsus paradoxus
194. TSH cannot be used for monitoring response to treatment in:
    a. Primary hypothyroidism   (Recent Pattern 2014-15)
    b. Secondary hypothyrodism
    c. Thyroprivic hypothyroidism
    d. Iodine deficiency
195. Least likely cardiac manifestations of Grave's disease in 25 year old female would include all of the following except?
    (Recent Pattern 2014-15)
    a. Sinus tachycardia   b. Atrial fibrillation
    c. Bounding pulses   d. Aortic systolic murmur
196. Replacement dose of Thyroxine per day is?
    (Recent Pattern 2014-15)
    a. 100 mcg   b. 200 mcg
    c. 300 mcg   d. 400 mcg
197. Used in thyroid crisis are A/E: (Recent Pattern 2014-15)
    a. Propranolol   b. Gradual warming
    c. Iodine   d. Corticosteroids
198. Most common presentation of sick euthyroid state:
    (Recent Pattern 2014-15)
    a. Low T_3 with normal T_4 b. Low T_3 with low T_4
    c. Low T_3 with high T_4 d. High T_3 with high T_4
199. In myxoedema which is not correct:
    (Recent Pattern 2014-15)
    a. Slow pulse   b. Hypertension
    c. Hypotension   d. Dry skin
200. Thyroid carcinoma with pulsatile vascular skeletal metastasis is seen in: (Recent Pattern 2014-15)
    a. Papillary   b. Follicular
    c. Medullary   d. Anaplastic
201. Myxoedema coma is treated with: (Recent Pattern 2014-15)
    a. Hydrocortisone   b. Liothyronine
    c. Levothyroxine   d. All of the above
202. Which one of the following clinical signs is not seen in ophthalmic Grave's disease?   (Recent Pattern 2014-15)
    a. Lid retraction   b. Frequent blinking
    c. Poor convergence   d. Upper lid "lad" on down gaze
203. Which is not seen in subacute thyroditidis:
    (Recent Pattern 2014-15)
    a. Raised T4 levels   b. Raised ESR
    c. Pain   d. High Radio iodine uptake
204. Radioiodine uptake in endemic goitre is:
    (Recent Pattern 2014-15)
    a. Normal   b. Increased
    c. Decreased   d. Erratic
205. Hung up ankle jerk is seen in?   (Recent Pattern 2014-15)
    a. Hypothyroidism   b. Thyrotoxicosis
    c. Sipple syndrome   d. Wermer syndrome
206. Which one of the following features may not be seen in hypothyroidism?   (Recent Pattern 2014-15)
    a. Cold intolerance
    b. Deafness
    c. Pericardial effusion
    d. Pretibial myxoedema
207. Goitrous hypothyroidism commonly occurs in all of the following except?   (Recent Pattern 2014-15)
    a. Hashimoto's thyroiditis
    b. Dyshoromonogenesis (Pendred syndrome)
    c. Thyroprivic hypothyroidism
    d. Iodine deficiency

208. Presentation of hypothyroidism is?
 (Recent Pattern 2014-15)
 a. Pretibial myxedema b. Hirusutism
 c. Easily brusiable skin d. Galactorrhoea
209. Gestational hyperthyroidism occurs due to:
 a. Beta hCG from placenta (Recent Pattern 2014-15)
 b. Transplacental TSH transfer
 c. T.P.O antibody
 d. Anti–thyroglobulin antibody
210. "Hour-glass" shape of the chest and "tri-radiate pelvis" are seen radio logically in: (Recent Pattern 2014-15)
 a. Thyrotoxicosis b. Myxedema
 c. Osteomalacia d. Hyperthyroidism
211. The laboratory screening test which suggests normal thyroid function is: (Recent Pattern 2014-15)
 a. TSH b. Free T4
 c. T3 d. Free T3
212. Which is true about Thyrotoxic Periodic paralysis.
 a. Sodium channel defect (Recent Pattern 2014-15)
 b. Hypokalemic periodic paralysis
 c. Precipitated by fasting
 d. Associated with myxedema coma
213. The most common differential diagnosis of hyperthyroidism in a young female is: (Recent Pattern 2014-15)
 a. Hysteria b. Essential tremor
 c. Anxiety neurosis d. Parkinsonism
214. Which of the following conditions is associated with Hypothyroidism: (AI 2011)
 a. Hashimoto's Thyroiditis b. Grave's Disease
 c. Toxic Multinodular Goiter d. Struma ovary
215. All of the following are features of thyrotoxicosis, EXCEPT-
 a. Diastolic murmur (AIIMS June 99)
 b. Soft non ejection systolic murmur
 c. Irregularly, irregular pulse
 d. Scratching sound in systole
216. Dancing carotid is seen in : (AIIMS Dec 98)
 a. Thyrotoxicosis b. Hypothyroidism
 c. AV Fistula d. Blow out carotid
217. All of the following are associated with Thyroid storm, except (AI 2002)
 a. Surgery for thyroiditis b. Surgery for thyrotoxicosis
 c. Stressful illness in thyrotoxicosis
 d. I131 therapy for thyrotoxicosis
218. Most common cause of Thyroiditis is: (AI 2000)
 a. Reidl's Thyroiditis
 b. Subacute Thyroiditis
 c. Hashimoto's Thyroiditis
 d. Viral Thyroiditis
219. All the following are true of DeQuervan's Thyroiditis except:
 a. Pain (AI 1996)
 b. Increased ESR
 c. Increased radioactive iodine uptake
 d. Fever
220. 'Hurthle cells' are seen in (AI 1995)
 a. Agranulomatous Thyroiditis
 b. Hashimoto's Thyroiditis
 c. Papillary carcinoma of the thyroid
 d. Thyroglossal cyst

221. The most common presentation of endemic goiter is
 (AI 1996)
 a. Hypothyroid b. Diffuse goiter
 c. Hyperthyroid d. Solitary nodule
222. Needle biopsy of solitary thyroid nodule in a young woman with palpable cervical lymph nodes on the same sides demonstrates amyloid in stroma of lesion. Likely diagnosis is (AI 2002)
 a. Medullary carcinoma thyroid
 b. Follicular carcinoma thyroid
 c. Thyroid adenoma
 d. Multi nodular goitre
223. Screening method for medullary carcinoma thyroid is:
 (AI 1997)
 a. Serum calcitonin b. S. calcium
 b. S. alkaline phosphate d. S. acid phosphatase

Disorders of Parathyroid Gland and Calcium Metabolism

224. A young female presents with complaints of bone pain and abdominal cramps and psychotic behaviour. A clinician is suspecting hyperparathyroidism in the patient. Which is the best imaging modality to arrive at the diagnosis?
 (AIIMS May 2017)
 a. Sestamibi scan b. MRI
 c. CT scan d. USG neck
225. A patient who is a known case of lung cancer came with complaints of weakness and serum calcium of 16.4mg%. What is the next step in the management of the patient?
 (AIIMS Nov 2016)
 a. IV Fluids and diuretics b. IV phosphate
 c. IV bisphosphonates d. Subcutaneous calcitonin
226. A patient with disseminated malignancy receiving palliative care presents at night with history of severe nausea and constipation. You make a provisional diagnosis of hypercalcemia which was confirmed with lab values. The next line of management is? (AIIMS May 2016)
 a. IV Fluid b. IV Steroids
 c. Thiazides d. IV Bisphosphonates
227. Match the following and choose the best combination

P	Fatty, fertile female of forty	U	Cholelithiasis
		V	Peptic ulcer
Q	Stones, bones, abdominal groans and psychic moans	W	Primary hyperparathyroidism
		X	Addison's asthma
R	They pant their way into old age	Y	Bronchial asthma
		Z	Hamman rich syndrome

 a. PQR = UWY
 b. PQR = UXZ
 c. PQR = VWZ
 d. PQR = VXY

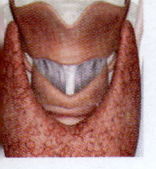

228. What is this sign called? **(APPG 2016)**

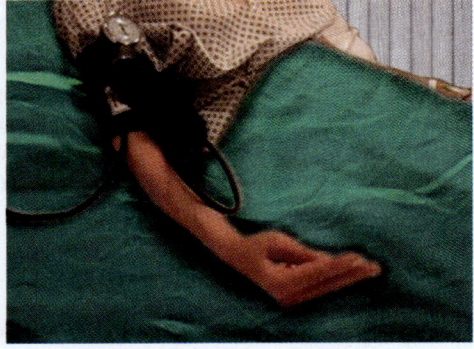

a. Chvostek sign b. Troisier sign
c. Trousseau's sign d. Lhermitte's sign

229. **An adult patient presents with systemic hypertension, renal calculus disease and severe peptic ulcer disease. Which one of the following is most likely occurrence in this case?**
a. Milk – alkali syndrome **(UPSC 2015)**
b. Hypervitaminosis – D
c. Primary hyperparathyroidism
d. Tubulo-interstitial Renal disease

230. **All the Following are helpful in the initial treatment of severe hypercalcemia associated with hyperparathyroidism except:**
a. Hydration with saline **(APPG 2015)**
b. Forced diuresis with loop diuretics
c. Glucocorticoids
d. Pamidronate

231. **Blade of grass lesion of found in?** **(APPG 2015)**
a. Osteoporosis b. Thalassemia
c. Paget's disease d. Carcinoma prostate

232. **Hypercalcemia is associated with all, except?**
a. Hyperparathyroidism **(Bihar Pg 2015)**
b. Sarcoidosis
c. Milk alkali syndrome
d. Celiac disease

233. **Osteoporosis is caused by all, except?** **(Bihar Pg 2015)**
a. Sarcoidosis b. Old age
c. Hypoparathyroidism d. Steroid therapy

234. **Hypercalcemia is caused by?** **(JIPMER May 2015)**
a. Adrenocortical insufficiency
b. Amyloidosis
c. Hyperthyroidism
d. Vitamin C intoxication

235. **Nutritional vitamin D deficiency has all except:**
(Recent Questions 2015-16)
a. Hypocalcemia b. Increased SAP
c. Increased PTH d. Hyperphosphataemia

236. **Which of the following finding shall be seen in patient with hyper-parathyroidism?** **(Recent Questions 2015-16)**
a. Hypophosphatemia b. Hyperphosphatemia
c. Hypermagnesemia d. Hypo magnesemia

237. **All are features of hyper-parathyroidism except:**
(Recent Questions 2015-16)
a. Increase serum calcium b. Decreased serum phosphate
c. Diarrhea d. Nephrocalcinosis

238. **Excess of calcium intake leads to:** **(AIIMS Nov 14)**
a. Cardiomyopathy b. Osteoporosis
c. Osteomalacia d. Milk alkali syndrome

239. **A middle aged female has a pathological fracture of clavicle, ribs and X-ray shows periosteal resorption of 2nd and 3rd metatarsals and phalanges. Most probable cause is?**
(AIIMS Nov 14)
a. Hyperparathyroidism b. Hypoparathyroidism
c. Renal Osteodystrophy d. Osteomalacia

240. **Features of hyperparathyroidism are all except?**
(Recent Pattern 2015-16)
a. Solitary adenoma b. Malignant
c. Thyroid malignancy d. Parathyroid hyperplasia

241. **Which of the following statements is not true?**
(AIIMS May 2013)
a. Parathyroid hormone-related protein is responsible for causing hypercalcemia in cancer patients.
b. The unionized fraction of calcium in the plasma is an important determinant of PTH secretion.
c. Mg^{2+} in influences PTH secretion in the same direction as Ca^{2+}, but is a less potent secret-agogue.
d. Ca^{2+} influences PTH secretion by acting on a calcium sensor G-protein coupled receptor located in the parathyroid gland.

242. **All of the following statements are true except:**
(Recent Pattern 2014-15)
a. 25-α-hydroxylation of vitamin D occurs in the liver
b. 1-α-hydroxylation of vitamin D occurs in the kidney
c. In the absence of sunlight, the daily requirement of Vitamin D is 400-600 IU
d. William's syndrome is characterized by precocious puberty, mental retardation and obesity

243. **70 year female is on treatment with Alendronate for severe osteoporosis. Now she complains of pain in right thigh. What is the next investigation to be performed:**
a. DEXA scan **(AIIMS Nov 2012)**
b. X-ray
c. Serum vitamin D levels
d. Serum alkaline phosphate levels

244. **Arrow headed finger on X-ray is suggestive of:**
(Recent Pattern 2014-15)
a. Acromegaly b. Hyperparathyroidism
c. Down syndrome d. Sarcoidosis

245. **Hypercalcaemia is caused by all except:**
(Recent Pattern 2014-15)
a. Multiple myeloma b. Hyperparathyroidism
c. Sarcoidosis d. Hypothyroidism

246. **Nephro-calcinosis is a feature of:** **(Recent Pattern 2014-15)**
a. Primary hyperparathyroidism
b. Medullary cystic kidney
c. Vitamin C intoxication
d. Pseudo-hypoparathyroidism

247. **Tufting of terminal phalanges is seen in:**
(Recent Pattern 2014-15)
a. Hypoparathyroidism b. Hyperparathyroidism
c. Hyperthyroidism d. Gallstone

248. **Imaging of choice in parathyroid pathology is:**
a. CT scan **(Recent Pattern 2014-15)**
b. Gallium scan
c. Thallium scan
d. Technetium-99 sestamibi scan

249. **Low serum alkaline phosphatase is seen with:**
    (Recent Pattern 2014-15)
    a. Hypoparathyroidism   b. Hypophosphatasia
    c. Hyperparathyroidism d. Pseudohypoparathyrodism
250. **Hypercalcemic crisis is seen in all except:**
    a. Metastatic carcinoma breast   *(Recent Pattern 2014-15)*
    b. Hyperparathyroidism
    c. Pancreatitis
    d. Hodgkin's lymphoma
251. **Hyperphosphataemia is seen in all except:**
    a. CRF   *(Recent Pattern 2014-15)*
    b. Prolonged phosphate intake
    c. Pseudo-pseudo-hypoparathyroidism
    d. Pseudo-hypoparathyrodism
252. **Increased urinary hydroxyproline is seen in?**
    (Recent Pattern 2014-15)
    a. Paget's disease   b. Ehler Danlos syndrome
    c. Hypo-parathyroidism d. Osteoporosis
253. **True about primary hyperparathyroidism is:**
    (Recent Pattern 2014-15)
    a. Hypotension   b. Recurrent abortion
    c. Neuropsychiatric changes d. Gallstone
254. **Most common cause of primary hyperparathyroidism:**
    a. Iatrogenic   *(AIIMS Nov 93)*
    b. Medullary carcinoma thyroid
    c. Parathyroid adenoma
    d. Parathyroid hyperplasia
255. **Subtle presentation of hyperparathyroidism is:**
    a. Psychiatric manifestation   *(AIIMS Dec 97)*
    b. Nephrocalcinosis
    c. Abdominal pain
    d. Asymptomatic hypercalcemia
256. **Which of the following is associated with secondary hyperparathyroidism**   *(AIIMS Dec 94)*
    a. Parathyroid adenoma
    b. Marked hypercalcemia
    c. Chronic renal failure
    d. Parathyroidectomy relieves the symptoms
257. **A 45 year old man, known case of chronic renal failure develops rugger jersy spine. The probable cause is:**
    a. Aluminium intoxication   *(AI 2000)*
    b. Secondary hyperparathyroidism
    c. Osteoporosis
    d. Osteomalacia
258. **Tufting of the terminal phalanges is seen in :**   *(AI 1995)*
    a. Hypoparathyroidism   b. Hyperparathyroidism
    c. Hyperthyroidism   d. Hypothyroidism
259. **Low calcium and high phosphate is seen in:**   *(AI 2010)*
    a. Hyperparathyroidism   b. Hypoparathyroidism
    c. Hyperthyroidism   d. Hypothyroidism
260. **Hypercalcemia is associated with all except:**   *(AI 2009)*
    a. Hyperparathyroidism   b. Sarcoidosis
    c. Milk alkali syndrome   d. Celiac disease
261. **Hypercalcemia is seen in all except:**   *(AIIMS May 93)*
    a. Acute pancreatitis   b. Hypervitaminosis D
    c. Addison's disease   d. Hyperparathyroidism

262. **Treatment of hypercalcemia includes, all, except:**
    (AIIMS Dec 97)
    a. Gallium nitrate   b. Plicamycin
    c. Etidronate   d. Thiazide
263. **All are used in treatment of hypercalcemia, except:**
    (AIIMS May 93)
    a. Phosphate   b. Mithramycin
    c. Vitamin D in high dose   d. Furosemide
264. **All of the following agents may be used in the management of Chronic Hypocalcemia, except:**   *(AI 2012)*
    a. Etidronate   b. Thiazides
    c. Elemental calcium   d. Vitamin D analogs
265. **Hypocalcemia with hyperphosphatemia are seen in:**
    (PGI Dec 2000)
    a. CRF   b. Pseudohypoparathyroidism
    c. Vit. D deficiency   d. Magnesium deficiency
266. **All of the following are seen in Ricket's except:**
    (AIIMS May 03)
    a. Bow legs   b. Gunstock deformity
    c. Pot belly   d. Cranio tabes
267. **Which is not true of hypocalcaemia:**   *(AI 1995)*
    a. Can occur in hypoparathyroidism
    b. Latent tetany is seen
    c. Prolonged QT interval
    d. Inverse relation with Mg^{++} levels
268. **During a routine check up, a 67-year-old man is found to have a level of serum alkaline phosphatase three times the upper limit of normal. Serum calcium and phosphorus concentrations and liver function test results are normal. He is asymptomatic. The most likely diagnosis is :**
    a. Metastatic bone disease   *(AIIMS Nov 99)*
    b. Primary hyperparathyroidism
    c. Paget's disease of bone
    d. Osteomalacia
269. **Alkaline phosphatase is elevated in all, except:**
    (AIIMS Dec 97)
    a. Rickets   b. Osteomalacia
    c. Hypoparathyroidism   d. Hypophosphatemia
270. **Osteoporosis may be seen in all except:**   *(AI 1998)*
    a. Hyperparathyroidism   b. Hypoparathyroidism
    c. Thyrotoxicosis   d. Heparin administration
271. **Osteoporosis is seen in:**   *(AI 1994)*
    a. Thyrotoxicosis   b. Cushing's disease
    c Menopause   d. All of the above
272. **Which one of the following is not a feature of vitamin D deficiency rickets?**   *(AIIMS Nov 2015)*
    a. Decrease in parathyroid hormone level
    b. Decrease in gut calcium absorption
    c. Increase in renal phosphate excretion
    d. Increase in serum alkaline phosphatase

Magnesium Metabolism

273. **1st sign of Magnesium sulphate toxicity is?**
    a. Drop in O_2 saturation   *(Recent Question 2016-17)*
    b. Loss of patellar reflex
    c. Decreased Respiratory Rate
    d. Hypotension refractory to vasopressors

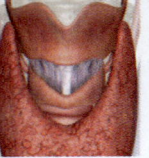

274. **Characteristic ECG change in hypomagnesemia is?**
     (Recent Question 2016-17)
     a. Increased PR interval   b. QRS widening
     c. T wave depression   d. QTC prolongation
275. **Hypomagnesaemia presents with all except:**
     (Recent Pattern 2014-15)
     a. Symptoms same as hypocalcaemia
     b. Development of torsades de pointes
     c. Potentiates hypocalcaemia
     d. Seen in diabetic ketoacidosis
276. **Hypomagnesemia is seen in all except:**
     (Recent Pattern 2014-15)
     a. Gitelman syndrome   b. Hungry bone syndrome
     c. Paget disease   d. Prolonged thiazide therapy
277. **Magnesium deficiency is seen in all except?**
     (Recent Pattern 2014-15)
     a. Hypercalcaemia   b. Tetany
     c. Starvation   d. Neurological abnormalities

M.E.N

278. **Which of the following is not seen in MEN1?**
     a. Posterior pituitary tumours   *(AIIMS Nov 2016)*
     b. Foregut carcinoids
     c. Parathyroid hyperplasia
     d. Pancreatic neuroendocrine tumours
279. **MEN 1 patient has urinary stones and increased serum calcium. Next investigation to be done is?**
     (JIPMER Nov 2015)
     a. Urinary metanephrine   b. Secretin study
     c. Serum calcitonin levels   d. 72 hour prolonged fasting
280. **All are associated with MEN4 except?** *(Recent 2014-15)*
     a. Parathyroid adenoma
     b. Pituitary adenoma
     c. Reproductive organ Tumors
     d. M.T.C
281. **All are features of MEN2B except ?** *(Recent 2014-15)*
     a. Mucosal neuroma
     b. Marfanoid Habitus
     c. Medullated corneal nerve fibres
     d. Meningioma
282. **Pancreatitis, pituitary tumor and pheochromocytoma may be associated with:** *(AI 2004, 2005)*
     a. Medullary carcinoma of the thyroid
     b. Papillary carcinoma of the thyroid
     c. Anaplastic carcinoma of the thyroid
     d. Follicular carcinoma of the thyroid

Disorders of GH, Vasopressin

283. **A 50 year old man presents with frontal bossing, enlarged tongue and spade like fingers. Which is of the following tests should be done in this patient?** *(AIIMS May 2017)*
     a. Insulin like growth factor
     b. Thyroid hormone assay
     c. Serum prolactin
     d. Serum Testosterone
284. **A 45 year old smoker and hypertensive patient is on enalapril and hydrochlorothiazide. He had an episode of hemoptysis and was found to be having lung cancer with metastasis to the brain. His current lab values are Sodium= 125mEq/dl, Blood sugar= 112mg/dl, Blood urea= 10mg/dl, serum osmolality =285mOsm and urine osmolality = 350mOsm. 24 hr urinary sodium is 100 mEq/day and BP= 150/90mmHg. Which of the following is the reason for low sodium values in the patient?** *(AIIMS May 2017)*
     a. SIADH
     b. Diuretic induced hyponatremia
     c. Cerebral salt wasting syndrome
     d. Pseudo-hyponatremia.
285. **True about SIADH is?** *(JIPMER Nov 2015)*
     a. Euvolemic hyponatremia
     b. Euvolemic hypernatremia
     c. Hypervolemic hypernatremia
     d. Hypervolemic hyponatremia
286. **All are true about Diabetes insipidus except?**
     a. Low urine osmolality   *(Recent Questions 2015-16)*
     b. Dilutional Hyponatremia
     c. Water deprivation test is used for diagnosis
     d. Polyuria
287. **All are correct about SIADH except:**
     (Recent Questions 2015-16)
     a. Normal KFT   b. Low uric acid
     c. Relative hypernatremia   d. Normal BP with gain of water
288. **All of following are seen in GH deficiency except:**
     (Recent Questions 2015-16)
     a. Hyperglycemia   b. Stunting
     c. Delayed bone age   d. High pitched voice
289. **The image shows?**

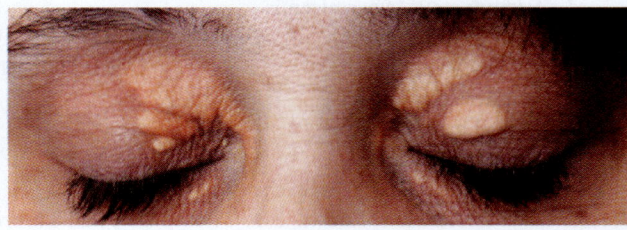

     a. Xanthelasma   b. Necrobiosis lipidoica
     c. Tuberous xanthoma   d. Orbital lipogranulomata
290. **The drug used in the management of medullary carcinoma thyroid is:** *(Bihar PG 2014)*
     a. Cabozantinib   b. Rituximab
     c. Tenofovir   d. Anakinra
291. **All are associated with pituitary apoplexy except:**
     (AIIMS May 07)
     a. Hyperthyroidism   b. Diabetes mellitus
     c. Sickle cell anemia d. Hypertension
292. **Which drug is essential in Sheehan's syndrome:** *(AI 1996)*
     a. Estrogen   b. Cortisone
     c. Thyroxin   d. Growth hormone
293. **SIADH secretion is seen in all except :** *(AI 1994)*
     a. Lung abscess
     b. Interstitial Nephritis
     c. Vinka alkaloids
     d. Bronchial adenoma

294. A 35 year old man presents with vomitings and confusion. On examination Na⁺ 120 m mol/L, K⁺ 4.2 m mol/L, Uric acid 2 mg/dl. Patient is not edematous. The diagnosis is:
    a. Cerebral toxoplasmosis with SIADH (AIIMS Nov 99)
    b. Hepatic failure
    c. Severe dehydration
    d. Congestive heart failure

295. All are true regarding SIADH except: (AIIMS Nov 93)
    a. Increased level of ADH
    b. Hyposmolar urine
    c. Hyponatremia
    d. Adequate hydration status

296. Which of the following is the drug of choice for the treatment of inappropriate anti-diuretic hormone secretion: (AIIMS Nov 05)
    a. Frusemide
    b. Hydrochlorothiazide
    c. Spironolactone
    d. Demeclocycline

297. All of the following conditions are known to cause diabetes insipidus, except: (AIIMS May 04) & (AI 2005)
    a. Multiple sclerosis
    b. Head injury
    c. Histiocytosis
    d. Viral encephalitis

298. Endocrinological causes of Carpal Tunnel syndrome include all of the following, except: (AI 2009)
    a. Diabetes Mellitus
    b. Hypothyroidism
    c. Acromegaly
    d. Addison's disease

Disorders of LH, FSH and Prolactin

299. A patient was prescribed bromocriptine for prolactinoma, and responded to her symptoms. What is it's mechanism of action? (AIIMS Nov 2017)
    a. D2 receptor partial agonist
    b. Increases prolactin levels
    c. Normalizes serum prolactin levels
    d. D2 receptor antagonist

300. Which of the following is not seen in hypogonadotropic hypogonadism? (AIIMS Nov 2017)
    a. Decreased FSH, LH
    b. Decreased testosterone
    c. Decreased prolactin
    d. Oligospermia

301. Which is the most common tumour of pituitary?
    a. Non-functioning adenoma (Recent Question 2016-17)
    b. Prolactinoma
    c. ACTH producing adenoma
    d. Oncocytoma

302. Which is the most common cell involved in non-functioning pituitary adenoma? (Recent Question 2016-17)
    a. Gonadotropin producing cell
    b. Prolactin producing cell
    c. GH producing cell
    d. TSH producing cell

303. Level of which hormone is likely to increase after hypothalamic ablation? (UPSC 2015)
    a. Growth hormone
    b. Prolactin
    c. FSH
    d. ACTH

304. For galactorrhea and amenorrhea syndromes, additional investigation apart from serum prolactin? (AIIMS May 2015)
    a. TSH
    b. LH
    c. Urinary Ketosteroids
    d. HCG

305. Laron dwarfism is due to? (Recent Pattern 2015-16)
    a. GH deficiency
    b. GHRH deficiency
    c. GH receptor resistance
    d. IGF-1 deficiency

306. Dilutional hyponatremia is seen in? (Recent Pattern 2014-15)
    a. Addison's disease
    b. Vincristine
    c. Diuretic therapy
    d. Craniopharyngioma

307. All of the following are true about SIADH except? (AIIMS Nov 2011)
    a. Vaptans are approved by FDA for its treatment
    b. Water-loading test can be used for diagnosis of the condition
    c. Urine sodium is usually normal in these patients
    d. Serum sodium may be as low as 125 mEq/L in these patients

308. All are true regarding ADH action except?
    a. Postoperative secretion is more (Recent Pattern 2014-15)
    b. ADH secretion occurs when plasma osmolality is low
    c. Acts on DCT
    d. Neuro-secretion

309. Which is NOT a side effect of GH administration?
    a. Gynecomastia (Recent Pattern 2014-15)
    b. Hypoglycemia
    c. Slipped capital femoral epiphysis
    d. Pseudotumor cerebri

310. Most common functioning tumour of pituitary is: (Recent Pattern 2014-15)
    a. Prolactinoma
    b. GH secreting adenoma
    c. ACTH secreting adenoma
    d. TSH secreting adenoma

311. Which of the following is under anterior pituitary control?
    a. Fluid and electrolyte balance (Recent Pattern 2014-15)
    b. Control of blood pressure
    c. Muscle activity
    d. Gonad function

312. All of the following causes hyperprolactinemia except: (Recent Pattern 2014-15)
    a. Methyldopa
    b. Phenothiazines
    c. Bromcriptine
    d. Metoclopramide

313. First drug to be started in Sheehan's syndrome is? (Recent Pattern 2014-15)
    a. Gonadotropins
    b. Oestrogen
    c. Thyroxine
    d. Corticosteroids

314. Investigation to be done for hyperprolactinaemia?
    a. Estradiol estimation (Recent Pattern 2014-15)
    b. LH estimation
    c. Diabetic status
    d. Thyroid status

315. Which is the first hormone to fall in the blood in Sheehan syndrome: (Recent Pattern 2014-15)
    a. GH
    b. ACTH
    c. prolactin
    d. TSH

316. Prolactinoma presents with: (Recent Pattern 2014-15)
    a. Inferior quadrantopia
    b. Superior quadrantopia
    c. Priapism
    d. Failure of lactation

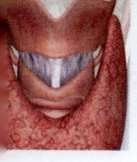

317. All are true regarding cranio-pharyngioma except:
    a. Derived from Rathke's pouch (Recent Pattern 2014-15)
    b. Contains epithelial cells
    c. Present in temporal or parietal lobes
    d. Causes visual disturbances
318. Acromegaly is characterized by all except: (AIPG 2011)
    a. Diabetes
    b. Muscular hypertrophy
    c. Enlarged nasal sinuses
    d. Increased heel pad thickness
319. The following are recognized features of panhypopituitarism except: (Recent Pattern 2014-15)
    a. Increased insulin sensitivity
    b. Pigmentation of the mucous membranes
    c. Low serum thyroxine and TSH levels
    d. Loss of secondary sex characters
320. Consider the following statements about acromegaly
    i. Impaired glucose tolerance (Recent Pattern 2014-15)
    ii. Galactorrhoea
    iii. Hypertension
    iv. Suppression of growth hormone with glucose
    Which of these statements are correct?
    a. i, ii & iv   b. ii, iii & iv
    c. i, iii & iv   d. i, ii & iii
321. All of the following are features of acromegaly except?
    a. Glucose intolerance (Recent Pattern 2014-15)
    b. Non-suppression of growth hormone by glucose ingestion
    c. Raised level of plasma somatomedin C
    d. Low serum phosphate
322. Paradoxical growth hormone response to TRH is seen in all except? (AIPG 2010)
    a. Malnutrition   b. Anorexia nervosa
    c. Prolactinoma   d. Acromegaly
323. A young woman comes with secondary amenorrhoea and galactorrhoea. MRI shows a tumor of < 10 mm diameter in the pituitary fossa. Treatment is: (Recent Pattern 2014-15)
    a. Hormonal therapy for withdrawal bleeding
    b. Chemotherapy
    c. Bromocriptine
    d. Surgery
324. A 33-year-old lady presented with polydipsia and polyuria. Her symptoms started soon after a road traffic accident 6 months ago. The blood pressure is 120/80 mmHg with no postural drop. The daily urinary output is 6-8 liter. Investigation showed Na = 130 mEq/L, K = 3.5 mEq/L urea = 15 mg/dl, sugar = 65 mg/dl the plasma osmolality = is 268 mosm/L and urine osmolality = 45 mosm/L. The most likely diagnosis is? (AIIMS Nov 2010)
    a. Central diabetes insipidus
    b. Nephrogenic diabetes insipidus
    c. Resolving acute tubular necrosis
    d. Psychogenic polydipsia
325. Consider the following statements: (Recent Pattern 2014-15)
    In nephrogenic diabetes insipidus the patient is likely to have:
    i. High vasopressin level
    ii. Poor or no response to desmopressin
    iii. High plasma osmolality.
    iv. Dilutional hyponatremia
    Which of these statements are correct?
    a. i, ii and iii   b. ii, iii and iv
    c. i and iv   d. i, ii, iii and iv
326. Polyuria with low fixed specific gravity urine is seen in?
    a. Diabetes mellitus (Recent Pattern 2014-15)
    b. Diabetes insipidus
    c. Chronic glomerulonephritis
    d. Potomania
327. Urine osmolality in diabetes insipidus is: (Recent Pattern 2014-15)
    a. <150 mOsm/L   b. <300 mOsm/L
    c. 600 mOsm/L   d. 900 mOsm/L
328. True about SIADH is all except: (Recent Pattern 2014-15)
    a. Hyponatraemia   b. Urine hyposmolar
    c. Increased ADH   d. Adequate hydration status
329. Central diabetes insipidus is characterized by: (Recent Pattern 2014-15)
    a. Low plasma and low urine osmolality
    b. High plasma and high urine osmolality
    c. Low plasma and high urine osmolality
    d. Low urine and high plasma osmolality
330. Syndrome of Inappropriate secretion of Anti-Diuretic hormone (SIADH) may be seen in the following except:
    a. Use of vincristine (Recent Pattern 2014-15)
    b. Oat cell carcinoma of lung
    c. Porphyria-acute attack
    d. Primary pulmonary emphysema
331. Pituitary diabetes insipidus is improved by: (Recent Pattern 2014-15)
    a. Water restriction   b. Lithium
    c. Chlorpropamide   d. Chlorthiazide
332. The syndrome of inappropriate ADH secretion is characterized by the following: (Recent Pattern 2014-15)
    a. Hyponatremia and urine sodium excretion > 20 mEq/L
    b. Hypernatremia and urine sodium excretion > 20 mEq/L
    c. Hyponatremia and hyperkalemia
    d. Hypernatremia and hyperkalemia
333. A 32-year-old female patient did not visit the physician for the last 6 year when she had given birth to her last daughter, which was her third child. She has currently come with complaints of vaginal pruritus. She also has history of cold intolerance and repeated skin infections. On examination, the skin is dry and coarse. The pubic and axillary hair is absent. All the following can be given for her treatment except: (AIPG 2010)
    a. Prednisolone   b. Thyroid hormone
    c. Ethinyl estradiol d. Insulin
334. Inappropriate ADH secretion is seen in all except: (Recent Pattern 2014-15)
    a. Head injury   b. Oat Cell carcinoma of Lung
    c. Acute encephalitis d. Chromophobe adenoma
335. All are causes of hyperprolactinemia, except (AIIMS May 94)
    a. Bromocriptine   b. Phenothiazine
    c. Methyldopa   d. Metoclopramide
336. All of the following are known to cause hyperprolactenemia except: (AI 1997)
    a. Methyldopa   b. Phenothiazines
    d. Bromocriptine   d. Metoclopramide

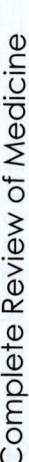

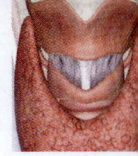

337. **Imaging of choice of hyper-prolactinemia:**
    (AIIMS Nov 93)
    a. TRH estimation   b. LH estimation
    c. Prolactin estimation   d. Estradiol estimation

338. **A 30 year old woman presented with secondary amenorrhoea for 3 years along with galactorrhoea. The most likely cause of her symptoms would be:** (AI 2004)
    a. Craniopharyngioma
    b. Prolactinoma
    c. Meningioma
    d. Sub-arachnoid haemorrhage

339. **Paradoxical response of GH release to TRH is seen in:**
    a. Prolactinoma   b. Acromegaly (AIIMS Dec 98)
    c. Malnutrition   d. Pituitary adenoma

340. **A combination of gynaecomastia, decreased serum testosterone and LH in a male patient is seen in:** (AIIMS Dec 97)
    a. Testicular failure   b. Sertoli cell tumor
    c. Gonadotrophins   d. Androgen resistant state

341. **The diagnosis of a patient presenting with familial Polyostosis, Precocious puberty and Pigmentation is:** (AI 1995)
    a. Tuberous sclerosis
    b. McCune Albright syndrome
    c. Klinefelter syndrome
    d. SLE

342. **Normal height with absent pubertal features?**
    a. Kallman syndrome   (AIIMS Nov 14)
    b. Pure gonadal dysgenesis
    c. Testicular feminising syndrome
    d. Turner syndrome

343. **Not a Cause of Gynaecomastia?** (Recent Pattern 2015-16)
    a. Hypothyroidism   b. Kallman
    c. Obesity   d. Klinefelter syndrome

344. **A patient has amenorrhea with hypothalamic lesion. The diagnosis is most likely to be?** (Recent Pattern 2014-15)
    a. Kallman's syndrome   b. Asherman's syndrome
    c. Stein Leventhal syndrome   d. Sheehans syndrome

345. **Gonadectomy is advised in:** (Recent Pattern 2014-15)
    a. Kallman's syndrome
    b. Testicular feminization syndrome
    c. Hemochromatosis
    d. Sexual precocity

Miscellaneous

346. **A 2-year-old child presents with precocious puberty. MRI shows a suprasellar mass attached to the mammillary body with a stalk. What is the diagnosis?** (Recent Questions 2016-17)
    a. Hypothalamic hamartoma
    b. Craniopharyngioma
    c. Pituitary adenoma
    d. Kallman syndrome

347. **Which of the following hormones are raised in Prader-Willi syndrome?** (Bihar Pg 2015)
    a. Growth Hormone (GH)
    b. Luteinizing Hormone (LH)
    c. Follicle Stimulating Hormone
    d. Ghrelin

348. **Which of the following drugs does not cause edema?**
    (UPSC 2015)
    a. Growth hormone   b. Beta blocker
    c. Anabolic steroids   d. Calcium-channel blockers

349. **Test to differentiate between anaphylaxis with anaphylactoid reaction?** (JIPMER Nov 2015)
    a. Serum Trytpase and C3a, C5a levels
    b. Urinary histamine and C3a, C5a levels
    c. Basophil count and C3 and C4 levels
    d. C3a, C5a levels and Absolute Basophil count

350. **In prolactinoma most common symptom other than galactorrhea is?** (Recent Questions 2015-16)
    a. Bitemporal hemianopia   b. Amennorhea
    c. Thyroid dysfunction   d. Headache

351. **Rib notching is found in all the following except:**
    (Recent Questions 2015-16)
    a. Neurofibromatosis   b. Coarctation of aorta
    c. Taussig bing operation   d. Hypoparathyroidism

352. **Obesity in children is seen in:** (Recent Questions 2015-16)
    a. Adrenal insufficiency
    b. Pseudo-hypo-parathyroidism
    c. Prader willi syndrome
    d. Soto syndrome

353. **True about obesity?** (Recent Questions 2015-16)
    a. Seen mostly in females
    b. Prevalence decrease upto 40 years of age
    c. No genetic predisposition
    d. Smoking is a risk factor

354. **Whipple's triad is useful for diagnosis of:**
    (Recent Questions 2015-16)
    a. Insulinoma   b. Glucagonoma
    c. Somatostatinoma   d. V.I.Poma

355. **Secretory diarrhea is caused by all except?**
    (Recent Questions 2015-16)
    a. Medullary thyroid tumor   b. Carcinoid Tumor
    c. Somatostinoma   d. Glucagonoma

356. **Which of the following is incorrect about this patient?**

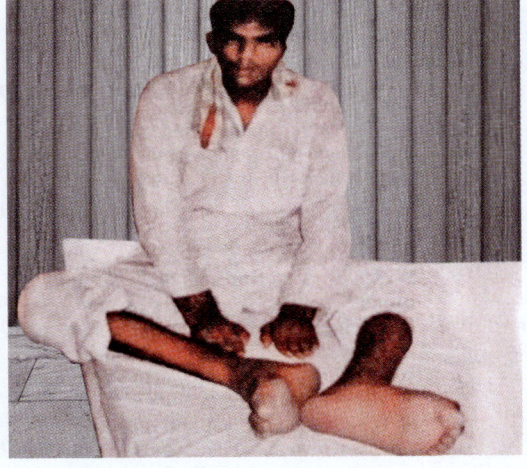

    a. Pegvisomant is used
    b. Homonymous hemianopia
    c. Acral enlargement
    d. Glucose tolerance test

357. **True about obesity?** *(Recent Pattern 2015-16)*
    a. Seen mostly in females
    b. Prevalence decrease upto 40 years of age
    c. No genetic predisposition
    d. Smoking is a risk factor

358. **An obese lady with BMI = 35. FBG is normal and PPBG is slightly elevated. Ideal management is?** *(JIPMER 2014)*
    a. Exercise   b. Insulin
    c. Metformin   d. Diet control

359. **Purtschner's retinopathy is seen in all except:** *(Recent Pattern 2014-15)*
    a. Fat embolism
    b. Pancreatitis
    c. Chest trauma
    d. Unilateral carotid artery occlusion

360. **Which is not seen in Allgrove syndrome:** *(Recent Pattern 2014-15)*
    a. ACTH excess leading to Cushing syndrome
    b. Achalasia
    c. Alacrimia
    d. Hyperpigmentation

361. **Prader-Willi syndrome is associated with an increase in which of the following hormones:** *(Recent Pattern 2014-15)*
    a. Ghrelin   b. GH
    c. FSH   d. LH

362. **Pinna calcification is seen in all except?** *(AIIMS Nov 2012)*
    a. Gout   b. Onchrnosis
    c. Frost bite   d. Addisons disease

363. **Age related deterioration of cognitive function is due to increase in following:** *(AIPG 2012)*
    a. Homocystiene   b. Cystiene
    c. Taurine   d. Methionine

364. **The most common presentation of cranio-pharyngioma:** *(Recent Pattern 2014-15)*
    a. Headache
    b. Visual field defects
    c. Endocrinal disturbance
    d. Cardiac disturbance

365. **Bony clival erosion with intra-cranial calcification is seen in:** *(Recent Pattern 2014-15)*
    a. Craniopharyngioma   b. Medulloblastoma
    c. Papilloma of the choroid plexus
    d. Sella chordoma

366. **Levodopa test is used to detect:** *(Recent Pattern 2014-15)*
    a. LH   b. ACTH
    c. FSH   d. GH reserve

367. **Adrenal reserve is best tested by means of infusion with:** *(Recent Pattern 2014-15)*
    a. Glucocorticoids   b. ACTH
    c. Hypothyroidism   d. Metyrapone

368. **A short stature patient with narrowed foramen magnum and rhizomelic limbs is seen in?** *(Recent Pattern 2014-15)*
    a. Achondroplasia   b. Laron dwarf
    c. Hypothyroidism   d. Morquio disease

369. **All are features of primary hemochromatosis except:** *(Recent Pattern 2014-15)*
    a. Chorea   b. Diabetes
    c. Arthritis   d. Skin pigmentation

370. **Clinical features of pancreatic cholera A/E:** *(AIPG 2010)*
    a. Hypokalemia   b. Achlorhydria
    c. Hypocalcemia   d. Glucose intolerance

371. **In Hemochromatosis iron deposition is found commonly at all sites except:** *(Recent Pattern 2014-15)*
    a. Heart   b. Joints
    c. Testes   d. Pancreas

372. **All the following statements about Wilson's disease are true except:** *(Recent Pattern 2014-15)*
    a. It is an autosomal recessive disorder
    b. Serum ceruloplasmin level is < 20 mcg/dl
    c. Urinary copper excretion is < 100 mcg/day
    d. Zinc acetate is effective as maintenance therapy

373. **Which of these is not an antihypertensive medication:** *(Recent Pattern 2014-15)*
    a. Clinidipine   b. Chlorthalidone
    c. Canagliflozin   d. Captopril

374. **Drug of choice for an attack of periodic paralysis with calcium channel defect is:** *(Recent Pattern 2014-15)*
    a. ACTH   b. Potassium chloride
    c. Calcium chloride d. Adrenaline

375. **Dancing carotid sign is seen in:** *(Recent Pattern 2014-15)*
    a. Thyrotoxicosis
    b. Papillary Ca
    c. Follicular Ca
    d. Hashimoto's disease

376. **Hypoglycemia is seen in** *(AIIMS May 01)*
    a. Acromegaly   b. Cushing's syndrome
    c. Hyperthyroidism   d. Hypopituitarism

377. **Hypoglycemia is a recognized feature of all of the following conditions, except:** *(AI 2002)*
    a. Uremia   b. Acromegaly
    c. Addison's disease d. Hepatocellular failure

378. **The triad originally described by Zollinger Ellison syndrome is characterized by:** *(AI 2002)*
    a. Peptic ulceration, gastric hypersecretion, non beta cell tumour
    b. Peptic ulceration, gastric hypersecretion, beta cell tumour
    c. Peptic ulceration, achlorhydria, non beta cell tumour
    d. Peptic ulceration, achlorhydria, beta cell tumour

379. **Carcinoid tumour is most common in** *(AIIMS May 04)*
    a. Esophagus   b. Stomach
    c. Jejunum   d. Appendix

380. **Carcinoid syndrome produces valvular disease primarily of the** *(AIIMS May 04)*
    a. Venous valves   b. Tricuspid valve
    c. Mitral valve   d. Aortic valve

381. **A male child with coarse facies, macroglossia, thick lips with hepatosplenomegaly presents with copious mucus discharge from nose. Probable underlying diagnosis is?**
    a. Hurler Disease   *(AIIMS May 2015)*
    b. Beckwith Wiedemann Syndrome
    c. Proteus Syndrome
    d. Hypothyroidism

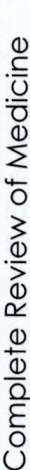

Answers with Explanations

Diabetes Mellitus & Insulinoma

1. Ans. (a) Acanthosis nigricans

Ref: Fitzpatrick Colour Atlas and synopsis of clinical dermatology, page 88

- The image shows presence of *asymmetric, velvety hyperpigmentation* at the back of the neck of the patient suggestive of diagnosis of acanthosis nigricans. It is seen in patients with impaired glucose tolerance and internal malignancy.
- Choice B is seen in patients with internal malignancy and but has multiple pigmented skin lesions.
- Choice C is a is a crusty, scaly growth caused by damage from exposure to ultraviolet (UV) radiation.
- Choice D has red inflamed lesions and is hence ruled out.

2. Ans. (c) Canagliflozin

Ref: Harrison 20th p 2867-68

- Sitagliptin is ruled out as DPP-4 inhibitors are associated with risk of pancreatitis
- Liraglutide is ruled out since it is available in injectable format and patient has refused to take injections.
- Pioglitazone has black box warning due to risk of bladder cancer.
- Canagliflozin will be the most suitable for the patient since it will help in reducing the weight of the patient as well.

3. Ans. (c) Metformin

Ref: Harrison 20th p 2865; Page 2413, Harrison 19th edition and Good man & Gillman 12 edition, pg. no. 1259

- Metformin should be discontinued in following settings in diabetics and insulin is used:
  1. Hospitalized patients
  2. Can't take orally
  3. Receiving Radiographic contrast material
- Metformin is excreted via the kidney and is contraindicated if GFR< 60ml/min/1.73 m2 BSA, level of serum creatinine is >1.4mg/dl in women and >1.5mg/dl in men.
- If metformin is erroneously prescribed, it would result in development of lactic acidosis in the patient.

4. Ans. (a) Immune mediated type 1

Ref: CMDT 2019 p 1220

Types of diabetes mellitus

Type 1 A	Immune mediated Diabetes mellitus (insulinopenia)
Type 1 B	Idiopathic mediated diabetes mellitus (insulinopenia)
Type 2	Due to insulin resistance
MODY	Maturity Onset Diabetes in Young
LADA	Latent Autoimmune Diabetes in Adults
MIDD	Maternally Inherited Diabetes and Deafness
Wolfram syndrome	Diabetes insipidus, diabetes mellitus, optic atrophy and deafness

5. Ans. (c) Type 1 diabetes mellitus

Ref: CMDT 2019 page 1221

Autoimmune markers for newly diagnosed type 1 diabetes mellitus

1. ICA antibody
2. Glutamic Acid Decarboxylase (GAD65)
3. Insulin islet cell antibody
4. Tyrosine phosphatase
5. Zinc transporter 8

6. Ans. (d) MODY5

Ref: CMDT 2019 page 1221

- HNF- 1β gene is involved in pathogenesis of MODY5.
- HNF- 1α gene is involved in pathogenesis of MODY 3.
- Most common type of MODY is MODY 3.

7. Ans. (a) MODY

Ref: CMDT 2019 page 1222

- Type 1 diabetes has insulinopenia due to reduced β cell mass
- Latent autoimmune diabetes in adults is a variant of type 1 diabetes mellitus
- MODY has impaired glucose induced insulin release due to autosomal dominant pattern of inheritance. The beta cell mass is normal. It involves mutations in nuclear transcription factor that regulates islet gene expression.
- Wolfram syndrome is an autosomal recessive condition neurodegenerative disorder leading to diabetes mellitus, diabetes insipidus, optic atrophy and deafness.

8. Ans. (d) Sarcoma

Ref: CMDT 2019, Table 27.3, page 1223

- In cirrhosis, blood sugar is elevated, due to reduced uptake of sugar by liver
- In myotonic dystrophy and lipodystrophy, there is tissue insensitivity to insulin leading to hyperglycemia.
- Sarcoma especially large retroperitoneal sarcomas secrete IGF-2 and lead to hypoglycaemia.

9. Ans. (d) Splenectomy

Ref: CMDT 2019 page 1225

HbA1C values are affected by conditions that affect RBC survival or mean erythrocyte age.

Falsely low HbA1C	Falsely elevated HbA1C
Recovery from acute blood loss Haemolytic anaemia IV iron EPO injections for CKD Vitamin C supplements Vitamin E supplements	Splenectomy Iron deficiency Anaemia

10. Ans. (a) Elevated uric acid; (b) Dense LDL; (c) Reduced HDL

Ref: CMDT 2019 page 1223

Syndrome X / metabolic syndrome is characterised by

1. Elevated BP
2. Impaired glucose tolerance
3. Dysbetalipoproteinemia
   a. Dense LDL which is highly atherogenic, though LDL may be normal
   b. Reduced HDL
   c. Elevated plasma triglycerides
4. Increased uric acid
5. Increased levels of plasminogen activator inhibitor type1 (pro-inflammatory state).

11. Ans. (b) Serum fructosamine

Ref: CMDT 2019 page 1226

- The patient is already diabetic at the time of conception. Since organogenesis occurs in first trimester, it is imperative to achieve good sugar control in T1. Hence serum fructosamine is recommended, because it accurately describes glycaemic control retrospectively for previous 1-2 weeks.
- Glycosylated haemoglobin gives information about retrospective control of diabetes mellitus for previous 8-12 weeks and is not suitable in the case given in the question.

12. Ans. (b) Serum fructosamine

Ref: CMDT 2019; page 1226

- Serum fructosamine is formed due to non-enzymatic glycosylation of serum proteins mainly albumin.
- It represents glycemic control for preceding 1-2 weeks.
- Normal values are 200-285mcmol/L

Advantages of serum fructosamine are:

1. Useful in Haemolytic states which affect interpretation of glycosylated haemoglobin.
2. Evaluation of glycemic control at the time of conception in a woman with pre-existing diabetes mellitus.

13. Ans. (d) Exercise

Ref: CMDT 2019; page 1225

- During exercise the muscles will consume sugar; hence sugar levels can be normal in a diabetic patient.
- However in malnourished patients, bedridden, infection state and severe emotional stress false positive OGTT is seen. It can be explained by catecholamine surge and release of counter-regulatory hormones.

14. Ans. (c) 70

Ref: CMDT 2019; page 1229

- High Glycemic index foods have values of 70 or greater and include baked potato, white bread and white rice.
- Low Glycemic index foods have values of 55 or lesser and include multi grain breads, pasta, legumes.

15. Ans. (a) Glyburide

Ref: CMDT 2019; page 1232

- Sulfonylureas act on receptors in pancreatic beta cells resulting in closure of potassium cells. This results in depolarization of Beta cell and release of insulin
- Glyburide has the highest affinity/ insulinotropic action while tolbutamide has least affinity.

16. Ans. (a) Glyburide

Ref: CMDT 2019; page 1232

- Glyburide should not be used in patients with liver disease and CKD due to risk of hypoglycaemia.
- Glipizide, Gliclazide and Glimepiride are metabolised by liver and hence can be used in patients with CKD.

17. Ans. (a) Hypoglycemia

Ref: CMDT 2019; page 1233

- Thiazolidinediones are contraindicated in patients with Cardiac status NYHA grade III and IV due to propensity cause fluid retention.
- Increased fracture risk is mentioned in women in both pre and post-menopausal women.
- Troglitazone the first medication from this class of drugs was withdrawn due to fatal liver failure.
- Like biguanides, Thiazolidinediones do not cause hypoglycaemia.

18. Ans. (a) Exenatide

Ref: CMDT 2019; page 1235

All GLP-1 receptor agonists are associated with increased risk of pancreatitis. Exenatide is documented to cause haemorrhagic/necrotising pancreatitis.

19. Ans. (c) Albiglutide

Ref: CMDT 2019; page 1235

GLP-1 Receptor agonists: exenatide, albiglutide, dulaglutide are available as once weekly administration by subcutaneous route. Liraglutide needs to be given once per day.

20. Ans. (d) 3% saline

Ref: CMDT 2019; page 1255

- A patient of type 1 Diabetes mellitus is on Continuous subcutaneous insulin infusion. Due to device malfunction/ tubing malfunction the delivery of insulin was halted.
- Since patients of type 1 diabetes are ketosis prone, she has gone into Diabetic ketoacidosis. The low bicarbonate points to acidosis.
- The patient's elevated blood sugar is drawing water into the intravascular compartment and hence volume expansion explains the sodium deficit. However there is no need of hypertonic saline as *correction of hyperglycemia by insulin shall suffice in managing sodium values.*
- Hypertonic saline is only given in acute onset hyponatremia with neurological features.
- *If severe hypophosphatemia can develop (<1mg/dl), phosphate should be replaced at no more than 3-4mmol/h via infusion.*
- *Potassium replacement should be started in 2nd to 3rd hour as acidosis begins to resolve.*

21. Ans. (b) Degludec

Ref: CMDT 2019; page 1238

Long acting insulin have onset of action after 30 minutes of administration and do not exhibit a peak action unlike other forms of insulin.

They are designed to provide constant values in blood for the entire day.

Insulin type	Onset of action	Peak action	Effective duration
Glargine	0.5-1 hr	Peakess/flat	24 hours
Detemir	0.5-1 hr	Peakless/flat	17 hours
Degludec	0.5-1 hr	Peakless/flat	42 hours

22. Ans. (d) DPP-4 inhibitors

Ref: CMDT 2019; page 1244

Effect of anti-diabetics on weight

- Metformin and DPP-4 inhibitors are weight neutral
- GLP-1 Agonists, SGLT2 inhibitors and Pramlintide promote weight loss
- Sulfonylureas, insulin and Pioglitazone are associated with weight gain

23. Ans. (b) Degludec

Ref: CMDT 2019; page 1240

Traditionally long acting insulins could not be mixed with short acting insulins due to different pH.

However insulin degludec preparation is now available as 70% insulin degludec and 30% insulin aspart and is injected once or twice per day.

24. Ans. (d) Molar ratio of insulin/C-peptide <1

Ref: CMDT 2019; page 1240

- Repeated injections of insulin at the same site can lead to lipo-hypertrophy.
- Excess injection can lead to blood sugar <50mg% and explains neuro-glucopenia.
- Excess bed time injection of long acting insulin will lead to 3am hypoglycaemia. This leads to release of counter-regulatory hormones and results in pre-breakfast hyperglycemia.
- *In case of exogenous insulin administration, the ratio of insulin/ C- peptide will be >1.0.*

25. Ans. (a) Kidney disease

(Ref: CMDT 2019; page 1247)

The most common cause of death in type 1 diabetes mellitus is end stage chronic kidney disease. In contrast in type 2 Diabetes mellitus macrovascular disease is more common leading to myocardial infarction and stroke.

26. Ans. (b) Myocardial disease

(Ref: CMDT 2019; page 1247)

The most common cause of death in type 1 diabetes mellitus is end stage chronic kidney disease. In contrast in type 2 Diabetes mellitus macrovascular disease is more common leading to myocardial infarction and stroke.

27. Ans. (a) Insulin

Ref: CMDT 2019; page 1240

The image shows an insulin pump which is appropriate for patients with type 1 diabetes who are motivated, mechanically inclined and educated about the disease.

The device shown is tubeless and delivers subcutaneous basal and bolus insulin from a wireless personal digital assistant.

Continuous subcutaneous insulin infusion pump

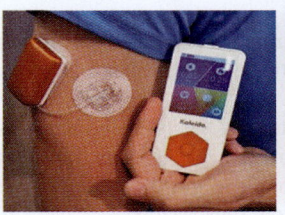 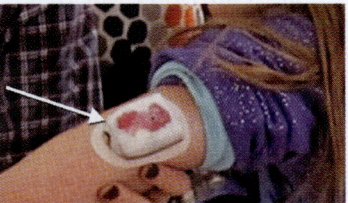

With catheter   No catheter

28. Ans. (b) Somogyi phenomenon

Ref: CMDT 2019; page 1243

- The patient is having 3am hypoglycaemia which is probably due to excess bed time insulin dose. This is triggering release of counter-regulatory hormones, resulting in pre-breakfast hyperglycemia. This is called as Somogyi phenomenon.
- It can be treated by giving lower dose of intermediate insulin at dinner time or more food at dinner time.
- Dawn phenomenon is due to reduced tissue sensitivity to insulin between 5am to 8am.

29. Ans. (a) Dawn phenomenon

Ref: CMDT 2019; page 1243

- There is reduced tissue sensitivity to insulin between 5 am to 8 am which leads to Pre-breakfast Hyperglycemia and is known as Dawn Phenomenon.
- Dawn phenomenon is found in 75% of Type 1 diabetes mellitus patients and can aggravate the hyperglycemia.

Pre-breakfast Hyperglycemia: Classification by Blood Glucose

	10PM	3AM	7AM
Somogyi effect	110mg%	40mg%	200mg%
Dawn Phenomenon	110mg%	110mg%	200mg%
Waning of insulin dose plus dawn phenomenon	110mg%	190mg%	220mg%

30. Ans. (a) Strict BP control

Ref: CMDT 2019; page 1245

The UKPDS (United Kingdom Prospective Diabetes Study group) regarding prevention of microvascular and macrovascular complications demonstrated that BP control is more significant than glycemic control in patients with type 2 Diabetes mellitus.

31. Ans. (a) Neuropathy

Ref: CMDT 2019; page 1248

- The most common complication in type 2 diabetes mellitus is neuropathy affecting 50% of patients.
- Distal symmetric polyneuropathy leading to loss of function in stocking glove pattern is the leading presentation of diabetic neuropathy.

32. Ans. (a) Semmes Weinstein filament test

Ref: CMDT 2019; page 1248

The image shows Semmes Weinstein filament test, which is performed to evaluate for diabetic neuropathy. It is a low cost, easy to apply, rapid test.

This assessment tool consists of a set of monofilaments that vary in thickness and diameter, the gradient forces of these monofilaments ranges from .086 gm to 448gm. These monofilaments are used to map out sensory loss.

Light touch	
• 10 g Semmes-Weinstein monofilament	• 2 × medial longitudinal arch
• Podiatrist test 10 sites	• Plantar heel
▪ Apex 1/3/5 toes	• Dorsum of foot
▪ Plantar MTPJ's of 1/3/5	

33. Ans. (c) Microalbuminuria correlates with nocturnal spike in Systolic blood pressure

Ref: CMDT 2019; page 1248

- Sensitive radioimmunoassay methods measure small amounts of urinary albumin in contrast to less sensitive dipstick strips. Hence choice A is wrong
- 24 hour urine albumin values are affected by exercise, dietary protein and sustained erect posture. This problem is circumvented with spot sample urine albumin to urine creatinine values. Hence choice B is wrong
- Most common cause of death in type 2 diabetes mellitus is myocardial infarction. Hence choice D is wrong.
- Microalbuminuria has been shown to correlate with elevated nocturnal blood pressure in diabetics. This can explain benefits of ACE inhibitors in reducing microalbuminuria.

34. Ans. (a) Pain in front of thigh

Ref: CMDT 2019; page 1249

Diabetic amyotrophy presents with severe pain in front of thigh. Subsequently weakness and wasting of quadriceps develops. Management involves analgesia and improved diabetes control. The symptoms improve over 6-18months.

35. Ans. (a) Dorsum of hands

Ref: Page 1252: Goodman and Gilman: 12th edition

The preferred sites for insulin administration are:
1. Abdomen
2. Anterolateral aspect of thigh
3. Dorsal Arm

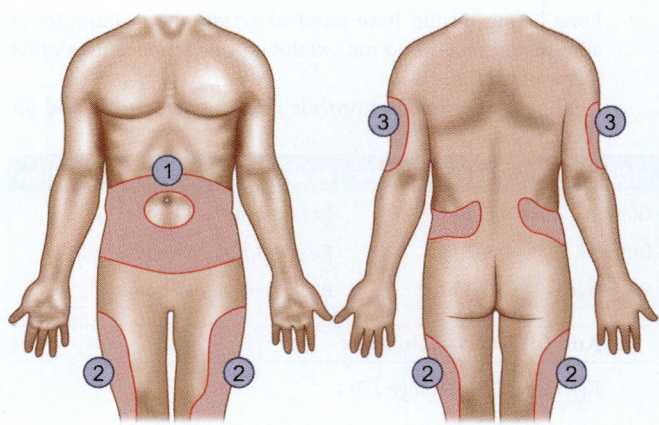

The route of administration is subcutaneous and abdominal wall has substantial subcutaneous fat. The site of injection can be rotated to prevent local site scarring. The rate of absorption from abdominal wall is fastest.

36. Ans. (c) Linagliptin

Ref: Page 2413 and table 418-5 page 2414: Harrison 19th edition

- Metformin is excreted via the kidney and hence urine MICRAL (Microalbuminuria) test and KFT should be done to estimate GFR of the kidney.
- Failure to perform these tests can result in accumulation of metformin and development of metabolic acidosis.
- Both Sitagliptin and Canagliflozin (SGLT-2 inhibitor acting on PCT) are metabolised by the kidney.
- Linagliptin has non-linear pharmacokinetics and unlike other DPP-4 inhibitors, has a largely non-renal excretion route. It is excreted unchanged in the faeces and urine. The effective half-life is 12 hours.

37. Ans. (a) Lumbar puncture

(Ref: Reference: Page 443e-6: Harrison 19th edition)

- Random blood sugar will help in evaluation of Non-ketotic Hyperosmolar coma versus hypoglycaemia as the cause of unconsciousness.
- Diabetics have accelerated atherosclerosis and NCCT will help in ruling out possibility of stroke
- ECG will help in evaluation of current status of atrial fibrillation as it can lead to embolic stroke. Hence, if required, rhythm control will be initiated.
- Lumbar puncture is contraindicated in patients with bleeding diathesis/novel anticoagulants. The most common site of bleeding after lumbar puncture in patients on anticoagulants is epidural space. This leads to neurological complications with very poor response to surgery.
- Moreover even if we are suspecting SAH, NCCT is the first investigation.

38. Ans. (c) Linagliptin

(Ref: Harrison 20th p 2866; Page 2413 and table 418-5 page 2414: Harrison 19th edition)

- Metformin is excreted via the kidney and hence urine MICRAL (Microalbuminuria) test and KFT should be done

to estimate GFR of the kidney. Failure to perform these tests can result in accumulation of metformin and development of metabolic acidosis.
- Both Sitagliptin and Canagliflozin (SGLT2 inhibitor acting on PCT) are metabolised by the kidney.
- Linagliptin has non-linear pharmacokinetics and, unlike other DPP-4 inhibitors, has a largely non-renal excretion route. It is excreted unchanged in the feces and urine. The effective half-life is 12 hours.

Diabetes with recurrent UTI	The gliflozins act by increasing urinary loss of sugar by blocking SGLT2. Hence they can increase urinary loss of sugar and promote development of UTI
Diabetic nephropathy with C.K.D	Glibenclamide is contraindicated in renal failure, hepatic dysfunction, pregnancy and diabetic ketoacidosis
Diabetes with heart failure	Thiazolidinediones cause fluid retention and oedema and are contraindicated in patients with NYHA grade III-IV.

39. Ans. (a) CTLA-4 Gene

(Ref: Harrison 20th p 2855; Harrison: 19th edition, Page 2403)

- Polymorphism in promoter region of insulin gene, CTLA-4 contributes to susceptibility to type 1 Diabetes mellitus.
- The most common cause of type 1 diabetes mellitus is autoimmunity. Most patients have DR3 and/ or DR4 haplotype
- Haplotype DQA1*0301 is strongly associated with type 1 DM.
- Concordance of type 1 DM in identical twins is 40-60%
- Chances of type 1 DM if single parent has type 1 DM is only 3-4%

40. Ans. (b) Type 2

(Ref: Harrison 20th p 2857; Harrison 19th edition, Page 2402)

The pancreatic beta cells secrete Islet amyloid polypeptide or amylin. It is found to be major component of *amyloid fibrils* found in islets of patients suffering from type 2 diabetes mellitus.

41. Ans. (d) Type B lactic acidosis due to linezolid

(Ref: Harrison 20th p 318; Harrison 19th edition, Page number 318)

The case given is of high anion gap metabolic acidosis with increased serum lactate and negative ketones. This rules out choice B and C

Lactic acidosis of type A variety occurs due to poor tissue perfusion and occurs due to
1. Shock or cardiac failure
2. Severe Anaemia
3. Mitochondrial enzyme defects
4. Carbon monoxide poisoning, Cyanide poisoning

Lactic acidosis of type B occurs due to
1. Malignancies
2. Diabetes mellitus
3. Renal or hepatic failure
4. Thiamine deficiency
5. Severe Infections (Cholera, Malaria)
6. Seizures
7. Drugs/toxins (biguanides, ethanol, methanol, propylene glycol, isoniazid, and fructose and Nucleoside analogue reverse transcriptase inhibitors in HIV and linezolid)

42. Ans. (a) PQR = YXW

(Ref: Harrison 20th p 2866)

43. Ans. (d) Airway, CT scan, Blood Sugar if <70 start dextrose

(Ref: Basic life support: Harrison 19th edition, Page 1768)

- For any trauma patient or any emergency, Airway is to be secured 1st.
- CT scan to rule out Intracranial bleed
- A diabetic patient found unconscious, always rule out hypoglycaemia

44. Ans. (a) Cerebral edema

(Ref: Harrison 20th p 2873; Harrison 19th Edition, Page 2431, 35)

- Prolonged hypoglycemia can damage the blood brain barrier and leads to cerebral edema.
- This also explains hemiplegia seen in hypoglycemic patients sometimes.
- Post ictal state is seen after hypoglycemic seizures.

45. Ans. (b) A, B and D

(Ref: Harrison 20th p 2851; Harrison 19th edition, page 2399-2400)

Endocrinopathies Leading to Diabetes	Diseases of the Exocrine Pancreas
1. Acromegaly	1. Pancreatitis
2. Cushing's	2. Pancreatectomy
3. Glucagonoma	3. Neoplasia
4. Pheochromocytoma	4. Cystic fibrosis
5. Hyperthyroidism	5. Hemochromatosis
6. Somatostatinoma	6. Fibrocalculous pancreatopathy
7. Aldosteronoma	

46. Ans. (b) Portal vein

(Ref: Atlas of organ transplantation, Page: 135, 3rd edition)

Islet cell transplantation involves the extraction of islets of Langerhans from organ donors through a complex purification process. These are the cells responsible for the production of insulin. These cells are then injected into the recipient, usually into the portal vein. They then engraft into the parenchyma of the liver and secrete insulin.

47. Ans. (b) Insulinoma

(Ref: Harrison 20th p 2883; Harrison 19th edition, Page 2430)

Whipple's triad is based on three criteria on which hyper-insulinism is due to pancreatic islet-cell disease is diagnosed:

1. Neuromuscular signs with fasting or exercise
2. Low blood glucose levels associated with clinical signs
3. Reversal of clinical signs with the administration of glucose.

Whipple's operation: Carcinoma pancreas
Whipple's disease: Malabsorption caused by Trophyerma Whipelli

48. Ans. (b) Immediately

(Ref: Harrison 20th p 2877; Harrison 19th, page 2424)

- Since the age of the patient is 50 years, it is highly likely that the patient has type II diabetes mellitus, which is insidious in onset. Hence though patient has no ocular complaints the fundus examination for retina evaluation should be done immediately.
- The significance of this problem is highlighted by the finding that individuals with DM are 25 times more likely to become legally blind than individuals without DM.
- Blindness is primarily the result of progressive diabetic retinopathy and clinically significant macular edema.

49. Ans. (c) Glucokinase

(Ref: CMDT 2019; page 1221)

Genetic defects of pancreatic cell function

MODY 1	HNF 4 alpha
MODY 2	Glucokinase
MODY 3	HNF 1 alpha
MODY 4	PDX 1
MODY 5	HNF 1 beta
MODY 6	Neuro D1

50. Ans. (d) E.U.S (Endoscopic ultrasound)

(Ref: Harrison 20th p 2887; Harrison 19th ed. page 2434)

For PETs in the pancreas, EUS is highly sensitive, localizing 77–100% of insulinomas, which occur almost exclusively within the pancreas.

Tests for location of pNET:
1. Somatostatin Receptor Scintigraphy is the initial imaging modality but is less available.
2. Helical CT scan has a sensitivity of 80%
3. Gadolinium based MRI has sensitivity of 85%
4. If above scans are negative, then Endoscopic ultrasound will be able to pick up the insulinoma which is usually <1.5 cm in size, with 90% sensitivity
5. If all the above tests turn negative then calcium stimulated angiography can be used to localise the tumour.
6. The intra-arterial calcium test also allows differentiation of the cause of the hypoglycaemia and indicates whether it is due to an insulinoma or a nesidioblastosis.

51. Ans. (d) Serum Bicarbonate > 15 mmol/L

(Ref: Harrison 20th p 2871; Harrison 19th edition, Page 2418)

- In diabetic ketoacidosis, the elevated blood sugar due to osmotic diuresis leads to polyuria. The stimulation of osmoreceptors will lead to increased thirst.
- DKA can lead to early presentation of type 1 DM but more frequently occurs in patients with pre-existing diabetes.
- In DKA serum ketones are present and detectable at dilutions of 1:8. Urine dipstick using sodium nitroprusside can help in detection but plasma beta hydroxybutyrate is preferred.
- Serum bicarbonate levels in DKA are <10mmol/L.

52. Ans. (c) Contain Haemoglobin with sugar moiety

(Ref: Harrison 20th p 2862; Harrison 19th edition, Page 2401)

- Glycosylated haemoglobin is not a reliable test in patients with hemoglobinopathies like thalassemia and sickle cell anemia.
- It is an excellent test indicating poor glycemic control in diabetics and higher values are associated with microvascular complications.
- It is a retrospective test indicating glycemic control for 8-12 weeks

53. Ans. (a) Hyperglycemia; (c) Dehydration; (d) Coma

(Ref: Harrison 20th p 2871-72; Harrison 19th/2417,2420)

Hyperglycemic Hyperosmolar State
- Hyperglycemia > 600 mg/dl
- Serum osmolality > 310 mosm
- No acidosis
- Bicarbonate > 15 meq/L
- Normal anion gap

Lactic Acidosis
- Acidosis with hyperventilation
- Blood pH <7.3
- Serum bicarbonate < 15meq/L
- High anion gap
- Serum lactate > 5mmol/L
- Absent serum ketones

54. Ans. (a) Sodium increase

(Ref: Harrison 20th p 2871)

- Sugar draws water into intravascular compartment and leads to reduction in sodium levels. For every 100mg% rise in sugar sodium valves reduce by 1.6 meq/L.
- In hyperosmolar coma seen with diabetes mellitus, Serum sodium concentration is usually decreased because of the osmotic flux of water from the intracellular to the extracellular space in the presence of hyperglycemia.
- Hence sodium and blood sugar follow inverse relation in diabetes mellitus

> **Must Know Points**
>
> Diagnostic criteria for nonketotic hyperglycaemic hyperosmotic syndrome (HHS)
> - Profound dehydration (decreased skin turgor, postural changes in blood pressure and pulse rate)
> - Neurological symptoms (ranging from mental confusion to coma)
> - Plasma glucose levels > 600 mg/dL (36 mmol/L)
> - Plasma osmolality (Posm) >310 mOsm/kg
> - Arterial pH > 7.3
> - Plasma bicarbonate levels > 15 mmol/L
> - Normal anion gap (< 14 mEq/L)
> - Absence of ketones

55. Ans. (d) Urine albumin > 30 mg/dl

(Ref: Harrison 20th p 2878)

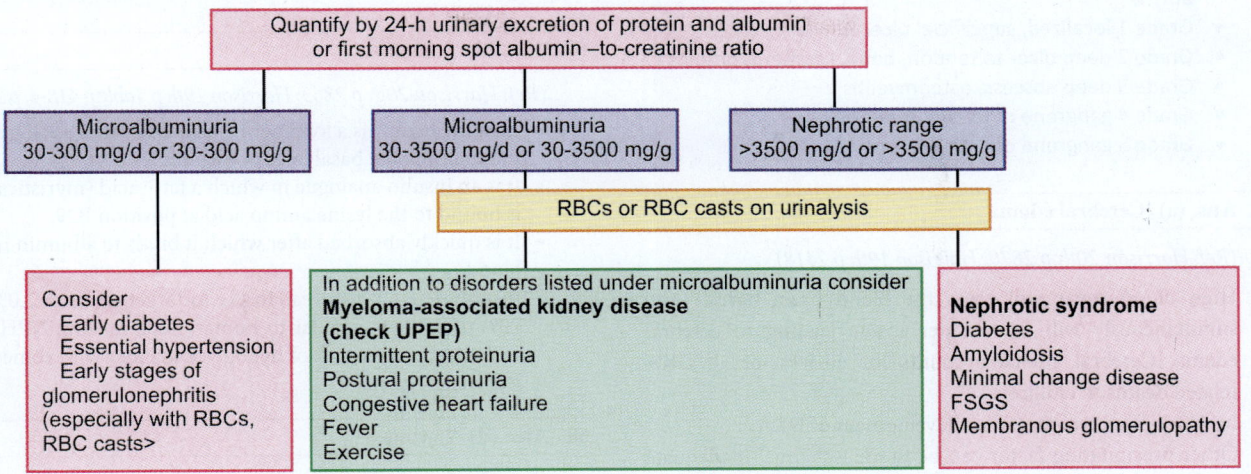

56. Ans. (d) Aldosterone

(Ref: page 613: Pathophysiology of disease: Lange: 2015 edition)

- Hypoglycemia in Addison disease is managed with hydrocortisone/dexamethasone.
- Administration of I.V. glucose in Addison leads to development of fever and is called as glucose fever.
- The etiology however remains unknown.

57. Ans. (c) Chromium

(Ref: Harrison 20th p 2319; Harrison 19th p 96e-10)

Chromium acts as a cofactor for insulin at insulin receptors and dietary deficiency of chromium would thus lead to impaired glucose tolerance

58. Ans. (c) Hypothyroidism

(Ref: Harrison 20th p 2851; Harrison 19th p 2399)

Cortisol, growth hormone and catecholamines increase the blood sugar levels leading to impaired glucose tolerance or diabetes mellitus.

59. Ans. (a) Candida

(Ref: Harrison 20th p 2882; Harrison 19th p 2429)

Individuals with DM have a greater frequency and severity of infection. Hyperglycemia aids the colonization and growth of a variety of organisms (Candida and other fungal species). Rhinocerebral mucormycosis occurs exclusively in diabetics but incidence is lesser than cardide infections.

60. Ans. (c) 180

(Ref: William's obstetrics 24th edition, table 52.4)

With OGTT using 100 gm glucose

1 hour value > 180 mg %
2 hour value > 155 mg%
3 hour value > 140 mg %

61. Ans. (b) Diabetes mellitus

(Ref: Diabetic neuropathy clinical management page 319, 2nd edition)

- Aldose reductase catalyzes the NADPH-dependent conversion of glucose to sorbitol, the first step in polyol pathway of glucose metabolism.
- Aldose reductase inhibitors are a class of drugs being studied as a way to prevent eye and nerve damage in people with diabetes mellitus.
- Examples of aldose reductase inhibitors include:
  - Tolrestat (withdrawn from market)
  - Epalrestat
  - Ranirestat
  - Fidarestat

62. Ans. (a) Decreased Immunity

(Ref: Harrison 20th p 2881; Harrison 19th p 2428)

The reasons for the increased incidence of foot ulcers in DM involve the interaction of several pathogenic factors:

1. Neuropathy (Microvascular complication) Motor and sensory neuropathy lead to abnormal foot muscle mechanics and to structural changes in the foot (hammertoe, claw toe deformity, prominent metatarsal heads, Charcot joint).
2. Autonomic neuropathy results in anhidrosis and altered superficial blood flow in the foot, which promote drying of the skin and fissure formation. PAD and poor wound healing impede resolution of minor breaks in the skin, allowing them to enlarge and to become infected.
3. Abnormal foot biomechanics
4. P.A.D (Macrovascular complication) leads to occlusive arterial disease that results in ischemia in the lower extremity and an increased risk of ulceration in diabetic patients. It is associated with, poor wound healing.

Grades of Diabetic Foot Ulcers

- Grade 0 skin intact but bony deformities produce a "foot at risk"
- Grade 1 localized, superficial ulcer
- Grade 2 deep ulcer to tendon, bone, ligament, or joint
- Grade 3 deep abscess, osteomyelitis
- Grade 4 gangrene of toes or forefoot
- Grade 5 gangrene of entire foot

63. Ans. (a) Cerebral edema

(Ref: Harrison 20th p 2870; Harrison 19th p 2418)

High blood sugar will cross the blood brain barrier and simultaneously will draw water inside leading to cerebral edema. Cerebral edema accounts for 60-90% of all DKA related deaths in children.

Infection is a precipitator for development of DKA.

Other precipitating factor can be tissue ischemia, inadequate insulin administration, drugs (Cocaine) and pregnancy.

64. Ans. (a) 126 mg/dl

(Ref: CMDT 2019 p 1225; Harrison 19th p 2399)

65. Ans. (d) Cardiomegaly

(Ref: William's Textbook of Endocrinology. 12th ed. P-976: Normal and Aberrant Growth)

Mauriac syndrome is a severe form of growth retardation seen in patients with poorly controlled type 1 diabetes mellitus. It is often referred to as diabetic dwarfism.

- It is characterized by growth failure, delayed puberty, hepatomegaly and Cushingoid features.
- The actual cause is unknown but is probably a combination of factors including inadequate glucose in the tissues, decreased IGF-1 and growth hormone levels, impaired bioactivity of the hormones, a circulating hormone inhibitor, or resistant or defective hormone receptors.
- The hepatomegaly seen in Mauriac syndrome is not seen in newly diagnosed patients who have been severely insulin deficient because it appears that periods of supraphysiologic insulin levels are associated with the hepatomegaly.
- Mauriac syndrome was much more common before long-acting insulin and knowledge of glycemic control (including monitoring of hemoglobin A1c) was available and is relatively rare today because of these treatments.
- It occurs in males and females equally and is most common in adolescence although there are reports in children as young as toddlers and in adults.
- Improved glycemic control helps to reverse the process, but catch-up growth may not be complete.

66. Ans. (a) Bromocriptine

(Ref: Harrison 20th p 2868; Diagnosis and management of Type 2 diabetes mellitus R.Henry, p 154)

Quick-release formulation of bromocriptine is thought to act on circadian neuronal activities within the hypothalamus to reset abnormally elevated hypothalamic drive for increased plasma glucose, triglyceride, and free fatty acid levels in fasting and postprandial states in patients with insulin-resistance.

67. Ans. (d) Detemir

(Ref: Harrison 20th p 2863; Harrison 19th p Table p 418-4, p 2411)

- Insulin detemir is a long-acting human insulin analogue for maintaining the basal level of insulin.
- It is an insulin analogue in which a fatty acid (myristic acid) is bound to the lysine amino acid at position B29.
- It is quickly absorbed after which it binds to albumin in the blood
- Insulin detemir reduces HbA1c to target levels of 7.0% for 70% of patients, similar to human basal insulin, NPH, but without the same risk of hypoglycemia and with somewhat less weight gain.

68. Ans. (d) 25 times

(Ref: Harrison 20th p 2877; Harrison 19th p 2424)

Individuals with DM are 25 times more likely to become legally blind than individuals without DM. Blindness is primarily the result of progressive diabetic retinopathy and clinically significant macular edema

69. Ans. (b) The level of fasting glucose is > 126 mg/dL and that of post-prandial glucose is > 199 mg/dL

(Ref: CMDT 2019, p 1225; Harrison 19th p 2399)

	Normal	IGT	Diabetes Mellitus
Fasting	<100 mg%	100-125 mg%	>126 mg%
2 hour value	<140 mg%	140-200 mg%	>200 mg%
HBA1c	<5.6%	5.6-6.4%	>6.5%

70. Ans. (c) Biguanides

(Ref: Harrison 20th p 2866; Harrison 19th p 2416)

Drug	Mechanism of Action	Examples	HbA1c Reduction (%)
Biguanides	↓ Hepatic glucose production	Metformin	1-2
α-Glucosidase inhibitors	↓ GI glucose absorption	Acarbose, Miglitol	0.5-0.8
Dipeptidyl peptidase IV inhibitors	Prolong endogenous GLP-1 action	Saxagliptin, Sitagliptin Vildagliptin	0.5-0.8
Insulin secretagogues: Sulfonylureas	↑ Insulin secretion	Glipizide Glyburide	1-2
Insulin secretagogues: Non-sulfonylureas	↑ Insulin secretion	Repaglinide Nateglinide	1-2
Thiazolidinediones	↓Insulin resistance, ↑ glucose utilization	Rosiglitazone, Pioglitazone	0.5-1.4

Biguanides are first line drugs for Type 2 DM but effect is delayed by several weeks.
- Alpha glucosidase inhibitors (acarbose and miglitol) reduce postprandial hyperglycemia by delaying glucose absorption; they do not affect glucose utilization or insulin secretion.
- Postprandial hyperglycemia, secondary to impaired hepatic and peripheral glucose disposal, contributes significantly to the hyperglycemic state in type 2 DM.
- These drugs, taken just before each meal, reduce glucose absorption by inhibiting the enzyme that cleaves oligosaccharides into simple sugars in the intestinal lumen. Therapy should be initiated at a low dose (25 mg of acarbose or miglitol) with the evening meal and may be increased to a maximal dose over weeks to months (50–100 mg for acarbose or 50 mg for miglitol with each meal).

This class of agents is not as potent as other oral agents in lowering the HbA1C but is unique because it reduces the postprandial glucose rise even in individuals with type 1 DM.

71. Ans. (a) Amphotericin B

(Ref: Harrison 20th p 1539; Harrison 19th p 2429)

- Primary antifungal therapy for Mucormycosis should be based on a polyene antibiotic except perhaps for mild localized infection (e.g., isolated suprafascial cutaneous infection) in immune competent patients, which has been eradicated surgically.
- Amphotericin B deoxycholate remains the only licensed antifungal agent for the treatment of mucormycosis.
- However, lipid formulations of AmB are significantly less nephrotoxic, can be administered at higher doses, and may be more efficacious than AmB deoxycholate for this purpose

72. Ans. (c) Lower limb ischemia

(Ref: CMDT 2015, p 1251; Harrison 19th p 2428)

- Atherosclerosis causes peripheral vascular disease incidence of which is 100 times higher in diabetic as compared to non-diabetic population.
- The incidence of amputation in diabetics is 15-40 times higher as compared to non diabetics.
- Chances for MI is observed to be 2 to 3 fold greater in diabetics
- Chances for cerebrovascular accidents/stroke is 3 times higher in diabetics
- Microvascular complications (predominantly indicated by the need for laser photocoagulation of retinal lesions) are reduced by 25% when mean HbA1c is 7%, compared with 7.9%.

73. Ans. (b) Plasma osmolality 380 mOsm

(Ref: Harrison 20th p 2870; Harrison 19th p 2416)

- Plasma osmolality in DKA is in range of 300-320mosm. Higher than 320mosm and upto 380mosm is seen with non ketotic hyperosmolar coma.
- In setting of insulin deficiency during diabetic ketoacidosis, the value of serum potassium is normal or increased. During course of treatment while the insulin drip is initiated, the level of potassium begins to fall
- Rothera test : A test for ketone bodies; 5 ml of fresh urine are saturated with solid ammonium sulfate and mixed with 10 drops of freshly prepared 2% sodium nitroprusside solution, which is then mixed with 10 drops of concentrated ammonia water and allowed to stand for 15 min; the presence of acetoacetic acid, or of larger concentrations of acetone, is indicated by the development of a blue-purple colour.
- Urine Benedict's test is positive in presence of sugar, which in setting of Random sugar exceeding 180 mg will definitively be positive.

74. Ans. (b) Ataxia telangiectasia

(Ref: Harrison 19th p 2399)

Hemochromatosis is associated with Bronze diabetes
Genetic syndromes sometimes associated with diabetes are

Wolfram's syndrome	Down's syndrome
Klinefelter's syndrome	Turner's syndrome
Friedreich's ataxia	Huntington's chorea
Laurence-Moon-Biedl syndrome	Myotonic dystrophy
Porphyria	Prader-Willi syndrome

75. Ans. (b) Addison's disease

(Ref: Harrison 19th Table 417-1, 2399)

- Diseases of the exocrine pancreas leading to diabetes—pancreatitis, pancreatectomy, neoplasia, cystic fibrosis, hemochromatosis, fibrocalculous pancreatopathy
- Endocrinopathies associated with diabetes —acromegaly, Cushing's syndrome, glucagonoma, pheochromocytoma, hyperthyroidism, somatostatinoma, aldosteronoma

76. Ans. (a) Increase in utilization of glucose

(Ref: Harrison 20th p 2870; Harrison 19th p 2418)

- Diabetic ketoacidosis is a characterized by insulin deficiency leading to cellular starvation and increase subcutaneous fat oxidation leading to ketone production.
- The resultant ketones lead to increase in anion gap.
- DKA occurs in setting of medical illness like stroke, MI, pneumonia and all these illnesses lead to enhancement of catabolic process.

77. Ans. (b) Low BUN

(Ref: Harrison 20th p 2870; Harrison 19th p 2418)

- DKA is characterized by hyperglycemia, ketosis, and metabolic acidosis (increased anion gap) along with a number of secondary metabolic derangements
- Nausea and vomiting are often prominent and lead to volume depletion.
- Elevated blood urea nitrogen (BUN) and serum creatinine levels reflect intravascular volume depletion.

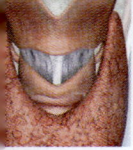

- Interference from acetoacetate may falsely elevate the serum creatinine measurement.

78. Ans. (b) Insulin antibodies are a hallmark for diagnosis of insulin resistance

(Ref: Harrison 20th p 2855-56; Harrison 19th p 2404)

- Insulin based antibodies can lead to development of latent autoimmune antibodies. It is damage to insulin receptors that causes development of insulin resistance. Another reason for insulin resistance can be mutations in insulin receptors.
- In DKA, bolus of IV (0.1 units/kg) short-acting insulin should be administered immediately. In mild episodes of DKA, short-acting insulin analogues can be used SC. IV insulin should be continued until the acidosis resolves and the patient is metabolically stable.
- As ketoacidosis improves, beta-hydroxybutyrate is converted to acetoacetate. Ketone body levels may appear to increase if measured by laboratory assays that use the nitroprusside reaction, which only detects acetoacetate and acetone. The improvement in acidosis and anion gap, a result of bicarbonate regeneration and decline in ketone bodies, is reflected by a rise in the serum bicarbonate level and the arterial pH. *Thus the marker for improvement after successful treatment for DKA is rise of bicarbonate and not the disappearance of ketones in urine.*
- Neuroglycopenic symptoms include weakness, tiredness, or dizziness; inappropriate behavior, difficulty with concentration; confusion; blurred vision; and, in extreme cases, coma and death.

79. Ans. (c) Insulin

(Ref: Harrison 20th p 2870; Harrison 19th p 2419)

Since patient is having DKA, the best option shall be insulin. In case of mild presentation short acting insulin can also be used subcutaneously.

80. Ans. (a) IDDM of 5 years duration

(Ref: Harrison 20th p 2877; Harrison 19th p 2424)

Complication of Retinopathy/nephropathy takes 5 years to develop in type 1 diabetes..
Complication of Retinopathy/nephropathy takes 15-20 years to develop in type 2 diabetes.

81. Ans. (a) Type 1.5 Diabetes Mellitus

(Ref: CMDT 2019 p 1221)

Type 1.5 diabetes mellitus is known as latent autoimmune diabetes and is treated with insulin replacement.

82. Ans. (c) Autonomic neuropathy

(Ref: Harrison 20th p 2879; Harrison 19th p 2426)

- Symtoms of hypoglycemia are those of sympathomimetic stimulation like palpitations tremors, sweating, anxiety, anger and decreased concentration.
- These symptoms are protective and prevent neuroglucopenia but in diabetics due to autonomic neuropathy, these symptoms will not appear and a diabetic may be unaware of his low sugar status as the nerves responsible for firing are damaged.
- This can lead to seizures and possible death in these patients too thought the most common cause of sudden death in diabetics is SILENT MI.

83. Ans. (c) Pre-tibial

(Ref: Harrison 20th p 2882; Harrison 19th p 2429)

- Necrobiosis lipoidica is a disorder of collagen degeneration with a granulomatous response, thickening of blood vessel walls, and fat deposition. The main complication of the disease is ulceration, usually occurring after trauma
- Most cases of necrobiosis lipoidica occur on the pretibial area, but cases have been reported on the face, scalp, trunk, and upper extremities, where the diagnosis is more likely to be missed

84. Ans. (c) >180 mg/dl

(Ref: Harrison 20th p 2870; Harrison 19th p 2419)

Obese patient age 45 years with presentation of diabetic ketoacidosis points to hyperglycemia.
Usually in DKA the value of blood sugar is around 300mg%.

85. Ans. (c) Glipizide

(Ref: Harrison 20th p 1232; Harrison 19th p 2413)

The basic principles of sulfonylurea metabolism can be summarized as follows:

- Chlorpropamide is eliminated almost exclusively by the kidney.
- Glyburide has weak active metabolites that are excreted in the urine and accumulate in patients with impaired kidney function.
- *Glipizide and tolbutamide are metabolized by the liver and primarily excreted in the urine as inactive metabolites. However, each has one metabolite that may have weak hypoglycemic activity.*

86. Ans. (b) Inferior wall MI

(Ref: Harrison 20th p 2880; Harrison 19th p 2427)

- Diabetics have accelerated atherosclerosis due to which they have 3 times more chances of MI as compared to non-diabetics
- The future development of autonomic neuro-pathy will mask findings of MI like chest pain and sweating leading to silent MI and this patient has only symptoms of dizziness which is due to decreased Cardiac output due to the silent / painless MI developed in this patient
- In inferior wall MI, the blockage of Right coronary artery leads to less supply to SAN (SA nodal artery ischemia) and leads to bradycardia severe enough to warrant a Temporary pacemaker insertion.

87. Ans. (b) Increased anion gap

(Ref: Harrison 20th p 2870; Harrison 19th p 2418)

88. Ans. (b) Insulin dose should be decreased in patients with ESRD

(Ref: Harrison 20th p 2878; Harrison 19th p 2426)

Among patients who are treated with insulin, *the starting dose of insulin may need to be lower* than would ordinarily be used for patients with normal kidney function.

Guidelines for adjustment of dose of insulin in patient of ESRD
- No dose adjustment is required if the GFR is >50 mL/min.
- The insulin dose should be reduced to approximately 75 percent of baseline when the GFR is between 10 and 50 mL/min
- The dose should be reduced by as much as 50 percent when the GFR is <10 mL/min

89. Ans. (c) I.V. insulin

(Ref: Harrison 20th p 2870; Harrison 19th p 2419)

IV insulin should be continued until the acidosis resolves and the patient is metabolically stable. As the acidosis and insulin resistance associated with DKA resolve, the insulin infusion rate can be decreased (to 0.05–0.1 units/kg per hour).
- Ketoacidosis begins to resolve as insulin reduces lipolysis, increases peripheral ketone body use, suppresses hepatic ketone body formation, and promotes bicarbonate regeneration. However, the acidosis and ketosis resolve more *slowly* than hyperglycemia.
- Soda-bicarbonate has no role in management of DKA
- I.V. fluids correct the water deficit and sodium deficit primarily.

90. Ans. (c) Fluroscein dye leak

(Ref: Harrison 20th p 2877; Harrison 19th p 2423)

The Diabetes Complications and Control Trial demonstrated that improvement of glycemic control reduced
- Non-proliferative and proliferative retinopathy (47% reduction)
- Micro-albuminuria (39% reduction), clinical nephropathy (54% reduction),
- Neuropathy (60% reduction).

The results of the DCCT predicted that individuals in the intensive diabetes management group would gain 7.7 additional years of vision, 5.8 additional years free from ESRD, and 5.6 years free from lower extremity amputations. If all complications of DM were combined, individuals in the intensive diabetes management group would experience 15.3 more years of life without significant microvascular or neurologic complications of DM, compared to individuals who received standard therapy.
- Choice A: Amyotrophy is an alternative term for lumbosacral plexopathy seen in diabetics and associated with pain in thigh and quadriceps wasting. Good sugar control reduces nerve damage
- Choice B. Good sugar control reduces nerve damage.
- *Choice C. fluroscein dye leakage implies macular edema and one it is developed then moderate visual loss will occur. The point is that the damage already has been done and good sugar control does not change angiography findings once they are developed. Also remember that macular edema causes visual loss while blindness in diabetics is due to vitreous haemorrhage and tractional retinal detachment.* Good sugar control reduces neovascularization and will reduce retinal detachment chances but not Dye leakage on FFA.
- Choice D. Progression to ESRD is reduced by good sugar control.

91. Ans. (a) Congenital malformations

(Ref: Harrison 20th p 3443; Harrison 19th p 2400)

- Congenital malformations are not seen in gestational diabetes as it develops by second trimester when the organogenesis has occurred already.
- Congenital malformations are seen in babies born to mothers with pre-existing uncontrolled diabetes mellitus
- Metformin has been shown to be as effective and having better compliance as compared to insulin in management of gestational diabetes mellitus.

92. Ans. (a) 30-300 mg/24 hours

(Ref: Harrison 19th p 2425)

Proteinuria	Description
Normal protein in urine	< 150 mg /24 hours
Normal albumin in urine	<30 mg/24 hours
Micro-albuminuria	30-300 mg/24 hours
Overt proteinuria	>550 mg/24 hours
Sub-nephrotic proteinuria	1-3 gram/24 hour
Nephrotic range	>3.5 gram/24 hours
Multiple myeloma	6-10 gram/24 hours

- In current edition of Harrison, albuminuria term is used and microalbuminuria has been removed. Albuminuria in a spot sample is defined as urinary albumin to creatinine ratio of $> \frac{30 \text{ mg}}{\text{g}}$ creatinine.

93. Ans. (d) Peripheral vascular disease

(Ref: Harrison 20th p 1227-28; Harrison 19th p 2423)

- Tight glycemic control improves the micro-vascular complications but has no effect on macrovascular complications.

Complication	% Reduction with good sugar control
Retinopathy	47%
Microalbuminuria	39%
Nephropathy	54%
Neuropathy	60%

94. Ans. (c) Diabetes mellitus

(Ref: Harrison 20th p 2882; Harrison 19th p 2429)

- Necrobiosis lipoidica is a necrotising skin condition that usually occurs in patients with diabetes but can also be associated with Rheumatoid Arthritis.
- It is a disorder of collagen degeneration with a granulomatous response, thickening of blood vessel walls, and fat deposition. The main complication of the disease is ulceration, usually occurring after trauma. Infections can occur but are uncommon

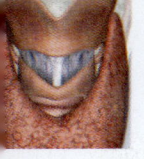

95. Ans. (a) **Type I Diabetes**

    (Ref: Harrison 20th p 2855; Harrison 19th p 2426)

96. Ans. (c) **DM type II > (a) MODY**

    (Ref: CMDT 2019, 1221; 'Clinical Endocrinology and Diabetes Mellitus' by Sachdev & Gupta 1st/916; 'Hand book of Diabetes' by Williams 3rd/72, Harrison 19th p 2404, 2406)

    - Since patient is on oral hypoglycemic drugs both T2DM and MODY are possible.
    - Indian patients with T2DM don't exhibit characteristic weight gain.
    - T2DM has positive family history but it may not be expressed in every generation.
    - MODY has autosomal dominant inheritance and can be expressed in every generation.

97. Ans. (a) **Family history is present in 90% of cases**

    (Ref: CMDT 2019, 1220)

98. Ans. (b) **Hydrochlorthiazide**

    (Ref: K.D.T 5th/532, Harrison 19th p 2426)

99. Ans. (c) **D-Xylose test**

    (Ref: CMDT 2019, p 1225; Harrison 19th p 2410)

100. Ans. (d) **Glycosylated Haemoglobin (HbA1C) > 6.5%**

     (Ref: Harrison 20th p 2850; Harrison 19th p 2399)

101. Ans. (b) **Long term status of blood sugar**

     (Ref: Harrison 20th p 2862)

102. Ans. (c) **Distal sensory neuropathy**

     (Ref: Harrison 20th p 2879; Harrison 19th p 2426)

103. Ans. (c) **c-DNA of pancreatic cell**

     (Ref: Harrison 20th p 2854; Harrison 19th p 2411)

104. Ans. (b) **D-Xylose test**

     (Ref: CMDT 2019, 1262; Harrison 19th p 2434)

105. Ans. (a) **Diabetes mellitus**

     (Ref: Harrison 20th p 2858)

106. Ans. (b) **Adrenal insufficiency**

     (Ref: Harrison 20th p 2733; Harrison 19th p 2324)

107. Ans. (a) **Serum fructosamine**

     (Ref: Harrison 20th p 1226; Evidence based diabetes care 2nd ed./229)

- Serum fructosamine is a retrospective test that tells you gives the fluctuations in blood sugar in the previous 2-3 weeks.
- In contrast glycosylated hemoglobin gives fluctuations in blood sugar value over the previous 6-8 weeks.
- **Also remember:** severity of bronze diabetes is determined by GLYCATED albumin.

108. Ans. (a) **Phenformin**

     (Ref: Harrison 20th p 1223; K.D. Tripathi 7th ed. / 275)

     - Phenformin was withdrawn from the market as it causes lactic acidosis
     - Metformin is the drug of choice for management of type 2 diabetes mellitus with obesity.
     - Rosiglitazone was withdrawn as it causes coronary artery thrombosis
     - Pioglitazone has a black box warning as it causes bladder cancer.

109. Ans. (c) **< 180 mg/dl**

     (Ref: Harrison 20th p 2860)

TABLE: Treatment goal for adults with diabetes

Parameters	Goal
HbA1C	< 7%
Preprandial capillary plasma glucose	70 – 130 mg/dl
Peak post prandial capillary plasma glucose	< 180 mg/dl
Blood pressure	< 140/90
Lipids	
LDL	< 70 mg/dl
HDL	> 40 mg/dl in men > 50 mg/dl in women
Triglycerides	< 150 mg/dl

*BP goal of <130/80 mm Hg for younger patients or those with cardiovascular risk factors.

Disorders of Adrenal Cortex

110. Ans. (c) **Hyperkalemia**

     (Ref: Harrison 20th p 2725; Harrison, 19th edition, Page 308)

     The image shows a patient of Cushing syndrome which presents with hypokalemic alkalosis due to partial mineralocorticoid activity of cortisol.

111. Ans. (d) **24 hour urinary chloride**

     (Ref: Harrison 20th p 2738; Harrison 19th edition, Page 2328)

     - The image shows clitoromegaly, labial fusion of a virilised female child. Inguinal folds don't exhibit any mass or swelling. Leading cause of it will be congenital adrenal hyperplasia.

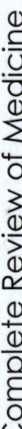

- Deficiency of 21-hydroxylase, resulting from mutations or deletions of CYP21A, is the most common form of CAH, accounting for more than 90% of cases

Choice A	Useful for determining bone age which is advanced in CAH due to sex steroids
Choice B	Useful to identify CAH where a girl child is having ambiguous genitilia
Choice C	Useful due to salt wasting and elevated potassium secondary to decreased aldosterone levels.

24 hour urinary chloride is useful in renal tubular disorders like Bartter syndrome and Gitelman syndrome.

112. Ans. (c) Hyperkalemia

(Ref: Page 521, William's textbook of endocrinology 12edition.

- Hyperkalemia is seen due with mineralocorticoid deficiency.
- It has been documented that ACTH via steroids can supress Interleukin-1 production. Vice versa in glucocorticoid deficiency, IL-1 will be elevated and can reset the thermostat leading to fever as presentation of glucocorticoid deficiency. This is usually mentioned as unexplained fever in textbook.
- Postural hypotension is explained by hyponatremia which occurs due to loss of feedback inhibition of AVP release due to deficiency of glucocorticoids.

Signs and Symptoms Caused by Glucocorticoid Deficiency	Signs and Symptoms Caused by Mineralocorticoid Deficiency
• Hyponatremia (due to loss of feedback inhibition of AVP release) • Postural hypotension/ Low BP • Unexplained Fever • Fatigue • Weight loss, anorexia • Myalgia, joint pain • Anaemia, lymphocytosis, eosinophilia • Slightly increased TSH (due to loss of feedback inhibition of TSH release) • Hypoglycaemia (more frequent in children)	• Hyponatremia (due to aldosterone deficiency) • Hyperkalemia (due to aldosterone deficiency) • Abdominal pain, nausea, vomiting • Dizziness, postural hypotension • Salt craving • Low blood pressure, postural hypotension • Increased serum creatinine (due to volume depletion)

113. Ans. (c) Distal myopathy

(Ref: Harrison 20th p 2725; Harrison 19th edition, page 2271, 2313)

- Cushing syndrome is characterized with proximal muscle weakness resulting in difficulty in climbing stairs.
- Lemon on sticks results in centripetal obesity. The weight gain leads to insulin resistance coupled with effects of cortisol leading to impaired glucose tolerance.

114. Ans. (d) Hermansky-pudlak syndrome

(Ref: Harrison 20th p 345; Harrison 19th edition, Page 375e-2 and page 730)

Busulfan administration	Busulfan, cyclophosphamide, 5-fluorouracil, and inorganic arsenic induce pigment production and cause diffuse hyperpigmentation
Nelson's syndrome	Increased ACTH (which has partial MSH activity) due to bilateral adrenalectomy
Addison's disease	Increased ACTH (which has partial MSH activity) due to destruction of adrenal cortex and low cortisol
Hermansky-pudlak syndrome	Autosomal recessive disorder which results in oculo-cutaneous albinism (decreased pigmentation), bleeding problems due to a platelet abnormality (platelet storage pool defect).

115. Ans. (a) Hyperglycemia

(Ref: Harrison 20th p 2734; Harrison 19th edition, Page 2324)

- The clinical features of primary adrenal insufficiency are characterized by the loss of both glucocorticoid and mineralocorticoid secretion.
- Therefore hypotension with hyponatremia is seen.
- Low aldosterone explains Hyperkalemia
- In secondary adrenal insufficiency, only glucocorticoid deficiency is present, as the adrenal itself is intact and thus still amenable to regulation by the RAA system.
- Remember adrenal androgen secretion is disrupted in both primary and secondary adrenal insufficiency.
- Hyperpigmentation is seen in primary Addison disease due to excess of POMC based derivatives.
- Hypopigmentation is seen in secondary Addison disease due to depletion of POMC based derivatives.

116. Ans. (d) Iatrogenic Steroids

(Ref: Harrison 20th p 2723-24; Harrison 19th edition, Page 2271)

- Overall, the medical use of glucocorticoids for immunosuppression, or for the treatment of inflammatory disorders, is the most common cause of Cushing's syndrome.
- Most common cause of ACTH Dependant Cushing syndrome is Cushing Disease (Pituitary Adenoma)
- Most common cause of ACTH independent Cushing Syndrome is Adrenal Adenoma

117. Ans. (a) Renin aldosterone ratio

(Ref: Harrison 20th p 2729; Harrison 19th edition, page 2319)

- The presence of hypertension and hypokalemia incriminates increased aldosterone values. For evaluation of primary hyper-aldosteronism plasma renin/aldosterone ratio is useful.
- ACTH stimulation test is done for Addison disease that presents with postural hypotension with hypokalemia
- 24 hour urinary catecholamines is used for diagnosis of pheochromocytoma.
- Octreo-scan is used for locating carcinoid tumour and primitive neuro-ectodermal tumours.

118. Ans. (a) Pituitary adenoma; (d) Pheochromocytoma

(Ref: Harrison 20th p 2724; Harrison 19th/2314)

ACTH dependent Cushing syndrome	ACTH Independent Cushing syndrome

• ACTH producing pituitary adenoma
• Ectopic ACTH
  ▪ Bronchial or pancreatic carcinoid
  ▪ Small cell cancer of lung
  ▪ Medullary carcinoma of thyroids
  ▪ Phaeochromocytoma
	• Adrenocortical adenoma/ carcinoma
	• Primary pigmented nodular adrenal disease
	• Adrenal hyperplasia
	• McCune Albright Syndrome

119. Ans. (d) ACTH

(Ref: Harrison 20th p 345; Harrison 19th ed. / 401e-4)

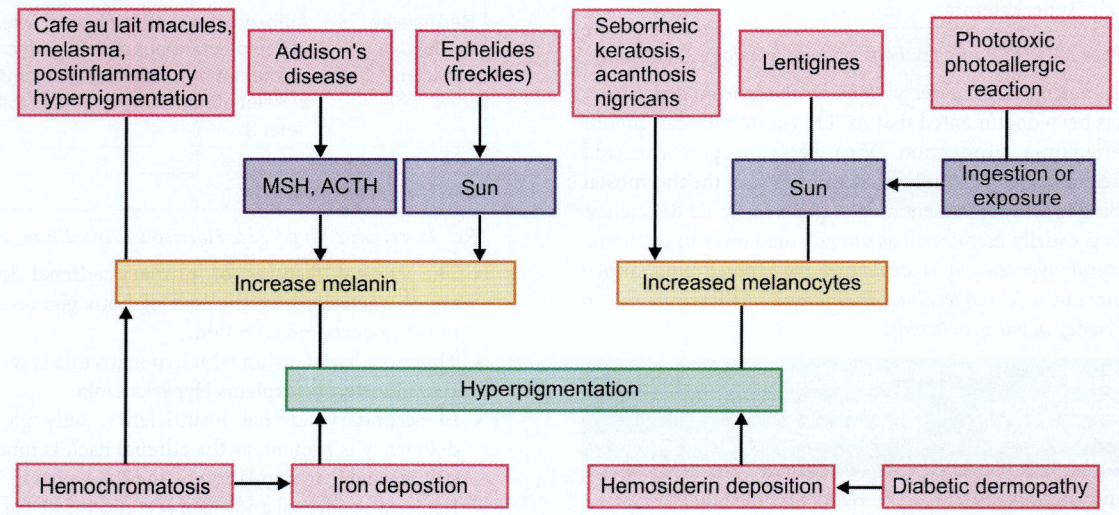

120. Ans. (d) Metabolic alkalosis

(Ref: Harrison 19th ed. / 2324)

- Metabolic alkolosis is seen with excess of aldosterone while choices a, b, c are seen with addison disease.

121. Ans. (a) Metabolic acidosis

(Ref: Harrison 20th p 2767; Harrison 19th ed. / 2327)

11 beta Hydroxylase Deficiency, is Characterized by:
- 11-deoxycortisol excess which can activate ENa_c and hence hypertension can be seen
- Mineralocorticoid excess leads to hypokalemia and metabolic alkalosis.
- Glucocorticoid deficiency leads to hypoglycemia plus excess of ACTH leads to hyperpigmentation around genitals
- Excess of adrenal androgens leads to Virilization.

Variant	Gene	Impact on Steroid Synthesis	Diagnostic Marker in Serum (and Urine)
21-Hydroxylase deficiency (21OHD)	CYP21A2	Glucocorticoid deficiency, mineralocorticoid deficiency, adrenal androgen excess	17-Hydroxyprogesterone
11-Hydroxylase deficiency (11OHD)	CYP11B1	Glucocorticoid deficiency, mineralocorticoid excess, adrenal androgen excess	11-Deoxycortisol
17-Hydroxylase deficiency (17OHD)	CYP17A1	Glucocorticoid deficiency, mineralocorticoid excess, androgen deficiency	11-Deoxycorticosterone
3-Hydroxysteroid dehydrogenase deficiency	HSD3B2	Glucocorticoid deficiency, mineralocorticoid deficiency, adrenal androgen excess	17-Hydroxypregnanolone

Contd...

122. Ans. (a) CFTR mutation

(Ref: Harrison 20th p 1988; Harrison 19th p 1697)

- Some individuals with polymorphisms of both CFTR genes have few or no CF manifestations until adolescence or adulthood, when they present with pancreatitis, sinusitis, diffuse bronchiectasis, or male infertility.

- In >95% of males, the body and tail of the epididymis, the vas deferens, and the seminal vesicles are obliterated or atretic.
- More than 95% of males are azoospermic because of failure of development of Wolffian duct structures, but sexual function is generally unimpaired. The incidence of inguinal hernia, hydrocele, and undescended testis is higher than expected

123. Ans. (a) Pigmentation

(Ref: Harrison 19th p 2324)

- In Secondary adrenal insufficiency mineralocorticoid secretion is intact. It manifests more insidiously with lack of skin hyperpigmentation.
- Hyponatremia is seen with gluco-corticoid deficiency because of loss of control of inhibition of vasopressin.
- Fatigue, hyponatremia, and hypoglycemia are some of the clinical manifestations in secondary adrenal insufficiency.

124. Ans. (d) Sipple syndrome

(Ref: Harrison 20th p 2752; Harrison 19th p 2340)

Sipple syndrome/ MEN 2A has a pheochro-mocytoma which is associated with weight loss due to sympathomimetic activity secondary to increased catecholamines.

125. Ans. (a) Adrenocortical carcinoma

(Ref. Harrison 20th p Table 379-5, 2731)

The most common cause of adrenal tumors is metastasis from another solid tumor like breast cancer and lung cancer.

Malignant	Percentage
Adrenocortical carcinoma	2-5%
Malignant pheochromocytoma	<1%
Adrenal neuroblastoma	<0.1%
Lymphomas (incl. primary adrenal lymphoma)	<1%
Metastases (most frequent: Breast, lung)	< 1-2%

126. Ans. (b) Metabolic acidosis present

(Ref: Harrison 19th p 2319)

- Most patients have hypertension, usually not very severe, and headaches. Malignant hypertension is rare. The hypertension is due to the increased sodium reabsorption and extracellular volume expansion. ECG and CXR signs of LVH are, in part, secondary to the hypertension. However, the LVH is disproportionate to the level of BP when compared to individuals with essential hypertension.
- Patients with primary aldosteronism characteristically do not have edema, *since they exhibit an "escape" phenomenon from the sodium-retaining aspects of mineralocorticoids.*
- Hypersecretion of aldosterone increases the renal distal tubular exchange of intratubular sodium for secreted potassium and hydrogen ions, with progressive depletion of body potassium and development of hypokalemia. Potassium depletion is responsible for the muscle weakness and fatigue and is due to the effect of potassium depletion on the muscle cell membrane. The polyuria results from impairment of urinary concentrating ability (secondary to hypokalemia) and is often associated with polydipsia.
- Metabolic alkalosis and elevation of serum bicarbonate are a result of hydrogen ion loss into the urine and migration into potassium-depleted cells. The alkalosis is perpetuated by potassium deficiency, which increases the capacity of the proximal convoluted tubule to reabsorb filtered bicarbonate.

127. Ans. (a) Dexamethasone

(Ref: Nelson 20th pg 817)

- Recommendations for pregnancies at risk consist of administration of dexamethasone, a steroid that readily crosses the placenta, in an amount of 20 µg/kg pre-pregnancy maternal weight daily. This suppresses secretion of steroids by the fetal adrenal, including secretion of adrenal androgens.
- If started by 6 wk of gestation, it reduces virilization of the external genitals in affected females. Chorionic villus biopsy is then performed to determine the sex and genotype of the fetus; therapy is continued only if the fetus is an affected female.
- DNA analysis of fetal cells isolated from maternal plasma for sex determination and CYP21 gene analysis may permit earlier identification of the affected female fetus.

128. Ans. (c) Ectopic adrenal hormone production

(Ref: Harrison 20th p 2724)

Ectopic site production is 15% while the adrenal adenoma is 10% while the incidence of adrenal carcinoma is 1%.

Causes of Cushing's Syndrome	%
ACTH-Dependent Cushing's	90
Cushing's disease (Pituitary adenoma)	75
Ectopic ACTH syndrome (due to ACTH secretion by Bronchial or pancreatic carcinoid tumors, oat cell lung cancer, medullary thyroid carcinoma, pheochromocytoma)	15
ACTH-Independent Cushing's	10
Adrenocortical adenoma	5-10
Adrenocortical carcinoma	1%
Primary pigmented nodular adrenal disease; McCune-Albright syndrome	<1%

129. Ans. (d) Iatrogenic steroids

(Ref: Harrison 20th p 2723; Harrison 19th p 2314)

Overall the most common cause of Cushing's syndrome is iatrogenic steroids but if asked regarding ACTH dependent cause then answer should be given as pituitary adenoma.

130. Ans. (a) Hypoglycemia

(Ref: Harrison 20th p 2725; Harrison 19th p 2315)

- Cushing syndrome causes impaired glucose tolerance and hyperglycemia. The majority of patients also experience psychiatric symptoms, mostly in the form of anxiety or depression, but acute paranoid or depressive psychosis may also occur.

- Due to partial mineralocorticoid activity of cortisol, hypertension and hypokalemia is explained.

131. Ans. (b) Plasma cortisol

(Ref: Harrison 20th p 2725; Harrison 19th p 2315)

- Weight gain with oligomenorrhea points to Cushing syndrome. Cortisol inhibits gonadotropin release that explains the amenorrhea.
- Hypertension in these patients is secondary to increased cortisol that has some mineralocorticoid activity also.
- Excess glucocorticoids also interfere with central regulatory systems, leading to suppression of gonadotropins with subsequent hypogonadism and amenorrhea, and suppression of the hypothalamic-pituitary-thyroid axis, resulting in decreased TSH (thyroid-stimulating hormone) secretion.
- Weight gain with menorrhagia and isolated diastolic hypertension in the question would have prompted thyroid dysfunction as the first answer.

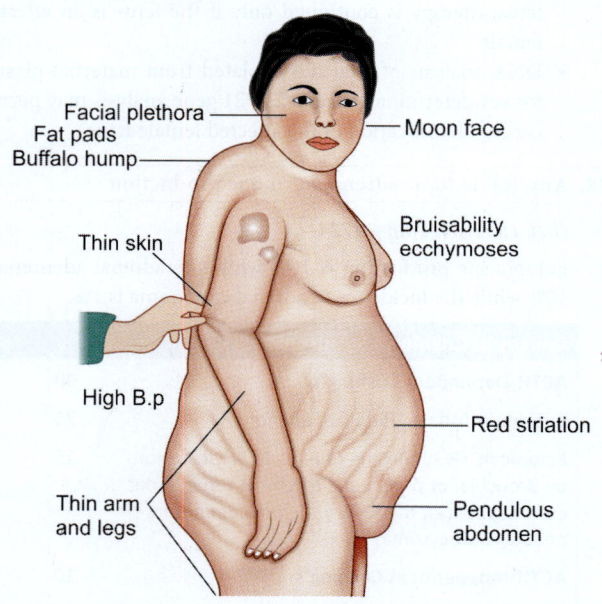

132. Ans. (d) Ectopic ACTH production > CA lung

(Ref: Harrison 20th p 2723; Harrison 19th p 2315)

- Ectopic ACTH production is predominantly caused by occult carcinoid tumors, most frequently in the lung, but also in thymus or pancreas.
- About 25% of patients with pulmonary carcinoid tumors are asymptomatic at the time of discovery. In symptomatic patients of pulmonary carcinoids, the most common clinical findings are those associated with bronchial obstruction, such as persistent cough, hemoptysis, and recurrent or obstructive pneumonitis. Wheezing, chest pain, and dyspnea also may be noted. Although uncommon, various endocrine or neuroendocrine syndromes can be initial clinical manifestations of either typical or atypical pulmonary carcinoid tumors.
- Small cell lung cancer can cause ectopic ACTH production. Since the term small cancer of lung is not mentioned in MCQ hence it should be the second best answer

133. Ans. (d) Anasarca

(Ref: Harrison 20th p 2729; Harrison 19th p 2319; CMDT 2019 pg 1188)

- Anasarca or swelling is not seen in CONN syndrome due to salt escape mechanism.
- Though there is gain of salt and water due to aldosterone excess, the increased preload will stretch the right atrium and cause release of A.N.F.
- This increase in ANF will cause natriuresis –salt and water loss and will cancel the gain caused by aldosterone.
- This natriuresis or salt loss shall be associated with water loss and leads to polyuria. The resultant polyuria will lead to polydipsia.
- The weakness is explained by hypokalemia.

134. Ans. (a) Association with MEN 2 syndrome

(Ref: Harrison 19th edition, Page 2315)

- Ectopic ACTH syndrome is due to ACTH secretion by *bronchial* carcinoid tumors which are seen with MEN 1 in 2% cases.
- *Excess glucocorticoid secretion* overcomes the ability of 11 beta-HSD_2 to rapidly inactivate cortisol to cortisone in the kidney, thereby exerting mineralocorticoid actions, manifest as diastolic hypertension, *hypokalemia*, and edema.
- Due to atherosclerosis and hypertension, coronary events have been described in these patients in Harrison.

135. Ans. (d) Hydrocortisone

(Ref: Harrison 20th p 2767; Harrison 19th p 2328)

- Most common type of CAH (21 hydroxylase deficiency) presents with hypoglycemia with hypotension and virilization. Hydrocortisone injection after birth will help in stabilizing the child by increasing blood sugar and increasing salt absorbtion from the kidney.
- Methylprednisolone and dexamethasone have negligible mineralocorticoid effects. Therefore, if the patient is hypovolemic, hyponatremic, or hyperkalemic, large dosages of hydrocortisone are preferred because of its mineralocorticoid effect.

136. Ans. (a) Deoxycorticosterone

(Ref: Harrison 20th p 2738; Harrison 19th p 2328)

- Two forms of adrenal hyperplasia (ie, 11-hydroxylase [CYP11B1] and 17-hydroxylase [CYP17] deficiency) result in hypertension due to the accumulation of supraphysiologic concentrations of deoxycorticosterone.
- This weak mineralocorticoid has little consequence at physiologic concentrations but causes sodium retention and hypertension at the suprphysiologic concentrations that occur in these conditions.

137. Ans. (a) Primary hyperaldosteronism

(Ref: Harrison 20th p 2728; Harrison 19th p 2318)

Primary hyperaldosteronism is due to bilateral adrenal hyperplasia or due to adrenal adenoma. Both these conditions are autonomous and lead to aldosterone production in excess.

The R.A.A.S system negative feedback will result in decrease in renin production.

Low renin Hypertension is a feature of primary hyperaldosteronism.

> **Causes of low renin hypertension**
> - Liddle syndrome
> - Conn's syndrome
> - Mineralocorticoid receptor mutation
> - Apparent mineralocorticoid excess (AME)
> - Glucocorticoid resistance
> - Gordon syndrome
> - Congenital adrenal hyperplasia (CAH)

138. Ans. (a) Hypoglycemia

(Ref: Harrison 20th p 2767; Harrison 19th p 2328)

139. Ans. (a) Hemochromatosis

(Ref: Harrison 20th p 2980; Harrison 19th p 2516)

140. Ans. (a) Chronic alcoholism

(Ref: Harrison 20th p 2726; Harrison 19th p 2316)

- In alcoholics there is increased urinary excretion of steroids, absent diurnal variation of plasma steroids with positive overnight dexamethasone test. All of these biochemical derangements decrease on alcohol discontinuation.
- High MCV and gamma glutamyl transferase will be indicative of alcoholism.

141. Ans. (b) Hypokalemia

(Ref: Harrison 20th p 2735; Harrison 19th p 2324)

- In Addison disease, the absence or less amount of aldosterone will lead to hypotension, salt craving and hyperkalemia
- Damage to zona fasiculata will lead to hypo-glycemia while damage to zona reticularis will lead to loss of axillary and pubic hair.
- Hypokalemia is seen with CONN syndrome.

142. Ans. (b) Maternal virilising tumor

(Ref: Harrison 20th p 2738, 2765; Harrison 19th p 2362, 2366)

Androgen insensitivity syndrome	Female appearance with internal male genitalia
Maternal virilizing tumour	Ambiguous genitalia with female internal genitalia
CAH	Ambiguous genitalia in a female with hyperpigmentation around genitals
5 alpha reductase deficiency	Ambiguous genitalia with male internal genitalia

Maternal virilizing tumour
- Causes masculinization of a female fetus.
- Thus, the findings would be ambiguous genitalia with female internal genitalia including uterus (Mullerian structures) and no testis (no inguinal masses as seen in AIS).
- The BP and pigmentation would not be affected

AIS (Androgen Insensitivity Syndrome)
- In this case, the androgen receptors do not respond to the androgens.
- Hence, there will be feminization of a masculine fetus.
- There is normal breast development, short vagina and absence of uterus (since the person is a male)
- Testis usually does not descend completely (cryptorchidism) and present as masses in the inguinal region.

Congenital Adrenal Hyperplasia
- This is due to deficient steroidogenesis.
- In 17-a and 11-P enzyme deficiencies, there is mineralocorticoid excess leading to hypertension
- In 21-a deficiency, adrenal hyperplasia with normotension, ambiguous genitalia with clitoris enlargement and labial fusion, and hyperpigmentation are the presenting features.

5-a-reductase deficiency
- This condition occurs in males.
- Hence, there is ambiguous genitalia and male internal genitalia (testis in the normal position and absence of Mullerian structures).

143. Ans. (d) Edema

(Ref: CMDT 2019, pg 1188; Harrison 19th p 2319)

In Conn's syndrome there is operation of salt escape mechanism that leads to absence of pedal edema. The logic is that though aldosterone is sky high in Conn's and therefore salt and water retention should cause development of edema, the volume expansion leads to dilatation of right side heart causing release of A.N.P (Atrial Natri-Ureteric Peptide). This product will cause of loss of water and will balance the gain made by aldosterone.

144. Ans. (c) ESRD (End Stage Renal Disease)

(Ref: Harrison 20th p 306; Harrison 19th p 1817)

- Cushing syndrome has increased cortisol that exhibits partial aldosterone activity. Therefore the increased aldosterone explains hypertension and potassium deficit.
- Liddle's syndrome, also called and Pseudoaldosteronism, is an autosomal dominant disorder characterized by dysregulation of an epithelial sodium channel (ENaC) due to a genetic mutation at the 16p13-p12 locus. This results in excess reabsorption of sodium and loss of potassium from the renal tubule, and is treated with a combination of low sodium diet and potassium-sparing diuretic drugs (e.g., amiloride)
- In hyperaldosteronism the increased levels of aldosterone will cause more sodium and water to enter the body leading to hypertension while the K loss occurring at ENac receptor due to aldosterone action explains hypokalemia.
- *In patients of ESRD the increased renin explains hypertension while the damage to kidney will reduce potassium excretion and will lead to hyperkalemia*

145. Ans. (b) Pituitary adenoma

(Ref: Harrison 20th p 2724; Harrison 19th p 2314)

146. Ans. (b) Increased adrenaline

(Ref: Harrison 20th p 2725; Harrison 19th Table 406-2, p 2315)

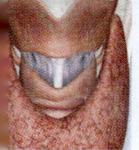

147. Ans. (c) Ca lung with ectopic ACTH production

(Ref: Harrison 20th p 2725; Harrison 19th p 2315)

148. Ans. (d) Ectopic ACTH secreting tumor

(Ref: Harrison 20th p 2725; Harrison 19th p 2315)

149. Ans. (a) Loss of Diurnal variation

(Ref: Harrison 20th p 2725; Harrison 19th p 2316)

Disorders of Adrenal Medulla

150. Ans. (a) Urinary V.M.A is most specific

(Ref: Harrison 20th edition, Page 2741)

- Paraganglioma is a term used to describe catecholamine producing tumors in the skull base and neck.
- The classic rule of tens is valid for pheochromocytoma (page 2740, Harrison 20th edition).
- Organ of Zuckerkandl is a collection of chromaffin cells near the origin of the inferior mesenteric artery or near the aortic bifurcation. It is the most common extra-adrenal site of pheochromocytoma.
- Urinary VMA is used for diagnosis of neuroblastoma and not pheochromocytoma. The *most sensitive test* for pheochromocytoma is urinary fractionated metanephrine.

151. Ans. (c) Neuroblastoma

(Ref: Nelson 20th edition, page 2463)

Vanillyl mandelic acid is a metabolic by-product of norepinephrine and epinephrine. *It is used for detection of tumors of neural crest origin*:

1. Neuroblastoma
2. Pheochromocytoma
3. Ganglioblastoma
4. Ganglioneuroma
5. Severe anxiety

For diagnosis of pheochromocytoma, fractionated metanephrine level in urine and stool are preferred.

152. Ans. (c) Surgery is mainstay of treatment; **(d)** Prior α blocker is given; **(e)** Prior β blocker is given

(Ref: Harrison 20th p 2743; Harrison 19th/2329-31; Robbins 9th/1134-36)

- 90% of pheochromocytomas are benign and 10% are malignant. For preoperative localization MRI abdomen is done. If scan turns out be negative then MIBG scan is done.
- Surgery is the treatment of choice. For pre-operative management of hypertension, alpha plus beta blockage should be given.
- If non selective beta blocker is given first, then unopposed alpha blocker action will lead to hypertensive crisis.

153. Ans. (a) Phenoxybenzamine

(Ref: Harrison 20th p 2743; pg 2963, Harrison 19th p 2331)

- Preoperative patient preparation is essential for safe surgery. alpha-Adrenergic blockers (phenoxybenzamine) should be initiated at relatively low doses (e.g., 5–10 mg orally three times per day) and increased as tolerated every few days.
- Adequate alpha blockade generally requires 7 days, with a typical final dose of 20–30 mg phenoxybenzamine three times per day

154. Ans. (d) FNAC

(Ref: Harrison 19th p 2330)

This is a simple logical question where putting a needle in a tumor which is deep inside the medulla produces Catechamines which is like a volcano waiting to explode. Tests for Pheochromocytoma.

> Screening test: 24 hour urinary fractionated metanephrine levels
> - IOC: plasma total free metanephrine test
> - M.I.B.G scan is done to evaluate whether the tumour is an adrenal or and extra-adrenal tumour (located at Organ of Zuckerlandt)

155. Ans. (d) Hypocalcemia

(Ref: Harrison 20th p 2740; Harrison 19th p 2329)

- Phaeochromocytoma produces norepinephrine (80% cases) leading to hypertension but since the catecholamines act for short duration and are released in bursts abnormally, the BP increases for some hours a day referred to as episodic hypertension.
- This catecholamine excess in future will lead to a persistent vasoconstriction, referred to as volume contracted state. This explains the postural hypotension as well as the relative increase in packed cell volume in this patient.
- Episodes of palpitations, headaches, and profuse sweating are typical and constitute a classic triad. The presence of all three symptoms in association with hypertension makes pheochromocytoma a likely diagnosis. However, a pheochromocytoma can be asymptomatic for years, and some tumors grow to a considerable size before patients note symptoms.
- Hypercalcemia is seen with phaeochromocytoma. Parathyroid hormone-like peptide isolated from the tumour explains hypercalcaemia.

156. Ans. (a) Norepinephrine

(Ref: Harrison 20th p 2740; Harrison 19th p 2329)

- The major catecholamine secreted in a phaeochromocytoma is norepinephrine in 80% cases.
- The term paraganglioma is used to describe catecholamine-producing tumors in the head and neck. These tumors may secrete little or no catecholamines.
- If size of phaeochromocytoma is < 5cm, then the major catecholamine produced is epinephrine.
- If phaeochromocytoma is seen with MEN 2A, then the major catecholamine produced is epinephrine.

157. Ans. (b) Café au lait spots

(Ref: Harrison 20th p 2744; Harrison 19th p 2331)

- About 25–33% of patients with a pheochromocytoma or paraganglioma have an inherited syndrome.
- Neurofibromatosis type 1 (NF 1) was the first described pheochromocytoma-associated syndrome.
- The NF1 gene functions as a tumor suppressor by regulating the Ras signaling cascade. Classic features of neurofibromatosis include multiple neurofibromas, café au lait spots, axillary freckling of the skin, and Lisch nodules of the iris. Pheochromocytomas occur in only about 1% of these patients and are located predominantly in the adrenals.

158. Ans. (d) Weight gain

(Ref: Harrison 20th p 2740; Harrison 19th p 2329)

- Due to increased sympathomimetic stimulation, phaeochromocytoma has a weight loss.
- Phaeochromocytoma produces norepinephrine (80% cases) leading to hypertension but since the catecholamines act for short duration and are released in bursts abnormally, the BP increases for some hours a day referred to as episodic hypertension.
- This catecholamine excess in future will lead to a persistent vasoconstriction, referred as volume contracted state. This explains the postural hypotension

159. Ans. (d) MIBG

(Ref: Harrison 19th p 2331)

- The first line treatment for scintigraphically documented metastasis is ^{131}I-M.I.B.G in 100–300 mci doses over 3-6 cycles.
- Averbuch's chemotherapy protocol includes dacarbazine (600 mg/m^2 days 1 and 2), cyclophosphamide (750 mg/m^2 day 1), and vincristine (1.4 mg/m^2 day 1), repeated every 21 days for three to six cycles.

160. Ans. (b) Atenolol

(Ref: Harrison 20th p 2743; Harrison 19th p 2330)

- Beta blockers will lead to unopposed alpha action leading to worsening of pre-existing vasoconstriction in phaeochromocytoma.
- Thus the correct way to manage phaeochro-mocytoma patients is first initiate alpha blockade and then follow up with beta blockade.
- Meytrosine inhibits catecholamine production and is useful in malignant phaeochromocytoma.
- Adequate alpha blockade generally requires 7 days, with a typical final dose of 20–30 mg phenoxybenzamine three times per day. HTN crisis might require sodium nitroprusside.
- Oral prazosin or intravenous phentolamine can be used to manage paroxysms while awaiting adequate alpha blockade. Before surgery, blood pressure should be consistently below 160/90 mmHg, with moderate orthostasis. Beta blockers (e.g., 10 mg propranolol three to four times per day) can be added after starting alpha blockers and increased as needed if tachycardia persists. Other antihypertensives, such as calcium channel blockers or angiotensin-converting enzyme inhibitors, have been used when blood pressure is difficult to control with phenoxy-benzamine alone.

161. Ans. (b) Norepinephrine

(Ref: Harrison 20th p 2740; Harrison 19th p 2330 Cecil's essentials of medicine, E-book 8th/e pg 689)

162. Ans. (d) Wheezing

(Ref: Harrison 20th p 2740; Harrison 19th p 2330)

163. Ans. (c) Low cortisol level

(Ref: Harrison 20th p 2740; Harrison 19th p 2330)

Carcinoid Tumor and Syndrome

164. Ans. (a) 24 hour urinary 5H.I.A.A

(Ref: Harrison 20th p 604; Harrison 19th ed. / 564-65)

- 5-HIAA is the major urinary metabolite of serotonin, a ubiquitous bioactive amine. Serotonin, and consequently 5-HIAA, are produced in excess by most carcinoid tumors, especially those producing the carcinoid syndrome of flushing, hepatomegaly, diarrhea, bronchospasm, and heart disease.

165. Ans. (b) Serotonin

(Ref: Harrison 20th p 604; Harrison 19th ed./564-65)

- Argentaffin cells in Carcinoid produce 5HT derivatives like serotonin. Epinephrine and norepinephrine are produced by chromaffin cells which are seen in phaeochromocytoma.

166. Ans. (d) Kulchitsky Cell

(Ref: Harrison 20th p 603-4; Harrison 19th p 563)

Enterochromaffin (EC) cells, or "Kulchitsky cells", are a type of entero-endocrine and neuro-endocrine cell occurring in the epithelia lining the lumen of the digestive tract and the respiratory tract that release serotonin.

Lung NETs are classified into four categories:

- Typical carcinoid [also called bronchial carcinoid tumor, Kulchitsky cell carcinoma I (KCC-I)]
- Atypical carcinoid [also called well-differentiated neuroendocrine carcinoma (KC-II)],
- Intermediate small cell neuroendocrine carcinoma
- Small cell neuro-endocarcinoma

167. Ans. (b) Tricuspid valves

(Ref: Harrison 20th p 603; Harrison 19th p 564)

- Carcinoid syndrome is associated with development of valvular defects on the right side of the heart.
- The Mnemonic to be remembered is T.I.P.S= Tricuspid insufficiency and Pulmonic stenosis.
- The Dense fibrous deposits are seen on ventricular aspect of Tricuspid value and less commonly on cusps of pulmonary value.

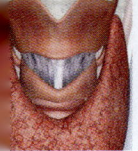

Prevalence of Heart disease in carcinoid syndrome

Tricuspid insufficiency	97%
Tricuspid stenosis	59%
Pulmonary insufficiency	50%
Pulmonary stenosis	25%
Left side lesion	11%

168. Ans. (a) Inflow tract of RV

(Ref: Harrison 20th p 603; Harrison 19th p 564)

The carcinoid syndrome occurs in approximately 5% of carcinoid tumors and becomes manifest when vasoactive substances from the tumors enter the systemic circulation escaping hepatic degradation. If the primary tumor is from the GI tract (hence releasing serotonin into the hepatic portal circulation), carcinoid syndrome generally does not occur until the disease is so advanced that it overwhelms the liver's ability to metabolize the released serotonin.

- *Secondary restrictive cardiomyopathy: About 50% of patients have cardiac abnormalities classically of the restrictive-type caused by serotonin-induced fibrosis of the valvular endocardium, notably the tricuspid and pulmonary valves, called cardiac fibrosis. This results in a heart with normal rhythm and contractility, but reduced preload and end-diastolic volume. "TIPS" is an acronym for Tricuspid Insufficiency, Pulmonary Stenosis (fibrosis of tricuspid and pulmonary valves*

169. Ans. (c) VMA in urine

(Ref: Harrison 20th p 603; Harrison 19th p 564)

- Vaniyl mandelic acid (V.M.A) is an end product of catecholamine metabolism and is used for screening for phaeochromocytoma.
- In carcinoid syndrome, the 5HT derivative bradykinin results in flushing episodes
- Neuroendocrine tumors along the GI tract use tryptophan as the source for serotonin production, which limits the available tryptophan for niacin synthesis. In normal patients, only one percent of dietary tryptophan is converted to serotonin; however, in patients with carcinoid syndrome, this value may increase to 70%. Carcinoid syndrome thus may produce Niacin deficiency and clinical manifestations of pellagra
- 5HT derivative histamine released by carcinoid causes bronchospasm and rhonchi.

Disorders of Thyroid Gland

170. Ans. (a) Myxedema coma

Ref: Harrison 20th edition, page 2702

- The past medical history of dry skin with constipation points to hypothyroidism. Patients of hypothyroidism can go into myxedema coma which presents with mild to moderate hypothermia with bradycardia and hypotension. A stressful event like infection, drugs, coronary event or CVA can trigger development of myxedema coma. Management is with levothyroxine and liothyronine intravenously.
- Both choices B and D will lead to tachycardia. Past medical history will have triggers for development of septic and cardiogenic shock respectively.

171. Ans. (b) Inadequate preoperative preparation

Ref: Harrison 20th ed, page 2707; SRB, 5th edition, page 494

Factors that trigger thyroid storm:
- Acute illness (Stroke, infection, trauma or DKA)
- Surgery (Inadequate preparation of patient)
- Radio-iodine treatment of partially treated or untreated hyperthyroidism.

Since the question mentions surgery hence the answer is inadequate preparation. It presents with worsening of thyrotoxicosis and fever, delirium, seizures, heart failure and jaundice. Death occurs due to heart failure, arrythmias or hyperthermia.

Burch-Wartofsky Point Scale for the Diagnosis of Thyroid Storm

Scores totaled
>45 Thyroid storm
25–44 Impending storm
<25 Storm unlikely

172. Ans. (b) Hyperthyroidism

(Ref: 76 e-16:Harrison 19th edition)

- The image shows presence of pre-tibial myxedema which is seen in hyperthyroidism. It is a non inflamed in durated plaque with orange skin appearance.
- Sarcoidosis will lead to skin involvement called as lupus pernio. It presents as violaceous plaques over nose, cheeks and ears.
- Diabetes mellitus leads to development of necrobiosis lipoidica diabeticorum. This is the closest choice in the question. It presents with lesions on the shin with *central yellow color*, transparency of skin, *telangiectasias* and red to red-brown border.

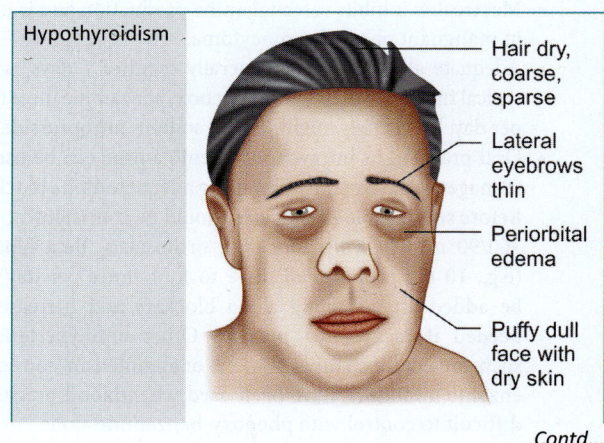

Contd...

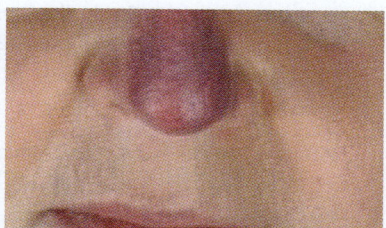
Sarcoidosis (lupus pernio)

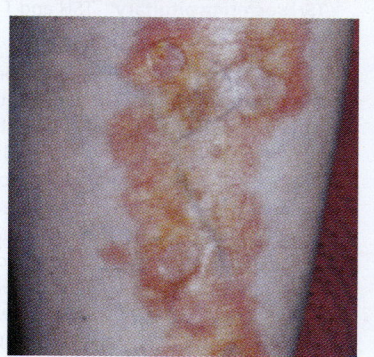
Diabetes (Necrobiosis lipoidica diabeticorum)

173. Ans. (a) Primary Hypothyroidism

(Ref: Harrison 20th p 2697; Harrison 19th edition, Page 2288)

High TSH is seen in:

1. Primary hypothyroidism due to feedback mechanism
2. Secondary thyrotoxicosis due to pituitary adenoma

Hypothyroidism will have low T4 and T3. Hence answer is choice A.
Hyperthyroidism will have increased T4 and T3. Hence choice B is ruled out.
Choice C: Subclinical hypothyroidism will have normal T4.
Choice D: Secondary hypothyroidism will have low TSH.

174. Ans. (a) Start anti-thyroid drugs, and do urgent MRI brain

(Ref: Harrison 20th p 2705; Harrison 19th edition, Page 2295-2296)

- The clinical setting of high TSH with tremors and diarrhea signifies hyperthyroidism due to either a TSH secreting pituitary tumor (secondary hyperthyroidism) or elevated TRH secretion from hypothalamus (tertiary hyperthyroidism).
- The presence of the catch in the MCQ "Bitemporal hemianopia" localizes the lesion to Pituitary mass compressing the optic chiasma.
- Hence, the diagnosis is most likely TSH secreting Pituitary Adenoma.
- A combination of trans-sphenoidal surgery, sella irradiation, and octreotide may be required to normalize TSH, because many of these tumors are large and locally invasive at the time of diagnosis.
- Radioiodine or anti-thyroid drugs can be used to control thyrotoxicosis.

175. Ans. (c) T3 increased, T4 increased, TSH decreased

(Ref: Harrison 20th p 2705)

The presentation given is of patient of Grave's disease and is characterised by supressed TSH and elevated T3, T4, FT3 and FT4.

176. Ans. (d) Hair loss

(Ref: Harrison 20th p 2703; Harrison 19th edition p 2290, 2292)

Hyperactivity	Due to increased BMR
Palpitations	Due to increased sympathomimetic activity by thyroid hormones
Diarrhea	Various reasons for diarrhea in thyrotoxicosis • Increased appetite and excessive fat-rich food intake may contribute to excessive fecal fat. • Moreover, diarrhea may be related to a hypersecretory state within the intestinal mucosa. • The adrenergic system may contribute to diarrhea as suggested by correction of transit in hyperthyroid patients treated with the β-adrenergic antagonist propranolol.

177. Ans. (c) Myasthenia Gravis

(Ref: Harrison 20th p 3237)

Disorders associated with Myaesthenia Gravis

Disorders of the thymus: Thymoma, thymic hyperplasia
Other autoimmune disorders: Hashimoto's thyroiditis, Graves' disease, rheumatoid arthritis, lupus erythematosus, skin disorders, family history of autoimmune disorder
Disorders or circumstances that may exacerbate myasthenia gravis: hyperthyroidism or hypothyroidism, occult infection, medical treatment for other conditions
Disorders that may interfere with therapy: tuberculosis, diabetes, peptic ulcer, gastrointestinal bleeding, renal disease, hypertension, asthma, osteoporosis, obesity

178. Ans. (d) Weight gain

(Ref: Harrison 20th p 2703; Harrison 19th ed. / 152)

- T3 and T4 have sympatho-mimetic activity and they affect basal metabolic rate. Hence in thyrotoxicosis the increase in BMR will lead to weight loss. The sympatho-mimetic activity leads to anxiety palpitations and tachycardia.

179. Ans. (b) Excessive iodine

(Ref: Harrison 20th p 2710; Harrison 19th ed. / 2285, 2297)

- Excess iodide transiently inhibits thyroid iodide organification, a phenomenon known as the *Wolff-Chaikoff effect*
- Thyroid hormone synthesis becomes excessive as a result of increased iodine exposure (Jod-Basedow phenomenon which is opposite of Wolf Chaikoff effect.)
- Iodine deficiency increases thyroid blood flow and upregulates the iodine trapping, stimulating more efficient iodine uptake.
- Ingestion of excess thyroid hormone or thyroid tissue is known as thyrotoxicosis factitia. In the first and second statements of this explanation iodine intake was affected but in Throtoxicosis factitia is due to the ingestion of hormone.

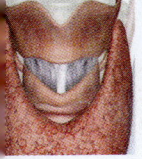

180. Ans. (d) Menorrhagia

(Ref: Harrison 20th p 2703; Harrison 19th ed. / 2293)

- Thyrotoxicosis is characterized by increased sympathomimetic action causing palpitations, anxiety and increased BMR causing weight loss. The menstrual abnormality in Grave's disease is oligo-menorrhea.
- **Remember:** Weight gain with menorrhagia is seen in hypothyroidism. Weight gain with hirusutism with oligomenorrhea is seen in Cushing syndrome.

181. Ans. (d) Hypothyroidism

(Ref: Harrison 20th p 2704, 189; Harrison 19th ed. / 2289)

Choices	Logic
Primary thyrotoxicosis	Cytokines appear to play a major role in thyroid-associated ophthalmopathy. There is infiltration of the extraocular muscles by activated T cells; the release of cytokines such as IFN-alpha and TNF results in fibroblast activation and increased synthesis of glycosaminoglycans that trap water, thereby leading to characteristic muscle swelling.
Sarcoidosis	Approximately 20% of patients with ophthalmic findings of sarcoid have soft tissue involvement of the orbit or lacrimal gland and present as a mass lesion with proptosis, ptosis, or ophthalmoplegia.
Pituitary adenoma	Pituitary adenoma if a Macroadenoma is associated with pituitary apoplexy and can lead to Proptosis.

182. Ans. (d) EEG is normal

(Ref: Harrison 20th p 2700; Harrison 19th p 2291)

- Hashimoto encephalopathy is included in differential diagnosis of any neuro-psychiatric illness not responding to conventional management. Though there is no shared antigen between the brain and thyroid gland but manifestations occur due to overtly aggressive immune system.
- The patients of hashimoto thyroiditis will develop myoclonus, seizures, psychosis.
- Electroencephalography is abnormal in more than 90% of cases. Typically, the EEG shows nonspecific, intermittent slow wave activity.
- CSF abnormalities in form elevated protein but normal glucose is seen
- Mainstay of treatment is methylprednisolone iv and then oral.

183. Ans. (a) Steroids

(Ref: Harrison 20th p 2700; Harrison 19th p 2291)

184. Ans. (d) Primary hypothyroidism

(Ref: Harrison 20th p 2697, 2699; Harrison 19th p 2287, 2292)

The clinical picture of short stature with low T4 and elevated TSH suggests primary hypothyroidism. *The enlarged pituitary can be explained by the feedback provided by low T4 in the blood. Many hypothyroid women develop galactorrhea due to pituitary enlargement.*

Now we will rule out other choices

Pituitary adenoma	Can produce any hormone and if it produces TSH, then T_4 should be elevated
TSH secreting pituitary tumor	TSH and T_4 both should be elevated
Thyroid target receptor insensitivity	<ul><li>Autosomal dominant disorder insensitivity</li><li>Characterized by elevated thyroid hormone levels and inappropriately normal or elevated TSH.</li><li>*Individuals with resistance to thyroid hormone do not, in general, exhibit signs and symptoms that are typical of hypothyroidism because hormone resistance is partial and is compensated by increased levels of thyroid hormone.*</li><li>The clinical features of RTH can include goiter, attention deficit disorder, mild reduction in IQ, delayed skeletal maturation.</li></ul>

185. Ans. (c) 0.004 mU/L

(Ref: Harrison 20th p 2697; Harrison 19th p 2288)

Extremely sensitive assays can detect TSH levels upto 0.004 mU/L.

186. Ans. (b) Jod-Basedow effect

(Ref: Harrison 20th p 2710; Harrison 19th p 2300)

- The Jod-Basedow effect is hyperthyroidism following administration of iodine or iodide, either as a dietary supplement or as contrast medium.
- This phenomenon is an iodine-induced hyper-thyroidism, due to increase in process of iodine trapping due to increased availability of daily iodine in micro-dosages over a large number of years
- In contrast Wolf Chaikoff effect is hypothyroidism due to decrease in iodine trapping due exposure to mega dosages of iodine in blood circulation.

Effect	Basis	Iodine Trapping	Net Result
Jod Basedow effect	Exposure to micro dosages of iodine over large number of years	Increases iodine trapping	Resulting in thyrotoxicosis
Wolf Chaikoff effect	Exposure to mega dosages of iodine over few weeks	Decreases iodine trapping	Resulting in hypothyroidism

187. Ans. (b) Treatment is done by monitoring to TSH level in plasma

(Ref: Harrison 20th p 2701)

- **Choice A:** Craniopharyngiome can expand an lead to central hypothyroidism.
- **Choice B:** is wrong as TSH is already low and can never normalize since pituitary is already damaged.
- TSH levels may be normal, reduced or even increased in secondary hypothyroidism. The is due to secretion of *immunoactive, bioinactive forms of TSH*. Hence choice C is correct.
- Adrenal insufficiency is always addressed first

188. Ans. (d) All of above

(Ref: Harrison 20th p 2707; Harrison 19th p 2265)

Causes of thyroid storm are:

- Sepsis
- Surgery
- Anesthesia induction
- Radioactive iodine (RAI) therapy
- Drugs (anticholinergic and adrenergic drugs such as pseudoephedrine; salicylates; non-steroidal anti-inflammatory drugs [NSAIDs]; chemotherapy) and iodinated contrast agent
- Excessive thyroid hormone (TH) ingestion
- Withdrawal of or noncompliance with anti-thyroid medications
- Diabetic ketoacidosis
- Direct trauma to the thyroid gland
- Vigorous palpation of an enlarged thyroid
- Toxemia of pregnancy and labor in older adolescents; molar pregnancy

189. Ans. (b) Acromegaly

(Ref: Harrison 20th p 2678; Harrison 19th p 2269)

- Heel pad thickness greater than 23 mm may indicate acromegaly. The overabundance of growth hormone in acromegaly causes, among other things, gradual enlargement of hands, feet, and exaggeration of facial features. Not limited to the bones, however, enlargement of other parts of the body, such as the soft tissues of the heel may help to diagnose acromegaly.

190. Ans. (d) Thromboembolism

(Ref: Harrison 20th p 2699; Harrison 19th p 2290)

- In hypothyroidism the weight gain is usually modest and due mainly to fluid retention in the myxedematous tissues.
- Libido is decreased in both sexes, and there may be oligomenorrhea or amenorrhea in long-standing disease, but menorrhagia is also common.
- Fertility is reduced, and the incidence of miscarriage is increased.
- Prolactin levels are often modestly increased and may contribute to alterations in libido and fertility and cause Galactorrhea.

191. Ans. (a) Retrosternal goiter

(Ref: Harrison 20th p 2711; Harrison 19th p 2301)

Pemberton's sign refers to symptoms of pre-syncope with evidence of facial congestion and external jugular venous obstruction when the arms are raised above the head, a maneuver that draws the thyroid into the thoracic inlet in case of a large retrosternal goiter.

192. Ans. (b) Hypothyroidism

(Ref: *William's Endo.* pg. 410)

Causes of Reversible dementia

1. Hypothyroidism
2. Normal pressure hydrocephalus
3. Depression
4. Drugs
5. Alcohol
6. Vitamin B_{12} deficiency

193. Ans. (b) Type III hyperlipoproteinemia

(Ref: Harrison 19th p 2291)

- In hypothyroidism, Massive Pericardial effusion is seen but since it develops over large period of time, pulsus paradoxus is absent. Coronary atherosclerosis is seen due to increased serum cholesterol and warrants a need for statins.
- Type III hyperlipo-proteinemia is due to high chylomicrons and IDL (intermediate density lipoprotein). It is also known as dysbetalipoproteinemia, the most common cause for this form is the presence of ApoE E2/E2 genotype. It is due to cholesterol-rich VLDL (β-VLDL).
  - The receptor defect causes levels of chylomicron remnants and IDL to be higher than normal in the blood stream.

194. Ans. (b) Secondary hypothyroidism

(Ref: Harrison 20th p 2701; Harrison 19th p 2288)

- In choices A,C,D all imply primary hypothyroidism where the defect lies at the level of the gland and the pituitary is normal. Hence in these patients TSH is elevated, and when levothyroxine will be started in these patients the levels of TSH will start coming back to normal.
- In contrast, in secondary hypothyroidism the pituitary is defective and produces less TSH leading to Low T_3 and T_4. Even after starting these patients on levothyroxine, though T_3 and T_4 will normalize, the TSH values will be unaffected due to defective pituitary.
- Thyroprivic hypothyroidism is another term for primary hypothyroidism.
- Trophoprivic hypothyroidism is another term for secondary hypothyroidism

195. Ans. (b) Atrial fibrillation

(Ref: Harrison 20th p 2704; Harrison 19th p 2294)

CVS finding in thyrotoxicosis

- The most common cardiovascular manifestation is sinus tachycardia, often associated with palpitations, occasionally caused by supra-ventricular tachycardia. *Atrial fibrillation is seen in patients > 50 years.*

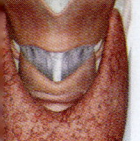

- The high cardiac output produces a bounding pulse, widened pulse pressure and Aortic systolic murmur
- Pleuro-pericardial scratch or Means Lerman scratch results from the rubbing of the pericardium against the pleura in the context of hyperdynamic circulation and tachycardia

196. Ans. (a) 100 mcg

(Ref: Harrison 20th p 2701; Harrison 19th p 2292)

Levothyroxine supplementation guidelines:
- Usual initial dose: 12.5-25 mcg PO qDay
- May adjust dose by 12.5-25 mcg q4-6weeks until patient becomes euthyroid and serum TSH concentration is normalized; adjustments q6-8 weeks also used
- Dose range: 100-125 mcg PO qDay

197. Ans. (b) Gradual warming

(Ref: Harrison 20th p 2707; Harrison 19th p 2297)

The patient is in thyroid storm and is having hyperthermia. Ice packs/cooling will reduce metabolic stress.

Management of thyroid storm

1. High-dose propylthiouracil (PTU) is preferred because of its early onset of action and capacity to inhibit peripheral conversion of T_4 to T_3
2. Administer iodine compounds (Lugol iodine or potassium iodide) orally or via a nasogastric tube to block the release of THs (at least 1 h after starting antithyroid drug therapy). If available, intravenous radiocontrast dyes such as ipodate and iopanoate can be effective in this regard. These agents are particularly effective in preventing peripheral conversion of T_4 to T_3.
3. Administer glucocorticoids to decrease peripheral conversion of T_4 to T_3. This may also be useful in preventing relative adrenal insufficiency due to hyperthyroidism.
4. Dextrose solutions are the preferred intravenous fluids to cope with continuously high metabolic demand

198. Ans. (a) Low T_3 with normal T_4

(Ref: Harrison 20th p 2709; Harrison 19th p 2299)

- The most common hormone pattern in *sick Euthyroid syndrome* is a decrease in total and unbound T_3 levels (low T_3 syndrome) with normal levels of T_4 and TSH.
- The magnitude of the fall in T_3 correlates with the severity of the illness. T_4 conversion to T_3 via peripheral deiodination is impaired, leading to increased reverse T_3 (rT_3).
- Despite this effect, decreased clearance rather than increased production is the major basis for increased rT_3. Also, T_4 is alternately metabolized to the hormonally inactive T_3 sulfate. It is generally assumed that this low T_3 state is adaptive, because it can be induced in normal individuals by fasting.

199. Ans. (c) Hypotension

(Ref: Harrison 20th p 2699; Harrison 19th p 2291)

Patients of hypothyroidism exhibit hypertension due to increased peripheral resistance secondary to increase in weight and myxedema. Myxedema characterized by deposition of GAG explains the weight gain as well as coarse dry skin. Bradycardia is seen in hypothyroidism patients with low voltage ECG.

200. Ans. (b) Follicular

(Ref: Harrison 20th p 2715; Harrison 19th p 2305)

- Follicular Thyroid Cancer tends to spread by hematogenous routes leading to bone, lung, and central nervous system metastases.
- The reason for high vascularity of metastatic lesion with thyroid carcinoma is postulated as an increase in vascular endothelial growth factor (VEGF) or V.E.G.F receptor expression by tumour tissue particularly in papillary and follicular thyroid carcinoma.
- The treatment for osseous metastases with thyroid carcinoma include I-131 radioablation localised resection and sometimes radiotherapy.

201. Ans. (d) All of the above

(Ref: Harrison 19th p 2293)

- Levothyroxine is given as a iv bolus dose followed by daily oral dose since conversion of T_4 into T_3 is impaired.
- Patients presenting with myxedema coma/crisis may have adrenal insufficiency, and stress doses of IV steroids must be administered along with initial thyroid replacement until adrenal function has been determined to be normal.

202. Ans. (b) Frequent blinking

(Ref: Harrison 20th p 2704; Harrison 19th p 2294)

- In thyrotoxicosis the increase in sympathetic activity due to increased T_3 and T_4 leads to *contraction of Muller's muscle*. These patients hence would have *infrequent blinking* and infact some of them might sleep with their eyes open leading to corneal erosions.
- Lid retraction, causing a staring appearance, can occur in any form of thyrotoxicosis and is the result of sympathetic overactivity. However, Graves' disease is associated with specific eye signs that comprise Graves' ophthalmopathy.
- The earliest manifestations of ophthalmopathy are usually a sensation of grittiness, eye discomfort, and excess tearing.
- The most serious manifestation is compression of the optic nerve at the apex of the orbit, leading to papilledema; peripheral field defects; and, if left untreated, permanent loss of vision

203. Ans. (d) High radio iodine uptake

(Ref: Harrison 20th p 2708; Harrison 19th p 2299)

- The patient usually presents with a painful and enlarged thyroid, sometimes accompanied by fever. There may be features of thyrotoxicosis or hypothyroidism, depending on the phase of the illness.
- The patient typically complains of a sore throat, and examination reveals a small goiter that is exquisitely tender. Pain is often referred to the jaw or ear.
- The patient characteristically evolves through three distinct phases over about 6 months: (1) thyrotoxic phase, (2) hypothyroid phase, and (3) recovery phase.

- In the thyrotoxic phase, T_4 and T_3 levels are increased, reflecting their discharge from the damaged thyroid cells, and TSH is suppressed.
- The T_4/T_3 ratio is greater than in Graves' disease or thyroid autonomy, in which T_3 is often disproportionately increased.
- The diagnosis is confirmed by a high ESR and low radioiodine uptake

204. Ans. (b) Increased

(Ref: Harrison 20th p 2698; Harrison 19th p 2288)

Causes of increased uptake in Radioactive iodine include the following

- Hyperthyroidism
- Iodine deficiency
- Pregnancy
- Recovery phase of subacute, silent, or postpartum thyroiditis (Not illness phase of subacute thyroiditis)
- Rebound after withdrawal of antithyroid medication
- Lithium carbonate therapy
- Hashimoto thyroiditis

205. Ans. (a) Hypothyroidism

(Ref: Harrison 20th p 2699; Harrison 19th p 2291)

Myxedema of the Achilles tendon leads to delayed relaxation of ankle jerk and is called hung up ankle jerk.

206. Ans. (d) Pretibial myxedema

(Ref: Harrison 20th p 2699; Harrison 19th p 2291)

- Pretibial myxedema is a feature of thyrotoxicosis.
- Decrease in BMR will lead to cold intolerance.
- Deafness is seen with congenital hypothyroidism.
- Pericardial effusions are seen with myxedema heart.

207. Ans. (a) Hashimoto's thyroiditis

(Ref: Harrison 20th p 2699; Harrison 19th p 2290)

- *Thyroprivic hypothyroidism* is another term for primary hypothyroidism.
- *Trophoprivic hypothyroidism* is another term for secondary hypothyroidism.
- The question mentions goitrous hypothyroidism where the gland is increased in size and is a result of iodine deficiency, dyshormonogenesis. Both these are causes of primary hypothyroidism which is also known as thyroprivic hypothyroidism.

Hypothyroidism phase in Hashimoto thyroiditis is usually insidious in onset, with signs and symptoms slowly progressing over months to years. The presentation of patients with hypo-thyroidism may be subclinical, without any symptoms, and may be found simply from routine screening of thyroid function. The usual finding is an elevated TSH level. The early compensatory increase in TSH tends to maintain a nearly normal thyroid function and keeps the patient in a euthyroid state.

208. Ans. (d) Galactorrhoea

(Ref: Harrison 20th p 2700; Harrison 19th p 2291)

In primary hypothyroidism, the feedback leads to increased production of TRH. The increased TRH stimulates the lactotrophs in anterior pituitary to cause production of prolactin and hence galactorrhea.

209. Ans. (a) Beta hCG from placenta

(Ref: Harrison 20th p 2694; Thyroid function in pregnancy, Harrison 19th p 2300)

- β-hCG, is capable of stimulating TSH receptor.
- The rise in circulating hCG levels during the first trimester is accompanied by a reciprocal fall in TSH that persists into the middle of pregnancy.
- Human chorionic gonadotropin-induced changes in thyroid function can result in transient gestational hyperthyroidism. Antithyroid drugs are rarely needed, and parenteral fluid replacement usually suffices until the condition resolves.

210. Ans. (c) Osteomalacia

(Ref: Oxford text book of rheumatology 4th ed. pg 1254, by R.A watts)

Radiological features of osteomalacia is A.D.U.L.T

Acetabuli protrusio
Decreased bone density
Under mineralization of osteoid
Looser's zone (pseudofracture)
Triradiate pelvis (females)

211. Ans. (a) TSH

(Ref: Harrison 20th p 2697; Harrison 19th p 2288)

- The enhanced sensitivity and specificity of TSH assays have greatly improved laboratory assessment of thyroid function.
- Because TSH levels change dynamically in response to alterations of T4 and T3, a logical approach to thyroid testing is to first determine whether TSH is suppressed, normal, or elevated.
- With rare exceptions, a normal TSH level excludes a primary abnormality of thyroid function.
- This strategy depends on the use of immuno-cheluminometric assays (ICMAs) for TSH that are sensitive enough to discriminate between the lower limit of the reference range and the suppressed values that occur with thyrotoxicosis. Extremely sensitive assays can detect TSH levels 0.004 mU/L, but, for practical purposes, assays sensitive to 0.1 mU/L are sufficient

212. Ans. (b) Hypokalemic periodic paralysis

(Ref: Harrison 20th p 3251, 305; Harrison 19th p 444e)

- Thyrotoxicosis periodic paralyses (TPP) are the most common secondary hypokalemic PP.
- T.P.P is most common in adults aged 20-40 years.
- Hyper-insulinemia, a carbohydrate load, and exercise are responsible for in precipitating paralytic attacks.
- The hypokelemia occurs due to direct and indirect activation of Na-K ATPase by thyroid hormones leading to K^+ influx into the muscles.

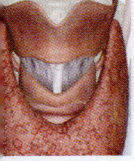

213. Ans. (c) *Anxiety neurosis*

(Ref: Harrison 20th p 2704; Harrison 19th p 2294)

- Hyperthyrodism features include hyperactivity, nervousness, and irritability, ultimately leading to a sense of easy fatigability in some patients. Insomnia and impaired concentration are common leading to anxiety neurosis like presentation.
- Apathetic thyrotoxicosis may be mistaken for depression in the elderly. Fine tremor is a frequent finding, best elicited by having patients stretch out their fingers while feeling the fingertips with the palm.

214. Ans. (a) *Hashimoto's Thyroiditis*

(Ref: Harrison 20th p 2698; Harrison 19th p 2290)

215. Ans. (a) *Diastolic murmur*

(Ref: Harrison 20th p 2704; Harrison 19th p 2294)

216. Ans. (a) *Thyrotoxicosis*

(Ref: Kundu 3rd/357; MRCP Paces handbook page 133)

217. Ans. (a) *Surgery for thyroiditis*

(Ref: Harrison 20th p 2707; Bailey and Love 24th/796; Harrison 19th p 2297)

218. Ans. (c) *Hashimoto's Thyroiditis*

(Ref: Harrison 20th p 2699; Harrison 19th p 2290)

219. Ans. (c) *Increased radioactive Iodine uptake*

(Ref: Harrison 20th p 2698; Harrison 19th 2298)

220. Ans. (b) *Hashimoto's Thyroiditis*

(Ref: Harrison 20th p 2699; Bailey 24th/803, 804, Harrison 19th p 2298)

221. Ans. (b) *Diffuse Goiter*

(Ref: Bailey & Love 22nd / 511; Robbins 6th / 1138)

222. Ans. (a) *Medullary Carcinoma thyroid*

(Ref: Harrison 20th p 2717; Harrison 19th p 2305)

223. Ans. (a) *Serum Calcitonin*

(Ref: Harrison 20th p 2717; Bailey 24th/801, 802, Harrison 19th p 2305-06)

Disorders of Parathyroid Gland and Calcium Metabolism

224. Ans. (a) *Sestamibi scan*

(Ref: Harrison 20th p 2928; Harrison 19th edition, page 2474)

- PTH action on bone will lead to bone resorption and resultant hypercalcemia can be life threatening.
- The leading cause of hyperparathyroidism is *parathyroid adenoma*.
- Hence minimally invasive approach to remove parathyroid adenoma is warranted.
- Pre-operative 99mTc Sestamibi scan with single photon emission CT can be used to predict the location of abnormal gland and intra-operative sampling.
- Rapid fall of PTH values (>50%) after removal of adenoma indicates successful surgery.
- The question also describes the traditional presentation of primary hyperparathyroidism: abdominal groans, psychic moans and renal stones (not described in the question).

225. Ans. (a) *IV Fluids and Diuretics*

(Ref: Harrison 20th p 2935; Harrison: 19th edition, Page 610)

- The patient is having acute hypercalcemia crisis which can lead to development of systolic arrest of the heart. Hence it is imperative to reduce serum calcium of the patient with administration of normal saline and subsequently furosemide drip.
- Normal saline will cause hydration and once the rehydration is complete then initiate furosemide drip. This will lead to urinary loss of calcium.
- Subsequently bisphosphonates and intranasal calcitonin are given. In case of renal shut down haemodialysis is required.

226. Ans. (a) *IV Fluid*

(Ref: Harrison 20th p 2935; Harrison: 19th edition, Page 610)

Refer to the explanation of the above question

227. Ans. (a) *PQR = UWY*

(Ref: Harrison 20th p 2927)

Fatty, fertile female of forty = Cholelithiasis	Incidence of gall stones is higher in women with obesity being a risk factor. The presence of concomitant insulin resistance and type 2 diabetes mellitus increases the risk. Presence of hypertriglyceridemia in syndrome X impairs gall bladder motility.
Stones, bones, abdominal groans and psychic moans= Primary hyperparathyroidism	Increased serum PTH in hyperparathyroidism leads to: • Calcium oxalate nephrocalcinosis= Stones • Increased PTH increases bone resorption= Bone pain • Constipation= abdominal pain • Neuropsychiatric manifestation like insomnia, irritability and depression= psychic moans
They pant their way into old age= Bronchial asthma	Adult onset intrinsic asthma worsens with age whereas the paediatric onset extrinsic asthma will improve with age.

228. Ans. (c) *Trousseau's sign*

(Ref: Harrison 20th p 314; Harrison 19th Edition, Page 315)

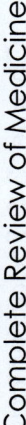

The image shows presence of trousseau sign/Carpo-pedal spasm seen in patients of Hypocalcemia.

Chvostek sign	Elicited by tapping over anterior border of parotid gland and seen in tetany
Troisier Sign	Left supraclavicular lymphadenopathy in metastatic abdominal malignancy
Lhermitte's sign	The Barber chair phenomenon is the name which describes an electric shock-like sensation that occurs on flexion of the neck. This sensation radiates down the spine, often into the legs, arms, and sometimes to the trunk

229. Ans. (c) Primary hyperparathyroidism

(Ref: Harrison 20th p 2930, 2932; Harrison 19th edition, page 2470-2472)

Milk alkali syndrome	Occurs due to *excessive ingestion of calcium and absorbable antacids* such as milk or calcium carbonate.
Hyper-vita-minosis D	Occurs with *Chronic ingestion of 40–100 times the normal physiologic requirement of vitamin D* (amounts >40,000–100,000 U/d) is usually required to produce significant hypercalcemia in normal individuals. In the question since there is no history of intake of any supplements this choice is ruled out. For treatment of Hyper-vitaminosis, however hydrocortisone is used.
Primary hyper-parathyroidism	• PTH increase will lead to increase in serum calcium • This calcium is deposited in blood vessels leading to hardening of blood vessels and resultant hypertension • In MEN 1 patients with hyperparathyroidism, duodenal ulcer may be the result of associated pancreatic tumors that secrete excessive quantities of gastrin (Zollinger-Ellison syndrome) • Increase calcium deposition in kidney tubules explains nephrocalcinosis
Tubulo-interstitial renal disease	Leads to salt wasting and polyuria with Fanconi's syndrome.

230. Ans. (c) Glucocorticoids

(Ref: Harrison 20th p 2935; Harrison 19th edition Page 2480-82)

- Glucocorticoids are used in management of hypercalcemia due to sarcoidosis, vitamin D intoxication, vitamin A application.

Management of dangerous hypercalcemia

1. Hydration with saline
2. Saline can be administered with furosemide and can be given twice daily to depress the tubular reabsorptive mechanism for calcium (Avoid dehydration or it will worsen hypercalcemia).
3. IV use of pamidronate and zolendronate is approved for the treatment of hypercalcemia; between 30 and 90 mg pamidronate, given as a single IV dose over a few hours, returns serum calcium to normal within 24–48 hours with an effect that lasts for weeks in 80–100% of patients.
4. Calcitonin nasal spray for its rapid onset of action.

231. Ans. (c) Paget's disease

(Ref: Rheumatology secrets page 401, chapter 53, 3rd edition)

Osteoporosis	Decreased bone density can be appreciated by decreased cortical thickness, loss of bony trabecula on X ray.
Thalassemia	• Squaring of metacarpal bones • Crew cut appearance
Paget disease	• The blade of grass sign is characteristic of Paget disease of bone. • Early in the disease course, the area of osteolysis that occurs in the diaphysis of the tibia or femur appears wedge-shaped and produces the blade of grass sign. • When there is calvarial involvement, the area of osteolysis appears more rounded and is termed osteoporosis circumscripta 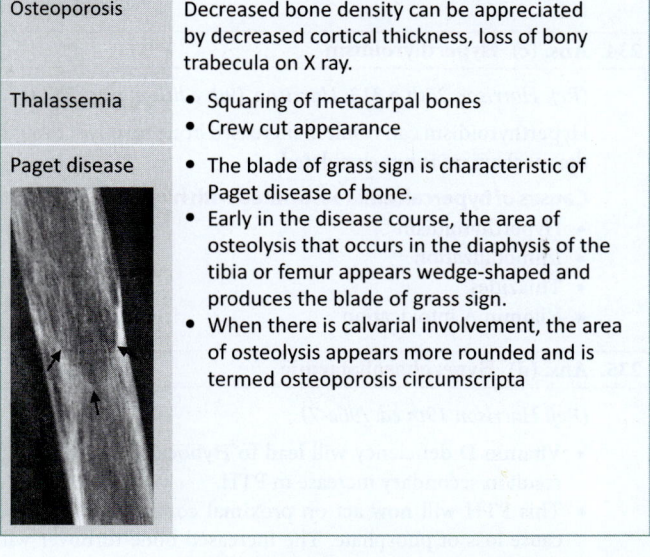

232. Ans. (d) Celiac Disease

(Ref: Harrison 20th p 313, 2930, 2932; Harrison 19th edition, page 2469)

- Hyperparathyroidism leads to increased bone resorption and leads to hypercalcemia.
- The non caseating granulomas in Sarcoidosis lead to increased Vitamin D3 synthesis. This increased GI absorption of calcium and explains the hypercalcemia.
- The milk-alkali syndrome is due to excessive ingestion of calcium and absorbable antacids such as milk or calcium carbonate. It is much less frequent since proton-pump inhibitors and other treatments became available for peptic ulcer disease.
- Recently the use of calcium carbonate in the management of secondary hyperparathyroidism led to reappearance of the syndrome which features hypercalcemia, alkalosis, and renal failure. The chronic form of the disease, termed *Burnett's syndrome*, is associated with irreversible renal damage

233. Ans. (c) Hypoparathyroidism

(Ref: Harrison 20th p 2947; Harrison 19th edition, Page 2489)

- In sarcoidosis the osteoporosis process is usually due to use of steroids. This means choice a and choice c are correct.
- Osteoporosis occurs more frequently with increasing age as bone tissue is lost progressively.
- In women, the loss of ovarian function at menopause (typically about age 50) precipitates rapid bone loss.

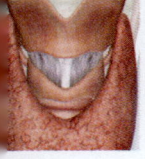

Endocrine disorders leading to osteoporosis and asked in various examinations

- Acromegaly
- Adrenal insufficiency
- Cushing's syndrome
- *Hyperparathyroidism*
- Thyrotoxicosis
- Type 1 diabetes mellitus

234. Ans. (c) Hyperthyroidism

(Ref: Harrison 20th p 313; Harrison 19th edition, page 2478)

Hyperthyroidism can result in increased bone turnover though the mechanism is not elucidated.

Causes of hypercalcemia associated with high bone turnover
- Hyperthyroidism
- Immobilization
- Thiazides
- Vitamin A intoxication

235. Ans. (d) Hyperphosphataemia

(Ref: Harrison 19th ed. /96e-7)

- Vitamin D deficiency will lead to Hypocalcemia. This will result in secondary increase in PTH.
- This PTH will now act on proximal convoluted tubule to cause loss of phosphate. The increased bone turnover will cause increase in serum alkaline phosphate.
- Important calcium/phosphate and SAP fluctuations which are asked.

Condition	Rickets	Hyper-parathyroidism	Osteoporosis	Paget Disease	Chronic Renal Failure
Serum calcium	Less	Increased	Normal	Normal	Less
Serum phosphate	Less	Less	Normal	Normal	Increased
SAP	Increased	Increased	Normal	Disproportionate Increased	Increased
PTH	Increasing	Increased	normal	normal	Increased

236. Ans. (a) Hypophosphatemia

Refer to above table

237. Ans. (c) Diarrhea

(Ref: Harrison 20th p 2927; Harrison 19th ed. / 2342)

- Hyperparathyroidism leads to increase PTH. PTH increases serum calcium by increasing dietary absorption of vitamin D3. It also ensures that the proximal convoluted tubule start loosing phosphate in urine leading to decreased serum phosphate.
- The increase serum calcium leads to deposition in kidney parenchyma forming calcium phosphate stones. The increased level of calcium also leads to constipation. Therefore abdominal pain are a feature of hyperparathyroidism. Renal Colic is due to stones and severe constipation. Diarrhea is not seen with hypercalcemia/hyperparathyroidism.

238. Ans. (d) Milk alkali syndrome

(Ref: Harrison 20th p 2933; Harrison 19th p 2479)

- The milk-alkali syndrome is due to excessive ingestion of calcium and absorbable antacids such as milk or calcium carbonate.
- The chronic form of the disease, termed Burnett's syndrome, is associated with irreversible renal damage. The acute syndromes reverse if the excess calcium and absorbable alkali are stopped.
- Calcium absorption is completed within 4 hours of intake. Avid absorption of large doses may lead to suppression of parathyroid hormone (PTH), which then leads to enhanced bicarbonate retention by the kidney.

239. Ans. (a) Hyperparathyroidism

(Ref: Harrison 19th p 2472)

- The distinctive bone manifestation of hyperparathyroidism is osteitis cystica fibrosa, which Histologically, shows and increase in the giant multinucleated osteoclasts in scalloped areas on the surface of the bone (Howship's lacunae) and a replacement of the normal cellular and marrow elements by fibrous tissue.
- X-ray changes include resorption of the phalangeal tufts and replacement of the usually sharp cortical outline of the bone in the digits by an irregular outline (subperiosteal resorption).

240. Ans. (c) Thyroid malignancy

(Ref: Harrison 20th p 2925; Harrison 19th p 2472)

Hyperparathyroidism is usually due to a solitary adenoma. It can also be due to MEN Type 1 which accounts for about 90% of parathyroid cancers which do not include thyroid malignancies in the group of the multiple endocrine neoplasms. Parathyroid hyperplasia can also lead to hyperparathyroidism.

241. Ans. (b) The unionized fraction of calcium in the plasma is an important determinant of PTH Secretion

(Ref: Ganong's Review of Medical Physiology'; 25th ed., page 379-380)

- *Circulating ionized calcium acts directly on the parathyroid glands in a negative feedback fashion to regulate the secretion of PTH.* The key to this regulation is a cell membrane Ca^{2+} receptor. This receptor is coupled via a G protein to phosphoinositol turnover and is found in many tissues. In the parathyroid, its activation inhibits PTH secretion.
- Parathyroid hormone-related protein is responsible for causing hypercalcemia in cancer patients. The hypercalcemia in the remaining 80% is due to the elevated circulating levels of parathyroid hormone-related protein or PTHrP (humoral hyper calcemia of malignancy). The tumors responsible for the hypersecretion include cancers of the breast, kidney, ovary and skin.
- Magnesium is required to maintain normal para-thyroid secretory responses. Impaired PTH release along with

diminished target responses to PTH, account for the hypocalcemia that occasionally occurs in magnesium deficiency.

242. Ans. (d) Williams' syndrome is characterized by precocious puberty, mental retardation and Obesity

(Ref: Harrison 20th p 2932; Harrison 19th p 2477)

- William syndrome is due to defect on chromosome 7 and is characterized by child with failure to thrive, elfin facies, Supra-valvular aortic stenosis and idiopathic hypercalcemia.
- Mental retardation and precocious puberty given in choice D is seen in William syndrome but not a characteristic feature. Obesity is not seen and all children exhibit ELFIN FACIES.
- Choices A and B are very logical on synthesis of vitamin D active metabolite in the kidney.
- Some Studies recommend 15 µg/day (600IU) while other have estimated that 12.5 µg/day (500 IU) is sufficient in the absence of sunlight. According to Park 21st ed Daily requirement of vitamin D is:

Adults	2.5 mcg or 100 IU
Infants and children	5.0 mcg or 200 IU
Pregnancy and lactation	10.0 mcg or 400 IU

243. Ans. (b) X-ray

(Ref: Harrison 20th p 2955; Harrison 19th p 2501)

Atypical femoral fracture in subtrochanteric femoral region or across femoral shaft are side effects of prolonged bisphosphonate use.

In this question patient is complaining of pain in right hip and thigh. Thus differential diagnosis of the patient can be
1. Fracture of neck of femur or shaft of femur.
2. Chronic pain probably not bony in origin; instead, it is related to abnormal strain on muscles, ligaments, and tendons and to secondary facet-joint arthritis associated with alterations in thoracic and/or abdominal shape.
3. Lumbar spinal canal stenosis resulting in nerve compression
   - Fracture neck of femur is the first differential and requires evaluation by X-RAY.

244. Ans. (b) Hyperparathyroidism

(Ref: Pg 66, Radiology secrets, E-book, 4th edition)

Radiological feature in X-ray hand of hyperparathyroidism
There is sub-periosteal resorption along the radial aspects of the middle phalanges of the index, middle and ring fingers, a finding virtually pathognomonic for hyperparathyroidism. The cortex appears spiculated. There is acro-osteolysis of several of the terminal phalanges leading to arrow headed fingers.

Radiological picture of X ray hand of acromegaly
Terminal phalangeal tufts become hypertrophied and have a "spade appearance" which is called spade phalanx sign. Joint spaces may be minimally enlarged. Premature osteoarthritis can set in the advanced stages of acromegaly.

245. Ans. (d) Hypothyroidism

(Ref: Harrison 20th p 2932; Harrison 19th p 2470)

246. Ans. (a) Primary Hyperparathyroidism

(Ref: Harrison 20th p 2927; Harrison 19th p 2472)

247. Ans. (b) Hyperparathyroidism

(Ref: Harrison 20th p 2927; Harrison 19th p 2472)

- Bone resorption may be classified as subperio-steal, intracortical, trabecular, endosteal, subchondral, subligamentous, or subtendinous.
- Subperiosteal bone resorption is an early and virtually pathognomonic sign of hyperpara-thyroidism, and this finding is marked by marginal erosions with adjacent resorption of bone and sclerosis.
- Although subperiosteal bone resorption can affect many sites, the most common site in hyperparathyroidism is the middle phalanges of the index and middle fingers, primarily on the radial aspect

248. Ans. (d) Technetium -99 sestamibi scan

(Ref: Harrison 20th p 2928; Harrison 19th p 2474)

Nuclear medicine scanning with radiolabeled sestamibi is also a widely used technique for imaging parathyroid glands. Sestamibi is commonly used in cardiac imaging and was found serendipitously to accumulate in parathyroid adenomas. This radionuclide is concentrated in thyroid and parathyroid tissue but usually washes out of normal thyroid tissue in under an hour. It persists in abnormal parathyroid tissue.

249. Ans. (b) Hypophosphatasia

(Ref: Harrison 20th p 2964; Harrison 19th p237, 426e-1)

The following conditions or diseases may lead to reduced levels of bone specific alkaline phosphatase:

- Hypophosphatasia, an autosomal recessive disease
- Postmenopausal women receiving estrogen therapy because of osteoporosis
- Men with recent heart surgery, malnutrition, magnesium deficiency, hypothyroidism, or severe anemia
- Pernicious anemia
- Aplastic anemia
- Chronic myelogenous leukemia
- Wilson

Hypophosphatasia is a rare and fatal metabolic bone disease. Clinical symptoms are heterogeneous ranging from the rapidly fatal perinatal variant, with profound skeletal hypomineralization and respiratory compromise to a milder, progressive osteomalacia later in life. Tissue non-specific alkaline phosphatase (TNSALP) deficiency in osteoblasts and chondrocytes impairs bone mineralization, leading to rickets or osteomalacia.

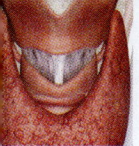

250. Ans. (c) Pancreatitis

(Ref: Harrison 20th p 313; Harrison 19th p 2470, Table 424-1)

Causes of Hypercalcemia

- *Parathyroid-related*
  - Primary hyperparathyrodism Adenoma
  - Lithium
  - Familial hypocalciuric hypercalcemia
- *Malignancy-related*
  - Solid tumor with metastases (breast)
  - Solid tumor with humoral mediation of hypercalcemia (lung, kidney)
  - Hematologic malignancies (multiple myeloma, lymphoma, leukemia)
- *Vitamin D-related*
  - Vitamin D intoxication
  - ↑1,25(OH)2D; sarcoidosis
- *Associated with high bone turnover*
  - Hyperthyroidism
  - Immobilization
  - Thiazides
  - Vitamin A intoxication
- *Associated with renal failure*
  - Severe secondary hyperparathyroidism
  - Aluminum intoxication
  - Milk-alkali syndrome

251. Ans. (c) Pseudo-pseudo-hypoparathyrodism

(Ref: Harrison 20th p 2915; Harrison 19th p 2461)

- **Choice A:** CRF will lead to retention of phosphate due to low GFR
- **Choice B:** Can considered due to increased intake
- PHP leads to reduction in normal phosphate loss via kidney tubules.
- PPHP is a term used to describe a patient whose appearance is same as patient of PHP, but is biochemically normal.

252. Ans. (a) Paget's disease

(Ref: Harrison 19th p 426-e)

Since *hydroxyproline is an amino-acid derived from collagen, increased amounts in urine is indicative of increased collagen breakdown* and seen in mainly Paget's disease, hyperparathyrodism, burns, acromegaly and psoriasis.

253. Ans. (c) Neuropsychiatric changes

(Ref: Harrison 20th p 2927; Harrison 19th p 2470)

Neuromuscular and psychologic manifestations of primary hyperparathyroidism include proximal myopathy, weakness and easy fatigability, depression, inability to concentrate, and memory problems or subtle deficits that are often characterized poorly and may not be noted by the patient.

The clinical syndrome of primary hyperpara-thyroidism can be easily remembered as "Bones, stones, abdominal groans, and psychic moans."

254. Ans. (c) Parathyroid Adenoma

(Ref: Harrison 20th p 2925; Harrison 19th p 2471-2472)

255. Ans. (d) Asymptomatic hypercalcemia

(Ref: Harrison 20th p 2925; Harrison 19th p 2472)

256. Ans. (c) Chronic renal failure

(Ref: Harrison 20th p 2939; Harrison 19th p 2478)

257. Ans. (b) Secondary hyperparathyroidism

(Ref: Harrison 20th p 2939; Harrison 19th p 2478)

258. Ans. (b) Hyperparathyroidism

(Ref: Harrison 20th p 2938; Harrison 19th p 2478)

259. Ans. (b) Hypoparathyroidism

(Ref: Harrison 20th p 2938; Harrison 19th p 2483)

260. Ans. (d) Celiac disease

(Ref: Harrison 20th p 313; Harrison 19th p Table 424-1, p 2470)

261. Ans. (a) Acute Pancreatitis

(Ref: Harrison 20th p 313; Harrison 19th p 2470)

262. Ans. (d) Thiazides

(Ref: Harrison 20th p 2935; Harrison 19th Table 424-4, p 2480)

263. Ans. (c) Vitamin D in high doses

(Ref: Harrison 20th p 2935; Harrison 19th p 2480)

Furosemide promotes urinary excretion of calcium. Thiazides reduces urinary excretion of calcium.

264. Ans. (a) Etidronate

(Ref: Greenspan's Endocrinology 8th/316; Clinical Review of USMLE Step 2 (Surgisphere) 2008/499; Spiral Manual of Endocrinology & Metabolism 4th/360, 361, Harrison 19th p 2488)

265. Ans. (a) CRF and (b) Pseudohypoparathyroidism

(Ref: Harrison 20th p 2939, 2940)

266. Ans. (b) Gunstock deformity

(Ref: OP Ghai 6th/128-129; 188, Harrison 19th p 2465)

267. Ans. (d) Inverse relation with Mg^{++} levels

(Ref: Harrison 20th p 314; Harrison 19th p 2457)

268. Ans. (c) Paget's disease of bone

(Ref: Harrison 20th p 2960-61; Harrison 19th p 426e)

269. Ans. (c) Hypoparathyroidism

(Ref: Chandrasoma Taylor 3rd/965)

270. Ans. (b) Hypoparathyroidism

(Ref: Harrison 20th p 2993; Harrison 19th p 2490)

271. Ans. (d) All of the above

(Ref: Harrison 20th p 2993; Harrison 19th p 2490)

272. Ans. (a) Decrease in parathyroid hormone level

(Ref: Harrison 20th p 2939; Page number 2465-66: Harrison 19th edition)

- Vitamin D deficiency leads to low serum calcium, and increased PTH levels.
- Increased PTH leads to bone resorption increasing bone turnover and increased SAP.
- PTH acts on proximal tubule of kidney to lead to loss of phosphate in urine leading to hypophosphatemia.
- Vitamin D3 promotes calcium absorption from the gut. In setting of vitamin D deficiency, calcium absorption from the gut is reduced.

Magnesium Metabolism

273. Ans. (d) Hypotension refractory to vasopressors

(Ref: Harrison 20th p 2917; Harrison: 19th edition, Page 2463)

- The most significant features of elevated magnesium are vasodilation and neuromuscular blockage.
- At values in excess of >2mmol/dl *hypotension refractory to vasopressors and volume expansion is an early diagnostic clue.*
- Nausea and vomiting develops progressing to respiratory failure.
- At values of 4 mmol/L hypoactive tendon reflexes will appear.
- Gastrointestinal hypomotility and ileus and facial flushing occurs
- In terminal stages paradoxical bradycardia and pupil dilatation is noted.
- At values of 10 mmol/L asystole occurs

274. Ans. (d) QTc prolongation

(Ref: Harrison 20th p 2917; Harrison 19th edn. Page 2462)

- Normal serum magnesium = 0.8–1.0 mmol/L.
- Hypomagnesaemia = <0.8 mmol/L

ECG Changes
- The primary ECG abnormality seen with hyomagnesaemia is a prolonged QTc.
- Atrial and ventricular ectopy, atrial tachyarrhythmias and torsades de pointes are seen in the context of hypomagnesaemia, although whether this is a specific effect of low serum magnesium or due to concurrent hypokalaemia is uncertain.

275. Ans. (d) Seen in Diabetic Ketoacidosis

(Ref: Harrison 20th p 2917; Harrison 19th Table 423-4 2462)

- Hypomagnesemia is seen during *treatment phase* of diabetic ketoacidosis.
- Hypomagnesemia often leads to hypocalcemia, a phenomenon largely explained by inhibition of parathyroid hormone bioactivity. Hypocal-cemia does not resolve until the magnesium deficiency has been corrected.
- The total body magnesium content of an average adult is 25 g, or 1000 mmol. Approximately 60% of the body's magnesium is present in bone, 20% is in muscle, and another 20% is in soft tissue and the liver. Approximately 99% of total body magnesium is intracellular or bone-deposited, with only 1% present in the extracellular space.
- Normal serum magnesium = 1.7-2.1mg/dl

Causes of Hypomagnesemia

More frequently asked causes
• Starvation
• Alcohol dependence
• Total parenteral nutrition
Redistribution of magnesium from extracellular to intracellular space includes:
• Hungry bone syndrome
• Treatment of diabetic ketoacidosis
• Alcohol withdrawal syndromes
• Refeeding syndrome
• Acute pancreatitis
Gastrointestinal magnesium loss includes:
• Diarrhea
• Vomiting and nasogastric suction
• Gastrointestinal fistulas and ostomies
Causes related to renal magnesium loss include the following, including inherited renal tubular defects
• Gitelman syndrome
• Classic Bartter syndrome

276. Ans. (c) Paget disease

(Ref: Harrison 20th p 2960-61; Harrison 19th p 2462)

277. Ans. (a) Hypercalcaemia

(Ref: Harrison 20th p 2917; Harrison 19th p 2462)

M.E.N

278. Ans. (a) Posterior pituitary tumours

(Ref: Harrison 20th p 2747; Harrison 19th edition, Page 2336)

Multiple Endocrine Neoplasia (11q13)/Intron 4 ss
1. Parathyroid adenoma (90%)- Most common presentation
2. Entero-pancreatic tumours- Most common is gastrinoma and least common is V.I.Poma in MEN1
3. Pituitary adenoma- most common is Prolactinoma and least common is non-functioning adenoma in MEN1
4. Associated tumours
   A. Adrenal cortical tumour
   B. Neuroendocrine tumours- thymus, lungs
   C. Lipoma
   D. Angiofibroma- Most common skin manifestation in MEN 1 (Angiofibroma>collagenoma)

E. Brain tumour- meningioma
F. Phaeochromoctoma (<1%)

279. Ans. (b) Secretin study

(Ref: Harrison 20th p 2748)

- Patient of MEN 1 have
  - Pituitary adenoma
  - Parathyroid adenoma
  - Pancreatic adenoma (Gastrinoma>insulinoma)
- In diagnosed cases of MEN1 where nephro-calcinosis is documented, evaluation of pancreatic adenoma is important.
- The *most common pancreatic adenoma in MEN 1 is ZES* and hence for evaluation of ZES, secretin study is done.
- Subsequently 72 hours fasting test and endoscopic ultrasound will be useful for evaluation of insulinoma
- The incidence of ZES in MEN I is 70% versus insulinoma being 10%.
- *If the same question is asking about MEN IIA, then calcitonin levels and urinary metanephrine levels shall be performed. In MEN IIA incidence of medullary carcinoma thyroid (90%) is more than that of pheochromocytoma(20-35%)*

280. Ans. (d) M.T.C

(Ref: Harrison 20th p 2747; Harrison 19 e, page 2336)

MEN4
- Chromosome location of defect in MEN4 is 12p13.
- Parathyroid adenoma
- Pituitary adenoma
- Reproductive organ tumors (e.g. Testicular cancer, neuro-endocrine cervical carainoma)

281. Ans. (d) Meningoma

(Ref: Harrison 20th p 2747; Harrison 19e., Page 2336)

MEN2B
- M.T. C pheochromocytoma associated abnormalities
  - Mucosal neuroma
  - Marfanoid Habitus
  - Medullated corneal nerve fibres
  - Megacolon

282. Ans. (a) Medullary Carcinoma of Thyroid

(Ref: Harrison 20th p 2747; Harrison 19th p 2340)

Disorders of GH, Vasopressin

283. Ans. (a) Insulin like growth factor

(Ref: Harrison 20th p 2679; Harrison 19th edition, page 2269)

- The *somatic growth* in the given clinical presentation is seen in acromegaly. Screening test to identify Acromegaly is Insulin like growth factor 1 levels and confirmation is done with oral glucose tolerance test.
- Due to pulsatile nature of GH secretion, measurement of single level is not useful.

- Hence the diagnosis is confirmed with demonstration of failure of GH level suppression to <0.4µg/L within 1-2 hours of oral glucose load.
- Prolactin may be elevated due to loss of inhibitory control secondary to mass effects of pituirary adenoma. However it would not be diagnostic in acromegaly.

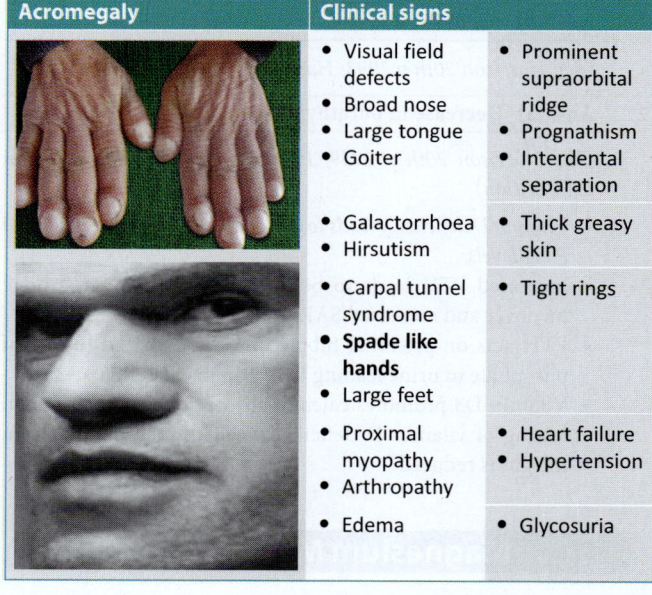

Acromegaly	Clinical signs	
	• Visual field defects • Broad nose • Large tongue • Goiter	• Prominent supraorbital ridge • Prognathism • Interdental separation
	• Galactorrhoea • Hirsutism	• Thick greasy skin
	• Carpal tunnel syndrome • **Spade like hands** • Large feet	• Tight rings
	• Proximal myopathy • Arthropathy	• Heart failure • Hypertension
	• Edema	• Glycosuria

284. Ans. (a) SIADH

(Ref: Harrison 20th p 2690; Harrison 19th edition page 229: CMDT 2019 page 899)

- Choice D: Pseudo-hyponatremia is ruled out as it is seen with conditions like hypertriglyceridemia, hyperproteinemia.
- Choice C: Cerebral salt wasting syndrome is ruled out as it is associated with *hypotension* as patients are *hypovolemic*. It occurs in setting of Subarachnoid haemorrhage
- Choice B: Thiazide induced hyponatremia will lead to hypovolemic status and elevated BUN.
- Important lab values in the question to be considered

	Normal	Value given in question	Interpretation
BUN	8-20mg/dl	10	Lower side
Plasma osmolality	285-295mosm	285	Lower side
Serum sodium	135-145meq/dl	125	Low
24 hour urine sodium	40-220meq	100	Normal

Points in favour of diagnosis of SIADH in this patient

1. Clinical *history of association with lung cancer*
2. *Plasma osmolality on lower side* (normal 285-295 mosm)
3. Urine osmolality >100msom during hypotonicity
4. Urine sodium >40meq/dl with normal salt intake
5. Low BUN

Etiologies of Hypo-osmolar Hyponatremia

Hypervolemia	Euvolemia	Hypovolemia

• Heart failure
• Cirrhosis
• Nephrotic syndrome
• Anaphylaxis
• Renal failure
• Sepsis
• Pregnancy
	• SIADH
	  ■ Tumors
	  ■ CNS disorders/injury
	  ■ Drug induced
	  ■ Pulmonary diseases
	  ■ Other
	• Glucocrticoid deficiency
	• Hypothyroidism
	• Primary polydipsia
		• Third space loss
		• Thiazide diuretics
		• Cerebral salt wasting
		• Mineralocorticoid deficiency
		• Salt-wasting nephropathy

Euvolemic hyponatremia does not mean total body water is normal.

	Total body water	Total Body Sodium
Hypovolemic hyponatremia	Decrease	Decrease
Euvolemic hyponatremia	Increase	Normal
Hypervolemic hyponatremia	Disproportionate increase as compared to increase of sodium	Increase

285. Ans. (a) Euvolemic hyponatremia

(Ref: CMDT 2019, page 900)

In SIADH, Excess of ADH leads to gain of water leading to excess of water. However subsequently, gain of water stimulates the baroreceptors leading to release of atrial natriuretic peptide. The ANP leads to loss of salt and water.

The loss and gain of water reaches a steady state based on osmo-receptor drive but urinary loss of salt continues to occur explaining hyponatremia.

Hypotonic Hyponatremia

Hypovolemic Hyponatremia	Euvolemic Hyponatremia	Hypervolemic Hyponatremia
• Dehydration • Diarrhea • Vomiting • Diuretics • ACE inhibitors • Cerebral salt wasting syndrome^Q	• SIADH • Post-Operative hyponatremia • Hypothyroidism • Psychogenic polydipsia	• Heart failure • Liver disease • Nephrotic syndrome • Advanced kidney disease

286. Ans. (b) Dilutional hyponatremia

(Ref: Harrison 20th p 2685; Harrison 19th ed./303-304)

- Diabetes insipidus has either low levels of vasopressin or it is not able to act. Therefore these patients pass a large amount of dilute urine (Polyuria and resultant polydipsia develops). The result is that due to loss of water from body these patients will develop relative hypernatremia.
- *The diagnostic test is water deprivation test*

Drugs
- Neurogenic diabetes inspidus is treated with desmopressin nasal spray.
- Nephrogenic diabetes inspidus is treated with thiazide diuretics.
- Remember: Dilutional hyponatremia is seen with S.I.A.D.H and test used for diagnosis is water

287. Ans. (c) Relative Hypernatremia

(Ref: Harrison 20th p 2689; Harrison 19th ed./2280)

- SIADH is characterized by gain of water and hence dilutional hyponatremia sets in. The gain of water explains low uric acid.
- Since in SIADH most of the water is reabsorbed via the CD, the low urine output prompts a physician to possibility of renal parenchymal disorder for which KFT must be done and must be normal.
- In the absence of a single laboratory test to confirm the diagnosis, SIADH is best defined by the classic *Bartter-Schwartz criteria*, which can be summarized as follows

> - Hyponatremia with corresponding hypo-osmolality
> - Continued renal excretion of sodium
> - Urine less than maximally dilute
> - Absence of clinical evidence of volume depletion
> - Absence of other causes of hyponatremia
> - Correction of hyponatremia by fluid restriction

288. Ans. (a) Hyperglycemia

(Ref: Harrison 20th p 2667; Harrison 19th ed./2257-58)

- From late in the first year until mid teens, poor growth and/or shortness is the *hallmark* of childhood GH deficiency.
- It tends to be accompanied by delayed physical maturation so that bone maturation and puberty may be delayed by several years.
- Severe GH deficiency in early childhood also results in slower muscular development, so that gross motor milestones may be delayed.
- Some severely GH-deficient children have recognizable, cherubic facial features characterized by maxillary hypoplasia and forehead prominence. These children have a high pitched voice and are stunted. GH deficiency is associated with hypoglycemia. In contrast, gigantism or acromegaly is associated with impaired glucose tolerance.

289. Ans. (a) Xanthelasma

(Ref: Harrison 20th p 328; Harrison 19th ed./365)

The image shows Bilateral Xanthelasma, which are yellow plaques depositions of yellowish cholesterol-rich material. They are more common on upper eyelid as compared to lower lids.

290. Ans. (a) Cabozantinib

(Ref: Harrison 20th p 2753; Harrison 19th p 2342)

- For metastatic or inoperable MTC, T.K.R inhibitors like vandetanib and cabozantinib are used.
- In adults with MTC >1 cm in size, metastases to regional lymph nodes are common (>75%).
- Total thyroidectomy with central lymph node dissection and selective dissection of other regional chains provides the best chance for cure. In patients with extensive local metastatic disease in the neck, external radiation may prevent local recurrence or reduce tumor mass but is not curative.
- Chemotherapy with combinations of adriamycin, vincristine, cyclophosphamide, and Dacarbazine may provide palliation.
- Clinical trials with small compounds (tyrosine kinase inhibitors) that interact with the ATP-binding pocket of the RET, vascular endothelial receptor, and type 2 and epidermal growth factor receptors and prevent phosphorylation have shown promise for treatment of hereditary and sporadic MTC.

291. Ans. (a) Hyperthyroidism

(Ref: Harrison 20th p 2665; Harrison 19th p 2257)

- An acute intrapituitary hemorrhagic vascular events can cause substanial pituitary damage and is called as pituitary apoplexy causes can be sheehan syndrome, diabetes, hypertension, sickle cell anemic shock.

292. Ans. (b) Cortisone

(Ref: Harrison 20th p 2665; Harrison 19th p 2257)

- Ist drug to be supplemented in Sheehan's syndrome is cortisol.
- Ist hormone to fall in Sheehan syndrome is GH.

293. Ans. (b) Interstitial nephritis

(Ref: Harrison 20th p 2690; Harrison 19th p 2281)

294. Ans. (a) Cerebral toxoplasmosis with SIADH

(Ref: Harrison 20th p 2690; Harrison 19th p 2282)

295. Ans. (b) Hyposmolar urine

(Ref: Harrison 20th p 2690; Harrison 19th p 2282)

296. Ans. (d) Demeclocycline

(Ref: Harrison 20th p 2690; Harrison 19th p 2282)

297. Ans. (a) Multiple sclerosis

(Ref: Harrison 20th p 2690; Harrison 19th p 2281)

298. Ans. (d) Addison's disease

(Ref: Harrison 20th p 2639, 2700; Harrison 19th p 2221)

Disorders of LH, FSH and Prolactin

299. Ans. (c) Normalizes serum prolactin levels

(Ref: Harrison 20th p 2676-77; Harrison 19th edition page 2268)

The ergot alkaloid bromocriptine is a dopamine receptor agonist that *suppresses prolactin secretion*. In micro adenomas, bromocriptine lowers serum prolactin levels up to 70% of patients.

Management of Prolactinoma

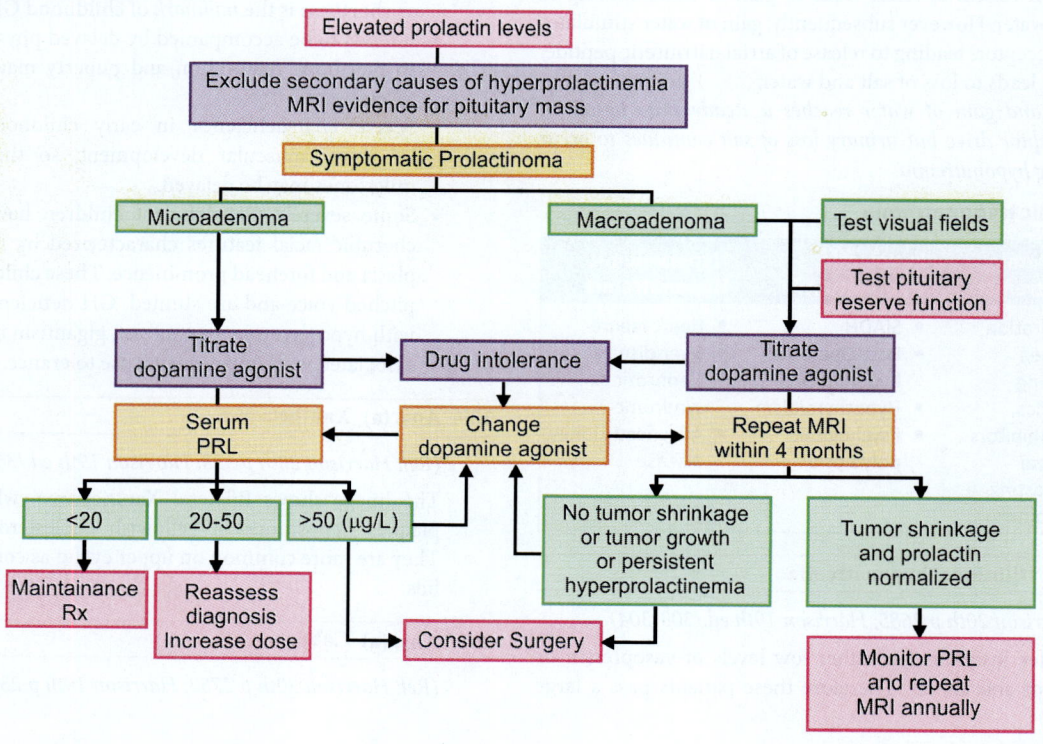

300. Ans. (c) Decreased prolactin

(Ref: Harrison 20th p 2664; Harrison 19th edition page no. 2261)

- LH and FSH are trophic hormones for testis and their impaired secretion results in secondary hypogonadism. The values of LH, FSH and testosterone are low leading to complete absence of pubertal development, micro-penis/sexual infantilism and undescended testis.
- Females present with primary amenorrhea and failure of secondary sexual development.

301. Ans. (a) Non-functioning adenoma

(Ref: Harrison 20th p 2674; Harrison:19th edition Page 2265; UICC manual of oncology: 2015 edition, page 611)

- The majority of pituitary adenomas (33-40%) are clinically non-functioning and produce no distinct clinical hyper-secretory syndrome.
- Most of them arise from gonadotrope cells and may secrete small amounts of alpha- and beta-glycoprotein hormone subunits or, very rarely, intact circulating gonadotropins.
- The most common secretory adenoma is prolactinoma.
- The least common secretory adenoma is TSH secreting tumours. The UICC manual of oncology 2015 edition mentions it as rare (<1%). This is followed by LH/FSH secreting tumour whose prevalence is mentioned as 1%.

302. Ans. (a) Gonadotropin producing cell

(Ref: Harrison 20th p 2674; Harrison: 19th edition, Page 2265)

Refer to the explanation of the above question

303. Ans. (b) Prolactin

(Ref: Harrison 20th p 2675; Harrison 19th, page 401e-1t)

- Prolactin secretion from the pituitary is normally inhibited by hypothalamic inhibitory factors, one of which is dopamine.
- Histamine also inhibits prolactin secretion, whereas serotonin and thyrotropin releasing hormone (TRH) stimulate its release.

Causes of Hyperprolactinemia may result from

1. Lesions obstructing the inhibitory influence from the hypothalamus (e.g. craniopharyngioma, sarcoidosis, surgical ablation)
2. Increased stimulation (elevated TRH in primary hypothyroidism)
3. Prolactin-secreting pituitary adenomas.
4. Exogenous sex steroids, phenothiazines, certain antidepressants, and antihypertensive may also cause hyperprolactinemia.

304. Ans. (a) TSH

(Ref: Harrison 20th p 2675; Harrison 19th edition, page 2267)

- TRH thus stimulates secretion of both TSH and PRL. Thus, in severe hypothyroidism elevated levels of TRH stimulates TSH as well as PRL, which is the cause of galactorrhea and amenorrhea sometimes seen in hypothyroidism.
- "In hyperprolactenemia, hypothyroidism should be should be excluded by measuring TSH and T4 levels."

Etiology of Hyperprolactinemia

1. **Physiologic hypersecretion**
   - Pregnancy
   - Lactation
   - Chest wall stimulation
   - Sleep
   - Stress
2. **Pituitary hypersecretion**
   - Prolactinoma
   - Acromegaly
3. **Systemic disorders**
   - Chronic renal failure
   - Hypothyroidism
   - Cirrhosis
   - Pseudocyesis
   - Epileptic seizures
4. **Drug-induced hypersecretion**
5. **Hypothalamic-pituitary stalk damage**

305. Ans. (c) GH receptor resistance

(Ref: Harrison 20th p 2667; Chapter 558: Nelson 18th edition, Harrison 19th p 2258)

Growth hormone insensitivity syndrome is also known as Laron dwarfism which is characterised by the receptor anomalies and immunological suppression seen in these patients

306. Ans. (b) Vincristine

(Ref: Goodman and Gillman ch. 25 Regulation of Renal function)

- Vincristine is documented to cause SIADH which leads to gain of water and resultant dilutional hyponatremia
- Addison will have hyponatremia due to aldosterone deficiency
- Diuretics will cause loss of salt due to inhibition of sodium chloride cotransporter.
- Craniopharyngioma can lead to diabetes insipidus of central origin.

Also Know: 3 Drug classes most commonly implicated in drug induced SIADH are:
1. Psychoprophic medication (Ex-SSRI, Halopendol and TCA)
2. Sulfonylureas (chlorpropamide)
3. Vinca Alkaloids (Vincristine, vinblastine)

307. Ans. (c) Urine sodium is usually normal in these patients

(Ref: Harrison 20th p 2689-90; Harrison 19th p 2416 Table 404-3, 2282)

SIADH is the most common cause of Euvolemic Hypo-osmolality, and it is also the single most common cause of hypo-osmolality encountered in clinical practice.

The clinical criteria necessary to diagnose SIADH are:

1. Decreased effective osmolality of the extra-cellular fluid (Posm <275 mOsm/kg H_2O).
2. Inappropriate urinary concentration at some level of hypoosmolality. This does not mean urine osmolality is greater than plasma osmolality, only less than maximally dilute (i.e., urine osmolality >100 mOsm/kg H_2O).
3. Patients of SIADH elevated urinary sodium excretion while on a normal salt and water intake.

- When patients are hyponatremic, values of uric acid are reported to be <4 mg/dL (<0.24 mmol/L).
- A water-loading test is the investigation of choice for SIADH.
- In acute SIADH, the keystone to treatment of hyponatremia is to restrict total fluid intake to less than the sum of insensible losses and urinary output.
- In chronic SIADH: Demeclocycline, fludrocortisone and Conivaptan are used, with vaptans being preferred

308. Ans. (b) ADH secretion occurs when plasma osmolality is low

(Ref: Harrison 20th p 2689-90; Harrison 19th p 2276-77)

- ADH causes water re-absorbtion and dilutes the plasma. Hence ADH secretion will not occur when plasma osmolality is low and the second choice of the question is wrong statement.
- ADH is produced from supraoptic nucleus of neurohypophysis or posterior pituitary.
- ADH acts on distal convoluted tubules and medullary collecting ducts of the kidney to reduce water loss by concentrating the urine. This antidiuretic effect is achieved by increasing the hydro-osmotic permeability of cells that line the distal tubule and medullary collecting ducts of the kidney.

- ADH secretion is regulated primarily by the effective osmotic pressure of body fluids. This control is mediated by specialised hypothalamic cells known as osmo-receptors, which are extremely sensitive to small changes in plasma concentration of sodium and certain other solutes.
- When plasma osmolarity increases, ADH secretion increases in direct proportion to plasma osmolarity quickly reaching levels sufficient to effect maximum diuresis.

309. Ans. (b) Hypoglycemia

(Ref: Harrison 19th p 2260)

- GH leads to increased blood sugar

Adverse reactions of GH

1. Reversible dose-related fluid retention.
2. Joint pain, and carpal tunnel syndrome, myalgias and paresthesia.
3. Hyperglycemia - GH is a potent counter-regulatory hormone for insulin action. Patients with type 2 diabetes mellitus initially develop further insulin resistance. Glycemic control improves with the sustained loss of abdominal fat associated with long-term GH replacement.
4. Headache, benign intracranial hypertension, Hypertension, atrial fibrillation, and tinnitus
5. Pituitary tumor regrowth and potential progression of skin lesions
6. Gynaecomastia
7. Acromegaly
8. Cardiomyopathy
9. Slipped Capital Femoral Epiphysis,Turner syndrome, and other known causes of short stature are more likely to develop SCFE before or during GH treatment than children with idiopathic short stature.

310. Ans. (a) Prolactinoma

(Ref: Harrison 20th p 2674; Harrison 19th p 2266)

Type of adenomas	Secretion	Staining	Pathology	Percentage of hormone production cases
Lactotrophic adenomas (prolactinomas)	Secrete prolactin	Acidophilic	Galactorrhea, hypogonadism, amenorrhea, infertility, and impotence	30%
Somatotrophic adenomas	Secrete growth hormone (GH)	Acidophilic	Acromegaly in adults; gigantism in children	15%
Corticotrophic adenomas	Secrete adenocorticotropic hormone (ACTH)	Basophilic	Cushing's disease	10%
Gonadotrophic adenomas	Secrete luteinizing hormone (LH), follicle stimulating hormone (FSH) and their subunits	Basophilic	Usually doesn't cause symptoms	10%
Thyrotrophic adenomas (rare)	Secrete thyroid-stimulating hormone (TSH)	Basophilic to chromophobic	Occasionally hyperthyroidism, usually doesn't cause symptoms	Less than1%
Null cell adenomas	Do not secrete hormones	May stain positive for synaptophysin		25% of pituitary adenomas are nonsecretive

*MC pituitary tumor overall is non functioning pituitary adenoma

311. **Ans. (d) Gonad function**

(Ref: Harrison 19th p 2358)

312. **Ans. (c) Bromocriptine**

(Ref: Harrison 20th p 2677; Harrison 19th 2266, 2268)

Bromocriptine is a dopamine agonist. Since dopamine inhibits prolactin synthesis, bromocriptine is used for inhibiting prolactin synthesis

313. **Ans. (d) Corticosteroids**

(Ref: CMDT 2019, pg 1120; Harrison 19th p 2257)

- Sheehan syndrome leads to acute presentation of hypopituitarism with severe secon drug adrenal insufficiency.
- Treatment of young women with hypopituitarism due to Sheehan syndrome usually includes replacement of hydrocortisone first and then replacement of thyroid hormone and estrogen with or without progesterone.
- Hydrocortisone is replaced first because thyroxine therapy can exacerbate glucocorticoid deficiency and theoretically induce an adrenal crisis.
- The standard dose of hydrocortisone is 20 mg/d for an adult (15 mg every morning and 5 mg every evening). Both thyroxine replacement and gonadotropin replacement are common, and doses are titrated to each individual.
- Replacement of growth hormone is necessary in children with hypopituitarism but is controversial in adults

314. **Ans. (d) Thyroid status**

(Ref: Harrison 20th p 2676; Harrison 19th p 2267)

- The predominant signal for control of release of prolactin is inhibitory, thereby preventing prolactin release, and is mediated by the neurotransmitter dopamine. The stimulatory signal is mediated by the hypothalamic hormone thyrotropin-releasing hormone. The balance between the 2 signals determines the amount of prolactin released from the anterior pituitary gland. Furthermore, the amount cleared by the kidneys influences the concentration of prolactin in the blood.
- Now in primary hypothyroidism patients the levels of T3,T4 are less and TSH, TRH would be elevated. This explains why some patients with hypothyroidism develop galactorrhea.
- The best answer in this question where MRI and serum prolactin is not given is thyroid function test.

315. **Ans. (a) GH**

(Ref: Harrison 19th p 2265)

- The pituitary enlarges during pregnancy and has a single arterial supply which makes it vulnerable in setting of shock after delivery.
- The cells producing GH exhibit significant hyperplasia and constitute a large part of the gland. As growth hormone (GH)-secreting cells are situated in the lower and lateral regions of the pituitary gland and are most likely to be damaged by ischemic necrosis, it is not surprising that GH is one of the first hormones to be lost
- Hence the largest part with the most critical blood supply is the maximum affected leading to fall in levels of GH earliest.

- Failure to lactate or difficulties with lactation are common initial symptoms of Sheehan syndrome.
- Treatment of young women with hypopituitarism usually includes replacement of hydrocortisone first and then replacement of thyroid hormone and estrogen with or without progesterone depending on whether she has a uterus. Hydrocortisone is replaced first because thyroxine therapy can exacerbate glucocorticoid deficiency and theoretically induce an adrenal crisis.

316. **Ans. (b) Superior quadrantopia**

(Ref: Harrison 19th p 2262)

- If a lesion is originating superior to the optic chiasm, like in a craniopharyngoma, the visual field defect will first appear as Bitemporal inferior quadrantanopia.
- If originating inferior to the optic chiasma like a prolactinoma, the visual field defect will first appear as bitemporal superior quadrantanopia.
- Lateral expansion of a pituitary adenoma can also compress the abducens nerve, causing a lateral rectus palsy.
- Usually the defect produced is bitemporal hemianopia in proalactinoma as the size of tumor increases.

317. **Ans. (c) Present in temporal or parietal lobes**

(Ref: Harrison 20th p 648; Harrison 19th p 2264)

- Craniopharyngiomas are benign, suprasellar cystic masses that present with headaches, visual field deficits, and variable degrees of hypopituitarism.
- They are derived from Rathke's pouch and arise near the pituitary stalk, commonly extending into the suprasellar cistern.
- Craniopharyngiomas are often large, cystic, and locally invasive. Many are partially calcified, exhibiting a characteristic appearance on skull X-ray and CT images.
- MRI is generally superior to CT for evaluating cystic structure and tissue components of craniopharyngiomas. CT is useful to define calcifications and evaluate invasion into surrounding bony structures and sinuses.

318. **Ans. (b) Muscular hypertrophy**

(Ref: Harrison 20th p 2678; Harrison 19th p 2269)

Clinical features of acromegaly are:

- *The Proximal muscle weakness and fatigue*
- Acral bony overgrowth results in frontal bossing, increased hand and foot size
- Mandibular enlargement with prognathism
- *Soft tissue swelling results in increased heel pad thickness, increased shoe or glove size, ring tightening,*
- Characteristic coarse facial features, and a large fleshy nose.
- Other commonly encountered clinical features include hyperhidrosis, a deep and hollow-sounding voice, oily skin, arthropathy, kyphosis, carpal tunnel syndrome
- Acanthosis nigricans, and skin tags.
- Generalized Visceromegaly occurs, including cardiomegaly, macroglossia, and thyroid gland enlargement.
- The paranasal sinuses and mastoid air cells in patients with acromegaly are typically enlarged. In addition, the bones of the calvarium are thickened and hyperostosis frontalis interna is common. The pituitary fossa may be normal or enlarged
- Increase of GH can lead to I.G.T

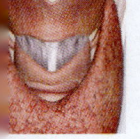

319. Ans. (b) Pigmentation of the mucous membranes

(Ref: Harrison 20th p 2735; Harrison 19th p 2324)

- Since ACTH has a partial MSH like activity and levels of ACTH in pan-hypopituitarism will fall, the hyperpigmentation cannot occur.
- In contrast diseases with increased ACTH like primary Addison disease will show hyperpigmentation.
- Insulin sensitivity implies hypoglycemia.
- LH/FSH fall will cause loss of secondary sex features.

320. Ans. (d) i, ii, iii

(Ref: Harrison 19th p 2269)

- Acromegaly leads to elevation of growth hormone which causes increase in level of blood glucose to levels of IGT.
- The enlarged pituitary tumor can press on the stalk leading to loss of inhibition for release of prolactin. This explains the galactorrhea
- The increased in somatomedins will cause increase in size of body tissues and organs. This will also lead to increase in peripheral tissues and explains the hypertension in these patients.
- The pituitary adenoma does not respond to glucose stimulation test (oral glucose 75gms) with failure to suppress GH production to <0.4 microgram/dl.
- About 20% of patients exhibit a paradoxical GH rise after glucose. PRL should be measured, as it is elevated in 25% of patients with acromegaly. Thyroid function, gonadotropins, and sex steroids may be attenuated because of tumor mass effects.

321. Ans. (d) Low serum phosphate

(Ref: Harrison 20th p 2678; Harrison 19th p 2269)

- GH increases the absorption of phosphate from the tubules leading to increased serum phosphate levels.
- GH increases the level of glucose leading to impaired glucose tolerance.
- Because GH secretion is inhibited by glucose measurement of glucose non-suppressibility may be useful. Patients with active acromegaly are unable to suppress GH concentration below 0.4 µg/L after a 75-g oral glucose load. A paradoxic rise in GH concentration is seen in 15-20% of patients with acromegaly following oral glucose administration.
- In acromegaly IGF-1 is produced primarily by the liver as an endocrine hormone as well as in target tissues in a paracrine/auto-crine fashion. Production is stimulated by growth hormone (GH) and can be retarded by undernutrition, growth hormone insensitivity, lack of growth hormone receptors.

322. Ans. (a) Malnutrition

(Ref: Harrison's 18th ed. ch. 339, 340, 350)

- The somatotrophs in pituitary exhibit abnormal receptors to TRH. Thus TRH infusion will cause stimulation of somatotrophs in pituitary adenoma to increase GH level which is referred to as paradoxical response to TRH infusion.
- The somato-lactotrophs also exhibit receptors to TRH and hence the same results can be seen in patients with prolactinoma.
- Anorexia nervosa patients have significant hypothalamic pituitary dysfunction with similar results.

323. Ans. (c) Bromocriptine

(Ref: Harrison 19th p 2267)

- Oral dopamine agonists (cabergoline and bromocriptine) are the mainstay of therapy for patients with micro- or macroprolactinomas. Dopamine agonists suppress PRL secretion and synthesis as well as lactotrope cell proliferation. In patients with microadenomas who have achieved normoprolactinemia and significant reduction of tumor mass, the dopamine agonist may be withdrawn after 2 years. These patients should be monitored carefully for evidence of prolactinoma recurrence.
- Indications for surgical adenoma debulking include dopamine resistance or intolerance and the presence of an invasive macroadenoma with compromised vision that fails to improve after drug treatment. Initial PRL normalization is achieved in about 70% of microprolactinomas after surgical resection, but only 30% of macroadenomas can be resected successfully.
- Radiotherapy for prolactinomas is reserved for patients with aggressive tumors that do not respond to maximally tolerated dopamine agonists and/or surgery.

324. Ans. (d) Psychogenic polydipsia

(Ref: Harrison 19th p 2276, 2279)

In setting of RTA followed by polyuria and polydipsia the probable diagnosis points to vasopressin related cause. This is further enhanced by mention of normal BP and 8 liters of urine per day.

Lab interpretation

Sodium	Low (normal = 135-145 meq/dl)
Potassium	Normal (normal = 3.5-5.5meq/dl)
Plasma osmolality	Low (285-295 mosm)
Urine osmolality	Low (100-900 mosm)
Urea	Normal (15- 40 mg%)

Interpretation

- In DI, urine osmolality is low while plasma osmolality is high. Thus choice A and B are ruled out.
- Resolving ATN is ruled out on clinical grounds as no history suggestive of Rhabdomyolysis is given.
- By exclusion and clinical plus lab picture psychogenic polydipsia explains the lab picture of low osmolality plasma and low osmolality urine.

325. Ans. (a) i, ii, iii

(Ref: Harrison 19th p 2278, fig 404.4)

Dilutional hyponatremia is seen with SIADH.

326. Ans. (c) Chronic glomerulonephritis

(Ref: Harrison 19th p 2276, 1811)

- Polyuria can be seen with choices A, B and D but fixed low specific gravity is a feature of chronic glomerulonephritis.
- Isosthenuria refers to the excretion of urine whose specific gravity (concentration) is neither greater (more concentrated) nor less (more dilute) than that of protein-free plasma, typically 1.008-1.012. Isosthenuria reflects renal tubular damage/failure of renal medullary function.
- Potomonia is known as beer drinkers hyponatremia and hypo-osmolality syndrome, related to massive consumption of beer.

327. Ans. (b) <300 mOsm/L

(Ref: Harrison 19th p 2278)

- Diabetes insipidus, is a syndrome characterized by the production of abnormally large volumes of dilute urine. The 24-hour urine volume is >50 mL/kg body weight, and the osmolarity is <300 mosmol/L.
- The polyuria produces symptoms of urinary frequency, enuresis, and/or nocturia, which may disturb sleep and cause mild daytime fatigue or somnoloscence. It also results in a slight rise in plasma osmolarity that stimulates thirst and a commensurate increase in fluid intake (polydipsia). Overt clinical signs of dehydration are uncommon unless fluid intake is impaired.

328. Ans. (b) Urine hyposmolar

(Ref: Harrison 19th p 2278)

The urine is concentrated and plasma is dilute in SIADH.

329. Ans. (d) Low urine and high plasma osmolality

(Ref: Harrison 19th p 2276-77)

Condition	Usual Clinical Setting MCQ Wise	Plasma osmolality	Urine Osmolality	Sodium Concentration
Central diabetes insipidus	Craniopharyngioma Idiopathic Sarcoidosis	Concentrated	Dilute	Relative hypernatremia
Nephrogenic DI	Lithium, scleroderma	Concentrated	Dilute	Relative hypernatremia
SIADH	Head injury, meningitis, vincristine	Dilute	Concentrated	Dilutional hyponatremia
Psychogenic polydipsia	RTA, pyschogenic	Dilute	Dilute	Normal
Adipsic hypernatremia	Pseudotumour cerebri SAH, psychogenic	Concentrated	Concentrated	Normal

330. Ans. (d) Primary pulmonary emphysema

(Ref: Harrison 19th Table 404-2, p 2281)

Asthma, pneumothorax and positive pressure ventilation are the respiratory causes of SIADH. Oat cell cancer is responsible for para-neoplastic syndrome of SIADH.

331. Ans. (c) Chlorpropamide

(Ref: Harrison 19th p 2278)

This anti-diabetic drug was withdrawn from market as it causes SIADH. So theoretically, it can be used in diabetes insipidus.

332. Ans. (a) Hyponatremia and urine sodium excretion >20 mEq/L

(Ref: Harrison 19th p 2282)

- In SIADH, the excessive retention of water expands extracellular and intracellular volume, increases glomerular filtration and atrial natriuretic hormone, suppresses plasma renin activity, and increases urinary sodium excretion.
- This natriuresis reduces total body sodium, and this serves to counteract the extracellular hypervolemia but aggravates the hyponatremia.

- The osmotically driven increase in intracellular volume results in swelling of brain cells and increases intracranial pressure; this is probably responsible for the symptoms of acute water intoxication.
- Within a few days, this swelling may be counteracted by inactivation or elimination of intracellular solutes, resulting in the remission of symptoms even though the Hyponatremia persists.

333. Ans. (d) Insulin

(Ref: Harrison 19th p 2257)

- The clinical presentation is that of Sheehan syndrome. In these patients GH deficiency develops and leads to hypoglycemia and therefore insulin is not required.
- Prednisolone will improve blood sugar and maintain sodium levels.
- Levothyroxine will improve cold intolerance
- Ethinyl estradiol will reduce symptoms related to deficiency of gonadotropins.

334. Ans. (d) Chromophobe adenoma

(Ref: Harrison 19th p 2281)

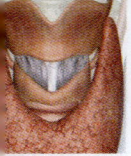

Chromophobe adenoma is a *nonfunctional pituitary tumor of the pars distalis and is hormonally inactive* but commonly causes clinical signs by compression of the pituitary gland and other nearby structures. Clinical signs include incoordination, weakness and exercise intolerance, muscle atrophy, sexual inactivity, blindness and dilatation and fixation of the pupils. It does not result in development of SIADH.

335. Ans. (a) Bromocriptine

(Ref: Harrison 20th p 2676; Harrison 19th Table 403-5 2266, 2268)

336. Ans. (c) Bromocriptine

(Ref: Harrison 20th p 2676)

337. Ans. (c) Prolactin estimation

(Ref: Harrison 20th p 2675)

338. Ans. (b) Prolactinoma

(Ref: Harrison 20th p 2675)

339. Ans. (b) Acromegaly

(Ref: Harrison 20th p 2678)

340. Ans. (b) Sertoli cell tumour

(Ref: Harrison 19th p 567, 2367)

341. Ans. (b) McCune Albright syndrome

(Ref: Harrison 19th p 2632)

342. Ans. (a) Kallman syndrome > **(b)** Pure gonadal dysgenesis

(Ref: Nelson text book of Pediatrics 19th edition page no: 1941, 1944)

- Height for age is normal in Kallman syndrome, distinguishing them during adolescence from individuals with constitutional delay in growth and development because adolescents in the latter group tend to be short for chronological age.
- Men with Kallmann syndrome or congenital idiopathic hypogonadotropic hypogonadism have prepubertal testes (< 4 mL) and lack scrotal pigmentation
- Lack of breast development is observed in women with Kallmann syndrome or congenital idiopathic hypogonadotropic hypogonadism.

Features	CAIS/ Testicular Feminization Syndrome	Pure Gonadal Dysgenesis
Karyotype	XY	XY
At birth, external genitalia	Highly variable	Mostly female
Mullerian structures	Absent	Present
Vagina	Blind vaginal pouch	Present
Internal gonads	No ovary. Testes are usually intra-abdominal but may descend into the inguinal canal; they consist largely of seminiferous tubules. Can have inguinal hernias containing testes	Undifferentiated streaks. Produces androgens
At puberty	There is normal development of breasts, and the habitus is female. Amennorhea and sexual hair is absent	No puberty Amennorhea and sexual hair is absent
Stature	Adult heights of these women are commensurate with those of normal males despite profound congenital deficiency of androgenic effects. Tall females	Normal stature and a female phenotype. Normal females

Contd...

343. Ans. (a) Hypothyroidism

(Ref: Harrison 19th p 2366)

Causes of gynecomastia
- Androgen insensitivity disorders
- Klinefelter's syndrome
- Sertoli cell tumors in isolation or in association with Carney complex.
- Tumors that produce hCG, including some testicular tumors.
- Increased conversion of androgens to estrogens can be a result of increased availability of substrate (androstenedione) for extra-glandular estrogen formation (CAH, hyperthyroidism)
- Diminished catabolism of androstenedione (liver disease) so that androgen precursors are shunted to aromatase in peripheral sites.
- Obesity is associated with increased aromatization of androgen precursors to estrogens.
- Extraglandular aromatase activity can also be increased in tumors of the liver or adrenal gland.
- Drugs can cause gynecomastia by acting directly as estrogenic substances (e.g., oral contraceptives, phytoestrogens, digitalis), inhibiting androgen synthesis (e.g., ketoconazole), or action (e.g., spironolactone).

344. Ans. (a) Kallman's syndrome

(Ref: Harrison 20th p 2776; Harrison 19th p 2256)

- Kallman syndrome is Hypogonadotropic hypogonadism (a lack of the pituitary hormones Luteinising Hormone and Follicle-Stimulating Hormone) and is a rare cause of amenorrhea with anosmia.
- Ashermann syndrome is characterized by adhesions and/or fibrosis of the endometrium most often associated with dilation and curettage of the intrauterine cavity.
- Stein Leveinthal syndrome will have hirusutism with weight gain and insulin resistance along with menstrual abnormalities

- Sheehan involves damage to anterior pituitary and not the hypothalamus.

345. Ans. (b) Testicular feminization syndrome

(Ref: Harrison 20th p 2765; Harrison 19th p 2354)

- Mutations in the androgen receptor cause resistance to androgen (testosterone, DHT) action or the androgen insensitivity syndrome.
- XY individuals with complete AIS (formerly called testicular feminization syndrome) have a female phenotype, normal breast development (due to aromatization of testosterone), a short vagina but no uterus (because MIS production is normal), scanty pubic and axillary hair, and a female psychosexual orientation.
- Gonadotropins and testosterone levels can be low, normal, or elevated, depending on the degree of androgen resistance and the contri-bution of estradiol to feedback inhibition of the hypothalamic-pituitary-gonadal axis.
- Most patients present with inguinal hernias (containing testes) in childhood or with primary amenorrhea in adulthood.
- Gonadectomy sometimes is performed, as there is a low risk of malignancy, and estrogen replacement is prescribed. Alternatively, the gonads can be left in situ until breast develop-ment is complete. The use of graded dilators in adolescence is usually sufficient to dilate the vagina and permit sexual intercourse.

Miscellaneous

346. Ans. (a) Hypothalamic hamartoma

(Ref: Nelson 20th edition Page 2658)

- Precocious puberty is caused by hamartoma of tuber cinerium and leads to excess production of LH.
- Craniopharyngioma presents with growth retardation and visual field defects.
- Kallman leads to hypogonadism and is ruled out
- Pituitary adenoma in children is mainly prolactin or ACTH secreting tumours

347. Ans. (d) Ghrelin

(Ref: Page 415-e4, Harrison 19th edition; pg 307 Nelson 20th ed)

- Prader-Willi syndrome (PWS) is a genetic syndrome that results from lack of expression of paternal (imprinted) genes located on chromosome 15q11-q13.
- *Prader has no Papa (i.e paternal chromosome deleted) angelMan has no Mama (i.e., as in mother: maternal chromosome deleted)*
- In the newborn period, children with PWS have hypotonia, poor suck, decreased arousal, and failure-to-thrive and often require tube feedings for several weeks to months. By 1-6 years of age, such patients develop insatiable appetite, progressive weight gain, short stature, hypogonadism, cognitive and motor delayed development, behavioural difficulties and sleep disturbances
- Adolescents and adults with PWS have high circulating concentrations of ghrelin, an orexigenic hormone produced by the stomach and it probably triggers the switch from a state of failure-to-thrive during infancy to that of insatiable appetite and morbid obesity in later childhood.

348. Ans. (b) Beta blocker

(Ref: Harrison 19th edition, page 252, 253t)

- GH and anabolic steroids cause water and salt retention.
- CCB decreases arteriolar resistance with little effect on veins. This increases the hydrostatic pressure leading to increased interstitial fluid.

349. Ans. (a) Serum Trytpase and C3a, C5a levels

(Ref: Harrison 19th edition, page 2116)

- Anaphylaxis requires a *pre-sensitization and IgE mediated degranulation of mast cells*. Due to degranulation of mast cells serum mature tryptase levels will increase.
- Anaphylactoid reaction is *non IgE based, direct complement mediated degranulation of mast cells*. Since it is complement mediated, the levels of anaphylatoxins C3a and C5a will decrease.

Anaphylaxis	Anaphylactoid

• Exaggerated response to a foreign substance
• Previous exposure/ sensitisation necessary
• Subsequent exposure triggers massive degranulation by mast cells, mediated by specific IgE antibodies
• Response is not related to quantity of the triggering allergen
• Investigation of Choice: Serum Tryptase Levels.
	• Triggered by direct stimulation on mast cells, causing histamine release
	• Complement activation (classical or alternative pathways)
	• No prior exposure necessary
	• No IgE antibody involvement
	• Example of anaphylactoid reaction
	  ▪ Common in reactions to contrast media
	  ▪ Drug directly acting on mast cells
	  ▪ Atracurium
	  ▪ Mivacurium
	  ▪ Morphine
	  ▪ Meperidine

350. Ans. (b) Amennorhea

(Ref: Harrison 19th ed. /2267)

- Most common symptom in females with prolactinoma (after galactorrhea) is menstrual - abnormalities.
- Most common symptom in men is: loss of libido followed by headache.

351. Ans. (d) Hypoparathyroidism

- The inferior notching of ribs is seen due to pulsation of collaterals in coarctation of aorta.
- Taussig bing operation is done for tetralogy of fallot and is a shunt surgery where the shunt pulsations can cause inferior rib notching.
- **Remember**: Inferior rib notching *(Roesler sign)*
  ▪ Enlarged collateral vessels -Coarctation of the aorta
  ▪ Interrupted aortic arch
  ▪ Subclavian artery obstruction-Takayasu disease
  ▪ Blalock-Taussig shunt : involves only upper 2 rib spaces

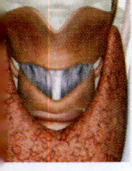

- AVM of the chest wall
- SVC obstruction with enlarged venous collaterals
- Neurogenic tumours - schwannoma (usually single)
- Neurofibromatosis type 1 (rarely can be superior if neurofibroma is very large)
- Superior notching of ribs is seen in Marfan syndrome, rheumatoid arthritis, SLE and hyperparathyroidism.

352. Ans. (c) Prader Willi syndrome

(Ref: Harrison 19th ed. / 415e-4; Nelson 20th/ed pg 307)

Adrenal insufficiency	Salt and water loss leads to weight loss
Pseudo-hypoparathyroidism	PTH receptor defect leads to hypocalcemia and hyperphosphatemia
Soto syndrome	Soto's syndrome aka cerebral gigantism is a rare genetic disorder characterized by excessive physical growth during the first 2 to 3 years of life. Patients with Soto's syndrome tend to be large at birth and are often taller, heavier, and have macrocephaly.

Prader Willi Syndrome
- Neonatal hypotonia with normal growth immediately after birth
- Small hands and feet, mental retardation
- Hypogonadism
- Some have partial deletion of chromosome 15 and loss of paternally expressed genes
- Hyperphagia leading to severe childhood obesity; ghrelin paradoxically elevated.

353. Ans. (d) Smoking is a risk factor

(Ref: Harrison 19th ed./2392)
- The prevalence of obesity is same for men and women at 36%.
- Prevalence increases with age.
- Genetic pre-disposition plays an important role.

Bmi (kg/m²)	Weight Status	Bmi Percentile for Children	Weight Status
<18.5	Underweight	<5th percentile	Underweight
18.5–24.9	Normal weight	5th–84th percentile	Normal weight
25–29.9	Overweight	85th–94th percentile	At risk for overweight
30–34.9	Obese	≥95th percentile	Overweight
35–39.9	Moderately obese		
40–49.9	Morbid obesity		
≥50	Super morbid obesity		

354. Ans. (a) Insulinoma

(Ref: Harrison 20th p 608; Harrison 19th ed./569)
- Whipple's triad is used for diagnosis of insulinoma. The findings seen are:
  - Fasting hypoglycemia (sympathomimetic symptoms)
  - Relief of symptoms with oral/iv sugar
  - Rebound hypoglycemia
- IOC for insulinoma is 72 hour prolonged fasting test
- Imaging modality is P.E.T scan
- *Drug of choice is Octreotide > diazoxide*

355. Ans. (c) Somatostinoma

(Ref: Harrison 19th ed./570)
- In Secretory diarrhea, the epithelial cells' ion transport processes are turned into a state of active secretion. Now since somatostatin is the inhibitory hormone of the GIT therefore secretory diarrhea cannot be seen in these patients.

Causes of Secretory Diarrhea
- The most common cause of acute-onset secretory diarrhea is a bacterial infection of the gut.
  - Features of secretory diarrhea include a high purging rate, a lack of response to fasting, and a normal stool ion gap (ie, 100 mOsm/kg or less), indicating that nutrient absorption is intact.
- Zollinger Ellison syndrome
- VIPoma
- Glucagonoma
- Insulinoma

356. Ans. (b) Homonymous Hemianopia

(Ref: Harrison 20th p 2678-79; Harrison 19th edition, Page 2267)

This patient of acromegaly would be having a pituitary tumour which can compress the optic chiasma leading to bitemporal hemianopia.
Note the large feet size and square hands. The nose appears big in a very tall stout patient
Investigation of choice is glucose tolerance test where failure to supress GH levels is seen.
X-ray foot lateral view shows increased heel pad thickness (>22 mm).

357. Ans. (d) Smoking is a risk factor

(Ref: Harrison 19th p 2392)
- The prevalence of obesity is same for men and women at 36%.
- Prevalence increases with age.
- Genetic pre-disposition plays an important role.

BMI (kg/m²)	Weight Status
<18.5	Underweight
18.5–24.9	Normal weight
25–29.9	Overweight
30–34.9	Obese

Contd...

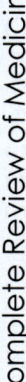

BMI (kg/m²)	Weight Status
35–39.9	Moderately obese
40–49.9	Morbid obesity
≥50	Super morbid obesity

358. Ans. (a) Exercise

(Ref: Harrison 19th p 2395)

- Hyperinsulinemia and insulin resistance are pervasive features of obesity, increasing with weight gain and diminishing with weight loss.
- Insulin resistance is more strongly linked to intraabdominal fat than to fat in other depots.
- Obesity, however, is a major risk factor for diabetes, and as many as 80% of patients with type 2 diabetes mellitus are obese.
- Weight loss and exercise, even of modest degree, increase insulin sensitivity and often improve glucose control in diabetes.
- Before prescribing a weight-loss diet, it is important to emphasize that it takes a long time for a patient to achieve an expanded fat mass; thus, the correction need not occur quickly. On the basis of ~3500 kcal = 1 lb of fat, ~500 kcal restriction daily equates to weight reduction of 1 lb per week. Diets restricted in carbohydrate typically provide a rapid initial weight loss. However, after 1 year, the amount of weight reduction is usually unchanged.

359. Ans. (d) Unilateral carotid artery occlusion

(Ref: Harrison 19th p 40e-4)

Purtscher retinopathy is seen in

- Head and chest trauma.
- Pancreatitis
- Long bone fractures are at risk for developing fat embolization
- Post partum
- Amniotic fluid embolization
- PIH
- Protein C and protein S deficiency have been reported.
- Thrombocytopenia purpura, cryoglobulinemia, hemolytic uremic syndrome, juvenile derma-tomyositis, and multiple myeloma.
- Unexplained vision loss in patients with these conditions (e.g., systemic lupus erythematosus, dermatomyositis, Scleroderma) should raise the possibility of Purtscher-like retinopathy.

Fundus findings of Purtscher retinopathy: Multiple cotton-wool spots surround the optic disc and hemorrhages around macula due to occlusion of posterior retinal artery with aggregated leucocytes.

360. Ans. (a) ACTH excess leading to Cushing syndrome

(Ref: William's Textbook of Endocrinology 12th ed. P-841-842-Endocrinology of fetus)

- Allgrove syndrome has Adrenal insensitivity to ACTH leading to cortisol deficiency in combination with Achalasia and Schirmer's test showing reduced tear production.
- Skin examination of patients may reveal abnormal findings that assist in confirming diagnosis.
- Hyperpigmentation is common but may be observed less frequently than in other forms of primary adrenal failure. Hyperkeratosis and fine fissuring of the palms of the hands and soles of the feet represent a unique feature of this syndrome.

361. Ans. (a) Ghrelin

(Ref: Nelson 20th edition pg 307)

- The role of ghrelin in the satiety defect found in Prader-Willi syndrome is a subject of active investigation.
- Affected patients develop extreme obesity associated with uncontrollable and voracious appetite.
- Ghrelin is a hunger-stimulating peptide and hormone that is produced mainly by P/D_1 cells lining the fundus of the human stomach and epsilon cells of the pancreas.
- Ghrelin levels increase before meals and decrease after meals. It is considered to be the counterpart of the hormone leptin, produced by adipose tissue, which induces satiation when present at higher levels.
- In some bariatric procedures, the level of ghrelin is reduced in patients, thus causing satiation before it would normally occur

362. Ans. (a) Gout

(Ref: Harrison's 18th edition Chapter 54. Skin Manifestations of Internal Disease and www.nejm.org/doi/full/10.1056/NEJMicm1000193)

- In gout the tophi are present adjacent to skin of joints, particularly those of the hands and feet. Additional sites of tophi formation include the helix of the ear and the olecranon and prepatellar bursae. The lesions are firm, yellow in color, and occasionally discharge a chalky material. But there is no mention of calcification in any text.
- Although rare, calcification and even true ossification of the auricular cartilages have been described in association with:
  - Mechanical tissue injury
  - *Exposure to cold*
  - Inflammatory conditions
  - *Alkaptonuria*
  - Endocrinopathies: Recognition of the association between auricular calcification and adrenal insufficiency can be an important step toward the identification of a life-threatening cortisol deficiency

363. Ans. (a) Homocystiene

(Ref: McCaddon et al 2006: Homocysteine and cognitive impairment)

- Homocysteine levels predict cognitive decline in healthy elderly, and hyperhomocysteinaemia is an independent risk factor for the development of dementia, including AD.
- Potential mechanisms by which homocysteine might influence cognition include a direct toxicity on glutamate neurotransmission and cerebrovascular endothelium, an indirect inhibition of transmethylation reactions in brain, potentiation of amyloid neurotoxicity and promotion of tau phosphorylation.

- Vitamin B_{12} is essential for two mammalian metabolic reactions-the conversion of methyl-malonyl-CoA to succinyl-CoA, and of homo-cysteine to methionine.
- Serum levels of methylmalonic acid rise in B_{12} deficiency, whereas homocysteine levels rise in both folate and B_{12} deficiency.
- Of these two metabolites, homocysteine has recently attracted interest with regard to cognitive function and aging.
- Elevated plasma homocysteine is associated with an increased risk of vascular disease and vascular dementia.
- There are also widely confirmed reports of elevated blood levels in patients with Alzheimer's disease and mild cognitive impairment.

364. Ans. (a) Headache

(Ref: Harrison 19th p 2264)

Craniopharyngioma typically is a slow-growing tumor. Symptoms frequently develop insidiously and usually become obvious only after the tumor attains a diameter of about 3cm. Clinical features: *The most common presenting symptoms are headache (55-96%), endocrine dysfunction (66-90%), and visual disturbances (37-68%).*

- Headache is slowly progressive, dull, continuous, and positional; it becomes severe in most patients when endocrine symptoms become obvious.
- On presentation, 40% of patients have symptoms related to hypothyroidism (eg, weight gain, fatigue, cold intolerance, constipation).
- Almost 25% have associated signs and symptoms of adrenal failure (eg, orthostatic hypotension, hypoglycemia, hyperkalemia, cardiac arrhythmias, lethargy, confusion, anorexia, nausea and vomiting), and 20% have diabetes insipidus (e.g., excessive fluid intake and urination).
- Most young patients present with growth failure and delayed puberty. Eighty percent of adults complain of decreased sexual drive, and almost 90% of men complain of impotence, while most women complain of amenorrhea.
- Visual manifestations depend on location
  - *Prechiasmal localization* - Typically results in associated findings of optic atrophy (eg, progressive decline of visual acuity, constriction of visual fields)
  - *Retrochiasmal location* - Commonly associated with hydrocephalus with signs of increased intracranial pressure (e.g., papilledema, horizontal double vision)
  - *Intrasellar craniopharyngioma* - Usually manifests as headache and/or endocrinopathy

365. Ans. (d) Sella chordoma

(Ref: Harrison 20th p 2673; Harrison 19th p 2264)

- Sella chordomas usually present with bony clival erosion, local invasiveness, and, on occasion, calcification. Normal pituitary tissue may be visible on MRI, distinguishing chordomas from aggressive pituitary adenomas. Mucinous material may be obtained by fine-needle aspiration.
- Anatomically clivus sits posterior to the sphenoid sinuses. Just lateral to the clivus bilaterally is the foramen lacerum which contains the internal carotid artery, proximal to its anastamosis with the Circle of Willis. Posterior to the clivus is the basilar artery.

366. Ans. (d) GH reserve

(Ref: Pediatric endocrinology Mark A. Sparling, table 10.9, 4th ed.)

367. Ans. (b) ACTH

(Ref: Harrison 19th p 2310)

ACTH stimulation test/ Cosyntropin test
- During the test, a small amount of synthetic ACTH is injected, and the amount of cortisol, that the adrenals produce in response is measured. This test may cause mild to moderate side effects in some individuals.
- This test is used to diagnose or exclude primary and secondary adrenal insufficiency.
- In addition to quantifying adrenal insufficiency, the test can distinguish whether the cause is adrenal (low cortisol and aldosterone production) or pituitary (low ACTH production).The ACTH stimulation test is recognized as the gold standard assay of adrenal insufficiency, although this test is primarily used to determine the presence of Addison's disease and pituitary impairment. The test is extremely sensitive (97% at 95% specificity) to primary adrenal insufficiency, but less so to secondary adrenal insufficiency.

368. Ans. (a) Achondroplasia

(Ref: Harrison 20th p 2965-66; Harrison 19th p 426e-7)

- Achondroplasia is evident at birth as a disproportionate short-limb dwarfing condition. Characteristics include an enlarged neurocranium, frontal bossing, flattening of the nasal bridge, midface hypoplasia, and a relatively prominent mandible
- *Abnormal development of the base of the skull results in a foramen magnum that is smaller than in average individuals.* The narrowing of the foramen magnum compresses the cervicomedullary region, causing symptoms of respiratory insufficiency, apnea, cyanotic episodes, feeding problems, quadriparesis, and sudden death
- *The upper extremity involvement is rhizomelic, with the proximal segments more severely affected than the distal segments.* The shoulders appear broad due to normal development of clavicle and well-developed musculature.
- A trident hand is common and is characterized by a persistent space between the long and ring fingers when approximation of the fingers is attempted in full extension. The fingertips reach the level of the hips, which causes difficulty with hygiene and dressing.
- Lower extremity involvement is rhizomelic, with hip flexion contractures, ligamentous laxity and external rotation of the extremity, and genu recurvatum before walking age.
- IQ is normal though not mentioned in the question.

369. Ans. (a) Chorea

(Ref: Harrison 19th p 2512)

370. Ans. (c) Hypocalcemia

(Ref: Harrison 19th p 570)

- A diagnosis of VIPOMA is made when watery diarrhea, hypokalemia, and achlorhydria are present in the setting of elevated serum vasoactive intestinal polypeptide (VIP) concentrations.
- Stool volumes of less than 700 mL virtually exclude the diagnosis, with typical stool volumes in the presence of VIPOMAS being more than 3 L daily.
- Evaluation for persistence of diarrhea when fasting and analysis of stool for electrolytes and osmolality may be useful diagnostic approaches in the evaluation of secretory diarrhea.
- Hypercalcemia occurs in the 25-50% patients of VIPOMA. The mechanism of action is not clear but is believed to be through increased bone resorption
- Hyperglycemia may be caused by the direct glycogenolytic effect of VIP on the liver and by the inhibitory effect of hypokalemia on pancreatic islet cell insulin release.

371. Ans. (c) Testes

(Ref: Harrison 20th p 2980; Harrison 19th p 2512)

Hemochromatosis is characterized pathologically by tissue damage produced by iron deposition that often manifests in middle age as a slowly progressive and symmetric arthropathy. Specific clinical manifestations relate to the site of abnormal iron accumulation.

1. Iron within the parenchymal cells of the liver is associated with liver cirrhosis
2. Iron deposits in the pancreas result in diabetes
3. Iron and melanin accumulations in the skin produce abnormal pigmentation (bronzing of skin)
4. Cardiac deposition of iron results in heart failure due to Restrictive cardiomyopathy
5. Arthropathy
6. The damage to pituitary manifests as hypogonadism

372. Ans. (c) Urinary copper excretion is <100 mcg/day

(Ref: Harrison 20th p 2983; Harrison 19th p 2519)

- *The urinary copper excretion* rate is greater than 100 mcg/d (reference range, < 40 mcg/d) in most patients with symptomatic Wilson disease. The rate may also be elevated in other cholestatic liver diseases.
- *Liver biopsy* is regarded as the criterion standard for diagnosis of Wilson disease. A liver biopsy with sufficient tissue reveals levels of more than 250 mcg/g of dry weight even in asymptomatic patients.
- *Mutation analysis* is an especially valuable diagnostic strategy for certain well-defined populations exhibiting a limited spectrum of ATP7B mutations.
- *Radiolabeled copper testing* directly assays hepatic copper metabolism. Blood is collected at 1, 2, 4, 24, and 48 hours after oral ingestion of radiolabeled copper (64 Cu or 67 Cu) for radioactivity in serum. In all individuals, radioactivity promptly appears after absorption, followed by hepatic clearance. In healthy people, reappearance of the radioactivity in serum occurs as the labeled copper is incorporated into newly synthesized ceruloplasmin and released into the circulation. In wilson disease this is delayed.

- *MRI of the brain* appears to be more sensitive than CT scanning in detecting early lesions of Wilson disease. MRI studies have identified focal abnormalities in the white matter, pons, and deep cerebellar nuclei. These lesions, measuring 3-15 mm in diameter, are typically bilateral, appearing with low signal intensity on T1-weighted images and with high signal intensity on T2-weighted images, representing cell loss and gliosis. Other studies describe decreased signal intensity in the putamen and other parts of the basal ganglia, which may represent either copper or iron ferritin deposition. A characteristic *"face of the giant panda"* sign has been described, formed by high signal intensity in the tegmentum (except for the red nucleus), preserved signal intensity of the lateral portion of the pars reticulata of the substantia nigra, and hypointensity of the superior colliculus.

373. Ans. (c) Canagliflozin

(Ref: Harrison 20th p 2866; Harrison 19th p 2415)

- Canagliflozin is an inhibitor of subtype 2 sodium-glucose transport protein (SGLT2), which is responsible for at least 90% of the glucose reabsorption in the kidney (SGLT1 being responsible for the remaining 10%).
- Blocking this transporter causes about 50 to 80 grams of blood glucose per day to be eliminated through the urine, corresponding to 200–300 kilocalories.
- Additional water is eliminated by osmotic diuresis, resulting in a lowering of blood pressure.
- Two thirds of the resulting weight loss are caused by the body using up fat tissue to replace the lost glucose, and the rest is mostly water.

374. Ans. (b) Potassium chloride

(Ref: Harrison 19th p 444e)

- Hypokalemic periodic paralysis is a calcium channel defect.
- During attacks, oral potassium supplementation is preferable to IV supplementation. The latter is reserved for patients who are nauseated or unable to swallow. Potassium chloride is the preferred agent for an acute attack (assuming a normal renal function).
- A reasonable initial dose for a 60-120 kg man (ie, 0.5-1 mEq/kg) is 60 mEq. Aqueous potassium is favored for quicker results. If there is no response in 30 minutes, an additional 0.3 mEq/kg may be given.
- Oral K.C.L (0.2-0.4) mm or/kg should be given every 30 minutes

375. Ans. (a) Thyrotoxicosis

(Ref: Bedside cardiology A. Sarkar, 1st ed. pg. 85)

Dancing carotids are seen in aortic regurgitation due to hyperdynamic circulation and since thyrotoxicosis can lead to Aortic Regurgitation, choice A is the answer.

Do not confuse with carotid thrill seen with aortic stenosis.

376. Ans. (d) Hypopituitarism

(Ref: Harrison 19th p 2257)

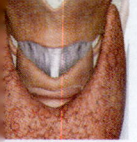

377. Ans. (b) Acromegaly

(Ref: Harrison 19th p 2269)

378. Ans. (a) Peptic Ulceration, Gastric Hypersecretion, Non beta Cell Tumour

(Ref: Harrison 19th p 2336)

379. Ans. (d) Appendix

(Ref: Harrison 19th p 564)

380. Ans. (b) Tricuspid valve

(Ref: Harrison 19th p 564)

381. Ans. (a) Hurler Disease

(Ref: Nelson's text book of Paediatrics, 19th, Page 510)

Hurler Disease	MPS I Hurler syndrome often presents in infancy or early childhood with <ul><li>Chronic rhinitis</li><li>Clouding of the cornea</li><li>Hepatosplenomegaly</li><li>Coarse facies</li><li>Macroglossia</li></ul>
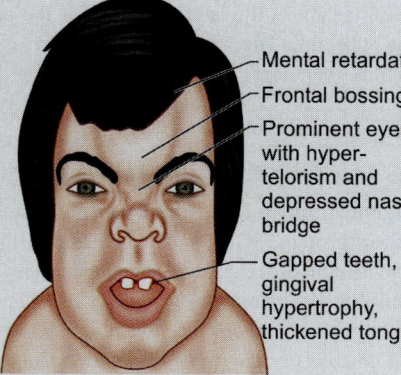 Mental retardation; Frontal bossing; Prominent eyes, with hypertelorism and depressed nasal bridge; Gapped teeth, gingival hypertrophy, thickened tongue	
Beckwith Wiedemann Disease 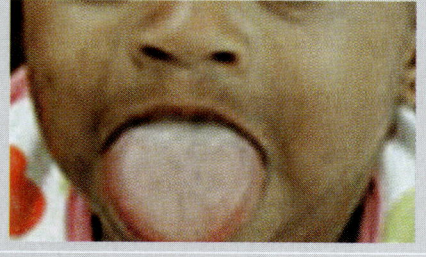	Presents with *Macroglossia* with hemi-hypertrophy, hypoglycaemia and genitourinary anomalies
Proteus Syndrome 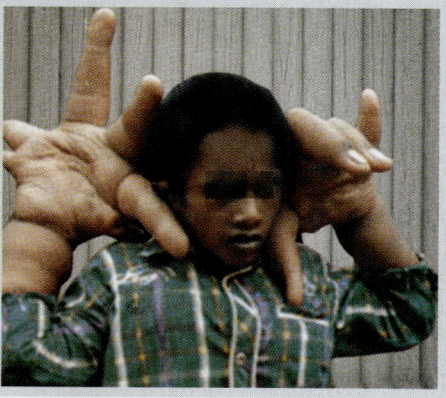	<ul><li>Proteus syndrome is a progressive condition wherein children are usually born without any obvious deformities.</li><li>Tumors of skin and bone growths appear as they age.</li><li>The severity and locations of these asymmetrical growths vary greatly but typically the skull, one or more limbs, and soles of the feet will be affected.</li></ul>
Hypothyroidism	Presents with short stature with coarse facies and large tongue but lips are normal. Hepatosplenomegaly is not seen. Chronic rhinitis is not seen.

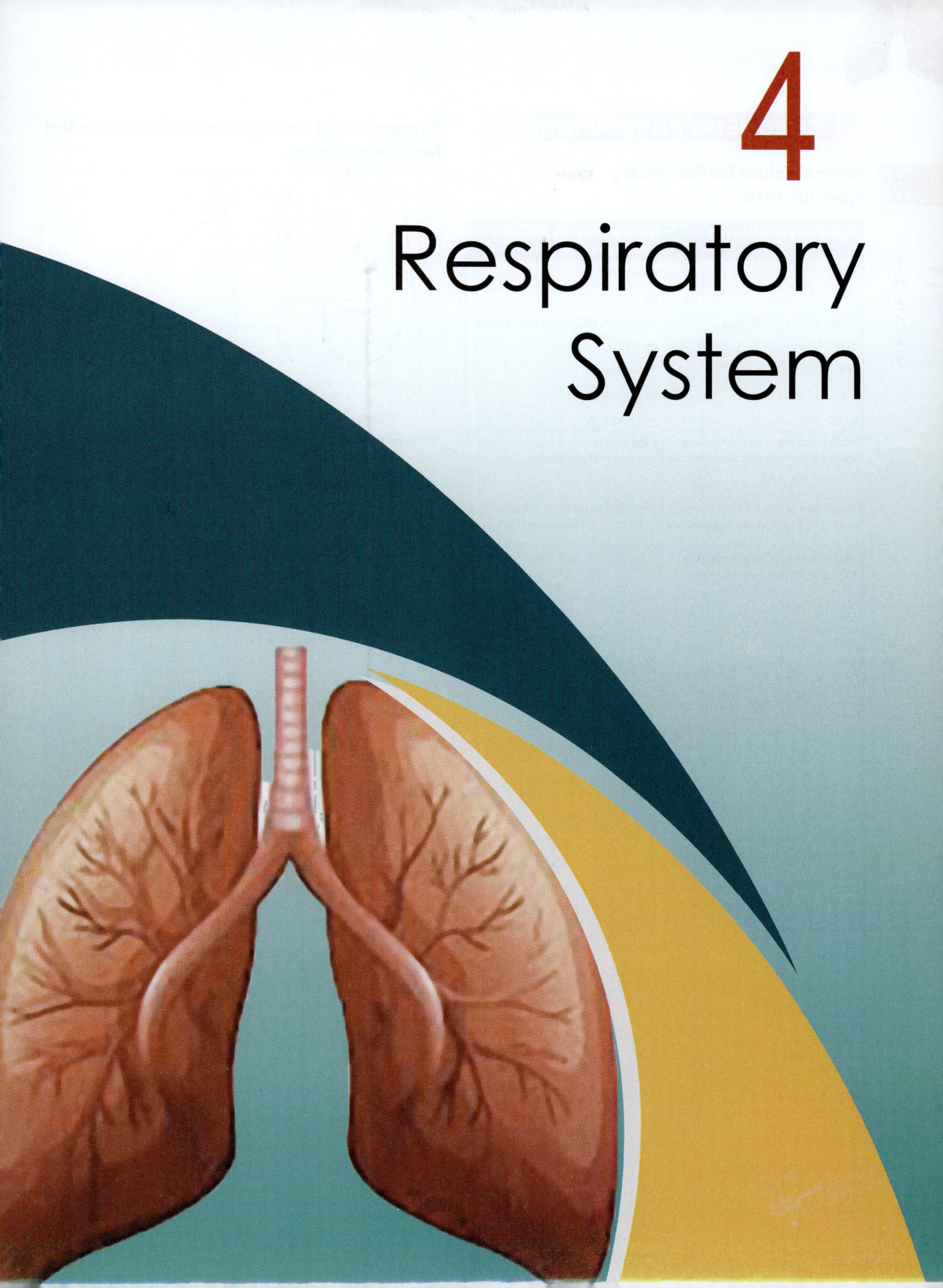

4
Respiratory System

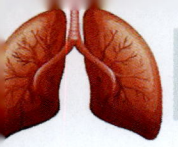

SPIROMETRY INTERPRETATION

Normal Values for Pulmonary Function Tests

Pulmonary function test	Normal value (95 percent confidence interval)
FEV_1	80 – 120%
FVC	80 – 120%
Absolute FEV_1/FVC ratio	Within 5% of the predicted ratio
TLC	80 – 120%
FRC	75 – 120%
RV	75 – 120%
DLCO	>60 – <120%

Residual volume cannot be measured by spirometry.
Residual volume can be best measured by body plethysmography.

Comparison of Normal versus Obstructive and Restrictive Curves

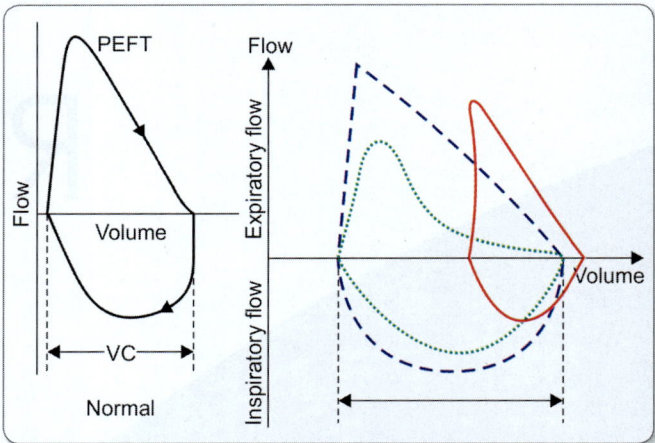

The dotted green pattern shows a prolonged expiration suggestive of asthma. The red line shows reduced TLC and RV in pulmonary fibrosis leading to pointed cap appearance of the curve. The inspiratory part of curve is smaller in restrictive lung disease due to smaller vital capacity.

Variable extra thoracic pattern Example: Retrosternal goiter	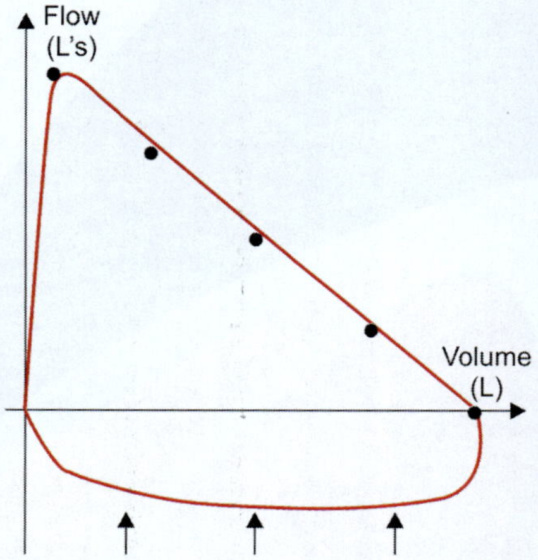	During inspiration, the retrosternal goiter moves downwards and compresses the airways leading to the inspiratory part being flat. However, during expiration, the retrosternal goiter moves up allowing airways to expel the air
Variable intrathoracic pattern Example: Laryngeal tumor	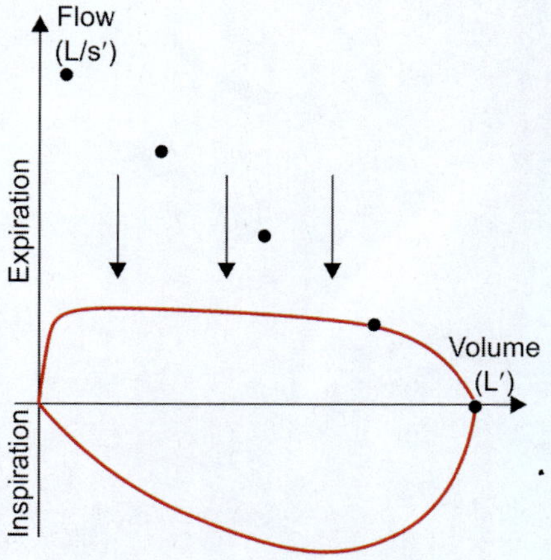	The expiratory pattern is flat During inspiration the force of inspiration moves the tumor to allow inflow. But during expiration, the tumor creates a ball valve effect leading to flattening of expiratory part

Contd...

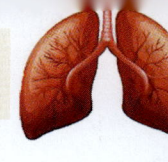

Fixed large airway obstruction
Example: Tracheal stenosis

Both inspiration and expiration becomes flat.
Example: Tracheal stenosis (due to prolonged intubation)

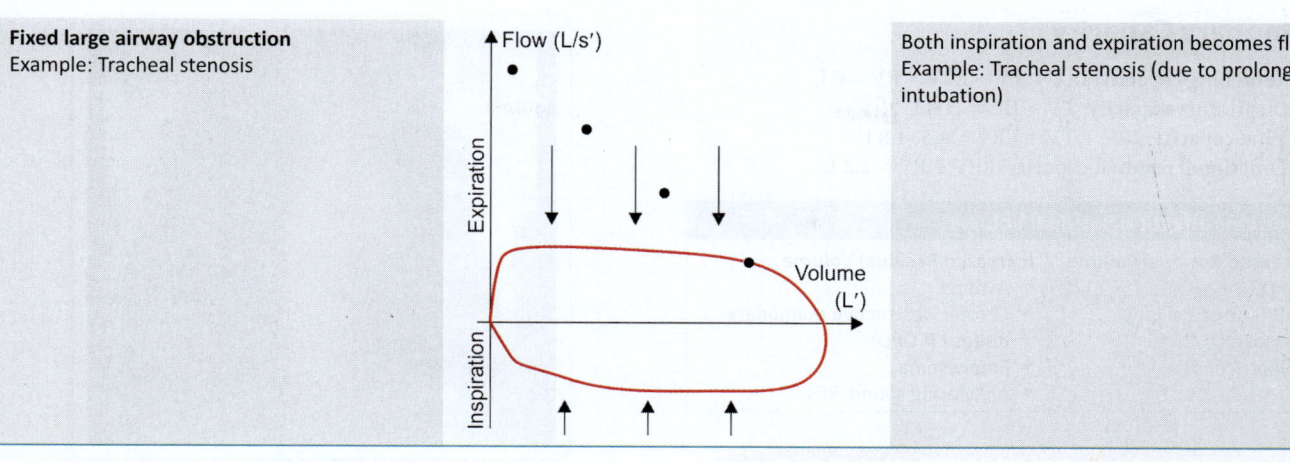

Steps to be followed for Spirometry Report Assessment

1. The inferior part of Y axis is the inspiration and superior side of Y axis is the expiration.
2. Imagine filling up your lungs from RV to TLC and then exhaling from TLC to RV.
3. In obstructive diseases, the expiratory part of curve is prolonged. The curve may shift rightward due to increase of Residual volume.
4. *In restrictive diseases, the inspiratory part of curve is very small and the whole recording shifts leftward due to decrease in TLC and RV.*
5. In tracheal stenosis, both inspiratory and expiratory patterns flatten out. This is called **fixed large airway obstruction**.
6. If only inspiratory part is flat, it indicates a lesion like retrosternal goiter compressing airways during respiration when it moves downwards. This is called extrathoracic obstruction as the lesion is outside the chest cavity primarily.
7. If only expiratory part is flat, it indicates a laryngeal tumor, which acts like a ball valve and obstructs expiration. This is called **variable intrathoracic obstruction**.

TABLE 4.1: Classification of Ventilatory Abnormalities by Spirometry

	Obstructive	Restrictive	Mixed
FEV_1	↓	↓ or Normal	↓
FVC	↓ or Normal	↓	↓
FEV_1/FVC	↓	Normal or ↑	↓

Features of Obstructive Pattern on Spirometry

- During an obstruction in airways, there is decrease in expiratory flow, which becomes more pronounced when expiration is more forceful.
- Hallmark is decrease in expiratory flow rates.
- FEV1 is *markedly reduced* and FVC is mildly reduced so that *ratio of FEV1/FVC is highly reduced*.
- Asthma has a reversible airflow obstruction where reversibility of airflow obstruction is defined as *change of FEV1 > 12% on salbutamol inhalation*.
- Diffusion capacity is normal except in emphysema, where it is reduced.

Features of Restrictive Pattern on Spirometry

- Hallmark is decrease in TLC and VC (Reduced lung volume).
- FEV1 is mildly reduced but FVC is highly reduced so that ratio of *FVC is normal or increased*.
- Diffusion capacity is *reduced*.

Causes of Restrictive Lung Disease

Restrictive – parenchymal	Restrictive – extra-parenchymal
• Sarcoidosis • Idiopathic pulmonary fibrosis • Pneumoconiosis • Drugs (Amiodarone) • Radiation • Acute respiratory distress syndrome (ARDS) in resolution phase	• Guillain Barre syndrome • Myasthenia gravis • Diaphragmatic paralysis • Cervical spine injury • Kyphosis • Obesity • Ankylosing spondylosis

- Restrictive lung diseases are characterized by decreased compliance and normal or increased FEV1/FVC
- Compliance decreases in restrictive lung disease. Compliance is usually unaffected in obstructive lung disease except emphysema where it is increased.
- Emphysema is associated with an increased static compliance.
- Surfactant deficiency leads to atelectasis that causes reduced compliance.

Diffusion Capacity of Lung (DL_{CO})

Decrease value of DL_{CO} is seen in	Increased level of DL_{CO} is seen in
• Emphysema • Interstitial lung disease • Recurrent pulmonary emboli • Anemia • Severe CHF • Pulmonary artery hypertension	• Mild CHF (due to increased pulmonary flow) (Note: It is increased in mild CHF and reduced in severe CHF) • Alveolar hemorrhage/ Good's Pasture syndrome • Polycythemia • Left to right shunts

* DL_{CO} in asthma is normal to mildly elevated.

Pulmonary Capacity

- **Total lung capacity**: IRV + TV + ERV + RV = **6 L**
- **Inspiratory capacity**: TV + IRV = **3.8 L**
- **Vital capacity**: IRV + TV + ERV = **4.5–4.8 L**
- **Functional residual capacity**: ERV + RV = **2.2 L**

Conditions affecting Residual Volume	
Decreased Residual volume	**Increased Residual Volume**
• ARDS • ILD (interstitial lung disease) • Kyphoscoliosis	• Asthma • Chronic obstructive pulmonary disease (COPD) • Emphysema • Ankylosing spondylitis

PULMONARY TUBERCULOSIS

TB Transmission

1. **Droplets**: TB transmission via droplets affects lungs and tonsils. Seeding of tonsils leads to cervical lymphadenopathy. *(MC form of extrapulmonary tuberculosis is TB lymphadenitis)*. The best test for TB lymphadenitis is FNAC. Any delay can result in development of cold abscess which is best managed by ATT with anti-gravity drainage. Sites of extrapulmonary TB in decreasing order are lymph nodes > pleura > genitourinary TB
2. **Ingestion**: Swallowing of *Mycobacterium tuberculosis* can lead to ileocecal TB. In rural India, *M.Bovis* affects GIT when unpasteurized milk is consumed by a person.
3. **Vertical transmission** occurs due to transplacental spread. *Ghon's focus is formed in the liver of the baby during the intrauterine life.*
4. **Direct contact**: It manifests as lupus vulgaris (skin TB)

Primary Tuberculosis

- This is usually clinically and radiographically silent. In most persons with intact cell-mediated immunity, T cells and macrophages surround the organisms in granulomas that limit their multiplication and spread. The infection is contained but not eradicated, since viable organisms may lie dormant within granulomas for years to decades. Reactivation of TB starts from the apex because of high ventilation/perfusion ratio.
- *Most common site of primary tuberculosis is lower part of upper lobe or upper part of lower lobe.* Due to subpleural location, it can lead to pleural effusion.
- As *M. tuberculosis* enters the lungs, it first forms **Ghon's focus**, after a while when bacterial presence generates inflammatory response causing enlargement of the hilar lymph node. This is referred to as **GHON complex**.
- In an immune patient, GHON complex is calcified preventing further spread of the infection and is called Ranke complex.
- In case of failure of formation of Ranke complex, primary progressive tuberculosis develops which includes following entities:
    1. Primary caseous pneumonia
    2. Tuberculous bronchopneumonia
    3. Miliary TB
- Reactivated TB bacteria migrate from the middle of the lungs to the apex due to higher ventilation/perfusion ratio.

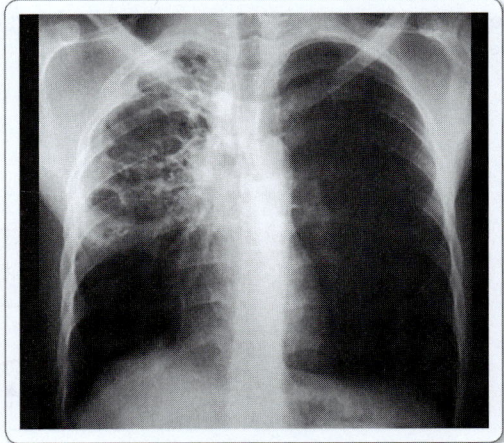

Figure 4.1: Pulmonary tuberculosis with large cavity in right upper zone

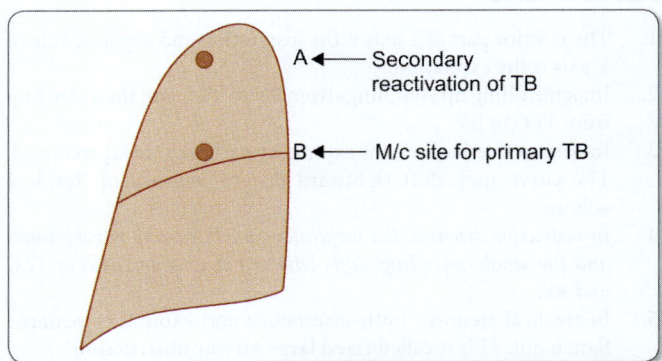

Figure 4.2: Sites for pulmonary TB

- Bacteria at the apex can form supraclavicular or infraclavicular lesions. If it is supraclavicular, it is known as **Puhl's lesion** and if it is infraclavicular it is known as **Assman focus**.

Puhl lesion	Supraclavicular focus in chronic pulmonary TB
Assman focus	Infraclavicular focus in chronic pulmonary TB
Weigert focus	Caseating metastatic focus in wall of pulmonary vein
Rich focus	TB meningitis
Simon focus	Calcified focus in apex
Simmond's focus	Tubercular foci in liver
Poncet's disease	Tubercular arthritis

Latent Tuberculosis Infection

- This does not have active disease and cannot transmit the organism to others. However, reactivation of disease may occur if the host's immune defenses are impaired.
- Active tuberculosis will develop in approximately 6% of individuals with latent tuberculosis infection, who are not given preventive therapy.

Clinical Features of TB

1. Chronic cough is the most common symptom
2. Fatigue, weight loss, fever, night sweats
3. Low grade fever with evening rise of the temperature
4. Chest pain: *due to pleurisy*
5. Hemoptysis is the last manifestation (*Source*: Bronchial artery)
6. When cavity erodes into the bronchus the sputum in this scenario will be positive for AFB. However, small cavity can also produce a similar symptom but it is negative for AFB because of the minimal erosion of the bronchus.
7. Further invasion can lead to involvement of veins, which then causes spread of infection via heart to multiple organs and causes disseminated TB.

Miliary or Disseminated TB

- Miliary TB is due to hematogenous spread of tubercle bacilli. Although in children it is often the consequence of primary infection, in adults it may be due to either recent infection or reactivation of old disseminated foci. The lesions are usually yellowish granulomas 1–2 mm in diameter that resemble millet seeds, thus the term *miliary*.
- Miliary TB ultimately spreads via artery to other organs in the body.
- *Eye examination may reveal choroidal tubercles, which are pathognomonic of miliary TB, in up to 30% of cases.*
- Meningismus occurs in <10% of cases. A high index of suspicion is required for the diagnosis of miliary TB. Frequently, chest radiography reveals a miliary reticulonodular pattern (more easily seen on underpenetrated film), although no radiographic abnormality may be evident early in the course and among HIV-infected patients.

Organs/Tissues Not Affected by Tuberculosis
- Cornea
- Pancreas
- Vagina
- Myocardium

Risk Factors for MTB Infection

- Age (late adolescence and early adulthood, elderly)
- HIV co-infection
- Silicosis
- Lymphoma: Leukemia
- Hemophilia
- Chronic renal failure and hemodialysis
- Type I- DM
- Malnutrition
- Old self-healed, fibrotic tuberculosis lesion
- Immunocompromised state

- MC cause of recurrent hemoptysis is bronchial adenoma.
- MC cause of hemoptysis in world as well as India is TB
- Hemoptysis in TB is due to rupture of bronchial artery and pulmonary artery.
- Damage to *pulmonary artery* in TB is known as *Rasmussen aneurysm*.
- MC cause of endemic hemoptysis is Paragonimus Westermani
- Pseudohemoptysis is seen with *Serratia marcescens*
- Spurious hemoptysis is seen with epistaxis.

Investigations for TB

1. **For demonstrating the presence of AFB:**
   - **By microscopy:** 10^4 bacilli /mL sputum
   - **BACTEC:** Radiolabeled palmitic acid C^{14} growth in 5–8 days
   - **SEPTICHECK:** Biphasic media (solid egg + liquid broth)
   - **MGT** (mycobacteria growth indicator tube)
   - Showing increased fluorescence on using O_2 by bacteria
2. **T-cell interferon γ-release assay**: In vitro test for cellular immunity, which measures cell mediated immune response by quantifying IFN-γ release by T-cells in response to stimulation by MTB antigens.
   - **Currently two ex-vivo assays are available**: The **T-SPOT TB** that directly counts the number of IFN-γ secreting T-cells and the whole blood **QuantiFERON- TB Gold In-Tube** that measures concentration of IFN-γ secretion.
3. **AMPLICOR:** PCR based, quick (within 7 hours)
4. **Tuberculin skin test/Mantoux test**
   - 0.1 mL (PPD RT 23 with Tween 80) **5U** is used to raise wheal by 6–10 mm. Read the induration (transverse) after 48–72 hrs
     ◆ 0–4 mm: –ve
     ◆ 5–9 mm: +ve in
       – HIV +ve
       – Close contact with TB patient
       – Patient on immunosuppressive treatment (>15 mg/d prednisolone for >1 month)
       – Radiograph consistent with old Koch's
     ◆ ≥ 10 mm +ve

Mantoux test is a prognostic test not a diagnostic test.

False positive	False negative
• BCG vaccine • Exposed to atypical Mycobacterium • Leprosy	• AIDS • Steroids usage • Chemotherapy • Measles • Recent blood transfusion

5. **Xpert MTB/RIF**: Nucleic acid amplification technology. It has sensitivity of 98% in acid fast bacilli (AFB) ⊕ cases, WHO recommends it as initial diagnostic test in Multidrug-resistant (MDR)-TB or HIV associated TB.

HIV-associated Tuberculosis

- TB has rapidly progressive and fatal course in HIV +ve patients as HIV increases reactivation of latent infection
- Extrapulmonary TB more common
- Cavity size: Small
- More lymphadenopathy (intrathoracic)
- Less smear positive cases
- **Mantoux test:** False negative
- **CXR**: Normal
- TBM more frequent (Extrapulmonary TB is more common than pulmonary TB in HIV with TB)
- Mycobacteremia more frequent
- Lack of granuloma formation
- Response to short course chemotherapy similar
- Severe skin reaction to **thioacetazone**
- IOC: Xpert MTB/RIF (pg 1113 Harison 19/e)
- **Rx**: HAART + ATT
- **Rifampicin** is **not** given with protease /non-nucleoside reverse transcriptase inhibitors. Rifabutin is substituted.

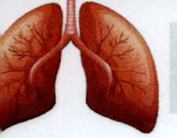

> **EXTRA MILE**
>
> In a patient diagnosed with HIV + TB together, *which drug should be given first ATT or ART?*
> - ATT should be started first, because of IRIS (immune reconstitution inflammatory syndrome).
> - If ART is started first, it may improve CD4 cells at first, but later a previously acquired infection (TB, Herpes), responds with an overwhelming inflammatory response that paradoxically makes the symptoms of infection worse.
> - Therefore, starting of ATT ~ 2 weeks before ART, have shown to decrease the incidence of immune reconstitution inflammatory syndrome (IRIS) (pg 1119, Harison 19/e).

Drug-Resistant TB

Strains of *M. tuberculosis* resistant to individual drugs arise by spontaneous point mutations in the mycobacterial genome that occur at low but predictable rates. Because there is no cross-resistance among the commonly used drugs, the probability that a strain will be resistant to two drugs is the product of the probabilities of resistance to each drug and thus is low.

- The development of drug-resistant TB is invariably the result of monotherapy—i.e., the failure of the healthcare provider to prescribe at least two drugs to which tubercle bacilli are susceptible or of the patient to take properly prescribed therapy. Drug-resistant TB may be either primary or acquired.
- **Primary drug resistance** is that which develops in a strain infecting a patient who has not previously been treated.
- **Acquired resistance** develops during treatment with an inappropriate regimen.

> Gene mutation responsible for
> - Rifampicin resistance: rpoB
> - Pyrazinamide resistance: pncA gene
> - INH Resistance: inhA gene.

OBSTRUCTIVE SLEEP APNEA SYNDROME (OSAS)

- OSAS occurs in around 1–4% of middle-aged males and is about half as common in women
- This disorder is characterized by intermittent closure/collapse of the pharyngeal airway which causes apneic episodes during sleep. These are terminated by partial arousal.
- By **convention, sleep apnea is defined as breath cessation of at least 10 seconds**
- OSAS is often identified when it is associated with a ≥ 3% drop in O_2 saturation and/or brain cortical arousal.
- OSAS leads to systemic hypertension to the tune of 5–10 mm Hg.
- This rise probably results from a combination of surges in blood pressure accompanying each arousal at apnea/hypopnea termination and from the associated 24-h increase in sympathetic tone.
- Epidemiologic data in normal populations indicate that this rise in blood pressure would *increase the risk of myocardial infarction by around 20% and that of stroke by about 40%.*

Whom to Treat?

- Epworth Sleepiness Score >11
- Troublesome sleepiness while driving or working
- >15 apneas + hypopneas per hour of sleep
- For those with similar degrees of sleepiness and 5–15 events per hour of sleep, RCTs indicate improvements in symptoms, including subjective sleepiness, with less strong evidence indicating gains in cognition and quality of life.

Complications of OSAS

1. Pulmonary hypertension
2. Cor pulmonale
3. Type II respiratory failure
4. Systemic hypertension
5. MI
6. Stroke
7. Arrhythmia-like atrial fibrillation

Investigations

Polysomnography which monitors
1. Oxygen saturation
2. Airflow at the nose and mouth
3. ECG: To demonstrate tachycardia seen during apneic event
4. EMG: Measured at chin and leg
5. EEG: To demonstrate cortical awakening
6. EOG: To record ocular movements.

Grading of Severity of OSAHS (Obstructive Sleep Apnea-Hypopnea Syndrome)

Mild OSAHS: 5–14 AHI events/hour
Moderate OSAHS: 15–29 AHI events/hour
Severe OSAHS: > 30 AHI events/hour

*AHI = Apnea–hypopnea index

Treatment

- Quit smoking
- Weight loss of at least 10% body weight
- Continuous positive airway pressure (CPAP) therapy works by blowing the airway open during sleep, usually with pressures of 5–20 mm Hg. CPAP has been shown in randomized placebo-controlled trials to improve breathing during sleep, sleep quality, sleepiness, blood pressure, vigilance, cognition, and driving ability as well as mood and quality of life in patients with OSAS.

PNEUMONIA

- Microorganisms gain access to the lower respiratory tract in several ways. The most common is by aspiration from the oropharynx. Small-volume aspiration occurs frequently during sleep (especially in the elderly) and in patients with decreased levels of consciousness.

Pneumonia is typically classified as
- **Community-acquired (CAP):** Streptococcus pneumoniae
- **Ventilator-associated (VAP).**
  - Non MDR: Streptococcus pneumoniae
  - MDR: Pseudomonas aeruginosa

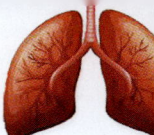

Community-acquired Pneumonia

- The causative agent is *Streptococcus pneumoniae*.
- On chest X-ray, lung consolidation with air bronchogram and infiltrations is observed. The radiological resolution of these findings takes 6 weeks.

Essentials of Diagnosis

- Fever or hypothermia, tachypnea, cough with or without sputum, dyspnea, chest discomfort, sweats or rigors
- *Bronchial breath sounds*^{Q} or inspiratory crackles on chest auscultation.
- Parenchymal opacity on chest radiograph. This opacity is also known as consolidation/ infiltration.
- Occurs outside of the hospital or within 48 hours of hospital admission in a patient not residing in a long-term care facility.

Scoring system for admitting patients with pneumonia
CURB 65 Score
- **C** – Confusion
- **U** – Uremia
- **R** – Respiratory rate (>30 per min)
- **B** – Blood pressure (90/60 mm Hg)
- **65** – Age (>65 yrs)

Score	Treatment
0–1	Outpatient/Inpatient for special cases
2	In Patient
3	In Patient (ICU care)

Treatment

1. Previously healthy and no antibiotics in last 3 months: Start Macrolides^Q.
2. Comorbidity/antibiotics in last 3 months: Levofloxacin, β lactams.

Healthcare-associated Pneumonia

Pneumonia that develops after 48 hrs of hospital stay is referred to as nosocomial pneumonia.
- **Causative agent** for this condition is *S. aureus* (MRSA).
- **Chest X-ray reveals:** Pneumatocele^Q, these are cystic lesions and can rupture leading to pneumothorax.

Clinical conditions associated with Healthcare associated Pneumonia
- Hospitalization > 48h
- Hospitalization for >2 days in prior 3 months
- Nursing home or extended care facility
- Chronic hemodialysis
- Home infusion therapy

Causative organisms for pneumonia

Risk factor	Etiology
Alcoholism	*Streptococcus pneumoniae*
Alcoholic with red currant jelly sputum	*Klebsiella pneumoniae*
Structural lung disease e.g. cystic fibrosis	*P. aeruginosa*
Dementia; stroke	Oral anaerobes
Lung abscess	CA MRSA, oral anaerobes
Ventilator associated pneumonia (Non MDR) (MDR)	*S. pneumoniae* *Pseudomonas*
COPD/Smoking	*Haemophilus influenzae*

HIV-associated Pneumonia

- Causative agent for this condition is *Pneumocystis jirovecii/carinii*. This is an interstitial pneumonia where pus is formed in the interstitial space. Hence the crepitations are unaltered by coughing.
- **Investigation of choice:** Bronchoalveolar lavage stained with Giemsa.
- **Treatment:** Co-trimoxazole^Q
- **Prophylaxis:** Co-trimoxazole^Q

Pneumonia in Alcoholics with Red Currant Jelly Sputum^Q

- Causative agent for this condition is **Klebsiella pneumoniae**. This is also known by an alternate name, Friedlander's pneumonia
- Chest X-ray: Bulging fissure sign *(due to pus in the interlobar fissure)*.
- Treatment: IV Cefotaxime + IV Amikacin.

Bird-Handler's Pneumonia

- This is known by an alternate name Psittacosis. Causative agent responsible for this condition is **Chlamydia psittaci**. This is an example of interstitial pneumonia.
- **Treatment:** Azithromycin, first line. Antibiotic treatment should be continued for 10–14 days post defervescence.

Features of Pneumonia Caused by Specific Organisms

Legionella Pneumophila

- Legionnaire's disease/PONTIAC fever (milder version)
- Inhalation, more common in summer through air conditioning plants and piped hot water systems

- Bilateral lower lobes[Q]
- Relative bradycardia[Q]
- **Can cause SIADH**: Leading to activation of V2 receptor → gain of H_2O → Dilutional hyponatremia. The patient will have disorientation, confusion and seizures.
- Macrolides (erythromycin + rifampicin is DOC)

Mycoplasma Pneumoniae

- Smallest free living organisms
- Young patients (5–15 yrs) in late summer
- Atypical pneumonia
- Lower lobe involvement
- Complications: Autoimmune hemolytic anemia[Q], erythema multiforme, Steven Johnson's syndrome
- Macrolide (erythromycin) - DOC. Penicillin group of drugs is ineffective.

Anaerobic Organisms + Aspiration

- **GNB**: Bacteroides fragilis
- **GPC**: Peptostreptococci, anaerobic and micro-aerophilic streptococci
- When pH <2.4 of aspirated contents it can lead to chemical lung injury and ARDS
- Necrotizing pneumonia leading to lung abscess formation
- Penicillin + metronidazole, clindamycin.
- MC cause of lung abscess in patients with impaired airway reflexes in anaerobes.

> **EXTRA MILE**
> - Clinical pulmonary infection score is used for diagnosis of ventilator associated pneumonia. The components are fevers, leukocytosis, oxygenation, CXR findings, Tracheal aspirate. The maximal score = 12.
> - Biomarkers of severe inflammation are
>   - CRP
>   - Procalcitonin
> - To be adequate for culture, sputum sample should have > 25 neutrophils and < 10 squamous epithelial cells/HPF

PLEURAL EFFUSION

Normal pleural fluid is 5–15 ml.

Types of Pleural Effusion

- **Transudative pleural effusion**: This condition is due to imbalance of pressure between hydrostatic pressure and oncotic pressure.
- **Exudative pleural effusion**: This condition results from inflammation.

Clinical Features

1. Dyspnea on account of large effusion, cough, respirophasic chest pain, bulging intercostals spaces.
2. Stony dullness on percussion with diminished breath sounds

Investigations

Pleural Tap (USG Guided)

Transudate	Exudate
Glucose equal to serum glucose pH same as body fluids 1000 WBC/ μL	- Sugar low - Protein elevated - *Pleural fluid protein to serum protein ratio >0.5* - *Pleural fluid LDH to serum LDH ratio >0.6* - *Pleural fluid LDH > 2/3rd URL of serum LDH*

* Italicised data is called as Light's criteria

Causes of Pleural Effusion

Transudate	Exudate
Causes	**Causes**
- CHF (90%) - Cirrhosis - Nephrotic syndrome - Peritoneal disease - SVC syndrome	- MC cause bacterial pneumonia - Metastatic cancer - Pulmonary embolism - TB - Connective tissue disorders like RA - Uremia - Meigs syndrome - Post MI

Malignant Pleural Effusion

- Lung cancer and breast cancer account for about 50–65% of malignant pleural effusions. Other common causes include pleural mesothelioma and lymphoma.

Characteristics of Important Exudative Pleural Effusions

Type	Gross appearance	Glucose	Others
Malignant effusion	Turbid to bloody	<60 mg%	Cytology shows abnormal cells; Treatment with **pleurodesis** with doxycycline or asbestos free talc
TB effusion	Serous	Low	High protein
Rheumatoid effusion	Turbid greenish	Low	High LDH RA factor positive; Cholesterol crystals
Pancreatitis	Turbid	Equal to serum glucose levels	S. amylase levels elevated
Empyema	Pus	Polymorphs	Needs intercostal drainage

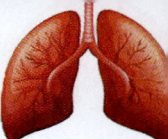

Causes of Left Sided Effusions	Causes of Right Sided Effusions
1. *Acute pancreatitis* (Sympathetic effusion) 2. Pericardial inflammation 3. Esophageal rupture 4. Left sided sub-diaphragmatic abscess 5. Thoracic duct involvement above D5 level.	1. Amoebic liver abscess, subphrenic abscess 2. Meig's syndrome 3. Thoracic duct involvement below D5 level

Causes of B/L Effusion

LVF, Pulmonary infarction, Hypoalbuminemia, Malignancy

Features of tubercular pleural effusion	Conditions associated with glucose < 60 mg/dL seen in Pleural fluid
All features of exudative effusion plus • Hemorrhagic effusion • Presence of high level of TB markers • Elevated adenosine deaminase levels • Interferon γ >140 pg/mL • Positive PCR • Glucose level equal to serum level mostly, occasionally <60 mg% • WBC ↑, predominantly small lymphocyte	• Parapneumonic effusion • Malignant disease • Rheumatoid arthritis **Increased levels of amylase seen in pleural fluid** • Pancreatitis • Malignant tumor • Esophageal rupture • Ruptured ectopic pregnancy

Comparison of Pneumonia Versus Pleural Effusion Versus Pneumothorax

	Pneumonia	Pleural effusion	Pneumothorax
Trachea	Central in position	Deviated to the opposite side	Deviated to the opposite side
Percussion	Dull	Stony dull	Hyper-resonant
Breath sounds	Bronchial breathing	Vesicular breathing	Absent

* Tracheal shift to same side is seen in collapse and idiopathic pulmonary fibrosis.

ASTHMA/REVERSIBLE AIRWAY DISEASE

- Narrowing of the airways is usually reversible, but in some patients with chronic asthma there may be an element of irreversible airflow obstruction. It is a Type I Hypersensitivity reaction.

Essentials of Diagnosis

1. Episodic or chronic symptoms of airflow obstruction
2. Reversibility of airflow obstruction, either spontaneously or following bronchodilator therapy. Change of FEV1 value between before and after salbutamol inhalation should reflect a increment of at least or > **12%**.^{Q}
3. Symptoms frequently worse at night or in the early morning.
4. Prolonged expiration and diffuse wheezes on physical examination.

Risk Factors and Triggers involved in Asthma

Triggers	
• Allergens • Upper respiratory tract viral infections • Exercise and hyperventilation • Cold air	• Sulfur dioxide and irritant gases • Drugs (β-blockers, aspirin) • Stress • Irritants (household sprays, paint fumes)

Occupational asthma is triggered by various agents in the workplace and may occur weeks to years after initial exposure and sensitization. Women may experience catamenial asthma at predictable times during the menstrual cycle.

Exercise-induced bronchoconstriction begins during exercise or within 3 minutes after its end, peaks within 10–15 minutes, and then resolves by 60 minutes. This phenomenon is thought to be a consequence of the airways' attempt to warm and humidify an increased volume of expired air during exercise.

Cardiac asthma is wheezing precipitated by decompensated congestive heart failure.

Drug induced asthma: COX 1 inhibitors precipitate asthma as they facilitate increased production of LOX enzyme resulting in increase in permeability and bronchoconstriction.
e.g.: Aspirin, diclofenac, ketorolac etc.

Symptoms	Physical Examination Findings
1. Episodic wheezing 2. Difficulty in breathing 3. Chest tightness 4. Cough 5. Excessive sputum production	1. Nasal mucosal swelling 2. Increased nasal secretion 3. Nasal polyps are often seen in intrinsic (adult onset) asthma 4. Hunched shoulders with expiratory Rhonchi

Investigations

1. Spirometry:
   - ↓FEV_1 (forced expiratory volume)

FEV1	Classification
50–80%	Mild
30–50%	Moderate
<30%	Severe

   - ↓PEFR (peak expiratory flow rate)
   - Increased residual volume
   - Increased total lung capacity
   - Increased functional residual capacity
2. Absolute Eosinophil count: Increased in childhood (extrinsic asthma)
3. IgE: increased
4. CXR: Evidence of hyperinflation with flattened diaphragmatic domes.

Evaluation of Asthma Exacerbation Severity

	Mild	Moderate	Severe	Subset: respiratory arrest imminent
Symptoms				
Breathlessness	While walking can lie down	While at rest prefers sitting	While at rest sits upright	
Talks in	Sentences	Phrases	Words	Cannot talk^Q
Alertness	May be agitated	Usually agitated	Usually agitated	Drowsy or confused
Signs				
Respiratory rate	Increased	Increased	Often > 30/min	
Use of accessory muscles; suprasternal retractions	Usually not	Commonly	Usually	Paradoxical thoraco^Q-abdominal movement
Wheeze	Moderate, often only end expiratory	Loud; throughout exhalation	Usually loud; throughout inhalation and exhalation	Absence of wheeze^Q
Pulse/minute	<100	>100	> 120	Bradycardia^Q
Pulses paradoxus	Absent <10 mm Hg	May be present 10 – 25 mm Hg	Often present > 25 mm Hg	Absence suggests respiratory muscle fatigue
Functional Assessment				
PEF percent predicted or percent personal best	> 70 %	Approx. 40 – 69 % or response lasts < 2 hours	< 40 %	< 25 % Note: PEF testing may not be needed in very severe attacks
PaO$_2$ (on air) and/or PCO$_2$	Normal (test not usually necessary)	> 60 mm Hg (test not usually necessary)	< 60 mm Hg: possible cyanosis	
	< 42 mm Hg (test not usually necessary)	≤ 42 mm Hg (test not usually necessary)	≥ 42 mm Hg: possible respiratory failure	
SaO$_2$ percent (on air) at sea level	>95% (test not usually necessary)	90–95 % (test not usually necessary)	< 90 %	

Treatment

- DOC Acute asthma exacerbation: Salbutamol nebulization
- Recurrent attacks: Inhaled steroids: E.g. Budesonide, fluticasone + LABA
- Chronic persistent asthma: e.g. Omalizumab
- *Brittle asthma: Subcutaneous adrenaline*
- Used for prophylaxis:
  - Leukotriene modifiers: E.g. Zileuton, montelukast
  - Mast cell stabilizers: E.g. Nedocromil, sodium cromoglycate, ketotifen

Status Asthmaticus / Severe Acute Asthma

1. Patient speaks in monosyllables
2. Breathing fast and shallow with use of accessory muscles
3. Loud Rhonchi (Inspiratory + Expiratory)
4. Pulsus paradoxus
5. **pO$_2$ decreased with pCO$_2$ >45 mm Hg → Type II respiratoy failure** [blood gas analysis shows respiratory acidosis]

Treatment

1. Oxygen driven salbutamol nebulization
2. Parenteral terbutaline if no improvement with salbutamol
3. Intravenous Hydrocortisone
4. Intravenous aminophylline (limited efficacy, high toxicity) is now not recommended, (page 267, CMDT 2019).
5. Mucolytics worsen cough and anxiolytics are contraindicated.
6. Intravenous magnesium sulphate may produce a clinically detectable improvement especially when FEV$_1$ < 25%.

Stepwise Approach to Asthma Therapy

Category	Treatment modality based
Mild intermittent	Inhaled short acting beta 2 agonist on SOS basis
Mild persistent	Inhaled low dose steroids + Inhaled short acting beta 2 agonist
Moderate persistent	Inhaled high dose steroids + theophylline + Inhaled short acting beta 2 agonist
Severe persistent	Oral steroids + theophylline + Inhaled short acting beta 2 agonist

Brittle Asthma

- Some patients show chaotic variations in lung function despite taking appropriate therapy, with diurnal variation in PEFR ≥ 40%
- Some show a persistent pattern of variability and may require oral corticosteroids or, at times, continuous infusion of Beta-2 agonist **(type I brittle asthma)**
- Whereas others have generally normal or near-normal lung function but *precipitous, unpredictable falls in lung function* that may result in death **(type 2 brittle asthma)**
- The latter patients are difficult to manage as they do not respond well to corticosteroids and the worsening of asthma does not reverse well with inhaled bronchodilators.
- **The most effective therapy is subcutaneous epinephrine, which suggests that the worsening is likely to be a localized airway anaphylaxis with edema.**
- In some of these patients, there may be allergy to specific foods.

PULMONARY EMBOLISM

Etiology

- Venous stasis due to immobility – post op, stroke and obesity
- Hyperviscosity: Polycythaemia
- Increased venous pressure: pregnancy
- Orthopaedic surgery and pelvic surgery
- Medications: OCP, HRT
- Malignancy
- Hyper-homocystinemia
- Antiphospholipid antibodies
- Factor V Leiden mutation: resistance to activated protein C (most inherited hypercoagulable state)
- Deficiency of protein C, protein S, anti-thrombin III

Massive PE: 5–10% cases, affects half of lung vasculature
Submassive PE: 20–25% cases, RV dysfunction with normal BP
Low risk PE: MC type, 70–75% cases, has best prognosis

Clinical Features

- Known as "Great Masquerader"
- Most common symptom is unexplained breathlessness. (page 296: CMDT 2017)
- Most reliable sign in tachypnea (especially in setting of post-operative patient of THR/TKR) [Page 296: CMDT 2017]
- Massive PE leads to RV failure and leads to dysnea, syncope, **hypotension** and cyanosis
- Sub-massive PE presents with respiratory distress, chest pain with breathing, RV malfunction but **normal BP**.
- Lower limb DVT presents as muscle cramp and pain in calf. Subsequently thigh swelling, tenderness and erythema develop.
- Upper limb DVT is seen after putting central lines, ICD, pacemakers and likelihood increases with increase in catheter diameter and number of lumens. It presents with asymmetry in supraclavicular fossa or in circumference of upper limbs.

Clinical Prediction Rule

Clinical variable	PE score
Signs and symptoms of DVT	3.0
Alternative diagnosis other than DVT	3.0
Heart rate >100/min	1.5
Immobilization >3 days. Surgery in previous 4 weeks	1.5
Prior PE or DVT	1.5
Haemoptysis	1.0
Cancer	1.0

If score >4 : PE likely
If score <4 : PE less likely

Investigations

- D-Dimer assay is a screening test to be done in case PE score is less than 4 (sensitivity 95% for PE and can be false positive in MI, pneumonia, sepsis)
- Imaging should be done immediately if PE score > 4
- ECG
  - Most *specific* ECG finding is S1 Q3 T 3 pattern (deep S in lead I, Deep Q in lead III and inverted T waves in lead III).
  - *Most common ECG abnormality* seen in PE is sinus tachycardia and non-specific ST segment abnormalities.
  - *RC strain* leads to T wave inversion in V1 to V4
- Venous ultrasonography reveals loss of vein compressibility and loss of respiratory variation. If venous USG is equivocal, MR venography can be done.
- CXR

Hampton Hump	Wedge shaped density above the diaphragm
Westermark sign	Focal oligemia
Palla sign	Enlarged right descending pulmonary artery

- CT chest with contrast/CTPA is imaging modality of choice. (Page 1666: Harrison 19th edition)
- Lung scan

Small particulate aggregates of albumin labelled with gamma emitting radionuclide are injected intravenously and are trapped in pulmonary bed	Perfusion assessment
Inhaled Xenon or Krypton	Ventilation assessment
Interpretation Two or more segmental perfusion defect in presence of normal ventilation has high probability for diagnosis of PE	

- Echocardiography:
  - Helps to rule out MI, aortic dissection, cardiac tamponade that may mimic PE.
  - McConell Sign: Hypokinesia of RV with Hyperkinesia of RV apex.
- ABG shows respiratory alkalosis
- Pulmonary angiography: Gold standard investigation.

Algorithm of Management

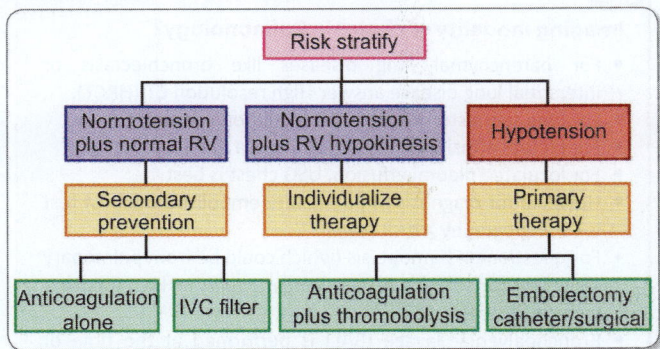

Management of Massive PE with Hypotension

- Replete volume with NS 500 mL
- Dopamine and dobutamine are first line inotropic agents for management of PE related shock.
- Fibrinolysis: tPA 100 mg infusion over 2 hours. Upper limit of use is 14 days after PE has occurred.

Treatment of choice
- Pharmacomechanical catheter directed therapy can pulverise the thrombus and requires lesser dose of fibrinolytic drugs
- Pulmonary embolectomy

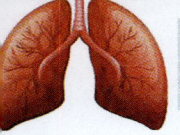

Management of Sub-massive PE with Normal BP and Normal RV

- Anticoagulation
  - Heparin/LMWH bridged to warfarin
  - Heparin/LMWH bridged to Novel oral anticoagulants like Dabigatran
  - Anti Xa agents like rivorabaxan

Duration of anticoagulation

DVT *provoked* by surgery, trauma, oestrogen or indwelling catheter	3 months
Proximal leg DVT *provoked* by trauma, oestrogen or indwelling catheter	3–6 months
Unprovoked DVT (idiopathic)	Lifelong
Long distance air travel	Lifelong

In life long anticoagulation aim is to have INR of 2–3 for first 6 months and 1.5 to 2 for next 6 months

- IVC filter indications
  - Bleeding that precludes anticoagulation
  - Recurrent venous thrombosis despite intensive anticoagulation

PESI (Pulmonary Embolism Severity Index)	
Age > 65 yr	1
Cancer	1
Chronic cardiopulmonary disease	1
Systolic BP <100 mmHg	1
Oxygen saturation	1

Low risk: 0 points: 30 day mortality: >1%
High risk: >1 points: 30 day mortality: 10%

Imaging modality of choice in Pulmonology?

- For parenchymal lung diseases like bronchiectasis or interstitial lung disease answer High resolution CT (HRCT).
- For lung sequestration, the IOC is pulmonary angiography.
- For pleural effusion or pneumothorax, a CXR is sufficient.
- For loculated pleural effusion, USG chest is best.
- However for diagnosis of pulmonary embolism, the best test is CT angiography > V/ P scan.
- For question on hemoptysis (which could be from pulmonary TB or lung cancer), the *first imaging modality* is HRCT followed by bronchoscopy.
- Bronchoalveolar lavage (BAL) is performed at the time of bronchoscopy in:
  1. Suspected malignancy
  2. Pneumonia in immunosuppressed (especially HIV)
  3. Suspected TB (if sputum negative)
  4. Interstitial lung diseases (e.g. extrinsic allergic alveolitis, histiocytosis).

Air Embolism

Conditions Resulting in Air Embolism

1. Neurosurgery: Trauma to cerebral venous sinuses with patient in sitting position
2. Trauma to internal jugular vein
3. Central line insertion (via the subclavian vein)
4. **Caisson / Decompression sickness**: This condition is observed in deep sea diving where air tank contains compressed air. Due to rapid ascent **nitrogen bubbles** are precipitated in the blood stream.

Clinical Features of Air Embolism

1. Respiratory distress
2. Syncope
3. Decreased systolic blood pressure
4. Mill wheel murmur (this is due to mixing of air with blood)

Investigation

1. **Transesophageal echocardiography (TEE):** To estimate the air in the right side of the heart
2. ET_{CO_2} suddenly decreasing to zero intra-operatively during neurosurgery.

Minimal amount of air required to cause air embolism: 100 mL

Treatment

1. Change the position of patient to the left lateral decubitus position (to dislodge the bubble) and finally into Trendelenburg's position *(head low, feet high)*.
2. Aspiration of air via cardiac catheterization (Definitive Management)

Fat Embolism

- It occurs following fracture of long bones. The released fat globules set up an inflammatory cascade, causing damage to lung and brain circulation.

Major criteria for diagnosing FES are as follows:
- Symptoms and radiologic evidence of respiratory insufficiency
- Cerebral sequelae unrelated to head injury or other conditions
- Petechial rash

Minor criteria are as follows:
- Tachycardia (heart rate >110 beats/min)
- Pyrexia (temperature >38.5°C)
- Retinal changes of fat or petechiae
- Renal dysfunction
- Jaundice
- Acute drop in hemoglobin level
- Sudden thrombocytopenia
- Elevated erythrocyte sedimentation rate
- Fat microglobulinemia

Investigation

1. Urine/Sputum: Microscopic examination using sudan black stain: check for fat globules

Treatment

1. High flow oxygen (TOC)
2. Heparin
3. Intermittent positive pressure ventilation
4. Steroids.

CHRONIC OBSTRUCTIVE PULMONARY DISEASE (COPD)

- COPD as a disease state is characterized by airflow obstruction, which is generally progressive, may be accompanied by airway hyper-reactivity, and may be partially reversible.
- Most patients with COPD have features of both emphysema and chronic bronchitis.
- Chronic bronchitis is more common than emphysema.

Chronic Bronchitis

- Chronic bronchitis is a clinical diagnosis defined by excessive secretion of bronchial mucus and is manifested by daily productive cough for 3 months or more in at least 2 consecutive years. *It leads to Type 2 respiratory failure [$\downarrow pO_2$, $\uparrow pCO_2$].*
- **Smoking being a major risk factor**, damages ciliated columnar epithelium of the respiratory tract, which leads to stasis of tracheobronchial secretions.
- This stasis facilitates the bacterial growth leading to bronchorrhea.
- In addition, inflamed and damaged airways cause turbulence in air flow, which causes rhonchi.

Clinical Features

1. Most of the patients observed in this condition are elderly in 50–60's chronic smoker and are obese.
2. Grade III dyspnea *(minimal activity like going to washroom or changing clothes causes breathlessness)*.
3. Central cyanosis (hence referred to as Blue bloaters)
4. Presence of Rhonchi.

Investigations

1. Spirometry: Decreased FEV1
2. Chest X-ray: Increased bronchovascular markings
3. DL_{CO}: Normal
4. ABG: Decreased pO_2, increased pCO_2

Treatment

1. Nicotine buccal spray > varenicline is DOC for nicotine dependence
2. Antibiotics in chronic bronchitis
3. Theophylline
4. Steroids for severe conditions
5. **Main stay of treatment: Low flow oxygen at 1 liter/min x 16 hours.**

Emphysema

- Elastase release from irritated alveolar macrophages leads to destruction of small airways like respiratory bronchioles.
- Macrophages accumulate in respiratory bronchioles of essentially all young smokers. Bronchoalveolar lavage fluid from such individuals contains roughly five times as many macrophages as lavage from non-smokers.
- Emphysema patients usually present with type-I respiratory failure [$\downarrow pO_2$, $\downarrow pCO_2$] → **Respiratory Alkalosis**

- In chronic bronchitis: Type-II respiratory failure ($\downarrow pO_2$, $\uparrow pCO_2$) → *Respiratory acidosis*
- In emphysema: Type-I respiratory failure ($\downarrow pO_2$, $\downarrow pCO_2$) → *Respiratory Alkalosis*

Classification

1. Centriacinar (MC in smokers and overall)
2. Panacinar (common in alpha-1-antitrypsin deficiency)
3. Irregular
4. Mixed

Centriacinar Emphysema

- This type of emphysema is most frequently associated with cigarette smoking, and leads to formation of blebs/bulla.
- Centriacinar emphysema is usually most prominent in the upper lobes and superior segments of lower lobes and is often quite focal.

Panacinar Emphysema

- This condition refers to abnormally large air spaces evenly distributed within and across acinar units.
- Panacinar emphysema is usually observed in patients with α1-AT deficiency, which has a predilection for the lower lobes.

Clinical Features of Emphysema

1. Effort intolerance
2. Increased respiratory rate
3. Use of accessory muscles for repiration
4. Barrel-shaped chest^Q
5. **Pink puffers**

Investigations

1. Spirometry: Decreased FEV_1
2. Chest X-ray: Air trapping, flat diaphragm and hyperinflation
3. Diffusion capacity of lung for carbon monoxide (DLco): Decreased
4. Arterial blood gas (ABG): Respiratory alkalosis

Treatment

- Single or bilateral lung transplantation
- Quit smoking: **Nicotine Buccal spray** > Varenicline is **DOC for nicotine dependence**.
- **VATS:** Video-assisted thoracoscopic surgery for Bullectomy

Complications of Emphysema

1. Spontaneous pneumothorax, which results from rupture of bulla. *This is the most common life threatening complication.* This condition is managed by intracostal drainage in the 5th intercostal space along the mid axillary line.
2. *Cor pulmonale*, is the overall *most common complication of emphysema* resulting due to hypoxia, which eventually leads to right ventricular failure.

Gold criteria for severity of airflow obstruction in COPD	
I: $FEV_1/FVC < 0.7$ and $FEV_1 \geq 80\%$ predicted	III: $FEV_1/FVC < 0.7$ and FEV_1 : 30–50% predicted
II: $FEV_1/FVC < 0.7$ and FEV_1 : 50–80% predicted	IV: $FEV_1/FVC < 0.7$ and $FEV_1 < 30\%$ predicted

Modified Medical Research Council Dyspnea Scale

Grade 0	No dyspnea	Not troubled by breathlessness except with strenuous exercise
Grade 1	Slight dyspnea	Troubled by shortness of breath when hurrying on a level surface or walking up a slight hill
Grade 2	Moderate dyspnea	Walks slower than normal based on age on a level surface due to breathlessness or has to stop for breath when walking on level surface at own pace
Grade 3	Severe dyspnea	Stops for breath after walking 100 yards or after a few minutes on a level surface.
Grade 4	Very severe dyspnea	Too breathless to leave the house or becomes breathless while dressing or undressing.

Categories of COPD

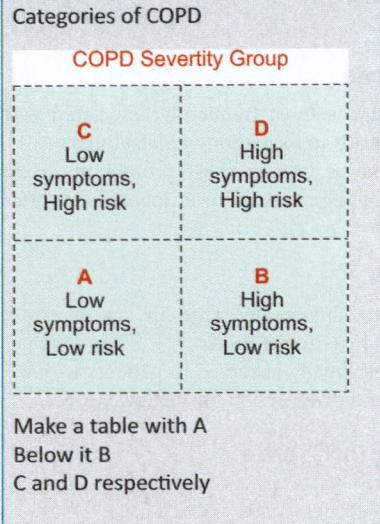

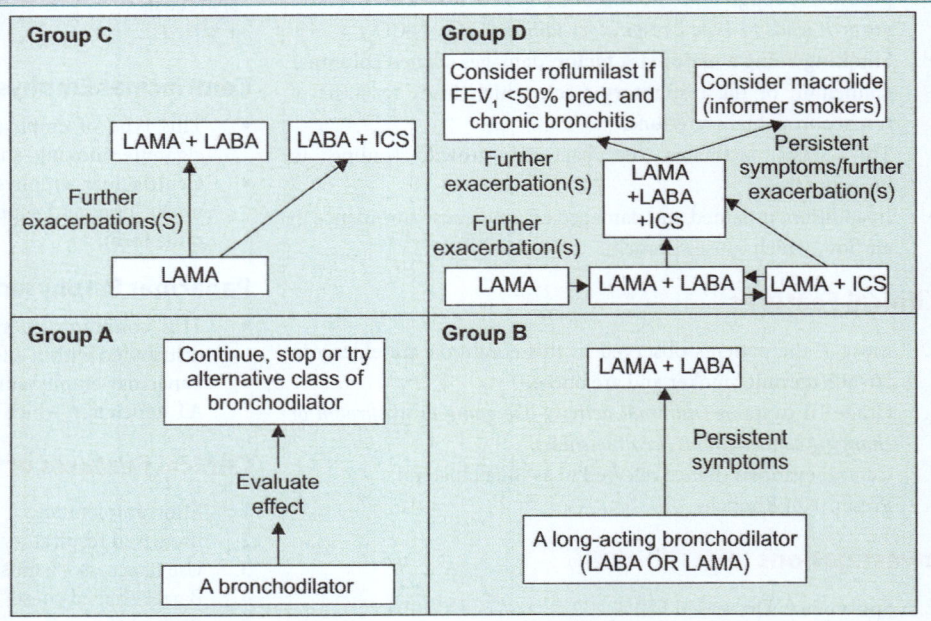

PDE4 Inhibitors

The selective phosphodiesterase 4 (PDE4) inhibitor roflumilast has been demonstrated to reduce exacerbation frequency in patients with severe copd, chronic bronchitis, and a prior history of exacerbations; its effects on airflow obstruction and symptoms are modest.

Bronchiectasis

Bronchiectasis refers to an irreversible airway dilatation that involves the lung in either a focal or a diffuse manner and that classically has been categorized as cylindrical or tubular (the most common form), varicose, or cystic.

Pattern of lung involvement by bronchiectasis	Etiology by categories (with specific examples)
Focal	Obstruction (e.g., aspirated foreign body, tumor mass)
Diffuse	• Infection (e.g., bacterial, nontuberculous mycobacterial)

Pattern of lung involvement by bronchiectasis	Etiology by categories (with specific examples)
	• Immunodeficiency (e.g., hypogammaglobulinemia, HIV infection, bronchiolitis obliterans after lung transplantation)
	• Genetic causes (e.g., cystic fibrosis, Kartagener's syndrome, α_1 antitrypsin deficiency)
	• Autoimmune or rheumatologic causes (e.g., rheumatoid arthritis, Sjogren's syndrome, inflammatory bowel disease); immune-mediated disease (e.g., allergic bronchopulmonary aspergillosis)
	• Recurrent aspiration
	• Miscellaneous (e.g., yellow nail syndrome; traction bronchiectasis from post-radiation fibrosis or idiopathic pulmonary fibrosis)
	• Idiopathic

Contd...

Clinical Manifestations

1. The most common clinical presentation is a persistent productive cough with ongoing production of thick, tenacious sputum. (MC site Bronchiectasis is left lower lobe.)
2. Physical findings often include crackles and wheezing on lung auscultation.
3. Some patients with bronchiectasis exhibit clubbing of the digits.
4. Traction bronchiectasis is dilated airways arising from parenchymal distortion as a result of lung fibrosis.
5. *Bronchiectasis sicca is seen with TB and involves upper lobe.*
6. *Most common site of bronchiectasis is left lower lobe.*

Diagnosis

- The diagnosis is usually based on presentation with a persistent chronic cough and sputum production accompanied by consistent radiographic features.
- While chest radiographs lack sensitivity, the presence of **"tram tracks"** indicating dilated airways is consistent with bronchiectasis.
- Chest CT is more specific for bronchiectasis and is the imaging modality of choice for confirming the diagnosis.
- CT findings include airway dilatation *(detected as parallel "tram tracks" or as the "signet-ring sign").*

Treatment

- Antibiotics
- Mucolytics
- Chest physiotherapy.

CYSTIC FIBROSIS (CF)

- CF is a monogenic autosomal recessive disorder that presents as a multisystem disease. The first signs and symptoms typically occur in childhood.
- CF is characterized by chronic bacterial infection of the airways that leads to bronchiectasis and bronchiolectasis, exocrine pancreatic insufficiency and intestinal dysfunction, abnormal sweat gland function, and urogenital dysfunction.
- It results from **mutations in the CFTR** gene located on **chromosome 7, ΔF 508 mutation (deletion)**, which leads to improper maturation and intracellular degradation of the mutant CFTR protein.

Clinical Features

1. **Meconium ileus:** Neonatal presentation which is diagnosed as well as treated with the help of gastrograffin enema.
2. **Recurrent pneumonia:** Thick and viscid mucous remains stagnant allowing the infection which manifests as pneumonia. *Earliest pathological lesion in lung is that of bronchiolitis*
    - Over all most common presentation^Q
    - It is also the most common cause of death.^{Q}
    - *Bronchiectasis mainly involving upper lung fields.*
3. **Secondary biliary cirrhosis:** Thick and viscid bile juice leads to cholestasis jaundice, which manifests as secondary biliary cirrhosis.
4. **Osmotic diarrhea:** Pancreatic juice contains amylase which is responsible for sugar absorption. As pancreatic juice becomes thick there is fall in amylase production leading to decrease in sugar absorption.
5. Sugar is an osmotic particle, which draws a lot of water from the surrounding tissues resulting in osmotic diarrhea.
6. **Infertility:** In males, azoospermia is caused due to *agenesis of vas deferens* and in females infertility is caused due to increased cervical mucous thickness. Most pregnancies if they occur, produce viable infants and breast feed normally.

Diagnostic criteria for cystic fibrosis

- >1 phenotypical finding or
- Positive neonatal screening
- Positive family history
  PLUS
  Lab evidence of CFTR dysfunction
- Two elevated sweat chloride tests
- Identification of 2CF mutations
- An abnormal nasal potential difference measurement

Essentials of Diagnosis

1. Chronic or recurrent productive cough, dyspnea, and wheezing.
2. Recurrent airway infections or chronic colonization of the airways with *H. influenzae, P. aeruginosa, S. aureus,* or *Burkholderia cepacia.* Bronchiectasis and scarring on chest radiographs.
3. Airflow obstruction on spirometry.
4. Earliest CXR finding is hyperinflation.
5. Pancreatic insufficiency, recurrent pancreatitis, distal intestinal obstruction syndrome, chronic hepatic disease, nutritional deficiencies, or male urogenital abnormalities.
6. Sweat chloride concentration >60 mEq/L on two occasions (False positive in Addison disease)^Q
7. Investigation of choice is CFTR mutation analysis using exonic sequencing.^{Q}
8. Trans epithelial nasal potential difference test is also performed.

RESPIRATORY FAILURE

Respiratory failure is one of the most common reasons patients are admitted to the ICU.

Accordingly, four different types of respiratory failure can be described, based on these pathophysiologic derangements.

Classification

- **Type 1 (Hypoxemic):** PO_2 <60 mm Hg on room air and PCO_2 is normal or decreased. Usually seen in patients with acute pulmonary edema or acute lung injury. These disorders interfere with the lung's ability to oxygenate blood as it flows through the pulmonary vasculature.
- **Type 2 (Hypercapnic/Ventilatory):** pO_2 is < 60 mm Hg, PCO_2 > 50 mmHg. This is usually seen in patients with an increased work of breathing due to airflow obstruction or decreased respiratory system compliance, with decreased respiratory muscle power due to neuromuscular disease, or with central respiratory failure and decreased respiratory drive.

- **Type 3 (Perioperative):** This is generally a subset of type 1 failure but is sometimes considered separately because it is so common. It occurs due to post operative atelectasis.
- **Type 4:** Secondary to cardiovascular instability. It occurs due to hypoperfusion of respiratory muscles. Seen with cardiogenic shock, lactic acidosis and anemia.

Approach to Hypoxemia

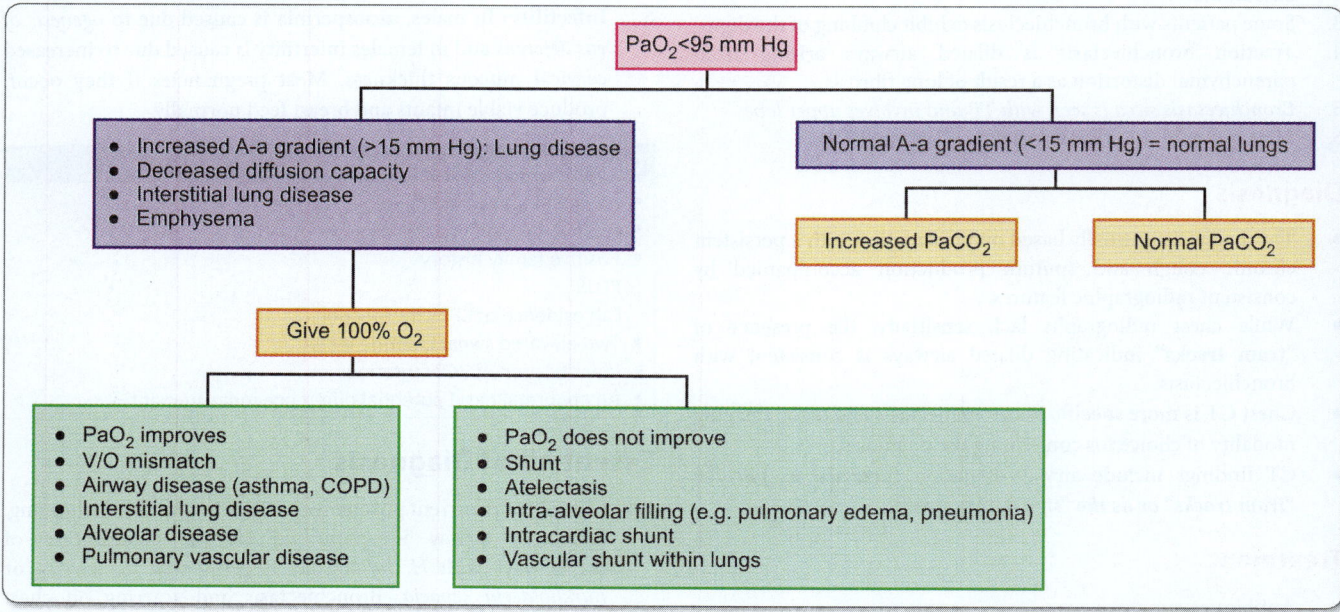

Management of Acute Respiratory Failure[Q]

Type 1 Respiratory failure	Low volume ventilation (Tidal volume of 6 mL/kg instead of 12 mL/kg)
Type 2 Respiratory failure	Noninvasive ventilation or assisted controlled mechanical ventilation
Type 3 Respiratory failure	Noninvasive ventilation with tight fitting face mask
Type 4 Respiratory failure	Treat the cause and intubate to reduce the work load of respiratory muscles.

Devices for Oxygenation

Almost all patients with ARF require supplemental oxygen. All should be placed on a pulse oximeter and oxygen saturation should generally be maintained above 90%.

Low flow nasal O_2	: 24–40%
Standard face mask	: 35–50%
Partial rebreather mask	: 40–70%
Nonrebreather mask	: 60–80%
Venturi/Air Entrainment mask	: 24–50%
High flow nasal O_2	: 21–100%

- **Nasal cannula**; Low-flow, low oxygen concentration, open device. 100% oxygen is delivered through cannulae at 0.5 – 6 L/min.
- **Venturi masks:** These are variable oxygen concentration, low to moderate flow, open devices. These air entrainment masks deliver 100% oxygen through a jet-mixing device that causes a controlled entrainment of air and thus allows for delivery of precise oxygen concentrations from 24 to 50 %. These masks are useful in patients with COPD in whom a precise titration of oxygen concentration may be desirable in order to minimize an increase in PCO_2.
- **Reservoir face masks:** These are high flow, high oxygen, open devices designed to minimize entrainment of air in patients with high inspiratory flow demands.
- **Resuscitation bag-mask-valve unit.** High oxygen, high flow device. The oxygen flow should be kept high (15 L/min) when this device is used. When the mask is held firmly over the face with a good facemask seal, entrainment of room air is minimized.

LUNG CANCER

- Lung cancer is the leading cause of cancer deaths in both men and women.[Q]
- Cigarette smoking causes 85–90% of cases of lung cancer.
- Other environmental risk factors for the development of lung cancer include exposure to environmental tobacco smoke, radon gas (among uranium miners[Q] and in areas where radium in the soil causes significant indoor air contamination), asbestos (60- to 100-fold increased risk in smokers with asbestos exposure), metals (arsenic, chromium, nickel, iron oxide) and industrial carcinogens (bis-chloromethyl ether).

Subtypes of Lung Cancer

Squamous cell carcinoma	Adenocarcinoma
• Most common variant in India • Smoking is a risk factor • **Central in location** • Local growth is surgically resected • Cavity formation seen	• MC variant of lung CA overall • Most common lung cancer among non-smokers • **Peripheral in location** • Transbronchial spread i.e., it arises at one lobe and spreads to the another
Small cell carcinoma / Oat cell carcinoma	**Large cell carcinoma**
• Most aggressive variant among these CA • Smoking is a risk factor • **Central in location** • It exhibits micrometastasis • It has worst prognosis	• This variant is observed in non-smokers • **Peripheral in location** • This is associated with estrogen production which manifest as gynecomastia.

Clinical Features of Lung Carcinoma

1. **Local central growth:**
   Cough, hemoptysis, wheeze and stridor, dyspnea, and post-obstructive pneumonitis (fever+cough)
2. **Peripheral growth:**
   Chest pain, cough, dyspnea, symptoms of lung abscess.
3. **Lymph node metastasis and compressive symptoms:**
   Tracheal obstruction, esophageal compression with dysphagia, recurrent laryngeal nerve palsy leading to hoarseness, phrenic nerve palsy leading to dyspnea, sympathetic neve paralysis leading to Horner's syndrome
4. **Pancoast tumor:** Adenocarcinoma > Squamous cell carcinoma growing in apex of lung with C_8, T_1, T_2, involvement and first and second rib erosion. Its features are:
   - Shoulder and arm pain
   - **Horner's syndrome:** When tumor crushes on sympathetic ganglia following features are seen: *(Mn: Post MEAL)*

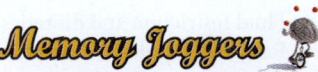

- **P**tosis: due to paralysis of Muller muscle
- **M**iosis
- **E**nopthalmos
- **A**nhidrosis
- **L**oss of ciliospinal reflex

5. **Metastasis:** To brain^Q, bone, kidney, liver, spinal cord.
6. **Paraneoplastic syndrome:**
   - **Endocrine manifestations**

SIADH	Small cell cancer *(SIADH is most common paraneoplastic manifestation of oat cell cancer)*
Ectopic ACTH	Small cell cancer
Hypercalcemia	Squamous cell cancer
Cushing's syndrome	Small cell cancer
Gynecomastia	Large cell cancer

> SIADH is the most common paraneoplastic manifestation of oat cell cancer.

- Neurological manifestations
  - Myopathy, myositis
  - Neuropathy
  - Lambert Eaton syndrome: Antibodies start damaging N_M junction → Ach↓
- Migratory venous thrombophlebitis is seen with adenocarcinoma (Trousseau's sign)
- Hypertrophic pulmonary osteoarthropathy Adenocarcinoma

Local Effects of Lung Tumor Spread

Clinical Features	Pathologic Basis
Pneumonia, abscess, lobar collapse	Tumor obstruction of airway
Lipid pneumonia	Tumor obstruction; accumulation of cellular lipid in foamy macrophages
Pleural effusion	Tumor spread into pleura
Hoarseness	Recurrent laryngeal nerve invasion
Dysphagia	Esophageal invasion
Diaphragm paralysis	Phrenic nerve invasion
Rib destruction	Chest wall invasion
SVC syndrome	Superior vena caval (SVC) compression by tumor
Horner's syndrome	Sympathetic ganglia invasion
Pericarditis, tamponade	Pericardial involvement

Investigation

1. **Sputum:** ≥ 5 sputum samples (69% sensitivity, 96% specificity)
2. **CXR:** Hilar enlargement, collapse, pleural effusion, rib erosion, mediastinal widening, elevated hemidiaphragm
   - **Central lesion:** Squamous cell CA, small cell CA
   - **Peripheral lesion:** Adenocarcinoma, large cell CA
3. **IOC for central tumors:** Bronchoscopy + Biopsy
4. **HRCT:** To evaluate size of tumor, spread of tumor and destruction by the tumor.
5. **Tumor markers**
   - **CEA** (carcinoembryonic antigen): Metastatic cancer
   - **NSE** (neuron-specific enolase): Prognostic marker in small cell carcinoma

Management

- **Small cell lung cancers:** Chemotherapy and radiotherapy
  - **Chemotherapy:** Etoposide + cisplatin/carboplatin

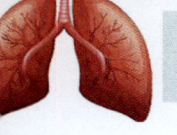

- **Non-small cell lung cancers:**
  - Surgical resection best
  - Fixation of tumor to vital structures like aorta, heart, esophages, nerves implies in resectability
  - **Chemotherapy:** (Paclitaxel + carboplatin)/(paclitaxel + vincristine + cisplatin)

Most Common (MC) for Lung Tumors

MC benign tumor of lung	Hamartoma
MC cause of recurrent hemoptysis	Bronchial adenoma
MC cause of cancer death	Lung cancer
MC type of cancer	Adenocarcinoma
MC type of cancer in India	Squamous cell carcinoma
MC risk factor	Smoking
MC natural risk factor	Radon gas (environmental pollutant)
MC central location	Squamous cell cancer (other: small cell cancer)
MC peripheral location	Adenocarcinoma (other: large cell /anaplastic)
MC rib destroyed in pancoast tumor	First rib
MC symptom of lung cancer	Cough
MC site of metastasis	Liver
MC nerve roots involved in pancoast tumor	C_8, T_1, T_2

ACUTE RESPIRATORY DISTRESS SYNDROME (ARDS)

The diagnosis of ARDS is made on clinical grounds on the following criteria.

1. Acute onset
2. Bilateral pulmonary infiltrate on chest X-ray
3. Pulmonary artery wedge pressure <18 mm Hg (i.e. LA pressure is normal)
4. A partial pressure of arterial oxygen to fractional inspired oxygen concentration (P_aO_2/F_iO_2) < 200 mm Hg.

Causes of ARDS

- MC cause of ARDS overall is sepsis
- MC cause of direct lung injury leading to ARDS is pneumonia.
- MC cause of indirect lung injury leading to ARDS is sepsis.

Pathophysiology of ARDS

1. *MC cell damaged in ARDS is endothelial cells.*
2. Diffuse alveolar damage
3. Reduced surfactant (injury to type II pneumocyte)
4. Increased permeability of alveolar capillary membrane
5. Due to damage to the normally tight alveolar barrier, edema fluid rich in protein, accumulates in the interstitial and alveolar spaces (non cardiogenic pulmonary edema).
6. The protein that aggregates in air spaces with cellular debris and dysfunctional pulmonary surfactant to form hyaline membrane whorls.

All of the above damage results in **reduced compliance** (Stiff lung), **diminished tidal volume, hypoxemia** (worsened gas exchange due to pulmonary shunting), **hypocapnia**.

Diagnostic Criteria (According to 18th edition of Harrison)	ALI	ARDS
PaO_2/FiO_2	< 300 mm Hg	<200 mm Hg
Onset	Acute	Acute
Chest radiograph	Bilateral alveolar or interstitial infiltrates	Bilateral alveolar or interstitial infiltrates
Absence of left atrial hypertension	PCWP <18 mm Hg No clinical evidence of increased left atrial pressure	PCWP <18 mm Hg No clinical evidence of increased left atrial pressure

Severity of ARDS

Mild: < $PaO_2/FiO_2 \leq 300$
Moderate: < $PaO_2/FiO_2 \leq 200$
Severe: < $PaO_2/FiO_2 \leq 100$

* Symptoms start within first 12–36 hours after initial insult. Exudative phase encompasses first 7 day of illness.

Treatment of ARDS

1. Fluid restriction and diuretics to keep PCWP low.
2. Early neurological blockage and low tidal volume ventilation.^{Q}
3. Keep $FiO_2 < 0.6$, PEEP < 10 cm H_2O, SpO_2 = 88–95%
4. Inverse ratio ventilation, Inspiration > Expiration time, I: E > 1: 1
5. High frequency jet ventilation: Disappointing results
6. Partial liquid ventilation using perfluorocarbons: Disappointing results
7. Extracorporeal membrane oxygenation: Limited utility.

Remember for ARDS

- Most common cause of ARDS is Sepsis
- Normal pulmonary capillary wedge pressure
- Non-cardiogenic pulmonary edema
- High protein pulmonary edema
- Intrapulmonary shunting
- PaO_2/FiO_2 ratio < 200
- CXR shows bilateral white out
- Treatment of choice is low volume ventilation using CPAP

INTERSTIAL LUNG DISEASE

- Interstitial lung disease (ILDs) represent a diverse group of chronic progressive lung disease associated with alveolar inflammation^Q and/or potentially irreversible pulmonary fibrosis^Q.
- A classification scheme proposed by the American Thoracic Society and European Respiratory Society includes these subtypes:
  - Known causes (environment, occupational, or drug-associated disease).
  - Rare lung disease (e.g., pulmonary histiocytosis, lymphangioleiomyomatosis)
  - Iodiopathic interstitial pneumonias
- Based on clinical, radiologic, and histologic features, IIPs are further subclassified into the following diagnoses:
  1. Idiopathic pulmonary fibrosis (IPF) characterized by progressive dyspnea, cough, restrictive lung disease, and a specific histopathologic pattern.
  2. IIPs other than IPF (including nonspecific interstitial pneumonia [INSIP], respiratory bronchiolitis associated ILD [RBILD], acute interstitial pneumonia [AIP], cryptogenic organizing pneumonia [COP], etc.

Risk Factors

1. Environmental or occupational exposure to inorganic or organic dusts.
2. Sixty-six to seventy-five percent of patients with ILD have a history of smoking.
3. Due to diversity of disease, age is not a reliable predictor or pathology:
   - Most patients with connective tissue disease-related pathology and inherited subtypes present between ages of 20 and 40 years.
   - Median age of patients with IPF is 66 years.

Pathophysiology

1. Alveolar inflammation may progress into irreversible fibrosis.
2. Varying degrees of ventilatory dysfunction occur among the ILD subtypes.
3. ILD associated with collagen vascular disease and systemic connective disorders can manifest involvement of skin, joints, muscular, and ocular systems.

Etiology

Some types of ILD are associated with specific exposures:
1. Medications (amiodarone, antibiotics [especially nitrofurantoin], chemotherapy agents, gold, illicit drugs)
2. Inorganic dusts (silicates, asbestos, talc, mica, coal dust, graphite)
3. Organic dust (moldy hay, inhalation of fungi, bacteria, animal proteins)
4. Metals (tin, aluminium, cobalt, iron, barium)
5. Gases, fumes, vapors, aerosols.
6. Collagen vascular disease
7. Sarcoidosis
8. Amyloidosis
9. Goodpasture syndrome
10. Churg-Strauss syndrome
11. Wegener's granulomatosis

History

1. Symptoms may include progressive exertional dyspnea and nonproductive cough.
2. Patient may also present with hemoptysis (due to idiopathic alveolar hemosiderosis)
3. Obtaining a history of illness: Duration (acute vs, chronic) potential environmental/occupational exposure travel, medical conditions (including systemic disease) and medication intake is important.
4. Some cases of lung disease may occur weeks to years after discontinuation of an offending agent (e.g. carmustine).

Physical Examination

Physical findings are usually nonspecific some common features include:
1. Fine bi-basiliar crepitation (typically present upon auscultation of lung bases on posterior axillary line)
2. Rales
3. Inspiratory 'Squeaks'
4. Clubbing of the digits and cyanosis in advanced disease.
5. Loud P_2 and wide fixed split S_2^Q (PAH)
6. Holosystolic TR murmur
7. Pedal edema

Diagnosis Tests and Interpretation

1. 6-minute walk test with SpO_2 monitoring to obtain global evaluation of submaximal exercise capacity
2. Arterial blood gas (ABG) shows Type 1 respiratory failure^Q (End stage lung disease leads to Type 2 respiratory failure)
3. If a systemic disorder is suspected consider antinuclear antibody (ANA), rheumatoid factor (RF), ESR, and antineutrophil cytoplasmic antibodies (ANCA).
4. Plasma ACE inhibitor concentration (sarcoidosis).
5. Chest X-ray (CXR); Most commonly reticular pattern^Q, less commonly nodular or mixed pattern. (*It is the first imaging modality to be done.*)
6. HRCT of the chest is the *most useful tool*^{Q} for distinguishing among ILD subclasses, especially if normal CXRs.
   - Characteristic changes on HRCT may help to distinguish between subtypes:
     - Reticulonodular, ground glass opacities and in later stages, honeycombing may be seen.
     - Associated hilar and mediastinal adenopathy are characteristic of stage I and II sarcoidosis.
7. **Other diagnostic procedures**
   - Pulmonary function testing demonstrates a restrictive defect (decreased vital capacity and total lung capacity)
   - DL_{co} reducing on exercise
   - Bronchoalveolar lavage (BAL) idiopathic pulmonary fibrosis shows *absence of lymphocytosis with increased neutrophils and eosinophils.*
   - Bronchoscopic transbronchial lung biopsy may help diagnose sarcoidosis

- Thorascopic surgery for lung biopsy has the greatest diagnostic specificity for ILDs^Q (pg 1710: Harrison 19th edition)

Treatment

Evidence does not support the routine use of any specific therapy for ILD.
1. No survival benefit of home oxygen use in ILD
2. No evidence that any pharmacologic therapies improve survival or quality of life
3. Corticosteroids have a role in some ILD subtypes

Medication

First Line

- Corticosteroids are most effective for certain ILDs, especially exacerbations of sarcoidosis, NSIP, COP, and hypersensitivity pneumonitis. However, response rates have been variable across and within subtype. The optimal dose and duration of therapy are unknown.
- Common starting dose of prednisone is 0.5 – 1 mg/kg/d for 4–12 weeks, with potential up titration to 0.5 mg/kg based on patient response.

Second Line

Second line agents have been used for IPF alone or in combination with steroids, with limited success rates:
1. Azathioprine
2. Pirfenidone, an orally active antifibroblast agent, currently submitted for FDA approval
3. Cyclophosphamide is commonly used in treatment of Wegener's granulomatosis. It is given 1.5–2 mg/kg/d PO for 3–6 months.
4. Methotrexate has been used in treatment of mild Wegener's granulomatosis in combination with corticosteroids.
5. Definitive management of end stage lung disease is lung transplantation.

- MC ILD is idiopathic pulmonary fibrosis (Ref: Page 1711, Harrison 19th edition)
- ILD in smokers is called desquamative interstitial pneumonitis
- ILD which is common in young women and responds to steroids, is nonspecific interstitial pneumonitis
- Reticular opacities are not linear but curvilinear markings predominantly at lung bases in CXR.
- Honey combing is a coarse reticular pattern and associated with lower lobe volume loss, visible on HRCT.
- Hammon Rich syndrome/Acute interstitial pneumonia presents similar in presentation to ARDs.
- Nonspecific interstitial pneumonia has a good prognosis, and is seen in nonsmoker young females.

Miliary opacities on CXR
- TB/VZ pneumonia
- Pulmonary hemosiderosis
- Silicosis/Pneumoconiosis
- Hypersensitivity pneumonitis
- Pulmonary Alveolar Proteinosis
- Metastasis: Thyroid/Renal/Breast

Image-Based Questions

1. The pattern shown on flow volume loop is?

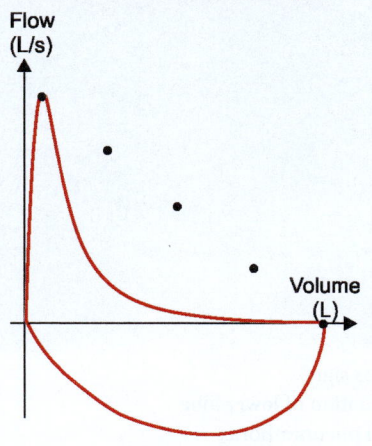

   a. Obstructive
   b. Restrictive
   c. Normal curve
   d. Mixed pattern

3. The image shows?

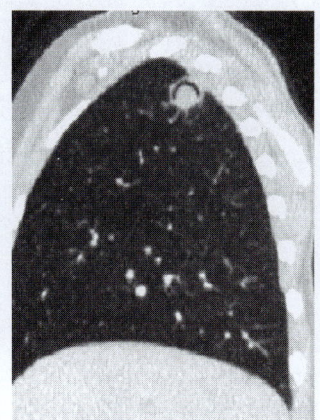

   a. Air Crescent Sign
   b. Silhouette sign
   c. Degenerating Rheumatoid nodule
   d. Military tuberculosis with Cavity

2. The flow volume curve shows?

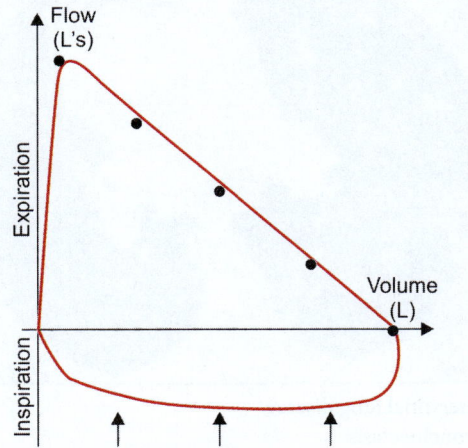

   a. COPD
   b. Interstitial lung disease
   c. Variable extrathoracic obstruction
   d. Variable intrathoracic obstruction

4. 45-year old diabetic and alcoholic presents with severe respiratory distress. The X ray chest was performed. The best antibiotic to be given to the patient is?

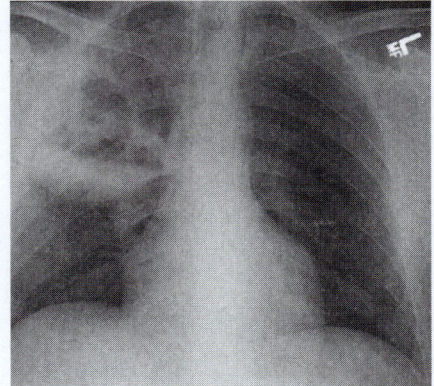

   a. Levofloxacin
   b. Cefotaxime plus Amikacin
   c. Penicillin
   d. Aztreonam plus Meropenem

5. The CXR shows?

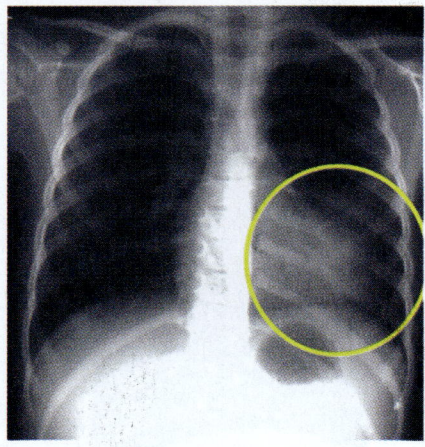

   a. Lingular pneumonia
   b. Left sided pleural effusion
   c. Left sided atelectasis
   d. Left sided pulmonary infarction

7. The CXR shows

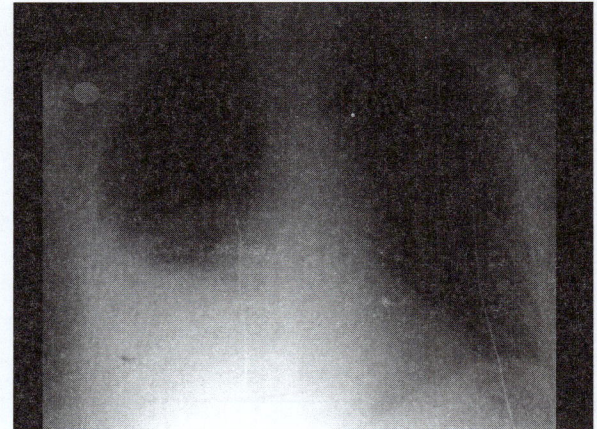

   a. Meniscus sign
   b. Consolidation of lower lobe
   c. Bilateral pneumothorax
   d. Pulmonary artery hypertension

6. The image shows presence of?

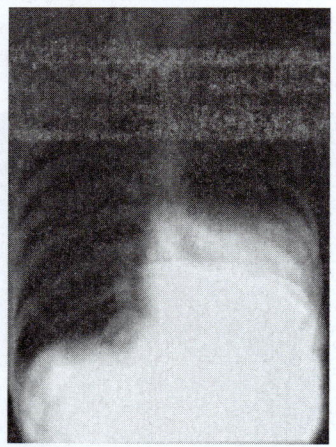

   a. Pleural effusion
   b. Hydropneumothorax
   c. Pneumothorax
   d. Pneumonia

8. The image shows presence of?

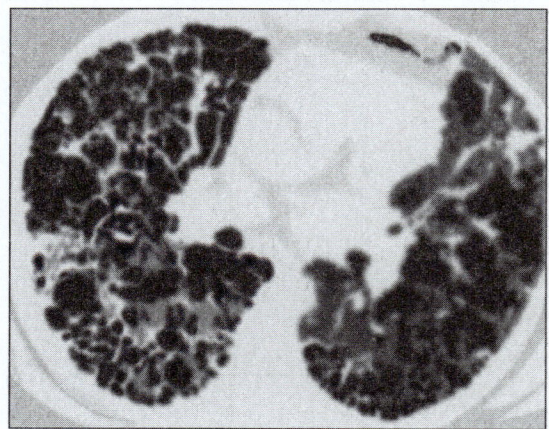

   a. Interstitial lung disease
   b. Bronchiectasis
   c. Aspergillosis
   d. Pulmonary alveolar proteinosis

9. The CXR shows presence of?

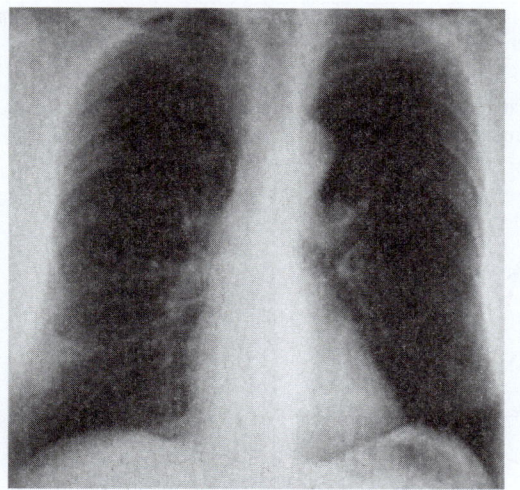

a. Westermark sign b. Hampton Hump
c. Pneumothorax d. Emphysema

10. Which of the following is a diagnostic criterion for this patient of acute pancreatitis with severe respiratory distress?

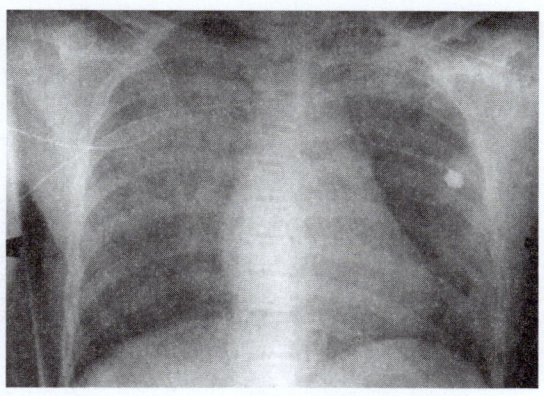

a. PaO_2/FiO_2 ratio < 200 and PCWP < 18 mm Hg
b. PaO_2/FiO_2 ratio < 200 and PCWP > 18 mm Hg
c. PaO_2/FiO_2 ratio < 300 and PCWP < 18 mm Hg
d. PaO_2/FiO_2 ratio < 300 and PCWP > 18 mm Hg

11. An asthmatic presents with brownish plugs in sputum. CT chest was performed. Probable diagnosis is?

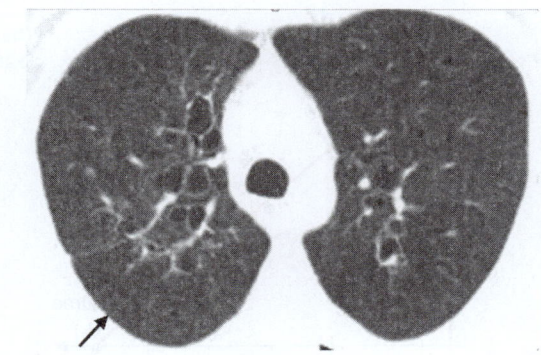

a. Wegener's granulomatosis
b. Cryptogenic organizing pneumonia
c. ABPA
d. Reconsider diagnosis of asthma

Answers of Image-Based Questions

1. **Ans. (a) Obstructive**
   - The image shows a *concave* prolonged flow during expiration which is suggestive of obstructive lung disease.
   - In restrictive pattern, due to reduction of TLC and RV the area under curve is reduced

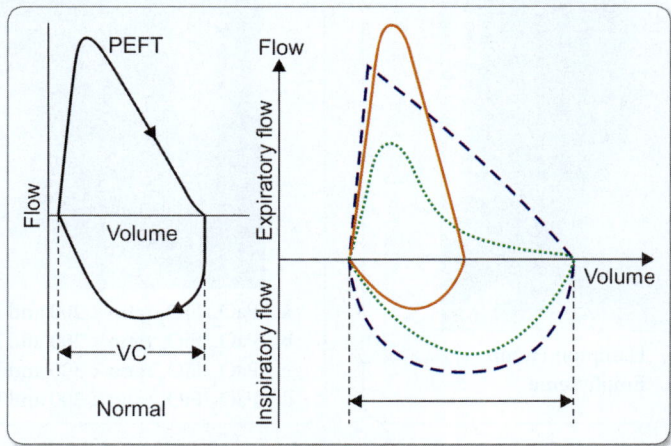

2. **Ans. (c) Variable extrathoracic obstruction**
   - The image shows the expiratory curve of the loop to be normal but the *inspiratory part is flat*.
   - This can occur with an obstructive lesion like retrosternal goiter.
   - The lesion is being sucked inwards along with the trachea during inspiration leading to partial obstruction and flattening of the inspiratory part of the flow-volume loop. During expiration, passive expiration occurs.
   - Hence the answer is extrathoracic obstruction

Variable extrathoracic pattern	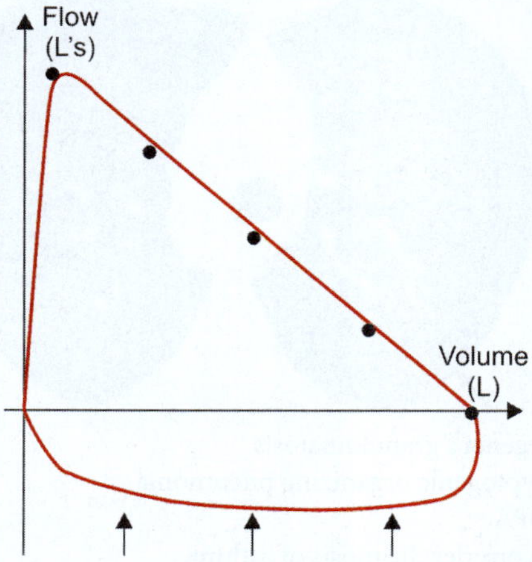 Flow (L's) vs Volume (L) graph	The inspiratory part is flat. Example : Retrosternal goiter
Variable intrathoracic pattern	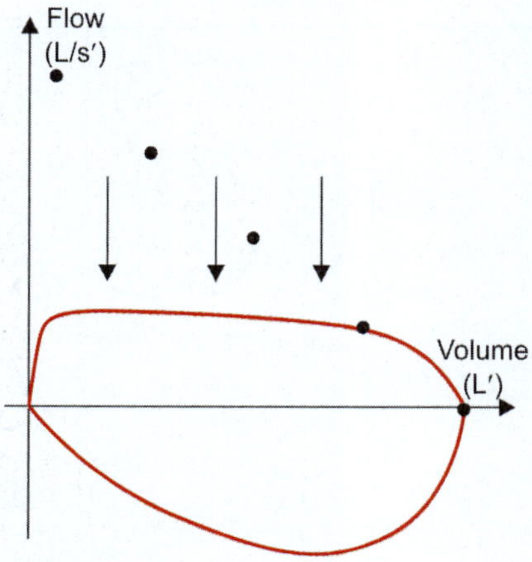 Flow (L/s') vs Volume (L') graph	The expiratory pattern is flat Example: Laryngeal tumor

Contd...

Fixed large airway obstruction	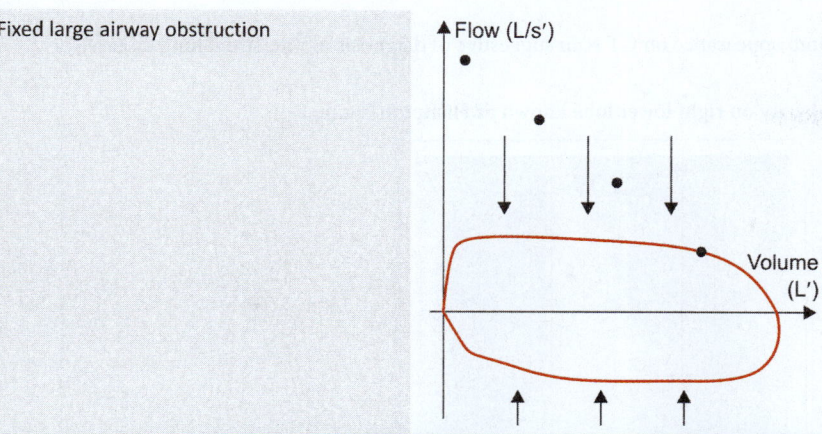	Both inspiration and expiration becomes flat. Example: Tracheal stenosis (due to prolonged intubation)

Pulmonary function test	Normal value (95 percent confidence interval)
FEV_1	80 – 120%
FVC	80 – 120%
Absolute FEV_1/FVC ratio	Within 5% of the predicted ratio
TLC	80 – 120%
FRC	75 – 120%
RV	75 – 120%
DLCO	>60 – <120%

3. **Ans. (a) Air crescent sign**
 In angioinvasive fungal infection, when neutrophil count recovers and the patient mounts an immune response, peripheral reabsorption of necrotic tissue causes the retraction of the infarcted center and air fills the space in between. *This creates an air crescent within the nodules and is a good prognostic finding because it marks the recovery phase of the infection.*

4. **Ans. (b) Cefotaxime plus Amikacin**
 - The image shows presence of bulging fissure sign indicating possible *Klebsiella pneumoniae*.
 - Third generation cephalosporins are highly effective for *K. pneumoniae* and other *Klebsiella* infections. They exhibit higher efficacy against resistant organisms. The antibiotic arrests bacterial growth by binding to one or more penicillin-binding proteins.

5. **Ans. (a) Lingular pneumonia**
 The CXR shows presence of silhouette sign, which is an obscured left heart border due to lingular pneumonia.

6. **Ans. (b) Hydropneumothorax**
 - The image shows a standing upright X-Ray with pleural reflection and straight level with absence of meniscus sign.
 - The CXR in pleural effusion will show meniscus sign (marked by arrows)

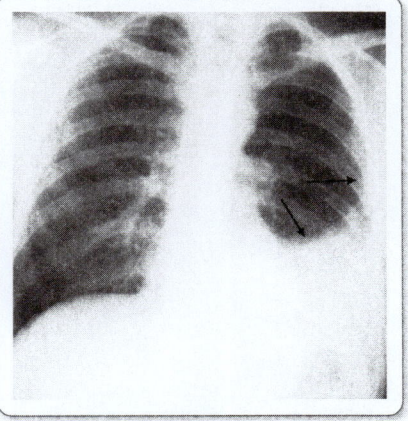

7. **Ans. (a) Meniscus sign**
 The CXR shows pleural effusion as both costophrenic and cardiophrenic angles are obliterated in a CXR and also notice the smooth concavity of fluid rising up in a S shape. This differentiates pleural effusion from pneumonia.

8. **Ans. (a) Interstitial lung disease**
   The image shows CT chest with honey comb appearance on CT scan suggestive of diagnosis of interstitial lung disease.
9. **Ans. (b) Hampton hump**
   The image shows presence of triangular opacity on right lower lobe known as Hampton Hump.

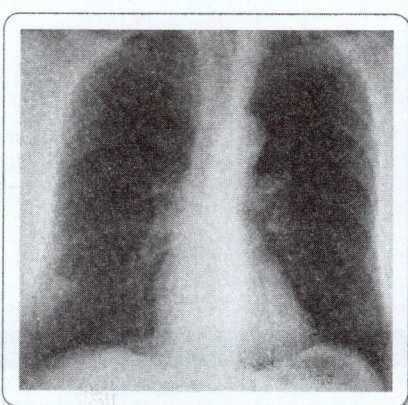

   It indicates pulmonary infarction *due to blockage of right descending pulmonary artery*.
10. **Ans. (a) PaO_2/FiO_2 ratio < 200 and PCWP < 18 mm Hg**
    - The chest X ray shows non cardiogenic pulmonary edema due to ARDS, which has normal PCWP.
    - The *diagnostic criteria of ARDS is PaO_2/FiO_2 ratio < 200 and PCWP < 18 mm Hg* and presence of bilateral lung infiltrates.
11. **Ans. (c) ABPA (allergic bronchopulmonary aspergilloma)**
    The CT chest shows presence of central bronchiectasis. With presence of concomitant asthma and brown sputum plugs, the diagnosis is allergic bronchopulmonary aspergilloma.

Conceptual Diagnostic Algorithm

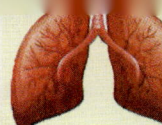

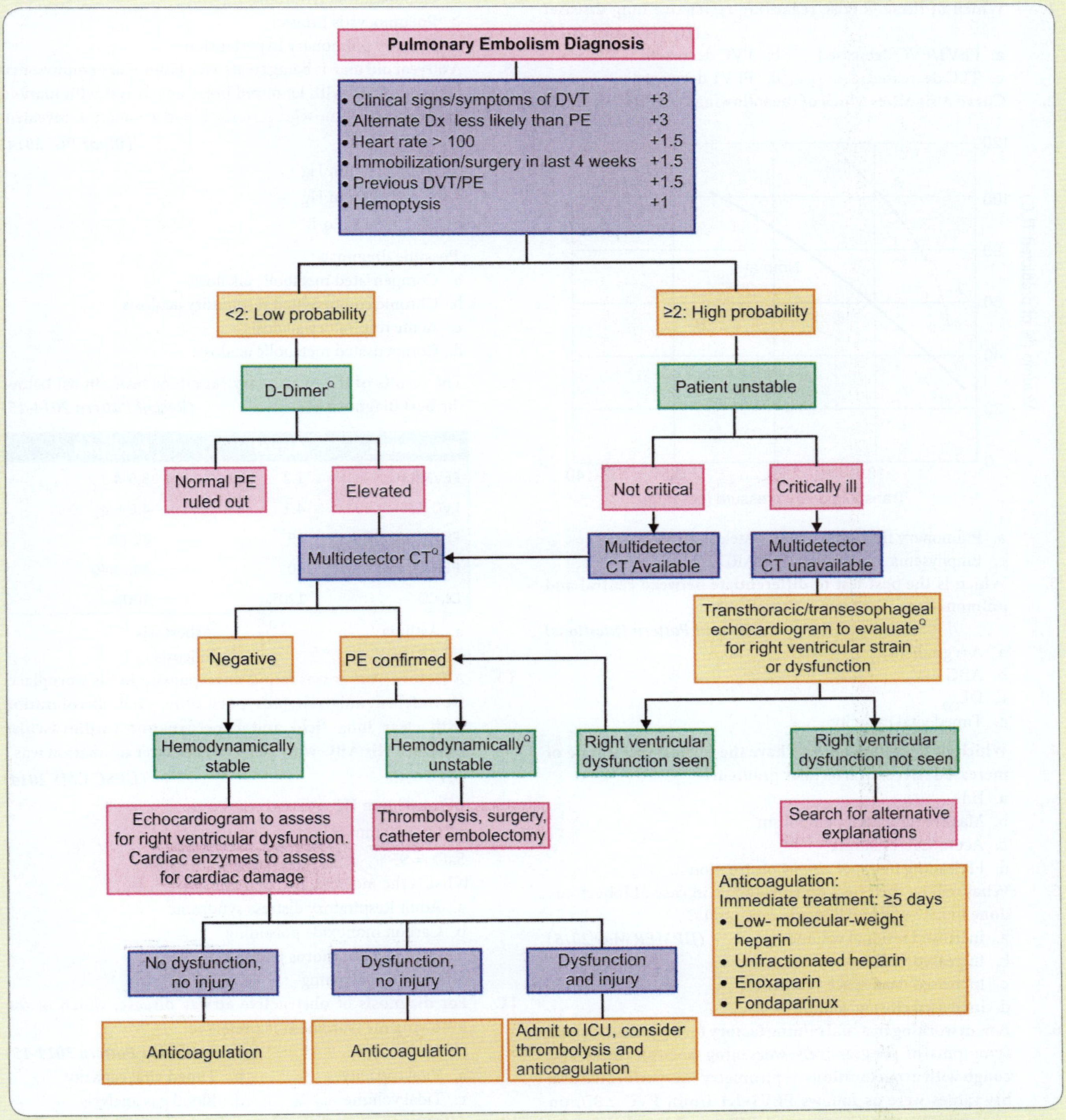

Pulmonary Embolism Diagnosis

• Clinical signs/symptoms of DVT	+3
• Alternate Dx less likely than PE	+3
• Heart rate > 100	+1.5
• Immobilization/surgery in last 4 weeks	+1.5
• Previous DVT/PE	+1.5
• Hemoptysis	+1

<2: Low probability
- D-Dimer
  - Normal → PE ruled out
  - Elevated → Multidetector CT
    - Negative
    - PE confirmed
      - Hemodynamically stable → Echocardiogram to assess for right ventricular dysfunction. Cardiac enzymes to assess for cardiac damage
        - No dysfunction, no injury → Anticoagulation
        - Dysfunction, no injury → Anticoagulation
        - Dysfunction and injury → Admit to ICU, consider thrombolysis and anticoagulation
      - Hemodynamically unstable → Thrombolysis, surgery, catheter embolectomy

≥2: High probability
- Patient unstable
  - Not critical → Multidetector CT Available → Multidetector CT
  - Critically ill → Multidetector CT unavailable → Transthoracic/transesophageal echocardiogram to evaluate for right ventricular strain or dysfunction
    - Right ventricular dysfunction seen → PE confirmed
    - Right ventricular dysfunction not seen → Search for alternative explanations

Anticoagulation:
Immediate treatment: ≥5 days
- Low-molecular-weight heparin
- Unfractionated heparin
- Enoxaparin
- Fondaparinux

* In MCQ if RV dyskinesia is mentioned with collapsing patient, Thrombolysis is the treatment of choice
* If RV dyskinesia is mentioned with normotension, anticoagulation is the mainstay of treatment.

Multiple Choice Questions

Spirometry, DL_{CO}, Alveolar-Arteriolar Gradient

1. Which of these is false regarding restrictive lung disease?
   (JIPMER May 2018)
   a. FEV1/FVC decreased
   b. FVC decreased
   c. TLC decreased
   d. FEV1 decreased

2. Curve A signifies which of the following? *(AIIMS Nov 2018)*

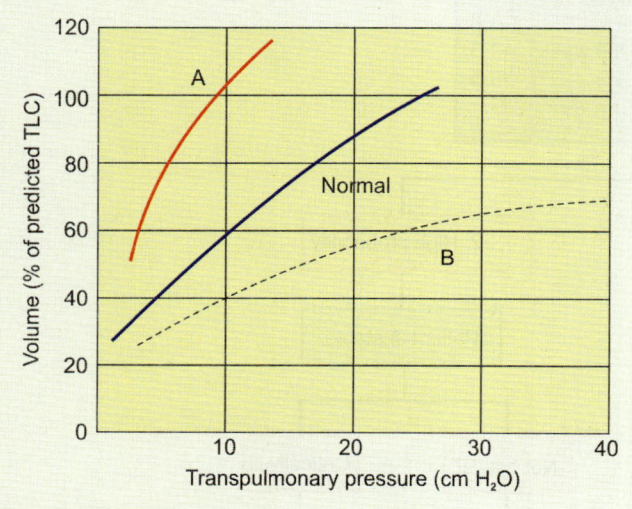

   a. Pulmonary fibrosis
   b. Atelectasis
   c. Emphysema
   d. ARDS

3. Which is the best test to differentiate between central and pulmonary cause of hypoventilation?
   (Recent Pattern Questions)
   a. A-a gradient
   b. ABG
   c. DL_{CO}
   d. Timed vital capacity

4. Which of the following will have the highest magnitude of increased Alveolar arteriolar gradient?
   a. ILD
   b. Massive pulmonary embolism
   c. Acute severe asthma
   d. FB leading to upper airway obstruction

5. What will be the effect on spirometry in case of lobectomy done in case of bronchogenic carcinoma?
   a. Increased residual volume *(JIPMER May 2015)*
   b. Increased vital capacity
   c. Increased dead space ventilation
   d. Increased closing volume

6. A man working in a coal mining factory for 16 years develops symptoms of progressively worsening breathlessness and cough with expectorations a spirometry was performed and his values were as follows FEV1-1.4 l/min FVC 2.8l/min and with FEV1/FVC ratio of 50. What could be the cause?
   a. Silicosis *(UPSC CMS 2015)*
   b. Hypersensitivity pneumonitis
   c. COPD
   d. Idiopathic pulmonary fibrosis

7. The diffusion capacity of lung is decreased in all of the following conditions except: *(Recent Pattern 2014-15)*
   a. Interstitial lung disease
   b. Goodpasture's syndrome
   c. Pneumocystis Jiroveci
   d. Primary pulmonary hypertension

8. A 60 year old man is being treated for pulmonary emphysema. He is admitted with laboured breathing at rest with marked use of accessory muscles. Arterial blood gas analysis revealed:
   pH 7.33 *(Bihar PG. 2014)*
   $PaCO_2$ 64 mm Hg
   PaO_2 50 mm Hg
   HCO_3 34 mEq/L
   Possible diagnosis
   a. Compensated metabolic alkalosis
   b. Chronic compensated respiratory acidosis
   c. Acute respiratory acidosis
   d. Compensated metabolic acidosis

9. The results of the pulmonary functions tests shown below, the best diagnosis is : *(Recent Pattern 2014-15)*

Parameters	Actual	Predicted
FEV1 (L)	1.2	3.5-4.3
FVC (L)	4.1	4.6-5.4
FEV1/FVC (%)	29	72-80
PEF (L/min)	80	440-540
DL CO	120%	100%

   a. Asthma
   b. Asbestosis
   c. ARDS
   d. Silicosis

10. A factory worker was found unresponsive in his workplace. He is afebrile anicteric, tachypneic drowsy pale discoloration with clear lung field and hyperdynamic cardiovascular findings. His ABG with 100% oxygen after intubation was
    pH = 7.45 *(UPSC CMS 2014)*
    pO_2 = 80 mm Hg
    pCO_2 = 30 mm Hg
    SaO_2 = 95%
    What is the most likely diagnosis?
    a. Adult Respiratory distress syndrome
    b. Carbon monoxide poisoning
    c. Organo-phosphorus poisoning
    d. Cyanide poisoning

11. For diagnosis of obstructive airway disease, which of the following measurement is preferred:
    (Recent Pattern 2014-15)
    a. Vital capacity
    b. Timed vital capacity
    c. Tidal volume
    d. Blood gas analysis

12. All show increased alveolar-arterial O_2 gradient except?
    a. Bronchiectasis *(Recent Pattern 2014-15)*
    b. ARDS (acute respiratory distress syndrome)
    c. Interstitial fibrosis
    d. Central hypoventilation

13. A patient with blood chemistry of pH 7.3, CO_2 of 60 and HCO_3 of 28 mEq/dl are indicative of:
    (Recent Pattern 2014-15)
    a. Partially compensated respiratory acidosis
    b. Uncompensated respiratory acidosis
    c. Fully compensated respiratory alkalosis
    d. Metabolic alkalosis with respiratory alkalosis

14. A patient presents with breathlessness. He has bilateral basal crepitations, lung function tests reveal decrease in total lung capacity (TLC) and vital capacity (VC) with normal FEV1/VC ratio. The most likely diagnosis is:
    a. Chronic bronchitis *(Recent Pattern 2014-15)*
    b. Idiopathic pulmonary fibrosis
    c. Cystic fibrosis
    d. Allergic bronchopulmonary aspergillosis

15. On an ABG, pH of 7.2, pO_2 of 46, pCO_2 of 80 are indicative of:
    (Recent Pattern 2014-15)
    a. Acute exacerbation of COPD
    b. Adult respiratory distress syndrome
    c. Interstitial pneumonitis
    d. Acute asthma

16. Which of the following is not true in obstructive lung disease?
    (Recent Pattern 2014-15)
    a. FEV1↓
    b. TLC↓
    c. FVC↓
    d. Reduced timed vital capacity

17. Residual volume is best measured by?
    a. Body plethysmography *(Recent Pattern 2014-15)*
    b. Helium dilution method
    c. Spirometry
    d. All of above

18. In restrictive lung disease: *(AIPG 2010)*
    a. FEV1/FVC decreased, compliance normal
    b. FEV1/FVC increased, compliance increased
    c. FEV1/FVC decreased, compliance increased
    d. FEV1/FVC increased, compliance decreased

19. If FEV1 is 1.3 L, FVC is 3.1 L in an adult man, the pattern is suggestive of:
    (Recent Pattern 2014-15)
    a. Normal lung function
    b. Restrictive lung disease
    c. Obstructive lung disease
    d. None of the above

20. All the following lung volumes can be measured by a simple spirometer except:
    (Recent Pattern 2014-15)
    a. Vital capacity
    b. Residual volume
    c. Tidal volume
    d. Forced vital capacity

21. Alveolar-arterial tension gradient increases in all except:
    a. Diffusion defects *(Recent Pattern 2014-15)*
    b. Central hypoventilation
    c. R-L shunt
    d. Ventilation perfusion abnormality

22. FEV1/FVC ratio is decreased in all except:
    a. Bronchiectasis *(Recent Pattern 2014-15)*
    b. Emphysema
    c. Chronic bronchitis
    d. Interstitial lung disease

23. Following pulmonary changes are seen in restrictive lung disease except:
    (Recent Pattern 2014-15)
    a. ↑FEV1/FVC
    b. ↓TLC
    c. ↓RV
    d. ↑VC

24. A patient presents with decreased vital capacity and total lung volume. What is the most probable diagnosis?
    (AI 2007)
    a. Bronchiectasis
    b. Sarcoidosis
    c. Cystic fibrosis
    d. Asthma

25. All are decreased in infiltrative lung disease, except:
    a. Vital capacity *(AIIMS Feb 97)*
    b. Alveolar arterial difference in PaO_2
    c. Total lung capacity
    d. Lung compliance

26. Decreased maximum mid-expiratory flow rate indicates obstruction in:
    (AIIMS May 95)
    a. Small airways
    b. Trachea
    c. Large airways
    d. Trachea and Bronchi both

27. In an emphysematous patient with bullous lesions, which is the best investigation to measure lung volume:
    a. Body Plethysmography *(AIIMS Nov 08)*
    b. Gas dilution
    c. Transdiaphragmatic pressure
    d. DLco

28. Pulmonary Compliance is decreased in all of the following conditions, Except:
    (AI 2011)
    a. Pulmonary Congestion
    b. COPD
    c. Decreased Surfactant
    d. Pulmonary Fibrosis

Types of Respiratory Failure

29. A 17-year-old boy presents with complaints of difficulty in breathing. There was venous congestion of face and neck. A clinical diagnosis of SVC syndrome was made. The X-ray showed mediastinal widening. What is the next step?
    (AIIMS Nov 2017)
    a. CT scan of chest
    b. Peripheral smear
    c. IV Cyclophosphamide
    d. Initiate Radiation Therapy

30. Maximum oxygen concentration can be delivered by?
    (AIIMS Nov 2017)
    a. Venturi Mask
    b. Nasal Cannula
    c. Face mask
    d. Face mask with reservoir

31. Which of the following is not an etiology for peripheral cyanosis?
    (Recent Pattern Questions)
    a. Cold exposure
    b. Deep vein thrombosis
    c. Methemoglobinemia
    d. Peripheral vascular disease

32. Crescendo- decrescendo breathing pattern is seen in?
    (Recent Pattern Questions)
    a. Central sleep apnea
    b. Obstructive sleep apnea
    c. NREM sleep
    d. REM sleep

33. A 55 year old female with morbid obesity presents to the ER with increased breathlessness, cough and orthopnea for 2 days. She has pulse rate of 96/minute, BP 136/90 mmHg, RR= 30/min and spO_2=76%. ABG report shows pO_2 =76 mm Hg, PCO_2= 24 mmHg and pH= 7.28. The next step is?
    (AIIMS May 2016)
    a. Intubation with low tidal volume ventilation
    b. Continuous positive pressure ventilation
    c. IV diuretics with digoxin
    d. High flow oxygen through non rebreathing face mask

34. Which is the best treatment of type 4 Respiratory failure? (Recent Question 2016-17)
    a. Non-invasive ventilation with tight fitting face mask
    b. Intubation with mechanical ventilation
    c. Continuous positive pressure ventilation
    d. High frequency jet ventilation
35. Which of the following is the common cause of respiratory failure Type 2? (Recent Question 2015-16)
    a. Chronic bronchitis exacerbation
    b. Acute attack asthma
    c. ARDS
    d. Pneumonia
36. Type II respiratory failure is seen in:
    a. Chronic bronchitis with cor-pulmonale
    b. Chronic renal failure
    c. Adult respiratory distress syndrome
    d. Pulmonary alveolar proteinosis
37. Type 3 respiratory failure occurs due to: (Recent Pattern 2014-15)
    a. Post-operative atelectasis   b. Kyphoscoliosis
    c. Flail chest   d. Pulmonary fibrosis
38. In type II respiratory failure there is:
    a. Low pO_2 and Low pCO_2 (Recent Pattern 2014-15)
    b. Low pO_2 and High pCO_2
    c. Normal pO_2 and High pCO_2
    d. Low pO_2 and Normal pCO_2
39. Respiratory failure type I consists of: (Recent Pattern 2014-15)
    a. Low PaO_2, normal or low $PaCO_2$
    b. Raised $PaCO_2$, low PaO_2
    c. Normal PaO_2, low PO_2
    d. Normal PaO_2 and $PaCO_2$ high
40. All of the following are true about type I respiratory failure except: (Recent Pattern 2014-15)
    a. Decreased PaO_2 b. Decreased $PaCO_2$
    c. Normal $PaCO_2$ d. Normal A-a gradient
41. Alveolar hypoventilation is observed in: (Recent Pattern 2014-15)
    a. Guillain-Barre syndrome   b. Acute asthma
    c. Bronchiectasis   d. CREST syndrome
42. Paradoxical breathing is characteristic of: (Recent Pattern 2014-15)
    a. Pneumonia   b. Pneumothorax
    c. Atelectasis   d. Flail chest
43. Prolonged hyperventilation may lead to all except: (Recent Pattern 2014-15)
    a. Paraesthesia   b. Alkalosis
    c. Tetany   d. Somnolence
44. PO_2 decreases on exercise in all except:
    a. COPD   (Recent Pattern 2014-15)
    b. Interstitial Fibrosing alveolitis
    c. Acute CCF
    d. Bronchiectasis
45. Acute respiratory failure does not occur with: (Recent Pattern 2014-15)
    a. Porphyria   b. Myasthenia gravis
    c. Polio   d. Lead poisoning
46. In type - II respiratory failure, there is: (AIIMS Nov 02)
    a. Low pO_2 and low pCO_2
    b. Low pO_2 and high pCO_2
    c. Normal pO_2 and high pCO_2.
    d. Low pO_2 and normal pCO_2.

Bronchial Asthma

47. A one-year old child presents with the following lesion on the face. His mother has a history of bronchial asthma. What is the diagnosis? (Recent Question 2019)

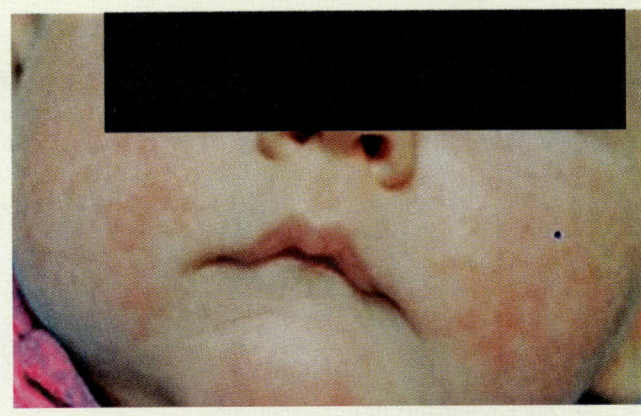

    a. Eczematous dermatitis   b. Seborrheic dermatitis
    c. Atopic dermatitis   d. Contact dermatitis
48. A known asthmatic, presented to the emergency with severe exacerbation not relieved by Salbutamol. The patient was given corticosteroids and aminophylline. What is the rationale of giving corticosteroids? (AIIMS Nov 2017)
    a. Corticosteroids facilitate the action of β2 agonists
    b. Corticosteroids sensitize adenosine receptors to xanthines
    c. Direct bronchodilator action of corticosteroids
    d. Increase mucociliary clearance
49. Which of the following is not required in case a second puff is to be taken from an inhaler? (AIIMS Nov 2016)
    a. Wash your mouth between 2 puffs
    b. Shake again
    c. Wait for one minute before taking second puff
    d. Keep the mouth piece dry
50. The following are indications for assisted ventilation in acute severe asthma EXCEPT? (APPG 2016)
    a. PEFR 50-60% of predicted value
    b. Rising paCo2> 6kPa (45 mm Hg)
    c. Diminishing level of consciousness
    d. Falling paO2< 8kPa (60 mm Hg)
51. Which of the following features of severity are used in in immediate assessment of acute severe asthma? (UPSC 2015)
    1. Pulse rate >110 per min
    2. Pulsus paradoxus
    3. Unable to speak in sentences
    Select the correct answer using the code given below:
    a. 1 only   b. 2 and 3 only
    c. 1 and 3 only   d. 1, 2 and 3
52. Which one of the following is not recommended in immediate treatment of acute severe asthma? (UPSC 2015)
    a. Oxygen supplementation
    b. High doses of inhaled B2–adrenoreceptor agonists
    c. Systemic corticosteroids
    d. Intravenous aminophylline
53. Which one of the following values is not a feature of Acute severe asthma? (APPG 2015)
    a. Pulsus Paradoxus
    b. PaO_2 of less than 8 kPa
    c. Heart rate of more than 110/min
    d. PEF of 60 to 70% of expected

54. The following are main diagnostic criteria for allergic bronchopulmonary aspergillosis except: (APPG 2015)
    a. Distal bronchiectasis   b. Peripheral eosinophilia
    c. Bronchial asthma   d. Pulmonary infiltrates
55. FEV_1/FVC is reduced in case of? (Bihar PG 2015)
    a. Pleural effusion   b. Lung fibrosis
    c. Asthma   d. All of the above
56. Thickening of pulmonary alveolar capillary membrane is seen in? (Bihar PG 2015)
    a. Asthma   b. Bronchitis
    c. Pulmonary fibrosis d. Emphysema
57. All are true about Aspirin sensitive asthma except?
    a. Nasal polyposis   (Recent Question 2015-16)
    b. Treatment with inhaled corticosteroids
    c. Rhinosinusitis
    d. Increased prostaglandins
58. Which of the following is given in the maintenance of severe persistent asthma: (Recent Question 2015-16)
    a. Oral steroids   b. Leukotriene agonist
    c. Ipratomium bromide   d. Long acting beta 2 agonist
59. What is the full form of ARIA (Recent Question 2015-16)
    a. Allergic Rhinitis Induced Asthama
    b. Allergic Rhinitis and its Impact on Asthma
    c. Allergy Rheumatology Immunology and Asthma
    d. Acetycholine Receptor Inducing Activity
60. Allergic broncho-pulmonary Aspergillosis presents with all except: (Recent Question 2015-16)
    a. Eosinophiluria
    b. Occurs in asthmatics
    c. Brownish plugs in sputum
    d. Central bronchiectasis
61. Central bronchiectasis is seen with (Recent Question 2015-16)
    a. Cystic adenomatoid malformation
    b. Cystic fibrosis
    c. Broncho carcinoma
    d. Tuberculosis
62. Which drugs are not used in severe persistent Asthma:
    a. Short acting beta 2 agonist (Recent Question 2015-16)
    b. Oral corticosteroids
    c. Long acting beta 2 agonist
    d. Inhaled high dose Steroids
63. Drug of choice for treatment of type 2 Brittle Asthma is? (Recent Question 2015-16)
    a. β-adrenergic agonist   b. Inhaled corticosteroids
    c. Antileukotrines DM   d. Subcutaneous epinephrine
64. Child known case of bronchial asthma comes with respiratory rate 48/min, cannot speak 2 words, occasional wheeze and oxygen saturation of 95%. You give 3 doses of salbutamol nebulisation then he started to speak a sentence but saturation falls to 85%. Cause is? (AIIMS Nov 2014)
    a. Bronchomalacia
    b. Right to left shunt
    c. VP mismatch with dead space ventilation
    d. Faulty pulse oxy-meter
65. One of the following is not an indicator of the severity of asthma exacerbation: (Recent Pattern 2014-15)
    a. Use of accessory muscles   b. Pulsus paradoxus
    c. Cyanosis   d. Systolic BP
66. ABPA complicates: (Recent Pattern 2014-15)
    a. Cystic fibrosis   b. TB cavity
    c. Bronchiectasis   d. Pneumoconiosis
67. Consider the following statements: (UPSC 2010)
    Life threatening features of acute-severe asthma in children include?
    1. Altered sensorium
    2. Pulsus paradoxus
    3. Audible wheeze in both inspiration and expiration
    4. Oxygen saturation 92-95%
    Which of these statements is/ are correct?
    a. 1 only   b. 2 and 4
    c. 1 and 2   d. 1, 2, 3 and 4
68. Bronchial asthma is associated with raised levels of: (Recent Pattern 2014-15)
    a. Leukotrienes   b. PGI2
    c. PGE2   d. Thromboxane
69. Aspirin sensitive asthma is associated with:
    a. Extrinsic asthma   (Recent Pattern 2014-15)
    b. Usually associated with urticaria
    c. Associated with nasal polyp
    d. Obesity
70. A pediatric asthmatic patient presents with a severe attack of acute wheezing and breathlessness and drowsiness. Arterial blood gas analysis done after one hour of treatment with oxygen, nebulised salbutamol and intravenous corticosteroids show pH 7.26, PaO_2 of 60 mm Hg and $PaCO_2$ of 60 mm Hg. The next step in treatment should be:
    a. Mechanical ventilation
    b. Intravenous bicarbonate
    c. Intravenous salbutamol   (AIPG 2011)
    d. Increase in rate of oxygen delivery
71. Consider the following statement: (UPSC 2014)
    Early onset extrinsic episodic asthma is characterized by:
    1. Family history of eczema or rhinitis
    2. Development of an early and late asthmatic reaction mediated by mast cells
    3. T lymphocytes that release cytokine like interleukin-4
    Which of these statements are correct?
    a. 1, 2 and 3   b. 1 and 2
    c. 2 and 3   d. 1 and 3
72. In bronchial asthma following pulmonary function abnormalities are present except: (Recent Pattern 2014-15)
    a. Decreased FEV1
    b. Decreased maximum expiratory flow rate
    c. Increased residual volume
    d. Increased inspiratory capacity
73. Consider the following statements: (UPSC 2013)
    The features of severe asthma include
    1. Central cyanosis
    2. Agitated behaviour
    3. Pulsus paradoxus
    4. Heart rate less than 60/minute
    Which of these statements are correct?
    a. 2, 3 and 4   b. 1, 3 and 4
    c. 1, 2 and 3   d. 1, 2 and 4
74. Best for treatment of Exercise induced asthma?
    a. Montelukast   (Recent Pattern 2014-15)
    b. Salbutamol
    c. Ipratropium
    d. Low dose Inhaled corticosteroids

75. **True about bronchopulmonary aspergillosis are A/E:**
    (Recent Pattern 2014-15)
    a. Central bronchiectasis
    b. Pleural effusion
    c. Asthma
    d. Eosinophilia

76. **In severe bronchial asthma, true is:**
    (Recent Pattern 2014-15)
    a. Inspiratory and expiratory rhonchi with reduced air entry
    b. Hyper-resonant chest
    c. Increased fremitus and absent breath sounds
    d. Decreased fremitus and crackles

77. **All of the following are useful for treating acute bronchial asthma in children except:** *(Recent Pattern 2014-15)*
    a. 100% Oxygen
    b. Hydrocortisone
    c. Salbutamol
    d. Sodium Cromglycate inhalation

78. **All of the following diseases are associated with peripheral blood eosinophilia except:** *(Recent Pattern 2014-15)*
    a. Allergic Bronchopulmonary Aspergillus (ABPA)
    b. Loeffer's syndrome
    c. Chronic bronchitis
    d. Churg's strauss syndrome

79. **The major diagnostic criteria for Allergic Bronchopulmonary Aspergillosis would include all the following except:**
    a. Peripheral eosinophilia *(Recent Pattern 2014-15)*
    b. Central bronchiectasis
    c. Bronchial asthma
    d. Culture of A. Fumigatus from the sputum

80. **Diagnostic features of Allergic Bronchopulmonary Aspergillosis (ABPA) include of all the following except:**
    (Recent Pattern 2014-15)
    a. Changing pulmonary infiltrates
    b. Peripheral eosinophilia
    c. Serum precipitins against Aspergillus fumigatus
    d. Occurrence in patients with old cavitatory lesions

81. **Commonly used route of administration for Omalizumab in asthma in:** *(Recent Pattern 2014-15)*
    a. Subcutaneous   b. Inhalational
    c. Intradermal   d. Intramuscular

82. **Bronchial asthma patient on artificial ventilation requires:**
    a. High frequency jet ventilation *(Recent Pattern 2014-15)*
    b. An equal IE ratio of 1:1
    c. Low volume ventilation
    d. An IE ratio 1:2.5

83. **Curschmann's Spirals in sputum is seen in:**
    (Recent Pattern 2014-15)
    a. Tuberculosis cavity   b. Asthma
    c. Bronchitis   d. Bronchiectasis

84. **Aspirin-sensitive asthma is associated with:** *(AI 1995)*
    a. Obesity   b. Urticaria
    c. Nasal polyp   d. Extrinsic asthma

85. **Universal finding in Asthma is** *(PGI June 02)*
    a. Hypoxia   b. Hypercarbia
    c. Respiratory acidosis   d. Metabolic Acidosis

86. **All are used in bronchial asthma, except:** *(AIIMS June 97)*
    a. Salbutamol   b. Morphine
    c. Aminophylline   d. Steroid

C.O.P.D

87. **Gold Criteria for *very severe* COPD is defined as?**
    (Recent Pattern 2018)
    a. FEV1/FVC < 0.7 and FEV1 < 80% predicted
    b. FEV1/FVC < 0.7 and FEV1< 70% predicted
    c. FEV1/FVC < 0.7 and FEV1< 50% predicted
    d. FEV1/FVC < 0.7 and FEV1< 30% predicted

88. **Which is correct about ILD?** *(Recent Pattern Questions)*
    a. Type I Respiratory failure, respiratory alkalosis
    b. Type II Respiratory failure, respiratory acidosis
    c. Type III Respiratory failure, respiratory alkalosis
    d. Type IV Respiratory failure, respiratory acidosis

89. **The following CT chest shows presence of?**
    (Recent Question 2016-17)

    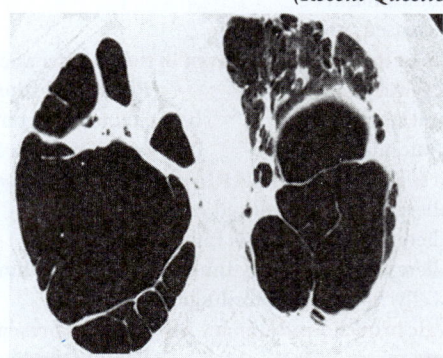

    a. Emphysema
    b. Artifact
    c. Silicosis
    d. Pneumo-ultra-microscopic silico-volcanosis

90. **Increased Reid index is classically associated with?**
    (APPG 2016)
    a. Chronic Bronchitis   b. Emphysema
    c. Brochiectasis   d. Interstitial lung disease

91. **Which are the drugs used for smoking cessation?**
    (Bihar PG 2015)
    a. Clonidine   b. Bupropion
    c. Varenicline   d. All of the above

92. **Which of the following features favour emphysema rather than interstitial fibrosis:** *(PGI May 2015)*
    a. ↑FEV1   b. ↓FEV1/FVC
    c. ↑RV   d. ↑TLC
    e. ↓Peak expiratory flow

93. **In a patient with COPD, with low spo_2 at rest best management option is?** *(Recent Question 2015-16)*
    a. Quit smoking   b. Bronchodilators
    c. Low flow Oxygen   d. Mucolytics

94. **In a patient with smoking history, which is important?**
    a. Duration of smoking *(Recent Question 2015-16)*
    b. Number of smoking
    c. Brand of Cigarette
    d. Filter of cigarette

95. **Emphysema presents with all except:**
    a. Cyanosis *(Recent Question 2015-16)*
    b. Barrel shaped chest
    c. Associated with smoking
    d. Type 1 respiratory failure

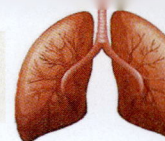

96. Which component of cigarette smoke is responsible for CAD?
    a. Nicotine   (Recent Question 2015-16)
    b. Tar
    c. Polycyclic aromatic hydrocarbons
    d. Benzene
97. Smoking causes all cancers EXCEPT?
                                (Recent Question 2015-16)
    a. Primary brain cancer   b. Oral cancer
    c. Kidney cancer   d. Bladder cancer
98. Central bronchiectasis is seen with?
                                (Recent Pattern 2015-16)
    a. Cystic Adenomatoid Malformation
    b. Cystic fibrosis
    c. Broncho carcinoma
    d. Tuberculosis
99. Bronchiectasis sicca is seen with: (Recent Pattern 2014-15)
    a. TB   b. Pertussis
    c. Cystic fibrosis   d. Kartaneger syndrome
100. All are complications of bronchiectasis except:
                                (Recent Pattern 2014-15)
    a. Cerebral abscess   b. Lung abscess
    c. Amyloidosis   d. Bronchogenic carnicoma
101. All are seen in emphysema except: (Recent Pattern 2014-15)
    a. Decreased vital capacity b. Hyperinflation
    c. Rhonchi   d. Reduced DLco
102. Emphysema presents with all except:
                                (Recent Pattern 2014-15)
    a. Cyanosis   b. Barrel shaped chest
    c. Associated with smoking d. Type 1 respiratory failure
103. Investigation of choice to distinguish between COPD with emphysema and bronchial asthma is?
                                (Recent Pattern 2014-15)
    a. Allergy test to pollens
    b. Non reversible airflow obstruction
    c. Chest X-ray
    d. Arterial blood gas analysis
104. The drug varenicline is used in: (Recent Pattern 2014-15)
    a. Pulmonary Hemosiderosis
    b. Sleep apnoea
    c. Anti-trypsin deficiency
    d. Nicotine dependence
105. False about emphysema is: (Recent Pattern 2014-15)
    a. Decreased FEV1
    b. Decreased timed vital capacity
    c. Increased residual volume
    d. Increased diffusion capacity
106. All are seen in chronic bronchitis except?
                                (Recent Pattern 2014-15)
    a. Cough > 3 months   b. Bronchorrea
    c. Hoover sign   d. Haemoptysis
107. The complication least likely to occur in a case of chronic bronchitis is: (Recent Pattern 2014-15)
    a. Pulmonary hypertension b. Spontaneous Pneumothorax
    c. Respiratory acidosis   d. Amyloidosis
108. Chronic Cor pulmonale is seen in all except:
    a. Massive Pulmonary embolization   (PGI-Dec-04)
    b. COPD
    c. Cystic fibrosis
    d. Primary pulmonary hypertension
109. The most common cause for chronic cor pulmonale is
    a. Recurrent pulmonary embolization   (PGI Dec 05)
    b. COPD
    c. Cystic fibrosis
    d. Bronchial Asthma
110. Bilateral Rhonchii may be seen in all of the following Except
                                (PGI June 08)
    a. Pulmonary Edema   b. Bronchiectasis
    c. Pulmonary Embolism   d. Chronic Bronchitis

Bronchiectasis and Suppurative Lung Diseases

111. A 40-year-old male alcoholic presents with features of fever and productive cough that increases with posture change. CXR of the patient is given below. Which of the following is the most appropriate management of this patient?
                                (AIIMS Nov 2016)

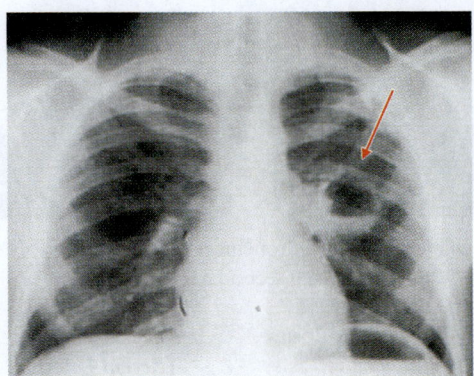

    a. Clindamycin   b. Gentamycin and paclitaxel
    c. Lobectomy   d. ATT
112. Which of the following is correct clinical finding in patients with post tubercular bronchiectasis?   (AIIMS May 2016)
    a. Mixed (fine and coarse) Crackles
    b. Bibasilar Crackles
    c. Crackles are essentially late inspiratory
    d. Tubular type of bronchial breathing is heard
113. A 43-year-old diabetic male presents with cough, fever and weight loss with loss of appetite since 2 months. CT chest shows?   (Recent Question 2016-17)

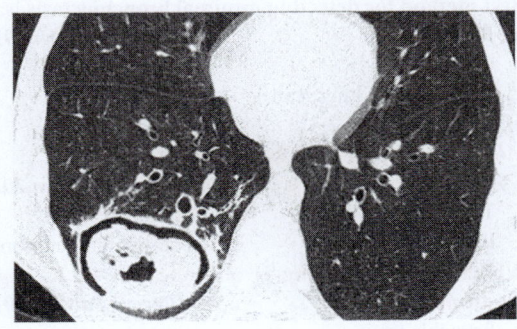

    a. Bronchiectasis
    b. Cavity
    c. Chronic Bronchitis
    d. Consolidation with Syn-pneumonic Effusion

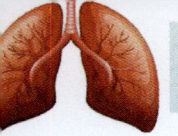

114. **Most common type of bronchiectasis?**
     (Recent Question 2016-17)
     a. Cylindrical   b. Varicose
     c. Cystic   d. Irregular

115. **Mid lung field bronchiectasis is seen with?**
     (Recent Question 2016-17)
     a. M.A.I   b. ABPA
     c. TB   d. Post radiation fibrosis

116. **This patient came with chronic productive cough and clubbing and coarse rales. What is the diagnosis of the CT scan above?**
     (APPG 2015)

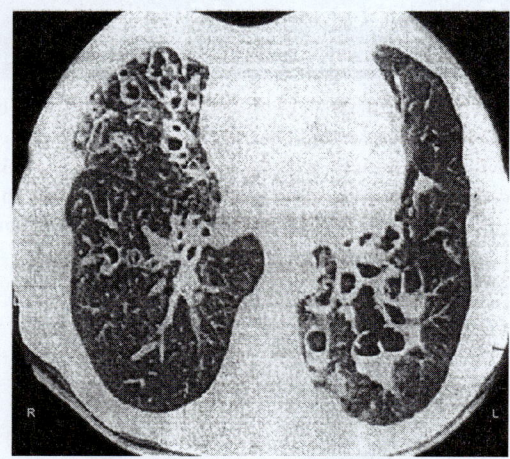

     a. Bilateral varicose Bronchiectasis
     b. Multiple cavitating secondaries
     c. Interstitial fibrosis
     d. Miliary tuberculosis

117. **IOC for Bronchiectasis:** *(Recent Question 2015-16)*
     a. HRCT scan   b. Spiral CT
     c. Bronchoscopy d. Pulmonary angiography

118. **Most common cause of lung abscess in comatose patient?**
     (Recent Pattern 2015-16)
     a. Staph aureus b. Oral anaerobes
     c. Klebsiella   d. Tuberculosis

119. **Chest X-ray in a 45 yr old patient shows cavity in upper lobe of lung. Next investigation for diagnosis is:**
     (Recent Pattern 2014-15)
     a. CT chest   b. USG chest
     c. MRI chest   d. BAL and biopsy

120. **Best method for detecting minimal bronchiectasis is:**
     a. Bronchogram   *(Recent Pattern 2014-15)*
     b. CT scan
     c. Radionuclide lung scan
     d. Chest X-ray

121. **Most likely precursor to bronchiectasis is:**
     (Recent Pattern 2014-15)
     a. Tuberculosis b. Carcinoma
     c. Bronchial adenoma d. Necrotising pneumonia

122. **Which of the following is not a feature of Kartagener's syndrome:** *(Recent Pattern 2014-15)*
     a. Bronchiectasis
     b. Pancreatic insufficiency
     c. Sinusitis
     d. Situs inversus

123. **Ultrastructural abnormalities reported in immotile cilia syndrome are:** *(Recent Pattern 2014-15)*
     a. Dynein in arm deficiency
     b. Absence of radial spokes
     c. Absence of central microtubule
     d. All of the above

124. **Parents of a child with bronchiectasis may give a past history of:** *(Recent Pattern 2014-15)*
     a. Chickenpox   b. Mumps
     c. Whooping cough d. Typhoid

125. **Not a CT finding in bronchiectasis:**
     a. Tree in bud appearance *(Recent Pattern 2014-15)*
     b. Crazy paving appearance
     c. Signet ring appearance
     d. Traction bronchiectasis with lung fibrosis

126. **Bronchiectasis is most common in:**
     (Recent Pattern 2014-15)
     a. Right middle lobe b. Right upper lobe
     c. Left lower lobe   d. Left upper lobe

127. **Which of the following is NOT a complication of bronchiectasis :** *(AIIMS Sept 96, AI 1998)*
     a. Lung abscess b. Lung cancer
     c. Amylodosis   d. Empyema

Cystic Fibrosis

128. **Infertility in kartagener syndrome is due to?**
     (AIIMS Nov 2018)
     a. Oligospermia b. Blockage of epididymis
     c. Asthenospermia d. Undescended testis

129. **Which of the following organisms is *unlikely* to be found in sputum of patients with cystic fibrosis?**
     (Recent Pattern Questions)
     a. Hemophilus influenzae
     b. Acinetobacter baumannii
     c. Burkholderia cepacia
     d. Aspergillus fumigatus

130. **Most common presentation in cystic fibrosis:**
     (Recent Pattern 2014-15)
     a. Lung infections b. Meconium ileus
     c. Malabsorbtion   d. Infertility

131. **An infant has a positive newborn screening test for cystic fibrosis. What cut off of sweat chloride confirms cystic fibrosis?** *(Recent Pattern 2014-15)*
     a. Sweat Chloride >30 mEq/dL
     b. Sweat Chloride > 40 mEq/dL
     c. Sweat Chloride > 50 mEq/dL
     d. Sweat Chloride > 60 mEq/dL

132. **Cystic fibrosis characteristically has following features except:** *(Recent Pattern 2014-15)*
     a. Skin frosting   b. Diabetes mellitus
     c. Chronic constipation d. Bronchiectasis

133. **The CFTR gene associated with cystic fibrosis is located on chromosome:** *(Recent Pattern 2014-15)*
     a. 5   b. 12
     c. 4   d. 7

134. True in mucoviscidosis are A/E: *(Recent Pattern 2014-15)*
    a. Meconium ileus
    b. Steatorrhoea
    c. Sinusitis
    d. Glomerulonephritis
135. Kartagener's syndrome is *not* associated with:
    (Recent Pattern 2014-15)
    a. Situs inversus
    b. Subluxation of lens
    c. Bronchiectasis
    d. Sinusitis
136. In cystic fibrosis the most frequent pulmonary pathogen causing recurrent pneumonia is? *(Recent Pattern 2014-15)*
    a. Pseudomonas
    b. Enterococci
    c. Staphylococci
    d. Klebsiella

Interstitial Lung Disease

137. A 45-year patient working in a factory for past 20 years presents with breathlessness. HRCT chest shows pleural thickening and fibrosis. Histopathology of the lesion shows? *(AIIMS May 2018)*

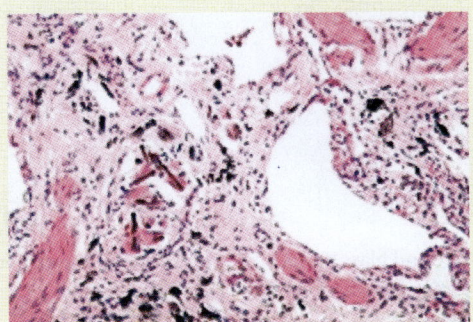

    a. Asbestosis
    b. Cotton fiber
    c. Coal worker pneumoconiosis
    d. Silicosis
138. ILD is seen in all of the following except?
    (Recent Pattern Questions)
    a. Tuberous sclerosis
    b. Sturge Weber syndrome
    c. Gaucher's disease
    d. Desquamative interstitial pneumonitis
139. Which of the following diseases results in granuloma formation in lungs? *(Recent Pattern Questions)*
    a. Hypersensitivity pneumonitis
    b. SLE
    c. Usual interstitial pneumonia
    d. Asbestosis
140. What is the first investigation to be done for suspected interstitial lung disease patient? *(Recent Pattern Questions)*
    a. Chest X-ray
    b. HRCT
    c. MDCT
    d. Spirometry
141. A 25-year-old female presents with progressive dyspnea for one year. CXR shows interstitial opacities and spirometry shows obstructive pattern. What is the diagnosis?
    (Recent Pattern Questions)
    a. Non-specific interstitial pneumonitis
    b. Pulmonary Lymphangioleiomyomatosis
    c. Idiopathic pulmonary fibrosis
    d. Pulmonary alveolar Proteinosis

142. Which subtype of ILD can present like ARDS?
    (Recent Pattern Questions)
    a. Desquamative interstitial pneumonitis
    b. Hamman Rich Syndrome
    c. Usual interstitial pneumonitis
    d. Cryptogenic organising Pneumonia
143. Which of the following ILD is not associated with smoking? *(Recent Pattern Questions)*
    a. Cryptogenic organising pneumonia
    b. Desquamative interstitial pneumonia
    c. Respiratory bronchiolitis
    d. Pulmonary Langerhan cell Histiocytosis
144. Which is not used in management of IPF?
    (Recent Pattern Questions)
    a. Thalidomide
    b. Pantoprazole
    c. Lung transplantation
    d. Acebrophylline
145. BAL of a patient shows foamy macrophages with decreased CD4: CD8 ratio. What is the diagnosis?
    a. Sarcoidosis *(Recent Pattern Questions)*
    b. Hypersensitivity pneumonitis
    c. Organising pneumonia
    d. Diffuse alveolar haemorrhage
146. Periodic acid (Schiff) stain positive intra-alveolar material is seen in? *(Recent Pattern Questions)*
    a. Alpha 1 antitrypsin deficiency
    b. Pulmonary alveolar Proteinosis
    c. Abetalipoproteinemia
    d. Lipoid pneumonia
147. Bronchocentric granulomatosis commonly occurs due to?
    (Recent Pattern Questions)
    a. Hypersensitivity reaction to Aspergillus
    b. Immunological reaction to HIV
    c. Damage by c-ANCA
    d. Damage by p-ANCA
148. Which subtype of interstitial lung disease is seen in patients of Sjogren syndrome? *(Recent Pattern Questions)*
    a. Usual interstitial pneumonia
    b. Non-specific interstitial pneumonia
    c. Acute interstitial pneumonia
    d. Cryptogenic organising pneumonia?
149. Comment on the diagnosis *(Recent Question 2016-17)*

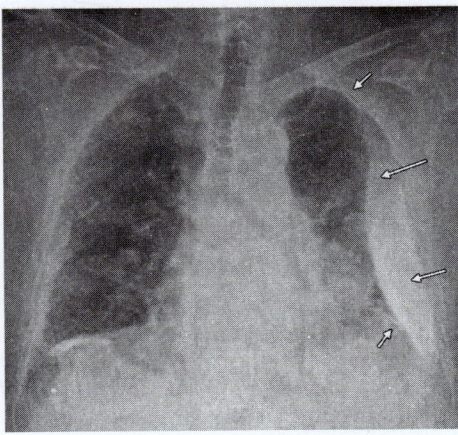

    a. Pleural calcification
    b. Pleural effusion
    c. Pulmonary consolidation
    d. Loculated effusion

150. The following CT chest shows presence of?
    (Recent Question 2016-17)

    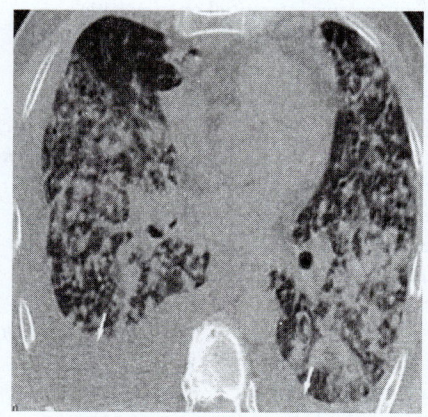

    a. Pneumoconiosis
    b. Primary Carcinoma of lung
    c. Bronchiectasis
    d. Chronic Bronchitis

151. Which one of the following is not likely to be associated with pulmonary fibrosis? *(UPSC 2015)*
    a. Coal Miners' Lung
    b. Primary biliary cirrhosis
    c. Asbestosis
    d. Ankylosing spondylitis

152. Cavitating pulmonary lesions can be seen in the following except? *(UPSC 2015)*
    a. Sarcoidosis
    b. Tuberculosis
    c. Carcinoma of lung
    d. Histoplasmosis

153. Investigation of choice for interstitial lung disease is?
    (Bihar PG 2015)
    a. Chest X-ray
    b. HRCT
    c. Gallium-67 DTPA scan
    d. MRI

154. Which of the following lung disease is shown in the image below?

    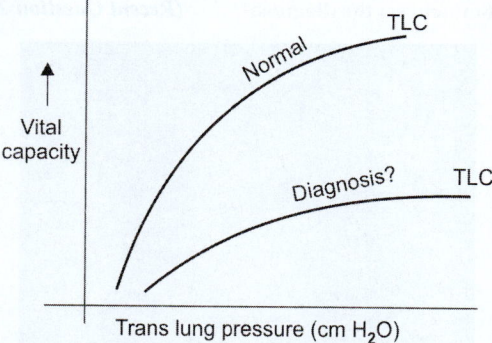

    a. Emphysema
    b. Asthma
    c. Interstitial Fibrosis
    d. Normal

155. Conglomerate nodules are found in? *(JIPMER Nov 2015)*
    a. Pulmonary Lymphangioleiomyomatosis
    b. Round pneumonia
    c. Silicosis
    d. Hypersensitivity pneumonitis

156. 35 year old Coal worker presents with difficulty in breathing on exertion for last 2 years. CXR was performed. It shows?

    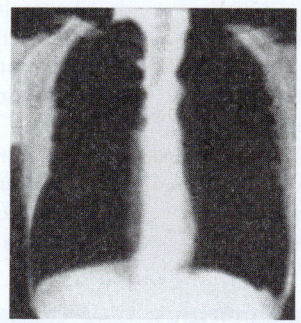

    a. Emphysema
    b. Reticulo-nodular infiltrates
    c. Pulmonary Fibrosis
    d. Cardiac atrophy

157. The CT chest of patient shows ?

    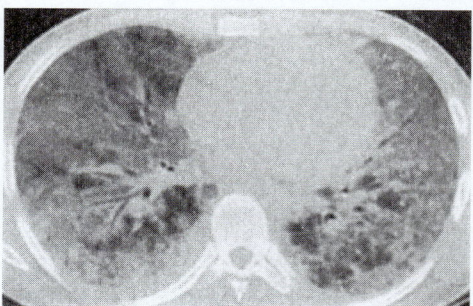

    a. Ground glass pattern
    b. Honey comb pattern
    c. Crazy pavement pattern
    d. Normal scan

158. The chest CXR of patient shows?

    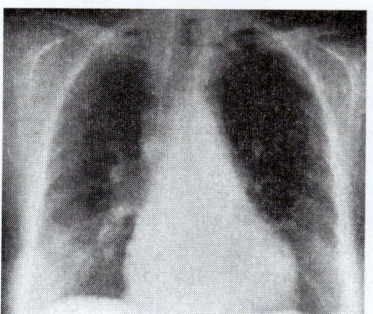

    a. Emphysema
    b. Reticular shadows
    c. Bat wing Edema
    d. Kerley B lines

159. Which of the following is the diagnosis of this patient with history of smoking?

    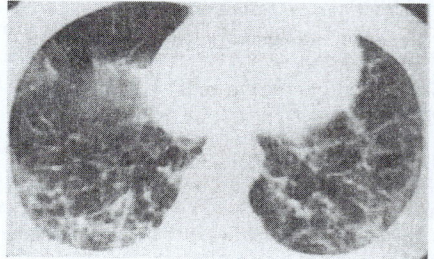

    a. Emphysema
    b. Idiopathic pulmonary fibrosis
    c. Progressive primary Tuberculosis
    d. bronchiectasis

160. Which of the following is true regarding Idiopathic Non specific interstitial pneumonia? *(AIIMS Nov 2014)*
    a. Honey combing on CT
    b. Male predominant
    c. Elderly age
    d. Good prognosis
161. A patient with bilateral hilar lymphadenopathy on CXR was suspected to have Sarcoidosis. What is the next step? *(JIPMER 2014)*
    a. CT thorax
    b. Lymph Node Biopsy
    c. Serum ACE
    d. Gallium scan
162. Asbestos causes all except? *(Recent Pattern 2015-16)*
    a. Mesothelioma
    b. Pleural effusion
    c. Bronchial cancer
    d. Atelectasis
163. Asbestosis causes all except? *(Recent Pattern 2014-15)*
    a. Shaggy heart borders
    b. Honeycombing
    c. Hilar lymphadenopathy
    d. Basal peribronchial fibrosis
164. Which one of the following is not correct regarding silicosis? *(Recent Pattern 2014-15)*
    a. Egg shell calcification is seen on chest X-ray
    b. It is more marked in the lower zone
    c. May lead to progressive massive fibrosis
    d. Increased timed vital capacity
165. Restrictive lung disease is associated with all except?
    a. High residual lung volume *(Recent Pattern 2014-15)*
    b. High PCO_2
    c. FEV1 below 50%
    d. Very low pO_2
166. All the following are features of interstitial lung disease except: *(Recent Pattern 2014-15)*
    a. Exertional dyspnoea
    b. Cyanosis
    c. Digital clubbing
    d. Coarse crepitations
167. Heerfordt's syndrome consists of fever, parotid enlargement, facial palsy and: *(Recent Pattern 2014-15)*
    a. Arthralgia
    b. Bilateral hilar lymphadenopathy
    c. Erythema nodosum
    d. Anterior uveitis
168. Recognized features of asbestosis *do not* include:
    a. Calcification of pleura *(Recent Pattern 2014-15)*
    b. Egg shell calcification of hilar lymph nodes
    c. Clubbing of fingers
    d. Restrictive pattern of ventilatory defect shown by pulmonary function
169. What is *true* regarding byssinosis: *(Recent Pattern 2014-15)*
    a. Dyspnea resolves after cessation of exposure
    b. Similar to chronic bronchitis and emphysema
    c. Present as mediastinal fibrosis
    d. Eosinophils are prominent in BAL
170. The typical feature of interstitial lung disease is: *(Recent Pattern 2014-15)*
    a. End Inspiratory rales
    b. Expiratory rales
    c. Inspiratory rhonchi
    d. Expiratory rhonchi
171. The following are interstitial lung disease except: *(Recent Pattern 2014-15)*
    a. Sarcoidosis
    b. Fibrosing alveolitis
    c. Bronchial asthma
    d. Pneumoconiosis
172. Cotton dust is associated with: *(Recent Pattern 2014-15)*
    a. Byssinosis
    b. Asbestosis
    c. Bagassosis
    d. Silicosis
173. The following does not occur with asbestosis: *(Recent Pattern 2014-15)*
    a. Atelectasis
    b. Pneumoconiosis
    c. Pleural mesothelioma
    d. Pleural calcification
174. Caplan Syndrome is Pneumoconiosis with
    a. Lymphadenopathy
    b. Congestive Cardiac Failure
    c. Rheumatoid Arthritis
    d. HIV
175. Serum ACE may be raised in all of the following *except*:
    a. Sarcoidosis
    b. Silicosis *(AI 2005)*
    c. Berylliosis
    d. Bronchogenic carcinoma

Pneumonia

176. CSF gram stain of a child suffering with meningitis is shown below. What is the causative agent? *(Recent Question 2019)*

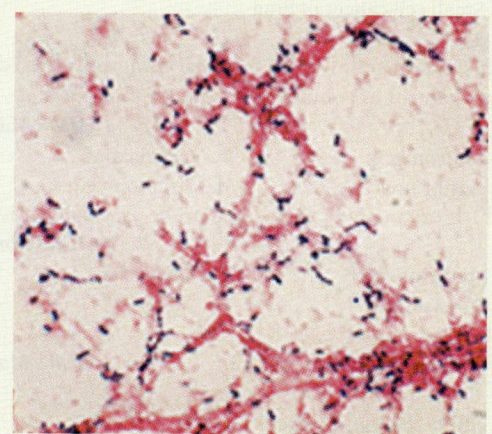

    a. Streptococcus pneumoniae
    b. H. Influenzae
    c. Klebsiella pneumonia
    d. Staphylococcus aureus
177. DOC for following infection (as shown in image) in a HIV patient: *(Recent Question 2019)*

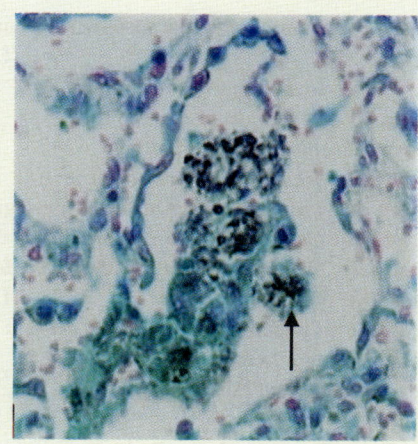

    a. INH+ Rifampicin
    b. Cotrimoxazole
    c. Doxycycline
    d. Azithromycin

178. A middle aged immunocompromised male presents with fever and breathlessness. HRCT shows a middle lobe lesion with infiltration. Lung biopsy from the lesion is shown in the imagae. The clinical diagnosis is? (AIIMS May 2018)

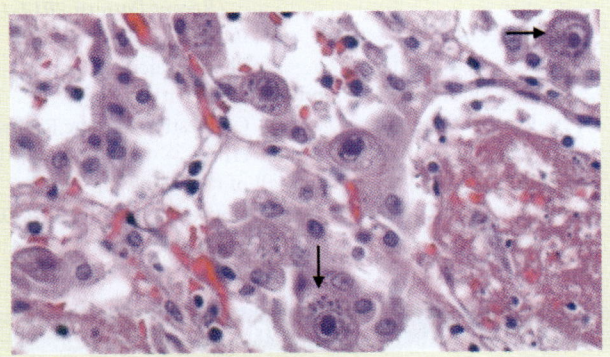

   a. CMV pneumonia
   b. Cryptogenic organizing pneumonia
   c. Small cell cancer of lung
   d. TB

179. Which of the following is the most commonly used drug for management of community acquired pneumonia?
 (AIIMS May 2018)
   a. Vancomycin   b. Ceftriaxone
   c. Azithromycin   d. Streptomycin

180. Which organism is most likely to be associated with VAP?
 (AIIMS May 2018)
   a. Acinetobacter   b. Klebsiella
   c. Clostridium   d. MTB

181. All are true about CURB 65 score except?
   a. Respiratory rate of >30/min   (AIIMS May 2017)
   b. BUN of >7 mmol/L
   c. SBP >100 mmHg
   d. Confused state

182. Which of following associations is correctly paired?
 (Recent Pattern Questions)
   a. Aspiration pneumonia: Streptococcus pyogenes
   b. Heavy alcohol use: Atypical pathogens
   c. Poor dental hygiene: Chlamydia and Klebsiella pneumoniae
   d. Structural lung disease: Burkholderia

183. Klebsiella pneumonia has the following characteristics except: (UPSC 2015)
   a. Upper lobes are frequently involved
   b. Pneumatocoele may occur commonly
   c. Empyema is much more common
   d. Lung abscess formation is very uncommon

184. A 28-year-old woman presented with high grade fever, cough, diarrhea and mental confusion for 4 days. X-ray chest revealed bilateral pneumonitis. Search for etiology will most likely reveal? (UPSC 2015)
   a. Streptococcus pneumoniae
   b. Staphylococcus aureus
   c. Legionella pneumophila
   d. Pseudomonas aeruginosa

185. Drug of choice for mycoplasma pneumonia is?
 (Bihar Pg 2015)
   a. Penicillin   b. Tetracycline
   c. Cefuroxime   d. Erythromycin

186. Pneumonia with confusion and diarrhoea?
 (JIPMER Nov 2015)
   a. Legionella   b. Mycoplasma
   c. Chylamydia   d. Pneumocystis carinii

187. In HIV positive patient with pneumocysti jiroveci infection, which of the following is used for prevention?
   a. Azithromycin   (Recent Question 2015-16)
   b. Acyclovir
   c. Levofloxacin
   d. Sulfomethoxazole+ trimethoprim

188. CURB 65 criteria includes all EXCEPT:
 (Recent Question 2015-16)
   a. Age more than or equal to 65 years
   b. Respiratory rate more than 30/min
   c. Systolic Blood pressure is more than 90 mmHg
   d. BUN level is >7 mmol/L

189. Which is correct about pneumonia?
 (Recent Pattern 2015-16)
   a. Bronchophony   b. Decreased vocal fremitus
   c. Shifting of trachea   d. Amphoric breathing

190. Unipolar flagellate organism that causes pneumonia?
 (Recent Pattern 2015-16)
   a. Pseudomonas   b. Mycoplasma
   c. Aeromonas   d. Klebsiella pneumonia

191. Pneumatocele is caused by: (Recent Pattern 2014-15)
   a. Streptococcus pneumonia   b. Haemophilus influenza
   c. Serratia marcescens   d. Klebsiella pneumonia

192. Round pneumonia is seen with: (Recent Pattern 2014-15)
   a. Streptococcal pneumonia   b. Kerosene oil aspiration
   c. Lung cancer   d. Mendelson syndrome

193. Which is not correct about aspiration pneumonia?
   a. 5-15% of community acquired pneumonia is due to aspiration pneumonia (AIIMS May 2013)
   b. Anaerobic infection is most common
   c. Superior segment of apex of lung is commonly involved in recumbent position
   d. 20-25ml of fluid less than pH 2.5 is required for aspiration pneumonia

194. Breath sounds are decreased in following except:
 (Recent Pattern 2014-15)
   a. Lobar pneumonia   b. Pneumothorax
   c. Pleural effusion   d. Atelectasis

195. X-ray finding of Staphylococcus pneumonia are A/E:
 (Recent Pattern 2014-15)
   a. Pneumatocele   b. Hilar lymphadenopathy
   c. Empyema   d. Visible air bronchogram

196. Tubular breathing is seen in: (Recent Pattern 2014-15)
   a. Pleural effusion   b. Consolidation
   c. Pleurisy   d. Tuberculous cavity

197. A 28 year female, has diarrhoea, confusion, high grade fever with bilateral pneumonitis. The diagnosis is: (AI 2000)
   a. Legionella   b. Neisseria meningitis
   c. Streptococcus pneumoniae
   d. H. influenza

198. All of the following features are seen in the viral pneumonia except: (AI 2005)
   a. Presence of interstitial inflammation
   b. Predominance of alveolar exudates
   c. Bronchiolitis
   d. Multinucleate giant cells in the bronchiolar wall

199. All of the following statements about Pneumocystis Jiroveci are true Except: (AI 2008)
    a. Usually associated with CMV infection
    b. May be associated with Pneumatocele
    c. Usually diagnosed by sputum examination
    d. Causes disease only in the immunocompromised host

200. Drug of choice for *Mycoplasma pneumoniae* is : (AIIMS Dec 94, May 94)
    a. Penicillin   b. Tetracycline
    c. Cefuroxime   d. Erythromycin

201. Commonest sign of aspiration pneumonitis is : (AIIMS Dec 94)
    a. Cyanosis   b. Tachypnea
    c. Crepitations d. Rhonchi

Tuberculosis

202. A 56-year-old presents with history of massive haemoptysis. Chest X-ray of patient is normal. Which of the following is not recommended for the patient? (AIIMS May 2017)
    a. Pulmonary artery embolization
    b. Bronchial artery embolization
    c. Surgical removal of the involved lobe
    d. Pro-coagulant drugs

203. All are differential diagnosis of the condition shown in the CT chest except? (Recent Question 2016-17)

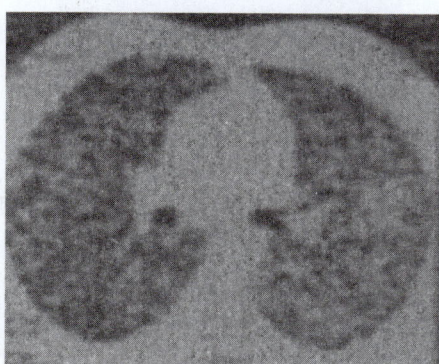

    a. Hemosiderosis
    b. Tropical pulmonary eosinophilia
    c. Collagen vascular disorders
    d. Diffuse pulmonary Lymphangioleiomyomatosis

204. CT scan chest shows presence of? (Recent Question 2016-17)

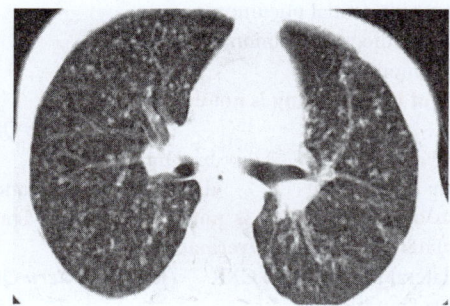

    a. Miliary TB   b. Endobronchial TB
    c. Bronchocele   d. Central Bronchiectasis

205. This Miliary pattern in CT scan can occur due to spread from? (Recent Question 2016-17)

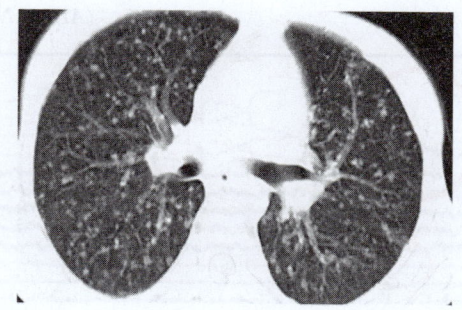

    a. Lymphatics
    b. Bronchial Vein
    c. Pulmonary artery
    d. All of the above

206. Systemic Miliary TB spreads via? (Recent Pattern 2015-16)
    a. Artery
    b. Vein
    c. Bronchus
    d. Lymphatic

207. Patient diagnosed with HIV and Tuberculosis. How to start ATT and c-A.R.T? (Recent Pattern 2015-16)
    a. Start ATT first
    b. Start cART first
    c. Start both simultaneously
    d. Start cART only

208. Persistent coarse crepitations in the chest is diagnostic of:
    a. Pulmonary TB (Recent Pattern 2014-15)
    b. Pulmonary oedema
    c. Cavity lesion
    d. Bronchiectasis

209. Miliary mottling of lung is seen in all except:
    a. Silicosis (Recent Pattern 2014-15)
    b. Aspergillosis
    c. Haemosiderosis
    d. Tuberculosis

210. False-negative tuberculin test is seen in *all except*:
    a. After 4-6 weeks of measles attack (AI 1996)
    b. Immunodeficiency state
    c. Miliary tuberculosis
    d. Atypical mycobacterial infection

211. A man presents with fever, wt loss and cough; Mantoux reads an induration of 17 x 19 mm; Sputum cytology is negative for AFB. Most likely diagnosis is: (AI 2001)
    a. Pulm tuberculosis
    b. Fungal infection
    c. Viral infection
    d. Pneumonia

212. A 60-year-old man is suspected of having bronchogenic carcinoma, TB has been ruled out in this patient. What should be the next investigation? (AI 01)
    a. CT guided FNAC
    b. Bronchoscopy and biopsy
    c. Sputum cytology
    d. X-Ray chest

Obstructive Sleep Apnea

213. Identify the sleep stage in the following Polysomnograph.
     (AIIMS Nov 2017)

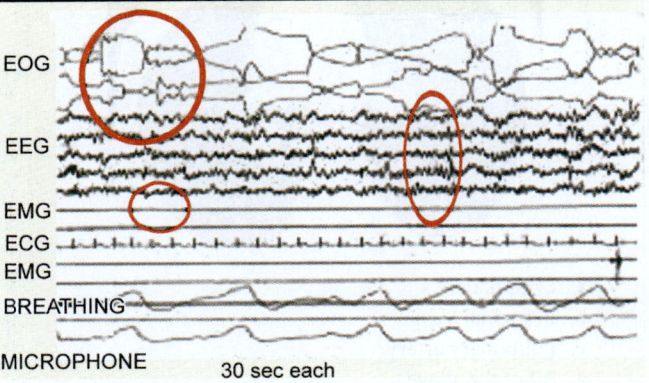

a. NREM stage 1   b. NREM stage 2
c. NREM stage 3   d. REM

214. Severe obstructive sleep apnea is defined as apnea-hypopnea index of greater than? *(Recent Question 2016-17)*
     a. 10 events/ hour   b. 15 events/ hour
     c. 20 events/ hour   d. 30 events/ hour

215. 'Sleep apnea' is defined as temporary pause in breathing during sleep lasting at least? *(Bihar PG)*
     a. 40 seconds   b. 30 seconds
     c. 20 seconds   d. 10 seconds

216. All of the following criteria are required for diagnosis of obesity hypoventilation syndrome EXCEPT
     (Recent Question 2015-16)
     a. Hypertension   b. Sleep disorder breathing
     c. BMI ≥ 30 kg/m^2 d. PaCO$_2$ ≥ 45 mmHg

217. False about obstructive sleep apnea *(AIIMS Nov 2014)*
     a. It affects more women
     b. Associated with hypertension
     c. Day time sleepiness
     d. >5 episodes/hour

218. 40-year-old smoker, obese, hypertension patient is having loud snoring. On sleep study patient had >5 episodes of apnea per hour of sleep at night. After control of BP and quitting smoking what is the next best management for improvement of symptoms of the patient?
     a. C.P.A.P   *(Recent Pattern 2014-15)*
     b. Uvulopalatoplasty
     c. Weight reduction and diet control
     d. Mandibular reposition surgery

219. Not true of obstructive sleep apnoea:
     (Recent Pattern 2014-15)
     a. Nocturnal asphyxia   b. Alcoholism is a cofactor
     c. Prone to hypertension   d. Spirometry is diagnostic

220. Obstructive sleep apnoea may result in all of the following except: *(Recent Pattern 2014-15)*
     a. Systemic hypertension   b. Pulmonary hypertension
     c. Heart block   d. Impotence

221. Most common cause of obstructive sleep apnea
     (Recent Pattern 2014-15)
     a. Craniofacial abnormalities   b. Hypothyroidism
     c. Alcoholism   d. Acromegaly

222. Duration of apnea in obstructive sleep apnea is
     (Recent Pattern 2014-15)
     a. <10 sec   b. >20 sec
     c. >30 sec   d. >60 sec

223. Obstructive sleep apnea is defined as _____ number of apnea events/hour? *(Recent Pattern 2014-15)*
     a. 2   b. 3
     c. 4   d. 5

224. The Epworth scale is used for assessing:
     a. Body mass index   *(Recent Pattern 2014-15)*
     b. Vital capacity in post-operative patients
     c. Sleep apnea
     d. Risk of embolism in perioperative patient

ARDS

225. 65-year-old alcoholic is admitted to the ICU with diagnosis of acute pancreatitis. After 48 hours he is unconscious and has the following findings: sP02= 60%, p02= 60 mmHg, pCO2 =30mm Hg and HR= 120 bpm. CXR was performed. Diagnosis is? *(Recent Question 2019)*

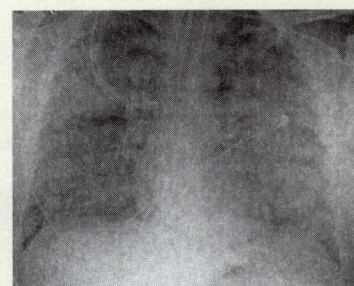

a. Mendelson syndrome   b. Shock lung
c. Nosocomial pneumonia   d. Sympathetic pleural effusion

226. Mild ARDS diagnostic criteria is? *(JIPMER May 2018)*
     a. PaO$_2$/FiO$_2$ less than 200 mm Hg
     b. PaO$_2$/FiO$_2$ less than 300 mm Hg
     c. PaO$_2$/FiO$_2$ more than 200 mm Hg
     d. PaO$_2$/FiO$_2$ more than 300 mm Hg

227. All of the following are correct about ARDS except?
     (Recent Pattern 2018)
     a. pAO$_2$/ FiO$_2$ <300   b. Acute onset illness
     c. PCWP >18 mm Hg   d. Bilateral alveolar infiltrates

228. A 23-year-old medical student develops extreme shortness of breath and develops blue fingertips and bilateral crackles after trekking in Ladakh. What is the probable diagnosis?
     a. Frost bite   *(Recent Pattern Questions)*
     b. Acute interstitial pneumonia
     c. Non cardiogenic pulmonary oedema
     d. Pneumonia

229. Which of the following is not done in TRALI?
     (Recent Pattern Questions)
     a. IVF   b. Diuretics
     c. Stop transfusion   d. Improve oxygenation

230. Which of the following is not correct about Transfusion Associated Circulatory Overload (TACO)?
     a. Bilateral infiltrates on CXR   *(Recent Pattern Questions)*
     b. Give Diuretics
     c. Normal PCWP
     d. Elevated BNP levels

231. A 35-year-old paraplegic male develops fever and dyspnea over last one week with fever, cough, rusty sputum and diffuse rales. BP is 70/50 mmHg with heart rate of 120/min. CXR shows diffuse alveolar infiltrates. Which is best for diagnosis? *(Recent Pattern Questions)*
    a. D-Dimer Assay
    b. Spiral CT
    c. VP scan
    d. Measurement of PCWP

232. Severe ARDS is defined as paO_2/FiO_2 ratio less than? *(Recent Question 2016-17)*
    a. 50
    b. 100
    c. 200
    d. 300

233. What is the most common cause of death in ARDS? *(Recent Question 2016-17)*
    a. V/P mismatch
    b. Non pulmonary causes
    c. Baro-trauma
    d. Chemical pneumonitis

234. ARDS is associated with all except? *(JIPMER May 2015)*
    a. Pulmonary embolism
    b. Acute pancreatitis
    c. Sepsis
    d. Aspiration

235. ARDS is characterised by all except?
    a. Decreased surfactant *(Recent Question 2015-16)*
    b. Alveolar transudate
    c. Decreased lung compliance
    d. pAO_2/FiO_2 ratio <200

236. ARDS includes all EXCEPT? *(Recent Question 2015-16)*
    a. Hypoxia
    b. Hypercapnia
    c. Non cardiogenic pulmonary edema
    d. Normal P.C.W.P

237. A patient on ventilator is having bilateral crepitations in all lung fields. CXR shows presence of?

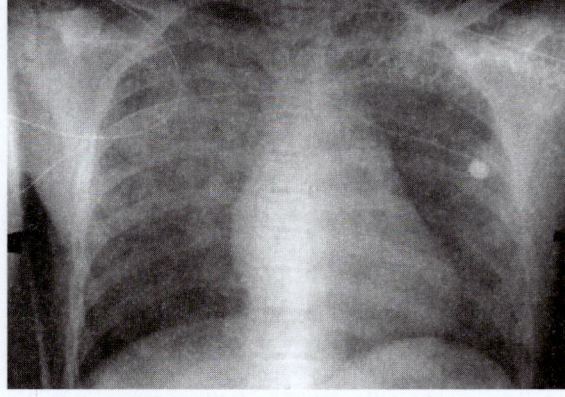

    a. Cardiogenic pulmonary edema
    b. Non cardiogenic pulmonary edema
    c. Neurogenic pulmonary edema
    d. Chemical pneumonitis

238. A construction worker had a cement slab falling on his chest. He was rescued but he develops difficulty in breathing with cyanosis. CXR shows:

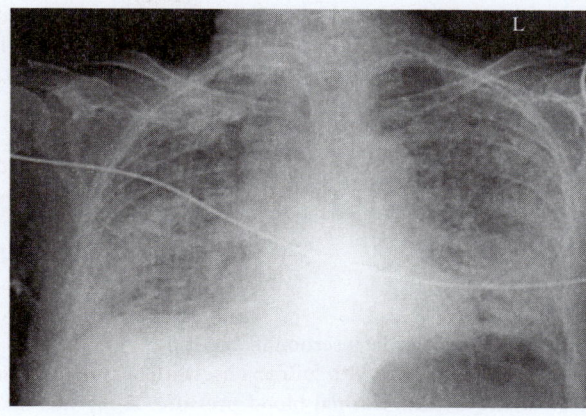

    a. ARDS
    b. Fat embolism
    c. Air embolism
    d. Pneumothorax

239. The following are features of adult respiratory distress syndrome except: *(Recent Pattern 2014-15)*
    a. Hypoxia
    b. Hypocapnia
    c. Low protein Pulmonary edema
    d. Stiff lungs

240. All of the following are well recognized predisposing factors for adult respiratory distress syndrome, except:
    a. Multiple blood transfusions *(Recent Pattern 2014-15)*
    b. Septicemia
    c. Status asthmaticus
    d. Toxic gas inhalation

241. True about adult respiratory distress syndrome except:
    a. paO_2/FiO_2 ratio < 200 *(Recent Pattern 2014-15)*
    b. PCWP < 18 mm Hg
    c. Hypoxia
    d. Low protein pulmonary edema

242. Correct about ARDS is: *(Recent Pattern 2014-15)*
    a. Low tidal volume ventilation
    b. High lung compliance
    c. Low protein pulmonary edema
    d. High pulmonary capillary pressure

243. All are correct regarding ARDS except?:
    a. Stiff lungs *(AIPG 2010)*
    b. Hypoxaemia without hypercapnea
    c. Increase in pulmonary capillary wedge pressure
    d. Intrapulmonary right to left shunt

244. The point which distinguishes ARDS from cardiogenic pulmonary edema is: *(Recent Pattern 2014-15)*
    a. Normal PO_2
    b. Normal pulmonary capillary wedge pressure
    c. Normal arterial alveolar gradient
    d. Normal PCO_2

245. ARDS includes all except: *(Recent Pattern 2014-15)*
    a. Hypoxia
    b. Hypercapnia
    c. Non cardiogenic pulmonary edema
    d. Normal P.C.W.P

246. All are seen in ARDS, *except*: *(AIIMS May 95)*
    a. Pulmonary edema
    b. Decreased tidal volume
    c. Hypercapnia
    d. Decreased compliance

Pleural Effusion, Pneumothorax and Pneumomediastinum

247. A patient with Staphylococcal pneumonia develops acute breathlessness. Probable cause is? *(JIPMER May 2018)*
    a. Pericarditis
    b. Pneumothorax
    c. Acute respiratory failure
    d. Parapneumonic effusion

248. A patient came with a chest trauma and difficulty in breathing. On examination a hyper-resonant note in the chest is found with BP = 90/60 mm Hg. What is the next best step in the management of this patient?
    a. Intubate *(AIIMS Nov 2018)*
    b. CXR
    c. IVF
    d. Wide bore needle insertion in 2nd ICS

249. A patient presented with sudden onset difficulty in breathing with RR 28/min, normal blood pressure. X-ray was taken which is given below. What is the diagnosis?
    (AIIMS Nov 2017)

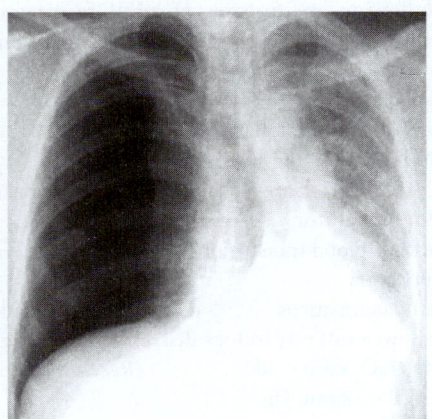

    a. Pneumothorax
    b. Hydro-pneumothorax
    c. Pleural effusion
    d. Consolidation

250. A car accident patient complains of breathlessness. On examination BP is 110/70 mmHg with GCS of 15/15. On examination, trachea shows deviation in suprasternal notch, with reduced breath sounds in left infra-axillary area and inframammary areas. S1 and S2 are normal in intensity and splitting. CXR is shown below. What is the best step in management of the patient? *(AIIMS May 2017)*

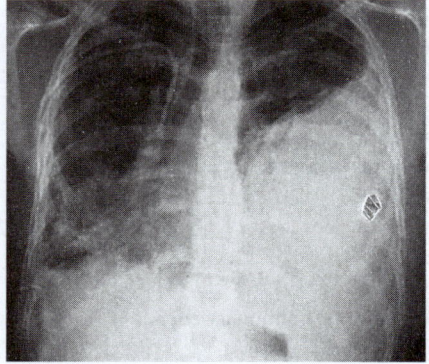

    a. Needle aspiration
    b. Pericardiocentesis
    c. Chest tube insertion
    d. Immediate thoracotomy

251. A patient is having right sided pleural effusion. On thoracocentesis, pleural fluid does not clot on standing. What is the possible cause? *(Recent Pattern Questions)*
    a. Meig's syndrome
    b. CHF
    c. Malignant pleural effusion
    d. TB

252. Which of the following conditions is managed with tube thoracotomy with instillation of tissue plasminogen activator? *(Recent Pattern Questions)*
    a. Malignant pleural effusion
    b. Para-pneumonic effusion
    c. Effusion secondary to pulmonary embolism
    d. Hemothorax

253. For diagnosis of pleural effusion as an exudate, more than _____ modified Light's criteria should be positive? *(Recent Pattern Questions)*
    a. 1
    b. 2
    c. 3
    d. All

254. All are true about Tension pneumothorax except? *(Recent Pattern Questions)*
    a. Leading cause is mechanical ventilation
    b. Positive pressure in pleural space throughout the respiratory cycle
    c. Needle aspiration of air
    d. Inadequate cardiac output

255. A young male met with Road traffic accident and is brought to the casualty. He complains of chest pain. His BP = 130/80 mm Hg, pulse rate = 88/min and RR = 22/min. On auscultation decreased air entry on left side with absent breath sounds is noted. X-ray chest is given below. Diagnosis is? *(AIIMS Nov 2016)*

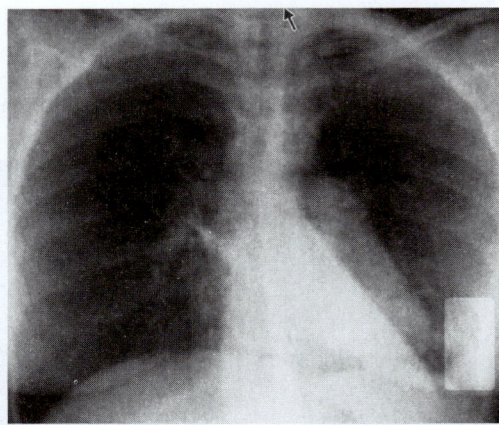

    a. Cardiac Tamponade
    b. Tension pneumothorax
    c. Flail chest due to fracture of ribs (5, 6, 7 and 8th ribs)
    d. Esophageal rupture and pneumo-mediastinum

256. A 16-year-old tall and thin built patient came to the emergency room with hypotension and severe dyspnea. On examination breath sounds are absent on left hemithorax with shift of trachea to the right side. The percussion note on the left side is hyper-resonant. What is the next line of management for the patient? *(AIIMS May 2016)*
    a. Send patient for urgent X-ray
    b. Put the patient on positive pressure ventilation for hypoxia
    c. Needle thoracotomy
    d. Start vasopressors for low BP

257. A 16 year old boy is admitted with difficulty in breathing. All are true about the CXR shown except?*(AIIMS May 2016)*

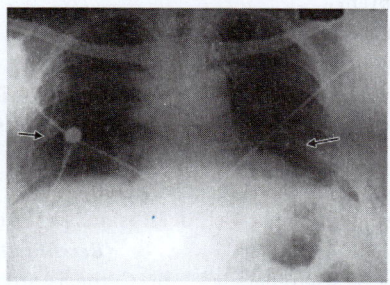

a. Pleural effusion
b. Mediastinum shifted to right
c. Pneumothorax
d. Bilateral ICD tubes

258. Therapeutic thoracocentesis should be performed if the free fluid in the lung separates the chest wall by greater than? *(Recent Question 2016-17)*
a. 5 mm
b. 10 mm
c. 15 mm
d. 20 mm

259. This patient came with acute dyspnea. Which of the following statements is TRUE? *(APPG 2016)*

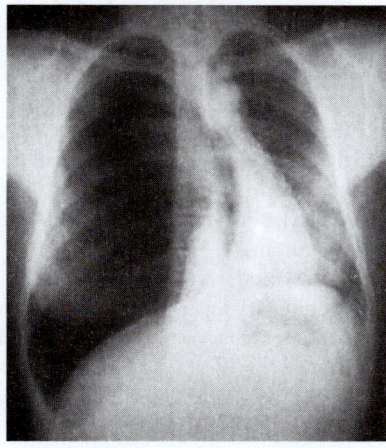

a. X-ray shows Westermark's sign on right side
b. A needle should be inserted into the chest wall in the second right intercostal space as an emergency
c. It is due to old tuberculosis and fibrosis of left lung
d. The patient needs emergency bronchoscopy to remove possible FB in left side

260. The CXR given shows presence of? *(AIIMS Nov 2015)*

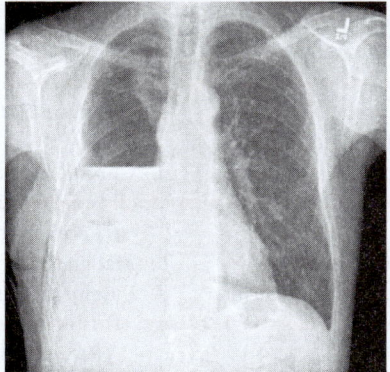

a. Hydropneumothorax
b. Pleural Effusion
c. Lung abscess
d. Collapse

261. A young man presents to the emergency department with shortness of breath and chest pain. Vitals show a HR of 120, Blood pressure is 80/50 and JVP is elevated with trachea shifted to left side. His oxygen saturation is 70% in spite of supplemental oxygen. What is the next step of management?
a. Insert a large bore needle on right side
b. Insert a large bore needle on left side *(JIPMER Nov 2014)*
c. Arrange for an urgent chest x ray and meanwhile give high doses of inhaled oxygen
d. Emergency tracheostomy to secure airway

262. Chylous pleural effusion occurs in: *(PGI 2018)*
a. TB
b. Malignancy
c. SLE
d. Thoracic duct injury
e. Congestive heart failure

263. Which is correct regarding the CXR? *(Recent Question 2015-16)*

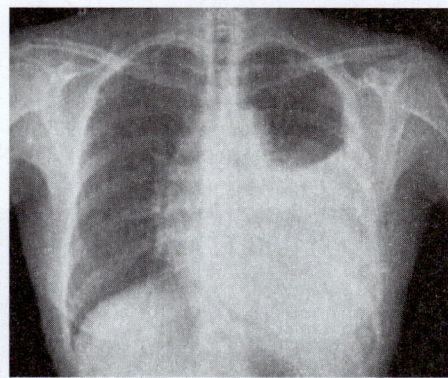

a. Pleural thickening
b. Segmental collapse
c. Ellis curve
d. Hypertranslucency

264. The image shows presence of?

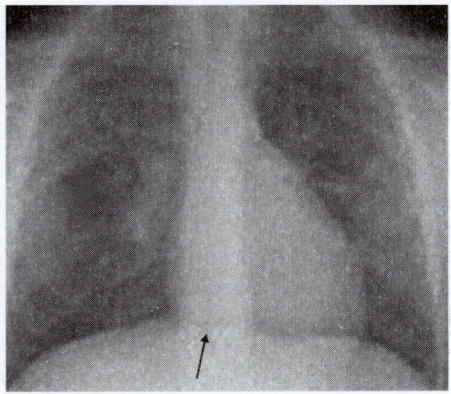

a. Pneumomediastinum
b. Hiatus hernia
c. Rolling Hernia
d. Hampton hump

265. Which is incorrect regarding the condition being managed in the picture?

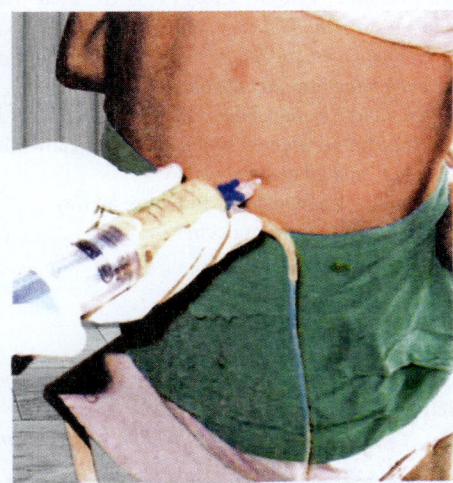

- a. S shaped Ellis curve in axilla
- b. Skodiac resonance
- c. Bronchial breathing
- d. Air entry is normal

266. The following X-ray was taken after Staph Aureus pneumonia. Diagnosis is ?

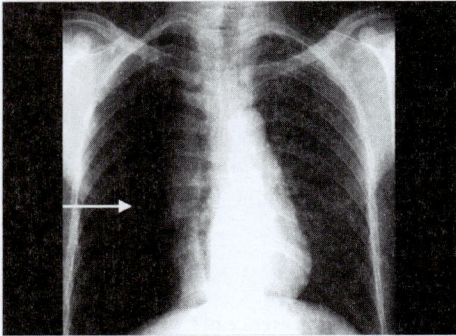

- a. Pneumothorax
- b. Lung abscess
- c. Empyema
- d. Increased Broncho-vascular markings

267. Light criteria for pleural effusion are all except? *(Recent Pattern 2015-16)*
- a. Effusion protein/serum protein ratio greater than 0.5
- b. Effusion lactate dehydrogenase (LDH)/serum LDH ratio greater than 0.6
- c. Effusion LDH level greater than two-thirds the upper limit of the laboratory's reference range of serum LDH
- d. Effusion sugar is less than 2/3 rd of blood sugar

268. Treatment of spontaneous pneumothorax is:
- a. IPPV *(Recent Pattern 2014-15)*
- b. Closed drainage
- c. Simple needle aspiration
- d. Thoractomy

269. Incorrect regarding chylous pleural effusion?
- a. Most common cause is trauma *(Recent Pattern 2014-15)*
- b. Milky white fluid
- c. High cholesterol
- d. Octreotide is used

270. Low glucose in pleural effusion is seen in all except:
- a. Rheumatoid arthritis *(Recent Pattern 2014-15)*
- b. Empyema
- c. Malignant pleural effusion
- d. Dressler's syndrome

271. Pleural fluid low in glucose is seen in all except: *(Recent Pattern 2014-15)*
- a. CHF
- b. Tuberculosis
- c. Mesothelioma
- d. Empyema

272. Transudative type of pleural effusion is a feature of: *(Recent Pattern 2014-15)*
- a. Variceal sclerotherapy
- b. Coronary artery bypass
- c. Peritoneal dialysis
- d. Radiation

273. Which of the following conditions may lead to exudative pleural effusions: *(Recent Pattern 2014-15)*
- a. Cirrhosis
- b. Nephrotic syndrome
- c. Congestive heart failure
- d. Bronchogenic carcinoma

274. Bilateral pleural effusion is seen in: *(Recent Pattern 2014-15)*
- a. Nephrotic syndrome
- b. Constrictive pericarditis
- c. Congestive cardiac failure
- d. All of the above

275. Pleural effusion in rheumatoid arthritis is typically associated with the following features except:
- a. Glucose > 620 mg/dl *(Recent Pattern 2014-15)*
- b. Protein > 3 gm/dl
- c. Pleural fluid protein to serum protein ratio of > 0.5
- d. Pleural fluid LDH to serum LDH ratio of >0.6

276. Pneumothorax occurs in all except:
- a. Langhans cell histiocytosis *(Recent Pattern 2014-15)*
- b. Marfan's syndrome
- c. Assisted ventilation
- d. Bronchopulmonary aspergillosis

277. All of the following are causes of hemorrhagic pleural effusion except: *(Recent Pattern 2014-15)*
- a. Pulmonary embolism
- b. Rheumatoid arthritis
- c. Pancreatitis
- d. TB

278. Most common cause for acute mediastinitis is:
- a. Esophageal perforation *(Recent Pattern 2014-15)*
- b. Cervical spondylitis
- c. Osteomyelitis of sternum
- d. Osteomyelitis of clavicle

279. Which statement is true regarding pneumothorax:
- a. Absent breath sounds *(Recent Pattern 2014-15)*
- b. Decreased percussion note
- c. Always needs chest tube insertion
- d. Tracheal tug

280. Transudative pleural effusion is present in all except: *(Recent Pattern 2014-15)*
- a. Meig's syndrome
- b. CCF
- c. Nephrotic syndrome
- d. Chronic liver disease

281. A high amylase level in pleural fluid suggests a diagnosis of: *(Recent Pattern 2014-15)*
- a. Tuberculosis
- b. Malignancy
- c. Rheumatoid arthritis
- d. Pulmonary infarction

282. Causes of haemorrhagic pleural effusion are all except: *(Recent Pattern 2014-15)*
- a. Pulmonary infarction
- b. Mesothelioma
- c. Bronchial adenoma
- d. Tuberculosis

283. The most common cause of spontaneous pneumothorax is:
    a. Tuberculosis (Recent Pattern 2014-15)
    b. Rupture of a sub-pleural bleb
    c. Bronchogenic carcinoma
    d. Bronchial adenoma
284. Hamman's crunch sign is seen in: (Recent Pattern 2014-15)
    a. Hamman rich syndrome b. Aortic aneurysm
    c. Pneumomediastinum   d. Pneumothorax
285. Tuberculous pleural effusion is characterized by A/E:
    a. Haemorrhage (Recent Pattern 2014-15)
    b. LDH more than 60%
    c. Protein is increased
    d. Mesothelial cells
286. Tension pneumothorax results in all except:
     (Recent Pattern 2014-15)
    a. Respiratory alkalosis   b. Decreased cardiac output
    c. Decreased venous return d. Absent breath sounds
287. In tension pneumothorax first line of management is:
    a. CXR (AIIMS May 2013)
    b. Needle in 2nd intercostal space
    c. Emergency thoracotomy
    d. ICD tube in 5th interostal space mid axillary line
288. The antibiotic commonly used for chemical pleurodesis is:
     (Recent Pattern 2014-15)
    a. Amoxicillin   b. Doxycycline
    c. Co-trimoxazole   d. Rifabutin
289. The organism most frequently related to mediastinal fibrosis is: (Recent Pattern 2014-15)
    a. Actinomyces   b. Histoplasma
    c. Hansen bacillus d. Staphylococcus
290. Most common cause of empyema is: (AIIMS Dec 97)
    a. Bronchopleural fistula b. Tubercular pneumonia
    c. Bacterial pneumonia   d. Pleurisy
291. Tuberculous pleural effusion is characterised by all of the following features except effusion : (AI 1997)
    a. Hemorrhagic effusion
    b. Pleural fluid LDH more than 60% that of serum LDH.
    c. Increased adenosine deaminase
    d. Increased mesothelial cells
292. Pleural fluid having low glucose is seen in all, except-
     (AIIMS May 93)
    a. Tuberculosis   b. Empyema
    c. Mesothelioma   d. Rheumatoid arthritis
293. All of the following show low glucose in pleural fluid, except- (AIIMS Dec 94)
    a. Empyema   b. Malignant pleural effusion
    c. Rheumatoid arthritis d. Dressler's syndrome
294. A high amylase level in pleural fluid suggests a diagnosis of (AIIMS May 03)
    a. Tuberculosis   b. Malignancy
    c. Rheumatoid arthritis d. Pulmonary infarction
295. While inserting a central venous catheter, a patient develops respiratory distress. The most likely cause is: (AI 2002)
    a. Hemothorax   b. Pneumothorax
    c. Pleural effusion d. Hypovolumia

Pulmonary Embolism

296. The image shows? (AIIMS Nov 2018)

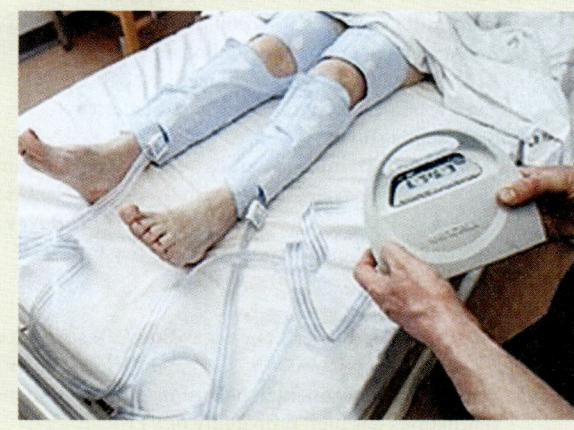

    a. Pneumatic compression stockings
    b. Anti-shock garment
    c. Alginate dressings
    d. Compression stockings (Unna boot)
297. Which of the following drugs is used for treatment of cancer associated thromboembolism? (AIIMS May 2018)
    a. LMW heparin
    b. Anti- thrombin III inhibitors
    c. Direct factor Xa inhibitors
    d. Warfarin
298. A patient had a femur fracture for which internal fixation was done. 2 days later, patient developed sudden onset shortness of breath with low grade fever. What is the likely cause? (AIIMS May 2017)
    a. Pneumothorax   b. Fat embolism
    c. Pleural effusion d. ARDS
299. A 20 year old boy is admitted to the casualty with history of breathlessness following a leg massage by his mother. He had a history of hairline ankle fracture and was on a below knee cast for 4 weeks which was removed recently. What is the most probable diagnosis? (AIIMS May 2017)
    a. Pulmonary Thromboembolism
    b. Pneumonia
    c. Fat embolism
    d. Air embolism
300. A 40 year old female patient of nephrotic syndrome presents to the ER, with complaints of acute onset of breathlessness after prolonged air travel for 16 hours. On clinical examination, pulse rate is 120/min with BP=130/80mm Hg. SpO_2 = 85% and bedside echo shows right ventricular dilation with interventricular septum deviation to left side. The next step in management is? (AIIMS May 2016)
    a. Intravenous plasminogen activator
    b. Unfractionated heparin
    c. Thrombectomy
    d. IVC filter

301. Which one of the following conditions is most likely to occur in a patient with the following hemodynamic data? Pressures: RA = 12 mm Hg, RV= 50/12 mm Hg, PA=50/15 mm Hg, PA wedge prWWessure = 8 mm Hg, Aorta=80/60, Cardiac Index = 1.4, SVR= 1800, PVR=500. *(APPG 2016)*
    a. Acute massive pulmonary embolism
    b. Acute MI with LVF and cardiogenic shock
    c. Hypovolemic shock following gastroenteritis
    d. Early septic shock

302. Postoperative patient with signs of deep vein thrombosis develops pulmonary embolism with dyspnoea. Next step is?-
    a. UFH iv   *(JIPMER Nov 2015)*
    b. Subcutaneous Low molecular weight heparin
    c. Spiral CT scan
    d. Angiography

303. All are the following are true regarding V/P scan except?
                                       (JIPMER Nov 2014)
    a. Two or more segmental perfusion defects with normal ventilations has high probability of PTE
    b. VP scan contraindicated in pregnancy
    c. An abnormal ventilation and perfusion is usually due to conditions other than PTE
    d. Normal scan rules out clinically significant pulmonary thromboembolism

304. Which is the best test to be done for Pulmonary embolism?
    a. D Dimer Assay   *(Recent Question 2015-16)*
    b. MRI
    c. Ventilation perfusion scan
    d. CT with IV contrast

305. In case of Pulmonary embolism, Right ventricle hypokinesia and decreased output, which Drug therapy is most helpful:
                                   (Recent Question 2015-16)
    a. Thrombolytic   b. LMW heparin
    c. Warfarin   d. Heparin

306. A 65-year-old woman after total knee implant surgery complains of calf pain and swelling in the leg from last 2 days. Later she complains of breathlessness and dies suddenly in the ward. Probable cause?   *(Recent Question 2015-16)*
    a. Pulmonary embolism   b. Myocardial infarction
    c. Stroke   d. ARDS

307. Characteristic ECG finding of pulmonary embolism:
                                    (Recent Pattern 2014-15)
    a. Sinus tachycardia   b. S1Q3T3
    c. T wave inversion   d. Epsilon waves

308. Most common ECG finding for pulmonary embolism?
                                    (Recent Pattern 2014-15)
    a. Sinus tachycardia   b. S1Q3T3
    c. T wave inversion   d. Epsilon waves

309. A patient undergoing surgery suddenly develops hypotension. The monitor shows that the end-tidal carbon dioxide has decreased abruptly by 15 mm Hg. What is the probable diagnosis?   *(Recent Pattern 2014-15)*
    a. Hypothermia   b. Pulmonary embolism
    c. Massive fluid deficit
    d. Myocardial depression due to anaesthetic agents

310. A patient had acute pulmonary embolism. Echocardiography showed right ventricular hypokinesia with tricuspid regurgitation with hypotension. The treatment to be given is: *(AIIMS Nov 2013)*
    a. LMWH   b. Thrombolytic therapy
    c. IVC filters   d. Anticoagulants

311. All are seen in massive pulmonary embolism except?
                                    (Recent Pattern 2014-15)
    a. Inter-ventricular septum deviation
    b. Fall of SBP
    c. Pulmonary plethora
    d. Elevated JVP

312. Most common clinical sign of pulmonary embolism is:
                                    (Recent Pattern 2014-15)
    a. Tachypnea   b. Tachycardia
    c. Cyanosis   d. Sweating

313. Most diagnostic of pulmonary emboli is:
                                    (Recent Pattern 2014-15)
    a. CTA   b. V/P scan
    c. HRCT   d. D- Dimer Assay

314. Pulmonary embolism causes all except:
    a. Bradycardia   *(Recent Pattern 2014-15)*
    b. Decreased cardiac output
    c. Arterial hypoxaemia
    d. Acute right ventricular strain

315. Most common source of pulmonary embolism is:
                                    (Recent Pattern 2014-15)
    a. Atherosclerosis   b. Fracture fixation
    c. Pelvic surgery   d. Cardiothoracic surgery

316. All of the following are true of pulmonary embolism except?   *(Recent Pattern 2014-15)*
    a. Sudden onset of pleuritic pain and haemoptysis and hypotension
    b. ECG shows evidence of acute left ventricular stress
    c. Blood LDH and SGOT levels are raised
    d. Isotope perfusion ventilation scan is diagnostic

317. Pulmonary embolism is seen in all except:
    a. Fanconi anemia   *(Recent Pattern 2014-15)*
    b. Paroxysmal nocturnal haemoglobinuria
    c. Oral contraception
    d. Old age

318. All of the following conditions may predispose to pulmonary embolism except: *(Recent Pattern 2014-15)*
    a. Protein S deficiency b. Malignancy
    c. Obesity   d. Progesterone therapy

319. Air embolism is diagnosed by: *(Recent Pattern 2014-15)*
    a. ↓End tidal CO_2 b. ↓End tidal N_2
    c. Doppler study   d. Ultrasound

320. Most common symptoms of pulmonary embolism:
                                    (Recent Pattern 2014-15)
    a. Chest pain   b. Dyspnea
    c. Haemoptysis   d. Cough

321. The dome of the diaphragm is elevated in:
                                    (Recent Pattern 2014-15)
    a. Typhoid fever   b. Pulmonary infarction
    c. Emphysema   d. Cirrhosis

322. All are true about pulmonary embolism, except:
    a. Chest pain is the most common symptom *(AIIMS May 94)*
    b. Most commonly presents within 2 weeks
    c. More is the survival time, more is the chance of recovery
    d. Arises from leg veins

323. In acute pulmonary embolism, the most frequent ECG finding is :   *(AIIMS May' 06)*
    a. S1Q3T3 pattern   b. P. pulmonale
    c. Sinus tachycardia   d. Right axis deviation

Hypersensitivity Pneumonitis

324. A patient presents with cough with expectoration. Diagnosis of farmers lung is suspected. Which statement is true regarding this condition? *(JIPMER May 2018)*
    a. May to June seasonal
    b. Persistent cough with expectoration
    c. X-ray features upper lobe predominant in chronic HP
    d. Pleural effusions are common

325. Match List I with List II and select the correct answer using the code given below the lists: *(UPSC 2015)*
    List-I (Disease) List-II (Antigen leading to hypersensitivity pneumonitis)
    a. Bagassosis   1. Oak, Cedar, Pine dust
    b. Byssinosis   2. Moldy hay
    c. Farmer's lung   3. Cotton
    d. Wood worker's lung   4. Sugarcane dust
    Code: A B C D
    a. 4 3 2 1   b. 4 2 3 1
    c. 1 3 2 4   d. 1 2 3 4

326. Which of the following is not a common feature of hypersensitivity pneumonitis? *(UPSC 2015)*
    a. Raised C-Reaction Protein
    b. Chest X-ray may be normal
    c. Lung biopsy may be diagnostic
    d. Systemic Eosinophilia

327. "Loeffler's syndrome" is characterized by? *(UPSC 2015)*
    a. Transient, migratory pulmonary infiltrations
    b. Fibrosis in the pulmonary apices
    c. Fibrosis in the base of one or both lungs
    d. Miliary mottling

Lung Cancer

328. A 65 year old uranium miner presents with muscle cramps, early morning headache. CXR and NCCT scan done shows? *(Recent Question 2016-17)*

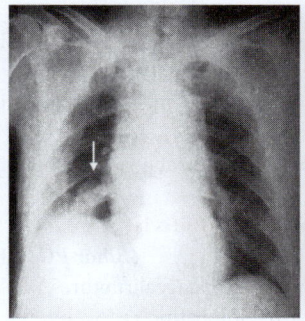 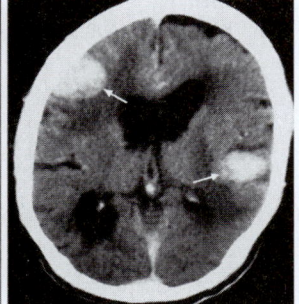

    a. SCLC, Brain metastasis
    b. NSCLC, Brain metastasis
    c. Pleural and intracranial calcification
    d. Gliobastoma multiforme, extracranial spread

329. Most common bronchogenic carcinoma is *(AIIMS June 2000)*
    a. Small cell carcinoma   b. Squamous cell carcinoma
    c. Mixed cell carcinoma   d. Adenocarcinoma

330. All of the following statements about small cell carcinomas are true, except *(PGI-June- 06)*
    a. Commonest Malignancy of lung
    b. Associated with paraneoplastic syndrome
    c. Cause SVC obstruction
    d. Chemosensitive
    e. Commonly metastasize to brain

331. In a chronic smoker, a highly malignant aggressive and metastatic lung carcinoma is: *(AIIMS May 01)*
    a. Squamous cell Carcinoma   b. Small cell Carcinoma
    c. Adenocarcinoma   d. Large cell carcinoma

332. Type of lung carcinoma producing superior vena cava syndrome: *(AIIMS June 97)*
    a. Squamous cell carcinoma   b. Adenocarcinoma
    c. Small cell carcinoma   d. Anaplastic carcinoma

333. Clubbing is least common in: *(AIIMS Dec 97)*
    a. Squamous cell carcinoma   b. Adenocarcinoma
    c. Small cell carcinoma of lung
    d. Mesothelioma

334. Mr X 40 yrs male patient presenting with polyuria, pain abdomen, nausea, vomiting, altered sensorium was found to have bronchogenic carcinoma. The electrolyte abnormality seen in him would be: *(AIIMS May 02)*
    a. Hypokalemia   b. Hyperkalemia
    c. Hypocalcaemia   d. Hypercalcemia

335. A 60 year old male presented to the emergency with breathlessness, facial swelling and dilated veins on the chest wall. The probable diagnosis is?
    a. Thymoma   b. Lung cancer
    c. Hodgkin's lymphoma
    d. Superior vena caval obstruction

336. All are cavitating lesions in the lungs, except- *(AIIMS May 94)*
    a. Caplan's syndrome   b. Hamartoma
    c. Wegner's granuloma   d. Squamous cell carcinoma

Miscellaneous

337. Maximum oxygen concentration can be delivered by? *(Recent Question 2019)*

    a. 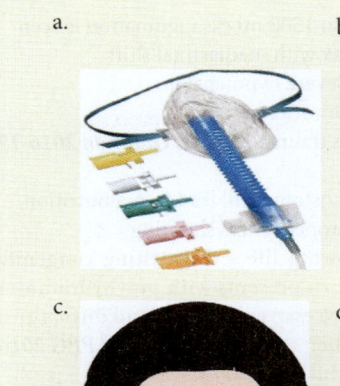   b.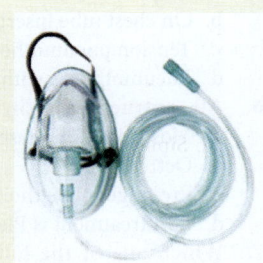

    c. 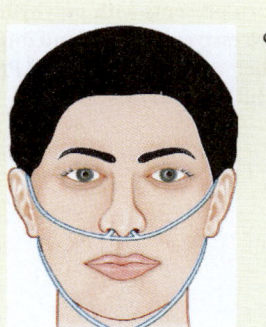   d.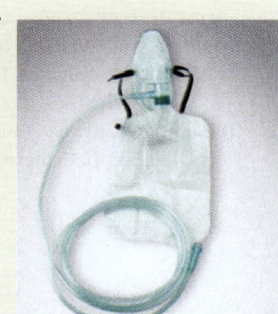

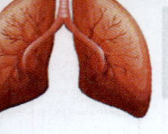

338. **Which drug is given to prevent acute mountain sickness?**
 (AIIMS Nov 2018)
   a. Acetazolamide
   b. Dexamethasone
   c. Digoxin
   d. Diltiazem

339. **Functioning of an intercostal drainage tube is best assessed by?** (AIIMS Nov 2017)
   a. Water column movement in the bottle
   b. Water column movement in the tube
   c. Bubbling in the underwater seal
   d. Auscultation of chest

340. **Orthopnea is seen in?** (Recent Pattern Questions)
   a. Myasthenic Crisis
   b. Massive pleural effusion
   c. Atrial Myxoma
   d. Stiffness of Costochondral junction

341. **Which of these does not support the diagnosis of Streptococcal Pharyngitis?** (Recent Pattern Questions)
   a. Cough
   b. Fever
   c. Pharyngeal Exudates
   d. Tender cervical lymphadenopathy

342. **Which variety of shock has elevated CVP and PCWP?** (Recent Pattern Questions)
   a. Cardiogenic Shock
   b. Hypovolemic shock
   c. Neurogenic shock
   d. Hypoadrenal shock

343. **A 25-year-old lady in third trimester of pregnancy wants to fly to Chennai for delivery. Her pregnancy has been uneventful. Which of these is the correct advise by her physician?** (Recent Pattern Questions)
   a. She can fly with no risk to her or fetus
   b. She cannot fly as she is in advanced stage of labour
   c. She can fly only with consent of airlines
   d. Multigravida can safely take this risk

344. **Which of the following investigations in not useful for diagnosis of mediastinal masses?** (Recent Pattern Questions)
   a. CT chest
   b. USG chest
   c. Iodine -131 Scan
   d. Barium GI series

345. **Which of the following is indication for emergency thoracotomy?** (Recent Question 2016-17)
   a. Empyema
   b. On chest tube insertion 1500 ml exsanguination is seen
   c. Tension pneumothorax with mediastinal shift
   d. Pneumothorax with Severe hypotension

346. **All are true about Chylothorax except?**
   a. Most common cause is trauma (Recent Question 2016-17)
   b. Octreotide
   c. Prolonged tube thoracostomy will lead to malnutrition
   d. Best treatment is Pleuroperitoneal shunting

347. **Which one of the following life - threatening congenital anomalies in the new-born presents with polyhydramnios, aspiration pneumonia, excessive salivation and difficulty in passing a nasogastric tube?** (APPG 2016)
   a. Tracheoesophageal fistula
   b. Gastroschisis
   c. Choanal atresia
   d. Diaphragmatic hernia

348. **Read the following two statements and select the correct answer –** (APPG 2016)
   Statement A (Assertion) = Lungs in respiratory distress syndrome of the premature infant are airless and atelectatic, looking like liver
   Statement B (Basis) = There is deficiency of surfactant, a substance, which reduces surface tension and prevents alveoli from collapsing.
   a. Statement A is False and Statement B is True
   b. Statement A and Statement B are both True and B is the Basis / Explanation for A
   c. Statement A and Statement B are both True but B is Not the Basis / Explanation for A
   d. Statement A is True and Statement B is False

349. **Chronic mountain sickness DOES NOT produce?**
   a. Erythrocytosis (APPG 2016)
   b. Hyperventilation
   c. Right Ventricular enlargement
   d. Cyanosis

350. **A patient presents with recurrent episodes of sinusitis, throat pain, epistaxis and bilateral cavitatory lesions in the lungs and renal failure, what is the diagnosis and next step?**
   a. Systemic fungal infection, Biopsy (AIIMS Nov 2015)
   b. Miliary TB, Mantoux Test
   c. Vasculitis, ANCA
   d. Multiple Metastasis

351. **Which of the following statements is true regarding H_1N_1?**
 (AIIMS May 2015)
   a. Pregnant woman with sore throat can be started immediately on oseltamivir without diagnostic testing under category B
   b. People on long term steroids can't receive Oseltamivir
   c. Category B concerns with low risk cases
   d. Category B patients have to undergo immediate testing

352. **A 35 year old 40kg male patient was diagnosed to be a case of pulmonary tuberculosis. The appropriate conventional regimen of anti-tubercular drugs would be:** (UPSC 2015)
   a. Rifampicin 450 mg + Isoniazid 300 mg + Pyrazinamide 1500 mg
   b. Rifampicin 600 mg + Isoniazid 300 mg + Pyrazinamide 1000 mg
   c. Rifampicin 450 mg + Isoniazid 200 mg + Pyrazinamide 1000 mg
   d. Rifampicin 450 mg + Isoniazid 200 mg + Pyrazinamide 1500 mg

353. **The most common cause of Mediastinitis is?**
 (Bihar PG 2015)
   a. Tracheal rupture
   b. Esophageal rupture
   c. Drugs
   d. Idiopathic

354. **Biot breathing is seen in?** (Recent Question 2015-16)
   a. Flail chest
   b. Uremia
   c. High altitude
   d. Lesion in the brain

355. **Pop-corn calcification is seen with?**
 (Recent Question 2015-16)
   a. Pulmonary Hamartoma
   b. Aspergillosis
   c. Broncho-Alveolar cancer
   d. Pulmonary Embolism

356. A 45-year-old with trauma presents after 4 hours with cheek swelling and urine not passed. On examination crepitus is palpated with periorbital swelling. What is your diagnosis?
(Recent Question 2015-16)

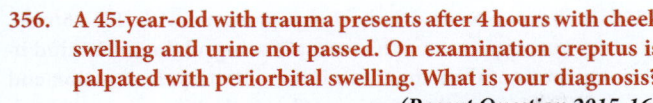

   a. Renal shut down
   b. Lung laceration
   c. Gas gangrene
   d. Base of skull fracture

357. Female patient with bilateral hilar lymphadenopathy and joint pain. ACE levels are elevated. Diagnosis is?
(Recent Question 2015-16)
   a. Sarcoidosis
   b. Silicosis
   c. Hodgkin's lymphoma
   d. Non Hodgkin's lymphoma

358. Finger in glove sign is seen in *(Recent Question 2015-16)*
   a. Pulmonary alveolar proteinosis
   b. Pneumocystis carinii
   c. Tuberculosis
   d. Bronchocele

359. Aspergillosis can present with all except:
   a. Lung cavity *(Recent Question 2015-16)*
   b. Eye infection
   c. Normal component in sputum
   d. Rhinocerebral involvement

360. A 65-year-old man presented with hemoptysis and grade III clubbing. The probable diagnosis of the patient is?
(Recent Question 2014-15)
   a. Non small cell lung Ca
   b. Small cell cancer of lung
   c. Tuberculosis
   d. Sarcoidosis

361. Hypersensitivity pneumonitis is consistent with the following findings except? *(Recent Question 2015-16)*
   a. Decreased DLCO
   b. Precipitating antibodies to causative antigens
   c. Granuloma on lung biopsy
   d. Eosinophilic alveolitis

362. The following CXR shows *(Recent Question 2015-16)*

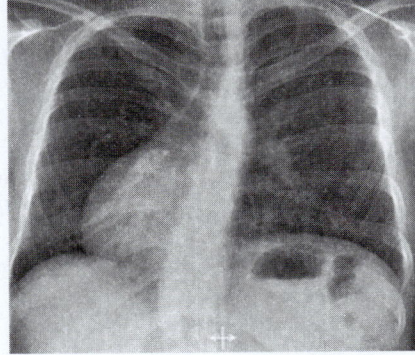

   a. Dextrocardia
   b. Pneumothorax
   c. Pneumomediastinum
   d. Pulmonary hamartoma

363. The CXR shows markings near the Costophrenic angle. Which of the following is the cause of these markings?

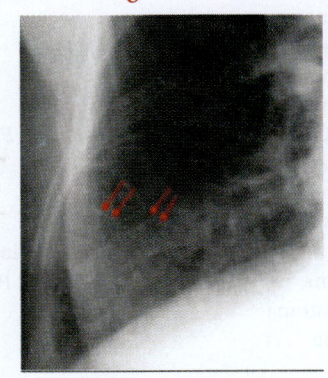

   a. Lymphangitis Carcinomatosis
   b. Pulmonary alveolar Proteinosis
   c. Lung abscess
   d. Pneumatocele

364. The image shows presence of?

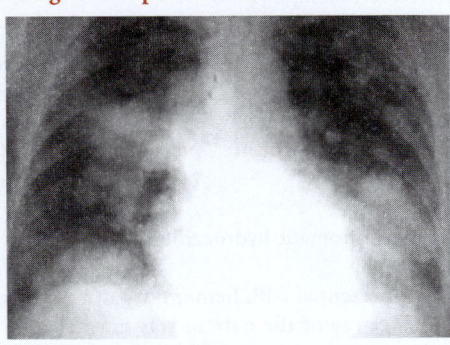

   a. Canon Ball metastasis
   b. Cardiogenic Pulmonary oedema
   c. Lingular Pneumonia
   d. Diffuse histoplasmosis

365. Highest likelihood of O_2 delivery to lungs? *(JIPMER 2014)*
   a. Face mask
   b. Nasal cannula
   c. Non-rebreathing mask
   d. Oxygen hood

366. Pseudohemoptysis is seen mostly with?
(Recent Pattern 2014-15)
   a. Streptococcus
   b. E.coli
   c. Serratia Marcescens
   d. R.S.V

367. The histologic hallmark of Langerhan's cells is:
   a. Dendritic cell processes *(Recent Pattern 2014-15)*
   b. Giant mitochondria
   c. Birbeck granules
   d. Eosinophilic granules

368. Which one of the following is common to all forms of shock?
   a. Decrease in tissue perfusion *(Recent Pattern 2014-15)*
   b. Decrease in pulmonary blood flow
   c. Decrease in P.C.W.P
   d. Decrease in right atrial pressure

369. All are true about hyaline membrane disease except:
   a. Wide spread atelectasis *(Recent Pattern 2014-15)*
   b. Absence of air bronchograms
   c. X-ray shows ground glass mottling
   d. High maternal sugar inhibits surfactant production

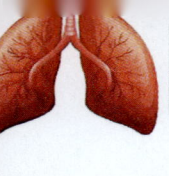

370. **The most common posterior mediastinal mass:**
    a. Neurogenic tumor *(Recent Pattern 2014-15)*
    b. Lymph nodes
    c. Neurogenic parasitic cyst
    d. Teratoma

371. **First treatment for anaphylactic shock is:**
    a. Subcutaneous adrenaline *(Recent Pattern 2014-15)*
    b. IV Corticosteroid
    c. Theophylline
    d. Anti-histaminic

372. **The following are located in anterior mediastinum except:**
    a. Thymoma *(Recent Pattern 2014-15)*
    b. Neurofibroma
    c. Teratoma
    d. Cyst

373. **Hypersensitivity pneumonitis is associated with:**
    a. Hilar lymphadenopathy *(Recent Pattern 2014-15)*
    b. Raised IgE
    c. Raised serum precipitins
    d. Increased eosinophils

374. **Rib notching is found in all the following except:**
    (Recent Pattern 2014-15)
    a. Neurofibromatosis   b. Coarctation of aorta
    c. Taussig Bing operation d. Hypoparathyroidism

375. **Which product of cigarette smoke is responsible for CAD?**
    a. Nicotine *(Recent Pattern 2014-15)*
    b. Tar
    c. Polycyclic aromatic hydrocarbons
    d. Benzene

376. **A patient presented with hemoptysis and persistent cough. The chest X-ray of the patient was normal. The next best investigation is?** *(Recent Pattern 2014-15)*
    a. Helical CT   b. High resolution CT
    c. Bronchoscopy   d. Angiography

377. **Subcutaneous Emphysema may be found in the following conditions:** *(Recent Pattern 2014-15)*
    a. Tracheostomy   b. Hemilich maneuver
    c. Chest injury   d. All of the above

378. **Bronchoalveloar lavage is beneficial in the evaluation of:**
    (Recent Pattern 2014-15)
    a. Squamous cell cancer lung
    b. Bronchiectasis
    c. Bronchopleural fistula
    d. Pulmonary alveolar Proteinosis

379. **The most common cause of bronchiolitis is:**
    a. Respiratory syncytial virus *(Recent Pattern 2014-15)*
    b. Adenovirus
    c. Herpes virus
    d. Influenza virus

380. **Most common lesion in middle mediastinum:**
    (Recent Pattern 2014-15)
    a. Congenital cyst   b. Lipoma
    c. Aneurysm   d. Neurogenic tumours

381. **In Kartagener's syndrome all are seen except:**
    (Recent Pattern 2014-15)
    a. Cystic fibrosis   b. Dextrocardia
    c. Sinusitis   d. Absence of cilia

382. **A 32 weeks new born baby presents with RR-86/min, grunting present with no nasal flaring, abdomen behind in movement than chest, minimum intercostal retraction and no Xiphisternal retraction. What is the Silverman scoring?**
    (Recent Pattern 2014-15)
    a. 1   b. 4
    c. 3   d. 6

383. **Miliary shadow on X-ray is seen in all except:**
    (Recent Pattern 2014-15)
    a. Tuberculosis   b. Loeffler's pneumonia
    c. Klebsiella   d. Varicella pneumonia

384. **Which is not a side effect of high dose inhaled beclomethasone dipropionate:** *(Recent Pattern 2014-15)*
    a. Dysphonia
    b. Thin skin
    c. Atrophic rhinitis
    d. Pituitary adrenal suppression

385. **Causes of hypersensitivity pneumonitis is?**
    (Recent Pattern 2014-15)
    a. Silicosis   b. Farmer's lung
    c. Anthracosis   d. Asbestosis

386. **SARS causative agent?** *(Recent Pattern 2014-15)*
    a. Corona-virus   b. Picorna-virus
    c. Myxovirus   d. Paramyxovirus

387. **Differential diagnosis of a solitary pulmonary nodule includes all of the following except:**
    (Recent Pattern 2014-15)
    a. Neurofibroma   b. Hamartoma
    c. Tuberculoma   d. Bronchial adenoma

388. **Least common cause of clubbing is:**
    (Recent Pattern 2014-15)
    a. Adenocarcinoma   b. Squamous cell CA
    c. Small cell CA   d. Mesothelioma

389. **A 30-year-old worker in chemical plant presents with stupor, cyanosis. Blood drawn for sampling shows brownish red color. Diagnosis:** *(Recent Pattern 2014-15)*
    a. Carbon monoxide poisoning
    b. Organophosphate poisoning
    c. Meth-hemoglobinaemia
    d. G-6-P-deficiency

390. **Cavitatory lesions in lung are seen in:** *(AI 2010)*
    a. Primary pulmonary Tuberculosis
    b. Staphylococcal pneumonia
    c. Preumoconiosis
    d. Interstitial Lung disease

391. **All are correct regarding sarcoidosis *except*:**
    a. Often cavitate *(AIIMS Dec 98)*
    b. Spontaneous remission is usual
    c. Tuberculin test is negative
    d. B/L hilar lymphadenopathy

392. **Pulmonary hypertension may occur in all of the following conditions except-** *(AIIMS Nov 06)*
    a. Toxic oil syndrome
    b. Progressive systemic sclerosis
    c. Sickle cell anemia
    d. Argemone mexicana poisoning

393. All are true about bilateral diaphragmatic paralysis, *except*: (AIIMS May 95)
    a. Sniff test is positive
    b. Causes normocapnic failure
    c. Diaphragmatic pacing is useful if any nerve is intact
    d. Seen in transverse myelitis

394. Most common cause of Mediastinitis is: (AIIMS 97)
    a. Tracheal rupture   b. Esophageal rupture
    c. Drugs   d. Idiopathic

395. All of the following are true about Kartagener's syndrome, Except (PGI-Dec-04)
    a. Dextrocardia   b. Infertility
    c. Mental retardation   d. Bronchiectasis

396. Causes of pulmonary renal syndrome: (PGI June 07)
    a. Leptospirosis   b. Hanta virus
    c. Paraquat poisoning   d. All of the above

397. 3.5 kg term male baby, born of uncomplicated pregnancy, developed respiratory distress at birth, not responded to surfactant, ECHO finding revealed nothing abnormal, X-ray showed ground glass appearance and culture negative. Apgars 4 and 5 at 1 and 5 minutes. History of one month female sibling died before. What is the diagnosis?
    a. TAPVC (AIIMS Nov 07)
    b. Meconium aspiration
    c. Neonatal pulmonary alveolar proteinosis
    d. Diffuse herpes simplex infection

Answers with Explanations

Spirometry, DL_{co}, Alveolar-Arteriolar Gradient

1. Ans. (a) FEV1/FVC decreased

Ref: Harrison 20th edition, Page 1949

- Timed vital capacity of FEV1/FVC is reduced in obstructive lung disease and increased to normal in restrictive lung disease.
- FEV1 is reduced in *both* restrictive and obstructive lung disease.

2. Ans. (c) Emphysema

Ref: Ganong review of medical physiology: 25th edition, Page 630

The image shows compliance curve of lungs with the curve A showing increased compliance which is a feature of emphysema. Choices B, C and D represent reduced compliance and would follow curve B.

3. Ans. (a) A-a gradient

Ref: Fishman pulmonary diseases: 5th edition, Page 2153

- In central causes of hypoventilation A-a gradient is normal. This is because pAO_2 and paO_2 reduce by the same magnitude. Minute ventilation is reduced.
- In pulmonary causes of hypoventilation A-a gradient is increased. Minute ventilation is normal to increased.
- Choice B, C and D will be affected in similar fashion in both types of hypoventilation.

4. Ans. (a) ILD

(Ref: Harrison 19th Page 1710, Massachusetts General Hospital Handbook, 6th edition pg 218, Cecil Essentials of medicine, 9th edition, Page 242)

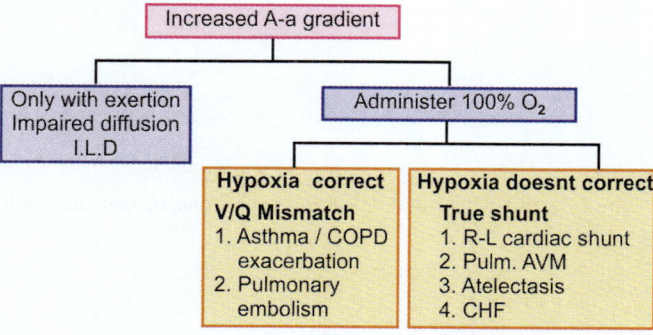

Remember in acute severe asthma, hypoventilation leads to normal A-a gradient

5. Ans. (c) Increased Dead space ventilation

(Ref: Textbook of pulmonary and critical care medicine volume 1: 2nd edition, page 362)

- In case of lobectomy since the remaining lung tissue is lesser, all parameters like vital capacity, residual volume and closing volume will reduce.
- Hence due to hypoxic stimulus post-operative patients of lobectomy will take *rapid shallow breaths*. This will lead to increased Dead space ventilation.

6. Ans. (c) COPD

(Ref: Harrison 20th edition page 1979; Harrison 19th edition page 1704t)

The FEV1/FVC ratio of the patient is low indicating obstructive airway disease. Coal workers pneumoconiosis is associated with effects of coal dust on alveolar macrophages leading to development of chronic bronchitis and COPD. Most people here mistake of answering as pulmonary fibrosis.

Interpretation of Spirometry Data

Spirometry	COPD	Restrictive lung disease
FEV1	Low ++	Low+
VC	Low+	Low ++
FEV1/FVC	Low	Normal/high
RV	High	Low
FRC	High	Low

7. Ans. (b) Goodpasture's syndrome

(Ref: Harrison 20th edition page 1951; Harrison 19th p 1715, 1710)

- DLCO is increased in Goodpasture as the basement membrane is damaged, thereby increasing the chances of diffusion of CO across lesser number of anatomical layers.
- DLCO is decreased in pulmonary artery hypertension since the fibrosis in pulmonary vessels will reduce the diffusion of CO across the anatomical layers.
- Causes of increased DL_{co}
  1. CHF
  2. Asthma
  3. Goodpasture
  4. Polycyathemia

8. Ans. (b) Chronic compensated respiratory acidosis

(Ref: Harrison 20th edition page 315; Harrison 19th p 322-323)

Since a patient of emphysema is having respiratory distress and muscle fatigue on clinical grounds he is probably having respiratory acidosis.

- pH of blood =7.33, interpretation is acidosis
- pCO_2 is 64 mm Hg (average of 40 mmHg), interpretation is increased pCO_2 and explains the acidosis
- HCO_3 is increased and indicates compensation (N = 22–26 mEq)
  - The diagnosis is compensated respiratory acidosis. Next step is to find out acute versus chronic compensation
  - The rule to be followed for acute compensation is for every 10mmHg rise of pCO_2, HCO_3 rises by 1meq
  - The rule to be followed for chronic compensation is for every 10 mmHg rise of pCO_2, HCO_3 rises by 4meq or more
  - Since the rule mentioned just above this statement is mathematically satisfied, the diagnosis is chronic compensated respiratory acidosis.

9. Ans. (a) Asthma

(Ref: Harrison 20th edition page 1963; Harrison 19th p 1679)

- All expiratory parameters are reduced in the data given with timed vital capacity of 29%.
- FEV1/ FVC is reduced in obstructive airway disease with lowering of peak expiratory flow rates. Due to air trapping in asthma the DLco may be normal or increased.

10. Ans. (b) Carbon Monoxide poisoning

(Ref: Harrison 20th edition p 511; Harrison 19th p 248)

- Points in favor are setting of industrial accident with hyperdynamic CVS in a drowsy patient with normal oxygen saturation. Cherry red lips are a post mortem finding and is not seen ante-mortem.
- The use of a *regular pulse oximeter is not effective in the diagnosis of carbon monoxide poisoning* as people suffering from carbon monoxide poisoning may have a normal oxygen saturation level on a pulse oximeter. *This is due to the carboxyhemoglobin being misrepresented as oxyhemoglobin.*
- Industrial workers at pulp mills, steel foundries, and plants producing formaldehyde or coke are at risk for exposure, as are personnel at fire scenes and individuals working indoors with combustion engines or combustible gases.
- Hence SaO_2 is falsely normal. Hyperventilation explains low pCO_2.

11. Ans. (b) Timed vital capacity

(Ref: Harrison 20th edition p 1949, 1971; Harrison 19th p 306e-2)

12. Ans. (d) Central hypoventilation

(Ref: Harrison 19th, pg. 2171)

In central hypoventilation, pAO_2 and paO_2 both are reduced leading to normal alveolar arteriolar gradient.

Remember
- Alveolar-arterial O_2 gradient is raised in alveolar hypoventilation
- Alveolar-arterial O_2 gradient is normal in central hypoventilation

13. Ans. (a) Partially compensated respiratory acidosis

(Ref: Harrison 20th p 315; Harrison 19th p 322-23)

- Since the pH is reduced and CO_2 is increased, the primary change in the patient is respiratory compromise.
- Now increase in CO_2 will lead to increase in H_2CO_3 leading to H^+ generation
- The increased H^+ will lead to acidosis which will trigger the compensation to kick in
- The compensation implies increase in HCO_3 to neutralize the increased H^+. Now since the value of HCO_3 is increased (Normal= 22-26 meq), it implies that compensation has been initiated.
- But since pH has not reverted to normal and is still 7.3, it implies compensation has not been completed.
- Final conclusion is partially completely respiratory acidosis.

14. Ans. (b) Idiopathic pulmonary fibrosis

(Ref: Harrison 20th p 1951; Harrison 19th p 1711)

- The presence of reduced TLC points to restrictive pattern, and is confirmed by normal FEV1/VC ratio.
- Choices A, C cause obstructive airway disease. ABPA causes central bronchiectasis and is a Suppurative lung disease.

15. Ans. (a) Acute exacerbation of COPD

(Ref: Harrison 19th p 1676-77)

- ABG shows severe hypoxia with hypercarbia with acidosis suggestive of type 2 respiratory failure.
- ARDS and acute asthma both have type 1 failure and are ruled out
- So we have to select between options A and C. Interstitial Pneumonitis on routine presentation will not have such low oxygen values but an acute exacerbation of chronic bronchitis will definitely present with low oxygen values.

16. Ans. (b) TLC reduction

(Ref: Harrison 20th p 1951; Harrison 19th p 306e)

Parameter	Obstructive	Restrictive
FEV1	Reduced	Reduced
TLC	Normal/Increased	Reduced
FVC	Reduced	Reduced
FEV1/FVC Ratio	Reduced	Normal/Increased
Residual Volume	Increased	Decreased

17. Ans. (a) Body plethysmography

(Ref: Harrison 20th p 1963; Harrison 19th p 306e)

- Pulmonary plethysmographs are commonly used to measure the functional residual capacity (FRC) of the lungs—the volume in the lungs when the muscles of respiration are relaxed—and total lung capacity
- The difference between full and empty lungs can be used to assess diseases and airway passage restrictions. An obstructive disease will show increased FRC because some airways do not empty normally, while a restrictive disease will show decreased FRC. Body plethysmography is particularly appropriate for patients who have air spaces which do not communicate with the bronchial tree; in such patients helium dilution would give an incorrectly low reading.
- *Do not confuse with Impedance plethysmography which is a non-invasive method used to detect venous thrombosis in these areas of the body.*

18. Ans. (d) FEV1/FVC increased, compliance decreased

(Ref: Harrison 20th p 1951; Harrison 19th p 306e)

- In restrictive lung disease, parenchymal involvement will lead to pulmonary fibrosis and hence it will be difficult to inflate the lung leading to reduction in lung compliance.
- The FEV1/ FVC ratio is increased in restrictive lung disease because the numerator and denominator in the ratio, both are reduced in restrictive lung disease with FVC decreasing disproportionately.

19. Ans. (c) Obstructive lung disease

(Ref: Harrison 20th p 1951)

- In obstructive lung disease, the FEV1 is reduced due to obstruction of air escaping from the lungs. Thus, the FEV1/FVC ratio will be reduced.
- Hence in this question 1.3/3.1 mathematically is about 40% in contrast to normal of > 80%

- More specifically, according to the National Institute for Clinical Excellence, the diagnosis of COPD is made when the FEV1/FVC ratio is less than 60%.
- According to the European Respiratory Society (ERS) criteria, when the patient's FEV1% is less than 88% of the predicted value for men, or less than 89% for women a diagnosis of COPD is made.
- In restrictive lung disease, the FEV1 and FVC are equally reduced due to fibrosis or other lung pathology (not obstructive pathology). Thus, the FEV1/FVC ratio should be approximately normal, or even increased.

20. Ans. (b) Residual volume

(Ref: Harrison 20th p 1951; Harrison 19th p 306e)

21. Ans. (b) Central hypoventilation

(Ref: Harrison 20th p 2012; Harrison 19th p 2171; Washington Manual of Critical Care p 191)

Alveolar arteriolar gradient = $pAO_2 - paO_2$
- Choices A,C, D will alter only paO_2 leading to increase in gradient. Higher the gradient more severe is the disease and requires ventilator support.
- *Causes of increase alveolar arteriolar mismatch are:*
  - V/Q Mismatch (eg: PNA, CHF, ARDS, atelectasis)
  - Shunt (eg: PFO, ASD, PE, pulmonary AVMs)
  - Alveolar Hypoventilation (eg: interstitial lung disease, environmental lung disease)

Remember that hypoventilation due to CNS diseases or neuromuscular disease will reduce the ventilatory drive and will lead to reduction in both pAO_2 as well as paO_2.

22. Ans. (d) Interstitial lung disease

(Ref: Harrison 20th p 1951; Harrison 19th p 1709-11)

23. Ans. (d) Increased vital capacity

(Ref: Harrison 20th p 1951)

Vital capacity is a sum of IRV + TV+ ERV and all these lung volumes are reduced in restrictive lung disease.

Parameter	Obstructive	Restrictive
FEV1	Reduced	Reduced
TLC	Normal/Increased	Reduced
FVC	Reduced	Reduced
FEV1/FVC Ratio	Reduced	Normal/Increased
Residual Volume	Increased	Decreased

24. Ans. (b) Sarcoidosis

(Ref: Harrison 19th p 2205-06)

Sarcoidosis affects lung prenchyme and can lead to lung fibrosis. This will lead to development of restrictive pattern. Remember that if it will lead to lymphadenopathy compressor on the airway then it can also result in obstructive pattern.

25. Ans. (b) Alveolar arterial difference in PaO_2

(Ref: Harrison 20th p 1951; Washington Manual of Critical Care p 191)

26. Ans. (a) Small airways

(Ref: Harrison 17th/1588)

27. Ans. (a) Body Plethysmography

(Ref: Harrison 20th p 1963; Harrison 19th p 2081)

28. Ans. (b) COPD

(Ref: Harrison 19th p 1704)

Types of Respiratory Failure

29. Ans. (a) CT scan of chest

Ref: Harrison 20th p 511; Harrison 19th edition, page 1788
- CT chest provides the most reliable view of mediastinal anatomy. The main feature is diminished opacification of central venous structures with prominent collateral venous circulation. Subsequently an endobronchial or USG guided biopsy can be done to establish the cause.
- The diagnosis of SVCS is a clinical one. CXR shows superior mediastinal widening with pleural effusion in 25% cases.
- The clinical sign of increased facial venous congestion on raising arms above the level of head is known as *Pemberton sign*.

30. Ans. (d) Face mask with reservoir

Ref: The ICU book Paul Merino, 4th edition, Page 64

System or Device	Oxygen delivery
Low flow nasal oxygen	24-40%
Standard face mask	35-50%
Partial rebreather mask (reservoir)	40-70%
Non rebreather mask (reservoir plus one way valves between the mask and reservoir bag and at exhalation ports)	60-80%
Venti-mask or Air Entrainment mask Used to deliver a fixed low concentration of oxygen irrespective of flow rates	24-50%

31. Ans. (c) Methemoglobinemia

Ref: Harrison 20th p 695; Harrison 19th edition, page 636
- *Methemoglobin* has such high oxygen affinity that virtually no oxygen is delivered to tissues and leads to central cyanosis. Levels >50–60% are often fatal.
- *All other causes will leads to peripheral cyanosis.*

32. Ans. (a) Central sleep apnea

Ref: Harrison 19th edition, page 1727
- Crescendo-decrescendo breathing pattern is known as *Cheyne stokes breathing*. It is characterised by hyperventilation alternating with apnea. It is also known as Central Apnea.
- It occurs due to prolonged circulation in CHF leading to delay between pulmonary capillaries and carotid chemoreceptors.
- Obstructive sleep apnea does not have hyperventilation and is hence ruled out.

33. Ans. (a) Intubation and low tidal volume ventilation

(Ref: Harrison 20th p 2026; Harrison 19th edition p 1731)

- The combination of morbid obesity with respiratory distress and orthopnea points to congestive heart failure as a possible etiology.
- The patient has low pO_2 with low PCO_2 which points to development of *type 1 respiratory failure*.
- The alveolar flooding is occurring due to elevated pulmonary microvascular pressures.
- The low CO_2 is explained by the hyperventilation in the patient.
- *For management of type 1 respiratory failure, low tidal ventilation is recommended for the patient.*
- Mechanical ventilation can lead to volutrauma, and is hence avoided in these patients.
- Choice B is useful in type II respiratory failure. Endotracheal intubation adds to the work of breathing in type 2 respiratory failure. Hence type II respiratory failure is managed with non-invasive ventilation.
- In Choice C intravenous diuretics are required in management of pulmonary oedema but digoxin is not used in acute CHF management in adults.
- Choice D is used in type II respiratory failure.

Type of Respiratory failure	Treatment recommended
I	Low volume ventilation
II	Non-invasive ventilation using tight fitting face mask. Avoid intubation in COPD Intubation only if respiratory failure is imminent.
III	Positioning and physiotherapy
IV	Intubation and mechanical ventilation

34. Ans. (b) Intubation with mechanical ventilation

(Ref: Harrison 20th p 2027; Harrison 19th edition p 1732)

- Type 4 respiratory failure occurs due to hypo-perfusion of respiratory muscles in patients of shock.
- Normally respiratory muscles consume <5% of total cardiac output and oxygen delivery.
- Patients in shock may have as much as 40% of cardiac output, distributed to respiratory muscles.
- Intubation and ventilator assisted breathing will allow redistribution of cardiac output away from respiratory muscles.
- Non-invasive ventilation with tight fitting face mask is used in management of type 2 Respiratory failure like in cases of exacerbations of COPD.

35. Ans. (a) Chronic bronchitis exacerbation

(Ref: Harrison 20th p 2026; Harrison 19th ed./1731-32)

Type 2 respiratory failure occurs as a result of alveolar hypoventilation and results in the inability to eliminate carbon dioxide effectively.

1. Increased resistive loads e.g., bronchospasm in COPD
2. Loads due to reduced lung compliance [e.g., alveolar edema, atelectasis, intrinsic positive end-expiratory pressure).
3. Diminished CNS drive to breathe due to drug overdose, brainstem injury, sleep-disordered breathing, and hypothyroidism.
4. Reduced strength can be due to impaired neuromuscular transmission (e.g., myasthenia gravis, Guillain-Barré syndrome, amyotrophic lateral sclerosis, phrenic nerve injury)
5. Respiratory muscle weakness (e.g., myopathy, electrolyte derangements, fatigue).
6. Loads due to reduced chest wall compliance (e.g., pneumothorax, pleural effusion, abdominal distention), and loads due to increased minute ventilation requirements (e.g., pulmonary embolus with increased dead space fraction, sepsis).

36. Ans. (a) Chronic bronchitis with cor-pulmonale

(Ref: Harrison 20th p 2026; Harrison 19th p 1736-38)

- Acute hypercapnic respiratory failure is usually caused by defects in the central nervous system, impairment of neuromuscular transmission, mechanical defect of the ribcage and fatigue of the respiratory muscles.
- The pathophysiological mechanisms responsible for chronic carbon dioxide retention is based on fact that patient has to push hard in order to maintain normal arterial carbon dioxide and oxygen tensions at the cost of eventually becoming fatigued and exhausted or to breathe at a lower minute ventilation, avoiding dyspnoea, fatigue and exhaustion but at the expense of reduced alveolar ventilation
- In chronic bronchitis exacerbation the overwork of respiratory muscles leads to fatigue of respiratory muscles and build up of carbon dioxide.

37. Ans. (a) Post-operative atelectasis

(Ref: Harrison 20th p 2026; Harrison 19th p 1736-40)

Type 3 respiratory failure can be considered as a subtype of type 1 failure. However, acute respiratory failure is common in the post-operative period with atelectasis being the most frequent cause. Thus measures to reverse atelectasis are paramount. In general residual anesthesia effects, post-operative pain, and abnormal abdominal mechanics contribute to decreasing FRC and progressive collapse of dependant lung units.

Causes of post-operative atelectasis include:

1. Decreased FRC
2. Supine/obese/ascites
3. Anesthesia
4. Upper abdominal incision
5. Airway secretions

Therapy is directed at reversing the atelectasis.
- Turn patient q1-2h
- Chest physiotherapy
- Incentive spirometry
- Treat incisional pain (may include epidural anesthesia or patient controlled analgesia)
- Ventilate at 45 degrees upright
- Drain ascites
- Re-expansion of lobar collapse
- Avoid overhydration

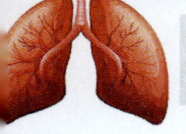

38. Ans. (b) Low pO$_2$ and High pCO$_2$

(Ref: Harrison 20th p 2026; Harrison 19th p 1736-40)

Type 1 respiratory failure	Type 2 respiratory failure
Low pO$_2$	Low pO$_2$
Normal or low pCO$_2$	High pCO$_2$
A-a gradient is increased	A-a gradient is normal (Reason: Hypoventilation leads to reduction of both pAO$_2$ as well as paO$_2$.)

39. Ans. (a) Low PaO$_2$, normal or low PaCO$_2$

(Ref: Harrison 20th p 2026; Harrison 19th p 1736-38)

40. Ans. (d) Normal A-a gradient

(Ref: Harrison 19th p 1736-38)

- A-a gradient is increased in type 1 respiratory failure as it affects only paO$_2$ only.
- A-a gradient is normal in type 2 respiratory failure as it lowers both pAO$_2$ and paO$_2$

41. Ans. (a) Guillain-Barre syndrome

(Ref: Harrison 20th p 2026; Harrison 19th p 2694-95)

- Neuromuscular diseases that can cause alveolar hypoventilation include myasthenia gravis, amyotrophic lateral sclerosis, Guillain-Barré syndrome, and muscular dystrophy. Patients with neuromuscular disorders have rapid, shallow breathing secondary to severe muscle weakness or abnormal motor neuron function. The central respiratory drive is maintained in patients with neuromuscular disorders. Thus, hypoventilation is secondary to respiratory muscle weakness.

42. Ans. (d) Flail chest

(Ref: Bailey 26th p 355)

- Breathing movements in which the chest wall moves in on inspiration and out on expiration, in reverse of the normal movements. Crush injuries of the chest, with fractured ribs and sternum, can lead to a severe degree of paradoxical breathing.
- It may be seen in children with respiratory distress of any cause, which leads to indrawing of the intercostal spaces during inspiration.
- Patients with chronic airways obstruction also show indrawing of the lower ribs during inspiration, due to the distorted action of a depressed and flattened diaphragm.

43. Ans. (d) Somnolence

(Ref: Harrison 19th p 1722-23)

- Hyperventilation leads to CO$_2$ washout from the body leading to respiratory alkalosis.
- The H$^+$ on buffer base are hence mobilized to neutralize the alkalosis.
- This leaves a few vacant sites on the buffer base which are now taken up by calcium.
- Since calcium exists in two forms the bound and the ionized calcium, due to increased binding of calcium to vacant sites on the protein, the level of ionized calcium falls. This leads to tetany.
- *Somnolence or drowsiness is a feature of Carbon dioxide narcosis and is seen with respiratory acidosis/hypoventilation.*

44. Ans. (c) Acute CCF

(Ref: CMDT 2015 pg. 398)

45. Ans. (d) Lead poisoning

(Ref: Harrison 20th p 2026; Harrison 19th p 2607-08; 472e)

- Polio and M.Gravis can lead to diaphragmatic paralysis.
- In acute intermittent porphyria, the clinical manifestation of acute attacks include vomiting, hypertension and tachycardia, acute abdominal pain (incidence estimated at 85%–95%), and peripheral neuropathy with muscle weakness (42%–68%). Respiratory failure is less common and less known (9%–20%). The exact mechanism through which these signs and symptoms occur remains unknown

46. Ans. (b) Low pO$_2$ and high pCO$_2$

(Ref: Harrison 20th p 2026; Harrison 19th p 1736-38)

Bronchial Asthma

47. Ans. (c) Atopic dermatitis

Ref: Fitzpatrick Dermatology in general practice: 7th edition, Page 497

- The image shows an eczematous lesion with xerosis on the face of the child whose mother is an asthmatic. This points to diagnosis of atopic dermatitis.
- The essential features (which must be present) are as follows:
  - Pruritus
  - Eczema with typical morphology and age-specific patterns (facial/neck/extensor involvement in children, flexural involvement in any age group, sparing the groin and axillary regions)
  - Chronic or Relapsing history

48. Ans. (a) Corticosteroids facilitate the action of β2 agonists

Ref: Harrison 20th p 1966; Harrison 19th edition Page 1677

- Corticosteroids do not have any bronchodilator activity and have no impact on mucociliary clearance. Hence choice C and D are ruled out.
- Sensitization of Adenosine receptors would lead to increase in bronchospasm, inflammation and mucus secretion.
- Mechanism of action of Corticosteroids in asthma is:

1. ICS reduce eosinophils in airways and sputum
2. Upregulation of Beta 2 receptors
3. Decrease in recruitment of inflammatory cells
4. Reduction of mucus production
5. Reduction of microvascular permeability.

Hence they would facilitate the action of bronchodilators

*Inhaled steroids are the **most effective controllers** in management of asthma and benefit athamatics of any age and severity.*

49. Ans. (a) Wash your mouth between 2 puffs

(Ref: G.I.N.A inhaler use check-list)

Recommendation for correct inhaler technique:

1. Remove cap
2. Check dose counter (if applicable)
3. Hold inhaler upright and shake well
4. Breathe out gently, away from the inhaler
5. Put mouthpiece between teeth without biting and close lips to form good seal
6. Start to breathe in slowly through mouth and, at the same time, press down firmly on canister
7. Continue to breathe is slowly and deep
8. Hold breath for about 5 seconds or as long as comfortable
9. While holding breath, remove inhaler
10. Breathe out gently, away from the inhaler
11. If an extra dose is needed, repeat steps
12. Replace cap
13. When the patient has finished taking all the dosage, then rinse the mouth with water and spit out the water. This is important especially in case of steroid inhaler..

50. Ans. (a) PEFR 50-60% of predicted value

(Ref: NAEPP3 guidelines, CMDT 2018 p 255, CMDT 2019, 266)

- PEFR of 50-60% indicates moderate asthma.
- Indication for intubation in asthma exacerbation is poor response to oxygen with salbutamol ebulisation and oral steroids. The definition of poor response is
    1. FEV1< 40%
    2. pCO_2 > 45mmHg
    3. Features of carbon dioxide narcosis
    4. Hypoxia defined as pO_2<60mm Hg

51. Ans. (d) 1, 2 and 3

(Ref: Harrison 20th, British thoracic society asthma guidelines 2018, page 1968)

"Pulsus paradoxsus may be present in acute severe asthma but is rarely a useful clinical sign". (Harrison 20th ed, Page 1968)

Guidelines for Assessment of Severity of Asthma Exacerbations in Adults

	Mild	Moderate	Severe	Respiratory arrest Imminent
Symptoms				
Breathlessness	while walking	At rest, limits activity	At rest, interferes with conversation	While at rest, mute
Talks in	Sentences	Phrases	Words	Silent
Alertness	May be agitated	Usually agitated	Usually agitated	Drowsy or confused
Signs				
Respiratory rate	Increased	Increased	Often > 30/minute	>30/minute
Body position	Can lie down	Prefers sitting	Sits upright	Unable to recline
Use of accessory muscles; suprasternal retractions	Usually not	Commonly	Usually	Paradoxical thoracoabdominal movement
Wheeze	Moderate, often only end expiratory	Loud; throughout exhalation	Usually loud; throughout inhalation and exhalation	Absent
Pulse/minute	<100	100-120	>120	Bradycardia
Pulsus paradoxus	Absent < 10 mm Hg	May be present 10-25 mm Hg	Often present > 25 mm Hg	Absence suggest respiratory muscle fatigue
Functional Assessment				
PEF or FEV_1 % predicted or % personal best	≥ 70%	40-69%	<40%	<25%
PaO_2 (on air, mm Hg)	Normal	≥60	<60: possible cyanosis	< 60: possible
PCO_2 (mm Hg)	< 42 mm Hg	< 42 mm Hg	≥ 42	

52. Ans. (d) Intravenous aminophylline

(Ref: CMDT 2015, page 251 and 253)

Methylxanthines are not recommended for therapy of acute severe asthma exacerbation owing to limited efficacy. In fact the toxicity caused by the drug in patients already on theophylline is more often seen rather than beneficial effects.

FEV_1 or PEF <40% (Severe)	Impending or Actual Respiratory Arrest
• Oxygen to achieve SaO_2 ≥ 90% • High-dose inhaled SABA plus ipratropium by nebulizer or MDI plus valved holding chamber, every 20 minutes or continuously for 1 hour • Oral systemic corticosteroids	• Intubation and mechanical ventilation with 100% oxygen • Neublized SABA and ipratropium • Intravenous corticosteroids • Consider adjunct therapies

* Mucolytics worsen cough – Anxiolytic drugs are contraindicated in severe asthma exacerbations.

53. Ans. (d) PEF of 60 to 70% of expected

(Ref: Harrison 19th edition, Page 1679)

In acute severe asthma, PEF/FEV$_1$/ is <40%.

54. Ans. (a) Distal bronchiectasis

(Ref: Harrison 20th edition, p 1975, Harrison 19th edition, p 1346t)

ABPA represents a hypersensitivity reaction to A. fumigatus and occurs in ~1% of patients with asthma and 15% of adults with cystic fibrosis. *Central bronchiectasis is characteristic*, but patients may present before it becomes apparent.

Clinical features of ABPA
- Bronchial obstruction with mucous plugs leading to breathlessness and repeated bouts of prolonged coughing.
- **Thick sputum casts, usually brown or clear.**
- *Eosinophilia*
- Chest X ray shows presence of pulmonary infiltrates
- CT chest shows central bronchiectasis
- The cardinal diagnostic tests include an
  - Elevated serum level of total IgE (usually >1000 IU/mL),
  - **Positive skin-prick test to A. fumigatus extract**
  - **Detection of Aspergillus-specific IgE and IgG (precipitating) antibodies.**

55. Ans. (c) Asthma

(Ref: Harrison 20th edition Page 1963, Harrison 19th edition, Page 1675)

- In asthma spirometry confirms airflow limitation with a reduced FEV1, FEV1/FVC ratio, and PEF. (Reversibility is demonstrated by a >12% and 200-mL increase in FEV1 15 minutes after an inhaled short-acting beta2-agonist or in some patients by a 2 to 4 week trial of oral corticosteroids.) (prednisone or prednisolone 30–40 mg daily)
- Most forms of ILD have FEV1/FVC ratio which is normal or increased. In Restrictive defects total lung capacity (TLC), functional residual capacity, and residual volume are reduced.

56. Ans. (a) Asthma

(Ref: Harrison 19th edition, 1963, Page 1671)

- Alveolar membrane thickening/remodelling is seen in asthma.
- Reid's index in chronic bronchitis is based on thickness of glands in airway wall to airway wall thickness.

57. Ans. (d) Increased prostaglandins

(Ref: Harrison 20th edition, p 1969; Harrison 19th ed. / 1680)

- Aspirin-sensitive asthma is associated with severe rhinosinusitis and recurrent nasal polyposis.
- The complex pathogenesis of aspirin-sensitive asthma involves chronic eosinophilic inflammatory changes, with evidence of increased mast cell activation.
- Aspirin-sensitive asthma is an underdiagnosed condition affecting up to 20% of the adult asthmatic population.
- It is associated with more severe asthma, requires increased use of inhaled and oral corticosteroids, more presentations to hospital and a risk of life- threatening reactions with aspirin.
- The cyclo-oxygenase pathways play a major role in the respiratory reactions that develop after aspirin ingestion.

58. Ans. (d) Long acting beta 2 agonist

(Ref: Harrison 19th edition.)

- LABA improve asthma control and reduce exacerbations when added to ICS, which allows asthma to be controlled at lower doses of corticosteroids.
- LABAs should not be given in the absence of ICS therapy as they do not control the underlying inflammation.
- This observation has led to the widespread use of fixed combination inhalers that contain a corticosteroid and a LABA, which have proved to be highly effective in the control of asthma.

Mild intermittent	Mild persistent	Moderate persistent	Severe persistent	Very severe persistent
				OCS
			LABA	LABA
		LABA	ICS	ICS
ICS Low dose	ICS Low dose	ICS Low dose	High dose	High dose
Short –acting B2-agonist as required for symptom relief				

59. Ans. (a) Allergic Rhinitis Induced Asthma

(Ref: Pubmed. nl)

ARIA stands for Allergic Rhinits Induced Asthma

60. Ans. (a) Eosinophiluria

(Ref: Harrison 20th edition, p 1975; Harrison 19th ed. / 1346-47)

- A.B.P.A allergic brochopulmonary Aspergillosis is hypersensitivity to the antigens on cell wall of aspergillus fumigatus. The clinical profile is an asthmatic patient presenting with passage of browinish plugs in the sputum.
- CXR shows fleeting pulmonary opacities and absolute eosinophil count is increased. Eosinophilia is a feature of asthma anyway but not eosinophiluria
- HRCT shows presence of central bronchiectasis.
- Treatment of choice for ABPA is steroids.
- REMEMBER: Eosinophiluria is a feature of allergic interstitial nephritis

61. Ans. (b) Cystic fibrosis

(Ref: Harrison 20th edition, p 1975; Harrison 19th ed. / 1681, 1686)

- ABPA represents a hypersensitivity reaction to A. fumigatus; and leads to central bronchiectasis.
- *ABPA occurs in ~1% of patients with asthma and in up to 15% of adults with cystic fibrosis; occasional cases are reported in patients with neither of the latter.*
- The cardinal diagnostic tests include an elevated serum level of total IgE (usually >1000 IU/mL), a positive skin-prick test

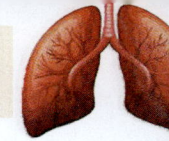

to A. fumigatus extract, or detection of Aspergillus-specific IgE and IgG (precipitating) antibodies.

62. Ans. (b) Oral corticosteroids

(Ref: Harrison 20th edition, p 1967; Harrison 19th ed. / 1676)

- Oral corticosteroids are given in very severe persistent asthma and not severe persistent asthma.
- L.A.B.A with inhaled high dose steroids is used for management of severe persistent asthma. S.A.B.A is used as and when required.

63. Ans. (d) Subcutaneous epinephrine

(Ref: Harrison 20th edition, p 1968; Harrison 19th ed. / 1680)

- Type 2 Brittle asthma, are symptom free patients developing sudden onset acute attack of asthma requiring mechanical ventilation or even death. These patients should ideally keep an autoinjector of epinephrine.
- Type 1 Brittle asthma is characterized by >40% variation in P.E.F.R for >50% of time. It is managed with L.A.B.A + high dose inhaled corticosteroids and oral steroids. Long term continuous subcutaneous infusion of β_2 agonists like terbutaline is also given.

64. Ans. (c) VP mismatch with dead space ventilation

(Ref: Rogers handbook of Pediatric intensive Care – fourth edition page no : 183.

- Oxygen saturation (SaO_2) levels may not reflect progressive alveolar hypoventilation, and the SaO_2 may initially fall during therapy *because β_2-agonists produce both bronchodilation and vasodilation and may initially increase intrapulmonary shunting.*
- The main catch point in this question is that salbutamol is given without oxygen. (Nebulization without oxygen which is a common practice).
- It is always essential to give salbutamol nebulization through high flow oxygen. (Standard practice).
- In status asthmaticus most children will have some degree of mucus plugging, atelectasis, ventilation perfusion mismatch and hypoxemia. In those lung segments with atelectasis, compensatory hypoxic pulomary vasoconstriction is often present. Treatment with inhaled beta agonists may induce generalized pulmonary vasodilation and as a result exacerbate ventilation perfusion mismatch and worsen hypoxemia. Oxygen should be a part of management for all children with status asthmaticus.
- Inference: Giving only salbutamol nebulization without oxygen can aggravate hypoxemia because of increase in dead space ventilation and VP mismatch.

65. Ans. (d) Systolic BP

(Ref: CMDT 2019 pg. 256, Harrison 19th p 1675)

66. Ans. (a) Cystic fibrosis

(Ref: Harrison 20th edition, p 1975, Harrison 19th p 1346-47)

67. Ans. (a) 1 only

(Ref: British Asthma guidelines 2015., Harrison 19th p 1679)

In a child with severe asthma any one of the following features is considered Life Threatening:
• PEF <33% best or predicted • SpO_2 <92% • PaO_2 <8 kPa • Normal $PaCO_2$ (4.6-6.0 kPa) • Silent chest • Cyanosis • Poor respiratory effort • Arrhythmia • *Exhaustion, altered conscious level*

68. Ans. (a) Leukotrienes

(Ref: Harrison 20th edition, p 1962; Harrison 19th p 1669)

69. Ans. (c) Associated with nasal polyp

(Ref: Harrison 20th edition, p 1969; Harrison 19th p 1680)

- 10% of asthmatics have negative skin tests to common inhalant allergens and normal serum concentrations of IgE.
- These patients, with non-atopic or intrinsic asthma, usually show later onset of disease (adult-onset asthma) commonly have concomitant nasal polyps, and may be aspirin-sensitive. They usually have more severe, persistent asthma.

70. Ans. (a) Mechanical ventilation

(Ref: Harrison 20th edition, p 1968; Harrison 19th p 807-809)

- The child is drowsy with pCO_2 of 60 mm Hg inspite of 1 hour of treatment and is progressing to impending respiratory failure.
- Nelson says "Mechanical ventilation aims to achieve adequate oxygenation while tolerating mild to moderate hypercapnia (pCO_2 50–70 mm Hg) to minimize barotrauma".
- Volume-cycled ventilators, using short inspiratory and long expiratory times, 10–15 mL/kg tidal volume, 8–15 breaths/min, peak pressures <60 cm H_2O, and without positive end-expiratory pressure are starting mechanical ventilation parameters that can achieve these goals. Considering the nature of asthma exacerbations leading to respiratory failure, those of rapid or abrupt onset tend to resolve quickly (hours to 2 days).

71. Ans. (a) 1, 2 and 3

(Ref: Harrison 20th edition, p 1959; Harrison 19th p 1679-80)

IL-4 mediates proinflammatory functions in asthma, including induction of IgE isotype switch and promotion of eosinophil transmigration across endothelium.

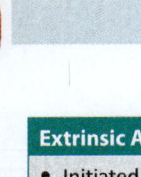

Extrinsic Asthma	Intrinsic Asthma
• Initiated by type I hypersensivity reaction induced by exposure to extrinsic antigen.	• Initiated by diverse, non-immune immune mechanism,s including ingestion of aspirin, pulmonary infections, cold, inhaled irritant, stress and exercise.

• Subtypes include:
  ■ Atopic (allergic) asthma
  ■ Occupational asthma
  ■ Allergic bronchopulmonary
	• No personal or family history of allergic reaction.
	• Develop later in life.

• Develop early in life	

72. Ans. (d) Increased inspiratory capacity

(Ref: Harrison 19th p 1679-80)

A prototype obstructive airway disease is acute asthma where the, luminal narrowing due to smooth muscle constriction and inflammation and thickening within the small- and medium-sized bronchi raise frictional resistance and reduce airflow. The following changes are seen in pulmonary function testing for these patients.
1. Total lung capacity (TLC) usually remains normal (although elevated TLC is sometimes seen in long-standing asthma), but FRC may be dynamically elevated.
2. RV is often increased due to exaggerated airway closure at low lung volumes, and this elevation of RV reduces FVC and insiratory capacity
3. Because central airways are narrowed, airways resistance is usually elevated. Mild arterial hypoxemia is often present due to perfusion of relatively underventilated alveoli distal to obstructed airways (and is responsive to oxygen supplementation).

73. Ans. (c) 1, 2 and 3

(Ref: Harrison 19th p 1697-98)

In severe exacerbations patients may be so breathless that they are unable to complete sentences and may become cyanotic. Examination usually shows
- Increased ventilation, hyperinflation, and tachycardia.
- Pulsus paradoxus may be present, but this is rarely a useful clinical sign. There is a marked fall in spirometric values and PEF.
- Arterial blood gases on air show hypoxemia and pCO_2 is usually low due to hyperventilation.
- A normal or rising pCO_2 is an indication of impending respiratory failure and requires immediate monitoring and therapy.
- A chest roentgenogram is not informative, but may show pneumonia or pneumothorax.

74. Ans. (d) Low dose inhaled corticosteroids

(Ref: Harrison 19th p 1671)

- Exercise induced asthma may be prevented by prior administration of beta2-agonists and antileukotrienes, but is best prevented by regular treatment with ICS, which reduce the population of surface mast cells required for this response

- The mechanism of exercise induced asthma is linked to hyperventilation, which results in increased osmolality in airway lining fluid and triggers mast cell mediator release, resulting in bronchoconstriction.
- Exercise-induced asthma (EIA) typically begins after exercise has ended, and recovers spontaneously within about 30 minutes. EIA is worse in cold, dry climates than in hot, humid conditions. It is, therefore, more common in sports such as cross-country running in cold weather, overland skiing, and ice hockey than in swimming.

75. Ans. (b) Pleural effusion

(Ref: Harrison 19th p 1695)

76. Ans. (a) Inspiratory and expiratory rhonchi with reduced air entry

(Ref: Harrison 19th p 1675, 1679)

In severe exacerbations, the greater extent of airways obstruction causes labored breathing and respiratory distress manifested as
1. Inspiratory and expiratory wheezing
2. Increased prolongation of exhalation
3. Poor air entry
4. Suprasternal and intercostal retractions
5. Nasal flaring
6. Accessory respiratory muscle use.
7. Sometimes, airflow may be so limited that wheezing cannot be heard.

77. Ans. (d) Sodium Cromoglycate inhalation

(Ref: Harrison 19th p 1679)

Cromolyn sodium inhibits the release of histamine, leukotrienes, and other mediators from sensitized mast cells exposed to specific antigens. It has no intrinsic anti-inflammatory, antihistamine, or vasoconstrictive effects.

78. Ans. (c) Chronic bronchitis

(Ref: Harrison 20th edition, p 1973)

Choice A is associated with asthma which is an allergic condition.
Choice B is associated c̄ parasites and hence eosinophilia is seen
Choice D is called eosinophilic granulomatosis with polyangitis.

79. Ans. (d) Culture of A. Fumigatus from the sputum

(Ref: Harrison 20th edition, p 1975; Harrison 19th edition, page 1681, 86)

Allergic bronchopulmonary aspergillosis
ABPA is defined by abnormalities including the following:

1. Asthma
2. Eosinophilia
3. A positive skin test result for A fumigatus
4. Serum IgE level > 1000 IU/dL
5. Positive test results for Aspergillus precipitins (primarily IgG but also IgA and IgM)
6. Minor criteria for diagnosis include positive Aspergillus radioallergosorbent assay test results and sputum culture

Other investigations
- Chest radiography results in ABPA may vary from fleeting pulmonary infiltrates to mucoid impaction to central bronchiectasis.
- CT scanning is helpful for better defining bronchiectasis, and images may show that apparent lobulated masses are mucus-filled dilated bronchi. Areas of atelectasis related to bronchial obstruction from mucoid impaction may be present.

80. Ans. (d) Occurrence in patients with old cavitatory lesions

(Ref: Harrison 20th edition, p 1975; Harrison 19th p 1681, 86)

81. Ans. (a) Subcutaneous

(Ref: Harrison 20th edition, p 1967; Harrison 19th p 1678)

Omalizumab is indicated for moderate-to-severe persistent asthma in patients with a positive skin test or in vitro reactivity to a perennial aeroallergen and symptoms that are inadequately controlled with inhaled corticosteroids 150-375 mg SC q2-4 Weeks

82. Ans. (d) An IE ratio 1:2.5

(Ref: CMDT 2018 pg. 242)

83. Ans. (b) Asthma

Ref: Harrison 19th p 1675-76)

Curschmann's spirals refers to spiral shaped mucus plugs in airways of asthmatics. They are often seen in association with Creola bodies and Charcot-Leyden crystals.

84. Ans. (c) Nasal polyp

(Ref: Harrison 20th edition, p 1969; Harrison 19th p 1680)

85. Ans. (a) Hypoxia

(Ref: Harrison 20th edition, p 1968; Harrison 19th p 1669-70)

86. Ans. (b) Morphine

(Ref: Harrison 20th edition, p 1968; Harrison 19th p 1669-70)

C.O.P.D

87. Ans. (d) FEV1/FVC < 0.7 and FEV1< 30% predicted

Ref: Harrison 20th edition, p 1991; Harrison 19th edition, page 1704:
Gold Criteria for Severity of Airflow Obstruction in COPD

GOLD Stage	Severity	Spirometry
I	Mild	FEV_1/FVC <0.7 and FEV_1 ≥80% predicted
II	Moderate	FEV_1/FVC <0.7 and FEV_1 ≥50% but <80% predicted
III	Severe	FEV_1/FVC <0.7 and FEV_1 ≥30% but <50% predicted
IV	Very severe	FEV_1/FVC <0.7 and FEV_1 <30% predicted

Abbreviation: COPD: chronic obstructive pulmonary disease; GOLD, Global Initiative for Lung Disease

88. Ans. (a) Type I Respiratory failure, respiratory alkalosis

Ref: Harrison 20th edition, p 2001; Harrison 19th edition, page 1710

- In ILD, oxygen levels are normal to reduce because of diffusion defect. The levels fall on 6-minute walk test further.
- Carbon dioxide washout leads to respiratory alkalosis due to hyperventilation.

89. Ans. (a) Emphysema

(Ref: Oxford handbook of medical imaging, Page 46)

CT chest shows large Bullae in bilateral lung fields diagnostic of emphysema.

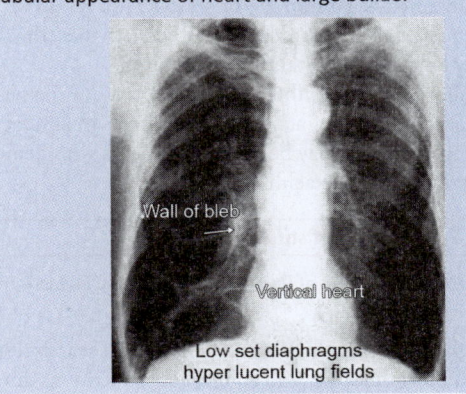

Also not the X-Ray finding of emphysema which shows tubular appearance of heart and large bullae.

90. Ans. (a) Chronic Bronchitis

(Ref: Harrison 19th edition, page 244)

Reid's index is a ratio between the thickness of the submucosal mucus secreting glands and the thickness between the epithelium and cartilage that covers the bronchi
A normal Reid Index should be smaller than 0.4, the thickness of the wall is always more than double the thickness of the glands it contains. Chronic smoking causes submucosal gland hypertrophy and hyperplasia, leading to a Reid Index of >0.5 indicating chronic bronchitis

91. Ans. (d) All of the above

(Ref: Harrison 20th edition, p 3294)

Effective Pharmacologic Interventions

First-line therapies (Number in brackets indicates efficacy)	
• Nicotine gum (1.5)	• Nicotine lozenge (2.0)
• Nicotine patch (1.9)	• Bupropion (2.1)
• Nicotine nasal inhaler (2.7)	• Varenicline (2.7)
• Nicotine oral inhaler (2.5)	
Second-line therapies	
• Clonidine (2.1)	• Nortriptyline (3.2)

92. **Ans. (b)** ↓FEV1/FVC; **(c)** ↑RV; **(d)** ↑TLC **and (e)** ↓Peak expiratory flow

(Ref: Harrison 20th edition, p 1951, 1991; Harrison 19th/1662)

93. **Ans. (c)** Low flow oxygen

(Ref: Harrison 19th ed. / 1707, 1740)

- In COPD, Ventilation/perfusion matching leads to under-ventilated lung which usually has low oxygen content which leads to localized vasoconstriction limiting blood flow to that lung tissue.
- Supplemental oxygen abolishes this constriction, leading to improved ventilation/perfusion matching.
- High flow oxygen is not tolerated as it leads to crusting, dryness and epistaxis.
- The treatment is guided by PaO_2 which should be maintained at 60 mm Hg or so (SaO_2 of 85-90%). During the period of exercise, sleep or other activities, the flow rate may be increased by another 1-2 L/min.
- While continuous therapy is required for patients who show hypoxaemia at rest, intermittent treatment during specific periods may be used for patients who demonstrate intermittent hypoxaemia

94. **Ans. (a)** Duration of smoking

(Ref: IASLC Textbook of Prevention and Early Detection of Lung Cancer: 2015 Review)

Though this is a highly debatable topic, most search results and discussion with faculty and google books mentions duration of smoking to be more important that the number of cigarettes smoked.

95. **Ans. (a)** Cyanosis

(Ref: Harrison 20th edition, p 1995; Harrison 19th ed. / 1664f)

- Emphysema is characterized by damage to respiratory bronchioles **leading to bleb formation**. The air gets trapped in the lungs causing hypoxia. However these patients do not have cyanosis and are called as **PINK PUFFERS.**
- Cigarette smoking is the most common cause of emphysema and the type seen is known as centri-acinar emphysema. **These patients develop type 1 respiratory failure** and the resultant hypoxia causes causes a **barrel shaped chest in** these patients.

96. **Ans. (d)** Benzene

(Ref: Harrison 19th ed. / 447t, 663)

Cigarette smoke product	Effects on human body
Aceta-aldehyde/anabasine	Addictive
Benzene	Carcinogenic + Cardio-toxic + reproductive potential toxicity
Benzopyrine	Carcinogenic
Carbon monoxide	Reproductive potential toxicity
Vinyl chloride	Carcinogenic

97. **Ans. (a)** Primary brain cancer

(Ref: Harrison 20th edition, p 3293)

- Smoking DOES NOT cause primary brain cancer.
- Kidney and bladder cancer are associated with smoking.
- Tobacco smoking causes cancer of lip, oral cavity, nasopharynx oropharynx, nasal cavity, stomach, esophagus, pancreas colon, rectum, genitourinary system and acute myeloid leukaemia.

98. **Ans. (b)** Cystic fibrosis

(Ref: Harrison 20th edition, p 1975; Harrison 19th p 1694-95)

- Central bronchiectasis is commonly reported with ABPA followed by cystic fibrosis.
- Bronchiectasis in cystic fibrosis is central and involves mainly the upper lobes in contrast to post infectious bronchiectasis which is seen in lower lobes.
- Adult CF involves disease that is more extensive than idiopathic Bronchiectasis(5 or 6 lobes involved).
- In syndromes with impaired mucociliary clearance, a lower-lobe involvement is more predominant.

99. **Ans. (a)** TB

(Ref: CMDT 2019 pg. 274, Harrison 19th p 1694-95)

Bronchiectasis sicca or dry bronchiectasis is a rare condition in which there are all the features of bronchiectasis except for the absence of copious amount of sputum which is usually a hall mark of bronchiectasis. HRCT shows abnormal dilatation bronchial tree is without infective sputum and occurs due to tuberculosis.

100. **Ans. (d)** Bronchogenic carcinoma

(Ref: Harrison 20th edition, p 1985; Harrison 19th p 1696)

In view of presence of infection in lung hematogenous dissemination of infection leading to cerebral or lung abscess can occur. Since it is a chronic infection, hence AA type of amyloidosis develops.

101. **Ans. (c)** Rhonchi

(Ref: Harrison 20th edition, p 1995; Harrison 19th p 1664, 1701)

- Rhonchi are seen in chronic bronchitis and not in emphysema where the blebs in airways lead to air trapping.
- Hyper-inflated chest is the norm in emphysema. The damage to alveoli in emphysema leads to reduced DLCO.

102. **Ans. (a)** Cyanosis

(Ref: Harrison 20th edition, p 1995; Harrison 19th p 249, 1740-41)

Emphysema is characterized by damage to respiratory bronchioles leading to bleb formation. The air gets trapped in the lungs causing hypoxia. However these patients do not have cyanosis and are called as PINK PUFFERS.

Cigarette smoking is the most common cause of emphysema and the type seen is known as centri-acinar emphysema. These patients develop type 1 respiratory failure and the resultant hypoxia causes a barrel shaped chest in these patients.

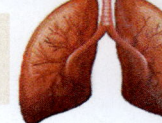

103. Ans. (b) Non reversible airflow obstruction

(Ref: Harrison 20th edition, p 1995; Harrison 19th p 1676)

104. Ans. (d) Nicotine Dependence

(Ref: Harrison 20th edition, p 3294; Harrison 19th p 507; 1705, 273)

- Varenicline is a partial agonist of the α4β2 subtype of the nicotinic acetylcholine receptor. In addition it acts on α3β4 and weakly on α3β2 and α6-containing receptors.
- Acting as a partial agonist varenicline binds to, and partially stimulates, the α4β2 receptor without producing a full effect like nicotine. Due to its competitive binding on these receptors, varenicline blocks the ability of nicotine to bind and stimulate the mesolimbic dopamine system.
- Varenicline also acts as an agonist at 5-HT$_3$ receptors, which may contribute to mood altering effects of varenicline

105. Ans. (d) Increased diffusion capacity

(Ref: Harrison 20th edition, p 1951; Harrison 19th p 306e)

Increased diffusion capacity is seen in:
- Acute congestive heart failure
- Asthma
- Polycythemia
- Pulmonary hemorrhage/Good Pasture syndrome

Decreased diffusion capacity is seen in:
- Pulmonary fibrosis
- Emphysema
- Pulmonary hypertension

106. Ans. (d) Haemoptysis

Ref: Harrison 20th edition, p 1995; Harrison 19th p 1701-04

The three most common symptoms in COPD are cough, sputum production, and exertional dyspnea. Many patients have such symptoms for months or years before seeking medical attention. Although the development of airflow obstruction is a gradual process, many patients date the onset of their disease to an acute illness or exacerbation.

Some patients with advanced disease have paradoxical inward movement of the rib cage with inspiration (Hoover's sign), the result of alteration of the vector of diaphragmatic contraction on the rib cage as a result of chronic hyperinflation.

107. Ans. (b) Spontaneous pneumothorax

(Ref: Harrison 20th edition, p 1995; Harrison 19th p 1701-04)

- Spontaneous pneumothorax is a complication of rupture of a bulla in a emphysematous patient.
- The chronic hypoxia in chronic bronchitis leads to pulmonary artery hypertension and cor pulmonale. The CO_2 retention leads to respiratory acidosis.
- The chronic nature of illness leads to AA type of amyloidosis.

108. Ans. (a) Massive pulmonary embolism

(Ref: Harrison 20th edition, p 1768; Harrison 19th p 1505-06)

Massive pulmonary embolism leads to acute cor pulmonale.

109. Ans. (b) COPD

(Ref: Harrison 20th edition, p 1768; Rubin's pathology 5th/231, Harrison 19th p 1505-06)

110. Ans. (c) Pulmonary embolism

(Ref: Harrison 19th p 1631)

Pulmonary embolism leads to cor-pulmonale with findings like loud P$_2$, murmur of TR, S$_3$ gallop, RV heave and ascites lungs have pulmonary oligaemia with no specific finding.

Bronchiectasis and Suppurative Lung Disease

111. Ans. (a) Clindamycin

(Ref: Harrison 20th edition, p 920; Harrison 19th edition, Page 815)

- The CXR shows an *air fluid level* diagnostic of lung abscess. The history of alcoholism predisposes to suppression of the protective airway reflexes under the influence of alcohol. Hence the anaerobic organism in the saliva can enter the airway and can cause development of suppurative lung abscess.
- The main clinical pointer in the question indicating presence of lung abscess is postural change in purulent sputum.
- The best antibiotic to treat anaerobic lung abscess is Clindamycin.
- Metronidazole does not work in this case.
- TB causes cavity usually in the RUZ.

112. Ans. (a) Mixed (Fine and coarse) Crackles

(Ref: Macloed's Clinical Examination: 13th edition, Page 154)

- Bronchiectasis is sequelae of pulmonary TB (primary and post primary) and occurs due to endobronchial TB. Crackles are heard when air bubbles through the secretions in major dilated bronchi in bronchiectasis. These crackles sound coarse and have a gurgling quality.
- Secondary tubercular bronchiectasis occurs as a result of lung parenchymal destruction with damage in upper lobes. (Bronchiectasis Sicca). In this condition haemoptysis occurs but sputum is not present since the secretions are not able to drain, leading to fine crackles.

Early inspiratory crackles	Bronchiolitis, chronic bronchitis and asthma
Mid-inspiratory crackles bilateral in lower lung fields	Pulmonary oedema
Late inspiratory crackles	Interstitial lung Disease, atelectasis, resolving pneumonia
Bibasilar crackles (both phases of respiration)	Interstitial pulmonary Fibrosis
Bronchial breathing (I:E Ratio=1:1)	Pneumonia

113. **Ans. (b) Cavity**

(Ref: Oxford Handbook of Clinical Imaging, Page 42)

The CT scan shows a thick walled cavity in right lung in clinical setting of diabetes which probably is fungal infection.

114. **Ans. (a) Cylindrical**

(Ref: Harrison 20th edition, p 1983; Harrison 19th edition, page 1694)

Most common type of bronchiectasis is cylindrical type.

115. **Ans. (a) M.A.I**

(Ref: Harrison 20th edition, p 1983; Harrison: 19th edition, page 1694)

Upper lobe bronchiectasis	TB Cystic Fibrosis ABPA Post radiation fibrosis
Mid lung bronchiectasis	M.A.I (Mycobacterium Avium intercellulare) Immotile cilia syndrome
Lower lung bronchiectasis	Chronic recurrent aspiration End stage fibrotic lung disease Recurrent immunodeficiency associated infections
Central bronchiectasis	ABPA Cystic fibrosis Mounier Kuhn Syndrome(Cartilage deficiency leading to tracheomegaly) William Campbell Syndrome

Bronchiectasis Sicca: Only hemoptysis is present without sputum production. It has upper lobe involvement.

116. **Ans. (a) Bilateral varicose Bronchiectasis**

(Ref: Harrison 20th edition, p 1984; Harrison 19th edition, page 308e-3f, 1694)

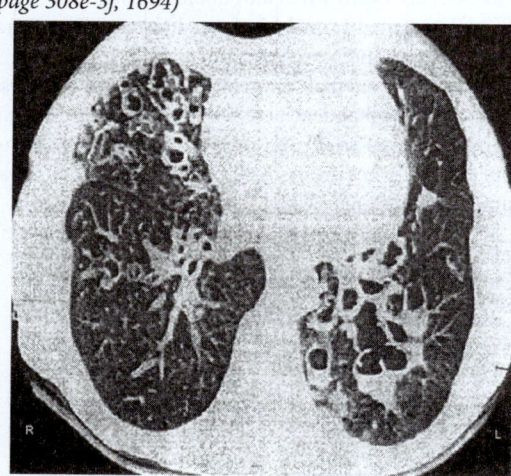

- The image shows multiple cystic cluster of thin-walled cystic spaces in lung parenchyma bilaterally and can be seen to bigger on left side as left lower lobe is more commonly involved in bronchiectasis.
- Fluid-filled bronchi are revealed as tubular or branching structures when they course horizontally.
- Varicose bronchiectasis term implies non-uniform bronchial dilatation.

Multiple Cavitating secondaries	Cavitation occurs in about 4% of total metastasis to lung and history does not give any information about the primary source of malignancy, hence the choice is ruled out.
Interstitial fibrosis	Presents with chronic cough, clubbing but fine crepitations and CT characterized by patchy and predominantly peripheral, subpleural, and bibasilar reticular opacities. The distribution is predominantly posterior. Honey combing is seen along with ground glass appearance.
Miliary tuberculosis	CT shows millet seed appearance and is grossly different from the image provided in the question.

117. **Ans. (a) HRCT scan**

(Ref: Harrison 20th edition, p 1984; Harrison 19th ed. / 308e-3f, 16940)

- The best test to evaluate the destruction and dilatation of large airways which are filled with pus in Bronchiectasis is HRCT
- Spiral CT is preferred for pulmonary embolism
- Pulmonary angiography is done for lung sequestration and is gold standard for pulmonary embolism.

118. **Ans. (b) Oral Anaerobes**

(Ref: Harrison 20th edition, p 920; Harrison 19th p 813, 1098)

- The term *lung abscess* refers to a microbial infection of the lung which results in necrosis of the pulmonary parenchyma.
- In the given choices almost all cause lung abscess. However Harrison's mentions: **Most lung abscesses in moribund intubated patients are due to anaerobic bacteria, like pepto streptococcus, Bacteroides etc.**

119. **Ans. (a) CT chest**

(Ref: Harrison 19th, page 1664)

- The CT scan allows better delineation of parenchymal processes, pleural disease, masses or nodules, and cavity.

120. **Ans. (b) CT scan**

(Ref: Harrison 20th edition, p 1920; Harrison 19th p 308e; 1694)

Chest CT is more specific for bronchiectasis and is the imaging modality of choice for confirming the diagnosis

121. Ans. (d) Necrotising pneumonia

(Ref: Harrison 20th edition, p 1983; Harrison 19th p 1694-95)

Bronchiectasis may be the sequela of a variety of necrotizing infections that are either inadequately treated or not treated at all. Primary infection is a particularly common cause of bronchiectasis.

122. Ans. (b) Pancreatic insufficiency

(Ref: Nelson 20th edition, p 2115)

123. Ans. (d) All of the above

(Ref: Nelson 20th edition p 2113)

Structures that make up the cilia including inner and/or outer dynein arms, central apparatus, radial spokes, etc. are missing or dysfunctional and thus the axoneme structure lacks the ability to move. Axonemes are the elongated structures that make up cilia and flagella. The underlying cause, dysfunction of the cilia begins during and impacts the embryologic phase of development, in immotile cilia syndrome.

124. Ans. (c) Whooping cough

(Ref: Nelson 20th edition, p 2095; Harrison 19th p 1694-95)

Typical offending organisms that have been known to cause bronchiectasis include the following

1. Pertussis
2. Influenza virus
3. Herpes simplex virus
4. Certain types of adenovirus
5. Measles virus
6. Mycobacterium tuberculosis/Mycoplasa pneumoniae

These organisms lead to progressive bronchial wall damage and dilation.

125. Ans. (b) Crazy paving appearance

(Ref: Harrison 20th edition, p 1920; Harrison 19th p 308e; 1694-95)

- While chest radiographs lack sensitivity, the presence of "tram tracks" indicating dilated airways is seen with bronchiectasis.
- Chest CT is more specific for bronchiectasis and is the imaging modality of choice for confirming the diagnosis. CT findings include airway dilation detected as parallel "tram tracks" or as the "signet-ring sign"—a cross-sectional area of the airway with a diameter at least 1.5 times that of the adjacent vessel.
- The crazy-paving pattern is seen in pulmonary alveolar proteinois and also can be observed in exogenous lipoid pneumonia, sarcoidosis, mucinous bronchoalveolar cell carcinoma, and acute respiratory distress syndrome.

126. Ans. (c) Left lower lobe

(Ref: Hammar's pulmonary pathology, p 141)

- Idiopathic bronchiectatic lesions are most commonly found in the lower lobes, probably because mucociliary clearance is facilitated by gravity in the upper lobes.
- The lesions are identified most commonly in the left lower lobe, followed by the right lower lobe and left upper lobe
- Bronchiectasis due to primary ciliary dyskinesia in the middle lobe, and bronchiectasis due to hypogammaglobulinemia in the lower/middle lobe and lingual segment
- The most common organisms are Haemophilus influenza (15%), Staphylococcus aureus (13%), Streptococcus pneumonia (5%), Pseudomonas aeruginosa (5%), and Mycoplasma pneumonia (5%).

127. Ans. (b) Lung cancer

(Ref: Harrison 20th edition, p 1985; API 8th / 374, 375, Harrison 19th p 1694-95)

Cystic Fibrosis

128. Ans. (c) Asthenospermia

Ref: Webster's Dictionary: 3rd edition, Page 231

- *Asthenospermia* or poor sperm motility is due to missing dynein arms, which is the basic defect of *Kartagener's syndrome*.
- It is a ciliopathic, autosomal recessive genetic disorder.
- Triad consists situs inversus, chronic sinusitis and bronchiectasis.

129. Ans. (b) Acinetobacter baumannii

Ref: Harrison 20th edition, p 1986; Harrison 19th edition, page 1699

- In patients with cystic fibrosis, Hemophilus influenzae and Staphylococcus aureus are responsible for early colonization.
- Later pseudomonas is the main organism colonizing the airways in 50% of patients followed by Burkholderia cepacia.
- Aspergillus fumigatus is the most common fungus that can colonise airways with/ without causing any lung disease. It can be found in airways of normal people as well as cystic fibrosis.

130. Ans. (a) Lung infections

(Ref: Nelson 20th p 2102-03; Harrison 19th p 1697-98, 1686)

Feature	%
Acute or persistent respiratory symptoms	50.5
Failure to thrive, malnutrition	42.9
Abnormal stools	35.0
Meconium ileus, intestinal obstruction	18.8
Family history	16.8
Electrolyte, acid-base abnormality	5.4
Rectal prolapse	3.4
Nasal polyps, sinus disease	2.0
Hepatobiliary disease	0.9

131. Ans. (d) Sweat chloride >60 mEq/dl

(Ref: Nelson 20th p 2104; Harrison 19th p 1698-99)

- The diagnosis of CF rests on the combination of clinical criteria and abnormal CFTR function as documented by sweat tests, nasal PD measurements, and CFTR mutation analysis.
- More than 60 mEq/L of chloride in sweat is diagnostic of CF when 1 or more other criteria are present.

132. Ans. (c) Chronic constipation

(Ref: Nelson 20th p 2103)

- In cystic fibrosis the excessive loss of salt in the sweat predisposes young children to salt depletion episodes, especially during episodes of gastroenteritis and during warm weather. These children present with hypochloremic alkalosis. Frequently, parents notice salt "frosting" of the skin or a salty taste when they kiss the child
- In addition to exocrine pancreatic insufficiency, evidence for hyperglycemia and glycosuria including polyuria and weight loss may appear, especially in the 2nd decade of life. Eight percent of 11–17 yr old patients and 18% of 18–24 yr olds have insulin-dependent diabetes.
- Exacerbations of lung symptoms, presumably owing to more active airways infection, eventually require repeated hospitalizations for effective treatment. Cor pulmonale, respiratory failure, and death eventually supervene unless lung transplantation is accomplished. Colonization with Burkholderia cepacia and other multidrug-resistant organisms may be associated with particularly rapid pulmonary deterioration and death.
- *(Instead of constipation, steatorrhea due to pancreatic exocrine insufficiency is a common presentation leading to malnutrition and weight loss.)*

133. Ans. (d) 7

Ref: Harrison 20th edition, p 1986; Harrison 19th p 1697-98, 435

- One thousand mutations have been described that can affect the CFTR gene.
- In patients with cystic fibrosis the blockage of the movement of ions and, therefore, water into and out of cells leads to the production of thick mucus.
- Absent vas deferens in males explains infertility in cystic fibrosis.
- In people with mutations giving rise to cystic fibrosis, the blockage in ion transport occurs in epithelial cells that line the passageways of the lungs, pancreas, and other organs. This leads to chronic dysfunction, disability, and a reduced life expectancy.
- The most common mutation, ÄF508 results from a deletion (Ä) of three nucleotides which results in a loss of the amino acid phenylalanine (F) at the 508th position on the protein. As a result the protein does not fold normally and is more quickly degraded.

134. Ans. (d) Glomerulonephritis

(Ref: Nelson 20th p 2102)

135. Ans. (b) Subluxation of lens

(Ref: Nelson 20th p 2115)

- Kartagener syndrome/immotile ciliary syndrome, is a rare, ciliopathic, autosomal recessive genetic disorder that causes a defect in the action of the cilia lining the respiratory tract lower and upper, sinuses, Eustachian tube, middle ear, flagella of sperm in males and situs inversus.
- *Triad includes bronchiectasis, sinusitis and situs inversus.*
- The main consequence of impaired ciliary function is reduced or absent mucus clearance from the lungs, and susceptibility to chronic recurrent respiratory infections, including sinusitis, bronchitis, pneumonia, and otitis media. Progressive damage to the respiratory system is common, including progressive bronchiectasis beginning in early childhood, and sinus disease.
- In males, immotility of sperm can lead to infertility.
- There is a marked reduction in fertility in female sufferers of Kartagener's Syndrome.
- Many affected individuals experience hearing loss and show symptoms of glue ear.

136. Ans. (a) Pseudomonas

(Ref: Harrison 20th edition, p 1988; FISHMAN pulmonary diseases 2008 edition, ch. 400, pg. 866, Harrison 19th p 1697)

- Cystic fibrosis has a high prevalence of airway colonization with Staphylococcus aureus, Pseudomonas aeruginosa and Burkholderia cepacia.
- The CF airway epithelial cells or surface liquids provide a favorable environment for harboring these organisms. CF airway epithelium may be compromised in its innate defenses against these organisms, through either acquired or genetic alterations.
- Another problem is the propensity for P. aeruginosa to undergo mucoid transformation in the CF airways. The complex polysaccharide produced by these organisms generates a biofilm that provides a hypoxic environment and thereby protects Pseudomonas against antimicrobial agents

Interstitial Lung Disease

137. Ans. (a) Asbestosis

Ref: Harrison 20th edition. page 1978: Robbins 9th edition, page 691

The image shows alveoli at 3'o clock position surrounded by cellular infiltrate and beaded or fusiform basophilic rods at 9'o clock position. Coupled with history of pleural thickening the diagnosis is asbestosis. Pleural thickening and calcification are a feature of asbestosis.

138. Ans. (b) Sturge Weber syndrome

Ref: Harrison 19th edition, page 1708

Inherited diseases leading to ILD

1. Tuberous sclerosis
2. Neurofibromatosis
3. Niemann Pick disease
4. Gaucher's disease
5. Hermansky- pudlak Syndrome

139. Ans. (a) Hypersensitivity pneumonitis

Ref: Harrison: 19th edition, page 1708

Granulomatous lung response is seen in

Known causes	Unknown causes
1. Hypersensitivity pneumonitis (organic dusts) 2. Beryllium 3. Silicosis	1. Sarcoidosis 2. Granulomatosis Vasculitides 3. Wegener's Granulomatosis 4. Churg Strauss 5. Bronchocentric Granulomatosis 6. Lymphomatoid Granulomatosis

Choice B, C and D lead to alveolitis and interstitial inflammation.

140. Ans. (a) Chest X-ray

Ref: Harrison 20th edition, p 2001; Harrison 19th edition, page 1710

ILD may be first suspected on basis of abnormal CXR. Findings seen are:

1. Bibasilar reticular pattern
2. Nodular opacities
3. Honeycombing

- Subsequently HRCT is done for assessment of extent of disease, mediastinal adenopathy and determining site for Biopsy.
- Lung biopsy is the most effective method for confirming diagnosis of ILD (page 1710: Harrison 19th).
- MDCT is used in pulmonary embolism. Hence choice C is ruled out.
- Spirometry findings show restrictive pattern but in some cases obstructive pattern is seen. Hence choice D is ruled out.

141. Ans. (b) Pulmonary Lymphangioleiomyomatosis

Ref: Harrison 20th edition, p A12; Harrison 19th edition, page 1716

- Interstitial lung disease leads to restrictive pattern on spirometry.
- However tuberous sclerosis and Lymphangioleiomyomatosis are *exceptions* and *lead to an obstructive pattern*.
- Pulmonary LAM presents in young females with emphysema, recurrent pneumo-thorax and chylous pleural effusion.

142. Ans. (b) Hamman Rich Syndrome

Ref: Harrison 20th edition, p 2004; Harrison 19th edition, page 1712

Hamman rich syndrome is a rare subset of ILD that can present dramatically like ARDS. It begins as a prodromal illness lasting a week followed by ARDS like symptoms. Mortality rate hits 60% with patients dying within 6 months of presentation.

143. Ans. (a) Cryptogenic organising pneumonia

Ref: Harrison 20th edition, p 2004; Harrison 19th edition, page 1712

Cryptogenic organising pneumonia has unknown etiology and has predilection for lower lobe of lung.

There are three ILD which are associated with cigarette smoking

1. DIP (Desquamative interstitial pneumonia) shows response to smoking cessation and histologically characterised by accumulation of macrophages in intra-alveolar spaces.
2. Respiratory bronchiolitis is a subset of DIP with cellular infiltrate in respiratory bronchioles. It resolves with cessation of cigarette smoking.
3. Pulmonary Langerhan cell Histiocytosis has presence of reticular or nodular opacities and upper lobe cysts. That explains development of pneumothorax. It improves with cessation of cigarette smoking.

144. Ans. (d) Acebrophylline

Ref: Harrison 20th edition, p 2002-3; Harrison 19th edition, page 1712

- Thalidomide reduces cough in patients of IPF.
- Chronic micro-aspiration may play a role in pathogenesis of IPF. Hence therapy of GER is beneficial.
- Lung transplantation referral should be done earlier due to unpredictable nature of progression of disease.
- Bronchodilators have no role in progression or management of IPF.
- Steroids and warfarin (due to risk of thrombotic vascular events) worsen mortality rates.

145. Ans. (c) Organising pneumonia

Ref: Harrison 19th edition, Page 1711

Organising pneumonia	Foamy macrophages in BAL with low CD4:CD8 ration
Hypersensitivity pneumonitis	Marked Lymphocytosis
Sarcoidosis	Marked lymphocytosis with CD4 : CD8 ratio of >3.5
Diffuse alveolar haemorrhage	Hemosiderin laden macrophages

146. Ans. (b) Pulmonary alveolar Proteinosis

Ref: CMDT 2019 p. 304, Harrison 19th edition, page 1711 and 1714

- PAS material in alveoli is accumulated surfactant due to decreased turnover in pulmonary alveolar proteinosis.
- It is characterised by dysfunction of alveolar macrophages which results in decreased surfactant clearance.
- The same material may be coughed up by patients and described as chunky gelatinous plugs.
- Lipoid pneumonia will show fat globules in macrophages.

147. Ans. (a) Hypersensitivity reaction to Aspergillus

Ref: Harrison 19th edition, Page 1716

Bronchocentric Granulomatosis is characterised by peri-bronchial necrotizing granulomatous inflammation. It occurs due to:

1. Hypersensitivity reaction to aspergillus in patients with asthma
2. In patients without asthma, rheumatoid arthritis and infections like TB are associated.

Immunological reaction to HIV virus leads to lymphocytic interstitial pneumonitis.

148. Ans. (b) Non-specific interstitial pneumonia

Ref: Harrison 20th edition, p 2003; Harrison 19th edition, page 1714

- Fibrotic NSIP is the most common subtype of ILD seen in patients of Sjogren syndrome.
- NSIP is also the most common subtype of ILD seen in patients of connective tissue disorders.
- Usual interstitial pneumonitis is found in idiopathic pulmonary fibrosis.
- Cryptogenic organising pneumonia has unknown etiology.
- Acute interstitial pneumonitis/ Hamman rich syndrome presents as ARDS like illness.

149. Ans. (a) Pleural calcification

(Ref: Harrison 20th edition, p 1978; Harrison: 19th edition, page 1689)

- The CXR shows thickened pleural plaques, and calcification along the parietal pleura, particularly along the lower lung fields and the diaphragm on the right side. Lateral to the left heart border another plaque is seen.
- Without additional manifestations, pleural plaques imply only exposure, not pulmonary impairment. Loss of lung volume due to fibrosis is seen on the left side. Tracheal position cannot be commented due to rotation in the film.

150. Ans. (a) Pneumoconiosis

(Ref: Oxford Handbook of medical imaging, Page 80)

- The CT chest shows presence of multiple small, discrete nodules more in posterior areas in bilateral lung fields, suggestive of pneumoconiosis.
- Lung cancer will *not have a diffuse involvement* and is ruled out.
- Bronchiectasis has dilated deformed airways filled with pus which are not visualised in this CT scan.

151. Ans. (a) Coal miner's lung

(Ref: Harrison's 19th edition, 1708; chapter 13 Robbins 8th edition, page 494)

- Much of the symptomatology associated with simple CWP is due to the effects of coal dust on the development of chronic bronchitis and C.O.P.D . The effects of coal dust are additive to those of cigarette smoking.
- *Choice D, Ankylosing spondylitis has pulmonary manifestations of the disease include fibrosis of the upper lobes, interstitial lung disease, and ventilatory impairment due to chest wall restriction, sleep apnea.*
- Choice C, Asbestosis leads to alveolitis and pulmonary fibrosis
- Choice B, is an autoimmune disease that may be associated with pulmonary fibrosis

152. Ans. (a) Sarcoidosis

(Ref: 2206, Harrison 19th edition, Page 1332)

Cavity is gas-filled space within a zone of pulmonary consolidation or within a mass or nodule, produced by the expulsion of a necrotic part of the lesion via the bronchial tree.

Between the two dose choices sarcoidosis and histoplasmosis, sarcoidosis is the correct answer. This is so because cavitation in sarcoidosis is not mentioned in harrison but only in medical journals.

Sarcoidosis	Lung findings are: • Peri-bronchial thickening and reticular nodular changes, which are predominantly subpleural. • 50% patients have obstructive airway disease with remaining developing restrictive lung disease. • CXR can show infiltrates, fibrosis and hilar lymphadenopathy.
Tuberculosis	• *Mycobacterium tuberculosis* generally has the highest prevalence of cavities among persons with pulmonary disease of any infection, probably because this pathogen causes extensive caseous necrosis. • In the case of *M. tuberculosis*, the tendency to form cavities is clearly advantageous to the propagation of the organism because cavities contain large numbers of organisms, which can then be efficiently aerosolized and transmitted to other susceptible hosts
Carcinoma lung	Cavitation is more frequently found among cases of squamous cell carcinomas than other histological type. Furthermore, the presence of cavitation in a lung tumor has been associated with a worse prognosis. Other primary tumors in the lung, such as lymphoma and Kaposi's sarcoma, may also present with cavitary lesions
Histoplasma	Lung manifestations of pulmonary histoplasmosis are: • Chest radiographs usually show signs of pneumonitis with hilar or mediastinal adenopathy. • Pulmonary infiltrates may be focal with light exposure or diffuse with heavy exposure. • *Chronic cavitary histoplasmosis is seen in smokers who have structural lung disease*

153. Ans. (b) HRCT

(Ref: Harrison 20th edition, p 2001; Harrison 19th edition, page 1710)

- Ideally lung biopsy should be done but is not given in the choices.High-resolution computed tomography is superior to the plain chest x-ray for early detection and confirmation of suspected ILD.
- In addition, HRCT allows better assessment of the extent and distribution of disease. Coexisting disease is often best recognized on HRCT scanning, e.g., mediastinal adenopathy, carcinoma, or emphysema.
- *In the appropriate clinical setting HRCT may be sufficiently characteristic to preclude the need for lung biopsy*

154. Ans. (c) Interstitial Fibrosis

(Ref: Page 287, Essentials of Medical Physiology, Leonard, 3rd edition)

- The curve is shifted downwards and to the right (Compliance is decreased) by pulmonary oedema and interstitial pulmonary fibrosis. There is stiffening and scarring of lung which leads to reduced lung compliance.

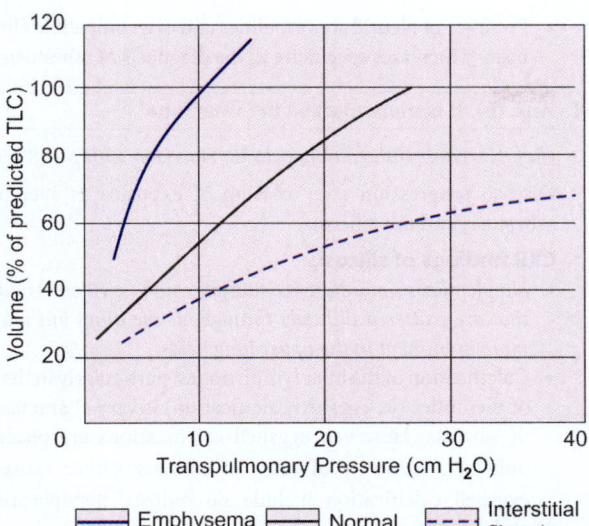

- In emphysema, the curve is shifted upward and to the left (compliance is increased).

155. Ans. (c) Silicosis

(Ref: Harrison 20th edition, p 1979; Harrison 19th edition, 1689-90)

- Conglomerate shadows are seen in silicosis
- Silicosis is the most prevalent occupational disease in the world caused by the inhalation of crystalline silica Quartz.
- On continued dust exposure, the nodules increase in size and number ultimately covering most parts of the lungs.
- The ILO classifies these large opacities as A, B based on size or on total cross-sectional area relative to the size of right upper zone.
- With coalescence of the nodules, the upper lobes become fibrotic and contract making the conglomerate nodules to migrate towards the hilar areas.
- Summary of Chest X ray findings in Silicosis

  1. Snow storm appearance of lung fields
  2. Hilar lymphadenopathy
  3. Egg-shell calcifications of the lymph nodes is strongly suggestive of silicosis
  4. The nodular opacities can enlarge and coalesce forming conglomerate shadows
  5. Progressive massive fibrosis PMF is seen when these nodules enlarge to more than 1 cm in diameter with associated fibrosis of lung

156. Ans. (a) Emphysema

(Ref: Harrison 20th edition, p 1979; Harrison 19th edition, page 308e-5)

The CXR of Coal worker patient shows presence of hyperinflation in lungs with a tubular appearance of heart. The lungs appear to be relatively more black with flattening of diaphragm on both sides. The heart appears smaller as lungs are hyper-inflated. These findings are suggestive of emphysema.

Coal worker pneumoconiosis is exposure to carbon and leads to findings of obstructive airway disease and not interstitial lung disease.

157. Ans. (a) Ground Glass pattern

(Ref: Harrison 20th edition, p 1978-79; Harrison 19th edition and page 2120: Nelson 20th edition, page 1710)

The image shows CT Chest with hazy appearance of increased attenuation with ground glass appearance and with preserved bronchial and vascular markings. This pattern suggest Interstitial lung Disease.

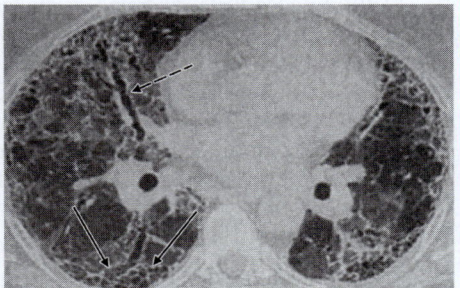

Honey comb pattern seen in usual interstitial pneumonitis. (Choice B)

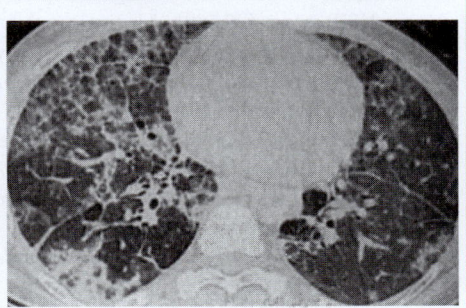

Crazy pavement pattern is seen mainly with pulmonary alveolar proteinosis. (Choice C)

158. Ans. (b) Reticular shadows

(Ref: Harrison 20th edition, p 1978; Harrison 19th edition, page 1712-13)

- The CXR shows presence of reticular nodular shadows in both lung fields.
- Choice A is ruled out as emphysema shows hyperinflation with flattening of diaphragm.
- Choice C and D are associated with increased CT ratio and cardiac borders can be ruled out. Hence answer by exclusion is choice B.
- The various reticular patterns seen are:

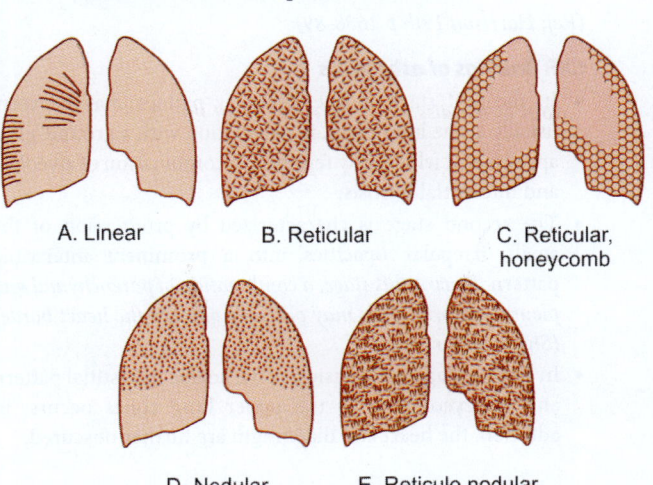

A. Linear   B. Reticular   C. Reticular, honeycomb

D. Nodular   E. Reticulo nodular

159. Ans. (b) Idiopathic pulmonary fibrosis

(Ref: Harrison 20th edition, p 2002; Harrison 19th edition, page 1712-13)

The CT image shows honey combing of lung and is seen in IPF. Two-thirds to 75% of patients with *IPF* and familial lung fibrosis have a history of smoking. Patients with *PLCH, respiratory bronchiolitis/desquamative interstitial pneumonia (DIP), Goodpasture's syndrome, respiratory bronchiolitis, and pulmonary alveolar proteinosis* are usually current or former smokers.

Areas of honeycomb change are composed of cystic fibrotic air spaces that frequently are lined by bronchiolar epithelium and filled with mucin. Smooth-muscle hyperplasia is commonly seen in areas of fibrosis and honeycomb change.

160. Ans. (d) Good prognosis

(Ref: Harrison 20th edition, p 2003; Harrison 19th p 1712, 1255)

- NSIP is a subacute restrictive process with a presentation similar to that of idiopathic pulmonary *fibrosis but usually at a younger age, most commonly in women who have never smoked.*
- The majority of patients with NSIP have a *good prognosis* (5-year mortality rate estimated at <15%), with most showing improvement after treatment with glucocorticoids, often used in combination with azathioprine
- Investigations = HRCT shows bilateral, subpleural ground-glass opacities, often associated with lower lobe volume loss. Patchy areas of airspace consolidation and reticular abnormalities may be present, but honeycombing is unusual.

161. Ans. (b) Lymph Node Biopsy

(Ref: Harrison 20th edition, p 2605; Harrison 19th p 2209-2210)

162. Ans. (d) Atelectasis

(Ref: Harrison 20th edition, p 1978; Harrison 19th p 1689-90)

Asbestos is known to cause mesotheliomas and bronchial cancers which can lead to pleural effusions.

163. Ans. (c) Hilar lymphadenopathy

(Ref: Harrison 19th p 1688-89)

CXR findings of asbestosis

- In the first stage, a fine, reticular pattern may be seen, usually at the lung bases, in association with a ground-glass appearance, which may represent a combination of alveolitis and interstitial fibrosis.
- The second stage is characterized by progression of the small, irregular opacities into a prominent interstitial pattern. *During this stage, a combination of parenchymal and pleural abnormalities may partially obscure the heart border (Shaggy Heart Sign)*
- In the last stage, progression of the coarse interstitial pattern and honeycombing to the upper lung zones occurs; in addition, the heart and diaphragm are further obscured.
- Presence of pleural abnormalities and of a compatible clinical history increases specificity in the diagnosis of asbestosis.

164. Ans. (b) It is more marked in lower zone

(Ref: Harrison 20th edition, p 1978; Harrison 19th p 1689-90)

Disease progression after ceasing of exposure is seen with asbestosis and not silicosis.

CXR findings of silicosis

- *Simple silicosis manifests as multiple small (< 10 mm) nodules that are scattered diffusely throughout the lungs but may be more prominent in the upper lung fields.*
- Calcification of the hilar lymph nodes, particularly in the rim of the nodes (ie, eggshell calcification) is very characteristic of silicosis. However, eggshell calcifications are observed only in a minority of cases of silicosis. Other causes of eggshell calcification include sarcoidosis, histoplasmosis, and irradiation.
- Progressive massive fibrosis manifests as bilateral upper lobe masses, which are formed by the coalescence of nodules.
- Cavitation may be seen.
- As these masses retract toward the hilum because of fibrosis, the lower lung fields may appear overinflated.
- Hilar calcifications may be present

165. Ans. (a) High residual lung volume

(Ref: Harrison 20th edition, p 1946)

Residual volume is increased in:

1. Asthma
2. COPD
3. Myasthenia Gravis
4. Normal in obesity but increased in morbid obesity

166. Ans. (d) Coarse crepitations

(Ref: Harrison 20th edition, p 2001; Harrison 19th p 1708)

- In I.L.D patients frequently are Dyspneic, which may be more pronounced with activity and generally is associated with an accompanying tachypnea.
- Central cyanosis may be present if significant hypoxemia and arterial oxygen desaturation are present.
- Fine end-inspiratory pulmonary rales (Velcro rales) are a common finding and may be difficult to distinguish from those auscultated in patients with congestive heart failure.
- Wheezes may be heard and reflect airway involvement, as in sarcoidosis.
- A right-sided gallop (S3), an accentuated second heart sound (P2) with fixed or paradoxic splitting, and a right ventricular lift may be present. These indicate the presence of Cor pulmonale.
- Digital clubbing is seen in I.L.D.

167. Ans. (d) Anterior uveitis

(Ref: Harrison 20th edition, p 2601)

Heerfordt syndrome is a variant of sarcoidosis and comprises of
1. **P**arotid enlargement
2. Ocular involvement (anterior **U**veitis)
3. **F**ever
4. **F**acial palsy
(mnemonic: **PUFF**)

Lofgren syndrome consists of
1. Hilar **l**ymphadenopathy
2. **O**steoarthropathy
3. **F**ever
4. **G**ranulomatous uveitis
5. **E**rythema **N**odosum
(mnemonic: **LOFGREN**)

168. Ans. (b) Egg shell calcification of hilar lymph nodes

(Ref: Harrison 20th edition, p 1978; Harrison 19th p 1689)

Causes of egg shell calcification in CXR

1. Silicosis
2. Treated lymphoma: (post irradiation Hodgkin disease) usually 1-9 years following treatment
3. Coal workers' pneumoconiosis (CWP)
4. Scleroderma
5. Amyloidosis
6. Blastomycosis

169. Ans. (a) Dyspnea resolves after cessation of exposure

(Ref: Harrison 20th edition, p 1977)

- Byssinosis presents with Monday Chest tightness which resolves with cessation of cotton dust exposure
- Byssinosis presents as hypersensitivity pneumonitis with honey-comb lung.
- In broncho-alveolar lavage of hypersensitivity pneumonitis patients lymphocytes are present and not eosinophils.

170. Ans. (a) End inspiratory Rales

(Ref: Harrison 20th edition, p 2001; Harrison 19th p 1709-10)

171. Ans. (c) Bronchial asthma

(Ref: Harrison 20th edition, p 1977; Harrison 19th p 1708-10)

172. Ans. (a) Byssinosis

(Ref: Harrison 20th edition, p 1977; Harrison 19th p 1688, 1691)

173. Ans. (a) Atelectasis

Ref: Harrison 20th edition, p 1978; Harrison 19th p 1689-90)

According to the American Thoracic Society (ATS), the general diagnostic criteria for asbestosis are:
- Evidence of structural pathology consistent with asbestosis, as documented by imaging or histology
- Evidence of causation by asbestos as documented by the occupational and environmental history, markers of exposure (usually pleural plaques), recovery of asbestos bodies, or other means
  - More than 50% of people affected with asbestosis develop *plaques in the parietal pleura*. Once apparent, the radiographic findings in asbestosis may slowly progress or remain static, even in the absence of further asbestos exposure. *Rapid progression suggests an alternative diagnosis.*
- Asbestosis resembles many other diffuse interstitial lung diseases, including other pneumoconioses. The differential diagnosis includes Idiopathic Pulmonary Fibrosis (IPF), Hypersensitivity pneumonitis, sarcoidosis, and others. Although lung biopsy is usually not necessary, the presence of *asbestos bodies in association with pulmonary fibrosis* establishes the diagnosis

174. Ans. (c) Rheumatoid Arthritis

(Ref: Harrison 20th edition, p 1979; Harrison 19th p 1690, 2138)

175. Ans. (d) Bronchogenic carcinoma

(Ref: Harrison 20th edition, p 2605; Harrison 19th p 506; 511-12, 1688, 2206)

Pneumonia

176. Ans. (a) Streptococcus pneumoniae

Ref: Jawetz medical microbiology 26th edition, Page 218

Streptococcus pneumoniae in sputum are seen as lancet-shaped gram-positive diplococci. The leading cause of meningitis in children is streptococcus pneumoniae.

177. Ans. (b) Cotrimoxazole

Ref: Harrison 20th edition, Page 1432

The image shows exudate in alveoli of lung stained with silver stain. The black organisms are Pneumocystis jiroveci. The drug used for Pneumocystis Jiroveci is co-trimoxazole.

178. Ans. (a) CMV pneumonia

Ref: Harrison 20th edition, page 1363; Robbins 9th edition, page 687

- Immunocompromised state narrows down the choices to A and D.
- The image depicts infected cells in alveoli of lungs with prominent basophilic nuclear inclusions, with a clear halo, and smaller basophilic cytoplasmic inclusions.
- Choice B is a presentation of Interstitial Lung Disease and presents gradually.
- Choice C would have a history of weight loss, cough, hemoptysis and the slide would show multiple small cells with scant cytoplasm, ill defined borders and finely granular nuclear chromatin.

179. Ans. (c) Azithromycin

Ref: Harrison 20th edition, Page 913

- For management of patients of CAP who are previously healthy and have not received antibiotics in the previous 3 months a macrolide like clarithromycin or azithromycin should be used.
- In setting of co-morbidities or having received antibiotics in the previous 3 months respiratory fluoroquinolones are used.

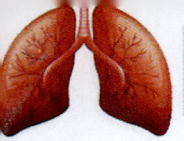

180. Ans. (a) Acinetobacter

Ref: Harrison 20th edition, page 915

- The leading cause of Ventilator associated pneumonia (MDR pathogens) is Pseudomonas aeruginosa > MRSA > Acinetobacter.
- The leading cause of Ventilator associated pneumonia (MDR pathogen) is Streptococcus Pneumoniae > Hemophilus influenzae.

Microbiologic Causes of Ventilator-Associated Pneumonia

NON-MDR Pathogens	MDR Pathogens

• Streptococcus pneumoniae
• Other Streptococcus spp.
• Haemophilus influenzae
• Methicillin-sensitive Staphylococcus aureus
• Antiobiotic-sensitive Enterobacteriaceae
  ■ Escherichia coli
  ■ Klebsiella pneumoniae
  ■ Proteus spp.
  ■ Enterobacter spp.
  ■ Serratia marcescens
	• Pseudomonas aeruginosa
	• Methicillin-resistant S. aureus
	• Acinetobacter spp.
	• Antibiotic-resistance Enterobacteriaceae
	  ■ ESBL-positive stains
	  ■ Carbapenem-resistant strains
	• Leguibella pneumophila
	• Burkholderia cepacia
	• Aspergillus spp.

181. Ans. (c) SBP >100 mmHg

Ref: Harrison 20th edition, p 911; Harrison 19th edition, page 806-807

CURB-65 Criteria

C: Confusion
U: urea >7 mmol/L
R: Respiratory rate >30/min
B: SBP <90 mmHg or DBP <60 mmHg
65: Age >65 years

182. Ans. (d) Structural lung disease: Burkholderia

Ref: Harrison 20th edition, p 910; Harrison: 19th edition, page 805

- Choice A aspiration pneumonia occurs in depressed level of consciousness and the commonest organism is oral anaerobes and gram negative bacteria.
- Choice B heavy alcohol use also leads to depressed level of consciousness.
- Choice C poor dental hygiene leads to Streptococcus mutans contributing to dental caries.
- In structural lung disease pseudomonas and Burkholderia are common causative organisms.

Factor	Possible pathogen(s)
Alcoholism	Streptococcus pneumoniae, oral anaerobes, Klebsiella pneumoniae, Acinetobacter spp., Mycobacterium tuberculosis
COPD and/or smoking	Haemophilus influenzae, Pseudomonas aeruginosa, Legionella spp., S. pneumoniae, Moraxella catarrhalis, Chlamydia pneumoniae

Contd...

Factor	Possible pathogen(s)
Structural lung disease (e.g., bronchiectasis)	P. aeruginosa, Burkholderia cepacea, Staphylococcus aureus
Dementia, stroke, decreased level of consciousness	Oral anerobes, gram-negative enteric bacteria
Lung abscess	CA-MRSA, oral anerobes, enemic fungi, M. tuberculosis, atypical mycobacteria

183. Ans. (d) Lung abscess formation is very uncommon

(Ref: CMDT 2019, Page 278)

- Klebsiella pneumonia is common in alcoholics and immunocompromised patients and presents as upper lobe involvement.
- CXR shows homogenous non segmental lobar consolidation showing bulging fissure sign and lung abscess in 50% of cases.
- Mass within a mass or air crescent sign occur secondary to sloughed lung parenchyma.
- Hence CT chest shows poorly marginated lowly attenuated areas with and without small air containing cavities called as pneumatoceles
- *Pulmonary necrosis, pleural effusion, and empyema can occur with disease progression.*

184. Ans. (c) Legionella pneumophila

(Ref: Harrison 20th edition, p 910; Harrison 19th edition, page 1016)

- The clinical profile of fever, cough and X-Ray revealing bilateral pneumonitis and presence of diarrhea and confusion indicates presence of atypical pneumonia.
- *The organism causing atypical pneumonia out of the four choices is Legionella pneumophila.*
- The presence of confusion can be explained by hyponatremia due to SIADH.

Clinical clues suggestive of legionnaires' Disease

Diarrhea
High fever (>40°C; >104°F)
Numerous neutrophils but no organisms revealed by Gram's staining of respiratory secretions
Hyponatremia (serum sodium level <131 mg/dL)
Failure to respond to β-lactam drugs (penicillins or cephalosporins) and aminoglycoside antibiotics
Occurrence of illness in an environment in which the potable water supply is known to be contaminated with Legionella
Onset of symptoms within 10 days after discharge from the hospital

185. Ans. (d) Erythromycin

(Ref: Harrison 18th edition, Table 175-2)

Organism	Drug(s)
M. pneumonia	Azithromycin, clarithromycin, erythromycin
U. urealyticum, U. Parvum	Azithromycin, clarithromycin

186. Ans. (a) Legionella

(Ref: Harrison 20th edition, p 1472; Harrison 19th edition, page 1016)

The Clinical manifestations often considered classic for Legionella pneumophila/Legionnaires' disease may suggest the following diagnosis:
- High fever (>40°C; >104°F)
- Diarrhoea
- Numerous neutrophils but no organisms revealed by Gram's staining of respiratory secretions
- Hyponatremia (serum sodium level <131 mg/dL)
- Failure to respond to beta -lactam drugs (penicillins or cephalosporins)
- Occurrence of illness in an environment in which the potable water supply is known to be contaminated with Legionella
- Onset of symptoms within 10 days after discharge from the hospital

187. Ans. (d) Sulfomethoxazole and trimethoprim

(Ref: CMDT 2019 p 1361; Harrison 19th ed. / 492)

- Prophylaxis with trimethoprim-sulfamethoxazole (TMPS-MZ) prevents many opportunistic infections, including infection with P. carinii, Toxoplasma gondii, and community-acquired respiratory, gastrointestinal, and urinary tract pathogens.
- Intolerance of TMP-SMZ is common; desensitization is useful less often in transplant patients than in patients with AIDS. Alternative agents provide a narrower spectrum of protection than does TMP-SMZ and less adequate protection against Pneumocystis species

188. Ans. (c) Systolic Blood pressure is more than 90 mmHg

(Ref: Harrison 20th edition, p 911)

- CURB 65 also known as the CURB criteria is a clinical prediction rule that has been validated for predicting mortality in Community Acquired Pnemonia.
- The CURB-65 criteria includes five variables:

  - Confusion
  - Urea >7 mmol/L
  - Respiratory rate > 30/min
  - Blood pressure, systolic < 90 mmHg or diastolic < 60 mmHg; and
  - Age >65 years

- Each criteria has one point which predicts the mortality in CAP.
  - Score 0–1: 30-day mortality rate is 1.5%- can be treated outside the hospital.
  - Score 2: 30-day mortality rate is 9.2%, and patients should be admitted to the hospital.
  - Score 3: mortality rates are 22% overall; these patients may require admission to an ICU.

189. Ans. (a) Bronchophony

(Ref: Harrison 20th edition, p 1944; Harrison 19th p 803-805)

- *Bronchophony* is the phenomenon of the patient's voice remaining loud at the periphery of the lungs or sounding louder than usual over a distinct area of consolidation, such as in pneumonia. This is a valuable tool in physical diagnosis used by medical personnel when auscultating the chest
- *Egophony* is the auscultation of the sound "AH" instead of "EEE" when a patient phonates "EEE." This change in note is due to abnormal sound transmission through consolidated lung and will be present in pneumonia but not in IPF.
- Similarly, areas of alveolar filling have increased *whispered pectoriloquy* as well as transmission of larger airway sounds (i.e., bronchial breath sounds in a lung zone where vesicular breath sounds are expected).

190. Ans. (a) Pseudomonas

(Ref: Harrison 20th edition, p 1167; Harrison 19th p 1044-45)

- *Pseudomonas aeruginosa is a Gram-negative, aerobic, rod-shaped and polar-flagella bacterium with unipolar motility.*
- The coliforms and proteus are gram negative bacteria and only klebsiella is non-flagellated.
- Furthermore, it is an opportunistic pathogen responsible for ventilator-acquired pneumonia (VAP). VAP due to P. aeruginosa is usually multidrug-resistant and associated with severe infection and increased mortality.

191. Ans. (a) Streptococcus pneumonia

(Ref: Harrison 20th edition, p 911, 1075)

- Most often, they occur as a sequelae to acute pneumonia, commonly caused by Staphylococcus aureus.
- Choices A, B and D are also mentioned in textbook as causes of pneumatocele. However the name of strep pneumonia is mentioned first. Pulmonary pneumatoceles are thin-walled, air-filled cysts that develop within the lung parenchyma. They can be single emphysematous lesions but are more often multiple, thin-walled, air-filled, cyst like cavities.

192. Ans. (a) Streptococcal pneumonia

(Ref: Harrison 20th edition, p 910; Harrison 19th p 951)

- S pneumoniae infection is characterized by homogenous parenchymal lobar opacities with air bronchograms. This condition can occasionally manifest as a round opacity stimulating a pulmonary mass, called round pneumonia.
- The proposed theory about why children develop round pneumonia and adults do not relates to the development of inter-alveolar communication and collateral airways. These are called *pores of Kohn* and *canals of Lambert* and when they develop, they allow air-drift between the parenchymal subsegments. In adults, these allow lateral dissemination of infection throughout a lobe, leading to lobar pnemonia. In children, where these have not developed, the limited spread of infection results in round pneumonia.

193. Ans. (c) Superior segment of apex of lung is commonly involved in recumbent position

(Ref: Fishman's pulmonary disease and disorders, 4th edition, pg 2136))

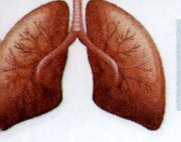

Position of patient while aspiration	Lobe of lung involved
Supine	Superior segment of right lower lobe
Standing/sitting	Posterobasal segment of right lower lobe
Lying on right side	Right middle lobe or posterior segment of right upper lobe
When aspiration occurs in a recumbent patient	The posterior segment of the upper lobes and the superior segment of the lower lobes are most commonly involved lung sites

- Small amounts of material from the buccal cavity, particularly during sleep, is not an uncommon event. No disease ensues in healthy persons, because the aspirated material is cleared by mucociliary action and alveolar macrophages.
- The acidity of gastric contents results in chemical burns to the tracheobronchial tree involved in the aspiration. If the pH of the aspirated fluid is less than 2.5 and the volume of aspirate is greater than 0.3 mL/kg of body weight (20-25 mL in adults), it has a greater potential for causing chemical pneumonia. The initial chemical burn is followed by an inflammatory cellular reaction fueled by the release of potent cytokines, particularly tumor necrosis factor (TNF)–alpha and interleukin (IL)–8.

194. Ans. (a) Lobar pneumonia

(Ref: Harrison 20th edition, p 1944)

The entry of air in pneumonia is normal and hence breath sounds are normal in intensity but have a tubular character where the ratio of I:E = 1:1 with expiration louder than inspiration.

Breath sounds are reduced in
1. Atelectasis
2. Pleural effusion
3. Pneumothorax [can be absent also]

195. Ans. (b) Hilar lymphadenopathy

(Ref: Harrison 20th edition, p 911; Harrison 19th p 805-06)

- In S aureus pneumonia, lobar enlargement with bulging of interlobular fissures can be seen in severe cases.
- Abscesses, cavitations (with air-fluid levels), and pneumatoceles are commonly seen, and 30-50% of patients develop pleural effusions, half of which are empyemas. Note that cavitation and associated pleural effusions are also observed in cases of anaerobic infections, gram-negative infections, and tuberculosis.

196. Ans. (b) Consolidation

(Ref: Harrison 20th edition, p 1944; Harrison 19th p 950-51)

Bronchial breathing anywhere other than over the trachea, right clavicle or right interscapular space is abnormal. Presence of bronchial breathing would suggest:

1. Consolidation
2. Cavitation
3. Complete alveolar atelectasis with patent airways
4. Mass interposed between chest wall and large airways
5. Massive pleural effusion with complete atelectasis of lung
   In all these conditions, there are no ventilation into alveoli and the sound that is heard originates from bronchi and is transmitted to the chest wall.

197. Ans. (a) Legionella

(Ref: Harrison 20th edition, p 1472; Harrison 19th p 1014-16)

198. Ans. (b) Predominance of alveolar exudates

(Ref: Robbins 7th/751, Harrison 19th p 1207-10)

199. Ans. (a) Usually associated with CMV infection

(Ref: Washington manual of Pulmonary Medicine (2006)/ 104 ; Jawetz 24th/ 648, 649,Harrison 19th p 372e, 756, 1358)

200. Ans. (d) Erythromycin

(Ref: Harrison 19th p 1163-64)

201. Ans. (b) Tachypnea

(Ref: Clinical/Anesthesiology 3rd/ 250, Harrison 19th p 1098)

Tuberculosis

202. Ans. (d) Pro-coagulant drugs

Ref: Harrison 20th edition, p 234; Harrison 19th edition, page 247
Management of large volume, life threatening haemoptysis

1. Patency of airway to be maintained using intubation with dual lumen endotracheal tubes
2. Chest imaging
3. Bronchoscopy (Rigid preferred)
4. Put bleeding site in dependant position
5. Bronchoscopy guided cauterization and laser therapy
6. If no respite, angiographic embolization of bleeding bronchial artery branch (can lead to paraplegia as spinal artery supply is compromised).
7. Lobectomy is last resort if everything else fails.

203. Ans. (d) Diffuse pulmonary Lymphangioleiomyomatosis

(Ref: Harrison: 19th edition, Page 1714-15; Oxford Handbook of Clinical Imaging, page 86)

The CT chest shows miliary mottling. The causes of miliary mottling are

1. Miliary TB
2. Loffler Pneumonia
3. Bronchopneumonia
4. Interstitial lung disease
5. Hemosiderosis
6. Sarcoidosis (confluent)
7. Histiocytosis-X

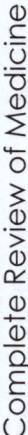

Diffuse pulmonary Lymphangioleiomyomatosis affects pre-menopausal women and presents with *Emphysema, recurrent pneumothorax and chylous pleural effusion*. The disease accelerates in pregnancy and abates after oophorectomy. HRCT shows multiple small thin walled cysts surrounded by normal lung without zonal predominance. Median survival is 10 years and is managed with sirolimus.

204. Ans. (a) Miliary TB

(Ref: Oxford Handbook of Clinical Imaging, Page 86)

The image shows multiple lesions of consolidation scattered through the lung parenchyma diagnostic of Miliary Tuberculosis.

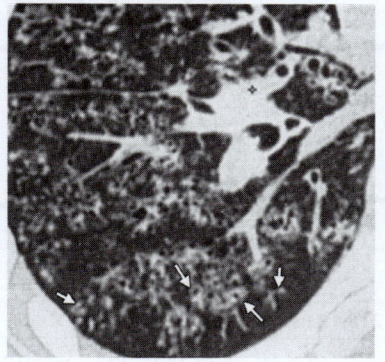

Endobrochial TB

Axial CT scan shows tree-in-bud appearance due to severe changes of bronchiolar dilatation and impaction.

205. Ans. (d) All of the above

(Ref: Harrison 20th edition, p 1245; Harrison 19th edition, page 1108f.)

Miliary pulmonary disease	Miliary systemic disease
It occurs in primary *progressive pulmonary TB* when organisms in the draining lymph nodes *can erode into the pulmonary arteries*. This will distribute the infection to both lung fields.	Once the infection in the lung reaches the *pulmonary vein* the bacteria can reach the left side heart Subsequently they can seed organs like liver and spleen.

206. Ans. (a) Artery

(Ref: Robbins 9th edition chapter 13., Harrison 19th p 1112)

- Systemic miliary ensues when infective foci in the lungs seed the pulmonary venous return to the heart; the organisms subsequently disseminate through the systemic arterial system.
- Almost every organ in the body may be seeded. Lesions resemble those in the lung.
- Miliary is most prominent in the liver, bone marrow, spleen, adrenals, meninges, kidneys, fallopian tubes, and epididymis
- *Robbins mentions that* **Miliary pulmonary disease** *occurs when organisms drain through lymphatics into the lymphatic ducts, which empty into the venous return to the right side of the heart and thence into the pulmonary arteries.*

207. Ans. (a) Start ATT first

(Ref: Harrison 20th edition, p 1246; Harrison 19th p 1112)

- Initiation of cART and/or anti-TB therapy may be associated with clinical deterioration due to immune reconstitution inflammatory syndrome (IRIS) reactions.
- These are most common in patients initiating both treatments at the same time, may occur as early as 1 week after initiation of therapy, and are seen more frequently in patients with advanced HIV disease.
- For these reasons it is often *recommended that initiation of cART be delayed in antiretroviral-naïve patients until 2–8 weeks following the initiation of treatment for TB.*

208. Ans. (d) Bronchiectasis

(Ref: Harrison 20th edition, p 1944; Harrison 19th p 1694-95)

- *Fine crackles* are soft, high-pitched, and very brief. This sound can be simulated by rolling a strand of hair between one's fingers near the ears, or by moistening one's thumb and index finger and rubbing them near the ears. Their presence usually indicates an interstitial process, such as pulmonary fibrosis or congestive heart failure.
- The sounds from interstitial pulmonary fibrosis been described as sounding like opening a Velcro fastener.
- *Coarse crackles* are somewhat louder, lower in pitch, and last longer than fine crackles. Their presence usually indicates an airway disease, such as bronchiectasis

209. Ans. (b) Aspergillosis

(Ref: Oxford Handbook of Clinical Imaging, 3rd/e, Page 86)

210. Ans. (d) Atypical mycobacterial infection

(Ref: Ananthnarayan 6th / 333; Park 18th/150, Harrison 19th p 1131, 1114, 1121)

211. Ans. (a) Pulmonary tuberculosis

(Ref: Harrison 19th p 1113)

212. Ans. (b) Bronchoscopy and biopsy

(Ref: Harrison 20th edition, p 542, Harrison 19th p 511-12)

The diagnostic yield of Bronchoscopy with biopsy is 85–90% as compared to other methods.

Obstructive Sleep Apnea

213. Ans. (d) REM

Ref: Harrison 20th edition, p 2015-16; Harrison 19th edition, page 1726, figure 319-2.

- The *EEG* shows Low amplitude, random fast waves (similar to awake state) called as *saw-tooth waves*.
- Also notice that *EOG* is showing rapid eye movement
- *EMG* is showing minimal muscle activity
- These indicate REM Sleep

Polysomnography interpretation is definitely a future AIIMS question and you can practice the table below.

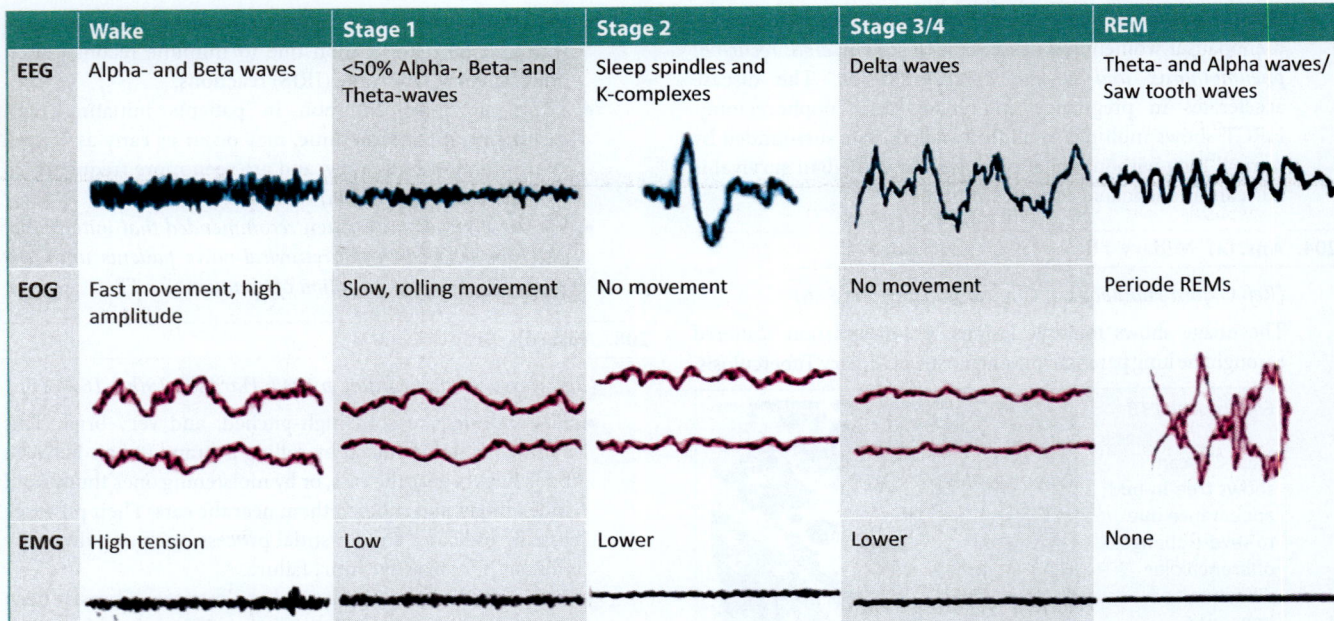

214. Ans. (d) 30 events/ hour

Ref: Harrison 20th ed., p 2015; Harrison 19th ed., p 1725)

Obstructive sleep apnea/ hypopnea syndrome quantification and severity scale is graded according to number of apena-hypopnea index events per hours

Mild OSAHS	5-14 events/ hour
Moderate OSAHS	15-29 events/ hour
Severe OSAHS	>30 events/ hour

215. Ans. (d) 10 seconds

(Ref: Harrison 20th edition, p 2015; Harrison 19th edition, 1724)

Apneas in OSA are defined in adults as breathing pauses lasting >10 s and hypopneas as events >10 s in which there is continued breathing but ventilation is reduced by at least 50% from the previous baseline during sleep.

216. Ans. (a) Hypertension

(Ref: Harrison 20th edition, p 2015; Harrison 19th ed. / 1724-25)

217. Ans. (a) It affects more women

(Ref: Harrison 20th edition, p 2014-15; Harrison 19th p 1723-1725)

- OHS is approximately 3–4% in middle-aged men and 2% in middle-aged women.
- It is defined by an apnea hypopnea index >5 and daytime sleepiness.
- The diagnosis of obesity hypoventilation syndrome (OHS) requires:
  - Body mass index (BMI) >30 kg/m^2
  - Sleep-disordered breathing
  - Chronic daytime alveolar hypoventilation, defined as $PaCO_2$>45 mmHg, and PaO_2< 70 mmHg in the absence of other known causes of hypercapnia.

218. Ans. (a) C.P.A.P

(Ref: Harrison 20th edition, p 2017; Harrison 19th p 1727)

Indications for treatment of OSAHS

1. Epworth Score >11 (scoring pattern for sleepiness, example sleepiness while watching TV or while talking is graded)
2. Troublesome sleepiness while driving or working
3. More than >15 apneas + hypopneas per hour of sleep.
4. For those with similar degrees of sleepiness and 5–15 events per hour of sleep, improvements in symptoms, including subjective sleepiness, with less strong evidence indicating gains in cognition and quality of life

- CPAP and MRS (Mandibular Repositioning Surgery) are the two most widely used and best evidence-based therapies. *Direct comparisons in RCTs indicate better outcomes with CPAP in terms of apneas and hypopneas, nocturnal oxygenation, symptoms, quality of life, mood, and vigilance. Adherence to CPAP is generally better than that to an MRS, and there is evidence that CPAP improves driving*, whereas there are no such data on MRSs. Thus, CPAP is the current treatment of choice.
- *Weight loss looks like a close answer but CMDT states than minimum weight loss to achieve any improvement is >10% and goes to state that this magnitude is not maintained.*
- Harrison states that" There is no evidence that pharyngeal surgery, including uvulo-palato-pharyngoplasty (whether by scalpel, laser, or thermal techniques) helps OSAHS patients". It is more successful at eliminating snoring rather curing obstructive sleep apnea.
- Also remember that *Polysomnography includes – EEG, EOG, EMG, ECG, pulse oximetry and airfow evaluation.* If the episodes of apnea are more than 15 per hour or 5-15 with sleepiness then CPAP is best treatment.

219. Ans. (d) Spirometry is diagnostic

(Ref: Harrison 20th edition, p 2015; Harrison 19th p 1724-25)

- An overnight sleep study, or polysomnography, is required to diagnose OSA. PSG is a multichannel recording of sleep and breathing and usually involves in-laboratory measurement of sleep architecture and electroence phalographic (EEG) arousals, eye movements, chin movements, airflow, respiratory effort, oximetry, electrocardiographic tracings, body position, snoring, and leg movements
- OSAHS raises 24-h mean blood pressure. The increase is greater in those with recurrent nocturnal hypoxemia, and is at least 4–5 mmHg. It may be as great as 10 mmHg in those with >20% arterial oxygen desaturation per hour of sleep. This rise probably results from a combination of surges in blood pressure accompanying each arousal at apnea/hypopnea termination and from the associated 24-h increases in sympathetic tone.
- Epidemiologic data in normal populations indicate that this rise in blood pressure would increase the risk of myocardial infarction by around 20% and that of stroke by about 40%.

220. Ans. (c) Heart block

(Ref: Harrison 20th edition, p 2015; Harrison 19th p 1724-25)

- OSAHS raises 24-h mean blood pressure. The increase is greater in those with recurrent nocturnal hypoxemia, and is at least 4–5 mmHg. It may be as great as 10 mmHg in those with >20% arterial oxygen desaturation per hour of sleep.
- The resultant hypoxia also leads to pulmonary artery constriction leading to PAH.
- Others effects of OSAHS are Personality and mood changes, including depression and anxiety/Sexual dysfunction, including impotence and decreased libido/Gastro-esophageal reflux
- Atrial fibrillation and stroke are also reported

221. Ans. (a) Craniofacial abnormalities

(Ref: Harrison 20th edition, p 2015; Harrison 19th p 1724-25)

- Craniofacial abnormalities are common in O.S.A in non-obese patients and children.
- Factors predisposing to OSAHS by narrowing the pharynx include obesity—with a body mass index (BMI) >30 kg/m²—and shortening of the mandible and/or maxilla. This change in jaw shape may be subtle and can be familial.
- Hypothyroidism and acromegaly predispose to OSAHS by narrowing the upper airway with tissue infiltration.
- Other predisposing factors for OSAHS include male sex and middle age (40–65 years), myotonic dystrophy, Ehlers-Danlos syndrome, and, perhaps, smoking.
- Nonstructural risk factors for OSA include the following:
  - Obesity
  - Central fat distribution
  - Male sex
  - Age
  - Postmenopausal state
  - Alcohol use
  - Sedative use
  - Smoking
  - Habitual snoring with daytime somnoloscence
  - Supine sleep position
  - Rapid eye movement (REM) sleep

222. Ans. (a) <10 sec

(Ref: Harrison 20th edition, p 2015; Harrison 19th p 1724)

OSAHS is defined as the coexistence of unexplained excessive daytime sleepiness with at least five obstructed breathing events (apnea or hypopnea) per hour of sleep. This event threshold may have to be increased in the elderly. Apneas are defined in adults as breathing pauses lasting less than 10 s

223. Ans. (d) 5

(Ref: Harrison 20th edition, p 2015; Harrison 19th p 1724-25)

OSAHS is defined as the coexistence of unexplained excessive daytime sleepiness with at least five obstructed breathing events (apnea or hypopnea) per hour of sleep. This event threshold may have to be increased in the elderly. Apneas are defined in adults as breathing pauses lasting less than 10 s and hypopneas as events less than 10 s in which there is continued breathing but ventilation is reduced by at least 50% from the previous baseline during sleep

224. Ans. (c) Sleep Apnea

(Ref: Harrison 20th edition, p 2011; Harrison 19th p 1725)

- The Epworth sleepiness scale has been validated primarily in obstructive sleep apnea, though it has also shown success in detecting narcolepsy and idiopathic hypersomnia.
- It is used to measure excessive daytime sleepiness and is repeated after the administration of treatment (e.g., CPAP) to document improvement of symptoms.
- In narcolepsy, the Epworth sleepiness scale has both a high specificity (100%) and sensitivity (93.5%).

ARDS

225. Ans. (b) Shock lung

Ref: Harrison 20th edition, Page 2031

- The CXR shows a bilateral white out. CP angles are normal. CT ratio can't be commented as it is a rotated film. Blood gases show type 1 respiratory failure.
- The combination of clinical history of Acute pancreatitis with type 1 respiratory failure and bilateral infiltrates points to diagnosis of ARDS which is also called as Shock lung.
- Choice A should have history of aspiration of stomach contents. Choice C is a possibility but a transtracheal culture would be required. Choice D is ruled out as bilateral CP angles are normal.

226. Ans. (b) PaO$_2$/FiO$_2$ less than 300 mm Hg

Ref: Harrison 20th edition, page 2031

Severity: Oxygenation	Onset	Chest radiograph	Absence of left atrial hypertension
Mild: 200 mmHg < PaO_2/FiO_2 ≤ 300 mmHg Moderate: 100 mmHg < PaO_2/FiO_2 ≤ 200 mmHg Severe: PaO_2/FiO_2 ≤ 100 mmHg	Acute	Bilateral alveolar or interstitial infiltrates	PCWP ≤18 mmHg or no clinical evidence of increased left atrial pressure

227. Ans. (c) PCWP >18 mmHg

Ref: Harrison 20th edition, p 2031; Harrison 19th edition, page 1736.

Since ARDS is a cause of non-cardiogenic pulmonary oedema, PCWP is <18 mmHg.

Diagnostic criteria for ARDS

Severity oxygenation	Mild : pAO_2/ FiO_2 <300 mm Hg Moderate: pAO_2/ FiO_2 <200 mm Hg Severe: pAO_2/ FiO_2 <100 mm Hg
Onset	Acute onset illness
CXR findings	Bilateral alveolar
Left atrial pressure values	PCWP < 18 mm Hg

228. Ans. (c) Non cardiogenic pulmonary oedema

Ref: Harrison 20th edition, p 3334; Harrison 19th edition, page 47e-4

- Visit to remote pilgrimage sites at high altitude can lead to development of high altitude pulmonary edema (HAPE).
- Oxygen scarcity at high altitude leads to hypoxic damage to endothelial cells of lungs
- It leads to non-cardiogenic pulmonary oedema and the resultant dysfunction of surfactant lining leads to alveoli to collapse at low lung volumes.
- Pneumonia is ruled out as there is no fever, purulent sputum or any evidence of lung infection given in the question.

229. Ans. (b) Diuretics

Ref: Harrison 20th edition, p 813; page 1749: Haematology basic principles and Practice E-Book

- TRALI is a non-cardiogenic pulmonary oedema and does not respond to diuretics.
- The reason for pulmonary oedema in TRALI is cytokine induced damage to microvasculature of lungs which leaks into alveoli.
- Diuretics are useful in pulmonary oedema that occurs due to congestive heart failure.
- IVF can be used for management of dangerous hypotension that occurs after TRALI. It must be *used extremely cautiously* with CVP monitoring. The pressure should be kept on lower side of normal(2-10cm H20).

230. Ans. (c) Normal PCWP

Ref: Harrison 20th edition, p 814; Harrison 19th edition, 138e-5

Blood products are excellent volume expanders and hence fast transfusion can suddenly worsen the patient with development of Transfusion associated circulatory overload.

Patient will develop:

1. Dyspnea with pAO_2 < 90% on room air
2. Bilateral infiltrates on CXR
3. Systolic hypertension

Administration of diuretics and regulating the flow rates can easily minimise the problem.

231. Ans. (d) Measurement of PCWP

Ref: Harrison 20th ed., p 2031; Harrison 19th ed., p 1736

- Not every bed ridden patient will develop pulmonary embolism.
- The paraplegic patient has developed a pneumonia episode and is going into septic shock.
- Rusty sputum and fever with dyspnea points to diagnosis of pneumonia.
- Sepsis is a leading cause of ARDS and for diagnosis of ARDS, PCWP should be less than 18mm Hg.
- Choices A, C and D point to diagnosis of pulmonary embolism in which CXR is normal or shows classical signs like Hampton hump, Palla sign.

232. Ans. (b) 100

(Ref: Harrison 20th edition, p 2031; Harrison 19th edition, page 1736)

Severity of ARDS is graded on the basis of fall in levels of oxygenation-

Mild: PaO_2/FiO_2 < 300
Moderate: PaO_2/FiO_2 < 200
Severe: PaO_2/FiO_2 < 100

233. Ans. (b) Non pulmonary causes

(Ref: Harrison 20th edition, p 2034; Harrison 19th edition, page 1739)

The question is a direct quote from Harrison saying "The major risk factors for ARDS mortality are non- pulmonary. Advanced age is an important risk factor"

Direct lung injury (like pulmonary contusion, pneumonia and aspiration) has higher mortality than indirect causes like TRALI.

234. Ans. (a) Pulmonary embolism

(Ref: Harrison 20th edition, p 2031; Harrison 19th edition, page 1736)

ARDS is associated with disorders that lead to *alveolar damage*. In pulmonary embolism however there is perfusion defect leading to *pulmonary oligemia*.

Causes of ARDS

Direct lung injury
• Pneumonia • *Mendelson syndrome (aspiration of stomach contents)* • Contusion of lung • Near drowning • Inhalation (toxic gas)

Contd...

Indirect lung injury
- Sepsis
- Poly-trauma with flail chest
- Burns
- Multiple transfusion (especially FFP> blood transfusion/ packed RBC)
- Drug overdose
- Post cardio-pulmonary bypass
- *Pancreatitis*

235. Ans. (b) Alveolar Transudate

(Ref: Harrison 20th edition, p 2031; Harrison 19th ed. / 1736-38)

- ARDS is characterised by high protein pulmonary edema and an exudate. The natural history of ARDS is marked by three phases—exudative, proliferative, and fibrotic—each with characteristic clinical and pathologic features.
- The presence of alveolar and interstitial fluid and the loss of surfactant can lead to a marked reduction of lung compliance.
- Without an increase in end-expiratory pressure, significant alveolar collapse can occur at end-expiration, impairing oxygenation.
- In most clinical settings, positive end-expiratory pressure (PEEP) is empirically set to minimize FiO_2 and maximize PaO_2.

236. Ans. (b) Hypercapnia

(Ref: Harrison 20th edition, p 2031; Harrison 19th ed. / 1736)

- ARDS is characterized by type 1 respiratory failure which has only hypoxia but the value of CO_2 is normal. ARDS has non cardiogenic pulmonary edema with normal PCWP.
- PCWP (Normal is 8-12mm Hg) is increased in Cardiogenic pulmonary edema.
- Remember hypercapnia/hypercarbia is a feature of type 2 respiratory failure.

237. Ans. (b) Non-cardiogenic pulmonary edema

(Ref: Harrison 20th edition, p 2031; Harrison 19th edition, page 1736)

Cardiogenic pulmonary edema

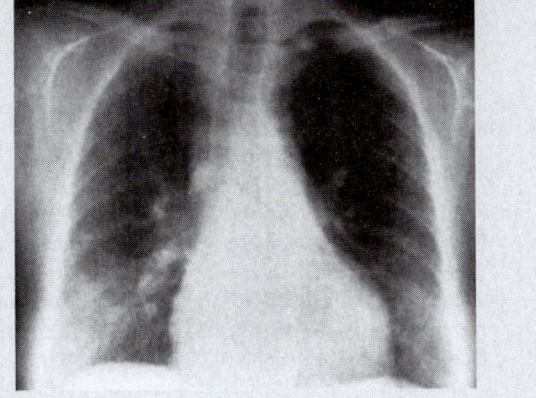

- Increased CT ratio
- Kerley B lines
- Bat wing configuration

Non-cardiogenic pulmonary edema

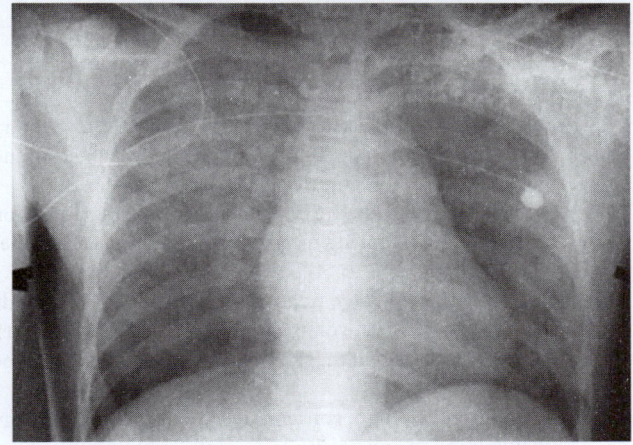

- Normal CT ratio
- Diffuse bilateral infiltrates sparing Costo-phrenic angle
- Absent Kerley B lines

238. Ans. (a) ARDS

(Ref: Harrison 20th edition, p 2031; Harrison 19th edition, page 1736)

The patient would have sustained a pulmonary contusion at construction site accident which has resulted in development of ARDS. The chest radiograph usually reveals alveolar and interstitial opacities involving atleast three quarters of the lung fields.

239. Ans. (c) Low protein pulmonary edema

(Ref: Harrison 19th p 1736-37)

- ARDS has type 1 respiratory failure and hence choice A and B are correct.
- Stiff lungs are explained by increased lung compliance.
- Since ARDS is an exudate, it is characterized by high protein pulmonary edema.

240. Ans. (c) Status asthmaticus

(Ref: Harrison 20th edition, p 2031)

Status asthmaticus is an example of type 2 respiratory failure while ARDS is type 1 respiratory failure. All other choices lead to cytokine release and damage the alveoli leading to ARDS.

241. Ans. (d) Low protein pulmonary edema

(Ref: Harrison 20th edition, p 2031)

- In ARDS alveolar capillary endothelial cells and type 1 pneumocytes (alveolar epithelial cells) are injured, leading to the loss of the normally tight alveolar barrier to fluid and macromolecules. *(Edema fluid that is rich in protein accumulates in the interstitial and alveolar spaces.)* Significant concentrations of cytokines (e.g., interleukin 1, interleukin

8, and tumor necrosis factor α) and lipid mediators (e.g., leukotriene B4) are present in the lung in this acute phase.

242. Ans. (a) Low tidal volume ventilation

(Ref: Harrison 20th edition, p 2033; Harrison 19th p 1736)

- Mechanical ventilation of patients with acute lung injury and ARDS may propagate lung injury. Cyclical collapse and reopening of alveoli may be partly responsible for this.
- Studies have suggested that stretching and overdistention of injured alveoli during mechanical ventilation can further injure the lung.
- On comparison of large tidal volume (12 mL/kg ideal body weight) to a low tidal volume (6 mL/kg ideal body weight), dramatic reduction in mortality rate in the low tidal volume group was seen.
- In addition, a "fluid conservative" management strategy [maintaining a relatively low central venous pressure (CVP) or pulmonary capillary wedge pressure (PCWP)] is associated with the need for fewer days of mechanical ventilation compared with a "fluid liberal" management strategy (maintaining a relatively high CVP or PCWP) in acute lung injury and ARDS

243. Ans. (c) Increase in pulmonary capillary wedge pressure

(Ref: Harrison 20th edition, p 2031; Harrison 19th p 1736-37)

- Increased PCWP is a feature of cardiogenic pulmonary edema while ARDS is a non-cardiogenic pulmonary edema.
- ARDS has type 1 respiratory failure which leads to hypoxia with normal or reduced pCO_2.
- The damage to alveoli lead to ventilation perfusion mismatch leading to intrapulmonary shunting.
- Non cardiogenic pulmonary edema has normal PCWP. Causes are
  - ARDS
  - Heroin inhalation
  - High altitude pulmonary edema

244. Ans. (b) Normal pulmonary capillary wedge pressure

(Ref: Harrison 19th p 1763)

245. Ans. (b) Hypercapnia

(Ref: Harrison 20th edition, p 2031; Harrison 19th p 1736-37)

- ARDS is characterized by type 1 respiratory failure which has only hypoxia but the value of CO_2 is normal. ARDS has non cardiogenic pulmonary edema with normal PCWP.
- PCWP (Normal is 8-12mm Hg) is increased in Cardiogenic pulmonary edema.
- Remember hypercapnia/hypercarbia is a feature of type 2 respiratory failure.

246. Ans. (c) Hypercapnia

(Ref: Harrison 20th edition, p 2031; Harrison 19th p 1736-38)

Pleural Effusion, Pneumothorax Pneumomediastinum

247. Ans. (b) Pneumothorax

Ref: Harrison 20th edition, Page 1075

Patients with Staphyloccocal pneumonia have a tendency to develops pneumatocele. The pneumatocele can rupture leading to respiratory distress.

248. Ans. (d) Wide bore needle insertion in 2nd ICS

Ref: Harrison 20th edition, Page 2009

The findings of hyper-resonant note in the chest with hypotension points to diagnosis of Tension pneumothorax. A Large bore needle should be inserted into the pleural space through second intercostal space to allow escape of air and improvement in hemodynamic status of the patient. The needle should be left in place until a thoracostomy tube can be placed.

249. Ans. (a) Pneumothorax

Ref: Harrison 20th edition, p 2009; Harrison 19th edition, 308e

The CXR shows:
1. Absent vascular markings in right lung field (Red markings)
2. Deep sulcus sign (blue arrow)
3. Pleural reflection (Yellow line)

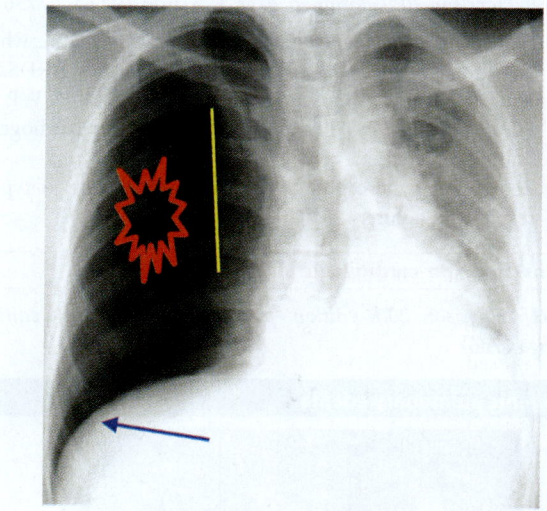

250. Ans. (c) Chest tube insertion

Ref: Harrison 19th edition, Page 1719

- The image shows blunting of left side costophrenic angle (dotted red markings). In setting of trauma it indicates development of *hemothorax*.
- This explains the reduced air entry, tracheal deviation to right (red arrow) and breathlessness in the patient. Rib fracture cannot be visualised.

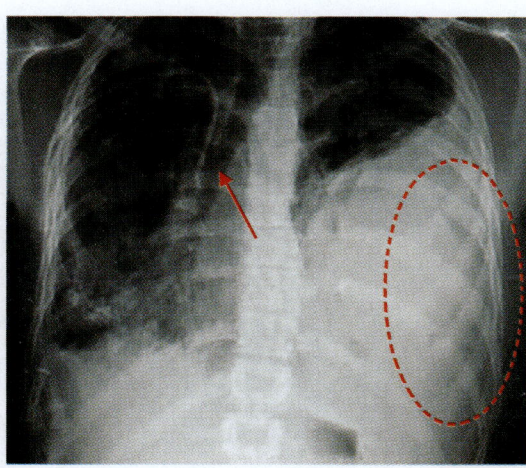

- Chest tube drainage is indicated with aggressive monitoring of vitals as they may get compromised anytime.
- Cardio-thoracic ratio looks normal (limitation AP view) and Heart sounds are also normal. This rules out cardiac tamponade and choice B
- Needle aspiration is done for pneumothorax.
- Immediate Thoracotomy is not required in the case.

251. Ans. (b) CHF

Ref: Harrison 20th edition, p 2006; Harrison 19th edition, page 1716

The pleural fluid that does not clot is a transudate and the only cause of transudate out of these four options is CHF. Choice A, C and D lead to exudative pleural effusion

252. Ans. (b) Para-pneumonic effusion

Ref: Harrison 20th edition, p 2007; Harrison 19th edition, page 1717

- In case of para-pneumonic effusion, therapeutic thoracentesis is recommended. However if the fluid recurs or is loculated then a chest tube is inserted with instillation of fibrinolytic agent.
- Usually tissue plasminogen activator and deoxyribonuclease is used.
- If this fails then thoracoscopy with breakdown of adhesions is performed.
- Decortication is the last resort if all above measures fail

253. Ans. (a) 1

Ref: Harrison 20th edition, p 2006; Harrison 19th edition, page 1716

Transudative and exudative pleural effusions are distinguished by measuring the lactate dehydrogenase (LDH) and protein levels in the pleural fluid. Exudative pleural effusions meet at least one of the following criteria, whereas transudative pleural effusions meet none:
1. Pleural fluid protein/serum protein >0.5
2. Pleural fluid LDH/serum LDH >0.6
3. Pleural fluid LDH more than two-thirds the normal upper limit for serum.

254. Ans. (c) Needle aspiration of air

Ref: Harrison 20th edition, p 2009; Harrison: 19th edition, page 1719

- Tension pneumothorax occurs mostly during mechanical ventilation or resuscitative efforts.
- The positive pressure is transmitted to mediastinum decreasing the venous return and cardiac output.
- A large bore needle should be inserted into pleural space through second intercostal space to allow air to escape.
- Needle aspiration using syringe is done for primary spontaneous pneumothorax.

Types of pneumothorax and primary management

Primary spontaneous pneumothorax	Simple needle aspiration followed by Thoracoscopy with pleural abrasion
Secondary pneumothorax	Tube thoracotomy Followed by thoracostomy with stapling of blebs.
Traumatic pneumothorax	Supplemental oxygen or aspiration followed by tube thoracotomy.
Tension pneumothorax	Large bore needle in 2nd I/C space followed by tube thoracostomy

255. Ans. (d) Esophageal Rupture and Pneumomediastinum

(Ref: Harrison 20th edition, p 2010; Harrison 19th edition, page 1720)

The CXR shows the following findings of pneumomediastinum

1. Air shadows below the heart are present indicating continuous diaphragm sign.
2. Presence of air at lateral 1/3rd of the clavicle, adjacent to left head of humerus indicating subcutaneous emphysema.
3. Left CP angle blunting due to pleural effusion. *The reduced air entry can be explained by left sided pleural effusion.*

Traditionally *Naclerio's V sign* is seen in pneumomediastinum
- It is presence of V shaped gas shadow near Cardiophrenic angle and diaphragm on left side as is seen in patients of Boerhaave syndrome.

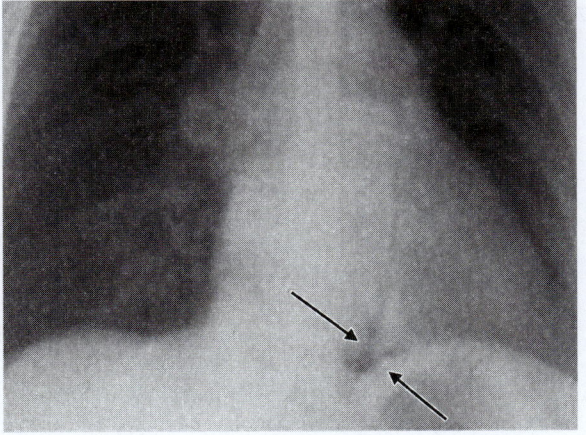

- *Mackler's triad* is chest pain, vomiting and subcutaneous emphysema seen in barotrauma esophagus.

- *Tension pneumothorax is ruled out as bronchovascular markings are seen and deep sulcus sign is absent. Cardiac tamponade should have increased CT ratio and hemodynamic compromise while in this patient BP= 130/80 mmHg.*

Pneumomediastinum	Pneumothorax	Flail chest
Continous diaphragm sign. Subcutaneous air seen near the left clavicle. Triangular shadow created due to displacement of heart and contents of esohagus into the mediastinum. In lateral view air around the heart and trachea is seen.	Absent vascular shadows on left side with tracheal shift. Deep Sulcus Sign on left side.	Fractured ribs with increased bronchovascular markings indicating pulmonary contusion and development of ARDS

256. Ans. (c) Needle thoracotomy

(*Ref: Harrison 20th edition, p 2009; Harrison 19th edition, page 1719*)

- The clinical features of sudden onset dysnea with mediastinal shift, hyper-resonant percussion note and absent breath sounds point to diagnosis of tension pneumothorax.
- Hence a needle thoracotomy using a large bore needle should be done in the pleural space through second intercostal space. This is followed by insertion of ICD, tube

257. Ans. (c) Pneumothorax

(*Ref: Harrison 20th edition, p 2009; Harrison, 19th edition, page 308e-13-14f:*)

Interpretation of Chest X-ray:
1. Left-sided pleural effusion
2. Trachea shifted because of pleural effusion
3. Bilateral ICD-for drainage of rapidly accumulating pleural effusion as mentioned in the question
4. There is no pneumothorax in the picture

Chest X-ray feature of pneumothorax are:
1. Visible visceral pleural edge see as a very thin, sharp white line
2. No lung markings are seen peripheral to this line
3. The peripheral space is radiolucent compared to adjacent lung
4. The lung may completely collapse
5. The mediastinum should not shift away from the pneumothorax unless it is a tension pneumothorax.

258. Ans. (b) 10 mm

(*Ref: Harrison 20th edition, p 2007; Harrison 19th edition, page 1717*)

- The possibility of para-pneumonic effusion should be considered in patients with bacterial pneumonia.
- If the free fluid separates the lung from the chest wall by >10mm, therapeutic thoracocentesis should be done.

Factors indicating need for a procedure more invasive than thoracocentesis are as follows

1. Loculated pleural effusion
2. Pleural fluid pH<7.20
3. Pleural fluid glucose of <60mg/dl
4. Positive culture of pleural fluid
5. Presence of gross pus

The data is mentioned in increasing order of importance

259. Ans. (b) A needle should be inserted into the chest wall in the second right intercostal space as an emergency

(*Ref: Harrison 20th edition, p 2009*)

- **The given CXR shows right sided pneumothorax with:**
  - Radiolucent costophrenic sulcus called deep sulcus sign
  - Jet black lung without any vascular shadows

- Straight visceral pleural line on medial border of left lung
- The presence of mediastinal air and mediastinal shift is seen
- For management of tension pneumothorax, a Lumbar puncture needle needs to be inserted in second intercostal space on right side to relieve the tension. A 3 way stop cock can then be attached to the needle for intermittent decompression while chest tube insertion is done on the right 5 intercostal space in mid axillary line.
- Westermark sign presents a triangular opacity in pulmonary infarction.

260. Ans. (a) Hydropneumothorax

(Ref: Chest-X ray Interpretation, Clarke, 3rd edition, Page 58)

Hydro-Pneumothorax	On erect chest radiography, it shows an air fluid level. On supine radiograph, sharp pleural line is bordered by increased opacity lateral to it within the pleural space.
Pleural effusion	Blunting of CP angle and presence of meniscus sign
Lung Abscess	Cavity with air fluid level usually in superior segment of right lower lobe.
Collapse	Direct signs include displacement of fissures and opacification of the collapsed lobe. Indirect signs include the following: Displacement of the hilum Mediastinal shift toward the side of collapse Loss of volume in the ipsilateral hemithorax Elevation of the ipsilateral diaphragm Crowding of the ribs Compensatory hyperlucency of the remaining lobes

261. Ans. (a) Insert a large bore needle on right side

(Ref: Harrison 20th edition, p 2009; Harrison's 19th edition, 1719)

Points in favor of diagnosis of tension pneumothorax
1. Chest pain and Shortness of breath
2. Oxygen saturation not improving with supplemental oxygen
3. Tracheal shift to opposite side
4. Hypotension due to mediastinal shift and kinking of great veins
5. JVP elevated

Management:
- If intercostal tube is not readily available a large bore needle can be inserted into the pleural space through the second anterior intercostal space
- The needle should be left in place until an I.C.D tube can be inserted.

Other findings in tension Pneumothorax (not given in question though)
- Unilateral chest expansion no or little movement on the involved side
- Diminished breath sounds on affected side
- Decreased tactile fremitus
- Hyper-resonance to percussion

262. Ans. (a) TB; (b) Malignancy; (d) Thoracic duct injury

(Ref: Kundu 4th/55; Harrison 19th/1718; P.J.M 20th/142

263. Ans. (c) Ellis curve

(Ref: Harrison 19th edition, Page 308e-14)

Ellis curve is seen in pleural effusion. It has a S shaped border in axilla where fluid accumulates in pleural cavity. You can see the transverse border of fluid on right lung field in this X ray. Pneumonia does not have a sharp border.

264. Ans. (a) Pneumomediastium

(Ref: Fundamentals of Diagnostic Radiology, Bryant 3rd edition, Page 411)

- The black arrow points to presence of continuous Diaphragm sign indicating presence of pneumo-mediastinum.
- Pneumo-mediastinum occurs after alveolar rupture as gas travels along the Broncho-vascular interstitial sheaths into the mediastinum.

265. Ans. (d) Air entry is normal

(Ref: Harrison 20th edition, p 1944, 2007)

The image shows a pleural tap being performed. Air entry is reduced in pleural effusion.

Skodiac resonance is hyper-resonant sound generated by percussion of chest just above the pleural effusion. Bronchial breathing can be heard, just above the level of effusion.

266. Ans. (a) Pneumothorax

(Ref: Harrison 20th edition, p 2009; Harrison 19th edition, page 308e-13)

Staph aureus pneumonia can lead to formation of Pneumatoceles. These are cystic cavities that can rupture leading to formation of pneumothorax.

267. Ans. (d) Effusion sugar is less than 2/3 rd of blood sugar

(Ref: Harrison 20th edition, p 2006; Harrison 19th p 1716-17)

Transudative and exudative pleural effusions are distinguished by measuring the lactate dehydrogenase (LDH) and protein levels in the pleural fluid. Exudative pleural effusions meet at least one of the following criteria, whereas transudative pleural effusions meet none:

- Pleural fluid protein/Serum protein >0.5
- Pleural fluid LDH/Serum LDH >0.6
- Pleural fluid LDH more than two-thirds normal upper limit for serum

These criteria misidentify ~25% of transudates as exudates.

268. Ans. (c) Simple needle aspiration

(Ref: Harrison 20th edition, p 2009; Harrison 19th p 1719)

- The initial recommended treatment for primary spontaneous pneumothorax is simple aspiration.
- Primary spontaneous pneumothoraxes occur almost exclusively in smokers; this suggests that these patients have

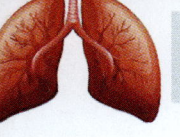

subclinical lung disease.
- If the lung does not expand with aspiration or if the patient has a recurrent pneumothorax, thoracoscopy with stapling of blebs and pleural abrasion is indicated. Thoracoscopy or thoracotomy with pleural abrasion is almost 100% successful in preventing recurrences.

269. Ans. (c) High cholesterol

(Ref: Harrison 19th p 1718)

- A chylothorax occurs when the thoracic duct is disrupted and chyle accumulates in the pleural space. *The most common cause of chylothorax is trauma (most frequently thoracic surgery)*, but it also may result from tumors in the mediastinum.
- Patients with chylothorax present with dyspnea, and a large pleural effusion is present on the chest radiograph.
- *Thoracentesis reveals milky fluid, and biochemical analysis reveals a triglyceride level that exceeds 1.2 mmol/L (>110 mg/dL).*
- Patients with chylothorax and no obvious trauma should have a lymphangiogram and a mediastinal CT scan to assess the mediastinum for lymph nodes. *The treatment of choice for most chylothoraxes is insertion of a chest tube plus the administration of octreotide.*
- If these modalities fail, a pleuroperitoneal shunt should be placed unless the patient has chylous ascites. An alternative treatment is ligation of the thoracic duct.

270. Ans. (d) Dressler's syndrome

(Ref: Harrison 19th p 1716-18)

Causes of low pleural fluid sugar
1. Malignant effusion
2. Tuberculous pleuritis
3. Esophageal rupture
4. Lupus pleuritis.
5. Rheumatoid pleurisy
6. Empyema

271. Ans. (a) C.H.F

(Ref: Harrison 20th edition, p 2006; Harrison 19th p 1725-26)

272. Ans. (c) Peritoneal dialysis

(Ref: Harrison 20th edition, p 2007; Harrison 19th p 1716)

273. Ans. (d) Bronchogenic carcinoma

Ref: Harrison 20th edition, p 2007; Harrison 19th p 1716)

The more common causes of exudates include the following:
1. Parapneumonic effusion
2. Malignancy (most commonly, lung or breast cancer, lymphoma, leukemia; less commonly, ovarian carcinoma, stomach cancer, sarcomas, melanoma)
3. Pulmonary embolism

Contd...

4. Collagen-vascular conditions (rheumatoid arthritis, systemic lupus erythematosus)
5. Tuberculosis
6. Pancreatitis
7. Trauma
8. Postcardiac injury syndrome
9. Esophageal perforation
10. Radiation pleuritis
11. Sarcoidosis
12. Pancreatic pseudocyst
13. Status-post coronary artery bypass graft surgery
14. Meigs syndrome (benign pelvic neoplasm with associated ascites and pleural effusion)
15. Ovarian hyperstimulation syndrome
16. Asbestos-related pleural disease
17. Yellow nail syndrome (yellow nails, lymphedema, pleural effusions)
18. Uremia

274. Ans. (d) All of the above

(Ref: Harrison 19th p 1716-18)

275. Ans. (a) Glucose > 620 mg/dl

(Ref: Harrison 20th edition, p 2006-7; Harrison 19th p 1713-14)

- A low pleural glucose concentration (30-50 mg/dL) suggests malignant effusion, tuberculous pleuritis, esophageal rupture, or lupus pleuritis.
- A very low pleural glucose concentration (i.e., < 30 mg/dL) further restricts diagnostic possibilities, to rheumatoid pleurisy or empyema.
- **The fluid is considered an exudate if any of the following applies: (Lights criteria)**
  - Ratio of pleural fluid to serum protein greater than 0.5
  - Ratio of pleural fluid to serum LDH greater than 0.6
  - Pleural fluid LDH greater than two thirds of the upper limits of normal serum value

Normal pleural fluid has the following characteristics:
- Clear ultrafiltrate of plasma that originates from the parietal pleura
- A pH of 7.60-7.64
- Protein content of less than 2% (1-2 g/dL)
- Fewer than 1000 white blood cells (WBCs) per cubic millimeter
- Glucose content similar to that of plasma
- Lactate dehydrogenase (LDH) less than 50% of plasma

276. Ans. (d) Bronchopulmonary aspergillosis

(Ref: Harrison 20th edition, p 2009; Harrison 19th p 1346-47)

- Langhans cell histiocytosis is a smoking-related, diffuse lung disease that primarily affects men between the ages of 20 and 40 years. Most common clinical manifestation at presentation are cough, dyspnea, chest pain, weight loss, and fever. Pneumothorax occurs in ~25% of patients. HRCT that reveals a combination of nodules and thin-walled cysts is virtually diagnostic of PLCH.
- In Marfan syndrome due to defect of fibrillin, pulmonary symptoms are not a major feature but spontaneous

pneumothorax is common. In spontaneous unilateral pneumothorax, air escapes from a lung and occupies the pleural space between the chest wall and a lung.

277. Ans. (b) Rheumatoid arthritis

(Ref: Harrison 19th p 1713-14, 2138)

Hemorrhagic pleural fluid may result from

1. Trauma
2. Malignancy
3. Postpericardiotomy syndrome
4. Asbestos-related effusion
5. Pulmonary embolism

278. Ans. (a) Esophageal perforation

(Ref: Harrison 20th edition, p 2009; Harrison 19th p 1719)

- Most cases of acute mediastinitis either are due to esophageal perforation or occur after median sternotomy for cardiac surgery.
- Patients with esophageal rupture are acutely ill with chest pain and dyspnea due to the mediastinal infection.
- The esophageal rupture can occur spontaneously or as a complication of esophagoscopy or the insertion of a Blakemore tube.
- Appropriate treatment consists of exploration of the mediastinum with primary repair of the esophageal tear and drainage of the pleural space and the mediastinum.

279. Ans. (a) Absent breath sounds

(Ref: Page 151: Macleod's 13th/e; Harrison 19th p 1719, 1743)

- Tracheal Tug is a abnormal downward movement of Trachea during systole that can be indicate a aneurysm of aortic arch.
- *The diagnosis of pneumothorax made by physical examination showing an enlarged hemithorax with no breath sounds, hyperresonance to percussion, and shift of the mediastinum to the contralateral side.*
- Tension pneumothorax must be treated as a medical emergency. If the tension in the pleural space is not relieved, the patient is likely to die from inadequate cardiac output or marked hypoxemia.
- A large-bore needle should be inserted into the pleural space through the second anterior intercostal space.
- If large amounts of gas escape from the needle after insertion, the diagnosis is confirmed. The needle should be left in place until a thoracostomy tube can be inserted.

280. Ans. (a) Meig's syndrome

(Ref: Harrison 20th edition, p 2006; Harrison 19th p 1716)

281. Ans. (b) Malignancy

(Ref: Harrison 19th p 1717)

- Malignant pleural effusion usually results from pleural metastasis. Nearly half of all the patients with disseminated lung cancer eventually get pleural effusion. Though pleural fluid examination is an important tool for diagnosis of MPE, the initial cytology is positive only in about 60% of the patients. Pleural biopsy confirms the diagnosis in only about 50-60% of the cases.
- Amylase levels in various other pleural effusions have been found elevated e.g. in pancreatitis and in rupture of the oesophagus. When oesophageal perforation is not a consideration, the finding of salivary amylase isoenzyme in pleural fluid suggests presence of a malignancy.

282. Ans. (c) Bronchial adenoma

(Ref: Harrison 19th p 1717-1718)

Grossly bloody fluid may result from trauma, malignancy, postpericardiotomy syndrome, or asbestos-related effusion and indicates the need for a spun hematocrit test of the sample; a pleural fluid hematocrit level of more than 50% of the peripheral hematocrit level defines a hemothorax, which often requires tube thoracostomy.

283. Ans. (b) Rupture of sub-pleural Bleb

(Ref: Harrison 19th p 1719)

284. Ans. (c) Pneumomediastinum

(Ref: Harrison 20th edition, p 2010; Harrison 19th p 1720)

- Pneumomediastinum is gas in the interstices of the mediastinum. The three main causes are (1) alveolar rupture with dissection of air into the mediastinum, (2) perforation or rupture of the esophagus, trachea, or main bronchi, and (3) dissection of air from the neck or the abdomen into the mediastinum.
- Typically, there is severe substernal chest pain with or without radiation into the neck and arms. The physical examination usually reveals subcutaneous emphysema in the suprasternal notch and Hamman's sign, which is a crunching or clicking noise synchronous with the heartbeat and is best heard in the left lateral decubitus position.
- The diagnosis is confirmed with the chest radiograph. Usually no treatment is required, but the mediastinal air will be absorbed faster if the patient inspires high concentrations of oxygen. If mediastinal structures are compressed, the compression can be relieved with needle aspiration.

285. Ans. (d) Mesothelial cells

(Ref: Harrison 20th edition, p 2007; Harrison 19th p 1109-10, 1718)

Mesothelial cells are found in variable numbers in most effusions, but their presence at greater than 5% of total nucleated cells makes a diagnosis of TB less likely. *Markedly increased numbers of mesothelial cells, especially in bloody or eosinophilic effusions, suggests pulmonary embolism as the cause of effusion.*

286. Ans. (a) Respiratory alkalosis

(Ref: Harrison 19th p 1719, 1750)

Since in tension pneumo-thorax, there is reduced blood supply to heart as well as collapse of affected lung, the contralateral lung will not be able to do the work of both the lungs. The result will be carbon dioxide retention leading to respiratory acidosis.

287. Ans. (b) Needle in 2nd intercostal space

(Ref: Harrison 20th edition, p 2009; Harrison 19th p 1719, 1750)

- Emergent needle decompression for tension pneumothorax is carried out on the affected side by placing an *18-gauge needle or angio-catheter into the hemithorax* at the midclavicular line in the second anterior intercostal space. This emergency maneuver relieves the tension created within the thorax. It does not treat the pneumothorax; subsequent chest tube insertion is required.
- Tube thoracostomy (chest tube insertion) and underwater seal drainage are the mainstays of treatment for spontaneous pneumothorax.
- Full re-expansion of the lung, even in the presence of a continuous leak, usually can be achieved with the application of suction to the thoracostomy drainage system.

288. Ans. (b) Doxycycline

(Ref: Harrison 20th edition, p 2009)

Successful pleurodesis is defined as a complete response to the chemical agent, meaning the absence of re-accumulation of pleural effusion determined by clinical examination or chest radiograph.

Agents used are:
- Talc –success rate of 93%
- Doxycycline success rate of 72%
- Bleomycin success rate of 54%

289. Ans. (b) Histoplasma

(Ref: Harrison 20th edition, p 2009)

- The spectrum of chronic mediastinitis ranges from granulomatous inflammation of the lymph nodes in the mediastinum to fibrosing mediastinitis.
- Most cases are due to histoplasmosis or TB, but sarcoidosis, silicosis, and other fungal diseases are at times causative.
- Patients with granulomatous mediastinitis are usually asymptomatic. Those with fibrosing mediastinitis usually have signs of compression of a mediastinal structure such as the superior vena cava or large airways, phrenic or recurrent laryngeal nerve paralysis, or obstruction of the pulmonary artery or proximal pulmonary veins.

290. Ans. (c) Bacterial pneumonia

(Ref: Harrison 19th p 968, 1098-99)

291. Ans. (d) Increased Mesothelial cells

(Ref: Harrison 19th p 1109-10)

292. Ans. None

(Ref: Harrison 19th p 1109-10, 1716)

293. Ans. (d) Dressler's Syndrome

(Ref: Harrison 19th p 1716-19)

294. Ans. (b) Malignancy

(Ref: Harrison 19th p 1717)

295. Ans. (b) Pneumothorax

(Ref: Handbook Of Critical Care By Paul Ellis Marik / 469, Harrison 19th p 1719)

Pulmonary Embolism

296. Ans. (a) Pneumatic compression stockings

Ref: SRB, 5th edition, page 241 and 243

- The image shows pneumatic compression stockings to prevent deep vein thrombosis is patients of stroke or post-surgery. The compression of calf muscles reduces incidence of stasis.
- Compression stockings (Unna boot) is a three-layer gauze compression stocking for management of *varicose veins*.

297. Ans. (a) LMW heparin

Ref: Page 1916: Harrison 20th edition

Low dose UFH or LMWH is the most common form of prophylaxis strategy in cancer surgery including gynecological cancer surgery. Enoxaparin is given 40mg daily for one month. It is also used in major orthopedic and high risk non-orthopedic patients.

298. Ans. (b) Fat embolism

Ref: Harrison 20th edition, p 1912; Harrison 19th edition, page 368, 1632

The patient had fracture of long bone and developed respiratory distress after 48 hours which is characteristic of Fat embolism.

GURD criteria for diagnosis of Fat embolism

Major criteria for diagnosing FES are as follows:
• Symptoms and radiologic evidence of respiratory insufficiency
• Cerebral sequelae unrelated to head injury or other conditions
• Petechial rash
Minor criteria are as follows:
• Tachycardia (heart rate >110 beats/min)
• Pyrexia (temperature >38.5°C)
• Retinal changes of fat or petechiae
• Renal dysfunction
• Jaundice
• Acute drop in hemoglobin level
• Sudden thrombocytopenia
• Elevated erythrocyte sedimentation rate
• Fat microglobulinemia

One major criteria, four minor criteria and macroglobulinemia is used for diagnosis of FES.

299. Ans. (a) Pulmonary Thromboembolism

Ref: Harrison 20th ed., p 1911; Harrison 19th ed. p 1631

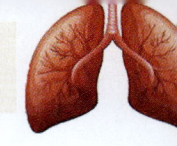

History of hair line fracture and below knee cast implies patient was immobilised. This could have resulted in development of thrombus in his calf veins. Following massage on the leg by his mother, clot would have embolised to lung circulation.

Fat embolism develops 24-36 hours after fracture of shaft of long bones.

300. Ans. (b) Unfractionated heparin

(Ref: Harrison 20th edition, p 1914; Harrison 19th edition, page 1634)

- Nephrotic syndrome is a hypercoagulable state. Prolonged air travel predisposes patient to development of stasis of blood in soleal veins. The thrombus in the deep veins can embolise to the heart and leads to pulmonary embolism.
- The echo shows RV dyskinesia with normo-tension. Hence the mainstay of treatment is UFH.
  Choice A: Thrombolysis is indicated as primary therapy in case of hypotension.
  Choice C: Embolectomy is also done in case of hypotension in PE.
  Choice D: Indications for insertion of an IVC filter are (1) active bleeding that precludes anticoagulation and (2) recurrent venous thrombosis despite intensive anticoagulation. The filter itself may fail by permitting the passage of small-to medium-size clots

Algorithm for PE Management

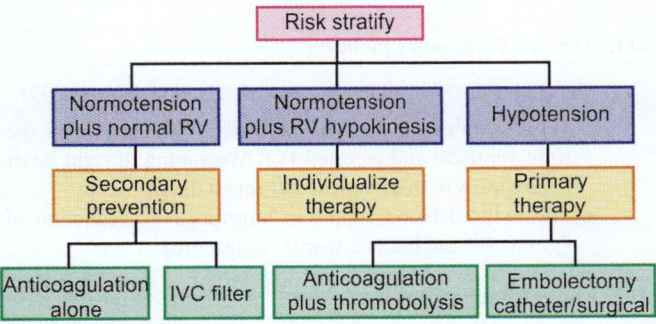

301. Ans. (a) Acute massive pulmonary embolism

(Ref: Harrison 20th edition, p 1914; Harrison 19th edition, page 1631)

Normal pressure	Value given (in mmHg)	Interpretation
RA= 2-6mmHg	12	Elevated
RV= 25/5 mmHg	50/12	Elevated
Pulmonary artery=25/10 mmHg	50/15	Elevated
PCWP=8-12mmHg	8	Normal
Aorta= <120/80	80/60	Hypotension

- The presence of normal PCWP rules out primary involvement of left side heart. Hence choice B is ruled out
- Choice C will lead to under-filling of right side of heart but this patient has elevated pressure values in right side of heart.
- Choice D will lead to increased cardiac output but this patient has hypotension.
- Increased RA, PV pressure with PAH indicates RV malfunction. Less flow to lungs will lead to systemic hypotension. Hence the patient has presentation of acute cor-pulmonale.

302. Ans. (b) Subcutaneous low molecular weight heparin

(Ref: Harrison 20th edition, p 1911)

- The clinical diagnosis of pulmonary embolism is already given in the question. Hence the choices with imaging are ruled out.
- Post-operative status by clinical prediction rule is 1.5 points.
- Presence of clinical signs of DVT is 3 points by clinical prediction rule
- Hence dichotomous clinical probability assessment score is > 4
- Anticoagulation is the foundation for successful treatment of DVT and PE.
- *For acute PE, the ACCP guidelines recommend starting low–molecular weight heparin (LMWH) or fondaparinux, preferred over unfractionated heparin (UFH)*

Clinical prediction rule for PE

Clinical variable	Points
Clinical symptoms or signs of DVT	3
Alternate diagnosis less likely than PE	3
HR>100	1.5
Immobilization > 3 days or surgery in previous 4 weeks	1.5
Previous PE or DVT	1.5
Haemoptysis	1
Cancer	1

Dichotomous clinical probability assessment
If score > 4: PE likely
If score < 4: PE unlikely

303. Ans. (b) V/P scan contraindicated in pregnancy

(Ref: Harrison 20th edition, p 1912; Harrison 19th edition, page 1631-32)

Choice A is correct	Pulmonary Embolism is diagnosed by V/P scan if two or more segmental perfusion defects are seen in the presence of normal ventilation.
Choice C is correct	Causes for ventilation perfusion defects other than acute PE: Asthma Chronic obstructive pulmonary disease.
Choice D is correct	The diagnosis of PE is very unlikely in patients with normal and nearly normal scans but is about 90% certain in patients with high-probability scans.

In ventilation perfusion scanning particulate albumin labelled with a gamma-emitting radionuclide are given intravenously.

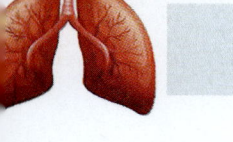

They are trapped in the pulmonary capillary bed and evaluated using a gamma camera. In setting of pulmonary embolism during pregnancy, it is a life threatening illness; hence V/P scan can be done.

304. Ans. (d) CT with IV contrast

(Ref: Harrison 20th edition, p 1912; Harrison 19th ed./1633-64)

- A definitive diagnosis of PE depends on visualization of an intraluminal filling defect in more than one projection.
- Chest CT with contrast has become the main test for diagnosis replacing the older invasive pulmonary angiography.
- Catheter-based diagnostic testing is used in case of an unsatisfactory chest CT and those patients where catheter-directed thrombolysis or embolectomy is planned

305. Ans. (a) Thrombolytic

(Ref: Harrison 20th edition, p 1913; Harrison 19th ed./1634-35)

- Anticoagulation with heparin has long been the standard treatment for normotensive patients with pulmonary embolism. By preventing clot propagation, heparin allows endogenous fibrinolysis to occur, with eventual resolution of thromboemboli. Presumably through this mechanism, heparin therapy has been shown to significantly reduce both the incidence of recurrent pulmonary embolism and patient mortality.
- However in the absence of an absolute contraindication, patients with pulmonary embolism induced hypotension or shock are usually treated with thrombolytic agents. The three thrombolytic agents used in treatment of pulmonary embolism- streptokinase, urokinase and recombinant tissue-type plasminogen activator (rt-PA).

306. Ans. (a) Pulmonary embolism

(Ref: Harrison 20th edition, p 1910; Harrison's 19th ed./1631)

- PE is the most common preventable cause of death among hospitalized patients. PE and DVT occurring after total hip or knee replacement is currently taken as unacceptable, and steps are taken to prevent it by giving subcutaneous fondaparinux.
- For patients who have DVT, the most common history is a cramp in the lower calf that persists for several days and becomes more uncomfortable as time progresses. For patients who have PE, the most common history is unexplained breathlessness.

307. Ans. (b) S1 Q3 T3

(Ref: Harrison 20th edition, p 1912; Harrison 19th p 1633, 101)

308. Ans. (a) Sinus tachycardia

(Ref: Harrison 20th edition, p 1912)

- The most common ECG abnormalities in the setting of pulmonary embolism are tachycardia and nonspecific ST-T wave abnormalities.
- The finding of $S_1 Q_3 T_3$ is nonspecific and insensitive in the absence of clinical suspicion for pulmonary embolism. The classic findings of right heart strain and acute cor pulmonale are tall, peaked P waves in lead II (P pulmonale); right axis deviation; right bundle-branch block; and $S_1 Q_3 T_3$ pattern.
- If electrocardiographic abnormalities are present, they may be suggestive of pulmonary embolism, but the absence of such abnormalities has no significant predictive value.

309. Ans. (d) Myocardial depression due to anaesthetic agents

(Ref: Harrison's 17th ed. pg. 1561)

A decrease in end tidal CO2 is seen with a decrease in cardiac output if ventilation remains same. Pulmonary embolism is more commonly seen *post operatively* and is hence ruled out.

310. Ans. (b) Thrombolytic therapy

(Ref: Harrison 20th edition, p 1913)

- Thrombolysis is indicated for hemodynamically unstable patients with pulmonary embolism. Thrombolysis dramatically improves acute cor pulmonale.
- Fibrinolytic regimens currently in common use for pulmonary embolism include 2 forms of recombinant tPA, alteplase and reteplase, along with urokinase and streptokinase. Alteplase usually is given as a front-loaded infusion over 90 or 120 minutes. Urokinase and streptokinase usually are given as infusions over 24 hours or more. Reteplase is a new-generation thrombolytic with a longer half-life; it is given as a single bolus or as 2 boluses administered 30 minutes apart

311. Ans. (c) Pulmonary plethora

(Ref: Harrison 20th edition, p 1911; Harrison 19th p 1631-33)

- Massive pulmonary embolism leads to congestion in the right ventricle and elevated JVP. Worsening of right heart failure leads to inter-ventricular septal deviation.
- The reduced blood supply to lungs leads to reduction of Systolic BP and hemodynamic compromise.

312. Ans. (a) Tachypnea

(Ref: Harrison 20th edition, p 1911)

In patients with recognized pulmonary embolism, the incidence of physical signs is
1. Tachypnea (respiratory rate >16/min) - 96%
2. Rales - 58%
3. Accentuated second heart sound - 53%
4. Tachycardia (heart rate >100/min) - 44%
5. Fever (temperature >37.8°C) - 43%

313. Ans. (a) CTA

(Ref: Harrison 20th edition, p 1912; Harrison 19th p 1632-34)

Computed tomography angiography (CTA) is the initial imaging modality of choice for stable patients with suspected pulmonary embolism. The American College of Radiology (ACR) considers chest CTA to be the current standard of care for the detection of pulmonary embolism.

Pulmonary angiography, CT scanning shows emboli directly, but CT is noninvasive, cheaper than pulmonary angiography, and widely available.

314. Ans. (a) Bradycardia

(Ref: Harrison 20th edition, p 1911; Harrison 19th p 1631-32)

Pulmonary embolism leads to right CHF and resultant tachycardia with normal to low Blood pressure.

315. Ans. (c) Pelvic surgery

(Ref: Harrison 19th p 1631-32)

316. Ans. (b) ECG shows evidence of acute left ventricular stress

(Ref: Harrison 20th edition, p 1911; Harrison 19th p 1633, 101)

The classic findings in pulmonary embolism are of right heart strain and acute cor pulmonale are tall, peaked P waves in lead II (P pulmonale); right axis deviation; right bundle-branch block; an $S_1 Q_3 T_3$ pattern; or atrial fibrillation

317. Ans. (a) Fanconi anemia

(Ref: Harrison 20th edition, p 1910; Harrison 19th p 1631-32)

- Old age will lead to prolonged immobilization post-surgery and increases the possibility of deep vein thrombosis.
- Estrogen based OCP increase thrombogenic potential.
- Thrombosis involves the venous system, and it usually occurs in hepatic, abdominal, cerebral, and subdermal veins. The tendency of patients with PNH to suffer thrombosis has been recognized as a major part of the syndrome and interpreted as a very bad prognostic sign and the most common cause of death in PNH.

318. Ans. (d) Progesterone therapy

(Ref: Harrison 20th edition, p 1910; Harrison 19th p 1631-32)

- Protein S, a vitamin K-dependent physiological anticoagulant, acts as a nonenzymatic cofactor to activated protein C in the proteolytic degradation of factor Va and factor VIIIa. Decreased (antigen) levels or impaired function (activity) of protein S leads to decreased degradation of factor Va and factor VIIIa and an increased propensity to venous thrombosis.
- Malignancy is a hypercoagulable state and predisposes to pulmonary embolism
- Obesity patients after surgery will be able to mobilize slower and therefore at risk for deep vein thromobosis
- Estrogen leads to hypercoagulable state and not progesterone.

319. Ans (c) Doppler Study

(Ref: CMDT 2014, page 311)

- Transesophageal echocardiography (TEE) has the highest sensitivity for detecting the presence of air in the right ventricular outflow tract or major pulmonary veins.
- It can detect as little as 0.02 mL/kg of air administered by bolus injection. It also has the added advantage of identifying paradoxical air embolism (PAE), and Doppler allows audible detection of venous air embolism (VAE). Echocardiography, both TEE and transthoracic echocardiography (TTE) not only allow for the diagnosis of VAE but also aid in the diagnosis of cardiac anomalies, assessment of volume status, pulmonary hypertension, and cardiac contractility, thereby allowing exclusion of other causes of hypotension, dyspnea, and aiding in further patient management.
- (Over all highest sensivity)T.E.E > doppler > E.T N_2 > E.T CO_2

320. Ans. (b) Dyspnea

(Ref: Harrison 20th edition, p 1912; Harrison 19th p 1632-33)

The common symptoms of pulmonary embolism are:
- Dyspnea (73%)
- Pleuritic chest pain (66%)
- Cough (37%)
- Hemoptysis (13%)

321. Ans. (b) Pulmonary infarction

(Ref: Page 474, Grainger and Allison Diagnostic Radiology; Harrison 19th p 1632)

Elevation of the Hemidiaphragm

- Subpulmonic effusion
- Pulmonary infarction
- Phrenic Nerve Paralysis= Breast Cancer/ Metastasis/ Iatrogenic-post CABG
- Subphrenic abscess (Right subhepatic-appendicitis) and (Left 2° ulcer perforation)
- Liver mass
- Interposition of the colon
- Distended stomach
- Congenital Diaphragmatic Hernia
- Traumatic Rupture of the Diaphragm
- Eventration of the Diaphragm

322. Ans. (a) Chest pain is the most common symptom

(Ref: Harrison 20th edition, p 1911; Harrison 19th p 1631-32)

323. Ans. (c) Sinus Tachycardia

(Ref: Harrison 20th edition, p 1911; Harrison 19th p 1633)

Hypersensitivity Pneumonitis

324. Ans. (c) X-ray features upper lobe predominant in chronic HP

Ref: page 2602: Harrison 20th edition

Hypersensitivity pneumonitis occurs due to inhalational exposure to variety of antigens leading to inflammatory response of alveoli and small airways. Choice A is ruled out as asthma attacks are seasonal in nature. Choice B is ruled out as major complaint of the patient in Hypersensitivity Pneumonitis is dyspnea associated with fever, chills and malaise. Choice D is ruled out as alveoli are involved in HP. The answer by exclusion is Choice C.

Causes of upper lobe involvement of lungs	

• Inhaled injurious gases
  ▪ Smoke inhalation
  ▪ Centrilobular emphysema
• Impaired mucociliary clearance
  ▪ Cystic fibrosis
• Inhaled particulates: pneumoconiosis
  ▪ Silicosis
  ▪ Coal worker pneumoconiosis
  ▪ Berylliosis
  ▪ Miscellaneous pneumoconioses (hard metal disease, kaolinosis, bauxite pneumoconio-sis, fuller's earth disease)
• Inhaled antigens
  ▪ Hypersensitivity pneumonitis
  ▪ Allergic bronchopulmonary aspergillosis
  ▪ Chronic eosinophilic pneumonia
• Granulomatous diseases
	• Granulomatous diseases
	  ▪ Tuberculosis
	  ▪ Sarcoidosis
	  ▪ Langerhans cell histiocytosis
	  ▪ Bronchocentric granulomatosis
	• Abnormal perfusion kinetics
	  ▪ Right-sided localized pulmonary edema in acute mitral regurgitation
	  ▪ Neurogenic pulmonary edema
	• Metabolic diseases
	  ▪ Metastatic pulmonary calcification
	• Increased mechanical stress
	  ▪ Ankylosing spondylitis

- Pathologic evidence on lung biopsy
  - Often evidence of poorly formed non-caseating granulomas
  - Mononuclear cellular infiltrates
  - Fibrotic scarring

Systemic eosinophilia is rather a hallmark laboratory feature in patient of eosinophilic granulomatosis with polyangiitis. It is not associated with HP.

327. Ans. (a) Transient, migratory pulmonary infiltrations

(Ref: Harrison 20th edition, p 1973; Harrison 19th edition, page 422)

Loeffler's syndrome is a transient, benign syndrome of migratory pulmonary infiltrates and peripheral blood eosinophilia of unknown cause

Pulmonary infiltrates with Eosinophila

- Allergic bronchopulmonary mycoses
- Parasitic infestations
- Drug reactions
- Eosinophilia-myalgia syndrome
- Loeffler's syndrome
- Acute eosinophilic pneumonia
- Churgstrauss
- Hyper-eosinophilic syndrome

Lung Cancer

328. Ans. (a) SCLC, Brain metastasis

(Ref: Harrison 20th edition, p 537; Harrison 19th edition, page 510 and 1687)

- The history of uranium mining means exposure to radon an inert gas that is a product of uranium decay.
- All types of lung cancer occur with increased frequency in uranium miners, but SCLC is the most common.
- The Chest X ray shows lesion in right para-cardiac area which is Small cell cancer of the lung exhibiting metastasis to brain.
- Muscle cramps can be explained by ectopic production of ACTH by SCLC leading to Hypokalemic Alkalosis.
- Most patients with this disease present with a short duration of symptoms, usually only 8-12 weeks before presentation. The clinical manifestations of SCLC can result from local tumor growth, intrathoracic spread, distant spread, and/or paraneoplastic syndromes.

329. Ans. (d) Adenocarcinoma

(Ref: Harrison 20th edition, p 538)

330. Ans. (a) Commonest Malignancy of lung

(Ref: Harrison 20th edition, p 538; Harrison 19th p 507-08)

331. Ans. (b) Small cell carcinoma

(Ref: Harrison 20th edition, p 538; Harrison 19th p 507-08)

332. Ans. (c) Small cell carcinoma

(Ref: Harrison 20th edition, p 538; Schwartz 8th 562, Harrison 19th p 507-08, 608-09)

325. Ans. (a) 4 3 2 1

(Ref: Harrison 20th edition, p 1970; Harrison 19th edition, p 1681)

Bagassosis	Sugar cane dust with Thermophilic Actinomycetes.
Byssinosis	Cotton dust
Farmer lung	Moldy hay with growth of Micropolysporafaeni
Wood worker lung	Oak cedar pine dust

326. Ans. (d) Systemic Eosinophilia

(Ref: Harrison 20th edition, p 1972; Harrison 19th edition, page 1682-83)

Clinical prediction rule for HP
1. Confirmed history of exposure (Strongest predictor) 2. Positive precipitating antibodies to the offending antigen 3. Recurrent episodes of symptoms 4. Symptoms occurring 4-8 hours after antigen exposure 5. Crackles on inspiration 6. Weight loss

WORK UP IN HP

- Radiographic evidence on chest radiograph is non-specific.
- HRCT: In subacute form of HP, ground glass opacities are characteristic as is presence of centri-lobular nodules. Sub-pleural honeycombing with sparing of lung bases.
- Bronchoscopic alveolar lavage (BAL) evidence: *Lymphocytes comprised the majority of the infiltrating cells with some plasma cells.*
- Mild elevations in erythrocyte sedimentation rate, C-reactive protein, and immunoglobulins of IgG, IgM, or IgA isotype may occur in all presentations of HP, reflecting acute or chronic inflammation.

333. Ans. (c) Small cell carcinoma of Lung

(Ref: Harrison 20th edition, p 538; Harrison 19th p 250, 507-08)

334. Ans. (d) Hypercalcemia

(Ref: Harrison 20th edition, p 542; Harrison 19th p 511-12)

335. Ans. (d) Superior Vena caval obstruction

(Ref: Harrison 20th edition, p 542; Harrison 19th p 1788, 608-09)

336. Ans. (b) Hamartoma

(Ref: Harrison 20th edition, p 547; Sutton 7th/138,140,123, Harrison 19th p 515)

Miscellaneous

337. Ans. (a)

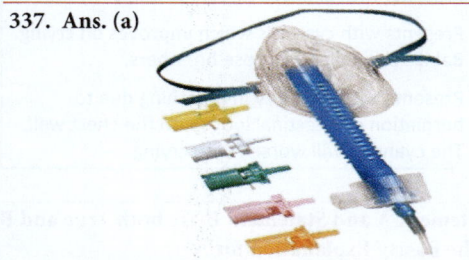

Ref: Morgan anaesthesia, 6th edition, Page 1333

- Choice D: Reservoir face mask is a high flow, variable performance device. At flow rate of 12-15L/min the delivered FiO_2 is in the range of 75-90%.
- Choice C is simple face mask while choice B is nasal cannula and both can deliver limited oxygen up to 40% due to diffusion and mixing with air.
- Choice A: Venturi mask is a high flow, fixed performance device. It can deliver up to 60% oxygen. When oxygen is pushed through a small jet orifice entering the mask, negative pressure is created which leads to room air to be entrained into the mask through apertures in the venturi barrel. The resultant air flow oxygen mixture can be varied by changing the interchangeable jet nozzles. (Notice the different colour nozzles in choice A). The high flow rates also flush out the expired carbon dioxide from the holes on the side of the mask. Hence there is no rebreathing or no increase in dead space.

338. Ans. (a) Acetazolamide

Ref: Harrison 20th edition, page 3336

Cold environment at high altitude coupled with exercise leads to increased pulmonary intravascular pressure and predisposes to high altitude pulmonary edema. Acetazolamide has been shown to blunt pulmonary hypoxic vasoconstriction.

339. Ans. (b) Water column movement in the tube

Ref: SRB, 5th edition, page 1121

- The functioning of chest tube is best assessed by movement of water column in ICD bag. Maximum movement is noted when the tube is first inserted. Progressively as the lung expands by resolution of pneumothorax, movement of column reduces. Absent movement indicates blocked tube.
- *Bubbling* in the bag indicates *development of bronchopleural fistula*. The smaller ones show a self-resolution but the bigger ones require a thoracotomy.
- Minor bubbling may be initially upon chest tube insertion for large pneumothorax which resolve spontaneously as the pneumothorax gets resolved.

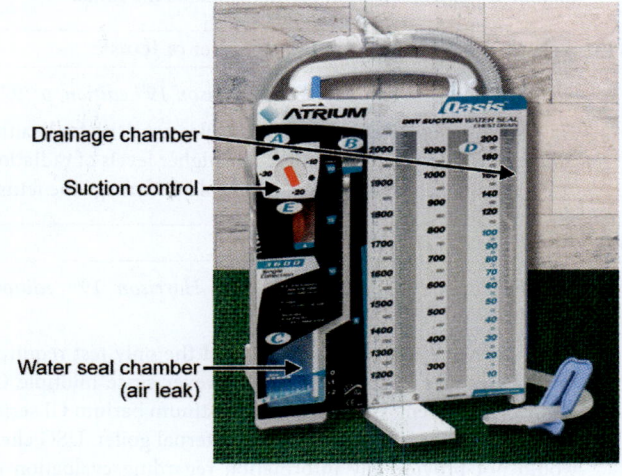

340. Ans. (a) Myasthenic Crisis

Ref: Fishman Manual of pulmonary disease and disorders, 3/e, page 551

- Orthopnea is classically seen in congestive heart failure. It is also seen in disorders of neuromuscular junction that lead to diaphragmatic paralysis. Hence orthopnea can be seen in disorders like M. Gravis, ALS, GBS and transverse myelitis.
- Massive unilateral pleural effusion leads to trepopnea (dyspnea in lateral decubitus position)
- Atrial myxoma leads to platypnea (dyspnea in sitting position)

341. Ans. (a) Cough

Ref: NMS Medicine case book: Lippincott, Page 574

Modified Centor Criteria for Pharyngitis and Tonsillitis

Clinical finding	Points
Absence of cough	1

Age
  3 to 14 years
  15 to 45 years
  Older than 45 years
	
	1
	0
	−1

Anterior cervical lymphadenopathy	1
Fever	1
Tonsillar erythema or exudates	1

Note: *Patients with a score of 1 or less do not require further testing or treatment, although contact with a person who has documented streptococcal infection should be considered in patients with a score of 1, and testing should be performed in these cases; those with a score of 2 or 3 should have rapid antigen detection testing and, if results are positive, should receive antibiotics; and those with a score of 4 or 5 should receive antibiotics.*

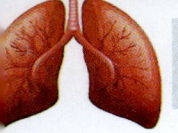

342. Ans. (a) Cardiogenic Shock

Ref: Harrison 20th edition, p 2053; Harrison 19th edition, page 1759

In all types of shock, CVP and PCWP are reduced with the exception of cardiogenic shock.

The prime reason for elevated CVP is poor forward flow with increased vascular resistance. The neuroendocrine mediated vasoconstriction further explains the same.

343. Ans. (a) She can fly with no risk to her or fetus

Ref: Harrison 20th edition, p 896; Harrison 19th edition, p 797

Harrison quotes: "Commercial air travel is not a risk for healthy pregnant women or to the fetus". The higher levels of radiation at higher altitude have also not been able to damage the fetus.

344. Ans. (b) USG chest

Ref: Harrison 20th edition, p 2009; Harrison 19th edition, p 1719

CT chest is the most valuable test and the only test required in all cases of mediastinal mass. However since multiple GI lesions can present in posterior mediastinum barium GI series is warranted. I-131 can scan for retrosternal goiter. USG chest would not provide any information regarding evaluation of mediastinal disorders.

345. Ans. (b) On chest tube insertion 1500 ml exsanguination is seen

(Ref: SRB surgery: 5th edition, Page 1114)

Indications for emergency thoracotomy

> **Penetrating thoracic injury** with the following conditions:
> - Previously witnessed cardiac activity (prehospital or in-hospital)
> - Unresponsive hypotension (systolic blood pressure [SBP] < 70 mm Hg) despite vigorous resuscitation
>
> **Blunt thoracic injury** with the following conditions:
> - Previously witnessed cardiac activity (prehospital or in-hospital)
> - Rapid exsanguination from the chest tube (>1,500 mL immediately returned)
> - Unresponsive hypotension (SBP < 70 mm Hg) despite vigorous resuscitation
> - Precordial wound in a patient with prehospital cardiac arrest
> - Trauma patient with cardiac arrest after arrival to ED

346. Ans. (d) Best treatment is pleuroperitoneal shunting

(Ref: Harrison 20th edition, p 2008; Harrison 19th edition, p 1718)

- The most common cause of chylothorax is trauma caused during thoracic surgery. It can also result from tumors in the mediastinum.
- The treatment of *choice for chylo-thorax* is insertion of a chest tube plus the administration of octreotide.
- If these modalities fail, a pleuro-peritoneal shunt should be placed unless the patient has chylous ascites. An alternative treatment is ligation of the thoracic duct.
- Patients with chylothoraxes should not undergo prolonged tube thoracostomy with chest tube drainage because this will lead to malnutrition and immunologic incompetence.
- Patients with chylo-thorax present with dyspnea, and a large pleural effusion is present on the chest radiograph.
- Thoracentesis reveals milky fluid with a triglyceride level that exceeds 110 mg/dL.

347. Ans. (a) Tracheoesophageal Fistula

(Ref: Rudolph paediatrics, page 1401: 22nd edition)

TEF	- Due to impaired swallowing of amniotic fluid: polyhydramnios - Aspiration due to fistula - Excessive salivation due to esophageal atresia - Difficulty in passing NG tube due to esophageal atresia
Gastroschisis	Presents with exposed intestinal loops
Choanal Atresia	Presents with cyanosis which improves on crying. Babies are obligatory nose breathers.
Diaphragmatic hernia	Presents with difficulty in breathing due to herniation of intestinal loops into the chest wall. The cyanosis will worsen with crying.

348. Ans. (b) Statement A and Statement B are both True and B is the Basis / Explanation for A

(Ref: Avery neonatology: 8th edition, Page 701)

349. Ans. (b) Hyperventilation

(Ref: Harrison 20th edition, p 3338; Harrison 19th edition, page 248)

- Chronic mountain sickness/ Monge's disease is characterised by development of polycythaemia and development of pulmonary artery hypertension in residents of high altitude areas. Due to PAH, Right ventricular enlargement and cyanosis can be explained.
- Venesection and acetazolamide are used.
- Hyperventilation is seen in acute mountain sickness with development of high altitude pulmonary oedema.

350. Ans. (c) Vasculitis, ANCA

(Ref: Harrison 20th edition, p 2578)

The patient has involvement of:
- Upper respiratory tract involvement= epistaxis and sinusitis
- Lower respiratory tract involvement = lung cavitation (multiple and bilateral)
- Kidney involvement= renal failure
  - These point to involvement of blood vessels of these three systems, diagnosis goes in favour of granulomatosis with angitis(Wegener's Granulomatosis). For diagnosis c-ANCA will be helpful along with biopsy findings of vasculitis.
  - The disease involves small arteries, arterioles, capillaries and leads to necrotizing granulomatous lesion involving both upper and lower respiratory tract and the kidney.

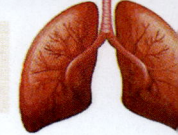

- The cytoplasmic pattern of immunofluorescence (c-ANCA) is caused by PR3-ANCA and has high specificity>90% for granulomatosis with angitis.
- Remissions can be obtained by use of cyclophosphamide with prednisolone.

Systemic fungal infection	Needs extreme immunosuppression to occur.
Miliary TB	Ruled out as lungs lesion are not cavities
Multiple metastasis	Involve lungs mainly but renal failure and epistaxis are unlikely

351. Ans. (a) Pregnant woman with sore throat can be started immediately on oseltamivir without diagnostic testing under Category B

(Ref: mohfw.nic.in)

Guidelines on categorization of Influenza A H_1N_1 cases requiring screening for home isolation, testing treatment, and hospitalization

Category- A
- Patients with mild fever plus cough/sore throat with or without body ache, headache, diarrhoea and vomiting will be categorized as Category-A. They do not require Oseltamivir and should be treated for the symptoms mentioned above. The patients should be monitored for their progress and reassessed at 24 to 48 hours by the doctor.
- No testing of the patient for H1N1 is required.
- Patients should confine themselves at home and avoid mixing up with public and high risk members in the family.

Category B
- **In addition** to all the signs and symptoms mentioned under Category-A, if the patient has **high grade fever** and **severe sore throat,** may require **home isolation and Oseltamivir**
- In addition to all signs and symptoms mentioned under Category-A, individuals having one or more of the following **high risk conditions** shall be treated with Oseltamivir
  - Children **with mild illness** but **with** predisposing risk factors.
  - Pregnant women
  - Persons aged 65 years or older
  - **Patients with** lung diseases, heart disease, liver disease, kidney disease, blood disorders, diabetes, neurological disorders, cancer and HIV/AIDS
  - **Patients on** long term cortisone therapy.
- No tests for H_1N_1 is required for Category-B
- All patients of Category-B should confine themselves at home and avoid mixing with public and high risk members in the family.

Category- C
- In addition to signs and symptoms of Category A and B, if patient has 1 or more of following:
- Breathlessness, chest pain, drowsiness, fall in blood pressure, sputum mixed with blood, bluish discolouration of nails
- Children with influenza like illness who had a severe disease as manifested by the red flag signs (Somnolence, high and persistent fever, inability to feed well, convulsions, shortness of breath, difficulty in breathing, etc).
- Worsenng of underlying chronic conditions.

All these patients mentioned above in Category-C require testing, immediate hospitalization and treatment.

352. Ans. (c) Rifampicin 450 mg + Isoniazid 200 mg + Pyrazinamide 1000 mg

(Ref: 6th edition K.D. Tripathi, page 746)

Recommended doses (per kg body weight) or essential anti-tuberculosis drug)			
Anti-tuberculosis drugs	Mode of action	Recommended dose (mg/kg)	
		Daily	3x per week
Isoniazid (H)	Bactericidal	5 (4-6)	10 (8-12)
Rifampicin (R)	Bactericidal	10 (8-12)	10 (8-12)
Pyrazinamide (P)	Bactericidal	25 (20-30)	35 (30-40)
Ethambutol (E)	Bacteriostatic	15 (15-20)	30 (25-35)
Streptomycin (S)	Bactericidal	15 (12-18)	15 (12-18)
Thioacetazone (T)	Bacteriostatic	2.5	Not applicable

353. Ans. (b) Esophageal Rupture

(Ref: Harrison 20th edition, p 2009; Harrison 19th edition, p 1719)

- Most cases of acute mediastinitis either are due to esophageal perforation or occur after median sternotomy for cardiac surgery.
- The esophageal rupture can occur spontaneously or as a complication of esophagoscopy or the insertion of a Blakemore tube.
- Patients with esophageal rupture are acutely ill with chest pain and dyspnea due to the mediastinal infection.
- Appropriate treatment consists of exploration of the mediastinum with primary repair of the esophageal tear and drainage of the pleural space and the mediastinum.
- The spectrum of chronic mediastinitis ranges from granulomatous inflammation of the lymph nodes in the mediastinum to fibrosingmediastinitis. Most cases are due to histoplasmosis or TB, but sarcoidosis, silicosis, and other fungal diseases are at times causative.
- Patients with granulomatous mediastinitis are usually asymptomatic. Those with fibrosingmediastinitis usually have signs of compression of a mediastinal structure such as the superior vena cava or large airways, phrenic or recurrent laryngeal nerve paralysis, or obstruction of the pulmonary artery or proximal pulmonary veins.

354. Ans. (d) Lesion in the brain

(Ref: Concepts in Medical Physiology, Johnson 5th edition, Page 295)

Biot's Breathing: Biot's Breathing is characterized by irregularly irregular breathing with sudden apnea and is seen in CNS lesions and is a sign of increased intracranial pressure.

Kussmaul's Respiration. Kussmaul Breathing is deep rapid respiration in metabolic acidosis and is classically associated with diabetic ketoacidosis

Cheyne-Stokes Respiration. Cheyne-Stokes Respiration is one of increasingly deep respiration followed by a steady diminution of breathing until an apneic episode occurs in neurologic diseases with raised ICP. Obesity may be present. Some patients will show pupillary dilation with rapid breathing and pupillary contraction with apnea.

The differential diagnoses are

CNS disease
CHF
Pneumonia
Carbon monoxide poisoning
Medications(eg, morphine).

Apneustic Breathing. Apneustic breathing is seen in severely ill patients with coma. The patient holds his or her breath at the end of inspiration until the Hering-Breuer (carotid body) reflex initiates exhalation. This breathing pattern suggests pontine disease.

355. Ans. (a) Pulmonary Hamartoma

(Ref: Harrison 20th edition, p 547; Harrison 19th ed. / 515-16)

- Popcorn calcification is virtually diagnostic on chest radiographs for pulmonary hamartoma.
- It characteristically appears as well-defined, solitary pulmonary nodules; they may show varying patterns of calcification, including an irregular popcorn, stippled, or curvilinear pattern, or even a combination of all 3 patterns.

356. Ans. (b) Lung Laceration

(Ref: Harrison 20th edition, p 2010)

- The image shows presence of subcutaneous emphysema which is also hinted in line 2 of the question where it mentions crepitus is palpated.
- Chest trauma, a major cause of subcutaneous emphysema, can cause air to enter the skin of the chest wall from the neck or lung.
- Most students mark it as renal shut down which is not the answer because it is unlikely within 4 hour of trauma insult.
- **Gas gangrene will again take time to develop and would lead to development of crepitus in the injured part.**

Causes of subcutaneous emphysema

- Trauma to parts of the respiratory system other than the lungs, such as rupture of a bronchial tube, may also cause subcutaneous emphysema
- May also occur with fractures of the facial bones, neoplasms, during asthma attacks.

When the alveoli of the lung are ruptured, as occurs in pulmonary laceration, air may travel beneath the visceral pleura (the membrane lining the lung), to the hilum of the lung, up to the trachea, to the neck and then to the chest wall

357. Ans. (a) Sarcoidosis

(Ref: Harrison 20th edition, p 2601; Harrison 19th ed. / 2206)

The clinical profile is compatible with diagnosis of sarcoidosis.

358. Ans. (d) Bronchocele

(Ref: Fundamentals of Diagnostic, Radiology, 3rd edition, Bryant, Page 375)

- A bronchocele is a mucous-filled dilated bronchi surrounded by aerated lung.
- CT chest can identify a bronchocele as a tubular intrapulmonary opacity distinct from vascular shadows
- Their appearance is similar to a"finger in glove"or the shape of the letters V or Y.

359. Ans. (d) Rhinocerebral involvement

(Ref: Harrison 20th edition, p 1534)

- Rhino-cerebral involvement is seen with mucormycosis in diabetics.
- A rapidly invasive Aspergillus infection in the lungs often causes cavity formation.
- Aspergillus fumigatus is found in sputum of normal people. Eye involvements occur in form of keratitis and endophthalmitis. Brain involvements in aspergillosis is via hematogenous dissemination.

360. Ans. (a) Non small cell lung Ca

(Ref: Harrison 19th ed. / 510-511)

- Most common cause of hemoptysis is tuberculosis but at 65 years of age it is more likely a presentation of lung cancer.
- Lung cancers can cause hemoptysis but clubbing is seen with non small cell cancer of the lung only. Remember that clubbing is absent in small cell cancer of the lung.

361. Ans. (d) Eosinophilic alveolitis

(Ref: Harrison 20th edition, p 1971; Harrison 19th ed./1681)

362. Ans. (a) Dextrocardia

- Situs solitus is the normal position, and situs inversus is the mirror image of situs solitus.
- Cardiac situs is determined by the atrial location.
- In situs inversus:
  - Morphologic right atrium is on the left, and the morphologic left atrium is on the right.
  - Normal pulmonary anatomy is also reversed so that the left lung has 3 lobes and the right lung has 2 lobes.
- Liver and gallbladder are located on the left
- Spleen and stomach are located on the right.

363. Ans. (a) Lymphangitis Carcinomatosis

(Ref: Harrison 19th edition, Page 476e-3, 1552)

The Chest X ray shows presence of kerley B lines perpendicular to the pleural reflections.

The following are causes of Kerley B lines

- Pulmonary edema
- Mitral stenosis
- Lymphangitis carcinomatosis
- Malignant lymphoma
- Congenital lymphangiectasia
- Viral and mycoplasma pneumonia
- Idiopathic pulmonary fibrosis
- Late stage hemosiderosis

364. Ans. (a) Canon Ball Metastasis

Large round circumscribed lesions are seen in right and left para-cardiac borders indicating presence of canon ball metastasis.

365. Ans. (c) Non Rebreathing Mask

(Ref: Synopsis of pediatric emergency, 4th edition)

Method	% of oxygen delivery
Face mask	35 - 65%
Nasal cannula	30-40%
Non rebreathing mask	90%
Oxygen hood	50%

366. Ans. (c) Serratia Marcesens

(Ref: john Hopkins internal medicine board review, box 22-3, 4th edition, Harrison 19th p 245-46 and 1661)

- Pseudo-hemoptysisis expectoration of blood other than respiratory tract. Like GIT or blood draining from larynx.
- Most common organism causing pseudo hemoptysis: Serratiamarcescens Serratia Marcescens has a predilection for growth on foodstuffs, especially of the starchy variety.

367. Ans. (c) Birbeck granules

(Ref: Harrison 19th p 135e-36)

Birbeck granules, also known as Birbeck bodies, are rod shaped or "tennis-racket" cytoplasmic organelles with a central linear density and a striated appearance. They are a characteristic microscopic finding in Langerhans cell histiocytosis

368. Ans. (a) Decrease in tissue perfusion

(Ref: Harrison 19th p 1729-31)

369. Ans. (b) Absence of air bronchograms

(Ref: Nelson 20th p 851)

- Chest radiographs of a newborn infant with respiratory distress syndrome reveal bilateral, diffuse, reticular granular or *ground-glass appearances*; air bronchograms; and poor lung expansion. The prominent air bronchograms represent aerated bronchioles superimposed on a background of collapsed alveoli
- Absence of air bronchograms is a feature of meconium aspiration syndrome

(Comparison of radiological features of HMD versus meconium aspiration versus Transient tachypnea of new born)

	HMD	MAS	TTNB
Lung volume	Small volume lung	Hyper-inflated lungs	Normal volume lungs
Lung Parenchyma	Fine granular opacities Air bronchogram	Coarse, linear and irregular opacities. No air bronchogram	Small effusion
Air leak	May to present post ventilation Pulmonary interstitial emphysema	Spontaneous pneumothorax and effusion 20%	Never
Interstitial shadows	None	None	Prominent interstitial markings and vessels. Thick septa

Contd...

370. Ans. (a) Neurogenic tumor

(Ref: Harrison 20th edition, p 2010; Harrison 19th p 1664-65)

- In the posterior mediastinum, neurogenic tumors, meningoceles, meningomyeloceles, gastroenteric cysts, and esophageal diverticula are commonly found.
- The most common lesions in the anterior mediastinum are thymomas, lymphomas, teratomatous neoplasms, and thyroid masses.
- The most common masses in the middle mediastinum are vascular masses, lymph node enlargement from metastases or granulomatous disease, and pleuropericardial and bronchogenic cysts.

371. Ans. (a) Subcutaneous adrenaline

(Ref: Harrison 20th edition, p 2501; Harrison 19th p 1749-50)

- Epinephrine maintains blood pressure, antagonizes the effects of the released mediators, and inhibits further release of mediators. Give 0.3–0.5 ml of 1 m (1:1000 dilution) with repeated dosages at 5–20 minutes.
- Administer an H1 blocker and an H2 blocker, because studies have shown the combination to be superior to an H1 blocker alone in relieving the histamine-mediated symptoms. Diphenhydramine and ranitidine are an appropriate combination. IV administration ensures that effective dosing is not impaired by hemodynamic compromise, which adversely affects gastrointestinal (GI) or IM absorption.
- Corticosteroids have no immediate effect on anaphylaxis

372. Ans. (b) Neurofibroma

(Ref: Harrison 19th p 1664-65)

373. Ans. (c) Raised serum precipitins

(Ref: Harrison 20th edition, p 2010; Harrison 19th p 1681)

- All forms of hypersensitivity may be associated with elevations in erythrocyte sedimentation rate, C-reactive protein, rheumatoid factor, lactate dehydrogenase, or serum immunoglobulins.
- Following acute exposure to an antigen, neutrophilia and lymphopenia are frequently present. Eosinophilia is not a feature.
- Examination for serum precipitins against suspected antigen, is an important part of the diagnostic workup and

should be performed on any patient with interstitial lung disease, especially if a suggestive exposure history is elicited. The occurrence of precipitins indicates sufficient exposure to the causative agent for generation of an immunologic response and is one of the major diagnostic criteria; however, the diagnosis of HP is not established solely by the presence of precipitins, as they are found in sera of many individuals exposed to appropriate antigens who demonstrate no other evidence of HP.

- Chest x-ray shows no specific or distinctive changes in HP. It can be normal even in symptomatic patients. The acute or subacute phases may be associated with poorly defined, patchy, or diffuse infiltrates; with discrete, nodular infiltrates; or with air-space consolidation. In the chronic phase, the chest x-ray usually shows a diffuse reticulonodular infiltrate. Honeycombing may eventually develop as the condition progresses. Apical sparing is common.
- High-resolution chest CT has become the procedure of choice for imaging of HP. Although pathognomonic features have not been identified, acute HP may appear with diffuse "ground-glass" infiltrates, a reticulonodular pattern, or confluent alveolar opacification.

374. Ans. (d) Hypoparathyroidism

(Ref: CMDT-2018 pg. 1135)

The inferior notching of ribs is seen due to pulsation of collaterals in coarctation of aorta. Taussig Bing operation is done for Tetralogy of Fallot and is a shunt surgery where the shunt pulsations can cause inferior rib notching.

Inferior rib notching (Roesler sign)
- Enlarged collateral vessels -Coarctation of the aorta
- Interrupted aortic arch
- Subclavian artery obstruction-Takayasu disease
- Blalock-Taussig shunt : involves only upper 2 rib spaces
- AVM of the chest wall
- SVC obstruction with enlarged venous collaterals
- Neurogenic tumours - Schwannoma (usually single)
- Neurofibromatosis type 1 (rarely can be superior if neurofibroma is very large)

Superior notching of ribs is seen in Marfan syndrome, rheumatoid arthritis, SLE and hyperparathyroidism.

375. Ans. (d) Benzene

(Ref: Harrison 19th p 663, 678)

Cigarette smoke product	Effects on human body
Aceta-aldehyde/anabasine	Addictive
Benzene	• Carcinogenic • Cardio-toxic • Reproductive potential toxicity
Benzopyrine	Carcinogenic
Carbon monoxide	Reproductive potential toxicity
Vinyl chloride	Carcinogenic

376. Ans. (b) High resolution CT scan

(Ref: Harrison 20th edition, p 234)

- For most patients, the first step in evaluation of hemoptysis should be a standard chest radiograph.
- If a source of bleeding is not identified on plain film, *a CT of the chest should be obtained*. CT allows better delineation of bronchiectasis, alveolar filling, cavitary infiltrates, and masses than does chest x-ray; it also gives further information on mediastinal lymphadenopathy, which may support a diagnosis of thoracic malignancy.
- If all of these studies are unrevealing, *bronchoscopy* should be considered. Bronchogenic carcinoma, and endobronchial lesions are often not reliably visualized on computed tomogram, bronchoscopy should be seriously considered to add to the completeness of the evaluation.

377. Ans. (d) All of the above

(Ref : www.nlm.nih.gov-google, Harrison 19th p 1703-04)

- Posterior tracheal wall laceration is another mechanism responsible for emphysema after Percutaneous Tracheostomy. After perforation of the posterior tracheal wall, the pleural space can be reached easily. This may result in a pneumothorax.
- Another mechanism for the development of emphysema is an imperfect positioning of the fenestrated cannula, whereby the fenestration is extra-luminal.
- Trauma to chest including after a vigorous Hemilich maneuver can lead to subcutaneous emphysema.

378. Ans. (d) Pulmonary Alveolar Proteinosis

(Ref: Harrison 20th edition, p 304-305; Harrison 19th p 1714)

- Pulmonary alveolar proteinosis can be diagnosed by Bronchoscopy with transbronchial biopsy and BAL may be helpful.
- Transbronchial biopsies of affected lung segments, coupled with findings on BAL, are sufficient to make the diagnosis. Use PAS reagent for BAL. Bronchoalveolar lavage fluid appears "milky." Papanicolaou staining may reveal green and orange globules that are diagnostic for PAP. Electron microscopy of BAL may reveal characteristic multi-lamellar structures.
- Non small cell cancer lung is diagnosed by bronchoscopy with biopsy
- Bronchiectasis is diagnosed with HRCT scan
- Bronchopleural fistula is diagnosed with bronchoscopy and is usually a complication of lung cancer surgery

379. Ans. (a) Respiratory syncytial virus

(Ref: CMDT 2019, p 1421)

380. Ans. (c) Aneurysm

(Ref: Harrison 20th edition, p 2010; Harrison 19th p 1664-65; 1719)

The most common masses in the middle mediastinum are vascular masses, lymph node enlargement from metastases or granulomatous disease, and pleuropericardial and bronchogenic cysts.

381. Ans. (a) Cystic fibrosis

(Ref: Nelson 20th p 2114)

382. Ans. (b) 4

(Ref: Maternity and Pediatric Nursing By Susan Scott Ricci, Terri Kyle, pg. 729-30; OP Ghai. 7/e, pg. 143])

Silverman - Anderson Index					
Score	Upper Chest Retraction	Chest Retraction	Xiphoid Retraction	Nares flaring	Grunt
0	Chest and abdomen rise together	No Intercostals retractions	No Xiphoid retractions	No nasal flaring	No expiratory grunt
1	Lag or minimal sinking of upper chest as abdomen rises	Minimal intercostals	Minimal xiphoid retractions	Minimal nasal falring	Expiratory grunt heard with stethoscope
2	Upper chest and abdomen"see-saw"	Marked intercostals retractions	Marked xiphoid retractions	Marked nasal flaring	Audible expiratory grunt

Now look at the values in the question

Upper chest	Lag on inspiration present	Score 1
Lower chest	Slight retraction present	Score 1
Xiphoid retraction	Not present	Score 0
Nares flaring	Not present	Score 0
Grunting	Audible grunting	Score 2
Total		Score 4

383. Ans. (c) Klebsiella

(Ref: Harrison 19th p 1108-1112, 1184)

- Miliary mottling or snow storm appearance on CXR is seen in Disseminated TB, Loffler pneu-monia, silicosis and chicken pox pneumonia.
- Klebsiella causes pneumonia and CXR shows bulging fissure sign due to accumulation of pus in inter-lobar fissure.
- The term miliary opacities refer to innumerable, small 1-4 mm pulmonary nodules scattered throughout the lungs. It is useful to divide these patients into those who are febrile and those who are not. Additionally, some miliary opacities are very dense, narrowing.

Common causes of Miliary picture on CXR

1. Infection
   - Tuberculosis (Disseminated)
   - Healed varicella pneumonia
2. Metastases - Miliary metastases
   - Thyroid carcinoma
   - Renal cell carcinoma
   - Breast carcinoma
   - Malignant melanoma
   - Pancreatic neoplasms
   - Osteosarcoma
   - Trophoblastic disease
3. Sarcoidosis
4. Pneumoconioses
   - Silicosis
   - Coal workers pneumoconiosis
5. Pulmonary haemosiderosis
6. Hypersensitivity pneumonitis
7. Langerhans cell histiocytosis (LCH)
8. Pulmonary alveolar proteinosis

384. Ans. (c) Atrophic rhinits

(Ref: CMDT 2019, p 271)

- Most of the side effects of steroids are mainly hoarseness, oro-pharyngeal candidiasis and decreased growth in children with adrenal suppression leading to skin thinning.
- The plausible explanation is that these drugs (since inhaled) avoid the first pass metabolism that orally administered steroids undergo and hence have preponderance to cause the usual manifestations of steroid toxicity.
- Inhaled corticosteroids are being given to more patients, at increasing doses and for longer periods of time.
- This has led to renewed concern about side-effects, particularly when higher doses (> 1 mg day-1) are used. The side-effects of particular concern are adrenocortical suppression, bone resorption, decreased growth in children, skin thinning and cataract formation. Changes in adrenocortical function are seen in a small proportion of patients given doses of 1-2 mg/day.

385. Ans. (b) Farmer's lung

(Ref: Harrison 20th edition, p 1970; Harrison 19th p 1681)

386. Ans. (a) Corona-virus

(Ref: CMDT 2019, p 1424, Harrison 19th p 1204)

SARS-associated coronavirus (SARS-CoV) caused epidemics of pneumonia from November 2002 to July 2003

387. Ans. (a) Neurofibroma

(Ref: CMDT 2019, p 297)

A solitary pulmonary nodule is defined as a discrete, well-marginated, rounded opacity *less than or equal to 3 cm in diameter* that is completely surrounded by lung parenchyma, does not touch the hilum or mediastinum, and is not associated with adenopathy, atelectasis, or pleural effusion. Lesions larger than 3 cm are considered masses and are treated as malignancies until proven otherwise. The differential diagnosis of a solitary pulmonary nodule is broad and management depends on whether the lesion is benign or malignant.

There are many causes of solitary pulmonary nodules, including:

- Malignant
  - Bronchogenic carcinoma
  - Solitary pulmonary metastasis
  - Lymphoma
  - Carcinoid tumours
    - Bronchial carcinoid tumour
    - Peripheral pulmonary carcinoid tumour
- Benign
  - Pulmonary hamartoma
- Inflammatory
  - Granuloma
  - Lung abscess
  - Rheumatoid nodule
  - Pulmonary inflammatory pseudotumour - plasma cell granuloma
  - Small focus of pneumonia - round pneumonia

388. Ans. (c) Small cell CA

(*Ref: Harrison 20th edition, p 237; Harrison 19th p 506-10*)

Clubbing is not seen/unlikely with

1. Small cell cancer of lung
2. Acute bacterial endocarditis
3. Chronic bronchitis

- Unidigital clubbing : Trauma/ gout/ sarcoidosis/ A-V fistula
- Fastest clubbing is seen with lung abscess

Condition	Type of breathing
Consolidation	Tubular breathing
Cavity	Cavernous breathing (akin to blowing air over empty coke bottle)
Tension pneumothorax	Amphoric breathing (metallic quality)

389. Ans. (c) Meth-hemoglobinaemia

(*Ref: CMDT 2019 pg. 1603*)

Meth-hemoglobinaemia: Symptoms are proportional to the fraction of methemoglobin. A normal methemoglobin fraction is about 1% (range, 0-3%). Symptoms associated with higher levels of methemoglobin are as follows:

- **3-15%** - Slight discoloration (eg, pale, gray, blue) of the skin
- **15-20%** - Cyanosis, though patients may be relatively asymptomatic
- **25-50%** - Headache, dyspnea, light headedness (even syncope), weakness, confusion, palpitations, chest pain
- **50-70%** - Abnormal cardiac rhythms; altered mental status, delirium, seizures, coma; profound acidosis
- **>70%** - Usually, death

Physical findings may include the following:

1. Discoloration of the skin and chocolate discoloration blood (the most striking physical finding)
2. Cyanosis – This occurs in the presence of 1.5 g/dL of methemoglobin (as compared with 5 g/dL of deoxygenated hemoglobin)
3. Seizures
4. Coma
5. Dysrhythmia (eg, brady - arrhythmia or ventricular dysrhythmia)

390. Ans. (b) Staphylococcal pneumonia

(*Ref: Robbins 7th/ed 383, 385; Oxford Hand book of Medicine 6th/ed 174, Harrison 19th p 805-806*)

391. Ans. (a) Often cavitate

(*Ref: Harrison 20th edition, p 2601-02; Harrison 19th p 2206, 09*)

392. Ans. (d) Argemone mexicana poisoning

(*Ref: Harrison 19th p 1658*)

393. Ans. (b) Causes normocapnic failure

(*Ref: Harrison 20th edition, p 2026*)

394. Ans. (b) Esophageal rupture

(*Ref: Harrison 20th edition, p 2009; Harrison 19th p 1719*)

395. Ans. (c) Mental retardation

(*Ref: Nelson 20th p 2114*)

396. Ans. (d) All of the above

(*Ref: Acute Renal failure in Practice' 1st/345; Oxford Textbook of clinical Nephrology 3rd/582*)

397. Ans. (c) Neonatal pulmonary alveolar proteinosis

(*Ref: Nelson 20th p 2119*)

5
Hepatology

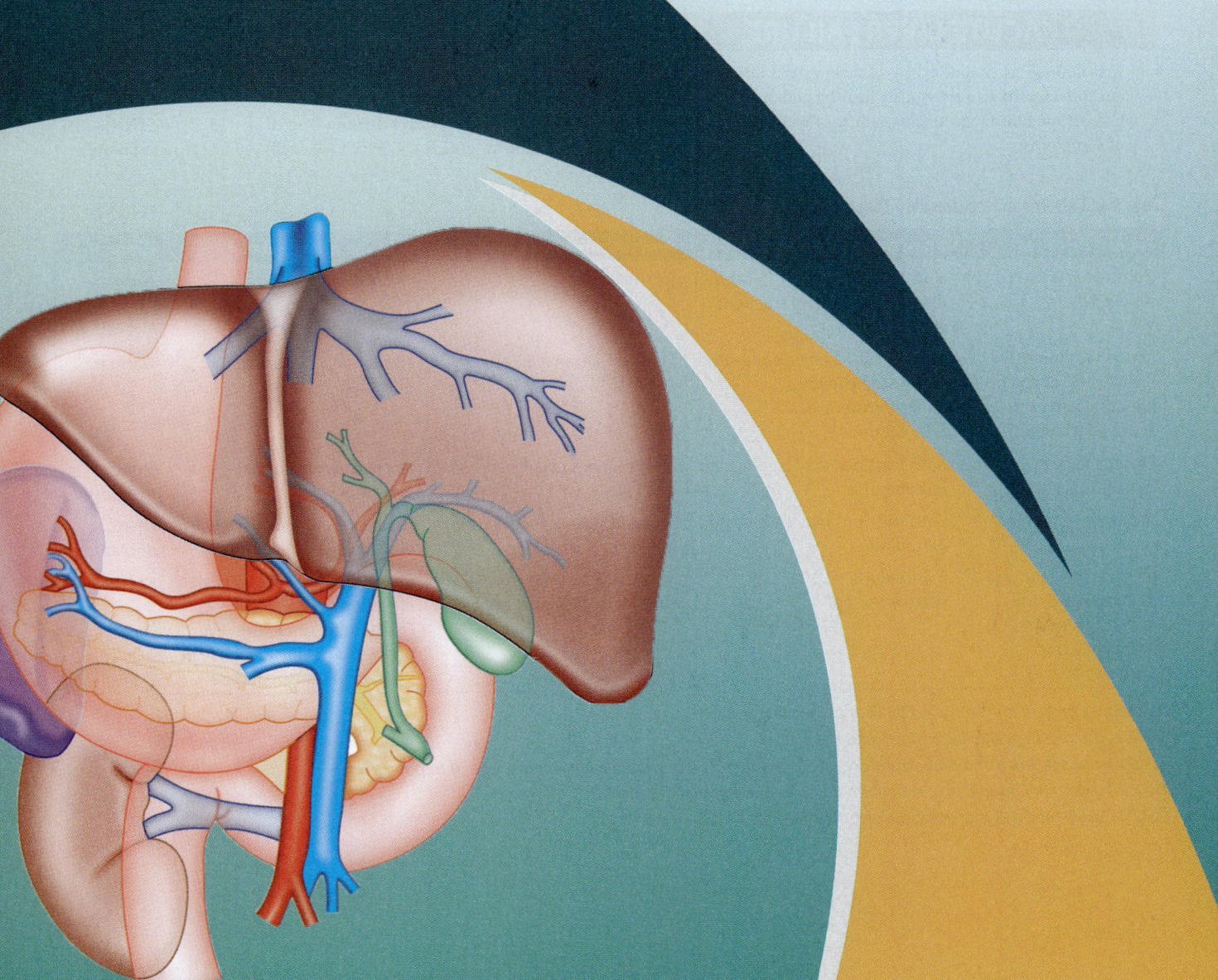

IMPORTANT SCORING PATTERNS IN LIVER DISEASE

Score	Done For?	Parameters Included
MELD SCORE	Liver transplantation	Bilirubin, international normalized ratio (INR), creatinine
PELD SCORE	Liver transplantation	Bilirubin, INR, albumin, age, nutritional status
Nazer index	Liver transplant in Wilson disease	Bilirubin, INR, SGOT
Maddrey's discriminant score	Guide to treatment in alcoholic hepatitis	Bilirubin, INR
Child Pugh classification	Grading of cirrhosis for survival rate determination and intervention	Bilirubin, albumin, ascites, INR, Asterixis

CMDT 2019, page 720 MELD- Na scoring system and incorporates serum sodium to increase accuracy

Child pugh score of ≥7 is an accepted criterion for listing a patient for liver transplantation

ACUTE LIVER FAILURE

- It is defined as coagulopathy (1.5 times the normal INR) and encephalopathy in a previously healthy person.
- Cut off for fulminant hepatic failure is within *8 weeks* of onset of symptoms.
- It is called subfulminant, if it occurs within 8–26 weeks of onset of symptoms.
- Most common cause of fulminant hepatic failure is Toxins in 50% of cases.

MELD Score (Model for End Stage Liver Disease)

- This score helps in deciding the need for liver transplantation.
- If MELD score > 17, listing for transplantation is done.

United Network for Organ Sharing (UNOS) Liver Transplantation Waiting List Criteria

Fulminant hepatic failure (including primary graft non-function and hepatic artery thrombosis within 7 days after transplantation as well as acute decompensated Wilson's disease).

The Model for End-Stage Liver Disease (MELD) score, on a continuous scale, determines allocation of the remainder of donor organs. This model is based on the following calculation:

3.78 x log **bilirubin** (mg/100 mL) + 11.2 x log INR **(international normalized ratio)** + 9.57 x log **creatinine** (mg/100 mL) + 6.43 (x 0 for alcoholics and cholestatic liver disease, x 1 for all other types of liver disease).

PELD Score (Pediatric End Stage Liver Disease)

PELD = 4.80 [log serum **bilirubin** (mg/dL)] + 18.57 [log **INR**] – 6.87 [log **albumin** (g/dL)] + 4.36 (<1 year old) + 6.67 (growth failure)

Liver Test Patterns in Hepatobiliary Disorders

Type of Disorder	Bilirubin	Aminotransferases	Alkaline phosphatase	Albumin
Hemolysis/Gilbert's syndrome	Normal to 86 μmol/L (5 mg/dL) 85% due to indirect fractions No bilirubinuria	Normal	Normal	Normal
Acute hepatocellular necrosis (viral and drug hepatitis hepatotoxins, acute heart failure)	Both fractions may be elevated Peak usually follows aminotransferases Bilirubinuria	Elevated, often > 500 IU, ALT > AST	Normal to <3x normal elevation	Normal
Chronic hepatocellular disorders	Both fractions may be elevated Bilirubinuria	Elevated, but usually <300 IU	Normal to <3x normal elevation	Often decreased
Alcoholic hepatitis, cirrhosis	Both fractions may be elevated Bilirubinuria	AST: ALT > 2 suggests alcoholic hepatitis or cirrhosis	Normal to <3x normal elevation	Often decreased
(Obstructive jaundice) Infiltrative diseases (tumor, granulomata); partial bile duct obstruction	Bilirubinuria Usually normal	Rarely >500 IU Normal to slight elevation	Elevated, often >4x normal elevation Fractionate, or confirm liver origin with 5'-nucleotidase or γ glutamyl transpeptidase	Normal

All clotting factors are produced by liver except factor 8
SGPT is the most specific liver function test
Alkaline phosphatase and 5'nucleotidase are found near the bile canalicular membrane of hepatocytes.
GGT is located in Endoplasmic reticulum and bile duct epithelial cells
SGOT / SGPT ratio > 2 is specific for alcoholic hepatitis and not GGT

LIVER TRANSPLANTATION

Indications for Liver Transplantation
- Chronic Hepatitis C > alcoholic liver disease: Most common indication
- Fulminant hepatic failure
- Wilson's disease and hemochromatosis
- Primary billiary cirrhosis and primary sclerosing cholangitis
- Hepatorenal syndrome
- Hepatopulmonary syndrome
- Autoimmune hepatitis

MELD score > 17 and child pugh score ≥7 has been the accepted criterion for listing a patient for liver transplantation

Contraindications to Liver Transplantation

Relative
1. Age > 70 years
2. Portal vein thrombosis
3. Severe obesity
4. HIV positive, with low CD_4 count (<100 μL)
5. Malnutrition
6. Severe hypoxia due to right → left intrapulmonary shunting
7. Pulmonary artery hypertension

Absolute
1. AIDS
2. Uncontrolled hepatobiliary infection
3. Sepsis
4. Alcohol abuse
5. Metastasis to liver/cholangiocarcinoma

Diseases that can Recur after Liver Transplantation
1. Autoimmune Hepatitis
2. Primary sclerosing cholangitis
3. Cholangiocarcinoma
4. Fulminant hepatitis A

HEPATITIS

Etiology of Viral Hepatitis

Viral strain	Most common route of transmission
Hepatitis-A	Feco-oral
Hepatitis-B	Heterosexual (Asia)
Hepatitis-C	Blood transfusion/IV drug abuse (Not transmitted by breast milk)
Hepatitis-D	Parenteral route
Hepatitis-E	Feco-oral

Viral Hepatitis in a Nutshell
- Most common cause of acute viral hepatitis in world is HEV with one third of world populations being infected (pg 2353: Harrison 20th edition) *(The same should be answer for India also).*
- Most common cause of chronic Hepatitis is Hepatitis C
- Most common cause of carriers in Hepatitis is Hepatitis B
- Virus that is NOT transmitted via breast milk: Hepatitis C
- Most common cause of fulminant hepatitis: Hepatitis D (Superinfection)
- Most common cause of fulminant hepatitis in pregnancy: Hepatitis E

Hepatitis-B
- It is a double-shelled DNA virus measuring roughly about 42 nm.
- Genome is 3.2 kb, circular DNA which is *partially single stranded, partially double stranded* and referred in textbook as ss/ds.

Mode of Transmission/Spread
1. Most common route of spread: Sexual contact (Heterosexual) in Asia and parenteral in western world
2. Blood transfusion
3. Vertical transmission
   - Occurs during delivery, through conjunctival inoculation on or through swallowing mother's blood.
   - If a mother is HBsAg and HBeAg positive during pregnancy, *(chances of vertical transmission are as high as 90%).*
   - To reduce the chances of transmission
     - Elective C-section is performed.
     - Passive immunity is provided to the baby in the form of HB-immunoglobulin within 24 hours of birth.
     - Active immunity with recombinant vaccine
4. Accidental needle stick injury
   - Majority during recapping of needle in clinical setting.
     - Chances of acquiring infection: 30%
     - Treatment to bring down the risk of Give HB-Ig within 6 hours of exposure.

Needle Stick Injury with HIV positive patient
- Occurs also during recapping of needles in clinical setting
- Chances of transmission are 0.3%
- Treatment: Post exposure prophylaxis (PEP)
  - Raltegravir + Emtricitabine + Tenofovir

Comparison of HIV vs. HBV Transmission Rate

	HIV	HBV	HCV
Vertical transmission	30%	90%	5%
Needle prick	0.3%	30%	3%

Antigens in Hepatitis B

HBsAg	1st to appear in the blood
HBcAg	Never appears in the blood

Contd...

HBeAg	Replication of the virus/infectivity
HBxAg	Hepatocellular cancer (HBV > HCV)
HBV-DNA	• PCR: If viral load is >2 X 10^4 viral copies IU/mL or ≥ 10^5 viral copies of DNA/mL *(indicative of high viral load)* and 2 times rise in SGPT level, then treat the patient for hepatitis B. • Currently drug of choice for hepatitis B is Tenofovir > Entecavir • Call for follow up and repeat PCR. • Successful treatment is said when < 300 viral copies DNA/ml are present

Significance of Antibodies in Hepatitis B

Anti-HBsAg	Seroconversion antibody
Anti-HBcAg	IgM → Window period / Acute hepatitis-B
	IgG → Chronic hepatitis-B
Anti-HBeAg	Decreased replication/decreased infectivity

Clinical Features of Acute Hepatitis B Infection

- Nausea/vomiting
- Mild weight loss (2–2.5 kg)
- Fever
- Icterus
- Pain in the right hypochondrium due to tender hepatomegaly *(normal liver span 12–15 cm)*
- Splenomegaly and cervical adenopathy in 20% of cases.

Investigations

1. Liver function test: Elevated SGPT *(most specific LFT)*
2. USG liver
   - Echotexture shows *starry sky liver*
   - Liver span is increased
3. Hepatitis-B antigen profile
   - HBsAg +
   - HBeAg +
   - IgM anti HBcAg +. The positive result of all three indicates acute hepatitis B with high infectivity.
   - Sequence of antigen antibody appearance is stated below:

HBsAg → HbeAg → Anti-HBcAg → (Elevated SGPT → Jaundice) → Anti-HBeAg → Anti-HBsAg

Serological Diagnosis of Hepatitis B

	HBsAg	Anti-HBsAg	HBeAg	Anti-HBcAg
Acute hepatitis	+	–	+	IgM
Window period	–	–	–	IgM
Chronic hepatitis	+	–	+	IgG
Recovery	–	+	–	IgG
Vaccinated	–	+	–	–

Treatment

- Acute hepatitis B requires only conservative management.
- Recovery is rule in 90% of hepatitis B patients, with anti-HBsAg being the **seroconversion antibody**
  - Bed rest
  - High carbohydrate diet (avoid oily/fatty food)
  - Itopride/mosapride: For nausea/vomiting
  - Cholestyramine for pruritus.
  - Remember that tenofovir entecavir/ alpha-interferon is used only for patients of chronic active hepatitis.

Indication of Hep B treatment
- High viral load 2 × 10^4 IU of DNA/mL plus doubling of SGPT
- DOC: Tenofovir > Entecavir > α-interferon

Fulminant Hepatic Failure Manifestations

(Incidence after Acute Hepatitis B = 0.1 – 1%)
1. Worsening of jaundice
2. Decreased liver span
3. Bleeding (because all clotting factors are synthesized in liver except factor 4).
4. **Hepatic encephalopathy** secondary to ammonia intoxication.

Symptoms of Hepatic Encephalopathy

1. Confusion with change of personality is an *early* feature (pg 2066: Harrison 19th ed.)
2. Visuospatial skill loss leading to constructional and dressing apraxia 2° to parietal lobe damage and is demonstrated by number connection test.
3. Asterixis. Not seen once patient is in coma.
4. Stupor → coma.
5. *It can be precipitated by excessive use of diuretics, abdominal paracentesis internal GIT bleeding, constipation, hypoxia, alkalosis.*
6. Cerebral herniation due to brain edema.

Investigations

1. Serum ammonia: Elevated
2. EEG: Markedly abnormal triphasic waves are seen in 3rd and 4th stage of hepatic encephalopathy.

- Rumack Matthew nomogram is used for PCM toxicity treatment decision making.
- Overall, most common cause of FHF is toxins.
- MC viral cause of FHF is hepatitis D
- MC viral cause of FHF in pregnancy: HEV.

Treatment

1. Mannitol
2. NG lactulose: DOC for treatment of hepatic encephalopathy

3. Topical antibiotic rifaximine through nasogastric tube *(previously Neomycin was used)*
4. L.O.L.A: infusion of L-ornithine and L-arginine
5. Maintain sugar via dextrose infusion
6. Maintain PT via fresh frozen plasma (FFP)
7. Orthoptic liver transplantation.

Hepatitis-C

- World wide, genotype 1 is most common
- Unlike hepatitis B, acute hepatitis C always progresses to cause chronic hepatitis.
- Most common cause of chronic hepatitis globally is Hepatitis C.
- It is transmitted through blood transfusion and sexual route.
- **Vertical transmission** rate: 5%.
- Screening test is Enzyme immunoassay: Anti-HCV antibody.
- If EIA: Anti-HCV antibody is negative, perform PCR HCV RNA.
- If HCV-RNA is positive, then treat even if SGOT/SGPT is normal.
- *Due to high rate of progression to chronic hepatitis C, it is most common cause of liver transplantation surpassing alcoholic hepatitis.*

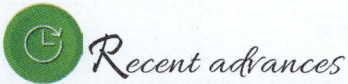

Management of Hepatitis C
- Genotype 1: Ledipasvir plus sofosbuvir for 12–24 weeks.
- Genotype 2: Sofosbuvir with ribavirin.
- Genotype 3: None of the drugs achieving sustained virological clearance.
- Acute flare of cryoglobulinemia: Rituximab, cyclophosphamide and methylprednisolone.
- If new drugs are not given, then answer is Pegylated interferon with ribavirin.
- All "asvirs" are NS5A inhibitors.
- Confirmation of diagnosis of hepatitis C is EIA anti HCV but in case of negative EIA, HCV RNA detection by PCR is done.
- Sustained virological response rate is negative HCV RNA in serum at 24 weeks of completion of therapy.

Hepatitis-D

- This is an incomplete delta virus with low multiplication rate.
- When HDV combines with HBV its multiplication rate increases dramatically, leading to significant damage to liver.
- HDV incidence decreases if there is 100% coverage with HBV vaccine.
- Pattern of Infection
  - **Co-infection:** In patients with acute hepatitis B, where they acquire infection with acute HDV leading to increased incidence **CHRONIC HEPATITIS**
  - **Superinfection:** In patients with chronic hepatitis B, there is pre-existing damage to liver and now in addition there is infection with HDV leading to **fulminant hepatic failure**.

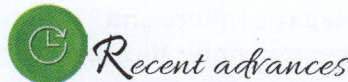

Fibrosure Test
- It is done in chronic hepatitis C patients to evaluate for severity of fibrosis.
- The test results are comparable to liver biopsy report.
- Calculation is based on combination of *five* serum biochemical parameters:
  1. α-2-macroglobulin
  2. Apolipoprotein A1
  3. Haptoglobin
  4. L-glutamyl transpeptidase
  5. Bilirubin.

Hepatitis A and E

	Hepatitis A	Hepatitis E
Infection route	Feco-oral	Feco-oral, *not transmitted by sexual, perinatal and percutaneous route*.
MC seen in	Children	Adults
Symptoms	Transient illness: URTI, nausea, vomiting, jaundice	Transient illness + cholestasis *(symptoms more severe here)*, mustard yellow urine, clay colored stool
Investigations	IgM anti HAV	IgM anti HEV
Treatment	Conservative	Conservative
Vaccine	Available: HAVRIX (GSK) Given > 1yrs 2 shots (First between 15 and 18 months and 2nd between 21 and 24 months)	Available *(as of now in China only)*

Extrahepatic Manifestations of Hepatitis B and Hepatitis C Viruses

Organs affected	HBV	HCV
Kidney	MGN: membranous glomerulopathy causes nephrotic syndrome	MPGN: Causes nephritic syndrome
Immunological	Serum sickness: Present with rash and joint pain	Essential **Cryoglobulinemia**: Presents with rash+joint pain+ stroke
Bone marrow	Aplastic anemia	Aplastic anemia
Blood vessel	PAN (polyarteritis nodosa)	None
Others	Guillain-Barré syndrome	Lichen planus, Sjogren's syndrome, porphyria cutanea tarda, type II DM, metabolic syndrome

Incidence of Fulminant Hepatic Failure and Chronic Hepatitis with Hepatotrophic Viruses

Hepatitis	A	B	C	D	E
Fulminant hepatic failure	+	+	+	+	+
Chronic hepatitis	–	+	+	+	–
Carriers	–	+	+	+	–

- Highest incidence of fulminant Hepatic failure is with Hepatitis D virus.
- In pregnant female with HEV infection, fulminant Hepatic failure incidence increases by 30%.
- Chronic hepatitis and carriers are seen in all EXCEPT Hep A & E.

Autoimmune Hepatitis

Type I autoimmune hepatitis	Lupoid features, ANA ⊕, p-ANCA ⊕
Type II autoimmune hepatitis	Chronic hep C, anti LKM_1 antibody
Type III autoimmune hepatitis	Chronic hepatitis D, anti LKM_3 antibody

- DOC: steroids (prednisolone).

(NOTE: Anti- LKM_2 antibody is associated with drug induced hepatitis). Anti- LKM_3 antibody is associated with hepatitis D).

ALCOHOLIC LIVER DISEASE (ALD)

- Most sensitive test: SGOT; SGOT/SGPT RATIO >1
- Most specific test: Carbohydrate deficient transferrin
- Gamma glutamyl transpeptidase is a non-specific test
- Prognosis in ALD is determined by *Maddrey's Discriminant Score*, which has two parameters, *Bilirubin, INR*.
- **Discriminant function ≥ 32 or MELD score > 21 in absence of comorbidity is treated with prednisolone 32 mg PO × 4 weeks followed by tapering for 4 week. Pentoxyphylline can be used.**

NON-ALCOHOLIC FATTY LIVER DISEASE (NAFLD)

It is associate with obesity/syndrome-X

Causes

1. Hepatitis C
2. Reye's syndrome (seen with VZ/influenza B)
3. Kwashiorkor
4. Drug-induced hepatitis
5. Fatty liver of pregnancy
6. HELLP syndrome
7. Inborn errors of metabolism

Recent advances

Non-Alcoholic Fatty Liver Disease

- It leads to macrovesicular steatosis (Reye syndrome leads to microvascular steatosis).
- Most patients are asymptomatic or complain of right upper quadrant pain.
- Antinuclear antibodies with elevated serum ferritin levels.
- Percutaneous liver biopsy is not recommended.
- **BARD score**: Serum bilirubin, AST/ALT >0.8 and diabetes mellitus has 96% negative predictive value.
- Vitamin E shows benefit. Previous approaches like metformin, thiazolidinediones, pentoxifylline and ursodeoxycholic acid have marked side effects.
- Liver transplantation is done in appropriate cases.

CIRRHOSIS (C.L.D)

- **MCC:** Alcoholic cirrhosis (micronodular cirrhosis)

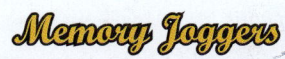

Mallory hyaline bodies are seen in
- **I**ntestinal bypass surgery
- **W**ilson's disease
- **B**iliary cirrhosis
- **A**lcoholic hepatitis
- **S**teatosis

Mnemonic: I Will Break Alcoholic Status

Clinical Features of Compensated cirrhosis

1. Spider nevi /angioma
2. Palmar erythema
3. Duputyren's contracture *(begins in ring finger)*
4. Clubbing of nails
5. Gynecomastia
6. Testis atrophy/ hypogonadism

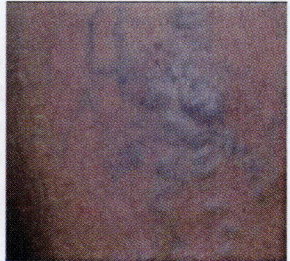

Spider Nevi | Caput Medusae

Contd...

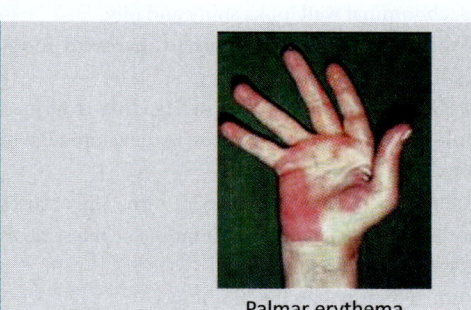

Palmar erythema

Cardiac Cirrhosis

- It is also known as **NUTMEG LIVER**.
- This occurs due to venous congestion, usually due to cardiac dysfunction like cor pulmonale.
- This congestion will stimulate hepatic stellate cells, which will initiate fibrosis leading to regressed liver size.
- **Investigation of choice**: USG guided liver biopsy
- **Treatment**: Orthoptic liver transplantation.

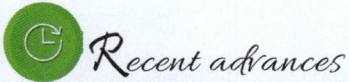

Ultrasound Elastography

Considering that liver biopsy is not a perfect reference standard, elastographic techniques based on shear waves generated by the acoustic beam are used for early detection of cirrhosis and has the advantage of being noninvasive.

Budd-Chiari Syndrome

- **Budd–Chiari syndrome** is a condition caused by occlusion of the hepatic veins that drains the liver.
- **Characterized by:**
  - Thrombosis of hepatic vein
  - Sudden congestion
  - Tender hepatomegaly with *USG showing enlarged caudate lobe of liver.*
- **Clinical features:** Acute abdomen and right hypochondriac pain, ascites and pedal edema.
- **On examination:** Tender hepatomegaly.

Causes of Budd-Chiari Syndrome

1. **Polycythemia vera: MCC of Budd chiari syndrome**
2. Paroxysmal nocturnal hemoglobinuria: 2nd MCC
3. **OCP**
4. Hepatic vein valves.

Investigations

1. USG abdomen
2. Doppler USG
3. **Investigation of choice:** Hepatic venography

Treatment

- Inj. Heparin: Causes gradual improvement

Decision Making for Cirrhosis

Done with the help of **Child–Pugh Classification of Cirrhosis**

Factor	Units	1 points	2 points	3 points
Serum bilirubin	Mmol/L	<34	34–51	>51
Serum albumin	g/L	>35	30–35	<30
	g/dL	>3.5	3.0–3.5	<3.0
Prothrombin time	Seconds	0–4	4–6	>6
	Prolonged INR	<1.7	1.7–2.3	>2.3
Ascites		None	Easily controlled	Poorly controlled
Hepatic encephalopathy		None	Minimal	Advanced

Interpretation

Points	Class	One year survival
5–6	A	100%
7–9	B	81%
10–15	C	45%

Score of > 8 is criterion to list for liver Transplantation

- Best marker for chronic liver disease: Albumin
- Clotting factor with shortest t1/2: Factor VII
- Clotting factor with longest t1/2: Factor 13
- First factor to decrease in blood in patients with chronic liver disease: Factor VII.
- Best management to control bleeding in chronic liver disease: FFP

Complications of Cirrhosis

Portal Hypertension (MC Complication of Cirrhosis)

- Normal portal pressure is 5–10 mmHg or 10–15 cm of water.
- Most common non alcoholic (overall is alcoholic cirrhosis) cause of portal hypertension is non-cirrhotic portal fibrosis.

Clinical Features

- **Splenomegaly**: 1st and most reliable clinical feature
- Ascites (Secondary to increased capillary bed hydrostatic pressure)
- Hematemesis secondary to esophageal varices

Investigations

IOC for portal hypertension: Doppler USG (to demonstrate increased pressure)

Classification of Portal HTN

Prehepatic portal HTN	Hepatic	Posthepatic
• Schistosomiasis • Thrombosis • Porta hepatis lymphadenopathy	• Fibrosis • Budd Chiari syndrome	• Budd Chiari syndrome

In all patients with portal hypertension, there is portosystemic collateral formation

Portosystemic Collaterals: 7 Sites

1. Esophageal varices: *(Source of bleeding: Coronary veins)*
2. Rectal hemorrhoids
3. Caput medusa
4. Bare area of liver
5. Retroperitoneal veins
6. Lumbar veins
7. Omental veins

- MCC of portal HTN in adults: Non-cirrhotic portal fibrosis
- MCC of portal HTN in pediatrics: Extrahepatic portal vein obstruction
- DOC for non-bleeding varices: Propranolol
- DOC for bleeding varices: Octreotide (IV with infusion pump)

Esophageal Varices

- In case of bleeding esophageal varices, two emergencies arise simultaneously:
  - Continuously decreasing SBP
  - Bleeding.
- To overcome this, following steps should be taken:

For ↓ SBP	For Bleeding
• IV crystalloids: normal Saline • Massive Blood transfusion: *immediate step*	• IV octreotide: **DOC** to ↓portal vein pressure • UGIE + banding/ sclerotherapy- **TOC**

- If a patient presents with recurrent hematemesis
- Definitive Rx: TIPS (Transjugular intrahepatic portosystemic shunt)

Ascites

- The term "ascites" denotes the pathologic accumulation of fluid in the peritoneal cavity.
- Healthy men have little or no intraperitoneal fluid, but women normally may have up to 20 mL depending on the phase of the menstrual cycle.

Threshold of Detection of Ascites

Puddle sign	>100 mL of fluid
Shifting dullness	500 mL of fluid
Massive ascites	Fluid thrill +
Tense ascites	Fluid thrill –

- In tense ascites, abdominal wall looks shiny and oily.
- Fluid thrill is absent in tense ascites due to increased intra-abdominal pressure.
- When this pressure becomes >12 mm of Hg, this is termed as intra-abdominal HTN, and progresses to development of abdominal compartment syndrome.
- Abdominal compartment syndrome (>25 mm Hg) causes kinking of mesenteric veins leading to gangrene of intestine as in the case of tense ascites.
- S.A.A.G. = Serum Albumin – ascites albumin

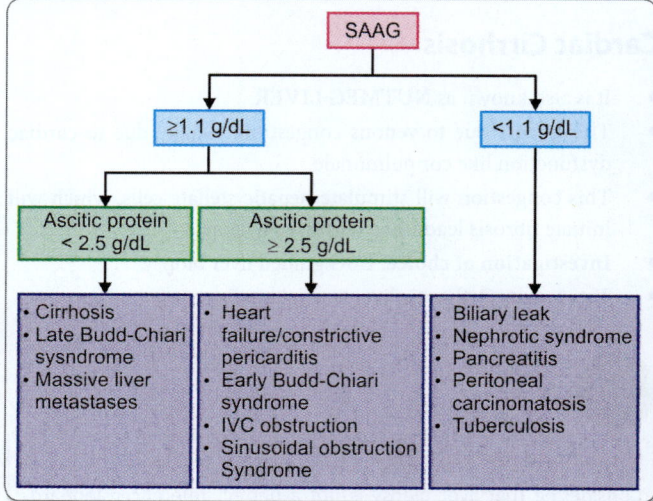

Types of Ascites

Investigations

IOC for ascites: USG abdomen

Treatment for Ascites with S.A.A.G. > 1.1

1. Salt restricted diet
2. Diuretics: Spironolactone
3. Massive ascites can lead to respiratory distress and can be managed by abdominal paracentesis after salt free IV albumin.
4. For recurrent ascites, TIPS is preferred.

- MCC of transudative ascites/ SAAG > 1.1: Portal HTN
- MCC of exudative ascites/ SAAG < 1.1: TB
- *Only transudative condition where SAAG< 1.1: Nephrotic syndrome*

Hepatorenal Syndrome

- Type 1 Hepatorenal syndrome: Doubling of serum creatinine or halving of creatinine clearance in less than 2 weeks.
- Type 2 Hepatorenal syndrome: Slowly progressive and chronic.

Clinical Features

1. Oliguria / anuria
2. **Uremia:** uremic fetor, uremic pericarditis and uremic melena.

3. Volume over load leads to swelling, weight gain and pulmonary edema.

Treatment
- Midodrine plus octreotide and IV albumin
- Hemodialysis
- Orthoptic liver transplantation

Hepatopulmonary Syndrome

Clinical Features
- Platypnea (dyspnea in sitting position)
- Orthodeoxia (change of oxygen saturation with position)
- Clubbing

Investigation
1. ABG
2. Bubble contrast echo (**IOC**)
3. Lung perfusion scan using macroaggregated albumin

Treatment
- IPPV
- Orthoptic liver transplant.

Obstructive Jaundice

Causes
1. Choledocholithiasis
2. Common bile duct strictures
3. Pancreatic cancer
4. Klatskin tumor (periampullary carcinoma)
5. Caroli cyst
6. Choledochal cyst
7. Biliary atresia
8. Primary sclerosing cholangitis
9. Primary biliary cirrhosis
10. Dubin-Johnson syndrome
11. Rotor syndrome.

Clinical Features of Obstructive Jaundice
1. Pruritus of palms and soles (due to excess of bile salts) *earliest presentation*
2. Mustard yellow urine (due to excretion of bilirubin through kidneys)
3. Clay-colored stools (due to absence of bile pigments in stool)
4. Yellow sclera.

Investigations
1. LFT
   - S. bilirubin: Elevated (conjugated)
   - SGOT and SGPT: Normal
   - S. alkaline phosphatase: Elevated 3x
   - 5'nucleotidase: Elevated
2. **USG abdomen:** IOC for obstructive jaundice
3. **MRCP:** To rule out any malignancy present
4. **Bromsulphalein test:** To rule out Dubin-Johnson syndrome

PRIMARY BILIARY CIRRHOSIS

- Abnormality in the intrahepatic as well as extrahepatic biliary tree leads to improper excretion of bile, presenting as obstructive jaundice.
- IOC: Anti-mitochondrial antibody^Q
- Definitive treatment is liver transplantation.

PRIMARY SCLEROSING CHOLANGITIS

- Abnormality in the intrahepatic biliary tree leading to improper excretion of bile, presenting as obstructive jaundice.
- This condition is characterized by p-ANCA positivity.
- *Periductal onion skin fibrosis is seen.*
- Definitive treatment is liver transplantation.

Primary biliary cirrhosis	Primary sclerosing cholangitis
Autoimmune disorder	Autoimmune disorder
Damage due to AMA (anti-mitochondrial Ab)	Damage due to p-ANCA antibody
IOC: AMA **Gold standard:** Liver biopsy — intrahepatic fibrosis seen	**IOC:** M.R.C.P Showing multiple strictures
Rx: Orthoptic liver transplantation	**Rx:** Stenting of biliary pathway Orthoptic liver transplantation

DUBIN-JOHNSON SYNDROME

- Autosomal recessive disorder caused by mutation in a gene responsible for a human canalicular organic anion transporter called MRP2 (multi drug resistance protein 2 or ABCC2).
- The color of the liver is black due to pigment deposition (epinephrine).
- This condition is characterized by improper excretion of conjugated bilirubin into bile duct.
- **Investigation of choice:** Bromsulphalein (BSP) test.

ROTOR SYNDROME

This is a milder version of Dubin-Johnson syndrome. In this condition, the color of liver is normal.

Expression of OATP1B1 and OATP1B3 (organic anion transport protein) is completely absent.

The functional consequence of this is that uptake of glucuronidase is hampered.

WILSON'S DISEASE

It is a rare, **autosomal recessive** disorder that usually occurs in persons under age 40.
- Excessive deposition of copper in the liver and brain.
- Serum ceruloplasmin, is low.
- Urinary excretion of copper and hepatic copper concentration are high.
- The genetic defect, localized to **chromosome 13**, has been shown to affect a copper-transporting **adenosine triphosphatase** (*ATP7B*) in the liver and leads to copper accumulation in the liver and oxidative damage of hepatic mitochondria.

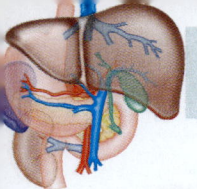

> For Menke's disease, gene responsible is: ATP 7A.

Clinical Features

1. Chronic hepatitis
2. Hemolytic anemia
3. Copper deposits in the basal ganglia damage the corpus striatum resulting in chorea. Copper deposition also occurs in pons, thalamus and cerebellum
4. Kayser-Fleischer ring (deposition of copper in descemet's membrane). They tend to decrease after 3–6 months of treatment and may disappear by 2 years.
5. Damaged proximal convoluted tubule leading to *Fanconi syndrome*.

Investigations

1. 24 hrs urine copper level: Screening test
2. Serum ceruloplasmin
3. Serum copper is low. Rises during hemolytic episodes.
4. Liver biopsy to estimate copper content (best test/IOC)
5. MRI head shows face of Panda appearance.

Other Causes of Decreased Ceruloplasmin

1. Malnutrition
2. Protein losing enteropathy
3. Nephrotic syndrome
4. Hepatic insufficiency
5. Hereditary hypoceruloplasminemia.

Treatment

- **DOC: Zinc acetate** (In presymptomatic/pediatric/pregnant/ hepatitis without decompensation)
- DOC in hepatic decompensation: **Trientene** (mild/moderate)
- Drug for management of CNS features of Wilson's disease *Tetrathiomolybdate*.

Kayser-Fleischer Rings

- Formed by the deposition of copper in the Descemet's membrane and seen at the limbus of the cornea.
- The color may range from greenish gold to brown.
- Well-developed rings may be readily visible to the naked eye or with an ophthalmoscope set at +40.
- When not visible to the unaided eye, the rings may be identified using slit-lamp examination or gonioscopy.
- Observed in up to 90% of individuals with symptomatic Wilson's disease and almost invariably present in those with neurologic manifestations.
- *No longer considered pathognomonic of Wilson's disease unless accompanied by neurologic manifestations, as they may also be observed in patients with chronic cholestatic disorders.*

- IOC for Wilson's disease: Liver biopsy with estimation of hepatic copper content.
- NAZER prognostic score used to guide treatment.
- NAZER prognostic score includes:
  - Serum bilirubin/SGOT/INR

HEMOCHROMATOSIS

- Hemochromatosis is an autosomal recessive disease caused in many cases by a mutation in the *HFE* gene on chromosome 6.
- **Primary hemochromatosis**: This is due to increased absorption of iron from the gut due to HFE gene mutation.
- **Secondary hemochromatosis**: This is due to recurrent blood transfusion as in the case of thalassemia.

Clinical Features

1. Liver is first organ to be affected and hepatomegaly is present in more than 95% symptomatic patients. (pg 2516, Harrison, 19th ed.)
2. Increased skin pigmentation leading to metallic or slate gray hue referred as Bronzing, from increased melanin.
3. Type 1 DM due to direct damage to β cells.
4. Arthropathy occurs in 25–50% of symptomatic patients and first involves 2nd/3rd metacarpophalangeal joints. Arthropathy progresses despite removal of iron by phlebotomy.
5. Cardiac involvement leads to restrictive cardiomyopathy and presents as CHF. MC arrhythmia seen in PSVT.
6. Hypogonadism due to pituitary damage may present as loss of libido, impotence.

- **Hemochromatosis triad**: Bronze skin, DM, Hepatomegaly
- **MC symptom of hemochromatosis**: Arthropathy (2nd/3rd MCP joint)

Investigations

1. Serum ferritin is elevated
2. **Screening test**: % saturation of transferrin
3. **Gold standard**: Liver biopsy.

Treatment

- **Primary hemochromatosis**: Phlebotomy
- **Secondary hemochromatosis**: Iron chelators – desferrioxamine & deferiprone (Preferred and DOC).

Comparison of Organs involved in Wilson's Disease and Hemochromatosis

Wilson's disease	Hemochromatosis
Liver damage	Liver damage
Hemolytic anemia	Restrictive cardiomyopathy
Basal ganglia damage (chorea)	Bronze diabetes
Fanconi syndrome	Pituitary damage (hypogonadism)

Image-Based Questions

1. 40-year-old intravenous drug abuser presents with vomiting, jaundice and right hypochondrium pain. USG abdomen shows presence of?

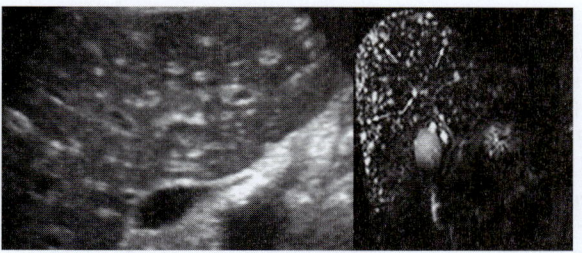

a. Amoebic liver abscess
b. Acute viral hepatitis
c. Acute cholecystitis
d. Hepatocellular carcinoma

2. Which is incorrect about the picture shown below?

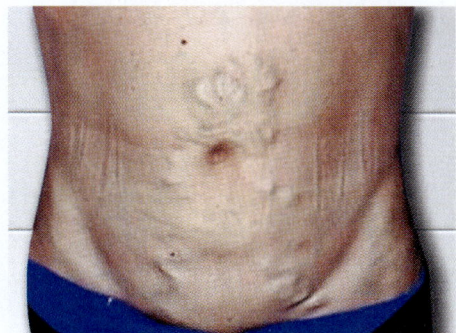

a. Flow of blood towards the umbilicus
b. Portal vein pressure > 15 cm water
c. Decompensated cirrhosis
d. Thrombocytopenia

3. The test being performed on the patient shows?

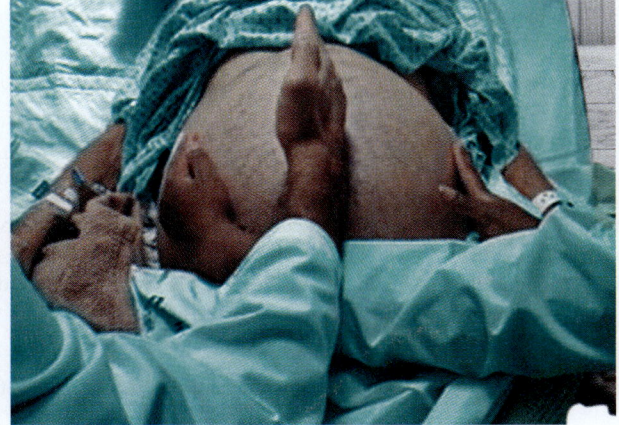

a. Fluid thrill
b. Shifting dullness
c. Puddle sign
d. Flank dullness

4. All are responsible for refractoriness of this condition to medical treatment except?

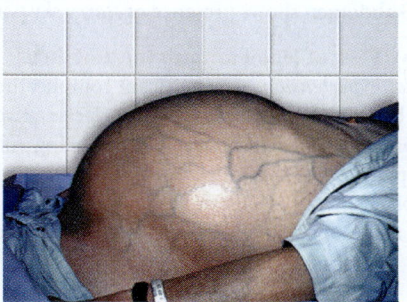

a. Non-compliance with salt intake
b. Hepatopulmonary syndrome
c. Hepatic vein thrombosis
d. Spontaneous bacterial peritonitis

5. A patient presents with choledocholithiasis. USG Liver shows?

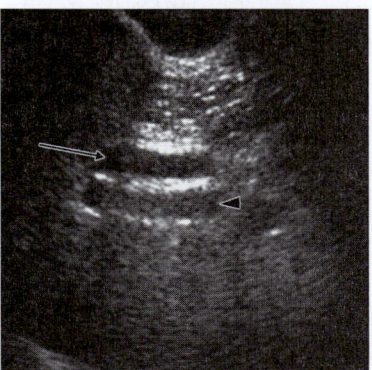

a. Double duct sign
b. Double barrel sign
c. Double bubble sign
d. Porcelain gall bladder

6. A 25-year-old shepherd presents with dragging discomfort in right hypochondrium and on examination shows presence of enlarged liver 5 cm below costal margins. The probable diagnosis is?

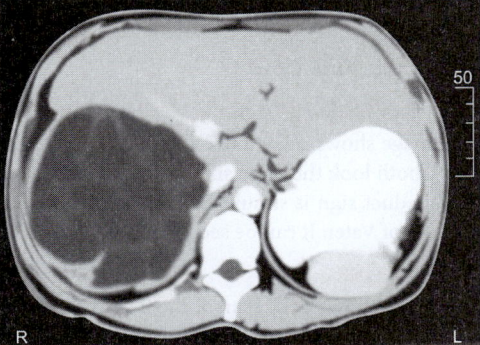

a. Amoebic liver abscess
b. Hydatid cyst
c. Pyogenic liver abscess
d. Hepatic adenoma

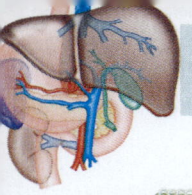

Answers of Image-Based Questions

1. **Ans. (b) Acute viral hepatitis**
   - USG abdomen shows presence of *starry sky pattern of the liver,* diagnostic of acute viral hepatitis

2. **Ans. (a) Flow of blood towards the umbilicus**
   - *Portal hypertension* is a significant complicating feature of *decompensated cirrhosis* and is responsible for the development of ascites and bleeding from esophagogastric varices, two complications that signify decompensated cirrhosis.
   - In patients with cirrhosis, who are being followed chronically, the development of portal hypertension is usually revealed by the presence of thrombocytopenia; the appearance of an enlarged spleen; or the development of ascites, encephalopathy, and/or esophageal varices with or without bleeding.
   - The thrombocytopenia is explained in case of development of hypersplenism in a congested spleen.

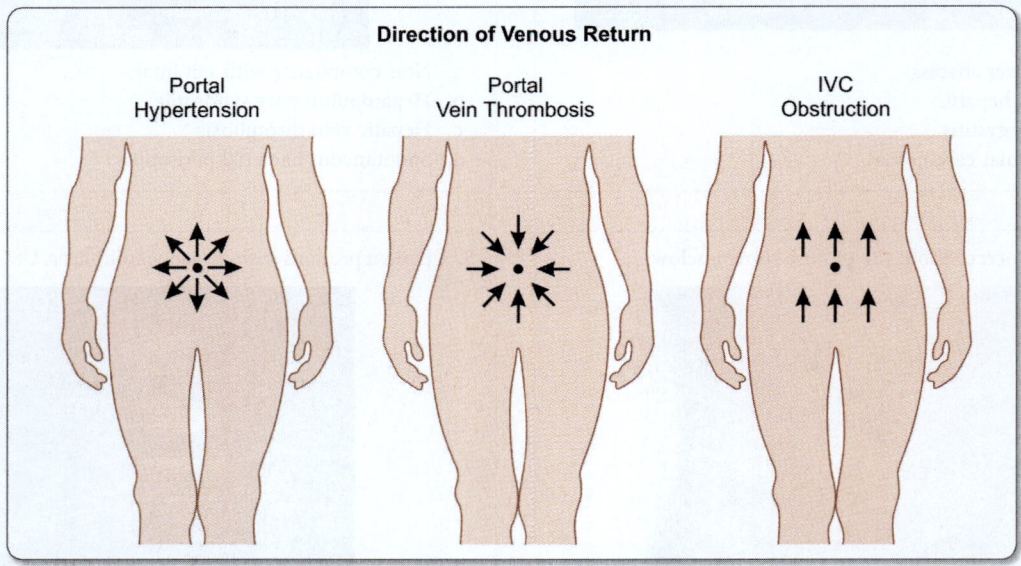

3. **Ans. (a) Fluid Thrill**
   - The test being done is fluid thrill while the assistant's hand in middle obliterates the transmission of impulse via the abdominal fat.
   - A fluid thrill or wave may be demonstrable in cases of tense ascites.
   - Flank dullness, which is present in about 90% of patients, is the most sensitive physical sign of ascites.
   - Shifting dullness on percussion is more specific but less sensitive than flank dullness for detection of ascites.
   - The puddle sign, can *detect as little as 120 mL of fluid clinically* requires the patient to be in knee-elbow position during examination.

4. **Ans. (b) Hepatopulmonary syndrome**
   Ascites is said to be refractory, if it persists inspite of maximal dose of diuretics (400–600mg of spironolactone) and 120–140mg of frusemide and salt restriction. The causes are:
   - Non-compliance with salt restriction
   - Hepatorenal syndrome
   - Infection or spontaneous bacterial peritonitis
   - GI bleeding
   - Hepatic vein thrombosis.

5. **Ans. (b) Double barrel sign**
   - The image shows dilated bile duct adjacent to the portal vein. The caliber of bile duct is much smaller than portal vein but in the image both look the same size and this makes it look like the double barrel of a rifle.
   - Double duct sign is simultaneous dilatation of pancreatic and biliary duct and is seen in carcinoma head of pancreas or cancer of ampulla of Vater. It can be seen in CT, MRI or ERCP.

6. **Ans. (b) Hydatid cyst**
   - The image shows a CT scan of the liver with classical cart wheel appearance, suggestive of multiple hydatid cysts. The calcified cysts are left alone as they are dead cysts.
   - Medical treatment with albendazole for 8 days is given and surgery is done in case of symptomatic cysts or asymptomatic patient with cyst >5 cm or a non-calcified infected cyst.

Multiple Choice Questions

Viral Hepatitis

1. A 40-year male patient who is a known smoker presents with fever, fatigue and complete aversion to cigarette smoking. On examination he has icterus with an enlarged tender liver. LFT shows: **(AIIMS May 2018)**

Total bilirubin	17.5 mg%
Direct bilirubin	5.5 mg%
SGOT	700 IU
SGPT	900 IU

   What investigations will you do for ruling out acute viral hepatitis?
   a. HBsAg, IgM antiHBc, AntiHCV, AntiHEV
   b. AntiHAV, HBsAg, IgM antiHBc, AntiHCV
   c. HBAg, IgM antiHBc, AntiHDV, AntiHCV, AntiHEV
   d. AntiHAV, IgM antiHBc, ANtiHCV, AntiHEV

2. Which of the following is used for laboratory diagnosis of alcoholic hepatitis? **(AIIMS Nov 2018)**
   a. ALP   b. AST
   c. LDH   d. GGT

3. Which is true regarding hepatitis C infection? **(JIPMER May 2018)**
   a. Most patients have severe symptoms when infected for the first time
   b. Highly likely to cause chronic ongoing infection
   c. Transmitted by eating raw oysters
   d. It is DNA virus

4. Cryoglobulinemia is seen with? **(Recent Pattern 2018)**
   a. Hepatitis C   b. Diabetes
   c. Leukemia   d. Ovarian cancer

5. There are 3 to 5% healthy hepatitis B carriers in India who are asymptomatic. They have the risk of developing HCC in future due to: **(AIIMS Nov 2017)**
   a. Inability to induce inflammation against the virus
   b. Integration of virus with host DNA
   c. Increased Liver Transaminases
   d. High rate of hepatocyte proliferation

6. Which of the following serum markers for liver fibrosis can replace the need for liver biopsy? **(AIIMS May 2017)**
   a. SGOT and SGPT
   b. Serum Hyaluronic acid
   c. GGT and Fibronectin
   d. Fibronectin and factor V levels

7. A patient is being evaluated for jaundice and liver fibrosis. His AST=87 IU/mL and ALT=81 IU/mL. His serological tests are given below. Which of the following is the next step in the diagnosis? **(AIIMS Nov 2016)**

IgM Anti- HbcAg	Non- reactive
Ig G Anti- HbcAg	Reactive
HbsAg	Non-Reactive
HBeAg	Non-Reactive
Anti-HCV	Reactive

   a. HBV DNA   b. Anti- HbsAg
   c. HCV RNA- RT PCR d. Liver biopsy

8. Which of the following virus is not transmitted by percutaneous transfer? **(Recent Question 2016-17)**
   a. Hepatitis A   b. Hepatitis B
   c. Hepatitis D   d. Hepatitis E

9. Which of the following viral markers signifies the ongoing viral replication in the case of Hepatitis-B infection? **(UPSC 2015)**
   a. Anti-HBs   b. Anti-HBc
   c. HBe Ag   d. HBs Ag

10. A person is HBsAg positive, but Anti-HBs Ab is negative. What should be the next step? **(AIIMS May 2015)**
    a. Repeat test after 6 months
    b. Check HBeAg, if positive start interferon
    c. Check HBV DNA load
    d. Reassure patient that he does not have any disease

11. Serology of the patient is given below. Diagnosis is? **(AIIMS Nov 2015)**

HbsAg	Non-reactive
IgG anti-HbcAg	Reactive
HbeAg	Non-reactive
HBV DNA	Undetectable

    a. Window period
    b. Chronic hepatitis inactive stage
    c. Recovery from remote infection
    d. Recovery from acute infection

12. Maximum chance of spread in accidental needle stick injury is? **(JIPMER Nov 2015)**
    a. Hepatitis B   b. HIV
    c. Hepatitis C   d. EBV

13. Why pre-transfusion testing does not decrease the incidence of hepatitis? **(JIPMER Nov 2014)**
    a. Most carriers do not have HBsAg
    b. Post transfusions hepatitis is caused by CMV
    c. Present screening test is not sensitive for HBsAg
    d. HCV not screened

14. All the following are used for treatment of chronic Hepatitis B except? **(AIIMS Nov 14)**
    a. Entecavir   b. Telbivudine
    c. Zidovudine   d. Lamivudine

15. Not seen in association with Hepatitis C virus: **(Recent Pattern 2014-15)**
    a. Lichen planus
    b. Cryoglobulinemia
    c. Porphyria cutanea tarda
    d. PAN

16. A 30-year-old man presented with nausea, fever and jaundice of 5 days duration. The biochemical tests revealed a bilirubin of 6.7 mg/dl, unconjugated 5.0 mg/dl with SGOT/SGPT (AST/ALT) of 1230/900 IU/ml. The serological tests showed presence of HbsAg IgM, anti HBc and HbeAg. The most likely diagnosis is: **(Recent Pattern 2014-15)**
    a. Chronic hepatitis B infection with high infectivity
    b. Acute hepatitis B infection with high infectivity
    c. Chronic hepatitis b infection with low infectivity
    d. Acute hepatitis B infection with low infectivity

17. **Drug of choice for hepatitis B:** *(Recent Pattern 2014-15)*
    a. Entecavir
    b. Sofosbuvir
    c. Simeprevir
    d. Tenofovir

18. **A patient has anti HBs without any other without any other antigen or antibody against HBV. This indicates:**
    (Recent Pattern 2014-15)
    a. Vaccinated state
    b. Chronic infection
    c. Persistent carrier
    d. Acute infection

19. **HbsAg Carrier state is not associated with:**
    (Recent Pattern 2014-15)
    a. Down's syndrome
    b. Chronic renal failure
    c. Poly-arteritis nodosa
    d. Infectious mononucleosis

20. **Most common route of transmission of hepatitis C:**
    (Recent Pattern 2014-15)
    a. I.V. drug abuse
    b. Sexual contact
    c. Factor 8 concentrate
    d. Feco-oral route

21. **Incubation period of hepatitis B is:** *(Recent Pattern 2014-15)*
    a. 6 weeks to 6 months
    b. 6 days to 6 weeks
    c. 6 months to 6 years
    d. More than 6 years

22. **Co-infection is essential for disease presentation in:**
    (Recent Pattern 2014-15)
    a. Hepatitis A
    b. Hepatitis B
    c. Non-A Non-B hepatitis
    d. Delta hepatitis

23. **Best site of giving hepatitis B vaccine is:**
    (Recent Pattern 2014-15)
    a. Subcutaneous
    b. Intradermal
    c. Intramuscular deltoid
    d. Intramuscular gluteal

24. **Which one of the following is not characteristic of Hepatitis-B?** *(Recent Pattern 2014-15)*
    a. Incubation period is 2-6 months
    b. Mode of infection is parenteral
    c. High fever is rare
    d. Anicteric hepatitis is not seen

25. **Patient comes for blood donation but he has Hbs Ag and HbeAg positive, and serum transminases level is normal. What would be the next management?**
    (Recent Pattern 2014-15)
    a. Treat with interferon
    b. HBV DNA estimation
    c. Liver biopsy
    d. Observation

26. **A 55-year-old male patient was diagnosed to have chronic hepatitis C. He responded to treatment with interferon. However, after one year of follow up he showed a relapse of disease. Which of the following would be the next most appropriate choice?** *(Recent Pattern 2014-15)*
    a. Ribavirin and pegylated interferon
    b. Lamivudine and interferon
    c. Nevirapine and lamivudine
    d. Indinavir and ribavirin

27. **A HBs Ag carrier mother with anti Hbe Antibody positive in blood the chances of hepatitis in newborn is:**
    (Recent Pattern 2014-15)
    a. 100%
    b. 90%
    c. 20%
    d. 0%

28. **Most common genotype of hepatitis B in cirrhosis in North India:** *(Recent Pattern 2014-15)*
    a. Genotype A
    b. Genotype B
    c. Genotype C
    d. Genotype D

29. **All of the following are true regarding chronic active hepatitis, except:** *(Recent Pattern 2014-15)*
    a. Common in females
    b. Progression to cirrhosis is not seen
    c. Remission with steroids
    d. May associate with autoimmune disease

30. **Which one of the following markers in the blood is the most reliable indicator of recent hepatitis B infection?**
    (Recent Pattern 2014-15)
    a. HbsAg
    b. IgG anti-HBs
    c. IgM anti-HBc
    d. IgM anti-Hbe

31. **In a patient with fever, nausea and pain in right hypochondrium for 6 hours. Liver is not palpable. Most probable diagnosis is:** *(Recent Pattern 2014-15)*
    a. Viral hepatitis
    b. Acute cholecystitis
    c. Gastritis
    d. Pleurisy

32. **Which statement is wrong regarding Hepatitis B?**
    a. It is due to RNA virus *(Recent Pattern 2014-15)*
    b. Blood is the main source of infection
    c. Chronicity is present
    d. It may turn into hepatocellular carcinoma

33. **Most common subtype of hepatitis B in Asia?**
    (Recent Pattern 2014-15)
    a. Ads
    b. Adw
    c. Ayr
    d. Ayw

34. **Not transmitted by percutaneous route:**
    (Recent Pattern 2014-15)
    a. Hepatitis A
    b. Hepatitis B
    c. Hepatitis C
    d. Hepatitis E

35. **Fulminant hepatitis is commonest seen with?**
    (Recent Pattern 2014-15)
    a. HAV
    b. HBV
    c. HCV
    d. HDV

36. **Which is not transmitted via breast milk?**
    (Recent Pattern 2014-15)
    a. Hepatitis A
    b. Hepatitis B
    c. Hepatitis C
    d. Hepatitis D

37. **The marker of hepatitis B in the window period is:**
    (Recent Pattern 2014-15)
    a. HBsAg
    b. Anti-HBs Ag
    c. IgM Anti-HBcAg
    d. IgG Anti-HbcAg

38. **Earliest manifestation of hepatitis B infection:**
    (Recent Pattern 2014-15)
    a. HbeAg
    b. HbsAb IgM
    c. Anti-Hbc IgM
    d. Anti-HbeAb IgM

39. **Which one of the following is transmitted non-parenterally:**
    (Recent Pattern 2014-15)
    a. HBV
    b. HCV
    c. HDV
    d. HEV

40. **A 30-year-old patient presents with H/O antibodies to HCV for 6 months duration and his AST/ALT is normal. There is no symptom or stigmata of liver disease. The most appropriate approach:** *(Recent Pattern 2014-15)*
    a. Re-assure the patient
    b. Repeat titer every 3 years
    c. Repeat enzymes yearly
    d. Do liver biopsy and start antiviral drugs accordingly.

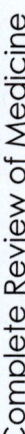

41. The commonest hepatotropic virus causing increased chronic carrier state is: *(Recent Pattern 2014-15)*
    a. HEV
    b. HAV
    c. HBV
    d. HCV

42. True about hepatitis with HCV is: *(Recent Pattern 2014-15)*
    a. Present with fulminant liver failure
    b. Chronicity is not seen
    c. Genotyping helps in treatment duration
    d. Feco/oral transmission

43. A 35-year-old male patient presented with history of jaundice for 15 days. The onset was preceded by a prodromal illness. His serum tested positive for HbsAg. A clinical diagnosis of acute hepatitis B was made. What should be the next best confirmatory investigation?
    a. Anti-HbeAg antibody *(Recent Pattern 2014-15)*
    b. Hbe antigen
    c. Anti-Hbe IgM antibody
    d. Anti-HbsAg antibody

44. A 45 day old infant developed icterus and two days later symptoms and signs of acute liver failure appeared. Child was found to be positive for HbsAg. The mother was also HbsAg carrier. The mother's hepatitis B serological profile is likely to be: *(Recent Pattern 2014-15)*
    a. HbsAg positive only
    b. HbsAg and HbeAg positivity
    c. HbsAg and anti Hbe antibody positivity
    d. Mother infected with mutant HBV

45. Vertical transmission of hepatitis C is: *(Recent Pattern 2014-15)*
    a. 5%
    b. 10%
    c. 25%
    d. 50%

46. The likelihood of becoming an HbsAg carrier after acute HBV infection is high in: *(Recent Pattern 2014-15)*
    a. Neonates
    b. Chronic hemodialysis patients
    c. Persons with Down's syndrome
    d. All of the above

47. HbsAg positive mother gives birth to live baby, plan of action for prevention of baby would consist of: *(Recent Pattern 2014-15)*
    a. Give hepatitis B vaccine to baby
    b. Give hepatitis B vaccine and immunoglobulin to baby
    c. No intervention require if baby is asymptomatic
    d. Prevent breastfeeding

48. Friction rub may not be heard in right upper quadrant in one of the following conditions: *(Recent Pattern 2014-15)*
    a. Fatty liver
    b. Recent biopsy
    c. Tumour
    d. Perihepatitis

49. True regarding, hepatitis B is? *(Recent Pattern 2014-15)*
    a. Circular single stranded
    b. Circular double stranded
    c. Circular Partial single stranded and partial double stranded
    d. Linear double stranded plus

50. Acute viral hepatitis is diagnosed by:
    a. HbsAg *(Recent Pattern 2014-15)*
    b. HbeAg
    c. HbsAg + IG M anti-HBc antibody
    d. HbsAg + HbcAg

51. Indicators of active multiplication of hepatitis B virus is: *(Recent Pattern 2014-15)*
    a. HbsAg
    b. HbcAg
    c. HbeAg
    d. Anti Hbs

52. The most common type of hepatitis associated with blood transfusion: *(Recent Pattern 2014-15)*
    a. Hepatitis C
    b. Hepatitis B
    c. Hepatitis A
    d. Hepatitis D

53. All of the following are correct about Hepatitis A virus except: *(Recent Pattern 2014-15)*
    a. Feco-oral transmission
    b. Short incubation period
    c. Single stranded RNA
    d. 3 to 4% carrier state

54. Antigen which does not appear in blood in hepatitis B: *(Recent Pattern 2014-15)*
    a. HbcAg
    b. HbeAg
    c. HbsAg
    d. None of the above

55. The most common presentation of hepatitis A is:
    a. Asymptomatic *(Recent Pattern 2014-15)*
    b. Fulminant hepatitis
    c. Chronic carrier state
    d. Transient illness with jaundice

56. In a patient with fulminant liver failure after viral hepatitis, which of the following will not change immediately? *(Recent Pattern 2014-15)*
    a. Serum albumin
    b. PT
    c. Serum bilirubin
    d. Serum ammonia

57. Granulomatosis hepatitis is not caused by: *(Recent Pattern 2014-15)*
    a. Blastomycosis
    b. Metastatic carcinoma
    c. Tuberculosis
    d. Cat scratch disease

58. Most common type of acute viral hepatitis in the world: *(Recent Pattern 2014-15)*
    a. Hepatitis A
    b. Hepatitis B
    c. Hepatitis C
    d. Hepatitis E

59. Severity in acute hepatitis is best estimated by: *(Recent Pattern 2014-15)*
    a. Serum bilirubin
    b. Prothrombin time
    c. α-glutaryl transferase
    d. Alkaline phosphatase

60. Dane particle pertains to: *(Recent Pattern 2014-15)*
    a. HAV
    b. HBV
    c. NANB
    d. None of the above

61. Occult hepatitis B is: *(Recent Pattern 2014-15)*
    a. HBV DNA <10^4 copies/ml with HBsAg negative
    b. HBV DNA <10^4 copies/ml with HBsAg positive
    c. HBV DNA <10^4 copies/ml with HBeAg negative
    d. HBV DNA <10^4 copies/ml with HBeAg positive

62. HCV is associated with: *(Recent Pattern 2014-15)*
    a. Autoimmune cirrhosis
    b. LKM antibody
    c. Antimitochondrial antibody
    d. None

63. Extrahepatic manifestations of HCV are all except: *(PGI Nov 2014)*
    a. Lichenoid eruptions
    b. Celiac disease
    c. Glomerulonephritis
    d. Cryoglobulinemia
    e. Arthritis

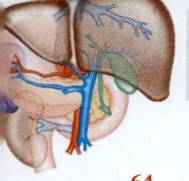

64. Early diagnosis of acute hepatitis-B infection is made by:
    a. Presence of HbeAg in serum   (Recent Pattern 2014-15)
    b. Presence of IgM anti HBc in serum
    c. Presence of HbsAg in serum
    d. Presence of IgG anti HBc in serum
65. The commonest hepatotropic virus progressing to chronicity is: (AIIMS May 01)
    a. HEV   b. HAV
    c. HBV   d. HCV
66. Non-parenteral hepatitis is: (AI 2000)
    a. Hepatitis E   b. Hep B
    c. Hep C   d. Hep D
67. Early diagnosis of acute hepatitis-B infection is made by
    a. Presence of Hbe Ag in serum   (AIIMS Nov 03)
    b. Presence of IgM anti-HBc in serum
    c. Presence of Hbs Ag in serum
    d. Presence of IgG anti-HBc in serum
68. Which of the following markers in the blood is the most reliable indicator of recent hepatitis B- infection?
                                        (AIIMS May 03)
    a. HBsAg   b. IgG anti – HBs
    c. IgM anti – HBc d. IgM anti – Hbe
69. A 35-year-old male patient presented with history of jaundice for 15 days. The onset was preceded by a prodromal illness. His serum tested positive for HBsAg. A clinical diagnosis of acute Hepatitis B was made. What should be the next best confirmatory investigation
                                        (AIIMS May 04)
    a. IgM Anti-HBcAg b. HBe antigen
    c. Anti-HBe IgM antibody d. HBV DNA by PCR
70. A thirty-year man presented with nausea, fever and jaundice of 5 days duration. The biochemical tests revealed a bilirubin of 6.7 mg/dl (conjugated 5.0 mg/dl) with SGOT/SGPT (AST/ALT) of 1230/900 IU/ml. The serological tests showed presence of HBs Ag. IgM anti-HBc and Hbe Ag. The most likely diagnosis is: (AIIMS Nov 02)
    a. Chronic hepatitis B infection with high infectivity
    b. Acute hepatitis B infection with high infectivity
    c. Chronic hepatitis infection with low infectivity
    d. Acute hepatitis B infection with low infectivity
71. A patient is found to be positive for HBs Ag on routine laboratory evaluation. Other serological tests for hepatitis are unremarkable. He is clinically asymptomatic and liver enzymes are within the normal range. Which of the following best describes his diagnosis: (AI 2010)
    a. Inactive HBV carrier   b. Acute Hepatitis B
    c. Chronic Hepatitis B   d. Active HBV carrier
72. All of the following are seen in active chronic hepatitis B except: (AIIMS Nov 07)
    a. IgM against core antigen
    b. Total core antibody
    c. HbeAg
    d. HbsAg
73. A patient is found to be positive only for Anti HBsAg. All other viral markers are negative. The likely diagnosis is:
                                        (PGI 2009)
    a. Vaccination   b. Chronic hepatitis B
    c. Acute hepatitis B d. Fulminant hepatitis B
74. All of the following should be included during preliminary evaluation of a case of suspected Acute viral hepatitis except: (AIIMS June 2000)
    a. Hbs Ag
    b. IgM anti HBc
    c. Anti-HCV
    d. IgM anti HBe
75. Hepatitis B infectivity is indicated by: (AI 1994)
    a. Anti-HBsAg
    b. HBsAg + HBeAg
    c. Anti-HBsAg – Anti-HBc
    d. Anti-HBeAg + Anti-Hbs Ag
76. A blood donor is not considered for safe transfusion, if he has: (AI 2000)
    a. Anti HBs Ag +ve
    b. Anti HBs Ag and HBc Ag +ve
    c. Hbs Ag +ve, & IgM anti HBc +ve
    d. Anti HBe +ve
77. Reserve transcriptase of hepatitis B virus is coded on the following gene: (AI 2000)
    a. C gene   b. S gene
    c. P gene   d. X gene
78. Which one of the following pairs regarding Hepatitis B is not correctly matched   (AIIMS Nov 2010)
    a. Acute Viral Hepatitis B - Supportive care
    b. Acute Viral Hepatitis B - Antiviral therapy
    c. Chronic Viral Hepatitis B - Supportive care
    d. Chronic Viral Hepatitis B - Antiviral therapy
79. HBs Ag positive person may have all of the following associated Renal lesions, Except: (PGI Dec 06)
    a. Membranous Glomerulonephritis
    b. Membrano proliferative Glomerulnephritis
    c. Mesangiocapillary Glomerulonephritis
    d. Focal Segmental Glomerulosclerosis
80. Interferon treatment is recommended in chronic hepatitis B in patients with: (PGI June 07)
    a. ↑ HBV DNA and Normal ALT
    b. ↑ HBV DNA and ↑ ALT
    c. ↑ HBV DNA and compensated cirrhosis
    d. ↑ HBV DNA and decompensated cirrhosis
81. Chronic liver disease is most commonly caused by:
                                        (AI 2000)
    a. Hepatitis B   b. Hepatitis A
    c. Hepatitis C   d. Hepatitis E
82. Hepatic C is associated with all except: (PGI June 08)
    a. PAN
    b. Dermatomyositis like syndrome
    c. Lichen Planus
    d. Psoriasis
83. During an epidemic of hepatitis E, fatality is maximum in
                                        (AI 2000)
    a. Pregnant women b. Infants
    c. Malnourished male d. Adolescents
84. Characteristic Auto antibodies of Autoimmune Hepatitis include all of the following, Except: (PGI Dec 06)
    a. Antinuclear Antibodies (ANA)
    b. Anti SLA
    c. Anti LKM1
    d. ANCA

85. **Features of Alcoholic hepatitis include all of the following except:** *(AI 1991)*
    a. Elevated bilirubin
    b. Prolonged prothrombin time
    c. Elevated serum albumin
    d. Anemia
86. **Ratio of AST/ALT > 1 is present in** *(AIIMS May 07)*
    a. Non alcoholic steatohepatitis
    b. Alcoholic hepatitis
    c. Wilson's disease
    d. All of the above
87. **Which is not true about alcoholic hepatitis:**
    a. Gamma glutamyl transferase is raised *(AIIMS May 95)*
    b. SGPT is raised > SGOT
    c. SGOT is raised > SGPT
    d. Alkaline phosphatase is raised
88. **All of the following statements about Non Alcoholic Fatty Liver disease are true, except:** *(PGI June 01)*
    a. Common in Diabetics
    b. Clofibrate provides effective treatment
    c. Commonest cause of cryptogenic cirrhosis
    d. Associated with elevated transaminases
89. **Micronodular cirrhosis is commonly seen in all except:**
    a. Chronic hepatitis B *(AIIMS Nov 07)*
    b. Alcoholic liver disease
    c. Hemochromatosis
    d. Chronic extrahepatic biliary obstruction
90. **Quantitative assessment of liver function can be done by:** *(PGI Dec 05)*
    a. Degree of ↑ Transaminases
    b. Degree of ↑ Alkaline phosphatase
    c. Degree of ↑ GGT
    d. Estimation of Galactose Elimination capacity
91. **Which one of the following serum levels would help in distinguishing an acute liver disease from chronic liver disease?** *(AI 2005)*
    a. Aminotransaminase
    b. Alkaline phosphatase
    c. Bilirubin
    d. Albumin

Jaundice

92. **A patient presents with serum bilirubin values of >40mg% and obstructive jaundice. This indicates?** *(AIIMS Nov 2016)*
    a. Carcinoma of gallbladder
    b. Concomitant renal failure
    c. Acute cholecystitis
    d. Complete obstruction of bile duct
93. **An 8th month primigravida presented with severe pruritis. Examination revealed mild icterus. Her serum bilirubin was 3mg/dl. She has elevated AST ALT and Alkaline phosphatase. Her RFT and coagulation profile were within normal limits. She could probably be having?**
    a. HELLP syndrome *(AP PG 2016)*
    b. Hepato renal syndrome
    c. Obstetric cholestasis
    d. Viral hepatitis
94. **In a child surgery was done for EHBO with hepatojejunal anastomosis. Post-operatively bilirubin level after 2 weeks was 6 mg/dl from a pre-operative level 12mg/dl. The reason for this could be?** *(AIIMS May 2015)*
    a. Normal lowering of bilirubin takes time
    b. Delta bilirubin
    c. Anastomotic stricture
    d. Mistake in lab technique
95. **Patient presents with icterus, urine urobilinogen is absent. This indicates?** *(AIIMS Nov 2015)*
    a. Hemolysis   b. Hepatitis
    c. Liver failure   d. Peri-hepatic obstruction
96. **Investigation of choice for biliary atresia in a 2 month old infant is?** *(AIIMS May 2015)*
    a. Hepatic scintigraphy   b. ERCP
    c. USG   d. CECT
97. **Which of the following is true regarding gamma glutamyl transferase?** *(JIPMER Nov 2014)*
    a. Elevated in carcinoma prostate with hepatic metastasis
    b. Highly specific to alcohol
    c. Exclusively found in liver
    d. Marker of infective hepatitis rather than cholestasis
98. **Vitamin K is given to patient of jaundice but PT remains unchanged. The probable cause is?** *(Recent Pattern 2014-15)*
    a. Obstructive jaundice   b. Cirrhosis
    c. Hemolytic jaundice   d. Biliary atresia
99. **Obstructive jaundice is best detected by:**
    a. Increased ALP *(Recent Pattern 2014-15)*
    b. Decreased ALP
    c. Increased AST
    d. Decreased AST
100. **Most common cause of obstructive jaundice in children:**
    a. Biliary atresia *(Recent Pattern 2014-15)*
    b. Criggler najjar syndrome
    c. Byler disease
    d. Caroli cyst
101. **A defect in which of the following processes give rise to bilirubinuria?** *(Recent Pattern 2014-15)*
    a. Conjugation of bilirubin to glucuronic acid
    b. Conversion of biliverdin to bilirubin
    c. Transport of conjugated bilirubin to bile canaliculi
    d. Transport of unconjugated bilirubin into hepatocytes
102. **A 40 year old lady has ALP of 550, SGOT of 75, total serum Bilirubin = 6.5mg% and conjugated serum bilirubin of 4.3mg%. The diagnosis of patient is:** *(AIIMS Nov 2013)*
    a. Dubin Johnson syndrome
    b. Obstructive jaundice
    c. Viral hepatitis
    d. Cholelithiasis
103. **Insulin resistance in liver disease is due to:**
    a. Steatosis *(AIIMS Nov 2012)*
    b. Hepatocyte damage
    c. Decreased release of insulin
    d. Decreased release of C – peptide
104. **Following is test marker of alcohol induced liver injury:**
    a. Gamma Glutamyl Transferase *(Recent Pattern 2014-15)*
    b. MCV
    c. SGPT/SGOT >2
    d. SGOT/SGPT >2

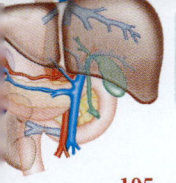

105. A patient presenting with jaundice is found to have 20 mg % of bilirubin, of which 9.3 is direct reacting & 85 U/L of alkaline phosphatase, the likely diagnosis is:
    a. Post hepatic obstructive lesion   *(Recent Pattern 2014-15)*
    b. Haemolytic jaundice
    c. Infective hepatitis
    d. Pre hepatic obstructive jaundice
106. Palmar erythema is seen in: *(Recent Pattern 2014-15)*
    a. CCF   b. ARF
    c. CRF   d. Hepatic failure
107. Raised unconjugated hyperbilirubinemia is seen in:
    a. Gilbert's Syndrome   *(Recent Pattern 2014-15)*
    b. Dubin Johnson syndrome
    c. Drug induced cholestasis
    d. Hepatocellular necrosis
108. Gilbert's syndrome all are true except?
    a. Mild conjugated bilirubinaemia *(Recent Pattern 2014-15)*
    b. Normal LFT
    c. Normal liver biopsy
    d. Ligandin defect
109. A patient presented with complaints of abdominal pain, melena, jaundice, and fever of 104°F; diagnosis will be: *(Recent Pattern 2014-15)*
    a. Carcinoma pancreas   b. CBD stones
    c. Hemobilia   d. Hepatitis
110. Initial investigation of choice in obstructive jaundice is: *(Recent Pattern 2014-15)*
    a. ERCP   b. Ultrasound
    c. Cholecystography   d. MRCP
111. Bilirubin is absent in urine because it is-   *(AIIMS Nov 99)*
    a. Distributed in the body fat
    b. Conjugated with glucoronidase
    c. Not filtered
    d. Lipophilic
112. A patient presents with unconjugated hyperbilirubinemia and presence of urobilinogen in urine. Which amongst the following is the least likely diagnosis: *(AI 2010)*
    a. Hemolytic jaundice
    b. Crigler Najjar syndrome
    c. Gilbert's syndrome
    d. Dubin Johnson syndrome
113. 5'-Nucleotidase activity is increased in: *(AI 2005)*
    a. Bone diseases
    b. Prostate cancer
    c. Chronic renal failure
    d. Cholestatic disorder
114. Abnormal excretory function of hepatocytes may be assessed by: *(PGI June 07)*
    a. Increased PT
    b. Increased ALT
    c. Increased Alkaline Phosphatase
    d. Increased gamma GT
115. True about Crigler Najjar type II syndrome is:
    a. Diglucuronide deficiency   *(PGI Dec 97)*
    b. Recessive trait
    c. Kernicterus is seen
    d. Phenobarbitone is not useful

Reye Syndrome

116. Micro-vesicular fatty liver in Reye's syndrome is?   *(AIIMS Nov 14)*
    a. Due to defect in beta oxidation of fatty acids
    b. Due to defect in oxidative phosphorylation
    c. Due to defect in fatty acid synthesis
    d. Defective synthesis of acyl COA synthesis
117. All of the following are true of Reye's syndrome except: *(Recent Pattern 2014-15)*
    a. It frequently complicates viral infections
    b. Prothrombin time is prolonged
    c. Disease may by precipitated by salicylates
    d. Deep jaundice is present
118. Microvascular steatosis is seen in all except:
    a. HELLP syndrome   *(Recent Pattern 2014-15)*
    b. Acute fatty liver of pregnancy
    c. Methotrexate toxicity
    d. Reye's syndrome

Budd-Chiari Syndrome

119. The following is the least likely manifestation of acute Budd-Chiari syndrome: *(Recent Pattern 2014-15)*
    a. Enlarged tender liver   b. Ascites
    c. Jaundice   d. Venous collaterals
120. In Budd-Chiari syndrome there is obstruction to:
    a. Inferior vena cava   *(Recent Pattern 2014-15)*
    b. Pulmonary artery
    c. Larger hepatic veins
    d. Portal vein
121. Budd-Chiari syndrome is commonly due to:
    a. Hepatic venous out flow obstruction
    b. Portal Cavernoma   *(Recent Pattern 2014-15)*
    c. Left Sided portal hypertension
    d. IVC thrombosis
122. Most common cause of Budd-Chiari syndrome is:
    a. Hepatic vein valves   *(Recent Pattern 2014-15)*
    b. Hypercoagulable state in Nephrotic syndrome
    c. PNH
    d. Polycythemia vera
123. In Budd Chiari syndrome, the site of venous thrombosis is:
    a. Infrahepatic inferior vena cava   *(AI 2004)*
    b. Infrarenal inferior vena cava
    c. Hepatic veins
    d. Portal veins

Hepatic Encephalopathy

124. Number Connection test is done in?   *(JIPMER 2014)*
    a. Cerebral Ataxia   b. Dementia
    c. Parkinsonism   d. Hepatic Encephalopathy
125. Milan criteria is used for: *Recent Pattern 2014-15)*
    a. Liver transplantation
    b. GERD staging
    c. Cirrhosis staging
    d. Hepatic encephalopathy staging

126. M.E.L.D score includes all except: *(Recent Pattern 2014-15)*
    a. Bilirubin   b. INR
    c. Serum creatinine d. Serum albumin
127. Which one of the following is least expected to precipitate hepatic encephalopathy in a liver cirrhosis patient:
    a. Peritoneal tap   *(Recent Pattern 2014-15)*
    b. Antibiotic treatment
    c. Variceal bleed
    d. Hypokalemia
128. Hepatic encephalopathy is aggravated by all except?
    a. Hyperkalemia   *(Recent Pattern 2014-15)*
    b. Anemia
    c. Hypothyroidism
    d. Barbiturates
129. Earliest sign in hepatic encephalopathy is:
    a. Asterixis   *(Recent Pattern 2014-15)*
    b. Alternate constriction and dilated pupil
    c. Constructional apraxia
    d. Psychiatric abnormalities
130. Most likely precipitating cause for acute hepato-cellular failure is: *(Recent Pattern 2014-15)*
    a. Oral lactulose
    b. Large IV albumin infusion
    c. Large carbohydrate meal
    d. Upper GI bleeding
131. Alzeheimer type II astrocyte are seen in:
    a. Hepatic encephalopathy *(Recent Pattern 2014-15)*
    b. Alzehiemer's
    c. Parkinsonism
    d. Biswanger disease
132. Acute hepatic encephalopathy is precipitated by:
    a. Lactulose   *(Recent Pattern 2014-15)*
    b. Potassium sparing diuretics
    c. Excessive use of diuretics
    d. Rifaximin
133. Which one of the following is not advocated in the management of hepatic encephalopathy?
    a. Oral Lactulose   *(Recent Pattern 2014-15)*
    b. I.V. Glucose drip
    c. High protein diet more than 60 grams/day
    d. If tests for blood in stool are positive then give colonic washout
134. First line management of portacaval Encephalopathy is?
    a. Lactulose   *(Recent Pattern 2014-15)*
    b. Large amounts of proteins
    c. Emergency portal systemic shunt surgery
    d. Diuretics
135. All the following drugs are used in hepatic encephalopathy except: *(Recent Pattern 2014-15)*
    a. LOLA   b. Rifaximin
    c. Lactulose   d. Phenobarbitone
136. Antibiotic of choice in cirrhotic patient to prevent encephalopathy: *(Recent Pattern 2014-15)*
    a. Neomycin
    b. Ampicillin
    c. Metronidazole
    d. Rifaximin
137. On a epidemic of hepatitis; fulminant hepatic failure is seen in: *(Recent Pattern 2014-15)*
    a. Malnourished child
    b. Pregnant female
    c. Old age
    d. Child < 15 year of age.
138. Which of the following is not a precipitating factor for hepatic encephalopathy in patients with chronic liver disease? *(AIIMS May 05)*
    a. Hypokalemia   b. Hyponatremia
    c. Hypoxia   d. Metabolic acidosis

Portal HTN

139. Cirrhosis of liver with portal hypertension occurs in all except: *(Recent Pattern 2014-15)*
    a. Cystic fibrosis
    b. Alpha 1 anti-trypsin deficiency
    c. Wilson's disease
    d. Inflammatory hepatosplenic schistosomiasis
140. Which is not characteristic of portal hypertension: *(Recent Pattern 2014-15)*
    a. Splenomegaly   b. Hypersplenism
    c. Ascites   d. Gynaecomastia
141. A patient presented to emergency ward with massive upper gastrointestinal bleed. On examination, he has mild splenomegaly. In the absence of any other information available. Which of the following is the most appropriate therapeutic modality? *(Recent Pattern 2014-15)*
    a. Intravenous propranolol
    b. Intravenous vasopressin
    c. Intravenous pantoprazole
    d. Intravenous somatostatin
142. Most common cause of congestive splenomegaly is: *(Recent Pattern 2014-15)*
    a. Chronic congestive cardiac failure
    b. Cirrhosis
    c. Hepatic vein occlusion
    d. Stenosis of splenic vein
143. A 45-year-old cirrhotic patient presented with severe haematemesis. The management of choice is: *(Recent Pattern 2014-15)*
    a. Whole blood transfusion
    b. Colloids are preferred over crystalloids
    c. Normal saline infusion
    d. IV fluid with diuretics
144. Which of the following is the most common presenting symptom of non-cirrhotic portal hypertension? *(AI 2006)*
    a. Chronic liver failure
    b. Ascites
    c. Upper gastrointestinal bleeding
    d. Encephalopathy
145. A man presents with history of hemetemesis of about 500 ml of blood. On examination, spleen is palpable 5 cms below the left costal margin. The most likely diagnosis is: *(AI 2012)*
    a. Portal Hypertension   b. Gastric ulcer
    c. Drug induced   d. Mallory Weiss Tear

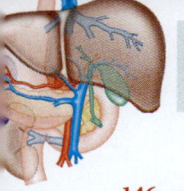

146. A 40 year old patient, a known case of cirrhosis develops acute episode of GI bleed. Initial therapy given for 6 hours. Which of the following procedure is useful?
    (AIIMS June 99)
    a. Nasogastric aspiration
    b. Urgent endoscopy
    c. Sedation
    d. Ultrasound

147. A 45 year old cirrhotic patient presented with severe haematemesis. The management of choice is:
    a. Whole blood transfusion is the best *(AIIMS June 99)*
    b. Colloids are preferred over crystalloids
    c. Normal saline infusion
    d. IV fluid with diuretics

148. Best treatment for refractory ascites
    a. AV shunt *(Recent Question 2016-17)*
    b. TIPS
    c. furosemide with paracentesis
    d. Distal splenorenal shunt

Ascites

149. SAAG > 1.1% is seen in all cases of ascites except?
    (AIIMS Nov 2017)
    a. Cirrhosis   b. Peritoneal tuberculosis
    c. Liver failure   d. Hepatic metastasis

150. Which one of the following statements is TRUE regarding the clinical sign being elicited here? *(AP PG 2016)*

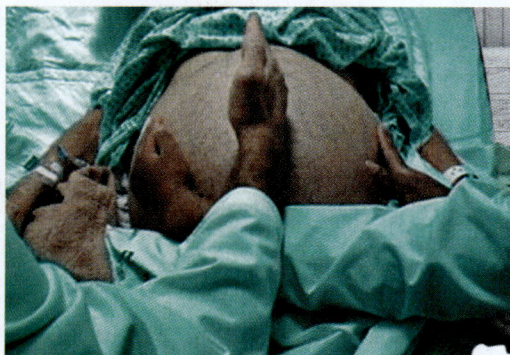

    a. This test helps to detect ascites
    b. This test is for eliciting shifting dullness
    c. The hand on the midline below the umbilicus will feel the vibrations in patients with ascites
    d. All these statements are True

151. Maximum dose of spironolactone is: *(APPG 2015)*
    a. 400 mg/day   b. 100 mg/day
    c. 160 mg/day   d. 50 mg/day

152. A chronic liver disease patient with ascites and non-bleeding varices presents with hematemesis and melena. What is the next step in management? *(Jipmer Nov 2014)*
    a. Inj vitamin K   b. Inj Tranexamic acid
    c. FFP transfusion   d. Platelet transfusion

153. Ascitic fluid with increased SAAG & ascitic protein > 2.5g/dL is/are found in: *(PGI May 2015)*
    a. T.B   b. CHF
    c. Cirrhosis   d. Pancreatitis
    e. Nephrotic syndrome

154. Best Treatment of refractory ascites is:
    a. AV shunt   *(Recent Pattern 2014-15)*
    b. TIPS
    c. Frusemide with paracentesis
    d. Distal splenorenal shunt

155. Child with S.A.A.G < 1.1 gm/dl: The probable diagnosis of the child is: *(Recent Pattern 2014-15)*
    a. Cirrhosis   b. Portal hypertension
    c. CHF   d. Nephrotic syndrome

156. Consider the following statements: *(Recent Pattern 2014-15)*
    Ascites in cirrhosis of liver is due to
    1. Portal hypertension
    2. Hypoalbuminaemia
    3. Inappropriate ADH secretion
    4. Secondary hyper-aldosteronism
    a. 1, 2 and 3 are correct   b. 1, 2 and 4 are correct
    c. 2, 3, 4 are correct   d. 1, 3 and 4 are correct'

157. Which finding suggests a SVC obstruction?
    a. Bulging flanks   *(Recent Pattern 2014-15)*
    b. Collateral flow towards umbilicus
    c. Everted umbilicus
    d. Pulsatile liver

158. Which one of the following is NOT true about Ascites?
    (Recent Pattern 2014-15)
    a. S.A.A.G > 1.1 is seen with portal hypertension
    b. S.A.A.G < 1.1 is seen with Nephrotic syndrome
    c. Pseudochylous ascites is seen with hypertriglyceridemia
    d. Black ascitic fluid is seen with pancreatic necrosis

159. First line of treatment in Ascites is: *(PGI June 96)*
    a. Salt Restriction b. Diuretics
    c. Paracentesis   d. Shunt

Hepatorenal Syndrome

160. Not a feature of hepatorenal syndrome:
    a. Normal GFR   *(Recent Pattern 2014-15)*
    b. Normal urinary sediments
    c. Low Na+ in urine
    d. Normal renal biopsy

161. Which of the following statement is incorrect with regard to Hepatorenal syndrome in a patient with cirrhosis
    a. Createnine clearance < 40 ml/min *(AI 2003)*
    b. Urinary sodium < 10mq/L
    c. Urine osmolality lower than plasma osmolality
    d. No sustained improvement in renal function after volume expansion.

Liver Cancer

162. Consider the following features *(AP PG 2016)*
    Asian Male.
    Alcoholic cirrhosis.
    Hypervascular lesion during arterial phase of CT
    Portal vein thrombosis.
    The above features are mostly suggestive of
    a. Hepatocellular carcinoma
    b. Metastatic colorectal carcinoma
    c. Cholangio carcinoma
    d. Neuroendocrine tumors

163. Which of the following is a vaccine preventable cancer?
    (JIPMER Nov 2014)
    a. Hepatocellular carcinoma
    b. Renal cell carcinoma
    c. Lymphoma
    d. Kaposi sarcoma
164. Best for management of 4 cm hepatocellular carcinoma in a cirrhotic patient with portal hypertension:
    a. Radiofrequency ablation   (Recent Pattern 2014-15)
    b. Transarterial catheter embolization (T.A.C.E)
    c. Percutaneous ethanol
    d. Orthoptic liver transplantation
165. Most common liver tumour associated with OCP:
    a. Focal nodular hyperplasia   (Recent Pattern 2014-15)
    b. Hemangioma
    c. Angiomyolipoma
    d. Hepatocellular adenoma
166. Best to diagnose a liver tumour?   (Recent Pattern 2014-15)
    a. CT
    b. USG
    c. MRI
    d. Sulphur colloid scan
167. Most common benign tumor of the liver:
    a. Focal nodular hyperplasia   (Recent Pattern 2014-15)
    b. Hemangioma
    c. Angiomyolipoma
    d. Hepatocellular adenoma
168. All of the following are risk factors for Hepatocellular carcinoma except: (All India 2010)
    a. Hepatitis C infection
    b. Alcoholism
    c. Alfatoxins
    d. Animal fat in diet
169. All of the following are important clinical manifestations of hepatocellular carcinoma except: (All India 2011)
    a. Jaundice
    b. Abdominal pain
    c. Abdominal mass
    d. Ascites
170. Increase in alpha-fetoprotein is seen in: (AIIMS June 2000)
    a. Hepatoblastoma   b. Neuroblastoma
    c. Thymoma   d. Angiosarcoma
171. About fibrolamellar carcinoma, what is TRUE:
    a. Diffuse in nature   (AIIMS May 94)
    b. Occurs after 60 years of age
    c. Cirrhosis is the most common presenting feature
    d. Has better prognosis

Wilson Disease

172. A 14-year-old boy with difficulty in walking and behavioral disturbance who recently recovered from prolonged jaundice, has bluish pigmentation over lunula. Which is the next investigation to be done?   (JIPMER May 2018)
    a. Nail fold capillaroscopy
    b. Slit lamp examination
    c. Biopsy of the pigmented area
    d. Ankle-Brachial Pressure Index

173. A 12 year old boy suffering from hepatitis presents with emotional lability. The paediatrician refers him to ophthalmologist (image of slit-lamp is given). What is the next investigation to be done?   (Recent Pattern 2018)

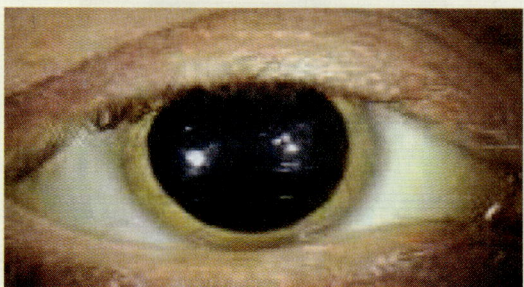

    a. MRI Brain
    b. Serum Ceruloplasmin
    c. PCR
    d. Serum ferritin

174. A 15 year old child presents with falling school grades and development of abnormal posture. On examination dystonia and increase muscle tone is noted. Slit lamp examination shows presence of KF ring. Liver biopsy for copper will be stained by which of the following stain?
    (Recent Question 2016-17)

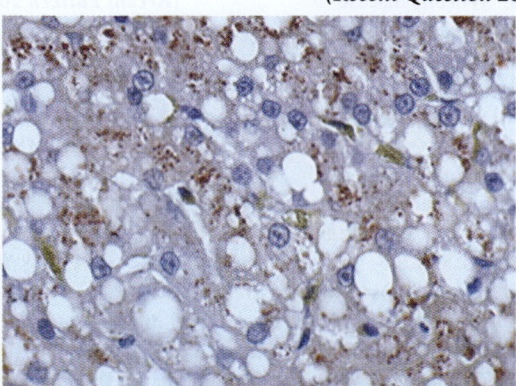

    a. Perl stain
    b. Rubeanic acid
    c. Supravital stain
    d. Schmorl's method

175. A 22 year old woman is evaluated in the emergency department for a 3 day history of dark urine and abdominal distension. On examination:- normal mental status, icterus present, Heart and Lungs normal, Hematocrit:- 26, Reticulocytes:- 5%, Platelets:- 1.3 lakhs, Alk.Phos:- 30 units/L, ALT:-110 units/L, AST:- 220 units/L, Total bilirubin:-13 (Direct:4 mg) HBsAg Positive and Hepatitis 'A' &'C' negative. Urine drug screen negative. Ultrasound abdomen shows a nodular appearing liver and enlarged spleen. Which is the most likely diagnosis?
    (APPG 2016)

    a. Acetaminophen intoxication
    b. Acute viral hepatitis
    c. Primary biliary cirrhosis
    d. Wilson disease

176. This young patient came with wing beating tremor and liver cell failure. The above is picture of his eye. What is the diagnosis? (APPG 2015)

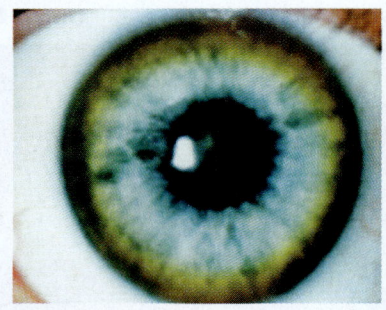

   a. Galactosemia
   b. Paralysis Agitans
   c. Hepatolenticular degeneration
   d. Primary Biliary Cirrhosis

177. Incorrect about Wilson disease (AIIMS Nov 2012)
   a. Decrease in urinary copper
   b. Decrease serum copper
   c. Decrease in serum ceruloplasmin
   d. Increase serum copper

178. Mallory hyaline changes seen in A/E:
   a. Wilson's disease (Recent Pattern 2014-15)
   b. Indian childhood cirrhosis
   c. Primary biliary cirrhosis
   d. Hepatitis E

179. All of the following are features of Wilson's disease, except- (AIIMS Dec 97)
   a. Hemolytic anemia   b. Testicular atrophy
   c. Chorea   d. Chronic active hepatitis

180. All of the following statements about. Wilson's disease are true, EXCEPT- (AIIMS May 04)
   a. It is an autosomal recessive disorder
   b. Serum ceruloplasmin level is < 20 mg/dl
   c. Urinary copper excretion is <100 µg/day
   d. Zinc acetate is effective as maintenance therapy

Hemochromatosis

181. A patient presents with Arthritis, hyperpigmentation of skin and hypogonadism, likely diagnosis is-
   a. Hemochromatosis (Recent Pattern 2017-18)
   b. Ectopic ACTH secreting tumour of the lung
   c. Wilson's disease
   d. Rheumatoid arthritis

182. Impotence and loss of libido in hemochromatosis is due to? (Recent Pattern 2014-15)
   a. Iron deposition in heart
   b. Iron deposition in pituitary
   c. Iron deposition in Liver and increased estrogen
   d. Iron deposition in the testis

183. Earliest phenotypic manifestation of Idiopathic hereditary hemochromatosis is- (AIIMS May 07)
   a. Post prandial increase in serum iron concentration
   b. Elevated serum ferritin level
   c. Slate grey pigmentation of skin
   d. Increased transferrin saturation

184. A 54 years, known diabetic patient develops cirrhosis. There is associated skin hyperpigmentation and restrictive cardiomyopathy which of the following is the best initial test to diagnose this case. (AIIMS Nov 2000)
   a. Percent transferrin saturation
   b. Serum ferritin
   c. Serum copper
   d. Serum ceruloplasmin

Miscellaneous

185. Which organ is not involved in hemochromatosis? (Recent Question 2016-17)
   a. Pituitary   b. Heart
   c. Pancreas   d. Testis

186. Which is the best guide to therapeutic treatment in alcoholic liver disease? (Recent Question 2016-17)
   a. Discriminant function   b. Child Pugh score
   c. Gamma GGT   d. SGOT/SGPT ratio

187. Which of the following is an absolute contraindication to liver transplantation? (Recent Question 2016-17)
   a. Age >70   b. Portal vein thrombosis
   c. Severe obesity   d. AIDS

188. Bile acid pool size is? (Recent Question 2016-17)
   a. 1g   b. 2g
   c. 3g   d. 4g

189. Niemann – Pick disease is due to deficiency of which of the following enzymes? (AP PG 2016)
   a. Acid Sphingomyelinase
   b. Hexosaminidase A
   c. Ceramidase
   d. Arylsulfatase B

190. A 48 year old lady presented with hepatosplenomegaly with pancytopenia. On microscopic examination of bone marrow cells, crumpled tissue paper appearance is seen. Which is the product likely to have accumulated? (AIIMS May 2015)
   a. Glucocerebroside   b. Sphingomyelin
   c. Sulfatide   d. Ganglioside

191. Which one of the following is implicated in the etiology of Fitz-Hugh-curtis syndrome? (APPG 2015)
   a. Chlamydial infection
   b. Perforation of dermoid cyst
   c. Gastric perforation
   d. Liver metastases in ovarian cancer

192. In hemochromatosis, all are affected EXCEPT: (Recent Question 2015-16)
   a. CNS   b. Bronze Pancreas
   c. Hyperpigmentation   d. Restrictive cardiomyopathy

193. Medical treatment of gallstone indicated in A/E:
   a. GB should be functioning (Recent Pattern 2014-15)
   b. Gallstone should be radiolucent
   c. Gallstone should be radiopaque
   d. Patient is unfit for surgery

194. Lady with cystic fibrosis with chronic pancreatitis will have deficiency of all except: (Recent Pattern 2014-15)
   a. Vitamin B12   b. Vitamin A
   c. Pancreatic cancer d. Niacin deficiency

195. **Spider naevi can occur in:** *(Recent Pattern 2014-15)*
    a. Rheumatoid arthritis
    b. Cirrhosis of the liver
    c. Pregnancy
    d. All of the above

196. **False statement regarding spontaneous bacterial peritonitis is:** *(Recent Pattern 2014-15)*
    a. Infection is preceded by ascites
    b. Clinical features are abdominal Pain, fever, leucocytosis and altered mental status
    c. Ascitic fluid protein of 1gm/dl
    d. Common organisms are Gram negative organisms

197. **Ranson's criteria includes all except:** *(Recent Pattern 2014-15)*
    a. Fall in hematocrit > 10%
    b. Calcium < 8 mg%
    c. WBC > 16, 000
    d. Base deficit > 2

198. **Incorrect about Mirrizi syndrome:** *(Recent Pattern 2014-15)*
    a. Jaundice
    b. Cystic duct obstruction
    c. MRCP for investigation
    d. Hemobilia

199. **Most common cause of hemobilia is:** *(Recent Pattern 2014-15)*
    a. Trauma
    b. Hemangioma
    c. Rupture of hepatic artery aneurysm
    d. Hepatitis

200. **The most common symptom of primary biliary cirrhosis is:** *(Recent Pattern 2014-15)*
    a. Pruritus
    b. Weakness
    c. Fever
    d. Pain abdomen

201. **CAGE scale is used in:** *(Recent Pattern 2014-15)*
    a. Alcohol Abuse
    b. Depression
    c. Suicidal intention
    d. Coma

202. **Grey Turner's sign is seen in:** *(Recent Pattern 2014-15)*
    a. Myocarditis
    b. Cholecystitis
    c. Pancreatitis
    d. Pleural effusion

203. **Maddrey discriminant score is used for determining mortality due to:** *(Recent Pattern 2014-15)*
    a. Alcoholic hepatitis
    b. Viral hepatitis
    c. Cryptogenic hepatitis
    d. Hepatic encephalopathy

204. **Following liver transplantation, recurrence of primary disease in the liver most likely occurs in:** *(Recent Pattern 2014-15)*
    a. Wilson's disease
    b. Autoimmune hepatitis
    c. Alpha-1-antitrypsin deficiency
    d. Primary biliary cirrhosis

205. **Medical treatment in gallbladder stone is amenable for:** *(Recent Pattern 2014-15)*
    a. Size of stone less than 10 mm
    b. Radiopaque
    c. Calcium bilirubinate oxalate
    d. GB non-functioning

206. **Causes of acute pancreatitis are A/E:** *(Recent Pattern 15)*
    a. Hypocalcemia
    b. Valproic acid therapy
    c. Biliary tract disease
    d. Blunt trauma

207. **Pencillamine is mostly used in:** *(Recent Pattern 2014-15)*
    a. Hepatolenticular disease
    b. Penicillin anaphylaxis
    c. Haemochromatosis
    d. Tertiary syphilis

208. **All of the following are true about Primary Biliary Cirrhosis except:** *(Recent Pattern 2014-15)*
    a. Increase 5'- nucleotidase
    b. Median age 50
    c. Second most common cause of cholangitis in children
    d. PBC frequently associated with CREST syndrome

209. **Normal liver microscopy is a feature of:** *(Recent Pattern 2014-15)*
    a. Wilson's disease
    b. Dubin-Johnson syndrome
    c. Gilbert's syndrome
    d. Criggler-Najjar

210. **Forrest classification is used for evaluating:** *(Recent Pattern 2014-15)*
    a. Upper GI bleeding
    b. Liver transplantation
    c. Lower GI bleeding
    d. Familial adenomatous polyposis

211. **HIDA scan is useful in:** *(Recent Pattern 2014-15)*
    a. Acute cholecystitis
    b. Meckel's diverticulum
    c. Colonic angio-dysplasia
    d. Diverticulitis

212. **All of the following are indications for liver transplantation except:** *(Recent Pattern 2014-15)*
    a. Hepatocellular carcinoma
    b. Criggler najar syndrome
    c. Gilbert disease
    d. Biliary atresia

213. **The following features differentiate Rotor syndrome from Dubin Johnson's syndrome except:** *(APPG 2014)*
    a. Liver patients with Rotor syndrome has no increased pigmentation and appears normal
    b. In Rotor syndrome Gall bladder is usually visualized on cholecystography
    c. Total urinary coproporphyrin is substantially increased in Rotor syndrome
    d. Fraction of corpophyrin I in urine is elevated usually more than 80% of the total in Rotor syndrome

214. **Which of the following finding is not suggestive of intrinsic hepatic fibrosis:** *(Recent Pattern 2014-15)*
    a. Bulging flanks
    b. Collateral flow toward umbilicus
    c. Everted umbilicus
    d. Venous hum

215. **Patient of acute pancreatitis developed sudden loss of vision the most likely cause is:** *(Recent Pattern 2014-15)*
    a. Purtscher's retinopathy
    b. Hyperglycemia
    c. Hypoxia
    d. CRVO

216. **Which is the diagnostic test in pancreatic steatorrhea:** *(Recent Pattern 2014-15)*
    a. Schilling test
    b. Serum lipase
    c. Serum amylase
    d. Fecal Elastase level

217. **Diabetic ketoacidosis mimics acute pancreatitis in all findings except:** *(Recent Pattern 2014-15)*
    a. Elevated amylase
    b. Elevated lipase
    c. Abdominal pain
    d. Hyperglycemia

218. **Low serum copper due to ATP 7A gene is due to?**
    a. Dubin-Johnson's syndrome *(Recent Pattern 2014-15)*
    b. Wilson disease
    c. Menke disease
    d. Gilbert's disease

219. **Major symptom of acute pancreatitis is:**
    a. Abdominal bloating *(Recent Pattern 2014-15)*
    b. Agonizing upper abdominal pain
    c. Jaundice
    d. Constipation

220. **Which is best in evaluating alcoholic hepatitis?**
    (Recent Pattern 2014-15)
    a. Carbohydrate deficient transferrin
    b. 5-nucleotidase
    c. SGPT raised
    d. MCHC

221. **Rockall score is used for prognosis of patients of:**
    a. Upper GI bleeding *(Recent Pattern 2014-15)*
    b. Lower GI bleeding
    c. Hepatic encephalopathy
    d. IBD

222. **Zieve syndrome is characterized by all except?**
    a. Alcohol abuse *(Recent Pattern 2014-15)*
    b. Hemolysis
    c. Hypertriglyceridemia
    d. Pancreatic lipase deficiency

223. **Purtscher's retinopathy results from:**
    a. Air embolism *(Recent Pattern 2014-15)*
    b. Chronic Pancreatitis
    c. Parasitic infections
    d. Compressive chest injury

224. **Ranson's criteria for acute pancreatitis include all except:**
    (Recent Pattern 2014-15)
    a. Hyperglycemia   b. LDH>250U
    c. Hypocalcemia   d. Hyperamylasia

225. **Which extraintestinal symptom of IBD worsens with exacerbation of disease activity?** *(Recent Pattern 2014-15)*
    a. Episcleritis
    b. Arthritis
    c. PSC
    d. Uveitis

226. **Pancreatic insufficiency is best diagnosed by:**
    a. Abnormal Schilling test corrected by pancreatic enzyme administration *(Recent Pattern 2014-15)*
    b. Ba meal study
    c. Amylase levels
    d. Lipase levels

227. **Gamma glutamyl transferase is elevated in:**
    a. Liver abscess *(Recent Pattern 2014-15)*
    b. Viral hepatitis
    c. Alcoholic liver disease
    d. Secondaries in liver

228. **All of the following are noticed in cirrhosis of liver, except:**
    a. Raised serum albumin *(Recent Pattern 2014-15)*
    b. Excessive urobilinogenuria
    c. Prolonged prothrombin time
    d. Raised serum globulin

229. **All of the following is associated with recurrent acute pancreatitis except:** *(Recent Pattern 2014-15)*
    a. Hypertriglyceridemia   b. Cystic fibrosis
    c. Pancreatic cancer   d. All of the above

230. **Investigation of choice in Hemobilia:**
    (Recent Pattern 2014-15)
    a. ERCP   b. Angiography
    c. Upper GI endoscopy   d. Barium study

231. **Hyperglycemia occurs after what % of beta cell mass is destroyed:** *(Recent Pattern 2014-15)*
    a. 20%   b. 40%
    c. 60%   d. 80%

232. **SGPT is found in:** *(Recent Pattern 2014-15)*
    a. Cytoplasm of hepatocytes
    b. Mitochondria of hepatocytes
    c. Nucleus of hepatocytes
    d. All of above

233. **Incorrect about liver transplantation:**
    a. University of winconsin solution for prolongation of cold ischemia time *(Recent Pattern 2014-15)*
    b. Done if MELD score > 17
    c. HLA matching not required
    d. Recurrence with Wilson disease

234. **In modified Pugh's classification score of 8, what to do?**
    a. Conservative management *(Recent Pattern 2014-15)*
    b. Orthotopic liver transplant
    c. Sclerotherapy
    d. Shunt surgery

235. **Leading association of non-alcoholic fatty liver disease?**
    (Recent Pattern 2014-15)
    a. Reye syndrome   b. Syndrome-X
    c. Coronary syndrome-X d. Pregnancy

236. **Best diagnosis of pancreatic disease:**
    (Recent Pattern 2014-15)
    a. Ultrasound   b. CT scan
    c. ERCP   d. PTC

237. **Serum amylase is raised in:** *(Recent Pattern 2014-15)*
    a. Rubella   b. Measles
    c. Mumps   d. Chickenpox

238. **Criteria for severity in acute pancreatitis includes all except:**
    (Recent Pattern 2014-15)
    a. 3 fold increase in serum lipase
    b. Serum creatinine > 2.0mg%
    c. PaO_2 < 60mmHg
    d. SBP<90

239. **Hand signs of liver cell failure are all except?**
    (Recent Pattern 2014-15)
    a. Palmar erythema   b. Clubbing
    c. Duputyren contracture   d. Splinter hemorrhages

240. **The most frequent location for spider angiomata in cirrhosis is:** *(Recent Pattern 2014-15)*
    a. Abdomen   b. Back
    c. Neck and shoulders   d. Upper & lower extremities

241. **Increased B12 level is seen in all, except:** *(AI 2000)*
    a. Cirrhosis
    b. Primary hepatocellular Cancer
    c. Hepatitis
    d. Cholestatic jaundice

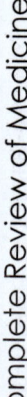

Answers with Explanations

Viral Hepatitis

1. (b) AntiHAV, HBsAg, IgM antiHBc, AntiHCV

(Ref: Harrison 20th edition p 2361)

LFT report shows elevated bilirubin with conjugated bilirubin >15% of total serum bilirubin. SGOT and SGPT elevation indicates cytopathic effect of probably a virus. For diagnosis of acute viral hepatitis *four* serological tests should be performed. **These are:**

1. HbsAg
2. IgM Anti- HBc
3. IgM Anti- HAV
4. Anti- HCV

- Absence of all of these serological markers is consistent with diagnosis of non-A, non-B and non-C hepatitis.
- Presence of positive test for only Anti- HCV confirms the diagnosis of acute hepatitis C.
- This is a source of confusion for most people since we read about chronic hepatitis C most of the time. However an early diagnosis of acute hepatitis C could prevent the patient from going into chronic hepatitis C and End stage liver disease.

2. Ans. (b) AST

(Ref: Harrison 20th edition p 2400)

- GGTP is not specific to alcohol since it is easily inducible and elevated in all forms of fatty liver.
- AST and ALT are increased 2-7 times with AST/ ALT ratio > 1 in alcoholic hepatitis
- ALP is used for evaluation of obstructive jaundice
LDH is elevated in hemolytic anemia and malignancy.

3. Ans. (b) Highly likely to cause chronic ongoing infection

(Ref: Harrison 20th edition p 2386)

Hepatitis C is an RNA virus and it presents as chronic hepatitis C. It is transmitted by parenteral route

4. Ans. (a) Hepatitis C

(Ref: Harrison 20th edition, p 2354; Harrison 19th edition p 2190-91)

Essential mixed cryoglobulinemia is characterised by cryoglobulins. They are cold precipitable monoclonal or polyclonal antibodies leading to systemic vasculitis. *It is associated with hepatitis C.* The features seen are:

1. Cutaneous vasculitis leading to palpable purpura (MC manifestation)
2. Arthralgia
3. Neuropathy leading to weakness
4. Glomerulonephritis

5. Ans. (b) Integration of virus with host DNA

(Ref: Harrison 20th edition, p 579; Harrison 19th edition p 544-545)

Integration of HBV DNA is seen in >90% of Hepatitis B related HCC. This can lead to truncation of HBx gene which happens to be a potent tumor activator. This explains the difficulty in achieving a cure as the viral inserts itself into host DNA and allows it to persist in the face of drugs that impair its replication. Harrison has used the term insertional mutagenesis.

6. Ans. (b) Serum Hyaluronic acid

(Ref: Trends in biomarkers in disease and pubmed index number: PMC5729599 p 57)

Serum Hyaluronic acid is a glycosaminoglycan and is a component of ECM that is produced by hepatic stellate cells. The degradation of same occurs in sinusoidal endothelial cells. The serum concentration of Hyaluronic Acid is elevated in patients of hepatic fibrosis and can serve as a non-invasive surrogate for liver biopsy.

1. Fibrosure/ Fibro Test
   - Incorporates haptoglobin, bilirubin, GGT and Apolipoprotein A-1 and α2macroglobulin.
   - High level of positive and negative predicitive values for diagnosing advanced fibrosis.
2. Fibroscan/ Transient Elastography
   Evaulates hepatic stiffness
3. Magnetic resonance Elastography

7. Ans. (c) HCV-RNA- RT PCR

(Ref: Harrison 20th edition p 2360; Harrison 19th edition p 2017)

- The serological status of this patient shows HCV infection since anti-HCV antibody is reactive.
- Hepatitis B surface antigen is negative and IgG Anti- HBcAg is reactive indicating remote infection with hepatitis B.
- Recovery is the rule in hepatitis B. In contrast hepatitis C results in development of cirrhosis. Even if transaminases are normal, hepatitis C results in long term damage to the liver.
- Hence the reason for elevated liver enzymes with development of liver fibrosis points to HCV being the culprit.
- The next step shall be to perform a PCR-HCV RNA and initiate treatment based on prevalent genotype in the area.
- Liver biopsy is ruled out as question says patient is already having fibrosis.

HBsAg	Anti-HBs	Anti-HBc	HBeAg	Anti-HBe	Interpretation
+	–	IgM	+	–	Acute hepatitis B, high infectivity
+	–	IgG	+	–	Chronic hepatitis B, high infectivity
+	–	IgG	–	+	Late acute or chronic hepatitis B, low infectivity HBeAg-negative ("precore-mutant") hepatitis B (chronic or, rarely, acute)
+	+	+	+/–	+/–	1. HBsAg of one subtype and heterotypic anti-HBs (common) 2. Process of seroconversion from HBsAg to anti-HBs (rare)
–	–	IgM	+/–	+/–	1. Acute hepatitis B 2. Anti-HBc window
–	–	IgG	–	+/–	1. Low-level hepatitis B carrier 2. Hepatitis B remote past
–	+	IgG	–	+/–	

8. Ans. (d) Hepatitis E

(Ref: Harrison 20th edition, p 2356; Harrison: 19th edition p 2013)

The following characteristics of Hepatitis E virus are enumerated in Table 332-2 of Harrison. Hepatitis E *does not* have a-
1. Percutaneous spread
2. Perinatal spread
3. Sexual route spread

9. Ans. (c) HBe Ag

(Ref: Harrison 20th edition, p 2360; Harrison 19th p 1993t)

- HBeAg, appearance coincides with high levels of virus replication and reflects the presence of circulating intact virions and detectable HBV DNA.(with the notable exception of patients with precore mutations who cannot synthesize HBeAg).
- In self-limited HBV infections, HBeAg becomes undetectable shortly after peak elevations in aminotransferase activity, before the disappearance of HBsAg, and anti-HBe then becomes detectable, coinciding with a period of relatively lower infectivity.

10. Ans. (c) Check HBV DNA load

(Ref: Harrison 20th edition, p 2361)

- In Chronic HBV infection, possibilities are:
  1. HBsAg remains detectable beyond six months
  2. Anti-HBc is primarily of the IgG class
  3. Anti-HBs is either undetectable or detectable at low levels
- During early chronic HBV infection, HBV DNA can be detected both in serum and in hepatocyte nuclei, where it is present in free or episomal form.
- **HBeAg is a qualitative marker and HBV DNA a quantitative marker of replicative phase**
- In chronic hepatitis B is the **degree of hepatitis B virus (HBV) replication is more** important than histology alone.
- In both HBeAg-reactive and HBeAg negative chronic hepatitis B, the **level of HBV DNA correlates with the level of liver injury and risk of progression.**
- The level of HBV replication is the most important risk factor for the ultimate development of cirrhosis and HCC in both HBeAg-reactive and HBeAg-negative patients.

11. Ans. (c) Recovery from remote infection

(Ref: Harrison 20th edition, p 2360; Harrison 19th edition p 2017)

Window period (Choice A)	Has presence of only IgM anti-HbcAg
Chronic hepatitis inactive state (Choice B)	Should have presence of HbsAg and IgG anti-HbcAg and HbeAg negative
Recovery from acute infection (Choice D)	Should have appearance of anti-HbsAg And Ig anti HbcAg simultaneously

Commonly encountered serologic patterns of hepatitis b infection

HBsAg	Anti-HBs	Anti-HBc	HBeAg	Anti-HBe	Interpretation
+	–	IgM	+	–	Acute hepatitis B, high infectivity
+	–	IgG	+	–	Chronic hepatitis B, high infectivity
+	–	IgG	–	+	Late acute or chronic hepatitis B, low infectivity HBeAg-negative ("precore-mutant") hepatitis B (chronic or, rarely, acute)
+	+	+	+/–	+/–	1. HBsAg of one subtype oand heterotypic ani-HBs (common) 2. Process of seroconversion from HBsAg to anti-HBs (rare)

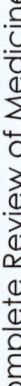

HBsAg	Anti-HBs	Anti-HBc	HBeAg	Anti-HBe	Interpretation
–	–	IgM	+/–	+/–	1. Acute hepatitis B 2. Anti-HBc "window"
–	–	IgG	–	+/–	1. Low-level hepatitis B cancer 2. Hepatitis B in remote past
–	+	IgG	–	+/–	Recovery from hepatitis B
–	+	–	–	–	1. Immunization with HBsAg (after vaccination) 2. Hepatitis B in the remote past 3. False-positive

12. Ans. (a) Hepatitis B

(Ref: Oxford handbook of emergency medicine, 4th edition p 418)

Percentage of chances of transmission of infection with accidental stick injury

HBsAg positive and HBeAg Positive	22-30%
HBsAg positive and HBeAg Negative	1-6%
Hepatitis C	1.8%
HIV	0.3%

13. Ans. (b) Post transfusions hepatitis is caused by CMV

(Ref: Pediatric Transfusion medicine volume 1 p 94

Choice C & D are ruled out as current screening tests are sensitive for detecting surface antigen and HCV testing is routinely done.

Possible reasons for post transfusion hepatitis in spite of screening:
1. CMV can cause asymptomatic infection
2. Transfusion transmitted CMV can cause problems in premature neonates, allograft recipients, splenectomized patients.
3. Leukocytes depleted blood use of frozen deglycerolized RBCs and screening of donors for the absence of antibody to CMV.
4. Inactive hepatitis B carrier does not mean patient is HBsAg negative. It means persistent HBV infection of liver with low or undetectable serum HBV DNA/levels with normal serum aminotransferase.

14. Ans. (c) Zidovudine

(Ref: Harrison 20th edition, p 2382)

Entecavir	Entecavir, an oral cyclopentyl guanosine analogue polymerase inhibitor, appears to be the most potent of the HBV antivirals.
Telbivudine	Telbivudine, a cytosine analogue, appears to be similar in efficacy to entecavir; however, it is slightly less potent in suppressing HBV DNA.
Lamivudine	Lamivudine inhibits reverse transcriptase activity of both HIV and HBV and is a potent and effective agent for patients with chronic hepatitis B. Although generally superseded by newer, more potent agents, Lamivudine is still used in regions of the world where newer agents are not yet approved are or not affordable

15. Ans. (d) PAN

(Ref: Harrison 20th edition, p 2356; Harrison 19th p 2044)

16. Ans. (b) Acute hepatitis B infection with high infectivity

(Ref: Harrison 20th edition, p 2360; Harrison 19th p 2081)

17. Ans. (d) Tenofovir

(Ref: Harrison 19th p 2033)

- Tenofovir is a first-line agent in the treatment of hepatitis B. It prevents the formation of 5' to 3' phosphodiester linkage essential for DNA chain elongation. Hence it causes premature termination of DNA transcription.

18. Ans. (a) Vaccinated state

(Ref: Harrison 20th edition, p 2360; Harrison 19th p 2033)

19. Ans. (d) Infectious mononucleosis

(Ref: Harrison 19th p 2031)

- Glomerulonephritis with the nephrotic syndrome is observed occasionally; HBsAg, immuno-globulin, and C3 deposition has been found in the glomerular basement membrane.
- While generalized vasculitis (polyarteritis nodosa) develops in considerably fewer than 1% of patients with chronic HBV infection, 20–30% of patients with polyarteritis nodosa have HBsAg in serum.
- Due to decreased humoral response and repeated admissions in hospital in childhood patients of Down's have a higher prevalence of hepatitis B infection.

20. Ans. (a) I.V. Drug abuse

(Ref: Harrison 20th edition, p 2357; Harrison 19th p 2041)

Transfusion of blood contaminated with HCV was once an important source of transmission. Since 1990, however, the screening of donated blood for HCV antibody has decreased the risk of transfusion-associated HCV infection to less than 1 case in 103, 000 transfused units

Persons who inject illegal drugs with non-sterile needles or who snort cocaine with shared straws are at highest risk for HCV infection. In developed countries, most new HCV infections are related to intravenous drug abuse (IVDA).

21. Ans. (a) 6 weeks to 6 months

(Ref: Harrison 20th edition, p 2356; Harrison 19th p 2031)

Incubation period of hepatotrophic viruses

Virus	Incubation period
Hepatitis A	2–7 weeks
Hepatitis B	30 – 180 days with average of 75 days
Hepatitis C	6–10 weeks
Hepatitis D	3–7 weeks
Hepatitis E	3–8 weeks

22. Ans. (d) Delta hepatitis

(Ref: Harrison 20th edition, 2385; Harrison 19th p 2031)

23. Ans. (c) Intramuscular deltoid

(Ref: Harrison 19th p 2031)

The fat in the buttock reduces the immunogenicity of the vaccine.

24. Ans. (d) Anicteric hepatitis is not seen

(Ref: Harrison 19th p 2035)

25. Ans. (b) HBV DNA estimation

(Ref: Harrison 20th edition, p 2383; Harrison 19th p 2035 and Chapter 53, API)

Since patient has voluntarily come for blood transfusion, it implies *clinically* his hepatitis B status is inactive disease. The patient in question is the first column of these AASLD guidelines and does not require any treatment. PCR DNA report will determine viral load. Serial monitoring of SGPT should be done for 3–6 months.

Recommendations for Treatment of Chronic Hepatitis B

HBeAg	Clinical	HBV DNA	ALT	Recommendation
Reactive	Inactive/mild disease	$>2 \times 10^4$	$<2 \times$ Upper limits of normal	No treatment; monitor. In patients >40, with family history of hepatocellular carcinoma, and/ or ALT persistently at the high end of the twofold range, liver biopsy may help in decision to treat
Reactive	Chronic hepatitis	$>2 \times 10^4$	$>2 \times$ Upper limits of normal	Treat
Reactive	Cirrhosis compensated	$>2 \times 10^3$	< or > Upper limits of normal	Treat with oral agents, not PEG IFN

26. Ans. (a) Ribavirin and pegylated interferon

(Ref: Harrison 20th edition, p 2391; Harrison 19th p 2059)

Retreatment is indicated for Relapsers after a previous course of standard interferon monotherapy or combination standard interferon/ribavirin therapy with a course of PEG IFN plus ribavirin.

A course of PEG IFN plus ribavirin—more likely to achieve a sustained virologic response in white patients without previous ribavirin therapy, with low baseline HCV RNA levels, with a 2-log10 reduction in HCV RNA during previous therapy, with genotypes 2 and 3, and without reduction in ribavirin dose. *However in current scenario ledipsavir + sofosbuvir for 12 weeks is indicated for genotype 1a and 1b.*

27. Ans. (c) 20%

(Ref: Harrison 19th p 2035)

- The proportion of babies that become HBV carriers is about 10-30% for mothers who are HBsAg-positive but HBeAg-negative. Now in this question anti-HBeAg is positive it implies that the viral replication has declined and HBeAg has become negative.
- However, the incidence of perinatal infection is even greater, around 70-90%, when the mother is both HBsAg-positive and HBeAg-positive.
- There are three possible routes of transmission of HBV from infected mothers to infants: transplacental transmission of HBV in utero; natal transmission during delivery; or postnatal transmission during care or through breast milk. Since transplacental transmission occurs antenatally, hepatitis B vaccine and HBIG cannot block this route.

28. Ans. (d) Genotype D

(Ref: National center for disease control jan-march 2014, vol. 3, issue 1)

- India has one of the largest pools of hepatitis B-infected patients.
- In a study reported from North India genotype-D was most common in patients suffering from chronic liver disease (CLD).
- The genotype-C was found to be only in one-tenth (10%) of the study population.

Country Wise Serotypes

Genotype A	North-West Europe, North America and Central Africa
Genotypes B and C	HBV genotypes in Eastern Asia, including Taiwan
Genotype D	Southern Europe, Middle East and India
Genotype F	American natives, Polynesia, Central and South America,
Genotype E	USA and France

- Genotype 3 is the most common type of hepatitis C in India.

29. Ans. (b) Progression to cirrhosis is not seen

(Ref: Harrison 20th edition, p 2375; Harrison 19th p 2030)

- Chronic hepatitis is defined as a chronic inflammatory reaction of the liver of more than 3-6 months duration, demonstrated by persistently abnormal serum aminotransferase levels and characteristic histologic findings
- The causes of chronic hepatitis include. HBV- HCV, and HDV, autoimmune hepatitis, chronic hepatitis associated with certain medications (particularly isoniazid), Wilson's disease, and á1-antiprotease deficiency.
- Autoimmune hepatitis responds to steroids.

30. Ans. (c) IgM anti-HBc

(Ref: Harrison 20th edition, p 2350; Harrison 19th p 2033)

31. Ans. (b) Acute cholecystitis.

(Ref: Harrison 20th edition, p 2427; Harrison 19th p 2080)

- Gastritis is ruled out on account of epigastric pain and pleurisy would present with inspiratory catch in respiration. *Since jaundice is not mentioned hence viral hepatitis is less likely.*
- Typical symptoms of acute hepatitis are fatigue, anorexia, nausea, and vomiting. Very high aminotransferase values (>1000 U/L) and hyperbilirubinemia are often observed. On examination hepatomegaly is seen with sharp edge of liver.
- The most common presenting symptom of acute cholecystitis is upper abdominal pain. The Signs of peritoneal irritation may be present, and the pain may radiate to the right shoulder or scapula.

32. Ans. (a) It is due to RNA virus

(Ref: Harrison 20th edition, p 2349)

- Hepatitis B is the only hepadna virus causing infection in humans
- It comprises capsule and a core containing DMA and DNA polymerase enzymes. Blood is the main source of infection
- Chronic HBV infection is marked by the presence of HBS Ag and Anti HBC IgG in the blood.

33. Ans. (b) adw

(Ref: Harrison 20th edition p 2348)

Genotype	Sub Type	Area
A	adw	USA, Europe
D	ayw	USA, Europe
B	adw	Asia
C	adr	Asia

34. Ans. (d) Hepatitis E

(Ref: Harrison 20th edition, p 2356)

Hepatitis E is not transmitted by percutaneous perinatal and sexual route.

35. Ans. (d) Hepatitis D virus

(Ref: Harrison 20th edition, p 2356; Harrison 19th p 2030)

Hepatitis D accounts for maximum number of fulminant cases of viral hepatitis, a sizable proportion of which are associated with HBV infection.

36. Ans. (c) Hepatitis C

(Ref: 1. Manual of neonatal care: 7th ed., Cloherty, ch. 48, Harrison 19th p 2030)

- Even if HCV RNA is present in breast milk, there is little evidence for its relevance to HCV transmission to children. Reasons are:
  1. High blood-to-milk gradient ranging from 103 to 107, and low concentrations of viral particles may be inactivated in the gastrointestinal tract . In addition, there may be a neutralizing effect of persisting maternal antibodies in nursed children.
  2. Noninfectious viral particles or viral concentrations that were too low to result in transmission.
  3. Presence of lactoferrin in mammalian breast milk, which has been described to inhibit the replication of viruses such as cytomegalovirus and HIV-1 in vitro
- The rate of vertical transmission of HCV from infected mothers to their children is 3%–5%.

37. Ans. (c) IgM anti-HBcAg

(Ref: Harrison 20th edition, p 2350; Harrison 19th p 2033)

38. Ans. (c) Anti-Hbc IgM

(Ref: Harrison 20th edition, p 2350; Harrison 19th p 2033)

- After a person is infected with HBV, the first virologic marker detectable in serum within 1–12 weeks, usually between 8–12 weeks, is HBsAg
- Circulating HBsAg precedes elevations of serum aminotransferase activity and clinical symptoms by 2–6 weeks and remains detectable during the entire icteric or symptomatic phase of acute hepatitis B and beyond.
- By contrast, anti-HBc is readily demonstrable in serum, beginning within the first 1–2 weeks after the appearance of HBsAg and preceding detectable levels of anti-HBs by weeks to months.

39. Ans. (d) HEV

(Ref: Harrison 20th edition, p 2356; Harrison 19th p 2030)

40. Ans. (d) Do liver biopsy and start antiviral drugs accordingly.

(Ref: Harrison 20th edition, p 2386; Harrison 19th p 2030)

- Chronic infection with hepatitis C is common even in those patients with return of amino-transferases to normal. There

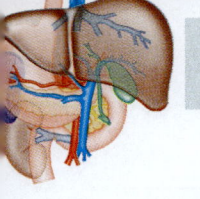

is 85% chances of chronic hepatitis C after acute hepatitis C. Amino-transferases continue to fluctuate and can be normal in patients with long-standing disease
- A pretreatment liver biopsy to assess histologic grade and stage provides substantial information about progression of hepatitis C in the past, and has prognostic value for future progression. It can identify such histologic factors such as steatosis and stage of fibrosis, which can influence responsiveness to therapy.
- Therefore final decision for therapy for these patients should be considered and the decision made based on such factors as patient motivation, genotype, stage of fibrosis, age, and comorbid conditions.

41. Ans. (c) HBV

(Ref: CMDT 2014, ch. 16, p 667)
- Globally, chronic HBV infection affects 350-400 million people, with disease prevalence varying among geographic regions, from 1-20%.
- The World Health Organization (WHO) estimates about 3% of the world's population has been infected with **HCV and that there are more than 170 million chronic carriers** who are at risk of developing liver cirrhosis and/or liver cancer.
- Most common cause of chronic hepatitis is hepatitis C *but carrier stage is seen higher with hepatitis B.*

42. Ans. (c) Genotyping helps in treatment duration

(Ref: Harrison 20th edition, p 2391; Harrison 19th p 203)
- Genotyping is helpful for predicting the likelihood of response and duration of treatment. Patients with genotypes 1 and 4 are generally treated for 12 months, whereas 6 months of treatment is sufficient for other genotypes.
- Genotyping can be performed by direct sequence analysis, reverse hybridization to genotype-specific oligonucleotide probes, or restriction fragment length polymorphisms (RFLPs).

43. Ans. (b) Hbe Antigen

(Ref: Harrison 19th p 2006)
- Since IgM anti-HBcAg is not given in the choices, the other readily detectable serologic marker of HBV infection, HBeAg, appears concurrently with or shortly after HBsAg.
- Its appearance coincides temporarily with high levels of virus replication and reflects the presence of circulating intact virions and detectable HBV DNA (with the notable exception of patients with precore mutations who cannot synthesize HBeAg. Its principal clinical usefulness is as an indicator of relative infectivity.
- In self-limited HBV infections, HBeAg becomes undetectable shortly after peak elevations in aminotransferase activity, before the disappearance of HBsAg, and anti-HBe then becomes detectable, coinciding with a period of relatively lower infectivity.

44. Ans. (b) HbsAg and HbeAg positivity

(Ref: Nelson 20th edition, p 1946; Harrison 19th p 2006)

45. Ans. (a) 5%

(Ref: Harrison 20th edition, p 2358; Harrison 19th p 2009)
- The chances of sexual and perinatal transmission have been estimated to be <5%, well below comparable rates for HIV and HBV infections.
- HCV potentially can be transmitted sexually and perinatally; however, both of these modes of transmission are inefficient for hepatitis C.

46. Ans. (d) All of above

(Ref: Harrison 19th p 2006)

47. Ans. (b) Give hepatitis B vaccine and immunoglobulin to baby

(Ref: Nelson 20th edition, p 1547; CMDT 2019 edition, p 695)

The following infants are considered "high-risk" and should receive both vaccine and HBIG.
1. Mother is HBsAg seropositive and HbeAg positive
2. Mother is HBsAg seropositive and HbeAg/anti-HBe negative
3. Mother is HBsAg seropositive and e markers are not available
4. Mother has acute hepatitis B in pregnancy
5. Mother is HBsAg seropositive and infant in born weighing 1500g or less

48. Ans. (a) Fatty liver

(Ref: Harrison 19th p 2053)

49. Ans. (c) Circular partial single stranded and partial double stranded

(Ref: Harrison 20th edition, p 2349; Harrison 19th p 2206, 2053)

50. Ans. (c) HbsAg + IG M anti-HBc antibody

(Ref: Harrison 20th edition, p 2360)

	HBsAg	Anti-HBs	Anti-HBcAg	HBeAg
Acute hepatitis B, high infectivity	+	-	IgM	-
Window period	-	-	IgM	-
Chronic hepatitis B	+	-	IgG	+
Cured	-	+	IgG	-
Vaccination	-	+	-	-

51. Ans. (c) HBeAg

(Ref: Harrison 20th edition, p 2350; Harrison 19th p 2006)

Hepatitis B surface antigen (HBsAg) and hepatitis B e antigen (HBeAg) (marker of infectivity) are the first markers that can be identified in the serum in acute disease. Hepatitis B core antibody (anti-HBc) immunoglobulin M (IgM) follows.

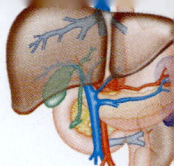

52. Ans. (b) Hepatitis B

(Ref: Wintrobe hematology 12th ed., Table 23.11)

Hepatitis B has higher chances of being transmitted via blood transfusion.

Organism	Estimated risk per unit of transmission
Hepatitis B	1:220, 000
Hepatitis C	1:1600, 000
HIV	1:1800, 000

53. Ans. (d) 3 to 4% carrier state

(Ref: Harrison 20th edition, p 2356; Harrison 19th p 2004)

Chronic hepatitis A does not occur & there is no carrier state.

54. Ans. (a) HBcAg

(Ref: Harrison 20th edition, p 2349; Harrison 19th p 2033)

- Because HBcAg is intracellular and, when in the serum, sequestered within an HBsAg coat, naked core particles do not circulate in serum and, therefore, HBcAg is not detectable routinely in the serum of patients with HBV infection.
- By contrast, anti-HBc is readily demonstrable in serum, beginning within the first 1–2 weeks after the appearance of HBsAg and preceding detectable levels of anti-HBs by weeks to months.

55. Ans. (d) Transient illness with jaundice

(Ref: CMDT 2019 edition, p 692)

- The patient's initial symptoms during the prodromal period include low-grade fever, nausea, vomiting, decreased appetite, and abdominal pain. Older children and adults are more likely to report pain in the right upper quadrant.
- Diarrhea may occur in young children, whereas constipation is more common in adults. If present, jaundice, dark urine, and light-colored stool develop several days to a week after the onset of systemic symptoms. Anicteric infections are common in young children

56. Ans. (a) Serum albumin

(Ref: CMDT 2019 edition, p 699)

Serum albumin has a half-life of 21 days and levels may be normal in fulminant hepatic failure and will take time to fall.

57. Ans. (b) Metastatic carcinoma

(Ref: www. Hepatitis Central.com, Harrison 19th p 2054)

Granulomatous hepatitis is a cause of pyrexia of unknown origin and granulomas are picked up on CT scan or USG abdomen. It is associated with infections like tuberculosis, cat scratch disease, blastomycosis, histoplasmosis.

58. Ans. (d) Hepatitis E

(Ref: Harrison 20th edition, p 2358; Harrison 19th ed p 2010)

Hepatitis E is most common cause of viral hepatitis in India, Asia and Africa. Harrison quotes "one third of world population appears to be infected".

59. Ans (b) Prothrombin time

(Ref: Harrison 20th edition, p 2359; Harrison 19th p 366e-1f)

- The level of elevation of AST/ALT does not correlate well with degree of lives cell damage.
- Prolonged PT reflects a severe biosynthetic defect and indicative of extensive hepatocellular necrosis.

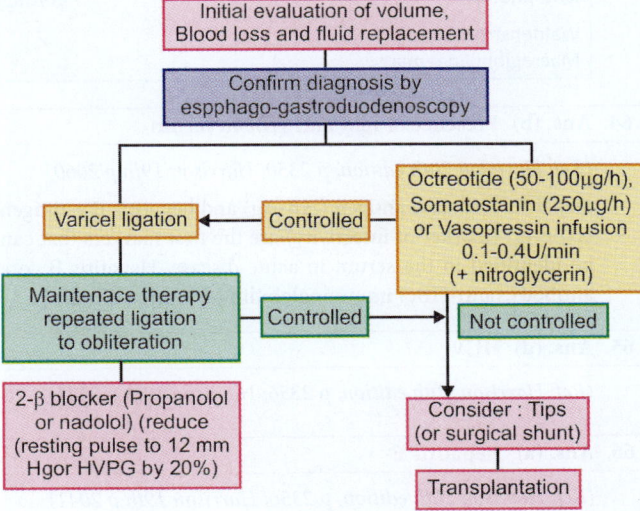

60. Ans. (b) HBV

(Ref: Harrison 19th p 2035)

61. Ans. (a) HBV DNA <10^4 copies/ml with HBsAg negative

(Ref: Harrison 19th p 2035)

- Occult hepatitis B is defined by the presence of HBV DNA in serum or liver in the absence of HBsAg. Serum HBV level is usually less than 10^4 copies/ml.
- Occult HBV infection has been found in patients with HCC, past HBV infection, or chronic hepatitis C, and individuals without HBV serological markers.

62. Ans. (b) LKM antibody

(Ref: Harrison 20th edition, p 2387; Harrison 19th p 2044)

Cross-reactivity between viral antigens (HCV NS3 and NS5A) and host autoantigens (cytochrome P450 2D6) has been invoked to explain the association between hepatitis C and a subset of patients with autoimmune hepatitis and antibodies to liver-kidney microsomal (LKM) antigen.

63. Ans. (b) Celiac disease

(Ref: Harrison 20th edition, p 2354; Harrison 19th p 2044)

Extra-hepatic manifestations of hepatitis C

Haematological	Systemic	Rheumatology	Dermatology	Organ dysfunction
Cryoglulinaemia	Arthralgia	Behcet's disease	Lichen myxoedematosus	Diabetes
Membranoproliferative glomerulonephritis	Arthritis	Vasculitis	Porphyria cutanea tarda	Cardiomyopathy
Multiple myeloma	Fatigue	Raynaud's syndrome	Pruritis	Idiopathic lung fibrosis
Neutropenia/thrombocytopenia	Fibromyalgia	Sialadenitis	Spider naevi	Peripheral neuropathy
Non-hodgkin's lymphoma	Corneal ulceration	Systemic lupus erythematous	Renal failure	Hypothyroidism
Waldenstrom Macroglobulinaemia			Vitiligo	

64. Ans. (b) Presence of IgM anti HBc in serum

(Ref: Harrison 20th edition, p 2350; Harrison 19th p 2060)

Hepatitis B surface antigen (HBsAg) and hepatitis B e antigen (HBeAg) (marker of infectivity) are the first markers that can be identified in the serum in acute disease. Hepatitis B core antibody (anti-HBc) immunoglobulin M (IgM) follows.

65. Ans. (d) HCV

(Ref: Harrison 20th edition, p 2356; Harrison 19th p 2041)

66. Ans. (a) Hepatitis E

(Ref: Harrison 20th edition, p 2356; Harrison 19th p 2041)

67. Ans. (b) Presence of IgM anti-HBc in serum

(Ref: Harrison 20th edition, p 2350; Harrison 19th p 215e-4t)

68. Ans. (c) IgM anti-HBc

(Ref: Harrison 20th edition, p 2350; Harrison 19th p 215e-4t)

69. Ans. (a) IgM Anti HBcAg

(Ref: Harrison 20th edition, p 2350; Harrison 19th p 215e-4t)

70. Ans. (b) Acute hepatitis B infection with high infectivity

(Ref: Harrison 20th edition, p 2350; Harrison 19th p 215e-4t)

71. Ans. (a) Inactive HBV carrier

(Ref: Harrison 19th p 2038f)

72. Ans. (a) IgM against core antigen

(Ref: Harrison 20th edition, p 2350; Harrison 19th p 2006)

73. Ans. (a) Vaccination

(Ref: Harrison 20th edition, p 2350; Harrison 19th p 2006)

74. Ans. (d) IgM anti HBe

(Ref: Harrison 20th edition, p 2350; Harrison 19th p 2008)

75. Ans. (b) HBs Ag + HBe Ag

(Ref: Harrison 20th edition, p 2350; Harrison 19th p 2006)

76. Ans. (c) Hbs Ag +ve and IgM anti-HBc +ve

(Ref: Harrison 20th edition, p 2350; Harrison 19th p 2007)

77. Ans. (c) P gene

(Ref: Harrison 20th edition, p 2348; Harrison 19th p 2006)

78. Ans. (b) Acute Viral Hepatitis B - Antiviral therapy

(Ref: Harrison 20th edition, p 2363; Harrison 19th p 2006)

79. Ans. (d) Focal Segmental Glomerulosclerosis

(Ref: Harrison 20th edition, p 2354; Harrison 19th p 2010)

80. Ans. (b) ↑HBV DNA and ↑ALT

(Ref: Harrison 20th edition, p 2383; Harrison 19th p 2007)

81. Ans. (c) Hepatitis C

(Ref: Harrison 20th edition, p 2350; Harrison 19th p 2084)

82. Ans. (b) Dermatomyositis like syndrome; (d) Psoriasis

(Ref: Dermatology byBurg dorf (Thieme Clinical companion Series) 2006/66, Harrison 19th p 2006t)

83. Ans. (a) Pregnant women

(Ref: Harrison 20th edition, p 2356; Park 18th /174: Harrison 19th p 1991)

84. Ans. (d) ANCA

(Ref: Harrison 20th edition, p 2397; Harrison 19th p 2050)

85. **Ans. (c)** *Elevated serum albumin*

(Ref: Harrison 20th edition, p 2400)

86. **Ans. (b)** *Alcoholic hepatitis*

(Ref: Harrison 20th edition, p 2400)

87. **Ans. (b)** *SGPT is raised > SGOT*

(Ref: Harrison 18th/p 2529)

88. **Ans. (b)** *Clofibrate provides effective treatment*

(Ref: Harrison 20th edition, p 2403-04)

89. **Ans. (a)** *Chronic hepatitis B*

(Ref: 'Pathology: Basic and systemic' by Woolfe (1998)/587, 597)

90. **Ans. (d)** *Estimation of Galactose Elimination capacity*

(Ref: 'Textbook of Hepatology' by Rodes 3rd / 475)

91. **Ans. (d)** *Albumin*

(Ref: Harrison 20th edition, p 2337)

Jaundice

92. **Ans. (b)** *Concomitant renal failure*

(Ref: SRB Surgery: 4th edition p 752)

- In patients of obstructive jaundice the value of serum bilirubin plateaus around 25-30mg% since the water soluble bilirubin is excreted via the urine. However *in setting of concomitant renal failure the concomitant loss of conjugated bilirubin via the kidney fails and leads to extremely high values.*
- Another reason can be a simultaneous overproduction of unconjugated bilirubin due to haemolysis, sepsis and sickle cell anaemia.

93. **Ans. (c)** *Obstetric Cholestasis*

(Ref: Harrison 20th edition, p 2340; Harrison 19th edition p 284, 2029, 2078)

- The presence of pruritus with jaundice points to presence of cholestatic component.
- The presence of SAP increasing the credibility of diagnosis of obstetric cholestatis
- HELLP syndrome is ruled out as coagulation profile is normal
- Hepato-renal syndrome is ruled out as RFT is normal.
- The closest choice is viral hepatitis which presents with jaundice with marked elevation of AST, ALT and SAP being mostly normal.

94. **Ans. (b)** *Delta bilirubin*

(Ref: Harrison 20th edition, p 277; Harrison 19th edition p 280)

Total serum bilirubin = Direct bilirubin + Indirect bilirubin + Delta Bilirubin

- **Delta bilirubin** is a part of the direct-reacting (conjugated) bilirubin that is covalently linked to albumin, is known as *delta fraction, or bili-protein.*
- Because of tight binding to albumin, the clearance rate of albumin-bound bilirubin from serum approximates the half-life of albumin, 12-14 days, rather than the short half-life of bilirubin, about 4 hours.
- It represents an important fraction of total serum bilirubin in patients with cholestasis & hepatobiliary disorders.
- The prolonged half-life of albumin-bound conjugated bilirubin explains why do?
1. Some patients with conjugated hyperbilirubinemia do not exhibit bilirubinuria during the recovery phase of their disease because the bilirubin is covalently bound to albumin and therefore not filtered by the renal glomeruli
2. Elevated serum bilirubin level declines more slowly than expected in some patients who otherwise appear to be recovering satisfactorily.
3. Late in the recovery phase of hepatobiliary disorders, all the conjugated bilirubin may be in the albumin-linked form. Its value in serum falls slowly because of the long half-life of albumin.

95. **Ans. (d)** *Peri-hepatic Obstruction*

(Ref: Harrison 20th edition, p 2342; Harrison 19th edition p 2000)

- Urobilinogen is formed by bacterial metabolism in the gut from conjugated bilirubin. Following secretion into bile, conjugated bilirubin reaches the duodenum and passes down the gastrointestinal tract without reabsorption by the intestinal mucosa.
- Hence it is absent in urine in obstructive jaundice.
- Urinary Urobilinogen is increased in haemolytic jaundice and decreased in hepatitis.
- Absence indicates post hepatic cause which from the above four choices are peri-heaptic obstruction.

	Normal	Haemolytic jaundice	Hepatitis	Obstruction
Urine urobilinogen	0-4mg/24 hrs	Increased	Decreased	Absent
Urine bilirubin	Absent	Absent	Present in case of micro-obstruction	present

96. **Ans. (a)** *Hepatic Scintigraphy*

(Ref: Nelson 19th p 1385-1387)

- The best test for diagnosis of biliary atresia is Percutaneous liver biopsy procedure and provides the most reliable discriminatory evidence.
- Since it is not in the choices Hepatobiliary scintigraphy is the best answer. It is a sensitive test but not specific

- Hepatobiliary scintigraphy with technetium-labelediminodiacetic acid derivatives is used to differentiate biliary atresia from non-obstructive causes of cholestasis.
- Although the uptake may be impaired in neonatal hepatitis, excretion into the bowel will eventually occur.
- USG shows small or absent gall bladder with non-visualization of the common duct and presence of triangular cord sign.

97. Ans. (a) Elevated in carcinoma prostate with hepatic metastasis

(Ref: Harrison 20th edition, p 2400; Harrison 19th edition p 1997, 2053)

- GGTP is not specific to alcohol and is elevated in all forms of fatty liver
- *Gamma glutamyl transferase is found in many different tissues including: Kidney, Pancreas, Spleen and heart.*

GGT Levels are increased in patients with liver diseases	Extrahepatic causes for GGT level elevations
1. Cirrhosis	Pancreatitis
2. Liver metastasis and carcinoma	Carcinoma of prostate
3. Cholestasis	Carcinoma of breast and lung
4. Chronic Hepatitis	Systemic lupus erythematous
5. Alcoholic liver disease	Alcoholism
6. Primary biliary cirrhosis	Congestive heart failure
7. Primary Sclerosing cholangitis	Chronic coronary artery disease

98. Ans. (b) Cirrhosis

(Ref: Harrison 20th edition, p 2406; Harrison 19th p 2058)

- The synthesis of vitamin K–dependent clotting factors is diminished because of a decrease in hepatic mass, and, under these circumstances, administration of parenteral vitamin K does not improve the clotting factors or the prothrombin time.

99. Ans. (a) Increased ALP

(Ref: Harrison 20th edition, p 2340; Harrison 19th p 283)

- Alkaline phosphatase is a marker of cholestasis, ie, elevation of alkaline phosphatase occurs in more than 90% of patients with cholestasis and suggests a reduction in bile flow.
- Because isozymes are found in the liver, bone, placenta, leukocytes, and small intestine, an elevated alkaline phosphatase is not specific for the biliary tract.
- Alkaline phocphatase levles of greater than four times normal are taken significant.

100. Ans. (a) Biliary atresia

(Ref: Lelson 20th edition, p 1933)

Incidence of biliary atresia is 1 in 10,000-15,000 live births.

- Biliary atresia is characterized by obliteration or discontinuity of the extrahepatic biliary system. *The disorder represents the most common surgically treatable cause of cholestasis seen during the newborn period*
- Progressive familial intrahepatic cholestasis type 1 (PFIC 1) (formerly known as Byler disease) is a severe form of intrahepatic cholestasis. Affected patients present with steatorrhea, pruritus, vitamin D–deficient rickets and gradually developing cirrhosis. The absence of bile duct paucity and extrahepatic features differentiate this disorder from Alagille syndrome
- Alagille syndrome (arteriohepatic dysplasia) is the most common syndrome with intrahepatic bile duct paucity. Bile duct "paucity" an absence or marked reduction in the number of interlobular bile ducts in the portal triads, with normal-sized branches of portal vein and hepatic arteriole.

101. Ans. (c) Transport of conjugated bilirubin to bile canaliculi

(Ref: Harrison 20th edition, p 2338)

102. Ans. (b) Obstructive jaundice

(Ref: Harrison 20th edition, p 2339)

Marker	Normal value	Interpretation
Alkaline phosphatase	20-140 IU/L	ELEVATED
SGOT	5-40 units per liter	Mild elevation
Total serum bilirubin	0.3-1mg/dl	Elevated
Conjugated serum bilirubin	0.1-0.4mg/dl	Elevated

1. If only serum bilirubin is elevated and conjugated serum bilirubin is > 15% of total bilirubin then suspect dubin johson and rotor syndrome
2. If ALP is elevated with serum bilirubin proceed to USG to evaluate for cause of obstructive jaundice.

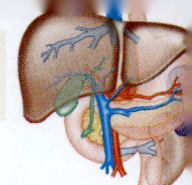

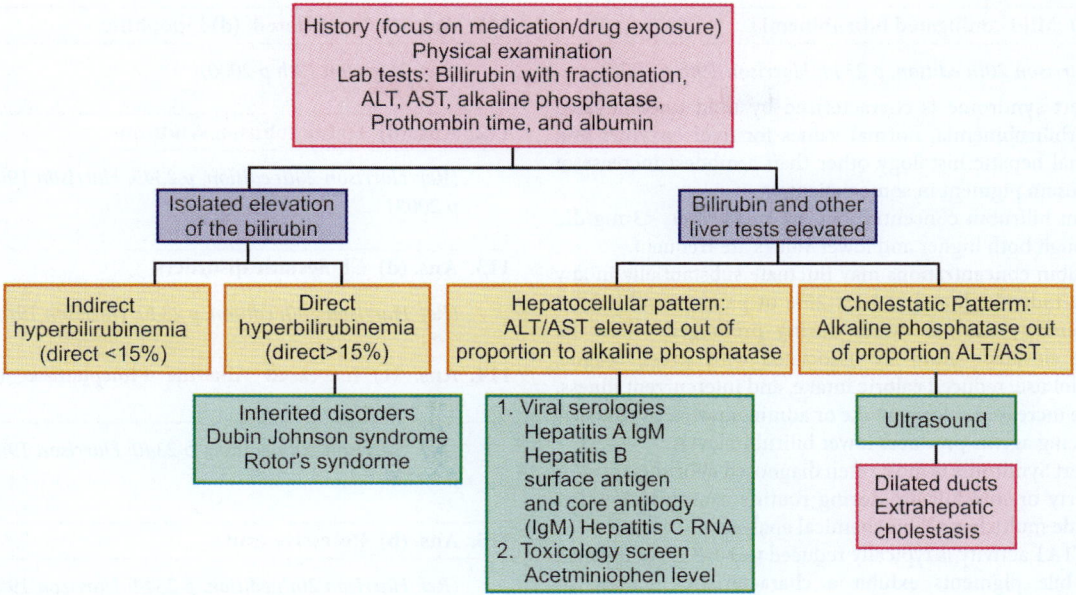

103. Ans. (b) Hepatocyte damage

(Ref: Comprehensive clinical hepatology, volume 1, p 202.)

- Increased insulin resistance is frequently associated with chronic liver disease and is a pathophysiological feature of **hepatogenous diabetes.** Distinctive factors including hepatic parenchymal cell damage, portal-systemic shunting and hepatitis C virus are responsible for the development of hepatogenous insulin resistance/diabetes
- Since blood glucose is delivered to the liver through the portal vein, hyperinsulinemia in patients with liver cirrhosis may be secondary to either hepatic parenchymal cell damage or to portal-systemic shunting. The rate at which insulin is degraded in the liver is reduced in patients with liver cirrhosis.

Finally liver transplantation rapidly normalises glucose tolerance and insulin sensitivity. Insulin secretagogues are not useful for medical treatment.

104. Ans. (d) SGOT/SGPT >2

(Ref: Harrison 20th edition, p 2341)

An SGOT: SGPT ratio>2:1 is suggestive while a ratio >3:1 is highly suggestive of alcoholic liver disease. The AST in alcoholic liver disease is rarely >300 U/L and the SGPT is often normal. A low level of SGPT in the serum is due to an alcohol-induced deficiency of pyridoxal phosphate.

105. Ans. (c) Infective hepatitis

(Ref: Harrison 20th edition, p 2341)

- Alkaline phosphatase (ALP): in females 42-98 U / L and males 53-120 U/L
- Since alkaline phosphatase is normal, obstructive jaundice is ruled out.
- A membrane-bound enzyme localized to the bile canalicular pole of hepatocytes, ALP is markedly elevated in persons with biliary obstruction.

- Elevated direct reacting bilirubin as well as elevated unconjugated bilirubin indicates hepato cellular jaundice. In hemolytic jaundice > 85% is due to indirect factions.

106. Ans. (d) Hepatic failure

(Ref: CMDT 2014, ch. 16, p 686)

A symmetrical and slightly warm area of erythema on the thenar and hypothenar eminences of the palm in chronic liver disease patients is referred to as palmar erythema.
1. May have a mottled appearance or blanch when pressed.
2. Not associated with pain, itch or scaling.
3. May involve the palmar aspect of the fingers and proximal nail folds

Causes of palmar erythema
Primary causes (where disease of pathological processes cannot be found)
- Hereditary – rare
- Pregnancy – common
- Senile

Secondary causes
- Chronic liver disease
- Autoimmune (e.g. Rheumatoid arthritis)
- Endocrinological – hyperthyroid
- Neoplastic

107. Ans. (a) Gilbert's syndrome

(Ref: Harrison 20th edition, p 2344; Harrison 19th p 2002)

Gilberts syndrome is characterized by mild unconjugated hyperbilirubinemia, normal values for standard hepatic bio-chemical tests, and normal hepatic histology other than a modest increase of lipofuscin pigment in some patients.
- Serum bilirubin concentrations are most often < 3 mg/dL.
- The clinical spectrum of hyperbilirubinemia fades into that of CN-II at serum bilirubin concentrations of 86 to 136 mmol/L /(5 to 8 g/dL).

108. Ans. (a) Mild conjugated bilirubinemia

(Ref: Harrison 20th edition, p 2344; Harrison 19th p 2002)

- Gilbert syndrome is characterized by mild unconjugated hyperbilirubinemia, normal values for liver enzymes and normal hepatic histology other than a modest increase of lipofuscin pigment in some patients.
- Serum bilirubin concentrations are most often <3 mg/dL, although both higher and lower values are frequent.
- Bilirubin concentrations may fluctuate substantially in any given individual, and at least 25% of patients will exhibit temporarily normal values during prolonged follow-up. More elevated values are associated with stress, fatigue, alcohol use, reduced caloric intake, and intercurrent illness, while increased caloric intake or administration of enzyme-inducing agents produces lower bilirubin levels.
- Gilbert Syndrome is most often diagnosed at or shortly after puberty or in adult life during routine examinations that include multichannel biochemical analyses.
- UGT1A1 activity is typically reduced to 10–35% of normal, and bile pigments exhibit a characteristic increase in bilirubin monoglucuronides. Defect in the hepatic uptake of other organic anions that at least partially share an uptake mechanism with bilirubin, such as sulfobromophthalein and indocyanine green, are observed in a minority of patients.

109. Ans. (c) Hemobilia

(Ref: Harrison 20th edition, p 273, 2431; Harrison 19th p 2089)

- Pain jaundice and fever are seen with CBD stone as well as hepatitis but melena is not seen and hence are ruled out.
- Carcinoma pancreas presents with painless obstructive jaundice. Patients with pancreatic cancer may present with the following signs and symptoms:
  1. Significant weight loss
  2. Midepigastric pain: Common symptom of pancreatic cancer, sometimes with radiation of the pain to the midback or lower-back region
  3. Often, unrelenting pain: Night time pain often a predominant complaint
  4. Painless obstructive jaundice: Most characteristic sign of cancer of head of the pancreas
  5. Pruritus: Often the patient's most distressing symptom
  6. Migratory thrombophlebitis (i.e, Trousseau sign) and venous thrombosis: May be the first presentation
  7. Palpable gallbladder (ie, Courvoisier sign)
- *Triad of abdominal pain jaundice and melena is suggestive of hemobilia.*

110. Ans. (b) Ultrasound

(Ref: Harrison 20th edition, p 2432)

Diagnostic Advantages of Hepatobiliary Ultrasound	Hepatobiliary Diagnostic Limitations of Ultrasound	Remarks
Rapid evaluation of liver and bile ducts Accurate identification of dilated bile ducts Not limited by pregnancy Guidance for fine-needle biopsy	Bowel gas Ascites Poor visualisation of distal C.B.D	Initial procedure of choice in biliary tract obstruction

111. Ans. (c) Not filtered; **(d)** Lipophilic

(Ref: Harrison 19th p 2000)

112. Ans. (d) Dubin Johnson syndrome

(Ref: Harrison 20th edition, p 2345; Harrison 19th edition p 2003)

113. Ans. (d) Cholestatic disorders

(Ref: Harrison 20th edition, p 2340; Harrison 19th edition p 284)

114. Ans. (c) Increased Alkaline Phosphatase; **(d)** Increased gamma GT

(Ref: Harrison 20th edition, p 2340; Harrison 19th edition p 1997)

115. Ans. (b) Recessive trait

(Ref: Harrison 20th edition, p 2344; Harrison 19th p 2001)

Reye Syndrome

116. Ans. (a) Due to defect in beta oxidation of fatty acids

(Ref: Nelson 20th edition, p 1960)

The most common secondary mitochondrial Hepatopathy is Reye syndrome
Recurrent Reye-like syndrome is encountered in children with genetic defects of fatty acid oxidation, such as
1. Deficiencies of the Plasmalemmal carnitine transporter
2. Carnitine palmitoyl transferase I and II
3. Carnitine acylcarnitine translocase
4. Medium- and long-chain acyl-CoA dehydrogenase multiple acyl-CoA dehydrogenase, and long-chain L-3 hydroxyacyl-CoA dehydrogenase or trifunctional protein.

117. Ans. (d) Deep jaundice is present

(Ref: Nelson 20th edition, p 1960)

The sign and symptoms of Reye syndrome include protracted vomiting, with or without clinically significant dehydration; hepatomegaly in 50%; *minimal or absent jaundice*; and lethargy progressing to encephalopathy, obtundation, coma, seizures, and paralysis. Notably, patients are afebrile.
The CDC developed the following diagnostic criteria for Reye syndrome:

- Acute noninflammatory encephalopathy with an altered level of consciousness
- Hepatic dysfunction with a liver biopsy showing fatty metamorphosis without inflammation or necrosis or a greater than 3-fold increase in alanine aminotransferase (ALT), aspartate aminotransferase (AST), or ammonia levels
- No other explanation for cerebral edema or hepatic abnormality
- Cerebrospinal fluid with a white blood cell count of 8 cells/μL.
- Brain biopsy with findings of cerebral edema without inflammation or necrosis

118. **Ans. (c)** *Methotrexate toxicity*

(Ref: CMDT 2019 p 699, 712)

> **Causes of Hepatic Steatosis**
> **Macrovesicular steatosis**
> - Excessive alcohol consumption
> - Hepatitis C (genotype 3)
> - Wilson's disease
> - Lipodystrophy
> - Starvation
> - Parenteral nutrition
> - Abetalipoproteinemia
> - Medications (e.g. tamoxifen, amiodarone, methotrexate, corticosteroids)
>
> **Microvesicular steatosis**
> - Reye's syndrome
> - Medications (valproate, anti-retroviral medicines)
> - Acute fatty liver of pregnancy
> - HELLP syndrome
> - Inborn errors of metabolism (e.g. LCAT deficiency, cholesterol ester storage disease, Wolman disease)

Budd-Chiari Syndrome

119. **Ans. (d)** *Venous collaterals*

(Ref: CMDT 2019 p 727)

Venous collaterals are formed in portal hypertension and require time to be formed and hence are unlikely to be seen in Budd Chiari syndrome

120. **Ans. (c)** *Larger hepatic veins*

(Ref: CMDT 2019 p 726; Harrison 19th p 673)
Budd-Chiari syndrome results from obstruction to the hepatic veins.

- Spontaneous thrombosis of the hepatic veins or neoplastic enlargements from other organs account for majority of cases.
- Syndrome is also associated with polycythemia, oral contraceptive usage.
- Few cases, presumably congenital are caused by obstruction of the suprahepatic portion of the inferior vena cava by a membranous web.
- Mild to moderate elevation in alkaline phosphatase level and prothrombin time prolongation are some times present.
- The AST level is typically mildly elevated but may be transiently very high following a period of marked systemic hypotension (shock liver), when the clinical picture can mimic acute viral or drug induced hepatitis.

121. **Ans. (a)** *Hepatic venous outflow obstruction*

(Ref: CMDT 2019 p 726, Harrison 19th p 673)

- Occlusion of a single hepatic vein is usually silent. Overt Budd-Chiari syndrome generally requires the occlusion of at least 2 hepatic veins. Venous congestion of the liver causes hepatomegaly, which can stretch the liver capsule and be very painful. Enlargement of the caudate lobe is common because blood is shunted through it directly into the inferior vena cava (IVC).
- Budd-Chiari syndrome is an uncommon condition induced by thrombotic or nonthrombotic obstruction of hepatic venous outflow and characterized by hepatomegaly, ascites, and abdominal pain

122. **Ans. (d)** *Polycythemia vera*

(Ref: CMDT 2019 p 727, Harrison 19th p 673)

The cause for the disease cannot be found in about half of the patients.

- Primary Budd-Chiari syndrome (75%): thrombosis of the hepatic vein
- Secondary Budd-Chiari syndrome (25%): compression of the hepatic vein by an outside structure (e.g. a tumor)
- Hepatic vein thrombosis is associated with the following in decreasing order of frequency:
  1. Polycythemia vera
  2. Pregnancy
  3. Post partum state
  4. Use of oral contraceptives
  5. Paroxysmal nocturnal hemoglobinuria
  6. Hepatocellular carcinoma
  7. Lupus anticoagulants

123. **Ans. (c)** *Hepatic vein*

(Ref: CMDT 2019 p 726)

Hepatic Encephalopathy

124. **Ans. (d)** *Hepatic encephalopathy*

(Ref: Harrison 20th edition p 2335; Sherlock diseases of liver and biliary tract, 12th edition, page 125, Harrison 19th p 441e-42f)

- Minimal hepatic encephalopathy describes a state of low-level cognitive dysfunction that is present in as many as 70% of patients with cirrhosis.
- It may be marked by decreased attention and executive function, as well as depressed psychomotor speed and visuomotor activity. Typically, the patient and those around the patient, including physicians, are not aware that the condition is present. Minimal hepatic encephalopathy is detected through psychometric testing

> - Number connection test
> - Digit symbol test
> - Block design test
> - Reaction times to light or sound, and the reaction time to interference in a task

125. **Ans. (a)** *Liver transplantation*

(Ref: Harrison 20th edition, p 584)

In transplantation medicine, the Milan criteria are applied as a basis *for selecting patients with cirrhosis and hepatocellular carcinoma for liver transplantation.*

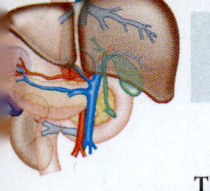

The Milan criteria state that a patient is selected for transplantation when he or she has:
- One lesion smaller than 5 cm.
- Up to 3 lesions smaller than 3 cm.
- No extrahepatic manifestations
- No vascular invasion
- MELD score is used for liver Transplantation in cases of fulminant hepatic failure

126. Ans. (d) Serum albumin

(Ref: Harrison 20th edition, p 2337; Harrison 19th p 1995)

Model for end stage liver disease

MELD = 3.78 × log[serum bilirubin (mg/dL)] + 11.2×log [INR] + 9.57 × log [serum creatinine (mg/dL)] + 6.43 × aetiology (0: cholestatic or alcoholic, 1- otherwise)

In interpreting the MELD Score in hospitalized patients, the 3 month mortality is
- 40 or more — 71.3% mortality
- 30–39 — 52.6% mortality
- 20–29 — 19.6% mortality
- 10–19 — 6.0% mortality
- <9 — 1.9% mortality

MELD score greater than 14 is an indication for liver transplantation.

127. Ans. (b) Antibiotic treatment

(Ref: Harrison 20th edition, p 2413; Harrison 19th p 252)

128. Ans. (a) Hyperkalemia

(Ref: Harrison 19th p 441e-42f)

Hyperkalemia	Hypokalemia is seen with overzealous of diuretics and this will lead to dehydration and increased hepatic encephalopathy
Anemia	Associated with GI bleeding that worsens hepatic encephalopathy
Hypothyroidism	Constipation in hypothyroidism will worsen hepatic encephalopathy by increasing bacterial load.
Barbiturates	Drugs like barbiturates and antipsychotics worsen hepatic encephalopathy

Common precipitating factors are as follows:
- Renal failure: Renal failure leads to decreased clearance of urea, ammonia, and other nitrogenous compounds.
- Gastrointestinal bleeding: The presence of blood in the upper gastrointestinal tract results in increased ammonia and nitrogen absorption from the gut. Bleeding may predispose to kidney hypoperfusion and impaired renal function. Blood transfusions may result in mild hemolysis, with resulting elevated blood ammonia levels.
- Infection: Infection may predispose to impaired renal function and to increased tissue catabolism, both of which increase blood ammonia levels.
- Constipation: Constipation increases intestinal production and absorption of ammonia.
- Medications: Drugs that act upon the central nervous system, such as opiates, benzo-diazepines, antidepressants, and antipsychotic agents, may worsen hepatic encephalopathy.
- Diuretic therapy: Decreased serum potassium levels and alkalosis may facilitate the conversion of NH4+ to NH3.

129. Ans. (d) Psychiatric abnormalities

(Ref: Harrison 20th edition, p 2413; Harrison 19th p 441e-42f)

Grading of the symptoms of hepatic encephalopathy is performed according to the so-called *West Haven classification system*

Grade 0: Minimal hepatic encephalopathy (also known as covert hepatic encephalopathy) lack of detectable changes in personality or behavior; minimal changes in memory, concentration, intellectual function, and coordination; asterixis is absent.
Grade 1: Trivial lack of awareness; shortened attention span; impaired addition or subtraction; hypersomnia, insomnia, or inversion of sleep pattern; euphoria, depression, or irritability; mild confusion; slowing of ability to perform mental tasks
Grade 2: Lethargy or apathy; disorientation; inappropriate behavior; slurred speech; obvious asterixis; drowsiness, lethargy, gross deficits in ability to perform mental tasks,.
Grade 3: Somnolent but can be aroused; unable to perform mental tasks; disorientation about time and place; marked confusion; amnesia; occasional fits of rage; present but incomprehensible speech
Grade 4: Coma with or without response to painful stimuli

130. Ans. (d) Upper GI bleeding

(Ref: Harrison 20th edition, p 2413; Harrison 19th p 739)

Upper GI bleeding will provide the bacteria in the gut with lots of nutrition to multiply and this will lead to increase in production of ammonia.

131. Ans. (a) Hepatic encephalopathy

(Ref: Harrison 20th edition, p 2413; Harrison 19th p 441e-42f)

- Hepatic failure and other situations associated with high blood ammonia such as porto-systemic shunts precipitate the syndrome of hepatic encephalopathy, characterized by confusion, drowsiness, stupor or coma.
- Ammonia taken up by astrocytes is converted to osmotically active glutamine, which causes cytotoxic astrocytic swelling. In addition to the rise in intracranial pressure, this process compromises astrocytic function.
- *Swollen astrocytes in hepatic encephalopathy are called Alzheimer type II astrocytes. Their nuclei are large and appear clear in H&E stains. They are also seen in Wilson disease.*

132. Ans. (c) Excessive use of diuretics

(Ref: Harrison 20th edition, p 2413; p 690, Harrison 19th p 441e-42f)

Common Precipitants of Hepatic Encephalopathy

Increased Nitrogen load	Drugs
Gastrointestinal bleeding	Narcotics, tranquilizers,
Excess dietary protein	Sedatives

Increased Nitrogen load	Drugs
Azotemia	Diuretics (excessive usage)
Constipation	
Electrolyte & metabolic imbalance	**Miscellaneous**
Hypokalemia	Infection, Surgery,
Alkalosis	Superimposed acute liver disease
Hypoxia	Progressive liver disease
Hyponatremia	Portal systemic disease
Hypovolemia	Shunts

133. Ans. (c) High protein diet more than 60 grams/day

(Ref: Harrison 20th edition, p 2413; Harrison 19th p 441e-42f)

Specific treatment of hepatic encephalopathy is aimed at
1. Elimination or treatment of precipitating factors and
2. Lowering of blood ammonia (and other toxin) levels by decreasing the absorption of protein and nitrogenous products from the intestine.
- In the setting of acute gastrointestinal bleeding, blood in the bowel should be promptly evacuated with laxatives (and enemas if necessary) in order to reduce the nitrogen load.
- *Protein should be excluded from the diet, and constipation should be avoided.*
- Ammonia absorption can be decreased by the administration of lactulose, a non-absorbable disaccharide that acts as an osmotic laxative.
- Metabolism of lactulose by colonic bacteria may also result in an acid pH that favors conversion of ammonia to the poorly absorbed ammonium ion.

134. Ans. (a) Lactulose

(Ref: Harrison 20th edition, p 2413)

135. Ans. (d) Phenobarbitone

(Ref: Harrison 19th p 441e-42f)

- LOLA is a stable salt of the 2 constituent amino acids. L-ornithine stimulates the urea cycle, with resulting loss of ammonia. Both L-ornithine and L-aspartate are substrates for glutamate transaminase. Their administration results increased glutamate levels. *Ammonia is subsequently used in the conversion of glutamate to glutamine by glutamine synthetase.*
- Rifaximin at a dose of 400 mg taken orally 3 times a day was as effective as lactulose or lactitol at improving hepatic encephalopathy symptoms. Similarly, rifaximin was as effective as neomycin and paromomycin.

136. Ans. (d) Rifaximin

(Ref: Harrison 20th edition, p 2414; Harrison 19th p 441e-42f)

Treatment of hepatic encephalopathy
1. The mainstay of treatment for encephalopathy, in addition to correcting precipitating factors, is to use lactulose, a nonabsorbable disaccharide, which results in colonic acidification.
2. Catharsis ensues, contributing to the elimination of nitrogenous products in the gut that are responsible for the development of encephalopathy. The goal of lactulose therapy is to promote 2–3 soft stools per day.
3. Poorly absorbed antibiotics are often used as adjunctive therapies for patients with alternating administration of neomycin and metronidazole. *More recently, rifaximin at 550 mg twice daily has been very effective in treating encephalopathy without the known side effects of neomycin or metronidazole.*
4. Zinc supplementation is sometimes helpful in patients with encephalopathy and is relatively harmless.

137. Ans. (b) Pregnant female

(Ref: Harrison 19th p 2018)

- Fulminant hepatitis is hardly ever seen in hepatitis C, but hepatitis E, as noted above, can be complicated by fatal fulminant hepatitis in 1–2% of all cases and in up to 20% of cases in pregnant women.
- The most feared complication of viral hepatitis is fulminant hepatitis (massive hepatic necrosis); fortunately, this is a rare event.
- Fulminant hepatitis is primarily seen in hepatitis B and D, as well as hepatitis E, but rare fulminant cases of hepatitis A occur primarily in older adults and in persons with underlying chronic liver disease, including, according to some reports, chronic hepatitis B and C.

138. Ans. (d) Metabolic acidosis

(Ref: Harrison 20th edition, p 2413)

The triggers for hepatic encephalopathy are hypokalemia, hypovelemia and *alkalosis*

Portal HTN

139. Ans. (d) Inflammatory hepatosplenic schistosomiasis

(Ref: Harrison 20th edition, p 2410; Harrison 19th p 2063)

- Wilson's disease is an inherited disorder of copper homeostasis with failure to excrete excess amounts of copper, leading to an accumulation in the liver and resultant cirrhosis.
- Alpha anti-trypsin deficiency results from an inherited disorder that causes abnormal folding of the alpha1AT protein, resulting in failure of secretion of that protein from the liver. It is unknown how the retained protein leads to liver disease. Patients with Alpha anti-trypsin AT deficiency at greatest risk for developing chronic liver disease have the ZZ phenotype.
- Cystic fibrosis leads to secondary biliary cirrhosis occurs.
- *Early inflammatory hepatosplenic schistosomiasis is caused by schistosoma eggs trapped in liver tissue.*

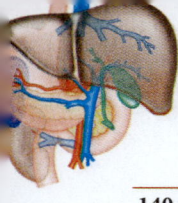

140. Ans. (d) Gynaecomastia

(Ref: Harrison 20th edition, p 2410; Harrison 19th p 2063)

Clinical features of portal hypertension: include hemorrhage from gastroesophageal varices, splenomegaly with hypersplenism, ascites & acute and chronic hepatic encephalopathy

141. Ans. (d) Intravenous somatostatin

(Ref: Harrison 20th edition, p 2411)

- This appears to be a case of variceal bleeding. About half of all episodes of variceal hemorrhage cease without intervention, although the, risk of rebleeding is very high.
- The medical management of acute variceal hemorrhage includes the use of vasoconstricting agents, usually somatostatin or Octreotide. Octreotide, a direct splanchnic vasoconstrictor, is given at dosages of 50–100 μg/h by continuous infusion.
- Vasopressin was used in the past but is no longer commonly used.
- Balloon tamponade (Sengstaken-Blakemore tube or Minnesota tube) can be used in patients who cannot get endoscopic therapy immediately or who need stabilization prior to endoscopic therapy.

142. Ans. (b) Cirrhosis

(Ref: Harrison 20th edition, p 2411)

- Congestive splenomegaly is common in patients with severe portal hypertension.
- Portal hypertension is the major complication of cirrhosis.

143. Ans. (a) Whole blood transfusion

(Ref: Harrison 20th edition, p 2043)

- Initial resuscitation requires rapid re-expansion of the circulating intravascular blood volume along with interventions to control ongoing losses.

- Continuing acute blood loss, with hemoglobin concentrations declining to <100 g/L (10 g/dL), should initiate blood transfusion, preferably as fully cross-matched recently banked (<14 days old) blood.
- Resuscitated patients are often coagulopathic due to deficient clotting factors in crystalloids and banked packed red blood cells (PRBCs). Early administration of component therapy during massive transfusion [fresh-frozen plasma (FFP) and platelets] approaching a 1:1 ratio of PRBC/FFP appears to improve survival. In extreme emergencies, type-specific or O-negative packed red cells may be transfused. Following severe and/or prolonged hypovolemia, inotropic support with norepinephrine, vasopressin, or dopamine may be required to maintain adequate ventricular performance.
- Once hemorrhage is controlled and the patient has stabilized, blood transfusions should not be continued unless the hemoglobin is <~7g/dL.

144. Ans. (c) Upper gastrointestinal bleeding

(Ref: Schwartz 7th/1420, 1421)

145. Ans. (a) Portal hypertension

(Ref: Harrison 20th edition, p 2410)

146. Ans. (b) Urgent endoscopy

(Ref: Harrison 20th edition, p 2411)

147. Ans. (a) Whole blood transfusion is the best

(Ref: Harrison 20th edition, p 2043)

148. Ans. (b) TIPS

(Ref: Harrison 20th edition, p 2412)

Ascites

149. Ans. (b) Peritoneal tuberculosis

(Ref: Harrison 20th edition, p 2412, 284; Harrison 19th edition p 287)

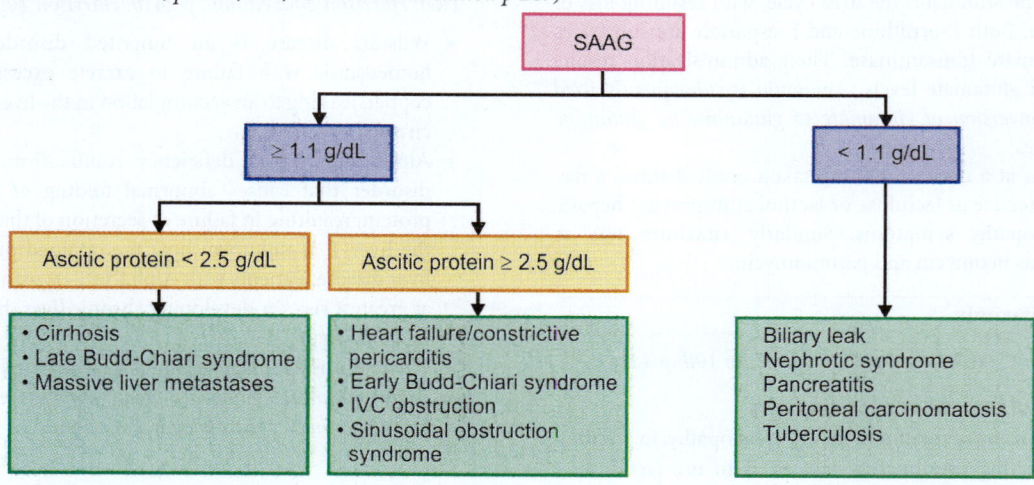

150. Ans. (a) This test helps to detect ascites

(Ref: Chamberlain clinical medicine, 13th edition p 124)

The test being done is fluid thrill for detection of ascites. The hand of second doctor in picture is to prevent transmission of vibrations by abdominal fat.

151. Ans. (a) 400 mg/day

(Ref: Harrison 20th edition, p 2412; Harrison 19th edition p 332e-9)

For management of Ascites, traditionally spironolactone is given at 100–200 mg/day single dose and furosemide is added at 40-80 mg/day. If ascitic fluid is not mobilized spironolactone can be increased to 400-600 mg/day.

152. Ans. (c) FFP transfusion

(Ref: Harrison 19th edition p 739)

In patient of chronic liver disease, the *total hepatocyte mass is lesser and thereby in these patients synthesis of clotting factors is reduced*. Since this patient does not have varices the cause of hematemesis in this patient is bleeding diathesis due to liver disease. Bleeding in such patients is treated with FFP in acute situations.

Abnormalities in coagulation in chronic liver diseases
1. Decreased synthesis of clotting factors and impaired clearance of anticoagulants
2. Thrombocytopenia from hypersplenism due to portal hypertension
3. Vitamin K requires biliary excretion for its subsequent absorption thus in patients with chronic cholestatic syndrome vitamin K absorption is frequently diminished

153. Ans. (b) CHF

(Ref: Harrison 20th edition, p 284)

Serum Albumin Ascites Gradient

>– 1.1 g/dL	< 1.1 g/dL
Cirrhosis	Peritoneal carcinomatosis
Alcoholic hepatitis	Peritoneal TB
CHF	Pancreatitis
Massive hepatic metastases	Serositis
Vascular occlusion	Nephrotic syndrome
Fatty liver disease of pregnancy	Bowel obstruction/ infarction/perforation
Myxedema	

154. Ans. (b) TIPS

(Ref: Harrison 20th edition p 2412; Harrison 19th edition p 288/2065)

Refractory ascites can be managed by
- Transjugular intrahepatic peritoneal shunt (TIPS), a radiologically placed portosystemic shunt to decompress the hepatic sinusoids.
- Serial large volume paracentesis (LVP) with albumin
- TIPS is superior to LVP in reducing the reaccumulation of ascites but is associated with an increased frequency of hepatic encephalo-pathy with no difference in mortality rates.

Diagnostic criteria for refractory ascites
1. Lack of response to maximal doses of diuretic for at least 1 week
2. Diuretic-induced complications in the absence of other precipitating factors
3. Early recurrence of ascites within 4 weeks of fluid mobilization
4. Persistent ascites despite sodium restriction
5. Mean weight loss <0.8 kg over 4 days
6. Urinary sodium excretion less than sodium intake

155. Ans. (d) Nephrotic syndrome

(Ref: Harrison 20th edition, p 284)

156. Ans. (b) 1, 2 and 4 are correct

(Ref: Harrison 20th edition, p 2412)

Ascites in cirrhosis is due to increased transudation from portal vein. The concomitant hypoalbuminemia decreases the oncotic pressure and worsens the ascites. Hyperaldosteronism contributes to resistance to loop diuretics. Therefore, the use of high doses of aldosterone antagonist (spironolactone up to 400 mg/day) is the main therapy to produce a negative sodium balance in cirrhotic patients with ascites.

157. Ans. (b) Collateral flow towards umbilicus

(Ref: Harrison 20th edition, p 511)

- Flow from upper abdomen towards the umbilicus point to SVC obstruction
- Flow from lower abdomen towards the umbilicus point to IVC obstruction
- Flow of blood away from the umbilicus points to Portal Hypertension.
- Ascites will always cause a stretched skin with everted umbilicus and bulging flanks
- Pulsatile liver is seen with severe tricuspid regurgitation

158. Ans. (c) Pseudochylous ascites is seen with hypertriglyceridemia

(Ref: Harrison 20th edition, p 283; Harrison 19th p 288)

- SAAG is calculated by subtracting the ascitic fluid albumin from the serum albumin and does not change with diuresis.
- A SAAG >1.1 g/dL reflects the presence of portal hypertension and indicates that the ascites is from an increased pressure in the hepatic sinusoids. Possible causes include cirrhosis, cardiac ascites, sinusoidal obstruction syndrome (venoocclusive disease), massive liver metastasis, or hepatic vein thrombosis (Budd-Chiari syndrome).
- A SAAG <1.1 g/dL indicates that the ascites is not related to portal hypertension as in tuberculous peritonitis, nephrotic syndrome, peritoneal carcinomatosis, or pancreatic ascites.
- White, milky fluid indicates the presence of triglycerides in levels >200 mg/dL (and often >1000 mg/dL), which is the

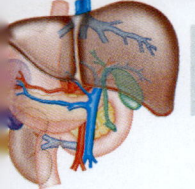

hallmark of chylous ascites. Chylous ascites results from lymphatic disruption that may occur with trauma, cirrhosis, tumor, tuberculosis, or certain congenital abnormalities.
- Dark brown fluid can reflect a high bilirubin concentration and indicates biliary tract perforation.
- Black fluid may indicate the presence of pancreatic necrosis or metastatic melanoma.

159. Ans. (a) Salt restriction

(Ref: Harrison 20th edition, p 2412)

Hepatorenal Syndrome

160. Ans. (a) Normal GFR

(Ref: Harrison 20th edition, p 2413; Harrison 19th edition p 1809)
- The hepatorenal syndrome is a form of functional renal failure without renal pathology that occurs in about 10% of patients with advanced cirrhosis or acute liver failure.
- There are disturbances in the arterial renal circulation in patients with HRS; these include an increase in vascular resistance accompanied by a reduction in systemic vascular resistance.
- The reason for renal vasoconstriction is most likely multifactorial. The diagnosis is made usually in the presence of a large amount of ascites in patients who have a stepwise progressive increase in creatinine.
- Type 1 HRS is characterized by a progressive impairment in renal function and a significant reduction in creatinine clearance within 1–2 weeks of presentation. Type 2 HRS is characterized by a reduction in glomerular filtration rate with an elevation of serum creatinine level, but it is fairly stable and is associated with a better outcome than that of Type 1 HRS.
- Patients are managed with midodrine, an alpha-agonist, along with octreotide and intravenous albumin. The best therapy for HRS is liver transplantation.
- In patients with either type 1 or type 2 HRS, the prognosis is poor unless transplant can be achieved.

161. Ans. (c) Urine osmolality is lower than plasma osmolality

(Ref: Harrison 20th edition, p 2413; Harrison 19h/2530- 2531)

Liver Cancer

162. Ans. (a) Hepatocellular carcinoma

(Ref: Harrison 20th edition, p 578-79; Harrison 19th edition p 544, 545)

HCC in the western world is mainly seen with hepatitis C but in developing world is related to chronic liver disease due to various conditions like alcoholic cirrhosis.

In clinical setting of
1. South Asian ethnicity
2. Presence of risk factor alcoholic cirrhosis
3. Presence of portal vein thrombosis malignant infiltration of portal vein radicles is considered. The presence of characteristic CT Scan finding confirms the diagnosis as hepatocellular carcinoma.

Triple-phase CT (including an arterial phase, a portal venous phase, and a late washout phase) has been found to be highly accurate in the diagnosis and characterization of HCC. CT findings are:
1. Hypervascular pattern with arterial enhancement and rapid washout during the portal venous phase. In contrast, regenerative nodules generally appear iso-attenuating or hypo-attenuating when compared to the remaining parenchyma.
2. Visualization of a tumor capsule
3. Demonstration of an internal mosaic resulting from variable attenuation within the tumor, and portal vein branch invasion.

> Choice B of metastasis is less likely as it has multiple lesions and large metastasis can outgrow their blood supply leading to central necrosis
>
> Choice C of cholangiocarcinoma will show no changes in liver parenchyma but involvement of biliary tree.
>
> Choice D is ruled out as more common NET arise in duodenum or pancreas.

163. Ans. (a) Hepatocellular carcinoma

(Ref: Harrison 20th edition, p 578; Harrison 19th edition p 544)
- Hepatitis B vaccinations can decreases the incidence of hepatitis B and thus hepatocellular carcinoma
- Another vaccine preventable cancer is human papilloma vaccine preventing cervical cancer.

164. Ans. (d) Orthoptic liver transplantation (OLT)

(Ref: Harrison 20th edition, p 584; ch. 39, p 1603, Harrison 19th p 545)
- Liver transplantation is first choice for cirrhotic patient with single tumors <5cm and portal hypertension chemoembolization/TACE is used for unresectable HCC.

165. Ans. (d) Hepatocellular adenoma

(Ref: Harrison 20th edition, p 590; Harrison 19th p 365)
- Hepatocellular adenoma (HCA) is rare, benign hepatic neoplasia that is usually identified as a well-defined, solitary lesion. Hepatocellular adenoma occurs predominantly in childbearing women and is related to endogenous or exogenous estrogen levels. High doses and long duration of OC, as well as pregnancy, are associated with a higher incidence of HCA, whereas discontinuation of OC is associated with regression of HCA
- An angiomyolipoma is a very rare hepatic tumor consisting of fat, epithelioid, and smooth muscle cells with thick-walled blood vessels.

166. Ans. (c) MRI

(Ref: Harrison 20th edition, p 582; Harrison 19th p 534)
- Ultrasound is usually the first investigation that detects the focal mass. It is a simple and noninvasive technique to differentiate solid from cystic lesions and may be sufficient to establish the diagnosis of small hemangiomas or hepatic

cysts. However, the diagnostic specificity for solid lesions is low even when improved by the use of color-flow Doppler or contrast US, which may add dynamic information regarding the lesions.
- Triple-phase CT is an excellent modality for characterizing lesions, yielding specific signs in cases of large hemangiomas or FNH, but in many cases, this single modality is not sufficient for establishing the correct diagnosis.
- Magnetic resonance imaging is the best imaging modality in terms of specificity for diagnosing hepatic lesions, particularly when liver-specific contrast agents are utilized

167. Ans. (b) Hemangioma

(Ref: Harrison 20th edition, p 590; Harrison 19th p 5)

- Cavernous hemangiomas are the most common Beningn Liver Tumour, with an incidence of up to 20% in the general population, depending on the ultrasound studies or autopsy series. This usually small lesion is a congenital hamartomatous proliferation of vascular endothelial cells and may be multiple in 10% of cases.
- Focal nodular hyperplasia (FNH) is the second most common solid BLT, occurring in up to 3% of the population. FNH is considered to be a nonneoplastic lesion that is caused by a hyperplastic response to a congenital vascular malformation or a disruption in blood supply.

168. Ans. (d) Animal fat in diet

(Ref: Harrison 20th edition, p 578)

169. Ans. (a) Jaundice

(Ref: Harrison 20th edition, p 581)

170. Ans. (a) Hepatoblastoma

(Ref: Harrison 20th edition, p 590)

171. Ans. (d) Has better prognosis

(Ref: Harrison 18th/p 590)

Wilson Disease

172. Ans. (b) Slit lamp examination

(Ref: Harrison 20th edition p 2982; Fitzpatrick color atlas, 8th edition p 834)

The combination of neuropsychiatric presentation with liver involvement points to possible diagnosis of Wilson disease. The main clue is blue pigmentation over the lunula. For work up and identification of KF ring, slit lamp examination should be done.

173. Ans. (b) Serum ceruloplasmin

(Ref: Harrison 20th edition, p 2982; Harrison 19th edition p 2519)

- The image shows a pale brownish ring at the limbus of cornea which is called as KF ring. Along with history of liver disease, it points to clinical diagnosis of Wilson disease.

- Hence Serum Ceruloplasmin levels should be evaluated.
- Ideally one should go for 24 hour urinary copper levels which are more reliable, followed by liver biopsy to estimate the copper content.

Investigations in Wilson disease and relative usefulness

Test	Usefulness
Serum ceruloplasmin	+
Kayser-Fleischer rings	++
Urine copper (24-h)	+++
Liver copper	++++
Haplotype analysis	++++ (siblings only)

KF ring tends to *decrease* after 3-6 months of treatment and *may disappear* by 2 years.

174. Ans. (b) Rubeanic acid

(Ref: Atlas of Liver pathology by Wright: 2nd edition p 107: figure 15.9)

- The rubeanic acid and rhodanine stains are utilized to detect the cytoplasmic accumulation of copper in the liver.
- Schmorl's method is used for detecting melanin and uses the reducing properties of melanin to stain granules blue-green. It is also used to detect lipofuscin.

175. Ans. (d) Wilson disease

(Ref: Harrison 20th edition, p 2982; Harrison 19th edition p 2519)

Points in favour of diagnosis of Wilson disease

1. Low haematocrit of 26% and increased reticulocyte count: This is due to hemolysis of RBC due to excess intracellular copper. Normal reticulocyte percentage in adults is 0.5-1.5%
2. Unconjugated jaundice due to haemolysis and defective conjugation in liver due to hepatocyte damage.
3. Mild elevation of enzymes unlike acute viral hepatitis where gross elevations in enzyme values.
4. Nodular liver with splenomegaly indicating a chronic process. Portal hypertension has already developed in the patient.
5. Hepatitis B positivity in the question was given to confuse you, since it can be an incidental finding.

Points against the diagnosis of acute viral hepatitis

1. Jaundice with mild elevation of AST/ALT
2. Nodular enlarged liver
3. Enlarged spleen

176. Ans. (c) Hepatolenticular degeneration

(Ref: Harrison 20th edition, p 2982; Harrison 19th edition p 2519)

- The image shows presence of Kayser Fleischer ring which along with combination of wing beating tremor (Asterixis) and liver cell failure favors diagnosis as Wilson disease.

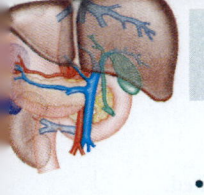

- They are seen in 99% of patients with neurological or psychiatric symptoms but only 30-50% patients with hepatic involvement.

Galactosemia	Inborn error of metabolism with Oil droplet cataracts and jaundice.
Paralysis agitans	It's another term for parkinsonism like features.
Primary biliary cirrhosis	Occurs due to Anti-Mitochondrial Antibodies and presents as cirrhosis of liver.

177. Ans. (a) Decrease in urinary copper

(Ref: Harrison 20th edition, p 2983; Harrison 19th p 2625)

- Wilson disease is characterized by paradoxically low serum copper due to deposition in tissues. However as levels of copper in RBC increases, hemolytic episodes explain the rise of serum copper during hemolytic episodes.
- The copper is excreted in urine leading to increased urinary copper and this is also the screening test for Wilson disease.
- Ceruloplasmin values are normal in Wilson initially but with cirrhosis, the values begin to fall. Since ceruloplasmin can also be low in PEM, cirrhosis, nephrotic syndrome it is not a screening test for Wilson

178. Ans. (d) Hepatitis E

(Ref: GI/Liver 4th edition, p 240)

Causes of Mallory hyaline bodies

- Intestinal bypass
- Wilson
- Biliary cirrhosis
- Indian childhood cirrhosis
- Cholestatic jaundice
- Focal nodular hyperplasia
- Hepatocellular carcinoma
- NASH

179. Ans. (b) Testicular atrophy

(Ref: Harrison 20th edition, p 2980)

180. Ans. (c) Urinary copper excretion is <100 µg/day

(Ref: Harrison 20th edition, p 2983)

Hemochromatosis

181. Ans. (a) Hemochromatosis

(Ref: Harrison 20th edition, p 2980)

182. Ans. (b) Iron deposition in pituitary

(Ref: Harrison 20th p 2980; Harrison 19th p 2514)

- Amenorrhea, loss of libido, impotence, and symptoms of hypothyroidism can be seen in patients with hereditary hemochromatosis. Although amenorrhea can occur in women, it is less frequent than hypogonadism in men.
- Hypogonadism is the most common endocrine abnormality causing decreased libido and impotence in men. It is usually due to pituitary iron deposition. Primary hypogonadism, presumably due to testicular iron deposition, can also occur but is much less common.
- The classic triad of cirrhosis, diabetes mellitus, and skin pigmentation occurs late in the disease, when total iron body content is 20g (i.e., > 5-times normal).

EXTRA MILE

- Symptoms from hemochromatosis usually begin between age 30 years and age 50 years, but they may occur much earlier in life.
- Most patients are asymptomatic (75%) and are diagnosed when elevated serum iron levels are noted on a routine chemistry screening panel or when screening is performed because a relative is diagnosed with hemochromatosis.
- Early symptoms include severe fatigue (74%), impotence (45%), and arthralgia (44%); fatigue and arthralgia are the most common symptoms prompting a visit to a physician. The most common signs at the time of presentation are hepatomegaly (13%), skin pigmentation, and arthritis.

Clinical manifestations include the following:
- Skin bronzing or hyperpigmentation (70%)
- Diabetes mellitus (48%)
- Liver disease (hepatomegaly, and later cirrhosis)
- Arthropathy
- Amenorrhea, impotence, hypogonadism
- Cardiomyopathy

183. Ans. (d) Increased transferrin saturation

(Ref: Harrison 20th edition, p 2981)

184. Ans. (a) Percent transferrin saturation

(Ref: Harrison 20th edition, p 2981)

Miscellaneous

185. Ans. (d) Testis

(Ref: Harrison 20th edition, p 2980; Harrison: 19th edition p 2517)

The clinical features of hemochromatosis are-
1. Hepatomegaly
2. Skin pigmentation
3. Diabetes mellitus
4. Restrictive cardiomyopathy
5. Arthritis
6. *Hypogonadism due to decreased production of gonadotropins due to impairment of hypothalamic pituitary function by iron deposition.*
7. Addison disease, hypothyroidism and hypoparathyroidism are rare manifestation of the disease.

186. Ans. (a) Discriminant function

(Ref: Harrison 20th edition, p 2406; Harrison: 19th edition p 2053)

- A discriminant score of >32 or MELD Score of >21(with absence of co-morbidity) is used to treat patients with alcoholic hepatitis.
- The drug used is prednisolone 32p.o daily for 4 weeks followed by tapering. An alternative is pentoxifylline.
- Discriminant function = 4.6 X (prolongation of PT above control in seconds) + Serum Bilirubin and can identify patients with poor prognosis in alcoholic liver disease.

187. Ans. (d) AIDS

(Ref: Harrison 20th edition, p 2416; Harrison 19th edition, Table 368-2: p 2069)

Absolute contraindications to liver transplantation
1. Uncontrolled hepatobiliary infections
2. Sepsis
3. Congenital anomaly (Un-correctable)
4. Active substance/ alcohol abuse
5. Advanced cardiopulmonary disease
6. Metastasis to liver
7. Cholangiocarcinoma
8. AIDS

Relative contraindications to liver transplantation
1. Age >70
2. Portal vein thrombosis
3. Severe obesity
4. HIV seropositivity with low CD4 counts
5. PAH
6. Psychiatric disorders

188. Ans. (d) 4g

(Ref: Harrison 20th edition, p 2423; Harrison 19th edition p 1934)

- Bile acids are not present in our diet but are synthesized in the liver by a series of enzymatic steps that represent catabolism of cholesterol. The rate limiting enzyme is 7 alpha hydroxylase.
- Bile acids are reabsorbed in the ileum, jejunum and colon. The total size of bile acid pool is 4g.
- In case of disease of the terminal ileum, the bile acids are not absorbed and lead to active chloride secretions in the colon. This leads to secretory bile acid diarrhoea.

189. Ans. (a) Acid sphingomyelinase

(Ref: Rudolph paediatrics 22nd edition p 637)

Acid Sphingomyelinase	Niemann pick disease
Hexosaminidase A	Taysachs disease
Ceramidase	Farber disease
Arylsulfatase B	Maroteaux-Lamy syndrome

190. Ans. (a) Glucocerebroside

(Ref: Robbin's Pathology 9th edition p 151-154)

- The key word in the question is crumpled tissue paper appearance of cytoplasm in bone marrow examination.
- In the setting of organomegaly and pancytopenia, the patient has a storage disorder.
- Lysosomal storage of glucocerebroside in cells of the monocyte-macrophage system leads to a characteristic cellular alteration of these cells.
- *Gaucher cells have a large cytoplasmic mass with a striated appearancethat has been likened to "wrinkled or crumpled tissue paper" or "crumpled silk".*
- GCs are present in the bone marrow, spleen, lymph nodes, hepatic sinusoids, and other organs and tissues in all forms of GD
- Gaucher's disease type 1 is a non-neuronopathic disease that can present in childhood to adulthood with slowly to rapidly progressive visceral disease. About 55–60% of such patients are diagnosed at <20 years. This pattern of presentation is distinctly bimodal, with peaks at <10 to 15 years and at >25 years.

191. Ans. (a) Chlamydial infection

(Ref: Harrison 20th edition, p 985, 1319; Harrison 19th edition p 877, 1169)

- The *Fitz-Hugh–Curtis syndrome is chlamydial infection leading to peri-hepatitis.*
- Peri-hepatitis should be suspected in young, sexually active women who develop right-upper-quadrant pain, fever, or nausea.
- Evidence of salpingitis may or may not be found on examination.
- Frequently, peri-hepatitis is strongly associated with extensive tubal scarring, adhesions, and inflammation observed at laparoscopy, and high titers of antibody to the 57-kDa chlamydial heat-shock protein have been documented.

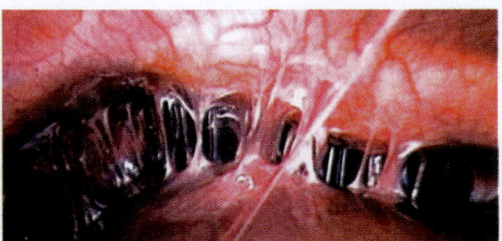

- Culture and/or serologic evidence of *C. trachomatis* is found in three-fourths of women with this syndrome.
- CDC recommends a broad spectrum treatment of this presentation though specific manangment is doxycycline.

CDC guidelines for management of OPD/IPD management of P.I.D
- Ceftriaxone/Cefoxitin intramuscularly (IM) once as a single dose **plus**
- Doxycycline 100 mg orally twice daily for 14 days
- Metronidazole 500 mg orally twice daily for 14 days can be added.

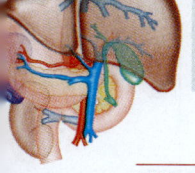

192. Ans. (a) CNS

(Ref: Harrison 20th edition, p 2980)

Organs Involved in Hemochromatosis are
- Liver (first organ to be affected) = 95%
- Excessive skin pigmentation
- Diabetes mellitus (bronze diabetes)
- Arthropathy
- Cardiac involvement (restrictive cardiomyopathy)
- Pituitary involvement (leading to hypopituitarism and hypogonadism) = mentioned in textbook as endocrine involvement.

193. Ans. (c) Gallstone should be radiopaque

(Ref: Harrison 20th edition, p 2427; Harrison 19th p 2076)

- For good results, medical therapy should be limited to radiolucent stones smaller than 10 mm in diameter. Stones larger than 15 mm in size rarely dissolve.
- The highest success rate (i.e., >70%) occurs in patients with small (<5 mm) floating radiolucent gallstones
- Pigment stones are not responsive to UDCA therapy to produce a lamellar liquid crystalline phase in bile that allows a dispersion of cholesterol from stones Ursodeoxycholic acid decreases cholesterol saturation of bile and also appears by physical-chemical means. UDCA may also retard cholesterol crystal nucleation.

194. Ans. (d) Niacin deficiency

(Ref: Harrison 20th edition, p 2446; Harrison 19th p 1699)

- Niacin is a water soluble vitamin and hence its absorption shall be unaffected.
- Incidence of pancreatic adenocarcinoma is 4% in patients with chronic pancreatitis
- B12 deficiency will occur as vitamin B12 will not be dissociated from cobalamin binding proteins due to pancreatic enzyme deficiency.
- Fat soluble vitamins absorption will be affected due to pancreatic lipase deficiency

195. Ans. (d) All of the above

(Ref: Harrison 20th edition, p 279; Harrison 19th p 2059)

- Spider angioma, is a common benign vascular lesion present in 10-15% of healthy adults and young children. They may appear as solitary or multiple lesions.
- It is characterized by a central red arteriole, or punctum, representing the body of the spider, surrounded by a radial pattern of thin-walled capillaries, resembling legs.
- While most lesions are unrelated to internal disease, spider angiomas have been associated with thyrotoxicosis, and frequently occur in the presence of estrogen-excess states, such as pregnancy or during the use of oral contraceptives.

196. Ans. (a) Infection is preceded by ascites

(Ref: Harrison 20th edition, p 953; Harrison 19th p 2065)

- SBP is a common and severe complication of ascites characterized by spontaneous infection of the ascitic fluid without an intraabdominal source.
- This implies pre-existing ascites is mandatory for SBP to develop with transmigration of bacteria into this transudative ascitic fluid
- Since the fluid is a transudate due to cirrhosis the protein is <2.5 g/dl
- Bacterial translocation is the presumed mechanism for development of SBP, with gut flora traversing the intestine into mesenteric lymph nodes, leading to bacteremia and seeding of the ascitic fluid.
- The most common organisms are Escherichia coli and other gut bacteria; however, gram-positive bacteria, including Streptococcus viridans, Staphylococcus aureus, and Enterococcus sp., can also be found. If more than two organisms are identified, secondary bacterial peritonitis due to a perforated viscus should be considered.
- The diagnosis of SBP is made when the fluid sample has an absolute neutrophil count >250/mL. Bedside cultures should be obtained when ascitic fluid is tapped.

197. Ans. (d) Base deficit > 2

(Ref: CMDT 2019 p 742)

198. Ans. (d) Hemobilia

(Ref: Harrison 20th edition, p 2427)

- Mirizzi's syndrome is a rare complication in which a gallstone becomes impacted in the cystic duct or neck of the gallbladder causing compression of the CBD, resulting in CBD obstruction and jaundice.
- Ultrasound shows gallstone lying outside the hepatic duct.
- Endoscopic retrograde cholangiopancreatography or magnetic resonance cholangiopancreatography (MRCP) will usually demonstrate the characteristic extrinsic compression of the CBD.

199. Ans. (a) Trauma

(Ref: Harrison 20th edition, p 2431; Harrison 19th p 2084)

Hemobilia present with abdominal pain, jaundice and melena.

Causes of hemobilia are:
1. Iatrogenic trauma- after cholecystectomy/ERCP/liver biopsy
2. Accidental trauma
3. Acalculous cholecystitis
4. Hepatocellular carcinoma>>Cholangio-carcinoma
5. Inflammatory conditions ranging from ascariasis to PAN
6. Vascular malformation
7. Coagulopathy

Most common site where bleed originates in Hemobilia: is liver> extra-hepatic biliary pathway> gallbladder>pancreas.

Investigations
- Once hemobilia is strongly suspected, the most useful study is angiography, which may reveal the precise source of bleed.
- It can also be combined with definitive therapy by radiological intervention.

Management: Angio-embolisation has now become the first line of treatment and involves selective occlusion with permanent embolic agents like microcoils and cyanoacrylate glue.

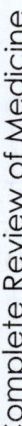

200. Ans. (a) Pruritus

(Ref: CMDT 2019 p 741; Harrison 19th p 366e-3f))

- Primary biliary cirrhosis is obstructive jaundice and is characterized by regurgitation of bile salts into circulation leading to pruritus as an initial manifestation.
- It is marked by the slow progressive destruction of the small bile ducts of the liver, with the intralobular ducts (Canals of Hering) affected early in the disease.
- Anti nuclear antibodies appear to be prognostic agents in PBC.

Signs & Symptoms of PBC include the following:
1. Fatigue (65% of patients)
2. Pruritus (55%)
3. Right upper quadrant discomfort (8-17%)
4. Physical examination findings depend on the stage of the disease. In the early stages, examination findings are normal. As the disease advances, the following signs may be noted:
   - Hepatomegaly (25%)
   - Hyperpigmentation (25%)
   - Splenomegaly (15%)
   - Jaundice (10%)
   - Xanthelasmata (10%):
   - Sicca syndrome (50-75%): Xerophthalmia xerostomia (i.e, dry mouth)

201. Ans. (a) Alcohol abuse

(Ref: Harrison 20th edition, p 2334; Harrison 19th p 1992)

CAGE scale: The CAGE scale is a 4-item questionnaire that assesses the presence of four indicators of problem drinking alcohol severity. An extensive body of research supports the reliability and validity of the CAGE scale.
> CAGE scores range from 0 to 4 depending on the number of problem drinking indicators endorsed, with higher scores reflecting more severe problem drinking patterns.

Acronym CAGE Questions:
- C - Have you ever felt you ought to Cut down on your drinking?
- A - Have people Annoyed you by criticizing your drinking?
- G - Have you ever felt Guilty or bad about your drinking?
- E - Have you ever had a drink first thing in the morning to steady your nerves or get rid of a hangover (Eye-opener)?
- One "yes" response should raise suspicion of an alcohol use problem, and more than one is a strong indication that abuse or dependence exists.

202. Ans. (c) Pancreatitis

(Ref: Bailey & Love 26th edition, p 945)

- *Grey Turner's sign is bruising developing in the flanks* due to retroperitoneal bleeding secondary to pancreatitis. It is produced by spread from the anterior pararenal space to between the two leaves of the posterior renal fascia and subsequently to the lateral edge of the quadratus lumborum muscle.
- *Cullen's sign is peri-umbilical bruising* that can be seen to be secondary to the tracking of liberated pancreatic enzymes to the anterior abdominal wall from the inflamed gastrohepatic ligament and across the falciform ligament.

203. Ans. (a) Alcoholic hepatitis

(Ref: Harrison 20th edition, p 2401)

The modified Maddrey's discriminant function is used to predict prognosis in alcoholic hepatitis. It is calculated by a simple formula

(4.6 x [PT test - control])+ S.Bilirubin in mg/dl

- Prospective studies have shown that, it is useful in predicting short term prognosis especially mortality within 30 days.
- A value more than 32 implies poor outcome with one month mortality ranging between 35% to 45%

204. Ans. (b) Autoimmune hepatitis

(Ref: Harrison 20th edition, p 2420; Harrison 19th p 207)

- Recurrence of Primary Disease occurs with autoimmune hepatitis, primary sclerosing cholangitis, and primary biliary cirrhosis overlap with those of rejection or post-transplantation bile-duct injury. Data support recurrent autoimmune hepatitis after liver transplantation.
- Hereditary disorders such as Wilson's disease and a 1-antitrypsin deficiency have not recurred after liver transplantation.
- Hepatic vein thrombosis (Budd-Chiari syndrome) may recur; this can be minimized by treating underlying lymphoproliferative disorders and by anticoagulation. Cholangiocarcinoma recurs almost invariably; therefore, few centers now offer transplantation to such patients. In patients with hepatocellular carcinoma, tumor recurrence in the liver is common after ~1 year, although better success has been reported

205. Ans. (a) Size of stone less than 10 mm

(Ref: Harrison 20th edition, p 2427)

In carefully selected patients with a functioning gallbladder and with radiolucent stones <10 mm in diameter, complete dissolution can be achieved in < 50% of patients within 6 months to 2 years.

206. Ans. (a) Hypocalcemia

(Ref: Harrison 20th edition, p 2438; Harrison 19th edition p 209)

Causes of Acute Pancreatitis	
Common Causes	**Uncommon Causes**
Gallstones (including microlithiasis)	Cystic fibrosis
Alcoholism Hypertriglyceridemia	Connective tissue disorders and thrombotic thrombocytopenic
Endoscopic retrograde cholangiopancreatography, especially after biliary manometry	T.T.P
Traum	Cancer of the pancreas
Postoperative	Hypercalcemia
Drugs (azathioprine, 6-mercaptopurine, sulfonamides, estrogens, tetracycline, valproic acid, anti-HIV medications)	Periampullary diverticulum
Sphincter of Oddi dysfunction	Pancreas divisum Hereditary pancreatitis Renal failure

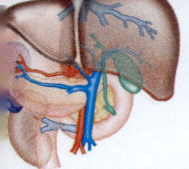

207. Ans. (a) Hepatolenticular disease

(Ref: Harrison 20th edition, p 2983)

208. Ans. (c) Second most common cause of cholangitis in children

(Ref: CMDT 2019, p 741)

- Primary biliary cirrhosis (PBC) is characterized by chronic inflammation and fibrous obliteration of intrahepatic bile ductules.
- PBC is frequently associated with a variety of disorders presumed to be autoimmune in nature, such as the syndrome of Calcinosis, Raynaud's phenomenon, Esophageal dysmotility, Sclerodactyly, Telangiectasia (CREST); the Sicca syndrome (dry eyes and dry mouth); Autoimmune thyroiditis; Type-1 Diabetes mellitus; and IgA deficiency
- Among asymptomatic patients 90% are women
- Age is 35-60 yrs
- Symptoms are: Pruritis, fatigue, jaundice, melanosis, steatorrhoea, xanthelasma, hepatomegaly, splenomegaly, clubbing, bony tenderness, ecchymosis, osteomalacia.
- Laboratory findings:
  1. Increased serum 5 nucleotidase activity
  2. Increased gamma-glutamyl transpeptidase activity
  3. Increased serum bilirubin levels
  4. Increased serum lipid levels
  5. Increased ALP
- Confirmation test is liver biopsy
- Best treatment of choice is liver transplantation.

209. Ans. (c) Gilbert's syndrome

(Ref: CMDT 2019, p 688; Harrison 19th edition p 2002)

210. Ans. (a) Upper GI bleeding

(Ref: Textbook of Clinical Gastroenterology and hepatology 2nd edition, p 1106)

Forrest classification is instrumental when stratifying patients with upper gastrointestinal hemorrhage into high and low risk categories for mortality. It is also a significant method of prediction of the risk of re-bleeding and very often is used for evaluation of the endoscopic intervention modalities

Acute hemorrhage
- Forrest I a (Spurting hemorrhage)
- Forrest I b (Oozing hemorrhage)

Signs of recent hemorrhage
- Forrest II a (Visible vessel)
- Forrest II b (Adherent clot)
- Forrest II c (Flat pigmented haematin on ulcer base)

Lesions without active bleeding
- Forrest III (Lesions without signs of recent hemorrhage or fibrin-covered clean ulcer base)

211. Ans. (a) Acute cholecystitis

(Ref: Harrison 20th edition, p 2425; Harrison 19th p 2080)

Acute Cholecystitis
- HIDA Scan: 99mTc hepatobiliary imaging (using iminodiacetic acid compounds), also known as the HIDA scan, is useful in demonstrating an obstructed cystic duct, which is the cause of acute cholecystitis in most patients.
- This test is reliable if the bilirubin in under 5 mg/dL and is contraindicated in pregnancy.

212. Ans. (c) Gilbert disease

(Ref: Harrison 20th edition, p 2416; Harrison 19th p 2072)

Indications for Liver Transplantation	
Childern	**Adults**
Biliary atresia	Primary biliary cirrhosis
Neonatal hepatitis	Secondary biliary cirrhosis
Congenital hepatic fibrosis	Primary sclerosing cholangitis
Alagille's syndrome	Autoimmune hepatitis
Byler's disease	Caroli's diseasec
a1-Antitrypsin deficiency	Cryptogenic cirrhosis
Inherited disorders of metabolism	Chronic hepatitis with cirrhosis
Wilson's disease	Hepatic vein thrombosis
	Fulminant hepatitis
	Alcoholic cirrhosis
	Chronic viral hepatitis
	Primary hepatocellular malignances
Crigler-Najjar disease type I	Hepatic adenomas
Familial hypercholesterolemia	Nonalcoholic steatohepatitis
	Familial amyloid polyneuropathy

213. Ans. (d) Fraction of corpophyrin I in urine is elevated usually more than 80% of the total in Rotor syndrome

(Ref: Harrison 20th edition, p 2346; Harrison 19th p 2004)

- Liver in patients with Rotor syndrome has no pigmentation and appears totally normal. The only abnormality in routine laboratory tests is an elevation of total serum bilirubin, due to a predominant rise in conjugated bilirubin. This is accompanied by bilirubinuria.
- In Rotor syndrome, the gallbladder is usually visualized on oral cholecystography, in contrast to the non-visualization that is typical of DJS.
- The pattern of urinary coproporphyrin excretion also differs. The pattern in Rotor syndrome resembles that of many acquired disorders of hepato-biliary function, in which coproporphyrin I, the major coproporphyrin isomer in bile, refluxes from the hepatocyte back into the circulation and is excreted in urine. *Thus, total urinary coproporphyrin excretion is substantially increased in Rotor syndrome, in contrast to the normal levels seen in DJS. Although the fraction of coproporphyrin I in urine is elevated, it is usually <70% of the total, compared with 80% in DJS.*
- The disorders also can be distinguished by their patterns of BSP excretion. Although clearance of BSP from plasma is delayed in Rotor syndrome, there is no reflux of conjugated BSP back into the circulation as seen in DJS.

214. Ans. (b) Collateral flow towards umbilicus

(Ref: Harrison 20th edition, p 282; Harrison 19th p 286)

In caput medusa the blood flows away from the umbilicus and is suggestive of portal hypertension. The increased flow results in a venous hum. The abdominal distention due to ascites explains flank fullness and everted umbilicus

215. Ans. (a) Purtscher's retinopathy

(Ref: H Harrison 20th edition, p 2444; Harrison 19th p 2091)

- Purtscher's retinopathy, a relatively unusual complication, is manifested by a sudden and severe loss of vision in a patient with acute pancreatitis.
- It is characterized by a peculiar funduscopic appearance with cotton-wool spots and hemorrhages confined to an area limited by the optic disc and macula; it is believed to be due to occlusion of the posterior retinal artery with aggregated granulocytes.

216. Ans. (d) Fecal elastase level

(Ref: Harrison 19th p 269)

- The fecal elastase-1 and small bowel biopsy are useful in the evaluation of patients with suspected pancreatic steatorrhea.
- The fecal elastase level will be abnormal and small bowel histology will be normal in such patients. A decrease of fecal elastase level to <100 g per gram of stool strongly suggests severe pancreatic exocrine insufficiency

217. Ans. (b) Elevated lipase

(Ref: Harrison 20th edition, p 2439; Harrison 19th p 2091)

- Diabetic ketoacidosis is often accompanied by abdominal pain and elevated total serum amylase levels, thus closely mimicking acute pancreatitis. *However, the serum lipase level is not elevated in diabetic ketoacidosis.*
- Hyperglycemia is common and is due to multiple factors, including decreased insulin release, increased glucagon release, and an increased output of adrenal glucocorticoids and catecholamines.

218. Ans. (c) Menke disease

(Ref: Harrison 20th edition, p 2982; Harrison 19th p 96e-10)

- Menkes disease, also known as kinky hair disease, is an X-linked neurodegenerative disease of impaired copper transport, due to ATP 7A gene.
- In Menkes disease, transport of dietary copper from intestinal cells is impaired, leading to the low serum copper levels. Abnormal copper transport in other cells leads to paradoxical copper accumulation in duodenal cells, kidney, pancreas, skeletal muscle, and placenta.
- Children with the classic form of Menkes disease usually present at 2-3 months of age with the following:
  1. Loss of developmental milestones
  2. Profound truncal hypotonia
  3. Epilepsy, divided into 3 periods: Early stage, median age 3 months, with focal clonic status; intermediate stage, median age 10 months, with intractable infantile spasms; late state, median age 25 months, with multifocal seizures, tonic spasms, and myoclonus
  4. Failure to thrive

219. Ans. (b) Agonizing upper abdominal pain

(Ref: Harrison 20th edition, p 2440; Harrison 19th p 2091)

Abdominal pain is the major symptom of acute pancreatitis. Pain may vary from a mild and tolerable discomfort and more commonly to severe, constant, and incapacitating distress. Characteristically, the pain, which is steady and boring in character, is located in the epigastrium and periumbilical region and often radiates to the back as well as to the chest, flanks, and lower abdomen. The pain is frequently more intense when the patient is supine, and patients may obtain some relief by sitting with the trunk flexed and knees drawn up. Nausea, vomiting, and abdominal distention due to gastric and intestinal hypomotility and chemical peritonitis are also frequent complaints

220. Ans. (a) Carbohydrate deficient transferrin

(Ref: CMDT 2014, ch. 16, p 680)

- Carbohydrate-deficient transferrin is perhaps the most reliable marker of chronic alcoholism, irrespective of the presence of liver disease. Carbohydrate-deficient transferrin has been proposed as a reliable biomarker in the differentiation of nonalcoholic steatohepatitis (NASH) from alcoholic hepatitis.

221. Ans. (a) Upper GI bleeding

(Ref: Gastrointestinal emergencies, 2nd edn., p 14)

- Rockall risk scoring system attempts to identify patients at risk of adverse outcome following acute upper gastrointestinal bleeding
- A convenient mnemonic is ABCDE - i.e. Age, Blood pressure fall (shock), Co-morbidity, Diagnosis and Evidence of bleeding.

Variable	Score 0	Score 1	Score 2	Score 3
Age	<60	60-69	>80	
Shock	No shock	Pulse > 100 BP>100 Systolic	SBP <100	
Co-morbidity	Nil major		CHF, IHD	Renal failure, liver failure, metastatic cancer
Diagnosis	Mallory-Weiss	All other diagnoses	GI malignancy	
Evidence of bleeding	None		Blood, adherent clot, spurting vessel	

* Comorbidity is scored as 0, 2, 3, and there is no score 1. This explains the blanks in the table..

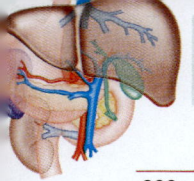

222. Ans. (d) Pancreatic lipase deficiency

(Ref: Harrison 20th edition, p 2406; Harrison 19th p 2059)
- Zieve syndrome occurs in severe alcoholic hepatitis and has hematlytic anaemia with spur cells and acanthocytes.

223. Ans. (d) Compressive chest injury

(Ref: Harrison 20th edition, p 2167)

Causes of purtschner retinopathy
1. Acute pancreatitis
2. Amniotic fluid embolism
3. Eclampsia and HELLP syndrome
4. Vasculitis like SLE, polymyositis, dermato-myositis
5. Traumatic chest compression and blunt head trauma are common causes. Chest trauma that is associated with Purtscher retinopathy ranges from mild to severe; the degree is not necessarily indicative of the risk of developing retinopathy. Compressive chest injuries often are seen with unrestrained drivers in motor vehicle accidents (MVAs).

224. Ans. (d) Hyperamylasia

(Ref: CMDT 2019, p 742; Harrison 19th edition p 2091)

Ranson Criteria:

At Admission:
1. Age in years > 55 years
2. White blood cell count > 16000 cells/mm^3
3. Blood glucose > 10 mmol/L (> 200 mg/dL)
4. Serum AST > 250 IU/L
5. Serum LDH > 350 IU/L

Within 48 hours:
1. Serum calcium < 2.0 mmol/L (< 8.0 mg/dL)
2. Hematocrit fall > 10%
3. Oxygen (hypoxemia PaO$_2$ < 60 mmHg)
4. BUN increased by 1.8 or more mmol/L (5 or more mg/dL) after IV fluid hydration
5. Base deficit (negative base excess) > 4 mEq/L
6. Sequestration of fluids > 6 L

225. Ans. (b) Arthritis

(Ref: Harrison 20th edition, p 2269)
- Arthritis develops in 15-20% patients of IBD and it worsens with disease activity. Control of bowel inflammation will reduce the arthritis symptoms.
- Uveitis can be seen in periods of remission of IBD
- Venous thromboembolism and erythema nodosum also worsens with disease activity.
- PSC may occur before symptoms of ulcerative colitis begin and may develop years after the proctocolectomy has been performed. 10% of PSC patients develop a cholangiocarcinoma.

226. Ans. (a) Abnormal Schilling test corrected by pancreatic enzyme administration

(Ref: Harrison 20th edition, p 2252; Harrison 19th p 269)

227. Ans. (c) Alcoholic liver disease

(Ref: Harrison 20th edition, p 2340)
- Gamma-glutamyltransferase (GGT) is primarily present in kidney, liver, and pancreatic cells. Small amounts are present in other tissues.
- Even though renal tissue has the highest level of GGT, the enzyme present in the serum appears to originate primarily from the hepatobiliary system, and GGT activity is elevated in any and all forms of liver disease.
- Elevated levels of GGT are noted not only in the sera of patients with alcoholic cirrhosis but also in the majority of sera from persons who are heavy drinkers.

228. Ans. (a) Raised serum albumin

(Ref: Harrison 20th edition, p 2337)

Damage to liver will result in low serum albumin levels.

229. Ans. (d) All of the above

(Ref: Harrison 20th edition, p 2444; Harrison 19th p 2091)

Recurrent Pancreatitis
1. Occult disease of the biliary tree or pancreatic ducts, especially microlithiasis, sludge
2. Drugs
3. Hypertriglyceridemia
4. Pancreas divisum
5. Pancreatic cancer
6. Cystic fibrosis

230. Ans. (b) Angiography

(Ref: Harrison 20th edition, p 2431; Harrison 19th p 2089)

Hemobilia is suspected if Upper GI endoscopy shows presence of blood in duodenum but confirmation of diagnosis is done only after angiography. Celiac axis angiography should always be accompanied with superior mesenteric arteriography because anomalous/accessory right hepatic artery may originate from the SMA.

231. Ans. (d) 80%

(Ref: Harrison 20th edition, p 2854)

Type 1 diabetes mellitus is characterized by an inability to produce insulin endogenously. Based on a series of histopathology studies, it is commonly stated that the onset of clinical symptoms corresponds to an 70-80% reduction in beta cell mass

232. Ans. (a) Cytoplasm of hepatocytes

(Ref: Table 16.2 Robbins, 8th ed.)
- SGPT and SGOT are found in cytoplasm of hepatocytes whereas SGOT is also found in mitochondria of hepatocytes.
- SGPT can be raised in other forms of tissue damage, such as myocardial infarction, muscle necrosis, renal disorders, cerebral disorders and intravascular hemolysis. In these diseases, serum SGOT levels are much higher than SGPT levels. However, in liver disease, generally SGPT increases more than SGOT.

233. Ans. (d) Recurrence with Wilson disease

(Ref: Harrison 20th edition, p 2420; Harrison 19th p 2042)

- Following perfusion with cold electrolyte solution, the donor liver is removed and packed in ice. The use of University of Wisconsin (UW) solution, rich in lactobionate and raffinose, has permitted the extension of cold ischemic time up to 20 hours; however, 12 hours may be a more reasonable limit
- *Recurrence after Wilson and alpha 1 anti-trysin deficiency is not seen*
- Tissue typing for human leukocyte antigen (HLA) matching is not required, and preformed cytotoxic HLA antibodies do not preclude liver transplantation.

234. Ans. (b) Orthotopic liver transplant

(Ref: Harrison 19th p 1994)

The Child-Pugh score is calculated by adding the scores of the five factors and can range from 5 to 15. Child-Pugh class can be A (a score of 5-6), B (7-9), or C (10 or above). Decompensation indicates cirrhosis with a Child-Pugh score of >7 (class B). This level has been the accepted criterion for listing liver transplantation.

Parameter	Point Assigned		
	1	2	3
Ascites	Absent	Slight	Moderate
Bilirubin, mg/dL	</=2	2-3	>3
Albumin, g/dL	>3.5	2.8-3.5	<2.8
Prothrombin time			
* Seconds over control	1-3	4-6	>6
* INR	<1.8	Grade 1-2	>2.3
Encephalopathy	None	Grade 1-2	Grade 3-4

A total score of 5-6 is considered grade A (well-compensated disease); 7-9 is grade B (significant functional compromise); and 10-15 is grade C (decompensated disease). These grade correlate with one-and two-year patient survival.

Grade	Points	One-year Patient Survival (%)
A: well-compensated disease	5-6	100
B: significant function compromise	7-9	80
C: decompen-sated disease	10-15	45

235. Ans. (b) Syndrome X

(Ref: Harrison 20th edition, p 2402; Harrison 19th p 2057)

- NAFLD is most commonly associated with metabolic syndrome. This includes carrying the diagnosis of type II diabetes, obesity, or hypertriglyceridemia.
- Other factors, such as drugs (eg, amiodarone, tamoxifen, methotrexate), alcohol, metabolic abnormalities (e.g., galactosemia, glycogen storage diseases, homocystinuria, and tyrosinemia), nutritional status (e.g., overnutrition, severe malnutrition, total parenteral nutrition [TPN], or starvation diet), or other health problems (e.g., celiac sprue and Wilson disease) may contribute to fatty liver disease

236. Ans. (b) CT scan

(Ref: Harrison 20th edition, p 2441; Harrison 19th p 2012)

237. Ans. (c) Mumps

(Ref: Harrison 19th p 2094t)

238. Ans. (a) 3 fold increase in serum lipase

(Ref: Harrison 20th edition, p 2439; Harrison 19th p 2093t)

- 3 fold increase in serum lipase is a diagnostic criteria and not used for severity of acute pancreatitis.
- The criteria for severity in acute pancreatitis was defined as organ failure of at least one organ system (defined as a
  1. Systolic blood pressure <90 mmHg,
  2. Pao2 < 60 mmHg,
  3. Creatinine >2.0 mg/dL after rehydration
  4. Gastrointestinal bleeding >500 mL/24 hours
  5. Local complication such as necrosis, pseudocyst, and abscess.
- The diagnosis of acute pancreatitis requires two of the following: typical abdominal pain, threefold or greater elevation in serum amylase and/or lipase level, and/or confirmatory findings on cross-sectional abdominal imaging. Although not required for diagnosis, markers of severity include hemoconcentration (hematocrit >44%), azotemia (BUN >22 mg/dL), and signs of organ failure.

239. Ans. (d) Splinter hemorrhages

(Ref: Harrison 20th edition, p 2406; Harrison 19th p 739)

The hand manifestations of chronic liver disease consist of spider nevi (invariably on the upper half of the body), palmar erythema (mottled redness of the thenar & hypothenar eminences), & Dupuytren's contractures.

240. Ans. (c) Neck and shoulders

(Ref: Harrison 20th edition, p 2406)

- Spider angiomata & palmar erythema occur in both acute and chronic liver disease and may be especially prominent in persons with cirrhosis, but they can occur in normal individuals and are frequently present during pregnancy.
- Spider angiomata are superficial, tortuous arterioles and, unlike simple telangiectases, typically fill from the center outwards. Spider angiomata occur only on the arms, face, and upper torso; they can be pulsatile and may be difficult to detect in dark skinned individuals.

241. Ans. (d) Cholestatic jaundice

(Ref: Harrison 19th p 284)

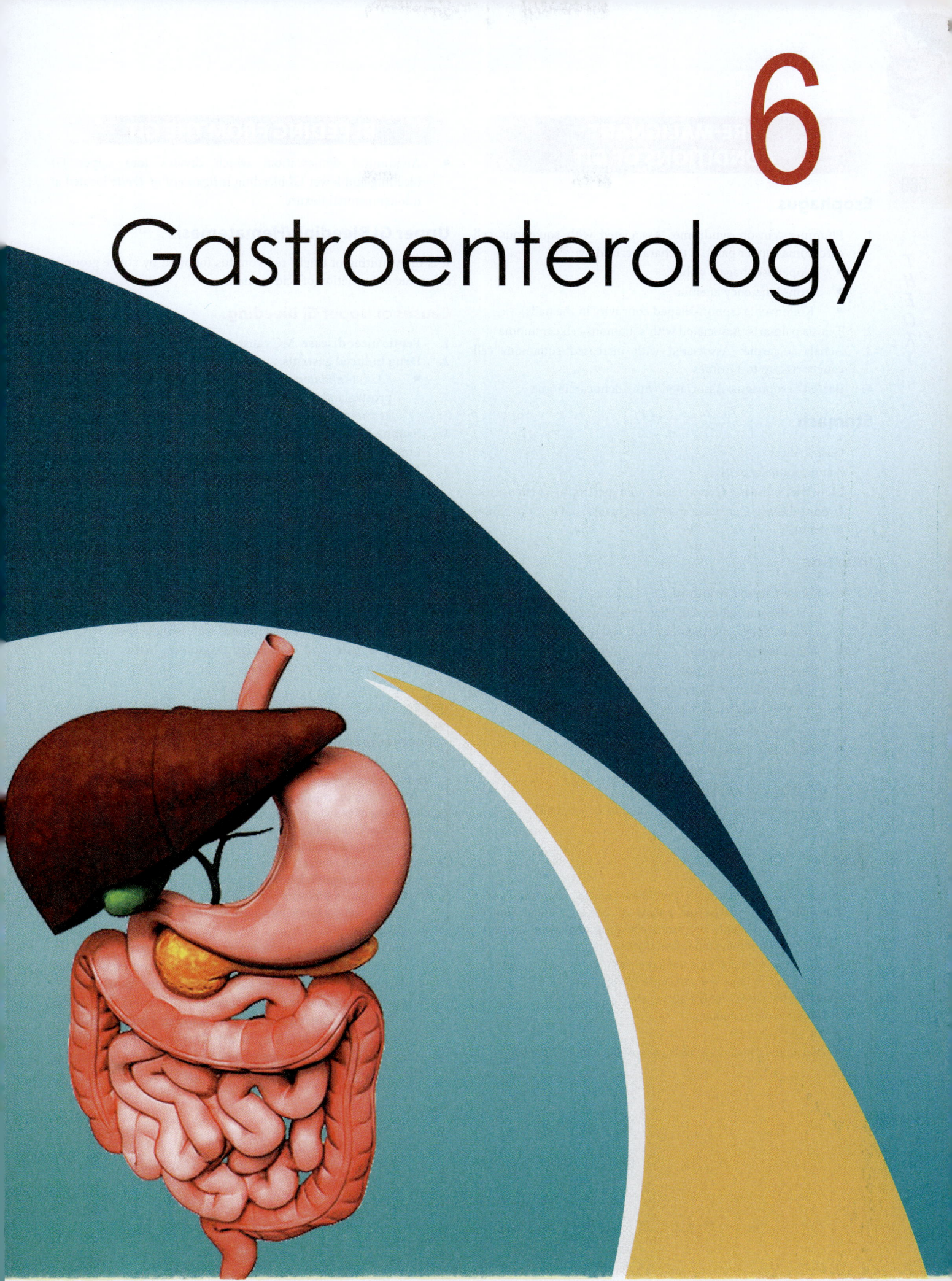

Gastroenterology

6

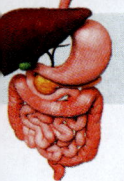

PRE-MALIGNANT CONDITIONS OF GIT

Esophagus

1. **Plummer Vinson syndrome:** Associated with squamous cell carcinoma (upper part). It is characterized by:
   - Upper esophageal webs
   - Iron-deficiency anemia
   - Koilonychia (spoon-shaped concavity in the nails)
2. **Tylosis palmaris:** Associated with squamous cell carcinoma
3. **Achalasia cardia:** Associated with increased squamous cell cancer risk up to 17 times
4. **Barrett's esophagus:** Associated with adenocarcinoma.

Stomach

1. Gastric ulcer
2. Autoimmune gastritis
3. **Menetrier's disease:** Hyperplasia and hypertrophy of rugosities
4. **Crohn's disease:** Can occur in any part of GIT, but most common in ileum.

Intestine

1. Cronkhite-Canada syndrome.
   - Ectodermal changes like hair loss from eyebrows, face and axillae. Skin hyperpigmentation and nail dystrophy
   - Onychoschizia (splitting of nails into layers)
   - Sessile/semipedunculated polyps in colon and small intestine [carpet-like polyposis]
2. Familial adenomatous polyposis
   - ≥ 100 polyps in colon
   - APC gene defective, on chromosome 5
   - Treatment: Prophylactic colectomy
3. Inflammatory bowel disease
   - Chances of malignancy are equal in UC and CD.

> - Gastrointestinal lesions in Cronkhite-Canada syndrome are hamartomatous polyps (or polyps of polyposis syndromes according to a newly proposed classification), histologically revealing pseudopolypoid-inflammatory changes.
> - Peutz-Jegher's syndrome is not a premalignant condition. Some authors say it is least likely to cause malignancy.
> - Peutz-Jegher's syndrome features are:
>   - Hamartomatous polyps
>   - MC site: Jejunum
>   - Oral mucosal melanosis: Blackening of skin around lips and anus

BLEEDING FROM THE GIT

- Anatomical demarcation, which divides into upper GI bleeding and lower GI bleeding is **ligament of Treitz** located at duodenojejunal flexure.

Upper GI Bleeding/Hematemesis

It is the vomiting of bright red vomitus followed by coffee grounds color due to formation of acid-hematin.

Causes of Upper GI Bleeding

1. **Peptic ulcer disease:** MC cause
2. **Drug induced gastritis:**
   - *COX-1 inhibitors* are responsible for gastritis as they inhibit prostaglandin synthesis. Example: Aspirin, diclofenac, ketorolac, piroxicam.
3. **Esophageal varices:** Due to portal hypertension. It is an important cause of upper GI bleed.
4. **Mallory-Weiss tear:** *It is a submucosal tear and the usual location of the tear is at cardia on the lesser curvature of the stomach (between 2 and 6 o' clock meridian on endoscopic viewing with the patient in the left lateral decubitus position).*
   - Endoscopic diagnosis of a Mallory-Weiss tear is readily made by identifying active bleeding, an adherent clot, or a fibrin crust over a mucosal split within or near the gastroesophageal junction. On an average, the split is 2–3 cm in length and a few millimeters in width.
   - Most patients (>80%) present with a single tear.
   - It is associated with binge alcoholism, hiatus hernia and hyperemesis gravidarium.

> **Boerhaave syndrome**
> This is most commonly associated with forceful vomiting and leads to esophageal rupture at lower 1/3 esophagus, posteriorly.
> - It presents as chest pain due to chemical mediastinitis with crashing of blood pressure.
> - Hamman Crunch sign (walking on fresh fallen snow with leather boots-on) is auscultated.
> - CT chest with contrast is used to confirm the tear
> - Usually gastrogaffin followed by thin barium is used.
> - NG suction, antibiotics with prompt surgical drainage and repair of non contaminated leaks is to be done.

5. **Dieulafoy's lesions** are characterized by a single large tortuous arteriole in the submucosa, which do not undergo normal branching or a branch with caliber of 1–5 mm (more than 10 times the normal diameter of mucosal capillaries). The lesion bleeds into the gastrointestinal tract through a minute defect in the mucosa, which is not a primary ulcer of the mucosa, but an erosion likely caused in the submucosal surface by protrusion of the pulsatile arteriole.

6. Gastric antral vascular ectasia: Water melon stomach

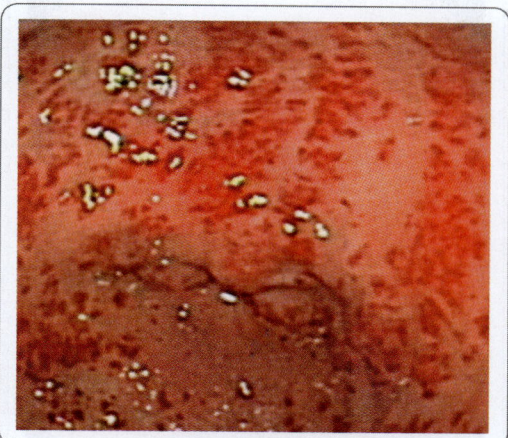

Water melon stomach

Hemobilia

Causes

1. Trauma: operative injury to liver, bile ducts
2. Intraductal rupture of hepatic abscess/aneurysm of hepatic artery
3. Tumor: erosion of blood vessels
4. Mechanical complications of choledocholithiasis
5. Hepatobiliary parasitism
6. Diagnostic procedures like liver biopsy

Clinical Features

1. Biliary pain
2. Obstructive jaundice
3. Melena
   IOC: CT angiography

Lower GI Bleeding

Cause of Hematochezia

1. Most common cause of hematochezia is Hemorrhoids > diverticulitis. Most common pediatric cause of hematochezia is rectal polyps > Meckel's diverticulum
2. Inflammatory bowel disease
   - **Ulcerative colitis**: *Presents with bloody diarrhea*
   - **Crohn's disease**: *Presents with colicky pain (because of stricture formation)*
3. Cancer colon
   - Bleeding most commonly seen with right colon Ca (cecum Ca) > left colon Ca (rectal Ca).
   - Left sided colon Ca most commonly presents with constipation.
4. **Acute mesenteric insufficiency:** Due to embolism of mural thrombus to SMA and/or IMA. It occurs after 2-3 days of MI.
   - **Investigation of choice:** Angiography
   - **Treatment**: Thrombolysis
5. Angiodysplasia of colon
   - Abnormal presence of submucosal bleeding

Black Tarry Stools (Melena)

- It is defined black tarry stools due to degradation of blood present in the stool over a duration of 6–8 hours.
- *Minimum amount of blood to cause melena:* **60 mL**.

Causes of Melena (All Causes of UGI Bleeding)

1. Most common cause: Peptic ulcer disease
2. Drug-induced gastritis
3. Portal hypertension
4. Mallory Weiss tear

- Investigation of choice: Upper GI endoscopy

Treatment

Gel embolization of bleeder

- **Superior mesenteric artery syndrome (SMA)** is an extremely rare life-threatening condition that can either be congenital and chronic, or induced and acute. SMA syndrome is characterized by compression of the duodenum between the abdominal aorta and the superior mesenteric artery.
- **Acute mesenteric insufficiency** can occur post MI due to embolism leading to presentation of acute abdomen, passage of maroon-colored stools and subsequent gangrene of the gut.

DISEASES OF ESOPHAGUS

- MC type of dysphagia is Oropharyngeal dysphagia and it results from neuromuscular disease in greater than three quarters of cases.
- The *upper esophageal sphincter* is commonly involved. This dysphagia is commonly *episodic*, although it may be unrelenting.
- Aspiration is frequent, and pain may occur.
- Specific diagnoses include cerebrovascular accident, Parkinson's disease, multiple sclerosis; bulbar poliomyelitis, diabetic neuropathy and mononeuritis multiplex; myasthenia gravis; and dermatomyositis, poliomyositis, and thyroid disease.

ZENKER'S DIVERTICULUM

- It is a pulsion diverticulum, where pharyngeal mucosa herniates through the **Killian's dehiscence**.
- It originates from the posterior wall of the pharynx.
- Herniation starts in the midline posteriorly, as out pouching enlarges, it localizes to one side of the esophagus and the most common side being the "left".
- It is an acquired and false diverticulum.

Killian's Dehiscence

It is a weak area between oblique fibers of superior constrictor superiorly and transverse fibers of cricopharyngeus inferiorly.

Clinical Features

1. Halitosis
2. Dysphagia
3. Regurgitation of previous day food particles.
4. In contrast schatzki's ring causes episodic dysphagia for solids especially meats (steakhouse syndrome).

Investigation of Choice

Barium swallow.

Treatment

1. Marsupialization procedure
2. Surgical diverticulectomy

EOSINOPHILIC ESOPHAGITIS

Etiology

1. GERD
2. Drug hypersensitivity
3. Connective tissue disorders
4. Hypereosinophilic syndrome
5. Infection
6. Dietary factors

Classification

1. Dysphagia and esophageal food impaction
2. Chest pain, aversion to food
3. Heart burn refractory to PPi
4. History of atopy

Diagnostic Criteria for Eosinophilic Esophagitis

Three criteria must be met to diagnose EoE:
1. Clinical symptoms of Esophageal dysfunction
2. Esophageal biopsy with a maximum eosinophil count of at least 15 eosinophils per high-power microscopy field.
3. Exclusion of other possible causes of esophageal eosinophilia, including proton-pump inhibitor responsive esophageal eosinophilia (PPI-REE)

Investigations

1. Endoscopic view shows corrugated appearance called as feline esophagus
2. Eosinophilia
3. Biopsy shows esophageal mucosal eosinophilia (>15 eosinophils/HPF)

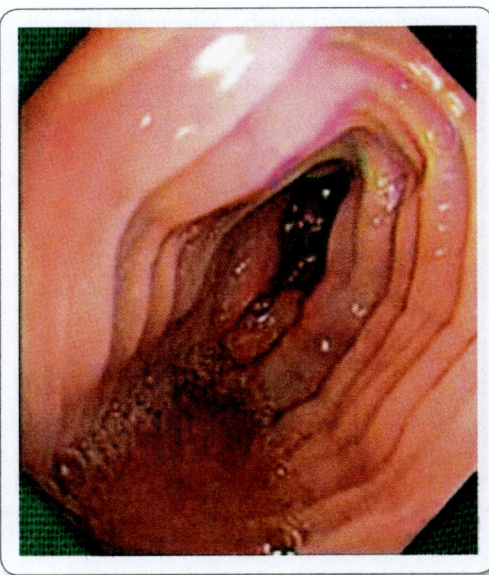

Treatment

1. PPI and elimination diets (remove milk, soy, wheat, nuts and seafood)
2. Elemental formula diets
3. Swallowed topical fluticasone or budesonide is highly effective
4. Esophageal dilatation

- Serpiginous ulcers in esophagus are seen in CMV esophagitis
- Volcano punched out ulcers in esophagus are seen in herpes simplex esophagitis
- CMV esophagitis can occur after solid organ transplantation
- Esophageal perforation is confirmed with contrast swallow usually gastrogaffin or barium. (Page 1910: Harrison 19th edition). CT chest is most sensitive in detecting mediastinal air.
- Radiation esophagitis is seen with treatment of breast and lung cancer.
- Pill esophagitis is common with doxycycline, tetracycline, quinidine, ferrous sulphate, NSAIDs and bisphophonates

MOTILITY DISORDERS OF ESOPHAGUS

- Achalasia cardia
- Diffuse esophageal spasm (cork screw esophagus).

Achalasia Cardia

- Loss of ganglia of myenteric plexus leading to increased tone of LES causing difficulty in swallowing.

Causes

1. Most common cause: Autoimmune (Harrison 20e, pg 2213)
2. Chagas disease: caused by *Trypanosoma cruzi* and transmitted by *Reduviid* bug.

Clinical Features

- Halitosis
- Regurgitation of previous day food
- Dysphagia *(more for liquids when compared to solids)*.

Investigations

1. **Investigation of choice**: Esophageal manometry
2. **Barium swallow**: Sigmoid esophagus or pencil tip appearance.

Treatment

1. Pneumatic dilatation: Efficacy 32–98%
2. Heller's myotomy performed with anti-reflux procedure (partial fundoplication): Efficacy 62–100% (pg 1905: Harrison 19e)
3. Botulinum toxin injected into LES, shows improvement for 6 months

Note: Achalasia cardia is a premalignant condition and can lead to squamous cell cancer. Pseudoachalasia due to tumor infiltration has to be ruled out by endoscopy.

AAA syndrome/Allgrove syndrome has alacrima, achalasia, adrenal insufficiency

Diffuse Esophageal Spasm/Esophageal Angina

Abnormal premature esophageal contraction with normal deglutitive LES relaxation.

Clinical Features

1. Chest pain: Non exertional, interrupts sleep, meal related
2. Dysphagia
3. Heart burn.

Investigations

1. ECG: to rule out cardiac causes of chest pain
2. *Investigation of choice*: Esophageal manometry
3. Barium swallow: Cork-screw appearance^Q/Rosary bead esophagus.

Algorithm for Evaluation of Dysphagia

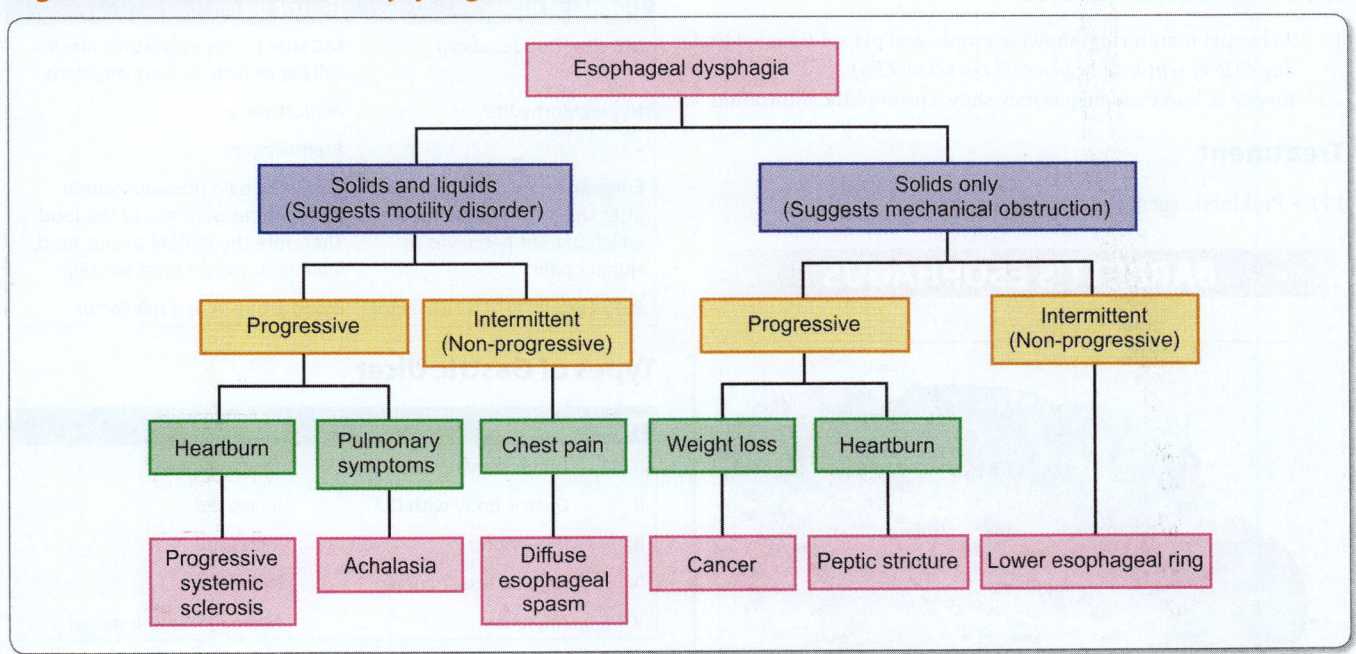

Treatment

- Only drugs showing efficacy are anxiolytic drugs. Nitrates, calcium channel blockers (CCB), and botulinum toxins are used. Surgical treatment with long myotomy and even esophagectomy is done in case of severe weight loss or unbearable pain.

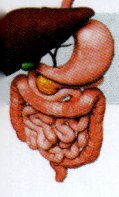

Diffuse esophageal spasm	Nutcracker esophagus	Hypertensive LES
Simultaneous non peristaltic contractions (>20% of wet swallows)	• Mean peristaltic amplitude of > 180 mm Hg for increased duration of contraction >7 seconds • Normal peristaltic sequence	• Elevated LES pressure > 26 mm Hg • Normal LES relaxation • Normal esophageal peristalsis

GASTROESOPHAGEAL REFLUX DISEASE (GERD)

Clinical Features

1. Retrosternal pain
2. Heart burn
3. Sour water brash
4. Chemical tracheitis leading to chronic nocturnal cough.

Investigation of Choice

1. 24 hrs pH monitoring, showing esophageal pH < 4.0 for > 4 hrs/day. *(Tip of sensor to be placed 5 cm below LES)*
2. Biopsy of lower esophagus may show eosinophilic infiltration.

Treatment

PPI + Prokinetic agent (Itopride/Mosapride)

BARRETT'S ESOPHAGUS

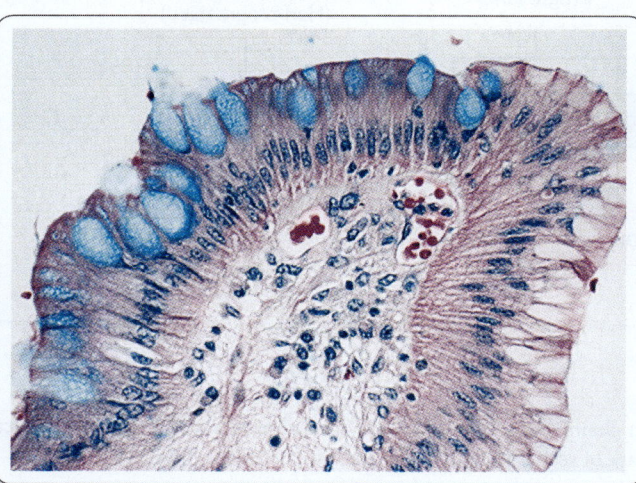

Alcian blue stain showing goblet cells

- Long-standing GERD leads to squamous epithelium getting converted into columnar epithelium (metaplasia).
- It is a premalignant condition for adenocarcinoma of esophagus.

Investigation of Choice

Upper GI endoscopy + punch biopsy.

Treatment

- Endoscopic mucosal resection
- Esophagectomy for high grade dysplasia however the procedure itself has mortality ranging from 3 to 10%. Esophageal resection of lower 1/3rd of esophagus with stomach mobilization.

PEPTIC ULCER DISEASE (PUD)

Damaging factors	Protective factors
Gastric acid	Mucus and bicarbonate
NSAIDS	Mucosal blood flow
H. pylori	Prostaglandin
Ischemia, smoking & alcohol	Epithelial regenerative capacity

- **Causes of PUD**: The most common cause is *H. pylori* infection followed by NSAIDS, smoking, steroids & stress.
- **Endocrine disorders leading to PUD**: Zollinger Ellison syndrome, Cushing's syndrome and hyperparathyroidism.

Duodenal ulcer	Gastric ulcer
MC site: Duodenal cap	**MC site**: Lesser curvature, specifically at or near incisura angularis
Hyperchlorhydria	Achlorhydria
–	Premalignant
Epigastric pain develops 2 hrs after the intake of the food which patient perceives as Hunger pain.	Epigastric pain develops within half-an-hour of intake of the food. Therefore the patient avoids food, leading to weight loss/ wasting
Blood group 'O' is a risk factor	Blood group 'A' is a risk factor

Types of Gastric Ulcer

Type	Location	Acid level
I	Lesser curve at incisura	Low to normal
II	Gastric body with DU	Increased
III	Pre-Pyloric	Increased
IV	High on lesser curve	Normal
V	Anywhere	Normal, NSAID induced

Investigations for H. Pylori

- **Investigation of choice**: Breath urea test
- **Gold standard**: Biopsy and stained with silver stain.
- Eradication of infection with H. Pylori is confirmed with Breath urea test > fecal antigen test

Treatment

Treatment Options for Peptic Ulcer Disease

Sequential quadruple therapy	Standard quadruple therapy	Standard triple therapy
Proton pump inhibitor twice daily • Days 1–5: amoxicillin 1 g • Days 6–10: Clarithromycin and metronidazole 500 mg	Proton pump inhibitor orally twice daily • Bismuth subsalicylate • Tetracycline • Metronidazole	Proton pump inhibitor • Clarithromycin 500 mg • Amoxicillin 1 g

- After completion of course of *H. pylori* eradication therapy, continue treatment with proton pump inhibitor once daily for 4–6 weeks if ulcer is large (>1 cm) or complicated.
- Confirm successful eradication of *H. pylori* with urea breath test, fecal antigen test, or endoscopy with biopsy at least 4 weeks after completion of antibiotic treatment and 1–2 weeks after proton pump inhibitor treatment.

Complications of PUD

1. Hemorrhage

Gastric Ulcer	Duodenal Ulcer
Source of bleeding here is left gastric artery *(MC vessel involved)*	Hemorrhage is more common posteriorly as compared to anteriorly and the source of bleeding is gastroduodenal artery

2. Perforation

Gastric Ulcer	Duodenal Ulcer
MC site of perforation- Lesser curvature → GI content goes to posterior of stomach → *lesser sac peritonitis*	It mostly perforates anteriorly, leading to *greater sac peritonitis*

3. Gastric and duodenal ulcers healing leads to fibrosis, which results in gastric outlet obstruction.

GASTRITIS

Type-A Gastritis (Autoimmune Gastritis)
- Antibodies against parietal cells, called anti-parietal cell antibodies
- Leads to Achlorhydria.
- Parietal cells are responsible for production of intrinsic factor (IF), which helps in the absorption of vit-B_{12}. Due to destruction of parietal cells, it leads to pernicious anemia.
- Premalignant condition for adenocarcinoma of stomach.

Type-B Gastritis
Occurs due to *H. pylori* infection and most commonly involves *antrum and stomach*. This is also a premalignant condition for adenocarcinoma of stomach.

Erosive Gastritis
- Cox-1 ⊖ inhibit prostaglandin production
  1. NSAIDS
  2. Curling ulcer Burn: 1st part of duodenum
  3. Cushing ulcer Raised ICP: Stomach

MENETRIERS DISEASE

- It is characterised by presence of large tortous mucosal folds giving a *cereberiform appearance to the stomach mucosa*.
- The folds are seen mostly in body and fundus and spare the antrum.
- Histologically *massive foveolar cell hyperplasia* and *reduction in oxyntic cells and parietal cells* is seen.

Clinical Features
1. Epigastric pain, nausea, vomiting
2. Occult GIT bleeding
3. *Protein losing enteropathy* due to hypersecretion of gastric mucus leading to hypoalbuminemia and edema.
4. Gastric acid secretion is *reduced*.

Investigations
1. UGIE shows large folds. Snare deep biopsy is mandatory to differentiate from gastric polyposis or infiltrative disorders like sarcoidosis. It is mentioned as premalignant by most authorities. (Page 1932: Harrison 19th edition).
2. CMV and H. Pylori serology
3. Serum albumin

Treatment
Cetuximab is now considered to be the first line of treatment and gastrectomy is done for medically refractory severe disease. Ulcers are managed with PPI.

ZOLLINGER ELLISON SYNDROME (ZES)

- Most common site is 2nd part of duodenum (D2) in gastrinoma triangle.
- This excessive acid production leads to peptic ulcer disease.

Clinical Features
1. Epigastric pain
2. Secretory diarrhea.
3. Investigation of choice is secretin study.[Q]
4. **Imaging modality of choice is Endoscopic ultrasound**.
5. For metastatic gastrinoma, imaging modality is Octreoscan

Treatment
- PPI is treatment of choice with octreotide.

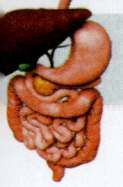

MALABSORPTION SYNDROME

Tests for Malabsorption Syndrome

Substance	Remarks
D-xylose test	Sugar malabsorption and tests jejunal damage or proximal enteropathy
14C triolein test	Fat malabsorption picked up by radiocarbon being tagged to the triglycerides
13C trioactanoin	Fat malabsorption due to pancreatic exocrine insufficiency
SeHCAT [usual name for 23-seleno-25-homo-tauro-cholic acid (selenium homocholic acid taurine or tauroselcholic acid)].	Used in a clinical test to diagnose bile acid malabsorption
Hydrogen breath test	For sugar malabsorption as unabsorbed sugar is degraded by bacteria
13C acetate breath tests	For stomach emptying
Urea breath test	For *H. pylori* that can split urea to CO_2, which is produced in breath. Due to the presence of *H. pylori*, in the plaque in teeth, erroneus results can be present.

The 14C-triolein breath test is used to investigate the absorption of fats from the small bowel. In principle, a 14C-labeled triglyceride is ingested, digested, absorbed and metabolized, releasing 14C-labeled carbon dioxide. The test may be performed in a day ward and requires laboratory facilities to detect the beta-emitting 14C. The test is unreliable in the following circumstances:
- Diabetes mellitus
- Gross obesity
- Thyroid disease

Results of Diagnostic Studies in Different Causes of Steatorrhea

	D-Xylose Test	Schilling Test	Duodenal Mucosal Biopsy
Chronic pancreatitis	Normal	50% abnormal; if abnormal, normal with pancreatic enzymes	Normal
Bacterial overgrowth syndrome	Normal or only modestly abnormal	Often abnormal; if abnormal, normal after antibiotics	Usually normal
Ileal disease	Normal	Abnormal	Normal
Celiac sprue	Decreased	Normal	Abnormal probably "flat"
Intestinal lymphangi-ectasia	Normal	Normal	Abnormal: "dilated lymphatics"

CELIAC SPRUE

- This condition is referred by the alternate name of **Gluten enteropathy**.
- Usual presentation of this condition is after the age of 6-months once the complimentary feeds are initiated such as cereals and fruits.
- Cereals like wheat, oat, rye and barley contain a protein named gliadin/gluten and a child suffering from celiac sprue is allergic to gluten.
- The antibodies against this will result in the damage of enterocytes and microvilli, which reduce the surface area of the small intestine.
- Since sugar remains unabsorbed, it will lead to osmotic diarrhea.

Clinical Features

A child > 6 months old presents with:
1. Failure to thrive
2. Anemia with delay in milestones
3. Loose motions (*Usually with intake of solid food items*).

Investigations

1. **Screening test**: According to American College of gastroenterology guidelines, immunoglobulin A anti-tissue transglutaminase antibody is the best first test for suspected celiac sprue. In children <2 years, the IgATTG test should be combined with testing for IgG-deaminated isolated gliadin peptides.
2. **IOC**: Small intestinal biopsy, repeated 4 weeks after gluten free diet is introduced. Villi are atrophic/absent with decreased villous/crypt ratio. (Normal ratio is 4–5 : 1)

Treatment

1. **Stop cereals** and start the child on maize or rice (*low cost option*)
   - Maize is considered as cereal of choice.
2. Iron + multi vitamin supplementation
3. Dietry restriction till 10 years of age. After that severity of condition decreases

- In celiac sprue damage to proximal small intestine is more than distal part of small intestine.
- Therefore, iron deficiency > Vit B12 deficiency.

Associated Diseases

- Dermatitis herpetiformis
- Insulin dependent DM (Type I DM)
- IgA deficiency
- Down's syndrome

Complications of Celiac Sprue

1. Development of cancer (both gastrointestinal and non-gastrointestinal lymphomas)
2. Intestinal ulceration
3. Collagenous sprue: It does not respond to gluten free diet and has a poor prognosis.

Refractory Celiac Sprue

1. Responds to 'Soy' protein restriction
2. Respond to glucocorticoids
3. Failure of all measures with fatal outcome.

Tropical Sprue

- This condition is due to infection of *Giardia, Yersinia* and *C. difficile*. These organisms damage the microvilli of the small intestine leading to malabsorption.
- As sugar remains unabsorbed in the intestine, it draws water from the surrounding leading to osmotic diarrhea.
- As fat is unabsorbed, it leads to deficiency of all fat soluble vitamin. *Fat soluble vitamins are A, D, E and K*

Investigations

- **Investigation of choice:** Upper GI endoscopy + biopsy. No improvement on gluten restriction.

Treatment

Tetracycline with folic acid for 6 months

BACTERIAL OVERGROWTH SYNDROME/ BLIND LOOP SYNDROME

- Colonic type bacterial proliferation in the small intestinal lumen secondary to either anatomic or functional stasis.
- These anaerobes use cobalamin leading to macrocytic anemia.

Clinical Features

- The diagnosis may be suspected from the combination of a low serum cobalamin level and an elevated serum folate level, as enteric bacteria frequently produces folate compounds that will be absorbed in the duodenum.
- Ideally, the diagnosis of the bacterial overgrowth syndrome is the demonstration of *increased levels of aerobic and/or anaerobic colonic-type bacteria in a jejunal aspirate obtained by intubation.*
- Breath hydrogen testing with lactulose (a non-digestible disaccharide) administration has also been used to detect bacterial overgrowth.

Investigation

Jejunal aspirate and culture (IOC).

Treatment

- *Tetracycline^Q* used to be the initial treatment of choice; due to increasing resistance, however, other antibiotics such as metronidazole, amoxicillin/clavulanic acid and cephalosporins have been employed.
- Primary treatment should be directed, if at all possible, to the surgical correction of an anatomic blind loop.
- Bacterial overgrowth secondary to strictures, one or more diverticula, or a proximal afferent loop can potentially be cured by surgical correction of the anatomic state.

WHIPPLE'S DISEASE

- Caused by *Tropheryma whipplei*, found in macrophages.
- This condition leads to malabsorption with CNS symptoms and migratory large joint arthropathy.

- **Investigation of choice:** Upper GI endoscopy + biopsy (stain with PAS).

Treatment

For management of symptomatic/ asymptomatic CNS disease or cardiac infection

1. Parenteral ceftriaxone or meropenem for 2 weeks
2. Oral doxycycline/ hydroxychloroquine for 1 year

Rates of relapse, particularly CNS disease was very high with oral tetracycline and TMP-SMX therapy and hence the use is not recommended.

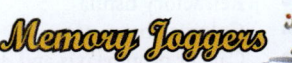

- Most common *heart valve* involved in whipple's disease is aortic valve
- Culture negative endocarditis is seen in whipple disease with duke' criteria not being satisfied.
- *CNS features* are in form of cognition defect progressing to dementia, supra-nuclear gaze palsy and oculofacial myorythmia
- MC extra-intestinal manifestation of whipple's disease is CNS feature of dementia.

INFLAMMATORY BOWEL DISEASE

IBD is a polygenic disorder and *not an autoimmune disorder.*

Crohn's Disease (Granulomatous Colitis)

- This condition involves entire gut with *ileum being the most common site whereas rectum is usually spared.*

Clinical Manifestations

1. **Colicky pain (due to multiple stricture formation):** Submucosal fibrosis leads to formation of Cobble-stone mucosa and stricture formation
2. Hematochezia
3. Toxic megacolon
4. Intra-abdominal abscess and intra-abdominal adhesions *(therefore surgery is avoided)*
5. Perianal fistula formation *(hallmark feature of CD).*

Investigations

1. ASCA (anti-saccharomyces cerevisae antibody): screening test
2. ESR elevated, CRP positive, TLC increased
3. Wireless capsule endoscopy allows direct visualization of entire small bowel. The diagnostic yield is higher than CT or MR enterography.

Treatment of Crohn's Disease

1. Glucocorticoids are useful in treatment of moderate to severe CD and induce remission. They have *no role in maintenance therapy.* Controlled ileal release budenoside is used for 2–3 months and then tapered.
2. Sulfasalazine will deliver antibiotic (sulfapyridine) and anti-inflammatory (5-ASA) to the site of active bowel disease in colon.

3. For distal ileal disease, delayed release mesalamine has be used.
4. 6-MP/Azathioprine/Infliximab/Natalizumab is used as a step-up treatment
5. Intravenous glucocorticoids are used before switching to TPN
6. Patients with small bowel CD have 80% chance of requiring surgery
7. It can range from perianal abscess drainage to balloon dilatation of small gut strictures or strictureplasty.
8. *Indications for surgery in Crohns' disease*
   - Stricture and obstruction unresponsive to medical therapy
   - Fulminant disease
   - Massive hemorrhage
   - Abscess formation
   - Refractory fistula
   - Colonic obstruction
   - Cancer prophylaxis and documented colon dysplasia

Ulcerative Colitis

- Involves colon only with the *most common site being RECTUM*.
- Ulcer in this condition develops very slowly, therefore regenerative activity of the epithelium kicks in leading to the formation of pseudopolyps.

Clinical Manifestations

Severity of Ulcerative Colitis

	Mild	Moderate	Severe
Bowel movements	<4 per day	4–6 per day	>6 per day
Bloody stools	Small	Moderate	Severe
Anemia	Mild	Present in majority	Present in majority
Tachycardia	None	Pulse rate <90	Pulse rate >90
Fever	Absent	Documented	Documented
Endoscopic findings	Fine granularity	Marked erythema and contact bleeding	Spontaneous bleeding and ulcerations

1. Painless bloody diarrhea anemia and hypoproteinemia
2. Extracellular plus intracellular bacteria found in the submucosa of gut
3. Toxic megacolon (UC>CD)
4. Incidence migratory large joint arthropathy.
5. Incidence of malignancy is equal in both ulcerative colitis and Crohn's disease.

Investigations

1. **P-ANCA**: Positive
2. **Investigation of choice**: Colonoscopy + biopsy
3. Barium enema: *Earliest radiological change is fine mucosal granularity*. This is followed by collar button ulcers and loss of Haustrations.
4. **Fecal lactoferrin levels is sensitive and specific marker for intestinal inflammation.**
5. Fecal calprotectin levels correlate with histological inflammation, predict relapse and detect pouchitis.

Treatment
- Sulfasalazine
- Azathioprine and 6-mercaptopurine (6-MP) are purine analogues commonly employed in the management of glucocorticoid-dependent IBD. Azathioprine is rapidly absorbed and converted to 6-MP, which is then metabolized to the active end product, thioinosinic acid, an inhibitor of purine ribonucleotide synthesis and cell proliferation. These agents also inhibit the immune response. Efficacy can be seen as early as 3–4 weeks but can take up to 4–6 months

Management of Mild-moderate UC

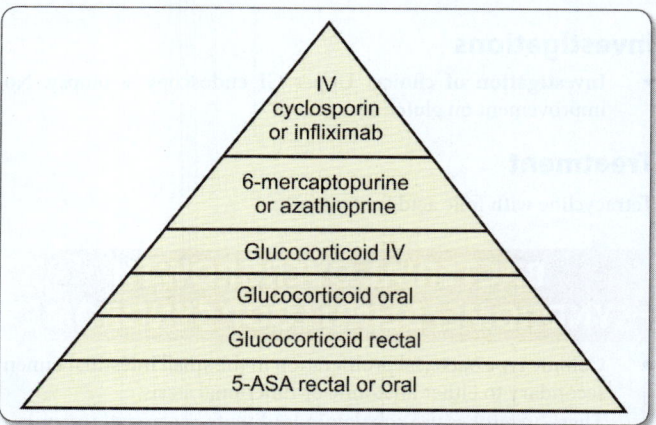

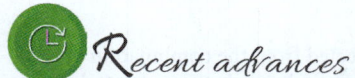

New Markers for Inflammatory Bowel Disease
- **Fecal calprotectin is a highly sensitive and specific marker for detecting histological inflammation**, predict relapses and detect pouchitis.
- Both fecal lactoferrin and calprotection are used to rule out active inflammation versus symptoms of irritable bowel syndrome or bacterial overgrowth.

These manifestations are seen more commonly in UC than CD
- Toxic megacolon
- Malignancy (According to older books, but pg 1965, Harrison 19/e, mentions equivalent risk in both UC and CD).
- Primary sclerosing cholangitis

Extraintestinal manifestation: CD > UC
1. Peripheral arthritis
   - Rheumatic migratory arthritis: large joints involved *(ankle, knee, elbow)*
2. Ankylosing spondylitis
3. Erythema nodosum
4. Uveitis
5. Parotitis
6. Osteoporosis

7. Clubbing
8. Pyoderma gangreosum

Incidence of peripheral arthritis is 15–20% of all IBD patients while incidence of Erythema Nodosum is 10–15%. Hence most common extra-intestinal manifestation of IBD is peripheral arthritis: Ref. Harrison 20th edition, page 2268

PSEUDOMEMBRANOUS COLITIS

- It is characterized by minimal inflammation or edema of colonic mucosa. In more severe cases, mucosa is covered with loosely adherent nodular or diffuse exudates.
- Symptoms include profuse, watery or mucoid, green foul smelling liquid stool which may contain small amounts of blood.
- Usually symptoms begin 3–9 days after antibiotics have been started. MC antibiotic responsible for causing pseudo-membranous colitis is Cephalosporins^Q > Clindamycin.

Investigations

1. Stool studies (*rapid enzyme immunoassays (EIAs) for toxins*): pathogenic strains of *C. difficile* produce two toxins. Toxin A is an enterotoxin and toxin B is a cytotoxin. Rapid enzyme immunoassays (EIAs) for toxins A and B have a 75–90% sensitivity.

   Until recently, EIA was the preferred diagnostic test in most clinical settings because it is inexpensive, easy to use, and results are available within 24 hours.
2. Nucleic acid amplification test (e.g., PCR assays) that amplify the toxin B gene have a 97% sensitivity and thus are superior to the EIA tests; these PCR assays are now preferred.
3. Assay for glutamate dehydrogenase (a common *C. difficile* antigen).

Immediate Treatment for Pseudomembranous Colitis

1. For patients with three or more relapses, updated guidelines recommend consideration of installation of a suspension of fecal bacteria from a healthy donor ('fecal microbiota transplant').
2. Treatment of choice is 'fecal transplantation' into the terminal ileum or proximal colon (by colonoscopy) or into the duodenum and jejunum (by nasoenteric tube), which results in disease remission after a single treatment in over 90% of patients with recurrent *C. difficile* infection.
3. Metronidazole, vancomycin, or fidaxomicin (a poorly absorbable macrolide antibiotic) should be initiated. *Metronidazole remains the preferred first-line therapy in patients with mild disease*, except in patients who are intolerant of metronidazole, pregnant women, and children. The duration of initial therapy is usually 10–14 days. Symptomatic improvement occurs in most patients within 72 hours.

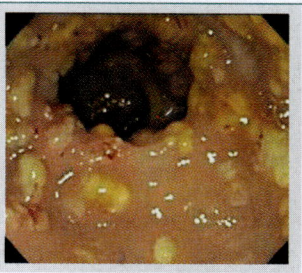
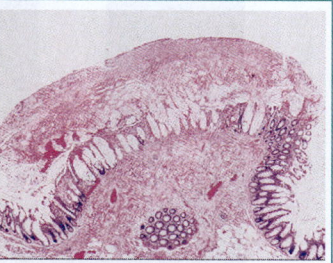
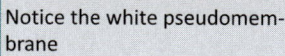

Notice the white pseudomembrane

Notice the mushroom shaped cloud emnating from debris due to damage by Clostridium difficile

Gastrointestinal Stromal Tumors

- Gastrointestinal stromal cell tumors (GISTs), were previously classified as gastrointestinal leiomyosarcomas and make up 1–3% of gastric neoplasms.
- Its cell of origin resembles the interstitial cell of Cajal, which controls peristalsis.
- *The majority of malignant GISTs have activating mutations of the c-kit gene that result in ligand-independent phosphorylation and activation of the KIT receptor tyrosine kinase, leading to tumorigenesis.*
- They most frequently involve the anterior and posterior walls of the gastric fundus and often ulcerate and bleed.
- These tumors rarely invade adjacent viscera and characteristically do not metastasize to lymph nodes, but they may spread to the liver and lungs. The treatment of choice is surgical resection.
- GISTs are unresponsive to conventional chemotherapy; yet 50% of patients experience objective response and prolonged survival when treated with imatinib mesylate (Gleevec) (400–800 mg PO daily), a selective inhibitor of the *c-kit* tyrosine kinase.
- Many patients with GIST whose tumors have become refractory to imatinib subsequently benefit from sunitinib (Sutent), another inhibitor of the c-kit tyrosine kinase.

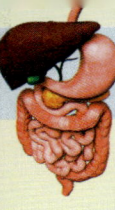

Image-Based Questions

1. The given barium swallow shows presence of?

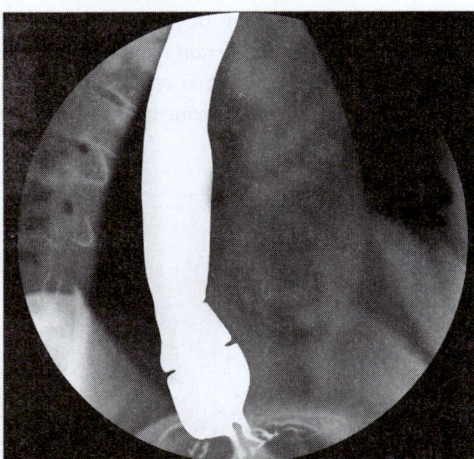

a. Apple core appearance
b. Schatzki's ring
c. Tapering of distal esophagus
d. Esophageal web

3. A 1-year-old child presents with failure to thrive and passage of bulky foul smelling stools. The image of intestinal biopsy and P. smear is suggestive of diagnosis of:

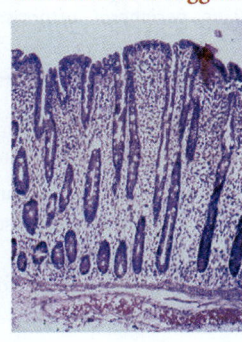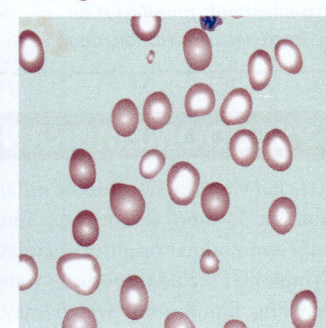

a. Celiac sprue
b. Bacterial overgrowth syndrome
c. Terminal ileitis
d. Crohn' disease

2. The following barium swallow shows presence of?

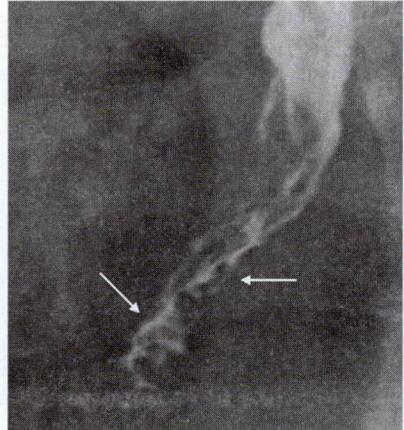

a. Eosinophilic esophagitis
b. Esophageal varices
c. Volcano ulcers in esophagus
d. Achalasia

4. A 45-year-old ulcerative colitis patient presents with a painful lesion on right leg. What is the diagnosis?

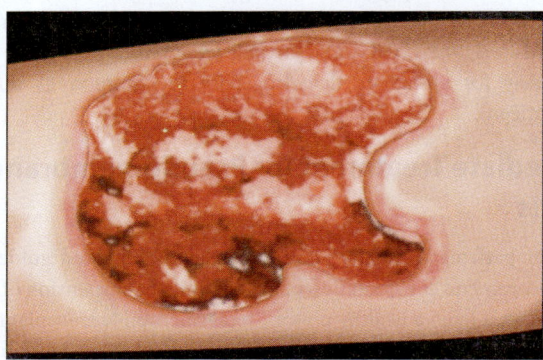

a. Pyoderma gangreosum
b. Febrile neutropenic dermatosis
c. Necrotizing fascitis
d. Granulomatosis with angitis

Answers of Image-Based Questions

1. **Ans. (b) Schatzki's ring**
   The image shows a Barium single contrast esophagoscopy showing indentation at lower part of Esophagus.

2. **Ans. (b) Esophageal varices**
   The image shows presence of worm-eaten appearance suggestive of esophageal varices. The classic textbook description is serpiginous thickening of folds, which appear as round, oval filling defects resembling beads of rosary. Point differentiating from malignancy of Esophagus is uniformity of the lesion.

3. **Ans. (a) Celiac sprue**
   - The image shows villous atrophy with flattening and peripheral smear shows microcytic hypochromic anemia suggestive of iron deficiency. This is likely in celiac sprue.
   - Choice B, C and D will affect terminal ileum and lead to vitamin B_{12} Deficiency. The peripheral smear will show macrocytes.

4. **Ans. (a) Pyoderma gangreosum**
   - The image shows an ulcer with granulation tissue in base in a patient of ulcerative colitis. This is diagnostic of pyoderma gangreosum. It is associated with inflammatory bowel disease, arthritis, and hematological malignancies.
   - Sweet syndrome will present with sudden onset of fever and erythematous, papular eruption. Patients have leucocytosis and skin biopsy shows a dense neutrophilic infiltrate.
   - Necrotizing fasciitis will usually not have any healing. It moves along the fascial planes and a deep crater is seen. It occurs due to mixed infection.

Multiple Choice Questions

Bleeding from GIT

1. The test shown below has been performed on a stool sample producing blue colour. Comment on the test being done. GIT/ bleeding from git *(Recent Question 2019)*

   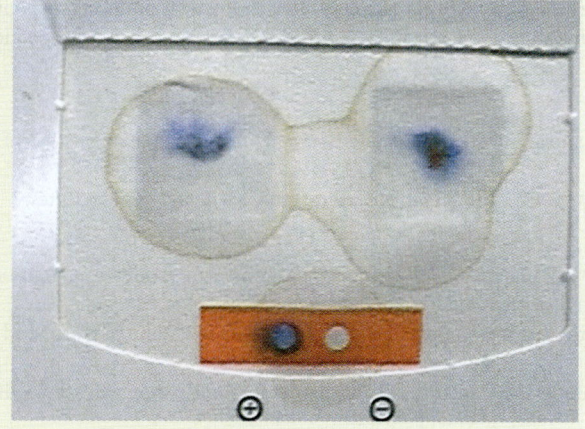

   a. Guaiac test
   b. Ehrlich test
   c. Fouchet's test
   d. Molisch test

2. Which is the most common site for chronic gastric ulcer?
   a. Lesser curvature at incisura *(Recent Pattern 2018)*
   b. High on lesser curvature
   c. Greater curvature
   d. Pre-pyloric

3. A patient presents with complaints of fever and abdominal distention. He is having history of bloody diarrhoea off and on for previous 6 months. X ray abdomen is shown below. What is the diagnosis? *(AIIMS May 2017)*

   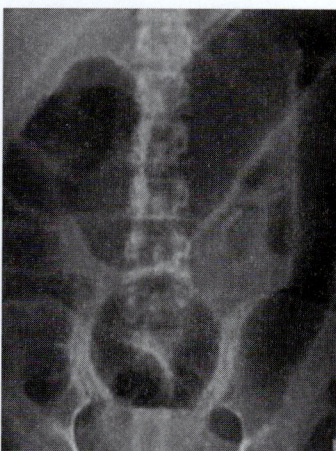

   a. Pneumatosis intestinalis
   b. Toxic megacolon
   c. Volvulus
   d. Intestinal perforation

4. All are true about persistent calibre artery except?
   a. Thermal coagulation *(Recent Question 2016-17)*
   b. Angiographic embolization
   c. Bleeds via pin point mucosal erosion
   d. Deep Enteroscopy

5. Among the following the least common cause of acute upper GI bleeding is? *(APPG 2015)*
   a. Mallory Weiss tear
   b. Ulcer
   c. Varices
   d. Vascular ectasia

6. 50 year old man became dizzy while passing stool and noticed fresh blood in stool. Previous stool examination for routine screening of carcinoma colon was normal. What is the most likely cause of bleed? *(AIIMS Nov 2014)*
   a. Early carcinoma colon
   b. Sigmoid diverticulitis
   c. Microscopic colitis
   d. Dilatation of veins of colon

7. Which indicates least chances of re-bleeding after hematemesis episode: *(Recent Pattern 2014-15)*
   a. Adherent clot on ulcer
   b. Clean based ulcer
   c. Gastric ulcer with AV malformation
   d. Visible bleeding vessel

8. Most common site of dieulafoys lesion is:
   a. Lesser curvature of stomach *(Recent Pattern 2015-16)*
   b. Greater curvature of stomach
   c. Pylorus
   d. Antrum

9. Most common cause of hematochezia in children?
   a. Rectal polyp *(Recent Pattern 2014-15)*
   b. Meckels diverticulum
   c. Necrotizing enterocolitis
   d. Acute gastritis

10. Rockall score is used for prognosis of patients of:
    a. Upper GI bleeding *(Recent Pattern 2014-15)*
    b. Lower GI bleeding
    c. Hepatic encephalopathy
    d. IBD

11. Massive bleeding per rectum in a 70 yr old patient is due to : *(AI 2010)*
    a. Diverticulitis
    b. Carcinoma colon
    c. Colitis
    d. Polyps

Diseases of Esophagus

12. Feline Oesophagus is seen in? *(Recent Pattern 2018)*
    a. GERD
    b. Stricture
    c. Eosinophilic esophagitis
    d. Radiation esophagitis

13. Which is the best investigation for Dysphagia Lusoria?
    a. Oesophageal manometry *(Recent Question 2016-17)*
    b. CT Scan
    c. Single contrast Barium swallow
    d. Digital CXR

14. Feline oesophagus is seen in? *(Recent Question 2016-17)*
    a. Eosinophilic esophagitis
    b. Schatzki ring
    c. GERD
    d. Herpes simplex esophagitis

15. Diffuse esophageal spasm is best diagnosed by? *(Bihar PG 2015)*
    a. Endoscopy
    b. Manometry
    c. Barium swallow
    d. CT

16. Diffuse oesophageal spasm treatment is?
    (JIPMER Nov 2015)
    a. Pneumatic dilatation   b. Oxybutynin
    c. Nitrates   d. Botulinum toxin

17. All of the following is true regarding G.E.R.D except?
    (JIPMER Nov 2014)
    a. Occurs during transient relaxation of L.E.S
    b. Can present with nocturnal cough
    c. Bicarbonate secreted by esophageal mucosa neutralizes the acid
    d. Normal esophageal mucosa on endoscopy excludes G.E.R.D

18. Incorrect about Zenkers diverticulum?
    (Recent Question 2015-16)
    a. Located in killian triangle
    b. Regurgitation of previous day food
    c. Premalignant
    d. Dysphagia

19. Identify the endoscopic image?   *(Recent Question 2017)*

    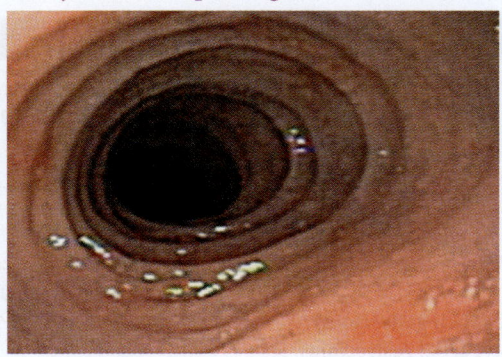

    a. Caustic burn
    b. Eosinophilic esophagitis
    c. Pseudomembranous Colitis
    d. Normal Esophagus

20. Gold standard test for achalasia cardia?   *(Recent 2015-16)*
    a. Esophageal manometry
    b. Barium swallow
    c. Endoscopy
    d. Endoscopic ultrasound

21. Which of the following is located in Laimer's triangle:
    a. Esophageal diverticulum   *(Recent Pattern 2014-15)*
    b. Colonic diverticulosis
    c. Meckel's diverticulum
    d. Peri-ampullary diverticulum

22. Esophageal tear is best detected with: *(Recent Pattern 2014-15)*
    a. CT   b. Angiography
    c. UGI endoscopy   d. Barium swallow

23. Most common complication of achalasia is:
    (Recent Pattern 2014-15)
    a. Recurrent pulmonary infections
    b. Stricture of esophagus
    c. Pleurisy
    d. Peptic ulcer

24. The most common cause of drug induced esophagitis is
    (Recent Pattern 2014-15)
    a. Metronidazole   b. Indomethacin
    c. Doxycyline   d. Steroids

25. Investigation of choice for dysphagia lusoria is?
    (Recent Pattern 2014-15)
    a. Barium studies   b. X-ray
    c. CT angiography   d. Esophageal manometry

26. Zenker's diverticulum presents with:
    (Recent Pattern 2014-15)
    a. Dysphonia   b. Reflux esophagitis
    c. Dysphagia   d. It is found in stomach

27. Which is true regarding Barrett's esophagus?
    (Recent Pattern 2014-15)
    a. Squamous metaplasia of lower esophagus
    b. Seen mainly in females
    c. Premalignant
    d. Responds to conservative management

28. Pseudoachalasia is seen with all except?
    (Recent Pattern 2014-15)
    a. Esophageal tumor   b. Paraneoplastic
    c. Carcinoma fundus   d. Rosary esophagus

29. Non progressive dysphagia in a lady with a sensation of something stuck in the throat and worsened by intake of cold drinks is suggestive of? *(Recent Pattern 2014-15)*
    a. Diffuse esophageal spasm
    b. Upper esophageal web
    c. Achalasia
    d. Scleroderma

30. Endoscopic mucosal resection in Barrett's esophagus results in: *(Recent Pattern 2014-15)*
    a. Stricture esophagus   b. Peptic ulceration
    c. Reflux esophagitis   d. Achalasia cardia

31. Which of the following staging is used for GERD?
    (Recent Pattern 2014-15)
    a. Ranson   b. Gleason
    c. Savary miller d. Hunter scale

32. Reflux esophagitis is defined as pH of esophagus to be less than: *(Recent Pattern 2014-15)*
    a. 1   b. 2
    c. 3   d. 4

33. Most common site of tear in Boerhaave syndrome:
    a. Lower end of oesophagus   *(Recent Pattern 2014-15)*
    b. At Gastroesophageal junction
    c. Upper esophagus
    d. Mild oesophagus

34. All of the following are correct statements regarding reflux esophagitis, except: *(Recent Pattern 2014-15)*
    a. Water brash   b. Weight gain
    c. Mediastinitis   d. Infant apnea

35. Most common site for iatrogenic rupture of esophagus:
    a. Cervical esophagus   *(Recent Pattern 2014-15)*
    b. Thoracic below aortic arch
    c. Thoracic above aortic arch
    d. Abdominal

36. All are true about Plummer-Vinson syndrome except:
    (Recent Pattern 2014-15)
    a. Esophageal webs
    b. Premalignant
    c. Common in elderly male
    d. Dysphagia

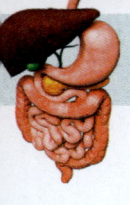

37. **True statement about a 6 cm Zenker's diverticulum is:**
    a. It is a true diverticulum *(Recent Pattern 2014-15)*
    b. Occurs in the mid oesophagus
    c. Treatment is CP myotomy
    d. It occurs in children

38. **A lady presented with non progressive dysphagia only for solids. Barium study showed proximal esophageal dilatation with distal constriction. The most likely diagnosis is.**
    (AI 2010)
    a. Peptic Stricture   b. Carcinoma Esophagus
    c. Achalasia Cardia   d. Lower Esophageal Ring

39. **Dysphagia lusoria is due to:** *(AIIMS Nov 03)*
    a. Oesophageal diverticulum
    b. Aneurysm of aorta
    c. Oesophageal web
    d. Compression by aberrant right subclavian artery

40. **Heller's operation is done for:** *(AIIMS Nov 93)*
    a. Achalasia cardia   b. Pyloric stenosis
    c. Peptic ulcer   d. CA Esophagus

41. **A male aged 60 years has foul breath; He regurgitates food that is eaten 3 days ago. A gurgling sound is often heard on swallowing : Likely diagnosis is:** *(AI 2001)*
    a. Zenker's diverticulum
    b. Meckel's diverticulum
    c. Scleroderma
    d. Achalasia cardia

42. **All of the following statements about Zenker's diverticulum are true Except:** *(AI 2009)*
    a. Acquired diverticulum
    b. Lateral X-rays on Barium swallow are often diagnostic
    c. False Diverticulum
    d. Out pouching of the anterior pharyngeal wall, just above the cricopharyngeus muscle

43. **Schatazki's ring is:** *(PGI Dec 98)*
    a. Mucosal ring at squamous columnar junction
    b. Muscular ring
    c. Dysphagia is the presenting symptom
    d. Inflammatory stricture

44. **Barret's esophagus is diagnosed by:** *(AIIMS Nov 06)*
    a. Squamous metaplasia
    b. Intestinal metaplasia
    c. Squamous dysplasia
    d. Intestinal dysplasia

45. **Barret's esophagus can lead to:** *(AIIMS June 98)*
    a. Stricture
    b. Reflux esophagitis
    c. Diffuse esophageal spasm
    d. Achalasia

46. **What is true regarding Barret's esophagus:** *(AIIMS Nov 94)*
    a. Seen in females
    b. Premalignant condition
    c. Responds to conservative management
    d. Squamous metaplasia is seen

47. **The most prevalent esophageal cancer world wide is:**
    a. Squamous cell cancer   *(AI 1991)*
    b. Adenocarcinoma
    c. Sarcoma
    d. Adenoid cystic carcinoma

48. **Hyperkeratosis of palm and sole is seen in:** *(AIIMS Dec 97)*
    a. Carcinoma colon   b. Hepatoma
    c. Adenocarcinoma lung d. Ca esophagus

49. **Adenocarcinoma of esophagus is commonly found in**
    a. Achlasia acardia   *(AI 1998)*
    b. Barret's oesophagus
    c. Plummer vinson syndrome
    d. Chronic smoking

50. **Best substitute of esophagus after esophagectomy is:**
    (AI 1996)
    a. Stomach   b. Jejunum
    c. Left colon   d. Right colon

51. **A patient on treatment with ketoconazole for a fungal disease develops Gastroesophageal Reflux Disease (GERD). Which of the following drugs should not be prescibed to him:** *(AI 2012)*
    a. Cisapride   b. Itopride
    c. Metoclopramide d. Domperidone

PUD and ZES

52. **Which is the best investigation for Metastatic Gastrinoma?**
    (Recent Question 2016-17)
    a. Selective arterial secretin injection
    b. Octreoscan
    c. MRI
    d. Endoscopic ultrasound

53. **What is the treatment of choice for Menetrier's disease?**
    (Recent Question 2016-17)
    a. Total gastrectomy
    b. Partial gastrectomy
    c. Cetuximab
    d. H_2 receptor antagonists

54. **Which of the following features are related to Zollinger Ellison syndrome?** *(UPSC 2015)*
    A. Aggressive and refractory peptic ulceration
    B. Unregulated gastrin release
    C. Beta islet cell tumor of pancreas
    D. Diarrhea present in upto 50% cases
    Select the correct answer using the code given below:
    a. A and B only   b. C and D
    c. A, B and C   d. A, B and D

55. **Consider the following statements with regard to duodenal ulcers?** *(UPSC 2015)*
    a. They occur most often in the second part of duodenum.
    b. Infection with H. pylori and NSAID–induced injury account for the majority of duodenal ulcers.
    c. Malignant duodenal ulcers are extremely rare.
    d. Eradication of H. pylori has greatly reduced the recurrence rates in duodenal ulcers.
    Which of the above statements is/are correct?
    a. A and C only   b. B, C and D only
    c. A, B and D only   d. A, B, C, and D

56. **Most sensitive test for diagnosis of H pylori?**
    a. Rapid urease test   *(JIPMER Nov 2014)*
    b. Demonstration of organism in gastric biopsy
    c. Breath urea test
    d. ELISA

57. **True about peptic ulcer:** *(PGI May 2015)*
    a. H. Pylori causes peptic ulcer
    b. Eradication therapy better than PPI therapy
    c. Eradication therapy also contain PPI
    d. Duodenum ulcer is more commonly associated with H. pylori than gastric ulcer
    e. Gastric ulcer is more commonly associated with H.pylori than duodenal ulcer

58. **H. pylori causes all except:** *(Recent Question 2015-16)*
    a. Peptic ulcer   b. Maltoma
    c. Carcinoid tumor   d. Gastric CA

59. **Prolonged intake of PPI does not cause** *(AIIMS Nov 14)*
    a. Hypothyroidism
    b. Pelvic fracture
    c. Clostridium difficile infection
    d. Increased community acquired pneumonia

60. **Bleeding from lesser curvature in gastric ulcer, source of bleeding is?** *(JIPMER 2014)*
    a. Right gastro-epiploic artery
    b. Right omento duodenal
    c. Pancreatoduodenal artery
    d. Left gastric artery

61. **Helicobacter pylori is associated with following except:**
    a. Type A gastritis   *(Recent Pattern 2014-15)*
    b. MALToma
    c. Gastric adenocarcinoma
    d. Hyperchlorhydria

62. **Eradication of infection by anti-H. pylori antibiotics is best determined by** *(Recent Pattern 2014-15)*
    a. S. ELISA   b. Breath urea test
    c. Rapid urease test   d. Biopsy

63. **A 60 year old male had a sudden fall in the toilet, his BP was 90/60 mm Hg and pulse was 100 per minute. His relatives reported that his stool was black/dark in color. Further careful history revealed that he is a known case of hypertension and coronary artery disease and was regularly taking aspirin, atenolol and sorbitrate. The most likely diagnosis is?** *(AIIMS May 2012)*
    a. Gastric ulcer with bleeding
    b. Acute myocardial infarction with cardiogenic shock
    c. Acute CVA
    d. Pulmonary embolism

64. **H. pylori causes:** *(Recent Pattern 2014-15)*
    a. Type A gastritis   b. Type B gastritis
    c. Autoimmune   d. Allergic gastritis

65. **A 70-year-old male patient presented to the emergency department with pain in epigastrium and difficulty in breathing for 6 hours. On examination, his heart rate was 56 per minute and the blood pressure was 106/60 mm Hg. Chest examination was normal. The patient has been taking omeprazole for gastroesophageal reflux disease for last 6 months. What should be the initial investigation:**
    a. An ECG   *(Recent Pattern 2014-15)*
    b. An upper GI endoscopy
    c. Urgent ultrasound of the abdomen
    d. An X-ray chest

66. **Which drug is not effective against H. pylori?** *(Recent Pattern 2014-15)*
    a. Colloidal bismuth   b. Metronidazole
    c. Amoxycilline   d. Erythromycin

67. **All of the following are indications for surgery in a case of duodenal ulcer except:** *(Recent Pattern 2014-15)*
    a. Acute perforation of ulcer   b. Pyloric stenosis
    c. Massive haemorrhage   d. Multiple large ulcers

68. **True about dumping syndrome is all except:**
    a. Caused by early emptying of stomach
    b. Medically managed   *(Recent Pattern 2014-15)*
    c. Controlled by small diets
    d. Needs re-surgery

69. **A 50-year-old lady presented with history of pain upper abdomen, nausea and decreased appetite for 5 days. She had undergone cholecystectomy 2 years back. Her bilirubin was 10 mg/dl, SCOT 900 IU/L, SGPT 700 IU/L and serum alkaline phosphatase was 280 IU/L. What is the most likely diagnosis?** *(AIPG 2011)*
    a. Acute pancreatitis
    b. Acute cholangitis
    c. Acute viral hepatitis
    d. Posterior penetration of peptic ulcer

70. **Which of the following statements about peptic ulcer disease is true?** *(Recent Pattern 2014-15)*
    a. Helicobacter pylori eradication increases the likelihood of occurrences of complication
    b. The incidence of complication has remained unchanged
    c. The incidence of Helicobacter pylori infection in India is very low
    d. Helicobacter pylori eradication does not alter the recurrence ratio

71. **Consider the following feature with reference to Zollinger Ellison syndrome:** *(Recent Pattern 2014-15)*
    1. Intractable peptic ulceration
    2. Secretory diarrhea
    3. Most common site is pancreas
    Which of these features are present in Zollinger-Ellison Syndrome
    a. 1 and 3   b. 2 and 3
    c. 1,2 and 3   d. 1 and 2

72. **Most common site of peptic ulcer:** *(Recent Pattern 2014-15)*
    a. 1st part of duodenum
    b. 2nd part of duodenum
    c. Antrum
    d. Terminal ileum

73. **All of the following are true regarding a patient with acid peptic disease except:** *(Recent Pattern 2014-15)*
    a. Misoprostol can prevent NSAID induced gastric injury
    b. DU is preventable by the use of night time H_2 blockers
    c. Omeprazole may help ulcers refractory to H_2 blockers
    d. Misoprostol is DOC in a pregnant lady

74. **Most common site of type 1 gastric ulcer:** *(Recent Pattern 2014-15)*
    a. Gastric body   b. Antrum
    c. Pylorus   d. Cardia

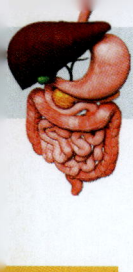

75. **Phlegmonous gastritis occurs due to:**
    (Recent Pattern 2014-15)
    a. H. pylori b. E. coli
    c. Drugs d. Reflux of acid
76. **Increased gastrin is seen in:** *(Recent Pattern 2014-15)*
    a. Zollinger-Ellison syndrome
    b. Iron deficiency anaemia
    c. Duodenal ulcer
    d. Gastric cancer
77. **Disabling paraumbilical pain within 10 minutes of eating food with history of weight loss. Past history is positive for Myocardial infarction in last year indicates.** *(New pattern)*
    a. Gastric ulcer
    b. Duodenal ulcer
    c. Abdominal angina
    d. Acute cholecytitis with stone impaction
78. **The most common complication of vagotomy is:**
    (Recent Pattern 2014-15)
    a. Diarrhoea b. Dryness of mouth
    c. Tachycardia d. Bleaching
79. **Most common viral cause of gastritis**
    (Recent Pattern 2014-15)
    a. H. Pylori b. CMV
    c. Hepatitis A d. Enterovirus
80. **Erosive gastritis commonly occurs at:**
    (Recent Pattern 2014-15)
    a. Cardia b. Fundus
    c. Greater curvature d. Antrum
81. **MC age of presentation of gastric ulcer is:**
    (Recent Pattern 2014-15)
    a. 3rd decade b. 4th decade
    c. 5th decade d. 6th decade
82. **Which of the following have hypergastrinemia with decrease acid output?** *(Recent Pattern 2014-15)*
    a. Peptic ulcer disease b. ZES
    c. G-cell hyperplasia d. Pernicious anemia
83. **Which one of the following is best for localization of Zollinger-Ellison syndrome?** *(Recent Pattern 2014-15)*
    a. EUS (Endoscopic ultrasound)
    b. Secretin injection test
    c. MRI
    d. Basal gastric acid output
84. **Not true in type A fundal gastritis is:**
    a. Low gastric PH *(Recent Pattern 2014-15)*
    b. Hyperchlorhydria
    c. Antibody against parietal cells and presence of autoimmunity
    d. Antibody against intrinsic factor
85. **Dumping syndrome is due to all except:**
    a. Motilin *(Recent Pattern 2014-15)*
    b. Small stomach
    c. Hypertonic fluid contents in bowel
    d. Neurotensin
86. **H. pylori is known to cause all of the following except:**
    (AI 1999)
    a. Gastric ulcer b. Duodenal ulcer
    c. Gastric lymphoma d. Fundal atrophic gastritis

87. **A patient with H. Pylori infection is treated with drugs. The best method to detect presence of residual H.pylori infection in this person is:** *(AI 2007)*
    a. Rapid urease test b. Urea breath test
    c. Endoscopy and biopsy d. Serum anti H.pylori titre
88. **Common sites for Cushing ulcers include all of the following except:** *(AI 1999)*
    a. Esophagus b. Stomach
    c. 1st part of duodenum d. Distal duodenum
89. **Commonest site of peptic ulcer is:** *(AI 1999)*
    a. Ist part of Duodenum
    b. IInd part of duodenum
    c. Distal 1/3 of stomach
    d. Pylorus of the stomach
90. **Artery to bleed in duodenal ulcer haemorrhage:**
    a. Splenic artery *(PGI Dec 2000)*
    b. Gastroduodenal artery
    c. Left gastric artery
    d. Superior mesenteric artery
91. **Dumping syndrome is due to:** *(AI 1999)*
    a. Diarrhoea
    b. Presence of hypertonic content in small intestine
    c. Vagotomy
    d. Reduced gastric capacity
92. **The best prognosis in carcinoma stomach is with:** *(AI 1995)*
    a. Superficial spreading type b. Ulcerative type
    c. Linitis plastica type d. Polyp
93. **All are true regarding Zollinger Ellison syndrome, except:**
    a. Diarrhoea *(AIIMS Dec 97)*
    b. Recurrence after operation
    c. Hypergastrinemia
    d. Decreased ratio of BAO to MAO
94. **Hypergastrinemia with hypochlorhydria is seen in:**
    a. Zollinger Ellison Syndrome
    b. VIPoma
    c. Pernicious anemia
    d. Glucagonoma

Inflammatory Bowel Disease

95. **What is the earliest radiological finding of ulcerative colitis on single contrast barium enema?**
    (Recent Question 2016-17)
    a. Loss of haustrations
    b. Fine mucosal granularity
    c. Pipe stem colon
    d. Collar button ulcer
96. **Treatment of Crohn's disease includes:** *(PGI May 2015)*
    a. Steroid b. 5-A.S.A
    c. Azathioprine d. Beta interferon
    e. Infliximab
97. **DOC of acute exacerbation of ulcerative colitis?**
    a. Sulfasalazine b. Steroids *(Recent 2015-16)*
    c. Infliximab d. Cyclosporine
98. **All are complications of ulcerative colitis, except:**
    (Recent Pattern 2014-15)
    a. Haemorrhage b. Stricture
    c. Malignant change d. Fistula

99. Best screening test for Crohn's disease is:
    a. A.S.C.A *(Recent Pattern 2014-15)*
    b. P-ANCA
    c. Fecal alpha 1 anti-trypsin
    d. Fecal calprotectin
100. A 41-year-old male patient presented with recurrent episodes of bloody diarrhea for 5 years. Despite regular treatment with adequate doses of sulfasalazine, he has had several exacerbations of his disease and required several weeks of steroids for the control of flares. What should be the next line of treatment for him?
    (Recent Pattern 2014-15)
    a. Methotrexate   b. Azathioprine
    c. Cyclosporine   d. Cyclophosphamide
101. Invariably involved site in ulcerative colitis:
    (Recent Pattern 2014-15)
    a. Sigmoid colon   b. Transverse colon
    c. Ileum   d. Rectum
102. Treatment of choice in intractable ulcerative colitis:
    (Recent Pattern 2014-15)
    a. Mucosal proctectomy + Ileoanal pouch anastomosis
    b. Proctectomy
    c. Colectomy with ileostomy
    d. Ileorectal anastomosis
103. Treatment of choice in ulcerative colitis is:
    (Recent Pattern 2014-15)
    a. 5 aminosalicylic acid   b. Azathioprine
    c. Metronidazole   d. Salicylates
104. Best treatment of refractory peri-anal fistula in crohn's disease: *(Recent Pattern 2014-15)*
    a. Fistulectomy   b. Infliximab
    c. Olasalazine   d. Mesalamine
105. Which of the following is the established biological therapy for Crohn's disease? *(Recent Pattern 2014-15)*
    a. Anti TNF α-antibody   b. IL-1 antagonist
    c. IL-6 antagonist   d. IL-8 antagonist
106. All are true about ulcerative colitis *except*:
    (Recent Pattern 2014-15)
    a. Smoking may prevent the disease
    b. 1:1 male female ratio
    c. Presents with bloody diarrhea
    d. Highly Associated with infertility
107. A highly sensitive and specific marker for detecting intestinal inflammation in ulcerative colitis is?
    (APPG 2014)
    a. CRP   b. Fecal lactoferrin
    c. Fecal calprotectin   d. Leukocytosis
108. Ulcterative colitis associated features include all, *except*:
    (Recent Pattern 2014-15)
    a. Iritis   b. Arthritis
    c. Urethritis   d. Pyoderma
109. Chronic inflammatory bowel disease is associated with:
    a. Chronic hepatitis   *(Recent Pattern 2014-15)*
    b. Fibrosis
    c. Cholangiosarcoma
    d. Primary sclerosing cholangitis
110. Skip granulomatous lesions are seen in: *(AI 1996)*
    a. Ulcerative colitis   b. Crohn's disease
    c. Whipple's disease   d. Reiter's disease

Premalignant Lesions of GIT

111. A 25 year old man has pigmented macules over the palms, soles and oral mucosa. He also has anemia and abdominal pain. Which one of the following is the most likely diagnosis? *(APPG 2015)*
    a. Cushing's syndrome
    b. Albright's syndrome
    c. Peutz-Jegher's Syndrome
    d. Incontinentia pigmenti
112. Not a pre-malignant lesion? *(AIIMS Nov 2014)*
    a. Peutz Jeghers
    b. Crohns disease
    c. Ulcerative colitis
    d. Barret esophagus
113. Mutation of STK 11 and LKB1 gene is associated with?
    a. Familial Adenomatous Polyposis   *(JIPMER 2014)*
    b. Hereditary nonpolyposis colorectal cancer
    c. Peutz – Jeghers syndrome
    d. Neurofibromatosis
114. Strong correlation with colorectal cancer is seen in:
    (AI 2003)
    a. Peutz-Jegher's polyp   b. Familial polyposis coli.
    c. Juvenile polyposis   d. Hyperplastic polyp.
115. In Peutz-Jeghers syndrome, polyps are seen in *(AI 1995)*
    a. Colon   b. Rectum
    c. Small bowel   d. Stomach
116. A girl presents with complaints of malena. On examination there are pigmented lesions involving her mouth and lips. Two of her sisters also had similar complaints. Which of the following is the most probable diagnosis:
    a. Cronkhite Canada syndrome   *(AIIMS Nov 2000)*
    b. Puetz Jagher's syndrome
    c. Gardner's syndrome
    d. Turcot's syndrome

Diarrhea

117. A known HIV positive patient on cART presents with diarrhea of 6months duration. Stoll microscopy shows cysts of 10-30um and kinyoun stain positive. What is the probable diagnosis? *(AIIMS May 2018)*

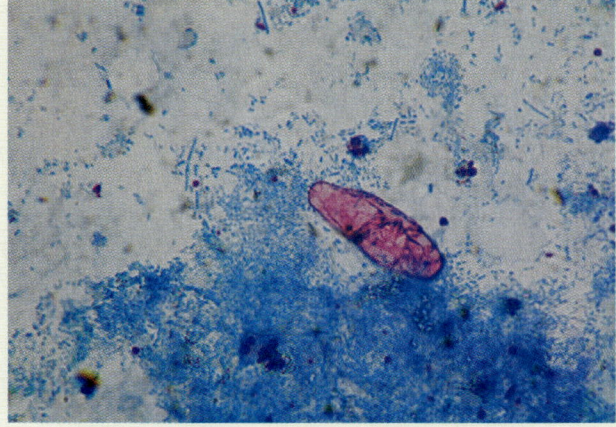

    a. Cystoisospora   b. Cryptosporidium
    c. Balantidium Coli   d. Strongyloides

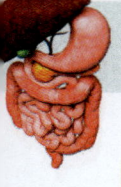

118. A 22-year old presents with diarrhea and intolerance to dairy products. On investigation he was found to have lactase deficiency. Agent least likely to cause lactose intolerance among these is? *(AIIMS May 2018)*
    a. Condensed milk
    b. Skimmed milk
    c. Yoghurt
    d. Ice cream

119. In a hospitalized patient on multiple antibiotics with diarrhea, the best method of diagnosis for Clostridium difficile infection is? *(AIIMS Nov 2017)*
    a. Pure strain isolation from culture
    b. Immunofluorescence
    c. Toxin detection by ELISA
    d. Toxin detection by NAAT

120. All are features of bile acid diarrhoea except?
    (Recent Question 2016-17)
    a. Fecal bile acid excretion increased
    b. Mild Steatorrhea
    c. Responds to low fat diet
    d. Responds to cholestyramine

121. All are diagnostic criteria for irritable bowel syndrome except? *(Recent Question 2016-17)*
    a. Pain improves with defecation
    b. Nocturnal episodes of colicky pain
    c. Onset associated with change in frequency of stool
    d. Onset associated with change in appearance/form of stool

122. Most common cause for diarrhoea in adults associated with intake of Shell fish? *(AIIMS Nov 2015)*
    a. Norovirus
    b. Calcivirus
    c. Rotavirus
    d. Filovirus

123. Which diarrhea decreases after prolonged fasting?
    a. Osmotic diarrhea
    b. Bloody *(Recent 2015-16)*
    c. Infective
    d. Secretory

124. A patient with chronic diarrhoea with abnormal D-xylose & Schilling test. What could be the diagnosis:
    a. Chronic pancreatitis *(Recent Pattern 2014-15)*
    b. Bacterial overgrowth syndrome
    c. Coeliac disease
    d. Gastric disease

125. Diabetes induced diarrhea is best managed by which of the following? *(Recent Pattern 2014-15)*
    a. Clonidine
    b. Octreotide
    c. Levosulpiride
    d. Clindinium

126. Patient with congenital lactose deficiency will experience distension, flatulence and diarrhea on ingestion of:
    (Recent Pattern 2014-15)
    a. Glucose
    b. Sucrose
    c. Milk
    d. Eggs

127. All cause diarrhea except? *(Recent Pattern 2014-15)*
    a. Diabetes
    b. Hypercalcemia
    c. Hyperthyroidism
    d. Irritable bowel syndrome

128. 30 year male with chronic diarrhoea, anemia. Most likely associated with: *(AIIMS May 07)*
    a. Antimitochondrial antibody
    b. Anti-endomysial antibody
    c. Anti-smooth muscle antibody
    d. Antinuclear antibody

Malabsorption Syndrome

129. Which test is recommended for this patient?
    (Recent Question 2019)

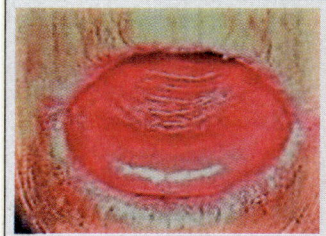 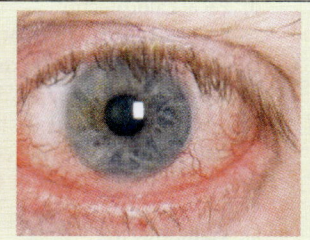

    a. Anti-endothelial cell antibodies
    b. Anti-endomysial antibodies
    c. RBC glutathione reductase levels
    d. Serum methylmalonic acid levels

130. Which is the most important complication of celiac sprue?
    (Recent Question 2016-17)
    a. Intestinal neoplasms
    b. Diabetes mellitus
    c. Dermatitis herpetiformis
    d. Bile acid diarrhea

131. The following conditions can cause protein-losing enteropathy except? *(UPSC 2015)*
    a. Ulcerative colitis
    b. Irritable bowel syndrome
    c. Celiac disease
    d. Lymphoma

132. The following tests can be used for diagnosing celiac disease except: *(UPSC 2015)*
    a. Anti-gliadin antibodies
    b. Anti-nuclear antibodies
    c. Anti-endomysial antibodies
    d. Anti-tissue transglutaminase antibodies

133. Which cereal is not to be given in celiac sprue?
    (Recent Question 2015-16)
    a. Wheat
    b. Maize
    c. Corn
    d. Rice

134. Malabsorption syndrome features include all, except:
    (Recent Pattern 2014-15)
    a. Anaemia
    b. Constipation
    c. Tetany
    d. Steatorrhoea

135. Anti-T.T.G antibodies are seen in: *(Recent Pattern 2014-15)*
    a. Giardia malabsorption
    b. Gluten enteropathy
    c. Lactose deficient
    d. Bile acid malabsorption

136. A 41-year-old patient presented with chronic diarrhea for 3 months. A D-xylose absorption test was order to look for:
    (Recent Pattern 2014-15)
    a. Carbohydrate malabsorption due to mucosal disease
    b. Carbohydrate malabsorption due to chronic pancreatitis
    c. Fat malabsorption due to mucosal disease
    d. Fat malabsorption due to chronic pancreatitis

137. Xylose absorption test is used to assess:
    a. Insulinoma *(Recent Pattern 2014-15)*
    b. Atypical carcinoid
    c. ZES
    d. Monosaccharide absorption

138. Protein losing enteropathy is characterized by all *except*: *(Recent Pattern 2014-15)*
    a. Decreased serum albumin and globulin
    b. Increased lymphatic flow
    c. 99mTc-dextran radionuclide study done
    d. Lymphangiectasia on biopsy
139. Alpha 1 anti-tryspin in stool is indicative of?
    a. Protein losing enteropathy *(Recent Pattern 2014-15)*
    b. Chronic pancreatitis
    c. Acute pancreatitis
    d. Whipple disease
140. Jejunal biopsy is diagnostic in: *(Recent Pattern 2014-15)*
    a. Coeliac sprue   b. Tropical sprue
    c. Whipple's disease   d. Radiation enteritis
141. True about tropical sprue are A/E: *(Recent Pattern 2014-15)*
    a. Protein losing enteropathy
    b. Steatorrhea
    c. Stomatitis
    d. Jejunal biopsy is specific
142. A 30-year-old lady presents with features of malabsorption and iron deficiency anaemia. Duodenal biopsy shows complete villous atrophy. Probable diagnosis is:
    a. Antiendomysial antibodies *(Recent Pattern 2014-15)*
    b. Anti-goblet cell antibodies
    c. Anti-Saccharomyces cerevisae antibodies
    d. Antineutrophil cytoplasmic antibodies
143. Jejunal biopsy is diagnostic in: *(Recent Pattern 2014-15)*
    a. Abetalipoproteinemia
    b. Giardiasis
    c. Tropical sprue
    d. Celiac sprue
144. Most common cause of malabsorption in our country is: *(Recent Pattern 2014-15)*
    a. Intestinal surgery   b. Gastric surgery
    c. Sprue   d. Intestinal parasite
145. Which of the finding is not a usual feature of Crohn's disease? *(Recent Pattern 2014-15)*
    a. Granulomas   b. Pseudopolyps
    c. Skip lesion   d. Right colon predominance
146. In celiac sprue there is a deficiency of all *except*: *(Recent Pattern 2014-15)*
    a. Vitamin A   b. Vitamin B_{12}
    c. Folic acid   d. Iron
147. Not included in armamentarium of tests for malabsorption syndrome *(AIIMS May 2013)*
    a. D- Xylose
    b. 14C Triolein breath test
    c. 13 C Trioctanoin breath test
    d. 13 C Triclosan breath test
148. Malabsorption syndrome does not result from:
    a. Parasite infestation   *(Recent Pattern 2014-15)*
    b. Small bowel diverticulae
    c. Post-gastrectomy
    d. Anterior resection of colon
149. Non-tropical sprue is characterized by:
    a. Elongation of intestinal villi *(Recent Pattern 2014-15)*
    b. Currant jelly stools
    c. Hypertriglyceridemia
    d. Poor absorption of lipids

150. Positive D – xylose test indicates all of the following, Except: *(AI 1992)*
    a. Pancreatic insufficiency
    b. Small intestinal mucosal disease
    c. Impaired carbohydrate absorption in small intestine
    d. Malabsorption
151. Best test for Small intestine malabsorption of carbohydrates is : *(AI 1997)*
    a. Lund meal test   b. Shilling test
    c. D-Xylose test   d. Follacin test
152. Which of the following statements about Schilling's test are true: *(PGI 2009)*
    a. Abnormal in pernicious anemia
    b. Normal in bacterial overgrowth syndrome
    c. Abnormal in ileal disease
    d. Normal in chronic pancreatitis
153. In which of the following conditions of malabsorption, an intestinal biopsy is diagnostic-: *(AIIMS May 05)*
    a. Celiac disease   b. Tropical sprue
    c. Whipple's disease   d. Lactose intolerance
154. Most common CNS manifestation of Whipple's disease is :
    a. Cerebellar ataxia   *(AI 1999)*
    b. Supranuclear ophthalmoplegia
    c. Seizure
    d. Dementia
155. Which of the following parasitic infestation can lead to malabsorption syndrome? *(AI 06)*
    a. Amoebiasis   b. Ascariasis
    c. Hookworm infestation   d. Giardiasis

Pediatric Gastroenterology

156. Consider the following: *(UPSC 2015)*
    a. Visible gastric peristalsis b. Bilious vomiting
    c. Palpable mass   d. Melena
    Which of the above is/are the feature/features of infantile hypertrophic pyloric stenosis?
    a. A, B and C   b. A and C only
    c. B and D   d. D only
157. A Term neonate with respiratory distress since birth. The CXR shows?

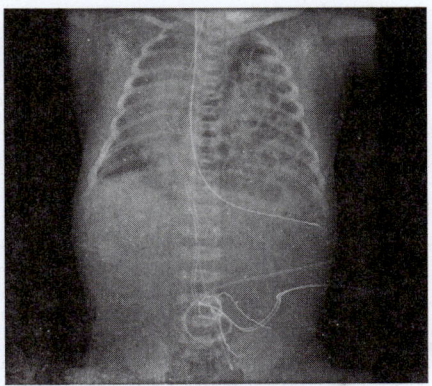

    a. Congenital diaphragmatic hernia
    b. Meconium aspiration syndrome
    c. Transient Tachypnea of New-born
    d. Pulmonary alveolar proteinosis

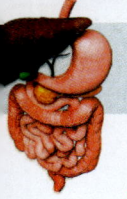

158. A neonate has been diagnosed with necrotizing enterocolitis with X ray abdomen showing gas in the portal vein. The correct staging of the patient is? *(Recent Pattern 2014-15)*
    a. Stage 1 b. Stage 2 A
    c. Stage 2 B d. Stage 3

159. Exposure to which of the following drugs is incriminated in IHPS (infantile hypertrophic pyloric stenosis): *(Recent Pattern 2014-15)*
    a. Erythromycin b. Lithium
    c. Warfarin d. Carbimazole

160. In a case of hypertrophic pyloric stenosis, the metabolic disturbance is *(AI 2002)*
    a. Respiratory alkalosis
    b. Metabolic acidosis
    c. Metabolic alkalosis with paradoxical aciduria
    d. Metabolic alkalosis with alkaline urine

MALT-oma

161. All of the following are true regarding primary gastric lymphoma, except? *(APPG 2016)*
    a. H.pylori is implicated especially in MALT type
    b. More amenable to treatment than gastric adenocarcinoma
    c. Mostly of B cell origin
    d. Can be easily differentiated clinically from gastric adenocarcinoma by the presence of early satiety and prominent lymph node metastases

162. Which is the most common site of MALT? *(AIIMS Nov 2014)*
    a. Stomach b. Ileum
    c. Duodenum d. Jejunum

163. What is wrong about GIST? *(AIIMS Nov 2014)*
    a. Originate from Cajal cells
    b. Common mesenchymal tumor of GIT
    c. Prognosis depends on size
    d. Associated with 'alk' mutation

Miscellaneous

164. Correct procedure of inserting the following equipment is? *(AIIMS May 2018)*

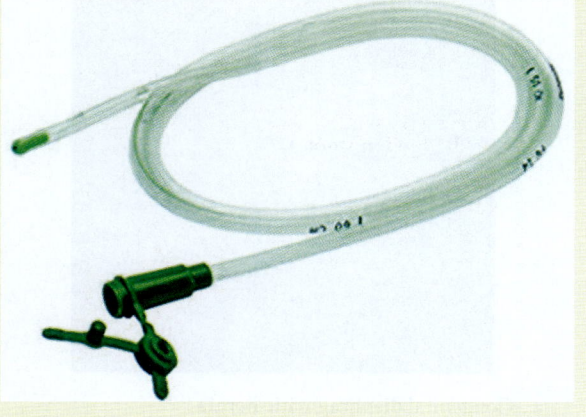

    a. Supine with neck flexed b. Supine with neck extended
    c. Sitting with neck flexed d. Sitting with neck extended

165. Which is the most common cause of chronic pancreatitis? *(Recent Pattern 2018)*
    a. Gall stones b. Alcohol
    c. Trauma d. E.R.C.P

166. Which of these has the highest sensitivity for detection of acute appendicitis? *(Recent Question 2016-17)*
    a. CT
    b. USG
    c. Barium meal follow through
    d. X ray Abdomen

167. Which one of the following statements is TRUE regarding Clostridium difficile diarrhoea? *(APPG 2016)*
    a. Penicillin / beta lactamase inhibitor combinations are currently the most commonly implicated drugs
    b. IV vancomycin is ineffective in the treatment of Clostridium difficile diarrhoea
    c. Grossly bloody diarrhoea with odorless stools and a normal leukocyte count is a characteristic feature
    d. Pseudo-membranes are characteristically present in the mucosa of the entire small intestine with duodenal sparing in 10% of patients

168. Carcinoid tumors commonly arise from? *(UPSC 2015)*
    a. G cells in pancreas
    b. Argentaffin cells of small intestine
    c. Pancreatic endocrine tumor
    d. Colon polyps

169. Which one on the following is the most likely diagnosis from this x-ray? *(APPG 2015)*

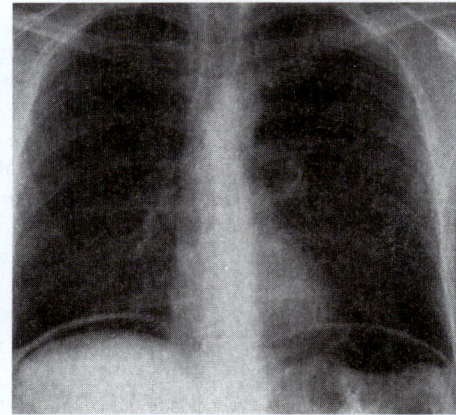

    a. Hydatid cyst right lung
    b. Right pleural effusion
    c. Right hydropneumothorax
    d. Perforated abdominal viscous

170. Which of the following is not associated with pancreatitis? *(JIPMER Nov 2014)*
    a. Raised serum amylase b. Raised serum lipase
    c. Hypocalcemia d. Hypoglycemia

171. A 45 year old male is brought to casualty after a night party with complaints of epigastric pain, penetrating towards back. Which is the best for diagnosis? *(Recent Question 2015-16)*
    a. Serum lipase b. CPK-MB
    c. ALP d. Gamma- GGT

172. Which of the following is seen on the image?
 (Recent Question 2015-16)

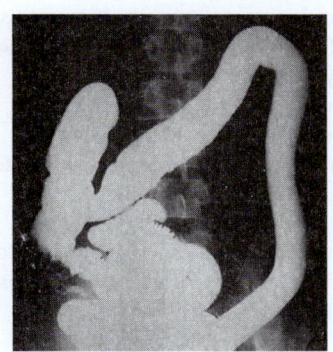

   a. Barium enema: Pipe stem colon
   b. Double contrast enema: apple core appearance
   c. Barium enema: Pseudo-polyps
   d. Double contrast enema: Thumb printing sign

173. Which of the following is the most probable diagnosis of this X ray abdomen? (Recent Question 2015-16)

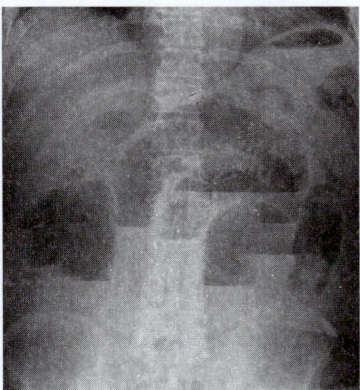

   a. Gas under diaphragm- peritonitis
   b. Multiple air fluid level- adhesions and bands
   c. Bird beak – volvulus
   d. Normal X ray PA view

174. Diagnosis: (Recent Question 2015-16)

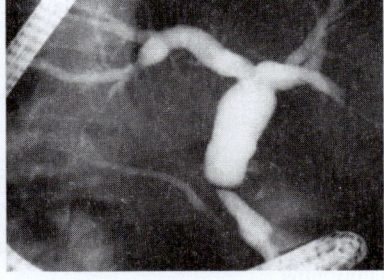

   a. CBD dilatation on ERCP
   b. CBD dilatation on PTC
   c. Cystic duct dilation on ERCP
   d. Cystic duct ectasia on ERCP

175. Traveler diarrhea is caused by? (Recent Question 2015-16)
   a. Campylobacter
   b. Aeromonas
   c. Actinobacillus
   d. Cryptosporidium

176. Aspirin is given for treatment of which cancer:
 (Recent Question 2015-16)
   a. Pancreatic cancer   b. Liver cancer
   c. Colon cancer   d. Stomach cancer

177. The following X Ray is suggestive of diagnosis of?

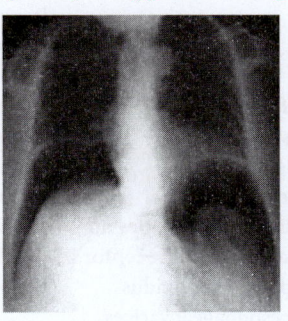

   a. Emphysema   b. Pneumoperitoneum
   c. Pneumo-mediastinum   d. Left sided Pneumothorax

178. Short bowel syndrome after extensive resection of intestine is mostly due to: (Recent Pattern 2014-15)
   a. Mesenteric artery occlusion
   b. Midgut volvulus
   c. Extensive Crohn's disease
   d. Inferior mesenteric vein occlusion

179. True in Menetrier's disease are A/E:
 (Recent Pattern 2014-15)
   a. Rugosities fold hypertrophy
   b. Foveolar hyperplasia
   c. Protein losing gastrophy
   d. Hyperchlorhydria

180. Paralytic ileus occurs in: (Recent Pattern 2014-15)
   a. Hypokalaemia   b. Hypomagnaesemia
   c. Hypocalcaemia   d. All of the above

181. Anti-diabetic drug causing hemorrhagic pancreatitis:
 (Recent Pattern 2014-15)
   a. Exenatide   b. Sitagliptin
   c. Saxagliptin   d. Canagliflozin

182. A 5 year child with history of barefoot walking and open air defecation presents with anemia and swelling around eyes. Which of the following infestation is most likely to be present. (AIIMS MAY 2014)
   a. Round worm   b. Hook worm
   c. Pin worm   d. Whip worm

183. Gastric mucosa in Meckel's diverticulum is diagnosed by:
 (Recent Pattern 2014-15)
   a. Endoscopy
   b. Occult blood in stool
   c. Technetium isotope scan
   d. Barium studies

184. All of the following are true regarding Acute pancreatitis except: (Recent Pattern 2014-15)
   a. Elevated serum amylase
   b. Alcoholics are more prone
   c. Ranson score is used to grade severity
   d. Raised serum calcium

185. Triple A syndrome is all except? (Recent Pattern 2014-15)
   a. Alacrymia   b. Addison disease
   c. Achlorhydria   d. Achalasia

186. **72 hour prolonged fasting test is used for?**
 (Recent Pattern 2014-15)
 a. Fat absorption
 b. Insulinoma
 c. Carbohydrate absorption
 d. Amino acid absorption

187. **Not a hormone causing early dumping?**
 (Recent Pattern 2014-15)
 a. VIP
 b. Neurotensin
 c. Motilin
 d. CCK

188. **Which of the following is/are associated with pancreatic exocrine insufficiency:** *(Recent Pattern 2014-15)*
 a. Hypertriglyceridemia
 b. Enterokinase deficiency
 c. Malabsorption
 d. All of the above

189. **A vasopressin analogue does not produce therapeutic effect through vasopressin V_2 receptor in which of the following**
 a. Central diabetes insipidus *(Recent Pattern 2014-15)*
 b. Bleeding esophageal varices
 c. Type I von Willebrand's disease
 d. Primary nocturnal enuresis.

190. **The area of colon which is least visualized by barium studies:** *(Recent Pattern 2014-15)*
 a. Sigmoid
 b. Hepatic flexure
 c. Splenic flexure
 d. Cecum

191. **A 25-year-old farmer presented with history of high grade fever for 7 days and altered sensorium for 2 days. On examination, he was comatosed and had conjunctival hemorrhage. Urgent investigations showed a hemoglobin of 11 gm/dl, serum bilirubin 8 mg/dl and urea 78 mg/dl. Peripheral blood smear was negative for malarial parasite. What is the most likely diagnosis?** *(Recent Pattern 2014-15)*
 a. Brucellosis
 b. Weil's disease
 c. Acute viral hepatitis
 d. Q fever

192. **A 25-year-old woman presents with recurrent abdominal pain and anemia. Peripheral blood smear shows basophilic stippling of the red blood cells. What is the most likely diagnosis?** *(Recent Pattern 2014-15)*
 a. Coeliac disease
 b. Hookworm infestation
 c. Sickle cell disease
 d. Lead poisoning

193. **A patient presents with lower gastrointestinal bleed. Sigmoidoscopy shows ulcers in the sigmoid. Biopsy from this area shows flask-shaped ulcers. Which of the following is the most appropriate treatment:** *(Recent Pattern 2014-15)*
 a. Intravenous ceftriaxone
 b. Intravenous metronidazole
 c. Intravenous steroids and sulphasalazine
 d. Hydrocortisone enemas

194. **Which of the following excludes a diagnosis of irritable bowel syndrome:** *(Recent Pattern 2014-15)*
 a. Relieved by defaecation
 b. Straining during stool passage
 c. Passage of blood per rectum
 d. Change of stool form

195. **Amongst the following, the most common site for Leiomyoma is** *(AI 1994)*
 a. Stomach
 b. Small Intestine
 c. Duodenum
 d. Colon

196. **Serum amylase level is raised in all except:** *(PGI June 98)*
 a. Blocked salivary duct
 b. Ruptured ectopic
 c. Appendicitis
 d. Pancreatitis

197. **Which of the following vitamin deficiencies is most commonly seen in short bowel syndrome:** *(AI 2012)*
 a. Vitamin B_{12}
 b. Biotin
 c. Vitamin B_1
 d. Vitamin K

198. **Which of the following features are associated with Irritable Bowel Syndrome:** *(AI 1992)*
 a. Weight loss
 b. Anorexia
 c. Abdominal distension
 d. Blood in stool

199. **Investigation of choice for invasive amebiasis is:** *(AI 02)*
 a. Indirect heamagglutination
 b. ELISA
 c. Counter immune electrophoresis
 d. Microscopy

200. **Most important prognostic factor for colorectal carcinoma is :** *(AI 2009)*
 a. Site of lesion
 b. Stage of lesion
 c. Age of patient
 d. Lymph node status

201. **All the following are causes of Acute Pancreatitis except:** *(AI 1994)*
 a. Gall stones
 b. Alcohol
 c. Hemochromatosis
 d. Hypercalcemia

202. **Cause of acute loss of vision in a patient of alcoholic pancreatitis is:** *(AI 95)*
 a. Purtscher's retinopathy
 b. Sudden alcohol withdrawal
 c. Acute congestive glaucoma
 d. CRAO

203. **Most common complication of acute pancreatitis is:** *(AIIMS May 95)*
 a. Pancreatic abscess
 b. Pseudocyst
 c. Phlegmon
 d. Pleural effusion

204. **Gold standard test for diagnosis of Insulinoma is:** *(AI 2009)*
 a. '72 hour' fast test
 b. Plasma Glucose levels < 3 mmol/l
 c. Plasma Insulin levels > 6mU/ml
 d. C- peptide levels < 50

205. **Which of the following statements about Cystic fibrosis (CF) is not true:** *(AI 2009)*
 a. Autosomal Recessive Disorder
 b. Abnormality in CFTR which leads to defective Calcium Transport
 c. Predisposition to pulmonary infection with Pseudomonas
 d. Cirrhosis is an established complication of CF

206. **Consider the following statements:** *(UPSC 2015)*
 Gastric lavage is contraindicated in children in case of
 a. Iron poisoning
 b. Kerosene poisoning
 c. Corrosive poisoning
 d. Aspirin poisoning
 Which of the above statements are correct?
 a. B, C and D
 b. A, B and D
 c. B and C only
 d. A and C

Answers with Explanations

Bleeding from GIT

1. Ans. (a) Guaiac test

Ref: Harrison 20th edition, page 574

The image shows a positive test for stool for occult blood also known as Guaiac test. The stool sample to be tested is applied on the strip followed by application of hydrogen peroxide. When the hydrogen peroxide is dripped on to the guaiac paper, it oxidizes the α-guaiaconic acid to a blue coloured quinone.

Guaiac test	Test for occult blood in stool/urine which produces blue colour if blood is present.
Ehrlich test	Test to identify indoles and urobilinogen
Fouchet's test	Test to identify bilirubin
Molisch test	Test to identify carbohydrates

2. Ans. (a) Lesser curvature at incisura

Ref: Sabiston 20th edition, pg 1208; Shackleford's surgery of alimentary tract, E-Book, pg 691

Type 1 Gastric ulcer is Located near the incisura on the lesser curvature and comprises 60% of all benign gastric ulcers. They are associated with normal to low acid production.

H. pylori have been found to be associated with these ulcers though it occurs even in those who have history of infection.

Modified Johnson classification for gastric ulcers

Type 1 Gastric ulcer is the most common type of gastric ulcer

TABLE: Gastric ulcer types

Type	Location	Acid level
I	Lesser curve at incisura	Low to normal
II	Gastric body with duodenal ulcer	Increased
III	Prepyloric	Increased
IV	High on lesser curve	Normal
V	Anywhere	Normal, NSAID-induced

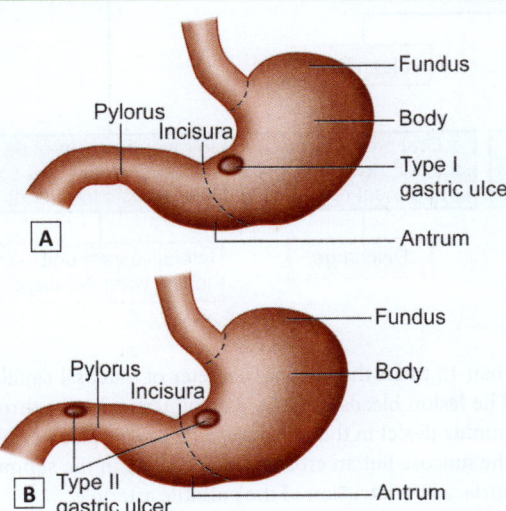

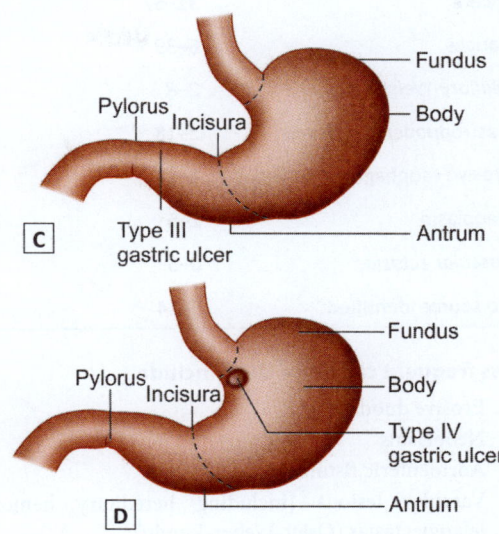

3. Ans. (b) Toxic megacolon

Ref: Abdominal X rays made easy page 65; Harrison 19th edition, page 1953

- The image shows peripheral placed bowel dilatations with loss of haustrations. It indicates large bowel dilatation.
- When transverse colon/ ascending colon diameter is >6cm it indicates development of toxic megacolon.
- It occurs in patients of UC and can be triggered by electrolyte abnormalities and narcotics.

Main causes of toxic megacolon:

1. Ulcerative colitis
2. Crohns' disease
3. Pseudomembranous colitis
4. Amoebic colitis
5. Chagas disease

Pneumatosis intestinalis is characterised by presence of intramural bowel gas and is seen in necrotising enterocolitis.

4. Ans. (d) Deep enteroscopy

(Ref: Harrison 20th edition, p 275; Harrison 19th edition, page 1891)

- Persistent calibre artery is called Dieulafoy's lesion. It is a large calibre arteriole that runs beneath the gut mucosa and bleeds via pinpoint mucosal erosion.
- For management of bleeding in Dieulafoy's lesion, endoscopic therapy like thermal coagulation or band ligation is effective.
- In case of failure to control bleeding with above methods, angiographic embolization is used.
- Deep enteroscopy is used in patients with diffuse small bowel bleeding like vascular ectasia.

5. Ans. (d) Vascular ectasia

(Ref: Harrison 20th edition, p 273; Harrison 19th edition, Page 276, Table 57.1)

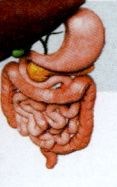

Sources of Bleeding	Proportion of Patients, %
Ulcers	31–67
Varices	6–39
Mallory-Weiss tears	2–8
Gastroduodenal erosions	2–18
Erosive esophagitis	1–13
Neoplasm	2–8
Vascular ectasias	0–6
No source identified	5–14

Less frequent causes of UGIB include

1. Erosive duodenitis
2. Neoplasms
3. Aortoenteric fistulas
4. Vascular lesions [including hereditary hemorrhagic telangiectasias (Osler-Weber-Rendu)
5. Gastric antral vascular ectasia ("watermelon stomach")
6. Dieulafoy's lesion (in which an aberrant vessel in the mucosa bleeds from a pinpoint mucosal defect)
7. Prolapse gastropathy (prolapse of proximal stomach into esophagus with retching, especially in alcoholics)
8. Hemobilia
9. Hemosuccus pancreaticus (bleeding from the bile duct or pancreatic duct)

6. **Ans. (d)** Dilatation of veins of colon

(*Ref: Harrison 19th p 1971*)

Choice A: Early carcinoma colon	1. Cancer of right side of colon present with occult bleeding while left side with obstructive symptoms. 2. Cancers arising in the rectosigmoid are often associated with hematochezia, tenesmus, and narrowing of the caliber of stool. (*Since recent screening was done, choice A is unlikely*).
Points in favour of choice B: Sigmoid diverticulitis	Mean age of presentation is 59 years. Diverticular bleeding is abrupt in onset, usually painless, sometimes massive, and often from the right colon. Lesions are easily picked up on sigmoidoscopy, hence choice B is unlikely.
Choice C: Microscopic colitis	1. Presents with watery non-bloody diarrhea and hence ruled out.
Dilatation of veins of colon	1. Angiodysplasia is a degenerative lesion of previously healthy blood vessels found most commonly in the cecum and proximal ascending colon. 2. Seventy-seven percent of angiodysplasias are located in the cecum and ascending colon, 15% are located in the jejunum and ileum, and the remainder is distributed throughout the alimentary tract. These lesions typically are non-palpable and small (< 5 mm). 3. Angiodysplasia is the most common vascular abnormality of the GI tract. After diverticulosis, it is the **second** leading cause of lower GI bleeding in patients older than 60 years.

7. **Ans. (b)** Clean based ulcer

(*Ref: Harrison 20th edition, p 274; Harrison 19th p 276*)

Most patients of hematemesis have a rebleed within the next 3 days of an episode. UGIE is diagnostic as well as prognostic as a clean based ulcer has a least chance of re-bleed while visible bleeding vessel has the highest chances.

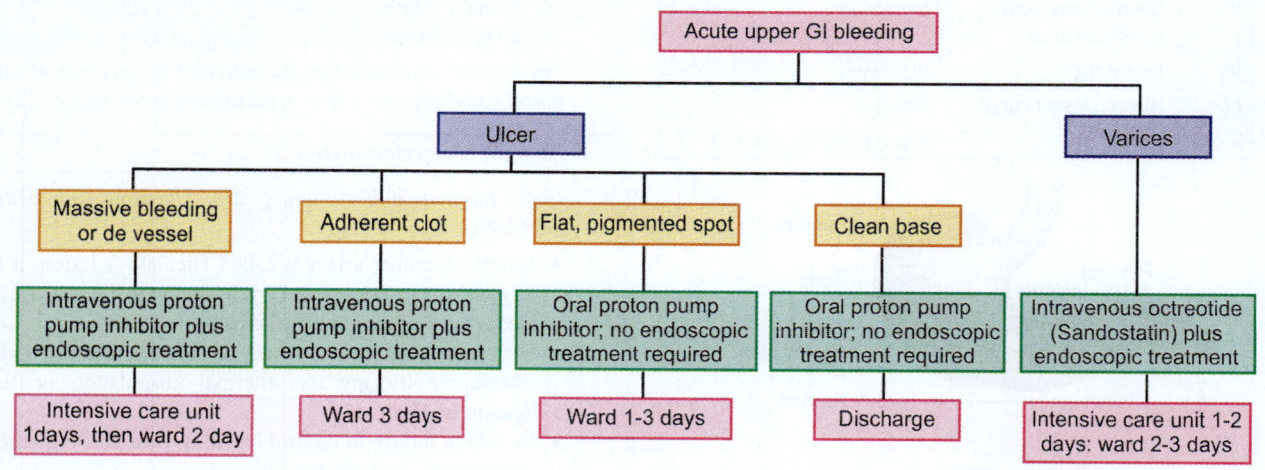

8. **Ans. (a)** Lesser curvature of stomach

(*Ref: Harrison 20th edition, p 2197; Harrison 19th p 277, 1891*)

- Dieulafoy's Lesions are characterized by a single large tortuous arteriole in the submucosa which does not undergo normal branching or a branch with caliber of 1–5 mm (more than 10 times the normal diameter of mucosal capillaries). The lesion bleeds into the gastrointestinal tract through a minute defect in the mucosa which is not a primary ulcer of the mucosa but an erosion likely caused in the submucosal surface by protrusion of the pulsatile arteriole.

- Approximately 75% of Dieulafoy's lesions occur in the upper part of the stomach within 6 cm of the gastroesophageal junction, most commonly in the lesser curvature.
- Extragastric lesions are seen in *duodenum (the most common location 14%)* followed by the colon (5%), surgical anastamoses (5%), the jejunum (1%) and the esophagus (1%).

9. Ans. (a) Rectal polyp

(Ref: Table 303.12 Nelson's 18th ed., Harrison 19th p 276, 1899)

Lower GI bleeding in children
- Neonate= anal fissure
- 1month- 1year= anal fissure
  - 1 year- 2 years= polyp
  - 2 years= polyp

10. Ans. (a) Upper GI bleeding

(Ref: Grading and staging in gastroenterology by tytgat pg. 110, Harrison's 19th p 276)

- Rockall risk scoring system attempts to identify patients at risk of adverse outcome following acute upper gastrointestinal bleeding
- The scoring system uses clinical criteria (increasing age, co-morbidity, shock) as well as endoscopic finding (diagnosis, stigmata of acute bleeding).
- A convenient mnemonic is ABCDE - i.e. Age, Blood pressure fall (shock), Co-morbidity, Diagnosis and Evidence of bleeding.

11. Ans. (a) Diverticulitis

(Ref: Harrison 19th p 1903)

Diseases of Esophagus

12. Ans. (c) Eosinophilic esophagitis

Ref: Harrison 20th edition, p 2203; Harrison, 19th edition, page 1895

- Narrowed oesophagus with linear furrows and multiple corrugated rings on endoscopy is a feature of feline oesophagus.
- This appearance should raise clinical suspicion of *eosinophilic esophagitis*.
- Diagnosis requires biopsy with histological findings of >15-20 eosinophils per HPF.
- This condition leads to recurrent dysphagia and food impaction.

13. Ans. (b) CT scan

(Ref: Grainger and Allison diagnostic Radiology: Sixth edition, page 34)

- Normally the aortic arch and left main bronchus cause smooth external indentation of oesophagus.
- However in case of dysphagia lusoria since the patient has aberrant right subclavian artery originating from the left sided aortic arch, the vessel will have to reach the right axilla by crossing the oesophagus at oblique angle.

- The diagnosis is best made in the arterial phase of CT chest where the vessel reading is observed.
- *Dysphagia aortica* is due to compression of distal esophagus by ectasia or aneurysm of the descending thoracic aorta.

14. Ans. (a) Eosinophilic esophagitis

(Ref: Harrison 20th edition, p 2203; Harrison 19th edition, page 1895)

- The presence of multiple corrugated rings and linear furrows all through a narrowed oesophagus is called feline oesophagus. This is seen in eosinophilic esophagitis.
- Histological confirmation of eosinophilic esophagitis is made with demonstration of 15 eosinophils per HPF.

15. Ans. (b) Manometry

(Ref: Harrison 20th edition, p 2214; Harrison 19th edition, p 1905)

- Manometry is used to diagnose motility disorders (achalasia, diffuse esophageal spasm) and to assess peristaltic integrity prior to the surgery for reflux disease.
- Esophageal manometry, or motility testing, entails positioning a pressure sensing catheter within the esophagus and then observing the contractility following test swallows.
- The upper and lower esophageal sphincters appear as zones of high pressure that relax on swallowing while the inter-sphincteric esophagus exhibits peristaltic contractions.

16. Ans. (c) Nitrates

(Ref: Harrison 20th edition, p 2214; Harrison 19th edition, page 1906)

Diffuse esophageal Spasm is managed with following interventions:
1. Nitrates and CCB
2. Hydralazine
3. Botulinum toxin
4. Anxiolytics
5. Long myotomy or esophagectomy for severe weight loss or unbearable pain

Diffuse oesophageal spasm	Nutcracker oesophagus	Hypertensive LES
Simultaneous non peristaltic contractions (>20% of wet swallows)	Mean peristaltic amplitude of > 180mm Hg for Increased duration of contraction >7 seconds Normal peristaltic sequence	Elevated LES pressure > 26mmHg Normal LES relaxation Normal oesophageal peristalsis

17. Ans. (c) Bicarbonate secreted by esophageal mucosa neutralizes the acid

(Ref: Harrison 20th edition, p 2216; Harrison's 19th edition, page 1906)

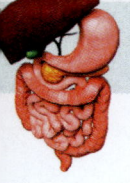

- Mechanisms of GERD:
  1. Transient LES relaxations
  2. LES hypotension
  3. Anatomic distortion of the esophagogastric junction inclusive of hiatus hernia
- The acid can reflux can lead to chemical tracheitis leading to nocturnal cough and bronchospasm.
- GERD is often diagnosed in the absence of endoscopic esophagitis, which would otherwise define the disease. In setting of partially treated disease ambulatory 24 hours pH monitoring is done and the outcome is expressed as the percentage of the day that the pH was less than 4 (indicative of recent acid reflux), with values exceeding 5% indicative of GERD

18. Ans. (c) Premalignant

(Ref: Harrison 20th edition, p 2211; Harrison 19th ed. / 1903)

- Zenker's diverticulum, aka pharyngoesophageal diverticulum is a diverticulum of the mucosa of the pharynx, just above the cricopharyngeal muscle. It is a false diverticulum.
- Pharyngo-oesophageal wall herniates through the point of least resistance (known as Killian's triangle).
- Zenker diverticulum often causes clinical manifestations such as dysphagia, and sense of a lump in the neck, regurgitation, cough, halitosis, infection, involuntary gurgling noises when swallowing.

19. Ans. (b) Eosinophilic esophagitis

(Ref: Harrison 20th edition, p 2203; Harrison 19th edition, page 1908)

The endoscopic view shows corrugation or rings appearance which is suggestive of diagnosis of eosinophilic esophagitis.
To confirm the diagnosis of eosinophilic esophagitis
1. Presence of 15 or more eosinophils per high power field (HPF) on esophageal biopsy
2. Exclusion of other disorders associated with similar clinical, histological, or endoscopic features, especially GERD

20. Ans. (a) Esophageal manometry

(Ref: Harrison 20th edition, p 2210; Bailey and love 26th edition, page 1014 and Harrison 19th p 1904)

- In long-standing achalasia, the esophagus may assume a sigmoid configuration. The diagnostic criteria for achalasia with esophageal manometry are impaired LES relaxation and absent peristalsis.
- High-resolution manometry has somewhat advanced this diagnosis; three subtypes of achalasia are differentiated based on the pattern of pressurization in the nonperistaltic esophagus.
- Because manometry identifies early disease before esophageal dilatation and food retention, it is the most sensitive diagnostic test.

21. Ans. (a) Esophageal diverticulum

(Ref: Harrison 20th edition, p 2211)

- Cervical esophageal diverticulum (Zenker Diverticulum) is located in Killian–Laimer triangle which is located inferior to the cricopharyngeus in the posterior midline above the confluence of the longitudinal layer of esophageal muscle. Laimer's triangle is covered only by the circular layer of esophageal muscle.

22. Ans. (c) UGI endoscopy

(Ref: Harrison 20th edition, p 2219)

- Endoscopy technique is the procedure of choice for both diagnosis and therapy of these lesions. Endoscopic diagnosis of a Mallory-Weiss tear is readily made by identifying active bleeding, an adherent clot, or a fibrin crust over a mucosal split within or near the gastroesophageal junction.
- A contact thermal modality, such as multipolar electrocoagulation (MPEC) or heater probe, with or without epinephrine injection, is typically used to treat an actively bleeding Mallory-Weiss tear.
- Angiotherapy with either selective vasopressin infusion or embolization of the left gastric artery can be performed in patients whose lesions have failed to respond to endoscopic therapy or who are at high risk of endoscopic complications.

23. Ans. (a) Recurrent pulmonary infections

(Ref: Harrison 20th edition, p 2213; Harrison 19th p 1904)

Achalasia is a rare motility disorder of the esophagus which results from lack of innervation of the lower esophageal sphincter muscles and leads to dilatation of proximal esophagus. Patients with achalasia presents typically with dysphagia, vomiting of undigested food and failure to thrive. Cough can be present in achalasia patients due to aspiration of food or due to airway compression by the dilated esophagus.

24. Ans. (c) Doxycycline

(Ref: Harrison 20th edition, p 2219; Harrison 19th p 1910)

Medications commonly implicated in pill induced esophagitis are doxycycline, tetracycline, quinidine, NSAIDS and bisphosphonates.

25. Ans. (c) CT angiography

(Ref: Harrison 20th edition, p 2213)

- Compression of the oesophagus by the aberrant right subclavian artery is known as dysphagia lusoria
- Barium study of the esophagus may show the indentation on the posterior esophageal wall by the artery.
- Chest x-ray can demonstrate enlargement of the superior mediastinum.
- *(CT angiography and MRI thorax are the best diagnostic modalities that could identify the arteria lusoria).*
- Most patients with aberrant right subclavian arteries do not have symptoms. Some present with mild dysphagia, while a small minority have a severe enough disturbance in swallowing that leads to inability to swallow and severe nutritional problems.
- In children, the most common presentations are stridor and recurrent chest infections, may be due to their tracheal softening comparing to adult population.

- The diagnosis of dysphagia lusoria is always difficult and late as the symptoms are often nonspecific and in the same time, diagnostic endoscopy is negative in more than 50% cases, and manometry has no diagnostic role.

26. Ans. (c) Dysphagia

(Ref: Harrison 19th p 1903)

While it may be asymptomatic, Zenker diverticulum often causes clinical manifestations such as dysphagia (difficulty swallowing), and sense of a lump in the neck; moreover, it may fill up with food, causing regurgitation, cough (as some food may be regurgitated into the airways), halitosis, potential infection of the pharyngeal areas due to food stuck, and involuntary gurgling noises when swallowing. It rarely, if ever, causes any pain.

27. Ans. (c) Premalignant

(Ref: Harrison 20th edition, p 2215; Harrison 19th p 1907)

- The average age of patients with Barrett esophagus is 55-65 years. The condition occurs in a 2:1 male-to-female ratio, with white males making up more than 80% of cases.
- It is causes columnar metaplasia of lower esophagus and does not respond to any treatment.
- It is a premalignant condition diagnosed with UGIE with biopsy. The goal of surveillance is the detection of dysplasia or early cancer. Currently, dysplasia is the best histologic marker for cancer risk. Surveillance involves repeated upper endoscopy with systematic 4-quadrant biopsies at 2cm intervals along the entire length of the segment of Barrett esophagus, with additional biopsy of any mucosal abnormalities.

28. Ans. (d) Rosary esophagus

(Ref: Harrison 20th edition, p 2213; Harrison 19th p 1904)

Causes of pseudo-achalasia
1. Tumor infiltration, most commonly seen with carcinoma in the gastric fundus or distal esophagus can mimic idiopathic achalasia.
2. Rarely, pseudoachalasia can result from a paraneoplastic syndrome with circulating antineuronal antibodies
   - Pseudoachalasia presents at young age, abrupt onset of symptoms (<1 year), and weight loss. Hence, endoscopy should be part of the evaluation of achalasia.
   - When the clinical suspicion for pseudoachalasia is high and endoscopy nondiagnostic, CT scanning or endoscopic ultrasonography may be of value.
   - Since barium swallow may not be able to differentiate achalasia from pseudoachalasia, UGIE and CT scan must be done for determining the cause as well as for staging.

Radiographically, a "corkscrew esophagus," "rosary bead esophagus," is indicative of diffuse esophageal spasm.

29. Ans. (a) Diffuse esophageal spasm

(Ref: Harrison 20th edition, p 2214; Harrison 19th p 1905)

- Non progressive dysphagia is seen in choice a and b while choice c and d have progressive dysphagia.
- Diffuse esophageal spasm presents with non cardiac chest pain and globus (something stuck in the throat). Pain may be associated with eating quickly or drinking hot, cold, or carbonated beverages. Patients with nutcracker esophagus or high-amplitude peristaltic contractions usually present with chest pain, as only 10% experience dysphagia.
- The hallmark symptom of esophageal rings and webs is dysphagia mainly to solid food usually is greater than dysphagia to liquid food. Since in this question cold drink is worsening and not improving the symptom of dysphagia, oeso-phageal web is a unlikely answer. When lumen diameter is less than 13 mm due to mucosal ring(Schatzki ring) episodic solid food dysphagia is seen

30. Ans. (a) Stricture esophagus

(Ref: Harrison 20th edition, p 2216; Harrison 19th p 1907)

Complications of endoscopic therapy in barret esophagus should be divided into immediate and delayed outcomes. Immediate complications include bleeding and perforation. Delayed complications from ablative therapy include stricture formation.

31. Ans. (c) Savary miller

(Ref: Grading and staging in gastroenterology by tytgat pg. 108)

Savary-Miller classification of reflux esophagitis. Grades 1, 2, 3, 4 and 5.

Grade 1:	Single erosion above gastro-esophageal mucosal junction.
Grade 2:	Multiple, non-circumferential erosions above gastro-esophageal mucosal junction.
Grade 3:	Circumferential erosion above mucosal junction.
Grade 4:	Chronic change with esophageal ulceration and associated stricture.
Grade 5:	Barrett's esophagus with histologically confirmed intestinal differentiation within columnar epithelium.

32. Ans. (d) 4

(Ref: Grading and staging in gastroenterology by page 108, Harrison's 19th p 1894)

- A reflux episode is defined as esophageal pH drop below four. Esophageal pH monitoring is performed for 24 or 48 hours and at the end of recording, patients tracing is analyzed and the results are expressed using six standard components.
- Of these 6 parameters a pH score called Composite pH Score or DeMeester Score has been calculated, which is a global measure of esophageal acid exposure. A DeMeester score > 14.72 indicates reflux.
- Components of 24-h Esophageal pH Monitoring (DeMeester scoring)
  1. Percent total time pH < 4
  2. Percent Upright time pH < 4
  3. Percent Supine time pH < 4
  4. Number of reflux episodes
  5. Number of reflux episodes > 5 min
  6. Longest reflux episode (minutes)

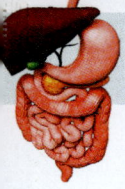

33. Ans. (a) Lower end of esophagus

(Ref: Harrison 20th edition, p 2219; Harrison 19th p 1910)

- Esophageal rupture in Boerhaave syndrome is due to be the result of a sudden rise in intraluminal esophageal pressure produced during vomiting, as a result of neuromuscular incoordination causing failure of the cricopharyngeus muscle to relax. The syndrome commonly is associated with overindulgence in food and/or alcohol.
- *The most common anatomical location of the tear in Boerhaave syndrome is at the left posterolateral wall of the lower third of the esophagus, 2-3 cm proximal to the gastro-esophageal junction, along the longitudinal wall of the esophagus.*
- The second most common site of rupture is in the subdiaphragmatic or upper thoracic area

34. Ans. (b) Weight gain

(Ref: Harrison 20th edition, p 2215; Harrison 19th p 1906)

Complications of esophagitis include the following:
1. Bleeding and stricture formation
2. Barrett esophagus occurs when the normal squamous epithelium of the esophagus is replaced with columnar epithelium; this condition is linked to the development of esophageal cancer; systematic review of patients with Barrett esophagus and colonic cancer also indicated a link between Barrett esophagus and colonic cancer.
3. Perforation with mediastinitis, although rare, is a serious complication
4. Volume depletion and weight loss may occur secondary to inability to swallow
5. Laryngitis, aspiration pneumonitis, and bronchospasm may occur if gastric contents are refluxed to the level of the larynx.
6. In infants, failure to thrive and apnea

35. Ans. (a) Cervical esophagus

(Ref: Harrison 20th edition, p 2219; Harrison 19th p 1910)

- The site of perforation varies depending upon the cause. (*Instrumental perforation is common in the pharynx or distal esophagus*). Spontaneous rupture may occur just above the diaphragm in the posterolateral wall of the esophagus. Perforations are usually longitudinal with the left side more commonly affected than the right.
- The esophagus *lacks a serosal layer* and is, therefore, more vulnerable to rupture or perforation. Once a perforation (i.e, full-thickness tear in the wall) occurs, retained gastric contents, saliva, bile, and other substances may enter the mediastinum, resulting in mediastinitis.
- The degree of mediastinal contamination and the location of the tear determine the clinical presentation. Within a few hours, a polymicrobial invasion of bacteria supervenes, which can lead to sepsis and, eventually, death if the patient is not treated with conservative management or surgical intervention. The *mediastinal pleura often ruptures, and gastric fluid is drawn into the pleural space by the negative intrathoracic pressure. Even if the mediastinal pleura is not violated, a sympathetic pleural effusion often occurs. This effusion is usually left-sided but can be bilateral.*

36. Ans. (c) Common in elderly male

(Ref: Harrison 20th edition, p 220; Harrison 19th p 237/532)

Plummer–Vinson syndrome or Sideropenic dysphagia, presents in postmenopausal women as a triad of post cricoid dysphagia from:
1. Esophageal webs,
2. Iron deficiency anemia with beefy-red tongue due to atrophic glossitis
3. Koilyonychia

It is a premalignant condition with increased risk of squamous cell carcinoma of esophagus.

37. Ans. (c) Treatment is CP myotomy

(Ref: Harrison 20th edition, p 2211-2212; Harrison 19th p 1903)

- Small lesions are satisfactorily treated with a cricopharyngeus (CP) myotomy with or without an invagination procedure. Intermediate and large diverticula (i.e., 2-6 cm) are best managed with open diverticulectomy with CP myotomy or by endoscopic diverticulotomy. (*Very large diverticula (i.e., >6 cm) are best managed with excision with CP myotomy or a diverticulopexy with CP myotomy, depending on the health of the patient*).
- The pathologic process in Zenker diverticulum involves herniation of the esophageal mucosa posteriorly between the cricopharyngeus (CP) muscle and the inferior pharyngeal constrictor muscles. Therefore, by definition, a Zenker diverticulum is a *false diverticulum*. The retention of food elements and secretions within the lesion's pouch frequently leads to halitosis, regurgitation, aspiration, and dysphagia in patients

38. Ans. (d) Lower esophageal ring

(Ref: Harrison 20th edition, p 2203; Harrison 19th p 1904)

39. Ans. (d) Compression by aberrant right subclavian artery

(Ref: Harrison 20th edition, p 2213; Bailey 24th/995; 23rd/859, Harrison 19th p 257)

40. Ans. (a) Achalasia cardia

(Ref: Harrison 20th edition, p 2213; Harrison 19th p 1904)

41. Ans. (a) Zenker's diverticulum

(Ref: Harrison 20th edition, p 2211; Harrison 19th p 1903)

42. Ans. (d) Out pouching of the anterior pharyngeal wall, just above the cricopharyngeus muscle

(Ref: Harrison 20th edition, p 2211; Current Diagnosis & Treatment in Otorhinology 2nd /490, Dhingra 4th/355, Harrison 19th p 1903)

43. Ans. (a) Mucosal ring at squamo-columnar junction; (c) Dysphagia is the presenting symptom

(Ref: Harrison 20th edition, p 2211; Oxford textbook of Medicine 4th/553, Harrison 19th p 257)

44. Ans. (b) Intestinal metaplasia

(Ref: Harrison 20th edition, p 2216; Harrison 19th p 1907)

45. Ans. (a) Stricture

(Ref: Manual of Gastroenterology 4th/132, Harrison 19th p 1907)

46. Ans. (b) Premalignant condition

(Ref: Harrison 20th edition, p 2216; Harrison 19th p 1907)

47. Ans. (a) Squamous cell cancer

(Ref: Harrison 20th edition, p 566; Current Diagnosis and Treatment in Gastroenterology/ 299, Harrison 19th p 532)

48. Ans. (d) Ca esophagus

(Ref: Harrison 20th edition, p 567; Harrison 19th p 532)

Hyperkeratosis of palms of soles is a feature of tylosis palmaris. It is associated with squamous cell cancer of esophagus.

49. Ans. (b) Barret's esophagus

(Ref: Harrison 20th edition, p 257; Harrison 19th p 532)

50. Ans. (a) Stomach

(Ref: Harrison 20th edition, p 567; Harrison 19th p 533)

51. Ans. (a) Cisapride

(Ref: Harrison 18th/46)

Cisapride has been withdrawn due to propensity to cause torsades de pointes.

PUD and ZES

52. Ans. (b) Octreoscan

(Ref: Harrison 20th edition, p 2240; Table 348-8: Harrison: 19th edition, page 1929)

- In case of *gastrinoma showing metastasis* the diagnostic sensitivity of octreoscan is 80-100%.
- In contrast in *primary gastrinoma*, Endoscopic ultrasound shows a sensitivity of 80-100% versus octreoscan which shows a sensitivity of 67-86%. (The given figures are quoted from Harrison page 2240, Harrison 20th ed.).

53. Ans. (c) Cetuximab

(Ref: Harrison 20th edition, p 2243; Harrison: 19th edition, page 1932)

- Cetuximab is the first line treatment for Menetrier's disease. Other agents like octreotide, H₂ receptor antagonists yield varying results.
- The rare gastropathy is characterised by foveolar cell hyperplasia and marked reduction in oxyntic cells, parietal cells and chief cells.

54. Ans. (d) A, B and D

(Ref: Harrison 20th edition, p 2240; Harrison 19th edition, page 568, 1927)

Zollinger Ellison Syndrome is a tumour of G cells. Due to presence of chronic hypergastrinemia there is a resultant marked gastric acid hypersecretion and growth of the gastric mucosa.

The gastric acid hypersecretion characteristically causes peptic ulcer disease, often refractory and severe, as well as diarrhea.

Clinical features:
1. Abdominal pain (70–100%)
2. Diarrhea (37–73%)
3. Gastroesophageal reflux disease (GERD) (30–35%)

Most common site of ZES (50–70%) is the duodenum, followed by the pancreas (20–40%) and other intraabdominal sites (mesentery, lymph nodes, biliary tract, liver, stomach, Ovary).

Work up:
1. The secretin provocative test is usually positive, with the criterion of a >120-pg/mL increase over the basal level having the highest sensitivity (94%) and specificity (100%).
2. Fasting hypergastrinemia, and Fasting stomach pH <2 when off anti-secretory drugs.
3. Plasma ionized calcium
4. Serum prolactin levels
5. Plasma PTH and GH levels
6. Increased Basal acid output

Tumour localisation in ZES: Endoscopic USG > portal venous sampling > octreo-scan. *Pointers to presence of ZES:*

> 1. Peptic ulcer disease (PUD); with diarrhea
> 2. P.U.D in an unusual location or with multiple ulcers
> 3. P.U.D refractory to treatment or persistent; PUD associated with prominent gastric fold
> 4. P.U.D associated with findings suggestive of MEN 1 (endocrinopathy, family history of ulcer or endocrinopathy, nephrolithiases)
> 5. P.U.D without Helicobacter pylori present.

55. Ans. (b) B, C and D only

(Ref: Harrison 20th edition, p 2227; Harrison 19th edition, page 1040)

- Majority of Duodenal ulcers occur due to H. pylori and NSAID-induced injury leading to decreased prostaglandins.
- DUs occur most often in the first portion of the duodenum (>95%), with ~90% located within 3 cm of the pylorus.
- They are usually <1 cm in diameter with depth at times reaching the muscularispropria.
- The base of the ulcer often consists of a zone of eosinophilic necrosis with surrounding fibrosis.
- The reason for the reduction in the frequency of DUs is likely related to the decreasing frequency of Helicobacter pylori due to eradication therapy.

56. Ans. (c) Breath urea test

(Ref: Harrison 20th edition, p 2234; Harrison 19th edition, page 1920)

ELISA test has sensitivity of 80% and has been replaced by C-13 urea breath test and fecal antigen immunoassay. Both have sensitivity of >90%.

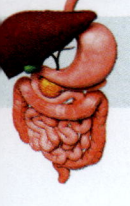

Endoscopy is not indicated to diagnose H. pylori in most circumstances. Hence though rapid urease test is having a comparable sensitivity and higher specificity, it is an *invasive test*

Sensitivity of various diagnosis tests

Test	Sensitivity in %
Rapid urease (INVASIVE)	80-95
Histology	80-90
Serology	>80
Urea breath test (NON INVASIVE)	>90
Stool antigen	>90

In assessment of response to treatment, non-invasive tests are preferred. Breath urea test will be done but can be false negative if done within 4 weeks of antibiotic treatment.

57. Ans. (a) H. pylori causes peptic ulcer; (b) Eradication therapy better than PPI therapy; (c) Eradication therapy also contain PPI; (d) Duodenum ulcer is more commonly associated with H. pylori than gastric ulcer

(Ref: Harrison 20th edition, p 2234-35; Harrison 19th/1911-21)

58. Ans. (c) Carcinoid tumor

(Ref: Harrison 19th ed. / 1039-1040)

- H. pylori releases urease enzyme which converts urea to ammonia and ammonia stimulates G cells of stomach which inturn stimulates parietal cells and cause excess secretion of acid. This acid travels into stomach & duodenum à causes peptic ulcers.
- H. pylori is a type 1 carcinogen, which, if present in stomach for long term can cause cancer called MALTOMA (Mucosa Associated Lymphoid Tumor), which is a B-type NHL.

59. Ans. (a) Hypothyroidism

(Ref: Harrison 20th edition, p 2230; Harrison 19th p 263/568)

Long-term acid suppression, especially with PPIs, has been associated with
1. A higher incidence of community-acquired pneumonia
2. Community and hospital acquired *Clostridium difficile-*associated disease.
3. A population-based study revealed that long-term use of PPIs was associated with the development of hip fractures in older women. The absolute risk of fracture remained low despite an observed increase associated with the dose and duration of acid suppression
4. PPIs may exert a negative effect on the anti-platelet effect of clopidogrel. The mechanism involves the competition of the PPI and clopidogrel with the same cytochrome p450 (CYP2C19).

60. Ans. (d) Left gastric artery

(Ref: Schwartz 9th edition page 917-921, Harrison 19th p 1925)

Ulcer located along the lesser curve of the stomach and posterior duodenal bulb are at greater risk for severe bleeding and rebleeding due to the proximity of the left gastric artery and gastro-duodenal artery, respectively. The mortality rate for bleeding peptic ulcers is approximately 6%-7%.

61. Ans. (a) Type A gastritis

(Ref: Harrison 20th edition, p 2242; Harrison 19th p 1039)

Type A is autoimmune gastritis with antibodies against parietal cells whereas the gastritis caused by H. Pylori is referred to as type B gastritis.

62. Ans. (b) Breath urea test

(Ref: Harrison 20th edition, p 2234; Harrison 19th p 1039)

- **Breath urea test**: The patient drinks a solution of urea labeled with the nonradioactive isotope 13C and then blows into a tube. If urease is present, the urea is hydrolyzed and labeled carbon dioxide is detected in breath samples.
- After first line course of antibiotics, breath urea test can be performed and if it turns negative that indicates eradication of infection.
- In case the test is still positive, second line antibiotics should be started.

63. Ans. (a) Gastric ulcer with bleeding

(Ref: Harrison 20th edition, p 1163)

- On examination of vitals where BP is low and pulse is increased, CVA is ruled out as stroke presents with cushing reflex (Bradycardia and hypertension).
- Pulmonary embolism develops in setting of hypercoagulable state which is unlikely as he is taking aspirin for long time
- Since patient is taking aspirin, it cuts the risk of MI and there is no history of chest pain or ECG findings given
- The diagnosis points to gastric ulcer with bleed in lieu of history of aspirin intake plus passage of black stools plus features of shock due to blood loss.

64. Ans. (b) Type B gastritis

(Ref: Harrison 20th edition, p 2242; Harrison 19th p 1039)

Helicobacter Pylori leads to type B gastritis characterized by hypergastrinemia and hyperchlorhydria.

65. Ans. (a) An ECG

(Ref: Harrison 20th edition, p 853)

- Geriatric age group presentation is a risk factor for coronary artery disease. Chest pain can be misleading. The breathlessness and bradycardia and hypotension point towards myocardial infarction.
- Hence the initial evaluation at presentation should be ECG.
- Second-degree heart block (intermittent AV block) may occur as a transient abnormality in inferior wall MI
- Although many patients have a normal pulse rate and blood pressure within the first hour of STEMI, about one-fourth of patients with anterior infarction have manifestations of sympathetic nervous system hyperactivity (tachycardia and/ or hypertension), and up to one-half with inferior infarction show evidence of parasympathetic hyperactivity (bradycardia and/or hypotension).

66. Ans. (d) Erythromycin

(Ref: Harrison 20th edition, p 1165; Harrison 19th p 1039)

The agents used with the greatest frequency include amoxicillin, metronidazole, tetracycline, clarithromycin, and bismuth compounds. Multiple drugs have been evaluated in the therapy of H. pylori. No single agent is effective in eradicating the organism. Combination therapy for 14 days provides the greatest efficacy. A shorter course administration (7–10 days), although attractive, has not proved as successful as the 14-days regimens.

67. Ans. (d) Multiple large ulcers

(Ref: Harrison 20th edition, p 2236; Harrison 19th p 1925)

Surgery is more often required for treatment of an ulcer-related complication.
1. Hemorrhage is the most common ulcer-related complication, occurring in ~15–25% of patients. Bleeding may occur in any age group but is most often seen in older patients (sixth decade or beyond). Patients unresponsive or refractory to endoscopic intervention will require surgery (~5% of transfusion-requiring patients).
2. Free peritoneal perforation occurs in ~2–3% of DU patients. Concomitant bleeding may occur in up to 10% of patients with perforation, with mortality being increased substantially. Peptic ulcer can also penetrate into adjacent organs, especially with a posterior DU, which can penetrate into the pancreas, colon, liver, or biliary tree.
3. Pyloric channel ulcers or DUs can lead to gastric outlet obstruction in ~2–3% of patients. This can result from chronic scarring or from impaired motility due to inflammation and/or edema with pylorospasm. If a mechanical obstruction persists, endoscopic intervention with balloon dilation may be effective. Surgery should be considered if all else fails.

68. Ans. (d) Needs re-surgery

(Ref: Harrison 20th edition, p 2237; Harrison 19th p 1926)

- Dietary modification is the cornerstone of therapy for patients with dumping syndrome.
- Small, multiple meals devoid of simple carbohydrates coupled with elimination of liquids during meals is important.
- Antidiarrheals and anticholinergic agents are complementary to diet. Pectin, which increases the viscosity of intraluminal contents, may be beneficial in more symptomatic individuals.
- Acarbose, an alpha-glucosidase inhibitor that delays digestion of ingested carbohydrates, has also been shown to be beneficial in the treatment of the late phases of dumping.
- The somatostatin analogue octreotide has been successful in diet-refractory cases

69. Ans. (c) Acute viral hepatitis

(Ref: Harrison 20th edition, p 2359; Harrison 19th p 2004, 2016)

Liver function tests: Normal values and changes in two types of jaundice

Tests	Normal values	Hepatocellular jaundice	Uncomplicated obstructive jaundice
Bilirubin			
Direct	0.1-.=0.3 mg/dL	Increased	Increased
Indirect	0.2-0.7 mg/dL	Increased	Increased
Urine bilirubin	None	Increased	Increased
Serum albumin/ total protein	Albumin, 3.5-5.5 g/dL	Albumin decreased Total protein, 6.5-8.4 g/dL	Unchanged
Alkaline phosphatase	30-115 units/L	Increased (+)	Increased (++++)
Prothrombin time	INR=1.0-1.4. After Vit. K, 10% increased in 24 hours	Prolonged if damage severe and does not respond to parenteral vitamin K	Prolonged if obstruction marked, but responds to parenteral vitamin K
ALT, AST	ALT, 5-35 units/L AST, 5-40 units/L	Increased in hepatocellular damage, viral hepatitis	Minimally increased

70. Ans. (b) The incidence of complications has remained unchanged

(Ref: Harrison 20th edition, p 1163-64; Harrison 19th p 1911)

- Helicobacter pylori eradication has reduced complications and recurrence of peptic ulcer. Due to low socio-economic status and Feco-oral contamination favoring spread of H. Pylori the incidence in India is high.
- The physician's goal in treating PUD is to provide relief of symptoms (pain or dyspepsia), promote ulcer healing, and ultimately prevent ulcer recurrence and complications. The greatest impact of understanding the role of H. pylori in peptic disease has been the ability to prevent recurrence. Documented eradication of H. pylori in patients with PUD is associated with a dramatic decrease in ulcer recurrence to <10–20% as compared to 59% in GU patients and 67% in DU patients when the organism is not eliminated. Eradication of the organism may lead to diminished recurrent ulcer bleeding

71. Ans. (d) 1 and 2

(Ref: Harrison 20th edition, p 2239; CMDT, ch. 15, pg. 619, Harrison 19th p 1927)

- Most gastrinomas (50–70%) are present in the duodenum, followed by the pancreas (20–40%) and other intraabdominal sites (mesentery, lymph nodes, biliary tract, liver, stomach, ovary).

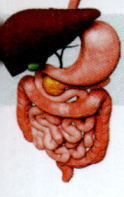

- The diagnosis of ZES requires the demonstration of inappropriate fasting hypergastrinemia, usually by demonstrating hypergastrinemia occurring with an increased basal gastric acid output (BAO) (hyperchlorhydria).
- Chronic unexplained diarrhea also should suggest gastrinoma.
- Approximately 20–25% of patients with ZES have MEN 1, and in most cases hyperparathyroidism is present before the gastrinoma. These patients are treated differently from those without MEN 1; therefore, MEN 1 should be sought in all patients by family history and by measuring plasma ionized calcium and prolactin levels and plasma hormone levels (parathormone, growth hormone).

72. Ans. (a) 1st part of duodenum

(Ref: Harrison 20th edition, p 2223; Harrison 19th p 1911)

73. Ans. (d) Misoprostol is DOC in a pregnant lady

(Ref: Harrison 20th edition, p 2234; CMDT, 2019 p 639, Harrison 19th p 1911)

Misoprostol can trigger uterine contractions and hence contraindicated in a pregnant lady.

74. Ans. (a) Gastric body

(Ref: SRB 5th ed., p 824; Harrison 19th p 1911)

Gastric Ulcers have been classified based on their location.

Type I	Occur in the gastric body and tend to be associated with low gastric acid production
Type II	Occur in the antrum and gastric acid can vary from low to normal
Type III	Occur within 3 cm of the pylorus and are commonly accompanied by duodenal ulcers and normal or high gastric acid production
Type IV	Are found in the cardia and are associated with low gastric acid production

75. Ans. (b) E. coli

(Ref: Harrison 20th edition, p 2241; Harrison 19th p 1930)

- Phlegmonous means a diffuse spreading inflammation of or within connective tissue. In the stomach, it implies infection of the deeper layers of the stomach (submucosa and muscularis).
- Phlegmonous gastritis is an uncommon form of gastritis caused by numerous bacterial agents, including streptococci, staphylococci, Proteus species, Clostridium species, and Escherichia coli.
- Phlegmonous gastritis usually occurs in individuals who are debilitated. It is associated with a recent large intake of alcohol, a concomitant upper respiratory tract infection, and AIDS.
- As a result, purulent bacterial infection may lead to gangrene. Phlegmonous gastritis is rare. The clinical diagnosis is usually established in the operating room, as these patients present with an acute abdominal emergency requiring immediate surgical exploration. Without appropriate therapy, it progresses to peritonitis and death.

76. Ans. (a) Zollinger- Ellison syndrome

(Ref: Harrison 20th edition, p 2239; Harrison 19th p 568, 1928)

- Most sensitive & specific method for identifying Zollinger-Ellison syndrome is demonstration of an increased fasting serum gastrin concentration (> 150 pg/mL)

77. Ans. (c) Abdominal angina

(Ref: GI/Liver secrets E-Book, pg. 406)

Abdominal angina is defined as the *(postprandial pain that occurs in individuals with mesenteric vascular occlusive disease such that blood flow cannot increase enough to meet visceral demands).* The classic feature is abdominal pain, which occurs a few minutes after eating and slowly subsides over next few hours. Gradually, most patients develop fear of eating and lose significant weight. A history of peripheral vascular disease and significant smoking is common.

78. Ans. (a) Diarrhea

(Ref: Harrison 20th edition, p 2237)

- 10% of patients may seek medical attention for the treatment of postvagotomy diarrhea. This complication is most commonly observed after truncal vagotomy
- This is due to a motility disorder from interruption of the vagal fibers supplying the luminal gut. Other contributing factors may include decreased absorption of nutrients, increased excretion of bile acids, and release of luminal factors that promote secretion. Diphenoxylate or loperamide is often useful in symptom control.

79. Ans. (b) CMV

(Ref: Harrison 20th edition, p 2241; Harrison 19th p 1930)

- Viral infections can cause gastritis. Cytomegalovirus (CMV) is a common viral cause of gastritis. It is usually encountered in individuals who are immunocompromised, including those with cancer, immunosuppression, transplants, and AIDS. Gastric involvement can be localized or diffuse.
- Fungal infections that cause gastritis include Candida albicans and histoplasmosis. Gastric phycomycosis is another rare lethal fungal infection. The common predisposing factor is immunosuppression.

80. Ans. (c) Greater curvature

(Ref: Shackle ford surgery of GIT, E-Book, pg 691; Harrison 19th p 1930)

- Because of gravity, the inciting agents lie on the greater curvature of the stomach. This partly explains the development of acute gastritis distally on or near the greater curvature of the stomach in the case of orally administered NSAIDs. However, the major mechanism of injury is the reduction in prostaglandin synthesis. Prostaglandins are chemicals responsible for maintaining mechanisms that result in the protection of the mucosa from the injurious effects of the gastric acid.

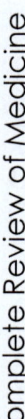

- H pylori gastritis typically starts as an acute gastritis in the antrum, causing intense inflammation, and over time, it may extend to involve the entire gastric mucosa resulting in chronic gastritis.

81. Ans. (d) **6th decade**

(Ref: Harrison 20th edition, p 2223; Harrison 19th p 1911)

GUs tend to occur later in life than duodenal lesions, with a peak incidence reported in the sixth decade. More than one-half of GUs occur in males and are less common than DUs, perhaps due to the higher likelihood of GUs being silent and presenting only after a complication develops

82. Ans. (d) **Pernicious anemia**

(Ref: Harrison 20th edition, p 2242; Harrison 19th p 568, 1927)

- Pernicious anemia is associated with auto-immune gastritis. The auto-antibodies against the parietal cells will lead to achlorhydria. This type of gastritis spares the antrum and involves mainly the body.
- Gastric acid plays an important role in feedback inhibition of gastrin release from G cells. Achlorhydria, coupled with relative sparing of the antral mucosa (site of G cells), leads to hyper-gastrinemia. Gastrin levels can be markedly elevated (>500 pg/mL) in patients with pernicious anemia. Hypergastrinemia and achlorhydria may also be seen in non-pernicious anemia–associated type A gastritis.

83. Ans. (a) **Endoscopic ultrasound (EUS)**

(Ref: Harrison 20th edition, p 2240; Harrison 19th p 568, 1927)

- Endoscopic ultrasound permits imaging of ZES with high degree of resolution (<5mm). This modality rules out small neoplasms in pancreas.
- In imaging modalities for ZES: best answer is EUS>octreoscan>MRI>USG
- The secretin provocative test is usually positive, with the criterion of a >120-pg/mL increase over the basal level having the highest sensitivity (94%) and specificity (100%).

84. Ans. (b) **Hyperchlorhydria**

(Ref: Harrison 20th edition, p 2242; Harrison 19th p 1931)

Type A gastritis is characterized by achlorhydria due to autoimmune destruction of parietal cells. The feedback leads to increased gastrin.

85. Ans. (b) **Small stomach**

(Ref: Harrison 20th edition, p 2237; Harrison 19th p 1926)

- Signs and symptoms arise from the rapid emptying of hyperosmolar gastric contents into the small intestine, resulting in a fluid shift into the gut lumen with plasma volume contraction and acute intestinal distention.
- Release of vasoactive GI hormones (vasoactive intestinal polypeptide, neurotensin, motilin) is also theorized to play a role in early dumping.
- Early dumping takes place 15–30 minutes after meals and consists of crampy abdominal discomfort, nausea, diarrhea, belching, tachycardia, palpitations, diaphoresis, light-headedness, and, rarely, syncope.
- Late phase of dumping is due to hypoglycemia from excessive insulin release.

86. Ans. (d) **Fundal atrophic gastritis**

(Ref: Harrison 19th p 1923)

87. Ans. (b) **Urea breath test**

(Ref: Harrison 20th edition, p 2234; Harrison 19th p 1923)

88. Ans. (d) **Distal duodenum**

(Ref: Harrison 20th edition, p 2241; Harrison 19th p 1918)

89. Ans. (a) **1st part of duodenum**

(Ref: Harrison 20th edition, p 2223; Robbins 7th/817, Harrison 19th p 1918)

90. Ans. (b) **Gastroduodenal artery**

(Ref: Bailey 24th/1026; CSDT 11th/550, Harrison 19th p 1925)

91. Ans. (b) **Presence of hypertonic contents in small intestine**

(Ref: Harrison 20th edition, p 2237; Love & Bailey 23rd / 913, Harrison 19th p 1926)

92. Ans. (a) **Superficial spreading type**

(Ref: Harrison 20th edition, p 568; Bailey 23rd/920, 921, Harrison 19th p 534)

93. Ans. (d) **Decreased ratio of BAO to MAO**

(Ref: Harrison 20th edition, p 2239; Harrison 19th p 1927)

94. Ans. (c) **Pernicious anemia**

(Ref: Harrison 20th edition, p 2242; Harrison 19th p 2346t)

Inflammatory Bowel Disease

95. Ans. (b) **Fine mucosal granularity**

(Ref: Harrison 20th edition, p 2263; Harrison 19th edition, page 1952)

- The earliest radiological change in UC on single contrast barium enema is fine mucosal granularity.
- Collar button ulcers and oedematous, thickened haustrations are seen with disease progression. Loss of haustrations is seen with long standing disease.

96. Ans. (a) **Steroid**; (b) **5-A.S.A**; (c) **Azathioprine**; (e) **Infliximab**

(Ref: Harrison 20th edition, p 2270; Harrison 19th/1959-64)

97. Ans. (b) **Steroids**

(Ref: Harrison 20th edition, p 2270; Harrison 19th p 1952)

- Ulcerative colitis is a chronic relapsing and remitting inflammatory disorder that can generally be managed successfully with maintenance oral medications.
- However, approximately 15% of patients with ulcerative colitis will develop a severe exacerbation and require

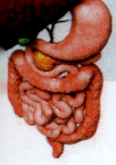

hospitalization. While many patients with acute severe ulcerative colitis will respond to a short course of intravenous corticosteroids like methylprednisolone once daily.
- In these patients with steroid-refractory colitis, the choice is between rescue medical therapy with cyclosporin or infliximab, or surgery. Well-timed rescue medical therapy is generally safe.
- Acute severe UC can be defined according to the original criteria set forth by Truelove and Witts:
  Six or more stools per day with either
  1. Body temperature of more than 37.8°C
  2. Pulse rate of more than 90 bpm
  3. Large amounts of blood per stool
  4. Hemoglobin level of less than 10.5 g/dl
  5. Erythrocyte sedimentation rate (ESR) of more than 30 mm/h

98. Ans. (d) Fistula

(Ref: Harrison 20th edition, p 2264; CMDT, ch. 15, pg. 646, Harrison 19th p 1953)

Fistula formation is a hallmark feature of Crohn's, since the transmural inflammation is the norm in Crohn's disease. In ulcerative colitis it is always a partial thickness involvement and hence the fistula is not formed.

99. Ans. (a) A.S.C.A

(Ref: Harrison 20th edition, p 2265; CMDT, ch. 15, pg. 642, Harrison 19th p 1954)

- ASCA-positive (anti-sacharomyces cerevisae antibody) seen with 70% of CD and 15% of UC patients.
- p-ANCA positivity is found in about 60–70% of UC patients and 5–10% of CD patients
- Fecal calprotectin levels correlate well with histologic inflammation, predict relapses, and detect pouchitis

100. Ans. (b) Azathioprine

(Ref: Harrison 20th edition, p 2274)

Azathioprine and 6-mercaptopurine (6-MP) are purine analogues commonly employed in the management of glucocorticoid-dependent IBD. Azathioprine is rapidly absorbed and converted to 6-MP, which is then metabolized to the active end product, thioinosinic acid, an inhibitor of purine ribonucleotide synthesis and cell proliferation. These agents also inhibit the immune response. Efficacy can be seen as early as 3–4 weeks but can take up to 4–6 months

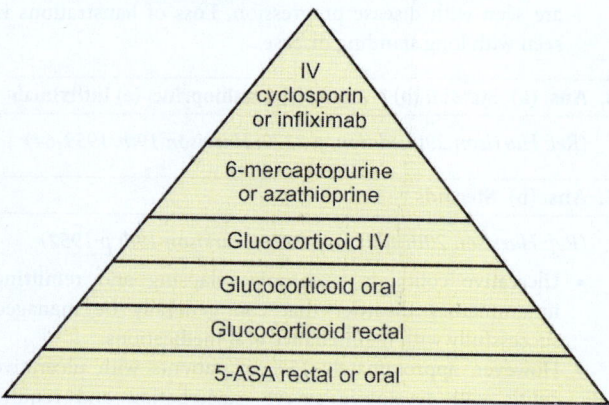

101. Ans. (d) Rectum

(Ref: Harrison 20th edition, p 2262; Harrison 19th p 1952)

Most common site involved in ulcerative colitis is the rectum. Rectum is usually spared in Crohn's disease

102. Ans. (a) Mucosal proctectomy + Ileoanal pouch anastomosis

(Ref: Harrison 20th edition, p 2274-75; Harrison 19th p 1962)

Since UC is a mucosal disease, the rectal mucosa can be dissected and removed down to the dentate line of the anus or about 2 cm proximal to this landmark. The ileum is fashioned into a pouch that serves as a neorectum. This ileal pouch is then sutured circumferentially to the anus in an end-to-end fashion. If performed carefully, this operation preserves the anal sphincter and maintains continence. The overall operative morbidity is 10%, with the major complication being bowel obstruction.

Indications for surgery in ulcerative colitis

1. Intractable disease
2. Fulminant disease
3. Toxic megacolon
4. Colonic perforation
5. Massive colonic hemorrhage
6. Extracolonic disease
7. Colonic obstruction
8. Colon cancer prophylaxis
9. Colon dysplasia or cancer

103. Ans. (a) 5 aminosalicyclic acid

(Ref: Harrison 20th edition, p 2270, Harrison 19th p 1962)

5-ASA is the active metabolite of sulfasalazine which exerts anti-inflammatory action. The mainstay of therapy for mild to moderate UC is sulfasalazine and the other 5-ASA agents. These agents are effective at inducing and maintaining remission in UC. They may have a limited role in inducing remission in CD but no clear role in maintenance of CD. The most convincing evidence for the use of sulfasalazine is treatment of active Crohn's disease involving the colon.

104. Ans. (b) Infliximab

(Ref: Harrison 20th edition, p 2274; Harrison 19th p 1963)

Infliximab is effective in CD patients with refractory perianal and enterocutaneous fistulas, with 68% response rate (50% reduction in fistula drainage) and a 50% complete remission rate. Reinfusion, typically every 8 weeks, is necessary to continue therapeutic benefits in many patients.

105. Ans. (a) Anti TNF α-antibody

(Ref: Harrison 20th edition, p 2274; Harrison 19th p 1963)

Tumor Necrosis Factor (TNF) is a key inflammatory cytokine and mediator of intestinal inflammation. The expression of TNF is increased in IBD. Infliximab is a chimeric mouse-human monoclonal antibody against TNF that is extremely effective in Crohn's disease. Recently adalimumab has also been approved for treatment of moderate to severe crohn disease.

Newer Immunosuppressive Agents for IBD

1. Tacrolimus
2. Mycophenolate mofetil
3. 6-Thioguanine
4. Thalidomide
5. The α4 integrin-specific humanized monoclonal antibody, natalizumab, prevents the migration of leukocytes into the parenchyma and blocks their activation in inflammatory sites.

106. Ans. (d) Highly associated with infertility

(Ref: Harrison 20th edition, p 2258; Harrison 19th p 1951)

Patients with quiescent UC and CD have normal fertility rates. *The fallopian tubes can be scarred by the inflammatory process of CD, especially on the right side because of the proximity of the terminal ileum.* In addition, perirectal, perineal, and rectovaginal abscesses and fistulae can result in dyspareunia. Infertility in men can be caused by sulfasalazine but reverses when treatment is stopped.

Comparison of epidemiological features of ulcerative colitis versus crohn's disease

Male/female ratio	1:1	1.1-8:1
Smoking	May prevent disease	May cause disease
Oral contraceptives	No increased risk	Odds ratio 1.4
Appendectomy	Protective	Not protective
Monozygotic twins	6% concordance	58% concordance
Dizygotic twins	0% concordance	4% concordance

107. Ans. (b) Fecal lactoferrin

(Ref: Harrison 20th edition, p 2263; Harrison 19th p 1954)

- Fecal lactoferrin is a highly sensitive and specific marker for detecting intestinal inflammation.
- Fecal calprotectin levels correlate well with histologic inflammation, predict relapses, and detect pouchitis.
- Leukocytosis may be present but is not a specific indicator of disease activity. Proctitis or procto-sigmoiditis rarely causes a rise in CRP.

108. Ans. (c) Urethritis

(Ref: Harrison 20th edition, p 2269; Harrison 19th p 1952)

Bloody diarrhea is the hallmark feature of ulcerative colitis.

Extracolonic manifestations: include:

1. Erythema nodosum
2. Pyoderma gangrenosum
3. Episcleritis
4. Iritis
5. Thrombo-embolic events
6. Oligo-articular, non-deforming arthritis. (Most common)

In patients who are HLA B27-seropositive, there may be anterior uveitis or ankylosing spondylitis which is independent of colitis activity.

109. Ans. (d) Primary sclerosing cholangitis

(Ref: Harrison 20th edition, p 2269)

The extra-intestinal involvement of ulcerative colitis is primary sclerosing cholangitis

Primary sclerosing cholangitis is a disorder characterized by both intrahepatic and extrahepatic bile duct inflammation and fibrosis, frequently leading to biliary cirrhosis and hepatic failure. PSC occurs less often in patients with CD.

110. Ans. (b) Crohn's disease

(Ref: Harrison 20th edition, p 2264; Harrison 19th p 1953)

Premalignant Lesions of GIT

111. Ans. (c) Peutz-Jegher's syndrome

(Ref: Harrison 20th edition, p 573; Harrison 19th edition, Page 359,538t)

Cushing syndrome	Presents with lemon on sticks with hypertension and anemia.
Albright syndrome	McCune-Albright syndrome (MAS) consists of at least 2 of the following 3 features: 1. Polyostotic fibrous dysplasia 2. Café-au-lait skin pigmentation 3. Autonomous endocrine hyperfunction (eg, gonadotropin-independent)
Peutz jehgers syndrome	The lentigines in patients with *Peutz-Jeghers syndrome* are located primarily around the nose and mouth, on the hands and feet, and within the oral cavity. This is associated with hamartomatous polyps. During the first 3 decades of life, anemia, rectal bleeding, abdominal pain, obstruction, and/or intussusception are common complications in patients with Peutz-Jeghers syndrome.
Incontinentia pigmenti	*The disease has a pediatric presentation* Major criteria are (1) typical neonatal vesicular rash with eosinophilia; (2) typical blaschkoid hyperpigmentation on the trunk, fading in adolescence; and (3) linear, atrophic hairless lesions. Minor criteria are (1) dental anomalies, (2) alopecia, (3) wooly hair, and (4) abnormal nails.

112. Ans. (a) Peutz Jegher's

(Ref: Harrison 20th edition, p 573; Bailey and Love 26th edition, page 1159)

Peutz–Jegher's	Malignant change in the polyps rarely occurs and, in general the polyps can be left alone. Resection may be indicated for heavy and persistent or recurrent bleeding or intussusception. Polyps may be removed by enterotomy, or, at laparotomy, snared via a colonoscope.
Crohn disease	Risk factors for developing cancer in Crohn's colitis are long-duration and extensive disease, bypassed colon segments, colon strictures, PSC, and family history of colon cancer. The cancer risks in CD and UC are probably equivalent for similar extent and duration of disease

Contd...

Ulcerative colitis	Patients with long-standing UC are at increased risk for developing colonic epithelial dysplasia and carcinoma
Barret esophagus	Patients with Barrett's esophagus generally undergo a surveillance program of periodic endoscopy with biopsies to detect dysplasia or early carcinoma.

113. Ans. (c) Peutz-Jegher syndrome

(Ref: Harrison 20th edition, p 573; Robbins 8th edition chapter 15, Harrison 19th p 536)

- *STK11* is a tumor suppressor gene, in that its over-expression can induce a growth arrest of a cell at the G1 phase of the cell cycle and that somatic inactivation of the unaffected allele of *STK11* is often observed in polyps and cancers from patients with Peutz-Jeghers syndrome.
- *The second gene involved in Peutz-Jegher's* polyps is caused by germ-line mutations in the *LKB1* gene.
- *Loss of the APC tumor suppressor gene in* FAP and Gardner syndrome give rise to hundreds of adenomas that progress to form cancers.
- MALT lymphoma a t(11;18) translocation is common (the translocation creates a fusion gene between the apoptosis inhibitor *BCL-2* gene in chromosome 11 and the *MLT* gene in chromosome 18.

114. Ans. (b) Familial polyposis coli

(Ref: Harrison 20th edition, p 573; Harrison 19th p 541)

115. Ans. (c) Small bowel

(Ref: Harrison 20th edition, p 573; Harrison 19th p 538t)

116. Ans. (b) Peutz Jehger syndrome

(Ref: Harrison 20th edition, p 573; Harrison 19th p 538t)

Diarrhea

117. Ans. (a) Cystoisospora

(Ref: Harrison 20th edition, page 1435-36)

- AIDS Positive patients usually have Cryptosporidium diarrhea.
- The pointer in the question against that diagnosis is size of sporulated cyst which is given to be 10-30 μm where as in cryptosporidium the sporulated oocyst is 4-6 μm. Hence the diagnosis is Cystoisospora which was formerly called as isospora.
- For treatment of cystoisospora cotrimoxazole is used whereas in cryptosporidium, nitazoxanide is used.

Property	Cryptosporidium	Cyclospora	Isospora
Infective form	Sporulated oocyst • Thick walled oocyst (80%) by contaminated food and water. • Thin walled (20%) Autoinfection	Sporulated oocyst (Contaminated food and water)	Sporulated oocyst (Contaminated food and water)
Sporulated oocyst	4–6 μm, round contains four sporozoites	8–12 μm, round contains 2 sporocyst, each having two sporozoites	23–26 μm contains 2 sporocyst, each having four sporozoites
Acid fastness Detection limit> 50,000 oocyst/ml stool	Uniformly acid fast	Variable acid fast	Uniformly acid fast

118. Ans. (d) Ice cream

(Ref: NCBI- NIH)

The amount of lactose in ice-cream is surprisingly lesser than yoghurt. Yoghurt is better tolerated than milk.

Food product	Amount of lactose per serving
Ice cream, 50 g	1.65
Ricotta cheese, 120 g	2.4
Yogurt (natural), 200 g	10.0*
Regular milk, 250 ml	15.75

119. Ans. (d) Toxin detection by NAAT

(Ref: Harrison 20th edition, p 966; Harrison 19th edition, Page 859, Table 161-1)

- Nucleic acid amplification test for C. Difficile toxin A or B gene in stool is more sensitive and specific than enzyme immunoassay toxin testing.
- NAAT for toxin and not for genes is used for diagnosis.
- Diagnosis of CDI is based on
  1. Diarrhea (> 3 unformed stools per day for > 2 days)
  2. Toxin A or B detected in stool by PCR or culture or pseudo-membranes seen in stool.

TABLE: Relative sensitivity and specificity of diagnostic tests for *Clostridium difficile* infection (CDI)

Type of test	Relative sensitivity[Q]	Relative specificity[Q]	Comment
Stool culture for C. difficile	++++	+++	Most sensitive test; specificity of ++++ if the C. difficile isolate tests positive for toxin; with clinical data, is diagnostic of CDI; turn around time too slow for practical use
Cell culture cytotoxin test on stool	+++	++++	With clinical data, is diagnostic of CDI; highly specific but not as sensitive as stool culture, slow turn around time

Contd...

Type of test	Relative sensitivity[Q]	Relative specificity[Q]	Comment
Enzyme immunoassay for toxin A or toxins A and B in stool	++ to +++	+++	With clinical data, is diagnostic of CDI; rapid results, but not as sensitive as stool culture or cell culture cytotoxin test
Enzyme immunoassay for *C. difficile* common antigen in stool	+++ to ++++	+++	Detects glutamate dehydrogenase found in toxigenic and non-toxigenic strains of *C. difficile* and other stool organisms; more sensitive and less specific than enzyme immunoassay for toxins; rapid results
Nucleic acid amplification tests for *C. difficile* toxin A and B gene in stool	++++	++++	Detect toxigenic *C. difficile* in stool; newly approved for clinical testing, but appears to be more sensitive than enzyme immunoassay toxin testing and at least as specific
Colonoscopy or sigmidoscopy	+	++++	Highly specific if pseudomembranes are seen; insensitive compared with other tests

120. Ans. (c) Responds to low fat diet

(Ref: Harrison 20th edition, p 2346; Table 349-2: Harrison 19th edition, page 1935)

- The primary functions of bile acids are to enhance the dietary lipid digestion by promoting the bile flow, solubilize cholesterol and phospholipids.
- In setting of ileal disease or ileal resection, bile acids are unabsorbed. These *bile acids lead to stimulation of chloride secretion and lead to bile acid diarrhea.* Hence the diarrhea will not respond to low fat diet.
- It is also called choleretic enteropathy and rather responds to cholestyramine.
- Steatorrhea does not occur in bile acid diarrhea since bile acid production increases to compensate for the rate of bile-acid losses.

121. Ans. (b) Nocturnal episodes of colicky pain

(Ref: Harrison 20th edition, p 2276; Harrison 19th edition, page 1965: Table 352-1)

The diagnostic criteria for irritable bowel syndrome is- Recurrent abdominal pain or discomfort for at least 3 days per month associated with >2 or more of the following features-

1. Pain improvement with defecation
2. Onset with change in form/appearance of stool
3. Onset with change in frequency of stool

Nocturnal diarrhea or pain is not a feature of irritable bowel syndrome and is seen with Diabetic neuropathy. Bleeding is also not a feature.

122. Ans. (a) Norovirus

(Ref: Harrison 20th edition, p 1463; Harrison 19th edition, page 1285-86)

Shellfish can accumulate large number of noroviruses, which can lead to outbreaks of diarrheal illness. Large outbreaks occur after intake of inadequately cooked shellfish, such as oyster and clams.

Bacteria	Viruses	Parasites
Bacillus Cereus	Noroviruses	Giardia
campylobacter	Hepatitis A	Paragonimus
Clostridium botulinism		Diphyllobotrium
Clostridium perfringens		
E.Coli		
Listeria		
Salmonella		
Shigella		
Vibrio Cholerae		
Vibrio Vulnificus		
Vibrio parahemolyticus		

123. Ans. (a) Osmotic diarrhea

(Ref: Harrison 20th edition, p 264; Harrison 19th p 269/303)

Osmotic diarrhea stops with fasting, has a low pH, and is positive for reducing substances.

124. Ans. (b) Bacterial overgrowth syndrome

(Ref: Harrison 20th edition, p 2252; Harrison 19th p 1944)

Since both are abnormal it indicates that there is a mucosal disease with impaired absorption of B12 which is a feature of bacterial overgrowth syndrome.

Result of Diagnostic Studies in Different Causes of Steatorrhea

	D-Xylose Test	Schilling Test	Duodenal Mucosal Biopsy
Chronic pancreatitis	Normal	50% abnormal; if abnormal, normal with pancreatic enzymes	Normal
Bacterial overgrowth syndrome	Normal or only modestly abnormal	Often abnormal; if abnormal, normal after antibiotics	Usually normal

Contd...

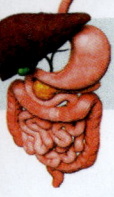

	D-Xylose Test	Schilling Test	Duodenal Mucosal Biopsy
Ileal disease	Normal	Abnormal	Normal
Celiac sprue	Decreased	Normal	Abnormal: probably "flat"
Intestinal lymphangiectasia	Normal	Normal	Abnormal: "dilated lymphatics"

125. Ans. (a) Clonidine

(Ref: Harrison 20th edition, p 267; Harrison 19th p 270, 272)

- Clonidine, an alpha-2-adrenergic agonist, increases colonic compliance, has antisecretory effects, and has been effective for treating diabetic diarrhea
- Diabetic diarrhea is a syndrome of unexplained persistent diarrhea in individuals with a longstanding history of diabetes. This may be due to autonomic neuropathy leading to abnormal motility and secretion of fluid in the colon. The most common is the irritable bowel syndrome.
- Fiber supplementation with bran, Citrucel, Metamucil, or high-fiber foods may also thicken the consistency of the bowel movement and decrease watery diarrhea.

126. Ans. (c) Milk

(Ref: Harrison 20th edition, p 264; CMDT, ch. 15, pg. 626, Harrison 19th p 272)

- Lactose intolerant individuals have insufficient levels of lactase, an enzyme that catalyzes hydrolysis of lactose into glucose and galactose, in their digestive system. In most cases this causes symptoms which may include abdominal bloating and cramps, flatulence, diarrhea, nausea, borborygmi, or vomiting after consuming significant amounts of lactose.
- Most accurate lactose intolerance test is a hydrogen breath test. After an overnight fast. 25 grams of lactose (in a solution with water) is swallowed. If the lactose cannot be digested, enteric bacteria metabolize it and produce hydrogen, which, along with methane, if produced, can be detected on the patient's breath by a clinical gas chromatograph or compact solid-state detector. The test takes about 2 to 3 hours to complete.

127. Ans. (b) Hypercalcemia

(Ref: Harrison 20th edition, p 261; Harrison 19th p 265)

- Hypercalcemia increases the tone of sphincters of the gut leading to refractory constipation.
- Autonomic dysfunction in diabetes explains the diarrhea.
- Thyrotoxicosis leads to secretary diarrhea. More over bile acid physiology is also affected in thyrotoxicosis due to autoimmune damage to liver in Graves.
- IBS has variable presentation between diarrhea and constipation.

128. Ans. (b) Anti-endomysial antibody

(Ref: Harrison 20th edition, p 2253)

Malabsorption Syndrome

129. Ans. (c) RBC glutathione reductase levels

Ref: Vasudevan Textbook of Biochemistry, 7th edition, page 479

The image shows presence of cheliosis, glossitis and circumcorneal vascularization. This is diagnostic of riboflavin deficiency. The test recommended is RBC glutathione reductase levels.

130. Ans. (a) Intestinal neoplasms

(Ref: Harrison 20th edition, p 2253; Harrison 19th edition, page 1942: and Harsh Mohan 7th edition, page 558)

The most important complication of celiac sprue is development of cancer both intestinal and non-intestinal neoplasms and lymphomas.

Complications of celiac sprue:
1. Intestinal neoplasms/ lymphoma
2. Refractory sprue
3. Collagenous sprue
Tropical sprue is associated with:
1. Dermatitis herpetiformis
2. Type 1 DM
3. IgA deficiency
4. Down and Turner syndrome

131. Ans. (b) Irritable bowel syndrome

(Ref: Harrison 20th edition, p 2256; Harrison 19th edition, page 1945:)

The causes of Protein losing enteropathy can be classified into three groups:

Disease process	Mechanism	Examples
Mucosal ulceration	Protein loss primarily represents exudation across damaged mucosa.	Ulcerative colitis Gastrointestinal carcinomas Peptic ulcer
Non-ulcerated mucosa	Loss across epithelia with altered permeability	Celiac disease Ménétrier's disease in the small intestine and stomach
Lymphatic dysfunction	Primary lymphatic disease or secondary to partial lymphatic obstruction.	Enlarged Lymph nodes Cardiac Disease

132. Ans. (b) Anti-nuclear antibodies

(Ref: Harrison 20th edition, p 2253; Harrison 19th edition, page 1940)

- Antibody testing, especially immunoglobulin A anti-tissue transglutaminase antibody (IgA TTG), is the best first test, although biopsies are needed for confirmation; in children younger than 2 years, the IgA TTG test should be combined with testing for IgG-deamidated gliadin peptides

- *The most sensitive and specific antibodies for the confirmation of celiac disease are tissue transglutaminase IgA, endomysial IgA, and reticulin IgA and correlate with the degree of mucosal damage.*
- Anti-gliadin antibodies were one of the first serological markers for coeliac disease. Problematic with Anti-gliadin antibodies is the typical sensitivity and specificity was about 85%.

133. Ans. (a) Wheat

(Ref: Harrison 20th edition, p 2253; Harrison 19th ed. / 1940)

- Coeliac disease is caused by a reaction to gliadin found in wheat, oats, rye and Barley. Upon exposure to gliadin, there is production of anti-tissue transglutaminase antibody which cross-reacts with small-bowel tissue, causing an inflammatory reaction.
- This leads to villous atrophy and leads to osmotic diarrhea.

134. Ans. (b) Constipation

(Ref: Harrison 20th edition, p 2249; Harrison 19th p 1946)

- Iron absorption occurs in duodenum which is affected in sprue.
- Due to fat malabsorption steatorrhea and vitamin D deficiency results.
- The symptoms & signs of malabsorption depend upon the length of small intestine involved & the age at which the patient presents.
- Infants (< 2 years) are more likely to present with typical symptoms of malabsorption, including diarrhea, weight loss, abdominal distention, weakness, muscle wasting, or growth retardation.
- However, they may also be watery and frequent in number (up to 10-12 daily).
- Most patients report chronic diarrhea or flatulence due to colonic bacterial digestion of mal-absorbed nutrients, but the severity of weight loss is variable.

135. Ans. (b) Gluten enteropathy

(Ref: Harrison 20th edition, p 2252; Harrison 19th p 1940)

- Serological blood tests are the first-line investigation required to make a diagnosis of coeliac disease.
- Anti-endomysial antibodies of the immuno-globulin A (IgA) type can detect coeliac disease with a sensitivity and specificity of 90% and 99%, respectively.
- Serology for anti-T.T.G antibodies was initially reported to have a higher sensitivity (99%) and specificity (>90%) for identifying coeliac disease.
- Modern anti-tTG assays rely on a human recombinant protein as an antigen. tTG testing should be done first as it is an easier test to perform.

136. Ans. (a) Carbohydrate malabsorption due to mucosal disease

(Ref: Harrison 20th edition, p 2249; Harrison 19th p 1938)

- D-Xylose is a monosaccharide, or simple sugar, that does not require enzymes for digestion prior to absorption.
- Its absorption requires an intact mucosa only. In contrast, polysaccharides require enzymes, such as amylase, to break them down so that they can eventually be absorbed as monosaccharides.
- In normal individuals, a 25 g oral dose of D-xylose will be absorbed and excreted in the urine at approximately 4.5 g in 5 hours. A decreased urinary excretion of D-xylose is seen in conditions involving the GI mucosa, such as small intestinal bacterial overgrowth and Whipple's disease. In cases of bacterial overgrowth, the values of D-Xylose absorption return to normal after treatment with antibiotics. In contrast, if the D-xylose urinary excretion is normal, then the problem must be due to a non-mucosal cause of malabsorption (i.e., pancreatic insufficiency).
- This test was previously in use but has been made redundant by antibody tests.

137. Ans. (d) Monosaccharide absorption

(Ref: Harrison 20th edition, p 2249; Harrison 19th p 1938)

Condition	Investigation of choice
Insulinoma	72 hour prolonged fasting
Atypical carcinoid	5 HTP (hydroxyl-tryptophan)
ZES	Secretin study
Monosaccharide malabsorption	D-Xylose absorption test

138. Ans. (b) Increased lymphatic flow

(Ref: Harrison 20th edition, p 2251; Harrison 19th p 1945)

Obstruction of lymphatics from any cause can produce increased pressure throughout the lymphatic system of the GI tract. This results in the *stasis of lymph* and, if the pressure is high enough, the loss of lymphatic fluid rich in albumin and other proteins from the lacteals in intestinal microvilli into the lumen of the GI tract. If the loss of albumin exceeds the rate of synthesis, hypoalbuminemia and, eventually, edema develop. In addition to the loss of albumin, other important components of lymph are also lost into the bowel, including lymphocytes, immunoglobulins, and hydrophobic molecules such as cholesterol, lipids, and fat-soluble vitamins.

139. Ans. (a) Protein losing enteropathy

(Ref: Harrison 20th edition, p 2256; Harrison 19th p 1945)

Alpha-1-antitrypsin (α-1-AT) is produced by the liver, intestinal macrophages, monocytes and mucous membrane cells of the gut. It belongs to the group of acute phase proteins and is one of the most important proteinase inhibitor. α-1-AT inhibits, beside others, the proteinases trypsin and the elastase of Neutrophils. Only a very small amount of α-1-AT is cleaved or resorbed in the gut. (*Therefore the measurement of α-1-AT in stool reflects the permeability of the gut during inflammatory processes*).

140. Ans. (c) Whipple's disease

(Ref: Harrison 20th edition, p 2251; CMDT, ch. 15, pg. 623, Harrison 19th p 1091, 1944)

Jujunal Biopsy in Whipple's disease shows macrophages in lamina propria, showing P.A.S (Schiff's reagent) positive

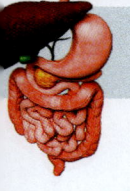

bacilli. The remaining choices show non specific findings of villous atrophy.

141. **Ans. (d)** *Jejunal biopsy is specific*

(Ref: Harrison 20th edition, p 2251; Harrison 19th p 1942)

Small intestinal mucosal biopsy is not pathognomonic and mimics fundings of celiac spreua.

142. **Ans. (a)** *Antiendomysial antibodies*

(Ref: Harrison 20th edition, p 2252)

The presence of anti-endomyosial A/b is 90–05%

143. **Ans. (a)** *Abetalipoproteinemia*

(Ref: Harrison 20th edition, p 2251; Harrison 19th p 2444)

- Abetalipoproteinemia, or Bassen-Kornzweig syndrome, is a rare autosomal recessive disorder that interferes with the normal absorption of fat and fat-soluble vitamins from food.
- It is caused by a mutation in microsomal triglyceride transfer protein resulting in deficiencies in the apolipoproteins B-48 and B-100, which are used in the synthesis and exportation of chylomicrons and VLDL respectively.
- On intestinal biopsy, vacuoles containing lipids are seen in enterocytes. This disorder may also result in fat accumulation in the liver (hepatic steatosis). Because the epithelial cells of the bowel lack the ability to place fats into chylomicrons, lipids accumulate at the surface of the cell, crowding the functions that are necessary for proper absorption.

144. **Ans. (d)** *Intestinal parasite*

(Ref: Harrison 20th edition, p 2249; Harrison 19th p 1946t)

145. **Ans. (b)** *Pseudopolyps*

(Ref: Harrison 20th edition, p 2263; Harrison 19th p 1954)

146. **Ans. (b)** *Vitamin B_{12}*

(Ref: Harrison 20th edition, p 2253; Harrison 19th p 1897f/1940)

- The proximal part of the gut is more involved in celiac sprue as compared to distal part. Hence vitamin B_{12} levels are rarely ever low.
- Due to maximum damage to duodenum and jejunum iron and folic acid deficiency is common
- Vitamin A deficiency can develop in celiac disease in the following ways. Upper digestive problems, such as low stomach acid, can fail to dissolve vitamin A out of food sources. Protein deficiency impairs absorption transport through the intestinal lining while fat malabsorption impairs vitamin A absorption into the lymph.

147. **Ans. (d)** *13 C triclosan breath test*

(Ref: Clinical biochemistry by William J. Marshall, 2nd ed. pg 240, Harrison 19th p 1946t)

D- Xylose test	Sugar malabsorption and tests jejunal damage or proximal enteropathy
14 C Triolein test	Fat malabsorption picked up by radiocarbon being tagged to the triglycerides
13 C Trioactanoin	Fat malabsorption due to pancreatic exocrine insufficiency
SeHCAT is the usual name for 23-seleno-25-homo-tauro-cholic acid (selenium homocholic acid taurine)	It is used in a clinical test to diagnose bile acid malabsorption
Hydrogen breath test	For sugar malabsorption as unabsorbed sugar is degraded by bacteria.
13C acetate breath tests	For stomach emptying

148. **Ans. (d)** *Anterior resection of colon*

(Ref: Harrison 19th p 1946t)

149. **Ans. (d)** *Poor absorption of lipids*

(Ref: Harrison 19th p 1940)

Nontropical sprue is alternative terminology to describe celiac sprue.

In non-tropical sprue (and to a lesser degree in tropical sprue), microscopic examination of the jejunum reveals
1. Blunting or absence of the villi
2. Substitution of cuboidal for columnar surface cells
3. Infiltration of the lamina propria with lymphocytes and plasma cells
4. Increased mitotic activity in the crypts of the unusually deep intestinal glands.

(The damage would lead to mal-absorption of carbohydrates and lipids).

150. **Ans. (a)** *Pancreatic insufficiency*

(Ref: Harrison 19th p 1938)

151. **Ans. (c)** *D-xylose test*

(Ref: Harrison 20th edition, p 2249; Harrison 19th p 1946t)

152. **Ans. (a)** *Abnormal in pernicious anemia;* **(c)** *Abnormal in ileal disease*

(Ref: Harrison 20th edition, p 2252; Harrison 19th p 1941t)

153. **Ans. (c)** *Whipple's Disease*

(Ref: Harrison 20th edition, p 2256; Harrison 19th p 1946t)

154. **Ans. (d)** *Dementia*

(Ref: Harrison 20th edition, p 2256; Harrison 19th p 1093)

155. Ans. (d) Giardiasis

(Ref: Harrison 20th edition, p 2253; Harrison 19th p 1946t)

Pediatric Gastroenterology

156. Ans. (b) A and C only

(Ref: Bailey and Love 26th edition, page 113:)

- Non-bilious vomiting is the initial symptom of pyloric stenosis. Choice B is wrong
- The vomiting may or may not be projectile initially but is usually progressive, occurring immediately after a feeding.
- In healthy infants, feeding can be an aid to the diagnosis. After feeding, there may be a visible gastric peristaltic wave that progresses across the abdomen. Choice A is correct.
- The diagnosis has traditionally been established by palpating the pyloric mass. Choice C is correct
- The mass is firm, movable, ≈2 cm in length, olive shaped, hard, best palpated from the left side, and located above and to the right of the umbilicus in the mid epigastrium beneath the liver edge.
- After the infant vomits, the abdominal musculature is more relaxed and the "olive" easier to palpate.
- The vomiting usually starts after 3 wk of age, but symptoms may develop as early as the 1st wk of life and as late as the 5th months.
- As vomiting continues, a progressive loss of fluid, hydrogen ion, and chloride leads to hypochloremic metabolic alkalosis.

157. Ans. (a) Congenital diaphragmatic hernia

(Ref: Current Pediatric Diagnosis and Treatment, 22nd edition, p 661)

- Notice the air filled loops of intestine in left lung. Respiratory distress is a cardinal sign in babies with CDH.
- This may occur immediately or there may be a "honeymoon" period of up to 48 hr when the baby is relatively stable.
- Early respiratory distress within 6 hr of life is thought to be a poor prognostic sign. The clinical signs of respiratory distress are characterized by tachypnea, grunting, use of accessory muscles, and cyanosis.
- Children with CDH will also have a scaphoid abdomen and increased chest wall diameter. Bowel sounds may also be heard in the chest with decreased breath sounds bilaterally.

158. Ans. (c) Stage 2B

(Ref: Ch. 102.2 Nelson's 18th ed., Harrison 19th p 99)

- The Bell system is the staging system most commonly used to describe necrotizing enterocolitis (NEC).
- Stage IIA shows ileus and pneumatosis intestinalis. Stage IIB shows portal vein gas. Stage IIIA shows features of stages IIB plus ascites.

159. Ans. (a) Erythromycin

(Ref: Nelson 20th edition, p 1380)

160. Ans. (c) Metabolic alkalosis with paradoxical aciduria

(Ref: Bailey 23rd / 917, Nelson: 19th p 1274)

MALT-oma

161. Ans. (d) Can be easily differentiated clinically from gastric adenocarcinoma by the presence of early satiety and prominent lymph node metastases

(Ref: Harrison 20th edition, p 570; Harrison 19th edition, page 703)

- Helicobacter pylori is a type A carcinogen incriminated in causing mucosa associated lymphoid tumour.
- Treatment with proton pump inhibitor (PPI) and antibiotics to eradicate H pylori is the most important modality used in the therapy of gastric MALTomas.
- Treatment with a combination of amoxicillin, clarithromycin, and PPIs results in eradication rates of 90%. This causes regression of low grade of MALToma.
- The traditional monotherapy regimens employed for MALTomas have included chlorambucil, cyclophosphamide, or fludarabine. The presence of t(11;18)(q21;q21) translocations has been shown to predict a poor response to therapy
- MALTOMA is a Non-Hodgkin lymphoma of B cell type.
- Median age of presentation is 65 years and non-specific features are seen. Early gastric cancer has no associated symptoms; however, some patients with incidental complaints are diagnosed with early gastric cancer. Most symptoms of gastric cancer reflect advanced disease.

162. Ans. (b) Ileum

(Ref: Harrison 20th edition, p 777; Harrison 19th p 703)

- MC site of MALT is ileum
- MALT lymphoma may occur in the stomach, orbit, intestine, lung, thyroid, salivary gland, skin, soft tissues, bladder, kidney, and CNS.

163. Ans. (d) Associated with Alk mutation

(Ref: Bailey and Love 26th edition, p 1160; Harrison 19th p 119 e-1)

- Gastrointestinal stromal cell tumors (GISTs), were previously classified as gastrointestinal leiomyosarcomas and make up 1–3% of gastric neoplasms.
- Its cell of origin resembles the interstitial cell of Cajal, which controls peristalsis.
- The majority of malignant GISTs have activating mutations of the c-kit gene that result in ligand-independent phosphorylation and activation of the KIT receptor tyrosine kinase, leading to tumorigenesis.
- They most frequently involve the anterior and posterior walls of the gastric fundus and often ulcerate and bleed.
- These tumors rarely invade adjacent viscera and characteristically do not metastasize to lymph nodes, but they may spread to the liver and lungs. The treatment of choice is surgical resection.

- GISTs are unresponsive to conventional chemotherapy; yet 50% of patients experience objective response and prolonged survival when treated with imatinib mesylate (Gleevec) (400–800 mg PO daily), a selective inhibitor of the *c-kit* tyrosine kinase.
- Many patients with GIST whose tumors have become refractory to imatinib subsequently benefit from sunitinib (Sutent), another inhibitor of the *c-kit* tyrosine kinase

Miscellaneous

164. Ans. (c) Sitting with neck flexed

(Ref: page 773: Oxford handbook of clinical medicine)

The image shows a Nasogastric tube which should be put in a conscious patient in sitting position with slight flexion of the neck.

Procedure for inserting NG tube

1. Examine the patient's nostril to check for septal deviation and identify the more patent nostril
2. Instil viscous lidocaine into the patent nostril
3. Estimate the length of insertion by measuring the distance from the tip of the nose, around the ear, and down to just below the left costal margin.
4. The estimated length falls in between the 2nd and 3rd pre-printed black lines on the tube
5. Position the patient sitting upright with the neck partially flexed. Ask the patient to hold a cup of water in his or her hand and put a straw in his or her mouth with instructions to sip water only when asked to.
6. Gently insert the NG tube along the floor of the nose, and advance it parallel to the nasal floor (i.e. directly perpendicular to the patient's head, not angled up into the nose) until it reaches the back of the nasopharynx, where resistance will be met (10-20 cm).

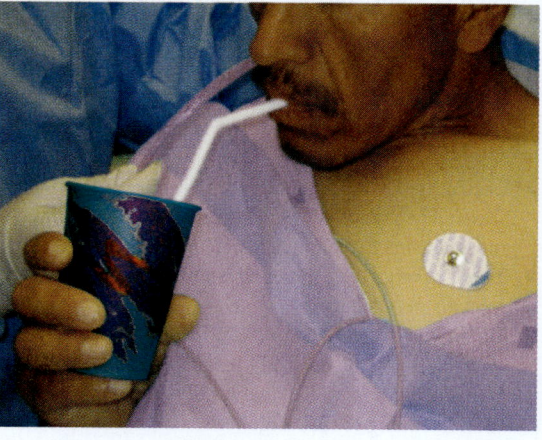

7. At this time, ask the patient to sip on the water through the straw and start to swallow (see the image).
8. Notice the flexion in the neck of the patient while the patient is swallowing water through a straw while the NG is advanced forwards.
9. Continue to advance the NG tube until the distance of the previously estimated length is reached.

165. Ans. (b) Alcohol

Ref: Harrison 20th edition, p 2445; page 2098: Harrison 19th edition

Most common cause of clinically apparent chronic pancreatitis in adults is alcoholism. Acute pancreatitis to caused by gall stones.

Most common cause of clinically apparent chronic pancreatitis in children is cystic fibrosis.

166. Ans. (a) CT

(*Ref: Harrison 20th ed., p 2301; Harrison 19th ed, page 1988*)

- The sensitivity of CT scan for detection of acute appendicitis is 0.94 and specificity is 0.95. Hence the negative predictive value of CT imaging is helpful in diagnosis.
- CT examination which shows dilatation of appendix>6mm with wall thickening and a lumen that does not fill with enteric contrast is diagnostic of inflammation of appendix.

167. Ans. (b) IV vancomycin is ineffective in the treatment of Clostridium difficile diarrhoea

(*Ref: Harrison 20th ed., p 967; Harrison 19th ed, page 855, 858*)

Choice A is false	Most common *antibiotic incriminated is Cephalosporins.*
Choice B is true	Oral vancomycin is used and not intravenous vancomycin. In 2013, The European Society of Clinical Microbiology and Infection released updated guidelines for the treatment of CDI • For patients with non-epidemic, non-severe CDI clearly induced by antibiotic use, with no signs of severe colitis, it may be acceptable to stop antibiotic treatment and observe the clinical response for 48 hours • For mild/moderate disease, oral metronidazole (500 mg 3 times daily for 10 days) is recommended as initial treatment • In patients for whom oral treatment is inappropriate, fidaxomicin may be used. • For patients with severe CDI, suitable antibiotic regimens include vancomycin (125 mg 4 times daily for 10 days; may be increased to 500 mg 4 times daily) or fidaxomicin (200 mg twice daily for 10 days) • Use of fidaxomicin is not supported in life-threatening CDI • Use of oral metronidazole in severe or life-threatening CDI is discouraged • Fecal transplantation is recommended for multiple recurrent CDI
Choice C is false	Presentation is *mild to moderate watery diarrhoea and rarely bloody.* Faecal leucocytes are present.
Choice D is false	Colonoscopy will show presence of raised, yellowish white, 2- to 10-mm plaques overlying an erythematous, edematous mucosa *in colon* and not the small intestine.

168. Ans. (b) Argentaffin cells of small intestine

(*Ref: Harrison 20th ed., p 603; Harrison 19th page 564*)

- Carcinoid tumor/NET originates from argentaffin cell. Historically, silver staining was used, and tumors were classified as showing an argentaffin reaction if they took up and reduced silver or as being argyrophilic if they did not reduce
- NETs generally are composed of monotonous sheets of small round cells with uniform nuclei, and mitoses are uncommon.

Shared general neuroendocrine cell markers for diagnosis
1. Chromogranins (A, B, C) .Chromogranin A is the most widely used.
2. Neuron-specific enolase (NSE) is the cytosolic marker of neuroendocrine differentiation.
3. Synaptophysin

169. Ans. (d) Perforated abdominal viscus

(Ref: Harrison 20th edition, p 953; Harrison 19th edition, page 847)

The X-Ray film shows an inspiratory film with gas under diaphragm diagnostic of perforation peritonitis.

Hydatid cyst right lung	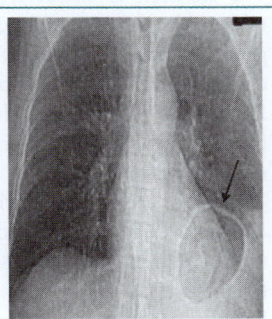 Water lily sign
Right pleural effusion	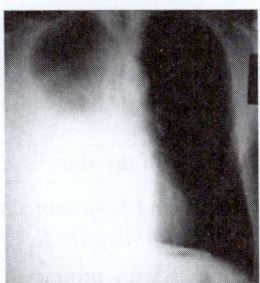 Meniscus sign with shifted trachea
Right hydro-pneumo-thorax	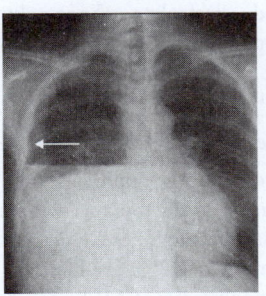

On an erect chest radiograph, recognition of hydro-pneumothorax can be rather easy - and is classically shown as an air-fluid level.
On the supine radiograph, this may be more challenging where a sharp pleural line is bordered by increased opacity lateral to it within the pleural space.

170. Ans. (d) Hypoglycemia

(Ref: Harrison 20th edition, p 2439; Harrison 19th edition, p. 1729-30:)

Pancreatitis is associated with the following lab parameters
1. Elevations of amylase and lipase
2. Leukocytosis
3. *Hyperglycemia*
4. Hypocalcemia
5. Hemo-concentration hematocrit >44%
6. Azotemia
7. Hyperbilirubinemia
8. LDH>500U/Dl
9. Hyperbilirubinemia
10. Hypoxia
11. Ascites
12. ECG ST-T wave changes simulating ischemia
13. CXR left pleural effusion

171. Ans. (a) Serum Lipase

(Ref: Harrison 20th edition, p 2439; Harrison 19th ed. / 2100)

- The cardinal symptom of acute pancreatitis is abdominal pain, which is characteristically dull, boring, and steady.
- *The pain radiates directly through the abdomen to the back in approximately one half of cases.*
- Lipase has a slightly longer half-life and its abnormalities may support the diagnosis if a delay occurs between the pain episode and the time the patient seeks medical attention.
- *Elevated lipase levels are more specific to the pancreas than elevated amylase levels. Lipase levels remain high for 12 days. In patients with chronic pancreatitis (usually caused by alcohol abuse and question mentions that the patient is back from a party), lipase levels may be elevated in the presence of a normal serum amylase level*

172. Ans. (a) Barium enema: Pipe stem colon

(Ref: Internal Medicine Guide 2e/36)

Lead pipe appearance of colon is the classical barium enema finding in chronic ulcerative colitis. There is complete loss of haustral markings in the diseased section of colon, and the organ appears smooth walled and cylindrical.

173. Ans. (b) Multiple air fluid level- adhesions and bands

(Ref: Manual of emergency medicine 5th ed/247)

- The X-ray abdomen shows bowel loops proximal to the point of obstruction will become dilated and fluid-filled.
- Absence of, or disproportionately smaller amount of, gas in the colon, especially the recto-sigmoid.
- Loops of small bowel may arrange themselves in a *step-ladder* configuration from the left upper to the right lower quadrant in a distal SBO
- Mostly fluid-filled loops of bowel may demonstrate a *string-of-beads sign* caused by the small amount of visible air in those loops

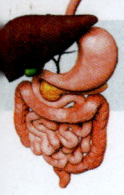

174. Ans. (a) CBD dilation on ERCP

(Ref: Cleveland Internal Medicine Case Reviews, 5e/93)

You can see the endoscope in left top half and right 5 o clock position which is radiopaque. It is advanced into D2 from where the ampulla of vater is located. The probe is advanced and dye injected which shows dilatation of whole biliary tree. A stricture is also noted proximal to which the biliary pathway is advanced.

175. Ans. (a) Campylobacter

(Ref: Harrison 20th edition, p 1184; Harrison 19th ed. p. 266)

- Diarrhea, the leading cause of illness in travelers, is usually a short-lived, self-limited condition; however, 40% of affected individuals need to alter their scheduled activities, and another 20% are confined to bed.
- The most frequently identified pathogens causing travelers' diarrhea are
  1. Toxigenic *Escherichia coli* and Enteroaggregative *E. coli* (Most common but not in choices)
  2. In Southeast Asia *Campylobacter* infections predominate
  3. *Salmonella, Shigella*
  4. Rotavirus
  5. Norovirus has caused numerous outbreaks on cruise ships

Except for giardiasis, parasitic infections are uncommon causes of travelers' diarrhea.

176. Ans. (c) Colon cancer

(Ref: Gastrointestinal Oncology 2nd ed/24)

- Aspirin has been shown to reduce the risk of colorectal cancer in latest studies in JAMA in September 2013. How it works is a matter of research but has shown a reduction in mortality.

177. Ans. (b) Pneumoperitoneum

(Ref: Harrison 20th edition, p 953; Harrison 19th edition p 847)

The image shows saddle back sign of pneumoperitoneum
Other signs diagnostic of pneumoperitoneum are

1. Anterior Subhepatic space Air
2. Doges Cap Sign (free Air in Morrison's Pouch)
3. Rigler's sign on supine AXR (also known as *double-wall* or *bas-relief sign*)
4. Falciform Ligament Sign
5. Football sign
6. *The cupola.* Air accumulation beneath the central tendon of the diaphragm

178. Ans. (a) Mesenteric artery occlusion

(Ref: Harrison 20th edition, p 2254; Harrison 19th p 1943)

- In healthy adults, the small intestine has an average length of approximately 6 meters (19.7 feet). Short bowel syndrome usually develops when there is less than 2 meters (6.6 feet) of the small intestine left to absorb sufficient nutrients.
- In mesenteric artery occlusion because thrombosis occurs at the origin of the vessel, the entire small bowel and proximal large bowel appear ischemic. In contradistinction, embolization of the SMA results in the proximal jejunum being spared, reflecting the more distal occlusion. But since a large part of gut is distal to jejunum and whole of colon is resected, short bowel syndrome will develop.
- **Other causes for short bowel syndrome**
  1. Crohn's disease
  2. Volvulus
  3. Tumors of the small intestine
  4. Injury or trauma to the small intestine
  5. Necrotizing enterocolitis
  6. Bypass surgery to treat obesity
  7. Surgery to remove diseases or damaged portion of the small intestine

179. Ans. (d) Hyperchlorhydria

(Ref: Harrison 20th edition, p 2243; CMDT, ch. 15, pg. 610)

- The stomach is characterized by large, tortuous gastric folds in the fundus and body of the stomach, with antrum generally spared, giving the mucosa a cobblestone or cerebriform (brain-like) appearance.
- Histologically, the most characteristic feature is massive foveolar hyperplasia (hyperplasia of surface and glandular mucous cells).
- The glands are elongated with a corkscrew-like appearance and cystic dilation is common. Inflammation is usually only modest, although some cases show marked intraepithelial lymphocytosis.
- Diffuse or patchy glandular atrophy, evident as hypoplasia of parietal and chief cells, is typical
- (*Twenty-four-hour pH monitoring reveals hypochlorhydria or achlorhydria, and a chromium-labelled albumin test reveals increased GI protein loss*). Serum gastrin levels will be within normal limits

180. Ans. (d) All of the above

(Ref: Bailey and Love 26th edition, p 1197; CMDT, ch. 15, pg. 627, Harrison 19th p 1982)

For patients with protracted ileus, mechanical obstruction must be excluded with contrast studies. Underlying sepsis and electrolyte abnormalities, particularly hypokalemia, hyponatremia, and hypomagnesemia, may worsen ileus

181. Ans. (a) Exenatide

(Ref: Harrison 20th edition, p 2867; Harrison 19th p 2090)

Exenatide is approved for monotherapy and for use as combination therapy with metformin, sulfonylureas, and thiazolidinediones. Some patients taking insulin secretagogues may require a reduction in those agents to prevent hypoglycemia. GLP-1 receptor agonists should not be used in patients taking insulin. The major side effects are nausea, vomiting, and diarrhea; hemorrhagic pancreatitis and reduced renal function have been reported.

182. Ans. (b) Hook worm

(Ref: Harrison 20th edition, p 1626; Harrison 19th p 1414)

In setting of open air defecation and barefoot walking with anemia hookworm infestation is likely. Though whip worm also cause blood loss of 5μl per worm but is spread by feco-oral route.

183. Ans. (c) Technetium isotope scan

(Ref: Harrison 20th edition, p 275; Harrison 19th p 277, 279)

- A Meckel scan uses 99m Tc pertechnetate to highlight the ectopic gastric mucosa
- Meckel diverticulum occurs in 2% of the population.
- The etiology of GI bleeding due to Meckel diverticulum is ileal ulceration caused by acid secretion from the ectopic gastric mucosa. Erosion into small arterioles leads to painless, brisk rectal bleeding. The site of ulceration is generally at the base of the diverticulum where the ectopic mucosa and the normal ileum join. More rarely, the ulcer appears distally in the ileum.

184. Ans. (d) Raised serum calcium

(Ref: CMDT 2019 p 742; Harrison 19th p 2090)

Lab findings of Acute pancreatitis:

- Elevated Pancreatic isoamylase, Lipase & Trypsin
- Leucocytosis (15,000 to 20,000/μl)
- Hyperglycemia
- Hypocalcemia
- Hyperbilirubinemia (> 4 mg/dl)
- LDH (< 8.5 μol/L)
- Serum albumin (< 3g/dl)
- Hypertriglyceridemia
- Proteinuria
- Granular casts, glycosuria (10- 20% cases)
- Elevated serum bilirubin
- Serum calcium of less than 8 mg/dl

185. Ans. (c) Achlorhydria

(Ref: CMDT 2019 p 1181; Harrison 19th p 2324t)

Triple-A syndrome (AAA), also known as Achalasia-Addisonianism-Alacrimia syndrome or Allgrove syndrome, is a rare autosomal recessive congenital disorder

- Triple-A syndrome is associated with mutations in the AAAS gene, which encodes a protein known as ALADIN (ALacrima Achalasia aDrenal Insufficiency Neurologic disorder), mapped the syndrome to a 6 cM interval on human chromosome 12q13 near the type II keratin gene
- Many cases of Allgrove (AAA) syndrome present with classic symptoms of primary adrenal insufficiency, including hypoglycemic seizures and shock.

186. Ans. (b) Insulinoma

(Ref: Harrison 20th edition, p 2749; Harrison 19th p 569)

187. Ans. (d) CCK

(Ref: Harrison 20th edition, p 2237; Harrison 19th p 1926)

- Release of vasoactive GI hormones (vasoactive intestinal polypeptide, neurotensin, motilin) is also theorized to play a role in early dumping.

188. Ans. (d) All of the above

(Ref: Harrison 20th edition, p 2251; Harrison 19th p 2090)

- Hypertriglyceridemia & Enterokinase deficiency are causes of Pancreatic Exocrine Insufficiency
- Triad of Pancreatic Exocrine Insufficiency include pancreatic calcification, steatorrhea, and diabetes mellitus.
- Pancreatic Exocrine Insufficiency shows symptoms/signs of malabsorption include weight loss & abnormal stools.

189. Ans. (b) Bleeding esophageal varices

(Ref: Harrison 19th p 276, 2063)

- In choice A and D vasopressin stimulates V2 receptors and leads to reduction in polyuria due to re-absorbtion of water via the water channels.
- DDAVP induces vWF secretion by binding to V2R and activating cAMP-mediated signaling in endothelial cells and controls bleeding in vWD.
- Vasopressin exerts vaso-constrictive effect on splanchnic circulation via V1 receptors.

	Receptor of vasopressin	Location	Action
V1	G protein-coupled, phosphalidylinositol/calcium	Vascular smooth muscle, platelet, hepatocytes, myometrium	Vasoconstriction, myocardial hypertrophy, platelet aggregation, glycogenolysis, uterin contraction
V3	G protein-coupled, phosphalidylinositol/calcium	Anterior pituitary gland	Releases ACTH, prolactin, endorphins
V2	Adenyl cyclase/cAMP	Basolateral membrane of collecting duct, vascular endothelium and vascular smooth muscle cell	Insertion of ACP-2 water channels into apical membrane, induction of AQP-2 synthesis, releases von Willebrand factor and factor VIII, vasodilation

190. Ans. (d) Cecum

(Ref: www.Hopkins Medicine.org, Harrison 19th p 590)

191. Ans. (b) Weil's disease

(Ref: Harrison 20th edition, p 1290; Harrison 19th p 1140)

- Severe leptospirosis, characterized by jaundice, renal dysfunction, and hemorrhagic diathesis, is referred to as Weil's syndrome.
- Leptospires are spirochetes belonging to the order Spirochaetales and the family Lepto-spiraceae.

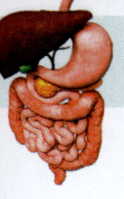

- Transmission of leptospires may follow direct contact with urine, blood, or tissue from an infected animal or exposure to a contaminated environment; human-to-human transmission is rare. Since leptospires are excreted in the urine and can survive in water for many months, water is an important vehicle in their transmission.
- The most common finding on physical examination is fever with conjunctiva suffusion. Less common findings include muscle tenderness, lymphadenopathy, pharyngeal injection, rash, hepatomegaly, and splenomegaly. The rash may be macular, maculopapular, erythematous, urticarial, or hemorrh-agic. Mild jaundice may be present.
- Severe Leptospirosis (Weil's Syndrome) Weil's syndrome, the most severe form of leptospirosis, is characterized by jaundice, renal dysfunction, hemorrhagic diathesis, and a mortality rate ranging from 5 to 15%.
- A definite diagnosis of leptospirosis is based either on isolation of the organism from the patient or on seroconversion or a rise in antibody titer in the microscopic agglutination test (MAT). For severe cases of leptospirosis, intravenous administration of penicillin G, amoxicillin, ampi-cillin, or erythromycin is recommended. In milder cases, oral treatment with tetracycline, doxycycline, ampicilhin, or amoxicillin should be considered.

192. Ans. (d) Lead poisoning

(Ref: Harrison 20th edition, p 3113; Harrison 19th p 2607, 472e-2t)

- Common symptoms include colicky abdominal pain, constipation, headache, and irritability. Severe poisoning may cause coma and convulsions. Chronic intoxication can cause learning disorders (in children) and motor neuropathy (e.g., wrist drop).
- Diagnosis is based on measurement of the blood lead level. Whole blood lead levels less than 10 µg/dL are usually considered nontoxic. Levels between 10 and 25 µg/dL have been associated with impaired neurobehavioral development in children. Levels of 25-50 µg/dL may be associated with headache, irritability, and sub-clinical neuropathy. Levels of 50-70 µg/dL are associated with moderate toxicity, and levels greater than 70-100 µg/dL are often associated with severe poisoning. Other laboratory findings of lead poisoning include microcytic anemia with basophilic stippling and elevated free erythrocyte protoporphyrin.
- Treatment: Edetate calcium disodium (EDTA) and an oral chelator succimer (dimercapto-succinic acid, DMSA)

193. Ans. (b) Intravenous metronidazole

(Ref: Harrison 20th edition, p 1569; Harrison 19th p 1366)

- The characteristic intestinal lesion is the amebic ulcer, which can occur anywhere in the large bowel (including the appendix) and sometimes in the terminal ileum but predominates in the cecum, descending colon, and the rectosigmoid colon ¾ areas of greatest fecal stasis. Trophozoites invade the colonic mucosa by means of their ameboid movement and proteo-lytic secretions and induce necrosis to form the characteristic flask-shaped ulcers. Ulcers are usually limited to the muscularis, but if penetration to the serous layer occurs, bowel perforation, local abscess, or generalized peritonitis may result. In fulminating cases, ulceration may be extensive, and the bowel becomes thin and friable.
- Metronidazole (or another nitroimidazole) plus a luminal amebicide is the treatment of choice

194. Ans. (c) Passage of blood per rectum

(Ref: Harrison 20th edition, p 2276; Harrison 19th p 1965)

The Rome III criteria for the diagnosis of irritable bowel syndrome requires that patients have had recurrent abdominal pain or discomfort at least 3 days per month during the previous 3 months that is associated with 2 or more of the following:
- Relieved by defecation
- Onset associated with a change in stool frequency
- Onset associated with a change in stool form or appearance
- Supporting symptoms include the following:
  - Altered stool frequency
  - Altered stool form
  - Altered stool passage (straining and/or urgency)
  - Mucorrhea
  - Abdominal bloating or subjective distention

195. Ans. (a) Stomach

(Ref: Harrison 20th edition, p 570; Bailey 21st / 892; Harrison 19th p 536)

196. Ans. (c) Appendicitis

(Ref: Harrison 19th p 1987)

197. Ans. (a) Vitamin B_{12}

(Ref: 'Clinical Nutrition in Gastrointestinal Disease' by Buchman (2006)/362, Harrison 19th p/362, 1943)

198. Ans. (c) Abdominal distension

(Ref: Harrison 19th p 1969)

199. Ans. (b) ELISA

(Ref: Harrison 20th edition, p 1572; Ghai 5th/221, Harrison 19th p 1363)

200. Ans. (b) Stage of lesion

(Ref: Harrison 20th edition, p 576; Robbins 7th / 866; Harrison 19th p 541)

201. Ans. (c) Hemochromatosis

(Ref: Harrison 20th edition, p 2436; Harrison 19th p 2091)

202. Ans. (a) Purtscher's retinopathy

(Ref: Harrison 20th edition, p 2167; Harrison 19th p 40e-4)

203. **Ans. (b) Pseudocyst**

(Ref: Harrison 19th p 2091)

204. **Ans. (a) 72 hour fast test**

(Ref: Harrison 20th edition, p 2749; Harrison 19th p 2338)

205. **Ans. (b) Abnormality in CFTR leads to defective Calcium Transport**

(Ref: Harrison 20th edition, p 1987; Harrison 19th p 1699)

206. **Ans. (c) B and C only**

(Ref: Harrison 19th edition, page 473e-6)

- According to the American Association of clinical Toxicology, gastric lavage should not be used routinely to manage patients who have been poisoned.
- This agency recommends considering gastric lavage only when the patient has ingested a potentially life-threatening amount of poison and only when lavage can be performed within 60 minutes from the time of ingestion.

Contraindications for gastric lavage include:

1. Ingestion of hydrocarbon with a high aspiration potential
2. Ingestion of a corrosive substance such as a strong acid or alkali, or absent airway protective reflexes unless that patient is intubated.
3. Assess relevant diagnostic data such as coagulation studies and verify the patient's history. Patients of craniofacial surgery or trauma, may require special insertion techniques or equipment (fluoroscopy).

Notes

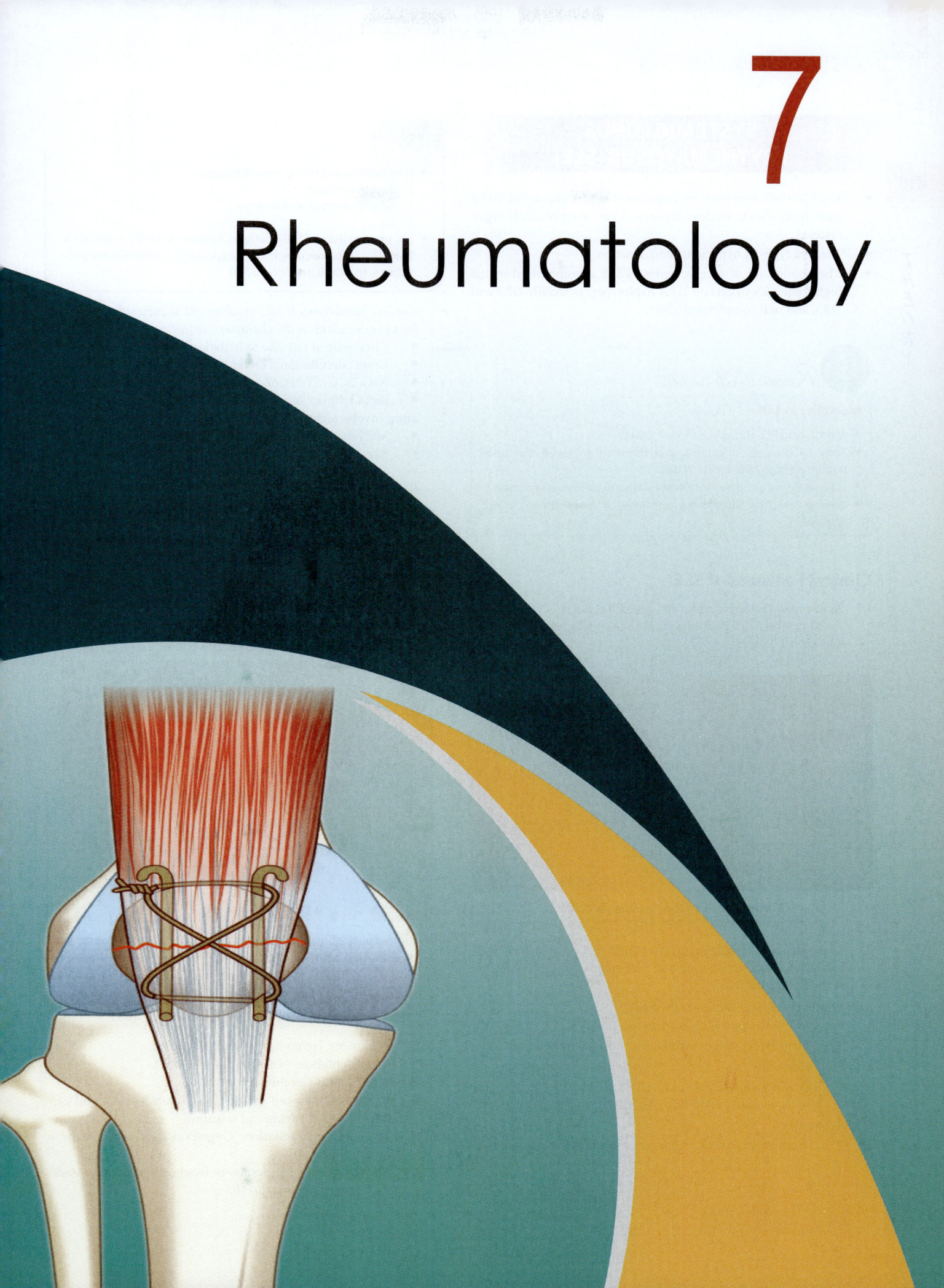

Rheumatology

7

SYSTEMIC LUPUS ERYTHEMATOSUS (SLE)

- SLE is an inflammatory autoimmune disorder characterized by auto-antibodies to nuclear antigens. It can affect multiple organ systems.
- This is a type-III hypersensitivity reaction
- The importance of specific genes in SLE is emphasized by the high frequency of certain HLA haplotypes, especially DR2 and DR3, and null complement alleles.

Recent advances

Mortality in SLE
- Mortality in SLE shows a bimodal pattern.
- Early in disease, infections are common followed by lupus nephritis (Page 856: CMDT 2019).
- Later in disease course, accelerated atherosclerosis is common.
- Overall infection should be answered if time frame is not specified.

Clinical Features of SLE

1. **Malar rash Butterfly rash** (MC acute SLE rash)
   Fixed erythema, flat or raised, over the malar eminences and sun exposed parts

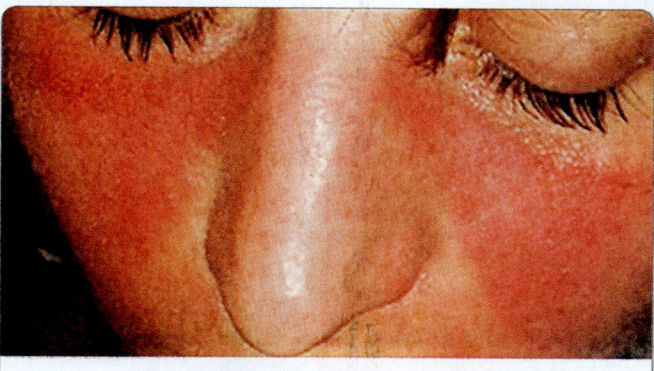

Butterfly rash sparing nasolabial folds

2. **Discoid rash:** Erythematous circular raised patches with adherent keratotic scaling and follicular plugging; atrophic scarring may occur
3. **Photosensitivity** (Ro/SS–A antibody)
   Exposure to sunlight leads to rash/sun burn
   Treatment: Hydroxychloroquine and sunscreen lotion
4. **Oral ulcers**
   - They are superficial small ulcers which are painless and occur on hard palate, buccal cavity and vermiform border.
5. **Synovitis**
   - This involves hands, wrists, knee joints and is non-erosive.

EXTRA MILE

- Non-erosive arthritis is seen in cases of:
  1. Rheumatic fever
  2. Inflammatory bowel disease
  3. SLE
- MC presentation of SLE is fatigue, malaise, fever and arthralgia: 95%. This is followed by hematological and cutaneous manifestations. (pg 2520, Harrison 20/e)

6. **Cardiac involvement:** MC involvement is pericarditis. Libman Sacks endocarditis *is the characteristic feature of cardiac SLE.*
   - Chest pain at rest due to irritation of phrenic nerve
   - Upon auscultation: Pericardial friction rub
   - IOC: ECG, ST ↑; Concave upwards in all leads except aVR.
   - Rx of Libman Sacks endocarditis: Valvuloplasty.
7. **Lung involvement**
   - MC lung involvement in SLE: Pleuritis
   - Rare involvement is **Shrinking lung syndrome and** intra-alveolar hemorrhage
8. **Kidney involvement:** Lupus nephritis
   - Present with hematuria *(cola-colored urine)*
   - *Investigations*:
     a. Urine m/e- >3 RBC/HPF and presence of RBC casts
     b. Urine protein concentration: 0.5 – 1g/24 hours
     c. KFT
     d. IOC: For lupus nephritis kidney biopsy. Upon HPE, *wire loop lesion* is characteristic finding. Most severe stage of lupus nephritis: Stage IV (diffuse lupus nephritis)

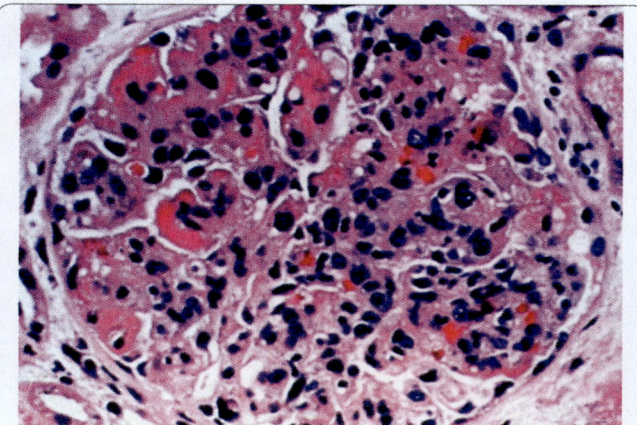

The glomerulus shown here is hypercellular due to mesangial cell proliferation and inflammatory cell infiltration. In addition, glomerular capillaries stain deep red and appear acellular and thickened due to heavy deposition of subendothelial immune complex deposits. This change is called the "wire loop" lesion.

   - Treatment: Hemodialysis if GFR < 30 mL
   - Transplantation if GFR < 15 mL (ESRD).
9. **Psychosis/ Lupus Cerebritis**
   - Lupus antibody can cross (blood brain barrier) and can cause cerebral edema and seizures.
   - MC CNS manifestation: Cognition defect *(antibody = Anti-neuronal Ab)*
   - MC psychiatric manifestation: Psychosis *[antibody = Anti-RNP (ribonucleoprotein)Ab]*

- Treatment: Haloperidol
- Spinal cord involvement in form of myelopathy

10. **Hematological manifestation**: Autoimmune hemolytic anemia because antibodies destroys own RBC.
    - These are warm antibodies: IgG → active at 37°C
    - On peripheral smear: Spherocytes seen
    - IOC: Direct Coomb's test
    - Treatment: Steroids
    - Lymphopenia and thrombocytopenia is also seen.

11. **Immunological manifestations in SLE**
    - ANA> upper reference limits
    - Anti-ds DNA
    - Anti-Smith antibody
    - Antiphospholipid antibody
    - Low serum complement
    - Positive direct Coombs test

4 features out of 11 should be present for the diagnosis of SLE, where at least one should be clinical and one should be a laboratory feature.

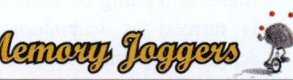

Mnemonic to remember features of SLE: SOSP BRAIN MA
4 out of 11 features for the diagnosis of SLE
S- Serositis (pleuritis, pericarditis w/o effusion)
O-Oral ulcers, Nasal ulcer
S- Synovitis ≥ 2 joints
P-Photosensitivity
B-Blood (hemolytic anemia, leucopenia, thrombocytopenia)
R-Renal (hematuria, proteinuria, HPN)
A-ANA (+ ANA)
I-Immunologic (+ double stranded anti-DNA)
N-Neurologic symptoms
M-Malar rash
A-Alopecia (Non scarring)

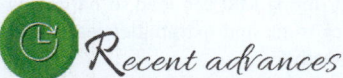

Drug induced Lupus
• It presents as SLE with fever, arthralgia, malar rash and serositis.
• Renal and CNS Involvement is rare/not seen.
• Gender ratio is equal.
• ANA is positive but dsDNA, Sm and RNP are absent.
• Complement level is normal.
• Most common drug leading to drug induced lupus is procainamide. (Ref: pg 2525: Harrison 20th edition)

Investigations

Most sensitive marker for SLE (used for screening)	Antinuclear antibody
Specific antibody for SLE	Anti-Smith antibody
Marker for drug induced SLE	Anti-histone antibody
Responsible for thrombus formation and recurrent abortions	Anti-phospholipid antibody
Antibody causing psychosis in SLE	Anti ribosomal P antibody
Predisposition to subacute cutaneous lupus, complete heart block in fetus	Ro/SSA
Antibody for CNS lupus	Anti-neuronal antibody/anti-glutamate antibody

Management of SLE

The mainstay of treatment for any inflammatory life-threatening or organ-threatening manifestation of SLE is systemic glucocorticoids (0.5–1 mg/kg per day PO or methylprednisolone sodium succinate IV daily for 3 days followed by 0.5–1 mg/kg of daily prednisone or equivalent).

Steroids are not useful in	Rx given in such situations
Libman Sacks endocarditis	Valvuloplasty
Anti-phospholipid antibody syndrome	Aspirin + heparin / warfarin
Photosensitivity	Hydroxychloroquine
Lupus nephritis with end stage renal disease	Transplantation
Psychosis	Haloperidol

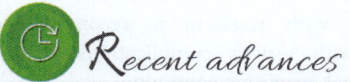

- DOC for SLE exacerbation *in pregnancy*: Hydroxychloroquine and steroids if necessary (Page no 2524: Harrison 20th edition)
- Preferred drug for management of *severe lupus nephritis*: Cyclophosphamide
- Preferred drug for management of *severe lupus cerebritis*: Dexamethasone

Pregnancy and SLE

- Flare up of SLE can occur during pregnancy. Active SLE in pregnant female is controlled with hydroxychloroquine and the lowest possible dose of prednisolone
- Recurrent abortions are due to thrombosis of uterine vessels, which results because of anti-phospholipid antibody (anti β2 glycoprotein).
- *Ro antibodies*, which are formed during pregnancy are of IgG class, they have the ability to cross placenta. These antibodies affect the AV node of the fetus resulting in complete heart block. This presentation is called neonatal lupus.

ANTIPHOSPHOLIPID ANTIBODY SYNDROME

A primary antiphospholipid syndrome is diagnosed in
- Patients who have venous or arterial occlusions or recurrent abortions or unexplained IUD (34 weeks)
- Diagnostic antiphospholipid antibodies are IgG or IgM anti-cardiolipin, or IgG or IgM antibodies to beta-2-glycoprotein, and lupus anticoagulant.

In < 1% of patients with antiphospholipid antibodies, a potentially devastating syndrome known as the "catastrophic antiphospholipid syndrome" occurs, leading to diffuse thromboses, thrombotic microangiopathy, and multiorgan system failure.

Laboratory Findings

- Three types of antiphospholipid antibodies are believed to contribute to this syndrome:
  1. Anti-cardiolipin antibodies
  2. Antibodies to beta-2 glycoprotein
  3. "Lupus anticoagulant" that prolongs certain phospholipid-dependent coagulation tests

- Antibodies to cardiolipin and to beta-2 glycoprotein are typically measured with enzyme immunoassays.
- *Anti-cardiolipin antibodies can produce a biologic false-positive test for syphilis*
- Presence of the lupus anticoagulant is a stronger risk factor for thrombosis or pregnancy loss than is the presence of antibodies to either beta-2-glycoprotein I or anticardiolipin.
- Testing for the lupus anticoagulant involves phospholipid dependent functional assays of coagulation, such as the *Russell viper venom time (RVVT)*. In the presence of a lupus anticoagulant, the RVVT is prolonged and does not correct with mixing studies but does with the addition of excess phospholipid: *Screening test.*

Treatment of APLAS (Antiphospholipid Antibody Syndrome)

- Lifelong anticoagulation with warfarin is recommended currently for patients with serious complications of this syndrome because recurrent events are common.
- In next pregnancy, treat patient with:
  - First trimester: Tab. aspirin + inj. heparin
  - Second trimester: Tab. aspirin + oral warfarin
- Treat patients with warfarin to maintain an INR of 2.0–3.0.
- Patients who have recurrent thrombotic events on this level of anticoagulation may require higher INRs (>3.0), but the bleeding risk increases substantially with this degree of anticoagulation.

SCLERODERMA (SYSTEMIC SCLEROSIS)

- Scleroderma (systemic sclerosis) is a rare chronic disorder characterized by *diffuse fibrosis of the skin and internal organs.*
- Symptoms usually appear in the third to fifth decades and *women are affected two to three times as frequently as men (F:M = 3:1)*

- Peak age for systemic scleroderma 30–50 years
- In children, localized scleroderma is more common than systemic scleroderma.

Clinical Features

1. *Raynaud's phenomena* is the earliest clinical feature of scleroderma.
2. Sclerodactyly
3. Hand contractures
4. *Leather-like skin* because of the extensive fibrosis under the skin. Salt and pepper skin in seen due to hyper and hypopigmentation in areas of fibrosis
5. Decreased saliva production due to fibrosis of salivary glands. This results in dryness of mouth, dysphagia and dental caries.
6. Esophageal dysmotility
7. Fibrosis of lower esophageal sphincter results in Gastroesophageal reflux disease (GERD).
8. Restrictive cardiomyopathy leading to Kussmaul's sign
9. Pulmonary fibrosis

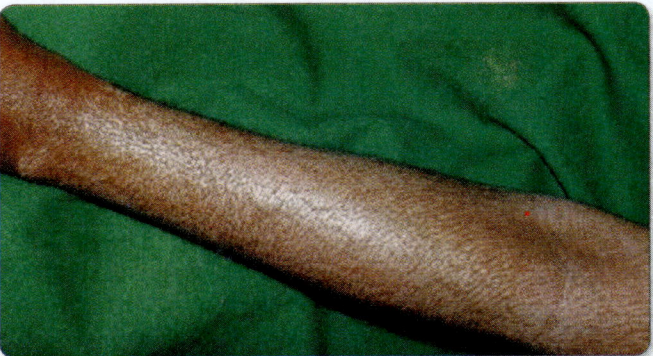

Salt and pepper skin seen in Scleroderma

10. Clubbing
11. Pulmonary artery hypertension (leading cause of mortality)
12. Renal fibrosis results in decline of GFR. The levels of renin increase leading to high levels of blood pressure. This event is termed as *scleroderma crisis.* Treatment of choice for scleroderma crisis: ACE Inhibitors.
13. Bilateral ureteric fibrosis resulting in renal failure.

- HTN crisis in eclampsia: Labetalol
- HTN crisis in stroke: Nicardipine
- Scleroderma crisis: ACE Inhibitors

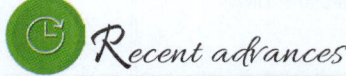

- Tendon friction rubs are seen in diffuse scleroderma.
- Gadolinium used as contrast during MRI can lead to hardening and thickening of the skin of trunk and extremities leading to nephrogenic fibrosing dermopathy.
- Mortality in Scleroderma is due to pulmonary artery hypertension. Harrison 20th edition, page 2560

Investigations

1. ESR normal/elevated indicates myositis or malignancy
2. ANA positive (Most common antibody positive)
3. **IOC**: Anti-topoisomerase antibody 1, anti-Scl-70 antibody and anti-RNA polymerase III.

Treatment

Steroids can worsen scleroderma crisis. For ILD, cyclophosphamide is used. No therapy can alter the course of disease.

RAYNAUD'S PHENOMENON

- Paroxysmal bilateral digital pallor and cyanosis followed by rubor. (White → Blue → Red)
- Precipitated by cold or emotional stress; relieved by warmth.

- Primarily affects young women.
- Primary form benign; secondary form can cause digital ulceration or gangrene.
- Can involve toes

Treatment of Raynaud's Phenomenon

- Avoid exposure to cold/use gloves
- DOC: CCB- can cause relief of spasm of bacterial vaginosis.

> - In female patients with Raynaud's, there is an increased incidence of Migraine, Stroke and Prinzmetal angina.
> - Raynaud's Disease: Idiopathic Raynaud's phenomenon

CREST SYNDROME

CREST syndrome, also known as the limited cutaneous form of systemic sclerosis is a multisystem connective tissue disorder.

- **C** – Calcinosis
- **R** – Raynauds phenomenon
- **E** – Esophageal dysmotility
- **S** – Sclerodactyly
- **T** – Telangiectasia *(abnormal blood vessel dilatation seen in conjunctiva)*

Investigation of Choice

Anti-centromere antibody, Th/To antibody and PM/SCL antibody

Treatment

Same as diffuse/systemic sclerosis

MIXED CONNECTIVE TISSUE DISORDER

- Patients who have localized Scleroderma coexisting with features of SLE, polymyositis, and rheumatoid arthritis may have mixed connective tissue disease (MCTD).
- This overlap syndrome is generally associated with the presence of high titers of autoantibodies to U1-RNP.
- The characteristic initial presentation is Raynaud's phenomenon associated with puffy fingers and myalgia. Gradually, features of sclerodactyly, calcinosis, and cutaneous telangiectasia develop. Skin rashes suggestive of systemic lupus erythematosus (malar rash, photosensitivity) or of dermatomyositis (heliotrope rash on the eyelids, erythematous rash on the knuckles) occur
- *Investigation of choice: U1 ribonucleoprotein antibody*
- Treatment: Steroids. In contrast to systemic sclerosis patients, MCTD shows a good response to steroids.

SJÖGREN'S SYNDROME/ SICCA SYNDROME

- Sjögren's syndrome is a systemic autoimmune disorder whose clinical presentation is usually dominated by dryness of the eyes and mouth due to immune-mediated *dysfunction of the lacrimal and salivary glands.*
- **Secondary Sjogren**: Dry mouth + dry eyes + rheumatoid arthritis
- **Minor salivary gland fibrosis** results in diminished salivary production which results in dental caries, halitosis and dysphagia. Bilateral parotid enlargement is observed in few patients.
- **Fibrosed lacrimal gland** hampers tear production resulting in dry eyes.
- Dry vagina due to involvement of Bartholin's glands results in development of dyspareunia.
- *MC extraglandular manifestation in primary Sjögren is arthralgia/arthritis. Least common involvement is myositis.*
- Xerotrachea/atrophic gastritis/subclinical pancreatitis occurs
- *Lymphoma can develop and is extranodal low grade marginal zone, B cell lymphomas.*^{Q}

Revised International Classification Criteria for Sjögren's Syndrome

1. Ocular symptoms
2. Oral symptoms
3. Ocular signs
    - Schirmer test performed without anesthesia (<5 mm in 5 minutes)
    - Rose Bengal dye score of >4 according to Van Bijsterveld score
4. Histopathology from labial biopsy shows focal lymphocytic sialadenitis
5. Salivary gland involvement (any one positive)
    - *Unstimulated whole salivary score (<1.5 mL in 15 minutes)*^{Q}
    - Parotid sialography
    - Salivary Scintigraphy
6. Antibodies in the serum to Ro/SS-A and La/SS-B antigens or both for diagnosis at least four of the six is positive, and histopathology and serology must be positive.

Composition of Saliva in Sjögren's Syndrome^Q

1. Increased salivary IgA
2. Increased salivary sodium
3. Decreased salivary phosphate
4. Reduced stimulated and unstimulated salivary flow rate. The normal flow rate of saliva is 1–2 mL/min. Reduced flow is defined as < 1.5 mL in 15 minutes.

Investigation of Choice

SS-A (Rho) and SS-B (La) antibody

Treatment

Treatment of Sicca symptoms is symptomatic and supportive.

Recent advances

SICCA Syndrome

Systemic involvement in sicca syndrome:
- Obstructive airway disease in absence of smoking
- Peripheral neuropathy
- Pancreatitis
- RTA type 1

Cevimeline^Q reduces xerostomia symptoms in sicca syndrome.

BEHCET'S SYNDROME

- It is also known as oro-oculogenital syndrome.
- Most commonly occurs among persons of Asian, Turkish, or Middle Eastern background, but may affect persons of any demographic profile. (Genetic HLA B51)
- *Recurrent, painful aphthous ulcers of the mouth are sine qua non for diagnosis*
- Erythema nodosum–like lesions; a follicular rash; pathergy phenomenon *(formation of a sterile pustule at the site of a needle stick).*

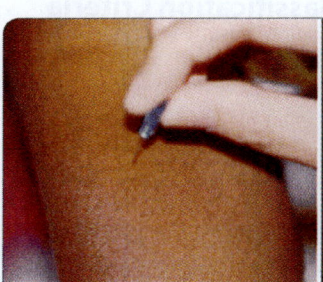
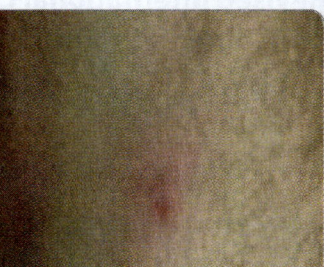

Positive pathergy test in Behcet's disease
Notice the sterile pustule

Signs/Symptoms	Points
Ocular injuries	2
Genital aphthous ulcers	2
Oral aphthosis	2
Skin injuries	1
Neurological manifestations	1
Vascular manifestations	1
Pathergy test*	1

Scoring for Behcet

- Either **anterior or posterior uveitis**. Posterior uveitis may be asymptomatic until significant damage to the retina has occurred.
- *The life expectancy is normal and the only serious complication is blindness. Nondeforming arthritis is seen. Superficial and deep vein thrombosis can occur. SVC obstruction can present dramatically. Pulmonary artery vasculitis involvement leads to hemoptysis.*

- **Treatment**: Topical steroids. Thrombophlebitis is managed with aspirin. Colchicine is useful for arthritis and cutaneous manifestations

DERMATOMYOSITIS

- Dermatomyositis is a systemic disorder of unknown cause whose principal manifestation is muscle weakness.

Clinical Features

1. Proximal muscle weakness (example: muscle around hip joint and shoulder joint). Ptosis is not seen
2. Gottron papules

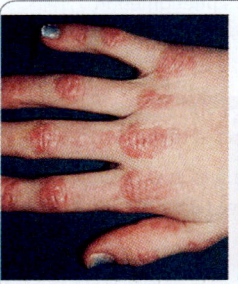
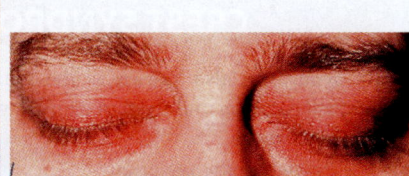

Gottron papules   Heliotrope Rash

3. Heliotrope rash and shawl sign
4. Photosensitivity
5. One in four patients of dermatomyositis possess increased risk of cancer. i.e cancer ovary, breast and lungs.

Investigations

1. Anti-Jo-1 antibody
2. IOC is muscle biopsy
3. CK-MB and EMG are not reliable for diagnosis.

Treatment

- Oral prednisone

POLYMYOSITIS

- **Polymyositis** may begin abruptly, but the usual presentation is one of gradual and progressive muscle weakness.
- The weakness chiefly involves proximal muscle groups of the upper and lower extremities as well as the neck.
- Skin lesions, Gottron papules, heliotrope rash is **absent**. Paraneoplastic association is not seen.

Investigation

- Muscle biopsy

Treatment

- Steroids

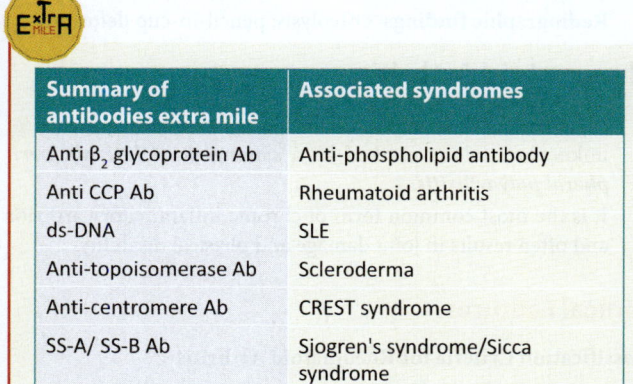

Summary of antibodies extra mile	Associated syndromes
Anti β₂ glycoprotein Ab	Anti-phospholipid antibody
Anti CCP Ab	Rheumatoid arthritis
ds-DNA	SLE
Anti-topoisomerase Ab	Scleroderma
Anti-centromere Ab	CREST syndrome
SS-A/ SS-B Ab	Sjogren's syndrome/Sicca syndrome
Anti-Jo-1 antibody	Dermatomyositis with lung involvement, Polymyositis

Recent advances

Anti-synthetase Syndrome

Seen in patients of dermatomyositis and polymyositis
- Fever, inflammatory arthritis
- Raynaud's phenomenon
- Mechanic hands
- Interstitial lung disease
- Anti-Jo-1 antibody

ARTHRITIS

Ankylosing Spondylitis

ASAS criteria for classification of Spondyloarthritis in patients with *Age of onset< 45 years presenting with low backache for > 3 months*

1. Sacroilitis on imaging with >1 SpA feature
   OR
2. HLA B-27 positive Plus >2 SpA features

SpA (Spondyloarthritis) features

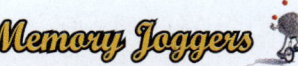

(Mnemonic: ABCDEFG- IP)
A= **A**rthritis
B= HLA-**B**27 positive
C= **C**RP positive
D= **D**actylitis
E= **E**nthesitis
F= **F**amily history of SPA
G= **G**ood response to NSAIDS
I= **I**nflammatory back pain
P= **P**soriasis

Clinical Features

1. Presents in adolescence or adulthood with low backache localized to lower lumbar or gluteal area
2. Nocturnal worsening of pain is seen. Bony tenderness is present in costosternal junctions, spinous processes, iliac crest and heels.
3. Monoarthritis of hip can limit movements and activity.
4. Loss of spinal motility with loss of lateral and anterior flexion of spine is seen. Modified Schober test is used to evaluate for lumbar spine flexion.
5. Chest expansion is restricted (normal >5 cm)
6. Cervical spine is last to be involved.
7. Most common extra-articular manifestation is uveitis.
8. *Most common cardiac lesion is aortic insufficiency and third degree heart block*

Investigations

1. HLA- B27+
2. RA factor is negative
3. CRP positive
4. Anti- CCP negative
5. X – Ray spine:
   - *Earliest feature is blurring of the cortical margins of subchondral bone* followed by erosions and sclerosis
   - Pseudowidening of joint space
   - *Squaring* of vertebra
   - Lumbar spine syndesmophyte formation resulting in enchondral bone formation and bamboo spine
6. MRI Spine: Intra- articular inflammation and marrow edema is seen
7. DEXA scan shows reduced bone density

Treatment

Exercise and NSAIDS. In case there is no response to NSAIDS, anti-TNF alpha monoclonal antibody like infliximab shows excellent response.

Acute Gout/Crystal Arthropathy

- Deposition of **urate crystals** in joints
- **Most common joint involved**: 1ˢᵗ MTP joint *leading to Podologia (swelling of 1ˢᵗ MTP joint)*
- Acute gouty arthritis is sudden in onset and frequently nocturnal. It may develop without apparent precipitating cause or may follow rapid increases or decreases in serum urate levels.

Investigation

- Joint aspiration → needle shaped crystals
  Serum uric acid often **Normal** during the attack

Drug of Choice

- Indomethacin (for 4–5 days till joint pain subsides). *Allopurinol is contraindicated in acute gout. It is DOC for chronic gout.*

Pseudo Gout

- Pseudo gout is an erosive arthritis mostly involving **knee joints**.
- Joint aspiration reveals **crystals of calcium pyrophosphate.**

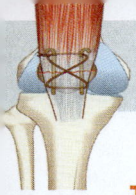

Treatment

Steroids

Osteoarthritis (OA)

- Osteoarthritis is observed in geriatric population.
- Most common joint involved in this condition is **knee joint**.
- Hands can also be involved, most common presentation is pain at the base of the thumb (*1st metacarpophalangeal joint*).
- **Heberden nodes** are present in DIP and **Bouchard nodes** are present in PIP.

Investigation

X-ray knee

Treatment

- NSAIDS followed by total knee replacement in case of severe OA.

Septic Arthritis

- Septic arthritis is the arthritis with the maximum joint damage.
- Causative agent for septic arthritis is *S.aureus*.
- *Most common joint involved: Hip joint in children and knee joint in adults*.

Psoriatic Arthritis

CASPAR Criteria for Psoriatic Arthritis

Presence of inflammatory articular disease (Joint, Spine, entheseal) with >3 points from the five mentioned below-

1. Evidence of current psoriasis
2. Typical nail dystrophy
3. Negative RA factor
4. Current dactylitis
5. Radiographic evidence of new bone formation in hand or foot

- Psoriasis precedes onset of arthritis in 80% of cases. Arthritis is usually asymmetric, with "sausage" appearance of fingers and toes of **DIP joints.**
- Ankylosis of the sacroiliac joints may occur.
- **Radiographic findings**: Osteolysis; pencil-in-cup deformity.

Rheumatoid Arthritis

- Rheumatoid arthritis is a chronic inflammatory disease of unknown etiology marked by a **symmetric (bilateral), peripheral polyarthritis**.
- It is the most common form of chronic inflammatory arthritis and often results in joint damage and physical disability.

Clinical Features

Classification Criteria for Rheumatoid Arthritis

		Score
Joint involvement	1 large joint (shoulder, elbow, hip, knee, ankle	0
	2–10 large joints	1
	1–3 small joints (MCP, PIP, thumb IP, MTP, wrists)	2
	4–10 small joints	3
	> 10 joints (at least 1 small joint)	5
Serology	Negative RF and positive anti-CCP	0
	Low-positive RF or low-positive anti-CCP antibodies (≤ 3 times ULN)	2
	High-positive RF or high-positive anti-CCP antibodies (> 3 times ULN)	3
Acute-phase reactants	Normal CRP and normal ESR	0
	Abnormal CRP abnormal ESR	1
Duration of symptoms	< 6 weeks	0
	≥ 6 weeks	1

- Morning stiffness for more than an hour.
- Bilateral wrist, PIP & MCP joints are involved.
- Presence of rheumatoid nodules on the extensor surface which are *nontender and firm due to adherence to periosteum*.

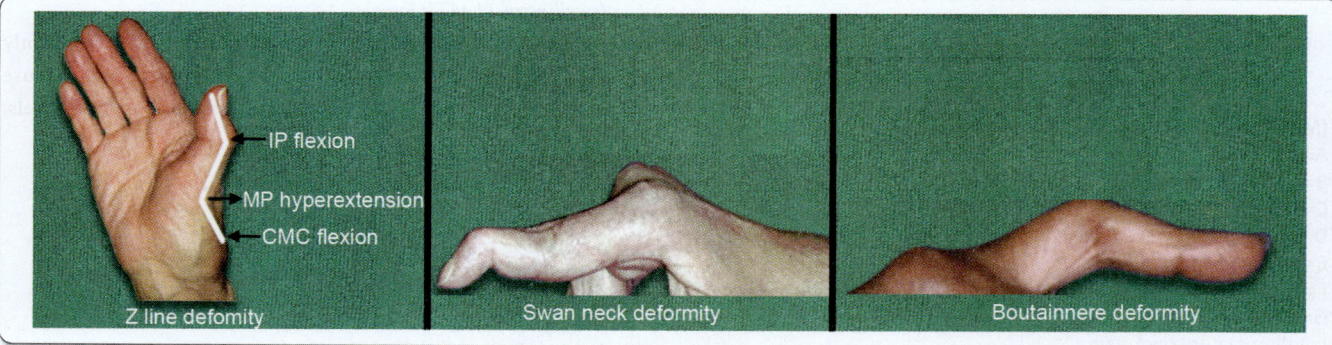

Z line deformity | Swan neck deformity | Boutainnere deformity

- **Atlantoaxial involvement** of the cervical spine may cause compressive myelopathy and neurologic dysfunction.
- **Screening test:** RA-factor (IgM linked to IgG)- *biologically false positive in 5% of population*
- **Investigation of choice:** Anti-cyclic citrulline phospholipid antibody (Anti-CCP Ab).
- **Treatment:** DMARD of choice is methotrexate. *Tofacitinib* is an inhibitor of Janus kinase 3. It is used to manage rheumatoid arthritis refractory to methotrexate.
- MC cause of death in RA is cardiovascular disease
- MC extra-articular manifestation is subcutaneous nodules
- MC hematological feature is NCNC anemia

Summary of Features seen is Rheumatoid Arthritis

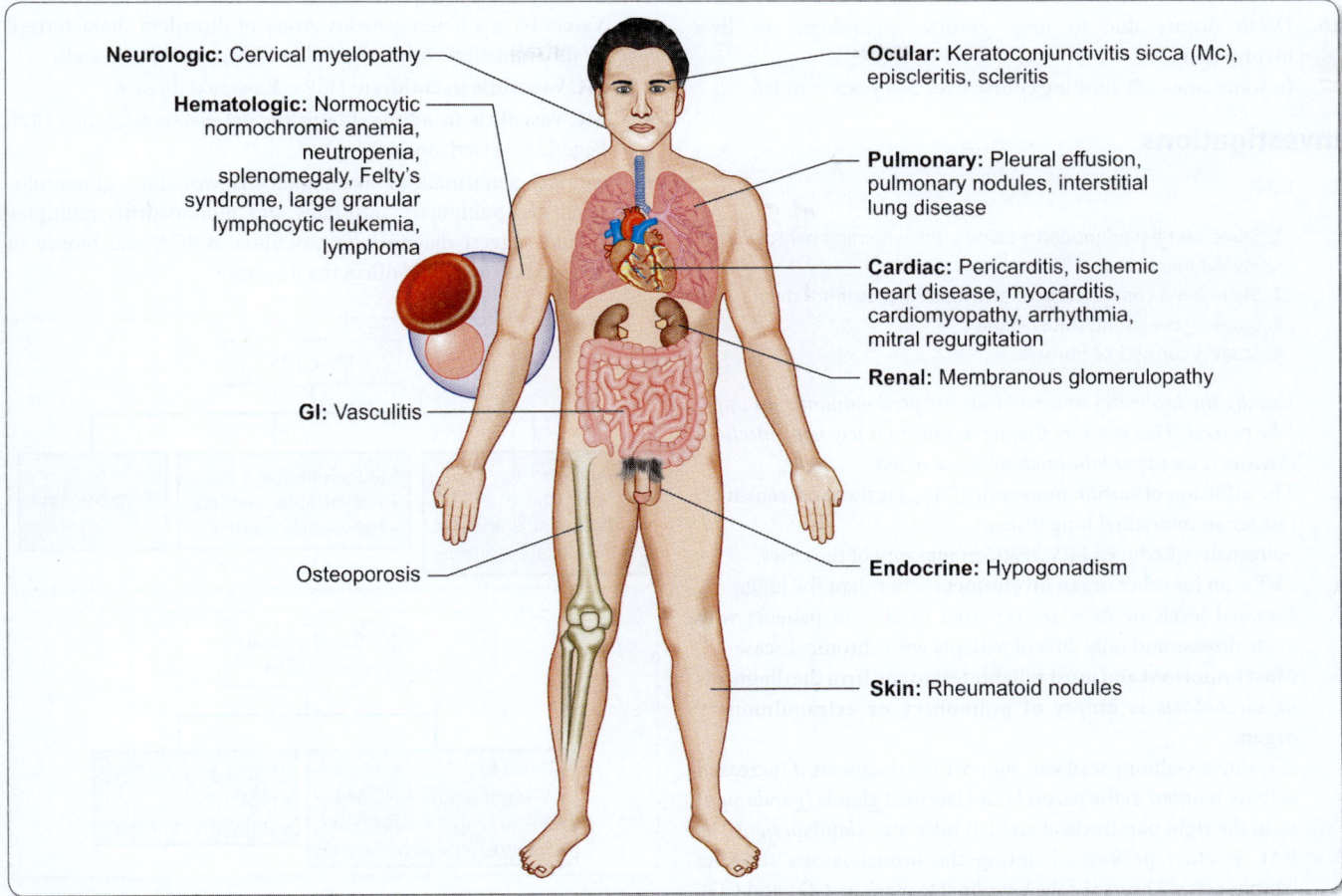

SARCOIDOSIS

It is a multisystem disorder requiring involvement of more than 2 systems for diagnosis. It is characterized by presence of noncaseating granulomas.

Clinical Features

1. It occurs in young previously healthy adults and second peak is seen after the age of 60 years
2. *Most common organ involved is the lung followed by the skin.*
3. *Least common organ involved is the heart*
4. Respiratory complaints including cough and dyspnea are the most common presenting symptoms.
5. 50% patients exhibit obstructive airway pattern with reduced FEV1/FVC ratio. 33% have normal spirometry and the rest exhibit features of ILD.
6. PAH is seen in 5% of total cases.
7. The classic skin lesions include erythema nodosum, maculopapular lesions, hyper- and hypopigmentation, keloid formation, and subcutaneous nodules. *A specific complex of involvement of the bridge of the nose, the area beneath the eyes, and the cheeks is referred to as lupus pernio.*
8. Most common eye manifestation is uvieitis. Some patients have posterior uveitis and pars planitis.
9. The most common abnormality of liver function is an elevation of the alkaline phosphatase level, consistent with an obstructive pattern. In addition, elevated transaminase levels can occur.
10. The most common hematologic problem is lymphopenia. Anemia occurs in 20% of patients. Bone marrow examination will reveal granulomas in about a third of patients.
11. Hypercalcemia and/or hypercalciuria occur in about 10% of sarcoidosis patients. *The mechanism of abnormal calcium metabolism is increased production of 1,25-dihydroxyvitamin D by the granuloma itself.*
12. Granulomas in the kidney and hypercalcemia both damage the kidney and lead to nephritis
13. Neurosarcoidosis
    - CSF findings include lymphocytic meningitis with a mild increase in protein; CSF glucose is usually normal but can be low.
    - Seventh cranial nerve involvement LMN type can occur.^{Q}
    - Myelopathy
    - Anterior hypothalamic disease with associated diabetes insipidus
    - Seizures and cognitive changes also occur.
14. Cardiac involvement is due to granulomas leading to CHF or heart blocks. Ventricular arrhythmias and *sudden death* due to ventricular tachycardia are common causes of death

15. Although sarcoidosis can affect any organ of the body, rarely does it involve the breast, testes, ovary, or stomach
16. *Death* occurs due to lung, cardiac, neurologic, or liver involvement.
17. In some cases self-limiting course over 2–5 years is noted.

Investigations

1. CXR

    1. Stage 1 is hilar adenopathy alone often with right paratracheal involvement.
    2. Stage 2 is a combination of adenopathy plus infiltrates
    3. Stage 3 reveals infiltrates alone
    4. Stage 4 consists of fibrosis.

    Usually the infiltrates in sarcoidosis are predominantly an upper lobe process. This is a rare finding as only in a few non-infectious diseases is an upper lobe predominance noted.

2. The diffusion of carbon monoxide (DL_{CO}) is the most sensitive^Q test for an interstitial lung disease.
3. Spirometry: Reduced FEV_1/FVC in majority of the cases.
4. PET scan for other organ involvement other than the lung.
5. Elevated levels of ACE are reported in 60% of patients with acute disease and only 20% of patients with chronic disease
6. **Most important and most reliable test to confirm the diagnosis of sarcoidosis is biopsy of pulmonary or extrapulmonary organ.**
7. A positive Gallium scan can support the diagnosis if increased activity is noted in the parotids and lacrimal glands (*panda sign*) or in the right paratracheal and left hilar area (*lambda sign*)
8. BAL is often performed during the bronchoscopy showing lymphocytes. The use of the lymphocyte markers CD4 and CD8 can be used to determine the CD4/CD8 ratio of these increased lymphocytes in the BAL fluid. A CD_4/CD_8 ratio of >3.5 in BAL is suggestive of diagnosis of sarcoidosis.
9. *Kveim-Siltzbach procedure- not used anymore*

Treatment

Treatment is mainly steroid based with steroid sparing agents.

Löfgren's syndrome, consists of
1. Erythema nodosum
2. Hilar adenopathy on chest roentgenogram
3. Uveitis
4. The recently proposed expansion of the term Lofgren's syndrome includes periarticular arthritis without erythema nodosum

*Löfgren's syndrome is associated with a good prognosis, with >90% of patients experiencing disease resolution within 2 years.
Elevations of ACE levels >50% of the upper limit of normal are seen in
1. Sarcoidosis
2. Leprosy
3. Gaucher's disease
4. Hyperthyroidism
5. Disseminated granulomatous infections such as Miliary tuberculosis.

VASCULITIS

- Vasculitis is a heterogeneous group of disorders characterized by inflammation within the walls of affected blood vessels.
- **MC vasculitis in children**: HSP > Kawasaki disease
- **MC vasculitis in adults**: Idiopathic cutaneous vasculitis (Ref: Page 2587: Harrison 20th ed.)
- Clinical abnormalities like cutaneous vasculitis, glomerulonephritis, pulmonary infiltrates and mononeuritis multiplex should suggest diagnosis of vasculitis. ANCA and biopsy of involved organ will confirm the diagnosis.

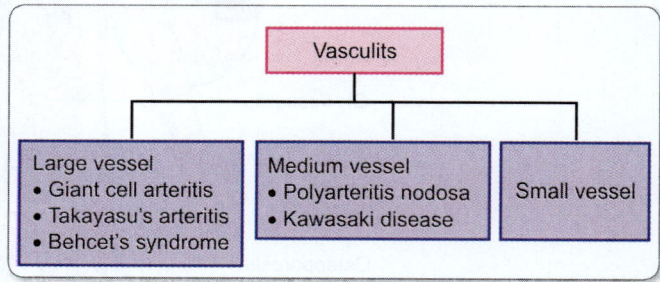

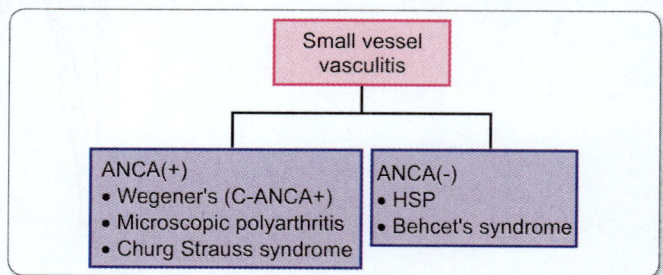

Giant Cell Arteritis

- Giant cell arteritis is a systemic pan-arteritis affecting medium-sized and large vessels in patients over the age of 50.
- Giant cell arteritis is also called temporal arteritis because the arteries that are frequently involved is *superficial temporal artery*.

Clinical Features

- Low grade fever
- Unilateral headache
- Jaw claudication
- Cord-like structure palpable at temporomandibular joint.

Investigation

1. ESR levels gross elevations up to 100 mm fall in 1st hour
2. Biopsy: Granulomatous vasculitis.

Treatment

Steroids.

Takayasu's Arteritis

- Inflammation of large blood vessels and is also known as *pulseless disease*
- **MC blood vessel usually involved** is left subclavian artery^Q

Clinical Features

1. Arm claudication
2. Unequal blood pressure *(BP in right arm is not the same as BP in left arm)*
3. Unequal radial artery impulse *(aka Radioradial delay)*
4. Renal artery ostial narrowing leading to renovascular hypertension.

Investigation

1. ESR ↑
2. Aortography shows ostial narrowing of blood vessels originating from arch of aorta.
3. MRI Aorta: IOC

Treatment

Steroids

- Unequal BP between left and right arm is seen in
  1. Takayasu's arteritis
  2. Coarctation of aorta
  3. Obstructive Aortoarteritis
  4. Supravalvular Aortic Stenosis
  5. Aortic dissection
- SBP of lower limb > SBP of upper limb, with difference > 20 mm Hg is seen in aortic regurgitation

- *Preductal coarctation of aorta: unequal BP between left and right arm.*
- *Preductal coarctation of aorta: SBP in upper limbs > SBP in lower limbs by >20 mmHg.*

Polyarteritis Nodosa (PAN)

- Involvement of small to medium-sized arteries.
- Characterized by presentation of necrotizing vasculitis.
- Lung is spared but kidney is often affected, causing renin-mediated hypertension.
- **Common features** include fever, abdominal pain, extremity pain, livedo reticularis, mononeuritis multiplex, anemia and elevated acute phase reactants (ESR or C-reactive protein or both).
- Associated with hepatitis B (10% of cases).

In cases of PAN –
- Pulmonary Artery is Not involved.
- Hemoptysis is never seen.
- NOT associated with renal artery stenosis.

Clinical Features

1. **Kidney:** Most commonly affected in this condition resulting in renin-mediated hypertension. (Vasculitis → hematuria → GFR↓ leading to ↑ renin → hypertension)
2. **Skin:** Livedo reticularis/mottling of the skin (fish net stocking)
3. Muscle weakness
4. Vasculitis of digital vessels leading to *asymmetrical gangrene*.
5. Coronary artery vasculitis leads to myocardial infarction.
6. Stroke

- **p-ANCA** *(perinuclear antigen)* is positive in:
  - Primary sclerosing cholangitis (PSC)
  - Ulcerative colitis
  - Microscopic polyangitis
  - Churg Strauss syndrome (Asthma + vasculitis)
- **c-ANCA** (cytoplasmic)
  - To diagnose Wegener's granulomatosis

Investigations

1. ESR: ↑
2. P-ANCA: Positive in 20% of cases
3. IOC: Skin biopsy

Treatment

- Steroids

Kawasaki Disease

- It occurs mainly in children between the ages of 3 months and 5 years but can occur occasionally in adults as well.
- It is an acute, self-limiting, mucocutaneous vasculitis characterized by the infiltration of vessel walls with mononuclear cells and later by IgA secreting plasma cells that can result in destruction of tunica media and aneurysm formation.
- It is also known as the *"mucocutaneous lymph node syndrome"*.

Clinical Features

High grade fever for more than 5 days with 4/5 features given below.
1. Unilateral cervical lymphadenopathy
2. Bilateral nonexudative conjunctivitis. Most common presentation
3. Strawberry tongue (white strawberry)
4. Peri-ungual peeling of skin or Beau lines in nails.
5. Polymorphous Rash

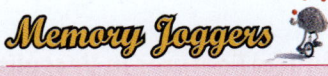

Mnemonic to remember KD- My HEART
- **M**ucosal changes: Oropharyngeal erythema, dry cracked lips, *strawberry tongue*
- **H**and and extremity changes: Reddened palms/soles, indurative edema, convalescent *desquamation from fingertips and toes* (after day 10)
- **E**ye changes: *Nonsuppurative conjunctival injection*
- **A**denopathy: *Cervical, unilateral of at least 1.5 cm*
- **R**ash: Polymorphous erythematous
- **T**emperature elevation: Often > **38°C** and lasting for >5 days

Investigations

Diagnosed usually clinically on basis of history and physical examination. Echocardiographs show large coronary artery aneurysms.

Treatment

IVIG plus aspirin. New drug for Kawasaki disease is Ulinastatin

Complications

- Major complications include arteritis and **aneurysms** of the coronary vessels, occurring in **about 25%** of untreated patients, on occasion causing myocardial infarction.

Granulomatosis with Angitis (formerly called Wegener's Granulomatosis)

- Wegener's granulomatosis is small vessel vasculitis. It is a granulomatous vasculitis.
- Granuloma contains well-defined multinucleated giant cell.
- **Clinical features:**
    - Most common site for vasculitis is upper respiratory tract, that presents with **epistaxis**.
    - Vasculitis of lower respiratory tract presents with **hemoptysis**.
    - Vasculitis of kidney presents as **hematuria**.
- **Investigation**: C-anti nuclear cytoplasmic antibody (c-ANCA)
- **Treatment**: Cyclophosphamide.

Henöch-Schonlein Purpura (HSP)

- Henoch-Schönlein purpura, the most common systemic vasculitis in children, occurs in adults as well.
- The purpuric skin lesions are typically located on the lower extremities but may also be seen on the hands, arms, trunk, and buttocks. *Most commonly on extensor surface known as extensor purpura.*
- This is an idiopathic disorder where *IgA is elevated abnormally.* This is also referred to as leucocytoclastic vasculitis / non-thrombocytopenic purpura.

Clinical Features

All the features of HSP are due to elevated IgA, which causes endothelial cell damage.
- Vasculitis of blood vessel in the skin manifests as purpura on the **extensor surface** *(palpable)*
- Vasculitis of synovial blood vessel manifests as arthralgia *(joint pain upon movement)*
- Vasculitis of G.I.T blood vessels manifests as hematochezia *(abdominal pain).*

Investigation

1. **IgA levels**: ↑
2. **Investigation of choice**: Skin biopsy showing evidence of biopsy.
3. **Platelet count**: Normal

Note: Thrombocytopenia is never seen in HSP

- Non-thrombocytopenic- extensor purpura: **HSP**
- Pinch Purpura: **Amyloidosis**
- Non-palpable Purpura: **Acute ITP**
- Red strawberry tongue: Scarlet fever
- Biomarkers of Kawasaki disease: Urine meprin A and urine filamin C

Treatment

Steroids.

Summary
Predominantly large-vessel vasculitides
• Takayasu's arteritis
• Giant cell arteritis (temporal arteritis)
• Behcet's disease
Predominantly medium-vessel vasculitides
• Polyarteritis nodosa
• Buerger's disease
• Primary angütis of the central nervous system
Predominantly small-vessel vasculitides
• Immune-complex mediated
• Cutaneous leukocytoclastic angütis ("hypersensitivity vasculitis")
• Henoch-Schönlein purpura
• Essential cryoglobulinemia
• "ANCA-associated" disorders
• Granulomatosis with polyangiitis (formerly Wegener's granulomatosis)
• Microscopic polyangiitis
• Churg-Strauss syndrome

Clinical Features in Vasculitis based on Vessel Involvement

Large vessel	Medium vessel	Small vessel
• **Constitutional symptoms**: Fever, weight loss, malaise, arthralgias/arthritis • Limb claudication • Asymmetric blood pressures[Q] • Absence of pulses[Q] • Bruits • Aortic dilation	• **Constitutional symptoms**: Fever, weight loss, malaise, arthralgias/arthritis • Cutaneous nodules • Ulcers • Livedo reticularis • Digital gangrene • Mononeuritis multiplex[Q] • Microaneurysms	• **Constitutional symptoms**: Fever, weight loss, malaise, arthralgias/arthritis • Purpura • Vesiculobullous lesions • Urticaria • Glomerulonephritis[Q] • Alveolar hemorrhage • Cutaneous extravascular necrotizing granulomas • Splinter hemorrhages[Q] • Uveitis • Episcleritis • Scleritis

Image-Based Questions

1. A 30-year old female patient presents with erythematous rash over the neck and involving the back. Her investigations reveal presence of anti-Mi-2 antibody. What is the diagnosis?

   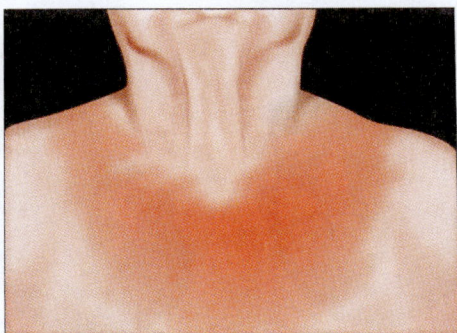

   a. Dermatomyositis b. SLE
   c. Inclusion body myositis d. Pyomyositis

2. A 35-year-old woman presents with lesion in genitals which recur frequently. Which of the following test is being done?

   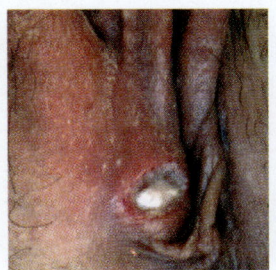 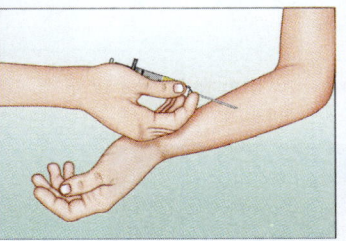

   a. Pathergy test
   b. Allergic skin testing
   c. Kveim Siltzbach test
   d. Pilocarpine intradermal test

3. The test shown below is done for diagnosis of?

   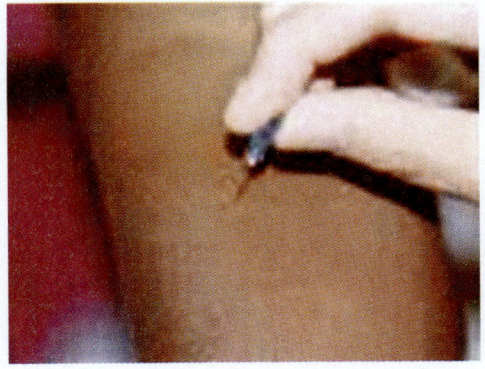

   a. Behcet's disease b. Tuberculosis
   c. Sarcoidosis d. Leprosy

4. Sample from joint aspiration was seen under a polarized microscope. The image shows?

   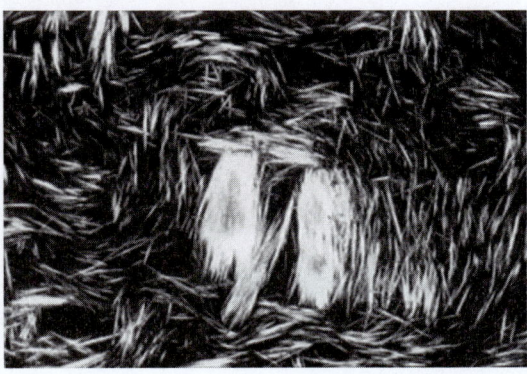

   a. Uric acid b. Calcium pyrophosphate
   c. Calcium phosphate d. Cystine

5. The image shows presence of? *(AIIMS Nov 2018)*

   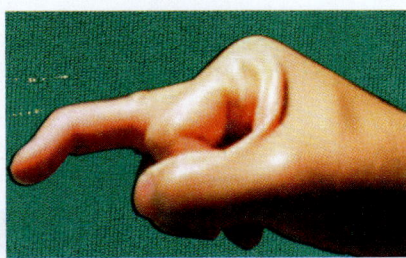

   a. Swan neck deformity
   b. Boutonniere deformity
   c. Mallet finger
   d. Duputyren's contracture

6. A 45-year-old crane operator at a construction site with pre-existing seropositive rheumatoid arthritis complains of progressive difficulty in breathing. Chest X-ray was performed. What is the diagnosis?

   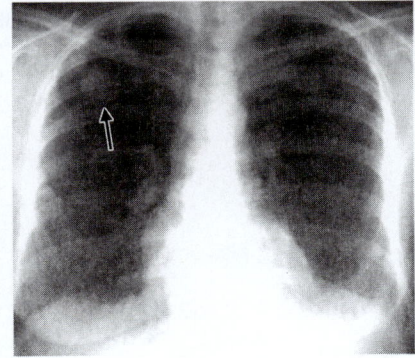

   a. Caplan syndrome
   b. Felty syndrome
   c. Bronchiolitis obliterans organizing pneumonia
   d. Lung cancer

7. A child presents with blotchy rash on legs, back and buttocks. All are true about the condition except?

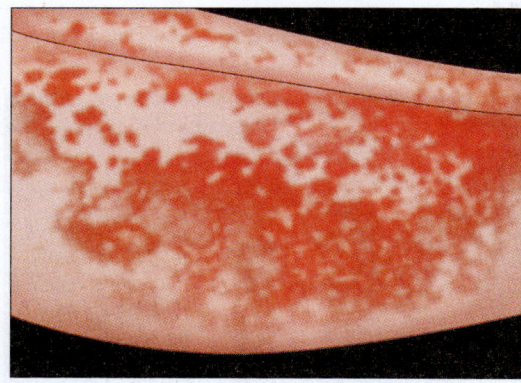

   a. Crops of palpable purpura
   b. Small vessel vasculitis
   c. Nephritis
   d. Low platelets

8. A 35-year-old woman with chronic sinusitis came for consultation due to an episode of hemoptysis. On examination, her eyelids were puffy and urine microscopic examination shows presence of RBC casts. CT chest was performed. What is the diagnosis?

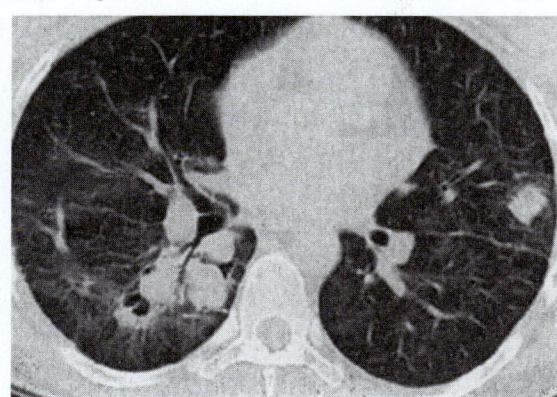

   a. Endobronchial TB
   b. Granulomatosis with angiitis
   c. Polyarteritis nodosa
   d. Pulmonary lymphangioleiomyomatosis

9. A patient with hypertension presents with following skin lesions. What is the diagnosis?

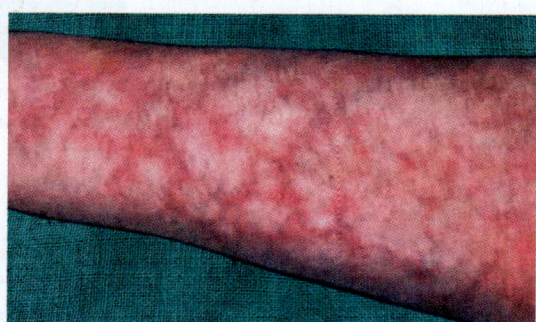

   a. Livedo reticularis
   b. Drug-induced rash
   c. Anaphylactoid purpura
   d. Erythromelalgia

Answers of Image-Based Questions

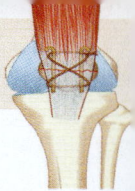

1. **Ans. (a) Dermatomyositis**
   The image shows presence of V sign which is erythematous rash seen over sun exposed part of the neck and seen in patients with dermatomyositis.

2. **Ans. (a) Pathergy test**
   - The image shows presence of an aphthous ulcer on the vulva, which according to history appears on recurrent basis. The test being performed is the pathergy test, which is a diagnostic criterion for Behcet's disease.
   - A 21 G hypodermic needle is blunted and inserted up to 1.5 mm depth, and the result is read after 24–48 hours. Positive result is taken as appearance of a sterile pustule.

3. **Ans. (a) Behçet's disease**
   - The pathergy test is a simple test in which the forearm is pricked with a small, sterile needle.
   - Occurrence of a small red bump or pustule at the site of needle insertion, 1 – 2 days after the test, constitutes a positive test. Although a positive pathergy test is helpful in the diagnosis of Behçet's disease, only a minority of Behçet's patients demonstrate the pathergy phenomenon.
   - Patients from the Mediterranean region are more likely to demonstrate a positive response to a pathergy test.

4. **Ans. (a) Uric acid**
   - The image shows presence of needle-shaped crystals of uric acid on polarized microscope.
   - Negative Birefringence: Urate crystals
   - Positive Birefringence: Calcium pyrophosphate crystals

5. **Ans. (c) Mallet finger**

Swan neck deformity	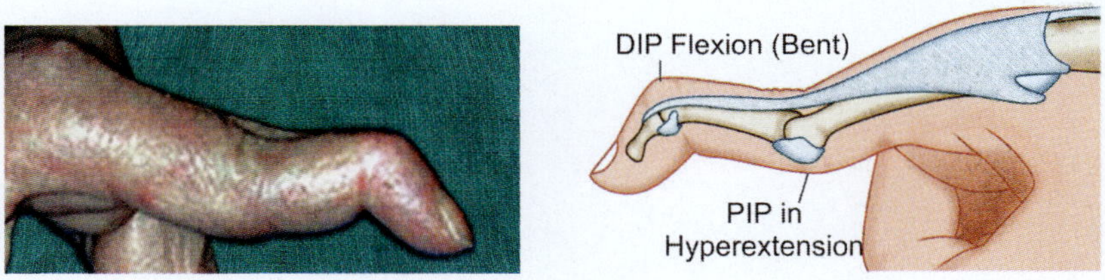
Boutonniere deformity	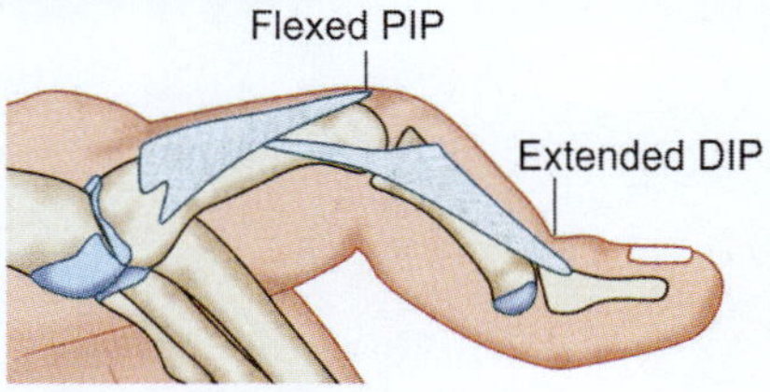
Mallet finger	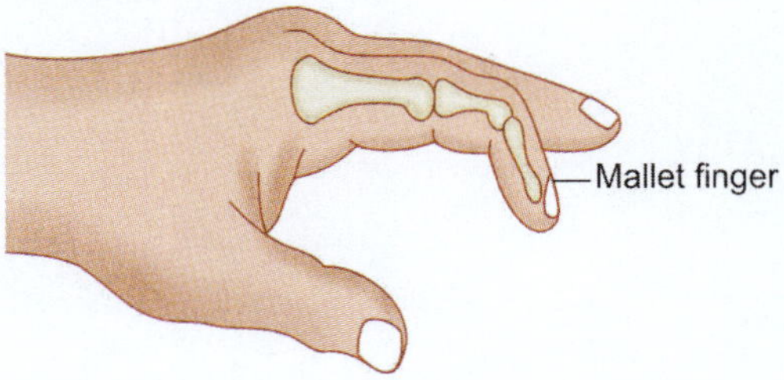
Duputyren's Contracture	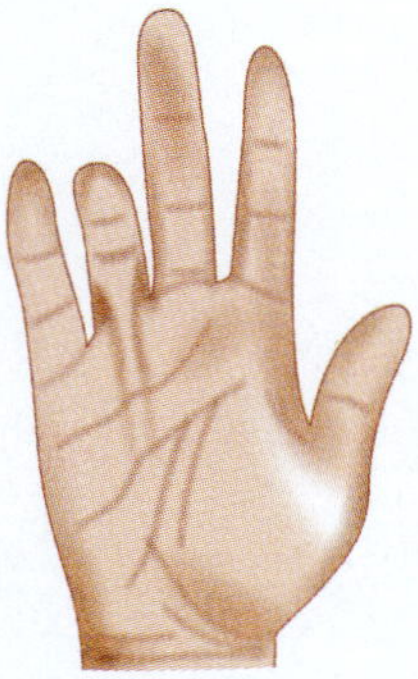

6. **Ans. (a) Caplan syndrome**
   The patient in this case is developing pneumoconiosis with rheumatoid nodule marked with arrow. This points to diagnosis of Caplan syndrome.

7. **Ans. (d) Low platelets**
   - *The image shows presence of pupura on the legs of a patient and considering the age of the patient, the first differential diagnosis is Henoch Schonlein Purpura.*
   - The first lesion is a skin lesion, which appears as a macule to progress to purpura and rash lasts for 3 weeks. It is a small vessel disease where kidney involvement can lead to hematuria. However, the hematochezia is due to vasculitis while the *platelet count is normal in HSP.*

8. **Ans. (b) Granulomatosis with polyangiitis**
   The CT shows nodules with cavitation (seen as small black dot in center of left sided nodule and right sided nodules). The presence of involvement of upper respiratory tract, lower respiratory tract with multiple cavitations and kidney involvement leads to probable diagnosis of granulomatosis with angiitis.

9. **Ans. (a) Livedo Reticularis**
   The image shows a reticular net-like appearance.

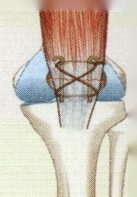

Conceptual Diagnostic Algorithm

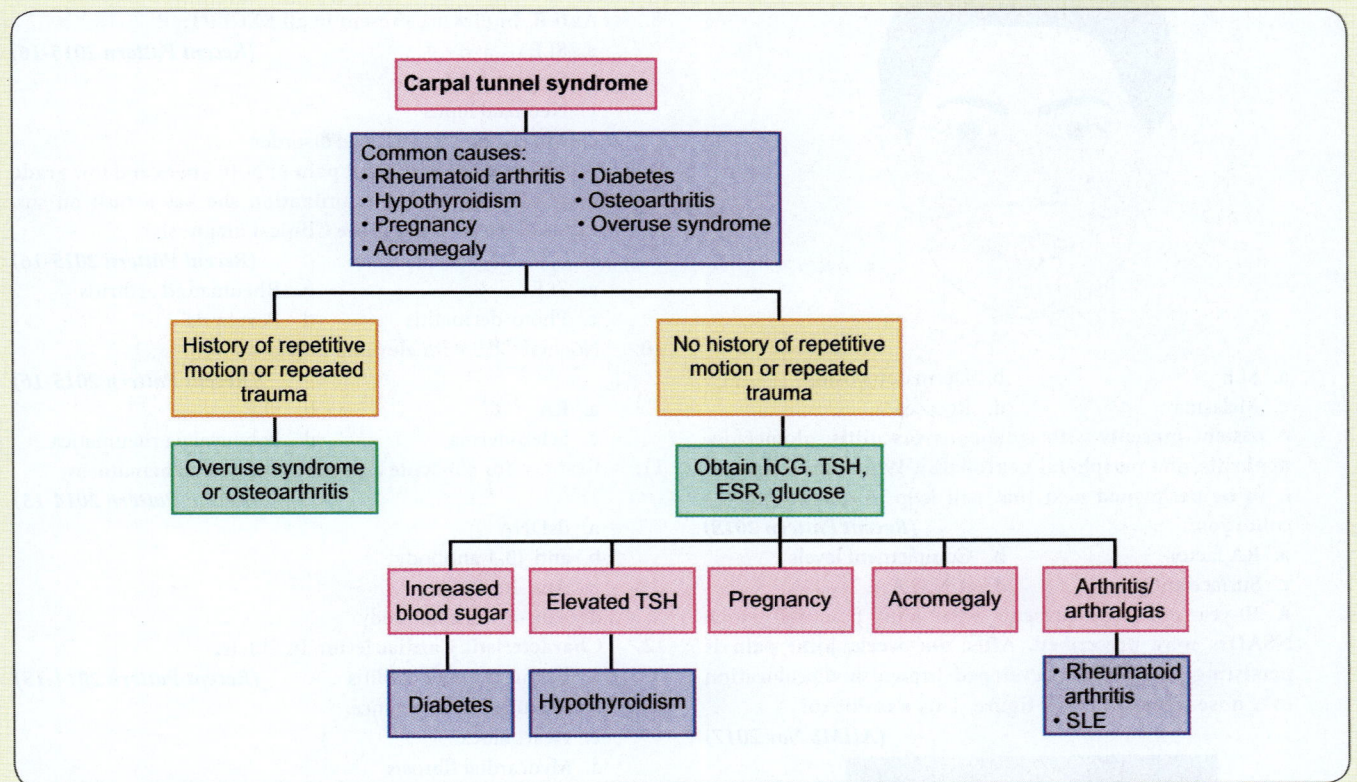

Multiple Choice Questions

SLE

1. Which of the following cannot be diagnosed without positive ANA? *(AIIMS Nov 2018)*
   a. SLE
   b. Sjogren Syndrome
   c. Drug induced lupus
   d. Scleroderma

2. A 25-year-old female presents with history of fever and oral ulcers and has developed erythematous lesions on her face. Comment on the diagnosis? *(Recent Pattern Jan 2019)*

   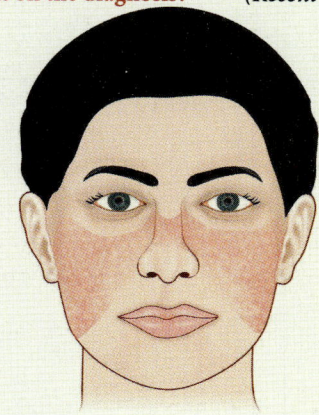

   a. SLE
   b. Dermatomyositis
   c. Melasma
   d. Rosacea

3. A patient presents with cutaneous vasculitis, glomerulonephritis, and peripheral neuropathy. Which investigation is to be performed next that will help in diagnosing the condition? *(Recent Pattern 2018)*
   a. RA factor
   b. Complement levels
   c. Surface antigen
   d. A.N.C.A

4. A 30-year-old male presents with joint pain for which NSAIDs were prescribed. After one week, joint pain is persisting and he has developed brownish discoloration over nose as shown in the figure. This was due to? *(AIIMS Nov 2017)*

   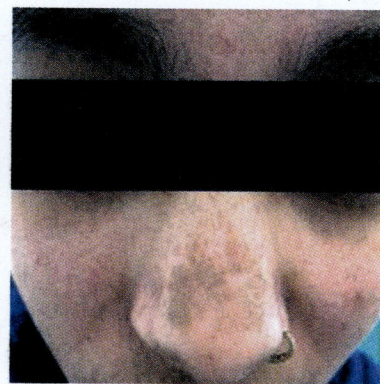

   a. Melasma
   b. Chikungunya
   c. Fixed drug eruption
   d. Dengue

5. Which of the following is not seen with SLE? *(Recent Question 2016-17)*
   a. Arthritis
   b. Alopecia
   c. Seizures
   d. Leucopenia

6. Which of the following is not an autoimmune disease? *(AIIMS Nov 2015)*
   a. SLE
   b. Grave's disease
   c. Ulcerative Colitis
   d. Rheumatoid Arthritis

7. All are true about SLE in pregnancy except? *(JIPMER Nov 2014)*
   a. Increased anti Ro and La implies low risk for congenital heart block
   b. Steroid can be continued in pregnancy
   c. Recurrent abortions
   d. Diseases worsens during pregnancy

8. Anti R_0 bodies are present in all EXCEPT: *(Recent Pattern 2015-16)*
   a. SLE
   b. Sjogren syndrome
   c. Neonatal lupus
   d. Mixed connective tissue disorder

9. A lady presents with joint pain in both knees and low grade fever off and on. On examination she has a rash on sun exposed parts. What is the Clinical diagnosis? *(Recent Pattern 2015-16)*
   a. SLE
   b. Rheumatoid arthritis
   c. Photo-dermatitis
   d. Porphyria

10. Normal CRP with elevated ESR is seen in? *(Recent Pattern 2015-16)*
    a. RA
    b. SLE
    c. Scleroderma
    d. Polymyalgia rheumatica

11. Best test for subacute cutaneous lupus Erythematosus: *(Recent Pattern 2014-15)*
    a. dsDNA
    b. anti-J0-1 antibody
    c. Anti-Ro/SS-A
    d. Anti-histone antibody

12. Characteristic Cardiac lesion in SLE is: *(Recent Pattern 2014-15)*
    a. Verrucous endocarditis
    b. Valvular incompetence
    c. Heart block
    d. Myocardial fibrosis

13. Antinuclear antibodies are seen in all except: *(Recent Pattern 2014-15)*
    a. Systemic sclerosis
    b. Morphea
    c. Pemphigus vulgaris
    d. SLE

14. A young girl is admitted with joint pains and butterfly rash and positive urine proteinuria. The best test for her diagnosis is? *(Recent Pattern 2014-15)*
    a. Anti ds-DNA antibody
    b. Anti-centromere antibody
    c. Antibodies to RNP
    d. Antibodies to tRNA synthetase

15. A 33-year-old woman has experienced episodes of fatigue, pleural effusion, pericardial effusion and carpal tunnel syndrome and macrocytic anemia. Best test for diagnosis shall be: *(Recent Pattern 2014-15)*
    a. Anti-beta 2 phospholipid antibodies
    b. Anti-smith antibody
    c. Antinuclear antibody
    d. Assay for thyroid hormones

16. **Butterfly rash in SLE involves all areas except**
    a. Cheeks   *(Recent Pattern 2014-15)*
    b. Nasolabial fold
    c. Lower eylids
    d. Bridge of nose

17. **Psychosis in SLE is caused by:** *(Recent Pattern 2014-15)*
    a. Anti-ribosomal P antibody
    b. Anti-glutamate acid decarboxylase antibody
    c. Anti-endomyosial antibody
    d. Anti-histone antibody

18. **Lupus anticoagulant causes all except:**
                                 (Recent Pattern 2014-15)
    a. Recurrent abortion   b. Arterial thrombosis
    c. Increase aPTT   d. Nephritis

19. **Most common presentation of cardiac lupus?** *(APPG 2014)*
    a. Myocarditis
    b. Pericarditis
    c. Aortic regurgitation
    d. Libman sacks endocarditis

20. **Most common cause of death in SLE in children**
    a. Lupus nephritis   *(Recent Pattern 2014-15)*
    b. Lupus cerebrits
    c. Libman sacks endocarditis
    d. Anemia and infections

21. **What is true regarding SLE in children?**
                                 (Recent Pattern 2014-15)
    a. Skin pigmentation more common
    b. No sex difference
    c. Presents with fever, fatigue and hematological abnormalities
    d. Cardiac involvement more common

22. **Lupus anti-coagulant is associated with all except:**
    a. Recurrent abortion   *(Recent Pattern 2014-15)*
    b. Polyhydramnios
    c. Intrauterine growth retardation
    d. Pre-eclampsia-early onset

23. **Most common presentation of S.L.E**
    a. Arthralgia   *(Recent Pattern 2014-15)*
    b. Erosive polyarthritis
    c. Butterfly rash
    d. Autoimmune hemolytic anemia

24. **All of the following are indicators for use of corticosteroids in SLE except:** *(Recent Pattern 2014-15)*
    a. Neuropsychiatric lupus
    b. Pericarditis
    c. Endocarditis
    d. Nephritic syndrome

25. **All are true about drug induced SLE except?**
    a. Female: Male ratio=9:1   *(Recent Pattern 2014-15)*
    b. Anti-histone Antibodies
    c. CNS involvement not common
    d. Renal involvement not common

26. **Cortiocosteroid are used in all except:**
    a. Lupus nephritis   *(Recent Pattern 2014-15)*
    b. Lupus cerebritis
    c. Libman sacks endocarditis
    d. Lupus pernio

27. **All are true about nervous system involvement in SLE except:** *(Recent Pattern 2014-15)*
    a. Seizures
    b. Antibodies against aquaporin-4 antibody
    c. Elevated protein level in CSF
    d. Pseudo-tumor cerebri

28. **Which of the following antibodies correlates with disease activity for S.L.E** *(Recent Pattern 2014-15)*
    a. Anti Smith antibody
    b. Anti dS DNA antibody
    c. Anti Histone antibody
    d. Anti Rho

29. **Bony erosion are seen in the following except?**
                                 (Recent Pattern 2014-15)
    a. Gout   b. Psoriasis
    c. SLE   d. Osteoarthritis

30. **Anti-double stranded DNA is highly specific for :**
                                 (AIIMS June 97)
    a. Systemic sclerosis   b. S.L.E.
    c. Polymyositis   d. Rheumatic sclerosis

31. **Best marker for drug induced lupus is :** *(AI 2007)*
    a. Antihistone antibodies
    b. Anti ds DNA
    c. ANA
    d. Anti smith Ab

32. **A 23-year-old woman has experienced episodes of myalgias, pleural effusion, pericarditis and arthralgias without joint deformity over course of several years. The best laboratory screening test to diagnose her disease would be:** *(AI 2003)*
    a. CD4 lymphocyte count
    b. Erythrocyte sedimentation rate
    c. Antinuclear antibody
    d. Assay for thyroid hormones

33. **Joint erosions are not a feature of :** *(AI 06)*
    a. Rheumatoid arthritis
    b. Psoriasis
    c. Multicentric reticulo-histiocytosis
    d. Systemic lupus erythematosus

34. **All of the following are true about SLE except:**
    a. Autoimmune Hematolytic Anemia   *(PGI Dec 06)*
    b. ↑ed ANA   c. Anti-ds DNA
    d. Raynaud's phenomenon e. Joint deformity

35. **Deposition of Anti ds DNA Ab in kidney, skin, choroid plexus and joints is seen in:** *(AI 2007)*
    a. SLE   b. Good pasture
    c. Scleroderma   d. Raynauds disease

36. **Autoimmune destruction of platelet is seen in :**
    a. SLE   *(AIIMS May 95)*
    b. Rheumatoid arthritis
    c. Reiter disease
    d. Polyarteritisnodosa

37. **All of the following are known to cause Lupus like syndrome, except** *(AIIMS Nov 2010)*
    a. INH   b. Penicillin
    c. Hydralazine   d. Sulphonamide

38. **In SLE, characteristic kidney lesion is:** *(PGI Dec 98)*
    a. Mesangial proliferation   b. Tubular fibrin deposits
    c. Wire loop lesions   d. IgG deposits

39. 30-year-old Basanti presents with light brown lesions involving both her cheeks. The lesions had never been erythematous. Which of the following is the most probable diagnosis: *(AIIMS Nov 2000)*
    a. SLE
    b. Chloasma
    c. Air borne contact dermatitis
    d. Photo sensitive reaction

40. Features of SLE include all of the following except:
    a. Recurrent abortion *(AI 1998)*
    b. Sterility
    c. Coomb's positive hemolytic anemia
    d. Psychosis

41. Lupus anticoagulants may cause all of the following except: *(AI 1998)*
    a. Recurrent abortion
    b. False +ve VDRL results
    c. Increase prothrombin time
    d. Arterial thrombosis

42. Indications of steroids in SLE are all except: *(AI 1998)*
    a. Myocarditis
    b. Endocarditis
    c. Thrombocytopenia
    d. Neuropsychiatric symptoms

43. Low doses of aspirin therapy is essentially advised for all of the following conditions except: *(AI 1997)*
    a. Rheumatoid Arthritis
    b. IUGR
    c. Post myocardinal infarction
    d. Pre ecclampsia

44. A 35-year-old lady complains dysphagia, Raynaud's phenomenon, sclerodactyly. Investigations show antinuclear antibody. The likely diagnosis is : *(AIIMS June 99)*
    a. Systemic lupus erythematosis
    b. Systemic sclerosis
    c. Mixed connective tissue disorder
    d. Rheumatoid arthritis

45. A 14-year-old girl on exposure to cold has pallor of extremities followed by pain and cyanosis. In later stages of life she is most prone to develop: *(AIIMS Nov 08)*
    a. SLE
    b. Scleroderma
    c. Rheumatoid Arthritis
    d. Dermatomyositis

Antiphospholipid Antibody Syndrome

46. What treatment should be given to pregnant female with A.P.L.A.S. to avoid abortion? *(AIIMS Nov 14)*
    a. IVIG
    b. Plasmapheresis
    c. Aspirin + LMW heparin
    d. Progesterone injections

47. A young female is suffering from, recurrent abortions and thrombosis of deep veins, thrombocytopenia, and a recent MI. The most likely diagnosis is: *(Recent Pattern 2014-15)*
    a. Catastrophic anti-phosphilpid antibody syndrome
    b. Primary anti-phospholipid antibody syndrome
    c. TTP
    d. Protein C deficiency

48. A lady presents with recurrent abortions and isolated prolongation of APTT. Which one of the following gives positive result?
    a. Prothrombin time *(Recent Pattern 2014-15)*
    b. Dilute Russell Viper Venom Time test
    c. Bleeding time
    d. Clot solubility test

49. All of the following statements about Antiphospholipid Antibody Syndrome (APLAb) are true, Except : *(AI 2010)*
    a. Single titre of Anticardiolipin is diagnostic
    b. Commonly presents with recurrent fetal loss
    c. May cause pulmonary hypertension
    d. Warfarin is given as treatment

50. Which of the following is recommended in a woman with Antiphospholipid Antibodies and history of prior abortions / still birth. *(AI 2010)*
    a. Aspirin only
    b. Aspirin + Low molecular weight Heparin
    c. Aspirin + Low molecular weight Heparin + Prednisolone.
    d. No Treatment

Scleroderma

51. All are true about scleroderma crisis except? *(Recent Question 2016-17)*
    a. Accelerated hypertension
    b. Onion skinning of renal vessels
    c. Anti-centromere antibody is a positive predictor of disease
    d. ACE inhibitors reduce mortality rate

52. Woman of 30-years presents with Raynaud's phenomenon, polyarthritis, dysphagia of 5-years and sclerodactyl. On work up Anti-centromere antibody is positive. The likely cause is? *(Recent Pattern 2014-15)*
    a. CREST
    b. Mixed connective tissue disorder
    c. SLE
    d. Rheumatoid arthritis

53. All of the following are features of Scleroderma except:
    a. Diffuse periosteal reaction *(Recent Pattern 2014-15)*
    b. Esophageal dysmotility
    c. Erosion of tip of phalanges
    d. Lung Nodular infiltrates

54. Anti-topoisomerase I is marker of:
    a. Systemic sclerosis *(Recent Pattern 2014-15)*
    b. Classic polyarteritis nodosa
    c. Nephrotic syndrome
    d. Rheumatoid arthritis

55. Screening test for sclerodema: *(Recent Pattern 2014-15)*
    a. Anti-nuclear antibody
    b. U1- Ribonucleoprotein antibody
    c. Anti- L.K.M antibody
    d. Anti- topoisomerase antibody

56. All are X-ray finding of scleroderma except? *(Recent Pattern 2014-15)*
    a. Dilatation due to aperistalsis of oesophagus
    b. Pseudo-obstruction
    c. Pneumatosis intestinalis
    d. Subperiosteal elevation

57. Recurrent aspiration pneumonia is caused by:
    a. Dermatomyostis/polymyositis *(Recent Pattern 2014-15)*
    b. Rheumatoid arthritis
    c. Progressive systemic sclerosis
    d. Systemic lupus erythrematosus
58. Indication of poor prognosis of systemic sclerosis is:
    a. Calcinosis cutis *(Recent Pattern 2014-15)*
    b. Renal involvement
    c. Alopecia
    d. Telangiectasia
59. All are features of scleroderma except?
    (Recent Pattern 2014-15)
    a. Decrease in tone of LES
    b. Restrictive cardiomyopathy
    c. Syndactyly
    d. Halitosis
60. Woman presented with dysphagia and stiff fingers and leather like skin is diagnosed to have?
    (Recent Pattern 2014-15)
    a. Buergers disease   b. Rheumatoid arthritis
    c. Sceleroderma   d. Osteoarthrosis
61. Which is not seen in scleroderma? *(Recent Pattern 2014-15)*
    a. Anti-scl 70 antibody   b. Bi-basiliar fibrosis
    c. Prayer sign   d. Ischemic stroke
62. All the following are features of Scleroderma *except* :
    a. Dysphagia *(AI 1995)*
    b. Raynaud's phenomenon
    c. Skin contracture
    d. Calcification in all the long bones

Sarcoidosis

63. Which of the following is seen in sarcoidosis:
    (Recent Pattern 2015-16)
    a. Hypercalcemia   b. Hypocalcemia
    c. Hyperphosphatemia d. Hypophosphatemia
64. The patient with breathlessness and skin lesions?

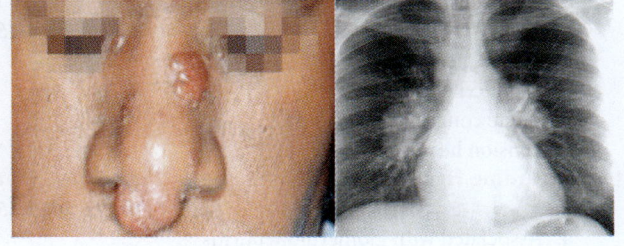

    a. Sarcoidosis
    b. Phakomatosis
    c. Pulmonary Lymphagiomatosis
    d. DRESS syndrome
65. Sarcoidosis is characterized by all except:
    a. Cavity *(Recent Pattern 2014-15)*
    b. Panda sign
    c. Hilar lymphadenopathy
    d. Egg shell calcification
66. Arthritis common with uveitis is: *(Recent Pattern 2014-15)*
    a. RA   b. Ankylosing spondylitis
    c. Still's disease   d. Reiter's disease
67. The most common cause of sudden death in sarcoidosis is?
    a. Pneumonia *(Recent Pattern 2014-15)*
    b. Cor pulmonale
    c. Arrythmias
    d. Liver failure
68. True about sarcoidosis? *(Recent Pattern 2014-15)*
    a. Causes large cavitatory lesions
    b. Spontaneous remission may occur
    c. Tuberculin test is negative
    d. Caseation and necrosis may occur
69. Most common cause of unilateral Hilar lymphadenopathy:
    a. Histoplasmosis *(Recent Pattern 2014-15)*
    b. Sarcoidosis
    c. Aspergillosis
    d. Tuberculosis
70. Sarcoidosis is least likely to be associated with:
    a. Uveitis *(Recent Pattern 2014-15)*
    b. Pericardial effusion
    c. Erythema nodosum
    d. Lymphadenopathy
71. Following cranial nerve is involved in patients with sarcoidosis: *(Recent Pattern 2014-15)*
    a. I cranial nerve   b. II cranial nerve
    c. III cranial nerve d. IV cranial nerve
72. The primary involvement of which organ is so far not reported to be affected by sarcoidosis is:
    (Recent Pattern 2014-15)
    a. Heart   b. Adrenals
    c. Kidney   d. Brain
73. Tufting of distal phalanx is characteristic of:
    a. Psoriatic arthropathy *(Recent Pattern 2014-15)*
    b. Sarcoidosis
    c. Hyperparathyroidism
    d. Hypoparthyroidism
74. All of the following are features of sarcoidosis except:
    (Recent Pattern 2014-15)
    a. Right paratracheal lymphadenopathy
    b. Cardiomyopathy
    c. Hypercalcemia
    d. Malabsorption syndrome
75. Heerfordt's syndrome consists of fever, parotid enlargement, facial palsy and: *(Bihar PG 2014)*
    a. Arthralgia   b. Bilateral hiladenopathy
    c. Erythema nodosum   d. Anterior uveitis
76. True about sarcoidosis is: *(Recent Pattern 2014-15)*
    a. Serum amyloid A is used as a marker for sarcoidosis
    b. Kveim test is diagnostic
    c. Hypocalcemia
    d. Pleural effusion is common
77. Lupus Pernio is a complication of: *(Recent Pattern 2014-15)*
    a. Sarcoidosis   b. Skin TB
    c. SLE complication d. DLE and SLE
78. Garland sign on CXR in sarcoidosis involves all except:
    a. Right paratracheal nodes *(Recent Pattern 2014-15)*
    b. Right hilar nodes
    c. Left hilar nodes
    d. Left pretracheal lymph nodes

79. In rheumatoid arthritis pathology starts in:
    a. Articular cartilage (Recent Pattern 2014-15)
    b. Capsule
    c. Synovium
    d. Muscle

80. Bilateral parotid gland enlargement is seen in all of the following except: (AI 1998)
    a. Sarcoidosis
    b. SLE
    c. Chronic pancreatitis
    d. Sjogern's syndrome

81. The following cranial nerve is most commonly involved in patients with sarcoidosis: (AIIMS Nov 02)
    a. II   b. III
    c. VII   d. IX

Vasculitis

82. A young female presents with rhinitis not subsiding with anti-histaminics, along with recurrent hemoptysis & glomerulonephritis. Which of the following is NOT an important differential diagnosis to be considered in the given scenario? (AIIMS Nov 2015)
    a. Goodpasture syndrome
    b. Wegener's granulomatosis
    c. Microscopic polyangitis
    d. Polyarteritis nodosa

83. A 45-year-old man presents with hematuria. Renal biopsy demonstrates a focal necrotizing glomerulonephritis with crescent formation. The patient gives history of intermittent hemoptysis and intermittent chest pain of moderate intensity. A previous chest X-ray had demonstrated multiple opacities, some of which were cavitated. The patient also has chronic cold like nasal symptoms. What is the most probable diagnosis? (UPSC 2015)
    a. Aspergillosis
    b. Polyarteritisnodosa
    c. Renal carcinoma metastatic to lung
    d. Wegener's granulomatosis

84. In Polyarteritis Nodosa, aneurysms are seen in all except? (Bihar PG 2015)
    a. Kidney   b. Lung
    c. Liver   d. Pancreas

85. Which antibody is incriminated in causing Henoch Schonlein Purpura? (Recent Pattern 2015-16)
    a. IgA   b. IgG
    c. IgM   d. IgD

86. Vasculitis seen only in childhood? (AIIMS Nov 2014)
    a. Kawasaki
    b. HSP
    c. Susac syndrome
    d. Giant cell

87. Incorrect about takayasu arteritis: (Recent Pattern 2014-15)
    a. Spares pulmonary artery
    b. Renovascular hypertension
    c. Blood pressure difference between left and right limbs
    d. Strongly positive mantoux

88. An 18-year-old boy presents with digital gangrene in third and fourth fingers for last 2 weeks. On examination the blood pressure is 170/110 mm of Hg and all peripheral pulses were palpable. Blood and urine examinations were unremarkable. Antinuclear antibodies, antibody to double stranded DNA and anti-neutrophil cytoplasmic antibody were negative. The most likely diagnosis is:
    a. Wegner's granulomatosis (Recent Pattern 2014-15)
    b. Polyarteritis nodosa
    c. Takayasu's arteritis
    d. Systemic lupus erythematosus (SLE)

89. All are true about Henoch Schonlein purpura except:
    a. Raised IgA (Recent Pattern 2014-15)
    b. Hematochezia
    c. Thrombocytopenia
    d. Joint pain

90. A 20-year-old woman presents with bilateral maxillary sinusitis, palpable purpura on the legs and hemoptysis. Radiograph of the chest shows a thin-walled cavity in left lower zone. Investigations reveal total leukocyte count 12000/mm³, red cells casts in the urine and serum creatinine 3 mg/dl. What is the most probable diagnosis?
    a. Henoch. Schonlein purpura (Recent Pattern 2014-15)
    b. Polyarteritis nodosa
    c. Wegener's granulomatois
    d. Disseminated tuberculosis

91. In Takayasu's arteritis there is: (Recent Pattern 2014-15)
    a. Intimal fibrosis
    b. Renal hypertension
    c. Coronary aneurysm
    d. All of the above

92. c-ANCA is pathogonomic of: (Recent Pattern 2014-15)
    a. Classical PAN
    b. Wegener's granulomatosis
    c. Crescentric nephritis
    d. SLE

93. A 35-year-old man present with episodes of vomiting, photophobia and unilateral Pulsatile headache. What is likely cause? (Recent Pattern 2014-15)
    a. Cluster headache
    b. Giant cell arteritis
    c. Acute congestive glaucoma
    d. Tension headache

94. Regarding Henoch Schönlein purpura all are true except? (Recent Pattern 2014-15)
    a. Associated with glomerulonephritis
    b. Non-Palpable purpura
    c. Decreased complement
    d. Normal platelet count

95. What is feature of temporal arteritis? (Recent Pattern 2014-15)
    a. Giant cell arteritis   b. Granulomatous vasculitis
    c. Necrotizing vasculitis d. Leucocytoclastic Vasculitis

96. Which of the following are true about findings of Poly-arteritis nodosa? (Recent Pattern 2014-15)
    a. There is tear in the lamina Dura
    b. Micro Aneurysm formation in the large blood vessel
    c. Nodules are formed in skin which are clinically palpable
    d. Chain of beads appearance

97. HLA-B*1502 is a genetic marker for:
    (Recent Pattern 2014-15)
    a. Systemic lupus erythematosus
    b. Polyarteritis nodosa
    c. Steven Johnson syndrome
    d. Seronegative spondy-arthritis syndrome

98. Giant cell arteritis causes which of the following in the eye:
    a. Episcleritis   *(Recent Pattern 2014-15)*
    b. Anterior ischemic optic neuropathy
    c. Neuroparalytic keratitis
    d. Band keratitis

99. A 30-year-old male patient presents with complaints of weakness in right upper and both lower limbs for last 4 months. He developed digital infarcts involving 2nd and 3rd fingers on right side and 5th finger on left side. On examination, BP was 160/140 mm Hg, all peripheral pulses were palpable and urine examination showed proteinuria and RBC-10-15/hpf with no casts. What is the most likely diagnosis?   *(Recent Pattern 2014-15)*
    a. Polyarteritis nodosa
    b. Systemic lupus erythematosus
    c. Wegener's granulomatosis
    d. Mixed cryoglobulemia

100. Kawasaki's disease has the following features except:
    a. Coronary artery aneurysm   *(Recent Pattern 2014-15)*
    b. Conjunctival suffusion
    c. Thrombocytopenia
    d. Desquamation of the skin of fingers and toes

101. Treatment of Kawasaki disease in children is?
    a. Oral steroids   *(Recent Pattern 2014-15)*
    b. IV steroids
    c. IV Immunoglobuin
    d. Mycophenolate mefentil

102. Treatment of choice in Wegner's granulomatosis is:
    (Recent Pattern 2014-15)
    a. Cyclosporine   b. Cyclophosphamide
    c. Steroids   d. Radiotherapy

103. True about Giant cell arteritis is all except:
    (Recent Pattern 2014-15)
    a. High dose of steroid is drug of choice
    b. ESR is usually raised
    c. Intracranial ICA is particularly susceptible
    d. Mainly affects people of >70 years

104. Consider the following statements regarding classic polyarteritis nodosa: *(Recent Pattern 2014-15)*
    I. It is multi-system necrotising vasculitis
    II. Small & medium vessels are involved
    III. Pulmonary artery involvement is a characteristic feature.
    IV. Up to 30% patient may show positive test for Hepatitis B surface antigen
    Which of these statements are correct?
    a. I and II   b. II and III
    c. I, II and IV   d. II, III and IV

105. Which of the following is an example of small-vessel vasculitis?   *(Recent Pattern 2014-15)*
    a. Takayasu arteritis   b. Microscopic polyangitis
    c. Giant cell arteritis   d. Polyarteritis nodosa

106. A 70-year-old male presents with left sided headache and generalized aches and pains of three months duration. The referring doctor has highlighted the remarkably elevated ESR and alkaline phosphatase. The most likely diagnosis is?   *(Recent Pattern 2014-15)*
    a. Multiple myeloma
    b. Disseminated carcinoma prostate
    c. Paget's disease
    d. Temporal arteritis

107. Cavitating lesion in lung is seen in: *(Recent Pattern 2014-15)*
    a. Wegner's granulomatosis   b. PAN
    c. SLE   d. Goodpasture's syndrome

108. Important feature in Henoch Schonlein purpura is?
    a. Raised IgA   *(Recent Pattern 2014-15)*
    b. Membranous glomerulonephritis
    c. Absent radial pulse
    d. Aneurysm of branching point

109. Hepatitis B virus is associated with: *(Recent Pattern 2014-15)*
    a. SLE   b. Polyarteritis nodosa
    c. Sjören's syndrome   d. Wegener's granulomatosis

110. Pulse absent in radial artery is seen in?
    (Recent Pattern 2014-15)
    a. Coarctation of aorta   b. Aortic regurgitation
    c. Takayasu arteritis   d. Dissection of Aorta

111. All of the following are small vessels vasculitis, Except:
    a. Classical PAN   *(PGI Dec 2000)*
    b. Wegner's granulomatosis   c. HSP
    d. Churg Strauss Syndrome   e. Microscopic Polyangitis

112. ANCA positive vasculitis include all of the following Except: *(PGI Dec 06)*
    a. Wegener's granulomatosis   b. Churgstrauss syndrome
    c. Microscopic PAN   d. Good pasture's syndrome

113. C-ANCA is associated with: *(PGI- June 08)*
    a. Wegener's Granulomatosis
    b. Microscopic Polyangitis
    c. Churg- Strauss Syndrome
    d. PolyarteritisNodosa (PAN)

114. p-ANCA is characteristic for: *(AIIMS Dec 92)*
    a. PAN
    b. Microscopic polyangitis
    c. Wegener's granulomatosis
    d. Henoch-Schonleinpurpura

115. All of the following condition are associated with granulomatous pathology, except: *(AI 2010)*
    a. Wegner's Granulomatosis (WG)
    b. Takayasu Arteritis (TA)
    c. Polyarteritis Nodosa (Classic PAN)
    d. Giant Cell Arteritis (GCA)

116. A 25 years old female develops serous otitis media of left ear with cough and occasional hemoptysis and hematuria and epistaxis for one and half months. Her Hemoglobin is 7 gm. B.P. > 170/100, ptoreinuria +++, RA positive (+ve) and ANCA positive (+ve), the likely cause is-   *(AIIMS June 99)*
    a. Wegener's granulomatosis
    b. Rheumatoid arthritis
    c. Rapidly proliferative glomerulonephritis
    d. Good pasteur's syndrome

117. A patient presents with melaena normal renal function, hypertension and mononeuritis multiplex. The most probable diagnosis is: *(AIIMS Nov 04)*
    a. Classical polyarteritis nodosa
    b. Microscopic polyangiitis
    c. Henoch-Schonleinpurpura
    d. Buerger's disease
118. Biopsy in PAN shows: *(PGI June 98)*
    a. Necrotizing arteritis   b. Atrophy
    c. Granulomatous lesion   d. Ring lesion
119. Which of the following is more frequently seen in Churg Strauss Syndrome in comparison to Wegener's Granulomatosis *(Recent Pattern Question)*
    a. Renal involvement
    b. Lower Respiratory Tract involvement
    c. Eye involvement
    d. Upper Respiratory Tract involvement
120. An elderly female presents to the emergency department with history of fever, headache and double vision. Biopsy of temporal artery revealed panarteritis. The most likely diagnosis is *(AIIMS Nov 09)*
    a. Nonspecific Arteritis
    b. Polyarteritis Nodosa
    c. Wegener's Granulomatosis
    d. Temporal Arteritis
121. Which of the following is the most frequent presenting symptoms in patients with giant cell arteritis
    a. Headache *(AI 1991, 1999)*
    b. Jaw claudication
    c. Polymyalgin Rheumatica
    d. Blindness
122. The investigation of choice for diagnosis of Giant cell Arteritis is *(AI-1990)*
    a. Temporal Artery biopsy
    b. Colour Doppler of Temporal Artery
    c. CT Angiography
    d. MRI
123. Bilateral upper limb pulse less disease is? *(Recent Pattern Question)*
    a. Giant cell Arteritis   b. Polyarteritis Nodosa
    c. Aortoarteritis   d. HSP
124. Reversed Coarctation is seen in: *(Recent Pattern Question)*
    a. Giant cell Arteritis   b. Polyarteritis Nodosa
    c. Takayasu Arteritis   d. Kawasaki Disease
125. A 24-year-old male presents with abdominal pain, rashes, palpable purpura and, arthritis. The most probable diagnosis is. *(AI 08)*
    a. Henoch Schonlein Purpura (HSP)
    b. Sweet syndrome
    c. Meningococcemia
    d. Hemochromatosis
126. A 5-year-old child presents with non-blanching purpura over the buttocks and lower limbs along with colicky abdominal pain. Further evaluation revealed deposition of IgA immune complexes. The most likely diagnosis is:
    a. Henoch Shonlein Purpura *(AIIMS 2011)*
    b. Kawasaki Disease
    c. Wegner's Granulomatosis
    d. Takayasu Disease

127. All of the following are true about HSP, Except: *(PGI Dec 2010)*
    a. Palpable Purpura   b. Kidney's commonly affected
    c. ANCA Negative   d. Thrombocytopenia
128. One of the following is a characteristic of Henoch–Schonlein Purpura: *(AI 2002)*
    a. Blood in stool   b. Thrombocytopenia
    c. Intracranial hemorrhage   d. Susceptibility to infection
129. Henoch–Schonlein Purpura is characterized by the deposition of the following immunoglobulin around the vessels : *(AIIMS Nov 05)*
    a. IgM   b. IgG
    c. IgA   d. IgE
130. A Ten-year-old boy presents to the pediatric emergency unit with seizures. Blood pressure in the upper extremity measured as 200/140 mm Hg. Femoral pulses were not palpable. The most likely diagnosis amongst the following is: *(AI 2010)*
    a. Takayasu Aorto arteritis   b. Renal parenchymal disease
    c. Grandmal seizures   d. Coarctation of Aorta
131. Renal artery stenosis may occur in all of the following, except : *(AI 06)*
    a. Atherosclerosis   b. Fibromuscular dysplasia
    c. Takayasu's arteritis   d. Polyarteritis nodosa

Ankylosing Spondylitis

132. Which of the following is true about "relapsing seronegative symmetric synovitis" with pitting edema? *(JIPMER May 2018)*
    a. Responsive to steroids   b. Malignant arthritis
    c. Poor prognosis   d. Causes deformities
133. A middle aged woman with history of back pain came to OPD. On examination she was positive for Schober test. Her nose and ears were hyperpigmented. What is your diagnosis? *(AIIMS May 2017)*

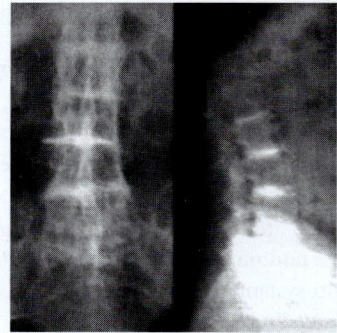

    a. Hypoparathyroidism   b. Ochronosis
    c. Fluorosis   d. Ankylosing Spondylitis
134. A 27-year-old male presents with back pain which is more in the morning and decreases in the evening. It is also relieved by bathing in warm water. What is the additional finding? *(AIIMS Nov 2015)*
    a. Liver enlargement
    b. Decreased chest expansion
    c. Interphalangeal joint swelling
    d. Marrow fibrosis

135. Which of the following is NOT true regarding anakinra?
    (APPG 2015 Medicine)
    a. Used in Muckle wells syndrome and Adult onset still's disease
    b. Not combined with anti TNF drugs due to the risk of serious infections
    c. Useful In familial cold urticaria
    d. Soluble IL-2 receptor antagonist

136. True about ankylosing spondylitis? (Jipmer May 2015)
    a. More in female
    b. 50% associated with HLA B27
    c. Heart is affected
    d. No association with plantar fasciitis

137. The following test is performed on the patient with low backache. All are true about the condition except?

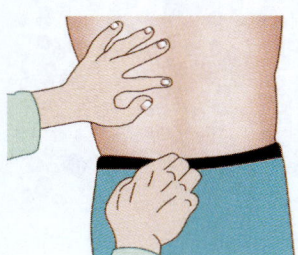
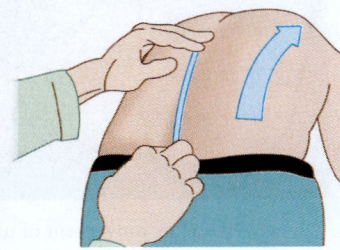

    a. Distance between two points increases by < 5 cm in lumbar flexion
    b. Chest wall expansion is < 4 cm
    c. Bone marrow edema
    d. Decreased FRC

138. HLA B27 has the maximum association with? (AIIMS Nov 14)
    a. Ankylosing spondylitis
    b. Rheumatoid arthritis
    c. Osteoarthritis
    d. Juvenile rheumatoid arthritis

139. The poly-arthritic condition that is NOT common in males:
    (Recent Pattern 2014-15)
    a. Gout
    b. Psoriatic arthritis
    c. Ankylosing spondylitis
    d. Systemic lupus erythematosus

140. In ankylosing spondylitis joint involvement is least in?
    (Recent Pattern 2014-15)
    a. Wrist and hand
    b. Sacroiliac joint
    c. Acromio-clavicular joint
    d. Costochondral junction

141. Schober's sign is used to evaluate: (Recent Pattern 2014-15)
    a. Flexion of lumbar spine
    b. Chest expansion
    c. Pain with motion of hip
    d. Neck pain and stiffness

142. In Seronegative spondyloarthritis, what will cause maximum reduction in pain and morning stiffness?
    (Recent Pattern 2014-15)
    a. Aspirin
    b. Indomethacin
    c. Corticosteroids
    d. Infliximab

143. A young male presents with joint pains and backache with relief of symptoms on movement/exercise. The most likely diagnosis is? (Recent Pattern 2014-15)
    a. Rheumatoid arthritis
    b. Ankylosing spondylitis
    c. Poly-articular juvenile arthritis
    d. Psoriatic arthropathy

144. All are seronegative (spondyloepiphyseal) arthritis with ocular manifestations, except- (AIIMS Nov 01)
    a. Ankylospondilitis
    b. Ritter's disease
    c. Rheumatoid arthritis
    d. Psoriatic arthritis

145. Treatment of choice in seronegative spondylarthritis is:
    a. Phenylbutazone (AIIMS Nov 93)
    b. Aspirin
    c. Indomethacin
    d. Corticosteroid

Rheumatoid Arthritis

146. Which of the following drugs is not used in management of Rheumatoid arthritis? (AIIMS May 2018)
    a. Etanercept
    b. Leflunomide
    c. Febuxostat
    d. Methotrexate

147. A woman presents with pain, swelling and redness of knee joint and hand. There were associated complaints of morning stiffness but the swelling spared the DIP joints. The image of the patient's hand is shown. What is the most likely diagnosis? (AIIMS May 2018)

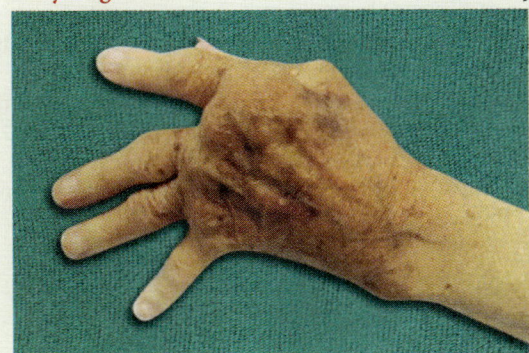

    a. Rheumatoid arthritis
    b. Heberden nodes and pre-existing osteo arthritis
    c. Tenosynovitis of extensor tendon of MCP joints
    d. Post traumatic dystrophy with complex regional pain syndrome

148. Which is not included in Polymyalgia rheumatic criteria (Healey criteria)? (JIPMER May 2018)
    a. Morning stiffness more than 1 hour
    b. Involvement of neck, shoulder, back for more than 6 months in a year
    c. ESR > 40 mm/hr
    d. Rapid response to prednisone < 20 mg/day

149. A 55-year-old female on methotrexate presents with continuous pain and swelling of bilateral hand joints. What is the best treatment plan for this patient?
 (Recent Pattern Jan 2019)

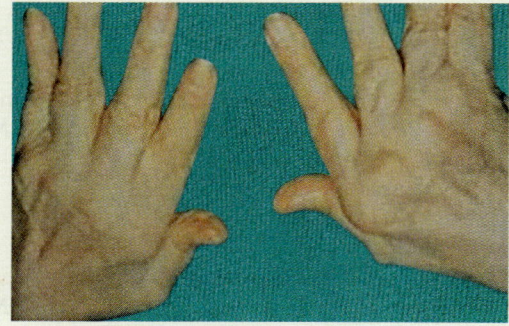

 a. Double the dose of methotrexate
 b. Methotrexate + high potency Oral steroids
 c. Methotrexate + Sulphasalazine + Hydroxychloroquine
 d. Stop methotrexate and start Monotherapy with anti-TNF-drugs

150. Which is the most common cause of death in rheumatoid arthritis? *(Recent Question 2016-17)*
 a. Cardiovascular complications
 b. Neurological complications
 c. Lung disease complications
 d. Haematological complications

151. Which is the most common valvular lesion seen in rheumatoid arthritis? *(Recent Question 2016-17)*
 a. Mitral regurgitation b. Tricuspid regurgitation
 c. Pulmonic regurgitation d. Aortic regurgitation

152. The most specific antibody for Rheumatoid arthritis is?
 a. Antinuclear antibody (ANA) *(AP PG 2016)*
 b. Rheumatoid factor
 c. Anti-cyclic citrullinated peptide (anti-CCP) antibody
 d. Anti-double stranded DNA antibody

153. Consider the following statements about poly-articular juvenile rheumatoid arthritis? *(UPSC 2015)*
 a. It is more common in girls
 b. Five or more joints are affected within the first six months of onset
 c. Uveitis occurs in 95% patients
 d. Rheumatoid factor may be negative
 Which of the statements given above are true?
 a. A and D only b. A, B and D
 c. B, C and D d. B and C only

154. The most common type of juvenile rheumatoid arthritis is:
 a. Rheumatoid factor positive polyarticular *(UPSC 2015)*
 b. Rheumatoid factor negative polyarticular
 c. Pauci-articular type
 d. Systemic onset type

155. Which part of the spine is most commonly affected in Rheumatoid arthritis? *(Bihar PG 2015)*
 a. Cervical b. Lumbar
 c. Thoracic d. Sacral

156. All are seen in Rheumatoid arthritis EXCEPT:
 a. Deformities *(Recent Pattern 2015-16)*
 b. Mononeuritis multiplex
 c. Periarticular osteoporosis
 d. Seronegative arthritis

157. In long standing rheumatoid arthritis which will be seen?
 (Recent Pattern 2015-16)
 a. Milk alkali syndrome b. Nephrolithiasis
 c. Paradoxical aciduria d. Secondary amyloidosis

158. Rheumatoid arthritis is seen with?
 (Recent Pattern 2015-16)
 a. HLA DR3 b. HLA DR4
 c. HLA DR 27 d. HLA B 27

159. Gold is used for management of? *(Recent Pattern 2015-16)*
 a. Ankylosing Spondylitis
 b. Rheumatoid Arthritis
 c. Psoriatic arthritis
 d. Rheumatic arthriitis

160. All are true about the condition except?

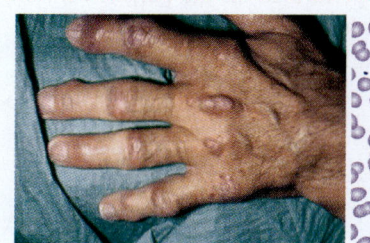 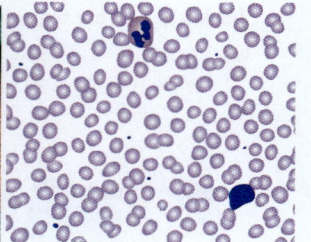

 a. Piano key movement of ulnar styloid
 b. Z line deformity
 c. Atlanto-axial deformity
 d. Tender nodules

161. Polyarticular onset JRA involves more than how many joints: *(Recent Pattern 2014-15)*
 a. 3 b. 4
 c. 5 d. 6

162. C V junction abnormalities are seen in all of the following except: *(Recent Pattern 2014-15)*
 a. Rheumatoid arthritis b. Ankylosing spondylitis
 c. Odontoid dysgenesis d. Basilar invagination

163. In rheumatoid arthritis the characteristic joint involvement is: *(Recent Pattern 2014-15)*
 a. Spine
 b. Knee
 c. Metacarpophalangeal joint
 d. Hip joint

164. The most common cardiac involvement in rheumatoid arthritis: *(Recent Pattern 2014-15)*
 a. Cardiomyopathy b. Pericarditis
 c. Myocarditis d. Endocarditis

165. Which of the following is the most specific test for rheumatoid arthritis? *(Recent Pattern 2014-15)*
 a. Anti- MCV antibody b. Anti cardiolipin antibody
 c. Anti Mi-2 antibody d. Anti Ro antibody

166. HLA-DR4 is a marker of: *(Recent Pattern 2014-15)*
 a. Rheumatoid arthritis
 b. Sarcoidosis
 c. Sero-negative gouty arthritis
 d. Psoriasis

167. Which type of anemia seen in Rheumatoid arthritis?
 a. Normocytic, normochromic *(Recent Pattern 2014-15)*
 b. Hyperchromic, Normocytic
 c. Hypochromic, normocytic
 d. Hypochromic, leucopenia

168. Clinical manifestation of Felty's syndrome are all except:
    a. Rheumatoid arthritis   (Recent Pattern 2014-15)
    b. Splenomegaly
    c. neutropenia
    d. Nephropathy

169. Rheumatoid arthritis commonly affects the:
    (Recent Pattern 2014-15)
    a. Cervical spine   b. Thoracolumbar spine
    c. Lumbar spine   d. Sacral spine

170. Caplan's syndrome is seen with ? (Recent Pattern 2014-15)
    a. COPD   b. Pneumoconiosis
    c. Pulmonary edema   d. Rheumatoid arthritis

171. A patient of rheumatoid arthritis develops sudden onset Quadriparesis increased muscle tone of limbs with exaggerated tendon jerks and worsening of gait. The investigation to be done? (Recent Pattern 2014-15)
    a. Flexion and extension Cervical area X-ray of neck
    b. MRI brain
    c. EMG and NCV
    d. Carotid angiography

172. Which is the most common site of subcutaneous nodules in rheumatoid arthritis? (Recent Pattern 2014-15)
    a. Elbow   b. Wrist
    c. Achilles tendon   d. Occiput

173. Not seen in rheumatoid arthritis is:
    (Recent Pattern 2014-15)
    a. Normal C.R.P   b. Juxtaarticular osteopenia
    c. Cervical myelopathy d. Hyperandrogenism

174. All may be true about Rheumatoid Arthritis except:
    a. Anti- MCV antibody (Recent Pattern 2014-15)
    b. RF positive
    c. Anti- CCP antibody
    d. Anti- Mi-2 antibody

175. All the following are true about Rheumatoid arthritis except: (AI 1994)
    a. Positive for Anti-IgG antibody
    b. Juxta-articular osteoporosis
    c. Morning stiffness
    d. C Reactive protein indicates better prognosis

176. A middle aged female presents with polyarthritis, elevated Rheumatoid factor and ANA levels. Which of the following features will help in differentiating Rheumatoid arthritis from SLE (AIIMS Nov 08)
    a. Soft tissue swelling in PIP Joint
    b. Juxta-articular osteoporosis on X-ray
    c. Articular erosions on X-ray
    d. Elevated ESR

177. True regarding Felty's syndrome is all, EXCEPT:
    (AIIMS Dec 97)
    a. Splenomegaly   b. Rheumatoid arthritis
    c. Neutropenia   d. Nephropathy

178. Which part of the spine is most commonly affected in Rheumatoid arthritis: (AI 1994) (AIIMS Feb 97)
    a. Cervical   b. Lumbar
    c. Thoracic   d. Sacral

179. Which of the following is the most specific test for Rheumatoid Arthritis (AIIMS Nov 06)
    a. Anti- ccp antibody b. Anti IgM antibody
    c. Anti IgA antibody   d. Anti IgG antibody

180. The following are rheumatoid disease modifying drugs except: (AI 1995)
    a. Chloroquine   b. Gold
    c. Penicillamine   d. BAL

181. Indication of systemic steroids in rheumatoid arthritis is:
    a. Mononeuritis multiplex (AI 1997)
    b. Carpul tunnel syndrome
    c. Presence of deformities
    d. Articular cartilage involvement

182. Hemophilia with Rheumatoid arthritis, analgesic of choice is: (PGI Dec 98)
    a. Ibuprofen   b. Asprin
    c. Acetaminophen   d. Phenylbutazone

183. Which of the following is not true about JRA? (AI 2009)
    a. Fever   b. Rheumatoid nodules
    c. Uveitis   d. Raynaud's phenomenon

Gout

184. This elderly male came with a history of recurrent attacks of pain and swelling in the great toe in the past. This is the present X-ray of the hands. The diagnosis can be confirmed by: (APPG 2015)

    a. Polarised microscopy of tissue fluid aspirate
    b. HLA B27
    c. Anti CCP antibodies
    d. X-ray of lumbosacral spine

185. Martel sign is seen in? (Recent Pattern 2015-16)
    a. Gout   b. Ankylosing spondylitis
    c. Osteoarthritis   d. Rheumatoid arthritis

186. Tophi in gout found in all regions except:
    (Recent Pattern 2014-15)
    a. Prepatellar bursae b. Muscle
    c. Helix of ear   d. Synovial membrane

187. Incorrect about diagnosis of a patient of Gouty arthritis?
    a. High synovial fluid protein (Recent Pattern 2014-15)
    b. High WBC count
    c. Urate crystal in synovial fluid
    d. Normal sugar in synovial fluid

188. All drugs used in treatment of acute gout except:
    (Recent Pattern 2014-15)
    a. Allopurinol   b. Aspirin
    c. Colchicine   d. Naproxen

189. The following statements are true regarding acute gout except: (Recent Pattern 2014-15)
    a. Acute gout is more common in males
    b. Serum uric acid is normal in acute gout
    c. First metatarsophalangeal joint is most commonly affected in acute gout
    d. Treatment with Allopurinol should be started immediately in the case of acute gout

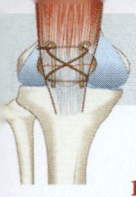

190. Prolonged allopurinol therapy in a patient with gout is NOT indicated for: *(Recent Pattern 2014-15)*
    a. Acute gouty arthritis
    b. Tophi
    c. Urate nephropathy
    d. Evidence of bone/joint damage

191. All of the following can be used to prevent gouty attack except: *(Recent Pattern 2014-15)*
    a. Allopurinol
    b. Aspirin
    c. Probenecid
    d. Sulfinpyrazone

192. Best treatment for gout with kidney impairment? *(Recent Pattern 2014-15)*
    a. Allopurinol
    b. Febuxostat
    c. Uricase
    d. Benzbromarone

193. All are true about pseudogout except?
    a. Calcium pyrophosphate crystals *(Recent Pattern 2014-15)*
    b. Most commonly idiopathic
    c. Hyperparathyroidism
    d. Most common joint involved is DIP

194. All joints are involved in acute gout except: *(Recent Pattern 2014-15)*
    a. MTP
    b. Glenohumeral joint
    c. Ankle joint
    d. Knee joint

195. Negatively Birefringent crystals in urine is seen with: *(Recent Pattern 2014-15)*
    a. Phosphaturia
    b. Uricosuria
    c. Cystinuria
    d. Struvite stones

Osteoarthritis and Psoriatic Arthritis

196. Glucosamine is prescribed in which of the following disease? *(AIIMS Nov 2017)*
    a. Arthritis
    b. Glaucoma
    c. Asthma
    d. Diabetes

197. An 85 years old woman presented with bilateral osteoarthritis of the knees she had no history of previous gastrointestinal disease. Which of the following is the most appropriate initial treatment for her? *(JIPMER Nov 2014)*
    a. Paracetamol
    b. Naproxen
    c. Celecoxib
    d. Dihydrocodeine

198. A 40-year-old patient presents with arthritis of PIP and DIP along with carpometacarpal joint of thumb and sparing of wrist and metacarpophalangeal joint, the most likely cause is: *(Recent Pattern 2014-15)*
    a. Psoriatic arthritis
    b. Osteoarthritis
    c. Rheumatoid arthritis
    d. Pseudogout

199. Least common site involved in osteoarthritis is?
    a. Hip joint *(Recent Pattern 2014-15)*
    b. Knee joint
    c. Carpometacarpal joint of thumb
    d. Distal carpophalangeal joint

200. All are radiological findings of OA except:
    a. Decreased Joint space *(Recent Pattern 2014-15)*
    b. Osteophytes formation
    c. Subchondral sclerosis
    d. Deposit of Calcium salts

201. Heberden nodes are seen in: *(Recent Pattern 2014-15)*
    a. Rheumatoid arthritis
    b. Rheumatic arthritis
    c. Osteoarthritis
    d. SLE

202. Which of the following is true of psoriatic arthritis? *(Recent Pattern 2014-15)*
    a. Involves distal joints of hand and foot
    b. Pencil in cup deformity
    c. Sacroilitis
    d. All of the above

Behçet's Disease Dermatomyositis and Polymyositis

203. In the revised guidelines for Behçet's disease, which criteria carries 2 points? *(JIPMER May 2018)*
    a. Ocular lesions
    b. Pathergy phenomenon
    c. Vasculitis
    d. Skin lesions

204. Among patients with polymyositis, which one of the following auto-antibodies is associated with an increased risk of interstitial lung disease?
    a. Anti-CCP antibody *(AP PG 2016)*
    b. Anti ds DNA antibody
    c. Anti cardiolipin antibody
    d. Anti-Jo-1 antibody

205. 9-year-old girl presents with 1 month difficulty in combing hair. She later developed maculopapular rash over metacarpophalangeal joints. Gower sign is positive. What is the next logical step? *(AIIMS Nov 2015)*
    a. Nerve conduction Study
    b. Rheumatoid Factor
    c. Creatinine Kinase levels
    d. NM junction study

206. The following features are suggestive of Behçet's syndrome except? *(UPSC 2015)*
    a. Orogenital ulcers
    b. Polyarthritis
    c. Uveitis
    d. Livedo reticularis

207. Primary idiopathic Polymyositis does not involve? *(Bihar PG 2015)*
    a. Pelvic girdle muscle
    b. Neck muscle
    c. Ocular muscle
    d. Pharyngeal muscle

208. In which of the causes of oral ulcer, Auto-antibodies are not seen? *(Recent Pattern 2015-16)*
    a. Behçet disease
    b. SLE
    c. Pemphigus
    d. Celiac disease

209. Incorrect about Behçet's syndrome is: *(Recent Pattern 2014-15)*
    a. There is a strong association with HLA-B7
    b. The skin may be hyperactive to minor injury such as venipuncture
    c. Inflammatory reaction around large blood vessels
    d. Cortiocosteroid therapy is of definite value

210. Keratoderma -Blenorrhagicum is pathognomonic of: *(Recent Pattern 2014-15)*
    a. Behçet's disease
    b. Reiter's disease
    c. Lyme's disease
    d. Glucagonoma

211. Recurrent oro-genital ulceration with arthritis is seen in: *(Recent Pattern 2014-15)*
    a. Behçet's syndrome
    b. Gonorrhoea
    c. Reiter's syndrome
    d. Syphilis

212. Not Seen in Bechet's syndrome is: *(Recent Pattern 2014-15)*
    a. Pyoderma gangrenosum
    b. Thrombophlebitis
    c. Glans penis Apthous ulceration
    d. Panuveitis
213. Lilac coloured (heliotrope) pigmentation over the face is characteristic of: *(Recent Pattern 2014-15)*
    a. Dermatomyositis
    b. Polymyositis
    c. Systemic lupus erythematosus
    d. Systemic sclerosis
214. All the following are features of Behçet's syndrome *except*: *(AI 1994)*
    a. Recurrent aphthous stomatitis
    b. Multi-system involvement
    c. Seen only in the tropics
    d. Common in youngsters
215. Recurrent Bilateral Hypopyon formation associated with thrombophlebitis is most consistent with which of the following: *(AI 2009)*
    a. HLA B 27 associated uveitis
    b. Behçet's syndrome
    c. Syphilis
    d. Herpes Zoster

Sicca/Sjogren Syndrome

216. Which of the following is wrong about Sjogren syndrome? *(AIIMS Nov 2016)*
    a. Saliva has increased concentration of IgA
    b. Saliva has increased concentration of sodium
    c. Saliva has increased concentration of phosphate
    d. Maximum amount of saliva secretion is <1.5ml in 15 min
217. Drug for management of Xerostomia? *(JIPMER Nov 2015)*
    a. Cevimeline
    b. 3, 4 aminopyridine
    c. Neostigmine
    d. Physostigimine
218. All are true about rheumatoid factor except:
    a. Also found in Sjogren Syndrome *(PGI May 2015)*
    b. May also present normally
    c. It is basically IgM
    d. Its presence is diagnostic of rheumatoid arthritis
219. Most common lymphoma associated with Sicca syndrome is: *(Recent Pattern 2014-15)*
    a. MALToma
    b. Burkitt lymphoma
    c. DLBCL
    d. Lymphoplasmacytic lymphoma
220. Sicca syndrome is associated with all except: *(Recent Pattern 2014-15)*
    a. Rheumatoid arthritis   b. Midline granuloma
    c. Sarcoidosis   d. Chronic active hepatitis
221. All of the following may be associated with Sjogren syndrome, *except* : *(AIIMS Dec 95)*
    a. Dry eyes
    b. Dry mouth
    c. Parotid gland enlargement
    d. Systemic manifestations

222. Sicca syndrome is associated with all, Except : *(AIIMS Feb 97)*
    a. Midline granuloma
    b. Chronic active hepatitis
    c. Rheumatoid arthritis
    d. Scleroderma

Kawasaki Disease

223. Kawasaki disease is associated with all of the following features *except*: *(AI 1996)*
    a. Erythema
    b. Posterior cervical Lymphadenopathy
    c. Thrombocytopenia
    d. Conjunctivitis
224. The treatment of choice for Kawasaki disease is: *(AIIMS May 2005)*
    a. Cyclosporine
    b. Prednisolone
    c. Immunoglobulins
    d. Methotrexate

Miscellaneous

225. Abnormalities in elastin protein can lead to all except? *(AIIMS May 2018)*
    a. Fractures
    b. Cutis Laxa
    c. Joint laxity
    d. Subluxation of lens
226. Patients with porphyria are highly sensitive to which wavelength? *(JIPMER May 2018)*
    a. 290-320 nm   b. 400-420 nm
    c. 320-400 nm   d. 250-290 nm
227. A 6-year-old child with abdominal pain and a rash is shown. Comment on the diagnosis? *(Recent Pattern Jan 2019)*

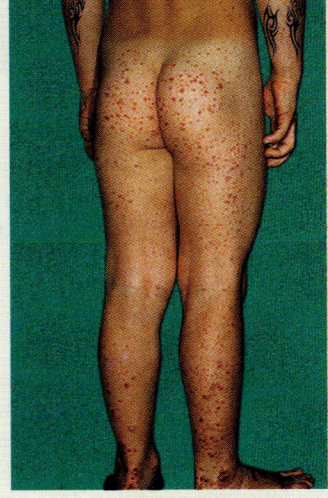

    a. Kawasaki
    b. Henoch Schonlein purpura
    c. Varicella
    d. Meningococcemia

228. A 75-year-female has chronic backache. X-ray spine is shown. What is the most likely diagnosis?
 (Recent Pattern Jan 2019)

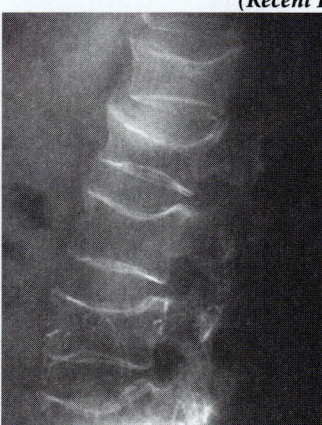

 a. Pott's spine b. Osteoporosis
 c. Spondylolisthesis d. Spondylodiscitis

229. A 7-year-old child is brought with fever, colicky abdominal pain and non-blanching palpable purpuric rash on buttocks and back of legs. What is the probable diagnosis?
 (Recent Question 2016-17)
 a. I.T.P b. H.S.P
 c. Meningococcemia d. Wegener's granulomatosis

230. Which one of the following statements is TRUE regarding the disease depicted in the pictures here (before & after treatment). *(AP PG 2016)*

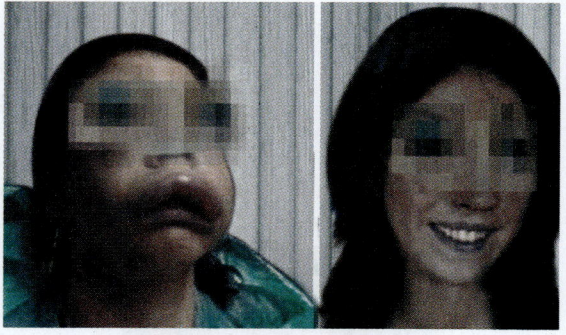

 a. All these statements are True
 b. Seen with ACEI but never seen with ARB
 c. Hereditary form is related to bradykinin deficiency
 d. Mostly due to degranulation of mast cells

231. What is not seen in Reiters syndrome? *(Bihar PG 2015)*
 a. Subcutaneous nodules
 b. Keratoderma blennorhagicum
 c. Circinate balanitis
 d. Oral ulcers

232. Which of the following is not an autoimmune disease?
 (AIIMS May 2015)
 a. SLE b. Graves disease
 c. Ulcerative Colitis d. Rheumatoid Arthritis

233. Which of the following condition does not cause multiple painful ulcers on tongue? *(Recent Pattern 2015-16)*
 a. TB b. Sarcoidosis
 c. Herpes
 d. Behçet disease

234. The child shown below has short stature with normal IQ. His siblings also exhibit similar findings. What is the probable diagnosis?

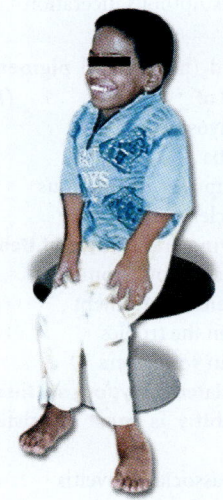

 a. Mucopolysaccharidosis
 b. Lysosomal storage disorder
 c. Gaucher's disease
 d. Nutritional rickets

235. DOC for *acute attack* of Hereditary angioneurotic edema?
 (Recent Pattern 2015-16)
 a. Danazol b. C1 inhibitor concentrate
 c. Icatibant d. methylprednisolone

236. Type 5 Hypersensitivity mimics? *(Recent Pattern 2015-16)*
 a. Type 1 b. Type 2
 c. Type 3 d. Type 4

237. MCTD includes all except? *(Recent Pattern 2015-16)*
 a. SLE b. Polymyositis
 c. Rheumatoid arthritis d. Inclusion body myositis

238. Which of the following disorders is least likely associated with progression to lymphoma? *(Recent Pattern 2014-15)*
 a. Sjogren's syndrome
 b. Ataxia telangiectasia
 c. Severe combined immunodeficiency
 d. Lynch II syndrome

239. Bilateral Painless parotid enlargement is seen in all except:
 (Recent Pattern 2014-15)
 a. Mumps b. Alcoholics
 c. Sarcoidosis d. Diabetes mellitus

240. A woman complaints of dyspnea at rest. Chest radiography reveals bihilar adenopathy with clear lung fields. All of the following investigations will be useful in differential diagnosis except: *(Recent Pattern 2014-15)*
 a. CD4/CD8 > 3.5 in B.A.L b. Serum ACE levels
 c. CECT of chest d. Gallium scan

241. A patient of chronic Left lung abscess with generalized edema, hypoproteinemia, hepato-splenomegaly without renal failure but reduced urine output. Diagnosis is?
 a. Amyloidosis *(Recent Pattern 2014-15)*
 b. Chronic cor-pulmonale with Rt. Heart failure
 c. Bronchiectasis
 d. Bronchogenic carcinoma

242. Neuropathic joint is seen in all except:
 (Recent Pattern 2014-15)
    a. Diabetes mellitus   b. Tabes dorsalis
    c. Syringomyelia   d. Frederich's ataxia
243. Following is characteristic neurologic finding in primary amyloidosis: (Recent Pattern 2014-15)
    a. Peripheral motor and sensory neuropathy
    b. Peripheral neuropathy associated with cerebral manifestation
    c. Guillain –Barre type of syndrome
    d. Spinal cord compression in thoracic region
244. Reactive arthritis is usually caused by:
 (Recent Pattern 2014-15)
    a. Shigella flexneri   b. Shigella boydii
    c. Shigella shiga   d. Shigella dysentriae
245. About fibromyalgia all are true except?
 (Recent Pattern 2014-15)
    a. Associated with EEG abnormalities
    b. More common in males than females
    c. Associated with low free cortisol levels
    d. Associated with decreased blood flow to brain
246. Photosensitivity is a feature of porphyria. All the following enzyme deficiencies have photo-sensitivity except?
    a. HMB synthase deficiency (Recent Pattern 2014-15)
    b. Uroporphyrinogen decarboxylase deficiency
    c. Protoporphyrinogen oxidase deficiency
    d. Coproporphyrinogen oxidase deficiency
247. Intravenous immunoglobulin is given in all except?
    a. Kawasaki disease (Recent Pattern 2014-15)
    b. Acute ITP
    c. Wegener's Granulomatosis
    d. Myasthenic Crisis
248. A young man develops tiny linear wheals on exposure to sun and exercise since 6 years. Most likely diagnosis is:
    a. Cholingeric urticaria (Recent Pattern 2014-15)
    b. Dermatographism
    c. Idiopathic chronic urticaria
    d. Pressure urticaria
249. Which of the following diabetes is associated with HLA?
    a. Type I (Recent Pattern 2014-15)
    b. Type II
    c. Fibro-calcific Diabetes mellitus
    d. MODY
250. The most common primary immunodeficiency is:
 (Recent Pattern 2014-15)
    a. Common variable immunodeficiency
    b. Isolated IgA immunodeficiency
    c. Wiskott-Aldrich syndrome
    d. AIDS
251. Which of the following regarding rheumatic nodules is false? (Recent Pattern 2014-15)
    a. Found over extensor surface
    b. Tender on palpation
    c. Associated with carditis
    d. Pea size nodules
252. Earliest valvular lesion in acute rheumatic fever:
 (Recent Pattern 2014-15)
    a. Mitral stenosis   b. Mitral insufficiency
    c. Aortic stenosis   d. Aortic regurgitation

253. The most characteristic murmur of rheumatic carditis is:
 (Recent Pattern 2014-15)
    a. Apical high-pitched early diastolic murmur
    b. Apical high-pitched holosystolic murmur
    c. Apical low-pitched mid-diastolic murmur
    d. Systolic ejection murmur along the left stenal border
254. In acute intermittent Porphyria, the metabolite which is elevated is: (Recent Pattern 2014-15)
    a. Uroblinogen   b. Porphoblinogen
    c. Coroporphyrin   d. Protoporphyrin
255. Onion skin spleen is seen in: (Recent Pattern 2014-15)
    a. ITP   b. Thalassemia
    c. SLE   d. Scleroderma
256. Consider the following clinicopathological changes in the Rheumatic Carditis: (Recent Pattern 2014-15)
    i. Mitral regurgitation   ii. Aortic regurgitation
    iii. ASLO rise   iv. Left atrial enlargement
    The correct chronological sequence of these events is
    a. iii, i, iv, ii   b. i, ii, iii, iv
    c. iv, ii, i, iii   d. iii, iv, i, ii
257. Lardaceous spleen is seen in: (Recent Pattern 2014-15)
    a. Alcoholic hepatitis   b. Chronic active hepatitis
    c. Focal amyloidosis   d. Diffuse amyloidosis
258. The defective platelet function is seen in all except:
    a. SLE (Recent Pattern 2014-15)
    b. Acute lymphoctic leukemia
    c. Myelofibrosis
    d. Henoch-Schölein purpura
259. Not associated with thymoma? (Recent Pattern 2014-15)
    a. Red cell aplasia
    b. Myasthenia gravis
    c. Hypergammaglobulinemia
    d. Compression of the mediastinum
260. Tietze's syndrome usually develops at .... costal cartilage: (Recent Pattern 2014-15)
    a. First and Second ribs   b. Second to fifth ribs
    c. Sixth to Eighth   d. All seven ribs
261. True in amyloidosis is all except: (Recent Pattern 2014-15)
    a. Multiple myeloma –AL type
    b. Secondary amyloidosis –AA type
    c. Renal amyloidosis is commonly present with hypertension
    d. Mild proteinuria
262. A patient suffering from lung abscess develops anasarca. The probable reason is: (Recent Pattern 2014-15)
    a. Cor-pulmonale   b. Good Pasture syndrome
    c. Pyelonephritis   d. Acute renal failure
263. The presence of small sized platelets on the peripheral smear is characteristic of: (Recent Pattern 2014-15)
    a. Idiopathic thrombocytopenic purpura
    b. Bernard Soulier syndrome
    c. Disseminated intravascular cogaulation
    d. Wiskott Aldrich syndrome
264. Features of rheumatic carditis are all except?
    a. Aschoff nodule (Recent Pattern 2014-15)
    b. Commisural involvement
    c. PR segment depression
    d. Fourth heart sound heard

265. **Ataxia telangiectasia is characterized by all of the following except?** *(Recent Pattern 2014-15)*
    a. Autosomal dominant inheritance
    b. Oculocutaneous telangiectasia
    c. Cerebellar ataxia
    d. Thymic hypoplasia

266. **The organism causing osteomyelitis in sickle cell anemia:** *(Recent Pattern 2014-15)*
    a. Salmonella   b. Staphylococcus
    c. H. influenzae   d. E. coli

267. **Good's syndrome is:** *(Recent Pattern 2014-15)*
    a. Thymic hyperplasia with myasthenia gravis
    b. Thymic hypoplasia
    c. Thymoma with hypogammaglobulinemia
    d. Thymoma with anti-basement membrane antibodies

268. **Recurrent giardiasis is a feature of:** *(Recent Pattern 2014-15)*
    a. C3 deficiency
    b. C1 inhibitor deficiency
    c. Di Georges syndrome
    d. Common variable immunodeficiency

269. **The most reliable investigation in amyloid disease is:**
    a. Rectal biopsy   *(Recent Pattern 2014-15)*
    b. Immunoglobulin assay
    c. Ultrasound
    d. Abdominal fat pad biopsy

270. **Best drug for bradykinin mediated Angioedema:** *(Recent Pattern 2014-15)*
    a. Icatibant   b. Levocetrizine
    c. Avil   d. Hydrocortisone

271. **HLA DRw 52 is associated with:** *(Recent Pattern 2014-15)*
    a. SLE   b. Scleroderma
    c. Sjogren   d. Behçet

272. **Amyloidosis occurs in all except:** *(Recent Pattern 2014-15)*
    a. Tuberculosis   b. Chronic bronchitis
    c. Lung abscess   d. Bronchiectasis

273. **Which of the following can be used for confirmation of anaphyalxis:** *(Recent Pattern 2014-15)*
    a. IgE levels   b. Basophil count
    c. Eosinophil count d. Serum tryptase

274. **Steroids are given in rheumatic fever when there is:**
    a. Carditis   *(Recent Pattern 2014-15)*
    b. Subcutaneous nodules
    c. Chorea
    d. All of the above

275. **Sclerema neonatarum affects all except:**
    a. Palms and soles *(Recent Pattern 2014-15)*
    b. Skin over thigh
    c. Skin over chest
    d. Skin over face

276. **A Carey-Coomb's murmur heard in a child with multiple joint pains is suggestive of:** *(Recent Pattern 2014-15)*
    a. Infective endocarditis   b. Rheumatoid arthritis
    c. Rheumatic fever   d. Libman-Sacs endocarditis

277. **Intra-cardiac calcifications indicate:** *(Recent Pattern 2014-15)*
    a. SBE   b. Rheumatic valves
    c. Old MI   d. Chronic pericarditis

278. **Partoid gland enlargement is seen in all except:** *(Recent Pattern 2014-15)*
    a. Sjogren's syndrome   b. Sarcoidosis
    c. Chronic pancreatitis d. SLE

279. **All of the following are seen in inflammatory polyarthritis, except** *(AIIMS May 94)*
    a. New bone formation
    b. Erythema
    c. Increased ESR
    d. Morning stiffness more than one hour

280. **Which of the organism most commonly causes reactive arthritis?** *(AIIMS Nov 08)*
    a. Ureaplasma urealyticum
    b. Group A beta hemolytic streptococci
    c. Borrelia burgdorferi
    d. Chlamydia

281. **A patient presents with Arthritis, hyperpigmentation of skin and hypogonadism, likely diagnosis is-** *(AI 2001)*
    a. Hemochromatosis
    b. Ectopic ACTH secreting tumour of the lung
    c. Wilson's disease
    d. Rheumatoid arthritis

282. **All of the following statements about hereditary hemochromatosis are true Except** *(AI 2008)*
    a. Arthropathy involving small joints of hands may be seen
    b. Skin pigmentation is a frequent presentation
    c. Desferroxamine is the treatment of choice
    d. Hypogonadism may be seen

283. **All are seen in hemochromatosis except-** *(AI 2008)*
    a. Hypogonadism
    b. Arthropathy
    c. Bronze diabetes
    d. Desferrioxamine is the treatment of choice

Answers with Explanations

SLE

1. Ans. (a) SLE

(Ref: Harrison 20th edition, p 2518)

- ANA> reference value is the first immunological manifestation mentioned in SLICC criteria for diagnosis of SLE. It is not a criterion for diagnosis of the remaining rheumatological diseases mentioned in choices b,c and d.
- This test is positive in 95% cases at the onset of disease and the remaining patients turn positive within one year of disease onset.
- ANA testing using immuno-fluorescent antibodies is more reliable than ELISA.

2. Ans. (a) SLE

(Ref: Harrison 20th edition, p 2518-2519)

- The image shows an erythematous rash sparing the nasolabial folds which coupled with clinical history points to diagnosis of SLE.
- Choice B leads to heliotrope rash involving the upper eye lid and proximal muscle weakness.
- Choice C presents as grey-brown patches, usually on the face on their cheeks, bridge of their nose, forehead, chin, and above their upper lip. It also can appear on sun-exposed parts of body, such as the forearms and neck.
- Choice D presents as redness can slowly spread beyond the nose and cheeks to the forehead and chin. There will be flushing, visible blood vessels and acne like breakouts.

3. Ans. (d) A.N.C.A

(Ref: Harrison 20th edition, p 2575; Harrison 19th edition, p 2179)

- Clinical abnormalities like palpable purpura, pulmonary infiltrates, microscopic hematuria, mononeuritis multiplex and glomerulonephritis that present in combination should suggest a diagnosis of vasculitis.
- Hence in the work up of these patients ANCA should be done.
- ANCA are antibodies directed against proteins in cytoplasmic granules of neutrophils and monocytes. They are seen in patients with:

1. Granulomatosis with angitis
2. Microscopic angitis
3. Churg strauss syndrome

Definitive diagnosis is made when biopsy report of afflicted organs is done.
When syndromes like PAN, Takayasu arteritis or CNS vasculitis are suspected then arteriogram of organs with suspected involvement should be performed.

4. Ans. (b) Chikungunya

(Ref: Harrison 20th edition, p 1498; Harrison 19th edition, p 381 and 1313)

	Post chikungunya Pigmentation	Fixed Drug eruption
Appearance	Macule, freckle like lesions with Addisonian type of palmar pigmentation.	Dull red to brown demarcated lesions with central bulla
Sensory complaints	Hyperpigmentation minus any sensory complaints	Hyperpigmentation with burning sensation
Sites	*Nose and cheeks* Develops after rash has subsided	Lips, hands, genitilia and oral mucosa

Points in favour of PCP:
1. History of high grade fever 2-4 weeks before onset
2. Acute onset of hypermelanosis
3. Persistent asthenia and joint pain even after defervescence of fever.

5. Ans. (a) Arthritis

(Ref: Harrison 20th edition, p 2518; Harrison 19th edition, p 2127)

According to the SLICC criteria, main lesion in SLE is synovitis and not arthritis.

Clinical manifestations in SLE
1. Skin- acute/subacute cutaneous LE
2. Oral ulcers
3. Alopecia
4. Synovitis
5. Renal lesions- proteinuria, RBC casts, biopsy proven
6. Neurological manifestations- seizures, psychosis, mono-neuritis, myelitis, peripheral neuropathy, cranial nerve involvement, confusional state
7. Haemolytic anemia
8. Leukopenia/ lymphopenia
9. Thrombocytopenia

Immunological manifestations
1. ANA> reference negative value
2. Anti-Sm
3. Anti-dsDNA
4. Antiphospholipid antibody
5. Low serum complement
6. Positive direct coombs test

Must have a total or 4 features with >1 clinical feature and 1 immunologic feature
or
Biopsy-proven LN with anti-dsDNA antibodies or ANA

6. Ans. (c) Ulcerative Colitis

(Ref: Robbins 9th edition, p 215-220)

DISEASES MEDIATED BY ANTIBODIES AND IMMUNE COMPLEXES
1. Autoimmune hemolytic anemia
2. Autoimmune thrombocytopenia
3. Myasthenia gravis
4. Grave's disease
5. Goodpasture syndrome
6. Systemic lupus erythematosus (SLE)

DISEAES MEDIATED BY T CELLS
1. Type 1 diabetes mellitus
2. Multiple sclerosis
3. Rheumatoid arthritis
4. Systemic sclerosis
5. Sjogren syndrome

DISEASES CAUSED BY AUTOIMMUNITY OR BY REACTIONS TO MICROBIAL ANTIGENS
1. *Inflammatory bowel disease (Crohn disease, ulcerative colitis)*
2. Inflammatory myopathies

7. Ans. (a) Increased anti Ro and La implies low risk for congenital heart block

(Ref: Harrison 20th edition, p 2517; Harrison 19th edition, p 2133)

Increased anti Ro and La implies low risk for congenital heart block	Wrong	Anti Ro antibody can be transmitted trans-placentally and can lead to complete heart block leading to neonatal lupus. The child will need a pacemaker for survival.
Steroids can be continued in pregnancy	Correct	Steroids can be given in pregnancy as they fall in category A with no evidence of teratogenicity. But a placental enzyme 11 dehydrogenase deactivates glucocorticoids.
Recurrent abortions	Correct	Presence of anti-cardiolipin antibody and anti beta2 glycoprotein antibody can lead to uterine artery or venous thrombosis leading to recurrent abortions.
Diseases worsens during pregnancy	Correct	All autoimmune diseases will worsen in pregnancy except rheumatoid arthritis.

8. Ans. (d) Mixed connective tissue disorder

(Ref: Harrison 20th edition, p 2560; Harrison 19th edition, p 2165)

- Anti-Rho or SS-A antibodies are seen in SLE, Sjogren syndrome and can be transmitted across the placenta resulting in neonatal lupus which presents as complete heart block.
- Mixed connective tissue disorder is associated with U_1 R.N.P. (Ribo-Nucleo-protein antibody).

9. Ans. (a) SLE

(Ref: Harrison 20th edition, p 2518; Harrison 19th edition, p 2126-27)

The diagnosis is based on joint pain in fever with rash and photosensitivity. Rheumatoid arthritis involves the small joints symmetrically and does not have presence of Rash.

The diagnostic criteria for SLE are as follows:

- Rash Fixed erythema, over the Malar Eminences
- Erythematous circular raised patches with adherent keratotic scaling and follicular plugging; atrophic scarring may occur
- Photosensitivity Exposure to UV light causes rash
- Oral ulcers Includes oral and nasopharyngeal ulcers
- Synovitis/Non-erosive arthritis of two or more peripheral joints
- Serositis: Pleuritis or pericarditis documented by ECG or rub or evidence of effusion
- Renal disorder Proteinuria >0.5 g/d or 3+, or cellular casts
- Neurologic disorder Seizures or psychosis without other causes
- Hematologic disorder Hemolytic anemia or leukopenia
- Immunological criteria like positive CRP, low C3, ELISA cardiolipin antibody
- ANA positivity

10. Ans. (b) SLE

(Ref: Harrison 19th edition, p 2124)

High ESR with normal CRP
1. SLE
2. Giant cell arteritis
3. Multiple myeloma
4. Leukemia
5. Ulcerative colitis

• RA	• Both CRP and ESR can be normal
• Scleroderma	• ESR normal; CRP elevated
• *SLE*	• *Normal CRP with elevated ESR*
• Polymyalgia Rheumatica	• ESR Elevated; CRP Elevated

11. Ans. (c) Anti-Ro/SS-A

(Ref: Harrison 20th edition, p 2517; Harrison 19th edition, p 375)

The question asked is not for SLE (systemic lupus erythematosus) but subacute cutaneous lupus erythematosus. Most patients with subacute cutaneous lupus erythematosus (SCLE) manifest a positive antinuclear antibody (ANA) and Anti-Ro (SS-A) autoantibodies.

Anti Ro antibody are seen in
1. Annular SCLE
2. Papulosquamous SCLE
3. SCLE with vasculitis, Sjögren syndrome, or C2d deficiency
4. Mothers of infants with neonatal lupus erythematosus (NLE)
5. Drug-induced SCLE

12. Ans. (a) Verrucous endocarditis

(Ref: Harrison 20th edition, p 2520; Harrison's 18th edition, ch.319)

- Libman-Sacks endocarditis (otherwise known as verrucous, marantic, or nonbacterial thrombotic endocarditis) is the most characteristic cardiac manifestation of the autoimmune disease systemic lupus erythematosus.
- The most common valve affected is mitral and then aortic, though all are involved.

13. Ans. (c) Pemphigus vulgaris

(Ref: CMDT 2019, page 854)

- The clinical features of localized scleroderma are three morphologic variants: morphea, genera-lized morphea, and linear scleroderma. The latter has been reported to have a higher frequency of antinuclear antibodies and has been associated with antibodies to single-stranded DNA (ssDNA).
- The frequency of positivity on ANA screening test (on Hep-2 cells) is as follows:

Mixed connective tissue disease : 100%
Drug-induced lupus erythematosus: 100%
Systemic lupus erythematosus : 95%-100%
Sjögren syndrome : 80%
Scleroderma : 60%-95%
Polymyositis-dermatomyositis : 49%-74%
Rheumatoid arthritis : 40%-60%
Normal : Less than 4%

14. Ans. (a) Anti ds-DNA antibody

(Ref: Harrison 20th edition, p 2517)

- Anti ds-DNA antibody is associated with increased risk of nephritis in cases of SLE.
- Anti centromere ab is associated with limited scleroderma.
- Antibodies to Ribosomal-Pantigen is associated with CNS lupus.
- Antibodies to tRNA synthetase are associated with, polymyositis with interstitial lung disease.

15. Ans. (d) Assay for thyroid Hormones

(Ref: Harrison 20th edition, p 2700; Harrison's 18th edition, ch. 319)

- Fatigue and serous cavity effusions is a feature of myxedema heart. Myxedema would lead to carpal tunnel syndrome and is also associated with macrocytic anemia.
- In SLE the anemia is autoimmune hemolytic anemia and this is a normocytic normochromic anemia while in the question the anemia mentioned is macrocytic anemia
- Carpal tunnel syndrome is not mentioned in features of SLE.
- The classic presentation of a triad of fever, joint pain, and rash in a woman of childbearing age should prompt investigation into the diagnosis of SLE.

16. Ans. (b) Nasolabial folds

(Ref: Harrison 20th edition, p 2519; Harrison 19th edition, p 2127)

17. Ans. (a) Anti-ribosomal P antibody

(Ref: Harrison 20th edition, p 2517; Harrison 19th edition, p 2126)

Anti- Ribosomal P antibody	CNS lupus
Anti – Glutamic acid decarboxylase antibody	Latent autoimmune diabetes
Anti- Endomyosial antibody	Celiac sprue
Anti-Histone antibody	Drug induced lupus

18. Ans. (d) Nephritis

(Ref: Harrison 20th edition, p 838; Harrison 19th edition, p 2254)

Lupus anticoagulant is an immunoglobulin due to phospholipids and proteins associated with the cell membrane. Lupus anticoagulant is a misnomer, as it is actually a pro-thrombotic agent. That is, Lupus anticoagulant antibodies in living systems cause an increase in inappropriate blood clotting. This leads to uterine venous and arterial thrombosis leading to recurrent abortions.

19. Ans. (b) Pericarditis

(Ref: Harrison 20th edition, p 2520)

- Pericarditis is the most common cardiac abnormality in systemic lupus erythematosus (SLE) patients, but lesions of the valves, myocardium and coronary vessels may all occur.
- In the past, cardiac manifestations were severe and life threatening, often leading to death. Echocardiography is a sensitive and specific technique in detecting cardiac abnormalities, particularly mild pericarditis, valvular lesions and myocardial dysfunction.
- Therefore, echocardiography should be performed periodically in SLE patients. Vascular occlusion, including coronary arteries, may develop due to vasculitis, premature athero-sclerosis or anti-phospholipid antibodies associated with SLE. Premature atherosclerosis is the most frequent cause of coronary artery disease (CAD) in SLE patients.

20. Ans. (a) Lupus nephritis

(Ref: OP ghai 7th edition, p 603)

21. Ans. (c) Presents with fever, fatigue and hematological abnormalities

(Ref: Nelson 20th editon, page 1177)

- Pediatric lupus contributes to 20% of all case load of SLE. Children present with more acute illness and have more frequent hematologic and central nervous system involvement at the time of diagnosis compared to adults with SLE.

- Almost all children require corticosteroids during the course of their disease, and many are treated with immunosuppressive drugs. Mortality rates remain higher with pediatric SLE compared to adult onset SLE.
- When directly comparing pediatric SLE to adult SLE the inflammatory rashes, including the typical malar erythema, are significantly more frequent in children than adults. Isolated discoid lupus erythematosus (DLE) is uncommon in childhood. *Since choice 'a' mentions the word skin pigmentation and not skin rash it has been ruled out.*
- **Gender issues with SLE**
  1. During the first decade of life to 4:1
  2. During the second decade to 9:1
  3. Decreases to 5:1 in SLE commencing after the age of 50 year

22. Ans. (b) Polyhydramnios

(Ref: Harrison 20th edition, p 2526)

- Anti-phospholipid antibodies are often but not always associated with adverse obstetric outcomes, including first trimester miscarriage, mid-trimester and later fetal loss, intrauterine death and stillbirth. However, the risk of pregnancy loss is greatest during the mid-trimester.
- Diagnostic criteria for APLS include:
  1. Unexplained deaths of a morphologically normal fetus (documented by ultrasound or direct examination of the fetus) at or beyond the 10th week of gestation
  2. Three or more unexplained consecutive spontaneous abortions before the 10th week of gestation, with maternal anatomic or hormonal abnormalities and paternal and maternal chromosomal causes excluded
  3. At least 1 premature birth of a morpho-logically normal neonate before the 34th week of gestation due to eclampsia or severe pre-eclampsia according to standard definitions, or recognized features of placental insufficiency.

23. Ans. (a) Arthralgia

(Ref: Harrison 20th edition, p 2520; Harrison 19th edition, p 2129)

- Most common presentation of SLE is arthralgia/ myalgia in 90% patients. Non-erosive polyarthritis is seen in 60% of patients.
- Most common hematological presentation of SLE is anaemia.
- Most common neurological presentation of SLE is cognitive disorder.
- Most common cardio-pulmonary presentation of SLE is pleurisy and not Libman Sacks Endocarditis.

24. Ans. (c) Endocarditis

(Ref: Harrison 20th edition, p 2531; Harrison 19th edition, p 2128)

- The pericardial friction rub of pericarditis resolves with steroids.
- Lupus cerebritis and lupus nephritis responds to steroids.
- No specific therapy is indicated for Libman-Sacks endocarditis. Valve surgery may be required for hemodynamically significant valvular dysfunction. Mechanical prostheses are usually implanted Manage heart failure due to valvular dysfunction according to usual guidelines. Medications may include vasodilators, beta blockers, diuretics, and digoxin

25. Ans. (a) Female male ratio = 9:1

(Ref: Harrison 20th edition, p 2525; Harrison 19th edition, p 2126)

Cerebritis, nephritis and episcleritis are rare features of drug induced LE while skin manifestations are more common. The age is about 50-70 years and features can occur up to 2 years of exposure to the drug.

Comparison of SLE and Drug Induced Lupus Erythematous

Findings	SLE	Drug induced lupus erythematosus
Clinical	Average age of onset is 20-30 y Female-to-male ratio of 9:1	Average age of onset is 50-70 y Female-to-male ratio of 1:1
Laboratory	• Antihistone antibodies in 50% • Anti-dsDNA present in 80% • C3/C4 levels decrease • Cutaneous findings in >75% • Raynaud phenomenon in 50% • Antinuclear antibodies in >95%	• Antihistone antibodies in >95% • Anti-ssDNA present • Anti-dsDNA rare • C3/C4 levels normal • Cutaneous findings in ~25% • Raynaud phenomenon in 25% • Antinuclear antibodies in >95%

26. Ans. (c) Libman Sacks Endocarditis

(Ref: Harrison 20th edition, p 2531; Harrison 19th edition, p 2129)

No specific therapy is indicated for Libman-Sacks endocarditis. Manage heart failure due to valvular dysfunction according to usual guidelines. Medications may include vasodilators, beta blockers, diuretics, and digoxin

27. Ans. (b) Antibodies against aquaporin 4 antibody

(Ref: Harrison 20th edition, p 3177; Harrison 19th edition, p 2128)

- Seizures are already known to occur in 14-25% of patients with lupus compared with 0.5-1% in the general population. Seizures may result from cerebral vasculitis (ischemic or hemorrhagic manifestations), cardiac embolism, opportunistic infection, drug intoxication, or associated metabolic derangements.
- Less common neurologic syndromes presenting in the patient known to have SLE include movement disorders (chorea, ataxia, Parkinsonism), pseudotumor cerebri, and venous sinus thrombosis.
- CSF can reflect increased central nervous system (CNS) lupus activity by showing elevated levels of white cells, protein,

immunoglobulin synthesis, or absolute immunoglobulin G (IgG). Anti-neuronal nuclear antibodies have some value in confirming CNS disease when performed on CSF, but these are less specific or sensitive than a serum test.

- *Aquaporin 4 antibody is used for diagnosis of Devic's disease (Neuromyelitis optica) which is a subset of multiple sclerosis.*

28. Ans. (b) Anti-ds DNA antibody

(Ref: Harrison 20th edition, p 2517; Harrison 19th edition, p 2126)

Test	Description
ANA	Screening test; sensitivity 95%; it cannot be diagnostic without clinical features
Anti-dsDNA	High specificity; sensitivity only 70%; levels vary based on disease activity
Anti-Sm	Specific antibody for SLE; only 30-40% sensitivity, *no definite clinical correlations*
Anti-SSA (Ro)	Present in 15% of patients with SLE
Anti-SSB (La)	Other connective-tissue diseases such as Sjögren syndrome; associated with neonatal lupus
Anti-RNP	Included with anti-Sm, SSA, and SSB in the ENA profile; may indicate mixed connective-tissue disease with overlap SLE, scleroderma.
Anticardiolipin	IgG/IgM variants measured with ELISA are among the antiphospholipid antibodies used to screen for antiphospholipid antibody syndrome
Lupus Anticoagulant	Multiple tests (eg, direct Russell viper Venom test) to screen for inhibitors in the clotting cascade in antiphospholipid antibody syndrome
Direct Coombs test	Coombs test–positive anemia to denote antibodies on RBCs
Anti-histone	Drug-induced lupus ANA antibodies are often of this type (eg, with procainamide or hydralazine; p-ANCA–positive in minocycline-induced drug-induced lupus)
Anti-ribosomal P	Uncommon antibodies that may correlate with risk for CNS disease, including increased hazards of psychosis in a large inception cohort, although the exact role in clinical diagnosis is debated

29. Ans. (c) SLE

(Ref: Harrison 19th edition, p 2124)

(Mn : SIR Ben Hen)

Non erosive arthritis is seen in

SLE
Inflammatory bowel disease
Rheumatic fever
Behçet disease
Henoch scholein purpura

Rarely deforming non-erosive arthropathy has been described in rheumatic fever and SLE.

30. Ans. (b) S.L.E.

(Ref: Harrison 19th edition, p 2131)

31. Ans. (a) Antihistone antibodies

(Ref: Harrison 20th edition, p 2517)

32. Ans. (c) Antinuclear antibody

(Ref: Harrison 20th edition, p 2517; Harrison 19th edition, p 2126)

33. Ans. (d) Systemic Lupus Erythematosus

(Ref: Harrison 20th edition, p 2518; Harrison 19th edition, p 2131)

34. Ans. (e) Joint Deformity

(Ref: Harrison 20th edition, p 2518; Harrison 19th edition, p 2131)

35. Ans. (a) SLE

(Ref: Harrison 20th edition, p 2518; Robbins 7th / 229, Harrison 19th edition, p 2131)

36. Ans. (a) SLE

(Ref: Harrison 20th edition, p 2518; Harrison 19th edition, p 2131)

37. Ans. (b) Penicillin

(Ref: Harrison 20th edition, p 2525; Harrison 19th edition, p 2152)

38. Ans. (c) Wire loop lesions

(Ref: Harrison 20th edition, p 2518; Harrison 19th edition, p 2131)

39. Ans. (b) Chloasma

(Ref: Behl/298)

40. Ans. (b) Sterility

(Ref: Harrison 20th edition, p 2518; Harrison 19th edition, p 2131)

41. Ans. (c) Increased Prothrombin Time

(Ref: Harrison 20th edition, p 2526; Harrison 19th edition, p 740)

Increased prothrombin time is seen with chronic liver disease. Antiphospholipid syndrome activates intrinsic system of clotting and leads to prolongation of aPTT.

42. Ans. (b) Endocarditis

(Ref: Harrison 20th edition, p 2531; Harrison 19th edition, p 2131)

43. Ans. (a) Rheumatoid Arthritis

(Ref: William's 20th/ 701, 849; Harrison 19th edition, p 2131)

44. Ans. (b) Systemic Sclerosis

(Ref: Harrison 20th edition, p 2552; Harrison 19th edition, p 2163)

45. Ans. (b) Scleroderma

(Ref: Harrison 20th edition, p 2552; Harrison 19th edition, p 1911)

Antiphospholipid Antibody Syndrome

46. Ans. (c) Aspirin + LMW heparin

(Ref: Harrison 20th edition, p 2527; Harrison 19th edition, p 2136)

- Pregnancy morbidity in anti-phospholipid antibody syndrome is prevented by a combination of heparin with aspirin 80 mg daily.
- Intravenous immunoglobulin (IVIg) 400 mg/kg qd for 5 days may also prevent abortions, while glucocorticoids are ineffective
- After the first thrombotic event, APS patients should be placed on warfarin for life aiming to achieve an international normalized ratio (INR) ranging from 2.5 to 3.5, alone or in combination with 80 mg of aspirin daily.

47. Ans. (b) Primary anti-phospholipid antibody syndrome

(Ref: Harrison 20th edition, p 2526; Harrison 19th edition, p 2135)

- *Three or more organ thromboses developing in less than a week is the cornerstone of C.A.P.S (Catastrophic anti-phospholipid antibody syndrome). However, in the question, no time frame is mentioned and this is there by ruled out.*
- Clinical manifestations of heterozygous protein C deficiency include Venous Thrombo-Embolism and warfarin-induced skin necrosis (WISN). Whether the risk of pregnancy loss is increased in this disorder is controversial. Heterozygous protein C deficiency does not appear to be associated with an elevated risk of arterial thrombosis and this patient had MI so is ruled out
- TTP should have features of kidney involvement and stroke like features.
- Primary anti-phospholipid antibody syndrome leads to hypercoagulability and recurrent thrombosis can affect virtually any organ system, including the following:
  1. *Peripheral venous system (deep venous thrombosis)*
  2. Central nervous system (cerebrovascular accident, sinus thrombosis)
  3. Hematologic (thrombocytopenia, hemolytic anemia)
  4. *Obstetric (pregnancy loss, eclampsia)*
  5. Pulmonary (pulmonary embolism, pulmonary hypertension)
  6. Dermatologic (livedo reticularis, purpura, infarcts/ulceration)
  7. *Cardiac (Libman-Sacks valvulopathy, Myocardial Infarction)*
  8. Ocular (amaurosis, retinal thrombosis)
  9. Adrenal (infarction/hemorrhage)
  10. Musculoskeletal (avascular necrosis of bone)

48. Ans. (b) Dilute russel viper venom time test

(Ref: Harrison's 19th edition, p 2791)

- Anti-phospholipid Syndrome–is an autoantibody mediated acquired thrombophilia.
- It is associated with Occurrence of arterial or venous thrombosis or recurrent miscarriage in association with laboratory evidence of persistent antiphospholipid antibody.
- *A prolonged clotting time of 30 seconds or greater that does not correct despite the mixing study suggests the presence of a lupus anticoagulant.*
- An abnormal result for the initial dRVVT assay should be followed by a dRVVT confirmatory test. In this test, the inhibitory effect of lupus anticoagulants on phospholipids in the dRVVT can be overcome by adding an excess of phospholipid to the assay. The clotting times of both the initial dRVVT assay and confirmatory test are normalized and then used to determine a ratio of time without phospholipid excess to time with phospholipid excess.
- In general, a ratio of greater than 1.2 is considered a positive result and implies that the patient may have antiphospholipid antibodies. The dRVVT test is more sensitive than the aPTT test for the detection of lupus anticoagulant, because it is not influenced by deficiencies or inhibitors of clotting factors VIII, IX or XI.
- Clot solubility test is done for factor 13 deficiency. Fibrin clots formed in the presence of factor XIII and thrombin are stable (as a result of crosslinking) for at least 1 h in 5 mol/l urea, whereas clots formed in the absence of factor XIII dissolve rapidly.

49. Ans. (a) Single titre of Anticardiolipin is diagnostic

(Ref: Harrison 20th edition, p 2526-2527; API Textbook of Medicine 8th/ed 306, 307; Harrison 19th edition, p 740)

50. Ans. (b) Aspirin + Low molecular weight Heparin

(Ref: Harrison 20th edition, p 2527; Harrison 19th edition, p 2135t)

Scleroderma

51. Ans. (c) Anti-centromere antibody is a positive predictor of disease

(Ref: Harrison 20th edition, p 2555-2556; Harrison 19th edition, p 1865)

- Scleroderma crisis occurs in 12% of cases with systemic sclerosis. It is characterised by accelerated hypertension and a rapid decline in kidney function.
- Histopathological examination shows arcuate artery intimal narrowing and medial proliferation.
- This is characteristically called onion skinning.
- Anti-U3-RNP may identify the young patients at risk for scleroderma crisis. *Anti-centromere is a negative predictor for scleroderma crisis.*
- Maximum mortality in scleroderma occurs due to Pulmonary artery hypertension and pulmonary fibrosis.

52. Ans. (a) CREST

(Ref: Harrison 20th edition, p 2546; Harrison 19th edition, p 2155)

Anti-centromere antibody is seen in CREST Syndrome

53. Ans. (a) Diffuse periosteal reaction

(Ref: Harrison 19th edition, p 2156)

- Scleroderma is a generalized connective tissue disease characterised by inflammatory, vascular and fibrotic changes of skin and a variety of internal organs.
- Pulmonary disease is estimated to occur in 70% to 85% of patients with scleroderma. Lung involvement is usually seen as diffuse and bilateral basilar reticulonodular infiltrates and *rarely pulmonary nodules.*
- Chest radiography is an insensitive imaging procedure that shows only late findings of pulmonary fibrosis, such as increased interstitial markings. Extremity radiography should be performed to reveal calcinosis and resorption of the distal tufts of the digits.
- *Esophageal dysmotility can be demonstrated using esophageal manometry.*
- Bone changes in scleroderma are acro-osteolysis, peri-articular osteoporosis, joint space narrowing and erosions.

54. Ans. (a) Systemic sclerosis

(Ref: Harrison 20th edition, p 2557; Harrison 19th edition, p 2163)

55. Ans. (a) Anti-nuclear antibody

(Ref: Harrison 20th edition, p 2557; CMDT 2013 p 838)

ANA is the screening method of choice for systemic rheumatic disease such as systemic lupus erthyematosus (SLE), mixed connective tissue disease, Sjögren syndrome, scleroderma, CREST syndrome, rheumatoid arthritis, polymyositis, and dermatomyositis.

56. Ans. (d) Subperiosteal elevation

(Ref: CMDT 2014 ch.20, p 838)

- At least 40-50% of patients with scleroderma experience esophageal symptoms such as heartburn and dysphagia, while up to 90% of patients have esophageal dysfunction on objective testing at some point in their disease. The disease results in smooth muscle dysfunction that causes esophageal aperistalsis and reduced lower esophageal sphincter pressures. Gastroesophageal reflux with poor acid clearance results with an increased incidence of complications such as peptic stricture and Barrett's esophagus.
- Scleroderma is a common cause of intestinal pseudo-obstruction, although the association with other connective tissue disorders, hypothyroidism, Chagas' disease, diabetes, Parkinson's disease and the use of narcotics. The lack of contractile activity at regular intervals results from atrophy and fibrosis of the muscularis layer of the small bowel. Plain radiographs of the abdomen show dilated loops of the small bowel with air fluid levels although this cannot exclude mechanical obstruction as a cause. A more characteristic sign of scleroderma intestinal pseudo-obstruction is a 'hide-bound' or 'accordion-like' appearance produced by closely packed valvulae resulting from excessive collagen deposition. This characteristic mucosal fold pattern is uniquely seen in scleroderma.
- Pneumatosis cystoides intestinalis (PCI) is a rare life-threatening gastrointestinal complication in the course of connective tissue disease (CTD). PCI is characterised by the appearance of intramural clusters of gas in the small and large bowel wall on X-ray or computed tomography and often is accompanied by free air in the peritoneal cavity.

57. Ans. (c) Progressive systemic sclerosis

(Ref: Harrison 20th edition, p 2554; CMDT 2014 ch.20, p 838)

Systemic sclerosis is characterized by fibrosis of lower esophageal sphincter leading to decrease in tone of LES and resultant GERD leads to recurrent aspiration pneumonia.

58. Ans. (b) Renal involvement

(Ref: Harrison 20th edition, p 2555-2556; Harrison 19th edition, p 2241)

- Patients with diffuse, rapid skin involvement have the highest risk (approximately 20-25%) of developing scleroderma renal crisis. Renal crisis occurs in about 10% of all patients with systemic sclerosis and is indicative of bad prognosis.
- Renal crisis presents as accelerated hyper-tension, oliguria, headache, dyspnea, edema, and rapidly rising serum creatinine levels.
- Renal crisis is observed within 4 years of diagnosis in about 75% of patients but may develop as late as 20 years after diagnosis. Renal crises are slightly more common in black than in whites, and men have a greater risk than women.
- Avoid high doses of corticosteroids since this is a significant risk factor for renal crisis.

59. Ans. (c) Syndactyly

(Ref: Harrison 19th edition, p 2182)

- Syndactyly is a condition wherein two or more digits are fused together. Scleroderma has sclerodactyly characterized by pitting scars present in tips of fingers.
- *Scleroderma leads to fibrosis in LES leading to decrease in tone of LES and resultant GERD.*
- The progressive fibrosis can involve the heart leading to restrictive cardiomyopathy and development of kussmual sign.
- The fibrosis of minor salivary glands reduces saliva production. Since saliva has bactericidal activity the resultant reduction in saliva production leads to halitosis.

60. Ans. (c) Scleroderma

(Ref: Harrison 19th edition, p 2164)

61. Ans. (d) Ischemic stroke

(Ref: Harrison 19th edition, p 2164)

In scleroderma, malignant hypertension is seen and this can lead to hemorrhagic but not ischemic stroke. For the rest of the choices the Classification criteria for systemic sclerosis will be helpful.

1. Autoantibodies to centromere proteins, Scl-70 (topo I) and fibrillrin
2. Bibasilar pulmonary fibrosis
3. Contractures of the digital joints or the prayer sign
4. Dermal thickening proximal to the wrists
5. Calcinosis cutis
6. Raynaud phenomenon (at least a 2-phase color change)
7. Esophageal distal hypomotility or reflux esophagitis
8. Sclerodactyly or nonpitting digital edema
9. Telangiectasias, which can be remembered by the abbreviation ABCDCREST.

Fulfilling 3 or more criteria indicates definite systemic scleroderma with a sensitivity and specificity as high as 99% and 100%, respectively.

Immune-mediated causes of uveitis

- Ankylosing spondylitis
- Behçet´s disease
- Drug or hypersensitivity reaction
- Inflammatory bowel disease
- Multiple sclerosis
- Psoriatic arthritis
- Reactive arthritis
- Rheumatic fever
- Sarcoidosis
- Sclerosing cholangitis
- Systemic lupus
- Vogt-Koyanagi-Harada Syndrome

62. Ans. (d) Calcification in all Long bones

(Ref: Harrison 19th edition, p 1911)

Sarcoidosis

63. Ans. (a) Hypercalcemia

(Ref: Harrison 20th edition, p 2603; Harrison 19th ed. / 313, 2208)

- Hypercalcemia is seen with sarcoidosis as the granulomas present in this disease synthesize vitamin D3. This increases the amount of absorption of calcium from the intestine and leads to hypercalcemia.

64. Ans. (a) Sarcoidosis

(Ref: Harrison 20th edition, p 2600)

65. Ans. (a) Cavity

(Ref: Harrison 20th edition, p 2601-2605; Harrison 19th edition, p 2205)

- The panda sign of sarcoidosis is a gallium-67 citrate scan finding. It is due to bilaeral involvement of parotid and lacrimal glands in sarcoidosis, superimposed on the normal uptake in the nasopharyngeal mucosa.
- CXR shows bilateral Hilar Adenopathy with pulmonary infiltrates. But cavity formation is extremely rare.
- Eggshell calcification refers to fine calcification seen at the periphery of a mass, and usually relates to lymph node calcification. The shell-like calcifications up to 2 mm thick must be present in the peripheral zone of at least two lymph nodes. In sarcoidosis calcification is uncommon but not mentioned as rare.

66. Ans. (b) Ankylosing spondylitis

(Ref: Harrison 20th edition, p 2566; Harrison 19th edition, p 2169)

Uveitis is the most common extra-articular manifestation of AS, occurring in 20-30% of patients. Of all patients with acute anterior uveitis, 30-50% have or will develop AS. The incidence is much higher in individuals who are HLA-B27 positive (84-90%). Uveitis is seen also with juvenile rheumatoid arthritis but in choices rheumatoid arthritis is mentioned.

67. Ans. (c) Arrhythmias

(Ref: Harrison 20th edition, p 2604; Harrison 19th edition, p 2208)

Cardiac involvement occurs initially with inflammation and granuloma formation followed by scarring. The initial inflammation can lead to triggered ventricular arrhythmias with subsequent scarring resulting in the substrate for reentrant monomorphic ventricular tachycardia.

68. Ans. (b) Spontaneous remission may occur

(Ref: Harrison 20th edition, p 2606; http://www.aafp.org/afp/2004/0715/p312.html; Harrison 19th edition, p 2205)

Acute sarcoidosis is more common in whites than in blacks and usually is associated with spontaneous remission within two years. Spontaneous remission also occurs in patients with Löfgren's syndrome, which consists of bilateral hilar lymphadenopathy, ankle arthritis, erythema nodosum, fever, myalgia, and weight loss

69. Ans. (d) Tuberculosis

(Ref: Harrison 19th edition, p 1102)

70. Ans. (b) Pericardial effusion

(Ref: Harrison 20th edition, p 2601; Harrison 19th edition, p 2207)

- Lung involvement is seen in 90% patients with bilateral hilar lymphadenopathy, peribronchial thickening and reticulo-nodular changes.
- *Non-Caseating granulomas are seen involving the eye, parotid gland, lymph nodes, liver spleen and lymph nodes.*
- The cutaneous symptoms vary, and range from rashes and nodules to erythema nodosum, granuloma annulare or lupus pernio

71. Ans. (b) IInd cranial nerve (optic nerve)

(Ref: Harrison 20th edition, p 2603; Harrison 19th edition, p 2209)

The first thing that we all have studied is that 7th cranial nerve is commonly involved in sarcoidosis and is not given in the choices.

CNS Manifestation of Sarcoidosis

1. These include cranial nerve involvement, basilar meningitis, myelopathy, and anterior hypothala-mic disease with associated diabetes insipidus.

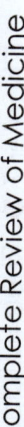

2. Seizures and cognitive changes also occur. Of the cranial nerves, seventh nerve paralysis can be transient and mistaken for Bell's palsy.
3. *Optic neuritis is another cranial nerve manifesta-tion of sarcoidosis.* This manifestation is more chronic and usually requires long-term systemic therapy. It can be associated with both anterior and posterior uveitis.
4. The MRI with gadolinium enhancement may demonstrate space-occupying lesions, but the MRI can be negative due to small lesions or the effect of systemic therapy in reducing the inflammation. The cerebral spinal fluid (CSF) findings include lymphocytic meningitis with a mild increase in protein. The CSF glucose is usually normal.

Löfgren's syndrome, consists of
1. Erythema nodosum,
2. Hilar adenopathy on chest roentgenogram
3. Uveitis.
4. Periarticular arthritis +/-

Löfgren's syndrome is associated with a good prognosis, with >90% of patients experiencing disease resolution within 2 years. A recently proposed expansion of the term Lofgren's syndrome includes periarticular arthritis without erythema nodosum

72. Ans. (b) Adrenals

(Ref: Harrison 20th edition, p 2601t; Harrison 19th edition, p 2010)

Involvement of the adrenal glands rarely occurs in sarcoidosis. The functional status of the adrenal gland in patients with sarcoidosis has nearly always been normal when evaluated after stimulation with exogenous ACTH, with the exception of patients with secondary adrenal failure due to hypothalamic-pituitary infiltration by sarcoid granulomas

Organ involved	%
Lung	95%
Skin	24%
Eye	12%
Liver	12%
Cardiac	2%

73. Ans. (c) Hyperparathyroidism

(Ref: Harrison 19th edition, p 1815)

Tufting of terminal phalanges is seen with:
1. Hyperparathyroidism
2. Acromegaly
3. Gigantism

74. Ans. (d) Malabsorption syndrome

(Ref: Harrison 20th edition, p 2603-2604; Harrison 19th edition, p 2211)

Right paratracheal lymphadenopathy is a feature of garland sign in sarcoidosis. The non-caseating granulomas are seen in the heart and this constitutes the most important cause of non-infectious dilated cardiomyopathy. The granulomas produce vitamin D_3 leading to hypercalcemia.

75. Ans. (d) Anterior uveitis

(Ref: Harrison: sarcoidosis, ch. 329)

Heerfordt syndrome (aka uveo-paratoid fever) is a variant of sarcoidosis and comprises of:
- Fever
- Parotid enlargement
- Facial palsy
- Ocular involvement

76. Ans. (a) Serum amyloid A is used as marker for sarcoidosis

(Ref: Harrison 19th edition, p 2209)

- Serum amyloid A is elevated and is a marker for granulomatous inflammation seen in sarcoidosis. The information on this marker is mentioned in medical journals only but the rest of the choices can be easily ruled out by logic
- The test is not commonly performed, and no substrate has been available since 1996. There is a concern that certain infections, such as bovine spongiform encephalopathy, could be transferred through a Kveim test.
- The levels of vitamin D3 are increased and lead to hypercalcemia as one of the findings of sarcoidosis.
- The X-ray findings seen are:

Stage 1 is hilar adenopathy alone, often with right paratracheal involvement.
Stage 2 is a combination of adenopathy plus infiltrates
Stage 3 reveals infiltrates alone.
Stage 4 consists of fibrosis

77. Ans. (a) Sarcoidosis

(Ref: Harrison 19th edition, p 2209)

Lupus pernio is the most characteristic cutaneous lesion of sarcoidosis. The lesion is typically described as red to purple (due to increased vasculature), swollen, with shiny skin changes right on the nose, cheeks, lips or ears. It is particularly resistant to both surgical and medical therapy.

78. Ans. (d) Left pretracheal lymph nodes

(Ref: Harrison 19th edition, p 2208)

Garland's triad (also known as the 1-2-3 sign or Pawnbrokers sign) is a lymph node enlargement pattern which has been described in sarcoidosis. It comprises of:
1. Right paratracheal nodes
2. Right hilar nodes
3. Left hilar nodes

79. Ans. (c) Synovium

(Ref: Harrison 19th edition, p 2145)

Synovial cell hyperplasia and endothelial cell activation are early events in the pathologic process that progresses to uncontrolled inflammation and consequent cartilage and bone destruction. Genetic factors and immune system abnormalities contribute to disease propagation.

80. Ans. (b) SLE

(Ref: Harrison 19th edition, p 2131)

81. Ans. (c) VII Cranial Nerve

(Ref: Harrison 19th edition, p 2212)

Vasculitis

82. Ans. (d) Polyarteritis nodosa

(Ref: Harrison 20th edition, p 2582-2583; Harrison 19th edition, p 2179-89)

Goodpasture syndrome	Disease where antibodies are directed against the alpha 3 NC1 domain of collagen IV produces an anti-GBM disease leading to hemoptysis and hematuria.
Wegener's granulomatosis	• Characterized by granulomatous vasculitis of the upper and lower respiratory tracts together with glomerulonephritis. • Lung involvement typically appears as multiple, bilateral, nodular cavitatory infiltrates, which on biopsy almost invariably reveal the typical necrotizing granulomatous.
Microscopic polyangitis	• Because of its predilection to involve the small vessels, microscopic polyangiitis and granulomatosis with polyangiitis (Wegener's) share similar clinical features • Diagnosis is based on histologic evidence of vasculitis or pauci-immune glomerulonephritis
Polyarteritis Nodosa	• Lungs are not involved in PAN. • The kidney presentation is that of renal failure and hypertension. • It is a necrotizing vasculitis of small and medium-sized muscular arteries in which involvement of the renal and visceral arteries is characteristic. • PAN does not involve pulmonary arteries, although bronchial vessels may be involved.

Also note that in the given case, a young female has presents with lung involvement as well as renal involvement in the form of glomerulonephritis, which suggests the possibility of a small vessel vasculitis. All of the given options are small vessel vasculitis except Polyarteritis Nodosa, which is a medium vessel vasculitis.

83. Ans. (d) Wegner's granulomatosis

(Ref: Harrison 20th edition, p 2578-2579)

The patient has involvement of:

1. Upper respiratory tract involvement= chronic cold symptoms suggestive of sinusitis
2. Lower respiratory tract involvement = intermittent hemoptysis due to bilateral lung cavitation

3. Kidney involvement= Hematuria with necrotizing vasculitis.
   - These point to involvement of blood vessels of these three systems, diagnosis goes in favor of granulomatosis with angitis (Wegener's Granulomatosis). For diagnosis c-ANCA will be helpful along with biopsy findings of vasculitis.
   - The disease involves small arteries, arterioles, capillaries and leads to necrotizing granulomatous lesion involving both upper and lower respiratory tract and the kidney.
   - The cytoplasmic pattern of immunofluorescence (c-ANCA) is caused by PR3-ANCA and has high specificity>90% for granulomatosis with angitis.

Aspergillosis	Will involve lungs in invasive aspergilloma but multiple cavity formation is not seen and neither is glomerulonephritis.
Polyarteritisnodosa	Ruled out as lung and pulmonary artery involvement is not seen. Hence intermittent hemoptysis is not seen in PAN
Rena cell carcinoma metastatic to lung	Ruled out as in first line itself it is mentioned that Renal biopsy shows segmental necrotizing glomerulonephritis

84. Ans. (b) Lung

(Ref: Harrison 20th edition, p 2582; Harrison 19th edition, p 2187)

Multiple organ systems are involved, and the clinicopathologic findings reflect the degree pulmonary arteries are not involved in PAN, and bronchial artery involvement is uncommon. The pathology in the kidney in classic PAN is that of arteritis without glomerulonephritis.

85. Ans. (a) IgA

(Ref: Harrison 20th edition, p 2586)

- The Presumptive pathogenic mechanism for Henoch-Schönlein purpura is immune-complex deposition.
- IgA is the antibody class most often seen in the immune complexes and has been demonstrated in the renal biopsies of these patients.
- A number of inciting antigens have been suggested including upper respiratory tract infections, various drugs, foods, insect bites, and immunizations.

86. Ans. (a) Kawasaki disease

(Ref: Harrison 20th edition, p 2588; Harrison 19th edition, p 2192)

Disease in choices	Age of presentation and findings
Kawasaki	The illness occurs predominantly in young children; 80% of patients are <5 yr, and, only occasionally, are teenagers or, more rarely, adults affected.
HSP	Henoch-Schönlein Purpura is usually seen in children; most patients range in age from 4 to 7 years; however, the disease may also be seen in infants and adults

Contd...

Susac's Syndrome	Susac's syndrome (SS) consists of the triad of encephalopathy, branch retinal artery occlusions (BRAO), and hearing loss. It usually affects women aged 20 to 40, but men are also affected, and the age range extends from 9 to 72 years (more details below)
Giant Cell Arteritis	Giant cell arteritis occurs almost exclusively in individuals >50 year

Susac's syndrome (SS) consists of the triad of Encephalopathy, branch retinal artery occlusions, and hearing loss. It usually affects women aged 20 to 40.

Investigations
1. **MRI** shows a white matter disturbance that is frequently confused with multiple sclerosis and acute disseminated encephalomyelitis. During the encephalopathy, the corpus callosum is always affected and shows central involvement, central callosal "holes" develop, a pathognomonic finding.
2. **Dilated fundus examination** will reveal branch retinal artery occlusions.
3. **The cochlear hearing loss,** sometimes associated with vertigo, is usually bilateral, and deafness becomes a major disabling problem.

Treatment
1. High-dose corticosteroid therapy is the mainstay, but additional therapies such as intravenous immunoglobulin, mycophenolate mofetil, and cyclophosphamide are often necessary.
2. Rituximab is the newest therapy.

87. Ans. (a) Spares pulmonary artery

(Ref: Harrison 20th edition, p 2585; OP Ghai 7th ed. p 605, Harrison 19th edition, p 2189)

Types of takayasu arteritis and its involvement:

Type 1- Aortic arch
Type 2- Descending aorta
Type 3- Aortic arch and descending aorta
Type 4- Aorta and pulmonary artery involvement

Takayasu is characterized by segmental inflammatory panarteritis resulting in stenosis of aorta and its branches causing weak peripheral pulses. Mantoux test is strongly positive in takayasu arteritis. Diagnosis is made by angiography. Treatment involves long term immunosuppression with prednisolone and methotrexate.

88. Ans. (b) Polyarteritis Nodosa

(Ref: Harrison 20th edition, p 2582-2583; Harrison 19th edition, p 2187)

- Since all peripheral pulses are palpable, hence Takayasu's arteritis is ruled out. The presence of gangrene in digits points to small blood vessel involvement.
- The presence of Hypertension further points to a vasculitis which is a feature of polyarteritis nodosa. Wegeners and SLE are ruled out as ANCA and dsDNA is negative.
- PAN can affect digital vessels leading to gangrene while the vasculitis component explains hypertension

89. Ans. (c) Thrombocytopenia

(Ref: Harrison 20th edition, p 2586; Harrison 19th edition, p 2190)

90. Ans. (c) Wegener's granulomatosis

(Ref: Harrison 20th edition, p 2578-2579; Harrison 19th edition, p 2184)

Wegeners granulomatosis/ granulomatosis with angitiis is characterized by

1. Upper respiratory tract symptoms- mentioned as maxillary sinusitis
2. Lower respiratory tract symptoms-mentioned as hemoptysis
3. Kidney involved – mentioned as hematuria
4. Skin involvement- mentioned as purpura

Clinical features of Granulomatosis with angitis
1. *Chronic sinusitis is the most common initial complaint in GPA,* occurring in 67% of cases; failure to respond to conventional treatment is suggestive. Other ENT manifestations are as follows: Rhinitis (22%)/Epistaxis (11%)/Serous otitis media and hearing loss/strawberry gingival hyperplasia
2. Pulmonary disease may cause any of the following: Pulmonary infiltrates (71%)/Cough (34%)/Hemoptysis (18%)
3. *Musculoskeletal manifestations:Myalgias/Arthralgias,* usually polyarticular and symmetrical, affecting small and medium joints
4. *Renal manifestations-Crescentic necrotizing glomerulonephritis* characterized by urinary sediment with more than 5 RBCs per HPF or erythrocyte casts
5. Nervous system manifestations-Mononeuritis multiplex/Sensorimotor polyneuropathy/Cranial nerve palsies
6. CNS manifestations include vasculitis of small to medium–sized vessels of the brain or spinal cord and granulomatous masses that involve the orbit, optic nerve, meninges, or brain.
7. *Cutaneous manifestations:Palpable purpura* or skin ulcers (45%); ulcerations may resemble pyoderma gangrenosum

91. Ans. (b) Renal hypertension

(Ref: Harrison 20th edition, p 2585; Harrison 19th edition, p 2189)

92. Ans. (b) Wegener's Granulomatosis

(Ref: Harrison 20th edition, p 2579; Harrison 19th edition, p 2184)

93. Ans. (c) Acute congestive glaucoma

(Ref: Harrison's 18th ed.ch.28)

Cluster headache ruled out	No history of retro-orbital pain, epiphora, nasal congestion
Giant cell arteritis ruled out	No History of temporal headache, F.U.O, young age of patient
Tension headache ruled out	Due to history of vomiting/ photophobia and unilateral headache

94. Ans. (b) Non palpable purpura

(Ref: Harrison 20th edition, p 2586; Harrison 19th edition, p 2190)

Non palpable purpura is a feature of acute idiopathic thrombocytopenic purpura.

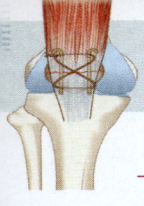

95. Ans. (a) Giant cell arteritis

(Ref: Harrison 20th edition, p 2583)

Giant cell arteritis, also referred to as cranial arteritis or temporal arteritis, is an inflammation of medium and large sized arteries. It characteristically involves one or more branches of the carotid artery, particularly the temporal artery. However, it is a systemic disease that can involve arteries in multiple locations, particularly the aorta and its main branches. Giant cell arteritis is closely associated with polymyalgia rheumatica, which is characterized by stiffness, aching, and pain in the muscles of the neck, shoulders, lower back, hips, and thighs. Most commonly, polymyalgia rheumatica occurs in isolation, but it may be seen in 40–50% of patients with giant cell arteritis. In addition, 10–20% of patients who initially present with features of isolated polymyalgia rheumatica later go on to develop giant cell arteritis. This strong clinical association together with data from pathophysiologic studies has increasingly supported that giant cell arteritis and polymyalgia rheumatica represent differing clinical spectrums of a single disease process.

96. Ans. (c) Nodules are formed in skin which are clinically palpable

(Ref: Harrison 20th edition, p 2582-2583)

- Inflammation in P.A.N may start in the vessel intima and progress to include the entire arterial wall, destroying the internal and external elastic lamina, resulting in fibrinoid necrosis.
- Vascular lesions in medium-sized muscular arteries occur mainly at bifurcations and branch points
- *Nodules in PAN usually occur on the lower extremities. Nodules are the least common skin manifestation of P.A.N.*
- Fibromuscular dysplasia, involves thickening of the media and collagen formation. It is typically reported as having the appearance of a 'string of beads' on angiographic review. "The 'bead' component is often larger than the normal arterial lumen, and in a subset of patients with FMD, aneurysms are present that may require treatment.

97. Ans. (c) Steven Johnson syndrome

(Ref: Harrison 20th edition, p 364)

Individuals who have HLA-B*1502 are more likely to experience a severe skin disorder called Stevens–Johnson syndrome in response to carbamazepine.

98. Ans. (b) Anterior ischemic optic neuropathy

(Ref: Harrison 20th edition, p 2584-2585)

99. Ans. (a) Polyarteritis nodosa

(Ref: Harrison 20th edition, p 2582-2583)

The diagnosis here is made on basis of presence of >3 out of 10 ACR criteria for diagnosis of PAN
1. *Hypertension (BP=160/140 mm Hg)*
2. *Kidney involvement without glomerulonephritis (RBC 10-15/HPF, but no casts seen)*
3. *Muscle weakness or myalgia*

The presence of digital gangrene further cements the diagnosis since small vessel involvement is there but the peripheral pulses are palpable.

- **Diagnostic criteria for PAN are mentioned below-(3 out of 10 should be present)**

1. Weight loss of 4 kg or more
2. Testicular pain/tenderness
3. Myalgia or muscle weakness/tenderness
4. Mononeuropathy or polyneuropathy
5. Diastolic blood pressure greater than 90 mm/Hg
6. Livedo reticularis

7. Elevated blood urea nitrogen (BUN) or creatinine level unrelated to dehydration or obstruction. Kidney involvement is due to vasculitis and not due to glomerulonephritis. Hence hematuria is seen but without RBC casts.
8. Presence of hepatitis B surface antigen or antibody in serum
9. Arteriogram demonstrating aneurysms or occlusions of the visceral arteries
10. Biopsy of small- or medium-sized artery containing polymorphonuclear neutrophils

100. Ans. (c) Thrombocytopenia

(Ref: Harrison 20th edition, p 2588; Harrison 19th edition, p 2179)

The acronym FEBRILE is used to remember the criteria as follows:
- Fever
- Enanthem
- Bulbar conjunctivitis
- Rash
- Internal organ involvement (not part of the criteria)
- Lymphadenopathy
- Extremity changes

The diagnostic criteria established by the American Heart Association (AHA) include fever lasting longer than 5 days (fever is an absolute criterion) and 4 of the 5 main clinical features, after diseases with similar findings have been excluded. The 5 major clinical findings are as follows:
1. Changes in the peripheral extremities: Initial reddening or edema of the palms and soles, followed by membranous desquamation of the finger and toe tips or transverse grooves across the fingernails and toenails (Beau lines)
2. Oropharyngeal changes: Erythema, fissuring, and crusting of the lips; strawberry tongue; diffuse mucosal injection of the oropharynx
3. Bilateral, nonexudative, painless bulbar conjunctival injection
4. Acute nonpurulent cervical lymphadenopathy with lymph node diameter greater than 1.5 cm, usually unilateral
5. Polymorphous rash (not vesicular): Usually generalized but may be limited to the groin or lower extremities

101. Ans. (c) Intravenous immunoglobulins

(Ref: Harrison 20th edition, p 2588; Harrison 19th edition, p 2193)

102. Ans. (b) Cyclophosphamide

(Ref: Harrison 20th edition, p 2580; Harrison 19th edition, p 2182)

103. Ans. (c) Intracranial Internal carotid artery is particularly susceptible

(Ref: Harrison 20th edition, p 2583-2584; Harrison 19th edition, p 2189)

GCA typically affects the superficial temporal arteries—hence the term temporal arteritis. In addition, GCA most commonly affects the ophthalmic, occipital, vertebral, posterior ciliary, and proximal vertebral arteries. GCA commonly affects arteries in the following pattern:
1. *Common, external, and internal carotid artery involvement is usually extracranial; rarely, proximal intracranial segments have been affected*
2. Intraorbital branches, especially the posterior ciliary and ophthalmic arteries, are commonly affected
3. Vertebral arteries are involved as frequently as the superficial temporal arteries in fatal cases, although basilar artery involvement is rare

104. Ans. (c) I, II and IV are correct

(Ref: Harrison 20th edition, p 2582-2583; Harrison 19th edition, p 2187)

Pulmonary artery is not involved in Polyarteritis Nodosa. It is a systemic vasculitis characterized by necrotizing inflammatory lesions that affect medium-sized and small muscular arteries, preferentially at vessel bifurcations, resulting in microaneurysm formation, aneurysmal rupture with hemorrhage, thrombosis, and, consequently, organ ischemia or infarction. 20-30% patients of PAN test positive for Hepatitis B surface antigen.

105. Ans. (b) Microscopic polyangitis

(Ref: Harrison 20th edition, p 2581; Harrison 19th edition, p 2186)

- Microscopic polyangitis affects capillaries, venules and arterioles besides affecting pulmonary vessels.
- In contrast small vessels and pulmonary vessels are not involved in polyarteritis nodosa.
- Takayasu affects aorta and its major branches.
- Giant cell arteritis affects cranial vessels, most commonly temporal artery.

106. Ans. (c) Paget's disease

(Ref: Harrison 20th edition, p 2960-2961; Harrison 19th edition, p 426e-2)

- Nonspecific headaches, impaired hearing, and tinnitus commonly result from skull involvement. The patient's hat size may increase (or, less commonly, decrease) as a result of skull enlargement or deformity.
- The most common cranial symptom is hearing loss, occurring in 30-50% of patients with skull involvement.
- The most common neurologic complication is deafness as a result of involvement of the petrous temporal bone.
- Hip pain is most common when the acetabulum and proximal femur are involved, especially in the sclerotic stage. Bowing of the femur and long bones or protrusion of the acetabulum causes pain that becomes worse with weightbearing and is relieved with rest. Knee and shoulder pain may occur because of altered mechanical forces across the articular joints from deformed bones.
- Other patients with Paget disease present with a range of manifestations related to complications. These include musculoskeletal, neurologic, and cardiovascular problems.
- Because of increased osteoblastic activity and bone formation, bone-specific alkaline phosphatase (BSAP) levels are elevated

107. Ans. (a) Wegner's granulomatosis

(Ref: Harrison 20th edition, p 2578-2579; Harrison 19th edition, p 2182)

Findings on chest radiography are abnormal in two thirds of adults with Wegener's granulomatosis (term not used) and referred to as Granulomatosis with angitis. T*he most common radiologic findings are single or multiple nodules and masses. Nodules are typically diffuse, and approximately 50% are cavitated.*

108. Ans. (a) Raised IgA

(Ref: Harrison 20th edition, p 2586; Harrison 19th edition, p 2190)

Henoch scholein purpura/ anaphylactoid purpura/**non-thrombocytopenic purpura**
1. Age of onset : 4-7 years
2. Immune complex deposition with IgA
3. Palpable EXTENSOR purpura with polyarthralgia
4. Colicky pain with nausea, vomiting, passage of blood per rectum
5. Renal glomerulonephritis with proteinuria and microscopic hematuria

109. Ans. (b) Polyarteritis Nodosa

(Ref: Harrison 20th edition, p 2583; Harrison 19th edition, p 2187)

110. Ans. (c) Takayasu arteritis

(Ref: Harrison 20th edition, p 2585; Harrison 19th edition, p 2189)

111. Ans. (a) Classical PAN

(Ref: Harrison 20th edition, p 2582; Refer text below, Harrison 19th edition, p 2187)

112. Ans. (d) Good pasture's syndrome

(Ref: Harrison 20th edition, p 2140; Refer text below, Harrison 19th edition, p 1839)

Goodpasture's syndrome is not classified as an ANCA positive vasculitis.

113. Ans. (a) Wegener's Granulomatosis

(Ref: Harrison 20th edition, p 2579; Harrison 19th edition, p 2182)

114. Ans. (b) Microscopic polyangitis

(Ref: Harrison 20th edition, p 2581; Harrison 19th edition, p 368e-1)

115. Ans. (c) Polyarteritis Nodosa (Classic PAN)

(Ref: Harrison 20th edition, p 2582-2583; Robbins 8th/ed; 'Vasculitis' by Ball & Bridges 2nd/286; Harrison 19th / 2187

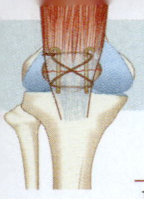

116. Ans. (a) Wegener's granulomatosis

(Ref: Harrison 20th edition, p 2579; Harrison 19th edition, p 2182)

117. Ans. (a) Classical polyarteritis nodosa

(Ref: Harrison 20th edition, p 2582-2583; Harrison 19th edition, p 2187)

118. Ans. (a) Necrotizing arteritis

(Ref: Harrison 20th edition, p 2583; Harrison 19th edition, p 2187)

119. Ans. (b) Lower Respiratory Tract involvement

(Ref: Harrison 20th edition, p 2581-2582; Oxford Desk (Ref: Nephrology (Oxford University Press) 2009/169, Harrison 19th edition, p 2186)

120. Ans. (d) Temporal Arteritis

(Ref: Harrison 20th edition, p 2583-2584; Robbins 8th/512; Harrison 19th edition, p 2188)

121. Ans. (a) Headache

(Ref: Harrison 20th edition, p 2584; Harrison 19th edition, p 2189)

122. Ans. (a) Temporal Artery Biopsy

(Ref: Harrison 20th edition, p 2584; Harrison 19th edition, p 2189)

123. Ans. (c) Aortoarteritis

(Ref: Harrison 20th edition, p 1922; Harrison 19th edition, p 1637)

124. Ans. (c) Takayasu Arteritis

(Ref: Harrison 20th edition, p 2585; API Textbook of Medicine 9th/ 754, Harrison 19th p 2190)

125. Ans. (a) Henoch Schonlein Purpura

(Ref: Harrison 20th edition, p 2586; Harrison 19th edition, p 1839)

126. Ans. (a) Henoch Shonlein Purpura

(Ref: Harrison 20th edition, p 2586; Harrison 19th edition, p 1839)

127. Ans. (d) Thrombocytopenia

(Ref: Harrison 20th edition, p 2586; Harrison 19th edition, p 1839)

128. Ans. (a) Blood in Stools

(Ref: Harrison 20th edition, p 2586; Harrison 19th edition, p 1839)

129. Ans. (c) IgA

(Ref: Harrison 20th edition, p 2586; Harrison 19th edition, p 1839)

130. Ans. (d) Coarctation of Aorta

(Ref: Harrison 20th edition, p 1837; Nelson's 18th/1900, 1901; Hurst 11th/ed 1809, Harrison 19th edition, p 1525)

131. Ans. (d) Polyarteritis nodosa

(Ref: Harrison 20th edition, p 2583; Harrison 19th edition, p 2187)

Ankylosing Spondylitis

132. Ans. (a) Responsive to steroids

(Ref: Rheumatology E-Book, 6th edition, p 168)

RS3PE, Relapsing, seronegative, symmetric synovitis with pitting edema is defined as seronegative arthritis with the following clinical features-

1. Clear pitting edema of hands (called boxing glove appearance of hands)
2. Polyarthritis with acute onset
3. Age > 50 years
4. Negative rheumatoid factor

It was earlier considered to be a subset of rheumatoid arthritis but is now regarded a different disease entity. This is because unlike rheumatoid arthritis there is absence of joint erosions and good response to steroids.

133. Ans. (b) Ochronosis

(Ref: Harrison 19th edition, p 434e-4)

Schober's test determines lumbar spine flexibility and motion. It can be positive in any condition leading to decreased lumbar spine mobility.

Ochronosis	Hyperpigmentation of nose and ears is a hallmark feature. Spine involvement is seen.
Hypoparathyroidism	Easily ruled out
Ankylosing spondylitis	It is more common in males. Hyperpigmentation is not explained by AS
Fluorosis	Hyperpigmentation is not explained by fluorosis. Dental symptoms are not present.

Clinical profile of Alkaptonuria

- Darkening of urine on air exposure
- May go unrecognised until middle life when degenerative joint disease may develop.
- Foci of gray brown scleral pigment and darkening of concha, anti-helix and finally helix develop before 30 years of age.
- Low back pain due to ochronotic arthritis develops. Hips, knee and shoulders may be involved between 30-40 years.
- *Cardiac involvement can be in the form of aortic stenosis requiring valve replacement.*
- Larynx, tympanic membranes, skin, pigmented renal or prostatic calculi can develop.

134. Ans. (b) Decreased chest expansion

- The clinical feature of young male waking up to a low back ache worse in morning and relieved on physical movement by eveningis suggestive of diagnosis of ankylosing Spondylitis.

- These patients in future can develop costochondritis leading to restriction in chest expansion
- The most specific findings involve loss of spinal mobility, with limitation of anterior and lateral flexion and extension of the lumbar spine and of chest expansion.
- Ankylosing Spondylitis presents with *bone marrow oedema*.
- Rheumatoid arthritis is more common in middle aged women (M:F=1:3) with peripheral polyarthritis involving the small joints in the hand symmetrically.

Clinical features of ankylosing spondylitis

1. **Early Diagnostic feature:** decreased chest expansion (<3.8 cm). Chest expansion is measured as the difference between maximal inspiration and maximal forced expiration in the fourth intercostal space in males or just below the breasts in females, with the patient's hands resting on or just behind the head. Normal chest expansion is >5 cm.
2. Patient walks in a stooped position and has essentially no motion in the spine.
3. Extra-articular features: iritis, cardiac conduction defects, aortic incompetence, spinal cord compression & amyloidosis.

Investigations

1. Rheumatoid factor and serologic tests: negative.
2. Radiographic appearance of the spine:
   a. **Early stages:** Lower lumbar disc degenerative condition with sacroiliac joint involvement.
   b. **End-stage disease:** Sacroiliac joints are fused.
   c. Squaring of vertebral bodies & development of delicate syndesmophytes.
   d. Complete fusion with a bamboo spine appearance
3. **HLA B27:** Positive

135. Ans. (d) Soluble IL-2 receptor antagonist

(Ref: Harrison 19th edition, p 372e-30)

Used in muckle wells syndrome and Adult onset still's disease	Anakinra is used for treatment of some rare syndromes dependent on IL-1 production 1. Neonatal-onset inflammatory disease 2. Muckle-Wells syndrome 3. Familial cold urticaria, 4. Systemic Juvenile-onset inflammatory arthritis 5. Adult-onset Still's disease.
Not combined with anti TNF drugs due to the risk of serious infections	Anakinra should not be combined with an anti-TNF drug due to the high rate of serious infections.
Useful In familial cold urticarial	Refer to first entry in the table
Soluble IL-2 receptor antagonist	The anakinra molecule is a *recombinant, nonglycosylated version of human IL-1 RA (RA here stands for receptor antagonist)* prepared from cultures of genetically modified *Escherichia coli* using recombinant DNA technology

136. Ans. (c) Heart is affected

(Ref: Harrison 20th edition, p 2566; Harrison 19th edition, page 2171)

- Ankylosing spondylitis is more common in men with M:F ratio of 2:1-3:1
- In western populations the prevalence of HLA B27 positivity is 90%
- *Heart involvement is in form of aortic regurgitation leading to CHF*
- It is associated with plantar fasciitis and enthesopathy

137. Ans. (d) Decreased FRC

- The image shows modified Schober test being done to evaluate for ankylosing Spondylitis.
- In cases with restriction of chest wall motion, decreased vital capacity and increased functional residual capacity are common.
- This distance increases by >5 cm and in the case of normal mobility and by <4 cm in the case of decreased mobility.
- Chest expansion is measured as the difference between maximal inspiration and maximal forced expiration in the fourth intercostal space in males or just below the breasts in females, with the patient's hands resting on or just behind the head. Normal chest expansion is <5 cm.

138. Ans. (a) Ankylosing spondylitis

(Ref: Harrison 20th edition, p 2564; Harrison 19th edition, p 2169)

AS shows a striking correlation with the histocompatibility antigen HLA-B27 and occurs worldwide roughly in proportion to the prevalence of B27 in 90% of patients with AS independent of disease severity.

139. Ans. (d) Systemic lupus erythematosus

(Ref: Harrison 20th edition, p 2515; Harrison 19th edition, p 2124)

- More than 90% of cases of SLE occur in women, frequently starting at childbearing age.
- The use of exogenous hormones has been associated with lupus onset and flares, suggesting a role for hormonal factors in the pathogenesis of the disease.
- The risk of SLE development in men is similar to that in prepubertal or postmenopausal women. Interestingly, in men, SLE is more common in those with Klinefelter syndrome (i.e, genotype XXY), further supporting a hormonal hypothesis.
- The female-to-male ratio peaks at 11:1 during the childbearing years. A correlation between age and incidence of SLE mirrors peak years of female sex hormone production
- AS, in general, is diagnosed more frequently in males; the male-to-female ratio is 3:1.

140. Ans. (a) Wrist and hand

(Ref: Harrison 20th edition, p 2565; Harrison 19th edition, p 2170)

In AS joint involvement tends to occur *most commonly in the hips, shoulders, and joints of the chest wall,* including the acromioclavicular and sternoclavicular joints, and often occurs in the first 10 years of disease. Involvement of the hips

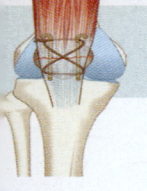

and shoulders may result in joint damage with radiographic changes. Involvement of the hips and shoulder joints is more common in persons with juvenile-onset AS than in adult patients with AS.

141. Ans. (a) Flexion of lumbar spine

(Ref: Harrison 20th edition, p 2565; Harrison 19th edition, p 2170)

Perform the Schober test by marking a 10-cm length of the lumbar spine (with the patient in the erect position), starting at the fifth lumbar spinous process. Instruct the patient to flex his or her spine maximally. Remeasure the distance between the marks. Normal flexion increases the distance by at least 5 cm

142. Ans. (d) Infliximab

(Ref: Harrison 20th edition, p 2567; Harrison 19th edition, p 2172)

Patients with AS treated with either infliximab, etanercept, adalimumab or golimumab (human anti-TNF-monoclonal antibodies) have shown rapid, profound, and sustained reductions in all clinical and laboratory measures of disease activity. Patients with long-standing disease and even some with complete spinal ankylosis have shown significant improvement in both objective and subjective indicators of disease activity and function, including morning stiffness, pain, spinal mobility, peripheral joint swelling, CRP, and ESR. MRI studies indicate substantial resolution of bone marrow edema, enthesitis, and joint effusions in the sacroiliac joints, spine, and peripheral joints

143. Ans. (b) Ankylosing spondylitis

(Ref: Harrison 20th edition, p 2564-2565; Harrison 19th edition, p 2169)

- Patients commonly experience morning stiffness lasting at least 30 minutes, improvement of symptoms with moderate physical activity, and diffuse nonspecific radiation of pain into both buttocks. Patients often experience stiffness and pain that awakens them in the early morning, a distinctive symptom not generally found in patients with mechanical back pain.
- Inflammatory back pain is the most common symptom and the first manifestation in approximately 75% of patients. The pain is typically dull and poorly localized to the gluteal and sacroiliac (SI) areas.
- The pain often begins unilaterally and intermittently, and generally begins in the lumbo-sacral region. However, as the disease progresses, it becomes more persistent and bilateral and progresses more proximally, with ossification of the annulus fibrosus that results in fusion of the spine (bamboo spine).

144. Ans. (c) Rheumatoid Arthritis

(Ref: Harrison 20th edition, p 2531; Harrison 19th edition, p 2145)

145. Ans. (c) Indomethacin

(Ref: Harrison 19th edition, p 2175)

Rheumatoid Arthritis

146. Ans. (c) Febuxostat

(Ref: Harrison 20th edition, p 2537)

- Choice A is a biological and Choice B and D are DMARDS used for management of RA.
- Febuxostat is a hypouricemic agent used for management of gout and has advantage of not requiring dose adjustment in setting of renal disease.

147. Ans. (a) Rheumatoid arthritis

(Ref: Harrison 20th edition, p 2528)

- The image shows subluxation at first metacarpophalangeal joint with extension of interphalangeal joints. Deformity at the wrist joint is noted. The history mentions sparing of DIP. These features point to diagnosis of Rheumatoid arthritis.

148. Ans. (b) Involvement of neck, shoulder, back for more than 6 months in a year

(Ref: Rheumatology Secrets: 3rd edition, p 193)

Healey Criteria for diagnosis of Polymyalgia Rheumatica

Diagnostic criteria – PMR (healey 1984)
- Age> 50 years
- Pain corresponding to proximal muscles of the limbs. 2 out of 3 regions: neck, shoulder and pelvic girdle. Symptoms > 1 month
- Morning stiffness > 1 hr
- Elevated ESR (>40 mm/hr)
- Rapid response to low dose of steroids

Do not confuse polymyalgia rheumatica with fibromyalgia.

149. Ans. (c) Methotrexate + Sulphasalazine + Hydroxychloroquine

(Ref: Harrison 20th edition, p 2539)

- The image shows subluxation at first MCP of both hands with deformity in fingers on right hand. Coupled with the clinical history, the diagnosis is Z line deformity of Rheumatoid arthritis with persistent disease activity.
- She is already on methotrexate and should now be put on triple therapy of methotrexate with sulphasalazine and hydroxychloroquine.
- Choice A will lead to higher side effects of methotrexate. Choice B will lead to increased incidence of osteoporosis. Choice D: anti- TNF drugs are used not alone but in conjunction with methotrexate.
- The original treatment pyramid for RA is now obsolete and aggressive approach to clinical remission is recommended. Failure to achieve remission with methotrexate calls for change in DMARD therapy as follows
  1. Oral triple therapy (Methotrexate + sulphasalazine + Hydroxychloroquine)
  2. Methotrexate and leflunomide
  3. Methotrexate and biologicals like certolizumab

150. Ans. (a) Cardiovascular complications

(Ref: Harrison 20th edition, p 2530; Harrison: 19th edition, p 2144)

- The overall mortality rate of RA is two times greater than general population, with ischemic heart disease being the most common cause of death.
- The life expectancy is reduced by 7 years for men and 3 years for women.

151. Ans. (a) Mitral regurgitation

(Ref: Harrison 20th edition, p 2529; Harrison 19th edition, p 2138)

Cardiac involvement in RA

1. Mitral regurgitation is the most common valvular abnormality in RA
2. Pericardium is the most frequent site of cardiac involvement in RA
3. Cardiomyopathy and diastolic malfunction
4. Coronary artery disease
5. Heart muscle may contain rheumatoid nodules or may be infiltrated with amyloid (Rare).

152. Ans. (c) Anti-cyclic citrullinated peptide (anti-CCP) antibody

(Ref: CMDT 2016 p 821)

- Anti-CCP is the most specific antibody for rheumatoid arthritis with specificity of 95%.
- 20% patients have elevated ANA and ESR. CRP levels are elevated proportional to disease activity.

153. Ans. (b) A, B and D

(Ref: Chapter 154: Nelson 18th edition)

- Poly-articular onset JIA (20-40%) *is common in girls* (3:1).
- Peak age of onset is at age 3 years.
- *It involves 5 or more joints during the first 6 months of the disease.*
- Poly-articular onset JIA commonly involves the small joints of the hand and, less frequently, the larger joints of the knee, ankle, or wrist.
- Asymmetric arthritis may be acute or chronic and may be destructive in 15% of patients.
- *Immunoglobulin M (IgM) rheumatoid factor (RF) is present in 10% of children with this JIA subgroup.*
- It is associated with subcutaneous nodules, erosions, and a poor prognosis. Approximately 40% of these patients test positive for ANA.
- Systemic symptoms, including anorexia, anemia, and growth retardation, are moderate.
- *An intermediate risk for uveitis exists.*

TABLE: Criteria for the Classification of Juvenile Rheumatoid Arthritis

Age at onset: <16 yr
Arthritis (swelling or effusion, or the presence of 2 or more of the following signs: Limitation of range of motion, tenderness or pain on motion.
Duration of disease: ≥6 wk
Onset type defined by type of articular involvement in the 1st 6 mo after onset:
Polyarthritis: ≥5 inflamed joints
Oligoarthritis: ≤4 inflamed joints
Systemic disease: arthritis with a characteristic intermittent fever
Exclusion of other forms of juvenile arthritis

154. Ans. (c) Pauci-articular type

(Ref: 8th edition, O.P.Ghai p 626)

Pauci-articular JRA
1. Onset is most frequent type of JRA accounting for 60% of patients.
2. Four or fewer joints are affected and the involvement is asymmetrical. Joint swelling rather than joint pain is usual complaint.

Pauci-articular onset type 1	Pauci-Articular type 2
This is common in young girls typically 3-5 years with knees elbows and ankles are affected. Small joints are not involved. Secondary glaucoma and cataract may also occur.	Pauci-Articular type 2 is more common in boys > 8 years of age. Many are HLAB 27 positive and some go on to develop ankylosing spondylitis later as adults.

Polyarticular onset JRA develops in 30% of patients and more common in girls. Five or more joints are affected within the first 6 months of onset of disease.

RA factor positive	RA factor negative
1. Symmetrical small joint arthritis with cervical spine involvement. 2. Rheumatoid nodules are present and represent most severe forms of disease	1. Knees, wrists and hips affected while small joints are less commonly involved. 2. Joint disease is less severe.

Systemic onset JRA
Occurs in 10% of cases with acute onset with quotidian fever, rash anywhere with central clearing, pericarditis and interstitial lung disease may be present. RA factor is negative

155. Ans. (a) Cervical

(Ref: Harrison 20th edition, p 2528; Harrison 19th edition, p 122, 2138)

Atlantoaxial involvement of the cervical spine is clinically noteworthy because of its potential to cause compressive myelopathy and neurologic dysfunction. Neurologic manifestations are rarely a presenting sign or symptom of atlantoaxial disease, but they may evolve over time with progressive instability of C1 on C2.

156. Ans. (d) Seronegative arthritis

(Ref: Harrison 20th edition, p 2535; Harrison 19th ed. /2136)

- Patients of rheumatoid arthritis harbor an antibody by the name of anti – C.C.P (cycliccitrulline phospholipid antibodies).
- The rheumatoid nodules in these patients can compress on various peripheral nerves leading to mono-neuritis multiplex. The joints are damaged with peri-articular erosions and osteoporosis.
- **The characterstic joint involvement is P.I.P, M.C.P and the wrist joint bilaterally.**

Sero-negative arthritis is a broad term and included within the group are the entities psoriatic arthritis, Reiter's syndrome, enteropathic arthritis, reactive arthritis, ankylosing spondylitis, undifferentiated seronegative arthritis, Whipple's disease, arthritis associated with pustular acne, post-intestinal bypass arthritis, and several forms of HIV associated arthritis.

157. Ans. (d) Secondary amyloidosis

(Ref: Harrison 19th ed. / 719, 723, 2458)

- Reactive amyloid A (AA) amyloidosis, one of the most severe complications of RA, is a serious, potentially life-threatening disorder caused by deposition of AA amyloid fibrils in multiple organs. These AA amyloid fibrils derive from the circulatory acute-phase reactant serum amyloid A protein (SAA), and may be controlled by treatment
- The introduction of biological therapies targeting specific inflammatory mediators revolutionised the treatment of rheumatoid arthritis (RA). Targeting key components of the immune system allows efficient suppression of the pathological inflammatory cascade that leads to RA symptoms and subsequent joint destruction.
- Milk alkali syndrome occurs due to abuse of calcium containing anta-acids leading to hypercalcemia

158. Ans. (b) HLA DR 4

(Ref: Harrison 19th ed. / 372e-1)

HLA allele	Diseases with increased risk
HLA-B27	Ankylosing spondylitis Post-gonococcal arthritis Acute anterior uveitis
HLA-B47	21-hydroxylase deficiency
HLA-DR2	Systemic lupus erythematosus
HLA-DR3	Autoimmune hepatitis Primary Sjogren syndrome Diabetes mellitus type 1 Systemic lupus erythematosus
HLA-DR4	Rheumatoid arthritis Diabetes mellitus type 1
HLA-DR3 and – DR4 combined	Diabetes mellitus type 1
HLA-DQ2 and HLA-DQB	Celiac disease

159. Ans. (b) Rheumatoid Arthritis

(Ref: Harrison 20th edition, p 2536-2539; Harrison 19th ed. / 2144-45)

- *Minocycline, gold salts, enicillamine, azathioprine, and cyclosporine have all been used for the treatment of RA with varying degrees of success; however, they are used sparingly now due to their inconsistent clinical efficacy or unfavorable toxicity profile.*
- Drugs used in Rheumatoid arthritis
- Hydroxychloroquine
- Lefluonomide
- Methotrexate
- Abatacept
- Anakinra
- Rituximab

160. Ans. (d) Tender nodules

(Ref: Harrison 20th edition, p 2528, 2528f; Harrison 19th ed. p 2146t)

- The image shows nodules on extensor distribution along with peripheral smear showing presence of normocytic anemia.
- The first differential to be considered is rheumatoid arthritis.
- The nodules are non-tender and are a late feature and hence not considered in diagnostic criteria for Rheumatoid arthritis.
- "Piano-key movement" of the ulnar styloid occurs due to inflammation about the ulnar styloid and tenosynovitis of the extensor carpi ulnaris.
- "Z-line deformity" is due to subluxation of the first MCP joint with hyperextension of the first interphalangeal (IP) joint due to damage to the tendons, joint capsule

161. Ans. (c) 5

(Ref: OP Ghai 7th ed. p 600.)

Poly-articular onset juvenile rheumatoid arthritis is characterized by *five or more joints (large and small)* are affected within the first 6 months.

162. Ans. (b) Ankylosing spondylitis

(Ref: MERCK MANUAL and Williams wilkins neurosurgery p 2732-2735)

- Axial involvement in RA is usually limited to upper cervical spine, on accession inflammation from synovial joints and bursae of the upper cervical spine leads to atlantoaxia subluxation.
- The most common acquired cause of cranio vertebral junction (CV) abnormality is RA (the Merck manual)
- Choice C and D are congenital malformations that lead to cranio-vertebral anomalies.
- *Best option is ankylosing spondylitis as it is least likely associated with CV junction anomaly.*

163. Ans. (c) Metacarpophalangeal joint

(Ref: Harrison 20th edition, p 2528)

- The hallmark feature of rheumatoid arthritis (RA) is persistent symmetric polyarthritis (synovitis) that affects the hands and feet, although any joint lined by a synovial membrane may be involved.
- In general, the small joints of the hands and feet are affected in a relatively symmetric distribution.
- In decreasing frequency, the metacarpophalan-geal (MCP), wrist, proximal interphalangeal (PIP), knee, metatars-ophalangeal (MTP), shoulder, ankle, cervical spine, hip, elbow, and temporomandibular joints are most commonly affected.

164. Ans. (b) Pericarditis

(Ref: Harrison 20th edition, p 2529)

- *Most frequent cardiac involvement in RA is pericarditis followed by cardiomyopathy.*

- Because of the heightened risk of premature atherosclerosis, adherence to primary prevention guidelines is mandatory. Because the prevalence of carotid atherosclerosis in RA is at least as high as in diabetes mellitus.

165. Ans. (a) Anti-MCV antibody (anti mutated citrullinated peptide antibody test)

(Ref: Harrison 19th edition, p 2281)

- The newly developed anti-mutated citrullinated vimentin (anti-MCV) assay has similar diagnostic performance as the anti-CCP2 ELISA. It's especially useful in the diagnosis of RA in anti-C.C.P2 seronegative patients. The combined application of anti-C.C.P2 and anti-M.C.V assays can improve the laboratory diagnostics of RA
- Main advantage of testing for anti-M.C.V is the early appearance of the anti-M.C.V antibodies, that allows for detection of early RA and submits adequate therapy just after the disease's onset. Moreover, anti-M.C.V titers show strong correlation to disease activity, disease severity and the success of therapy.
- Rheumatoid factor is an autoantibody, usually IgM directed against the Fc region of IgG (screening). Despite its name its name, rheumatoid factor is not specific for rheumatoid arthritis, it can also be seen in wide range of autoimmune disorders, inflammatory disease and chronic infections.
- Anticitrullinated peptide antibody test (anti ccp) test is more specific than rheumatoid factor for diagnosis of rheumatoid arthritis. It may be positive very early in the course of the disease. Hence it is considered as IOC.

166. Ans. (a) Rheumatoid arthritis

(Ref: CMDT 2013, p 826)

DR4 is associated with
1. Extra-articular rheumatoid arthritis
2. Hydralazine-induced female systemic lupus erythematosus
3. Pemphigoid gestationalis
4. Pemphigus foliaceus
5. Obstructive hypertrophic cardiomyopathy
6. IgA nephropathy

167. Ans. (a) Normocytic, normochromic

(Ref: Harrison 20th edition, p 2529; Harrison 19th edition, p 2138)

- Anemia of chronic illness traditionally encom-passed any inflammatory, infectious, or malig-nant disease of a long-standing nature. The modern definition includes rheumatoid arthritis, severe trauma, heart disease, or diabetes mellitus.
- In these conditions, there is primarily a decreased availability of iron, relatively decreased levels of erythropoietin, and a mild decrease in the lifespan of RBCs to 70-80 days.
- Early onset rheumatoid arthritis with positive rheumatoid factor is more likely to have Normo-cytic normochromic anemia

168. Ans. (d) Nephropathy

(Ref: Harrison 20th edition, p 2530; Harrison 19th edition, p 372e-15t)

- Felty's syndrome is characterized by Rheumatoid arthritis with splenomegaly and neutropenia
- Caplan syndrome is Rheumatoid arthritis in association with coal worker pneumoconiosis
- Felty Syndrome affects approximately 1-3% of all patients diagnosed with RA, and RA occurs in about 1% of the general population.
- Many years of aggressive destructive rheumatoid arthritis (RA) precede the onset of Felty syndrome (FS). On occasion, RA and FS develop simultaneously. The extra-articular manifestations of RA (e.g., rheumatoid nodules, pleuropericarditis, vasculitis, peripheral neuropathy, episcleritis, other forms of eye involvement, Sjögren syndrome, adenopathy, skin ulcers) are more common in patients who develop Felty Syndrome)

169. Ans. (a) Cervical spine

(Ref: Harrison 20th edition, p 2528)

- In decreasing frequency, the metacarpophalangeal (MCP), wrist, proximal interphalangeal (PIP), knee, metatarsophalangeal (MTP), shoulder, ankle, cervical spine, hip, elbow, and temporomandibular joints are most commonly affected.

170. Ans. (d) Rheumatoid arthritis

(Ref: Harrison 20th edition, p 2529; Harrison 19th edition, p 2138)

171. Ans. (a) Flexion and extension cervical area X-Ray of neck

(Ref: Harrison 19th edition, p 214)

- The clinical picture suggests atlanto axial subluxation due to rheumatoid arthritis. Thus the patient fits into Class IIIB ranawat classification of neurological deficit which is– Objective weakness and long-tract signs; patient no longer ambulatory.
- Therefore we need to decide whether the patient requires conservative management or surgical intervention. This is decided by MRI spine ideally which is not given in the choices.
- The textbook then mentions that on X-ray, the anterior atlantodental interval (AADI) has been used to monitor patients with rheumatoid arthritis over time. This measures the interval from the posterior margin of the anterior ring of C1 to the anterior surface of the odontoid.
- An interval of more than 3 mm in an adult or 4 mm in a child is considered abnormal. Various authors have recommended surgery for values of more than 8 mm, 9 mm, or 10 mm. Anterior atlantoaxial subluxation may also be assessed by the PADI measurement, as measured from the posterior aspect of the odontoid to the anterior margin of the lamina of C1.
- Rheumatoid arthritis (RA) of the cervical apophyseal joints produces neck pain, stiffness, and limitation of motion. In advanced RA, synovitis of the atlantoaxial joint may damage the transverse ligament of the atlas, producing forward displacement of the atlas on the axis (atlantoaxial subluxation).

- Surgery should be considered when myelopathy or spinal instability is present. MRI spine (NOT GIVEN IN CHOICES) is the imaging modality of choice.

172. Ans. (a) Elbow

(Ref: Harrison 19th edition, p 2145)

- Rheumatoid nodules occur in approximately 25% of patients with RA, but they occur in fewer than 10% of patients during the first year of the disease. These lesions are most commonly found on extensor surfaces or sites of frequent mechanical irritation.
- The olecranon process, the proximal ulna, the back of the heel, the occiput, and the ischial tuberosities are common periosteal sites for rheumatoid nodule development. Nodules may also form in subcutaneous tissues of the fingers, in toe and heel pads, in tendons, and in viscera.

173. Ans. (d) Hyperandrogenism

(Ref: Harrison 20th edition, p 2530; Harrison 19th edition, p 2144)

- Hypoandrogenism is seen in RA. *CRP can be either normal or elevated in RA.* Normal CRP and normal ESR are scored as 0 points.
- A score of ≥ 6 is a must for diagnosis of RA.

174. Ans. (d) Anti-Mi-2 antibody

(Ref: Harrison 20th edition, p 2534-35, 2592; Harrison 19th edition, p 2145)

Anti Mi-2 antibodies are useful of diagnosis of dermatomyositis Potentially useful laboratory studies in suspected RA fall into 3 categories—markers of inflammation, hematologic parameters, and immunologic parameters—and include the following:
- Erythrocyte sedimentation rate (ESR)
- C-reactive protein (CRP) level
- Complete blood count (CBC)
- Rheumatoid factor (RF) assay
- Antinuclear antibody (ANA) assay
- Anti cyclic citrullinated peptide (anti-CCP) and anti mutated citrullinated vimentin (anti-MCV) assays (currently used in the 2010 American College of Rheumatology [ACR]/European League Against Rheumatism [EULAR] classification criteria)

175. Ans. (d) C Reactive protein indicates better prognosis

(Ref: Harrison 20th edition, p 2534-35; Harrison 19th edition, p 2145)

176. Ans. (c) Articular erosions on X-ray

(Ref: Current Diagnosis & Treatment in Rheumatology 2nd/208; Harrison 19th edition, p 2145/2131)

177. Ans. (d) Nephropathy

(Ref: Harrison 20th edition, p 2530; Harrison 19th edition, p 411/418)

178. Ans. (a) Cervical

(Ref: Harrison 20th edition, p 2528; Harrison 19th edition, p 2145)

179. Ans. (a) Anti–ccp Antibody

(Ref: Harrison 20th edition, p 2535; Harrison 19th edition, p 2145)

180. Ans. (d) BAL

(Ref: Harrison 20th edition, p 2536-2539; Harrison 19th edition, p 2145)

181. Ans. (a) Mononeuritis Multiplex

(Ref: Harrison 19th edition, p 2145)

182. Ans. (c) Acetaminophen

(Ref: Rossi's principles of Transfusion Medicine p 350; Turek's 6th/164, Harrison 19th edition, p 734)

The question is based on acquired hemophilia which is seen with autoimmune disorders. For management of acquired factor VIII inhibitors, human factor VIII concentrate and recombinant factor VII concentrate is used. Aspirin and antiplatelet drugs are avoided and acetaminophen is recommended.

183. Ans. (d) Raynaud's phenomenon

(Ref: CSDT 16th/828)

Gout

184. Ans. (a) Polarised microscopy of tissue fluid aspirate

(Ref: Harrison 19th edition, p 2233-34)

- Notice the *eccentric juxta-articular lobulated* soft tissue mosses
- The clinical diagnosis favors development of chronic gout.
- HLA B27positive ankylosing spondylitis presents as low back ache.
- Rheumatoid arthritis mainly presents as bilaterally symmetrical small joint involvement.
- Other than the great toe, the most common sites of gouty arthritis are the instep, ankle, wrist, finger joints, and knee. In early gout, only 1 or 2 joints are usually involved.
- *Consider the diagnosis in any patient with acute monoarticular arthritis of any peripheral joint except the glenohumeral joint of the shoulder.*
- In gout, crystals of monosodium urate (MSU) appear as needle-shaped intracellular and extracellular crystals.
- When examined with a polarizing filter and red compensator filter, they are yellow when aligned parallel to the slow axis of the red compensator but turn blue when aligned across the direction of polarization (i.e, they exhibit negative birefringence).
- Negatively birefringent urate crystals are seen on polarizing examination in 85% of specimens. Microscopic analysis in pseudo-gout shows calcium pyrophosphate (CPP) crystals, which appear shorter than MSU crystals and are often rhomboidal.

Radiological Changes in Gout in Hands	Crystal of Uric Acid in Joint Aspiration
1. Eccentric juxta-articular lobulated soft-tissue masses 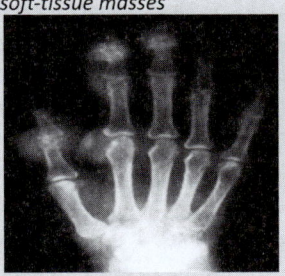 2. Preservation of joint space initially Absence of periarticular demineralization Erosion of joint margins with sclerosis Cartilage destruction late. 3. Bone findings "Punched-out" lytic bone lesion ± sclerosis of margin "Mouse / rat bite" from erosion of long-standing soft-tissue tophus "Overhanging margin" (40%) called as *Martel sign*.	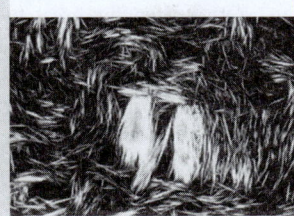

185. Ans. (a) Gout

(Ref: Harrison 20th edition, p 2631-2632; Harrison 19th ed. / 2233-34)

- In approximately 40% of cases, the gouty erosions have a raised margin or lip that radiologically is referred to as Martel's hook or Martel's Sign. No loss of bone density is expected
- The osteological signs of gout can be located on the joint surfaces, around the joint itself, or even at a distance from the joint.
- Lesions from gout have a diagnostic appearance on radiographs that radiologists refer to as a "punched out" appearance, and which can be seen as crescent-shaped erosions, with smooth, well remodelled margins, on dry bone
- Lesions vary in size, are usually rounded or oval, and may have a sclerotic border.

186. Ans. (b) Muscle

(Ref: CMDT 2014 ch.20, p 812)

- Although gout typically causes joint inflammation, it can also cause inflammation in other synovial-based structures, such as bursae and tendons. Tophi are collections of urate crystals in the soft tissues. They tend to develop after about a decade in untreated patients who develop chronic gouty arthritis. Tophi may develop earlier in older women, particularly those receiving diuretics.
- Tophi are classically located along the helix of the ear, but they can be found in multiple locations, including the fingers, the toes, the prepatellar bursa, and along the olecranon, where they can resemble rheumatoid nodules. Rarely, a creamy discharge may be present.
- The finding of an apparent rheumatoid nodule in a patient with a negative rheumatoid factor assay or a history of

drainage from a nodule should prompt consideration of gout in the differential diagnosis.

187. Ans. (a) High synovial fluid protein

(Ref: Harrison 19th edition, p 2236)

- When a patient presents with acute inflammatory monoarticular arthritis, aspiration of the involved joint is critical to rule out an infectious arthritis and to attempt to confirm a diagnosis of gout or pseudogout on the basis of identification of crystals.
- Crystals must be distinguished from birefringent cartilaginous or other debris. Debris may have fuzzy borders and may be curved, whereas crystals have sharp borders and are straight. Uric acid crystals exhibit negative birefrigence.
- Synovial fluid should also be sent for cell count. During acute attacks, the synovial fluid is inflammatory, with a WBC count higher than 2000/μL (class II fluid) and possibly higher than 50, 000/μL, with a predominance of polymorpho-nuclear neutrophils, though low WBC counts are occasionally found.
- Synovial fluid glucose levels are usually normal, whereas they may be depressed in septic arthritis and occasionally in rheumatoid arthritis. Measurement of synovial fluid protein has no clinical value.

188. Ans. (a) Allopurinol

(Ref: Harrison 19th edition, p 2233)

Xanthine oxidase inhibitor; inhibits conversion of hypoxanthine to xanthine to uric acid; decreases production of uric acid without disrupting synthesis of vital purines.

189. Ans. (d) Treatment with Allopurinol should be started immediately in the case of acute gout

(Ref: Harrison 19th edition, p 2233)

- Gout has a male predominance. Estrogenic hormones have a mild uricosuric effect, and gout is therefore unusual in premenopausal women. For pseudo-gout, the male-to-female ratio is approximately 50:50.
- Measurement of serum uric acid is the most misused test in the diagnosis of gout. The presence of hyperuricemia in the absence of symptoms is not diagnostic of gout. In addition, as many as 15% of patients with symptoms from gout may have normal serum uric acid levels at the time of their attack. Thus, the diagnosis of gout can be missed if the joint is not aspirated.
- The spontaneous onset of excruciating pain, edema, and inflammation in the metatarsal-phalangeal joint of the great toe is highly suggestive of acute crystal-induced arthritis. Podagra is the initial joint manifestation in 50% of gout cases; eventually, it is involved in 90% of cases. Podagra is not synonymous with gout, however: it may also be observed in patients with pseudogout, sarcoidosis, gonococcal arthritis, psoriatic arthritis, and reactive arthritis.
- Therapy to control the underlying hyperuricemia generally is contraindicated until the acute attack is controlled (unless kidneys are at risk because of an unusually heavy uric acid load). Starting therapy to control hyperuricemia during an acute attack may intensify and prolong the attack. If the patient has been on a consistent dosage of probenecid or

allopurinol at the time of the acute attack, however, the drug should be continued at that dosage during the attack.

190. Ans. (a) Acute gouty arthritis

(Ref: Harrison 19th edition, p 2233)

Allopurinol is the drug of choice in patients with
1. Severe tophaceous deposits
2. Uric acid nephropathy/nephrolithiasis.
3. The drug is also preferred as a pretreatment agent to protect against uric acid nephropathy in patients with lymphoproliferative or myelopro-liferative disorders.

Sudden Increase or decrease in serum levels of uric acid can trigger acute gout attack. Allopurinol initially mobilizes uric acid stored in the tissues and increase serum uric acid level, which can make the situation worse in an acute gouty attack or can trigger a gout attack in chronic hyperurecemic patients. Thats why its not indicated in an acute gout attack. When we start allopurinol as prophylactic in chronic hyper-urecemic patients, we should warn the patient about this and also give colchicine or NSAIDs with allopurinol for the first few weeks to avoid a flare of it.

191. Ans. (b) Aspirin

(Ref: CMDT 2014 ch.20, p 812)

- Allopurinol blocks xanthine oxidase and thus reduces the generation of uric acid.
- Probenecid is filtered at the glomerulus, secreted in the proximal tubule and reabsorbed in the distal tubule. Probenecid works by interfering with the kidneys' organic anion transporter (OAT), which reclaims uric acid from the urine and returns it to the plasma.
- Sulfinpyrazone works by competitively inhibiting uric acid reabsorption in the proximal tubule of the kidney.

192. Ans. (b) Febuxostat

(Ref: Harrison 19th edition, p 1871/2235)

- Febuxostat, a non-purine selective inhibitor of xanthine oxidase, is a potential alternative to allopurinol in patients with gout.
- Febuxostat is administered orally and is metabolized mainly in the liver. In contrast, allopurinol and its metabolites are excreted primarily by the kidney. Therefore, febuxostat can be used in patients with renal impairment with no dosage adjustment.

193. Ans. (d) Most common joint involved is DIP

(Ref: Harrison 19th edition, p 2235/372e-8t)

Many cases of pseudogout in elderly people are idiopathic, but pseudogout has also been associated with trauma and with many different metabolic abnormalities, the most common of which are hyperparathyroidism and hemochromatosis. Risk factors for pseudogout include use of loop diuretics (but not thiazide diuretics) and proton pump inhibitors, which cause hypomagnesemia. The most common joint involved is knee joint.

194. Ans. (b) Glenohumeral joint

(Ref: Harrison 19th edition, p 2145)

Other than the great toe, the most common sites of gouty arthritis are the instep, ankle, wrist, finger joints, and knee. In early gout, only 1 or 2 joints are usually involved. Consider the diagnosis in any patient with acute monoarticular arthritis of any peripheral joint except the glenohumeral joint of the shoulder.

195. Ans. (b) Uricosuria

(Ref: Harrison 19th edition, p 431e-5)

- In gout, crystals of monosodium urate (MSU) appear as needle-shaped intracellular and extracellular crystals. When examined with a polarizing filter and red compensator filter, they are yellow when aligned parallel to the slow axis of the red compensator but turn blue when aligned across the direction of polarization (ie, they exhibit negative birefringence). *Negatively birefringent urate crystals are seen on polarizing examination in 85% of specimens.*

Osteoarthritis and Psoriatic Arthritis

196. Ans. (a) Arthritis

(Ref: Harrison 20th edition, p 2631; Harrison 19th edition, p 2232)

- For patients with symptomatic knee or hip OA, who are unwilling to undergo total joint arthroplasty, opioid analgesics have shown modest efficacy. Duloxetine can also be used.
- Glucosamine or chondroitin supplementation has been used for OA but large publicly supported trials have failed to show any benefit.
- A pubmed search also reveals a meta-analysis conducted in 2017 stating no benefit of glucosamine in Osteoarthritis.

197. Ans. (a) Paracetamol

(Ref: Harrison 20th edition, p 2630; Harrison 19th edition, p 2231)

- NSAIDS are the most popular but Paracetamol is the initial analgesic of choice for patients with OA in knee hip or hands.
- The dose required may go up to 1-4 grams per day.
- Considering the age of the patient and increased rates of cardio-vascular events associated with COX-2 inhibitors and with some conventional NSAIDs such as diclofenac many of these drugs are not appropriate long term treatment choices for older persons with osteoarthritis especially those at high risk of heart diseases or stroke.

198. Ans. (b) Osteoarthritis

(Ref: Harrison 20th edition, p 2624; Harrison 19th edition, p 2226)

- Osteoarthritis predominantly involves the weight-bearing joints, including the knees, hips, cervical and lumbosacral spine, and feet. Other commonly affected joints include the distal interphalangeal (DIP), proximal interphalangeal (PIP), and carpometacarpal (CMC) joints.

- Heberden nodes, which represent palpable osteophytes in the DIP joints, are more characteristic in women than in men.

199. Ans. (d) Distal carpophalangeal joint

(Ref: Harrison 19th edition, p 2230)

200. Ans. (d) Deposit of calcium salts

(Ref: Harrison 19th edition, p 2230)

In the load-bearing areas, radiographs can depict
1. Joint-space loss
2. Subchondral bony sclerosis
3. Cyst formation.
4. Osteophytes form because of the increase in a damaged joint's surface area. This is most common from the onset of arthritis. Osteophytes usually limit joint movement and typically cause pain.

201. Ans. (c) Osteoarthritis

(Ref: Harrison 20th edition, p 2625f; Harrison 19th edition, p 2226f)

202. Ans. (d) All of above

(Ref: Harrison 20th edition, p 2571-2572; Harrison 19th edition, p 2175)

- Characteristics of peripheral Psoriatic arthritis include DIP involvement, including the classic "pencil-in-cup" deformity; marginal erosions with adjacent bony proliferation ("whiskering"); small-joint ankylosis; osteolysis of phalangeal and metacarpal bone, with telescoping of digits; and periostitis and proliferative new bone at sites of enthesitis.
- A total of five patterns of the disease are described
    1. Arthritis of the DIP joints
    2. Asymmetric oligoarthritis
    3. Symmetric polyarthritis similar to RA
    4. Axial involvement (spine and sacroiliac joints)
    5. Arthritis mutilans, a highly destructive form of disease

Behçet's Disease Dermatomyositis and Polymyositis

203. Ans. (a) Ocular lesions

(Ref: Textbook of Rheumatology E-book, 9th edition, p 1528)

- In the International criteria for Behçet disease, genital aphthous lesions and eye lesions have more diagnostic value than the others. They each get 2 points.
- The remaining 4 items (Oral aphthosis, Skin lesions, Vascular manifestations, Positive Pathergy test) get one point each.
- The patient has to *get 3 or more points* to be diagnosed/classified as having Behçet's Disease.

Criteria for diagnosis of Behçet disease

Sign/symptom	Points
Ocular lesions	2
Genital aphthosis	2
Oral aphthaosis	2
Skin lesions	1
Neurological manifestations	1
Vascular manifestations	1
Positive pathergy test*	1*

*Pathology test is optional and the primary scoring system does not include pathergy testing. However, where pathergy testing is conducted one extra point may be assigned for a positive result.

204. Ans. (d) Anti- Jo-1 antibody

(Ref: Harrison 19th edition, p 2199-2200)

Myositis Specific Antibodies

Anti Jo-1 and anti synthetase antibodies	Polymyositis and dermatomyositis with Interstitial lung disease, arthritis, mechanic's hands
Anti –Mi-2	Dermatomyositis with rash
Anti MDAS	Dermatomyositis with rapidly progressive lung disease
Anti -140	Juvenile dermatomyositis
Anti-Signal recognition particle	Severe acute necrotising myopathy

205. Ans. (c) Creatinine Kinase levels

(Ref: Harrison 20th edition, p 2591-2592)

The clinical diagnosis based on proximal muscle weakness, gottron papules over her knuckles is suggestive of diagnosis of dermatomyositis. Since the questions says next logical step it would be to perform CK levels.

Nerve conduction Study	Not useful in muscle disorders
RA factor	Screening for Rheumatoid arthritis and negative in Dermatomyositis
CK levels	Most sensitive enzyme is CK, which in active disease can be elevated as much as fiftyfold. It is sensitive and hence should be next investigation in this patient.
NM junction study	NM junction study would be a Single fiber EMG reduction of the motor unit action potentials in the proximal muscles and fibrillation potentials suggestive of fiber splitting, necrosis, and vacuolization

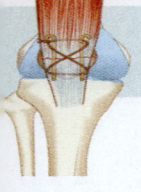

Investigations in case of juvenile dermatomyositis

1. *The most sensitive enzyme is CK, which in active disease can be elevated as much as fiftyfold. Along with the CK, the serum glutamic-oxaloacetic and glutamate pyruvate transaminases, lactate dehydrogenase, and aldolase may be elevated.*
2. Myositis-specific antibody assays such as antibodies against the aminoacyl t-RNA synthetases (i.e., anti-Jo-1 antibody), anti-signal recognition particle (anti-SRP antibody), and nuclear helicase (anti-Mi-2 antibody).
3. Nail-fold capillary microscopy may show end-row loop capillary loss and formation of bushy loops representing capillary dilatation and branching.
4. Magnetic resonance imaging (MRI) with T2-weighted fat suppression and short tau inversion recovery (STIR) is useful in the diagnostic workup because it reveals edema, a marker of muscle inflammation.
5. Electromyography (EMG) reveals a reduction of the motor unit action potentials in the proximal muscles and fibrillation potentials suggestive of fiber splitting, necrosis, and vacuolization.
6. *Muscle biopsy—in spite of occasional variability in demonstrating all of the typical pathologic findings—is the most sensitive and specific test for establishing the diagnosis of inflammatory myopathy and for excluding other neuromuscular diseases. Inflammation is the histologic hallmark for these diseases*

206. Ans. (d) Livedo Reticularis

(*Ref: Harrison 20th edition, p 2589-2590; Harrison 19th edition, p 2194*)

Orogenital ulcers (Choice A) Uveitis (Choice C)	Diagnosis of Behçet's disease is recurrent oral ulceration plus two of the following: 1. Recurrent genital ulceration 2. Eye lesions (most commonly uveitis) 3. Skin lesions 4. Pathergy test
Polyarthritis	Non-deforming arthritis or arthralgias are seen in a 50% of patients and affects the knees and ankles. The arthritis is non-deforming and asymmetric in nature and can assume a mono-articular, oligo-articular, or poly-articular pattern of involvement.
Livedo reticularis	It is a reddish-violet reticular discoloration of the skin that mainly affects the limbs. It is caused by an interruption of blood flow in the dermal arteries, either due to spasm, inflammation, or vascular obstruction, and is associated with diseases of varying etiology and severity which are given below and *do not include Behçet disease*

Secondary livedo reticularis is of known cause. It may be a sign of vasculitis (inflammation of the blood vessels) or of obstruction of the vessel by some circulating material. The following conditions may be responsible:

Vasculitis	Obstruction
1. Polyarteritisnodosa 2. Systemic lupus erythematosus 3. Dermatomyositis 4. Rheumatoid arthritis 5. Lymphoma 6. Pancreatitis 7. Tuberculosis	1. Cryoglobulinaemia 2. Antiphospholipid syndrome 3. Hypercalcaemia 4. Polycythaemiarubraverathrombo-cythaemia 5. Infections 6. Arteriosclerosis 7. Homocystinuria 8. Intra-arterial injection (drug addicts) 9. Amantadine

207. Ans. (c) Ocular Muscle

(*Ref: Harrison 19th edition, p 2194*)

Polymyositis is a subacute inflammatory myopathy affecting adults, and rarely children, who *do not have* any of the following:
1. Rash
2. *Involvement of the extraocular and facial muscles*
3. Family history of a neuromuscular disease,
4. History of exposure to myotoxic drugs or toxins,
5. Endocrinopathy, neurogenic disease, muscular dystrophy, biochemical muscle disorder
6. IBM as excluded by muscle biopsy analysis

208. Ans. (a) Behçet Disease

(*Ref: Harrison 20th edition, p 2589-2592; Harrison 19th edition, p 2194*)

- Although Behçet's disease is classified among the vasculitides laboratory diagnostic does not include regularly autoantibodies associated with vascular manifestations of systemic autoimmune diseases.
- The autoantigens for pemphigus vulgaris and pemphigus foliaceus are desmoglein 3 and desmoglein 1, respectively.
- The anti-desmoglein 1 antibodies in pemphigus foliaceus and anti-desmoglein 3 antibodies in pemphigus vulgaris are pathogenic.
- Anti- tissue transglutaminase antibodies are pathognomonic for celiac disease.
- Anti- nuclear antibody is seen in SLE
- Causes of Apthous Ulcers:

Infections:
- Viral (Herpes, CMV, EBV, HIV)
- Fungal (Candida)
- Bacterial (Vincent's infection, syphilis)

Dermatological:
- Pemphigus, pemphigoid, lichen planus

Drug :
- Chemotherapy drugs
- Erythema multiforme, Stevens-Johnson syndrome

Systemic diseases:
- Behçet's syndrome, SLE

Nutritional:
- Vitamin deficiency (Vitamin B and C), iron deficiency

Neoplasia:
- Leukemia, squamous cell carcinoma, Kaposi's sarcoma

Gastrointestinal:
- Crohn's disease, celiac disease

Traumatic
- Dentures

Chemical or thermal burns:
- Corrosives, hot liquids

209. Ans. (a) There is a strong association with HLA-B7

(Ref: Harrison 20th edition, p 2589; Harrison 19th edition, p 2194)

- HLA B7 is associated with sarcoidosis and with increased risk of cervical cancer.
- The main pathologic lesion in Behçet is systemic perivasculitis with early neutrophil infiltration and endothelial swelling. In some patients, diffuse inflammatory disease, involving all layers of large vessels and resulting in formation of pseudoaneurysms, suggests vasculitis of vasa vasorum
- Nonspecific skin inflammatory reactivity to any scratches or intradermal saline injection (pathergy test) is a common and specific manifestation.
- Uveitis and CNS-Behçet's syndrome require systemic glucocorticoid therapy (prednisone, 1 mg/kg per day) and azathioprine (2–3 mg/kg per day).

210. Ans. (b) Reiter's disease

(Ref: Harrison 20th edition, p 2560-2570; Harrison 19th edition, p 2174)

Reiter Syndrome is Associated with:
1. Conjunctivitis
2. Uveitis
3. Urethritis
4. Arthritis
5. Keratoderma blenorrhagicum

211. Ans. (a) Behçet's syndrome

(Ref: Harrison 20th edition, p 2589; Harrison 19th edition, p 2194)

212. Ans. (c) Glans penis Apthous ulceration

(Ref: Harrison 20th edition, p 2589-2590; Harrison 19th edition, p 2194)

- In Behçet's disease the genital ulcers are less common but more specific, are painful, do not affect the glans penis or urethra, and produce scrotal scars. Epididymitis is seen in 5% of patients. It is a connective tissue disorder where the males and females are affected equally, but males often have more severe disease.
- Skin involvement is observed in 80% of patients and includes folliculitis, erythema, Sweet's syndrome, and Pyoderma Gangrenosum.
- Superficial or deep peripheral vein thrombosis is seen in 30% of patients
- Eye involvement with scarring and bilateral panuveitis is the most dreaded complication, since it occasionally progresses rapidly to blindness. In addition to iritis, posterior uveitis, retinal vessel occlusions, and optic neuritis can be seen in some patients with the syndrome.

213. Ans. (a) Dermatomyositis

(Ref: Harrison 20th edition, p 2591; Harrison 19th edition, p 2202)

- Characteristic, possibly pathognomonic cutaneous features of dermatomyositis: Heliotrope, Gottron papules.
- Characteristic but not pathognomonic features of dermatomyositis:

  a. Malar erythema, poikiloderma in a photosensitive distribution
  b. Violaceous erythema on the extensor surfaces, and periungual and cuticular changes
  c. Flat, red rash involving the face and upper trunk or other body surfaces, including knees, elbows, neck, anterior chest (ie, v sign), or back and shoulders (i.e., shawl sign)

214. Ans. (c) Seen only in Tropics

(Ref: Harrison 20th edition, p 2589-2590; Harrison 19th edition, p 2194)

215. Ans. (b) Behçet's syndrome

(Ref: Harrison 20th edition, p 2590; Harrison 19th edition, p 2194)

Recurrent bilateral Hypopyon is a characteristic feature of Behçet's syndrome.

Behçet's syndrome is also associated with thrombophlebitis which is therefore the single best answer of choice.

Sicca/Sjogren Syndrome

216. Ans. (c) Saliva has increased concentration of Phosphate

(Ref: Harrison 20th edition, p 2560-2562; Harrison 19th edition, p 2168)

- Sjögren syndrome leads to reduced salivary flow with unstimulated whole salivary flow<1.5ml in 15 minutes.
- The normal pH of saliva is 6.0 to 7.5. The buffer systems responsible for human saliva buffer capacity include the bicarbonate, phosphate and protein systems. These systems protect the teeth against demineralization by maintaining optimal pH for hydroxyapatite.
- In Sjogren syndrome the value of phosphate in saliva is reduced leading to lower pH values and development of dental caries.
- Normal concentrations of total calcium, total protein and levels of amylase activity indicate that the remaining functional acinar cells are capable of synthesis and secretion of primary saliva with normal composition despite the marked lymphocytic infiltration and structural changes.

Sialo-metric analysis of saliva in Sjögren Syndrome

Contents increased	Contents reduced	Contents normal
Sodium Chloride IgA	Phosphate, bicarbonate buffer systems	Calcium Protein Amylase

217. Ans. (a) Cevimeline

(Ref: CMDT 2016 p 837)

Cevimeline hydrochloride is a cholinergic agent with muscarinic agonist activity prominently affecting the M1 and M3 receptors prevalent in exocrine glands. This increases the salivary secretions and reduced the dry mouth manifestations in Xerostomia. Other drug used is pilocarpine.

218. Ans. (a) Also found in Sjogren Syndrome; **(b)** May also present normally; **(c)** It is basically IgM

(Ref: Harrison 20th edition, p 2523; Harrison 19th edition, p 2143)
Anti CCP antibody is diagnostic of rheumatoid arthritis.

219. Ans. (a) MALToma

(Ref: Harrison 20th edition, p 2561t; Harrison 19th edition, p 2167t)

- Among patients with Sjögren syndrome, the incidence of non-Hodgkin lymphoma is 4.3% (18.9 times higher than in the general population), with a median age at diagnosis of 58 years. The mean time to the development of non-Hodgkin lymphoma after the onset of Sjögren syndrome is 7.5 years.
- *The most common histologic subtype of non-Hodgkin lymphoma in Sjögren syndrome is mucosa-associated lymphoid tissue (MALT) lymphoma, which can develop in any non-lymphoid tissue infiltrated by periepithelial lymphoid tissue—most commonly the salivary glands, but also the stomach, nasopharynx, skin, liver, kidneys, and lungs.*

220. Ans. (b) Midline granuloma

(Ref: Harrison 20th edition, p 2560-2562; Harrison 19th edition, p 2167t)

- Primary Sjögren syndrome occurs in the absence of another underlying rheumatic disorder, whereas secondary Sjögren syndrome is associated with another underlying rheumatic disease, such as systemic lupus erythematosus (SLE), rheumatoid arthritis (RA), or scleroderma.
- Sjögren like syndromes are seen in patients infected with HIV, HTLV-1, and hepatitis C.

221. Ans. (d) Systemic manifestations

(Ref: Harrison 20th edition, p 2561-2562; Harrison 19th edition, p 1857)

222. Ans. (a) Midline granuloma

(Ref: Harrison 20th edition, p 2560-2562; Table: 324.1, Harrison 19th edition, p 2167)

Kawasaki Disease

223. Ans. (c) Thrombocytopenia

(Ref: Harrison 20th edition, p 2588; Harrison 19th edition, p 2193)

224. Ans. (c) Immunoglobulins

(Ref: Harrison 20th edition, p 2588; Nelsons 18th/1038; Harrison 19th edition, p 2193)

Miscellaneous

225. Ans. (a) Fractures

(Ref: Harrison 20th edition, p 2976)

- Mutations in major structural components of elastic fibres, especially elastin, fibrillin and fibulin-5, cause severe, often life-threatening, heritable connective tissue diseases such as Marfan syndrome, Menkes Syndrome, and Cutis laxa
- Abnormalities in elastin are also found in patients with supravalvular aortic stenosis, Cutis laxa, Costello syndrome and Fragile X syndrome.
- Choices C and D are presentations of Marfan syndrome.
- Fractures are a feature of osteogenesis imperfecta which occurs due to collagen I structural mutations.

226. Ans. (b) 400-420 nm

(Ref: Fitzpatrick color atlas, 8th edition, p 211)

- Porphyrin are excited by visible light with a wavelength between 400 and 410 nm and emit an intense red fluorescence. The released energy reacts with oxygen to produce free radicals and singlet oxygen that damages tissues.

227. Ans. (b) Henoch Schonlein purpura

(Ref: Rudolph paediatrics 22nd edition, p 1537)

- The image shows presence of extensor purpura visible on buttocks and extensor part of thigh and ankles. The presence of concomitant joint pain indicates IgA dominant immune deposits involving skin, gut and glomeruli.

228. Ans. (b) Osteoporosis

(Ref: Differential diagnosis in conventional radiology: 3rd edition, p 3)

- The image shows X-Ray of lumbo-sacral spine showing *codfish or fish mouth vertebra* with *irregularly reduced intervertebral joint space.* This is a feature of osteoporosis.
- The bone softening leads to exaggeration of the normal concavity of the superior and inferior surfaces of one or more vertebral bodies

229. Ans. (b) H.S.P

(Ref: Harrison: 19th edition, p 2190)

- The combination of fever, extensor palpable purpuric rash and GIT symptoms favour diagnosis of Henoch Schonlein purpura in the child.
- ITP is ruled out as it has non palpable purpura.
- Meningococcemia will cause a rash on lower extremities but will not have a predilection for extensor sites.
- Wegeners' granulomatosis presents with epistaxis, haematuria and haemoptysis.

230. Ans. (d) Mostly due to degranulation of mast cells

(Ref: Harrison 19th edition, p 363 and 2117)

The image shows presence of angioedema and the transmitter involved is histamine and bradykinin. There is a fast increase in local vascular permeability in subcutaneous and submucosal tissue.

Choice B is wrong	ACE inhibitors and ARB both cause angioedema though the incidence with ARB is lesser. Cough is however only seen with ACE inhibitors.
Choice C is wrong	Hereditary angioedema is an autosomal dominant disease caused by low levels of the plasma protein C1 inhibitor (C1-INH). Deficiencies in C1-INH allow unchecked activation of the classic complement pathway and *increase in Bradykinin levels*

Acute episodes often involve the lip, eyes, and face; however, angioedema may affect other parts of body, including respiratory and gastrointestinal (GI) mucosa. Laryngeal swelling can be life-threatening.

Angioedema with identifiable etiologies include those caused by the following:
- Hypersensitivity (e.g. food, drugs, or insect stings)
- Physical stimuli (e.g. cold or vibrations)
- Autoimmune disease or infection
- ACE inhibitors and ARB (Lower incidence as compared to ACE inhibitor)
- NSAIDs
- C1-INH deficiency (hereditary and acquired)

231. Ans. (a) Subcutaneous nodules

(Ref: Harrison 19th edition, p 2173)

Clinical features of Reactive arthritis:
1. Arthritis is usually asymmetric and additive involving the joints of the lower extremities, especially the knee, ankle, and subtalar, metatarsophalangeal, and toe interphalangeal joints.
2. Tendinitis and fasciitis are particularly characteristic lesions, producing pain at multiple insertion sites (entheses), especially the Achilles insertion.
3. In males, urethritis may be marked or relatively asymptomatic.
4. Ocular disease is common, ranging from transient, asymptomatic conjunctivitis to an aggressive anterior uveitis that occasionally proves refractory to treatment and may result in blindness.
5. Oral ulcers tend to be superficial, transient, and often asymptomatic.
6. The characteristic skin lesions, *keratoderma blenorrhagica*, consist of vesicles that become hyperkeratotic, ultimately forming a crust before disappearing. They are most common on the palms and soles but may occur elsewhere as well.
7. Lesions may occur on the glans penis, termed *circinate balanitis*; these consist of vesicles that quickly rupture to form painless superficial erosions.

232. Ans. (c) Ulcerative Colitis

(Ref: Harrison 19th edition, p 1952-53; Robbins 9th edition p 215-220)

Diseases Mediated by Antibodies and Immune Complexes

DISEASES MEDIATED BY ANTIBODIES AND IMMUNE COMPLEXES
1. Autoimmune hemolytic anemia
2. Autoimmune thrombocytopenia
3. Myasthenia gravis
4. Grave's disease
5. Goodpasture syndrome
6. Systemic lupus erythematosus (SLE)

DISEAES MEDIATED BY T CELLS
1. Type 1 diabetes mellitus
2. Multiple sclerosis
3. Rheumatoid arthritis
4. Systemic sclerosis
5. Sjogren syndrome

DISEASES CAUSED BY AUTOIMMUNITY OR BY REACTIONS TO MICROBIAL ANTIGENS
1. *Inflammatory bowel disease (Crohn disease, ulcerative colitis)*
2. Inflammatory myopathies

233. Ans. (b) Sarcoidosis

(Ref: Harrison 19th edition, p 237, 417)

- Painful ulcers in mouth
- Apthous ulcers
- Behçet disease
- Denture stomatitis
- Thermal burns
- Tuberculosis
- Herpes
- Carcinoma tongue
- Arsenic poisoning

234. Ans (a) Mucopolysaccharidosis

(Ref: Harrison 19th edition, p 432e-1)

Notice the coarse facies with short stature and short stubby deformed fingers.

The diagnosis is MPS type IV (Morquio's) characterised by Orthopedic involvement (eg, spondyloepiphyseal dysplasia) as the primary finding; preservation of intelligence; genu valgum, short stature, spinal curvature, odontoid hypoplasia, ligamentous laxity, and atlantoaxial instability.

Remember the most common form of MPS is however type 3 MPS.

235. Ans. (b) C1 inhibitor concentrate

(Ref: Oxford handbook of medicine, 2nd edition, chapter 12, p 736-38, Harrison 19th edition, p 1874)

- In HAE types I and II, the **treatment of choice in acute attacks consists of replacement with commercially available C1 inhibitor (C1-INH) concentrates** or kallikrein inhibitor or, if those are unavailable, fresh-frozen plasma. In HAE type III, infusion of C1-INH has proven to be ineffective.
- For prophylaxis, attenuated androgens are currently the initial mode of treatment. Therapy should be minimized, balancing disease severity with minimizing adverse effects. The drug most commonly used is danazol, but all attenuated androgens are useful in treatment.
- Icatibant is a selective bradykinin B2 receptor antagonist approved for use in HAE
- The World Allergy Organization (WAO) issued the following 2013 recommendations for the management of hereditary angioedema types I and II (HAE-I/II)

Contd...

1. Consider on-demand treatment for all HAE attacks that (1) result in debilitation/dysfunction and/or (2) involve the face, neck, or abdomen; attacks affecting the upper airways must be treated
2. Treat all HAE attacks as early as possible with C1-INH, ecallantide, or icatibant; do not use oral anti-fibrinolytics as on-demand treatment
3. Consider intubation or tracheotomy early in progressive upper airway edema

236. Ans. (b) Type 2

(Ref: Clinical microbiology and Infectious Diseases, 2nd edition, p 30, Harrison 19th edition, p 232)

- Type V hypersensitivity reactions were additionally added to the scheme originally described by Coombs and Gell. Contrary to type IV and in agreement with types I, II, and III, respectively, they are mediated by antibodies too.
- The type V reactions are sometimes considered as a subtype of the type II hypersensitivity.
- **Graves disease** is characterised by production of antibodies directed against the TSH binding receptor that subsequently stimulate the thyroid gland, resulting in production of hormones (thyroxine and triiodothyronine). As antibodies increase the function of a target organ, this type of hypersensitivity is called stimulatory.
- Autoantibodies cannot only stimulate cells of a target organ/tissue, however, on the contrary, also to inhibit it (hence the designation–inhibitory hypersensitivity reactions). A prototype of such a situation is **myasthenia gravis**. It is an autoimmune disease characterised by production of autoantibodies directed against the acetylcholine receptors (AchR) present in neuro-muscular plates.
- **In some patients of Pernicious anemia** subgroup of antibodies to intrinsic factor are directly induced. Without intrinsic factor, the ileum can no longer absorb the B12 and the disease develops.

237. Ans. (d) Inclusion body Myositis

(Ref: Chapter 323, Harrison 19th edition, p 2154)

- Patients who have localized Scleroderma coexisting with features of SLE, polymyositis, and rheumatoid arthritis may have mixed connective tissue disease (MCTD).
- This overlap syndrome is generally associated with the presence of high titers of autoantibodies to U1-RNP.
- The characteristic initial presentation is Raynaud's phenomenon associated with puffy fingers and myalgia. Gradually, lcSSc features of sclerodactyly, calcinosis, and cutaneous telangiectasia develop.
- Skin rashes suggestive of systemic lupus erythematosus (malar rash, photosensitivity) or of dermatomyositis (heliotrope rash on the eyelids, erythematous rash on the knuckles) occur

238. Ans. (c) Severe combined immunodeficiency

(Ref: Harrison 19th edition, p 563)

Choice	Cancers associated
Sjogren syndrome	NHL mainly MALT-oma involving salivary glands>stomach.

Contd...

| Ataxia telengectasia | Elevated incidence of cancers, approximately 100-fold in comparison to the general population. In children, more than 85% of neoplasm cases are acute lymphocytic leukemia or lymphoma. in adults with ataxia-telangiectasia, solid tumors are more frequent |
| Lynch-II syndrome | Gastrointestinal cancer associated with endometrial/ovarian carcinoma. Early onset brain tumor and lymphoma also seen in children. |

- Severe combined immunodeficiency (SCID) is a disorder that results from any of a heterogenous group of genetic conditions affecting the immune system. Leading to severe T and B cell dysfunction.
- *Cellular hallmarks that help differentiate between various forms of SCID are as follows:*
- X-linked SCID. Lymphopenia occurs primarily from the absence or near absence of T cells (CD3+) and natural killer (NK) cells. Variable levels of B cells occur, which do not make functional antibodies.
- AK3 deficiency: Lymphopenia occurs primarily from the absence or near absence of T cells (CD3+) and NK cells. Normal or high levels of B cells occur, which do not make functional antibodies.
- ADA deficiency: Lymphopenia occurs from the death of T and B cells secondary to the accumulation of toxic metabolites in the purine salvage pathway. Functional antibodies are decreased or absent.
- ZAP-70 deficiency: Lymphopenia occurs because of the absence of CD8+ T cells. As in all types of SCID, no antibody formation is present.

239. Ans. (a) Mumps

(Ref: CMDT 2014 ch.32, p 1370)

240. Ans. (c) CECT of chest

(Ref: Harrison 19th edition, p 2236)

- The chest roentgenogram remains the most commonly used tool to assess lung involvement in patients of sarcoidosis and can identify hilar adenopathy with infiltrates and pulmonary fibrosis. CT scan is also used for better evaluation of alveolitis and resultant fibrosis but contrast study is not required.
- Patients with pulmonary sarcoidosis frequently have increased numbers of lymphocytes and a high ratio of CD4+ to CD8+ T-lymphocytes (CD4/CD8 ratio) in bronchoalveolar lavage (BAL) fluid
- The positive emission tomography (PET) scan has increasingly replaced gallium 67 scanning to identify areas of sarcoidosis in the chest and other parts of the body.
- Serum levels of angiotensin-converting enzyme (ACE) can be helpful in the diagnosis of sarcoidosis. However, the test has somewhat low sensitivity and specificity. Elevated levels of ACE are reported in 60% of patients with acute disease and only 20% of patients with chronic disease.
- Gross elevation of ESR is seen in

1. Sarcoidosis,
2. Leprosy,
3. Gaucher's disease,
4. Hyperthyroidism,
5. Disseminated granulomatous

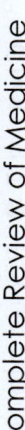

241. Ans. (a) Amyloidosis

(Ref: Harrison 19th edition, p 732)

- In amyloidosis, the typical organs involved include the kidney, liver, and spleen. AA type develops in setting of chronic inflammatory disease like bronchiectasis or lung abscess. The edema and hypoproteinemia is explained by nephrotic range proteinuria and hepato-splenomegaly by liver and spleen deposition
- Lung abscess can lead to Cor pulmonale with Right sided heart failure. This can explain hepatomegaly and development of edema but splenomegaly and hypoproteinemia is not a feature of CHF.

242. Ans. (d) Friedreich's ataxia

(Ref: Harrison 19th edition, p 2629)

Neuropathic joints refers to progressive degeneration of a weight bearing joint, a process marked by bony destruction, bone resorption, and eventual deformity. Onset is usually insidious. If this pathological process continues unchecked; it could result in joint deformity, ulceration and/or superinfection, loss of function, and in the worst-case scenario, amputation or death.

Causes of Neuropathic Joint

1. Diabetes mellitus neuropathy (the most common in the U.S. today, resulting in destruction of foot and ankle joints), with Charcot joints in 1/600-700 diabetics. Related to long-term poor glucose control.
2. Alcoholic neuropathy
3. Cerebral palsy
4. Leprosy
5. Syphilis (tabes dorsalis)
6. Spinal cord injury
7. Myelomeningocele
8. Syringomyelia
9. Intra-articular steroid injections
10. Congenital insensitivity to pain

243. Ans. (a) Peripheral motor and sensory neuropathy

(Ref: CMDT 2014 ch.13, p 530)

ATTR usually presents as a syndrome of familial amyloidotic polyneuropathy or familial amyloidotic cardiomyopathy. Peripheral neuropathy usually begins as a lower-extremity sensory and motor neuropathy and progresses to the upper extremities. Autonomic neuropathy is manifest by gastrointestinal symptoms of diarrhea with weight loss and orthostatic hypotension.

244. Ans. (a) Shigella Flexneri

(Ref: Harrison 19th edition, p 2173)

Organisms that have been associated with Reiter Arthritis include the following:
1. C trachomatis (L2b serotype)
2. Ureaplasma urealyticum
3. Neisseria gonorrhoeae
4. Shigella flexneri
5. Salmonella enterica serovars Typhimurium
6. Mycoplasma pneumoniae
7. Mycobacterium tuberculosis
8. Yersinia enterocolitica and pseudotuberculosis
9. Campylobacter jejuni
10. Clostridium difficile
11. Beta-hemolytic (example, group A) and viridans streptococci

245. Ans. (b) More common in males than females

(Ref: Harrison 19th edition, p 2238)

- The disordered sleep physiology in fibromyalgia has been identified as a sleep anomaly of alpha-wave intrusion, which occurs during NREM stage 4 sleep leading to EEG abnormalities (option'1')
- This intrusion into deep sleep causes the patient to awaken or to be aroused to a lighter level of sleep.
- Central pain modulatory systems in females are influenced by phasic alterations in reproductive hormone levels.
- Aversive stimuli and stressful tasks are more likely to evoke sympathetic nervous system, HPA axis, and psychological responses in females than in males; hence fibromyalgia is more common in females with **female : male ratio of 9:1.**

There are 5 main measurable neuroendocrine abnormalities are associated with dysfunction of the HPA axis seen in fibromyalgia. These include

1. Low free cortisol levels in 24-hour urine samples
2. Loss of the normal circadian rhythm, with an elevated evening cortisol level (when it should be at its lowest level)
3. Insulin-induced hypoglycemia associated with an overproduction of ACTH
4. Low levels of growth hormone
5. Stimulated ACTH secretion leading to insufficient adrenal release of glucocorticoids

246. Ans. (a) HMB synthase deficiency

(Ref: Harrisons's 18th edition, p 3168)

Acute intermittent porphyria	HMB synthase deficiency, does not exhibit photosensitivity.
Uroporphyrinogen decarboxylase deficiency	Porphyria cutanea Tarda
Protoporphyrinogen oxidase deficiency	Variegate porphyria
Coproporphyrinogen oxidase deficiency	Hereditary copro-porphyria

247. Ans. (c) Wegener's Granulomatosis

(Ref: CMDT 2013 p 848)

IVIG is an approved treatment for the following conditions:

1. ITP
2. Kawasaki disease
3. Guillain-Barré syndrome
4. Polymyositis/dermatomyositis.
5. Allogeneic bone marrow transplantation
6. Graft versus host disease
7. Chronic lymphocytic leukemia
8. Common variable immunodeficiency (CVID)
9. Chronic inflammatory demyelinating polyneuro-pathy (CIDP)
10. Kidney transplantation with a high antibody recipient or with an ABO incompatible donor
11. Primary immunodeficiency disorders associated with defects in humoral immunity.

248. Ans. (a) Cholinergic urticaria

(Ref: Harrison's 18th edition, ch.317, p 2711)

- Cholinergic urticaria typically presents with a number of small, short-lasting hives but may also involve cutaneous inflammation (wheals) and pain which develops usually in response to exercise, bathing, staying in a heated environment, or emotional stress.
- Although the symptoms subside rapidly, commonly within 1 hour, CU may significantly impair quality of life, especially in relation to sporting and sexual activities
- Traditionally, an intradermal injection of either 0.05 mL of 0.002% carbamylcholine chloride (carbachol) or 0.05 mL of 0.02% (0.01 mg) methacholine has been used to produce a flare-up of cholinergic urticaria containing characteristic wheals, often with satellites.

249. Ans. (a) Type 1 diabetes mellitus

(Ref: CMDT 2013, p 1193)

Type 1 diabetes mellitus is associated with HLA DR3-DQ2/DR4-DQ8 genotype is associated with the highest diabetes risk. This genotype is found in 20–30% of type 1 diabetic patients and in almost 50% of patients diagnosed in early childhood. Islet autoantibodies differ in their association with HLA haplotypes.

250. Ans. (a) Common variable immunodeficiency

(Ref: CMDT 2013, p 868)

- *Common variable immunodeficiency (CVID), one of the most prevalent primary immunodeficiency diseases, is a heterogeneous group of immunologic disorders of unknown etiology.*
- Recurrent pyogenic infections of sino-pulmonary tract have been reported in 94% of patients. Symptoms may appear during childhood or, more often, after puberty. Haemophilus influenzae, Moraxella catarrhalis, Streptococcus pneumoniae, and Staphylococcus aureus are the organisms most commonly involved.
- The most common autoimmune conditions in patients with common variable immuno-deficiency are cytopenia, idiopathic thrombo-cytopenic purpura (ITP) in particular, and hemolytic anemia or, more rarely, autoimmune neutropenia

251. Ans. (b) Tender on palpation

(Ref: Harrison's 18th edition, ch.322)

- Rheumatic nodules are non-tender and hence require no intervention. They should not be confused with rheumatoid nodules which are tender.
- Both are present in extensor distribution like occiput, olecranon process, tips of spinous process of vertebra.

252. Ans. (b) Mitral insufficiency

(Ref: Harrison's 18th edition, ch.322 p 2752)

253. Ans. (c) Apical low pitched mid diastolic murmur

(Ref: Harrison 19th edition, p 2150)

254. Ans. (b) Porphobilinogen

(Ref: Harrison's 18th edition, ch.358)

- AIP is an autosomal dominant disease that results from defects in the enzyme porphobilinogen-deaminase. This enzyme speeds the conversion of porphobilinogen to hydroxymethylbilane. In AIP, the porphyrin precursors, porphobilinogen and amino-levulinic acid (ALA), accumulate. The predominant problem appears to be neurologic damage that leads to peripheral and autonomic neuropathies and psychiatric manifestations.
- Urine porphyrin studies are the mainstay in the diagnosis of acute porphyria attacks. Establish the diagnosis promptly by testing for increased porphobilinogen in a single-void urine.
- Patients with acute exacerbations of porphyria have logarithmic increases (5-100 times) in metabolic precursors (ALA, PBG, etc). Minor elevations of these precursors are nondiagnostic and nonspecific.
- Significantly increased ALA and PBG in urine have 100% specificity (ie, rules in) for acute intermittent (hepatic) porphyria, variegate porphyria, and coproporphyria. A normal urine PBG result has a sensitivity of almost 100% (i.e., rules out) in the diagnosis of porphyria in acutely symptomatic patients.

255. Ans. (c) SLE

(Ref: Harrison 19th edition, p 2127)

Three histological lesions are most characteristic of SLE
1. Onion skin lesion of splenic artery
2. Libman sacks endocarditis
3. Hematoxylin bodies

> Onion skin patterns are seen in
> 1. Splenic artery in SLE
> 2. Ewing sarcoma
> 3. Charcot marie tooth disease
> 4. Primary sclerosing cholangitis
> 5. Malignant HTN

256. Ans. (a) iii, i, iv, ii

(Ref: Ch 322, Harrison's 18th ed.)

In rheumatic carditis, the preceding sore throat by Group A Beta hemolytic streptococcus results in rise of ASLO titer followed by development of mitral regurgitation. This will lead to left atrial enlargement. In future however aortic valve involvement can be seen where the aschoff nodules will cause damage to chordae tendinae of aortic valve leading to aortic regurgitation.

257. Ans. (d) Diffuse amyloidosis

(Ref: Robbins 8th edition, p 166-172)

258. Ans. (d) Henoch schölein purpura

(Ref: Harrison's 18th edition, ch.14)

259. Ans. (c) Hypergammaglobulinemia

(Ref: Harrison's 18th edition, ch.e20, p 839)

- A third of all people with a thymoma have symptoms caused by compression of the surrounding organs by an expansive mass. These problems may take the form of superior vena cava syndrome, dysphagia, cough, or chest pain.
- One-third of patients have their tumors discovered because they have an associated autoimmune disorder. As mentioned earlier, the most common of those conditions is myasthenia gravis (MG); 10–15% of patients with MG have a thymoma and, conversely, 30–45% of patients with thymomas have MG.
- Additional associated autoimmune conditions include pure red cell aplasia and Good's syndrome (thymoma with combined immunodeficiency and hypogammaglobulinemia). Other reported disease associations are with acute pericarditis, Addison's disease, agranulocytosis, alopecia areata, ulcerative colitis, Cushing's disease, hemolytic anemia, limbic encephalopathy, myocarditis, nephrotic syndrome, panhypopituitarism, pernicious anemia

260. Ans. (b) Second to fifth Ribs

(Ref: Harrison's 18th edition, p 2060)

Pain with palpation of affected costochondral joints is a constant finding in costochondritis. The second through the fifth costo-chondral junctions typically are involved. More than 1 junction is involved in more than 90% of patients.

261. Ans. (c) Renal amyloidosis is commonly present with hypertension

(Ref: Harrison 19th edition, p 732)

Renal amyloidosis is usually manifested as proteinuria, often in the nephrotic range and associated with significant hypoalbuminemia, secondary hypercholesterolemia, and edema or anasarca.

In some patients, tubular rather than glomerular deposition of amyloid can produce azotemia without significant proteinuria. The heart is the second most commonly affected organ and the leading cause of mortality

262. Ans. (a) Cor-pulmonale

(Ref: Harrison 19th edition, p 2632)

In setting of lung abscess, the resultant hypoxia leads to development of Cor-pulmonale. The resultant RVF can lead to hepatic congestion and development of edema.

263. Ans. (d) Wiskott Aldrich syndrome

(Ref: Harrison 19th edition, p 89e-3f)

- In Wiskott Aldrich syndrome, the WASp gene codes for the protein by the same name, which is 502 amino acids long and is mainly expressed in hematopoietic cells.
- Due to its mode of inheritance, the overwhelming majority of patients are male. The first signs of WAS are usually petechiae and bruising, resulting from thrombocytopenia. Spontaneous nose bleeds and bloody diarrhea are common. Eczema develops within the first month of life. Recurrent bacterial infections develop by three months. Splenomegaly is not an uncommon finding. The majority of WAS children develop at least one autoimmune disorder, and malignancies (mainly lymphoma and leukemia) develop in up to a third of patients.
- A numerical grading of severity for Wiskott Aldrich syndrome is

0.5:	Intermittent thrombocytopenia
1.0:	*Thrombocytopenia and small platelets (microthrombocytopenia)*
2.0:	Microthrombocytopenia plus normally responsive eczema or occasional upper respiratory tract infections
2.5:	Microthrombocytopenia plus therapy-responsive but severe eczema or airway infections requiring antibiotics
3.0:	Microthrombocytopenia plus both eczema and airway infections requiring antibiotics
4.0:	Microthrombocytopenia plus eczema continuously requiring therapy and/or severe or life threatening infections
5.0:	Microthrombocytopenia plus autoimmune disease or malignancy

- *In contrast Bernard Soulier syndrome is, characterized by giant platelets*, prolonged bleeding time, thrombocytopenia, increased megakaryocytes, and decreased platelet survival, Bernard–Soulier syndrome is associated with quantitative or qualitative defects of the platelet glycopotein complex GPIb/V/IX. The degree of thrombocytopenia may be estimated incorrectly, due to the possibility that when the platelet count is performed with automatic counters, giant platelets (which may be as frequent as 70–80% in occasional patients) may reach the size of red blood cells and, as a consequence, are not recognized as platelets by the counter.

264. Ans. (d) Fourth heart sound heard

(Ref: Harrison 19th edition, p 2150-51)

265. Ans. (a) Autosomal dominant inheritance

(Ref: Harrison 19th edition, p 2109)

The pattern of inheritance of Ataxia telengiectasia is autosomal recessive. The clinical features are:

1. Progressive cerebellar ataxia usually becomes clinically apparent when the child begins to walk. The ataxia affects station, gait, and intention.
2. Telangiectasia of the bulbar conjunctiva first appears at age 3-7 years and, subsequently, involves the malar areas, palate, ears, and antecubital and popliteal spaces.
3. Other features of this syndrome include retardation of growth, dysarthric speech, dry coarse hair and skin, and mental retardation after age 10 years.
4. The complete syndrome includes hypoplasia of the thymus associated with defective T-cell function and decreased levels of circulating immunoglobulin. Recurrent respiratory tract and sinus infections are common, frequently causing death in adolescence or young adulthood.
5. A high incidence of malignancies, particularly leukemia and Hodgkin lymphoma, occurs.

266. Ans. (a) *Salmonella*

(Ref: Harrison 19th edition, p 840t)

267. Ans. (c) *Thymoma with hypogammaglobulinemia*

(Ref: Harrison 19th edition, 1839)

Good's syndrome (thymoma with immunodeficiency) is a rare cause of combined B and T cell immuno-deficiency in adults. The clinical characteristics of Good's syndrome are increased susceptibility to bacterial infections with encapsulated organisms and opportunistic viral and fungal infections. The most consistent immunological abnormalities are hypo-gammaglobulinaemia and reduced or absent B cells. This disorder should be treated by resection of the thymoma and immunoglobulin replacement to maintain adequate trough of IgG values.

268. Ans. (d) *Common variable immunodeficiency*

(Ref: Harrison 19th edition, p 270)

Persistent diarrhea and malabsorption caused by Giardia lamblia infection occur in patients with CVID. Symptoms generally resolve after treatment with metronidazole. Infectious and autoimmune etiologies are the most likely causes for severe chronic diarrhea.

269. Ans. (d) *Abdominal fat pad biopsy*

(Ref: Harrison 19th edition, p 723)

The best sites from which to obtain a biopsy specimen in systemic amyloidosis are the abdominal fat pad and rectal mucosa (approaching 90% sensitivity for fat pad and 73-84% for rectal mucosa). While some imaging modalities can strongly suggest amyloidosis, a tissue sample showing birefringent material is still the criterion standard. This is definitely the case in terms of cardiac specific amyloid. While, endomyocardial biopsy is the best confirmatory test for local cardiac amyloid deposition, it can be very risk averse and requires a center of excellence with the full complement of immunohistochemical and molecular-based testing.

270. Ans. (a) *Icatibant*

(Ref: Harrison 19th edition, p 2117)

- Antihistamines do not work for patients with bradykinin-mediated angioedema, and corticosteroids have limited or no value in this type of angioedema. However, fresh frozen plasma (FFP), antifibrinolytics, C1 esterase inhibitor (C1-INH), ecallantide, and icatibant can be used to manage bradykinin-mediated angioedema.
- In histamine-mediated angioedema, second-generation antihistamines are often first-line treatment. Corticosteroids can be used in severe cases of this form of the disease, but long-term use of these agents should be avoided in outpatient treatment.

271. Ans. (c) *Sjogren syndrome*

(Ref: Harrison 19th edition, p 1857)

The frequency of HLA-DR52 in patients with primary Sjögren syndrome is estimated to be 87%, but it is also significantly increased in secondary Sjögren syndrome that occurs with rheumatoid arthritis or systemic lupus erythematosus.
HLA B5/HLA B51 is related to Behçet disease.

272. Ans. (a) *Tuberculosis*

(Ref: Harrison's 18th edition, ch.165)

Some of the conditions associated with AA include the following:
1. Rheumatoid arthritis (RA)
2. Alzheimer disease
3. Multiple myeloma
4. Juvenile idiopathic arthritis
5. Ankylosing spondylitis
6. Psoriasis and psoriatic arthritis
7. Still disease
8. Behçet syndrome
9. Familial Mediterranean fever
10. Crohn disease
11. Leprosy
12. Osteomyelitis
13. Tuberculosis
14. Chronic bronchiectasis
15. Castleman disease
16. Hodgkin disease and non-Hodgkin lymphoma
17. Renal cell carcinoma
18. Carcinoma of the gastrointestinal, lung, or urogenital tract
19. Cryopyrin-associated periodic syndromes (CAPS)

273. Ans. (d) *Serum tryptase*

(Ref: CMDT 2013 p 866)

Two of the most abundant and best-characterized preformed granule mediators released by these cells during anaphylaxis are tryptase and histamine. Elevations in tryptase and histamine can sometimes be detected in blood samples obtained shortly after the onset of symptoms. Also, elevated levels of histamine, histamine metabolites (N-methylhistamine and N-methylimidazole acetic acid) and the prostaglandin, 11-beta-PGF2-alpha (11β-PGF2α), can be measured in urine after an anaphylactic event.

274. Ans. (a) *Carditis*

(Ref: Harrison 19th edition, p 2153)

- Rheumatic carditis is treated with steroids. Though 18th edition of Harrison states that there is no evidence of benefit in meta-analysis trial.
- Rheumatic arthritis is treated with aspirin. In case of poor/no response steroids are used.
- Medications to control the abnormal movements do not alter the duration or outcome of chorea. Milder cases can usually be managed by providing a calm environment.
- In patients with severe chorea, carbamazepine or sodium valproate are preferred to haloperidol. A response may not be seen for 1–2 weeks, and a successful response may only be to reduce rather than resolve the abnormal movements. Medication should be continued for 1–2 weeks after symptoms subside.
- Subcutaneous nodules do not require any treatment.

275. Ans. (a) Palms and soles

(Ref: CMDT 2014 ch.20)

Physical findings of sclerema neonatorum appear suddenly, first on the thighs and buttocks and then, spreading rapidly, often affecting all parts of the body except the palms, soles, and genitalia. The involved skin is pale, waxy, and firm to palpation. The skin cannot be pitted or pinched up because it is bound to underlying subcutaneous tissue, muscle, and bone. The affected infant often displays flexion contractures at the elbows, knees, and hips.

Infants affected by sclerema neonatorum are premature, and the others are full term but have a serious underlying illness. They are often of low birth weight (< 2500 g) and have cyanosis and low Apgar score.

276. Ans. (c) Rheumatic fever

(Ref: Harrison 19th edition, p 2153)

Carey Coomb's murmur is a clinical sign which occurs in patients with mitral valvulitis due to acute rheumatic fever. It is described as a short, mid-diastolic rumble best heard at the apex, which disappears as the valvulitis improves. It is often associated with an S3 gallop rhythm, and can be distinguished from the diastolic murmur of mitral stenosis by the absence of an opening snap before the murmur. The murmur is caused by increased blood flow across a thickened mitral valve

277. Ans. (b) Rheumatic valves

(Ref: Harrison 19th edition, p 2138)

- Traditionally calcification in heart is related to atherosclerosis and endomyocardial fibrosis. However the question is about the calcification inside the heart related to rheumatic heart disease.
- In rheumatic carditis, calcified mitral stenosis is a long term sequalae which is treated with prosthetic valve.

278. Ans. (d) SLE

(Ref: Harrison 19th edition, p 2131)

Causes of Bilateral Parotid Enlargement

• Adenolymphoma	• Pancreatitis, chronic
• Amyloidosis	• Parotid adenoma
• Bulimia nervosa	• Parotid cancer
• Cirrhosis of liver	• Parotitis
• Chronic pancreatitis	• Pituitary tumour (growth hormone secreting)
• Cystic fibrosis	• Propylthiouracil
• Gamma heavy chain disease	• Sarcoidosis
• Adenoid cystic carcinoma	• Sicca syndrome
• Heerfordt-Waldenstroem syndrome	• Malabsorption syndrome
• HIV-1 disease	
• Mumps	
• Mikulicz syndrome	

279. Ans. None or A New bone formation

(Ref: Harrison 18th/p 2818, 2819)

280. Ans. (d) Chlamydia

(Ref: Harrison 19th edition, p 2175)

281. Ans. (a) Hemochromatosis

(Ref: Harrison 19th edition, p 2516)

282. Ans. (c) Desferroxamine is the treatment of choice

(Ref: Harrison 19th edition, p 2516)

283. Ans. (d) Desferroxamine is the treatment of choice

(Ref: Harrison 19th edition, p 2516)

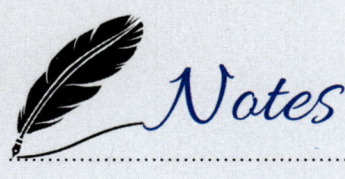

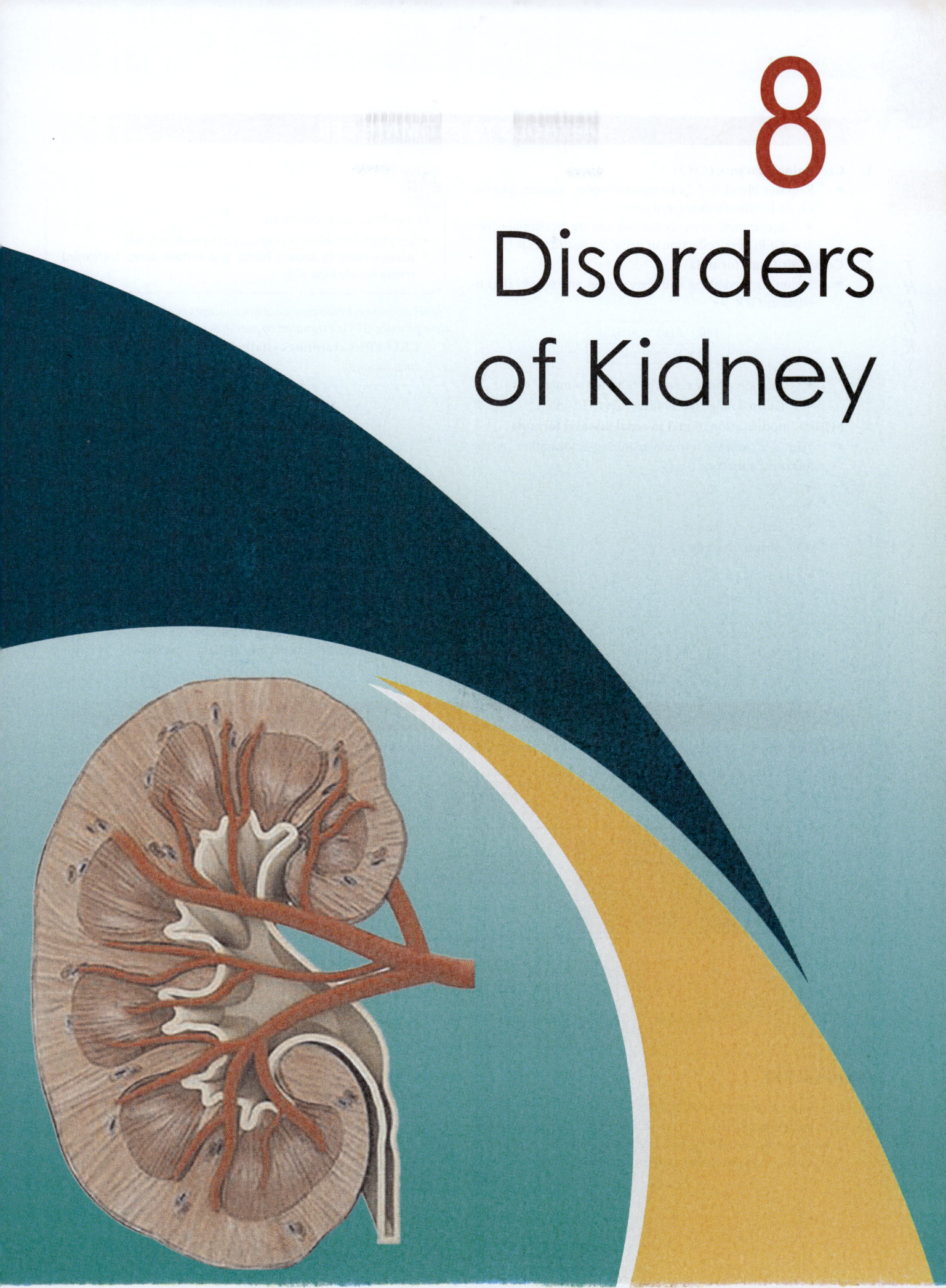

8
Disorders of Kidney

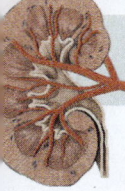

METHODS TO ESTIMATE GFR

1. **Creatinine clearance (CrCl)**
   - Requires blood and 24-hr urine samples; measure plasma Cr, 24-hr urine volume and urine Cr
     - Incomplete urine collection can underestimate true GFR; over-collection of urine overestimates it
2. **Cockcroft-Gault formula**
   - Serum Cr used along with age, gender and weight (kg) to estimate GFR

$$\frac{(140 - \text{Age}) \times \text{weight}}{72 \times \text{S. creatinine}}$$

   - Multiply above result by 0.85 for women
   - Normal range is >90 mL / min (>1.5 ml/s)
3. **MDRD (modification of diet in renal disease) formula**
   - This is a complex formula requiring information on the following variables:
     - Age
     - Gender
     - Serum creatinine
     - African descent

Errors in Cr measurement
- Very high bilirubin level causes [Cr] to be falsely low
- Acetoacetate (a ketone body) and certain drugs (cefoxitin) create falsely high [Cr]

*(PAH clearance, inulin clearance are concepts in physiology, but in real-time practice GFR is estimated by methods given above)

4. **CKD-EPI-Creatinine cystatin C method** (*Best method for GFR calculation*)

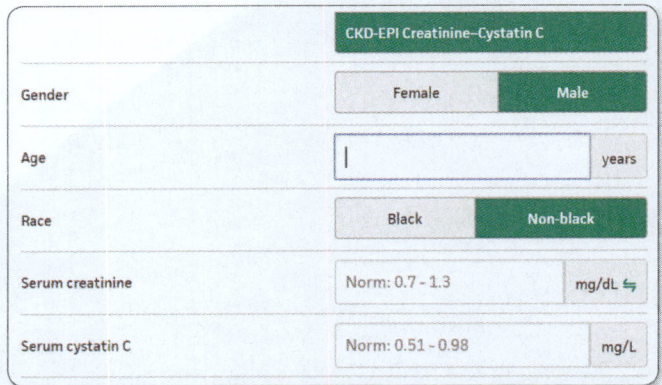

Online calculator to calculate GFR by CKD EPI- creatinine- cystatin C method

ACUTE KIDNEY INJURY (AKI)

AKI complicates 5–7% of acute care hospital admissions and up to 30% of admissions to the intensive care unit

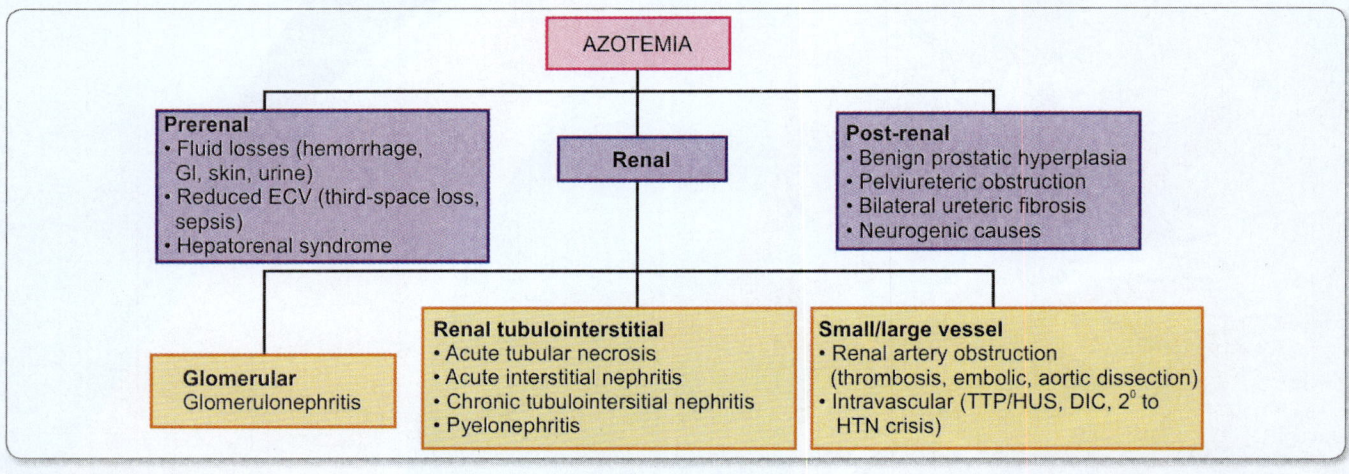

Prerenal AKI

- *It is the most common form of AKI.*
- It is the designation for a rise in SCr or BUN concentration due to inadequate renal plasma flow and intraglomerular hydrostatic pressure to support normal glomerular filtration.

- The most common clinical conditions associated with prerenal azotemia are:
  - Hypovolemia
  - Decreased cardiac output
  - Medications that interfere with renal autoregulatory responses such as NSAIDs and inhibitors of angiotensin II.

Renal AKI

The most common causes of intrinsic AKI are sepsis, ischemia, and nephrotoxins, both endogenous and exogenous.

- Endogenous toxins
  - Hemolysis
  - Rhabdomyolysis[Q]
  - Multiple myeloma
  - Intratubular crystals (calcium oxalate crystals due to ethylene glycol)
- Exogenous toxins
  - Iodinated contrast
  - Aminoglycosides[Q]
  - Cisplatin
  - Amphotericin B.

Non-oliguric acute kidney is caused by aminoglycoside antibiotics.

Postrenal AKI

- Postrenal AKI occurs when the normally unidirectional flow of urine is acutely blocked either partially or totally, leading to increased retrograde hydrostatic pressure and interference with glomerular filtration.
- Obstruction to urinary flow may be caused by functional or structural derangements anywhere from the renal pelvis to the tip of the urethra.
- For AKI to occur in healthy individuals, obstruction must affect both kidneys unless only one kidney is functional, "wherein" unilateral obstruction can cause AKI.

KDIGO Criteria for AKI

Stage	Serum Creatinine	Urine Output
1.	1.5–1.9 times baseline or ≥ 0.3 mg/dL increase	<0.5 mL/kg/h for 6 h
2.	2–2.9 time baseline	<0.5 mL/kg/h for 12 h
3	3 times baseline or Increase in serum creatinine to ≥4 mg/dL or Initiation of renal replacement therapy	<0.3 mL/kg/h for 24 h or Anuria for ≥ 12h

Biomarkers of AKI

1. Neutrophil gelatinase associated lipocalcin (NGAL) is a leading new biomarker of Acute kidney injury (AKI). *NGAL can bind to iron siderophore complexes and may have tissue protective effects in the proximal tubule. It is highly upregulated after inflammation and kidney injury and can be detected in urine within 2 hours* of cardiopulmonary bypass associated AKI
2. Urine Kidney injury molecule
3. Urinary IL-18

RIFLE criteria for acute renal damage

Class	GFR	Urinary obstruction
Risk	↑ SCr × 1.5 or ↓ GFR > 25%	<0.5 mL/kg/h × 6 h
Injury[Q]	↑ SCr × 2 or ↓ GFR > 50%	<0.5 mL/kg/h × 12 h
Failure[Q]	↑ SCr × 3 or ↓ GFR > 75% or if baseline SCr ≥ 353.6 µmol/L (≥4 mg/dL) ↑ SCr > 44.2 µmol/L (>0.5 mg/dL)	<0.3 mL/kg/h × 24 h or anuria × 12 h
Loss of kidney function	Complete loss of kidney function >4 weeks	
End-stage kidney disease	Complete loss of kidney function >3 months	

Clinical Features

1. A reduction in urine output (oliguria, defined as <400 mL/24 h) usually denotes more significant AKI (i.e., lower GFR).
2. Preserved urine output can be seen in nephrogenic diabetes insipidus characteristic of long-standing urinary tract obstruction, tubulointerstitial disease, or nephrotoxicity from cisplatin or aminoglycosides, among other causes.
3. Red or brown urine may be seen with or without gross hematuria; *if the color persists in the supernatant after centrifugation, then pigment nephropathy from rhabdomyolysis or hemolysis should be suspected.*
4. Nausea and vomiting.
5. Uremic encephalopathy.
6. Uremic pericarditis leading to chest pain
7. Puffy eyes and pedal edema.

Investigations

1. **Serum creatinine**: Contrast nephropathy leads to a rise in SCr within 24–48 hours, peak within 3–5 days, and resolution within 5–7 days. In comparison, atheroembolic disease usually manifests with more subacute rises in SCr, although severe AKI with rapid increase in SCr can occur in this setting. With many of the epithelial cell toxins such as aminoglycoside antibiotics and cisplastin, the rise in SCr is characteristically delayed for 4–5 days to 2 weeks after initial exposure
2. CBC for anemia and eosinophilia. *Eosinophilia and eosinophiluria indicate atheroembolic kidney disease*
3. Urine microscopy for casts
4. Potassium elevated
5. Serum calcium: Falls
6. Serum phosphate: Rises

7. **FENa**: The fractional excretion of sodium (FENa) is the fraction of the filtered sodium load that is reabsorbed by the tubules and is a measure of both the kidney's ability to reabsorb sodium as well as endogenously and exogenously administered factors that affect tubular reabsorption. With prerenal azotemia, the FENa may be below 1%, suggesting avid tubular sodium reabsorption
8. **Urine sodium**: In case of tubular necrosis urine sodium will be high since it cannot be reabsorbed back via the PCT
9. Imaging with USG or CT scan for postrenal causes.

Investigation in Prerenal AKI
- BUN/creatinine ratio above 20
- FENa <1%
- Hyaline casts in urine sediment
- Urine specific gravity >1.018
- Urine osmolality >500 mOsm/kg

Management

1. **Nephrotoxin-specific**
   - **Rhabdomyolysis**: Forced alkaline diuresis
   - **Tumor lysis syndrome**: Allopurinol or rasburicase
2. Volume overloading
   - Salt and water restriction
   - Diuretics
   - Ultrafiltration
3. Hyponatremia
   - Restriction of enteral free water intake, minimization of hypotonic intravenous solutions including those containing dextrose
4. Hyperkalemia
   - Restriction of dietary potassium
   - Stop potassium-sparing diuretics, ACE inhibitors, ARBs, NSAIDs
   - Loop diuretics to promote urinary potassium loss
   - Potassium binding ion-exchange resin (sodium polystyrene sulfonate)
   - Insulin (10 units regular) and glucose (50 mL of 50% dextrose) to promote entry of potassium intracellularly
   - Inhaled salbutamol to promote entry of potassium intracellularly
   - Calcium gluconate or calcium chloride to stabilize the myocardium (DOC)
5. **Metabolic acidosis**: Sodium bicarbonate (if pH <7.2 to keep serum bicarbonate >15 mmol/L)
6. **Hyperphosphatemia**: Phosphate binding agents (calcium acetate, sevelamer hydrochloride, aluminum hydroxide)
7. **Hypocalcemia**: Calcium carbonate or calcium gluconate, if symptomatic
8. **Hypermagnesemia**: Stop Mg^{2+} containing antacids
9. **Hyperuricemia**: Acute treatment is not required except in the setting of tumor lysis syndrome
10. **Nutrition**: Sufficient protein and calorie intake to avoid negative nitrogen balance
11. **Dialysis** is indicated
    - When medical management fails to control volume overload or hyperkalemia or acidosis or in some toxic ingestions
    - Complications of uremia (asterixis, pericardial rub or effusion, encephalopathy, uremic bleeding).

Distinguishing Prerenal from Intrarenal Disease in Acute Kidney Injury		
Index	Prerenal	Intrarenal (e.g. ATN)
Urine Osmolality	>500	<350
Urine Sodium (mmol/L)	<20	>40
FENa	<1%	3-6%
Plasma BUN /Cr (SI Units)	>80%	<40:1
Urinalysis	Normal	RBC, pigmented granular casts

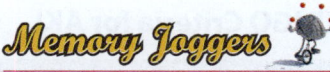

INDICATIONS FOR DIALYSIS IN AKI (HAVE PEE)
- **H**yperkalemia (refractory)
- **A**cidosis (refractory)
- **V**olume overload (refractory)
- **E**levated BUN (>35 mM)
- **P**ericarditis
- **E**ncephalopathy
- **E**dema (Pulmonary)

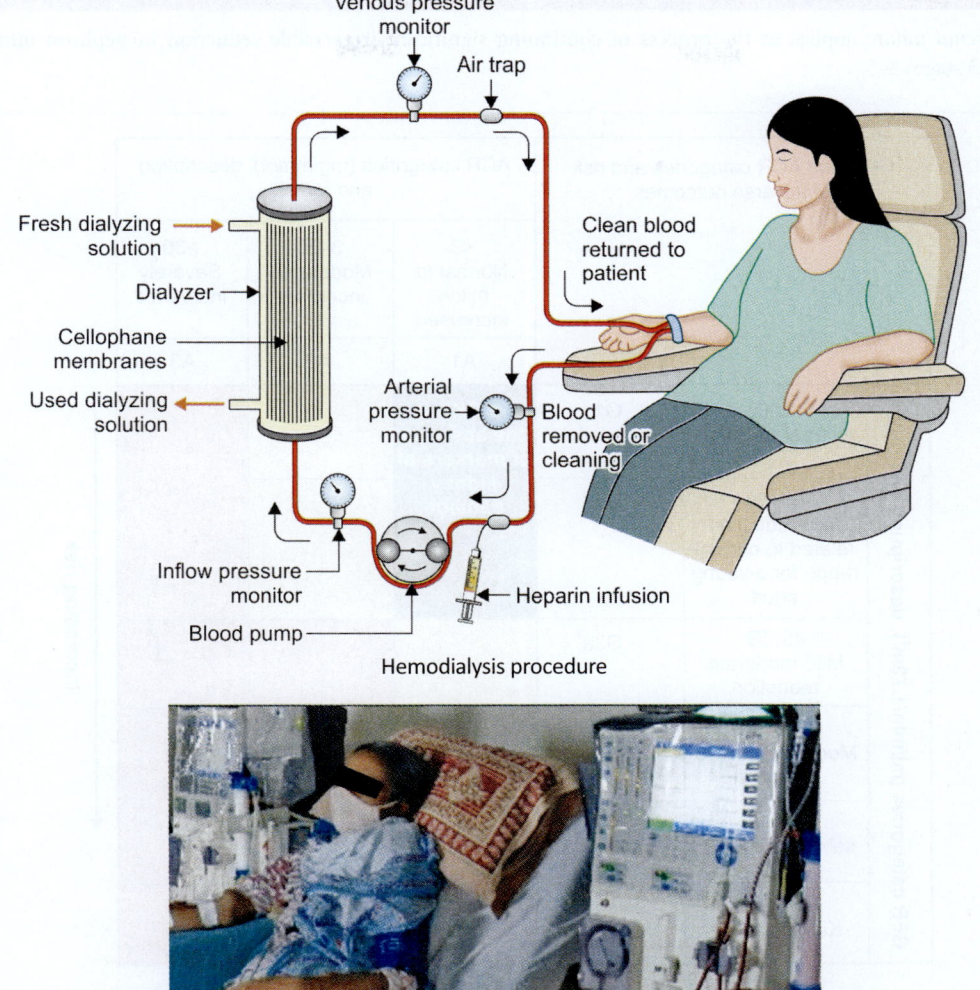

Hemodialysis procedure

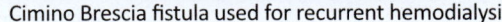

Cimino Brescia fistula used for recurrent hemodialysis

Functional[Q] biomarkers of kidney damage
1. Serum creatinine
2. Serum cystatin C
3. Urine albumin

Cystatin C is a 13KD cysteine protease inhibitor that gained popularity as an alternative of serum creatinine in measurement of GFR but has disadvantage of rising only when sufficient kidney damage is present. Higher levels are seen with male gender, greater height and weight which essentially is the limitation of creatinine as well.

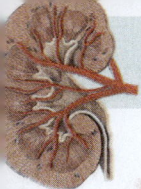

CHRONIC KIDNEY DISEASE

The term *chronic renal failure* applies to the process of continuing significant irreversible reduction in nephron number and typically corresponds to CKD stages 3–5.

GFR and ACR categories and risk of adverse outcomes			ACR categories (mg/mmol), description and range		
			<3 Normal to mildly increased	3–30 Moderately increased	>30 Severely increased
			A1	A2	A3
GFR categories (ml/min/1.73m²), description and range	≥90 Normal and high	G1	No CKD in the absence of markers of kidney damage		
	60–89 Mild reduction related to normal range for a young adult	G2			
	45–59 Mild-moderate reduction	G3a[1]			
	30–44 Moderate-severe reduction	G3b			
	15–29 severe reduction	G4			
	<15 Kidney failure	G5			

Increasing risk →

Albuminuria Categories in CKD		
Category	ACR (mg/g)	Terms
A1	< 30	Normal to mildly increased
A2	30–300	Moderately increased*
A3	> 300	Severely increased**

*Relative to young adult level. ACR 30–300 mg/g for > 3 months indicated CKD.
**Including nephrotic syndrome (albumin excretion ACR > 2220 mg/g)

Management

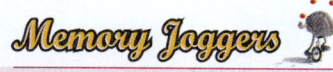

Management of CRF Patient = ABCDE
- Control of Hb**A**1c to < 7% to slow the progression to ESRD using insulin
- Control of **B**P using ACE inhibitors like ramipril
- **C**alcium for hypocalcemia as vit D3 is low
- Vitamin **D**3 supplementation to reduce damage to bones due to secondary hyperparathyroidism
- **E**rythropoeitin injections to raise hematocrit

- Torsemide for pedal edema/anasarca
- If GFR<30 mL/min/1.73 m² of BSA (CKD stage 4), hemodialysis is required
- If GFR<15 mL/min/1.73 m² of BSA (CKD stage 5), allogenic renal transplantation is required.
- Sevalemer and Lanathum are non-calcium containing polymers functioning as phosphate binders. (Harrison's 19th ed. p. 1816,)

INDICATIONS FOR DIALYSIS IN CHRONIC RENAL FAILURE
- **Absolute indications:**
  1. Uremic pericarditis
  2. Refractory accelerated hypertension
  3. Volume overload unresponsive to medications
  4. Hyperkalemia unresponsive to medications
  5. Severe metabolic acidosis unresponsive to medications
  6. Neurologic signs or symptoms of uremia (encephalopathy, neuropathy, seizures)
  7. Clinically significant bleeding diathesis
  8. Persistent severe nausea and vomiting,
  9. Plasma Cr >1060 μmol/L or BUN >36 mmol/L
- **Relative indications:** Anorexia, decreased cognitive functioning, profound fatigue and weakness, severe anemia unresponsive to erythropoietin, persistent severe pruritus, restless legs syndrome

Peritoneal Dialysis vs. Hemodialysis		
	Peritoneal Dialysis	**Hemodialysis**
Rate	Slow	Fast
Locations	Home	Hospital (usually)
Ultrafiltration	Osmotic pressure via dextrose dialysis	Hydrostatic pressure
Solute removal	Concentration gradient and convection	Concentration gradient and convection
Membrane	Peritoneum	Semipermeable artificial membrane
Method	Indwelling catheter in peritoneal cavity	Line from vessel to artificial kidney

- Most common complication of hemodialysis is hypotension/cardiovascular complications.
- Most common cause of CKD is diabetic nephropathy.

Urine Examination Findings

Eosinophils
- Detected using Wright's or Hansel's stain (not affected by urine pH)
- Consider allergic interstitial nephritis, *atheroembolic* disease.

Oval Fat Bodies
- Renal tubular cells filled with lipid droplets
- Seen in heavy proteinuria (i.e. nephrotic syndrome).

Casts
- Cylindrical structures formed by intratubular precipitation of *Tamm-Horsfall mucoprotein*; cells may be trapped within the matrix of protein.

Interpretation of Casts	
Hyaline casts	Physiologic (concentrated urine, fever, exercise)
Red blood cell casts	Glomerular bleeding (glomerulonephritis, vasculitis)
White blood cell casts	Infection (pyelonephritis) Inflammation (interstitial nephritis)
Pigmented granular casts (heme granular casts, muddy brown)	Acute tubular necrosis, glomerulonephritis, interstitial nephritis
Fatty casts	Heavy proteinuria (>3.5 g/day)

Crystals
- Uric acid: Consider acid urine, hyperuricosuria (e.g. gout)
- Calcium phosphate: Alkaline urine
- Calcium oxalate: Consider hyperoxaluria, ethylene glycol poisoning
- Sulfur: Sulfa-containing antibiotics.
- For shapes of crystals, *refer* to explanation of image-based question number 1 of this chapter

Urine Electrolytes
- Commonly measured: Na, K, Cl, osmolality and pH
- No 'normal' values; electrolyte excretion depends on intake and current physiological state
- Therefore, results must be interpreted in the context of a patient's current state, e.g.
  - A patient who is clearly ECF volume depleted should have a low urine Na (kidneys should be retaining Na); a high urine Na in this setting suggests a renal problem or a diuretic; urine Na <10 mmol/L suggests prerenal etiology
  - Daily urinary potassium excretion rate should be decreased (<20 mmol/d) in the setting of hypokalemia; if higher than 20 mmol/d, suggests renal etiology
- Osmolality is useful to estimate the kidney's concentrating ability
  - FENa refers to the fractional excretion of Na
  - FENa = Urine [Na] x Plasma [Cr] / (Plasma [Na] x Urine [Cr]) x 100
  - FENa <1% suggests the pathology is prerenal.

Examples of Common Urine Electrolyte Abnormalities
- **High urine Na (>20 mmol/L) in the setting of acute renal failure:** Intrarenal disease, presence of non-reabsorbable anions (e.g. ketones), or action of diuretic including osmotic diuresis from glucose
- **High urine Na (>40 mmol/L) in the setting of hyponatremia:** Diuretics, tubular disease (e.g. Bartter's syndrome) and SIADH
- Urine pH is useful to grossly assess renal acidification:
  - "Low" pH (<5.5) in the presence of low serum pH is an appropriate renal response
  - A high pH in this setting might indicate a renal acidification defect (e.g. renal tubular acidosis).

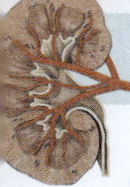

Proteinuria

- (N) proteinuria: < 150 mg/d
- (N) albuminuria: < 30 mg/d
- Microalbuminuria: 30–300 mg/d
- Glomerular proteinuria: > 2 g/d
- Tubular proteinuria: < 2 g/d.

Differences between Tubular and Glomerular Proteinuria

Tubular proteinuria	Glomerular proteinuria
Occurs in injury involving the tubulointerstitial region of kidney	Occurs due to injury of the renal glomerulus
Comprises • Low molecular weight proteins (β_2 microglobulin) filtered by the glomerulus and not reabsorbed by the tubules • Cellular enzymes secreted by renal tubules • Increased amount of Tamm-Horsfall protein	Comprises predominantly of albumin (low molecular weight protein)
Quantitative excretion of protein is usually < 2 g/d	Quantitative excretion of protein may be large (>3–3.5 g/d)
Urinary protein electrophoretic pattern (UPEP) shows more globulin than albumin	UPEP shows more albumin than globulin
Albumin: β_2 microglobulin ratio is 100:1 (normal ratio is 50–200:1).	Albumin: β_2 microglobulin ratio > 1000:1.

Selective proteinuria is said to occur when the ratio of clearance of IgG (1.6 lakh kd) to transferrin (88,000 kd) is less than 0.1. Minimal change disease in child produces selective proteinuria. Because of low molecular weight, there is selective excretion of albumin in urine.

Microalbuminuria

- Albumin is a non-glycosylated protein with a molecular weight of 66,000 daltons.
- It is synthesized in liver parenchymal cells at a rate of 14 g/day.
- Causes of microalbuminuria can be glomerular (e.g. due to diabetic microangiopathy, hypertension, minor glomerular lesion), tubular (inhibition of reabsorption) or postrenal. Albumin is also a marker protein for various forms of proteinuria.
- *The determination of the urinary albumin to urinary creatinine ratio is a more accurate measurement of albumin excretion, since it corrects for variations in urine volume.*
- This measurement *can be performed on a single random urine sample* and has shown a strong correlation with the 24 h urinary albumin loss.
- The urine albumin assay is an automated immunoturbidimetric assay.

Hematuria

- (N) RBC count is < 3 RBC/ HPF^Q (dysmorphic) or <5RBC/μL or < 8000 RBC/ mL or < 500,000 RBC/day (by Addis count)^Q
- Clots are not encountered in patients with glomerular disease
- Terminal hematuria is classical infestation of S. haematobium and bladder cancer (smoking, aniline dye exposure)
- Hematuria associated with hearing loss: Alport's syndrome
- Hematuria associated with hemoptysis: Good Pasture's syndrome
- Hematuria associated with tinnitus: Vasculitis
- Isothenuria is inability to concentrate the urine and is classical manifestation of CRF.
- Drugs causing nephrogenic diabetes inspidus
  - Demeclocycline
  - Lithium

Pyuria

- **Common microbial pathogen causing UTI**: *Escherichia coli* (50–90% cases)

Urinary Tract Infection (UTI)

The 2010 Infectious Disease Society of America (IDSA) consensus limits for cystitis and pyelonephritis in women are more than 1000 colony-forming units (CFU)/mL and more than 10,000 CFU/mL, respectively, for clean-catch midstream urine specimens.

Historically, the definition of UTI was based on the finding at culture of 100,000 CFU/mL of a single organism. However, this misses in up to 50% of symptomatic infections, so the lower colony rate of greater than 1000 CFU/mL is now accepted

Causes of Sterile Pyuria

1. Inadequately treated UTI
2. Infections like tuberculosis, atypical Streptococcus, corynebacteria, fastidious microorganisms
3. Calculi
4. Bladder tumors
5. Papillary necrosis
6. Interstitial nephritis
7. Polycystic kidneys

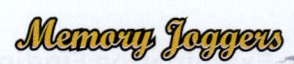

Causes of Papillary Necrosis
Mnemonic: **Post CARDS**
- **P**yelonephritis
- **O**bstruction of urinary tract
- **S**ickle cell anemia
- **T**B
- **C**irrhosis
- **A**nalgesic abuse
- **R**enal transplant rejection
- **D**iabetes mellitus (Most common)
- **S**ystemic vasculitis

GLOMERULAR DISEASES

- 1.6 million glomeruli (0.5–2.4 million) in 2 mature kidneys
- 120–180 L of ultra filtrate/d is produced
- (N) GFR = 80–125 mL/min

Cell	Function	Pathology
Endothelial cell	Maintains glomerular perfusion	ARF, diffuse proliferative GN
Mesangial cell	Controls GFR	Mesangio- proliferative GN
Basement membrane	Prevent filtration of plasma proteins	Membranous nephropathy
Visceral epithelial	Prevent filtration of plasma proteins	Minimal change disease (MCD), focal segmental glomerulo-sclerosis (FSGS)
Parietal epithelial cell	Maintain Bowman's space	Crescentic GN

- *Nephrotic syndrome:* (1, 2, 3 are essentials of diagnosis)
    1. > 3 g/24 h proteinuria
    2. Hypoalbuminemia
    3. Edema
    4. Hyperlipidemia and lipiduria
    5. Hypercoagulable state
- *Nephritic syndrome:*
    - Hematuria (active urine sediment)
    - Hypertension
    - Subnephrotic proteinuria
- Nephritic syndrome and rapidly progressive glomerulonephritis:
    - Patient develops renal failure over weeks to months
    - Crescentic glomerulonephritis is classical morphological finding.
    - Three Serological markers are serum C_3 level, anti-GBM antibodies and antineutrophil cytoplasmic antibody (ANCA)
    - Renal biopsy is gold standard for diagnosis.

Nephrotic Syndrome

Clinical Features

- Patient usually presents with insidious onset of generalized edema, without a decrease in urine output. Patient may complain of passing frothy urine due to presence of protein.

Minimal Change Disease

This occurs commonly in children below 16 years of age, accounting for about 70–80% of nephrotic syndrome in them and 20% in adults.
- Proteinuria in the nephrotic range is present. Selective proteinuria is seen (there is selective excretion of low molecular weight protein like albumin and absence of high molecular weight protein like globulin in the urine).
- **Renal biopsy**: Light microscopic examination is normal. Foot process fusion is seen under electron microscope.
- Remissions of proteinuria with glucocorticoids carry a good prognosis. 1–1.5 mg/kg/d of prednisolone for 4 weeks, followed by 1mg/kg/d on alternate days for 4 weeks. If therapy is extended upto 20–24 weeks, 90% of children enter remission.
- Cytotoxic therapy may be required for relapse.
- Progression to renal failure is uncommon.

Membranous Glomerulopathy

Causes of Membranous Glomerulopathy

Membranous glomerulonephritis

- Primary/idiopathic membranous glomemlonephritis
- Secondary membranous glomerulonephritis
- **Infection:** Hepatitis B and C, syphilis, malaria, schistosomiasis, leprosy, filariasis
- **Cancer:** Breast, colon, lung, stomach, kidney, esophagus, neuroblastoma
- **Drugs:** Gold, mercury, penicillamine, nonsteroidal anti-inflammatory agents, probenecid
- **Autoimmune diseases:** Systemic lupus erythematosus, rheumatoid arthritis, primary biliary cirrhosis, dermatitis herpetiformis, bullous pemphigoid, myasthenia gravis, Sygren's syndrome, Hashimoto's thyroiditis
- **Other systemic diseases:** Fanconi's syndrome, sickle cell anemia, diabetes, Crohn's disease, sarcoidosis, Guillain-Barre syndrome, Weber-Christian disease, angiofollicular lymph node hyperplasia

- This occurs commonly in adults, accounting for 30–40% of nephrotic syndrome in them.
- *In 70% of cases, auto antibodies against M-type phospholipase A2 receptor circulate and blind to epitope present in PLA_2R on human podocytes*
- Underlying disease such as SLE, hepatitis B, solid tumors, and intake of drugs such as captopril or penicillamine
- Hypertension, mild renal insufficiency and abnormal urine sediment may develop later.
- *Renal vein thrombosis is common.*
- Glucocorticoids may reduce the decline in renal function if given prior to renal insufficiency, but they do not correct proteinuria. Nonselective proteinuria is seen.
- Cyclophosphamide, chlorambucil and cyclosporine are shown to reduce proteinuria.

Membranoproliferative Glomerulonephritis (Mesangiocapillary Glomerulonephritis or Lobar Glomerulonephritis)

- This accounts for approximately 5% of idiopathic nephrotic syndrome.
- They present with microscopic to gross hematuria and selective or non-selective proteinuria depending on the severity of the disease, with hypertension.
- Type 1 is most common and associated with hepatitis C.

Causes of Membranoproliferative Glomerulonephritis

Type I Disease (Most Common)
- Idiopathic
- Subacute bacterial endocarditis
- Systmic lupus erythematosus
- Hepatitis C ± cryoglobulinemia
- Mixed cryoglobulinemia
- Hepatitis B
- Cancer: Lung, breast, and ovary (germinal)

Contd...

Type II Disease (Dense Deposit Disease)
- Idiopathic
- C_3 nephritic factor-associated
- Partial lipodystrophy

Type III Disease
- Idiopathic
- Complement receptor deficiency

Focal Segmental Glomerulosclerosis

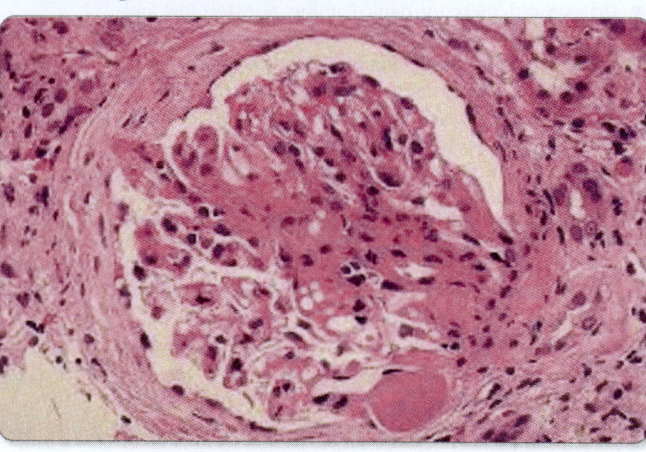

Normocellular glomerulus with segmental hyaline eosinophilic deposits

Causes of FSGS

Idiopathic or primary Disease

Secondary
- Hereditary (mutations on genes for podocyte proteins)
- **Virus:** HIV, parvovirus
- **Medication:** Heroin, interferon-alpha, lithium, pamidronate
- Adaptive changes (hyperfiltration)
  - **Loss of kidney mass:** Agenesis, vesicoureteral reflux, nephrectomy
  - Hypertension, diabetes, obesity, cyanotic cardiopathy
- **Tumours:** lymphoma
- Added to glomerular diseases
  - **Focal proliferative glomerulonephritis:** IgA, lupus nephritis, extracapillary proliferative GN
  - Alport's Syndrome
  - Membranous GN
  - Thrombotic microangiopathy

- Associated with HIV infection, DM, heroin use and oligonephropathies.
- This accounts for about 30–35%(1/3) of nephrotic syndrome in adults.
- Hyperlipidemia is severe in cases with focal sclerosis.
- Prognosis is variable. In steroid-responsive patients, prognosis is good, but in steroid unresponsive patients and in patients with heavy proteinuria rapid progression to end stage renal failure occurs within a few months.

> **EXTRA MILE**
> - MC type of nephrotic syndrome in adults is Focal segmental glomerulosclerosis.
> - MC type of nephrotic syndrome in children is Minimal change disease.

Evaluation of Nephrotic Syndrome
1. 24-hour urine for protein, creatinine clearance
2. Serum albumin, cholesterol, complement
3. Urine protein electrophoresis
4. Rule out SLE, diabetes mellitus
5. Review drug exposure
6. Renal biopsy
7. Consider malignancy (in elderly patient with membranous GN)
8. Consider renal vein thrombosis (if membranous GN or symptoms of pulmonary embolism are present).

Treatment
- Bed-rest.
- If GFR > 60 mL/min, no dietary restriction required. If GFR < 60 ml/min, dietary protein restriction of 0.8 gm/kg/d is required.
- Diuretics relieve edema but do not treat the underlying disorder. Overzealous use of diuretics should be avoided as the patients are often intravascularly depleted and may precipitate prerenal failure.
- Salt-free albumin infusion may help to alleviate the symptoms of edema temporarily.

Complications
- Venous thrombosis and pulmonary embolism (urinary loss of antithrombin III, low plasma volume, increased clotting factors II, V, VII, VIII, and X).
- Infections (pneumococcal peritonitis).
- Hypercholesterolemia (atherosclerosis, xanthomata).
- Hypovolemia and renal failure.
- Loss of specific binding proteins, e.g., transferrin, thyroid-binding protein.

Summary of Important Causes of Nephrotic Syndrome

	Minimal change	Membranous Glomerulopathy	Focal segmental Glomerulosclerosis	Membranoproliferative Glomerulonephritis
Secondary causes	DM, amyloidosis	HBV, SLE, malignancy (lung, breast, GI)	Reflux nephropathy, HIV, HBV	HCV, malaria, SLE, leukemia, lymphoma
Drug causes	NSAIDs	Gold, pencillamine	Heroin	N/A
Therapy	Steroids	Reduce BP, ACEI, steroids	Steroid, ACEI/ARB for proteinuria	Aspirin, dipyridamole

Glomerulonephritis

Acute Glomerulonephritis

It is a clinical syndrome consisting of hematuria, proteinuria, hypertension, and renal insufficiency. The Clinical severity ranges from asymptomatic microscopic or gross hematuria to a rapid loss of kidney function like in case of rapidly progressive GN.

Causes

1. Post-infectious GN.
   - Commonly follows group A beta-hemolytic *Streptococcus* infection
   - Onset occurs 1–3 weeks after an infection of either throat or skin
   - Most common cause of acute GN in children accounting for 80% of cases
2. IgA nephropathy:
   - (Most common form of primary acute GN in the 2nd and 3rd decades)^Q
3. Anti –GBM disease:
   - Also called Good Pasture's syndrome
   - Occurs commonly in the 2nd or 3rd decade
4. ANCA associated GN:
   - Rarely seen and often has a relapsing and remitting course.
   - 3 disease presentations
      - Granulomatosis with Angütis
      - Churg–Strauss disease
      - Microscopic Polyangütis
5. MPGN:
   - May present in the setting of systemic viral or rheumatic illness.
6. Lupus nephritis:
   - 30 – 70% of systemic lupus patients will have renal involvement.
   - Cryoglobulin-associated vasculitis: associated with hepatitis C infection.

Examination Findings

- Sinus disease: ANCA; associated GN
- Pharyngitis or impetigo: Postinfectious GN
- Pulmonary abnormality : Anti GBM disease or lupus nephritis
- Hepatomegaly or liver tenderness could pain to cryoglobulinemia-associated GN or IgA nephropathy
- Purpura may point to ANCA-associate: GN or Henoch Schonlein purpura GN.

Complications of Acute Glomerulonephritis

1. Hypertensive retinopathy and encephalopathy
2. Rapidly progressive GN
3. Microscopic hematuria
4. Chronic kidney disease
5. Nephrotic syndrome

Post-Infectious Glomerulonephritis

- Immune complex disease preceded by infection with certain strains of bacteria, most commonly streptococcus and staphylococcus.
- *The most common form of PIGN is post-streptococcal glomerulonephritis (PSGN).*
- PSGN occurs predominantly in children.
- The clinical presentation varies from asymptomatic to the acute nephritic syndrome, characterized by gross hematuria, proteinuria, edema, hypertension, and acute kidney injury.

Etiology

1. Glomerular immune complex causing complement activation and inflammation:
   - Nephritis-associated plasmin receptor (NAPIr): Activates plasmin, contributes to activation of the alternative complement pathway.
   - Streptococcal pyrogenic exotoxin B (SPE B): Binds plasmin and acts as a protease; promotes the release of inflammatory mediators.
2. Activation of the alternative complement pathway causes initial glomerular injury as evidenced by C3 deposition and decreased levels of serum C3.

History

- Patients present with sudden onset of hematuria associated with edema and hypertension 1 -2 weeks after an infection.
- A triad of edema, hematuria, and HTN
- PIGN in children usually follows group A β-hemolytic streptococcal (GAS) skin/throat infection.
- The latent period between GAS infection and PIGN depends on the site of infection: 1-3 weeks following GAS pharyngitis and 3-6 weeks following GAS skin infection.
- Adult PIGN most commonly follows staphylococcal infections (3 x more common than streptococcal infections) of the upper respiratory tract, skin, heart, lung, bone, or urinary tract.
- Skin and throat infections with particular M types of streptococci (nephritogenic) strains antedate glomerular disease.
- M types 47, 49, 55, 2, 60 and 57 are seen following impetigo.
- M types 1, 2, 3, 4, 25, 49, 12 are seen following pharyngitis.

Physical Examination

1. Edema due to sodium and water retention.
2. Gross hematuria: Urine described as "tea-colored" or "cola-colored".
3. Hypertension: Hypertensive encephalopathy is an uncommon, but serious complication.
4. Microscopic hematuria: Subclinical cases of PIGN
5. Respiratory distress: Due to pulmonary edema

Investigations

1. Urinalysis shows hematuria with/without RBC casts and pyuria.
2. Proteinuria present, but nephrotic range proteinuria is common in children
3. Culture: PSGN usually presents weeks after a GAS infection, only ~25% of patients will have either a positive throat or skin culture.
4. Complement: 90% of patients will have depressed C3 and CH50 levels in the 1st 2 weeks of the disease, whereas C2 and C4 levels remain normal, C3 and CH50 levels return to normal within 4-8 weeks after presentation.
5. Serum Creatinine
6. Serology: Elevated titers of antibodies support evidence of a recent GAS infection.
7. In pharyngeal infection. ASO, anti-DNAse B, anti-NAD, and AHase titers elevated.
8. In skin infection, only the anti - DNAse and AHase titers are typically elevated.
9. Renal biopsy should be done only when diagnosis is unsure
    - Light microscopy: Diffuse proliferative glomerulonephritis with prominent endocapillary proliferation and numerous neutrophils within the capillary lumen. Deposits may also be found in the mesangium ("*starry sky*"). Crescent formation is uncommon and is associated with a poor prognosis.
    - Immunofluorescence microscopy: Deposits of C3 and IgG distributed in a diffuse granular patter.
    - Electron microscopy: *Dome-shaped sub-epithelial electron-dense deposits* that are referred to as "humps." These deposits are immune complexes and they correspond to the deposits of IgG and C3 found on immunofluorescence.
10. Renal biopsy: Usually not performed as clinical history is highly suggestive and resolution of PIGN typically begins within 1 week of presentation.

Indications of renal biopsy in glomerular disorders[Q]

- Persistently low C3 levels beyond 6 weeks for possible diagnosis of membranoproliferative glomerulonephritis
- Recurrent episodes of hematuria are suggestive of IgA Nephropathy
- Progressive increase in serum Creatinine is not characteristic of PIGN

Treatment

- No specific therapy exists for PIGN and no evidence indicates that aggressive immunosuppressive therapy has a beneficial effect in patients with rapidly progressive crescentric disease.
- Management is supportive, with focus on treating the clinical manifestations of PIGN. These include HTN and pulmonary edema.
    - General measures include sodium and water restriction and loop diuretics
    - Calcium channel blockers/ACE inhibitors may be used in cases of severe HTN
- Patients with evidence of persistent bacterial infection should be given a course of antibiotic therapy.

Rapidly Progressive Glomerulonephritis

- This is characterized by hematuria, proteinuria and renal failure, which progresses over a period of weeks to months.
- Crescentic GN is usually found on renal biopsy.
- Fifty percent of patients require dialysis within 6 months of diagnosis.
- Combination of glucocorticoids in pulse doses, cytotoxic agents (azathioprine, cyclophosphamide) and intensive plasma exchange may be useful.

Causes of Rapidly Progressive Glomerulonephritis

Immune complex GN (45%)	
• Idiopathic proliferative GN	• Cryoglobulinemia
• MPGN	• Bacterial endocarditis
• Postinfectious GN	• IgA nephropathy
• Crescentic GN	• Henoch Schonlein purpura (HSP)
• Lupus nephritis	
Pauci-immune GN (45%)	
• Wegener's granulomatosis	• Drugs: ciprofloxacin
• Microscopic polyarteritis	
Anti GBM (10%)	
• Good Pasture's disease	

Good Pasture's Syndrome

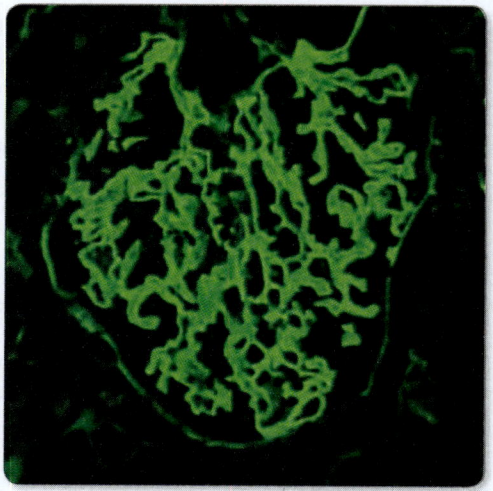

Linear pattern on immunofluorescence

- This is characterized by lung hemorrhage, GN, and circulating antibody to basement membrane, usually in young men. Hemoptysis may precede nephritis.
- α3 NCI domain of collagen IV is a target antigen
- Circulating antiglomerular basement membrane (GBM) antibody and linear immunofluorescence on renal biopsy establishes the diagnosis.
- Plasma exchange may produce remission.

Henoch-Schonlein Purpura

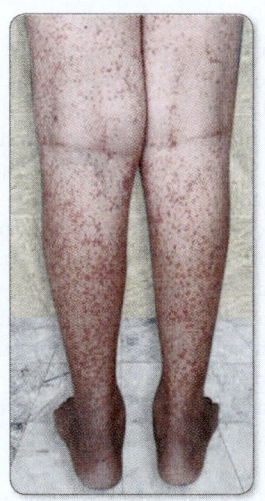

Extensor purpura

- It is a generalized vasculitis causing GN, purpura, arthralgias and abdominal pain, occurring mainly in children.
- Renal involvement is manifested by hematuria and proteinuria.
- Serum IgA is increased in half of patients.
- Mesangial IgA deposits on immunofluorescence.
- Treatment is symptomatic.

Most common cause of vasculitis in children is Henoch-Schonlein purpura.

IgA Nephropathy (Berger's Disease)

- *This is the most common form of primary glomerular disease in the world and most common cause of hematuria overall.*
- It progresses to end stage renal disease in 20–40% of patients affected over a 20-year period.
- Gross, intermittent hematuria, which is glomerular in origin, is the presenting symptom. *After 48 hours of an upper respiratory tract infection, the intermittent microscopic hematuria is upgraded to gross hematuria.*
- Mesangial IgA is present.
- No therapeutic regimen has been shown to clearly affect outcome in IgA nephropathy.
- However, warfarin and dipyridamole with or without cyclophosphamide may be of help.

Most common cause of microscopic hematuria is Berger's disease.

TUBULOINTERSTITIAL DISEASES OF KIDNEY

- Tubulointerstitial diseases constitute a diverse group of acute and chronic hereditary and acquired disorders involving renal tubules and supporting structures.
- Functionally, they may result in *nephrogenic diabetes insipidus*^{Q} with polyuria, nocturia, *non-anion gap acidosis,*^{Q} salt wasting, and hypo- or hyperkalemia.
- Azotemia is common.
- Proteinuria is modest, hypertension is less common, and anemia may be severe.

Most characteristic feature of tubular disorders of kidney is salt wasting.

Causes of Tubulointerstitial Disease

- **Toxins**
    - Exogenous toxins
        - Analgesic nephropathy
        - Lead nephropathy
        - Miscellaneous nephrotoxins (antibiotics, cyclosporine, radiographic contrast media, heavy metals)
    - Metabolic toxins
        - Acute uric acid nephropathy
        - Miscellaneous (hyperoxaluria, cystinosis)
- **Neoplasia**
    - Lymphoma
    - Leukemia
    - Multiple myeloma
- **Immune disorders**
    - Sjögren's syndrome
    - Amyloidosis
    - Transplant rejection
    - AIDS
    - Vascular disorders
    - Arteriolar nephrosclerosis
    - Atheroembolic disease
    - Sickle cell nephropathy
- **Hereditary renal diseases**
    - Hereditary nephritis (Alport's syndrome)
    - Polycystic kidney disease
- **Miscellaneous disorders**
    - Chronic urinary tract obstruction
    - Vesicourethral reflux.

UROLITHIASIS

- Medical expulsive therapy: *alpha 1-Antagonists (e.g., terazosin) and calcium channel blockers (e.g. Nifedipine) improve likelihood of spontaneous stone passage.*
- 75% of patients are successfully treated conservatively and pass the stone spontaneously.

- Stones that do not pass usually require surgical intervention.
- 30–50% of patients will have recurrent stones.
- The American Urological Association recommends patients with newly diagnosed ureteral stone <10 mm in distal ureter for medical expulsive therapy.

Etiology

1. Calcium oxalate and/or phosphate stones (80%):
   - MC cause is idiopathic hypercalciuria.
2. Hyperoxaluria:
   - Enteric hyperoxaluria:
     - Intestinal malabsorptive state associated with celiac sprue, or intestinal resection.
     - Bile salt malabsorption leads to formation of calcium soaps.
   - Primary hyperoxaluria: Autosomal-recessive
   - Dietary hyperoxaluria: Overindulgence in oxalate-rich food.
3. Hyperuricosuria:
   - Seen in 10% of calcium stone formers
   - Caused by increased dietary purine intake, systemic acidosis, myeloproliferative diseases, gout, chemotherapy, Lesch-Nyhan syndrome.
   - Thiazides, probenecid.
4. Hypocitraturia:
   - Caused by acidosis: Renal tubular acidosis, malabsorption, thiazides, enalapril, excessive dietary protein.
   - Uric acid stones (10-15%): Hyperuricemia causes as above.
   - Struvite stones (5-10%): Infected urine with urease-producing organisms (most commonly Proteus sp.)
   - Cystine stones (<1%): Autosomal-recessive disorder of renal tubular reabsorption of cystine.

Investigations

1. Urinalysis for RBCs, leukocytes, nitrates, pH (acidic urine <5.5 is associated with uric acid stones; alkaline >7 with struvite stones.
2. Midstream urine for microscopy, culture, and sensitivity.
3. Blood: Urea, creatinine, electrolytes, calcium, and urate
4. Parathyroid hormone levels
5. Non-contrast-enhanced CT scan of the abdomen and pelvis has replaced IV pyelogram as the *investigation of choice*
   - Stone is found most commonly at levels of ureteric luminal narrowing: Pelviureteric junction, pelvic brim, and VUJ.
   - Acute obstruction: Proximal ureter and renal pelvis are dilated to the level of obstruction, and perinephric stranding is possible on imaging.
6. X-ray of kidneys, ureter, and bladder to determine if stone is radiopaque or lucent.
   - Calcium oxalate/phosphate stones are radiopaque.
   - Uric acid stones are radiolucent.
   - Staghorn calculi (that fill the shape of the renal calyces) are usually struvite and opaque.
   - Cystine stones are faintly opaque (ground-glass appearance).
   - *Ultrasound has low sensitivity and specificity, but is often the first choice for pregnant women.*

Medical Treatment of Kidney Stones

- Uric acid stone dissolution therapy.
  - Alkaline urine with potassium citrate keep pH >6.5.
  - Allopurinol 100–300 mg/d PO
- Cystine stone dissolution:
  - Alkalinize urine with potassium citrate; keep pH >6.5.
  - Chelating agents: Alpha-mercaptopropionylglycine, D-penicillamine, Tiopronin
- Stop medications that increase risk of stone formation: Probenecid, loop diuretics, salicylic acid, salbutamol, indinavir, triamterene and acetazolamide.
- Manage hypercalciuria with thiazides on an acute basis only.
- Manage hypocitraturia with potassium citrate and high-citrate juices (e.g., orange, lemon)
- Manage enteric hyperoxaluria with oral calcium/magnesium, cholestyramine, and potassium citrate.
- Increased fluid intake
- Patients who form calcium stones should minimize high-oxalate foods such as green leafy vegetables, peanuts, chocolates, and beer.
- Decrease protein and salt intake.
- Lowering calcium intake is *not* advisable and even may increase urine calcium excretion.

Vascular Disease of the Kidney

Large Vessel	Small Vessel

- Renal artery occlusion
- Renal vein thrombosis
- Renal artery stenosis
  - Atherosclerosis
  - Fibromuscular dysplasia
	- Hypertension
	- Atheroembolic disease
	- Thrombotic microangiopathy
	  - HUS
	  - TTP
	  - DIC
	  - Scleroderma

RENAL ARTERY OCCLUSION

Etiology

1. Abdominal trauma, surgery, embolism, vasculitis, extrarenal compression, hypercoaguable state and aortic dissection
2. Kidney transplant more vulnerable

Signs and Symptoms (Depend on Presence of Collateral Circulation)

- Fever, nausea, vomiting, flank, pain
- Leukocytosis, elevated AST, LDH, ALP
- Acute onset hypertension (activation of RAAS) or sudden worsening of long standing hypertension
- Renal dysfunction (if bilateral, or solitary functioning kidney)

Investigations

1. Renal arteriography (more reliable but risk of contrast-mediated ATN, Atheroembolic renal disease)
2. Contrast-enhanced CT or magnetic resonance angiography, duplex Doppler studies (operator dependent)

Treatment

- Prompt localization of occlusion and restoration of blood flow
- Anticoagulation, thrombolysis, percutaneous angioplasty or clot extraction, surgical thromboembolectomy

RENAL ARTERY STENOSIS

- Chronic renal impairment secondary to hemodynamically significant renal artery stenosis or microvascular disease
- Significant cause of ESRD: 15% in patients over 50 years old (higher prevalence if significant vascular disease)
- Usually associated with large vessel disease elsewhere
- Causes:
  - Atherosclerosis- more common in elderly
  - Fibromuscular dysplasia – more common in females, age 30-50 years

Risk Factors

- > 50 years old smoking
- Other atherosclerotic disease
- Severe /refractory HTN and /or hypertensive crises

Treatment

- ACE ⊖ and CCB are used for management of Renovascular hypertension. In bilateral renal artery stenosis, percutaneous transluminal renal angioplasty with stenting is done.

RENAL VEIN THROMBOSIS

Etiology

1. Hypercoagulable state (e.g. membranous glomerulopathy), ECF volume depletion, extrinsic compression of renal vein, significant trauma, malignancy (i.e. RCC), sickle cell anemia.
2. Clinical presentation is determined by rapidity of occlusion and formation of collateral circulation
3. Acute: nausea /vomiting, flank pain, hematuria, elevated plasma LDH, rise in Cr, sudden rise in proteinuria
4. Chronic: increasing proteinuria and /or tubule dysfunction

Investigations

1. Renal venography (Gold standard), CT or MR angiography, duplex Doppler U/S

Treatment

- Anticoagulation with heparin then warfarin

THROMBOTIC THROMBOCYTOPENIC PURPURA

It occurs due to *accumulation of ultra-large multimers of von Willebrand factor* as a result of decreased activity of plasma protease ADAMTS13.

Causes of Reduced ADAMTS13 Activity

1. Upshaw–Schulman syndrome is a hereditary condition characterized by congenital deficiency of ADAMTS13 and can present with TTP after few weeks of life.
2. Drugs: Ticlopidine and quinine
3. Thrombotic microangiopathy with mitomycin-C, gemcitabine

Pentad of TTP shows

1. Fever
2. Renal failure
3. Neurological abnormalities
4. Microangiopathic hemolytic anemia
5. Thrombocytopenia

Treatment

- Plasma exchange with vincristine and rituximab.
- Plasma infusion is sufficient to replace deficiency of ADAMTS13 in Upshaw Schulman syndrome.

AUTOSOMAL DOMINANT KIDNEY DISEASE

- It is inherited as autosomal dominant disorder with *complete penetrance and variable expressivity.*
- 85% cases have PKD 1 gene on chromosome 16p13
- The remaining have PKD2 gene on 4q21-q23 and is associated with *milder* clinical course.

Clinical Features

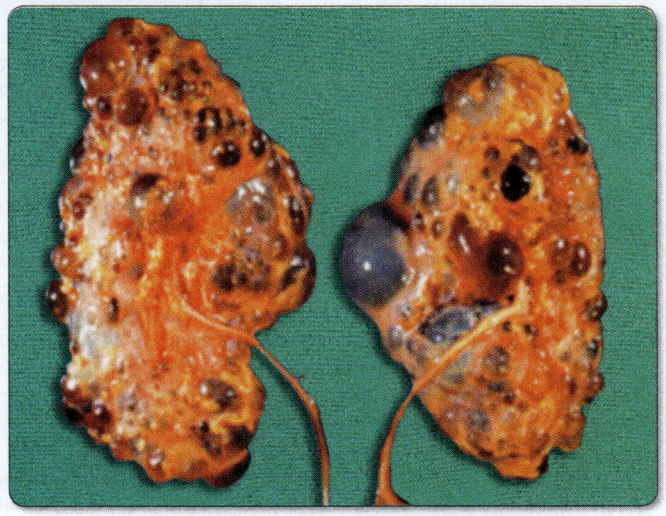

Bleeding in cysts is the reason for flank pain

Radiographic Diagnostic Criteria for ADPKD

Age (years)	Number of cysts
Ultrasonography (at-risk of ADPKD type 1)	
< 30	≥ 2 in one or both kidneys
30 to 59	≥ 2 in each kidney
≥ 60	≥ 4 in each kidney

- *Progressive formation of renal cysts and since they do not communicate with the excretory pathways the progressive increase in tension leads to flank pain in 60% cases. (Most common symptom).*
- The pain is due to renal cyst infection, hemorrhage or nephrolithiasis
- Gross hematuria in 40% cases
- High renin hypertension
- Increased incidence of infection and acute pyelonephritis.
- *Most common kidney stones seen in ADPKD are uric acid stones*
- RCC can develop but unlike routine presentation is bilateral, multi-centric and sarcomatoid type.
- *Most common cause of death is CVS complications due to uncontrolled hypertension.*

Extra-renal manifestations of ADPKD
- Liver cysts (most common Overall)
- Spleen and pancreatic cysts. Cysts are not seen in lung/brain
- Berry aneurysm
- Mitral valve prolapse
- Colonic diverticulosis

Investigations

The presence of at least 2 cysts in each kidney in the age group of 30–59 years and 4 cysts per kidney after age of 60 years is the diagnostic criteria.^{Q}

1. CT scan and T2W MRI are more sensitive than USG but expose the patient to radiation risk and risk of contrast induced nephropathy
2. USG
3. Genetic testing by linkage studies

Treatment
- BP control to <140/90mmHg
- Lipid soluble antibiotics for cyst infection.
- For pain control partial or total bilateral nephrectomy.
- Kidney transplantation
- Sirolimus or everolimus
- Tolvaptan slow decline of renal function

- Most common extrahepatic manifestations of ADPKD is liver cysts
- Most common extrahepatic manifestations of ARPKD is congenital hepatic fibrosis
- Most common renal lesion in tuberous sclerosis is Angiomyolipoma
- Hemorrhage into Angiomyolipoma in tuberous sclerosis is called Wunderlich syndrome

TUBULAR DISORDERS

Comparison of Bartter's and Gitelman's Syndrome

	Bartter's syndrome	Gitelman's syndrome
Defect	Defect in TAL. The proteins affected include the apical loop diuretic–sensitive sodium-potassium-chloride co-transporter NKCC2 (type 1), the apical potassium channel ROMK (type 2), and the basolateral chloride channel ClC-Kb (type 3)	Mutations in the thiazide-sensitive Na-Cl co-transporter, NCCT, in the DCT. Defects in NCCT in Gitelman's syndrome impair sodium and chloride reabsorption in the DCT and thus *resemble the effects of thiazide diuretics*. The involvement of TRPM6 and TRPM7 which are gate keepers of magnesium metabolism leads to magnesium wasting.
Clinical age of presentation	• Bartter's syndrome is a rare disease that most often presents in the neonatal period or early childhood with polyuria, polydipsia, salt craving, and growth retardation. Blood pressure is normal or low • Metabolic abnormalities include hypokalemia, hypochloremic metabolic alkalosis, decreased urinary concentrating and diluting ability, hypercalciuria with nephrocalcinosis, mild hypomagnesemia, and increased urinary prostaglandin excretion • In the antenatal period, fetal polyuria may cause maternal polyhydramnios and premature labor. Sensorineural deafness occurs in patients with Barttin gene mutations	*Gitelman's syndrome is more common than Bartter's syndrome and has a generally milder clinical course with a later age of presentation. It is characterized by* prominent neuromuscular symptoms and signs, including fatigue, weakness, carpopedal spasm, cramps, and tetany
Investigation for differentiation	24 Hr urinary chloride	24 Hr urinary chloride with *serum magnesium*
Treatment	• Lifelong therapy with potassium and magnesium supplements and liberal salt intake • High doses of spironolactone or amiloride treat the hypokalemia, alkalosis, and magnesium wasting • Nonsteroidal anti-inflammatory drugs (NSAIDs) reduce the polyuria and salt wasting in Bartter's syndrome but are ineffective in Gitelman's syndrome. They may be lifesaving in hyperprostaglandin E syndrome and can be given in the form of a COX-2 inhibitor to avoid the gastrointestinal side effects of long-term high-dose NSAIDs	• Same as Bartter's syndrome • In Gitelman's syndrome, magnesium repletion is essential to correct the hypokalemia and control muscle weakness, tetany, and metabolic alkalosis; however, it may prove difficult in patients wasting large amounts of magnesium

RENAL TUBULAR ACIDOSIS (RTA)

Proximal RTA (Type 2)

- Proximal RTA is caused by a failure of the proximal tubular cells to reabsorb filtered bicarbonate from the urine, leading to urinary bicarbonate wasting and subsequent acidemia.
- The distal intercalated cells function normally, so the acidemia is less severe than dRTA and the urine can acidify to a pH of less than 5.5.
- pRTA also has several causes, and may occasionally be present as a solitary defect, but is usually associated with a more generalized dysfunction of the proximal tubular cells called Fanconi syndrome, in which there is also phosphaturia, glycosuria, aminoaciduria, uricosuria, and tubular proteinuria.
- The principal feature of Fanconi syndrome is bone demineralization (osteomalacia or rickets) due to phosphate wasting

Distal RTA (Type 1)

It is the classical form of RTA, characterized by a failure of H^+ secretion into lumen of nephron by the alpha intercalated cells of the medullary collecting duct of the distal nephron.

- The intercalated cells apical H^+/K^+ antiporter is non-functional, resulting in proton retention and potassium excretion. Since calcium stones demonstrate a predisposition for deposition at higher pH (alkaline), the substance of the kidney develops stones bilaterally; this does not occur in the other RTA types
- Normal anion gap metabolic acidosis/acidemia
- Hypokalemia, hypocalcemia, hyperchloremia
- Urinary stone formation (related to alkaline urine, hypercalciuria, and low urinary citrate).
- Nephrocalcinosis (deposition of calcium in the substance of the kidney)
- **Bone demineralization (causing rickets in children and osteomalacia in adults)**
- The kidneys are unable to acidify the urine to pH < 5.5 in presence of systemic metabolic acidosis.

Distal RTA (Type 4)

- *MC type of RTA*
- It is characterized by hyperkalemic hyperchloremic acidosis. It occurs due to aldosterone deficiency or resistance.
- The hyperkalemia impairs NH_4^+ production in proximal tubule by inducing a state of intracellular alkalosis.

Types of Renal Tubular Acidosis

	Type 1	Type 2	Type 4
Location of defect	Distal tubule	Proximal tubule	Adrenal (aldosterone resistance)
Potassium Pathophysiology	Hypokalemia; Failure of H^+ secretion by the α (−) intercalated cells and inability to reclaim K^+	Hypokalemia; Failed HCO_3^- reabsorption from the urine by the proximal tubular cells	Hyperkalemia; Deficiency of aldosterone, or a resistance to its effects, (hypoaldosteronism or pseudohypoaldosteronism)

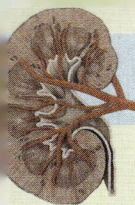

Image-Based Questions

1. Which urine crystals are shown in the figure below?

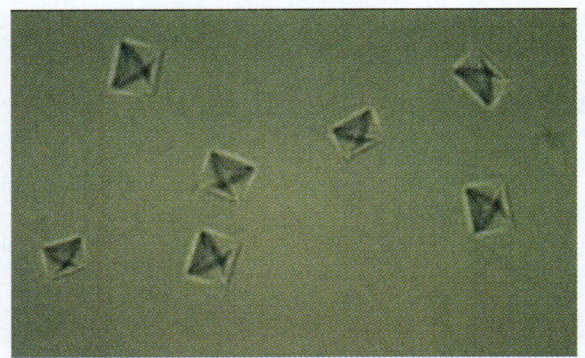

a. Calcium oxalate
b. Uric acid
c. Calcium phosphate
d. Cystine

2. IVU of the patient is diagnostic of?

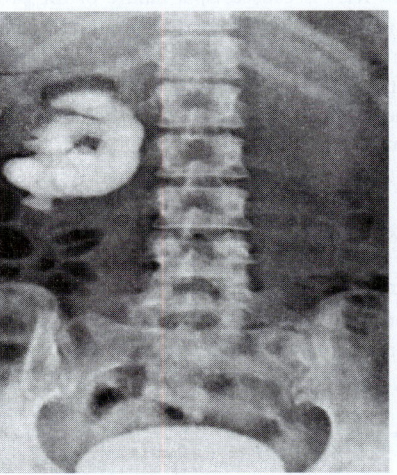

a. Duplication of renal collecting system
b. Hydronephrosis
c. Papillary necrosis
d. Vesicoureteric reflux

3. What is the most common location of this malformation?

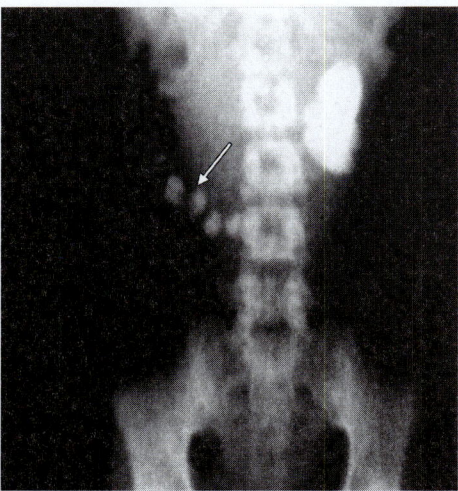

a. L1　　　　　　　　b. L2
c. L3　　　　　　　　d. L4

Answers of Image-Based Questions

1. **Ans. (a) Calcium oxalate**

Calcium oxalate (Envelope/Bipyramidal Shape)	
Uric acid — Amber color crystals variable in both size and shape and can look like barrels, rosettes, rhomboids, needles or hexagonal plates.	
Triple phosphate (Coffin Lid Appearance)	
Cystine (Hexagonal crystals)	
Calcium phosphate stone (Rosette Shaped)	

2. **Ans. (b) Hydronephrosis** *(Ref: Page 1871: Harrison 19th edition)*
   - The image shows *clubbing of calyces* and *dilatation of the pelvis* diagnostic of Hydronephrosis^Q
   - In duplication of renal system, drooping lily sign will have inferodisplacement of ureter.
   - Papillary necrosis will show ring sign due to sloughed papillae.
   - Since no reflux is seen from the bladder retrograde on either side, VUR is ruled out.

3. **Ans. (d) L4** *(Ref: Page 1003: SRB surgery: 5th edition)*
   The image shows medialization of calyxes. The classical curving of ureter is not seen in this image. The diagnosis is horse-shoe kidney. The fusion of lower poles occurs at lower border of 4th lumbar vertebra.

Conceptual Diagnostic Algorithm

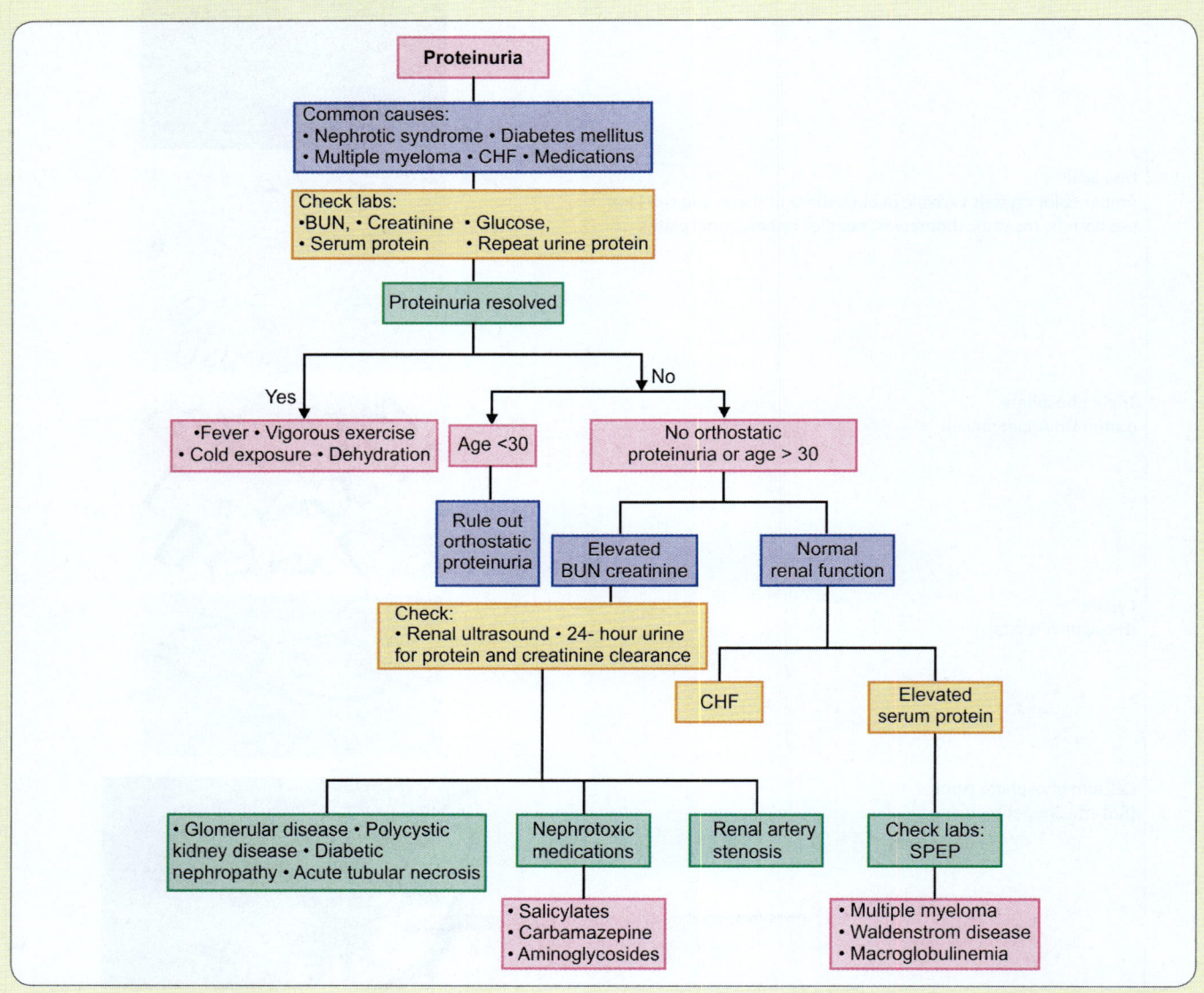

Anuria or oliguria
Common causes: obstruction, acute renal failure shock
Check Labs: Urinalysis, BUN, Creatinine
Catheterize bladder
Urine in bladder
No urine or very little
Bladder neck obstruction
Low BP
Normal or elevated BP
BPH tubor
Renal disease
Medications
Acute tubular necrosis, acute glomerulonephritis, acute renal failure, chronic renal failure
Aminoglycosides, gold amphotericin B, chemotherapy

Uremia
Common causes: chronic renal failure, obstructive uropathy, prerenal azotemia, medications
Acute renal failure
Chronic renal failure
Renal ultrasound
Diabetes mellitus, HTN, glomerulonephritis, Amyloidosis, SLE
Obstructive uropathy
No obstruction
BPH neoplasm
Prerenal azotemia
Renal azotemia
• Sepsis • CHF
• Shock
• Cirrhosis
Drug-induced renal failure
• Acute tubular necrosis
• Renal artery stenosis
• Collagen-vascular disease
• Rhabdomyolysis
• Aminoglycosides
• Sulfonamides
• Lithium
• ACE inhibitors
• NSAIDs
• Contrast media

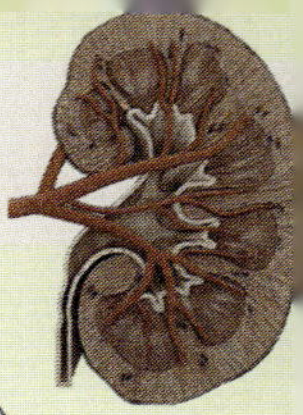

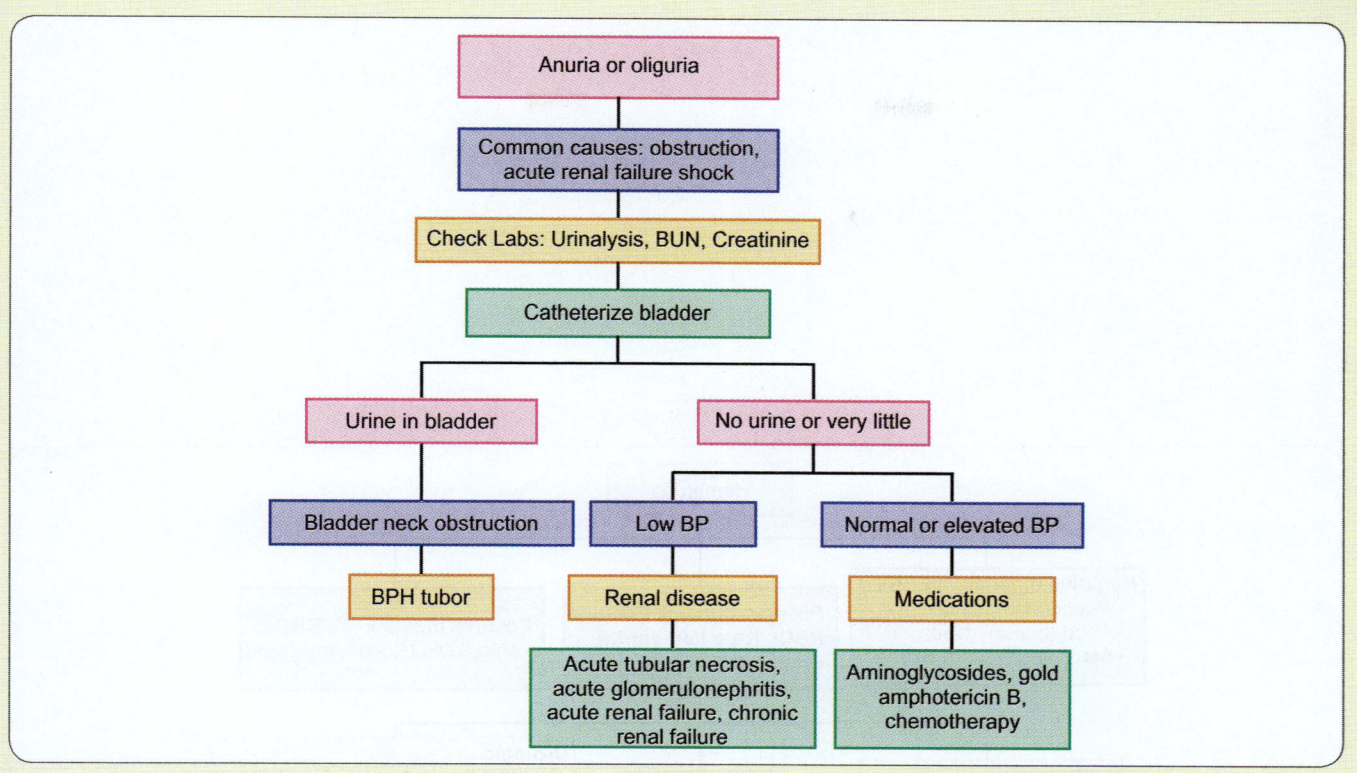

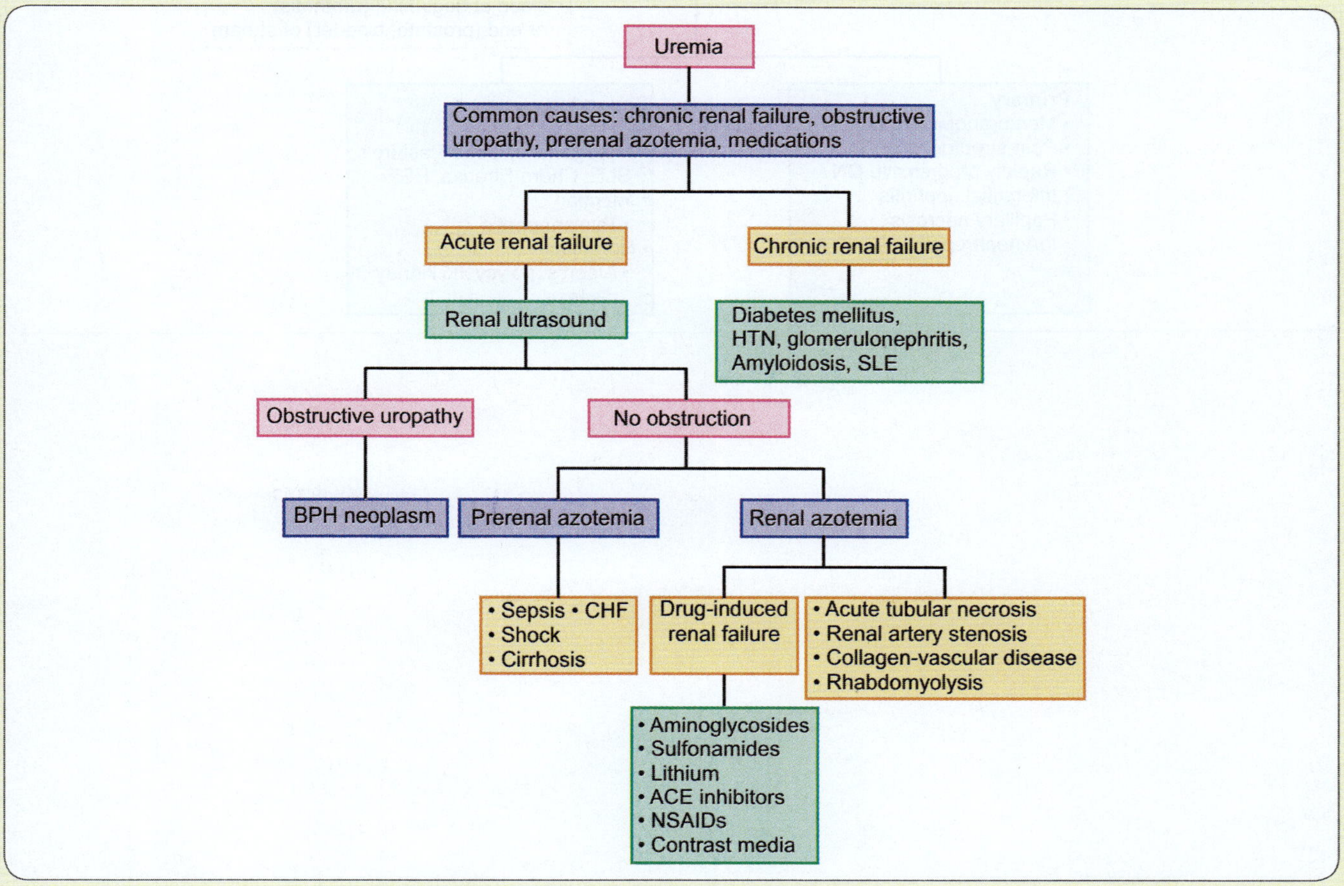

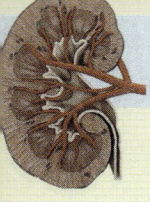
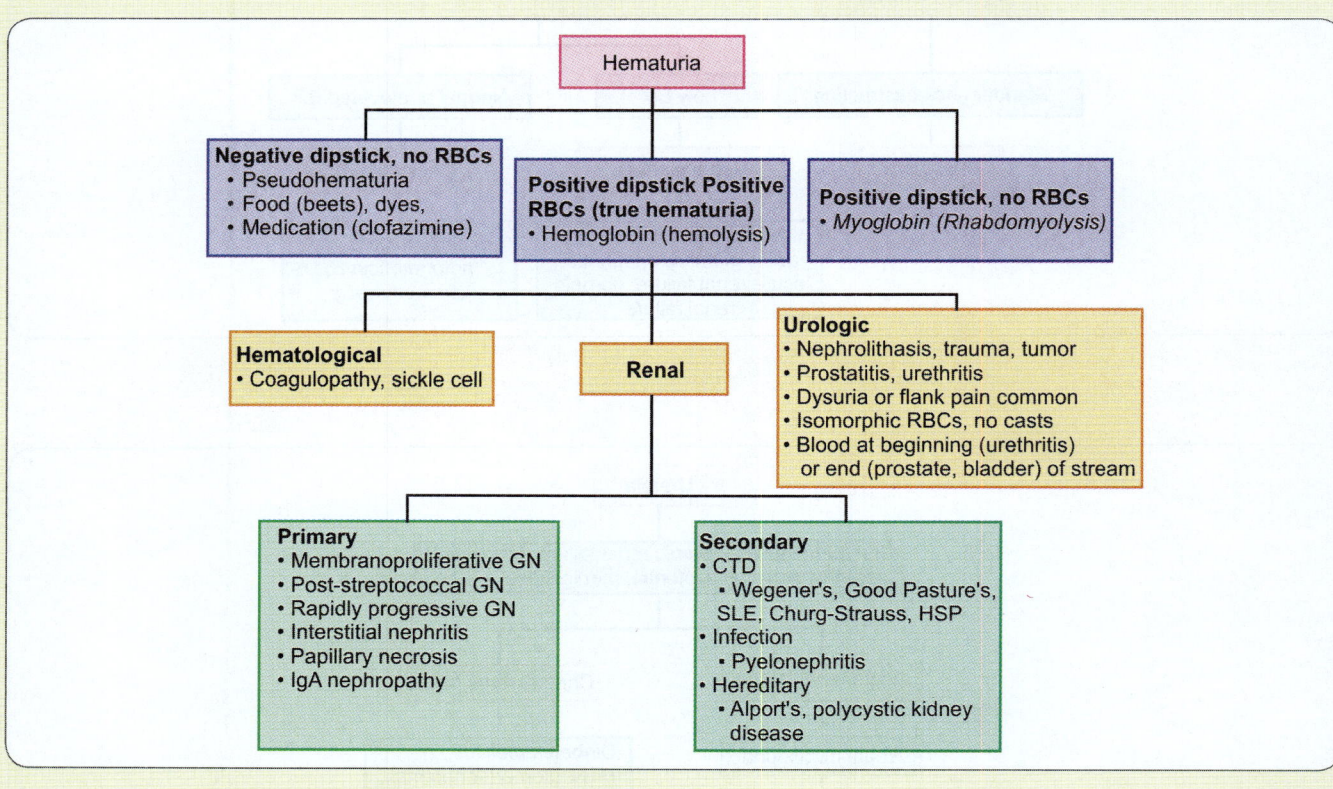

Multiple Choice Questions

Acute Kidney Injury

1. Polyuria is defined as? **(Recent Questions 2019)**
   a. >30 ml/kg/day   b. >40 ml/kg/day
   c. >50 ml/Kg/day   d. >60 ml/kg/day

2. Which of the following parameters is used to identify tubular damage in KDIGO criteria as compared to RIFLE criteria? **(AIIMS Nov 2018)**
   a. Uosm   b. Urinary Na+
   c. Urinary NGAL   d. Fe Na

3. A 70-year-old diabetic and hypertensive patient was being investigated for angina and a coronary angiogram was performed. Two days later, he developed fever and abdominal discomfort and dyspnea and a mottled skin rash. His great toe appeared black. His BP increased to 180/100. His creatinine was found to have risen from a pre-angiography level of 1.2 to 3.6 mg/dl. He has eosinophilia. Which one of the following statements is TRUE regarding this condition. **(Recent Pattern 2017-2018)**
   a. N-acetylcysteine would have prevented this condition
   b. This is contrast induced nephropathy
   c. Heparin is the treatment of choice
   d. Kidney biopsy will show micro-vessel occlusion with a cleft in the vessel

4. A 50-year-old patient develops cardiogenic shock following acute myocardial infarction. His urine output decreases in next few days. He has increased serum urea and creatinine, urine analysis reveals no glucose or protein but numerous hyaline casts are present. After few days he develops polyuria and serum creatinine levels fall. Histopathology of renal biopsy in this patient would reveal? **(JIPMER Nov 2014)**
   a. Immune complex   b. Glomerular crescents
   c. Patchy tubular necrosis d. Mesangial deposits

5. A 42-yrs old female present with diazepam and alcohol overdose She is comatose temperature is 34.5 degree Celsius BP 100/80 mm of Hg creatinine is 2.4 AST 500 GGT 35 IU. Urine dipstick showed 3 +blood but urine analysis was normal. USG abdomen was normal. What is the most likely diagnosis? **(JIPMER Nov 2014)**
   a. Hypothermia   b. Alcoholic hallucinosis
   c. Rhabdomyolysis   d. Acute interstitial nephritis

6. Acute renal failure results in **(Recent Question 2015-16)**
   a. Hyperkalemic alkalosis b. Hypokalemic alkalosis
   c. Hyperkalemic acidosis   d. Hypokalemic acidosis

7. All of the following causes acute renal failure except: **(Recent Question 2015-16)**
   a. Pyelonephritis   b. Snakebite
   c. Rhabdomyolysis   d. Analgesic nephropathy

8. Marker of acute kidney injury all except? **(Recent Pattern 2017-18)**
   a. Clusterin   b. Osteopontin
   c. Alanine aminopeptidase d. Acid phosphatase

9. Oliguric phase of ARF is characterized by A/E: **(Recent Pattern 2014-15)**
   a. Chest pain   b. Acidosis
   c. Hypertension   d. Hypokalemia

10. In renal failure, metabolic acidosis is due to?
    a. Increased H+ production **(Recent Pattern 2014-15)**
    b. Loss of HCO_3^-
    c. Decreased excretion of ammonia
    d. Use of diuretics

11. Biomarker not involved in acute kidney injury is? **(AIIMS Nov 2013)**
    a. NGAL   b. KIM 1
    c. Micro RNA 122   d. Cystatin C

12. The difference between sodium and chloride is low, the metabolic disorder in the patient would be? **(Recent Pattern 2014-15)**
    a. Metabolic acidosis b. Metabolic alkalosis
    c. Respiratory acidosis d. Respiratory alkalosis

13. Worsening of kidney function on contrast nephropathy is best evaluated with? **(AIIMS Nov 2013)**
    a. High serum creatinine b. Low serum creatinine
    c. High serum bilirubin   d. Low serum bilirubin

14. Anuria is defined as urine output less than? **(Recent Pattern 2014-15)**
    a. 4 ml /hr   b. 8ml/hr
    c. 12 ml/hr   d. 16 ml/hr

15. Monoclonal antibodies to the CD25 (IL-2α) receptors are being used for the treatment of : **(Bihar PG 2014)**
    a. Haematologic neoplasm
    b. Autoimmune diseases
    c. Bone marrow transplantation
    d. Kidney transplant rejection

16. In Hepatorenal syndrome, urine shows: **(Recent Pattern 2014-15)**
    a. Proteinuria   b. Hematuria
    c. A and b   d. No abnormality

17. Complication of diuretic phase of acute renal failure is: **(Recent Pattern 2014-15)**
    a. Convulsion
    b. Hyperkalemia
    c. Increased sodium excretion in urine
    d. Metabolic acidosis

18. Investigations in a patient of oliguria revealed: Urine osmolality: 800 mosm/kg. Urinary sodium 10 mmol/L. BUN: creatinine=20:1. The most likely diagnosis is?
    a. Prerenal acute renal failure **(Recent Pattern 2014-15)**
    b. Acute tubular necrosis
    c. Acute cortical necrosis
    d. Urinary tract obstruction

19. The differentiating factor between pre-renal and renal azotemia is: **(Recent Pattern 2014-15)**
    a. Sodium fraction excretion b. Creatinine clearance
    c. Serum creatinine level   d. Urine specific gravity

20. Non-oliguric renal failure is commonly seen in: **(Recent Pattern 2014-15)**
    a. Snake bite   b. Hypovolemic shock
    c. Aminoglycoside toxicity d. Multiple myeloma

21. Most unlikely cause of acute tubular necrosis amongst the following is : **(AI 1999)**
    a. Severe-bacterial-infection
    b. Massive burn
    c. Severe crush injury in the foot
    d. Rupture of aortic aneurysm

22. Which of the following values are suggestive of acute tubular necrosis : (AIIMS Nov 2000)
    a. Urine osmolality>500
    b. Urine sodium>40
    c. Blood urea nitrogen/plasma creatinine>20
    d. Urine creatinine /plasma creatinine>40
23. Fractional excretion of sodium <1 is seen in
    a. Prerenal azotemia (AIIMS Nov- 07)
    b. Acute tubular necrosis
    c. Acute ureteral obstruction
    d. Interstitial nephritis
24. Plasma urea / creatinine ratio of 20:1 may be seen in :
    a. Rhabdomyolysis (AI 2010)
    b. Ureteric calculi
    c. Prerenal failure
    d Chronic Glomerulonephritis
25. Prerenal and renal azotemia is differentiated on the basis of: (PGI Dec 99)
    a. Creatinine clearance   b. Serum creatinine level
    c. Sodium fraction excretion d. Urine bicarbonate level
26. All of the following are true about Oliguric ARF (AI-1993)
    a. Anemia   b. Metabolic Acidosis
    c. Uremia   d. Hypercalcemia
27. Which of the following statements is incorrect with regard to Hepatorenal syndrome in a patient with cirrhosis
    a. Createnine clearance < 40 ml/min (AI 2003)
    b. Urinary sodium < 10mq/L
    c. Urine osmolality lower than plasma osmolality
    d. No sustained improvement in renal function after volume expansion.
28. A 28-year-old boy met with on accident and sustained severe crush injury. He is most likely to develop: (AIIMS Nov 09)
    a. Acute Renal Failure   b. Hypophosphatemia
    c. Hypercalcemia   d. Acute Myocardial Infarction

Chronic Kidney Disease

29. Which of the following drug does not cause nephrotoxicity? (Recent Question 2016-17)
    a. Cisplatin   b. Cyclophosphamide
    c. Cyclosporine   d. Sirolimus
30. A 50-year-old diabetic patient is feeling unwell. On work up his serum creatinine = 5.0 mg% and blood urea = 125 mg%. Urine MICRAL test is positive. Which of the following will be useful for this patient?
    (Recent Question 2016-17)

    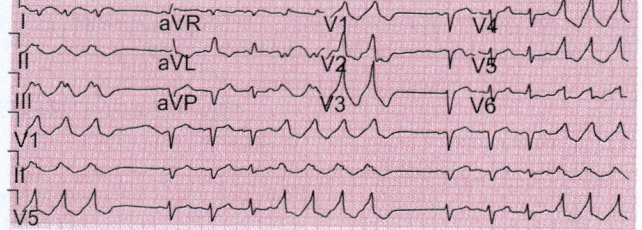

    a. Diuretics
    b. Cardio-selective beta blocker
    c. ACE inhibitor
    d. Amiodarone
31. Which of the following conditions typically has rickets with normal or low calcium, elevated phosphorus, elevated parathormone, and elevated alkaline phosphatase?
    (APPG 2016)
    a. Vitamin D deficiency
    b. Chronic kidney disease
    c. Dent's disease
    d. Fanconi syndrome
32. The triad of 'saturnine gout' + hypertension + renal failure is seen in? (APPG 2016)
    a. Diabetic nephropathy with hyporeninemic hypoaldosteronism
    b. Lead nephropathy
    c. Sickle cell nephropathy
    d. Aristolochic acid nephropathy
33. Which of the following statement on microalbuminuria is not true? (AIIMS Nov 2015)
    a. Cannot be detected by routine lab tests
    b. Urine protein less than 30-299 µg/day is called microalbuminuria
    c. Microalbuminuria is an independent risk factor for cardiovascular risk in diabetic patients
    d. Microalbuminuria is earliest marker of diabetic nephropathy.
34. All of the following may result in polyuria except:
    (UPSC 2015)
    a. Chronic renal failure   b. Hypoadrenalism
    c. Hypercalcemia   d. Lithium carbonate therapy
35. Regarding adult polycystic kidney disease, which one of the following statements is not correct? (UPSC 2015)
    a. Inherited as autosomal dominant with 100% penetrance
    b. Often associated with hepatic cysts
    c. Associated with increased incidence of subarachnoid hemorrhage
    d. Renal cell carcinoma is a frequent association
36. Which of the following is not a feature of chronic renal failure? (UPSC 2015)
    a. Hyperparathyroidism
    b. Osteomalacia
    c. Hyperthyroidism
    d. Decreased 1, 25(OH)2 vitamin D3 level
37. Patient on insulin in CKD stage 4. What is the dose adjustment of insulin required? (Recent Question 2015-16)
    a. Increased insulin   b. Decreased insulin
    c. Normal insulin   d. Add DPP-4 inhibitors
38. All are true about GFR except? (Recent Question 2015-16)
    a. 30-40% decrease after 70 years of age
    b. Best estimated by Creatinine clearance
    c. C.K.D is defied as GFR < 30 ml/min/1.73 m² for 4 weeks
    d. GFR is dependent on height in children
39. The most common neurological disorder seen in CRF patients: (Recent Pattern 2014-15)
    a. Dementia   b. Peripheral neuropathy
    c. Restless leg syndrome d. Encephalopathy
40. The term end-stage renal disease (ESRD) is considered appropriate when GFR falls to: (Recent Pattern 2014-15)
    a. 50% of normal   b. 25% of normal
    c. 10-25% of normal   d. 5-10% of normal

41. Patient with CRF is having a sodium level = 110 mEq/dl. Till what level should serum sodium be corrected in next 24 hours? *(Recent Pattern 2014-15)*
    a. 120 mEq/dl
    b. 130 mEq/dl
    c. 140 mEq/dl
    d. 150 mEq/dl
42. Not seen with uremic lung? *(Recent Pattern 2014-15)*
    a. Alveolar injury
    b. Pulmonary edema
    c. Interstitial fibrosis
    d. Fibrinous exudate in alveoli
43. Diagnostic feature of CRF is: *(Recent Pattern 2014-15)*
    a. Broad casts in urine
    b. Elevated blood urea
    c. Proteinuria
    d. Bleeding diathesis
44. Which one of the following studies is most sensitive for detecting diabetic nephropathy in early stage? *(Recent Pattern 2014-15)*
    a. Microalbuminuria
    b. Creatinine clearance test
    c. Ultrasonography
    d. Serum cretinine level
45. CRF shows all except: *(Recent Pattern 2014-15)*
    a. Hyperphosphataemia
    b. Hyperuricaemia
    c. Decreased half life of insulin
    d. Decreased Serum vitamin D3
46. Clinical features of CRF/uraemia appear when renal function is reduced to: *(Recent Pattern 2014-15)*
    a. 70%
    b. 50%
    c. 30%
    d. 20%
47. CRF changes are A/E: *(Recent Pattern 2014-15)*
    a. Hyperkalaemia
    b. Hypophosphatemia
    c. Hypocalcaemia
    d. Hypokalemia
48. Raised PTH is found in: *(Recent Pattern 2014-15)*
    a. Pseudopseudohypoparathyroidism
    b. Renal osteodystrophy
    c. Hypercalcaemia
    d. Osteogenesis imperfecta
49. An adult patient presents with normal or enlarged kidneys with massive proteinuria. Most likely cause is: *(Recent Pattern 2014-15)*
    a. Chronic pyelonephritis
    b. Chronic glomerulonephritis
    c. Amyloidosis
    d. Renal artery stenosis
50. A 28 yr old man has lenticonus and ESRD. His maternal uncle also died of similar illness. Diagnosis is: *(AIIMS May 2012)*
    a. ARPKD
    b. ADPKD
    c. Oxalosis
    d. Alport's syndrome
51. Central nervous system manifestations in chronic renal failure are a result of all of the following except: *(Recent Pattern 2014-15)*
    a. Hyperosmolarity
    b. Hypocalcemia
    c. Acidosis
    d. Hyponatremia
52. Dialysis disequilibrium occurs due to: *(Recent Pattern 2014-15)*
    a. Cerebral edema
    b. Hypertension
    c. Alumunium toxicity
    d. A Beta2 amyloid deposition
53. Normal sized to enlarged kidneys in a patient with chronic renal failure is indicative of: *(Recent Pattern 2014-15)*
    a. Benign Nephrosclerosis
    b. Chronic glomerulonephritis
    c. Chronic interstitial nephritis
    d. Primary amyloidosis
54. Chronic renal failure is often complicated by all of the following except: *(Recent Pattern 2014-15)*
    a. Myopathy
    b. Hemolytic uremic syndrome
    c. Peripheral neuropathy
    d. Ectopic calcification
55. Dementia in patient of chronic renal failure with chronic hemodialysis is due to: *(Recent Pattern 2014-15)*
    a. Aluminium toxicity
    b. Uremia
    c. Cerebral amyloid angiopathy
    d. A β amyloid deposition
56. In chronic renal failure there is: *(Recent Pattern 2014-15)*
    a. Decrease anion gap
    b. Normal anion gap
    c. Increased anion gap
    d. Metabolic alkalosis
57. Convulsions are commonly precipitated in terminal renal failure by: *(Recent Pattern 2014-15)*
    a. Hyperkalemia
    b. Hypokalemia
    c. Water intoxication
    d. Hypermagnesemia
58. Anaemia of advanced renal insufficiency is best treated by: *(Recent Pattern 2014-15)*
    a. Blood transfusions
    b. Recombinant human erythropoietin
    c. Parenteral iron therapy
    d. Folic acid supplementation
59. In uraemia all are reversed by dialysis except: *(Recent Pattern 2014-15)*
    a. Sexual dysfunction
    b. Pericarditis
    c. Uraemic lung
    d. Neuropathy
60. Restless leg syndrome (RLS) is seen in: *(AI 2009)*
    a. Hypercalcemia
    b. Hyperphosphatemia
    c. Chronic renal failure
    d. Hyperkalemia
61. Metabolic complication in CRF include all of the following except: *(AI 1998)*
    a. Hyperkalemia
    b. Hypophosphatemia
    c. Hypocalcemia
    d. Hypokalemia
62. Renal osteodystropy differs from nutritional and genetic forms of osesteomalacia in having: *(AI 2002)*
    a. Hypocalcaemia
    b. Hypercalcemia
    c. Hypophostaemia
    d. Hyperphosphatemia

Hemodialysis

63. Which of the following is an absolute indication for hemodialysis? *(Recent Question 2015-16)*
    a. Hypertension
    b. Hypokalemia
    c. Pericarditis
    d. Metabolic alkalosis
64. Which of the following Microorganism is incriminated in infection after Hemodialysis? *(Recent Question 2015-16)*
    a. Chlamydia
    b. Gram positive
    c. Gram negative
    d. Anaerobes
65. Hemodialysis can be performed for long periods from the same site because? *(Recent Question 2015-16)*
    a. Arteriovenous fistula reduces bacterial contamination of site
    b. Arteriovenous fistula results in arterialization of vein
    c. Arteriovenous fistula reduces chances of graft failure
    d. Arteriovenous fistula facilitates small bore needles for high flow rates

66. **Chronic hemodialysis in ESRD patient is done:**
    (Recent Question 2015-16)
    a. Once per week   b. Twice per week
    c. Thrice per week   d. Daily

67. **A patient of ESRD is undergoing hemodialysis. Central dialysis catheter is placed at which site?**

    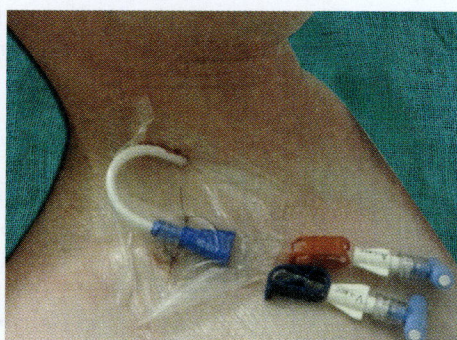

    a. Right internal jugular vein
    b. Left internal jugular vein
    c. Right subclavian vein
    d. Right subclavian artery

68. **The patient is scheduled for haemodialysis. The A-V fistula is known as?** *(Recent Question 2015-16)*

    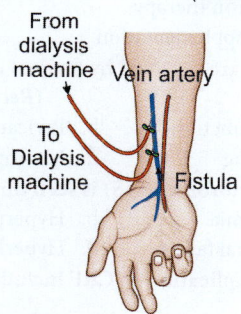

    a. Cimino- Brescia fistula
    b. Hughes fistula
    c. SLED (sustained Low efficiency dialysis)
    d. Continuous renal replacement therapy

69. **Chronic hemodialysis in ESRD patient is done?**
    (Recent Pattern 2015-16)
    a. Once per week   b. Twice per week
    c. Thrice per week   d. Daily

70. **The following are the complications of haemodialysis except:** *(Recent Pattern 2014-15)*
    a. Hypotension   b. Peritonitis
    c. Hypertension   d. Bleeding tendency

71. **Most common acute complication of dialysis is:**
    (Recent Pattern 2014-15)
    a. Hypotension   b. Bleeding
    c. Dementia   d. Muscle cramps

72. **Amyloidosis protein associated with hemodialysis?**
    (Recent Pattern 2014-15)
    a. A Beta2   b. A Beta
    c. A transthyretin   d. AL

73. **The absolute indications for dialysis include the following except:** *(Recent Pattern 2014-15)*
    a. Persistent Hyperkalaemia   b. Congestive cardiac failure
    c. Pulmonary edema   d. Hyperphosphatemia

74. **Most common complication causing death in patients on recurrent hemodialysis?** *(Recent Pattern 2014-15)*
    a. Cardiovascular
    b. Adynamic osteomalacia
    c. Dyselectrolytemia
    d. Encephalopathy

75. **All of the following uremic manifestations improve with dialysis except:** *(Recent Pattern 2014-15)*
    a. Metabolic acidosis
    b. Osteodystrophy
    c. Asterixis
    d. Nausea, vomiting and anorexia

76. **Following are absolute indication for hemo-dialysis except:**
    a. GI bleeding   *(Recent Pattern 2014-15)*
    b. Convulsions
    c. Pericarditis
    d. Hyperkalemia of 6.5 mEq/L

77. **Dialysis patients are prone to develop:**
    (Recent Pattern 2014-15)
    a. Lead toxicity   b. Iron toxicity
    c. Aluminium toxicity   d. Zinc toxicity

Kidney Transplantation

78. **Post kidney transplantation a patient presents with diarrhoea. The motility of the worms is shown in the figure. Correct statement about the organism is?**
    (AIIMS Nov 2018)

    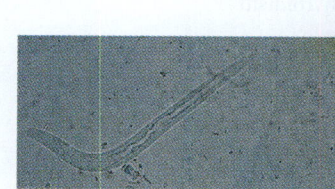 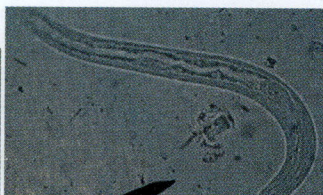

    a. Monoecious organism related with parthenogenesis
    b. Transmitted by intake of contaminated food and water
    c. Loeffler pneumonia is caused by the same organism
    d. Infection occurs by filariform larvae

79. **Which is true about the inclusion bodies seen in specimen of patient who underwent kidney transplantation?**
    (Recent Question 2016-17)

    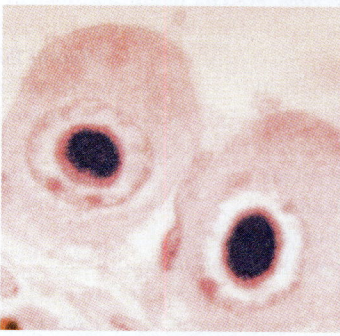

    a. Basophilic intranuclear inclusion
    b. Eosinophilic intranuclear inclusion
    c. Eosinophilic intracytoplasmic inclusion
    d. Basophilic intracytoplasmic inclusion

80. Which is the best test for detection of recent CMV infection?
 (Recent Question 2016-17)
 a. Urine microscopy showing owl eye inclusion
 b. IgM anti-CMV antibody
 c. Nucleic acid testing
 d. Immuno-fluorescence on urine specimen

81. Category 4 donation after cardiac death (DCD) is defined as? *(Recent Question 2016-17)*
 a. Donation after patient is brought dead
 b. Donation by donor who died to high creatinine
 c. Donation by donor who died due to CVA
 d. Donation after cardiac arrest following brain stem death

82. Life expectancy after living donor kidney transplantation is _____? *(Recent Question 2016-17)*
 a. 5 years b. 10 years
 c. 15 years d. 20 years

83. Select the FALSE statement regarding Kidney Transplantation? *(APPG 2016)*
 a. Selective renal angiogram in the recipient helps to know vascular anatomy for anastomosis
 b. Antithymocyte globulin (ATG) is used in induction therapy
 c. ABO compatibility between donor and recipient is a prerequisite
 d. Commonly used maintenance immunosuppression comprises prednisone & mycophenolate mofetil & Tacrolimus

84. Recurrence of lesions is seen after renal transplant in all except: *(Recent Pattern 2014-15)*
 a. SLE b. Diabetic nephropathy
 c. Alport's syndrome d. Goodpasture's syndrome

85. All are true for transplanted kidney except:
 (Recent Pattern 2014-15)
 a. Humoral antibody is responsible for rejection
 b. CMI is responsible for rejection
 c. Previous blood transfusion increases chances of rejection
 d. HLA identity similarity seen in 1:100 people

86. A 7-year-old child has steroid DEPENDENT Nephrotic syndrome. His weight is 30 kg and height of 106 cm. He is having truncal obesity with subcapsular bilateral cataracts. Best drug for this patient: *(AIIMS May 2013)*
 a. Mycophenolate b. Levamisole
 c. Cyclophosphamide d. Azathioprine

87. A patient recently under-went a renal allograft transplantation and on treatment with azathioprine and prednisolone he developed, fever and cough with thick sputum and left lower lung consolidation with a cavity. The culture specimen demonstrates gram+ve organism with beaded string appearance. Initial treatment will include:
 (Recent Pattern 2014-15)
 a. Penicillin b. Erythromycin
 c. Ceftazidime d. Sulfisoxazole

88. A 40-year-old man underwent kidney trans-plantation for end-stage renal disease. Two months after transplantation, he developed fever and features suggestive of bilateral diffuse interstitial pneumonia. Which one of the following is the most likely etiological agent?
 (Recent Pattern 2014-15)
 a. Herpes simplex virus b. Cytomegalovirus
 c. Epstein-Barr virus d. Legionella

89. Nephrotic syndrome associated with malaria is due to infection of? *(Recent Pattern 2014-15)*
 a. P. malariae b. P. ovale
 c. P. vivax d. P. falciparum

90. The most common ocular infection after renal transplantation is by: *(Recent Pattern 2014-15)*
 a. Cytomegalovirus b. Toxoplasma
 c. Herpes virus d. EB virus

91. Most common cancer after kidney transplanta-tion?
 (Recent Pattern 2014-15)
 a. Skin cancer b. Renal cell cancer
 c. NHL d. Hodgkins lymphoma

92. A renal transplant recurrence of the disease occurs mostly with: *(Recent Pattern 2014-15)*
 a. Lupus nephritis
 b. DM nephropathy
 c. Membranous glomerulonephritis
 d. Membranous proliferative glomerulonephritis

93. Disease, which does not recur in the kidney after renal transplant: *(AIIMS Feb 97)*
 a. Alport's syndrome
 b. Amyloidosis
 c. Good Pasteur's syndrome
 d. Diabetic nephropathy

94. A 7-year-old boy presented with generalized edema. Urine examination revealed marked albuminuria. Serum biochemical examinations showed hypoalbuminaemia with hyperlipidemia. Kidney biopsy was undertaken. On light microscopic examination, the kidney appeared normal. Electron microscopic examination is most likely to reveal –
 (AIIMS Nov-03)
 a. Fusion of foot processes of the glomerular epithelial cells
 b. Rarefaction of glomerular basement membrane
 c. Deposition of electron dense material in the basement membrane
 d. Thin basement membrane

95. True about Light microscopic changes in Minimal Change Glomerulonephritis is: *(AI 95)*
 a. No abnormality
 b. Fusion of foot process
 c. Absence of Immunoglobulins
 d. Absence of complement

96. A child presents with hematuria and nephrotic syndrome. A diagnosis of minimal change disease was made. Which of the following statements about the diagnosis is true:
 (AIPG 2010)
 a. Glomerular function is lost due to loss of polyanions around the foot processes
 b. Foot processes of podocytes in the Glomerular membrane are normal
 c. Glomerular function is lost due to deposition of IgA on the glomerular membrane
 d. Focal segmental changes are observed

97. All are steroid resistant except: *(AI 96)*
 a. Post-streptococcal glomerulonephritis
 b. Minimal change glomerulonephritis
 c. RPGN
 d. Recurrent hematuria

98. Which of the following drugs is not a part of the 'Triple Therapy' immunosuppression for post-renal transplant patients? *(AI 2006)*
    a. Cyclosporine
    b. Azathioprine
    c. FK 506
    d. Prednisolone

Nephrotic Syndrome

99. Most common nephropathy associated with malignancy?
    a. Membranous
    b. MCD *(AIIMS May 2015)*
    c. IgA
    d. FSGS

100. A 10-year-old child presents with oedema and decreased urine output. On evaluation, serum albumin is 2.5 g/dL, S. Creatinine is 0.5 mg/dl, Urine protein is 3+ with no RBC casts. Pathological change expected is? *(AIIMS May 2015)*
    a. Minimal change disease
    b. Interstitial nephritis
    c. IgA nephropathy
    d. FSGS

101. Which of the following is true about glomerular proteinuria?
    a. DM *(PGI Nov 2014)*
    b. Amyloidosis
    c. Multiple myeloma
    d. ACE inhibitors decreases proteinuria

102. All are true about most common cause of nephrotic syndrome in children except? *(Recent Question 2015-16)*
    a. It is not associated with hypertension
    b. Minimal change disease in children <10 year
    c. Massive Proteinuria > 3.5 gm%/24 Hours
    d. Low Complement Levels

103. Membranous Glomerulopathy is seen in? *(Recent Question 2015-16)*
    a. Diabetes
    b. HTN
    c. Renal failure
    d. Malignancy

104. All are seen in Nephrotic syndrome except: *(Recent Question 2015-16)*
    a. Atherosclerosis
    b. Thrombo-embolism
    c. Increased protein C levels
    d. Lipiduria

105. Type of glomerulopathy in HIV positive patient is: *(Recent Question 2015-16)*
    a. Focal segmental glomerulosclerosis
    b. Diffuse glomerulosclerosis
    c. Membranous glomerulopathy
    d. Mesangio-proliferative glomerulonephritis

106. Nephrotic syndrome patient after a bout of diarrhea presented with acute kidney injury and serum creatinine = 4.5. All are possible reasons except?
    a. Renal vein thrombosis *(AIIMS Nov 14)*
    b. Diarrhea water depletion
    c. Frusemide water depletion
    d. Steroid induced diabetes

107. Leprosy causes: *(Recent Pattern 2014-15)*
    a. Membranous GN
    b. Focal glomerulosclerosis
    c. Membranoproliferative GN
    d. Mesangioprolferative GN

108. Nephrotic syndrome is the hall mark of the following primary kidney diseases except: *(Recent Pattern 2014-15)*
    a. Membranous Glomerulopathy
    b. IgA nephropathy
    c. Minimal change disease
    d. Focal segmental Glomerulosclerosis

109. Muehrcke lines in nails are seen in: *(Recent Pattern 2014-15)*
    a. Nephrotic syndrome
    b. Barrter syndrome
    c. Nail patella syndrome
    d. Acute tubular necrosis

110. Non- selective proteinuria is seen in:
    a. Minimal change *(Recent Pattern 2014-15)*
    b. Mesangio-proliferative GN
    c. Membranous glomerulonephritis
    d. Focal segmental Glomerulosclerosis

111. Membranous GN with reduced complement level is seen in? *(Recent Pattern 2014-15)*
    a. Hepatitis B
    b. SLE
    c. Malaria
    d. Syphilis

112. Regarding complications of nephrotic syndrome incorrect is: *(Recent Pattern 2014-15)*
    a. Volume overload state
    b. Hypercoagulable state
    c. Hyperlipidaemia
    d. Hypocalcemia

113. In bronchogenic carcinoma patient presenting as a case of nephrotic syndrome, if kidney biopsy is done the most likely lesion will be? *(Recent Pattern 2014-15)*
    a. Membranous GN
    b. Focal proliferative GN
    c. Minimal change disease
    d. Focal segmental glomerulosclerosis

114. Renal vein thrombosis is associated with which underlying disease of kidney: *(Recent Pattern 2014-15)*
    a. Chronic glomerulonephritis
    b. Pyelonephritis
    c. SLE
    d. Nephrotic syndrome

115. All of the following are decreased in Nephrotic syndrome except *(Recent Pattern 2014-15)*
    a. Transferrin
    b. Ceruloplasmin
    c. Albumin
    d. Fibrinogen

116. Chronic reflux nephropathy causes:
    a. Membranous nephropathy *(Recent Pattern 2014-15)*
    b. Focal segmental GN
    c. MPGN
    d. Lipoid nephrosis

117. Hypercoagulation in Nephrotic syndrome is caused by:
    a. Loss of Antithrombin III *(AI 2010)*
    b. Decreased Fibrinogen
    c. Decreased Metabolism of Vitamin K
    d. Increase in protein C

118. A patient with nephrotic syndrome on longstanding corticosteroid therapy may develop all the following except: *(AI 2002)*
    a. Hyperglycemia
    b. Hypertrophy of muscle
    c. Neuropsychiatric symptoms
    d. Suppression of the pituitary adrenal axis

119. A patient who has been diagnosed with bronchiectasis 5 years ago presents with edema on legs and proteinuria. The most likely finding in his kidney will be: *(AI 2012)*
    a. Minimal Change Disease
    b. Amyloid Nephropathy
    c. Rapidly Progressive Glomerulonephritis (RPGN)
    d. Crescenteric Glomerulonephritis

120. **Reflux Nephropathy with proteinuria in the nephrotic range may be seen in patients with:** (AIIMS Nov 06)
    a. Membranous glomerulonephritis
    b. Focal segmental Glomerulosclerosis
    c. Nodular glomerulosclerosis
    d. Crescenteric glomerulonephritis

121. **Renal vein thrombosis is most commonly associated with:**
    a. Diabetic nephropathy (AI 2001)
    b. Membranous glomerulopathy
    c. Minimal change disease
    d. Membrano-proliferative glomerulonephritis

Nephritic Syndrome and Hematuria

122. **Which of the following immunological reactions occurs in Good-pasture syndrome?** (UPSC 2015)
    a. Type I atopy   b. Type II cytotoxic
    c. Type III immune complex   d. Type IV cell mediation

123. **Henoch schonlein purpura is characterized by the following except:** (APPG 2015 Medicine)
    a. Glomerulonephritis   b. Thrombocytopenia
    c. Hematochezia   d. Palpable purpura

124. **True statement regarding post streptococcal glomerulonephritis is?** (JIPMER Nov 2014)
    a. Renal biopsy is indicated in severe renal dysfunction
    b. Microscopic hematuria resolves within 2 weeks
    c. Serum C3 levels are normal
    d. Serum triglyceride levels are elevated

125. **Feature of RPGN are A/E:** (Recent Pattern 2014-15)
    a. Rapid recovery
    b. Crescent formation
    c. High blood pressure
    d. Non-selective proteinuria

126. **Type I membrano proliferative Glomerulo-nephritis is commonly associated with all except:**
    a. SLE (Recent Pattern 2014-15)
    b. Hepatitis C infections
    c. Captopril
    d. Neoplastic diseases

127. **Characteristic finding in AGN:** (Recent Pattern 2014-15)
    a. Red cell cast   b. Hematuria
    c. Proteinuria   d. Epithelial Cells

128. **RBC cast in the microscopic examination of the urine is an indicator of:** (Recent Pattern 2014-15)
    a. Acute glomerulonephritis
    b. Acute pyelonephritis
    c. Chronic glomerulonephritis
    d. Nephrotic syndrome

129. **What is the minimum number of red blood cells *per microliter* of urine required for diagnosis of hematuria?** (APPG 2014)
    a. 3   b. 5
    c. 8   d. 10

130. **Essential feature of nephritic syndrome is:** (Recent Pattern 2014-15)
    a. Proteinuria   b. Hypoalbuminaemia
    c. Hyperlipidaemia   d. Hematuria

131. **Manifestation of acute glomerulonephritis includes each of the following except:** (Recent Pattern 2014-15)
    a. Peri-orbital edema
    b. Hypertensive encephalopathy
    c. Acute renal failure
    d. Optic atrophy

132. **A female patient presents with upper respiratory tract infection. Two days after, she develops hematuria. Probable diagnosis:** (Recent Pattern 2014-15)
    a. IgA nephropathy
    b. Wegener's granulomatosis
    c. Henoch-Schnlein purpura
    d. Poststreptococcal glomerulonephritis

133. **Triad of glomerulonephritis pulmonary hemorrhages and antibody to basement membrane is called:** (Recent Pattern 2014-15)
    a. Goodpasture's syndrome
    b. Systemic Necrotising Vasculitis
    c. Mixed connective tissue disease
    d. Diabetic nephropathy

134. **The following type of glomerulonephritis should *not* be treated with prednisolone:** (Recent Pattern 2014-15)
    a. Minimal change disease
    b. Lipoid nephrosis
    c. Congenital Nephrotic Syndrome
    d. Post-streptococcal GN

135. **Presence of which of the following in the urine is diagnostic of glomerular injury:** (AIIMS- June 99)
    a. Bright red cells
    b. 20% dysmorphic RBC's
    c. 100 RBC per high power field
    d. beta 2 micro globulin

136. **In hematuria of glomerular origin the urine is characterized by the presence of all of the following except:** (AI 2004)
    a. Red cell casts   b. Acanthocytes
    c. Crenated red cells   d. Dysmorphic red cells

137. **Presence of which of the following correlates best with renal pathology:** (AIIMS June 2000)
    a. Hyaline cast   b. Coarse granular cast
    c. Broad cast   d. Epithelial cast

138. **Post-infective glomerulonephritis present as:** (AI 1996)
    a. ARF   b. Nephrotic syndrome
    c. Nephritic syndrome   d. Asymptomatic hematuria

139. **RPGN occurs in A/E:** (AIIMS Sep 96)
    a. SLE
    b. Post streptococcal glomerulonephritis
    c. Diabetic nephropathy
    d. Good pastures syndromes

140. **The prognosis of rapidly proliferating glomerulonephritis (Crescentric GN) depends upon:** (AIIMS Nov 01)
    a. Number of crescents   b. Size of crescents
    c. Shape of crescents   d. Cellularity of crescents

141. **True about Post-Streptococcal Glomerulonephritis is:**
    a. 50% of cases occur after pharyngitis (AI 2000)
    b. Early treatment of Pharyngitis eliminates the risk of P.S.G.N.
    c. Glomerulonephritis, secondary to skin infection, is more common in summer
    d. Recurrence is seen

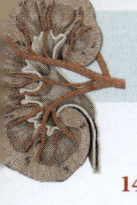

142. Wire loop lesions are often characteristic for the following class of lupus nephritis: (AIIMS May 04)
    a. Mesangial proliferative glomerulonephritis (WHO class II)
    b. Focal proliferative glomerulonephritis (WHO class III)
    c. Diffuse proliferative glomerulonephritis (WHO class IV)
    d. Membranous glomerulonephritis (WHO class V)

143. All of the following factors are associated with adverse prognosis and high risk of Renal progression in Lupus Nephritis, Except: (PGI Dec 03)
    a. High levels of Anti-ds DNA
    b. Persistant proteinuria (Nephrotic range > 3gm/day)
    c. Hypocomplementenemia
    d. Anti La (SSB)

144. Serum C3 is persistently low in the following except:
    a. Post streptococcal glomerulonephritis (AI/AIIMS 2008)
    b. Membranoproliferative glomerulonephritis
    c. Lupus nephritis
    d. Glomerulonephritis related to bacterial endocarditis

Hemolytic Uraemic Syndrome

145. Hemolytic-uremic syndrome true is A/E: (AIPG 2011)
    a. Uremia
    b. Hypofibrinogenemia
    c. Thrombocytopenia
    d. Positive Coomb's test

146. A young boy with skin rashes (Purpura), acute onset, oliguria, CNS manifestation after 5 days of diarrhea is suffering from: (Recent Pattern 2014-15)
    a. D+ HUS
    b. D- HUS
    c. Aplastic anemia
    d. TTP

147. Which is not a feature of Hemolytic-Uremic syndrome:
    a. Thrombocytosis (Recent Pattern 2014-15)
    b. Uraemia
    c. Hematuria
    d. Segmented RBC's in peripheral smear

148. Which of the following is not a feature of Hemolytic-Uremic syndrome? (Recent Pattern 2014-15)
    a. Encephalopathy
    b. Oliguria
    c. Thrombocytopenia
    d. Purpura

149. All are features of haemolytic uremic syndrome, except:
    a. Hyperkalemia (AIIMS Dec 95)
    b. Anaemia
    c. Renal microthrombi
    d. Neuropsychiatric disturbances

150. A 20-year-old male presents with features of acute renal failure 5 days after an episode of diarrhea. Blood examination shows thrombocytopenia and Hb-10 gm%. Likely cause is: (AIIMS June 99)
    a. Haemolytic uremic syndrome
    b. Hereditary spherocytosis
    c. Haemolytic crises
    d. Chronic glomerulonephritis

Interstitial Nephritis

151. The following conditions can cause interstitial nephritis except: (UPSC 2015)
    a. Infections   b. Hepatorenal syndrome
    c. Lymphoma   d. Sarcoidosis

152. Interstitial nephritis is common with (Recent Question 2015-16)
    a. NSAID   b. Black water fever
    c. Rhabdomyolysis   d. Tumor lysis syndrome

153. Which of the following DOES NOT cause Polyuria: (Recent Question 2015-16)
    a. Interstitial nephritis   b. Hypokalemia
    c. A.D.H insufficiency   d. Rhabdomyolysis

154. Salt losing nephritis is: (Recent Pattern 2014-15)
    a. Interstitial nephritis   b. Polycystic Kidney
    c. Lupus nephritis   d. R.P.G.N

155. Salt losing nephritis is a feature of: (AI 2000)
    a. Interstitial nephritis   (AIIMS 95)
    b. Renal Amyloidosis   (AIIMS May 94)
    c. Lupus nephritis
    d. Post Streptococcal Glomerulonephritis

Bartter and Gitelman Syndrome

156. All are true about Bartter syndrome except?
    a. Urinary calcium increased (JIPMER Nov 2015)
    b. Hypokalemia
    c. Mineralocorticoid antagonist can be used
    d. Metabolic alkalosis

157. All of following are features of Bartter's syndrome except: (Recent Pattern 2014-15)
    a. Hypertension   b. Periodic paralysis
    c. Alkalosis   d. Polyuria

158. Gitelman's Syndrome incorrect is: (Recent Pattern 2014-15)
    a. Hypokalemic metabolic alkalosis
    b. Mimics thiazide diuretics
    c. Hypercalciuria
    d. Generally milder clinical course

159. Gitelman's Syndrome differs from Bartter's Syndrome in all except: (APPG 2014)
    a. Less common
    b. Later age of presentation
    c. Prominent neuromuscular signs and symptoms
    d. Generally milder clinical course

160. All are true regarding Bartter syndrome except?
    a. Hypokalemic alkalosis (Recent Pattern 2014-15)
    b. Hypomagnesuria
    c. Congenital SN hearing defect
    d. Associated with Barttin mutation

Tumor Lysis Syndrome

161. Initial treatment of tumor lysis syndrome is: (Recent Pattern 2014-15)
    a. Rasburicase + hydration + urinary alkalization
    b. Allopurinol+ Hydration + urinary alkalization
    c. Hydration + urinary alkalization
    d. Hydration

162. Test predicting the return of renal function in a patient with tumour lysis syndrome is? *(Recent Pattern 2014-15)*
    a. Serum creatinine
    b. Serum phosphate
    c. Serum potassium
    d. Serum Uric acid

Papillary Necrosis

163. Renal papillary necrosis can be caused by: *(Recent Pattern 2014-15)*
    a. Phenacetin
    b. Sulphonamides
    c. Gentamicin
    d. Penicillin
164. Papillary necrosis is most commonly seen in: *(AIPG 2010)*
    a. Diabetes mellitus
    b. Sickle cell anemia
    c. Acute pyelonephritis
    d. Analgesic nephropathy
165. Papillary necrosis is seen with all except? *(Recent Pattern 2014-15)*
    a. Chronic alcoholism
    b. Sickle cell anemia
    c. Analgesic nephropathy
    d. Medullary sponge kidney

Cystic Kidney Disease

166. A 40-year-old man has been diagnosed with autosomal dominant polycystic kidney disease. How the cysts should be present in USG to call it ADPKD? *(Recent Question 2016-17)*
    a. 1 Cyst per kidney
    b. 2 cyst per kidney
    c. 3 cyst per kidney
    d. 4 cyst per kidney
167. The gross specimen section of kidney depicts: *(APPG 2015 Medicine)*

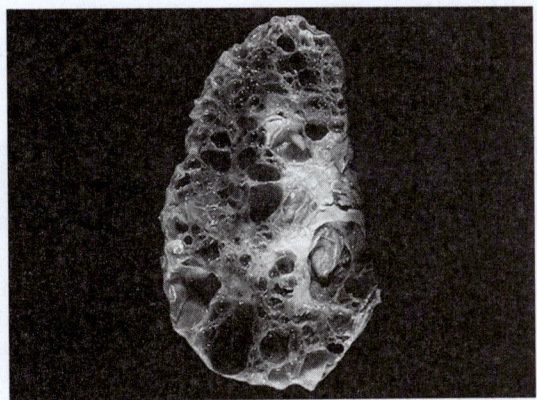

    a. Renal cell carcinoma
    b. Medullary sponge kidney
    c. Polycystic kidney
    d. Hydatid cyst
168. All can be manifestations of polycystic kidney except: *(Recent Pattern 2014-15)*
    a. Urine retention
    b. Renal hypertension
    c. Renal failure
    d. Haematuria
169. Autosomal dominant polycystic kidney is not associated with cysts in: *(Recent Pattern 2014-15)*
    a. Liver
    b. Pancreas
    c. Brain
    d. Lungs
170. Commonest Symptom of medullary sponge kidney disease: *(Recent Pattern 2014-15)*
    a. Anuria
    b. Anemia
    c. Azotemia
    d. UTI
171. True regarding chromosomal location of adult polycystic kidney disease I and II respectively is: *(Recent Pattern 2014-15)*
    a. Chr 16 and 5
    b. Chr 16 and 4
    c. Chr 11 and 5
    d. Chr 21 and 18
172. Medullary cystic kidney disease is best diagnosed by:
    a. Radio nucleotide scanning *(Recent Pattern 2014-15)*
    b. Biopsy
    c. USG
    d. CT Scan
173. True about adult polycystic kidney disease is all. except:
    a. Autosomal dominant inheritance *(AIIMS 2001)*
    b. Hypertension is rare
    c. Can be associated with cysts in liver, lungs and pancreas
    d. Pyelonephritis is common
174. Which of the following is associated with adult polycystic kidney disease? *(AIIMS 2001)*
    a. Berry Aneurysm in Circle of Willis
    b. Saccular aneurysms of aorta
    c. Fusiform aneurysms of aorta
    d. Leutic aneurysms
175. Polycystic disease of the kidney may have cysts in all of the following organs except: *(AI 2004)*
    a. Lung
    b. Liver
    c. Pancreas
    d. Spleen
176. Which of the following is the common extrarenal involvement in autosomal dominant polycystic kidney disease: *(AIIMS Nov 04)*
    a. Mitral valve prolapse
    b. Hepatic cysts
    c. Splenic cysts
    d. Colonic diverticulosis
177. Medullary cystic disease of the kidney is best diagnosed by: *(AI 2002)*
    a. Ultrasound
    b. Nuclear scan
    c. Urography
    d. Biopsy

Nephrocalcinosis (Kidney Stones)

178. Which of these is correct about Struvite stones?
    a. Present in alkaline urine *(Recent Question 2015-16)*
    b. Most common kidney disease
    c. Are Calcium pyrophosphate stones
    d. Most common kidney stones
179. IOC for ureteric stone? *(Recent Pattern 2015-16)*
    a. CT scan
    b. USG
    c. MIBG scan
    d. DMSA scan
180. All are indicated in a 30-year-old patient with increased serum cysteine and multiple renal stones except: *(AIIMS Nov 2012)*
    a. Cysteamine
    b. Increase fluid intake
    c. Alkalinisation of urine
    d. Pencillamine
181. A 35-year-old female with recurrent renal stone. Not advised is? *(AIIMS Nov 2012)*
    a. Increase water intake
    b. Restrict protein
    c. Restrict salt
    d. Restrict calcium
182. Nephrocalcinosis is seen in all except:
    a. Polycystic kidney *(Recent Pattern 2014-15)*
    b. Hyperparathyroidism
    c. Medullary sponge kidney
    d. Renal tubular acidosis

183. **Most common cause of calcium oxalate stones is?**
    a. Hyper-parathyrodism   (Recent Pattern 2014-15)
    b. Idiopathic Hypercalciuria
    c. Dietary intake of milk based products
    d. Renal tubular acidosis type 1

184. **Nephro-calcinosis is common in which type of renal tubular acidosis:**   (Recent Pattern 2014-15)
    a. Type I   b. Type II
    c. Type III   d. Type IV

185. **All of the following statement about Renal Calculi are true, Except:**   (AI 1993)
    a. Cystine stones form in acidic urine
    b. Struvite stones form in alkaline urine
    c. Oxalate stones are radiopaque
    d. Uric acid stones are resistant to ESWL

186. **Stone which is resistant to lithotripsy:**   (AIIMS May 07)
    a. Calcium oxalate   b. Triple phosphate stone
    c. Cystine stone   d. Uric acid stone

187. **Which of the following stones is hard to break by ESWL:**
    a. Calcium Oxalate Monohydrate   (AI 2010)
    b. Calcium Oxalate Dihydrate
    c. Uric acid
    d. Struvite

188. **All of the following types of Renal Stones are Radiopaque, Except:**   (AIIMS June 2000)
    a. Oxalate   b. Uric Acid
    c. Cystine   d. Mixed

189. **Renal Calculi associated with proteus infection:**   (AI 2009)
    a. Uric Acid   b. Triple Phosphate
    c. Calcium oxalate d. Xanthine

190. **Ureteric colic due to stone is caused by:**   (AI 2008)
    a. Stretching of renal capsule due to back pressure
    b. Increased peristalsis of ureter to overcome the obstruction
    c. Irritation of intramural ureter
    d. Extravasation of urine.

191. **Locate the renal stone with pain radiating to medial side of thigh and perineum due to slipping of stone in males:**
    a. At pelvic brim   (AIIMS June 2000)
    b. Intramural opening of ureter
    c. Junction of ureter and renal pelvis
    d. At crossing of gonadal vessels and ureter

192. **Referred pain from ureteric colic is felt in the groin due to involvement of the following nerve:**   (AI 2003)
    a. Subcostal   b. Iliohypogastric
    c. Ilioinguinal   d. Genitofemoral

193. **Treatment used for lower ureteric stone is:** (AIIMS June 98)
    a. Endoscopic removal
    b. Diuretics
    c. Drug dissolution
    d. Laser

194. **Nephrocalcinosis is seen in all except–**   (AIIMS May 07)
    a. Sarcoidosis   b. Distal RTA
    c. Milk alkali syndrome   d. Medullary cystic kidney

195. **A patient is known to have calcium nephrocalcinosis for the post 10 years. All of the following dietary recommendations should be suggested, Except:**   (AIIMS Nov 2010)
    a. Protein Restriction   b. Calcium Restriction
    c. Salt Restriction   d. All of the above

Renal Tubular Acidosis

196. **Hypokalemia is seen in:**   (Recent Question 2015-16)
    a. RTA- I   b. RTA- II
    c. RTA- III   d. RTA- IV

197. **Renal tubular acidosis are A/E:**   (Recent Pattern 2014-15)
    a. Impaired acid production
    b. Impaired bicarbonate resorbtion
    c. Inability to acidify urine
    d. Nephrolithiasis

198. **R.T.A shows all except:**   (Recent Pattern 2014-15)
    a. Urine pH always < 5.5   b. Anion gap normal
    c. Bicarbonaturia   d. Vitamin D deficiency

199. **In which renal tubular acidosis, is hyperkalemia a prominent feature:**   (Recent Pattern 2014-15)
    a. Type I   b. Type II
    c. Type III   d. Type IV

200. **Causes of low urinary calcium include:**
    a. Renal tubular acidosis   (Recent Pattern 2014-15)
    b. Cushing's syndrome
    c. Chronic glomerulonephritis/CKD
    d. Paget's disease

201. **True about renal tubular acidosis are A/E:**   (Recent Pattern 2014-15)
    a. Increased urinary anion gap   b. Bicarbonaturia
    c. Hyperchloremia   d. High urinary PH

202. **Type II RTA is associated with all of the following, except**
    a. Normal Anion Gap Acidosis   (AI-1990)
    b. Hyper calciuria
    c. Decreased urinary citrate
    d. Minimum urinary pH <5.5

203. **All are features of renal tubular acidosis type I, except:**   (AIIMS Sept 96)
    a. Stone in kidney   b. No anion gap
    c. Hypokalemia   d. Fanconi syndrome

Renovascular Hypertension and Renal Vein Thrombosis

204. **A 70-year-old male patient with uncontrolled hypertension has serum creatinine of 4.5 mg% and mild proteinuria. Renal ultrasound shows left kidney 9 cm and right kidney 7 cm in length (normal 10 cm). There was no evidence of obstruction. What is the next investigation of choice?**
         (JIPMER Nov 2014)
    a. I.V.P   b. MR Angiography
    c. Isotope Renogram   d. Retrograde pyelography

205. **The following angiogram in hypertension patient shows?**

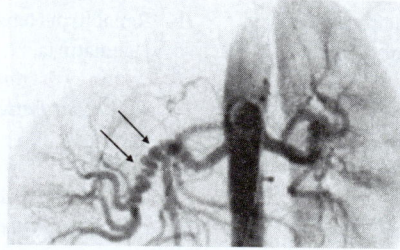

    a. Fibromuscular dysplasia   b. Atherosclerosis
    c. Takayasu arteritis   d. Non-specific arteritis

206. The accurate diagnostic aid in renal artery stenosis is:
    a. Selective renal angiography   (Recent Pattern 2014-15)
    b. Ultrasound
    c. CT scan
    d. IVU
207. Renal artery stenosis is associated with:
    a. High renin Hypertension   (Recent Pattern 2014-15)
    b. Normal renin hypertension
    c. Low renin hypertension
    d. Fibrinoid necrosis of vessels
208. Which is characteristic feature of malignant hypertension in kidney?   (Recent Pattern 2014-15)
    a. Hyaline necrosis   b. Fibrinoid necrosis
    c. Medical wall hyperplasia   d. Micro-aneurysm
209. Most common cause of renal artery stenosis in young boy in India: (AIPG 2010)
    a. Atherosclerosis   b. Fibromuscular hyperplasia
    c. Neurofibroma   d. Nonspecific aortoarteritis
210. Most common cause of renal artery stenosis in young adults in India is: (AIIMS Dec 97)
    a. Atherosclerosis   b. Nonspecific aortoarteritis
    c. Fibromuscular dysplasia   d. None of the above
211. Renal artery stenosis may occur in all of the following except: (AI 2006)
    a. Atherosclerosis   b. Fibromuscular dysplasia
    c. Takayasu's arteritis   d. Polyarteritis nodosa
212. A 10-year-old child develops hematuria after 2 days of diarrhoea. Blood film shows fragmented RBCs & thrombocytopenia. Ultrasound shows marked enlargement of both kidneys. The likely diagnosis is: (AIIMS June 99)
    a. Renal artery stenosis, bilateral
    b. Disseminated intravascular coagulopathy
    c. Haemolytic uremic syndrome
    d. Renal vein thrombosis

Miscellaneous

213. Birt-Hogg-Dube syndrome is associated with?   (JIPMER May 2018)
    a. Renal cell carcinoma   b. Lung Ca
    c. Stomach Ca   d. Ovarian Ca
214. All are true about Karyomegalic interstitial nephritis except?   (Recent Question 2016-17)
    a. Chronic tubulointerstitial nephritis
    b. Tubular atrophy
    c. Increased frequency of calcium phosphate stones
    d. Autosomal recessive pattern of inheritance
215. Best for prevention of struvite stone?   (Recent Question 2016-17)
    a. Urine alkaliniser   b. Acetohydroxamic acid
    c. Tiopronin   d. D-Penicillamine
216. Which of the following helps most in nephrolithiasis?   (Recent Question 2015-16)
    a. Low sodium diet   b. Low calcium diet
    c. High sodium diet   d. Low citrate diet
217. Positive dipstick for RBC with Red color urine and Red supernatant after centrifugation is due to: (Recent Question 2015-16)
    a. Porphyria   b. Hematuria
    c. Hemolysis   d. Rhabdomyolysis
218. RBC casts are seen in?   (Recent Question 2015-16)
    a. Acute tubular nephritis   b. Acute glomerulonephritis
    c. Acute Pyelonephritis   d. Acute interstitial nephritis
219. Identify the needle shown?

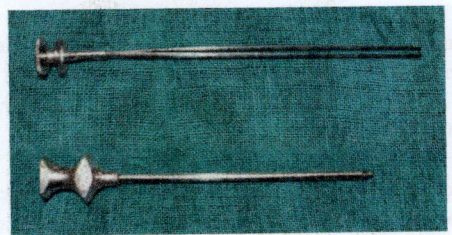

    a. Bone marrow biopsy needle
    b. Vim silverman needle
    c. Trucut biopsy needle
    d. Bone marrow aspiration needle
220. The following urinary bladder on MCU is diagnostic of?

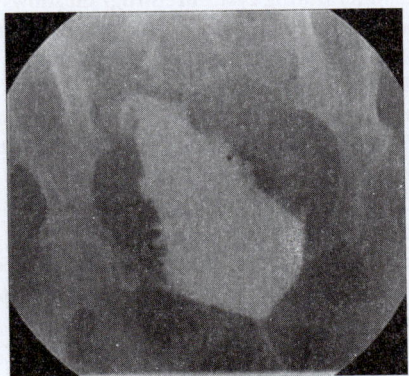

    a. V.U.R   b. Neurogenic Bladder
    c. Bladder Diverticula   d. Bladder outlet obstruction
221. Hypochromic-microcytic anemia occurs in all except:
    a. Iron deficiency   (Recent Pattern 2014-15)
    b. Thalassaemia
    c. Lead poisoning
    d. Chronic renal failure
222. The most likely diagnosis in the case of a patient with multiple pulmonary cavities, hematuria and red cell casts is: (Recent Pattern 2014-15)
    a. Anti-GBM disease
    b. Churg-Strauss
    c. Systemic lupus erythematosus
    d. Wegner's granulomatosis
223. Mosaic pattern of cement line is characteristically seen in: (Recent Pattern 2014-15)
    a. Hyperparathyroid   b. Paget's disease of bone
    c. Renal osteodystrophy   d. Osteomalacia
224. Iliac horns on X-ray pelvis is seen in: (Recent Pattern 2014-15)
    a. Alport's syndrome
    b. Nail-Patella syndrom
    c. Ehlers-danlos syndrome
    d. Marfan's syndrome
225. Recurrent hematuria in a deaf mute is seen in: (Recent Pattern 2014-15)
    a. Fanconi's anemia   b. Alport's syndrome
    c. Renal cysts   d. Nephrotic syndrome

226. **Dent's disease is characterised by all except?** *(AIPG 2011)*
    a. Chloride channel defect
    b. Males are affected
    c. Nephrolithiasis
    d. Defect in limb of Loop of Henle

227. **Osmotic demyelination syndrome develops due to rapid correction of hyponatremia at a level exceeding?**
    (Recent Pattern 2014-15)
    a. 0.5 mEq/hr   b. 2 mEq/hr
    c. 5 mEq/hr   d. 10 mEq/hr

228. **A child with bigger limbs (history suggestive of hemi-hypertrophy) and abdominal mass is suggestive of:**
    (AIIMS May 2013)
    a. Aldosteronoma   b. Neuroblastoma
    c. Rhabdomyosarcoma d. Wilm's tumor

229. **A 4-year-old girl presented with urinary infection with E. coli, pus cells in urine, dilatation of left ureter with hydro-ureter; micturating cysto-urethrogram shows filling defect in bladder, likely diagnosis is:** *(Recent Pattern 2014-15)*
    a. Sacrococcygeal teratoma   b. Ureterocele
    c. VUR   d. P.U.V

230. **Plasmapheresis is indicated for which of the following:**
    a. Wegener's granulomatosis *(Recent Pattern 2014-15)*
    b. Henoch-Schonlein purpura
    c. Goodpasture's syndrome
    d. Acute transplant rejection

231. **The kidney in sickle cell anemia is characterized by:**
    a. Pyuria *(Recent Pattern 2014-15)*
    b. Inability to concentrate urine
    c. Decrease in glomerular filtration
    d. Inability to acidify the urine

232. **Neonate with recurrent seizures with hypocalcemia, recurrent infections. Diagnosis is?** *(Recent Pattern 2014-15)*
    a. Di George syndrome   b. Barter syndrome
    c. Gitelman syndrome   d. Idiopathic hyercalciuria

233. **Which of the following are true regarding congenital nephrogenic diabetes insipidus:** *(Recent Pattern 2014-15)*
    a. ADH receptors are not sensitive
    b. It is associated with SIADH
    c. Serum ADH levels are normal
    d. Urine is hyperosmolar

234. **Hypercalciuria can be treated with:**
    (Recent Pattern 2014-15)
    a. Torsemide   b. Acetazolamide
    c. Frusemide   d. Indapamide

235. **Amyloid kidney is characterized by all except:**
    (Recent Pattern 2014-15)
    a. Hypercholesterolemia b. Normal sized kidney
    c. HTN   d. Heavy proteinuria

236. **Which one of the following statements regarding pyelonephritis is correct?** *(AIPG 2009)*
    a. Recurrent infection with the same strain usually occurring after one week of cessation of therapy.
    b. Xantho-granulomatous pyelonephritis is seen with diabetes mellitus
    c. Emphysematous pyelonephritis is seen with staghorn calculus
    d. 10,000 viable bacteria per ml in clean voided midstream urine is of significance

237. **A 35-year-old, 70 kg male present with sodium =160meq/dl. Calculate the free water deficit for this patient:**
    (Recent Pattern 2014-15)
    a. 5 L   b. 10 L
    c. 15   d. 20 L

238. **Rate of correction of hypernatremia is:**
    (Recent Pattern 2014-15)
    a. 0.5 mEq/dl   b. 1 mEq/dl
    c. 2 mEq/dl   d. 3 mEq/dl

239. **Immediate treatment for hyperkalemia with ECG changes:**
    a. Calcium chloride
    b. Calcium hydroxide
    c. K+ Binding Resin Enema
    d. Calcium carbonate

240. **In a child, non-functioning kidney is best diagnosed by:**
    (AI 2005)
    a. Ultrasonography.   b. IVU.
    c. DTPA renogram.   d. Creatinine clearance.

241. **Marker for the renal vasculitis in children is:** *(AI 98)*
    a. IgA level
    b. Low complement level
    c. Increased Antineutrophilic cytoplasmic antibody titre
    d. Increase antinuclear antibody

242. **Association of deafness & nephritis is seen in:**
    a. Pickwickian syndrome   *(AIIMS May 93)*
    b. Alport's syndrome
    c. Fabry's disease
    d. Lawrence Moon Biedl syndrome

243. **Positive Urinary Anion Gap helps to establish the diagnosis of:** *(AI 2009)*
    a. Alcoholic ketoacidosis   b. Diabetic ketoacidosis
    c. Renal tubular Acidosis   d. Acidosis in Diarrhea

244. **Which of the following changes does not occur in malignant hypertension:** *(AI 2008)*
    a. Peticheal Haemorrhages on cortical surface
    b. Fibrinoid necrosis of arterioles
    c. Intimal concentric thickening
    d. Hyaline arteriosclerosis

245. **Commonest histoloical finding in Benign Hypertension is:**
    (AI 2009)
    a. Proliferative endarteritis b. Necrotizing arteriolitis
    c. Hyaline arteriosclerosis   d. Cystic Medial Necrosis

246. **The most common cause of renal scarring in a 3-year-old child is:** *(AI 2005)*
    a. Trauma
    b. Tuberculosis
    c. Vesicoureteral reflux induced pyelonephritis
    d. Interstitial nephritis

247. **The most common histological variant of renal cell carcinoma is:** *(AIIMS Nov 2005)*
    a. Clear cell type   b. Chromophobe type
    c. Papillary type   d. Tubular type

248. **Classic triad in Renal cell carcinoma includes all of the following, except:** *(AI 1991)*
    a. Hematuria
    b. Hypertension
    c. Flank mass
    d. Abdominal Pain

249. All are associated with Wilm's tumor except:
    a. Anirida   (AIIMS Feb 1997)
    b. Male pseudohermaphrodite
    c. Arthogryposis multiplex congenita
    d. Hemihypertrophy
250. The most important determinant of prognosis in Wilm's tumor: (AI 2006)
    a. Stage of disease
    b. Loss of heterozygosity of chromsome 1p
    c. Histology
    d. Age less than one year at presentation
251. All of the following are true about Rhabdomyolysis, except: (PGI Dec 04)
    a. Hyperuricemia
    b. Hyperphosphatemia
    c. Hypercalcemia
    d. Creatine kinase
252. A 65-year-old male smoker presents with gross total painless hematuria. The most likely diagnosis is:
    a. Carcinoma of urinary bladder   (AI 2003)
    b. Benign prostatic hyperplasia
    c. Carcinoma prostate
    d. Cystolithiasis
253. A 60-year-old smoker came with a history of painless gross hematuria for one day. Most logical investigation would be:
    a. Urine routine   (AI 2007)
    b. Plain X ray KUB
    c. USG KUB
    d. Urine microscopy for malignant cytology
254. Urinary K+ excretion is increased in: (AIIMS Nov-04)
    a. Bronchiectasis   b. Meningitis
    c. Osteomyelitis   d. Hepatitis
255. Renal damage due to amphotericin B are all, except
                                              (AIIMS Nov 01)
    a. Azotemia   b. Renal tubular acidosis
    c. Glomerulonephritis   d. Hypokalemia

Answers with Explanations

Acute Kidney Injury

1. (b) >40 ml/kg/day

(Ref: Chapter 69, API Text Book of internal medicine)

- Polyuria is defined as urine output of > 40 ml/kg/day.
- Polydipsia is defined as water intake of >100 ml/kg/day.
- The question is a controversial one mathematically speaking but reference of API is given. Harrison has not given data in ml/kg.
- In children the cut off of polyuria is (urine output > 4 ml/kg/hr), polydypsia (water intake > 2 L/m^2/d)

2. (c) Urinary NGAL

(Ref: Harrison 20th edition, page 2108)

- Urinary neutrophil gelatinase associated lipocalcin is a novel biomarker of acute kidney injury. It is highly upregulated after inflammation and kidney injury and can be detected in plasma and urine after 2 hours of AKI onset.
- In RIFLE criteria Fractional excretion of sodium, urine osmolality were used to differentiate pre-renal from renal causes.

Comparison of RIFLE versus AKIN versus KDIGO criteria for AKI

RIFLE Criteria	RIFLE Creatinine definition	AKIN Criteria	AKIN Creatinine definition	KDIGO Criteria	KDIGO Creatinine definition	Urine output*
Risk	≥1.5-fold increase from baseline SCr or decrease in GFR ≥25%	Stage 1	≥0.3 mg/dL, increase or ≥15 fold increase from baseline SCr within 48 hrs	Stage 1	>0.3 mg/dL increase within 48 hrs or 1.5–1.9 times baseline within 7 days	<0.5 mL/kg/h for >6 hours
Injury	≥2-fold increase from baseline SCr or decrease in GFR ≥50%	Stage 2	≥2-fold increse from baseline SCr	Stage 2	2.0–2.9 times baseline within 17 days	<0.5 mL/kg/h for 12 hours
Failure	≥3-fold increase from baseline SCr ≥4 mg/dL or decrease in GFR ≥75%	Stage 3	≥3-fold increase from baseline SCr or increase to ≥4.0 mg/dL with an acute increase of >0.5 mg/dL or initiation of RRT	Stage 3	≥3 times baseline within 7 days or increase to ≥4.0 mg/dL with an acute increase of >0.5 mg/dL or initiation of RRT	<0.3 mL/kg/h for 24 hours or anuria for >12 hours

3. Ans. (d) Kidney biopsy will show micro-vessel occlusion with a cleft in the vessel

(Ref: Harrison 20th edition, p 2148; Harrison 19th edition, p 1835t, 1848)

- Diabetes and angina both point to atherosclerosis. In patients undergoing angiography, catheterization can lead to embolism of a vulnerable atherosclerotic plaque in descending aorta downstream to renal arteries leading to athero-embolic kidney disease.
- The symptoms of diabetic patient developed after angiography and since atherosclerotic lesion can involve the aorta, the athero-embolic event would explain the events.
- Presence of eosinophilia and mottling of toes and reduced kidney function confirm the diagnosis as choice D
- Contrast induced nephropathy can occur in diabetics with chronic kidney disease. However rash, toe discoloration with sudden rise of creatinine and eosinophilia are not seen in contrast induced nephropathy. Hence choice B is ruled out

- Choice A is ruled out as it is prevents contrast induced nephropathy
- Choice C is ruled as out as heparin will not manage cholesterol embolism

4. Ans. (c) Patchy tubular necrosis

(Ref: Harrison 20th edition, p 2102; Harrison 19th edition, p 1802)

Cardiogenic shock has resulted in development of acute kidney injury. The history given shows patient passing from initiation to maintenance and lastly recovery phase due to ischemic acute tubular necrosis.

Morphological features of ischemic ATN

- Focal tubular epithelial necrosis at multiple points along the nephron
- Large skip areas in between
- Rupture of basement membranes (Tubulorrhexis)
- Occlusion of tubular lumens by casts (Tamm Horsfall protein)

Clinical course of acute kidney injury

Initiation	• Dominated by the inciting medical surgical or obstetric event in the ischemic from of AKI • The only indication of renal involvement is a slight decline in urine output with a rise in BUN
Mantainence	• Sustained decreases in urine output to between 40 and 400 ml/day oliguria • Salt and water overload • Rising BUN concentrations • Hyperkalemia • Metabolic acidosis • Manifestations of uremia • With appropriate balance of water and blood electrolytes including dialysis the patient can be supported through this oliguric crisis
Recovery	• Steady increases in urine volume that may reach up to 3L/day • The tubules are still damaged so large amounts of water sodium and potassium are lost in the flood of urine • Hypokalemia rather than hyperkalemia becomes a clinical problems • There is a peculiar increased vulnerability to infection at this stages • Eventually renal tubular functions is restored and concentrating ability improves • BUN and creatinine levels begin to return to normal • Subtle tubular functional impairment may persist for months • Most patients who reach this phase eventually recover completely.

5. Ans. (c) Rhabdomyolysis

(Ref: Harrison 20th edition, p 2104-2105; Harrison 19th edition, 1804-5)

In the setting of drug overdose the patient has presented with hypothermia and deranged kidney function. The key word in the question is "urine dipstick is 3 + for blood but urine microscopy is normal." This implies that myoglobin in urine is giving false positive report for blood detected by urine dipstick.

Rhabdomyolysis causes
- Traumatic crush injuries
- Muscles ischemia during vascular or orthopedic surgery
- *Alcohol intoxication with prolonged immobility*
- Exposure hypothermia
- Compression during coma or immobilization
- Prolonged seizures activity
- Excessive exercise
- Heat stroke
- Malignant hyperthermia
- Infections
- Metabolic disorders hypophosphatemia severe hypothyroidism
- Myopathies drug induced metabolic or inflammatory

Clinical Manifestations
In adults Rhabdomyolysis is characterized by the triad of:
1. Muscle weakness
2. Myalgia
3. Dark urine

6. Ans. (c) Hyperkalemiac acidosis

(Ref: Harrison 20th edition, p 2108; Harrison 19th ed./1808, 1810)

- Acute kidney injury will cause inability to excrete H^+ and K^+ both leading to hyperkalemic acidosis.
- The acidosis seen is high anion gap metabolic acidosis.

7. Ans. (d) Analgesic Nephropathy

(Ref: Harrison 20th edition, p 2105; Harrison 19th ed./1861)

- AKI is a serious complication of snakebites by the viperidae family.
- Pyelonephritis can be hematogenously acquired and cause extensive necrosis of kidney parenchyma.
- Crush injury or Rhabdo-myolysis can result in myoglobinuria causing blockage of kidney tubules and resultant acute tubular necrosis.

Remember: Analgesic nephropathy causes chronic interstitial nephritis and presents with chronic kidney disease.

8. Ans. (d) Acid phosphatase

(Ref: Harrison 19th p 1799)

- Acid phosphatase is NOT a marker of AKI, instead it is alkaline phosphatase.
- List of markers for AKI
  1. Alanine aminopeptidase
  2. Alkaline phosphatase
  3. Glutamyltranspeptidse
  4. Glutamy S transferase
  5. Alpha 1 microglobulin
  6. Beta 2 microglobulin
  7. Kidney injury molecule 1
  8. Osteopontin
  9. Clusterin
  10. Neutrophil gelatinase associated lipocalcin

9. Ans. (d) Hypokalemia

(Ref: Harrison 19th p 1799)

Uremic pericarditis is characterized by chest pain. The failed kidneys fail to excrete H+. The decrease in GFR explains the increase of renin leading to hypertension. Hyperkalemia is always a feature of Oliguric phase of ARF.

10. Ans. (c) Decreased excretion of ammonia

(Ref: Harrison 19th p 1799, 1811)

- Metabolic acidosis can occur because of increased endogenous acid production (lactate and ketoacids), loss of bicarbonate or accumulation of endogenous acid (as seen in renal failure)
- Ammonia is excreted out linked to H^+ as ammonium ion and for every positive charge lost, to maintain electro-neutrality chloride is lost. In case of renal failure ammonia and protons both are retained leading to high anion gap acidosis as the positive charges in body are increased.

11. Ans. (c) Micro RNA 122

(Ref: Harrison 19th p 1799)

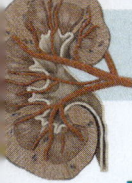

Marker	Significance
Neutrophil gelatinase induced lipocalcin	• In the case of acute kidney injury, NGAL is secreted in high levels into the blood and urine within 2 hours of injury. • Because NGAL is protease resistant and small, the protein is easily excreted and detected in the urine. • NGAL levels in patients with AKI have been associated with the severity of their prognosis and can be used as a biomarker for AKI. • NGAL can also be used as an early diagnosis for procedures such as chronic kidney disease, contrast induced nephropathy, and kidney transplant.
Kidney injury molecule	Tumor suppressor micro-RNA that regulates intrahepatic metastasis of hepato-cellular carcinoma
Micro RNA 122	In response to progressive injury, kidney cells produce the molecule, KIM-1, which maintains its expression over time in chronic kidney disease, and has been known as an early predictive molecule and a useful biomarker for kidney injury in preclinical trials and in patients
CYSTATIN C	Cystatin C is a member of the cystatin superfamily of cysteineprotease inhibitors and is produced at a relatively constant rate from all nucleated cells. Cystatin C has a low molecular weight (approximately 13.3 kilodaltons), and it is removed from the bloodstream by glomerular filtration in the kidneys. If kidney function and glomerular filtration rate decline, the blood levels of cystatin C rise. Serum cystatin C has been proposed to be a more sensitive marker of early GFR decline than is plasma creatinine; however, like serum creatinine, cystatin C is influenced by age, race, and sex and additionally is associated with diabetes, smoking, and markers of inflammation

12. Ans. (a) Metabolic acidosis

(Ref: Harrison 19th p 322)

- The question mentions that difference between sodium and chloride is low which mathematically is possible if serum chloride increases.
- Now physiologically speaking Chloride excretion occurs in urine along with ammonium in 1:1 ratio to maintain electroneutrality.
- If chloride in blood is more it means it was not lost in urine
- If chloride is not lost, H$^+$ are not lost in form of ammonium
- Hence there is increase of H$^+$ in body leading to HYPERCHLOREMIC METABOLIC ACIDOSIS
- This kind of presentation is seen with renal tubular acidosis type 1,2,4: ureterosigmoidostomy: alkali loss in urine.
- HYPOCHLOREMIC Metabolic alkalosis occurs with Chloride loss due to vomiting or due to fistula.

13. Ans. (a) High serum creatinine

(Ref: Harrison 19th p 289)

- S. Creatinine concentration usually begins to increase within 24 hours after contrast agent administration, peaks between days 3 and 5, and returns to baseline in 7-10 days. Serum cystatin C is also increased in patients with contrast induced nephropathy
- Nonspecific formed elements can appear in the urine, including renal tubular epithelial cells, pigmented granular casts, urate crystals, and debris. However, these urine findings do not correlate with severity.
- Urine osmolality tends to be less than 350 mOsm/kg. The fractional excretion of sodium (FENa) may vary widely. In the minority of patients with oliguric CIN, the FENa is low in the early stages, despite no clinical evidence of volume depletion.

14. Ans. (a) 4 ml/hr

(Ref: Harrison 19th p 292)

As per chapter 44, Harrison, oliguria <400 ml/day, anuria is < 100 ml/ day.

15. Ans. (d) Kidney transplant rejection

(Ref: Harrison 19th p 1829)

- (Antibodies to CD 25) -**Basiliximab** reduces the incidence and severity of acute rejection in kidney transplantation without increasing the incidence of opportunistic infections.

16. Ans. (c) A and B (Proteinuria and hematuria)

(Ref: Harrison 20th edition, p 2109; Harrison 19th p 1809)

Hepatorenal syndrome is characterized by pre-renal variety of acute kidney injury and the blood supply to the glomerulus is compromised.

Major criteria (All major criteria are required to diagnose HRS.)
- Low GFR, indicated by a serum creatinine level higher than 1.5 mg/dL or 24-hour creatinine clearance lower than 40 mL/min
- Absence of shock, ongoing bacterial infection and fluid losses, and current treatment with nephrotoxic medications
- No sustained improvement in renal function (decrease in serum creatinine to < 1.5 mg/dL or increase in creatinine clearance to >40 mL/min) after diuretic withdrawal and expansion of plasma volume with 1.5 L of plasma expander
- *Proteinuria less than 500 mg/d and no ultrasonographic evidence of obstructive uropathy or intrinsic parenchymal disease*

Additional criteria (Additional criteria are not necessary for the diagnosis but provide supportive evidence.)
- Urine volume less than 500 mL/d
- Urine sodium level less than 10 mEq/L
- Urine osmolality greater than plasma osmolality
- Serum sodium concentration less than 130 mEq/L
- *Urine red blood cell count of less than 50 per high-power field*

17. Ans. (c) Increased sodium excretion in urine

(Ref: Harrison 20th edition, p 2108; Harrison 19th p 1807)

The recovery phase of ATN is characterized by regeneration of tubular epithelial cells. *During recovery, an abnormal diuresis sometimes occurs, causing salt and water loss and volume depletion.*

1. The urine output gradually returns to normal, but serum creatinine and urea levels may not fall for several more days.
2. Tubular dysfunction may persist and is manifested by sodium wasting, polyuria unresponsive to vasopressin, or hyperchloremic metabolic acidosis.
3. The mechanism of the diuresis is not completely understood, but it may in part be due to the delayed recovery of tubular cell function in the setting of increased glomerular filtration. In addition, continued use of diuretics (often administered during initiation and maintenance phases) may also add to the problem.

18. Ans. (a) Prerenal acute renal failure

(Ref: Harrison 20th edition, p 2099-2101; Harrison 19th p 1807)

	Pre renal	Renal (ATN)	Post renal
Urine osmolality	>500 mosm	~300 mosm	<400
Urine sodium	<20 mmol/dl	>20 mmol/dl	Variable
FeNa	<1	>1	Variable
Urine microscopic findings	Hyaline casts	Muddy brown casts	Normal or RBC/WBC
BUN: creatinine ratio	>20:1 (normal 10:1)	<20:1	>20:1

19. Ans. (a) Sodium fraction excretion

(Ref: Harrison 20th edition, p 2108-2109; Harrison 19th p 1809)

20. Ans. (c) Aminoglycoside toxicity

(Ref: Harrison 19th p 938t)

Non oliguric renal failure is characterised by damage to collecting duct leading to inability to absorb water, and hence surprisingly urine flow is normal. This is seen with aminoglycoside antibiotics.

21. Ans. (d) Rupture of Aortic Aneurysm

(Ref: Harrison 20th edition, p 2105t; Harrison 19th p 1803)

22. Ans. (b) Urine sodium > 40

(Ref: Harrison 19th p 1803)

23. Ans. (a) Prerenal Azotemia

(Ref: Harrison 20th edition, p 2105t; Harrison 19th p 1809)

24. Ans. (c) Prerenal failure

(Ref: Harrison 20th edition, p 2105t; Harrison 19th p 1810)

25. Ans. (c) Sodium Fraction Excretion

(Ref: Harrison 20th edition, p 2105; Harrison 19th p 1809)

26. Ans. (d) Hypercalcemia

(Ref: Harrison 19th p 1755)

27. Ans. (c) Urine osmolality is lower than plasma osmolality

(Ref: Washington manual of Medical Therapeutics 32nd/506, Harrison 19th p 1809)

28. Ans. (a) Acute Renal Failure

(Ref: Harrison 20th edition, p 2103; Robbin's 7th/604, 605; Ghai 6th/574,Harrison 19th p 1799)

Acute Renal failure is an established complication of crush syndrome with myoglobin causing blockage of kidney tubules.

Chronic Kidney Disease

29. Ans. (d) Sirolimus

(Ref: Harrison 20th edition, p 2596; Harrison: 19th edition, p 1829)

Sirolimus is a non-nephrotoxic -TOR inhibitor with a long half-life of 62 hours. It was the first mTOR inhibitor to be developed in solid organ transplantation.

30. Ans. (a) Diuretics

(Ref: Harrison 20th edition, p 312; Harrison 19th edition, p 1815)

- The ECG shows a heart rate of 125 bpm with extreme axis deviation.
- P waves are absent with bizarre wide complex qRS in lead V4, V5 and V6
- Tall tented T waves which are seen with hyperkalemia are present in all the leads.
- The patient is a diabetic with deranged KFT. The patient is suffering from CKD and must be reaching stage 4-5 leading to hyperkalemia producing such pronounced ECG changes. He is at risk of diastolic arrest of the heart. Hence the control of potassium is of paramount importance in this patient.
- Hyperkalemia in CKD patients responds to-
  1. Dietary restriction of potassium with use of kaliuretic diuretics.
  2. Potassium binding resins like calcium resonium and sodium polystyrene can promote potassium loss via GI Tract.
  3. Intractable hyperkalemia requires dialysis. RTA component should be managed with alkali supplementation if bicarbonate falls below 20 mmol/L.

31. Ans. (b) Chronic Kidney Disease

(Ref: Harrison 20th edition, p 2114)

Vitamin D3 deficiency	Low serum calcium with low phosphate Elevated PTH
Chronic kidney disease	Low serum calcium (due to less synthesis of vitamin D3) Elevated Phosphate (due to less clearance in kidney dysfunction) Elevated PTH

Contd...

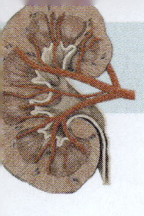

Dents disease	X Linked recessive defect due to defect in CLCN5 gene on chromosome Xp11.22. It leads to hypercalciuria leading to nephrocalcinosis. Other defects are same as that of Fanconi Syndrome.
Fanconi syndrome	Defect in Proximal convoluted tubule leading to urinary loss of bicarbonate, phosphate, sugar, amino-acids

32. Ans. (b) Lead nephropathy

(Ref: Harrison 20th edition, p 2163; Rheumatology Secrets: 3rd edition, p 342)

- The cause of saturnine gout is *lead toxicity*. The symptoms of lead toxicity precede the development of gout.
- Hence patient will have anemia, basophilic stippling of RBC, abdominal pain and nerve palsy
- The damage to kidney will lead to hypertension and progressive renal malfunction
- Knee joint involvement is more common than MTP involvement in saturnine gout.

33. Ans. (b) Urine protein less than 30-299 µg/day is called microalbuminuria

(Ref: : Harrison 19th edition, p1834)

Significance of microalbuminuria:

- Microalbuminuria is the finding of albumin in the urine not detectable by the urine dipstick which is sensitive to protein concentration > 1 gm%.
- It precedes the decline in GFR and indicates the presence of renal and cardiovascular complications.
- Microalbuminuria is a marker of greatly increased cardiovascular morbidity and mortality for patients with either type 1 or type 2 diabetes.
- Annual screening for microalbuminuria will allow the identification of patients with nephropathy at a point very early in its course.
- Improving glycemic control, aggressive antihypertensive treatment, and the use of ACE inhibitors or ARBs will slow the rate of progression of nephropathy.

Definition of abnormalities in albumin excretion

Category	24-hr urine albumin (mg/24h)	Dipstick analysis	Spot collection (µg/mg creatinine)
Normal	<30	Negative	<30
Microalbuminuria	30-299	Negative, trace, 1+	30-299
Clinical albuminuria	≥300	1+ to 3+	≥300

34. Ans. (a) Chronic renal failure

(Ref: Harrison 19th edition, p 294, 1861)

Hypoadrenalism	Aldosterone deficiency leads to Salt wasting and Polyuria
Hypercalcemia	Hypercalcemia can lead to reversible renal tubular defects, increased urination.
Lithium carbonate	Lithium accumulates in principal cells of the collecting duct by entering through the epithelial sodium channel (ENaC) and leads to nephrogenic diabetes insipidus manifesting as polyuria and polydipsia.

35. Ans. (d) Renal cell carcinoma is a frequent association

(Ref: Harrison 19th edition, page 185-51)

Adult polycystic kidney disease is autosomal dominant with 100% penetrance.

Autosomal dominant polycystic kidney disease	AD	16p13	PKD1	Polycystin-1	Cortical and medullary cysts	Cerebral aneurysms; liver cysts
	AD	4q21	PKD2	Polycystin-2	Cortical and medullary cysts	
Autosomal recessive polycystic kidney disease	AR	6p21	PKHD1	Fibrocystin (polyductin)	Distal tubule and collecting duct cysts	Hepatic fibrosis; Caroli's disease

- In 83% of patients aged 15–46 yrs, MRI shows an incidence of hepatic cysts. Most patients are asymptomatic with normal liver function tests, but hepatic cysts may bleed, become infected, rupture, and cause pain.
- ADPKD patients have an increased risk of subarachnoid or cerebral hemorrhage from a ruptured intracranial aneurysm compared with the general population. Saccular aneurysms of the anterior cerebral circulation may be detected in up to 10% of asymptomatic patients on magnetic resonance angiography (MRA) screening

36. Ans. (c) Hyperthyroidism

(Ref: Harrison 19th edition, page 1820)

Choice A and D	In CRF vitamin D3 production is low. This leads to low serum calcium and resultant secondary hyperparathyroidism. The increased PTH will increase the resorption of bones leading to osteitis cystica fibrosa.
Choice B	Due to hyperphosphatemia, the increased phosphate chelates with calcium leading to increased incidence of calcification of coronary arteries, heart valves and hence the less availability of calcium can explain the osteomalacia.

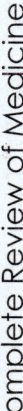

37. **Ans. (b) Decreased insulin**

(*Ref: Harrison 18th edition, Chapter 344:*)

- Exogenous insulin is normally metabolized by the kidney. However, when there is impairment of kidney function, the half-life of insulin is prolonged because of lower levels of degradation.
- This necessitates insulin dose reduction.
- **Also remember:** The clearance of both sulfonylureas and its metabolites is highly dependent on kidney function. In patients with Stage 3-5 CKD, first-generation sulfonylureas should be avoided. Of the second-generation sulfonylureas, glipizide is recommended because its metabolites are not active, and there is a lower potential for development of hypoglycemia.

38. **Ans. (c) CKD is defined as GFR < 30 ml/min/1.73 m² for 4 weeks**

(*Ref: Harrison 19th edition, p 290-91*)

- CKD is defined as GFR < 60ml/min/1.73m2 *for 12 weeks/3 months. Hence choice C is wrong.*
- The average rate of decline varies, but it averages about 0.8 mL/min/1.73 m²/ year after age of 30 years. The decline accelerates after about 65 to 70 years of age.
- In terms of GFR ranges for specific ages, an average 85-year-old male would be expected to have a glomerular filtration rate around 55–60 mL/min/1.73 m², depending on his GFR at age 30. *Hence choice A is correct.*
- Choice B is correct since GFR is best measured by creatinine clearance.
- Choice is d is correct in children.

$$eGFR = \frac{k \times height}{Serum\ Creatinine}$$

39. **Ans. (b) Peripheral neuropathy**

(*Ref: Harrison 19th edition, p 1811*)

40. **Ans. (d) 5-10% of normal**

(*Ref: Harrison 19th edition, p 1811*)

CKD Stage	GFR level (mL/min/1.73 m²)
Stage 1	< 90
Stage 2	60 – 89
Stage 3	30 – 59
Stage 4	15 – 29
Stage 5	<15 (End stage renal disease)

41. **Ans. (a) 120 mEq/dl**

(*Ref: Harrison 19th edition, p 1811*)

Three major considerations guide therapy for hyponatremia.
1. The presence and/or severity of symptoms determine the urgency and goals of therapy. Patients with acute hyponatremia present with symptoms that can range from headache, nausea, and/or vomiting to seizures, obtundation, and central herniation; patients with chronic hyponatremia that is present for >48 h are less likely to have severe symptoms.
2. Patients with chronic hyponatremia are at risk for ODS if plasma Na+ concentration is corrected by >8–10 mM within the first 24 h and/or by >18 mM within the first 48 h.
3. The response to interventions such as hyper-tonic saline, isotonic saline, and vasopressin antagonists can be highly unpredictable, and so frequent monitoring of plasma Na+ concentration during corrective therapy is imperative.

42. **Ans. (c) Interstitial fibrosis**

(*Ref: Harrison 19th edition, p 1796*)

- Its pathophysiology is based on uremia-induced increased permeability of pulmonary alveolo-capillary interfaces, leading to interstitial and intra-alveolar edema, atelectasis, alveolar hemorrhage, and pulmonary hyaline membrane formation.
- These changes are compounded by bleeding diathesis secondary to platelet dysfunction in advanced renal disease.
    - The pulmonary symptoms and radiographic findings are reversible with hemodialysis.

43. **Ans. (a) Broad casts in urine**

(*Ref: Harrison 20th edition, p 2144-2145; Harrison 19th p 1811*)

Broad casts in urine indicate that the tubules in the kidney are chronically damaged and hence the remaining tubules are trying to take over the function of the damaged ones. Hence these surviving tubules dilate and thereby produce casts bigger in size than the normal ones and are referred to as broad casts.

44. **Ans. (a) Microalbuminuria**

(*Ref: Harrison 20th edition, p 2145; Harrison 19th edition, p 2425*)

- Microalbuminuria is defined as excretion of 30–300 mg of albumin per 24 hours (or 20–200 mcg/min or 30–300 mcg/mg Creatinine) on 2 of 3 urine collections.
- The detection of low levels of albumin excretion (Micro-albuminuria) has been linked to the identification of incipient diabetic kidney disease. This phase calls for aggressive management to prevent or retard overt diabetic nephropathy.

45. **Ans. (c) Decreased half-life of insulin**

(*Ref: Harrison 19th edition, p 1811*)

The two primary sites for insulin clearance are the liver and the kidney. The liver clears most insulin during first-pass transit, whereas the kidney clears most of the insulin in systemic circulation. Degradation normally involves endocytosis of the insulin-receptor complex, followed by the action of insulin-degrading enzyme. In kidney damage *clearance of insulin is reduced* leading to elevated insulin levels.

46. **Ans. (b) 50%**

(*Ref: Harrison 19th p 1811*)

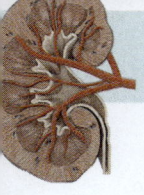

- Clinical features of uremia develop when more than 50% kidney parenchyma is destroyed.
- A normal kidney contains approximately 1 million nephrons, each of which contributes to the total glomerular filtration rate (GFR). In the face of renal injury (regardless of the etiology), the kidney has an innate ability to maintain GFR, despite progressive destruction of nephrons, as the remaining healthy nephrons manifest hyperfiltration and compensatory hypertrophy. This nephron adaptability allows for continued normal clearance of plasma solutes.
- Stage 1 and 2 of CKD are asymptomatic with symptoms beginning in stage 3

47. Ans. (b) Hypophosphatemia

(Ref: Harrison 19th p 1813)

CRF is always associated with hyperphosphatemia. The pathophysiology of secondary hyperpara-thyroidism and the consequent high-turnover bone disease is related to abnormal mineral metabolism through the following events:
1. Declining GFR leads to reduced excretion of phosphate and, thus, phosphate retention;
2. The retained phosphate stimulates increased synthesis of PTH and growth of parathyroid gland mass;
3. Decreased levels of ionized calcium, resulting from diminished calcitriol produc-tion by the failing kidney as well as phosphate retention, also stimulate PTH production.
4. Fibroblast growth factor 23 (FGF-23) is part of a family of phosphatonins that promotes renal phosphate excretion. Recent studies have shown that levels of this hormone, secreted by osteocytes, increases early in the course of CKD. High levels of FGF-23 are also an independent risk factor for left ventricular hypertrophy and mortality in dialysis patients. Moreover, elevated levels of FGF-23 may indicate the need for therapeutic intervention (e.g., phosphate restriction), even when serum phosphate levels are within the normal range.

48. Ans. (b) Renal osteodystrophy

(Ref: Harrison 20th edition, p 291/2933; Harrison 19th p 291/2478)

Secondary hyperparathyroidism is seen in chronic renal failure due to decrease in production of vitamin D_3.

49. Ans. (c) Amyloidosis

(Ref: Harrison 19th p723)

50. Ans. (d) Alport's Syndrome

(Ref: Harrison 20th edition, p 2977; Harrison 19th p 2513)

Four forms of Alport syndrome are:
1. Classic AS, which is inherited as an X-linked disorder with hematuria, sensori-neural deafness, and conical deformation of the anterior surface of the lens (lenticonus);
2. A subtype of the X-linked form associated with diffuse leiomyomatosis;
3. An autosomal recessive form; and
4. An autosomal dominant form. Both autosomal recessive and dominant forms can cause renal disease without deafness or lenticonus.

Molecular Defects

Most patients have mutations in four of the six genes for the chains of type IV collagen (COL4A3, COL4A4, COL4A5, and COL4A6).

Diagnosis: The diagnosis of classic AS is based on X-linked inheritance of hematuria, sensorineural deafness, and lenticonus. The lenticonus together with hematuria is pathognomonic of classic AS. The sensorineural deafness is primarily in the high-tone range. It can frequently be detected only by an audiogram and is usually not progressive. The hematuria usually progresses to nephritis and may cause renal failure in late adolescence in affected males and at older ages in some women. Renal transplantation is usually successful.

51. Ans. (b) Hypocalcemia

(Ref: Harrison 19th p 2049)

- Hypocalcemia in C.K.D is linked to development of secondary hyperparathyroidism with osteitis cystica fibrosa and Rugger jersey spine development. The concomitant hyper-phosphatemia leads to calcification of blood vessels which explains worsening atherosclerosis. *Hence Hypocalcemia in CKD patients leads to endocrinological and cardiovascular complications.*
- Hyperosmolarity occurs as urea is one of the parameters deciding serum osmolality. Sodium, potassium, glucose and urea determine plasma osmolality.
- Acidosis will damage Blood brain barrier and will worsen the urameic encephalopathy present in these patients
- Hyponatremia secondary to volume overload explains the seizures in these patients.

52. Ans. (a) Cerebral edema

(Ref: Harrison 19th p 250)

- Dialysis disequilibrium syndrome occurs in patients receiving hemodialysis.
  - Symptoms include headache, nausea, emesis, blurred vision, muscular twitching, disorientation, delirium, hypertension, tremors, and seizures.
  - The condition tends to be self-limited and subsides over several hours.
  - Dialysis disequilibrium syndrome is attributed to a reverse urea effect. *Urea is cleared more slowly from the brain than from the blood, an effect that causes an osmotic gradient leading to the net flow of water into the brain and to transient cerebral edema.*

53. Ans. (d) Primary amyloidosis

(Ref: Harrison 19th p 723)

Bilaterally enlarged kidneys seen in:
1. Diabetes mellitus
2. Amyloidosis
3. Polycystic kidneys
4. HIV nephropathy
5. Hydronephrosis bilateral

54. Ans. (b) Hemolytic uremic syndrome

(Ref: Harrison 20th edition, p 2111-2119; Harrison 19th p 1030)

- HUS is a cause of development of Acute kidney injury.
- The toxins in CRF cause myopathy and neuropathy while the hyperphosphatemia explains the ectopic calcification of tubules.

55. Ans. (a) Aluminium toxicity

(Ref: Harrison's 18th ed. ch. 371, 281 Table-371.5 DDx of Dementia)

- Patients undergoing long-term dialysis acquire dialysis encephalopathy (or dialysis dementia), which is a subacute, progressive, and often fatal disease.
- Aluminium toxicity either from aluminium phosphate salts or from aluminium in the dialysate were linked to the pathogenesis of dialysis dementia. Starting in the early 1980s, aluminum was actively removed from the dialysate with a large reduction in the incidence of dialysis dementia.

56. Ans. (c) Increased anion gap

(Ref: Harrison 20th edition, p 2114; Harrison 19th p 1807)

Causes of increased anion gap (>12 mEq/L; "MUDPILERS")

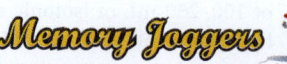

> **Memory Joggers**
> - **M**ilk-alkali syndrome
> - **U**remia
> - **D**iabetic ketoacidosis
> - **P**ropylene glycol
> - **L**actic acidosis
> - **I**soniazid intoxication
> - **E**thanol ethylene glycol
> - **R**habdomyolysis/renal failure
> - **S**alicylates

A normal anion gap (6-12 mEq/L) may indicate the following:
- Loss of bicarbonate (i.e., diarrhea)
- Recovery from diabetic ketoacidosis
- Ileostomy fluid loss
- Carbonic anhydrase inhibitors (acetazolamide, dorzolamide, topiramate)
- Renal tubular acidosis
- Arginine and lysine in parenteral nutrition

A decreased anion gap (< 6 mEq/L) may suggest the following:
- Hypoalbuminemia
- Plasma cell dyscaria
- Monoclonal protein
- Bromide intoxication

57. Ans. (c) Water intoxication

(Ref: Harrison 19th edition, p 332e-9)

In setting of terminal renal failure, the volume overload in combination with damage to blood brain barrier leads to cerebral edema which leads to seizures. The problem will be compounded by hypertensive state that leads to increase cerebral flow and resultant worsening of cerebral edema.

58. Ans. (b) Recombinant human erythropoeitin

(Ref: Harrison's 18th ed. ch. 280)

59. Ans. (a) Sexual dysfunction

(Ref: Harrison 20th edition, p 2113; Harrison 19th p 1823)

Choice	Improvement /persistence after Hemodialysis
Sexual dysfunction	PERSISTS
Pericarditis	Improves
Uremic lung	Improves
Neuropathy	Improves/persists both are mentioned

Hence from the two close answers, sexual dysfunction is a better answer to this question.

60. Ans. (c) Chronic Renal Failure

(Ref: Harrison 20th edition, p 2118; Harrison 19th p 192)

61. Ans. (b) Hypophosphatemia

(Ref: Harrison 20th edition, p 2114-2115; Harrison 19th p 2458)

62. Ans. (d) Hyperphosphatemia

(Ref: Harrison 20th edition, p 2115; Harrison 19th p 2460)

Hemodialysis

63. Ans. (c) Pericarditis

(Ref: Harrison 20th edition, p 2122; Harrison 19th edition, p 1810, 1822)

Indications for emergency dialysis is AEIOU
- **A**cidosis, especially if severe (pH < 7.2 and refractory to HCO_3 or unable to give HCO_3 due to volume overload) or symptomatic (arrhythmias).
- **E**lectrolytes, especially potassium with EKG changes. Temporize with Ca, D50, insulin, bicarb, kayexalate.
- **I**ngestions, especially those that cause renal failure such as salicylates or ethylene glycol.
- **O**verload, i.e. volume overload causing pulmonary edema. Temporize with nitrates and mega doses of Lasix (160–200 mg IV) – push slowly to avoid ototoxicity.
- **U**remia, i.e. confusion, pericarditis, seizures, platelet dysfunction with severe bleeding, intractable N/V.

When to start dialysis in CKD?
- Dialysis should be instituted whenever the glomerular filtration rate (GFR) is <15 mL/min and there is one or more of the following: symptoms or signs of uraemia, inability to control hydration status or blood pressure or a progressive deterioration in nutritional status.

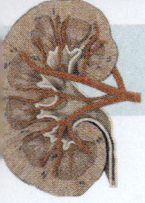

- In any case, dialysis should be started before the GFR has fallen to 6 mL/min/1.73 m², even if optimal pre-dialysis care has been provided and there are no symptoms

64. Ans. (b) Gram Positive Organisms

(Ref: Harrison 20th edition, p 2122-2123)

- Catheter-related bloodstream infections (CRBSIs) are a major complication of long-term catheter use in HD. Gram positive organism are seen followed by gram negative organisms.
- Similarly in peritoneal dialysis, the clinical presentation typically consists of pain and cloudy dialysate, often with fever and other constitutional symptoms. The most common culprit organisms are gram-positive cocci, including *Staphylococcus*, reflecting the origin from the skin. Gram-negative rod infections are less common; fungal and mycobacterial infections can be seen in selected patients, particularly after antibacterial therapy.
- In cases where peritonitis is due to hydrophilic gram negative rods (e.g., *Pseudomonas* sp.) or yeast, antimicrobial therapy is usually not sufficient, and catheter removal is required to ensure complete eradication of infection. Non-peritonitis catheter-associated infections (often termed *tunnel infections*) vary widely

65. Ans. (b) Arteriovenous fistula results in arterialization of vein

(Ref: Harrison 20th edition, p 2123; Harrison 19th edition, p 1822-23)

- The fistula, graft, or catheter through which blood is obtained for hemodialysis is often referred to as a *dialysis access*.
- A native fistula created by the anastomosis of an artery to a vein (e.g., the Brescia-Cimino fistula, in which the cephalic vein is anastomosed end-to-side to the radial artery) results in arterialization of the vein.
- This facilitates its subsequent use in the placement of large needles (typically 15 Gauge) to access the circulation.
- Fistulas have the highest long-term patency rate of all dialysis access options

- The most important complication of arteriovenous grafts is thrombosis of the graft and graft failure, principally due to intimal hyperplasia at the anastomosis between the graft and recipient vein.
- Many patients undergo placement of an arteriovenous graft (i.e., the interposition of prosthetic material, usually polytetrafluoroethylene, between an artery and a vein) or a tunneled dialysis catheter

66. Ans. (c) Thrice per week

(Ref: Harrison 20th edition, p 2124; Harrison 19th ed. / 1823)

For the majority of patients with ESRD, between 9 and 12 hours of dialysis are required each week, usually divided into three equal sessions.

Current Targets of Hemodialysis

- Urea reduction ratio (the fractional reduction in blood urea nitrogen per hemodialysis session) of >65–70%.
- Body water–indexed clearance x time product (KT/V) above 1.2 or 1.05.

Remember

Hypotension is the most common acute complication of hemodialysis. Since the introduction of bicarbonate-containing dialysate, dialysis-associated hypotension has become less common. The management of hypotension during dialysis consists of discontinuing ultrafiltration, the administration of 100–250 mL of isotonic saline or 10 mL of 23% saturated hypertonic saline, or administration of salt-poor albumin.

67. Ans. (a) Right internal Jugular Vein

(Ref: KDIGO 2012 guidelines)

Generally, for tunneled CDCs, the preferred veins for central access are the right internal jugular (RIJ), right external jugular (REJ), left internal jugular (LIJ), left external jugular (LEJ)—in that order.

The National Kidney Foundation's Kidney Disease Outcomes Quality Initiative Clinical Practice Guidelines for Hemodialysis Adequacy (K/DOQI Guidelines) state that subclavian vein (SCV) catheterization should be avoided in patients with end stage renal disease (ESRD) because of the risk for central venous stenosis, with subsequent loss of the entire ipsilateral arm for vascular access.

68. Ans. (a) Cimino- Brescia Fistula

	IHD	SLEDD	CRRT
Name	Intermittent hemodialysis	Slow (or sustained) low efficiency daily dialysis	Continuous renal replacement therapy
Mechanism and Molecules removed	Dilaysis–mostly low MWt	Small+middle molecules with SLEDD/F	Small+middle molecules with CVVHDF
Use	Ambulatory CRF Hyperkalemia	Critically ill Hyperkalemia	Critically ill Non-ambulatory
Blood flow	300-400 mL/min	200-300 mL/min	50-200 mL/min
Dialysate flow	500-800 mL/min	1-2L/h	2-3 L/h
Efficiency	High	Moderate	Low (but increased clearance of high VD molecules over time)

Contd...

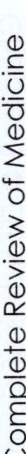

	IHD	SLEDD	CRRT
Hemodynamic Stability	Poor Hypotension common	Good	Good
Duration	3–4 h 3×/week	6–12 h daily	Continuous (24h/filter)
Access	Fistula of vascath (must be good)	Fistula of vascath (must be good)	Vascath only
Anticoagulation	Not needed	Usually not needed	Important

69. Ans. (c) Thrice per week

(Ref: Harrison 20th edition, p 2124; Harrison 19th p 1822)

For the majority of patients with ESRD, between 9 and 12 h of dialysis are required each week, usually divided into three equal sessions.

Current Targets of Hemodialysis
1. Urea reduction ratio (the fractional reduction in blood urea nitrogen per hemodialysis session) of >65–70%.
2. Body water–indexed clearance x time product (KT/V) above 1.2 or 1.05)

- Hypotension is the most common acute complication of hemodialysis. Since the introduction of bicarbonate-containing dialysate, dialysis-associated hypotension has become less common. The management of hypotension during dialysis consists of discontinuing ultrafiltration, the administration of 100–250 mL of isotonic saline or 10 mL of 23% saturated hypertonic saline, or administration of salt-poor albumin.

70. Ans. (b) Peritonitis

(Ref: Harrison 20th edition, p 2122-2124; Harrison 19th p 1822)

71. Ans. (a) Hypotension

(Ref: Harrison 20th edition, p 2124; Harrison 19th p 1824)

- Hypotension is the most common acute complication of hemodialysis, particularly among patients with diabetes mellitus.
- Numerous factors appear to increase the risk of hypotension, including excessive ultrafiltration with inadequate compensatory vascular filling, impaired vasoactive or autonomic responses, osmolar shifts, overzealous use of antihypertensive agents, and reduced cardiac reserve.
- Patients with arteriovenous fistulas and grafts may develop high output cardiac failure due to shunting of blood through the dialysis access; on rare occasions, this may necessitate ligation of the fistula or graft.

72. Ans. (a) A Beta2

(Ref: Harrison 19th edition, p 723)

Dialysis-related amyloidosis:
1. Accounts for approx. 50% of patients on hemodialysis between 8-12 years
2. Amyloid protein is Aβ2M-globulin
3. Occurs in association with chronic hemodialysis, almost never before 5 years of treatment
4. Visceral deposits are rare
5. Osteoarticular deposits are common; presenting complaints include carpal tunnel syndrome, flexor tenosynovitis, bone cysts, and pathologic fractures
6. Systemic manifestations usually only occur after 15 years of hemodialysis, and include cardiac, gastrointestinal, and renal involvement
7. As well as supportive treatment, therapy may involve use of high-flux biocompatible polyarylonitrile and polysulfone dialysis membranes, which enhance removal of β2M proteins
8. Renal transplantation may be considered

73. Ans. (d) Hyperphosphatemia

(Ref: Harrison 19th edition, p 1810)

74. Ans. (a) Cardiovascular

(Ref: Harrison 19th edition, p 1810)

- Cardiovascular disease constitutes the major cause of death in patients with ESRD. Cardiovascular mortality and event rates are higher in dialysis patients than in patients post transplantation, although rates are extraordinarily high in both populations.
- The underlying cause of cardiovascular disease is unclear but may be related to shared risk factors (e.g., diabetes mellitus, hypertension, atherosclerotic and arteriosclerotic vascular disease), chronic inflammation, massive changes in extracellular volume (especially with high interdialytic weight gains), inadequate treatment of hypertension, dyslipidemia, anemia, dystrophic vascular calcification, hyperhomocysteinemia, and, perhaps, alterations in cardiovascular dynamics during the dialysis treatment.

75. Ans. (b) Osteodystrophy

(Ref: Harrison 19th edition, p 291/2478)

The uremic milieu leads to uremic encephalopathy as urea can cross the Blood brain barrier. The urea irritates the stomach mucosa leading to Protracted nausea and vomiting in these patients. Due to inability of kidney to excrete protons, metabolic acidosis ensues. However when dialysis is performed it will lead to removal of urea and resultant improvement in condition of the patient.

However the bone changes due to secondary hyperparathyroidism in these patients leads to osteitis cystica fibrosa and Rugger jersey spine which cannot be reversed without kidney transplantation or calcitriol with calcium supplementation.

76. Ans. (d) Hyperkalemia of 6.5 mEq/L

(Ref: Harrison 19th edition, p 1823)

Hyperkalemia of 6.5 mEq/dl would not be life threatening and needs medical therapy. Only in case of refractory life threatening hyperkalemia hemodialysis is indicated.

There are a number of clinical indications to initiate dialysis in patients with CKD. These include:
1. Pericarditis or pleuritis *(urgent indication)*
2. Progressive uremic encephalopathy or neuropathy, with signs such as confusion, asterixis, myoclonus, wrist or foot drop, or, in severe cases, seizures *(urgent indication)*
3. A clinically significant bleeding diathesis attributable to uremia *(urgent indication)*
4. Persistent metabolic disturbances that are refractory to medical therapy; these include hyperkalemia, metabolic acidosis, hypercal-cemia, hypocalcemia, and hyperphosphatemia
5. Fluid overload refractory to diuretics
6. Hypertension poorly responsive to antihypertensive medications
7. Persistent nausea and vomiting
8. Evidence of malnutrition

The first five of the above indications are potentially acutely life-threatening and should not be allowed to develop prior to initiation of dialysis in patients with known CKD under medical care. The last two develop more insidiously and can also be due to other comorbidities or drug effects. They are no less dangerous.

77. Ans. (c) Alumunium toxicity

(Ref: Harrison's 19th edition, p 1810)

- In patients on long-term hemodialysis, osteo-malacia is associated with the accumulation of aluminum in bone.
- Studies have also shown that patients on hemodialysis who are exposed to dialysate containing high aluminum concentrations are at increased risk of osteomalacia.
- Typical presentations may include proximal muscle weakness, bone pain, multiple nonhealing fractures, acute or subacute alteration in mental status, and premature osteoporosis. These patients almost always have some degree of renal disease. Most patients are on hemodialysis or peritoneal dialysis.

Kidney Transplantation

78. (d) Infection occurs by filariform larvae

(Ref: Jawetz medical microbiology: 27th edition, p 730)
- The image shows rhabditiform larva of Strongyloides stercoralis.
- Choice A is ruled out as it is a dioecious organism related to parthenogenesis.
- Choice B is ruled out as it is transmitted by skin penetration of larva.

- Choice C is ruled out as Loeffler pneumonia is caused by ascariasis.

79. Ans. (a) Basophilic intranuclear inclusion

(Ref: Harrison 19th edition, p 1190)

CMV infection is commonly seen after solid organ transplantation. The image shows a cytomegalic large cell (infected with virus), containing 8-10 μm basophilic intranuclear inclusions which are eccentrically placed. This appearance is also called owl eye appearance. The risk is greatest 5-13 weeks after transplantation and the patient runs the risk of graft failure.

80. Ans. (c) Nucleic acid testing

(Ref: Harrison: 19th edition, p 1193)

- CMV infection cannot be diagnosed on clinical grounds alone and quantitative nucleic acid testing for CMV by PCR technology is best suited for diagnosis.
- The *virus continues to be shed in the urine* for months or years after recent infection and hence urine microscopy or immunofluorescence is not accurate for diagnosis
- IgM anti-CMV is used for diagnosis of recent infection but can be *false positive* due to Rheumatoid factor.
- The IgG anti-CMV antibody has a disadvantage that it takes 4 weeks to appear.

81. Ans. (d) Donation after cardiac arrest following brain stem death

(Ref: Harrison 20th edition, p 2126; Harrison, 19th edition, p 1826)

Donation after cardiac death

I:	Brought in dead
II:	unsuccessful Resuscitation
III:	Awaiting Cardiac Arrest
IV:	Cardiac arrest after Brainstem Death
V:	Cardiac arrest in a Hospital patient

Kidneys for transplantation can be used from categories II-V but are commonly used from categories III and IV

82. Ans. (d) 20 years

(Ref: Harrison 20th edition, p 2126; Harrison, 19th edition, p 1826)

The life expectancy from a living donor graft is 20 years whereas that of deceased donor graft is close to 14 years.

83. Ans. (a) Selective renal angiogram in the recipient helps to know vascular anatomy for anastomosis

(Ref: Harrison 20th edition, p 2126-2128; Harrison 19th edition, p 1827-28)

- *Selective renal arteriography is performed in **donors*** to rule out presence of multiple or abnormal renal arteries because of technical difficulty in removal of organ and increase in ischemia time of transplanted kidney.
- The donor kidney is anastomosed to the recipient external or internal iliac artery and is placed in right iliac fossa.

- *Hence the recipient renal angiogram mentioned in choice A is not required.*
- To minimise the risk of early acute rejection, induction therapy is given using antithymocyte globulin (Polyclonal antibody) as it will induce lymphocyte depletion. Monoclonal antibody alemtuzumab directed against CD52 antigen located on B and T cells will also be useful.
- Subsequently maintenance therapy is given comprising triple therapy
  - Prednisolone
  - Calcineurin inhibitor: Cyclosporine or tacrolimus
  - Antimetabolite: Azathioprine or mycophenolate mofetil

mTOR inhibitor can replace the last two agents(Calcineurin inhibitor and anti-metabolites): Sirolimus and everolimus are used.

> Rejection episode can present with fever, swelling and tenderness over the allograft though this is rarely seen. Most acute rejection episodes are associated with rise of only serum creatinine without significant reduction in urine output. **Management of acute episode of rejection is methylprednisolone for 3 days. In case of failure antithymocyte globulin can be used.**

84. Ans. (c) Alport's syndrome

(Ref: Harrison 20th edition, p 2977; Harrison 19th p 2513)

- Alport's syndrome is a genetically acquired disease with defect of type 4 collagen. In case the new kidney is deployed after transplantation, then new kidney does not have the defect carried by the host.
- SLE and Good-pasture are autoimmune diseases where the persistent antibody response will mount an offensive on the transplanted kidney. In diabetic patients the poor sugar control will also cause microvascular damage to the transplanted kidney.

85. Ans. (d) HLA identity similarity seen in 1:100 people

(Ref: Harrison 20th edition, p 2126-2128; Harrison 19th p 925)

- Both cellular and humoral (antibody-mediated) effector mechanisms can play roles in kidney transplant rejection. Antibodies can also initiate a form of antibody-dependent but cell-mediated cytotoxicity by recipient cells that bear receptors for the Fc portion of immunoglobulin.
- Cellular rejection is mediated by lymphocytes that respond to HLA antigens expressed within the organ. The CD4+ lymphocyte responds to class II (HLA-DR) incompatibility by proliferating and releasing pro-inflammatory cytokines that augment the proliferative response of both CD4+ and CD8+ cells.
- CD8+ cytotoxic lymphocyte precursors respond primarily to class I (HLA-A, -B) antigens and mature into cytotoxic effector cells. The cytotoxic effector ("killer") T cells cause organ damage through direct contact and lysis of donor target cells
- *Repeated blood tranfusions increase the chance of transplant rejection.* PRA (Percent Reactive Antibody) is the amount of HLA antibody present in a patient's serum. The patient could have HLA antibody as a result of transfusions, prior transplants, and/or pregnancies.
- *There are three general groups of HLA, they are HLA-A, HLA-B and HLA-DR. There are many different specific HLA proteins within each of these three groups. (For example, there are 59 different HLA-A proteins, 118 different HLA-B and 124 different HLA-DR).*

86. Ans. (c) Cyclophosphamide

(Ref: Nelson Textbook, 18th ed., ch. 527, Harrison 19th p 252)

- Steroid-dependent patients, frequent relapsers, and steroid-resistant patients may be candidates for alternative agents, particularly if the child suffers severe corticosteroid toxicity (cushingoid appearance, hypertension, cataracts, and/or growth failure).
- Cyclophosphamide prolongs the duration of remission and reduces the number of relapses in children with frequently relapsing and steroid-dependent nephrotic syndrome.
- The potential side effects of the drug (neutropenia, disseminated varicella, hemorrhagic cystitis, alopecia, sterility, increased risk of future malignancy) should be carefully reviewed with the family before initiating treatment. The dose of cyclophosphamide is 2–3 mg/kg/24 hr given as a single oral dose, for a total duration of 8–12 wk. Alternate-day prednisone therapy is often continued during the course of cyclophosphamide administration. During cyclophosphamide therapy, the white blood cell count must be monitored weekly and the drug should be withheld if the count falls below 5,000/mm^3.

87. Ans. (d) Sulfisoxazole

(Ref: Harrison 19th p 932)

- The two close possible clinical diagnoses for the patient are PNEUMOCYSTIS or NOCARDIA.
- *The first step in diagnosis is examination of sputum or pus for crooked, branching, beaded, gram-positive filaments 1 microm wide and up to 50 micron long which is diagnostic of Nocardia.*
- *In contrast pneumocystis on toluidine blue staining looks like crushed ping pong balls, and causes diffuse infiltrates on CXR.*
- Pneumonia, the most common form of nocardial disease in the respiratory tract, is typically subacute; symptoms have usually been present for days or weeks at presentation.
- The onset is occasionally more acute in immunosuppressed patients.
- Cough is prominent and produces small amounts of thick, purulent sputum that is not malodorous. Fever, anorexia, weight loss, and malaise are common; dyspnea, pleuritic pain, and hemoptysis are less common.
- Roentgenographic patterns vary, but some are highly suggestive of nocardial pneumonia. Infiltrates vary in size and are typically dense. Single or multiple nodules are common, sometimes suggesting tumors or metastases. Infiltrates and nodules tend to cavitate. Empyema is present in one-quarter of cases.
- Sulfonamides are the drugs of choice. The combination of sulfamethoxazole (SMX) and trimethoprim (TMP) is probably equivalent to a sulfonamide alone.

88. Ans. (b) Cytomegalovirus

(Ref: Harrison 20th edition, p 2130-2131; Harrison 19th p 1190)

- CMV is a common and dangerous DNA virus in transplant recipients. It does not generally appear until the end of the first post-transplant month.
- Tissue invasion of CMV is common in the gastrointestinal tract and lungs. CMV retinopathy occurs late in the course, if untreated.
- Valganciclovir is drug of choice that has been proved effective in both prophylaxis and treatment of CMV disease
- Treatment of active CMV disease with valganciclovir is always indicated. In many patients immune to CMV, viral activation can occur with major immunosuppressive regimens.

List of Organisms Causing Infection >1 Month After Kidney Transplant
- Pneumocystis carinii
- Cytomegalovirus
- Legionella
- Hepatitis B
- Hepatitis C

89. Ans. (a) P. Malariae

(Ref: Harrison 20th edition, p 2150; Net source PubMed, Harrison 19th p 252)

Epidemiologically P. Malariae has the best conclusive incidence of causing renal parenchymal disease like nephrotic syndrome

90. Ans. (a) Cytomegalovirus

(Ref: Harrison 20th edition, p 2130-2131; Harrison 19th p 1190)

91. Ans. (a) Skin cancer

(Ref: Harrison 20th edition, p 2131; Harrison 19th p 1831)

The incidence of tumors in patients on immuno-suppressive therapy is 5–6%, or approximately 100 times greater than that in the general population in the same age range. The most common lesions are cancer of the skin and lips and carcinoma in situ of the cervix, as well as lymphomas such as non-Hodgkin's lymphoma. The risks are increased in proportion to the total immunosuppressive load administered and the time elapsed since transplantation. Surveillance for skin and cervical cancers is necessary.

92. Ans. (d) MPGN (Membranous proliferative glomerulonephritis)

(Ref: Harrison 20th edition, p 2141; Harrison 19th p 1841)

Recurrence of kidney lesions after transplantation

Lesion	% of Recurrence
Lupus Nephritis	30%
Diabetic nephropathy	20%
MGN	30-50%
MPGN type II	100%

- Secondary causes of membranoproliferative (mesangiocapillary) glomerulonephritis (MPGN) (type I) include infections such as viral hepatitis B or C and systemic diseases. Treatment of these underlying causes may thus reduce the risk of recurrence. Recurrent disease should also be differentiated from de novo MPGN which occurs as part of the histological changes in patients with chronic transplant nephropathy.

93. Ans. (a) Alport's syndrome

(Ref: Harrison 20th edition, p 2977; API 6th/ 666, Harrison 19th p 2513)

94. Ans. (a) Fusion of foot processes of the glomerular epithelial cells

(Ref: Harrison 20th edition, p 2142)

95. Ans. (a) No abnormality

(Ref: Harrison 20th edition, p 2142; Harrison 19th p 1842)

96. Ans. (a) Glomerular function is lost due to loss of polyanions around the foot processes

(Ref: Harrison 20th edition, p 2142)

97. Ans. (b) Minimal Change Glomerulonephritis

(Ref: Harrison 20th edition, p 2142; Harrison 19th p 1842)

98. Ans. (c) FK 506

(Ref: NICE Guidelines 'Immunosuppression therapy for renal transplantation in adults' (www.nice.org.uk/pdf/TA085 guidance. pdf); KDT 5th/790)

Nephrotic Syndrome

99. Ans. (a) Membranous

(Ref: Harrison 20th edition, p 2144; Robbin's Pathology 9th edition, p 917-918)

Membranous nephropathy can be associated with tumors of the **colon, lung** and **hematological** malignancies like chronic lymphocytic leukemia.

100. Ans. (a) Minimal change disease

(Ref: Harrison 20th edition, p 2142; Nelson 19th edition, p 1799-1800 and OP Ghai 8th edition, p 477)

- The presence of edema and decreased urine output points to kidney lesion.
- All the three essential diagnosis of nephrotic syndrome i.e. presence of 3 + proteinuria, serum albumin on lower side of normal, and edema are present.
- Considering the age of the patient and preserved kidney function, the diagnosis of the patient is minimal change disease.

Dipstick detection of proteinuria
- Trace = 5–20 mg/dL
- 1 + = 30 mg/dL
- 2 + = 100 mg/dL
- 3 + = 300 mg/dL
- 4 + = Greater than 2000 mg/dL

- Interstitial nephritis of acute variety presents with fever, rash, peripheral eosinophilia, and oliguric renal failure occurring after 7–10 days of treatment with methicillin or another beta-lactam antibiotic.
- IgA nephropathy presents with recurrent episodes of gross hematuria following URTI.
- FSGS presents with ephritic syndrome with deranged KFT and is unlikely.

101. Ans. (a) DM; (b) Amyloidosis; (d) ACE inhibitors decreases proteinuria

(Ref: Harrison 19th/293; KDT 7th/505; Robbins 9th/ 898,262; O.P.Ghai 8th/473)

- Multiple myeloma is characterized by tubular proteinuria. The Bence jones proteins induce tubular damage and increased beta-2-micro-globulin levels in urine are a prognostic indicator of kidney function.
- ACE inhibitors dilate the efferent arteriole and reduce the glomerular proteinuria.
- DM and amyloidosis damage basement membrane of kidney.

102. Ans. (d) Low Complement Levels

(Ref: Harrison 20th edition, p 2142; Harrison 19th ed./1841)

- Nephrotic syndrome is kidney disease with proteinuria, hypoalbuminemia, and edema. Nephrotic-range proteinuria is 3 grams per day or more. On a single spot urine collection, it is 2 g of protein per gram of urine creatinine.
- Persistently low C3 levels are indicative of acute Glomerulonephritis
- Common primary causes of nephrotic syndrome include kidney diseases such as minimal-change nephropathy, membranous nephropathy, and focal glomerulosclerosis. Secondary causes include systemic diseases such as diabetes mellitus, lupus erythematosus, and amyloidosis. Congenital and hereditary focal glomerulosclerosis may result from mutations of genes that code for podocyte proteins, including nephrin, podocin, or the cation channel 6 protein

103. Ans. (d) Malignancy

(Ref: Harrison 20th edition, p 2144)

Autoimmune diseases	Infectious diseases	Malignancy
Ankylosing spondylitis	Filariasis	Carcinoma (solid organ)
Dermatomyositis	Hepatitis B	Leukemia
Graves	Hepatitis C	Lymphoma
Hashimoto	Leprosy	Melanoma
MCTD	Malaria	
Rheumatoid arthritis	Schistosomiasis	
Sjögren	Syphilis	
SLE		
Scleroderma		

Contd...

Autoimmune diseases	Infectious diseases	Malignancy
Drugs	**Miscellaneous**	
Captopril	De novo in renal allografts	
Gold	Kimura disease	
Lithium	Sarcoidosis	
Mercury-containing compounds	Sickle cell disease: This is uncommon. It usually produces focal segmental glomerulosclerosis.	
Penicillamine		
Probenecid	Systemic mastocytosis	

104. Ans. (c) Increased protein C levels

(Ref: Harrison 20th edition, p. 2135; Harrison 19th edition, 1841)

Essential features of diagnosis of nephrotic syndrome are:
- Proteinuria>3.5gms /24 hours period
- Hypo-albuminaemia< 2.5gm%
- Edema –peri-orbital edema- pedal edema

Non essential features are
- Hyperlidemia-increased cholesterol and increased triglycerides
- Lipiduria
- Loss of protein C/S/AT III in urine leading to hyper-coagulable state.

105. Ans. (a) Focal segmental glomerulosclerosis

(Ref: Harrison 20th edition, p 2142-2143; Robbins 8th edition, ch 14)

- HIV nephropathy is associated with development of focal segmental glomerulosclerosis. (also seen with reflux nephropathy). *It is also the commonest cause of nephrotic syndrome in adults.*

106. Ans. (d) Steroid induced diabetes

(Ref: Harrison 20th edition, p 2142; NELSON text book of Pediatrics 19th edition, p 1756 Harrison 19th edition, p 1841)

- In Nephrotic syndrome intravascular volume is already compromised due to hypoalbuminemia. In presence of diarrhea and dehydration there is further risk of compromise in intravascular volume and renal vein thrombosis which predisposes the patient to have acute kidney injury.
- Children with nephrotic syndrome are also at increased risk for thromboembolic events. The incidence of this complication in children is 2-5%. Both arterial and venous thromboses may be seen, including renal vein thrombosis, pulmonary embolus, sagittal sinus thrombosis, and thrombosis of indwelling arterial and venous catheters.
- The risk of thrombosis is related to increased prothrombotic factors (fibrinogen, thrombocytosis, hemoconcentration, relative immobilization) and decreased fibrinolytic factors (urinary losses of antithrombin ill, proteins C and S).

107. Ans. (b) Focal glomerulosclerosis

(Ref: Harrison 20th edition, p 2150; Harrison 19th p 1849)

- Renal involvement in leprosy is related to the quantity of backeria as kidney is the target organ during splanchic localization. The most common renal involvement is FSGS, mesangioproliferative glomerulonephritis.

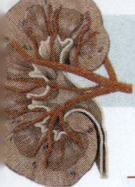

108. Ans. (b) IgA nephropathy

(Ref: Harrison 20th edition, p 2139-2142; Harrison 19th p 1841)

IgA nephropathy presents with microscopic/gross hematuria and not nephrotic syndrome.

109. Ans. (a) Nephrotic syndrome

(Ref: KDIGO 2012 guidelines pg. 128-29, Harrison 19th p 1841)

- Muehrcke's lines are white lines (leukonychia) that extend all the way across the nail and lie parallel to the lunula.
- The appearance of Muehrcke's lines is nonspecific, but they are often associated with decreased protein synthesis, which may occur during periods of metabolic stress (e.g., after chemotherapy) and in hypoalbuminemic states such as the nephrotic syndrome.
- **It should not be confused with Half-and-half nail syndrome, also known as Lindsay nails, is one of the most characteristic, but not pathognomonic, onychopathies seen in chronic renal failure.** Although the exact pathogenesis is unclear, it is speculated that acidosis and an increase in toxic uremic substances occurring subsequent to sudden renal decompensation may stimulate melanin formation by nail matrix melanocytes.
- While half-and-half nails affect an estimated 20% to 50% of chronic renal failure patients, a pattern has yet to be determined with regard to sex, age, and cause of the kidney disease.

110. Ans. (d) F.S.G.S (Focal segmental glomerulosclerosis)

(Ref: Harrison 20th edition, p 2142; Harrison 19th edition, p 1835t, 1842)

- In composite forms of glomerular inflammatory reactions, such as in membranous glomerulone phritis or diffuse proliferative glomerulonephritis, the loss of size selectivity and perhaps also charge selectivity might explain the pattern of non-selective proteinuria that is found in these disease.
- The most likely defect of glomeruli characteristic of minimal change nephropathy is loss of the charge selectivity of the glomerular capillary wall. As the size selectivity of the glomerular capillary wall is intact, molecules the size of IgG or larger are rejected while albumin is able to pass through the small pores, resulting in a preferential albuminuria, that is, that proteinuria is highly selective.
- Based on a comparison of the clearance of high-molecular-weight proteins to that of albumin, the pattern of glomerular proteinuria may be described as either selective or non-selective.
- The protein usually used as the high-molecular-weight marker is IgG, but others proteins such as haptoglobin, ceruloplasmin and α2-macroglobulin (α2M) have also been used.
- Patients with an IgG SI of 0.2 or higher are considered to have a non-selective proteinuria whereas patients with a ratio below 0.2 are considered to have a selective proteinuria.

111. Ans. (b) SLE

(Ref: Harrison 20th edition, p 2144; Harrison 19th edition, p 1843)

- Infection-Hep B and C, syphilis, malaria, schistomiasis leprosy. filariasis.
- Cancer-Colon CA, lung CA, Breast CA, renal CA Esophagus, neuroblastoma

112. Ans. (a) Volume overload state

(Ref: Harrison 20th edition, p 2142; Harrison 19th edition, p 252)

Metabolic consequences of the nephrotic syndrome include the following:
- Infection
- Hyperlipidemia and atherosclerosis
- Hypocalcemia and bone abnormalities
- Hypercoagulability
- Hypovolemia

113. Ans. (a) Membranous GN

(Ref: Harrison 20th edition, p 2144; Harrison 19th edition, p 1843)

- Neoplasm and nephrotic syndrome may occur concomitantly, although the time interval between them may be a year or more.
- If a nephrotic syndrome presents in an adult patient, underlying malignancy should be considered. It may be found in 10–22% of cases, being more prevalent in the older age group.
- Bronchogenic carcinoma is rarely associated with Nephrotic Syndrome, and may be encountered in 3% of patients initially presenting with Nephrotic syndrome.
- Though both MGN and MPGN can be associated with lung malignancy, on a comparative basis the more commonly seen is MGN and is hence the answer in the question.

114. Ans. (d) Nephrotic syndrome

(Ref: Harrison 20th edition, p 2167; Harrison 19th edition, p 252)

Although renal vein thrombosis (RVT) has numerous etiologies, it occurs most commonly in patients with nephrotic syndrome (i.e., >3 g/d protein loss in the urine, hypoalbuminemia, hypercholesterolemia, edema).

The syndrome is responsible for a hypercoagulable state. The excessive urinary protein loss is associated with decreased antithrombin III, a relative excess of fibrinogen, and changes in other clotting factors; all lead to a propensity to clot.

115. Ans. (d) Fibrinogen

(Ref: Harrison 20th edition, p 2142; Harrison 19th edition, p 252)

- Venous thrombosis and pulmonary embolism are well-known complications of the Nephrotic syndrome.
- Hypercoagulability in these cases appears to derive from urinary loss of anticoagulant proteins, such as antithrombin III and plasminogen, along with the simultaneous increase in clotting factors, especially factors I, VII, VIII, and X.
- Moreover, that risk appeared especially elevated during the first 6 months of Nephrotic syndrome, being at almost 10%. This high incidence may justify the routine use of preventive anticoagulation treatment during the first 6 months of a persistent nephrotic syndrome.
- There is also increased risk of arterial thrombotic events, including coronary and cerebrovascular ones, in nephrotic syndrome.

116. Ans. (b) Focal segmental GN

(Ref: Harrison 20th edition, p 2143, Table 308-5; Harrison 19th edition, p 1842)

Causes of Secondary FSGS
- **Drugs**
  - Intravenous heroin
  - Analgesics
  - Pamidronate
  - Lithium
  - Anabolic steroids
- **Viruses**
  - Hepatitis B
  - HIV
  - Parvovirus
- **Hemodynamic factors** - With reduced renal mass
  - Solitary kidney
  - Renal allograft
  - Renal dysplasia
  - Renal agenesis
  - Oligomeganephronia
  - Segmental hypoplasia
  - Vesicoureteric reflux
- **Hemodynamic causes** - Without reduced renal mass
- Massive obesity
- Sickle cell nephropathy
- **Malignancies**
  - Lymphomas
  - Other malignancies

117. Ans. (a) Loss of Antithrombin III

(Ref: Harrison 20th edition, p 2142; Harrison 19th edition, p 252)

118. Ans. (b) Hypertrophy of muscle

(Ref: KDT 5th/264, 265, Harrison 19th edition, p 252)

119. Ans. (b) Amyloid Nephropathy

(Ref: Harrison 19th edition, p 723)

120. Ans. (b) Focal segmental Glomerulosclerosis

(Ref: Harrison 20th edition, p 2143; Harrison 19th p 1842)

121. Ans. (b) Membranous Glomerulopathy

(Ref: Harrison 20th edition, p 2167)

Nephritic Syndrome and Hematuria

122. Ans. (b) Type II cytotoxic

(Ref: Harrison 19th edition, p 377e-4, 1839)

Type 2 Hypersensitivity	Type 3 Hypersensitivity	Type 4 Hypersensitivity
Autoimmune hemolytic anemia Autoimmune thrombocytopenic purpura	Systemic lupus erythematosus	Multiple sclerosis
Pemphigus vulgaris	Post-streptococcal glomerulonephritis	
Vasculitis caused by ANCA	Polyarteritis nodosa	Rheumatoid arthritis^Q
Goodpature syndrome	Reactive arthritis	Peripheral neuropathy, Guillain-Barre syndrome
Acute rheumatic fever	Serum sickness	Inflammatory bowel disease (Crohn's disease)
Myasthenia gravis	Arthus reaction	Contact dermatitis
Graves disease		
Insulin-resistant diabetes		
Pernicious anemia		

123. Ans. (b) Thrombocytopenia

(Ref: Harrison 20th edition, p 2586; Harrison 19th edition, p 2190)

Henoch schonlein purpura is known as non-thrombocytopenic purpura.

Clinical features of HSP
- Hallmark of HSP is rash, beginning as pinkish maculo-papules which later develop into petechiae or purpura, They present clinically as palpable purpura that evolve from red to purple.
- Arthritis, present in more than 2/3 of children with HSP, is usually localized to the knees and ankles
- Edema and damage to the vasculature of the gastrointestinal tract may also lead to intermittent colicky abdominal pain. There may be enlarged mesenteric lymph nodes and hemorrhage into the bowel.
- Renal involvement occurs in 25–50% of children and may manifest with hematuria, proteinuria, or both; nephritis or nephrosis; or acute renal failure.
- Hepatosplenomegaly and lymphadenopathy
- Neurological involvement is the development of seizures, paresis, or coma.
- Other rare complications include rheumatoid-like nodules, cardiac and/or eye involvement, mononeuropathies, pancreatitis, and pulmonary or intramuscular hemorrhage.

124. Ans. (a) Renal biopsy is indicated in severe renal dysfunction

(Ref: Harrison 20th edition, p 2137; Harrison 19th edition, p 1837)

Renal biopsy in P.S.G.N should be considered only in-
1. Presence of acute renal failure
2. Absence of evidence of streptococcal infections or normal complement levels
3. When hematuria and proteinuria leads to diminished renal function
4. Low C3 levels persist more than 2 months
- In the first week of symptoms 90% of patients will have a depressed CH50 and *decreased levels of C3 with normal levels of C4*

- Resolution of the hematuria and proteinuria in the majority of children occurs within 3-6 weeks of the onset of nephritis but 3-10% of children may have persistent microscopic hematuria non nephritic proteinuria or hypertensions
- Serum triglyceride levels are increased in nephrotic syndrome not in nephritis

125. Ans. (a) Rapid Recovery

(Ref: Harrison 20th edition, p 2134-2135; Harrison 19th p 1836)

- Rapidly progressive glomerulonephritis (RPGN) is characterized by a rapid loss of renal function (usually a 50% decline in the glomerular filtration rate (GFR) within 3 months with glomerular crescent formation seen in at least 50% or 75% of glomeruli seen on kidney biopsies.
- If left untreated, it rapidly progresses into acute renal failure and death within months.
- In 50% of cases, RPGN is associated with an underlying disease such as Goodpasture syndrome, systemic lupus erythematosus, or Wegener granulomatosis; the remaining cases are idiopathic.
- Most types of RPGN are characterized by severe and rapid loss of kidney function featuring severe hematuria, red blood cell casts in the urine, and proteinuria, sometimes exceeding 3 g protein/24 h, a range associated with nephrotic syndrome. Hypertension and edema is also seen. Severe disease is characterized by pronounced oliguria or anuria, which indicates a poor prognosis.
- The clinical picture is consistent with nephritic syndrome, although the degree of proteinuria may occasionally exceed 3 g/24 h, a range associated with nephrotic syndrome

126. Ans. (c) Captopril

(Ref: Harrison 20th edition, p 2141; Harrison 19th p 1843)

Membranoproliferative Glomerulonephritis

Type I Disease (Most Common)	Type II	Type III
• Idiopathic • Subacute bacterial endocarditis • Systemic lupus erythematosus • Hepatitis C ± cryoglobulinemia • Mixed cryoglobulinemia • Hepatitis B • Cancer: Lung, breast, and ovary • C3 nephritic factor–associated partial lipodystrophy	• Idiopathic • C_3 nephritic fctor-associated partial lipodystrophy	• Idiopathic • Complement receptor deficiency

127. Ans. (a) Red cell cast

(Ref: Harrison 20th edition, p 289)

RBC casts indicate glomerular bleeding and are seen with acute glomerulonephritis. Hematuria can be seen with even kidney stones or bladder cancer and hence not a characteristic finding of AGN.

128. Ans. (a) Acute glomerulonephritis

(Ref: Harrison 20th edition, p 289)

Casts—These urinary sediments are formed by coagulation of albuminous material in the kidney tubules. Casts are cylindrical and vary in diameter. Casts in the urine always indicate some form of kidney disorder and should always be reported. If casts are present in large numbers, the urine is almost sure to be positive for albumin.

There are seven types of casts. They are as follows:

1. **Hyaline casts** are the most frequently occurring casts in urine. Hyaline casts can be seen in even the mildest renal disease. They are colorless, homogeneous, transparent, and usually have rounded ends.
2. **Red cell casts** indicate renal hematuria. Red cell casts may appear brown to almost colorless and are usually diagnostic of glomerular disease. White cell casts are present in renal infection and in noninfectious inflammation. The majority of white cells that appear in casts are hyper-segmented neutrophils.
3. **Granular casts** almost always indicate significant renal disease. However, granular casts may be present in the urine for a short time following strenuous exercise. Granular casts that contain fine granules may appear grey or pale yellow in color. Granular casts that contain larger coarse granules are darker. These casts often appear black because of the density of the granules.
4. **Epithelial casts** are rarely seen in urine because renal disease that primarily affects the tubules is infrequent. Epithelial casts may be arranged in parallel rows or haphazardly.
5. **Waxy casts** result from the degeneration of granular casts. Waxy casts have been found in patients with severe chronic renal failure, malignant hypertension, and diabetic disease of the kidney. Waxy casts appear yellow, grey, or colorless. They frequently occur as short, broad casts, with blunt or broken ends, and often have cracked or serrated edges.
6. **Fatty casts** are seen when there is fatty degene-ration of the tubular epithelium, as in degene-rative tubular disease. Fatty casts also result from lupus and toxic renal poisoning. A typical fatty cast contains both large and small fat droplets. The small fat droplets are yellowish-brown in color.
7. **Broad casts** seen in C.K.D.

129. Ans. (b) 5

(Ref: Harrison 20th edition, p 2134; Harrison 19th p 1847)

>5 RBC/μL of centrifuged specimen

There are two cut off for hematuria

1. >3RBC/HPF
2. >5RBC/μL

130. Ans. (d) Hematuria

(Ref: Harrison 20th edition, p 2134; Harrison 19th p 1834)

Nephritic syndrome is characterized by inflammation of the kidney leading to hematuria with hypertension and sub-nephrotic proteinuria.

131. **Ans. (d)** Optic atrophy

    (Ref: Harrison 20th edition, p 2137)

    Sudden onset hypertension in AGN may be associated with LVF, hypertensive encephalopathy and papilledema but not optic neuritis.

132. **Ans. (a)** IgA nephropathy

    (Ref: Harrison 20th edition, p 2139-2140; Harrison 19th p 1839)

    - Eighty percent of episodes in IgA nephropathy are associated with upper respiratory tract infections, mainly acute pharyngotonsillitis. This synchronous association of pharyngitis and macroscopic hematuria is known as synpharyngitic nephritis.
    - Gross hematuria usually appears simultaneously or within the first 48-72 hours after the infection begins; persists less than 3 days; and, in about a third of patients, is accompanied by loin pain, presumably due to renal capsular swelling.
    - Urine is usually brown rather than red, and clots are unusual.
    - The presenting illness of episodic, grossly visible hematuria is more common in younger people, whereas that of abnormal urine sediment is more frequent in older individuals.

133. **Ans. (a)** Goodpasture's Syndrome

    (Ref: Harrison 20th edition, p 2139; Harrison 19th edition, p 1839)

    Good pasture syndrome is a rare autoimmune disease in which antibodies attack the lungs and kidneys, leading to bleeding from the lungs and to kidney failure. It may quickly result in permanent lung and kidney damage, often leading to death. It is treated with immuno-suppressant drugs such as corticosteroids and cyclophosphamide, and with plasmapheresis, in which the antibodies are removed from the blood.

134. **Ans. (d)** Post streptococcal GN

    (Ref: Harrison 20th edition, p 2137; Harrison 19th edition, p 1837)

    - By the time the child with acute post-streptococcal glomerulonephritis (PSGN) presents with symptoms, the glomerular injury has already occurred, and the healing process has begun. Thus, influencing the ultimate course of the disease by any specific therapy directed at the cause of the nephritis is not possible.
    - Only a small percentage of patients with acute glomerulonephritis require initial hospitalization, and most of those are ready for discharge in 2-4 days. As soon as the blood pressure is under relatively good control and diuresis has begun, most patients can be discharged and monitored as outpatients. Local skin infections will be treated with penicillin for 10 days but steroids are not warranted.

135. **Ans. (b)** 20% Dysmorphic RBC

    (Ref: Harrison 20th edition, p 294, 2134; Harrison 19th p 1831)

136. **Ans. (b)** Acanthocytes

    (Ref: Harrison 20th edition, p 294; Harrison 19th edition, p 294)

137. **Ans. (c)** Broad Cast

    (Ref: Harrison 20th edition, p 294; Harrison 19th edition, p 294)

138. **Ans. (c)** Nephritic syndrome

    (Ref: Harrison 20th edition, p 2137; Harrison 19th p 1837)

139. **Ans. (c)** Diabetic Nephropathy

    (Ref: Harrison 20th edition, p 2134-2135; Harrison 19th p 1836)

140. **Ans. (a)** Number of crescents

    (Ref: Robbins 6th /453, Harrison 19th p 1836)

141. **Ans. (c)** Glomerulonephritis secondary to skin infection is more common in Summer

    (Ref: Harrison 20th edition, p 2137; Harrison 19th p 1837)

142. **Ans. (c)** Diffuse Proliferative Glomerulonephritis (WHO class IV)

    (Ref: Harrison 18th/p 2727)

143. **Ans. (d)** Anti – LA (SSB)

    (Ref: Samter's Immunologic disease 6th/497; 'Systemic Lupus Erythematosis' 4th/894)

144. **Ans. (a)** Post streptococcal glomerulonephritis

    (Ref: Harrison 20th edition, p 2137; Harrison 19th edition, p 1837)

Hemolytic Uraemic Syndrome

145. **Ans. (d)** Positive Coomb's test

    (Ref: Harrison 20th edition, p 2105t, 717; Harrison 19th p 657)

    - *Positive Coomb's test is seen with auto-immune hemolytic anemia but in H.U.S the type of anemia seen is microangiopathic hemolytic anemia.*
    - The entrapment of platelets in micro-thrombi formed in small blood vessels leads to thrombocytopenia. The consumption of clotting factors due to initiation of coagulation cascade leads to hypo-fibrinogenemia.
    - Hemolytic uremic syndrome is primarily a disease of infancy and early childhood and is classically characterized by the triad of microangiopathic hemolytic anemia, thrombocytopenia, and acute renal failure which explains uraemia.

146. **Ans. (d)** TTP

    (Ref: Harrison 20th edition, p 827; Harrison 19th edition, p 377e-4)

    - Classically, the following five features ("pentad") are indicative of TTP

    1. Thrombocytopenia leading to bruising or purpura
    2. Microangiopathic hemolytic anemia (anemia, jaundice and a blood film featuring evidence of mechanical fragmentation of red blood cells)
    3. Neurologic symptoms (fluctuating), such as hallucinations, bizarre behavior, altered mental status, stroke, or headaches
    4. Kidney failure
    5. Fever

147. Ans. (a) **Thrombocytosis**

   (*Ref: Harrison 20th edition, p 2164-2165; Harrison 19th p 1030*)

   - H.U.S is characterized by the involvement of widespread occlusive microvascular thromboses resulting in thrombocytopenia, microangiopathic hemolytic anemia, and variable signs and symptoms of end-organ ischemia like kidney damage.
   - The hallmark of hemolytic uremic syndrome in the peripheral smear is the presence of schistocytes. These consist of fragmented, deformed, irregular, or helmet-shaped RBCs. They reflect the partial destruction of RBCs that occurs as they traverse vessels partially occluded by platelet and hyaline microthrombi. The peripheral smear may also contain giant platelets. This is due to the reduced platelet survival time resulting from the peripheral consumption/destruction.

148. Ans. (d) **Purpura**

   (*Ref: Harrison 20th edition, p 2164-2165; Harrison 19th p 1030*)

   - Uraemia in H.U.S explains encephalopathy.
   - Thrombotic microangiopathies are characterized by the involvement of widespread occlusive microvascular thromboses resulting in thrombocytopenia, microangiopathic hemolytic anemia, and variable signs and symptoms of end-organ ischemia like kidney damage.
   - The thrombocytopenia presents as GI bleed whereas Purpura presents in TTP.
   - The pathophysiology of thrombotic thrombo-cytopenic purpura is different in that, as opposed to endothelial cell injury, thrombotic thrombo-cytopenic purpura is thought to be caused by a deficiency in the metalloprotease ADAMTS13, which is involved in the regulation of von Willebrand factor. A lack of this protein results in spontaneous platelet aggregation and the widespread deposition of platelet-rich thrombi in the microvasculature of various organs, most notably the heart, brain, and kidneys.

149. Ans. (d) **Neuropsychiatric disturbances**

   (*Ref: Harrison 20th edition, p 2164-2165; Harrison 19th p 1030*)

150. Ans. (a) **Hemolytic uremic syndrome**

   (*Ref: Harrison 20th edition, p 2164-2165; Harrison 19th p 1030*)

Interstitial Nephritis

151. Ans. (b) **Hepatorenal syndrome**

   (*Ref: Harrison 20th edition, p 2413; Harrison 19th edition, p 1809-1810*)

Hepato-renal syndrome	It occurs due to various causes like fulminant hepatic failure, end stage liver disease, Weil's disease and leads to pre renal acute kidney injury. Type 1 hepato-renal syndrome presents with AKI while Type 2 presents with refractory ascites.
Infections	Inflammation or fibrosis of the renal interstitium and atrophy of the tubular compartment are seen with infections like *Streptococcus, Staphylococcus, Legionella, Salmonella, Brucella, Yersinia, EBV, CMV, hanta virus, polyoma virus*.
Lymphoma	Interstitial infiltration by malignant B lymphocytes is a common autopsy finding in patients dying of chronic lymphocytic leukemia and non-Hodgkin's lymphoma; however, this is usually an incidental finding. Rarely, such infiltrates may cause massive enlargement of the kidneys and oliguric acute renal failure.
Sarcoidosis	It leads to chronic hypercalcemia and resultant hypercalcemic nephropathy affecting interstitium.

152. Ans. (a) **NSAID**

   (*Ref: Harrison 20th edition, p 2157; Harrison 19th ed. / 1856*)

   Choices B,C,D lead to acute tubular necrosis and hence by exclusion the answer is A.

   Causes of Acute Interstitial Nephritis
   - Drugs like beta lactams, quinolones, NSAID, COX-2 inhibitors, phenytoin, valproate and P.P.I
   - Infections like streptococcus, staphylococcus
   - Connective tissue disorder like SLE, Sjogren
   - Light chain nephropathy
   - Urate nephropathy

   Causes of Chronic Interstitial Nephritis
   - V.U.R
   - Sickle cell disease
   - Hypokalemic nephropathy

153. Ans. (d) **Rhabdomyolysis**

   (*Ref: Harrison 19th edition, p 1804*)

   - Interstitial nephritis is characterized by tubular damage leading to polyuria.
   - Rhabdo-myolysis leads to myo-globinuria leads to blockage of tubules and thereby reduction of urine output.
   - Hypokalemic nephropathy in choice B and ADH insufficiency (diabetes insipidus) in choice C leads to Polyuria.

154. Ans. (a) **Interstitial nephritis**

   (*Ref: Harrison 20th edition, p 2158; Harrison 19th p 1856*)

   65% of the salt excreted from the body is reabsorbed via proximal convoluted tubule and hence in interstitial nephritis where the tubule is involved, salt loss will be seen.

155. Ans. (a) **Interstitial Nephritis**

   (*Ref: Harrison 20th edition, p 2158; Harrison 19th p 1856*)

Bartter and Gitelman Syndrome

156. Ans. (c) **Mineralocorticoid antagonist can be used**

   (*Ref: Harrison 20th edition, p 306; Harrison 19th edition, p number 295, 306*)

Contd...

- The defect in Bartter syndrome in thick ascending limb of Loop of Henle leads to increase urinary loss of calcium and development of Nephrocalcinosis.
- The salt wasting and polyuria leads to dehydration. This stimulates the R.A.A.S system leading to secondary hyperaldosteronism. This explains the hypokalemia. Moreover the ROMK receptors in TAL are also affected leading to urinary loss of potassium.
- Barter syndrome leads to increased intra-renal prostaglandins and hence indomethacin is prescribed
- Secondary Aldosteronism explains the development of metabolic alkalosis.

157. Ans. (a) Hypertension

(Ref: Harrison 20th edition, p 306; Harrison 19th edition, p 306)

- Bartter syndrome has presentation of normal BP due to down regulation of angiotensin II receptors.
- There is loss of sodium and water from thick ascending limb of loop of Henle while the resultant loss of salt and water from the body leads to secondary aldosteronism.
- The secondary Stimulation of ENac receptor leads to gain of salt and water from the collecting duct but the gain is counterbalanced by the loss occurring in thick ascending limb of loop of Henle leading to normal or low BP in Bartter syndrome.

158. Ans. (c) Hypercalciuria

(Ref: Harrison 20th edition, p 306; Harrison 19th edition, p 306)

Gitelman syndrome- GS is an inheritable renal disorder characterized by hypomagnesemia, hypokalemia and hypocalciuria linked to the gene encoding the thiazide sensitive Na⁻ Cl-cotransporter located on chromosome 16q.

159. Ans. (a) Less common

(Ref: Harrison 20th edition, p 306; Harrison 19th edition, p 306)

Defect	Bartter syndrome	Gitelman syndrome
Clinical age of presentation	Defect in TAL. The proteins affected include the apical loop diuretic–sensitive sodium-potassium-chloride co-transporter NKCC2 (type 1), the apical potassium channel ROMK (type 2), and the basolateral chloride channel ClC-Kb (type 3)	Mutations in the thiazide-sensitive Na-Cl co-transporter, NCCT, in the DCT. Features resemble the effects of thiazide diuretics.
Clinical features	• Bartter's syndrome is a rare disease that most often presents in the neonatal period or early childhood with polyuria, polydipsia, salt craving, and growth retardation. Blood pressure is normal or low. • Metabolic abnormalities include hypo-kalemia, hypochloremic metabolic alkalosis, decreased urinary concentrating and diluting ability, hypercalciuria with nephrocalcinosis, mild hypoma-gnesemia. • In the antenatal period, fetal polyuria may cause maternal polyhydramnios and premature labor. Sensorineural deafness occurs in patients with Barttin gene mutations	• Gitelman's syndrome is more common than Bartter's syndrome and has a generally *milder* clinical course. • It is characterized by prominent neuromuscular symptoms and signs, including fatigue, weakness, carpo-pedal spasm, cramps, and tetany.
Investigation of choice	24 hr Urinary chloride	24 hr Urinary chloride with hypomagnesemia
Treatment	• Lifelong therapy with potassium and magnesium supplements and liberal salt intake. • High doses of spironolactone or amilo-ride treat the hypokalemia, alkalosis, and magnesium wasting. • Nonsteroidal anti-inflammatory drugs (NSAIDs) reduce the polyuria and salt wasting in Bartter's syndrome but are ineffective in Gitelman's syndrome.	• Same as left side • In Gitelman's syndrome, magnesium repletion is essential to correct the hypokalemia and control muscle weak-ness, tetany, and metabolic alkalosis; however, it may prove difficult in patients wasting large amounts of magnesium

Conclusion: Gitelman's syndrome is more common than Bartter's syndrome and has a generally milder clinical course with a later age of presentation. It is characterized by prominent neuromuscular symptoms and signs, including fatigue, weakness, carpopedal spasm, cramps, and tetany.

160. Ans. (b) Hypomagnesuria

(Ref: Harrison 20th edition, p 306; Harrison 19th edition, p 306)

- Bartter's syndrome has *hypomagnesemia* secondary to loss in urine as a consequence of defect in TAL of loop of henle
- Bartter' syndrome is a rare disease that most often presents in the neonatal period or early childhood with polyuria, polydipsia, salt craving, and growth retardation. Blood pressure is normal or low.
- Metabolic abnormalities include hypokalemia, hypochloremic metabolic alkalosis, decreased urinary concentrating and diluting ability, hypercalciuria with nephrocalcinosis, mild hypomagnesemia, and increased urinary prostaglandin excretion.

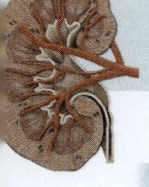

Tumor Lysis Syndrome

161. Ans. (b) Allopurinol + Hydration+ Urinary alkalinization

(Ref: Harrison 20th edition, p 519; Harrison 19th p 1795)

Tumor Lysis syndrome is characterized by:
1. Hyperuricemia
2. Hyperkalemia
3. Hyperphosphatemia
4. Hypocalcemia

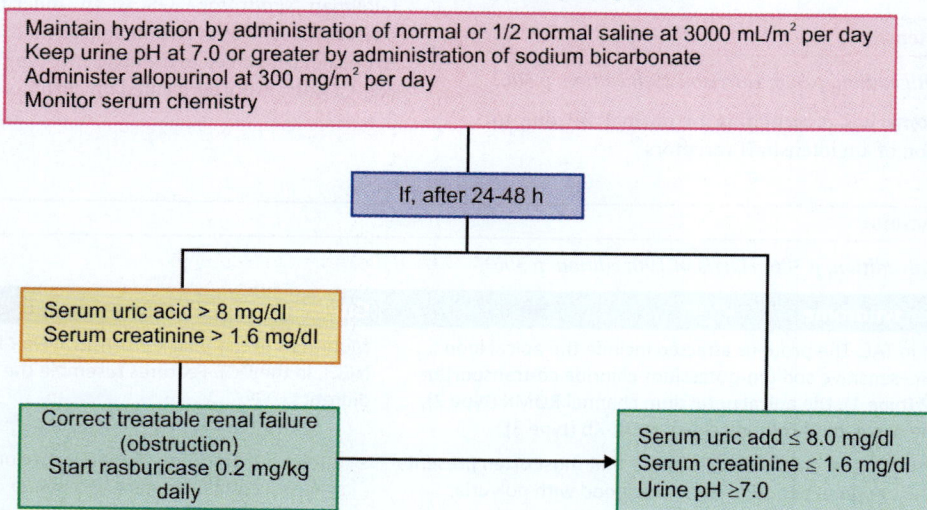

Management: The standard preventive approach consists of allopurinol, urinary alkalinization, and aggressive hydration.
1. Aggressive IV hydration not only helps to correct electrolyte disturbances by diluting extracellular fluid, it also increases intravascular volume.
2. Ideally, IV hydration in high-risk patients should begin 24-48 hours prior to initiation of cancer therapy and continue for 48-72 hours after completion of chemotherapy.
3. Continuous infusion rates as high as 4-5 L daily (or 3 L/m² daily), yielding urine volumes of at least 3L daily.
4. Intravenous allopurinol may be given in patients who cannot tolerate oral therapy. In some cases, uric acid levels cannot be lowered sufficiently with the standard preventive approach.
5. Rasburicase (recombinant urate oxidase) can be effective in these instances.

162. Ans. (d) Serum uric acid

(Ref: Harrison 19th p 1795)

- The prognosis of tumor lysis syndrome is excellent, and renal function recovers after the uric acid level is lowered to <10 mg/dL.
- If hyperuricemia develops, urine alkalinization prevents renal precipitation of uric acid but may increase the risks for nephrocalcinosis. If alkaline diuresis is employed, regular determinations of urine pH should guide the extent of therapy.
- Because increased urine flow rates help to inhibit crystal deposition in renal tubules, close monitoring of urine output is necessary to assess adequacy of hydration.
- Patients develop deposits of uric acid within the distal renal tubule, which cause intrarenal hydronephrosis. Uric acid crystals can also be seen within tubular epithelial cells and the medullary microcirculation. Uric acid precipitates may also occur in the renal pelvis and ureters, leading to hydronephrosis and acute renal failure from extrarenal sources.

Papillary Necrosis

163. Ans. (a) Phenacetin

(Ref: Harrison 20th edition, p 2162; Harrison 19th edition, p 477t)

164. Ans. (a) Diabetes mellitus

(Ref: Harrison 20th edition, p 2162; Harrison 19th p 1861; Uroradiology 2/e, pg 471)

Important causes of papillary necrosis is listed as
1. Diabetic nephropathy
2. Sickle nephropathy
3. Analgesic nephropathy
   - Papillary necrosis may result from ischemia due to sickling of red cells in the relatively hypoxemic and hypertonic medullary vasculature and present with gross hematuria and ureteric obstruction by sloughed ischemic papillae
   - Analgesic nephropathy results from the long-term use of compound analgesic preparations containing

phenacetin, aspirin, and caffeine. The major culprit is Phenacetin which has been withdrawn since 1983. Hence nowadays this is an unlikely cause.

- In its classic form, analgesic nephropathy is characterized by renal insufficiency, papillary necrosis attributable to the presumed concentration of the drug to toxic levels in the inner medulla, and a radiographic constellation of small, scarred kidneys with papillary calcifications best appreciated by computed tomography.

165. Ans. (d) Medullary sponge kidney

(Ref: Harrison 20th edition, p 2156; Harrison 19th edition, p 1855)

Renal papillary necrosis (RPN) is characterized by coagulative necrosis of the renal medullary pyramids and papillae brought on by several associated conditions and toxins that exhibit synergism toward the development of ischemia.

A useful mnemonic device for the conditions associated with renal papillary necrosis is **POSTCARDS**, which stands for the following:

- **P**yelonephritis
- **O**bstruction of the urinary tract
- **S**ickle cell hemoglobinopathies, including sickle cell trait
- **T**uberculosis
- **C**irrhosis of the liver, chronic alcoholism
- **A**nalgesic abuse
- **R**enal transplant rejection, radiation
- **D**iabetes mellitus
- **S**ystemic vasculitis

Cystic Kidney Disease

166. Ans. (b) 2 cysts per kidney

(Ref: Harrison 20th edition, p 2153; Harrison 19th edition, p 1852)

Diagnostic criteria for ADPKD

15-29 years	2 renal cysts (unilateral or bilateral)
30-59 years	2 cysts per kidney
>60 years	4 cysts per kidney

167. Ans. (c) Polycystic kidney

(Ref: Harrison 20th edition, p 2150-2154; Harrison 19th edition, p 1852-53)

The specimen shows an enlarged kidney with cysts of varying sizes in both cortex and medulla. Minimal normal kidney tissue is present.

	ADPKD	MSK
Pathology	AD 16p13 (PKD1) 4p21 (PKD2) Cortical and medullary cysts both are seen	AD 1q21 MKCD1 Ectasia of the papillary collecting ducts of one or both kidneys.
Gross specimen differentiating features	**Very large kidneys** composed solely of a mass of cysts of *varying sizes up to 3 or 4 cm in diameter with no intervening parenchyma*. The cysts are filled with fluid, which may be clear, turbid, or hemorrhagic	Pathologic features of medullary cystic disease include **small contracted kidneys**. Numerous small cysts lined by flattened or cuboidal epithelium are present, *typically at the cortico-medullary junction*
Clinical features	Abdominal discomfort Hematuria UTI Hypertension Abdominal mass S. Creatinine elevated	It is diagnosed incidentally during investigation of hematuria. Renal colic Nephrolithiasis Recurrent UTI
Significant IVP findings	Spider leg appearance	Paint brush appearance Bouquet of flowers
Complications	Cyst rupture or hemorrhage into a cyst Gross hematuria Nephrolithiasis occurs in about 20% of patients. Urinary tract infection, including acute pyelonephritis, occurs with increased frequency in ADPKD. Infection in a kidney cyst is a particularly serious complication. It is most often due to Gram-negative bacteria and presents with flank pain, fever, and chills.	Urinarystasis hypocitraturia Distal Renal Tubular acidosis leading to the formation of small calcium-containing calculi.
Extra renal manifestation	Hepatic, splenic and pancreatic cysts Mitral valve prolapse Colonic diverticulosis Saccular (berry aneurysm)	Congenital anomalies of the urinary tract Congenital hepatic ductal ectasia (Caroli's disease). Hemihypertrophy

Contd...

168. Ans. (a) Urine retention

(Ref: Harrison 20th edition, p 2152; Harrison 19th edition, p 477t)

Clinical features of ADPKD

1. Hypertension is common and often precedes renal dysfunction, perhaps mediated by increased activity of the renin-angiotensin system. There is only mild proteinuria, and impaired urinary concentrating ability manifests early as polyuria and nocturia.
2. Dull, persistent flank and abdominal pain and early satiety are common due to the mass effect of the enlarged kidneys or liver.
3. Cyst rupture or hemorrhage into a cyst may produce acute flank pain or symptoms and signs of localized peritonitis.
4. Gross hematuria may result from cyst rupture into the collecting system or from uric acid or calcium oxalate kidney stones.

5. Nephrolithiasis occurs in about 20% of patients. Urinary tract infection, including acute pyelonephritis, occurs with increased frequency in ADPKD

169. Ans. (c) Brain

(Ref: Harrison 20th edition, p 2152; Harrison 19th p 477t)

Extra- renal manifestations of ADPKD
1. Patients with ADPKD have a twofold to fourfold increased risk of subarachnoid or cerebral hemorrhage from a ruptured intracranial aneurysm compared with the general population. However brain cysts are not mentioned in any standard reference books.
2. Other vascular abnormalities include aortic root and annulus dilation. Cardiac valvular abnormalities occur in 25% of patients, most commonly mitral valve prolapse and aortic regurgitation.
3. In 83% of patients aged 15–46 years, the MRI shows an incidence of hepatic cysts. Most patients are asymptomatic with normal liver function tests. Cysts may also be seen in pancreas and spleen.
4. Colonic diverticulae are common, with a higher incidence of perforation in patients with ADPKD.
5. Abdominal wall and inguinal hernias also occur with a higher frequency than in the general population.

170. Ans. (d) UTI

(Ref: Harrison 20th edition, p 2156; Nelson 18th ed., ch. 529, Harrison 19th edition, p 1855)

Patients with this condition typically maintain normal renal function through adulthood, complications include nephrolithiasis, pyelonephritis, hyposthenuria (inability to concentrate urine), and distal RTA.

171. Ans. (b) Chromosome 16 and 4

(Ref: Harrison 20th edition, p 2151; Harrison 19th edition, p 1851)

In ADPKD, mutations in the PKD-1 gene on chromosome 16 (ADPKD-1) account for 85% of cases, and mutations in the PKD-2 gene on chromosome 4 (ADPKD-2) account for the remainder.

172. Ans. (d) CT Scan

(Ref: Harrison 20th edition, p 2153; Harrison 19th edition, p 1854)

- MCKD should be considered in young adults with a family history suggesting dominant inheritance of kidney disease who present with progressive renal failure, bland urinalysis with little or no proteinuria, and small dense kidneys with medullary cysts on radiographic imaging.
- Contrast enhanced thin section CT scan is the modality of choice. Multiple cysts are seen in MKCD in medulla and cortico-medullary regions.

173. Ans. (b) Hypertension is rare

(Ref: Harrison 20th edition, p 2151; Harrison 19th edition, p 1851)

174. Ans. (a) Berry Aneurysm in Circle of Willis

(Ref: Harrison 20th edition, p 2151; Harrison 19th p 1851)

175. Ans. (a) Lung

(Ref: Harrison 20th edition, p 2151; Harrison 19th edition, p 1851)

176. Ans. (b) Hepatic cysts

(Ref: Harrison 20th edition, p 2151; Urology secrets 3rd/134 Clinical pedicatric urology (2002)/ 657, Harrison 19th p 1851)

Hepatic cysts are the most common extra renal manifestations of Adult polycystic kidney Disease.

177. Ans. (c) Urography

(Ref: Harrison 20th edition, p 2153; Harrison 19th p 1854)

Since in choices CT scan is not given, best answer is urography

Nephrocalcinosis (Kidney Stones)

178. Ans. (a) Present in alkaline urine

(Ref: Harrison 20th edition, p 2172; Harrison 19th edition, p1871)

- These struvite stones are also known as triple-phosphate stone.
- Two conditions must coexist for the formation of struvite calculi.
- Alkaline urine (pH>7.2)
- The presence of ammonia in the urine.

179. Ans. (a) CT scan

(Ref: Harrison 20th edition, p 2175; Bailey and love 26th edition, p 1293) Harrison 19th edition, Ch 342, p 1866)

All of routine methods have become less useful with the advent of more sensitive and specific nonenhanced computed tomography (CT) scanning. When CT is available, it is now considered the examination of choice for the detection and localization of urinary stones.

180. Ans. (a) Cysteamine

(Ref: Harrison 20th edition, p 3022-3023; Harrison 19th p 1866)

The clinical diagnosis of profile given in question is CYSTINURIA. T*he clinical profile should not be confused with Cystinosis which is treated with cysteamine. A typical cystinotic patient is mostly a child and has pale blond hair and blue eyes, although the disease also occurs among dark-haired individuals with brown eyes*

- **Cystinuria** is an autosomal-recessive defect in re-absorptive transport of cystine and the dibasic amino acids ornithine, arginine, and lysine from the luminal fluid of the renal proximal tubule and small intestine. The only phenotypic manifestation of cystinuria is cystine urolithiasis, which often recurs throughout an affected individual's lifetime. Surgical intervention is necessary, but the cornerstones of treatment are dietary and medical prevention of recurrent stone formation.
- Homozygous cystinuria is characterized by lifelong, recurrent urolithiasis that is difficult to manage, either surgically or medically. Cystine is one of the sulfur-containing amino acids; therefore, the urine may have the characteristic odor of rotten eggs.

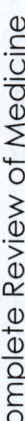

- Urinalysis may show typical hexagonal or benzene crystals, which are essentially pathognomonic of cystinuria. Microscopic crystalluria is present in 26%-83% of patients.
- The foundation of cystine stone prevention is adequate hydration and urinary alkalinization. When this conservative therapy fails, the addition of thiol drugs, such as D-penicillamine and captopril.
- Penicillamine combines chemically with cystine (cysteine disulfide) to form penicillamine–cysteine disulfide, which is more soluble than cystine and is readily excreted. As a result, urinary cystine concentrations are lowered and the formation of cystine calculi is prevented. With prolonged treatment, existing cystine calculi may be gradually dissolved.

Cystinosis

- Nephropathic cystinosis is an inherited (autosomal recessive) lysosomal storage disorder caused by defective transport of the amino acid cystine out of lysosomes. The stored cystine is poorly soluble and crystallizes within the lysosomes of many cell types, leading to widespread tissue and organ damage.
- Cystinosis is caused by mutations in the gene that encodes cystinosin, the cystine-lysomal exporter. Because of the defect in cystinosin, cystine cannot leave the lysosomes and is accumulated there as birefringent, hexagonal, or rectangular crystals within cells of various organ systems.
- A typical cystinotic patient has pale blond hair and blue eyes, although the disease also occurs among dark-haired individuals with brown eyes.
- Treatment: Cysteamine, blunts the decline in renal function and improves the linear growth of these children, despite the fact that it does not ameliorate the defect in renal tubule transport. Oral cysteamine therapy should be initiated as soon as the diagnosis is made. Cysteamine has to be administered orally every 6 hours, including the night, to prevent nocturnal accumulation of cystine.

181. Ans. (d) Restrict calcium

(Ref: Harrison 20th edition, p 2171-2172; Harrison 19th p 1866)

- Recent studies have shown that low-calcium diets *increase* the risk of incident stone formation. Low-calcium diets may lead to stone formation by reducing the amount of calcium to bind oxalate in the intestine, thereby increasing urine oxalate levels.
- If diet therapy is not sufficient to prevent stones, then thiazide diuretics may be used. Thiazide diuretics lower urine calcium and are effective in preventing the formation of stones

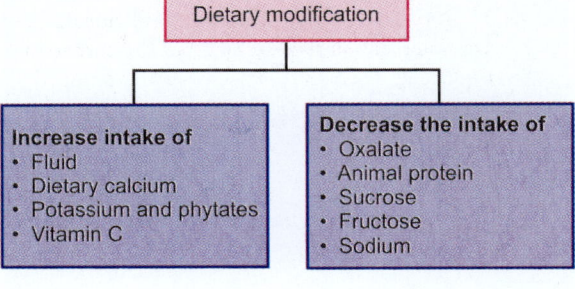

182. Ans. (a) Polycystic kidney

(Ref: Harrison 19th p 477t)

Causes of Nephrocalcinosis

1. Medullary sponge kidney
2. Hyperparathyroidism
3. Hypoparathyroidism
4. Renal tubular acidosis
5. Renal tuberculosis
6. Renal papillary necrosis
7. Hyperoxaluria
8. Immobilization
9. Milk-alkali syndrome
10. Hypervitaminosis D
11. Sarcoidosis

183. Ans. (b) Idiopathic hypercalciuria

(Ref: Harrison 20th edition, p 2171-2172; Harrison's table 281-7 Harrison 19th edition, p 2237)

Stone Type and Causes	Percent of all Stones	Percent Occurrence of Specific Causes
Calcium stones	75-85	
Idiopathic hypercalciuria		50-55
Hyperuricosuria		20
Primary hyperparathyroidism		3-5
Distal renal tubular acidosis		Rare
Dietary hyperoxaluria		10-30

184. Ans. (a) Type I

(Ref: Harrison 20th edition, p 320; Harrison 19th p 332e-7t)

- Distal RTA is characterized by a failure of acid secretion by the alpha intercalated cells of the cortical collecting duct of the distal nephron. This failure of acid secretion may be due to a number of causes, and it leads to an inability to acidify the urine to a pH of less than 5.3.
- Because renal excretion is the primary means of eliminating acid from the body, there is consequently a tendency towards acidemia. There is an inability to excrete protons while potassium cannot be reabsorbed, leading to acidemia and hypokalemia.
- In other words, the intercalated cells' apical H^+/K^+ antiporter is non-functional, resulting in potassium-wasting and proton retention. Since calcium stones demonstrate a proclivity for deposition at higher pHs, the substance of the kidney develops stones bilaterally; this does not occur in the other RTA types.
- Normal anion gap metabolic acidosis/acidemia
- Hypokalemia, hypocalcemia, hyperchloremia
- Urinary stone formation (related to alkaline urine, hypercalciuria, and low urinary citrate).
- Nephrocalcinosis (deposition of calcium in the substance of the kidney).
- Bone demineralisation (causing rickets in children and osteomalacia in adults)

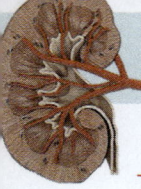

185. Ans. (d) **Uric acid stones are resistant to ESWL**

(Ref: Schwartz 8th/1547; Bailey 24th/1319)

186. Ans. (c) **Cystine stones**

(Ref: Schwartz 8th/1547; Bailey & Love 24th/131)

187. Ans. (a) **Calcium Oxalate Monohydrate**

(Ref: Smith's textbook of Endourology 1st (2007)/143, Harrison 19th edition, p 143)

188. Ans. (b) **Uric Acid**

(Ref: Bailey and Love 24th/1317; Smith's Urology 16th/262)

189. Ans. (b) **Triple phosphate**

(Ref: Bailey 24th/1316. 1319; Smith's Urology 16th/262; Schwartz 8th/1547)

190. Ans. (b) **Increased peristalsis of the ureter to overcome obstruction**

(Ref: Smiths Urology 17th /31)

191. Ans. (a) **At pelvic brim**

(Ref: S. Das 4th/408; Bailey & Love, 24th/1317; Smith's Urology 17th/31, Harrison 19th edition, p 2187)

192. Ans. (d) **Genitofemoral**

(Ref: Gray's Anatomy 38th/18, Bailey & Love's 25th ed p 1293)

193. Ans. (a) **Endoscopic removal**

(Ref: Bailey & Love's 25th ed p 1294)

194. Ans. (d) **Medullary cystic kidney**

(Ref: Harrison 19th p 477t)

195. Ans. (b) **Calcium Restriction**

(Ref: 'The Washington Manual Nephrology Subspecialty Consult' 2nd/245)

Renal Tubular Acidosis

196. Ans. (a) **RTA- 1**

(Ref: Harrison 20th edition, p 320; Harrison 19th ed. / 332e-7t)

- There are three forms of renal tubular acidosis (RTA). Types 1 and 2 may be acquired or primary whereas the **most common form, type 4 RTA,** is usually acquired in association with moderate renal dysfunction and is **characterized by hyperkalemia.**

TYPE-I Distal RTA (dRTA)

- In this type of RTA kidneys are unable to acidify the urine to pH <5.5 in the presence of systemic metabolic acidosis or after acid loading as a result of impaired hydrogen ion secretion or bicarbonate reabsorption in the distal nephron.
- Other features are: HYPOKALEMIA, hypocitraturia, hypercalciuria, nephrocalcinosis, and/or nephrolithiasis. Chronic untreated acidosis may cause rickets or osteomalacia.

TYPE-II Proximal RTA (pRTA)

- It is the result of impaired bicarbonate reabsorption in the proximal tubular where the bulk of filtered bicarbonate is recovered. It is most often secondary to various autoimmune, drug-induced, infiltrative, or other tubulopathies or a result of tubular injury from inherited diseases.
- Clinical features are: hyperphosphaturia, hyperuricosuria, hypercalciuria, nonselective amino aciduria and glycosuria.

197. Ans. (a) **Impaired acid production**

(Ref: Harrison 20th edition, p 320)

- Renal tubular acidosis type 2 is characterized by PCT damage and inability to reabsorb bicarbonate resulting in bicarbonaturia.
- The damage to DCT in RTA 1 leads to inability to acidify urine due to damage to $H^+ K^+$ antiporter. The concomitant calcium loss in urine leads to nephrolithiasis and rickets.

198. Ans. (d) **Vitamin D deficiency**

(Ref: Harrison 20th edition, p 320; Harrison's ch. 284, Harrison 19th edition, p 332e-7t)

- RTA is characterized by damage to tubules ranging from PCT to DCT. In case of PCT damage Bicarbonaturia is seen. In DCT damage inability to acidify urine is seen leading to urine pH always <5.5.
- RTA causes normal anion gap acidosis. Vitamin D deficiency is seen with Chronic Renal failure.

RTA 1 has calcium loss in urine leading to renal rickets but not nutritional deficiency of vitamin D_3

199. Ans. (d) **Type IV**

(Ref: Harrison 20th edition, p 320; Harrison 19th edition, p 332e-7t)

	RTA1	RTA2	RTA4
Site of lesion	DCT (damage to H+- K+ antiporter)	PCT	DCT (aldosterone resistance)
Causes	Genetic Inability to excrete H+ and resultant Hypokalemia due to potassium loss.	Wilson, expired tetracycline Bicarbonaturia Aminoaciduria and glucosuria	CRF Hyperkalemia and inability to excrete hydrogen.
Salient features MCQ based important point	Nephrocalcinosis Inability to acidify the urine to pH <5.5 in the presence of systemic metabolic acidosis	Fanconi syndrome	1. Administration of certain drugs, such as amiloride 2. Structural defects that inhibit active sodium reabsorption, such as sickle cell nephropathy 3. Severe limitation of sodium reabsorption in the distal tubule because of proximal sodium avidity, secondary to diseases such as cirrhosis 4. Increased epithelial permeability to chloride, causing increased reabsorption and preventing the formation of negative voltage linked to sodium reabsorption.
Treatment	Alkali replacement at doses equivalent to 1–3 mmol/kg per day of bicarbonate in divided doses will usually correct the, hypokalemia, and hypocitraturia, maintaining growth and preventing bone disease in early-onset dRTA.	Treatment of proximal RTA requires 5–15 mmol/kg per day of bicarbonate together with supplemental potassium.	Treat the cause

200. Ans. (c) Chronic glomerulonephritis/CKD

(Ref: Harrison 20th edition, p 2114)

- RTA 1 is associated with hypercalciuria and nephrolithiasis. In cushing syndrome increased cortisol increases bone turn over and increased urinary calcium is seen.
- In Paget's disease of bone, urinary calcium is normal or increased
- However in chronic glomerulonephritis, ESRD will ensue and the resultant decrease in vitamin D_3 will ensure hypocalcemia and low urinary calcium.
- *Causes of Hypocalciuria:*

  1. Drugs can decrease urine calcium, including thiazide diuretics.
  2. Hypo-parathyroidism, Pseudohypopara-thyroidism (a lack of response to PTH rather than decreased secretion of PTH)
  3. Rickets
  4. Hypothyroidism
  5. Steatorrhea
  6. Nephrosis/chronic kidney disease
  7. Familial hypocalciuric hypercalcemia (FHH), also known as familial benign hyper-calcemia.

201. Ans. (a) Increased urinary anion gap

(Ref: Harrison 20th edition, p 320; Harrison 19th p 332e-7t)

Causes of normal anion gap are:
- Loss of bicarbonate (i.e., diarrhea)
- Recovery from diabetic ketoacidosis
- Ileostomy fluid loss
- Carbonic anhydrase inhibitors (acetazolamide, dorzolamide, topiramate)
- Renal tubular acidosis
- Arginine and lysine in parenteral nutrition
- Normal variant

202. Ans. (c) Decreased Urinary citrate

(Ref: Harrison 20th edition, p 320; Harrison 19th p 332e-7t)

203. Ans. (d) Fanconi syndrome

(Ref: Harrison 20th edition, p 320; Harrison 19th p 332e-7t)

Renovascular Hypertension and Renal Vein Thrombosis

204. Ans. (c) Isotope Renogram

(Ref: Harrison 19th edition, p 1628)

Choice A, IVP is not done now days due to risk of anaphylaxis with the dye.
Choice B, Retrograde Pyelograph is used for vesicovaginal reflux.
Choice D, MR angiography is problematic in patient with C.K.D, due to risk of contrast nephropathy and nephrogenic systemic fibrosis.
- The most useful initial imaging study is a renal ultrasound
- A discrepancy >1 cm in kidney length suggests either a unilateral development abnormality or disease process or reno-vascular disease with arterial insufficiency affecting one kidney more than the other.

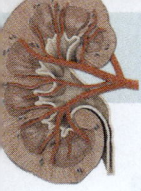

- The diagnosis of renovascular disease can be undertaken with Doppler sonography > isotope
- Renogram > MRI studies.

205. Ans. (a) Fibromuscular Dysplasia

(Ref: Harrison 20th edition, p 3085-3086; Harrison 19th edition, p 1617, 27)

206. Ans. (a) Selective renal angiography

(Ref: Harrison 20th edition, p 1906-1907; Harrison 19th p 1627)

- Gadolinium-contrast magnetic resonance angiography offers clear images of the proximal renal artery but may miss distal lesions.
- Potential risks include nephrotoxicity, particularly in patients with diabetes mellitus or pre-existing renal insufficiency.
- Some degree of renal artery obstruction may be observed in almost 50% of patients with atherosclerotic disease.
- Functionally significant lesions generally occlude more than 70% of the lumen of the affected renal artery. On angiography, the presence of collateral vessels to the ischemic kidney suggests a functionally significant lesion.
- *Contrast Arteriography is gold standard for comparing Doppler, isotope renal scan diagnostic accuracy.*

207. Ans. (a) High renin hypertension

(Ref: Harrison 20th edition, p 1906-1907; Harrison 19th p 1627)
Renal artery stenosis is associated with high renin hypertension.

208. Ans. (b) Fibrinoid necrosis

(Ref: Harrison 20th edition, p 1908-1909; Harrison 19th p 1615)
Fibrinoid necrosis is a form of necrosis, or tissue death, in which there is accumulation of amorphous, basic, proteinaceous material in the tissue matrix with a staining pattern reminiscent of fibrin. It is associated with conditions such as immune vasculitis (e.g. Henoch-Schönlein purpura), malignant hypertension, preeclampsia, or hyperacute transplant rejection.

209. Ans. (d) Nonspecific aortoarteritis

(Ref: http://www.indianpediatrics.net/jan2005/jan-47-54.htm Harrison 19th edition, p 1627)

- The commonest cause for renovascular hypertension in children reported in western literature is fibro-muscular dysplasia (FMD).
- However, in India Takayasu disease (idiopathic aortoarteritis) is the most important cause accounting for up to 87% of children with renovascular hypertension.
- Renal artery stenosis may also occur in association with neurofibromatosis, Williams syndrome, Marfan syndrome, rubella syndrome, Klippel Trenaunay Weber syndrome, linear sebaceous nevus syndrome, Kawasaki disease and Crohn disease.
- Bilateral renal artery disease is more common than unilateral, with or without intra-renal arterial involvement.

210. Ans. (b) Nonspecific aortoarteritis

(Ref: Harrison 20th edition, p 1906-1907; Disease of kidney and urinary tract 8th/1279, Harrison 19th edition, p 1618)

211. Ans. (d) Polyarteritis nodosa

(Ref: Harrison 20th edition, p 1906-1907; API 8th 541, Harrison 19th edition, p 1618)

- PAN will lead to aneurysm formation due to necrotising vasculitis, and not stenosis.

212. Ans. (d) Renal vein thrombosis

(Ref: Harrison 20th edition, p 2167; Harrison 19th edtion, p 1866)
Child has developed kidney enlargement in short duration within days after episode of diarrhea. The dehydration and sluggish circulation can lead to Renal vein Thrombosis.
Choice A is ruled out due to chronic nature and development of small kidneys
Choice B will lead to bleeding.
Choice C will have normal size kidney, and is ruled out.

Miscellaneous

213. (a) Renal cell carcinoma

(Ref: Fitzpatrick dermatology in general medicine, 8th edition, p 1356)

- Birt-Hogg-Dube syndrome is an autosomal dominant geno-dermatosis. The clinical features are-

> - Hair follicle hamartomas
> - Kidney tumors
> - Spontaneous pneumothorax

214. Ans. (c) Increased frequency of calcium phosphate stones

(Ref: Harrison 20th edition, p 2166; Harrison 19th edition, p 1855)

- Karyomegalic interstitial nephritis is an autosomal recessive condition due to FAN1 gene that shows karyomegaly with interstitial fibrosis and tubular atrophy.
- *Karyomegaly means enlargement of nucleus of cells.*
- It is seen in renal tubular cells after exposure with nephrotoxin.

215. Ans. (b) Acetohydroxamic acid

(Ref: Harrison 20th edition, p 2172-2173; Harrison: 19th edition, p 1871)

- Struvite stones are called triple phosphate stones and occur due to infection of upper urinary tract with urease producing bacteria like Proteus mirabilis, Klebsiella pneumoniae and Providencia species
- These organisms hydrolyse urea and elevate urine pH to >8.0. This causes precipitation of triple phosphate and the stone quickly fills the renal pelvis.
- Triple phosphate stones need complete extraction.
- In patients with surgically altered urinary drainage or spinal cord injury, urease inhibitor acetohydroxamic acid can be used.

- Choice C and D, tiopronin and penicillamine are used in medical management of cystine stones.

216. Ans. (a) Low sodium diet

(Ref: Harrison 20th edition, p 2171-2172; Harrison 19th edition, p 1870-71)

- Because calcium and sodium compete for reabsorption in the renal tubules, excess sodium intake and consequent excretion result in loss of calcium in the urine. High-sodium diets are associated with greater calcium excretion in the urine.
- Calcium intake in patients with kidney stones should be normal with adequate water intake.

217. Ans. (d) Rhabdomyolysis

(Ref: Harrison 20th edition, p 2106; Harrison 19th edition, ed. / 1804-05)

In haematuria, supernatant is clear and sediment is red.
In myoglobinuria, supernatant is red and sediment is clear.

- A urine dipstick test for blood that has positive findings in the absence of red blood cells (RBCs) suggests myoglobinuria. Myoglobin being a high molecular protein can block kidney tubules leading to acute tubular necrosis.
- In porphyria, gross examination of the urine can provide a valuable clue, since urine of porphyria cutanea tarda patients is red to brown in natural light and pink to red in fluorescent light. However since all types of porphyria do not have red color urine, hence it has been kept as second differential diagnosis in this question.
- In hemolysis state like paroxysmal nocturnal hemoglobinuria the color of urine is brown to black on account of presence of hemoglobinuria.

218. Ans. (b) Acute Glomerulonephritis

(Ref: Harrison 20th edition, p 2137)

Acute nephritic syndrome	Hematuria, RBC casts Azotemia, oliguria Edema, hypertension
Chronic renal failure	• Azotemia for >3 months • Prolonged symptoms or signs of uremia • Symptoms or signs of renal osteodystrophy • Kidneys reduce in size bilaterally • Broad casts in urinary sediment
Nephrotic syndrome	• Proteinuria > 3.5 g per 1.73 m² per 24 h • Hypoalbuminemia • Edema • Hyperlipidemia

219. Ans. (b) Vim Silverman Needle

The image shows a Vim Silver man needle. It is not a disposable needle and has been replaced by automatic biopsy needles but historically speaking revolutionised the kidney biopsy procedure. The prongs which are introduced into the trocar will collect the biopsy sample.

220. Ans. (b) Neurogenic Bladder

The image shows a conical urinary bladder with small diverticula on the surface and is called a Christmas tree bladder. This is seen in Neurogenic Bladder.

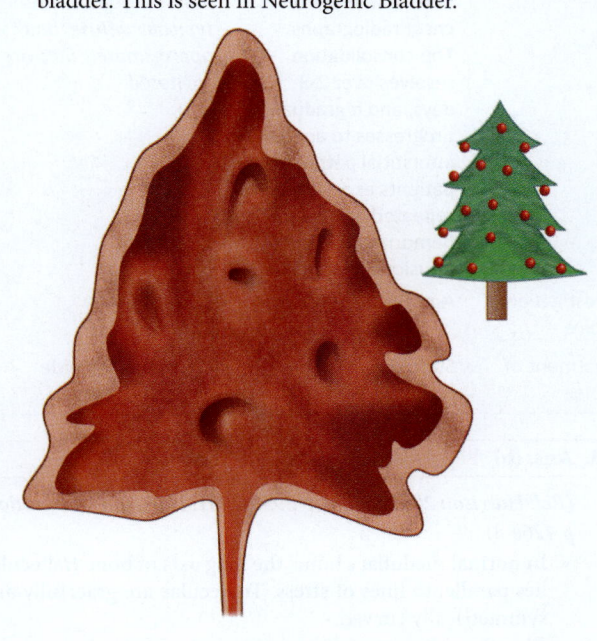

221. Ans. (d) Chronic renal failure

(Ref: Harrison 20th edition, p 2117; Harrison 19th edition, p 393)

The type of anemia in CRF is Normocytic Normo-chromic anemia

222. Ans. (d) Wegener's granulomatosis

(Ref: Harrison 20th edition, p 2578-2579; Harrison 19th p 2185)

	Goodpasture disease/Anti-GBM disease	Wegeners Granulomatosis (granulomatosis with angitis)
Pathology	Type 2 hypersensitivity	C-ANCA associated vasculitis
Clinical features	Hemoptysis plus hematuria	• Fever with constitutional symptoms seen with connective tissue disorder. • Epistaxis plus hemoptysis • Hematuria • Arthralgia • Mono-neuritis multiplex • Palpable purpura • Coronary arteritis.

Contd...

CXR findings	Patchy parenchymal consolidations, which are usually bilateral, symmetric perihilar, and bibasilar. The apices and costophrenic angles are usually spared. 18% of patients may have normal findings on chest radiographs. The consolidation resolves over 2-3 days, and it gradually progresses to an interstitial pattern as patients experience repeated episodes of hemorrhage. Pleural effusions are unusual.	Findings on chest radiography are abnormal in two thirds of adults with GPA. The most common radiologic findings are single or multiple nodules and masses. Nodules are typically diffuse, and approximately 50% are cavitated
Investigation of choice	Anti GBM antibody titer	C-ANCA
Treatment of choice	Steroids	Cyclophosphamide

223. Ans. (b) Paget's disease of bone

(Ref: Harrison 20th edition, p 2959-2961; Harrison 19th edition, p 426e-3)

- In normal medullary bone, the long axis of bone trabeculae lies parallel to lines of stress. Trabeculae are gracefully and symmetrically curved.
- *Blue-staining cement lines (representing successive waves of orderly accretion of new bone) are disposed concentrically with each other and with the surface of the trabeculae.*
- *In contrast, Paget's disease of bone shows trabeculae that are markedly and irregularly thickened; the cement lines are randomly arranged (the mosaic pattern).*
- Despite the increased quantity of bone, the incongruent arrangement of the collagen fibers (outlined by the cement lines) results in diminished tensile strength and increased susceptibility to fracture.

224. Ans. (b) Nail-Patella syndrome

(Ref: Harrison 20th edition, p 2147-2148; Harrison 19th p 1847)
Nail patella syndrome is an autosomal dominant defect on chromosome 9 leading to hypoplastic nails with hypoplastic patella and right iliac crest which shows a bony exostosis or posterior iliac horn.

Bony changes seen are:
1. Patellar involvement is present in approximately 90% of patients; however, patellar aplasia occurs in only 20%.
2. In instances in which the patellae are smaller or luxated, the knees may be unstable.
3. The elbows may have limited motion (e.g., limited pronation, supination, extension).
4. Subluxation of the radial head may occur.
5. Arthrodysplasia of the elbows is reported in approximately 90% of patients.
6. General hyperextension of the joints can be present.
7. Exostoses arising from the posterior aspect of the iliac bones ("iliac horns") are present in as many as 80% of patients; this finding is considered pathognomonic for the syndrome.
8. Other reported bone changes include scoliosis, scapular hypoplasia, and the presence of cervical ribs.
9. Kidney issues may arise such as proteinuria and nephritis. Proteinuria is usually the first sign of renal involvement and either rapidly or years after suffering from asymptomatic proteinuria, renal failure occurs in around 5% of NPS patients

225. Ans. (b) Alport syndrome

(Ref: Harrison 20th edition, p 2977; Harrison 19th edition, p 2513)

Diagnosis
1. The diagnosis of classic alport syndrome is based on X-linked inheritance of hematuria, sensorineural deafness, and lenticonus.
2. The lenticonus together with hematuria is pathognomonic of classic AS. The sensorineural deafness is primarily in the high-tone range. It can frequently be detected only by an audiogram and is usually not progressive.
3. Because of the X-linked transmission, women are generally underdiagnosed and are usually less severely affected than men.
4. The hematuria usually progresses to nephritis and may cause renal failure in late adolescence in affected males and at older ages in some women. Renal transplantation is usually successful.

Molecular Defects
Most patients have mutations in four of the six genes for the chains of type IV collagen (COL4A3, COL4A4, COL4A5, and COL4A6).

226. Ans. (d) Defect in limb of Loop of Henle

(Ref: Harrison 20th edition, p 2914)

- Dent disease, an *X-linked recessive disorder of proximal renal tubular dysfunction, is characterized by low molecular weight proteinuria, hypercalciuria, nephrocalcinosis, nephrolithiasis, and chronic kidney disease.*
- Males younger than age ten years may manifest only low molecular weight (LMW) proteinuria and/or hypercalciuria, which are usually asymptomatic. Thirty to 80% of affected males develop end-stage renal disease (ESRD) between ages 30 and 50 years.
- Rickets or osteomalacia are occasionally observed, and mild short stature, although underappreciated, may be a common occurrence. Disease severity can vary within the same family. Males with Dent disease 2 (caused by mutations in OCRL) are at increased risk for intellectual disability. Due to random X-chromosome inactivation, some female carriers may manifest hypercalciuria and, rarely, renal calculi.
- Diagnosis/testing. The diagnosis is based on renal findings and/or a family history consistent with X-linked inheritance. *A mutation in CLCN5 accounts for approximately 60% of those with Dent disease.*
- **Management. Treatment of manifestations:** Although thiazide diuretics can decrease urinary calcium excretion in boys with Dent disease, side effects limit their use. The

effectiveness of angiotensin-converting enzyme (ACE) inhibitors and angiotensin receptor blockers (ARB) in children with proteinuria to prevent or delay further loss of kidney function is unclear.

227. Ans. (a) 0.5 mEq/hr

(Ref: Harrison 20th edition, p 300; Harrison 19th edition, p 300)

- Harrison mention correction for hyponatremia in first 24 hours = 10 mM/24 hours
- Hence mathematically the closest Ans: 0.5 mEq/hour
- CMDT 2015 mentions correction rate of ≤ 0.5mEq/hour

228. Ans. (d) Wilms' tumor

(Ref: Nelson Textbook, 18th ed., ch. 492, Harrison 19th p 101e-6t)

Several syndromes and congenital abnormalities commonly are reported in patients with Wilms tumor.

1. **WAGR** syndrome is a contiguous gene deletion syndrome that consists of Wilms tumor, aniridia, genitourinary abnormalities (cryptorchidism, streak ovaries, bicornate uterus, ambiguous genitalia), and mental retardation. Patients with this syndrome have a constitutional deletion of chromosome 11p13 where the Wilms tumor gene, WT1, and the aniridia gene, PAX6, are located.
2. **Denys-Drash** syndrome is characterized by male pseudohermaphrodism, early-onset renal failure characterized by mesangial sclerosis, and an increased risk of Wilms tumor. Patients with this syndrome typically carry a missense mutation in the WT1 gene.
3. **Beckwith-Wiedemann syndrome** *is characterized by hemihypertrophy, macroglossia, and visceromegaly, with a 3–5% risk of developing Wilms tumor.* A variety of 11p15.5 abnormalities have been reported in patients with this syndrome, and it is postulated that a second Wilms tumor gene, WT2, is located in this region. Loss of imprinting of the insulin-like growth factor 2 gene, an epigenetic process, also is associated with Wilms tumor. The genitourinary anomalies most commonly associated with Wilms tumor are hypoplasia, fusion and ectopia of the kidney, duplications of the collecting systems, hypospadias, and cryptorchidism.

229. Ans. (b) Ureterocele

(Ref: Nelson ch. 540, Harrison 19th edition.)

- A ureterocele is a cystic dilatation of the terminal ureter and is obstructive because of a pinpoint ureteral orifice. Ureteroceles are much more common in girls than in boys.
- In girls, ureteroceles nearly always are associated with ureteral duplication, whereas in 50% of affected boys there is only one ureter.
- Ultrasonography is effective in demonstrating the ureterocele and whether the associated obstructed system is duplicated or single.
- VCUG usually shows a filling defect in the bladder, sometimes large, corresponding to the ureterocele, and often shows reflux into the adjacent lower pole collecting system with typical findings of a "drooping lily" appearance to the kidney. Nuclear renal scintigraphy is most accurate in demonstrating whether the affected renal moiety has significant function.

230. Ans. (c) Goodpasture's syndrome

(Ref: Harrison 20th edition, p 2139; Harrison 19th edition, p 1839)

Disorders for which apheresis is accepted as first-line therapy, either as a primary standalone treatment or in conjunction with other modes of treatment are as follows:
1. Guillain-Barre syndrome
2. Myasthenia gravis
3. Chronic inflammatory demyelinating polyneuro-pathy
4. Hyperviscosity in monoclonal gammopathies
5. Thrombotic thrombocytopenic purpura
6. Goodpasture syndrome
7. Hemolytic uremic syndrome (atypical, due to autoantibody to factor H)
8. Wilson disease, fulminant

231. Ans. (b) Inability to concentrate urine

(Ref: Harrison 20th edition, p 693; Harrison 19th edition, p 636)

- Depending on the predominant site of tubule involvement, clinical manifestations vary. Proximal tubule dysfunction generally impairs urinary concentration, while more distal tubule dysfunction may impair potassium excretion, leading to hyperkalemia
- The inner medulla's relatively hypoxic, hyper-tonic, and acidic environment is known to predispose to sickling of red blood cells, which significantly decreases renal medullary blood flow through vaso-occlusion.
- At the same time, hematuria, which is commonly seen in patients with sickle cell nephropathy, increases venous pressure, which further worsens ischemia of the renal medulla and predisposes the patient to further RBC sickling.

232. Ans. (a) Di George syndrome

(Ref: Harrison 20th edition, p 2937; Nelson 18th ed. ch. 430, Harrison 19th edition, p 2113)

- **Mnemonic: CATCH-22** is used to describe DiGeorge syndrome, with the 22 to remind one the chromosomal abnormality is found on the 22 chromosome:
- Cardiac Abnormality (especially tetralogy of Fallot) Abnormal facies
- Thymic aplasia = explains the recurrent infections
- Cleft palate
- Hypocalcemia/Hypoparathyroidism = explains recurrent seizures and tetany.

233. Ans. (a) ADH receptors are not sensitive

(Ref: Harrison 20th edition, p 303; Nelson 18th edition ch. 559, Harrison 19th edition, p 304)

- Vasopressin exerts its principal effect on the kidney via V2 receptors located primarily in the collecting tubule, the thick ascending limb of the loop of Henle, and the peri-glomerular tubules.

- The human V2 receptor gene is located on the long arm of the X chromosome (Xq28) at the locus associated with congenital, X-linked, vasopressin-resistant diabetes insipidus.
- Activation of the V2 receptor results in increases in intracellular cyclic adenosine mono-phosphate, which leads to the insertion of the aquaporin-2 water channel into the apical (luminal) membrane. This allows water movement along its osmotic gradient into the hypertonic inner medullary interstitium from the tubule lumen and excretion of concentrated urine.

234. Ans. (d) Indapamide

(Ref: Harrison's 18th ed. Goodman and Gillman 12th ed. ch.25, 284)

Hypercalciuria, or excessive urinary calcium excretion, is the most common identifiable cause of calcium kidney stone disease. Idiopathic hyper-calciuria is diagnosed when clinical, laboratory, and radiographic investigations fail to delineate an underlying cause of the condition. Secondary hyper-calciuria occurs when a known process produces excessive urinary calcium.

Thiazides, such as trichlormethiazide or indapamide, substantially reduce urinary calcium excretion, but they do not correct the primary defect, which is increased, uncontrolled intestinal calcium absorption.

235. Ans. (b) Normal sized kidney

(Ref: Harrison 20th edition, p 805; Harrison 19th edition, p 723)

- Patients typically present with proteinuria and/or hypertension followed by progressive renal failure. Both kidneys are enlarged in amyloidosis.
- The latter may evolve extremely slowly, and patients with hereditary apolipoprotein AI and lysozyme amyloidosis may not develop end-stage renal failure for several decades. In contrast to AL amyloidosis, orthostatic hypo-tension is unusual, probably because autonomic involvement and amyloid cardiomyopathy are rare in Familial Renal Amyloidosis.

236. Ans. (d) 10,000 viable bacteria per ml in clean voided midstream urine is of significance

(Ref: Harrison 19th edition, p 867)

- Recurrence of UTI occurs because of either a relapse or a reinfection. Women who have relapsing infection have recurrent bacteriuria with the same infecting microorganism that was present before initial treatment, and urine cultures show no growth in the usual 2-week interval between the initial and successive episode. Recurrence by this mechanism usually occurs within 2 weeks of stopping antibiotic therapy for a prior episode of cystitis. Hence choice A is wrong
- Xantho-granulomatous pyelonephritis is seen with staghorn calculus. Hence choice B is wrong.
- Emphysematous pyelonephritis is seen with diabetes mellitus. Hence choice C is wrong.
- *The 2010 Infectious Disease Society of America (IDSA) consensus limits for cystitis and pyelonephritis in women are more than 1000 colony-forming units (CFU)/mL and more than 10,000 CFU/mL, respectively, for clean-catch midstream urine specimens. Historically, the definition of UTI was based on the finding at culture of 100,000 CFU/mL of a single organism. However, this misses up to 50% of symptomatic infections, so the lower colony rate of greater than 1000 CFU/mL is now accepted.*

237. Ans. (a) 5 L

(Ref: CMDT pg. 875)

Water deficit = $\dfrac{\text{Total body water} \times (\text{current sodium} - 140)}{140}$

TBW (male) = 0.5 × weight = 35L for the patient mentioned in question

Water deficit = $\dfrac{35 \times (160 - 140)}{140}$

Water deficit = 5 liters

238. Ans. (b) 1 mEq/dl

(Ref: Harrison 20th edition, p 304; Harrison 19th edition, p 2279)

- The correction rate for hypernatremia is 1 mEq/dl
- The correction rate for hyponatremia is 0.5 mEq/dl
- For severe hypernatremia defined as >158 mEq/dl, administer free water or via NG tube if not obtunded. Else 5% dextrose in water can be given. N/2 hypotonic saline can also be given to reduce the sodium load.

239. Ans. (a) Calcium chloride

(Ref: Harrison 20th edition, p 310; Harrison 19th edition, p 312)

- *Calcium increases threshold potential, thus restoring normal gradient between threshold potential and resting membrane potential, which is elevated abnormally in hyperkalemia. One ampule of calcium chloride has approximately 3 times more calcium than calcium gluconate. Onset of action is <5 min and lasts about 30-60 min. Doses should be titrated with constant monitoring of ECG changes during administration; repeat dose if ECG changes do not normalize within 3-5 min.*
- Potassium binding resin exchanges Na^+ for K^+ and binds it in gut, primarily in large intestine, decreasing total body potassium. Onset of action after PO ranges from 2-12 h (longer when administered rectally). Lowers K^+ over 1-2 h with duration of action of 4-6 h. Potassium level drops by approximately 0.5-1 mEq/L
- Calcium hydroxide and calcium carbonate have no role in management of hyperkalemia.

240. Ans. (c) DTPA renogram

(Ref: Principles and Practice of Paediatric Nephrology by Nammalwar and Vijay Kumar/85)

241. Ans. (a) IgA levels

(Ref: Robbins 7th/990)

242. Ans. (b) Alport's syndrome

(Ref: Harrison 20th edition, p 2977; Harrison 19th edition, p 2513)

243. Ans. (c) Renal Tubular Acidosis

(Ref: Harrison 19th edition, p 332e-7t)

244. Ans. (d) Hyaline Arteriosclerosis

(Ref: Robbins 7th /1006, 1007, 1008)

245. Ans. (c) Hyaline Arteriosclerosis

(Ref: Robbins 7th / 1006, 1007, 1008)

246. Ans. (c) Vesicouretrial reflux induced pyelonephritis

(Ref: Harrison 20th edition, p 2160; Pediatr Nephrol. 1993 Aug; 7(4):361-4 The small scarred kidney in childhood; Risdon Ra.,Harrison 19th edition, p 1859)

247. Ans. (a) Clear cell type

(Ref: Harrison 20th edition, p 616; Harrison 19th edition, p 579)

248. Ans. (b) Hypertension

(Ref: Harrison 20th edition, p 616; Harrison 19th edition, p 579)

249. Ans. (c) Arthogryposis multiplex congenita

(Ref: Robbin's 7th/604, 605; Ghai 6th/574, Harrison 19th edition, p 101e-6t)

250. Ans. (c) Histology > (a) Stage of disease

(Ref: Devita 6th/2177, Harrison 19th edition, p 101e-6t)

251. Ans. (c) Hypercalcemia

(Ref: Primer on kidney disease 4th/310, 311, Harrison 19th edition, p 1810)

252. Ans. (a) Carcinoma of urinary bladder

(Ref: Bailey 23rd/1229, Harrison 19th edition, p 575)

253. Ans. (d) Urine microscopy for malignant cytology

(Ref: Bailey & Love 24th/1463, Harrison 19th edition, p 575)

254. Ans. (d) Hepatitis

(Ref: Critical care Medicine 3rd/236 Rudolph Pediatrics 21st/1711, Harrison 19th edition, p 283)

255. Ans. (c) Glomerulonephritis

(Ref: Harrison 20th edition, p 1438; KDT 5th/717, Harrison 19th edition, p 1330)

9

Hematology

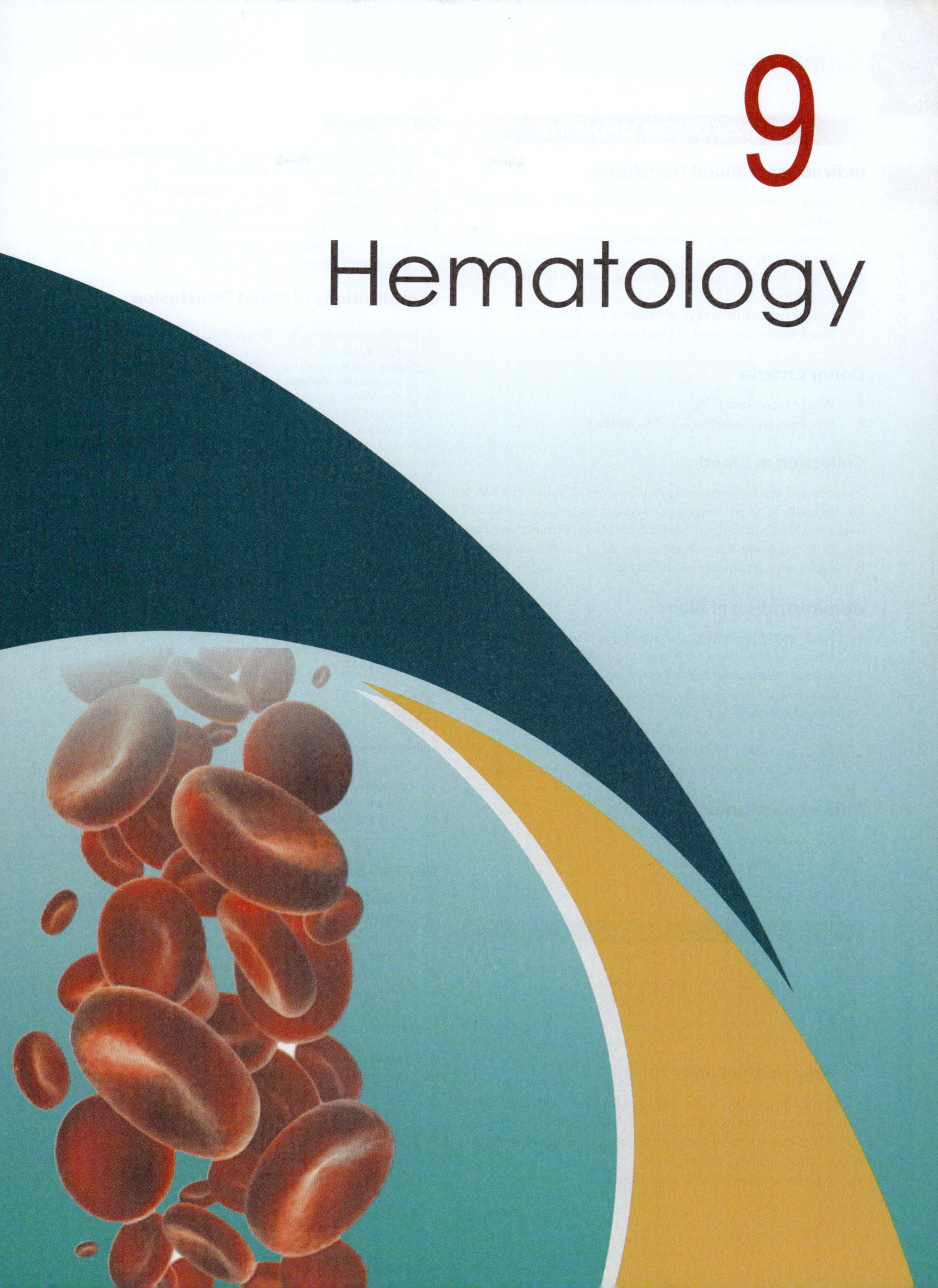

TRANSFUSION MEDICINE

Indications of Blood Transfusion

1. Acute blood loss following trauma with >15% of total body volume
2. During major surgery like abdomino-perineal surgery
3. Burns and sepsis
4. Whole blood is given to replace losses during surgery, hematemesis
5. Packed cells are used in severe anemia and thalassemia
6. Blood fractions are used in bleeding hemophiliacs

Donor Criteria

1. Weight more than 45 kg
2. Free from HIV, hepatitis B and C, Malaria

Collection of Blood

It is collected in a bag containing 75 mL of CPDA buffer. The RBC's lose the ability to release oxygen in 7 days though they survive up to 5 weeks in CPDA buffer. Hence ideally fresh blood taken within 7 days should be transfused. Platelets are destroyed in 24–48 hours. Stored blood does not contain factor 5 and factor 8

Administration of Blood

- After blood grouping and matching, *540 mL of blood is transfused at 40 drops per minute to administer the blood within 4 hours.* Since one unit of blood contains 350 mg of iron, recurrent transfusions can lead to iron overload. This can be managed with desferroxamine.
- The shelf life of blood in a blood bank is 21–42 days varying by the buffer with the CPD buffer leading to shelf life of 35 days.
- The storage temperature of blood in blood bank is 4 degrees.

Buffer Constitution

- C : Citrate
- P : Phosphate
- D : Dextrose
- A : Adenine

Buffer	Shelf life
ACD	21 days
CPD	28 days
CPDA	35 days
SAG–M	42 days

Function of the Buffer

- Citrate binds with calcium, which inhibits clot formation.
- Phosphate helps in shifting oxy-Hb dissociation curve towards right, which promotes oxygen delivery to the tissues.
- Dextrose helps in RBC nutrition.
- Adenine synthesizes ATP, extends shelf life

SAG-M Blood

- In some donations, made to blood bank, plasma is removed and a crystalloid solution of SAG-M is added.
- The main reason for this is good viability of RBC.
- The disadvantage is that it lacks any proteins.^{Q}
- Hence for each four units of SAG–M blood, one unit whole blood is required. For subsequent every 2 units of SAG–M blood, 4.5% albumin must be given.

Complications of Blood Transfusion

1. **Febrile non-hemolytic transfusion reaction**: Most common complication
2. Citrate toxicity leads to elevated bicarbonate levels in the body and **metabolic alkalosis**.
3. Citrate ion binds with ionized calcium ion resulting in decreased availability of calcium resulting in **tetany.** Death in tetany usually occurs due to laryngospasm.
4. Post-expiry date blood transfusion results in hemolysis resulting in hyperkalemia. This can trigger ventricular fibrillation.
5. Mismatched transfusion (type-II hypersensitivity reaction) can lead to development of acute tubular necrosis.
6. Infections (bacteria that can grow at 4°C: Pseudomonas, Yersinia and acinetobacter)
7. Recurrent blood transfusion results in graft versus host disease and secondary hemochromatosis.
8. Transfusion-related acute lung injury (TRALI). MC cause of death after blood transfusion.^{Q}
9. Viral infection risk^Q
   - HBV <1 in 82,000
   - HTLV <1 in 1,000,000
   - HCV <1 in 2,800,000
   - HIV <1 in 4,000,000

Management of mismatched blood transfusion
- Stop the transfusion
- IV normal saline
- IV hydrocortisone
- Anti-histaminics.

Massive Blood Transfusion

Blood transfusion of more than 5L over a period of 24 hrs is termed as massive blood transfusion. Current protocol is:

- 6 units of packed RBC
- 6 units of fresh frozen plasma
- 6 units of platelets.
- The recommended ratio of blood component is 1: 1: 1.^{Q}

Conditions Requiring Massive Blood Transfusion

- Gunshot injury with hemodynamic compromise
- Coronary artery by-pass graft surgery
- Ruptured aneurysm of abdominal aorta.

Complications of Massive Blood Transfusion

- Fast infusion of the blood (at 4°C) can cause **hypothermia** resulting in sluggish circulation.

- Citrate toxicity leading to **metabolic alkalosis**.
- **Bleeding** tendency due to dilutional hyponatremia.

BLOOD PRODUCTS

Packed Red Blood Cells

- Obtained by centrifugation of whole blood at 2000–2300 g for 15–20 minutes
- Stored at 4°C.
- Transfuse within 35 days of collection, otherwise cell lysis may result in hyperkalemia.
- Transfuse within 7 days of collection, if renal failure or hepatic failure is present to reduce solute load.
- Infuse each unit over max of 4 hours.

Indications for Packed RBC Transfusion

- Hb <7g/dL
- Maintain Hb between 70 and 100 g/L during active bleeds (7g/dL – 10g/dL)
- Consider maintaining a higher Hb for patients with:
  - CAD/unstable coronary syndromes
  - Uncontrolled, unpredictable bleeding
  - Impaired pulmonary function.

Selection of Red Cells for Transfusion

- When a need for RBC transfusion is anticipated, the following should be ordered:
  - *Group and screen*: Determines the blood group and Rh status of the recipient as well as the presence of autoantibodies vs. major/minor blood group antigens.
  - *Crossmatch*: Involves mixing the recipient's blood with potential donor blood and looking for clotting. *Takes 30-45 min.*
- When blood is required, several options are available:
  - **1st line**: Fully crossmatched blood (not always available in emergency situations)
  - **2nd line**: Donor blood of the same group and same Rh status as the recipient
  - **3rd line**: O– blood for fertile females; O+ blood for all others.

Platelet Products

Prepared by centrifugation of platelet rich plasma at 1200–1500g at 15–20 minutes. Start at 0.1 unit/kg, when platelets are less than 20,000 with evidence of bleeding.

Product	Indication
Random donor (pooled)	Thrombocytopenia with bleeding
Single donor platelets	Potential BMT recipients
HLA matched platelets	Refractory to pooled or single donor platelets

- Stored at 20–24°C (room temperature)^Q
- Random donor platelets are transfused in groups of 5 units; this should increase the platelet count by at least $15 \times 10^9/L$.
- Single donor platelets (transfused as single units) should increase the platelet count by $40–60 \times 10^9/L$.
- If an increase in the platelet count is not seen post-transfusion, alloantibodies, bleeding, sepsis or hypersplenism may be present.
- One single donor platelet is equal to 8 units of random donor plasma.^{Q}

Indications for Platelet Transfusion

Plt($\times 10^9$/L)	Indications
<10	Non-immune thrombocytopenia
<20	Procedures not associated with significant blood loss
<50	Procedures associated with blood loss or major surgery (>500 mL EBL)
<100	Pre-neurosurgery or head trauma
Any	Platelet dysfunction and marked bleeding

Plasma

- Obtained same way as packed RBCs
- The plasma is stored at minus 40 degrees.^{Q}
- It can be stored for 2 years^Q
- *1 unit of FFP can increase the clotting factors by 3%*^{Q}

Uses

1. Burns, hypoalbuminemia and severe protein loss
2. Severe liver disease with deranged PT and bleeding
3. Congenital clotting factor deficiency with bleeding
4. Deficiency following warfarin administration, DIC and MBT

Cryoprecipitate

- When FFP is allowed to *thaw* at 4 degrees, the supernatant layer develops and is called as cryoprecipitate. It is rich in factor 8, VWF but lacks factor 9.^{Q}
- It is stored at minus 40 degrees and can be kept for 2 years
- It can raise fibrinogen levels to achieve blood levels of 150 mg/dL

Prothrombin Complex Concentrates

Derived from pooled plasma and can be used in emergency reversal of warfarin therapy in uncontrolled bleeding. It contains factor II, IX and X.^{Q}

Autologous Blood Transfusion

A healthy patient with hematocrit >30% can donate blood few weeks prior to any elective surgery.

Artificial Blood

1. Perfluorocarbon is a substitute oxygen carrier with half-life of 7 days
   - High affinity to oxygen
   - Colorless and inert molecule never to be infused alone and is emulsified with albumin or lipids.
2. Stroma free hemoglobin: Biomimetic hemoglobin-based substitute

Blood Substitutes

Human albumin 4.5% is made by fractionation and heat extraction to produce albumin which is stored at 4 degrees for many months. It does not transmit hepatitis.

Transfusion Related Acute Lung Injury (TRALI)

- It occurs due to donor plasma antibody acting against leucoyte specific antigens of the recipient.
- This causes release of cytokines which damages pulmonary vasculature. This results in features of breathlessness and drop in SpO_2 values within 6 hours of transfusion
- *It is the most common cause of death after blood transfusion.*
- Estimates of the incidence of TRALI include:

  1 in 5000 units of packed RBC
  1 in 2000 plasma-containing components^Q
  1 in 400 units of whole-blood-derived platelet concentrates.

- The CXR of patient will show evidence of *non-cardiogenic pulmonary edema.*
- Clinical recovery can occur with supportive ventilator therapy over next one week. Resolution starts after 2–3 days.^{Q}
- The first event is the clinical condition of the patient, resulting in pulmonary endothelial activation and neutrophil sequestration, and the second event is the transfusion of biologically active mediators (lipids, cytokines) that activate adherent neutrophils leading to endothelial damage, capillary leak, and TRALI.
- In recent literature, *delayed TRALI syndrome occurs in up to 25% of critically ill patients receiving a blood transfusion, develops 6-72 hrs after the transfusion,* and is associated with a mortality of up to 40%. The risk of delayed TRALI increases with increasing numbers of transfused blood products. The management of both the classic and delayed TRALI syndromes is essentially supportive and includes a volume limited ventilator strategy.

Characteristics of Selected Blood Components

Component	Volume, mL	Content	Clinical response
PRBC	180–200	RBCs with variable leukocyte content and small amount of plasma	Increase hemoglobin 10g/L and hematocrit 3%
Platelets	50–70	5.5×10^{10}/RD unit	Increase platelet count 5000–10,000/µL
	200–400	$\geq 3 \times 10^{10}$/SDAP product	CCI $\geq 10 \times 10^9$/L within 1h and $\geq 7.5 \times 10^9$/L within 24h posttransfusion
FFP	200–250	Plasma proteins – coagulation factors, proteins C and S, antithrombin	Increase coagulations factors about 2%
Cryoprecipitate	10–15	Cold-insoluble plasma proteins, fibrinogen factor VII VWF	Topical fibrin glue, also 80 IU factor VIII

ANEMIAS

Anemia is present in adults if the hematocrit is < 41% (hemoglobin < 13.5 g/dL) in males or < 36% (hemoglobin < 12 g/dL) in females. The most common cause of anemia is iron deficiency in India and is due to nutritional factors.

Classification of Anemias by Mean Red Blood Cell Volume (MCV)

Microcytic	• Iron deficiency • Thalassemia • Anemia of chronic disease • Sideroblastic anemia
Macrocytic (Megaloblastic)	• Vitamin B_{12} deficiency • Folate deficiency • DNA synthesis inhibitors
Macrocytic (Nonmegaloblastic)	• Myelodysplasia • Liver disease • Reticulocytosis • Hypothyroidism • Bone marrow failure state (e.g., aplastic anemia, marrow infiltrative disorders, etc.)
Normocytic	• Kidney disease • Mild form of most acquired etiologies of anemia • Autoimmune hemolytic anemia

Iron Deficiency Anemia

- Iron deficiency is the most common cause of anemia worldwide. Apart from circulating red blood cells, the major location of iron in the body is the storage pool as ferritin or as hemosiderin in macrophages.
- About 10% of the dietary iron is absorbed in the stomach, duodenum and upper jejunum under acidic conditions. Dietary iron present as heme is efficiently absorbed (10–20%) but non-heme iron less so (1–5%), largely because of interference by phosphates, tannins, and other food constituents.
- The major iron transporter from the diet across the intestinal lumen is ferroportin, which also facilitates the transport of iron in macrophages to apotransferrin for delivery to erythroid cells prepared to synthesize hemoglobin.
- Hepcidin, produced during inflammation, negatively regulates iron transport by promoting the degradation of ferroportin.
- Small amounts of iron—approximately 1 mg/d—are normally lost through exfoliation of skin and mucosal cells.

- Serum ferritin < 12 ng/mL is seen in IDA
- Divalent metal transporter 1 (DMT1), is responsible for entry of iron into enterocytes. Ferroportin is for exit out of enterocytes to be transported with transferin.

Causes of Iron Deficiency

Dietary lack	Impaired absorption	Increased requirement	Chronic blood loss
• Infants • Children • Low socio-economic status • Elderly	• Steatorrhea • Sprue • Chronic diarrhea • Gastrectomy	• Growing infants and children • Pregnant females • Premenopausal women	• GIT (peptic ulcer, gastric cancer, hemorrhoids, hookworm disease) • Urinary tract (renal, pelvic or bladder cancers) • Genital tract (uterine cancer, menorrhagia)

Stages

It is characterized by the following stages.

Stage I or Stage of Negative Iron Balance

This is a stage characterized by decreased amount of storage iron manifesting as decreased serum ferritin concentration and reduced amount of bone marrow iron staining with Prussian blue stain. The serum iron and red cell protoporphyrin levels are absolutely normal. *Though TIBC is marginally increased, the red cell indices and morphology are normal.*

Stage II or Stage of Iron Deficient Erythropoesis

This is a stage of reduced circulating iron in addition to decrease in storage form of iron. So, this stage is characterized by deficient iron stores, reduced serum ferritin, decreased % saturation of serum transferring and increased TIBC. *The red cell morphology is normal.*

Stage III or Stage of Iron Deficiency Anemia

It is characterized by all features of stage II and in addition *abnormal morphology of the red cells*, i.e. the presence of microcytic and hypochromic cells.

Clinical Features

- Pallor and fatigue
- Subendocardial ischemia
- Palpitation
- Diaphoresis.

On Examination

- Pale appearance of conjunctiva, nail bed & palmar creases
- Pallor is best observed in palmar creases.

Investigations

1. Hb levels: < 11 gm%
2. Peripheral smear shows anisocytosis and poikilocytosis
3. **Screening test**: RCDW (red cell distribution width) & zinc protoporphyrin levels. RCDW > 14.5%
4. **Investigation of choice**: Iron studies

Serum iron	Decreased
TIBC	Increased
Ferritin	Decreased
Transferrin saturation	Decreased

*First to decrease in IDA is S. ferritin.

Treatment

- Oral iron supplementation + Vit-C
- Single administration of IV iron dextran
- Iron therapy should continue for 3–6 months after restoration of normal hematologic values to replenish iron stores.

Note: Severe IDA with CHF is treated with packed RBC.

Anemia of Chronic Disease

Etiology

1. Infection
2. Malignancy
3. Inflammatory and rheumatologic disease; chronic renal and liver disease
4. Endocrine disorders (e.g. diabetes mellitus, hypothyroidism, hypogonadism, hypopituitarism)

Pathophysiology

- An anemia of underproduction, due to impaired iron utilization.
- Trapping of iron in macrophages: Reduced plasma iron levels making iron relatively unavailable for new hemoglobin synthesis.
- Erythropoietin levels are normal or slightly elevated but the marrow is unable to respond with increase in erythropoiesis.
- A mild hemolytic component is often present.
- Red blood cell survival modestly decreased.

Investigations

1. Associated with elevation in acute phase reactants (ESR, CRP, fibrinogen)
2. "Classic" serum iron indices
   - Serum iron and TIBC low, % saturation normal
   - Serum ferritin is increased^Q
3. Peripheral blood
   - Mild: Usually normocytic and normochromic
   - Severe: May be microcytic and hypochromic
4. Absolute reticulocyte count is frequently low, reflecting overall decrease in RBC production
5. Bone marrow
   - Normal or increased iron stores in bone marrow^Q
   - Decreased or absent staining for iron in erythroid precursors.

Treatment

- Anemia resolves if underlying disease is treated.
- Only treat patients who can benefit from a higher hemoglobin level.

- Erythropoietin may normalize the hemoglobin value (the required dose of erythropoietin is higher than the dose required for patients with renal disease).

Lead Poisoning

L: Lead Lines on gingivae and epiphyses of long bones on X-ray
E: Encephalopathy and erythrocyte basophilic stippling
A: Abdominal colic and microcytic anemia (sideroblastic)
D: Drops -* Wrist and foot drop

Treatment: Dimercaprol and EDTA are first line agents.

Sideroblastic Anemia

- **Sideroblasts** are erythrocytes with Fe-containing (basophilic) granules in the cytoplasm
- **Normal**: Granules are small, randomly spread in the cytoplasm
- Found in healthy individuals
- **"Ring sideroblasts"**: Fe deposits in mitochondria, forming a ring around the nucleus

Etiology

1. Hereditary (rare)
2. X-linked, median survival 10 years
3. Idiopathic (acquired)
   - AKA refractory anemia with ringed sideroblasts: a subtype of MDS
   - May be a preleukemic phenomenon (10% transform to AML)
4. Reversible with exposure to drugs (isoniazid, chloramphenicol), alcohol, lead, copper deficiency, zinc toxicity, hypothyroidism.

Clinical Manifestations

- Standard anemia symptoms
- Hepatosplenomegaly, iron overload syndrome.

Investigations

1. Serum iron indices
2. Increased serum Fe, normal TIBC, increased ferritin, increased soluble transferring receptor (STfR)
3. Blood film/bone marrow biopsy
   - *Ringed sideroblasts (diagnostic hallmark)*
   - *RBCs are hypochromic, can be micro-, normo-, or macrocytic,*
   - *Anisocytosis, poikilocytosis, basophilic stippling.*

Treatment

Depends on etiology
- **X-linked**: High dose pyridoxine (vitamin B_6) in some cases
- **Acquired**: Epo and G-CSF
- **Reversible**: Remove precipitating cause
- Supportive transfusions for severe anemia

Must Know for Questions Pertaining to Comparison of IDA versus Sideroblastic Anemia versus Anemia of Chronic Disease

	Lab Tests				Blood Film
	Ferritin	Serum Iron	TIBC	RDW	
Iron-deficiency anemia	↓↓	↓	↑	↓(>15)	Hypochromic, microcytic
Anemia of chronic disease	N/↑	↓	↓	N	• Normocytic/microcytic • Dual population
Sideroblastic anemia	N/↑	↑	N	↑	Basophilic stippling
Thalassemia	N/↑	N/↑	N	N/↑	• Hypochromic, microcytic • Target cells • Poikilocytosis

β-Thalassemia

- This is usually caused by point mutations rather than deletions on chromosome 11. These mutations result in premature chain termination or in problems with transcription of RNA and ultimately result in reduced or absent β-globin chain synthesis.
- Defects that result in absent globin chain expression are termed β0, whereas those causing reduced but not absent synthesis are termed β+.
- The reduced β-globin chain synthesis in β-thalassemia results in a relative increase in the percentages of hemoglobins A2 and F compared to hemoglobin A on hemoglobin electrophoresis.
- In the presence of reduced β chains, the excess α chains are unstable and precipitate, leading to damage of red blood cell membranes. This leads to both intramedullary (bone marrow) and peripheral blood hemolysis.
- In cases of severe thalassemia, the marked expansion of the erythroid element in the bone marrow may cause severe bony deformities, osteopenia, and pathologic fractures.

	α-globin genes transcribed	Hb A	Hb A2	Hb F	Transfusions
Normal	Homozygous β	97–99%	1–3%	< 1%	
Thalassemia minor	Heterozygous β0	80–95%	4–8%	1–5%	None
Thalassemia intermedia	Homozygous β++ (mild)	0–30%	0–10%	6–100%	Occasional
Thalassemia major	Homozygous β0 β0	0%	4–10%	90–96%	Dependent

Clinical Features of β-Thalassemia Major

1. Severe anemia with CHF
2. Spleno-hepatomegaly
3. Frontal & maxillary bossing due to bone marrow expansion (Chipmunk facies).

Investigations

Investigations	Findings
Hemoglobin	Decreased
Peripheral smear	MCHC, target cells
Reticulocyte count	Increased
NESTROFT (Screenings)	Decreased osmotic fragility
HPLC > hemoglobin electrophoresis	Investigation of choice

(NESTROFT: Naked eye single tube red cell osmotic fragility test)

Diagnostic Criteria for Thalassemia

- Microcytosis disproportionate to the degree of anemia.
- Positive family history or lifelong personal history of microcytic anemia.
- Normal or elevated red blood cell count.
- Abnormal red blood cell morphology with microcytes, hypochromia, acanthocytes, and target cells.
- In β-thalassemia, elevated levels of hemoglobin A2 or F.
- Elevated HbA_2 alone suggest diagnosis of thalassemic trait.

Management of Thalassemia

- Treatment of choice is allogenic bone marrow transplantation.
- For transfusion dependent thalassemia major, packed RBC transfusions are given.
- Yersinia infections are common in iron overloaded patients following multiple transfusions.[Q]
- Patients who require more than 200–250 mL/kg of packed cells[Q] year to maintain hemoglobin may benefit from procedure of splenectomy. Splenectomy in thalassemic is deferred till the age of 7 yrs.

Sickle Cell Anemia

- Sickle cell anemia is an autosomal recessive disorder in which an abnormal hemoglobin leads to chronic hemolytic anemia.
- A single DNA base change leads to an amino acid substitution of valine for glutamine in the sixth position on the β-globin chain. Hemoglobin S is unstable and polymerizes in the setting of various stressors, including hypoxemia and acidosis, leading to the formation of sickled red blood cells.

Symptoms and Signs

1. The disorder has its onset during the first year of life, when hemoglobin F levels fall, since a signal is sent to switch from production of γ-globin to β-globin.
2. Chronic hemolytic anemia produces jaundice, pigment gallstones, splenomegaly and poorly healing ulcers over the lower tibia.
3. Acute painful episodes due to acute vaso-occlusion from clusters of sickled red cells. (MC presentation)
4. Acute vaso-occlusion may cause strokes due to sagittal sinus thrombosis and may also cause priapism.
5. Ischemic necrosis of bone occurs, rendering the bone susceptible to osteomyelitis due to salmonellae and staphylococci.
6. Pulmonary infarction and myocardial infarction leading to acute chest syndrome.
7. Avascular necrosis of the vertebrae, which appear as fish (fish vertebrae).
8. *Kidney involvement leads to papillary necrosis and isothemuria.*

Investigations

1. Hemoglobin
2. Peripheral smear
3. H.P.L.C : IOC

Treatment

- Allogeneic hematopoietic stem cell transplantation[Q] can cure more than 80% of children with sickle cell anemia who have suitable HLA-matched donors.
- Hydroxyurea reduces the frequency of painful crises in patients, whose quality of life is disrupted by frequent pain crises.

Sickle Cell Trait

- People with sickle cell trait may experience sudden cardiac death and rhabdomyolysis during vigorous exercise, especially at high altitudes
- They may also be at increased risk for venous thromboembolism.

Hereditary Spherocytosis

- Autosomal dominant disorder with ankyrin defect
- Ankyrin, spectrin provide most of the scaffolding for the red blood cell membranes.
- The net result is a decrease in surface-to-volume ratio that results in a spherical shape of the cell.
- These spherical cells are less deformable and unable to pass through the small fenestrations in the splenic red pulp. Hemolysis takes place because of trapping of red blood cells within the spleen and their removal by splenic macrophages.

Clinical Features

1. Anemia
2. Splenomegaly
3. Hemolytic jaundice
4. Pigmented gall stones
5. Non-healing ulcers on medial malleolus.

Investigations

Investigations	Findings
Hemoglobin	Decreased
Peripheral smear	Spherocytes (exhibit absence of central pallor)
Reticulocytes	Increased
Osmotic fragility test (most sensitive test)[Q]	Increased
Osmotic gradient ektacytometry	Limited availability and helps to differentiate from other causes.

Treatment

- Elective splenectomy with vaccination. Post-splenectomy RBC's exhibit Howell Jolly Bodies and cabot rings.[Q] Life long folic acid supplementation is must to prevent megaloblastic crisis.

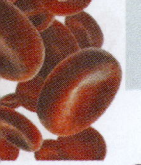

G6PD Deficiency

Definition

Deficiency in glucose-6-phosphate dehydrogenase (G6PD) leads to a sensitivity of RBCs to oxidative stress due to a lack of reduced glutathione.

Pathophysiology

X-linked recessive, more prevalent in black males.

Clinical Features

X-linked form frequently presents as episodic hemolysis precipitated by Oxidative stress caused by:

- Drugs (e.g. sulfonamide, antimalarials, nitrofurantoin)
- Infection
- Food (fava beans)
- In neonates, it can present as prolonged, pathologic neonatal jaundice.

Investigations

1. Neonatal screening of G6PD assay
2. Should not be done in acute crisis when reticulocyte count is high since reticulocytes have high G6PD levels
3. Heinz bodies^Q (granules in RBCs due to oxidized Hb); passage through spleen results in the generation of bite cells
4. Features of intravascular hemolysis (e.g. RBC fragments).

Treatment

- Transfusion in severe cases
- Stop offending drugs or food and avoid triggers.

Autoimmune Hemolytic Anemia

- Autoimmune hemolytic anemia is an acquired disorder in which an IgG autoantibody is formed that binds to the red blood cell membrane and does so most avidly at body temperature (i.e., a "warm" autoantibody).
- The antibody is most commonly directed against a basic component of the Rh system present on most human red blood cells.
- Autoimmune hemolytic anemia typically produces an anemia of rapid onset that may be life-threatening in severity.
- Patients complain of fatigue and dyspnea and may present with angina or congestive heart failure. On examination, jaundice and splenomegaly are usually present.

> - Acquired hemolytic anemia caused by IgG autoantibody
> - Spherocytes and reticulocytosis on peripheral blood smear
> - Positive antiglobulin (Coombs) test.

Treatment

Steroids

Hemolysis

Extravascular	Intravascular
Conditions	Conditions
• Sickle cell anemia • Hereditary spherocytosis • Thalassemia • G6PD	• PNH • PCH • G6PD (drug induced)

Microangiopathic Hemolytic Anemia (MAHA)

Etiology

1. Thrombotic thrombocytopenic purpura (TTP)/hemolytic uremic syndrome (HUS)
2. DIC
3. Eclampsia, HELLP syndrome
4. Malignant hypertension vasculitis
5. Malfunctioning heart valves

Investigations

1. **Blood film**: Evidence of hemolysis, schistocytes
2. Hemolytic work-up
3. **Urine**: Hemosiderinuria, Hemoglobinuria

MYELOPROLIFERATIVE DISORDERS

Polycythemia Vera

Polycythemia vera is an acquired myeloproliferative disorder that causes overproduction of all three hematopoietic cell lines, most prominently the red blood cells. Erythroid production is independent of erythropoietin and the serum erythropoietin level is low.

Essentials of Diagnosis

1. JAK2 (V617F) mutation^Q
2. Increased red blood cell mass
3. Splenomegaly
4. Normal arterial oxygen saturation
5. Usually elevated white blood count and platelet count.

Clinical Features

1. Hyperviscosity symptoms: Headache, dizziness, tinnitus, blurred vision, and fatigue
2. Budd Chiari syndrome
3. (Pruritus with hot water is due to histamine release from the basophils)^Q
4. Splenomegaly.

Investigation

1. Hb > 21 gm%
2. Hematocrit > 65%
3. *Urinary erythropoietin screening*
4. F.I.S.H to demonstrate JAK-2 mutation: IOC

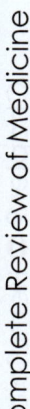

Treatment

1. Venesection or phlebotomy till hematocrit is < 45%
2. Ruxolitinib JAK-2 inhibitor
3. Low dose aspirin and allopurinol
4. Hydroxyurea: to reduce platelet count

ESSENTIAL THROMBOCYTOSIS

- Essential thrombocytosis is an uncommon myeloproliferative disorder of unknown cause in which marked proliferation of the megakaryocytes in the bone marrow leads to elevation of the platelet count.
- The disorder is often suspected when an elevated platelet count is found. Less frequently, the first sign is thrombosis, which is the most common clinical problem.
- The risk of thrombosis rises with age. Venous thromboses may occur in unusual sites such as the mesenteric, hepatic, or portal vein. Some patients experience erythromelalgia, painful burning of the hands accompanied by erythema; this symptom is reliably relieved by aspirin. Splenomegaly is present in at least 25% of patients.

- Elevated platelet count in absence of other causes.
- Normal red blood cell mass.
- Absence of bcr/abl gene (Philadelphia chromosome).

Investigations

1. An elevated platelet count is the hallmark of this disorder, and may be over 2,000,000/mcL.
2. The bone marrow shows increased numbers of megakaryocytes but no other morphologic abnormalities.

Treatment

- Aspirin
- Hydroxyurea (drug of choice)
- Anagrelide.

Platelet count increases in the following situations
- Trauma
- Polycythemia vera
- Essential thrombocytosis

PRIMARY MYELOFIBROSIS

- This is a myeloproliferative disorder characterized by fibrosis of the bone marrow, splenomegaly, and a leukoerythroblastic peripheral blood picture with teardrop poikilocytosis.Q
- Myelofibrosis can also occur as a secondary process following the other myeloproliferative disorders (e.g., polycythemia vera, essential thrombocytosis). It is believed that fibrosis occurs in response to increased secretion of platelet-derived growth factor (PDGF) and possibly other cytokines.
- In response to bone marrow fibrosis, extramedullary hematopoiesis takes place in the liver, spleen, and lymph nodes. In these sites, mesenchymal cells responsible for fetal hematopoiesis can be reactivated.

Clinical Features

1. Pallor
2. Recurrent infection
3. Petechiae occur mostly around the ankle. This can lead to purpura leading to epistaxis, hematuria and hematemesis
4. Splenohepatomegaly.
5. Hematopoiesis in liver leads to portal hypertension.
6. Transverse myelitis due to poiesis in epidural space.

Investigations

1. Complete blood count

Hemoglobin	Decreased
TLC	Decreased
Platelet	Decreased

2. Bone marrow biopsy
3. Bone marrow aspiration on examination reveals *dry tap*
4. Peripheral smear shows *tear drop* appearance of RBC.

- **Dry tap on bone marrow aspiration is seen in the following conditions**
  1. Myelopthisis
  2. Myelofibrosis
  3. Hairy cell leukemia

In aplastic anemia, bone marrow is readily aspirated but is dilute with hemopoietic cells occupying less than 25% of marrow space.

Treatment

Allogenic bone marrow transplantation

CHRONIC MYELOID LEUKEMIA (CML)

- CML is a myeloproliferative disorder characterized by overproduction of myeloid cells. These myeloid cells retain the capacity for differentiation, and normal bone marrow function is retained during the early phases. CML is characterized by a specific chromosomal abnormality and specific molecular abnormality.
- The Philadelphia chromosome is a reciprocal translocation between the long arms of chromosomes 9 and 22. A large portion of 22q is translocated to 9q, and a smaller piece of 9q is moved to 22q.
- The portion of 9q that is translocated contains abl. The abl gene is received at a specific site on 22q, the break point cluster (bcr). The fusion gene bcr/abl produces a novel protein that differs from the normal transcript of the abl gene as it possesses tyrosine kinase activity. Tyrosine kinase is responsible for uncontrolled multiplications of the cells.

Symptoms and Signs

1. Fatigue
2. Night sweats
3. Low-grade fever related to the hypermetabolic state caused by overproduction of white blood cells.
4. Patients may also complain of abdominal fullness related to splenomegaly.

On Examination

- Spleen is enlarged (often markedly so) and sternal tenderness may be present as a sign of marrow overexpansion.

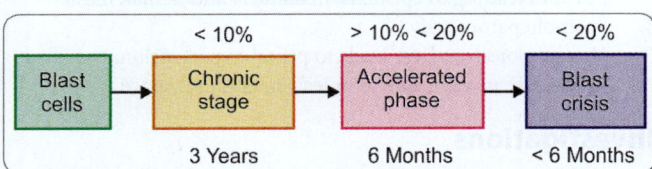

Investigations

1. **TLC**: Increased > 150, 000/mcL
2. **Peripheral smear**: Immature cells in peripheral smear are observed which is also known as shift to left myelopoiesis. Basophilia and eosinophilia are seen.
3. **Serum vitamin B_{12} levels**: Elevated as DNA synthesis increases
4. PCR in peripheral blood/FISH (fluorescent in situ hybridization): Investigation of choice

Treatment of CML

1. Treatment in CML is not an emergency with even cell counts of 20,000/mcL, as majority of circulating cells are mature myeloid cells.
2. Leukapheresis is warranted only if patient has symptoms of hyperleukocytosis like priapism, respiratory distress, blurring of vision, altered mental status.
3. Normalization of cell counts with regression of splenomegaly occurs in 3 months.
4. qPCR showing a 3 log reduction of bcr/abl transcript desired within 12 months as a molecular major response.^{Q}
5. Cytogenetic response is when less than 35% of metaphases contain philadelphia chromosome.^{Q}
6. Major molecular response comparison
   Imatinib = 30% at 1 yr
   Dasatinib = 71% at 2 yr
   Nilotinib = 64% at 2 yr
7. *If resistant to above tyrosine kinase inhibitors, Bosutinib is used.*^{Q}
8. *T315I mutation is resistant to all of above, hence third generation ponatinib is used.*^{Q}
9. In accelerated phase, the response to tyrosine kinase inhibitors is limited, hence allogenic stem cell transplantation should be done *(pg 525, CMDT 2017)*

- Chronic myeloid leukemia
- Elevated white blood count
- Markedly left-shifted myeloid series but with a low percentage of Promyelocytes and blasts
- Presence of bcr/abl gene (Philadelphia chromosome).

Diagnostic Comparison of Myeloproliferative Disorders Blood Indices

	White count	Hemato-crit	Platelet count	Red cell morphology
Polycythemia vera	N or ↑	↑	N or ↑	N
Essential thrombocytosis	N or ↑	N	↑↑	N
Primary myelofibrosis	N or ↑ or ↓	↓	N or ↑ or ↓	Abnormal
CML	↑↑	N	N or ↑	N

Clinical Indicators

Condition	Feature	IOC	Treatment
Polycythemia vera	Hb > 21 gm%	JAK-2 mutation and	Phlebotomy
CML	Massively enlarged spleen	PCR/FISH	Imatinib
Essential thrombo-cytosis	Clotting tendency	↑ Platelet count	Hydroxyurea >> Anagrelide
Myelofibrosis	Pancytopenia	Bone marrow biopsy	Bone marrow transplant

PLATELETS

Thrombocytopenia

Thrombocytopenia occurs when platelet count <150 x10^9/L.

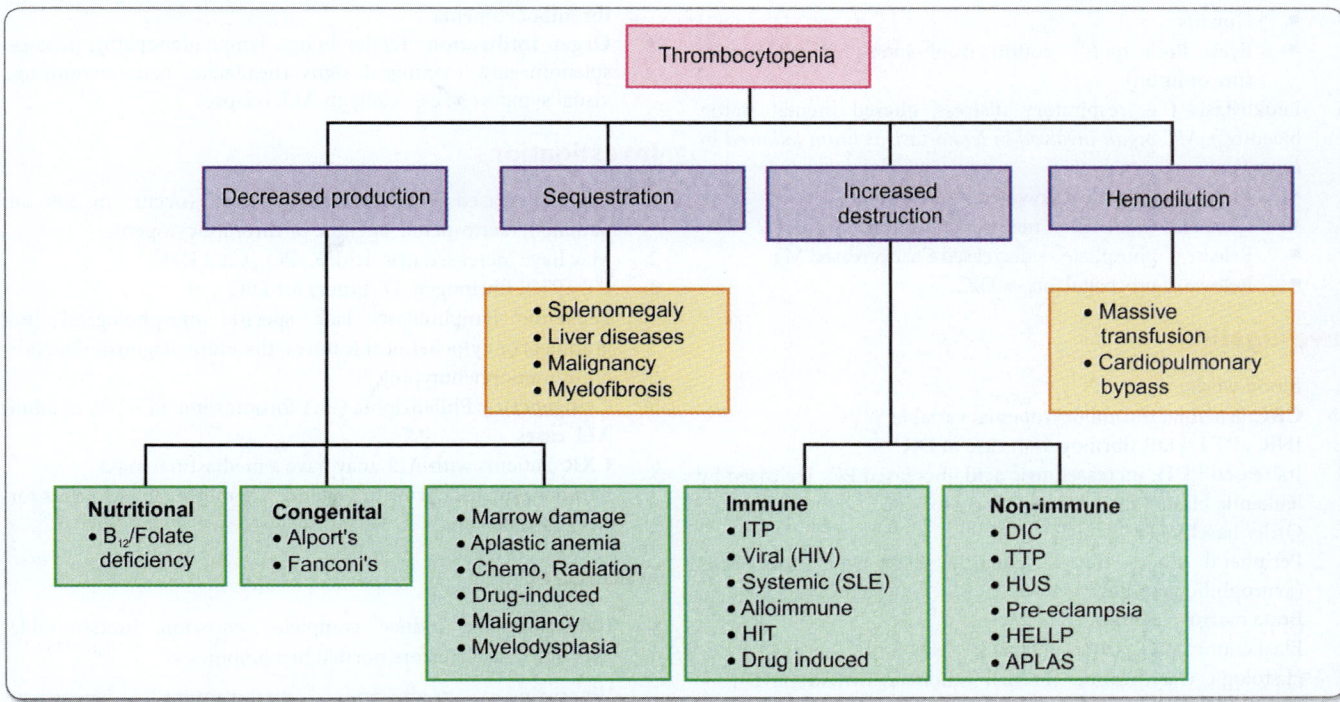

Thrombocytosis

- Platelet count >500 x10^9/L
- **Reactive thrombocytosis**: Acute phase reactant (e.g. surgery, inflammation, infection, trauma, bleeding, iron deficiency, neoplasms)
- **Autonomous thrombocytosis**: Thrombocytosis due to myeloproliferative or myelodysplastic disorders [e.g. CML, primary myelofibrosis, polycythemia vera (PV), myelodysplastic syndrome (MDS), AML]
- **Essential thrombocythemia**: one of the myeloproliferative disorders, diagnosis of exclusion

Immune Thrombocytopenic Purpura (ITP)

Features	Acute	Chronic ITP
Peak age	2–6 years	20–40 years
Sex predilection	None	F > M (3:1)
History of recent infection	Common	Rare
Onset of bleed	Abrupt	Insidious
Duration	Usually weeks	Months to years
Spontaneous remission	80% or more	Uncommon

HEMATOLOGIC MALIGNANCIES – MYELOID MALIGNANCIES

Acute Myeloid Leukemia (AML)

- Incidence increased with age, median age of onset is 65 years old
- Accounts for 10–15% of childhood leukemias.

Risk Factors

- Myelodysplastic syndromes (MDS)
- Benzene
- Radiation and alkylating agents for previous malignancy

Pathophysiology

Etiology subdivided into

- **Primary**: de novo
- **Secondary**: To hematologic malignancies (e.g. myeloproliferative disorders and MDS) or to previous chemotherapeutic agents (i.e. alkylating agents)

Uncontrolled growth of blasts in marrow leads to:
- Suppression of normal hematopoietic cells
- Appearance of blasts in peripheral blood
- Accumulation of blasts in other sites
- Metabolic consequences of a large tumor mass.

Clinical Features

1. Anemia
2. Thrombocytopenia (associated with DIC in promyelocytic leukemia)^Q
3. Neutropenia (even with normal WBC) → Infections, fever
4. Accumulation of blast cells in marrow leads to skeletal pain, bony tenderness, especially sternum

5. Organ infiltration with leukemic cells leads to
   - Gingival hypertrophy
   - Splenomegaly: Early satiety, left upper quadrant fullness
   - Hepatomegaly
   - Lymphadenopathy
   - Skin: Leukemia cutis
   - Gonads
   - Eyes: *Roth spots*^{Q}, cotton wool spots, vision changes (uncommon)
6. Leukostasis (i.e. respiratory distress, altered mental status, bleeding). *MC organ involved in leukostasis is brain followed by lungs.*^{Q}
   - Metabolic effects, aggravated by treatment
   - Increased uric acid → nephropathy, gout
   - Release of phosphate → decreased Ca, decreased Mg
   - Release of procoagulants → DIC.

Investigations

1. Blood work
2. **CBC**: Anemia, thrombocytopenia, variable WBC
3. INR, aPTT, FDP, fibrinogen in case of DIC
4. Increased LDH, increased uric acid, increased PO_4 (released by leukemic blasts), increased K, decreased Ca
5. Order baseline RFTs, LFTs
6. Peripheral blood film: Circulating blasts with Auer rods (azurophilic granules)
7. Bone marrow aspirate
8. Blast count: AML >20% (normal is <5%)
9. Histologic classification [French-American-British (FAB)] → (MO-M7): Based on stage at which cell differentiation stops
10. Cytogenetics, immunophenotyping
11. CXR to rule out pneumonia, EGG, MUGA scan prior to chemotherapy

Treatment

- Mainstay of treatment is chemotherapy with cytarabine and etoposide.
- All AML subtypes are treated similarly
  *Except promyelocytic variant with t(15:17) translocation: All – trans-retinoic acid (ATRA) added, to induce differentiation

On initiation of ATRA, differentiation syndrome develops leading to respiratory distress. CXR shows pulmonary infiltrates. It is managed with dexamethasone.

LYMPHOID MALIGNANCIES

Acute Lymphoblastic Leukemia (ALL)

Definition

- Malignant disease of the bone marrow in which early lymphoid precursors proliferate and replace the normal hematopoietic cells of the marrow.
- WHO subdivides ALL into two types depending on cell of origin
  - B cell: Precursor B lymphoblastic leukemia
  - T cell: Precursor T lymphoblastic leukemia.

Clinical Features

75% of ALL occurs in children <6 years old; second peak at age 40

Clinical symptoms usually secondary to

- **Bone marrow failure**: Anemia, neutropenia (50% present with fever; also infections of oropharynx, lungs, perianal region), thrombocytopenia
- **Organ infiltration**: Tender bones, lymphadenopathy, hepato-splenomegaly, meningeal signs (headache, nausea/vomiting, visual symptoms; especially in ALL relapse)

Investigations

1. **CBC**: increased leukocytes >10 x 10^9/L (occurs in 50% of patients); neutropenia, anemia, or thrombocytopenia
2. May have increased uric acid, K, PO_4, Ca, LDH
3. PT, aPTT, fibrinogen, D-dimers for DIC
4. Leukemic lymphoblasts lack specific morphological (no granules) or cytochemical features, therefore diagnosis depends on immunophenotyping
5. **Cytogenetics**: Philadelphia (Ph) chromosome in ~25% of adult ALL cases
6. **CXR**: Patients with ALL may have a mediastinal mass
7. Lumbar puncture prior to systemic chemotherapy to assess for CNS involvement.

Treatment

- **Induction**: To induce complete remission (undetectable leukemic blasts, restore normal hematopoiesis)

  Vincristine, prednisone, methotrexate, leucovorin L-aspariginase, intrathecal methotrexate and ara-c

  * In Philadelphia chromosome-positive ALL imatinib mesylate (Gleevec™, a bcr-abl tyrosine kinase inhibitor) can be added which is found to induce complete remission in up to 95% cases.

- **Consolidation and/or intensification chemotherapy:**
  - Consolidation: Continuing same chemotherapy to eliminate further subclinical leukemic cells
  - Intensification: High doses of different (non-cross-reactive) chemotherapy drugs to eliminate cells with resistance to primary treatment.
- **Maintenance chemotherapy**: Low dose intermittent chemotherapy over prolonged period (2–3 years) to prevent relapse.
- **Prophylaxis**: CNS with radiation therapy or methotrexate (intrathecal or systemic).
- **Hematopoietic stem cell transplantation**: Potentially curative (due to pre-implant myeloablative chemoradiation and post-implant graft-versus-leukemia effect) but relapse rates and non-relapse mortality is high.

Lymphomas

Definition

- Collection of lymphoid malignancies in which malignant lymphocytes accumulate at lymph nodes and lymphoid tissues, leading to lymphadenopathy, extranodal disease, and constitutional symptoms.

- Ann Arbor staging can be used for both Hodgkin's and non-Hodgkin's lymphoma, but grade/histology is more important for non-Hodgkin's lymphoma because it tends to present at more advanced stages.

Staging (Ann Arbor Staging System)

- **Stage I**: Involvement of a single lymph node region or extra-lymphatic organ or site
- **Stage II**: Involvement of two or more lymph node regions or an extralymphatic site and one or more lymph node regions on same side of diaphragm
- **Stage III**: Involvement of lymph node regions on both sides of the diaphragm; may or may not be accompanied by single extra lymphatic site or splenic involvement
- **Stage IV**: Diffuse involvement of one or more extralymphatic organs including bone marrow
- Subtypes:
  - A = Absence of B symptoms
  - B = Presence of B symptoms
  - Unexplained fever >38°C
  - Unexplained weight loss (>10% of body weight in 6 months)
  - Night sweats

Chromosome Translocations

Translocation	Gene Activation	Associated Neoplasm
t(8;14)	c-myc activation	Burkitt's lymphoma
t(14;18)	bcl-2 activation	Follicular lymphoma
t(9;22)	Philadelphia chromosome (bcr-abl hybrid)	CML, ALL in adults (25% of the time)
t(11;14)	Overexpression protein cyclin Dl	Mantle cell lymphoma

Hodgkin's Lymphoma

Definition

Malignant proliferation of lymphoid cells with Reed-Sternberg cells (thought to arise from germinal center B-cells)

Epidemiology

- Bimodal distribution with peaks at the age of 20 years and >50 years
- Association with Epstein-Barr virus in up to 50% of cases

Hodgkin's Lymphoma	Non – Hodgkin's Lymphoma
More often localized to single axial group of nodes (cervical, mediastinal, para-aortic)	More frequent involvement of multiple peripheral nodes
Orderly spread by contiguity	Non contiguous spread
Mesenteric nodes and Waldeyer ring rarely involved	Waldeyer ring and mesenteric nodes commonly involved
Extranodal involvement uncommon	Extranodal involvement common

WHO Classification of Hodgkin's Lymphoma

Nodular sclerosis	Mixed cellularity	Lymphocyte rich	Lymphocyte depleted	Lymphocyte predominant (non-classical HL)
MC type of HL	MC type of HL *in India*		Associated with HIV	
Incidence equal in M and F	M > F	M>F	M>F	M>F
RS cell variant in lacunar cell (clear space surrounding cell)	Has eosinophils and plasma cells. Maximum number of RS cell	Mononuclear and RS cell. Lowest number of RS cells	3 unique RS cell (pleomorphic, mummified, necrobiotic type). Maximum area of necrosis	LH cells (popcorn cells) in background. Other cells scanty or absence of B cells
Cells are CD 15 + CD30+	Cells are CD 15 + CD30+	Cells are CD15+ CD30+ and CD20-	Cells are CD 15+ CD30+	RS cell are CD 20+ CD 15-, CD30- BCL6 +, EMA+
No association with EBV	Associated with EBV	Associated with EBV	Associated with EBV	No association with EBV
Excellent prognosis	Prognosis very good	Good to excellent prognosis	Poor prognosis	Excellent prognosis
Adolescents and young adults	Biphasic incidence (young adults as well as > 55 years)	Old age group	Old age group	Young males

Clinical Features

1. Asymptomatic lymphadenopathy (70%)
2. Non-tender, rubbery consistency
3. Cervical/supraclavicular (60–80%), axillary (10–20%), inguinal (6–12%)
4. Splenomegaly (50%) + hepatomegaly
5. Mediastinal mass found on routine CXR, may be symptomatic (cough)
6. Rarely may present with SVC syndrome, pleural effusion
7. Systemic symptoms
   - B symptoms (especially in widespread disease; fever in 30%), pruritus
   - Alcohol-induced pain in nodes
   - Paraneoplastic manifestation in form of nephrotic syndrome

Investigations

1. CBC
2. Excisional lymph node biopsy confirms diagnosis (IOC)
3. Bone marrow biopsy to assess marrow infiltration (only necessary if B symptoms, stage III or IV, bulky disease or cytopenia)

Treatment

- **Stage I-II**: Chemotherapy (ABVD) followed by involved field XRT
- **Stage III-IV**: Chemotherapy (ABVD, BEACOPP), with XRT for bulky disease
- **Relapse, resistant to therapy**: High dose chemotherapy, bone marrow transplant.

Complications of Treatment

- **Cardiac disease**: Adriamycin is cardiotoxic
- **Pulmonary disease**: Secondary to bleomycin, which causes interstitial pneumonitis
- **Infertility**: Recommend sperm banking
- Secondary malignancy in irradiated field
- <2% risk of MDS, AML (secondary to treatment, usually within 8 years)
- Solid tumors of lung, breast, >10 years after treatment
- Non-Hodgkin's lymphoma
- **Hypothyroidism**: Post XRT
- **Infection**: Post splenectomy (give pneumovax, HiB, and pneumococcal conjugate vaccines) during treatment

Prognosis

Adverse prognostic factors:

- Serum albumin <4 g/L (4 gm/dL)
- Hemoglobin <105 g/L (10.5 gm/dL)
- Male
- Stage IV disease
- Age ≥45 years
- Leukocytosis (WBC >1.5x10^9/L)
- Lymphocytopenia (lymphocytes <0.06 x 10^9/L or <8% of WBC count or both)

- Each additional adverse prognostic factor decreases freedom from progression at 5 years.

Non-Hodgkin's Lymphoma (NHL)

Definition

Malignant proliferation of lymphoid cells without Reed-Sternberg cells.

Classification

- Multiple classification systems exist at present and may be used at different centers
- Can originate from both B (85%) and T-or NK-(15%) cells
- **B cell NHL**: Burkitt's lymphoma, mantle cell lymphoma, follicular lymphoma
- **T cell NHL**: Mycosis fungoides, anaplastic large cell lymphoma
- **WHO/REAL classification system**: 3 categories of NHLs based on natural history
  - Indolent (35–40% of NHL): Follicular lymphoma, small lymphocytic lymphoma/CLL, mantle cell lymphoma
  - Aggressive (50% of NHL): Diffuse large B-cell lymphoma
  - Highly aggressive (~5% of NHL): Burkitt's lymphoma.

Clinical Features

1. Painless superficial lymphadenopathy, usually >1 lymph region
2. Constitutional symptoms (fever, weight loss, night sweats) not as common as in Hodgkin's disease
3. **Cytopenia**: Anemia ± neutropenia ± thrombocytopenia if bone marrow fails
4. **Abdominal signs**:
   - Hepatosplenomegaly
   - Retroperitoneal and mesenteric involvement (2nd most common site of involvement)
5. Oropharyngeal involvement in 5–10% with sore throat and obstructive apnea
6. **Extranodal involvement**: Most commonly GI tract, also testes, bone, kidney
7. CNS involvement in 1% (often with HIV).

Treatment

- **Localized disease** (e.g. GI, brain, bone, head and neck)
  - Surgery (if applicable)
  - Radiotherapy to primary site and adjacent nodal areas
  - Adjuvant chemotherapy
  - Radiation therapy for localized disease
  - Chemotherapy (single agent, combination or rituximab/an anti-CD20 antibody)
- **Aggressive lymphoma**: Goal of treatment is curative
  - Combination chemotherapy: CHOP is mainstay, plus rituximab if B-cell lymphoma
  - Radiation for localized/bulky disease
  - CNS prophylaxis with high-dose methotrexate (intrathecal or systemic) if certain sites involved

Complications

- Hypersplenism
- Infection
- Autoimmune hemolytic anemia and thrombocytopenia
- Vascular obstruction (from enlarged nodes)
- Tumor lysis syndrome (particularly in very aggressive lymphoma).

Characteristics of Selected Non-Hodgkin's Lymphomas

	Follicular lymphoma	Diffuse large B-cell lymphoma (DL BCL)	Burkitt's lymphoma	Mantle cell lymphoma
Percentage of NHLs	22–30%	33%	<1% adult NHLs 30% childhood	6%
Genetic mutation	Bcl-2 activation	Bcl-2, Bcl-6, MYC rearrangements	NHLs c-myc activation	Overexpression of cyclin D1 (Bcl-1 activation)
Classification	Indolent	Aggressive (high-grade)	Very aggressive	Indolent
Risk factors	Middle-age – elderly	Previous CLL (Richter's transformation: 5% CLL patients progress to DLBCL}	*Endemic:* African origin, EBV-associated *Sporadic:* no EBV 3-HIV-related-AIDS-defining illness	Male (male:female = 4:1)
Clinical features	• Widespread painless LAD ± bone marrow involvement • Frequent transformation to aggressive lymphoma • Very responsive to chemoradiation tx	• Rapidly progressive LAD and extranodal infiltration	• Endemic form -massive jaw LAD • "Starry-sky" histology • High risk of tumor Lysis syndrome upon treatment	• Often presents at Stage IV, with palpable LAD • Involvement of GI tract (lymphomatosis polyposis), Waldeyer's ring • Extremely aggressive, 5-year survival 25%

Chronic Lymphocytic Leukemia (CLL)

Definition

Indolent disease characterized by clonal malignancy of mature B-cells.

Epidemiology

- **Most common leukemia in Western world**[Q]
- Mainly older patient; median age 65 years.

Pathophysiology

Accumulation of neoplastic lymphocytes in blood, bone marrow, lymph nodes and spleen.

Clinical Features

1. 25% asymptomatic (incidental finding)
2. 5–10% present with B symptoms (≥1 of: unintentional weight loss ≥10% of body weight within previous 6 months, fever >38°C or night sweats for >2 weeks without evidence of infection, extreme fatigue)
3. Lymphadenopathy (50–90%), splenomegaly, hepatomegaly
4. **Immune dysregulation**: Autoimmune hemolytic anemia (Coombs +), immune thrombocytopenia purpura (ITP), hypogammaglobulinemia ± neutropenia
5. **Bone marrow failure**: Late, secondary to marrow involvement by CLL cells.

Investigations

1. **CBC**: absolute lymphocytosis >5 x 10^9/L
2. **Peripheral blood film**: Lymphocytes are small and mature and called *smudge cells*
3. Flow cytometry
4. **Cytogenetics**: FISH
5. **Bone marrow aspiration**: aspirate shows infiltration of marrow by lymphocytes in 3 patterns: nodular (10%), interstitial (30%), diffuse (35%, worse prognosis), or mixed (25%).

Natural History and Treatment

- Natural history: Indolent but incurable, with slow progression; thus select gentlest treatment that will control symptoms
- Intermittent chlorambucil or *fludarabine* [DOC]
- Corticosteroids, IVIG: Especially for autoimmune phenomena
- Chemotherapy: Including rituximab (anti-CD20 mAb).

Complications

- Bone marrow failure
- Immune complications like autoimmune hemolytic anemia, immune thrombocytopenia (ITP), immune deficiency (hypogammaglobulinemia, impaired T-cell function)
- Polyclonal or monoclonal gammopathy (often IgM)
- Hyperuricemia with treatment
- **5% undergo richter's transformation (aggressive transformation to diffuse large B-cell lymphoma).**

BASIC PHYSIOLOGY OF HEMOPOEITIC SYSTEM

Erythrocyte

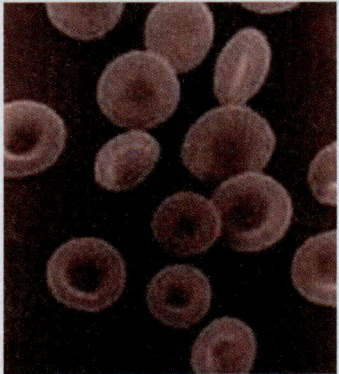

- Anucleate and biconcave
- Life span of 120 days
- **Life span of transfused RBC = 60–80 days**
- **Life span of fetal RBC = 100 days**
- Source of energy is glucose (90% used in glycolysis, 10% used in HMP shunt)
- Membrane contains chloride-HCO_3^- antiporter, which allows RBCs to export HCO_3^- and transport CO_2 from the periphery to the lungs for elimination

- Anisocytosis = varying sizes; Poikilocytosis = varying shapes
- Reticulocyte = immature erythrocyte, marker of erythroid proliferation
- **Reticulocytosis is a hallmark feature of all hemolytic anemias**

Platelet (Thrombocyte)

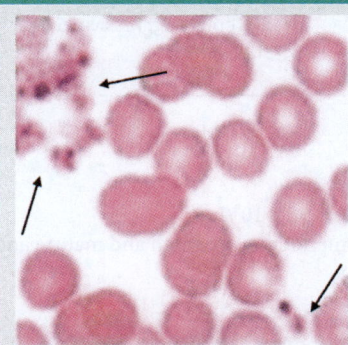

- Involved in 1° hemostasis. Small cytoplasmic fragment derived from megakaryocytes
- **Life span of 5 days**
- **Life span of transfused platelet = 24 hours**
- **Stored at room temperature of 20–24 degrees**
- Approximately 1/3 of platelet pool is stored in the spleen

- Thrombocytopenia or decreased platelet function leads to formation of petechiae
- vWF receptor is: GpIb
- Fibrinogen receptor is: GpIIb/IIIa
- Splenectomy leads to thrombocytosis
- Most radioresistant blood cell

Leukocyte

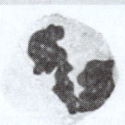
Granulocyte neutrophil

Monocyte
Lymphocyte

- Divided into granulocytes (neutrophil, eosinophil, basophil) and mononuclear cells (monocytes, lymphocytes). Responsible for defense against infections. Normally 4000–10,000 cells/mm^3
- WBC differential from highest to lowest
- Neutrophils (54–62%)
- Lymphocytes (25–33%)
- Monocytes (3–7%)
- Eosinophils (1–3%)
- Basophils (0–0.75%)

- Leucopenia is seen in typhoid
- Hyperleucocytosis is seen with leukemias
- Leukemoid reaction is seen in severe infection
- Lymphocyte is most radiosensitive blood cell

Neutrophil

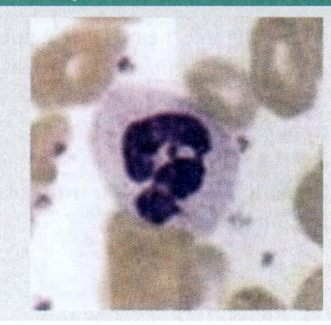

- Acute inflammatory response cell increased in bacterial infections
- Phagocytic. Multilobed nucleus, small, more numerous specific granules contain ALP, collagenase, lysozyme and lactoferrin
- Larger, less numerous azurophilic granules (lysosomes) contain proteinases, acid phosphatase, myeloperoxidase and β-glucuronidase

- Hypersegmented neutrophils (5 or more lobes) are seen in vitamin B_{12}/ folate deficiency
- Increased band cells (immature neutrophils) reflects states of increased myeloid proliferation (bacterial infection, CML)
- Neutropenia is defined as count < 1500/mcL (pg 517: CMDT 2017)
- *Severe neutropenia is defined as neutrophil count below 500/mcL (pg 517: CMDT 2016)*
- Cyclic neutropenia is due to problems in ELANE gene, neutrophil elastase gene.

Contd...

Monocyte

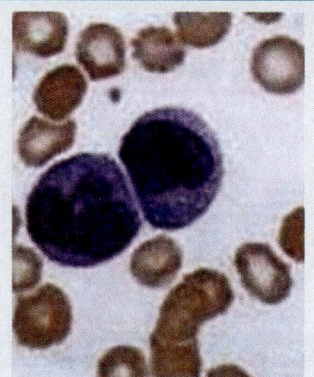

- Differentiates from macrophages in the tissues
- Large, kidney-shaped nucleus **and has an extensive "frosted glass" cytoplasm**
- Largest white blood cell

- Monocytosis is seen in malaria, Brucellosis, Bacterial endocarditis.
- Most striking increase in blood monocyte concentration occurs in clonal monocytosis (MDS) and monocytic, myelomonocytic leukemia.

Macrophage

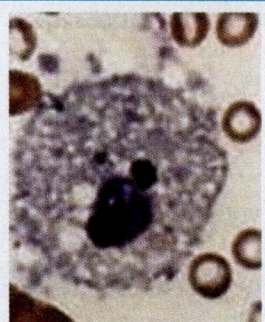

- Phagocytoses bacteria, cellular debris, and senescent RBCs and scavenges damaged cells and tissues
- Long life in tissues. Macrophages differentiate from circulating blood monocytes
- Activated by γ-interferon. Can function as antigen-presenting cell via MHC II. CD14 is a cell surface marker for macrophages

- Important component of granuloma formation (e.g., TB, sarcoidosis)
- Macrophage: in the tissue

Eosinophil

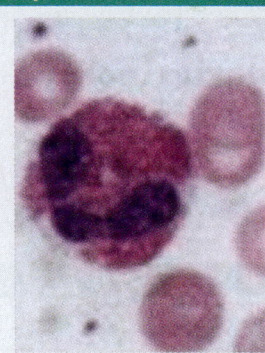

- Defends against helminthic infections (major basic protein)
- Bilobate nucleus
- Packed with large eosinophilic granules of uniform size
- Highly phagocytic for antigen-antibody complexes
- Produces histaminase and arylsulfatase (helps limit reaction following mast cell degranulation)

Causes of eosinophilia = NAACP:
- Neoplasia
- Asthma
- Allergic processes
- Connective tissue diseases
- Parasites (invasive)

Basophil

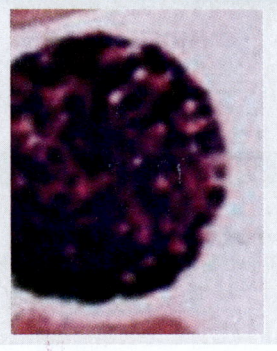

Mediates *anaphylaxis*. Densely basophilic granules containing heparin (anticoagulant), histamine (vasodilator) and leukotrienes

Isolated basophilia is uncommon, but can be a sign of myeloproliferative disease, particularly CML

Contd...

Mast cell

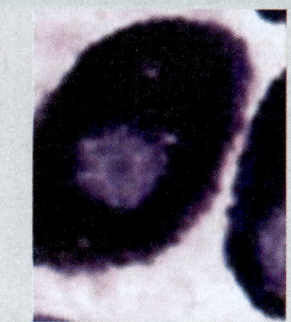

- Mediates allergic reaction in local tissues. Mast cells resemble basophils structurally and functionally but are not the same cell type
- Can bind the Fc portion of IgE to membrane
- IgE cross-links upon antigen binding, causing degranulation, which releases histamine, heparin, and eosinophil chemotactic factors

- Cromolyn sodium prevents mast cell degranulation (used for asthma prophylaxis)

Dendritic cell

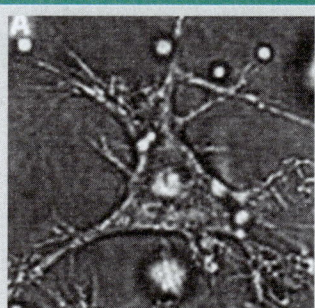

- Highly phagocytic antigen presenting cell. Functions as link between innate and adaptive immune systems
- Expresses MHC class II and Fc receptor on surface
- Called Langerhans cell in the skin

Lymphocyte

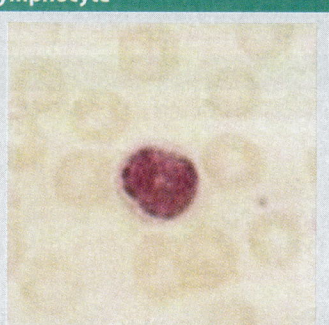

- Divided into B cells, T cells and NK cells
- B cells and T cells mediate adaptive immunity. NK cells are part of the innate immune response
- Round, densely staining nucleus with small amount of pale cytoplasm

B lymphocyte

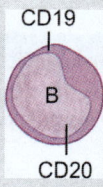

- Part of humoral immune response. Arises from stem cells in bone marrow. Matures in marrow
- Migrates to peripheral lymphoid tissue (follicles of lymph nodes, white pulp of spleen, unencapsulated lymphoid tissue)
- When antigen is encountered, B cells differentiate into plasma cells that produce antibodies, and memory cells. Can function as an APC via MHC II

- B is for bone marrow
- 85% of NHL is B cell type
- MALToma is B cell type NHL
- CLL is also of B cell origin

T lymphocyte

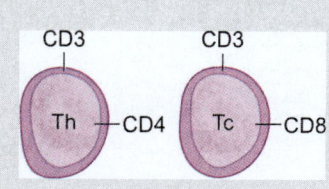

- Mediates cellular immune response
- Originates from stem cells in the bone marrow, but matures in the thymus. T cells differentiate into cytotoxic T cells (express CD8, recognize MHC I), helper T cells (express CD4, recognize MHC II), and regulatory T cells. CD28 (costimulatory signal) necessary for T-cell activation
- The majority of circulating lymphocytes are T cells (80%)

- T is for thymus
- CD is for cluster of differentiation
- CD4 + helper T cells are the primary target HIV

Contd...

Plasma cell

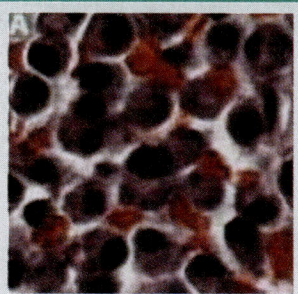

- Produces large amounts of antibody specific to a particular antigen
- Eccentric nucleus clock-face chromatin distribution, abundant RER, and well-developed Golgi apparatus

Multiple myeloma is a plasma cell cancer
Triad in multiple Myeloma
1. Bone marrow biopsy shows plasma cells > 10%
2. Serum electrophoresis showing a M-spike
3. Evidence of end organ damage

PATHOLOGY OF HEMOPOEITIC SYSTEM

Cell	Associated pathology	Remarks	Cell	Associated pathology	Remarks
Acanthocyte (Spur cell)	• Liver disease • Abetalipoproteinemia (states of cholesterol dysregulation)	Notice the spiny architecture of the RBC	**Elliptocyte**	Hereditary elliptocytosis	Defect of protein Spectrin in the cell wall of RBC. (Contrast from: ANKYRIN defect in cell wall of RBC in Hereditary spherocytosis)
Basophilic stippling of RBC	• Anemia of chronic disease • Alcohol abuse • Lead poisoning • Thalassemia		**Macro-ovalocyte**	Megaloblastic anemia	Also seen in pernicious anemia are hyper-segmented PMNs
Bite cell	G6PD deficiency	XLR pattern of inheritance, hence seen in boys and girls are carriers	**Ringed sideroblast**	Sideroblastic anemia	Excess iron in mitochondria is pathologic
Schistocyte, helmet cell	1. DIC 2. TTP/HUS, 3. Traumatic hemolysis (i.e., Mechanical heart valve prosthesis)	—	**Teardrop cell**	Bone marrow infiltration (e.g., myelofibrosis)	RBC "sheds a tear" because it's been forced out of its home in the bone marrow

Contd...

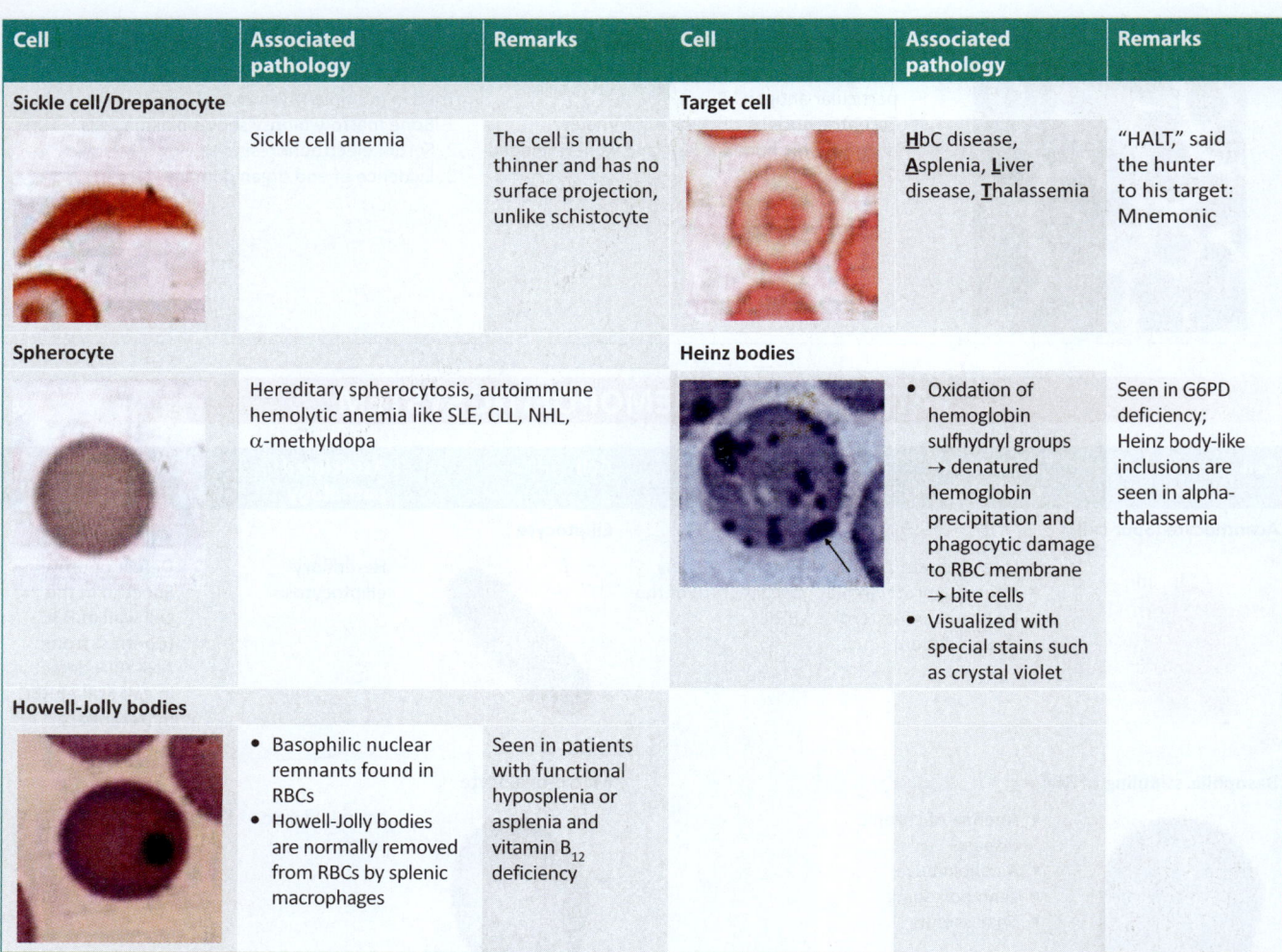

Cell	Associated pathology	Remarks	Cell	Associated pathology	Remarks
Sickle cell/Drepanocyte	Sickle cell anemia	The cell is much thinner and has no surface projection, unlike schistocyte	**Target cell**	HbC disease, Asplenia, Liver disease, Thalassemia	"HALT," said the hunter to his target: Mnemonic
Spherocyte	Hereditary spherocytosis, autoimmune hemolytic anemia like SLE, CLL, NHL, α-methyldopa		**Heinz bodies**	• Oxidation of hemoglobin sulfhydryl groups → denatured hemoglobin precipitation and phagocytic damage to RBC membrane → bite cells • Visualized with special stains such as crystal violet	Seen in G6PD deficiency; Heinz body-like inclusions are seen in alpha-thalassemia
Howell-Jolly bodies	• Basophilic nuclear remnants found in RBCs • Howell-Jolly bodies are normally removed from RBCs by splenic macrophages	Seen in patients with functional hyposplenia or asplenia and vitamin B_{12} deficiency			

Image-Based Questions

1. Which of the following explains the anemia shown in the P. smear of a neonate?

   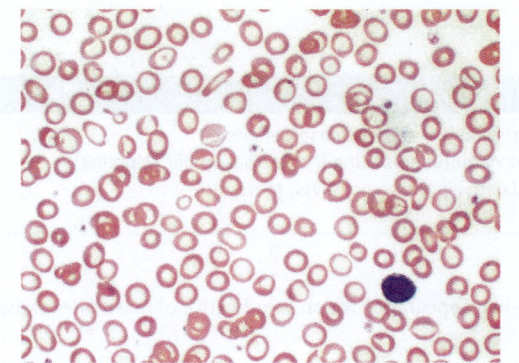

   a. DMT 1 mutation
   b. Ferroportin excess
   c. Low haptoglobin
   d. X-linked sideroblastic anemia

2. All are causes of arrow marked finding in RBC except?

   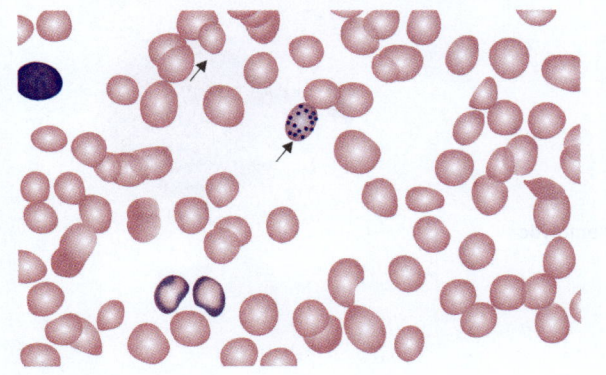

   a. Thalassemia
   b. Lead poisoning
   c. Myelodysplastic syndrome
   d. Asplenia

3. The following facies are seen in:

   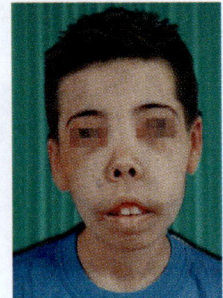

   a. Malnutrition   b. Thalassemia
   c. Scurvy   d. Leprosy

4. Identify the defect in the peripheral smear:

   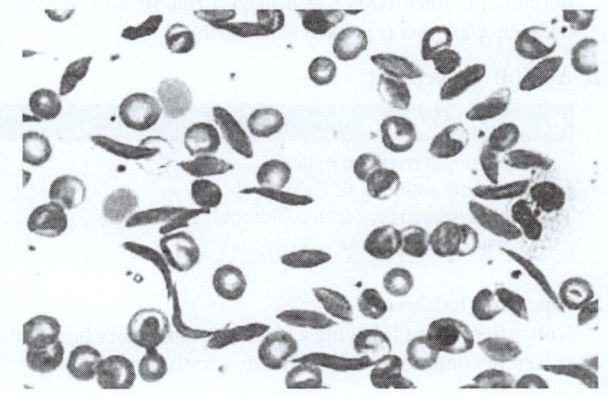

   a. Drepanocyte
   b. Acanthocyte
   c. Poikilocyte
   d. Elliptocyte

5. The image shows presence of?

   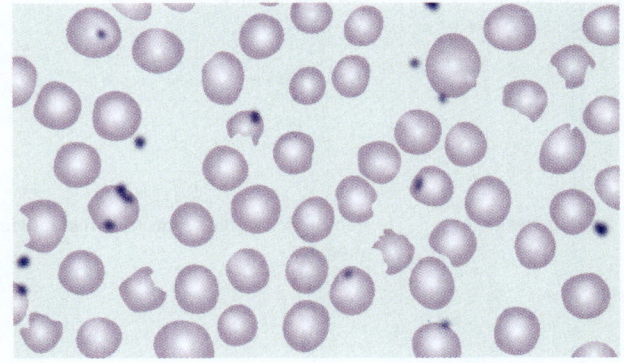

   a. Bite Cells
   b. Burr Cells
   c. Mott Cells
   d. Smudge Cells

Answers of Image-Based Questions

1. **Ans. (a) DMT 1 mutation**
   The image shows microcytic hypochromic anemia due to DMT 1 mutation. These patients will have inability to absorb iron from the duodenum. Since DMT1 also plays a role in iron transfer from endosomes into the cystosol of developing erythrocytes severe iron deficiency anemia is present since birth.

2. **Ans. (d) Asplenia**

Basophilic stippling	
• Thalassemia trait and major • Hemolytic anemia • Myelodysplastic syndrome/sideroblastic anemia • Megaloblastic anemia	• Pyrimidine 5' nucleotidase deficiency • Heavy metal poisoning (coarse basophilic stippling) ▪ Lead, zinc, arsenic, silver, mercury

3. **Ans. (b) Thalassemia**
   Notice the patient is having a prominent maxillary bone with chimpanzee-like appearance which is indicative of marrow expansion and is seen in conditions with ineffective erythropoiesis.

4. **Ans. (a) Drepanocyte**
   Peripheral blood smear shows the typical elongated, crescent-shaped RBCs called Drepanocyte (Sickle RBC). Patients with homozygous sickle cell disease have red blood cells (RBCs) that are less pliable and more "sticky" than normal RBCs. Vaso-occlusive crisis is often precipitated by infection, fever, excess: exercise, anxiety, abrupt changes in temperature, hypoxia, or hypertonic dyes. There is also a nucleated RBC at the bottom of the figure, which may be attributable to increased bone marrow production.

5. **Ans. (a) Bite cells**

Bite cell	G6PD deficiency	
Burr cell	Hemolytic uremic syndrome, microangiopathic hemolytic anemia	
Mott cell	Multiple myeloma	
Smudge cell	Chronic lymphocytic leukemia	

Conceptual Diagnostic Algorithm

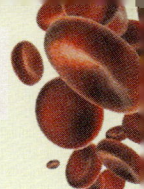

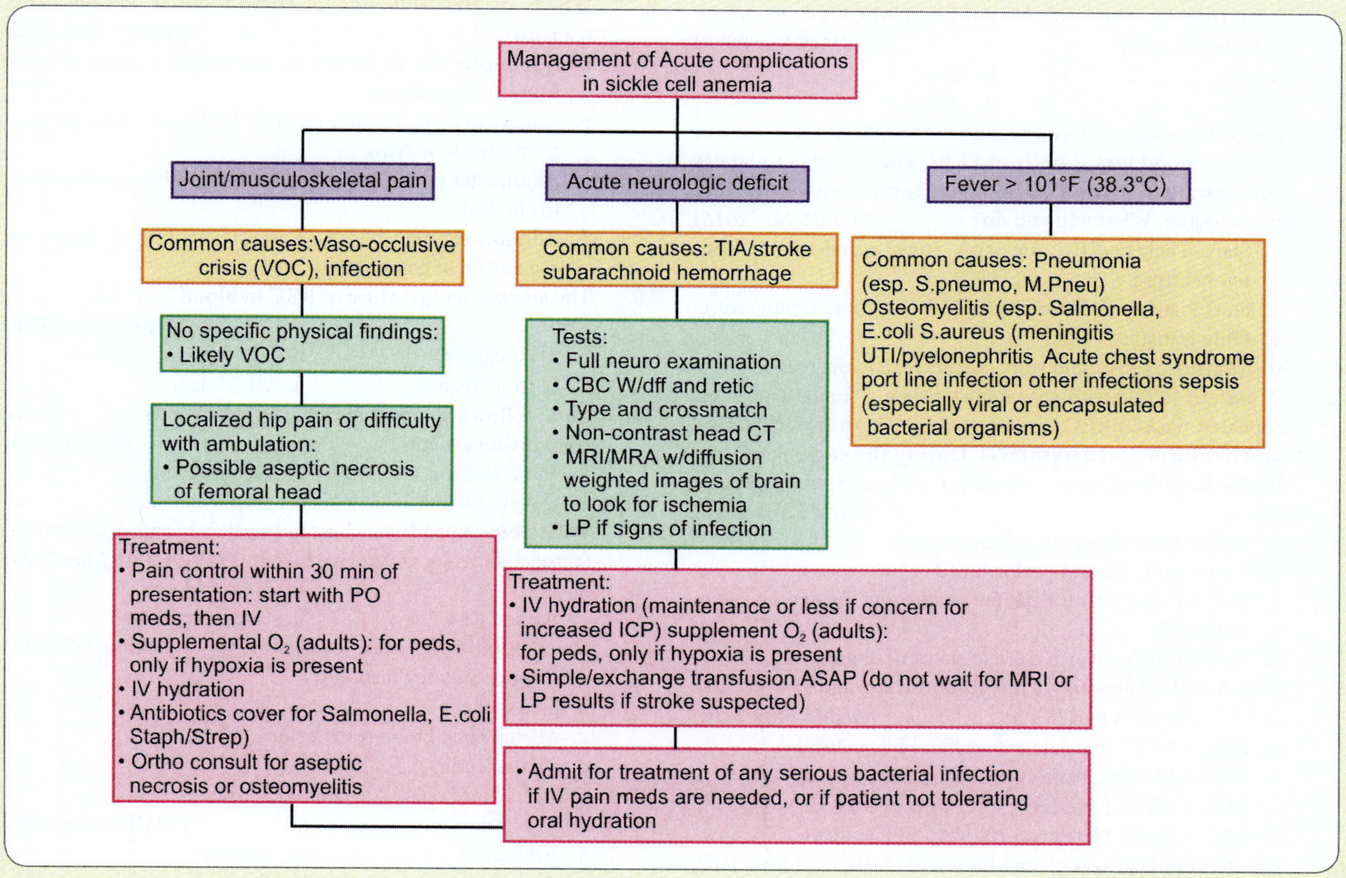

```
                    Management of Acute complications
                          in sickle cell anemia
    ┌───────────────────────────┼───────────────────────────┐
Joint/musculoskeletal pain   Acute neurologic deficit    Fever > 101°F (38.3°C)
```

Joint/musculoskeletal pain

Common causes: Vaso-occlusive crisis (VOC), infection

No specific physical findings:
- Likely VOC

Localized hip pain or difficulty with ambulation:
- Possible aseptic necrosis of femoral head

Treatment:
- Pain control within 30 min of presentation: start with PO meds, then IV
- Supplemental O_2 (adults): for peds, only if hypoxia is present
- IV hydration
- Antibiotics cover for Salmonella, E.coli Staph/Strep)
- Ortho consult for aseptic necrosis or osteomyelitis

Acute neurologic deficit

Common causes: TIA/stroke subarachnoid hemorrhage

Tests:
- Full neuro examination
- CBC W/dff and retic
- Type and crossmatch
- Non-contrast head CT
- MRI/MRA w/diffusion weighted images of brain to look for ischemia
- LP if signs of infection

Treatment:
- IV hydration (maintenance or less if concern for increased ICP) supplement O_2 (adults): for peds, only if hypoxia is present
- Simple/exchange transfusion ASAP (do not wait for MRI or LP results if stroke suspected)

- Admit for treatment of any serious bacterial infection if IV pain meds are needed, or if patient not tolerating oral hydration

Fever > 101°F (38.3°C)

Common causes: Pneumonia (esp. S.pneumo, M.Pneu) Osteomyelitis (esp. Salmonella, E.coli S.aureus (meningitis UTI/pyelonephritis Acute chest syndrome port line infection other infections sepsis (especially viral or encapsulated bacterial organisms)

Multiple Choice Questions

ABO System, Blood Transfusions and Blood Components

1. A patient on warfarin presents with major bleeding and is found to have INR of 15. How much fresh frozen plasma (FFP) is required to treat this situation? *(JIPMER May 2018)*
   a. 15 ml/kg
   b. 10 ml/kg
   c. 5 ml/kg
   d. 20 ml/kg

2. A trauma patient presents at emergency department. There is no time for cross matching. FFP of which group can be transfused safely? *(AIIMS Nov 2018)*
   a. O –
   b. O +
   c. AB –
   d. AB +

3. Following an RTA, A young man is brought into ER. Due to massive blood loss, 2 units of PRBC and 4 units of platelet concentrate is obtained from blood bank. Only one IV line is accessible. What will you do? *(AIIMS Nov 2018)*
   a. Start Packed RBC 1st and store platelets at room temperature
   b. Start Platelets and store Packed RBC at room temperature
   c. Only transfuse PRBC
   d. Transfuse PRBC and store platelets at 2-6 degrees

4. A patient is a known case of thalassemia major and is on repeated packed RBC transfusion. She is on iron chelators and has history of arrythmias. During the current BT, she has backache and looks very anxious. The next management is? *(AIIMS Nov 2018)*
   a. Observe for change in colour of urine
   b. Continuous BT and perform ECG
   c. Stop BT and wait for patient to become normal and then restart BT
   d. Stop BT and perform clerical check of blood group

5. Which of the following is correct about storage temperature of RBC, Platelets and FFP? *(AIIMS May 2018)*
   a. RBC = 2-6°C, Platelets = 20-24°C, FFP = -30°C
   b. RBC = 20-24°C, Platelets = 2-6°C, FFP = -30°C
   c. RBC = 2-6°C, Platelets = 30°C, FFP = 20-24°C
   d. RBC = 2-6°C, Platelets = 20-24°C, FFP = +30°C

6. A patient in ICU was given blood transfusion. 3 hours later SpO_2 is reduced to 75% with respiratory difficulty. CVP is 15 cm water and PCWP is 25 mm Hg. CXR is shown below. What is the diagnosis? *(Recent Pattern 2018)*

   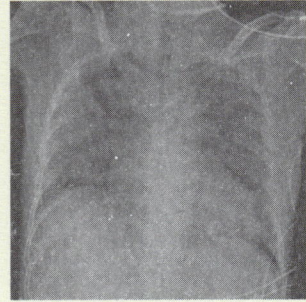

   a. Tension pneumothorax
   b. Transfusion related acute lung injury
   c. Transfusion associated circulatory overload
   d. Mismatched blood transfusion

7. Which of the following is incorrect about Transfusion associated circulatory overload? *(Recent Pattern 2018)*
   a. Elevated PCWP
   b. Diuretics
   c. IVF
   d. Elevated levels of BNP

8. Which of the following is not true about TRALI? *(AIIMS Nov 2016)*
   a. No role of steroids
   b. High mortality rate of 10%
   c. Supportive care is mainstay of treatment
   d. Resolves in 2-3 weeks

9. Which of the following is correct about Packed RBC transfusion? *(AIIMS May 2016)*
   a. Administer via 18-20 G cannula within 4 hours of issue from the blood bank
   b. Administer via 16-18G cannula within 4 hours of issue from the blood bank
   c. Administer via 18-20 G cannula within 4 hours of reaching the bedside
   d. Administer via 18-20G cannula within 4 hours of separation of components

10. The storage temperature of RBC in blood bank is? *(AIIMS May 2016)*
    a. 2- 6 degrees
    b. 1-2 degrees
    c. -2 to -6 degrees
    d. 20-24 degrees

11. The following are major complications of massive transfusion except? *(APPG 2016)*
    a. Hyperthermia
    b. Hyperkalemia
    c. Coagulopathy
    d. Hypocalcemia

12. Which blood product is best to be given in multiple clotting factor deficiency and active bleeding? *(AIIMS May 2015)*
    a. FFP
    b. Whole blood
    c. Packed RBC
    d. Cryoprecipitate

13. Haemoglobinuria does not occur in? *(Bihar PG 2015)*
    a. Copper Sulfate Poisoning
    b. Snake bite
    c. Mismatched blood transfusion
    d. Thalassemia

14. Carbohydrate related to blood grouping? *(JIPMER Nov 2015)*
    a. Arabinose
    b. Xylulose
    c. Xylose
    d. Fucose

15. Mismatched BT in a patient under General anaesthesia in Operation theatre presents with? *(JIPMER Nov 2015)*
    a. Dyspnea
    b. Hypotension
    c. Intraoperative bleeding
    d. Pulmonary oedema

16. A 30 years old male was given blood transfusion in the O.T. following which he develops tachycardia hypotension BP-70/40 mm of Hg and hematuria within 10 minutes of starting the transfusion. The most probable cause is? *(JIPMER Nov 2014)*
    a. Anesthetic drug hypersensitivity
    b. D.I.C
    c. G.V.H.D
    d. ABO incompatibility

17. Sugar responsible for ABO blood group expression? *(JIPMER 2014)*
    a. Fucose
    b. Galactose
    c. Glucose
    d. Ribose

18. All are complications of blood transfusion except?
    a. Hypomagensemia   (Recent Pattern 2015-16)
    b. Hypokalemia
    c. Hypocalcemia
    d. Metabolic alkalosis
19. Blood transfusion should be completed within _____ hours of initiation: (Recent Pattern 2014-15)
    a. 1-4 hours
    b. 3-6 hours
    c. 4-8 hours
    d. 8-12 hours
20. Most common complication of massive transfusion: (Recent Pattern 2014-15)
    a. Hypothermia   b. Acidosis
    c. Hyperkalemia   d. Hypocalcemia
21. Cryoprecipitate does not contain? (Recent Pattern 2014-15)
    a. Factor 8   b. Factor 9
    c. Von wilebrand factor   d. Fibrinogen
22. Which one of the following is the cause of non - cardiogenic pulmonary oedema seen in immunologic blood transfusion reaction: (Recent Pattern 2014-15)
    a. Antibody to IgA in donor plasma
    b. Antibody to donor leukocyte antigen
    c. Donor antibody to leukocyte of patient
    d. RBC incomapatibility
23. True about blood transfusion reaction: (Recent Pattern 2014-15)
    a. Complement mediated severe hemolysis
    b. Extravascular hemolysis
    c. Transfusion should not be stopped
    d. Death unlikely
24. Shelf life of blood in a blood bank in CPDA buffer: (Recent Pattern 2014-15)
    a. 21 days   b. 30 days
    c. 35 days   d. 42 days
25. Complication of blood transfusion can be all except: (Recent Pattern 2014-15)
    a. Hyperkalemia   b. Citrate toxicity
    c. Metabolic acidosis   d. Hypothermia
26. Not an Indicator of mismatched Blood transfusion in patient under general anesthesia: (Recent Pattern 2014-15)
    a. Fever with chills
    b. Hypotension
    c. Excessive oozing of blood from surgical site
    d. Passage of black urine
27. Most common cause of febrile non haemolytic transfusion reaction?   (Recent Pattern 2014-15)
    a. ABO mismatch   b. Rh mismatch
    c. HLA mismatch   d. All of the above
28. Most common complication of blood transfusion:
    a. Transfusion associated hepatitis (Recent Pattern 2014-15)
    b. Hyperkalemia
    c. Hemolysis
    d. Febrile non hemolytic transfusion reaction
29. Hypochromic microcytic anemia is seen in all, except:
    a. Thalassaemia   (Recent Pattern 2014-15)
    b. Tropical Sprue
    c. Ancylostomiasis
    d. Chronic inflammatory disease
30. There are more than 400 blood groups, we consider only ABO blood group, because: (Recent Pattern 2014-15)
    a. Presence of antibodies in the serum when the RBC lacks the corresponding antigen
    b. A &B antigens are secreted by cells which are not in the circulation only.
    c. Soluble blood group antigens cannot block binding of organisms to polysaccharides.
    d. These antigens are lipoproteins
31. True about Rh factor is   (Recent Pattern 2014-15)
    a. There are no natural anti-Rh antibodies in serum
    b. Seen only in females
    c. Approximately 15 % of Indians are Rh positive
    d. D is the least powerful Rh antigen
32. Wrong about FFP: (Recent Pattern 2014-15)
    a. Stored at minus 18 degrees
    b. Given for reversal of warfarin toxicity
    c. ABO matching is mandatory before transfusion
    d. Deficient in factor 5 and 8
33. Transfusing blood after prolonged storage could lead to:
    a. Citrate intoxication   (Recent Pattern 2014-15)
    b. Potassium intoxication
    c. Circulatory overload
    d. Haemorrhagic diathesis
34. Acute renal failure in a patient who received incompatible blood transfusion with hemolytic reaction is best managed by: (Recent Pattern 2014-15)
    a. 20% Mannitol
    b. IV fluids with K⁺ supplementation
    c. Alkalinizing the urine
    d. Stopping blood transfusion
35. Which of the following infection has highest chances of transmission by blood transfusion?
              (Recent Pattern 2014-15)
    a. HIV   b. HBV
    c. HTLV-1   d. HCV
36. Incorrect about platelet transfusion:
              (Recent Pattern 2014-15)
    a. Platelets carry the Rh antigen
    b. Platelets bear the antigens of ABO system
    c. Six units for healthy adult
    d. Transfuse to attain count of $50 \times 10^9/L$
37. Blood transfusion may be indicated in:
              (Recent Pattern 2014-15)
    a. Acute pulmonary oedema
    b. Epistaxis with hypertension
    c. Congestive cardiac failure
    d. Acute leukaemia
38. A 30-year-old female, RBC count 4.5 million, MCV 55fl, TLC 7000, no history of blood transfusion. Diagnosis is ?
    a. Iron deficiency anemia   (Recent Pattern 2014-15)
    b. Thalassemia major
    c. Thalassemia minor
    d. Megaloblastic anemia
39. MC blood transfusion reaction is-   (AI 2008)
    a. Febrile nonhemolytic transfusion reaction
    b. Hemolysis
    c. Transmission of infections
    d. Electrolyte imbalance

40. All of the following infections may be transmitted via blood transfusion, except: (AI 2002)
    a. Parvo B-19
    b. Dengue virus
    c. Cytomegalo virus
    d. Hepatitis G virus
41. Cryoprecipitate contains all except- (AIIMS Nov 07)
    a. Factor VIII
    b. Factor IX
    c. Fibrinogen
    d. VWF

Anemia and RBC Defects

42. A 25-year-old female presents to your OPD 1 year post-partum. She was treated for iron deficiency anemia when she was pregnant. Now she is pale and haemoglobin value is 5 gm%. Her reticulocyte count is 9%. Calculate her corrected reticulocyte count. (AIIMS May 2017)
    a. 1
    b. 3
    c. 4.5
    d. 6
43. All are causes of Coombs positive haemolytic anaemia except? (AIIMS May 2016)
    a. Haemolytic disease of new-born
    b. Drug induced autoimmune haemolytic anaemia
    c. Aplastic Anaemia
    d. Haemolytic Transfusion reaction
44. Severe aplastic anemia is defined as bone marrow cellularity less than _____? (Recent Question 2016-17)
    a. 5%
    b. 10%
    c. 20%
    d. 25%
45. All are essential for diagnosis of Aplastic anemia except? (Recent Question 2016-17)
    a. Bone marrow aspiration shows dry tap
    b. Bone marrow biopsy shows cellularity<25%
    c. Diminished CD34 antigen bearing cells
    d. Corrected reticulocyte count <1%
46. Match List-I with List-II and select the correct answer using the code given below the lists: (UPSC 2015)

List-I (Disease)	List-II (Cause)
A. Macrocytic anemia	1. Iron deficiency
B. Microcytic anemia	2. Hypothyroidism
C. Hemolytic anemia	3. Vitamin B_{12} deficiency
D. Megaloblastic anemia	4. Alpha methyldopa

Code:	A	B	C	D
a.	3	1	4	2
b.	3	2	1	4
c.	2	1	4	3
d.	1	4	3	2

47. Match List-I with List-II and select the correct answer using the code given below the lists: (UPSC 2015)

List-I (Blood picture)	List-II (Type of Anemia)
A. Microcytic, hypochromic red cells	1. Vitamin B_{12} deficiency anemia
B. Macrocytic, hypochromic red cells	2. Thalassemia major
C. Large number of early, intermediate and	3. Aplastic anemia late erythroblasts
D. Low reticulocyte count	4. Iron-deficiency anemia

Code:	A	B	C	D
a.	1	4	2	3
b.	2	3	4	1
c.	4	1	2	3
d.	3	1	2	4

48. Which one of the following is NOT associated with microcytic hypochromic anemia? (APPG 2015)
    a. Thalassemia
    b. Iron deficiency
    c. Hereditary spherocytosis
    d. Chronic lead poisoning
49. All of the following cause microcytic hypochromic anemia, except? (Bihar PG 2015)
    a. Lead poisoning
    b. Thalassemia
    c. Iron deficiency
    d. Fanconi's anemia
50. Diamond Blackfann anaemia is associated with? (JIPMER Nov 2015)
    a. Microcytic anaemia
    b. Aplastic anaemia
    c. Pure red cell aplasia
    d. Fanconi's anemia
51. A 45-year-old lady diagnosed to have anemia Hb-7.8, MCV = 70 and serum ferritin = 8 ng/dl. After 1 month of iron therapy with adequate dose Hemoglobin is still 8gm%. What is the most probable cause for treatment failure is?
    a. Non compliance (JIPMER Nov 2014)
    b. Acquired Sideroblastic anemia
    c. Inadequate intake of iron
    d. Folate deficiencies
52. In cobalamin deficiency which is not seen? (Recent Question 2015-16)
    a. Microcytic anemia
    b. Long tract signs
    c. Loss of proprioception
    d. Rhomberg Sign
53. Poikilocytosis and anisocytosis is seen in?
    a. Megaloblastic anaemia (Recent Question 2015-16)
    b. Iron deficiency anaemia
    c. Nutritional deficiency anaemia
    d. Thalassemia
54. Blood transfusion associated acute lung injury occurs due to? (Recent Question 2015-16)
    a. Nosocomial infections
    b. HLA mediated
    c. Auto-immune disorder
    d. Genetic susceptibility
55. Low serum iron and low serum ferritin is seen in: (Recent Question 2015-16)
    a. Iron deficiency anemia
    b. Chronic kidney disease
    c. Sideroblastic anemia
    d. Fanconi anemia
56. All are true about cross-matching of blood except: (Recent Question 2015-16)
    a. Mandatory in all cases except emergency
    b. Recipient serum is tested against donor packed cells
    c. Donor serum is tested against recipient packed cells
    d. Involves visible agglutination
57. The image shows presence of ?

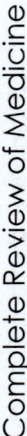

    a. Acanthocyte
    b. Schistocyte
    c. Echinocyte
    d. Stomatoctye

58. **In the treatment of megaloblastic anemia, vitamin B₁₂ and folic acid should be given together because:**
    (Recent Pattern 2014-15)
    a. Vitamin B_{12} acts as a cofactor for dihydrofolate reductase;
    b. Folic acid alone causes improvement of anemic symptoms but neurological dysfunction continues.
    c. Vitamin B_{12} deficiency may result in methylfolate trap
    d. Folic acid is required for conversion of methy-malonyl-CoA to succinyl Co-A.

59. **All the following are suggestive of iron-deficiency anemia except:** *(Recent Pattern 2014-15)*
    a. Koilonychia
    b. Pica
    c. Decreased serum ferritin
    d. Decreased total iron-binding capacity (TIBC)

60. **Hemolytic anemia are associated with all of the following, except:** *(Recent Pattern 2014-15)*
    a. Increased indirect bilirubin in the serum
    b. Decreased red cell survival
    c. Increased number of reticulocytes
    d. Increased fecal Urobilinogen

61. **A patient with microcytic hypochromic anemia, Hb-9%, serum iron is 20 g/dl, ferritin level 800 ng/ml, transferrin percentage saturation is 64. What is possible diagnosis:**
    (Recent Pattern 2014-15)
    a. Atransferrinemia   b. Iron deficiency anemia
    c. DMT 1 mutation   d. Hemochromatosis

62. **Seen in chronic inflammatory anemia is:**
    (Recent Pattern 2014-15)
    a. Serum iron↓ S. ferritin↑ and transferrin↓
    b. Serum iron↑ S. ferritin↑ and transferrin↑
    c. Serum iron↓ S. ferritin↓ and transferrin↓
    d. Serum iron↑ S. ferritin↓ and transferrin↑

63. **Reticulocyte count in Hemolytic jaundice is greater than?**
    (Recent Pattern 2014-15)
    a. 0.5%   b. 1%
    c. 1.5%   d. 2.5%

64. **Coombs negative hemolytic anemia is seen in:**
    (Recent Pattern 2014-15)
    a. Micro-angiopathic hemolytic anemia
    b. SLE
    c. CLL
    d. Rh incompatibility

65. **Coomb's positive hemolytic anemia associated with:**
    (Recent Pattern 2014-15)
    a. TTP   b. PAN
    c. SLE   d. HUS

66. **A patient with previously normal hemoglobin suffered a sudden massive acute hemorrhage. He is most likely to show all of the following except:** *(Recent Pattern 2014-15)*
    a. High reticulocyte count   b. High neutrophil count
    c. High packed cell volume   d. High MCV

67. **Spur cell anemia is seen in:** *(Recent Pattern 2014-15)*
    a. Drug induced anemia   b. Hepatocellular disease
    c. Renal disease   d. Alcoholism

68. **Low serum haptogloblin in hemolysis is masked by:**
    a. Liver disease   *(Recent Pattern 2014-15)*
    b. Pregnancy
    c. Bile duct obstruction
    d. Malnutrition

69. **Which causes aplastic anemia?** *(Recent Pattern 2014-15)*
    a. Hepatitis B   b. Hepatitis C
    c. Hepatitis A   d. EBV

70. **A young female has the following lab values: Hemoglobin= 9.8 gm%, MCV=70 serum iron= 60, serum ferritin =100, the diagnosis is:** *(Recent Pattern 2014-15)*
    a. Thalassemia trait
    b. Chronic iron deficiency anemia
    c. Megaloblastic anemia
    d. Anaemia of chronic infection

71. **Warm-antibody immune-hemolytic anemia is seen in all except:** *(Recent Pattern 2014-15)*
    a. SLE   b. α - Methyldopa ingestion
    c. Quinidine   d. Infectious mononucleosis

72. **Anemia of chronic disease is associated with:**
    (Recent Pattern 2014-15)
    a. Increased Fe, decreased Transferrin, increased Ferritin
    b. Decreased Fe, decreased Transferrin, increased Ferritin
    c. Decreased Fe, increased Transferrin, decreased Ferritin
    d. Increased Fe, increased Transferrin, decreased Ferritin

73. **Which of the following causes of Anemia is associated with a Hypoplastic marrow?** *(Recent Pattern 2014-15)*
    a. Fanconi's Anemia
    b. Paroxysmal Nocturnal Hemoglobinuria
    c. Hypersplenism
    d. Myelofibrosis

74. **Pernicious anemia is associated with all of the following, except:** *(Recent Pattern 2014-15)*
    a. Macrocythaemia
    b. Vitamin B_{12} deficiency
    c. Weakness, numbness & tingling of extremities
    d. Increased reticulocyte count

75. **A patient presented with splenomegaly, anemia & shows reticulocytosis & increased bone narrow cellularity. The diagnosis is:** *(Recent Pattern 2014-15)*
    a. Pernicious anemia   b. Hemolytic anemia
    c. Myelofibrosis   d. Hairy cell leukemia

76. **Iron requirement is determined from the equation:**
    (Recent Pattern 2014-15)
    a. 2.3 x wt (kg) x Hb deficit (g/dl) + 500
    b. 3.3 x wt. (kg) x Rb deficit (g/dl) + 1000
    c. 4 x wt. (kg) x Hb deficit (g/dl) + 1000
    d. 4.3 x wt. (kg) x Hb deficit (g/dl) + 1500

77. **Plasma ferritin levels may be reduced in all of the following conditions, except:** *(Recent Pattern 2014-15)*
    a. Iron deficiency   b. Vitamin C deficiency
    c. Liver disease   d. Hypothyroidism

78. **Which of the following types of anemia is associated with a Raised MCV and Normal MCHC?**
    (Recent Pattern 2014-15)
    a. Sideroblastic anemia
    b. Vitamin B_{12} and Folic acid deficiency
    c. Beta thalassemia
    d. Iron deficiency anemia

79. **Megalocytic anaemia is caused by all, except:**
    (Recent Pattern 2014-15)
    a. Goat milk ingestion   b. Type A gastritis
    c. Antimetabolites   d. Lead poisoning

80. **Iron is mainly absorbed in the:** *(Recent Pattern 2014-15)*
    a. Stomach b. Duodenum
    c. Jejunum d. Ileum
81. **A 20-year-old female presenting with anemia, mild jaundice for 2 years, peripheral smear showing spherocytes, the best investigation to be done is:** *(Recent Pattern 2014-15)*
    a. Reticulocyte count b. Osmotic fragility test
    c. Coomb's test d. Bone marrow aspiration
82. **Macrocytic anemia occurs in:** *(Recent Pattern 2014-15)*
    a. Hypothyroidism
    b. CRF
    c. Anemia of chronic disease
    d. Vitamin-C deficiency
83. **Oral iron supplements used for iron deficiency anemia:** *(Recent Pattern 2014-15)*
    a. Tolerable dose will deliver 40 to 60 mg of iron per day
    b. Mass of total salt is important in determining daily dose
    c. Treatment should be stopped as soon as normal hemoglobin level is reached
    d. Desired rate of hemoglobin improvement is 0.5 mg per day
84. **All of the following are true regarding B_{12} deficiency, except:** *(Recent Pattern 2014-15)*
    a. Pernicious anemia
    b. Sub-acute combined degeneration of cord
    c. Carpal tunnel syndrome
    d. Infertility
85. **All of the following are true about Congenital Haemolytic anemia, except:** *(Recent Pattern 2014-15)*
    a. Increased fragility b. Splenomegaly
    c. Splenectomy is useful d. Positive direct Coomb's test
86. **Which one of the following is true regarding Thalassemia Major?** *(Recent Pattern 2014-15)*
    a. Normocytic normochromic anemia
    b. Enlargement of medullary cavity
    c. Iron deficiency anemia
    d. Megaloblastic anemia
87. **All of the following are characteristic features of treatment of iron deficiency anemia with oral iron supplements, except:** *(Recent Pattern 2014-15)*
    a. Bioavailability is enhanced with vitamin C
    b. The proportion of iron absorbed reduces as hemoglobin improves
    c. The reticulocyte count should begin to increase in two weeks and peak in 4 weeks—this suggests good response to treatment
    d. The treatment should be discontinued immediately once hemoglobin normalizes to prevent side effects of iron.
88. **All of the following cause Microcytic Hypochromic anemia except:** *(AI 1995/AIIMS 1997)*
    a. Lead poisoning b. Thalassemia
    c. Iron deficiency anemia d. Fanconi's anemia
89. **Anemia of Chronic disease can be differentiated from Iron deficiency anemia by:** *(PGI 2009)*
    a. ↑ TIBC
    b. ↓ TIBC
    c. ↑ S.ferritin
    d. ↓ Fe store in marrow
    e. ↓ Ferritin
90. **A child has Hb-6.5 gm%, MCV-65, MCH-15 and protoporphyria with red cell distribution width much less is most likely to be suffering from :** *(AIIMS June 2000)*
    a. Thalassemia b. Iron deficiency anaemia
    c. Porphyria d. Megaloblastic anaemia
91. **Elevated serum ferritin, serum iron and percent transferrin saturation are most consistent with the diagnosis of :** *(AI 2004)*
    a. Iron deficiency anemia b. Anemia of chronic disease
    c. Hemochromatosis d. Lead poisoning
92. **All of the following are features of iron deficiency anemia, except:** *(AIIMS May 2013)*
    a. Increased RDW b. Decreased Serum Iron
    c. Decreased TIBC d. Decreased Serum Ferritin
93. **The earliest sign of iron deficiency anaemia:** *(AIIMS Feb 1997)*
    a. Increase in iron binding capacity
    b. Decrease in serum ferritin level
    c. Decrease in serum iron level
    d. All the above
94. **Most sensitive and specific test for diagnosis of iron deficiency is:** *(AI 2003, AI 2001)*
    a. Serum iron levels
    b. Serum ferritin levels
    c. Serum transferrin receptor population
    d. Transferrin saturation
95. **Iron overload occurs in all, except :** *(AIIMS Sept 96)*
    a. Thalassemia b. Myelodysplastic syndrome
    c. Polycythemia vera d. Sideroblastic anaemia
96. **Seen in chronic inflammatory anemia is:** *(PGI Dec 99)*
    a. Serum iron ↓, S. ferritin ↑ and transferrin ↓
    b. Serum iron ↑, S. ferritin ↑ and transferrin ↑
    c. Serum iron ↓, S. ferritin ↓ and transferrin ↑
    d. Serum iron ↑, S. ferritin ↓ and transferrin ↓
97. **Anemia of chronic disease is characterized by all, except**
    a. Decreased serum iron *(AIIMS May 94)*
    b. Increased total iron binding capacity (TIBC)
    c. Increased serum ferritin
    d. Increased macrophage iron in bone marrow
98. **Anemia in chronic renal failure (CRF) is due to:**
    a. Decreased erythropoietin production *(PGI June 01)*
    b. Iron deficiency
    c. Hypoplastic bone marrow
    d. Decreased Vit B12
    e. Decreased folate levels
99. **Not present in Sideroblastic anaemia is:** *(AIIMS Feb 97)*
    a. Microcytic anaemia
    b. Decreased transferrin saturation
    c. Sideroblast cells in blood smear film
    d. Ineffective erythropoiesis
100. **Macrocytic anemia may be seen with all of the following conditions except:** *(AI 1998, AIIMS 1996)*
    a. Liver disease b. Copper deficiency
    c. Thiamine deficiency d. Orotic aciduria
101. **Megaloblastic anemia in blind loop syndrome is due to:**
    a. Vitamin B_{12} malabsorption *(AI 99)*
    b. Bacterial overgrowth
    c. Frequent diarrhoea
    d. Decrease iron intake

102. **Haptaglobin levels are decreased in:** *(AI 1996)*
    a. A mismatched transfusion reactions
    b. Thalassemia
    c. G 6PD deficiency
    d. All of the above
103. **All are seen in Hemolytic anemia** *except:* *(AI 1996)*
    a. Hemosiderinuria   b. Reticulocytosis
    c. Spherocytosis   d. Increased haptoglobin
104. **All are features of hemolytic anaemia except:**
    (AIIMS Dec 95)
    a. Thrombocytopenia   b. Hemosiderinuria
    c. Decreased haptoglobin d. Raised indirect bilirubin
105. **Reticulocytosis is NOT a feature of:** *(AIIMS Dec 94)*
    a. Paroxysmal nocturnal hemoglobinuria
    b. Following acute bleeding
    c. Hereditary spherocytosis
    d. Anemia in CRF
106. **Cold haemagglutinin is associated with-** *(AI 97)*
    a. IgM   b. IgG
    c. IgA   d. Donath landsteiner antibody
107. **Autoimmune hemolytic anemia is seen in** *(AIIMS May 94)*
    a. Sickle cell anemia
    b. Chronic lymphocytic leukemia (CLL)
    c. Acute myelocytic leukemia (AML)
    d. Multiple myeloma
108. **Coomb's +ve Hemolytic Anaemia is seen in** *except:*
    a. Alcoholic cirrhosis   *(AI 2000)*
    b. Chronic active hepatitis
    c. Primary biliary cirrhosis
    d. Primary sclerosing cholangitis
109. **Microangiopathic Hemolytic anemia is seen in all Except:**
    a. TTP   *(AIIMS Nov 2009)*
    b. Metallic heart valve
    c. Microscopic polyangitis
    d. Anti-phospholipid syndrome
110. **All of the following statements about Fanconi's anemia are true, Except.** *(AI 2010)*
    a. Autosomal dominant inheritance
    b. Hypocellular Bone Marrow
    c. Congenital Anomalies
    d. Usually normocytic / macrocytic cell morphology

Thalassemia and Sickle Cell Anemia

111. **Haemoglobin electrophoresis can detect all except?**
    (Recent Question 2016-17)

    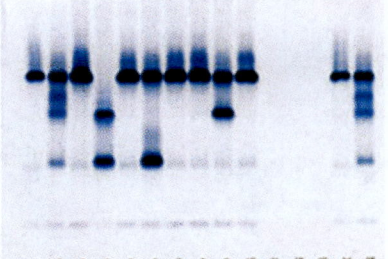

    a. Beta thalassemia intermedia
    b. Alpha thalassemia trait
    c. Sickle cell disease
    d. Hb E disease

112. **Golf ball inclusion bodies in RBCs are seen in?**
    (Recent Question 2016-17)
    a. Normal reticulocytes   b. HbH disease
    c. Pernicious anaemia   d. G6PD deficiency
113. **A 25-year-old lady came with anemia jaundice and recurrent joint pains. All of the following are true except:**
    a. HbA will be undetectable   *(APPG 2015)*
    b. She may have retinopathy
    c. She can present with pulmonary bleeds
    d. Hydroxyurea would help her
114. **The abnormality in X-ray skull shown can be seen in the following conditions except:** *(APPG 2015)*

    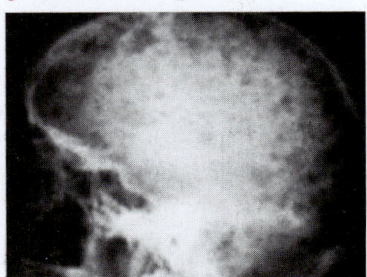

    a. Hyperparathyroidism   b. Paget's disease
    c. Multiple myeloma   d. Histiocytosis X
115. **Persistent priapism is due to:** *(Recent Pattern 2014-15)*
    a. Sickle cell anaemia   b. Hairy cell leukaemia
    c. Paraphimosis   d. Urethral stenosis
116. **Regarding to Thalassemia minor the following is incorrect:**
    a. Hypochromic microcytic cells *(Recent Pattern 2014-15)*
    b. Raised HbA2
    c. Severe anemia
    d. RBC count increased
117. **Basic defect in HbS is:** *(Recent Pattern 2014-15)*
    a. Altered function   b. Altered solubility
    c. Altered stability   d. Altered O_2 binding capacity
118. **In Beta thalassemia, the most common gene mutation is:**
    (Recent Pattern 2014-15)
    a. Intron 1 inversion   b. Intron 22
    c. 619 bp deletion   d. 3.7 bp deletion
119. **Fetal hemoglobin achieves adult values by**
    (Recent Pattern 2014-15)
    a. 6 months of age   b. 12 months of age
    c. 24 months of age   d. 36 months of age
120. **Sickle cell anemia is usually associated with all, except:**
    (Recent Pattern 2014-15)
    a. Shortened RBC life span
    b. Normal reticulocyte count
    c. Abnormality in Hemoglobin
121. **X-ray skull characteristically shows "Hair standing on end" appearance in one of the following disease:**
    a. Still's disease   *(Recent Pattern 2014-15)*
    b. Scurvy
    c. Thalassemia major
    d. Cirrhosis of liver
122. **Auto-splenectomy is associated with:**
    a. Systemic lupus erythematosus *(Recent Pattern 2014-15)*
    b. Trauma
    c. Sarcoidosis
    d. ITP

123. **HbH is characterized by:** *(Recent Pattern 2014-15)*
    a. Deletion of three alpha chain genes
    b. Deletion of three alpha chains and one beta chain genes
    c. Deletion of two alpha and two beta chain genes
    d. Deletion of four alpha chain genes

124. **Pancytopenia may occur in the following except:**
    a. Megaloblastic anemia *(Recent Pattern 2014-15)*
    b. Severe iron-deficiency anemia
    c. Hypoplastic anaemia
    d. Paroxysmal nocturnal haemoglobinuria

125. **Hemoglobin with zeta 2 and gamma 2 chains are seen in which of the following:** *(Recent Pattern 2014-15)*
    a. Gower 1
    b. Gower II
    c. Portland
    d. Fetal Gb

126. **The most appropriate drug used for chelation therapy in beta thalassemia major is:** *(Recent Pattern 2014-15)*
    a. Oral desferrioxamine
    b. Oral deferiprone
    c. Intramuscular EDTA
    d. Oral succimer

127. **Which of the following is not seen in a chronic case of Sickle cell anemia:** *(AI 1996)*
    a. Hepatomegaly
    b. Pulmonary hypertension
    c. Cardiomegaly
    d. Splenomegaly

128. **All are true for sickle cell anemia, except** *(AIIMS May 94)*
    a. Pulmonary arterial hypertension
    b. Fish vertebra
    c. Leukopenia
    d. Increased size of heart

129. **Commonest acute presentation of sickle cell anaemia is:**
    a. Priapism
    b. Bone pain *(AIIMS Dec 98)*
    c. Fever
    d. Splenomegaly.

130. **The mother has sickle cell disease; Father is normal; Chances of children having sickle cell disease and sickle cell trait respectively are:** *(AI 2001)*
    a. 0 and 100%
    b. 25 and 25%
    c. 50 and 50%
    d. 10 and 50%

131. **Crew haircut appearance in X-rays skull and Gandy gamma bodies are seen in:** *(AIIMS Nov 93)*
    a. G6-PD deficiency
    b. Hodgkin's lymphoma
    c. Hereditary spherocytosis
    d. Sickle cell anaemia

132. **All of the following are true about β thalassemia trait, Except:** *(PGI June 2008)*
    a. Microcytic hypochromic picture
    b. ↑ed HbA2
    c. ↑ed HbF
    d. Patient requires blood transfusion

133. **True about β-thalassemia trait:** *(PGI June 06)*
    a. Increased HbF
    b. Increased HbA2
    c. Microcytosis
    d. Severe anemia

134. **The peripheral blood smear of a patient shows features of thalassemia, also presented with anaemia. Family history is also +ve. The investigation done to establish the diagnosis is:** *(AIIMS 1999)*
    a. ESR estimation
    b. Blood spherocyte estimation
    c. Bone marrow aspiration
    d. Hb-electrophoresis

G6PD Deficiency and Hereditary Spherocytosis

135. **This is a peripheral blood smear of a patient with anaemia. What is the most likely diagnosis?** *(APPG 2016)*

    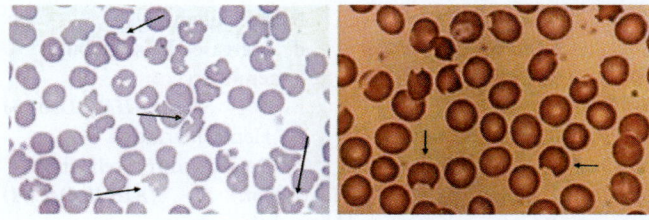

    a. Spherocytes & Howell Jolly bodies in Hereditary spherocytosis
    b. Echinocytes of Pyruvate kinase deficiency
    c. Ring cells & helmet cells in Malaria
    d. Bite cells of G-6-PD deficiency

136. **Hemolysis in G6PD (glucose 6 phosphate dehydrogenase) enzyme deficiency may occur with all of the following drugs except:** *(UPSC 2015)*
    a. Primaquine
    b. Phenacetin
    c. Probenecid
    d. Penicillin

137. **Which of the following conditions does not cause pancytopenia?** *(UPSC 2015)*
    a. Hypersplenism
    b. Aplastic anemia
    c. Cancer infiltrating the bone-marrow
    d. Hemolysis from G6PD enzyme deficiency

138. **True about G6PD?** *(JIPMER Nov 2015)*
    a. Autosomal dominant
    b. Does not protect against malaria
    c. Present as chronic haemolytic Anaemia
    d. Common cause of neonatal jaundice

139. **The following peripheral Smear shows presence of?**

    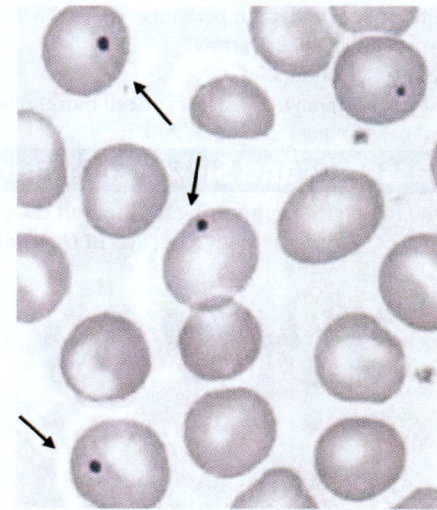

    a. Howell Jolly bodies
    b. Heinz bodies
    c. Pappenhiemer's Bodies
    d. Cabot Rings

140. Identify the inclusion body in RBCs in a patient with splenectomy 5 years ago after a motor vehicle crash: 4

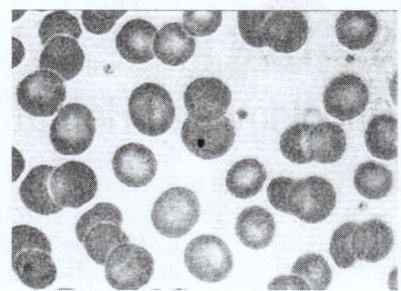

   a. Heinz bodies
   b. Toxic granules
   c. Howell jolly bodies
   d. Warthin finkeldy inclusion bodies

141. **All are true about G6PD except:** *(Recent Pattern 2014-15)*
   a. Bite cells
   b. Intravascular hemolysis
   c. Favism
   d. Confers protection against plasmodium vivax

142. **Incorrect about osmotic fragility test is:** *(Recent Pattern 2014-15)*
   a. Increased in hereditary spherocytosis
   b. Decreased in thalassemia
   c. Hemolysis on exposure to hypertonic saline environment
   d. Osmotic fragility decreased in iron deficiency

143. **Spherocytosis is associated commonly with:** *(Recent Pattern 2014-15)*
   a. Hypernatraemia   b. Hyperkalaemia
   c. Hyponatraemia   d. Hypokalaemia

144. **The following protein defects can cause hereditiary spherocytosis except :** *(AI 07)*
   a. Anykyrin   b. Palladin
   c. Glycophorin C   d. Anion transport protein

145. **Osmotic fragility is increased in:** *(PGI June 98)*
   a. Sickle cell anemia
   b. Thalassemia
   c. Hereditary spherocytosis
   d. Chronic lead poisoning

146. **Splenectomy is most useful in :** *(AI 1998)*
   a. Thrombocytopenia   b. Hereditary spherocytosis
   c. H.S. purpura   d. Sickle cell anemia

147. **Which doesn't cause hemolysis in G6 PD deficiency:** *(PGI Dec 99)*
   a. Oestrogen   b. Salicylates
   c. Primaquine   d. Nitrofurantoin

PNH and PCH

148. **A 5-year-old child presented with microcytic hypochromic anemia. Serum ferritin is low. All of the following condition will have low ferritin except?** *(UPSC 2015)*
   a. Celiac disease
   b. Thalassemia major
   c. Nutritional anemia
   d. Paroxysmal nocturnal Hemoglobinuria

149. **Which of the following causes of Anemia is associated with a Hypoplastic marrow?** *(Bihar PG 2015)*
   a. Fanconi's Anemia
   b. Paroxysmal Nocturnal Hemoglobinuria (PNH)
   c. Hypersplenism
   d. Myelofibrosis

150. **Pancytopenia with Cellular marrow is seen in all except?** *(Bihar PG 2015)*
   a. Megaloblastic anemia
   b. Myelodysplasia
   c. Paroxysmal nocturnal Hemoglobinuria
   d. G6PD Deficiency

151. **Urine Samples of the patient were collected. Probable diagnosis can be best evaluated by?**

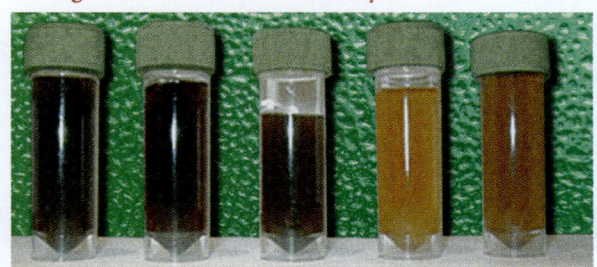

   a. Flow Cytometry
   b. Bone marrow examination
   c. 24 hour urinary Homogenetisic acid
   d. Urine myoglobin and serum creatinine

152. **Pancytopenia with cellular marrow is seen in all except:**
   a. Megaloblastic anemia   *(Recent Pattern 2014-15)*
   b. Myelodysplasia
   c. Paroxysmal Nocturnal hemoglobinuria
   d. G6PD deficiency

153. **P.N.H is associated with all of the following condition, except:** *(Recent Pattern 2014-15)*
   a. Aplastic anemia
   b. Increased LAP scores
   c. Venous thrombosis
   d. Iron deficiency anemia

154. **Reticulocytosis is seen in all except:**
   a. P.N.H   *(Recent Pattern 2014-15)*
   b. Hemolysis
   c. Nutritional anemia
   d. Dyserythropoietic syndrome

155. **Which of the following statements about paroxysmal cold hemoglobinuria is NOT true?** *(Recent Pattern 2014-15)*
   a. Chronic autoimmune form responds well to splenectomy
   b. Results from formation of Donath-Landsteiner antibody
   c. Attacks are associated with hemoglobinuria
   d. Can occur secondary to syphilis

156. **The gold standard test for the diagnosis of Paroxysmal Nocturnal Hemoglobinuria (PNH) is:** *(Recent Pattern 2014-15)*
   a. Flow cytometry   b. Sucrose hemolysis test
   c. HAM test   d. None

157. **PNH is associated with all of the following conditions, except** *(AI 2002)*
   a. Aplastic anemia   b. Increased LAP scores
   c. Venous thrombosis   d. Iron deficiency anemia

158. All of the following are true about PNH, Except:
    (PGI Dec 2000)
    a. Hypocellular marrow   b. Budd-chiari syndrome
    c. Thrombosis   d. LAP score low

159. Which of the following is NOT seen in Paroxysmal Nocturnal Hemoglobinuria: (AIIMS Nov 2000)
    a. Thrombosis   b. Hemosiderinuria
    c. Decreased LDH   d. Thrombocytopenia

160. Causes of Deep venous thrombosis include all of the following, Except. (AI 2009)
    a. Diabetes Mellitus
    b. Oral contraceptives
    c. Paroxysmal Nocturnal Hemoglobinuria (PNH)
    d. Prolonged surgery

161. Most common cause of Budd Chiari syndrome is:
    a. Idiopathic   (AIIMS May 94)
    b. Valves in hepatic veins
    c. Hepatocellular carcinoma
    d. Thrombosis of hepatic veins

Disorders of WBC & Leukemias

162. The following image shows   (AIIMS Nov 2018)

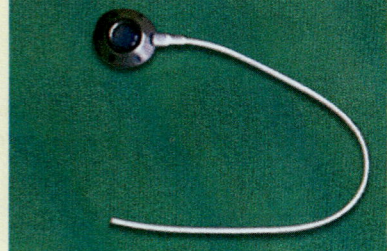

    a. Chemoport
    b. Ommaya reservoir
    c. Peripherally inserted Central catheter
    d. Thermo-probe

163. All of the following are associated with HHV8 except?
    (AIIMS May 2018)
    a. Kaposi sarcoma   b. Primary effusion lymphoma
    c. Castleman disease   d. Adult T-cell Leukemia

164. A young girl with APML on day 3 of treatment develops tachypnea, weight gain and fever. CXR shows bilateral pulmonary infiltrates. What is the best management for the patient? (AIIMS May 2017)
    a. Dexamethasone   b. Dacarbazine
    c. Cytarabine   d. Doxorubicin

165. L-Asparaginase is useful for treatment of?
    (AIIMS May 2016)
    a. ALL   b. CLL
    c. CML   d. AML

166. Which of the following has the least 5 year survival rate following allogenic bone marrow transplantation?
    (Recent Question 2016-17)
    a. Severe Combined Immunodeficiency state
    b. Aplastic Anemia
    c. Blast crisis in CML
    d. Chronic lymphocytic leukaemia

167. Leukostasis is common with which of the following?
    (Recent Question 2016-17)
    a. ALL   b. AML
    c. CML   d. CLL

168. Which organ is mainly affected in Leukostasis?
    (Recent Question 2016-17)
    a. Liver   b. Heart
    c. Kidney   d. Lung

169. Steroids are not indicated in the treatment of?
    (AIIMS Nov 2015)
    a. Kaposi Sarcoma   b. Hodgkin Lymphoma
    c. CLL   d. Multiple Myeloma

170. Most important best prognostic marker in ALL?
    a. Leucocyte count >50000 (AIIMS Nov 2015)
    b. Hyperploidy
    c. Response to treatment
    d. Organomegaly

171. Which of the following statements is true regarding juvenile chronic myeloid leukemia? (UPSC 2015)
    a. Philadelphia chromosome is negative.
    b. Thrombocytopenia is uncommon.
    c. The prognosis is better than the adult form of chronic myeloid leukemia.
    d. Single agent chemotherapy with Busulfan or Hydroxyurea can achieve remission

172. Treatment of choice in hairy cell leukemia is?
    (Bihar PG 2015)
    a. Steroid   b. Cladiribine
    c. Splenectomy   d. Pentostatin

173. 2-year-old child with ALL, which of the following has the best prognosis? (Recent Question 2015-16)
    a. Age between 1-10 years b. TLC >1 lac
    c. Petechiae   d. t(9:22)

174. Philadelphia chromosome refers:
    (Recent Question 2015-16)
    a. Long arm of chromosome 9 and long arm of chromosome 22
    b. Short arm of chromosome 9 and short arm of chromosome 22
    c. Short arm of chromosome 9 and long chromosome 22
    d. Long arm of chromosome 9 and short arm of chromosome 2

175. Vitamin B_{12} level in chronic myeloid leukemia is:
    (Recent Pattern 2014-15)
    a. Elevated   b. Decreased (slightly)
    c. Normal   d. Markedly decreased

176. Agranulocytosis is defined as neutrophil count less than:
    (Recent Pattern 2014-15)
    a. 100/ μL   b. 200/ μL
    c. 300/ μL   d. 500/ μL

177. What is the most effective treatment for chronic myeloid leukaemia? (Recent Pattern 2014-15)
    a. Allogeneic bone marrow transplantation
    b. Heterogeneic bone marrow transplantation
    c. Chemotherapy
    d. Hydroxyurea & interferon

178. What is the Neutrophil count for moderate neutropenia:
    (Recent Pattern 2014-15)
    a. < 500/mm³   b. 500-1000/mm³
    c. >1000/mm³   d. 100/mm³

179. Radiation exposure does not cause:
    (Recent Pattern 2014-15)
    a. ALL   b. AML
    c. CML   d. CLL
180. Filgrastim is used for the treatment of:
    (Recent Pattern 2014-15)
    a. Neutropenia   b. Anemia
    c. Polycythemia   d. Neutrophilia
181. Arsenic is used in treatment of: (Recent Pattern 2014-15)
    a. Acute Promyelocytic leukemia
    b. A.L.L
    c. CML
    d. Transient myeloproliferative disorder
182. Most common type of acute myeloid leukemia:
    (Recent Pattern 2014-15)
    a. M2   b. M3
    c. M4   d. M5
183. Which one of the following laboratory tests differentiates leukamoid reaction from chronic myeloid leukemia?
    (Recent Pattern 2014-15)
    a. LAP (leukocyte alkaline phosphatase)
    b. LCA (leukocyte common antigen)
    c. MPO (myelo-peroxidase)
    d. TRAP (tartrate resistant alkaline phosphatase)
184. DIC is seen in the following type of AML:
    (Recent Pattern 2014-15)
    a. M3   b. M4
    c. M2   d. M5
185. A 2-year-old child comes with ear discharge, seborrheic dermatitis, polyuria and hepatos-plenomegaly. Which of the following is the most likely diagnosis:
    a. Leukemia   (Recent Pattern 2014-15)
    b. Lymphoma
    c. Langerhan's cell histiocytosis
    d. Germ cell tumor
186. Gum hypertrophy is seen in which type of AML:
    a. Myelogenous leukaemia (Recent Pattern 2014-15)
    b. Myelomonocytic leukaemia
    c. Megakaryocytic leukaemia
    d. Erthroleukemia
187. 80-year-old, asymptomatic man present with a Total leucocyte count of 1 lakh, with 80% lymphocytes and 20% PMCs. What is the most probable diagnosis?
    (Recent Pattern 2014-15)
    a. HIV   b. CML
    c. CLL   d. TB
188. Treatment of choice of CNS leukemia is:
    a. Intrathecal methotrexate (Recent Pattern 2014-15)
    b. Vincristine and predinisolone
    c. Intrathecal vincristine
    d. Prednisolone
189. According to FAB classification, promyelocytic blood picture belongs to which type of AML?
    (Recent Pattern 2014-15)
    a. M0   b. M1
    c. M2   d. M3
190. Cis- Retinoic acid syndrome is used for?
    (Recent Pattern 2014-15)
    a. JMML   b. M3 AML
    c. M4 AML   d. CML

191. All of the following are features of juvenile CML except:
    a. Thrombocytopenia (Recent Pattern 2014-15)
    b. Fetal Hb is increased
    c. Philadelphia chromosome is positive
    d. Lymphadenopathy
192. A peripheral smear with increased neutrophils, basophils, eosinophils, and platelets is highly suggestive of:
    a. Actute myeloid leukemia (Recent Pattern 2014-15)
    b. Acute lymphoblastic leukemia
    c. Chronic myelogenous leukemia
    d. Myelodysplastic syndrome
193. Haemoglobin F is raised in: (AIIMS Dec 97)
    a. Juvenile chronic myeloid leukemia
    b. Hereditary spherocytosis
    c. Congenital red cell aplasia
    d. Myasthenia gravis
194. 'Which of the following is NOT used in treatment of hairy cell leukemia: (AIIMS Feb 97)
    a. Steroid   b. Pentostatin
    c. Splenectomy   d. Alpha-interferon
195. Chronic Lymphocytic Leukemia (CLL) is associated with:
    a. Individuals > 50 years of age (AI 2011)
    b. Mature small lymphocytes in peripheral smear
    c. Hepatosplenomegaly and lymphadenopathy
    d. All of the above
196. All of the following are features of juvenile CML except:
    a. Thrombocytopenia (AI 94)
    b. Fetal Hb is increased
    c. Philadelphia chromosome is positive
    d. Lymphadenopathy
197. Marker specific for myeloid lineage- (AIIMS Nov 95)
    a. CD33   b. CD14
    c. CD13   d. MPO
198. Which of the following is a good prognostic factor in ALL:
    (PGI 2008)
    a. High WBC count b. Male sex
    c. Age < 2 years d. Hyperdiploidy
199. Treatment of choice in intracranial ALL is: (PGI June 99)
    a. Intrathecal methotrexate
    b. Vincristine and prednisolone
    c. Intrathecal vincristine
    d. Prednisolon
200. While handling a febrile neutropenic patient all are essential except: (AI 1998)
    a. Repeated hand washing of hospital person
    b. White cell infusion
    c. Prophylactic antibiotic
    d. Colony stimulating factor for macrophages

Lymphomas

201. A 20-year-old boy presents with cervical Lymphadenopathy. Histology of lymph node biopsy shows RS cells with background reactive with T lymphocytes. The cells are positiive for CD20, LCA, EMA and negative for CD 15 and CD 30. What is the diagnosis? (AIIMS May 2017)
    a. Nodular lymphocytic predominant
    b. T cell rich B cell lymphoma
    c. Nodular sclerosis HL
    d. Chronic lymphocytic leukemia

202. Pop corn variant of Reed-Sternberg cell is seen in:
(Recent Pattern 2014-15)
a. Follicular center lymphoma
b. Lymphocyte depleted Hodgkin's disease
c. Nodular sclerosis Hodgkin's disease
d. Lymphocyte predominant Hodgkin's disease

203. Which of the following statements on lymphoma is not True? (Recent Pattern 2014-15)
a. A single classification system of Hodgkin's disease is almost universally accepted
b. HD tends to remain localized to a single group of lymph nodes and spreads by contiguity
c. Several types of Non-Hodgkin's lymphoma may have a leukemic phase
d. In general follicular NHL has worse prognosis compared to diffuse NHL

204. In Ritcher's transformation CLL transforms into:
a. Large B cell Lymphoma (Recent Pattern 2014-15)
b. Anaplastic carcinoma
c. Burkitt lymphoma
d. Lymphoproliferative lymphoma

205. Reedsternberg cells are: (Recent Pattern 2014-15)
a. B cells
b. T cells
c. Natural killer cells
d. All of above

206. 'ABVD' regimen is used in: (Recent Pattern 2014-15)
a. Chronic lymphocytic leukemia
b. Acute lymphoblastic leukemia
c. N.H.L
d. Hodgkin's disease

207. In lymphoplasmacytoid lymphoma which of the following monoclonal immunoglobulin is seen:
(Recent Pattern 2014-15)
a. IgA
b. IgD
c. IgG
d. IgM

208. Most common type of Hodgkin's lymphoma is: (AI 1996)
a. Nodular sclerosis
b. Lymphocyte predominance
c. Mixed cellularity
d. Lymphocyte depletion

209. Classical markers for Hodgkin's disease is- (AIPGMEE 08)
a. CD 15 and CD 30
b. CD 15 and CD 22
c. CD 15 and CD 20
d. CD 20 and CD 30

210. All of the following are good prognostic features of Hodgkin's disease except: (AI 04)
a. Haemoglobin>10 gm/dl
b. WBC count<15000/mm^3
c. Absolute lymphocyte count<600/μl
d. Age < 45 yrs

211. The classification proposed by the International Lymphoma Study Group for non-Hodgkin's lymphoma is known as:
a. Kiel classification (AI 2005)
b. REAL classification
c. WHO classification
d. Rappaport classification

212. Burkitt's Lymphoma is associated with: (AI 2010)
a. t (8:14)
b. t (11:14)
c. t (15:17)
d. t (14:18)

Platelet and Bleeding Disorders

213. A patient with ITP on steroids underwent splenectomy. Patient got fever on 3rd post-operative day. Next investigation is likely to reveal? (AIIMS May 2015)
a. Left lower lobe consolidation
b. Port site infection
c. Focal Intra-abdominal collection
d. UTI

214. Clotting factor activated on platelets? (JIPMER May 2015)
a. 8
b. 9
c. 10
d. 11

215. Which statement is most appropriate for DIC?
a. Increased fibrinogen (JIPMER Nov 2014)
b. Increased D dimer
c. Resolves if causative factor removed
d. Absence of bleeding abnormalities rules out DIC

216. Thrombocythemia is characterized by:
(Recent Question 2015-16)
a. Platelets elevation
b. Low Platelets
c. Neutrophilia
d. Monocytosis

217. A Patient has ecchymosis and petechiae all over the body with no hepato-splenomegaly. All are true except?
(Recent Pattern 2014-15)
a. Increased megakaryocytes in bone narrow.
b. Bleeding into the joints
c. Decreased platelet in blood
d. Disease resolves itself in 80% of Patients in 2-6 weeks.

218. Which of the following is given to treat thrombocytopenia secondary to anti-cancer therapy and is known to stimulate progenitor megakaryocytes? (Recent Pattern 2014-15)
a. Filgrastim
b. Oprelvekin
c. Erythropoietin
d. Anagrelide

219. Platelets transfusion must be completed in:
(Recent Pattern 2014-15)
a. 1 hours
b. 2 hours
c. 3 hours
d. 4 hours

220. Seen in D.I.C all except: (Recent Pattern 2014-15)
a. Hyperfibrinogenemia
b. Increase fibrin degradation products
c. Prolonged PT
d. Increased APTT

221. Which one of the following is not used in DIC?
(Recent Pattern 2014-15)
a. Heparin
b. Epsilon amino caproic acid
c. Blood transfusion
d. I.V. fluids

222. Platelets in stored blood do not live after:
(Recent Pattern 2014-15)
a. 24 hours
b. 48 hours
c. 72 hours
d. 96 hours

223. False statement regarding DIC is: (Recent Pattern 2014-15)
a. Thrombocytopenia
b. Decreased fibrinogen
c. Decreased aPTT
d. Increased PT

224. Anti-coagulant of choice for heparin induced thrombocytopenia is: (Recent Pattern 2014-15)
a. Lepirudin
b. Aprotinin
c. Abciximab
d. Plasminogen

225. **Disseminated intravascular coagulation can occur in all of the following except:** *(Recent Pattern 2014-15)*
    a. Snake bite
    b. Placenta praevia
    c. Falciparum malaria
    d. Haemophilia

226. **Which of the following drugs does not act by blocking Gp IIb/IIIa receptors?** *(Recent Pattern 2014-15)*
    a. Abciximab
    b. Eptifibatide
    c. Tirofiban
    d. Clopidogrel

227. **A 25-year-old female presented with history of recurrent abortions. The most relevant investi-gation to identify the cause is:** *(Recent Pattern 2014-15)*
    a. Bleeding time
    b. Prothrombin time
    c. Dilute russel viper venom time
    d. Clot solubility test

228. **Thrombotic event is seen in all of following except:**
    a. PNH   *(Recent Pattern 2014-15)*
    b. DIC
    c. ITP
    d. Heparin induced thrombocytopenia

229. **Purpura fulminans is seen in:** *(Recent Pattern 2014-15)*
    a. Protein C deficiency
    b. Protein S deficiency
    c. AT III deficiency
    d. Factor 5 leiden mutation

230. **Feature of hemorrhagic disease of new born is:**
    a. Prolonged prothrombin time   *(Recent Pattern 2014-15)*
    b. Defective platelet count
    c. Prolonged bleeding time
    d. Prolonged thrombin time

231. **Idiopathic Thrombocytopenic purpura is associated with:** *(Recent Pattern 2014-15)*
    a. Small megakaryoblasts
    b. Non palpable purpura
    c. Massive splenomegaly
    d. Evan syndrome

232. **Bleeding crisis in acute Idiopathic thrombo-cytopenic Purpura is managed by all except:** *(Recent Pattern 2014-15)*
    a. RhIG
    b. Prednisolone
    c. Intravenous immunoglobulin
    d. Eltrombopag

233. **The following is not true of platelet transfusion:**
    a. Useful in ITP   *(Recent Pattern 2014-15)*
    b. Used in D.I.C.
    c. Effective for 9-10 days
    d. Effect decrease with repeated usage

234. **Shelf life of platelets in blood bank is:** *(Recent Pattern 2014-15)*
    a. 5 days
    b. 7 days
    c. 10 days
    d. 21 days

235. **Bleeding tendencies are common in:**
    a. Chronic myeloid leukaemia   *(Recent Pattern 2014-15)*
    b. Chronic lymphocytic leukaemia
    c. Acute monocytic leukaemia
    d. None of the above

236. **All of the following are true about Warfarin therapeutic usage except** *(Recent Pattern 2014-15)*
    a. The INR is maintained between 2 & 3
    b. It is very useful in the prophylaxis of thrombo-embolism
    c. It's effect is monitored by observing the clotting time
    d. Used in DVT

237. **Storage temperature of platelets is:** *(Recent Pattern 2014-15)*
    a. - 4 degrees Celsius
    b. + 4 degrees Celsius
    c. - 20 degrees Celsius
    d. + 20-24 degrees Celsius

238. **Which of the following is the finding in functional defect in platelets?** *(Recent Pattern 2014-15)*
    a. Normal platelet counts and prolonged bleeding time
    b. Normal platelet count and bleeding time
    c. Prolonged bleeding time, prothrombin time and PTT
    d. Thrombocytopenia and prolonged bleeding time

239. **Pawn ball megakaryocytes are characteristic of:**
    a. Myelodysplastic syndrome   *(Recent Pattern 2014-15)*
    b. idiopathic thrombocytopenic purpura
    c. Thrombotic thrombocytopenic purpura
    d. Chloramphenicol toxicity

240. **Bleeding time is increased in all except:** *(Recent Pattern 2014-15)*
    a. Thrombocytopenia
    b. Thrombasthenia
    c. Renal failure
    d. Acquired hemophilia

241. **Which one of the following platelet counts is usually associated with increased incidence of spontaneous bleeding** *(Recent Pattern 2014-15)*
    a. Greater than 80,000/mm^3
    b. 40,000/mm^3
    c. 20,000 mm^3
    d. Less than 20,000 mm^3

242. **The presence of small sized platelets on the peripheral smear is characteristic of:** *(Recent Pattern 2014-15)*
    a. Idiopathic thrombocytopenic purpura
    b. Bernard soulier syndrome
    c. Disseminated intravascular coagulation
    d. Wiskott Aldrich syndrome

243. **DIC is most likely characterized by:** *(Recent Pattern 2014-15)*
    a. Significant numbers of schistocytes
    b. A brisk reticulocytosis
    c. Decreased coagulation factor levels
    d. Significant thrombocytopenia

244. **A patient is on aspirin, what will be the finding?** *(AI 2007)*
    a. Prolonged BT
    b. Prolonged PT
    c. Prolonged APTT
    d. Prolonged CT

245. **The commonest mode of inheritance of Von Willebrand's disease :** *(AIIMS Dec 97)*
    a. Codominant
    b. Autosomal recessive
    c. Autosomal dominant
    d. X-linked recessive

246. **The presence of small sized platelets on the peripheral smear is characteristic of:** *(AIIMS Nov 03)*
    a. Idiopathic thrombocytopenic purpura
    b. Bernard soulier syndrome
    c. Disseminated intravascular coagulation
    d. Wiskott Aldrich syndrome

247. **Thrombocytopenia occurs in all *except*:** *(AI 2001)*
    a. Henoch schonlein purpura
    b. TTP
    c. DIC
    d. Wiskott Aldrich syndrome

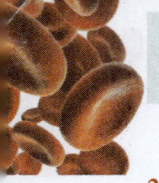

248. **Autoimmune destruction of platelet is seen in:**
    (AIIMS May 95)
    a. SLE
    b. Rheumatoid arthritis
    c. Reiter disease
    d. Polyarteritis nodosa

249. **Palpable purpura is seen in** *(AIIMS May 94)*
    a. Idiopathic thrombocytopenic purpura (ITP)
    b. Scurvy
    c. Henoch Sconlein Purpura
    d. Monoclonal cryoglubinemia

250. **Idiopathic thrombocytopenic purpura is associated with all of the following Except:** *(Recent Pattern Question)*
    a. Splenomegaly
    b. Mucosal bleeding
    c. Thrombocytopenia
    d. Increased megakaryocytes

251. **Platelet transfusion is not indicated in:** *(AI 1996)*
    a. Dilutional Thrombocytopenia
    b. Immunogenic Thrombocytopenia
    c. Aplastic Anemia
    d. DIC

252. **All of the following statements about Thrombotic thrombocytopenic purpura (TTP) are true, Except :**
    (Recent Pattern Question)
    a. Microangiopathic Hemolytic Anemia
    b. Thrombocytopenia
    c. Normal complement levels
    d. Grossly abnormal coagulation tests

Von Willebrand Disease and Clotting Factor Defects

253. **Which of the following is the best test to diagnose bleeding in DIC?** *(AIIMS May 2018)*
    a. Increased PT
    b. Increased aPTT
    c. Decreased fibrinogen
    d. Increased Fibrin degradation products

254. **Girl with mild vWF previous history of heavy bleeding during tooth extraction. What is the prophylaxis to be given before tooth extraction?** *(JIPMER Nov 2014)*
    a. Desmopressin
    b. Blood transfusion
    c. Fresh frozen plasma
    d. Cryoprecipitate

255. **Girl with von-willebrand disease. Prophylactic action to be taken before wisdom tooth extraction?** *(JIMPER 2014)*
    a. Epsilon aminocaproic acid
    b. Cryoprecipitate
    c. Desmopressin
    d. Abciximab

256. **Rarest type of von willebrand disease:**
    (Recent Pattern 2014-15)
    a. vWD type 1
    b. vWD type 2A
    c. vWD type 2N
    d. vWD type 3

257. **Most common cause of DIC is:** *(Recent Pattern 2014-15)*
    a. Sepsis
    b. Placenta previa
    c. Abruption placentae
    d. Snake bite

258. **A 45-year-old lady with normal PT and increased aPTT. About 2 year back, she was operated for cholecystectomy & did not have any bleeding episode. What is next investigation for clinical diagnosis** *(Recent Pattern 2014-15)*
    a. Factor VIII assay
    b. Dilute russel viper venom assay
    c. Platelet aggregation test
    d. Ristocetin Cofactor assay

259. **Most common inherited bleeding disorder:**
    a. Von wilebrand disease *(Recent Pattern 2014-15)*
    b. Bernard soulier
    c. Glanzmann thrombasthenia
    d. ITP acute

260. **In Hemophilia B what is most common cause of death?**
    a. Hemorrhage *(Recent Pattern 2014-15)*
    b. HIV,HBV, HCV due to transfusions
    c. Transfusion reactions
    d. Deep vein thrombosis

261. **Anti-factor VIII antibodies are seen in:**
    a. Postpartum *(Recent Pattern 2014-15)*
    b. Hemophilia who have received infusion of plasmaconcentrates
    c. Both A & B
    d. None

262. **The coagulation profile in a 13-year-old girl with Menorrhagia having von Willebrands disease is:**
    (Recent Pattern 2014-15)
    a. Isolated prolonged PTT with a normal PT
    b. Isolated prolonged PT with a normal PTT
    c. Prolongation of both PT and PTT
    d. Prolongation of thrombin time

263. **von Willebrand's disease is usually inherited as**
    (Recent Pattern 2014-15)
    a. Autosomal dominant
    b. Autosomal recessive
    c. X-linked recessive
    d. Multicentric

264. **Not useful for treatment of hemophilia B?**
    a. FFP *(Recent Pattern 2014-15)*
    b. Cryoprecipitate
    c. Factor 9 concentrates
    d. Prothrombin complex concentrates

265. **All are true about hemophilia,** *except* *(AIIMS May 94)*
    a. Increased Bleeding time (BT)
    b. Decreased factor VIII
    c. Decreased factor IX
    d. Increased partial thromboplastin time (PTT)

266. **False statement regarding DIC is:** *(AI 2001)*
    a. Thrombocytopenia
    b. Decreased fibrinogen
    c. Decreased PTT
    d. Increased PT

267. **The most sensitive test for DIC is:** *(AI 2001)*
    a. Serum fibrinogen levels
    b. Serum levels of fibrin degradation products (FDP)
    c. Prolonged PT and PTT
    d. Thrombocytopenia

268. **Predisposing factor for arterial thrombosis:** *(PGI Dec. 04)*
    a. AT III deficiency
    b. Protein S deficiency
    c. Protein C deficiency
    d. Homocystenemia

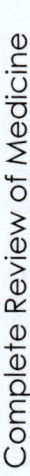

Multiple Myeloma

269. A 70-year-old male patient has single well-defined lytic lesion of skull. The patient had no other complaint and urine examination had no abnormality. What is the most likely diagnosis? *(Recent Pattern 2019)*

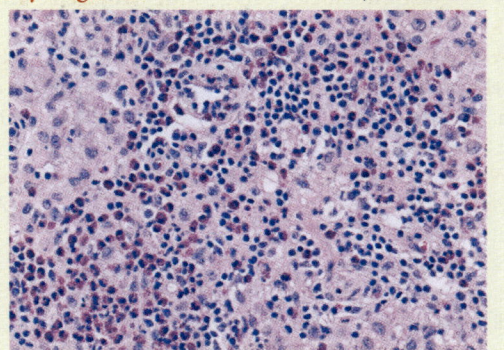

   a. Unifocal Langerhans cell histiocytosis
   b. Monoclonal Gammopathy of unknown significance
   c. Multiple myeloma
   d. Paget's disease

270. Commonest site of lytic lesion, in multiple myeloma is? *(Bihar PG 2015)*
   a. Vertebral column   b. Femur
   c. Clavicle   d. Pelvis

271. Bone scan of multiple myeloma shows? *(JIPMER Nov 2014)*
   a. Diffuse increased uptake
   b. Diffuse decreased uptake
   c. Hot spot
   d. Cold spot

272. Which of the following is the least common feature of Multiple Myeloma? *(Recent Pattern 2014-15)*
   a. Bone pain
   b. Normocytic Normochromic Anemia
   c. Susceptibility to bacterial Infection
   d. Hyperviscosity syndrome

273. Most common heavy chain disease is:
   a. Franklin disease   *(Recent Pattern 2014-15)*
   b. Seligmann disease (Alpha heavy chain disease)
   c. Mu heavy chain disease
   d. Waldenstrom cryoglobulinemia

274. Most common cause of kidney involvement in multiple myeloma: *(Recent Pattern 2014-15)*
   a. Hypercalcemia   b. Amyloid deposition
   c. Tubular proteinuria d. Hyperviscosity

275. Increased ESR is seen in all, except: *(Recent Pattern 2014-15)*
   a. Rheumatic fever   b. Multiple myeloma
   c. Sickle cell anaemia d. Tuberculosis

276. Which of the following is associated with Bence jones proteinuria? *(Recent Pattern 2014-15)*
   a. γ chain disease
   b. α chain disease
   c. λ chain disease
   d. mu chain disease

277. Immunoglobulin not affected in Multiple myeloma: *(Recent Pattern 2014-15)*
   a. IgG   b. IgA
   c. IgM   d. IgD

278. All of the following are true about multiple myeloma except: *(Recent Pattern 2014-15)*
   a. Lytic bone lesions   b. Back pain
   c. Polycythemia   d. Viscosity of blood

279. Most common cause of death in multiple myeloma is: *(Recent Pattern 2014-15)*
   a. Infection   b. Bleeding
   c. CHF   d. Kidney failure

280. Maximum ESR is seen in: *(Recent Pattern 2014-15)*
   a. CHF   b. Polycythemia vera
   c. Multiple myeloma   d. Sickle cell anemia

281. Kappa light chains in urine are seen in:
   a. Mu chain disease   *(Recent Pattern 2014-15)*
   b. Seligman disease
   c. Franklin disease
   d. Waldenstrom macroglobulinemia

282. Most common clinical feature of multiple myeloma: *(Recent Pattern 2014-15)*
   a. Bone pain   b. Anemia
   c. Hypercalcemia   d. Bleeding

283. Classical 'Rain drop' lesions seen in: *(Recent Pattern 2014-15)*
   a. Burkitt's lymphoma   b. Hodgkin's lymphoma
   c. Multiple myeloma   d. Haemophilia

284. Commonest site of lytic lesion in multiple myeloma is: *(Recent Pattern 2014-15)*
   a. Vertebral column   b. Femur
   c. Clavicle   d. Pelvis

285. Which of the following is the least common feature of Multiple Myeloma: *(AI 2012)*
   a. Bone pain
   b. Normocytic Normochromic Anemia
   c. Susceptibility to bacterial infection
   d. Hyperviscosity syndrome

286. All of the following are minor criteria for multiple Myeloma, Except *(AIIMS Nov 2010)*
   a. Plasmacytosis 20%   b. Multiple lytic lesions
   c. Plasmacytoma on tissue biopsy
   d. Monoclonal Ig spike < 2g/dl for IgA and < 3.5 for IgG

287. Commonest site of lytic lesion, in multiple myeloma is
   a. Vertebral column   b. Femur   *(AIIMS Dec 97)*
   c. Clavicle   d. Pelvis

288. Raised serum alkaline phosphatase is seen in all, *except* *(AIIMS Dec 94)*
   a. Paget's disease   b. Multiple myeloma
   c. Osteomalacia   d. Hyperthyroidism

289. An 80-year-old asymptomatic woman was detected to have a monoclonal spike on serum electrophoresis (IgG levels 1.5 g/dl). Bone marrow revealed plasma cells of 8%. The most likely diagnosis is: *(AI 2004)*
   a. Multiple myeloma   b. Indolent myeloma
   c. Monoclonal gammopathy of unknown significance
   d. Waldenstorm's macroglobulinemia

290. Franklin's disease is associated with: *(AIIMS May 95)*
   a. Gamma heavy chain disease
   b. Multiple myeloma
   c. Alpha heavy chain disease
   d. Waldenstorm's macroglobulinemia

Myeloproliferative and Other Bone Marrow Disorders

291. Match the following treatable causes, to be looked for, when the following haematological diseases are diagnosed and choose the best combination (APPG 2016)

    P Myelodysplastic syndrome   X Look for tuberculosis infection
    Q Myelophthisicanemia   Y Look for B19 parvovirus infection
    R Pure red cell aplasia   Z Look for B12/folate/B6 deficiency

    a. PQR = VXY   b. PQR = UXZ
    c. PQR = VWZ   d. PQR = ZXY

292. Polycythaemia is commonly seen in: (Recent Pattern 2014-15)
    a. Congestive cardiac failure b. Hereditary spherocytosis
    c. Chronic corpulmonale   d. Uncomplicated ASD

293. Polycythemia vera is absolute venous hematocrit of >: (Recent Pattern 2014-15)
    a. 45%   b. 55%
    c. 65%   d. 70%

294. Most common myeloproliferative disorder:
    a. Polycyathemia vera (Recent Pattern 2014-15)
    b. CML
    c. Chronic eosinophilic leukemia
    d. Myelofibrosis

295. Which one of the following is not commonly seen in polycythemia vera? (Recent Pattern 2014-15)
    a. Thrombosis
    b. Hyperuricemia
    c. Prone for acute leukemia
    d. Spontaneous severe infection

296. All of the following are true regarding myelo-fibrosis except: (Recent Pattern 2014-15)
    a. Tear drop poikilocytes
    b. Giant abnormal platelets
    c. Leucoerythroblastic blood picture
    d. Absent spleen

297. True about polycythemia rubra vera is all except:
    a. Bleeding (Recent Pattern 2014-15)
    b. Thrombosis
    c. ↓ed ESR
    d. Increased erythropoietin

298. Myeloproliferative diseases include all except:
    a. Myelofibrosis (Recent Pattern 2014-15)
    b. Chronic neutrophilic leukemia
    c. Acute myelogenous leukemia (AML)
    d. Systemic mastocytosis

299. Polycythaemia vera is associated with all except:
    a. Increased red cell mass (Recent Pattern 2014-15)
    b. Leukocytosis
    c. Splenomegaly
    d. Decreased platelet count

300. Not seen in Polycythemia Vera: (Recent Pattern 2014-15)
    a. Budd chiari syndrome   b. Hypertension
    c. Erythromelalgia   d. Infections

301. Essential WHO criteria for polycythemia vera:
    a. Tyrosine kinase JAK2 mutation (Recent Pattern 2014-15)
    b. Low levels of erythropoietin levels
    c. Thrombocytosis
    d. Increased MCV

302. A 59-year-old male came with Hb 18.0 gm/dl on three occasions. The resident doctor wants to exclude Polycythemia Vera. Which of the following is the most relevant investigation: (AIIMS May 04)
    a. Hematocrit   b. Total leukocyte count
    c. Red cell mass   d. Reticulocyte count

303. Which of the following is not commonly seen in Polycythemia Vera? (AI 2002)
    a. Thrombosis
    b. Hyperuricemia
    c. Prone for acute leukemia
    d. Spontaneous severe infection

304. In Polycythemia vera, all the following are seen except: (AIIMS May 01)
    a. Thrombocytopenia   b. Increased GI bleed
    c. Thrombosis   d. Transient visual loss

305. Which is not seen in polycythemia vera: (AIIMS Feb 97)
    a. Increased Vit B_{12} binding capacity
    b. Increase erythropoietin level
    c. Increase RBC count
    d. Ocular congestion

306. A pt. being investigated for anemia has a dry marrow tap; peripheral smear reveals tear drop cells; likely diagnosis is: (AI 2001)
    a. Leukemia   b. Lymphoma
    c. Myelofibrosis   d. Polycythemia rubra vera

Miscellaneous

307. Biopsy report of an 8-year-old child with leg swelling shows a round blue cell tumor consistent with diagnosis of Ewing's Sarcoma. What will be the best method to detect translocation t(11:22) in this malignancy? (AIIMS May 2018)
    a. Conventional karyotyping b. Next generation sequencing
    c. FISH   d. PCR

308. All of the following are correct about the procedure that is carried out with the instrument except? (AIIMS May 2016)

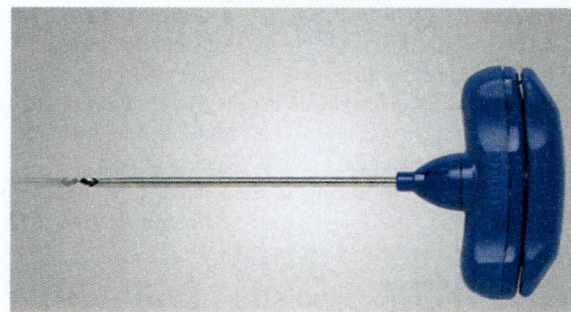

    a. Procedure carried out in lateral or prone position
    b. Useful in diagnosis of infiltrative and granulomatous conditions
    c. Platelet count of 40,000/cu.mm is a contraindication
    d. Breath holding is not necessary during this procedure

309. **RUNT disease is?** *(Recent Question 2016-17)*
    a. GVHD
    b. Hyper-acute rejection
    c. Acute rejection
    d. Chronic rejection
310. **Which is not seen in graft verus host disease?**
    (Recent Question 2016-17)
    a. Dermatitis
    b. Enteritis
    c. Hepatitis
    d. Nephritis
311. **Which is not a feature of HELLP syndrome?**
    a. Renal failure *(Recent Question 2016-17)*
    b. Sub-capsular liver hematomas
    c. Low platelets
    d. Rhabdomyolysis
312. **All of the following statements are true regarding Anti-lymphocyte Serum (ALS) except?** *(APPG 2016)*
    a. Unlike other mmune-suppressive agents, ALS is devoid of any action other than that on lymphocytes
    b. ALS acts only against lymphocytes in circulation and not on cells in the lymphoid organs
    c. ALS is a homologous antiserum raised against lymphocytes
    d. Effect of ALS decreases on repeated administration
313. **Consider the following features?** *(UPSC 2015)*
    a. X-linked recessive inheritance
    b. Atopic dermatitis
    c. Low serum levels of IgA
    d. Small platelets
314. **Schistocytes are seen in:** *(Recent Question 2015-16)*
    a. HUS
    b. TTP
    c. DIC
    d. All of the above
315. **All of the following are Vitamin-K deficiency features except** *(Recent Question 2015-16)*
    a. Associated thrombocytopenia with prolonged bleeding
    b. Deficiency is rarely seen, except in infants
    c. Factor X is first to be affected
    d. Warfarin causes Vitamin K deficiency
316. **60-year-old person presents with history of angina and shortness of breath for the past week. Blood withdrawn shows thick brownish red color. Diagnosis?**
    (Recent Question 2015-16)
    a. Sickle cell anemia
    b. Hemolytic anemia
    c. Meth-hemoglobinaemia
    d. G-6-P-deficiency
317. **Which organism causes infection after splenectomy:**
    (Recent Question 2015-16)
    a. H. Influenza
    b. Staph aureus
    c. E.coli
    d. Klebsiella
318. **Which of the following is NOT a hyper-coagulable state**
    (Recent Question 2015-16)
    a. Pregnancy
    b. MI
    c. Abruptio-placentae
    d. Cirrhosis
319. **Priapism can be due to?** *(Recent Question 2015-16)*
    a. C.M.L
    b. Myelo-fibrosis
    c. A.I.H.A.
    d. Thrombocytopenia
320. **Hairy cell leukemia is** *(Recent Question 2015-16)*
    a. B cell tumor
    b. T cell tumor
    c. NK cell tumor
    d. All of above
321. **Identify the RBC type in a patient awaiting liver transplantation:**

    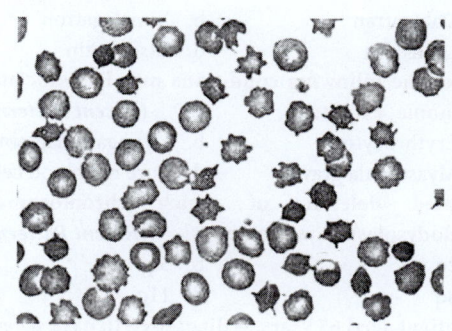

    a. Schistocyte
    b. Acanthocyte
    c. Starry sky pattern
    d. Tear drop RBC
322. **Identify the RBC in a patient with a mechanical prosthetic aortic valve because of aortic stenosis:**

    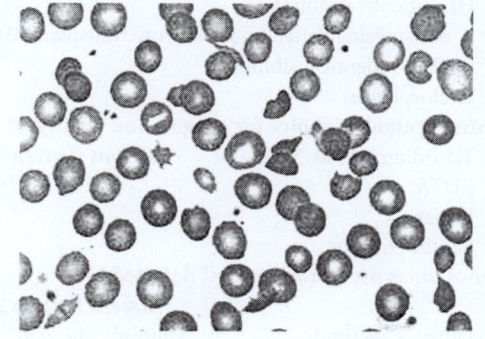

    a. Schistocyte
    b. Acanthocyte
    c. Poikiocytosis
    d. Spur cells
323. **A 20-year-old male has features of acute renal failure. Blood examination shows thrombocytopenia and Hb=10 gm%. Likely cause is:**

    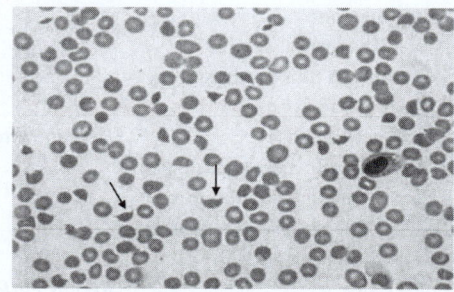

    a. HUS
    b. Hereditary spherocytosis
    c. Hemolytic crisis
    d. Chronic glomerulonephritis
324. **Pregnant lady on her ANC has family history of thromboembolism (factor v leiden deficiency) in heterozygous state. So next management is?**
    a. Warfarin *(JIPMER 2014)*
    b. Heparin
    c. Aspirin
    d. Observation and calf pain report ASAP
325. **Leukoerythroblastic picture may be seen in all of the following except:** *(Recent Pattern 2014-15)*
    a. Myelofibrosis
    b. Metastatic carcinoma
    c. Gaucher's disease
    d. Thalassemia

326. **Recent oral direct thrombin inhibitor which can be used for prevention of stroke is:** *(Recent Pattern 2014-15)*
    a. Dabigatran
    b. Ximelagatron
    c. Lepirudin
    d. Saxagliptin

327. **All of the following conditions may be associated with a thymoma, except:** *(Recent Pattern 2014-15)*
    a. Erythrocytosis
    b. Hypogammaglobulinemia
    c. Myasthenia gravis
    d. Pure red blood cell aplasia

328. **Isolated deletion of which chromosome causes myelodysplastic syndrome:** *(Recent Pattern 2014-15)*
    a. 2q
    b. 5q
    c. 8q
    d. 11q

329. **A patient aged 65 years, is diagnosed to have severe aplastic anemia. HLA compatible sibling is available. The best option of treatment is:** *(Recent Pattern 2014-15)*
    a. Anti-thymocyte globulin followed by cyclosporine
    b. A conventional bone marrow transplantation from the HLA identical sibling
    c. A non-myeloablative bone marrow transplant-ation from the HLA identical sibling
    d. Cyclosporine

330. **Anticoagulant of choice for coagulation testing is?**
    a. Trisodium citrate 3.2% *(Recent Pattern 2014-15)*
    b. EDTA
    c. Heparin
    d. Sodium oxalate

331. **Bence Jones proteinuria is best detected by?** *(Recent Pattern 2014-15)*
    a. Dipstick method
    b. Sulfosalicylic acid
    c. Heat test
    d. Electrophoresis

332. **Which is best to prevent rejection after bone marrow transplantation in aplastic anemia?** *(Recent Pattern 2014-15)*
    a. Anti-thymocyte globulin + cyclosporine
    b. Prednisolone
    c. Cyclosporine
    d. Tacrolimus plus prednisolone

333. **Anti-D (Rho) Ig is used for the prevention of:**
    a. Sickle cell disease *(Recent Pattern 2014-15)*
    b. Hemorrhagic disease of newborn
    c. Paroxysmal haemoglobinuria
    d. Hemolytic disease of newborn
    e. Small sized spleen

334. **Apheresis is:** *(Recent Pattern 2014-15)*
    a. Selective separation of components of blood
    b. Preventing blood transfusion infections (HIV, HBV)
    c. Separation of platelets from plasma
    d. Isolating organisms from mixed culture

335. **Which of the following is the most common organ of origin causing cancer related death in female <20 years?** *(Recent Pattern 2014-15)*
    a. Breast
    b. Cervix
    c. Bone marrow
    d. Lung

336. **Bone marrow transplantation indicated in all except:** *(Recent Pattern 2014-15)*
    a. Osteopetrosis
    b. Mucopolysaccharidosis
    c. Hemochromatosis
    d. Beta-Thalassemia

337. **Apixaban is a new drug that acts by:** *(Recent Pattern 2014-15)*
    a. Inhibiting TNF alpha
    b. Inhibiting coagulation factor Xa
    c. Inhibiting platelet aggregation
    d. Activating plasminogen

338. **Which of the following statements about erythropoietin is FALSE?** *(Recent Pattern 2014-15)*
    a. It is used for the treatment of anemia due to chronic renal failure
    b. It results in decrease in reticulocyte count
    c. It decrease the requirement of blood transfusions
    d. It can cause hypertension

339. **All of the following are WHO classified Myelodysplastic Syndromes except:** *(Recent Pattern 2014-15)*
    a. CML
    a. Refractory anemia with excess blasts
    c. Refractory anemia with ringed sideroblasts
    d. Refractory anemia

340. **All of the following statements regarding the lupus anticoagulant (LA) are true except:** *(Recent Pattern 2014-15)*
    a. Las typically prolong the activated partial thromboplastin time
    b. A 1:1 mixing study will not correct in the presence of Las
    c. Bleeding episodes in patients with Las may be severe and life threatening
    d. Female patients may experience recurrent midtrimester abortions

341. **All are true about warfarin, except:** *(Recent Pattern 2014-15)*
    a. It causes inhibition of vitamin K dependent clotting factors
    b. Its half-life is 36 hours
    c. It can cross placenta
    d. Its dose is increased in liver disease

342. **Pancytopenia is a feature of:** *(Recent Pattern 2014-15)*
    a. Dengue fever
    b. Enteric fever
    c. SLE
    d. All of the above

343. **Erythropoietin is increased in all of the following conditions except:** *(Recent Pattern 2014-15)*
    a. Hepatocellular carcinoma
    b. Renal cell carcinoma
    c. Cerebellar Hemangioblastoma
    d. Pancreatic carcinoma

344. **Which of the following drugs is not recommended in septic shock?** *(Recent Pattern 2014-15)*
    a. Normal saline
    b. Activated protein C
    c. Steroids
    d. Rituximab

345. **Reduction in neural tube defects with folic acid supplementation:** *(Recent Pattern 2014-15)*
    a. 40%
    b. 50%
    c. 60%
    d. 70%

346. **Direct Coomb's test detects the presence of antibodies on the surface of erythrocytes by using:**
    (Recent Pattern 2014-15)
    a. Sensitization of red cells with the antibody globulin
    b. Anti-human globulin antiserum
    c. Incomplete antibody
    d. Non-agglutinating antibody

347. **Thiamine deficiency is known to occur in all of the following *except*:** *(AI 2003)*
    a. Food Faddist
    b. Homocystinemia
    c. Chronic alcoholic
    d. Chronic heart failure patient on diuretics

348. **All of the following are the causes of relative polycythemia *except*:** *(AI 2005)*
    a. Dehydration
    b. Dengue haemorrhagic fever
    c. Gaisbock syndrome
    d. High altitude

349. **Feature of hemorrhagic disease of new born is-**
    a. Prolonged prothrombin time *(AIIMS June 97)*
    b. Defective platelet count
    c. Prolonged bleeding time
    d. Prolonged thrombin times

Answers with Explanations

ABO System, Blood Transfusions and Blood Components

1. Ans. (a) 15 ml/kg

(Ref: Harrison 20th edition, p 854 and Blood banking and transfusion medicine by Hillyer: 2nd edition, p 490)

- An FFP volume of 15 mL/kg (approximately 4 units in a 70 kg adult) is typically sufficient to reverse coagulopathy caused by warfarin toxicity.
- Ideally *prothrombin complex concentrates* at 50-100 units/kg IV at 12-hour interval is given for major bleeding episodes in warfarin toxicity. Recombinant factor VIIa is also used to reverse the coagulopathy in hours. Oral vitamin K1 is given in absence of serious/ life-threatening hemorrhage.

2. Ans. (d) AB +

(Ref: Crash course in Clinical hematology and immunology: 5th edition, p 204)

Group AB plasma does not contain any Anti-A or Anti- B or Anti-AB antibodies. Hence group AB plasma can be given to patients who are group AB, A, B or O. Hence, they are called universal FFP donor.

Universal Blood donor	O negative
Universal Blood Acceptor	AB positive
Universal FFP donor	AB positive
Universal FFP acceptor	O negative

3. Ans. (a) Start Packed RBC 1st and store platelets at room temperature

(Ref: Transfusion protocol in trauma: NCBI- NIH)

Massive blood transfusion encompasses giving blood components to the patient. Due to presence of blood loss, packed RBC are required on priority. Platelets are to be given after packed RBC as per the protocol steps mentioned below. (See the red box highlighted). Platelet units can be stored at room temperature 20-24 degrees for 5 to 7 days.

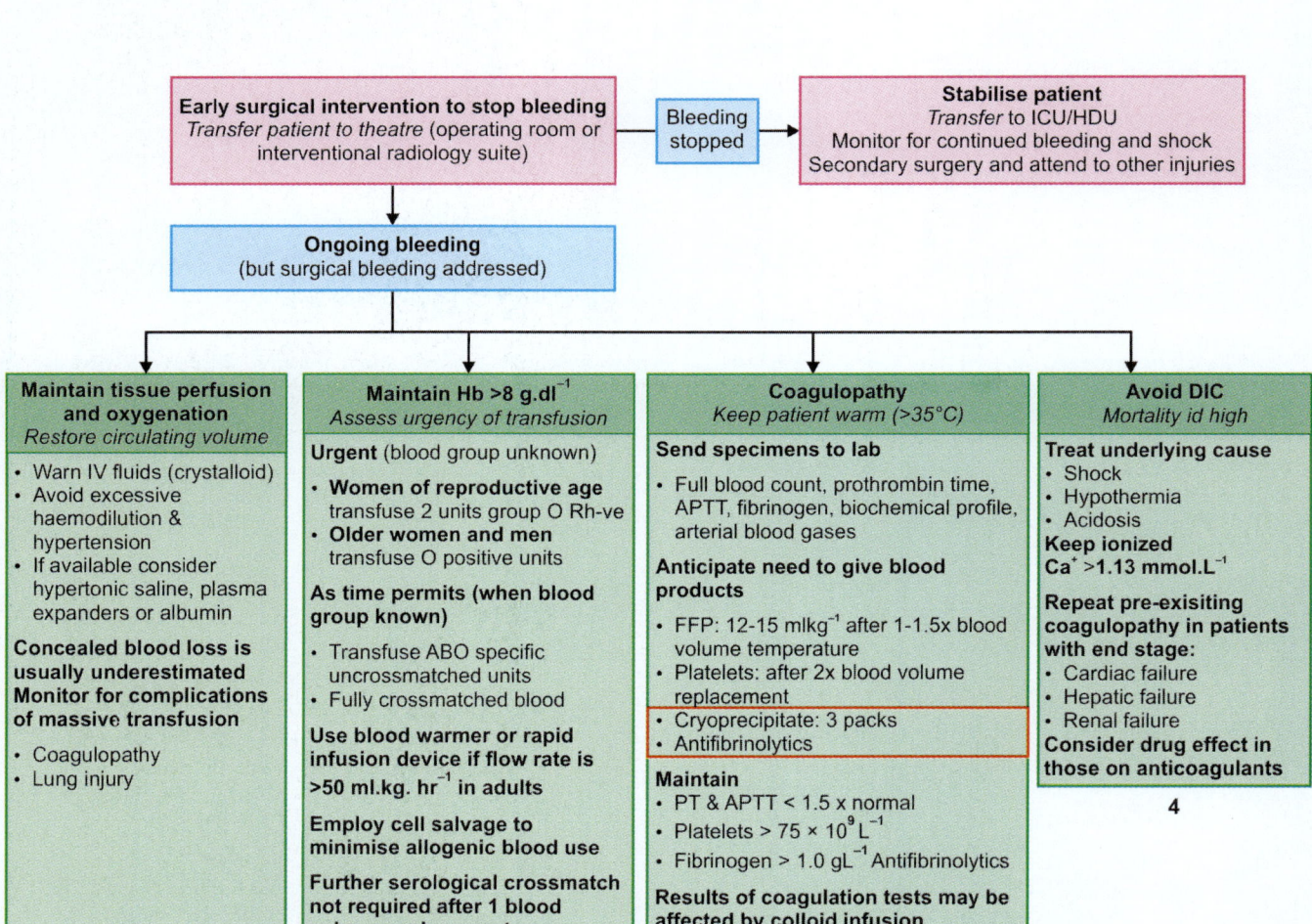

4. Ans. (d) Stop BT and perform clerical check of blood group

(Ref: Harrison 20th edition, p 812)

- The presentation of backache and anxious look points to development of a mismatched blood transfusion/acute hemolytic transfusion reaction. The alarming symptom here is backache/Flank pain which occurs when kidneys get involved due to immune mediated RBC lysis.
- This usually occurs due to a clerical error where the bag of blood has been marked wrongly as a particular blood group. The transfusion must be stopped immediately and the bag sent for evaluation of blood group.

5. Ans. (a) RBC = 2-6°C, Platelets = 20-24°C, FFP = -30°C

(Ref: Harrison 20th edition, p 811-812)

6. Ans. (c) Transfusion associated circulatory overload

Ref: Harrison 20th edition, p 814; Harrison 19th edition, 138e-5

The presence of respiratory distress after blood transfusion points to diagnosis of Transfusion associated circulatory overload since CVP and PCWP both are elevated.

TACO vs. TRALI	TACO	TRALI
EF	<40%	>40%
PCWP	>18 mm Hg	≤18 mm Hg
C × R	CTR > 0.55	CTR < 0.55
Fluid balance	Positive	Neutral
BNP	>1200 pg/mL	< 250 pg/mL
BP	↑	↓
T	Unchanged	Febrile
WBC	Unchanged	Transient ↓

7. Ans. (c) IVF

(Ref: Harrison 20th edition, p 814; Harrison 19th edition, 138e-5)

Since TACO (Transfusion associated circulatory overload) is associated with development of fluid overload, *IVF must be stopped and diuretics must be administered* to lower PCWP.

8. Ans. (d) Resolves in 2-3 weeks

(Ref: Harrison 20th edition, p 813-14; Harrison 19th edition, p 724 and Morgan Anaesthesia: 5th edition, p 1173)

- The incidence of TRALI is more with plasma containing products. It is caused by donor anti-granulocyte antibodies in the plasma targeting the leucocyte antigens on the neutrophils sequestered in the lungs of the patient.
- The resultant acute lung injury does not respond to steroids, diuretics and needs supportive management in the form of non-invasive ventilation or CPAP.
- TRALI starts within 6 hours of transfusion and leads to fever with bilateral radiographic infiltrates.

The mortality rate is 5-10% and in most cases begins to resolve in 2-3 days and not weeks.

9. Ans. (a) Administer via 18-20 G cannula within 4 hours of issue from the blood bank

(Ref: WHO Handbook of transfusion guidelines p 32)

Transfusion guidelines

Blood product	Start transfusion	Completion time
Whole blood/ Packed RBC	<30 minutes	<4 hours and discard if the time limit is discarded.
Platelet concentrate	Immediately	<30 min
FFP	Immediately	<30 min
Cryoprecipitate	Immediately	<30 min

Blood administration set:

- Use a new, sterile blood administration set containing an integral 170–200 µ filter.
- Change the set at least 12-hourly during blood transfusion.
- In a very warm climate, change the set more frequently and usually after every four units of blood, if given within a 12-hour period.
- Use a fresh blood administration set or special platelet transfusion set, primed with saline. All blood components can be slowly infused through small-bore cannulas or butterfly needles, e.g. 21 to 25 G. For rapid infusion, large-bore cannulas, e.g. 14 G, are needed.

10. Ans. (a) 2-6 degrees

(Ref: Clinical Transfusion protocol WHO, p 16)

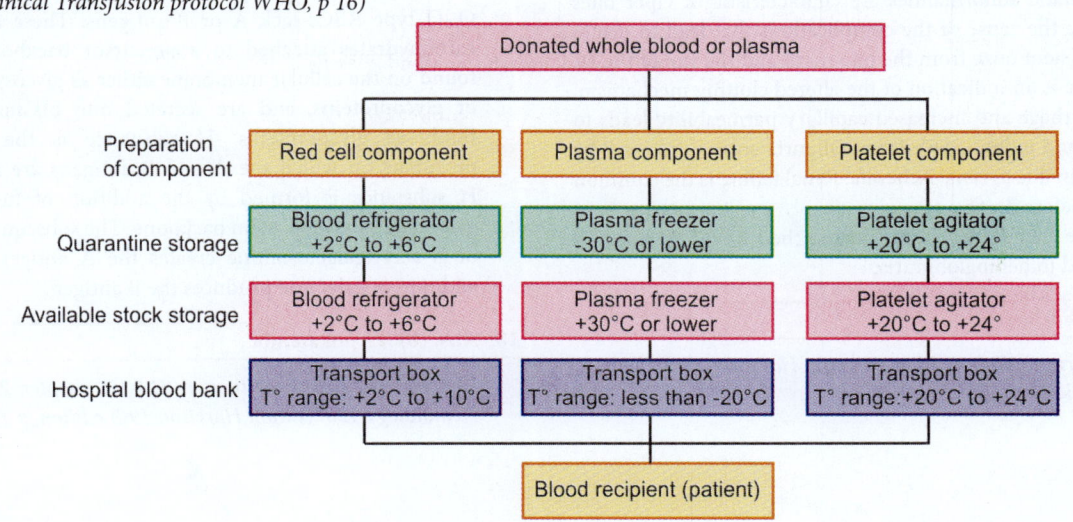

11. Ans. (a) Hyperthermia

(Ref: Harrison 20th edition, p 814-15; Harrison 19th edition, Chapter 138e-4)

- Massive blood transfusion involves up to 5 litres of blood in a 24 hours period.
- Due to need for quick transfusion, infusion of large volume at low temperature will lead to hypothermia. *Hypothermia is the most common complication of MBT.*
- The *presence of citrate toxicity will lead to hypocalcemia* as citrate and calcium will chelate.
- The *Dilutional thrombocytopenia explains the coagulopathy* component.

12. Ans. (a) FFP

(Ref: Harrison 20th edition, p 812; Wintrobe's hematology 12th edition, chapter 23; Harrison 19th edition, chapter 138e)

Whole blood on storage becomes deficient in factor V and VIII. Cryoprecipitate is deficient in factor 9. FFP is the best source of clotting factors.

Whole Blood	No elements removed
Packed RBC	Plasma, WBC, Platelets removed
Cryoprecipitate	Contact factors -VIII -XIII VWF Fibrinogen
FFP	Coagulation factors - II, VII, IX, X, XI, XII, XIII, heat labile V& VIII

13. Ans. (d) Thalassemia

(Ref: Harrison 19th edition, p 673 and 2733)

- The main complications of copper sulphate ingestion include intravascular haemolysis, met-hemoglobinaemia, acute kidney injury and rhabdomyolysis. The lethal dose can be as small as 10 grams.
- Viper bite is primarily vasculotoxic. It causes rapidly developing swelling of the bitten part. Local necrosis is mainly ischemic as thrombosis blocks the local blood vessels and causes a dry gangrene. Systemic absorption is slow; it occurs via the lymphatics and leads to lymphangitis. Hemostatic abnormalities are characteristic of viper bites and are the cause of the complications that lead to death. A persistent ooze from the bite mark and the site of the IV cannula is an indication of the altered clotting mechanism. Hemorrhage and increased capillary permeability leads to shock and pulmonary edema. Oliguria ensues, followed by loin pain due to renal ischemia. Renal failure is the common event before death
- Massive hemolysis due to mismatched blood transfusion will lead to hemoglobinuria.

14. Ans. (d) Fucose

(Ref: Harrison 20th edition, p 810; Harrison 19th edition, Chapter 138e)

Major blood group antigens

1. Blood group antigens are carbohydrates attached to a precursor backbone, may be found on the cellular membrane either as glycosphingolipids or glycoproteins, and are secreted into plasma and body fluids as glycoproteins.
2. H substance is the immediate precursor on which the A and B antigens are added.
3. *H substance is formed by the addition of fucose to the glycolipid or glycoprotein.*
4. Addition of N-acetylgalactosamine creates the A antigen, while the addition of galactose produces the B antigen.
5. Genes that determine the A and B phenotypes are found on chromosome 9p and are expressed in a Mendelian codominant manner.

15. Ans. (c) Intraoperative bleeding

(Ref: Chapter 138e-5: Harrison 19th edition)

Mismatched BT in patient under General anaesthesia will present in form increase oozing of blood from surgical site and hemoglobinuria leading to urine discoloration which can be noticed in the urobag.

16. Ans. (d) ABO incompatibility

(Ref: chapter 138-e-2: Harrison 19th edition)

Anesthetic drug hypersensitivity	In anesthetized patients tachycardia, Hypotension, is the usual presentation as most inhalational agents cause vasodilatation
DIC	Ruled out as it presents with bleeding from venipuncture sites GIT, lungs and skin and along with thrombosis of microcirculations and large vessels
GVHD	Ruled out as it presents with Fever and Maculopapular rash, Diarrhea and LFT abnormalities.
ABO incompatibility	Presents with Hypotension and Tachycardia along with development of fever and chills. *The patient develops intravascular hemolysis leading to hemoglobinemia and hemoglobinuria and resultant acute renal failure.*

17. Ans. (a) Fucose

(Ref: Harrison 19th edition, p 138e-1)

The major blood groups of this system are A, B, AB, and O. O type RBCs lack A or B antigens. These antigens are carbohydrates attached to a precursor backbone, may be found on the cellular membrane either as glycosphingolipids or glycoproteins, and are secreted into plasma and body fluids as glycoproteins. H substance is the immediate precursor on which the A and B antigens are added. This H substance is formed by the addition of fucose to the glycolipid or glycoprotein backbone. The subsequent addition of *N*-acetylgalactosamine creates the A antigen, while the addition of galactose produces the B antigen.

18. Ans. (b) Hypokalemia

(Ref: Harrison 20th edition, p 814-15; chapter 23, Wintrobe's Hematology 12th edition, Harrison 19th edition, p 138e-5)

- RBC leakage during storage increases the concentration of potassium in the unit. Neonates and patients in renal failure are at risk for hyperkalemia. Preventive measures, such as using fresh or washed RBCs, are warranted for neonatal transfusions because this complication can be fatal.
- Increased potassium and other solutes creates an environment of metabolic alkalosis
- Citrate, commonly used to anticoagulate blood components, chelates calcium and thereby inhibits the coagulation cascade. Hypocalcemia, manifested by circumoral numbness and/or tingling sensation of the fingers and toes, may result from multiple rapid transfusions. Because citrate is quickly metabolized to bicarbonate, metabolic alkalosis can ensue due to citrate toxicity.

19. Ans. (a) 1-4 hours

(Ref: Wintrobe's Hematology 11th edition, p 1679, Harrison 19th edition, p 138e-E)

One unit of red cells is often given in 1 to 4 hours, depending on the amount to be transfused and on the patient's cardiovascular status. Infusion of a unit for longer than 4 hours is not recommended, as there is a risk of bacterial proliferation because the opened unit is at room temperature. Drugs or medications should not be injected into the blood.

20. Ans. (a) Hypothermia

(Ref: Wintrobe Hematology: 11th edition, p 1708, Harrison 19th edition, p 138e-5)

- Hypothermia may occur if a large volume of cold blood is infused rapidly.
- *Hypothermia is one of the most common complications of massive transfusion and contributes to the associated coagulopathy.*
- Neonates and the elderly are particularly sensitive to this reaction. Hypothermia affects the way the liver metabolizes citrate, resulting in an increased risk of hypocalcemia.
- Rapid infusions of citrated blood products in such patients, especially through central venous lines, may lead to arrhythmias.
- Hypothermia interferes with platelet function and clotting, both of which are improved when the patient is warmed.
- One way of approaching this problem is with the use of warmed intravenous fluids or blood. Blood-warming devices are available that can warm adequately the blood administered even during a rapid and massive transfusion

21. Ans. (b) Factor 9

(Ref: Harrison 20th edition, p 812; Hematology in clinical practice. 4th edition, ch. 37)

- Cryoprecipitated AHF, or cryoprecipitate, is an extract of FFP that is enriched in high-molecular-weight plasma proteins, but lacks factor 9.
- It is prepared by thawing one unit of FFP at 1° to 6°C. Under these conditions, the high-molecular-weight proteins remain as a precipitate. The precipitated protein is concentrated by centrifugation, and all except approximately 15 ml of supernatant is removed.
- Each unit of this cryoprecipitate contains
  1. Approximately 80 to 120 units of factor VIII
  2. At least 150 mg of fibrinogen.
  3. Factor XIII and the high-molecular-weight multimers of vWF.
- Cryoprecipitate was originally developed for the treatment of hemophilia A. It is no longer the treatment of choice for that disorder because less infectious alternatives are available.
- At the present time, cryoprecipitate is most often used for correction of hypofibrinogenemia (<100 mg/dl), particularly in patients with disseminated intravascular coagulation or in those whose fibrinogen is depleted from prolonged exposure to cardiopulmonary bypass circuits.

22. Ans. (c) Donor antibody to leukocyte of patient

(Ref: Harrison 19th edition, p 138e-5)

23. Ans. (a) Complement mediated severe hemolysis

(Ref: Harrison 19th edition, p 138e-5)

Management of Hemolytic Reactions
- Once a hemolytic reaction is suspected, the transfusion should be stopped immediately.
- Blood should be drawn to identify hemoglobin in plasma to repeat compatibility testing and to obtain coagulation studies and platelet count.
- A urinary catheter should be inserted, and the urine should be checked for hemoglobin.
- Osmotic diuresis should be initiated with mannitol and i v. fluids.
- In the presence of rapid blood loss, platelets and F.F.P. are indicated

Hemolytic Transfusion Reactions

Immediate	Delayed
• Donor red cells are destroyed by the recipient's blood containing preformed IgM antibodies. • Complement fixation occurs • Occurs immediately	• Mild Reaction • Non complement fixing antibodies. • Occurs 4 days to 2 weeks after transfusion • Extravascular hemolysis

Symptoms in Awake Patients
- Chills, fever, nausea and chest and flank pain

Symptoms in Patients under general anesthesia
- Rise in temperature, unexplained tachycardia, hypotension, hemoglobinuria and diffuse oozing in surgical field

24. Ans. (c) 35 days

(Ref: Wintrobe's Hematology 11th ed. 1657-58, Harrison 19th edition, p 685)

- CPDA-1 is Citrate-Phosphate-Dextrose buffer supplemented with adenine. It was made available in the USA in 1978. CPDA-1 is now one of the standard anticoagulant-preservative solutions in clinical use.
- The shelf life of RBC concentrates in CPDA-1 is 35 days.
- In CPD buffer life span is 28 days. The Acid citrate dextrose buffer introduced at time of world war 2 also ensured a shelf life of 21 days.

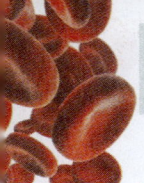

25. Ans. (c) Metabolic acidosis

(Ref: Harrison 19th edition, p 138e-5)

26. Ans. (a) Fever with chills

(Ref: Wintrobe Hematology: 11th ed. pg. 1701)

- Immediate intravascular Hemolytic Transfusion Reactions occur soon after the incompatible transfusion has begun.
- Occasionally, they are mild; more typically, there is a sudden change clinically.
- Fever with or without chills is one of the most common manifestations of such reactions. Other signs and symptoms include anxiety, chest or back pain, flushing, dyspnea, tachycardia, and hypotension.
- If the patient is under general anesthesia, these symptoms may not be recognized; only severe hypotension and evidence of oozing or hemoglobinuria serve as clues to the presence of a hemolytic reaction.
- Such reactions are life-threatening and include acute renal failure, shock, and intravascular coagulation. It has been estimated that a fatal immediate hemolytic reaction occurs in approximately 1/600,000 red transfusions. The mortality of a severe IHTR increases with the amount of blood transfused, with a 44% mortality rate in patients receiving more than 1 L of incompatible blood

27. Ans. (c) HLA mismatch

(Ref: Wintrobe: Hematology: 11th ed., Pg 1704; Harrison 19th edition, p 138e-4/5)

Causes of FNHTR
1. HLA antibodies are most commonly found, followed by platelet-specific antibodies; and Granulocyte-specific antibodies.
2. Another cause of FNHTRs is the transfusion of cytokines that have developed in vitro, especially in whole blood–derived platelet concentrates stored at room temperature
3. Recent studies have shown that during storage, the leukocytes in platelet concentrates release cytokines that may be responsible for the febrile reaction. The incidence of FNHTRs to platelet concentrates increases with the age of the platelet concentrate and the leukocyte concentration in the product.
4. The possibility of bacterial contamination of the product must be considered as a possible cause of FNHTR. Symptoms caused by transfusion of bacteria or their toxins can be mild or may be fatal.
Platelet components are involved more often because they are stored at room temperature. However, certain organisms such as Yersinia enterocolitica proliferate in red cells at storage temperatures of 1° to 6°C.

28. Ans. (d) Febrile non hemolytic transfusion reaction

(Ref: Harrison 19th edition, p 138e)

- Allo-immunization to antigen on leukocytes and platelets is one of the most common causes of nonhemolytic febrile transfusion reactions.

29. Ans. (b) Tropical Sprue

(Ref: Harrison 19th edition, p 673)

- Thalassemia and anemia of chronic disease are known causes of hypochromic microcytic anemia.
- Ancyclostomiasis a genus of hook worm leads to blood loss.
- Acute intestinal infection in tropical Sprue leads to jejunal and ileal mucosa injury; then intestinal bacterial overgrowth and increased plasma enteroglucagon results in retardation of small-intestinal transit. Central to this process is folate deficiency, which probably contributes to further mucosal injury.

30. Ans. (a) Presence of antibodies in the serum when the RBC lacks the corresponding antigen

(Ref: Harrison 20th edition, p 809; Harrison 19th edition, p 138e-1)

- Preformed ABO antibodies are present in person's serum, when his RBC's lack the corresponding antigen
- In other blood groups preformed antibodies are not present
- The ABO blood group system is important because essentially all individuals produce antibodies to the ABH carbohydrateantigen that they lack.
- The first blood group antigen system recognized in 1900, was ABO, the most important in transfusion medicine.
- The major blood groups of this system are A, B, AB, and O. O type RBC's lack A or B antigens.
- These antigens are carbohydrates attached to a precursor backbone, and may be found on the cellular membrane either as glycosphingolipids or glycoproteins, and are secreted into plasma and body fluids as glycoproteins.
- In most people, A and B antigens are secreted by the cells and are present in the circulation.

31. Ans. (a) There are no natural anti-Rh antibodies in serum

(Ref: Harrison 20th edition, p 810)

- Approximately 15% of the population lacks this antigen.
- In patients lacking the antigen, anti-D antibodies are not naturally present but the antigen is highly immunogenic.
- The Rh system is the second most important blood group system in pre-transfusion testing. The Rh antigens are found on a 30- to 32-kDa RBC membrane protein that has no defined function. Although >40 different antigens in the Rh system have been described, five determinants account for the vast majority of phenotypes.
- The Rh antigens together are proteins of 417 amino acids. These proteins cross the red cell membrane 12 times. There are only small loops of the protein on the exterior of the cell membrane.
- Therefore the Rh antigens are not as available to react with their specific antibodies and there are fewer antigen sites than ABO. Unlike the ABO system the Rh antigens are not soluble and are not expressed on the tissues. They are well developed at birth and therefore can easily cause hemolytic disease of the newborn if the baby has a Rh antigen that the mother lacks. Besides the antigens being well-developed at birth, they are very good immunogens. This is especially true to D, which if the most immuno-genic after A and B antigens

32. Ans. (d) Deficient in factor 5 and 8

(*Ref: Harrison 20th edition, p 812; Hematology in clinical practice. 4th ed. ch. 37 and ch. 33*)

- FFP may be stored at -18°C or below for up to 1 year.
- Each unit of FFP prepared from whole blood contains approximately 200 ml of plasma. Apheresis plasma may be packaged into 200 or 400-ml bags. A typical dose of 10 to 15 ml/kg would constitute approximately 25 to 30% replacement therapy for coagulation factors.
- FFP must be ABO compatible with the recipient's red cells
- *Under these conditions, there is minimal loss of activity of the labile coagulation factors V and VIII.* One ml of FFP contains approximately one unit of coagulation factor activity.
- After thawing, FFP may be stored in the refrigerator for up to 24 hours before use. FFP is indicated for use in patients who are bleeding or having an invasive procedure and who are deficient in multiple coagulation factors or in a single factor for which there is no specific factor concentrate available.
- It is also indicated for replacement of clotting factors during massive transfusion, for reversal of warfarin (if immediate reversal is necessary), and as the replacement fluid for plasma exchange procedures in patients with TTP
- It should not be used as a volume expander, because alternative products with lower risk of infectious diseases and allergic reactions are available for this purpose (e.g., crystalloid, albumin, starch).

33. Ans. (b) Potassium intoxication

(*Ref: Harrison 19th edition, p 138-e*)

Prolonged storage can lead to hemolysis and thereby hyperkalemia.

34. Ans. (d) Stopping blood transfusion

(*Ref: Harrison 19th edition, p 138e-5*)

- Microvascular thrombosis and deposition of haemoglobin in the distal renal tubule can result in acute renal failure.
- The extent of precipitation is inversely related to urine flow. I.V. fluids, vasopressors and diuretics should be given to maintain renal perfusion pressure, and to produce a diuresis.
- If acute renal failure develops, haemofiltration should be considered.

35. Ans. (b) HBV

(*Ref: Wintrobe Hematology 11th edition, p 1712: Table 24.11, Harrison 19th edition, p 138e-3*)

Agent	Window Period (Days)	Incidence of New Infections in Repeat Donors (per 100,000 Person-Years)	Estimated Risk/Unit Transfused
Hepatitis B	59	3.016	1:171,000
Hepatitis C	10	1.889	1:1,613,000
Human immunodeficiency virus	11	1.554	1:1,779,000

36. Ans. (a) Platelets carry the Rh antigen

(*Ref: Wintrobe Hematology 11th ed. pg. 1681, Harrison 19th edition, p 138e*)

- Platelets bear both intrinsic and adsorbed antigens of the ABH system. Transfusion of ABO-incompatible platelets may be associated with decreased post transfusion platelet recovery and normal survival. The reduction in recovery is variable and may be related to the isohemagglutinin titer of the recipient
- Platelets do not carry the Rh antigen.
- Transfusion to achieve a platelet count of 50×10^9/L is generally recommended for bleeding patients. However, hemostasis may be achieved through repeated platelet transfusion even in the absence of a demonstrable rise in platelet count.
- Transfusion is indicated in bleeding patients with platelet dysfunction regardless of the platelet count. Dilutional thrombocytopenia may occur after massive transfusion of red cells and plasma volume expanders. However, a platelet count of less than 50×10^9/L is not generally seen unless more than two blood volumes have been replaced.

37. Ans. (d) Acute leukaemia

(*Ref: Harrison 19th edition, p 138e-5*)

38. Ans. (c) Thalassemia minor

(*Ref: Harrison 19th edition, p 637*)

- Since MCV is reduced this indicates microcytic anemia, which rules out choice D.
- No history of blood transfusion rules out thalassemia major.
- Hence we have to choose between iron deficiency anemia and thalassemia minor
- A mathematical index known as Mentzer index is used to differentiate between these two conditions
- Mentzer index = MCV/RBC count
  If mentzer index
  < 13 → thalassemia minor
  > 13 → Iron deficiency

The Mentzer index in the given question is ~ 12 thus it is most likely a case of thalassemia minor.

- The key point in the differential diagnosis of these two conditions is the R.B.C. count
- In thalassemia minor the R.B.C. count is near normal only the hemoglobin is reduced.
- In this condition the R.B.C. count is not reduced as much as the hemoglobin and hematocrit in fact it is usually normal.
- This due to the fact that the marrow can keep on producing the cell at normal rate but it cannot fill them with hemoglobin.

39. Ans. (a) Febrile nonhemolytic transfusion reaction

(*Ref: Harrison 18th edition, p 953*)

40. Ans. (b) Dengue virus

(*Ref: Harrison's 18th edition, ch. 113*)

41. Ans. (b) Factor IX

(*Ref: Harrisons 18th edition, ch. 113*)

Anemia and RBC Defects

42. Ans. (b) 3

Ref: Clinical Haematology by Turgeon p 35

Reticulocyte is defined as RBC containing 2 or more dots of precipitated RBC

Corrected reticulocyte count

$$= \text{Reticulocyte count} \times \frac{\text{Hemoglobin in gm\%}}{15}$$

Hence corrected reticulocyte count $= \frac{9 \times 5}{15} = 3\%$

43. Ans. (c) Aplastic anemia

(Ref: Harrison 19th edition p 337e-4 and 658)

- Aplastic anemia is due to marrow defect where pancytopenia is seen.
- Haemolytic disease of new-born occurs due to Rh incompatibility.
- Alpha-methyl-dopa results in warm antibody mediated haemolytic anaemia
- Mismatched blood transfusion is due to type II hypersensitivity reaction leading to haemolysis significant enough to cause acute tubular necrosis.

44. Ans. (d) 25%

(Ref: Wintrobe hematology:12th edition Table 42.4)

TABLE Classification of Aplastic anemia Based on severity of Pancytopenia

- Severe aplastic anemia (SAA)
  - Bone marrow cellularity < 25%
  - Two of three peripheral blood criteria:
    1. Absolute neutrophil count <500/mm³
    2. Platelet count < 20,000/mm³
    3. Reticulocyte count <60,000/mm³ or < 1% corrected reticulocyte count
- Very severe aplastic anemia (VSAA)
  - Same as SAA with absolute neutrophil count < 200/mm³
- Nonsevere (moderate) aplastic anemia
  - Bone marrow cellularity <25%
  - Peripheral blood cytopenias do not fulfil criteria for SAA

45. Ans. (a) Bone marrow aspiration showing a dry tap

(Ref: Harrison 20th edition, p 727; Harrison 19th edition, p 663)

- The bone marrow is usually readily aspirated but dilute on smear, and the fatty biopsy specimen may be grossly pale on withdrawal; a "dry tap" instead suggests fibrosis or myelophthisis.
- In severe aplasia the smear of the aspirated specimen shows only red cells, residual lymphocytes, and stromal cells; the biopsy (which should be >1 cm in length) is superior for determination of cellularity and shows mainly fat under the microscope, with *hematopoietic cells occupying <25% of the marrow space*; in the most serious cases the biopsy is virtually 100% fat.

- Cells bearing the *CD34 antigen*, a marker of early hematopoietic cells, *are greatly diminished,* and in functional studies, committed and primitive progenitor cells are virtually absent; in vitro assays have suggested that the stem cell pool is reduced to <1% of normal in severe disease at the time of presentation.

46. Ans. (c) 2 1 4 3

(Ref: Harrison 19th edition, p 398)

Macrocytic anemia	Hypothyroidism due to hypo-metabolic state
Microcytic anemia	Iron deficiency
Hemolytic anemia	Alpha methyldopa leads to development of autoimmune hemolytic anemia
Megaloblastic anemia	Vitamin B12 deficiency

47. Ans. (c) 4 1 2 3

(Ref: Harrison 19th edition, p 663)

Microcytic, hypochromic red cells	Iron Deficiency Anemia
Macrocytic, hypochromic red cells	Vitamin B12 anemia
Large number of early, intermediate and late erythroblasts	Thalassemia will have large number of these cells due to ineffective erythropoiesis.
Low reticulocyte count	Aplastic Anemia

48. Ans. (c) Hereditary spherocytosis

(Ref: Harrison 20th edition, p 712; Harrison 19th edition, p 651-52)

Causes of Microcytic hypochromic anemia:
1. Sideroblastic anemia (INH, Lead poisoning)
2. Iron deficiency anemia
3. Thalassemia
4. Anemia of chronic disease

49. Ans. (d) Fanconi's anemia

(Ref: Harrison 20th edition, p 723-25; Harrison 19th edition, p 434, 664)

The causes of microcytic hypochromic anemia is
S= Sideroblastic Anemia
I= Iron deficiency Anemia
T= Thalassemia
A= Anemia of chronic disease

50. Ans. (c) Pure Red cell aplasia

(Ref: Harrison 20th edition, p 729, Table 98-4; Chapter 43, Wintrobe's Hematology 12th edition)

Diamond blackfann syndrome is an inherited bone marrow failure syndrome leading to pure red cell aplasia. The diagnostic criteria are:
1. Normochromic, usually macrocytic anaemia
2. Reticulocytopenia
3. Normocellular bone marrow with selective deficiency of erythroid precursors

4. Normal or only slightly decreased granulocyte count
5. Normal or slightly increased platelet count

DBA	
Pure red cell aplasia	Present
Age	< 1 year
Inheritance	Sporadic and dominant or possibly but unlikely recessive inheritance Mutation analysis available for DBA1 (RPS19; RPS24; RPS17)
Congenital anomalies	Present
Mean corpuscular volume	Elevated
Fetal hemoglobin	Elevated
I RBC antigen	Present
Erythrocyte ADA activity	Elevated

51. Ans. (a) Non-compliance

(Ref: Harrison 19th edition, p 628-29)

The patient has presence of microcytic anemia with low serum ferritin. Oral iron was started but hemoglobin has increased by 0.2gm% only. The most probable cause of the same is:
1. Non compliance
2. Intolerance to oral iron leading to patient not taking medicine or avoiding for most of the days
3. Consumption of less dose of iron which is consumed post meals

Responses to iron Therapy
1. The response to iron therapy varies depending on the erythropoietin stimulus and the rate of absorption.
2. The reticulocyte count should begin to increase within 4-7 days after initiation of therapy and peak at 7-10 days.
3. A useful test in the clinic to determine the patient's ability to absorb iron is the iron tolerance test two iron tablets are given to the patient on an empty stomach and the serum iron is measured serially over the subsequent 2 hours.
4. Normal absorption will result in an increase in the serum iron of at least 100g/dl.

52. Ans. (a) Microcytic anemia

(Ref: Harrison 20th edition, p 698, 702; Harrison 19th edition, p 640, 645)

B12 deficiency is characterised by:
- Loss of vibratory and position sense (Rhomberg sign)
- Abnormal gait
- Dementia
- Impotence
- Loss of bladder and bowel control
- Macrocytic anemia

53. Ans. (b) Iron deficiency anaemia

(Ref: Harrison 20th edition, p 683; Harrison 19th ed./627-28)

- Initially the anemia is normocytic normochromic and subsequently hypochromic and microcytic. There is mild to moderate anisocytosis (variation in size) and poikilocytosis (Variation and shape).
- The long, thin elliptocytes of iron deficiency are sometimes referred to as pencil cells.
- Target cells are uncommon and anisochromasia is characteristic. There are two features that can be useful in making the distinction from thalassaemia trait.
- Subsequently there is a fall in the MCV and the MCH and, when it is measured by a sensitive technique, a fall in the MCHC as well.

54. Ans. (b) HLA mediated

(Ref: Harrison 20th edition, p 813-14)

- Transfusion-Related Acute Lung Injury (TRALI) is a syndrome characterized by acute respiratory distress following transfusion.
- TRALI usually results from the donor plasma that contains high-titer anti-HLA antibodies that bind recipient leukocytes.
- The leukocytes aggregate in the pulmonary vasculature and release mediators that increase capillary permeability.
- Testing the donor's plasma for anti-HLA antibodies can support this diagnosis.
- The implicated donors are frequently multiparous women, and transfusion of their plasma component should be avoided.
- All plasma-containing blood products have been implicated including rare reports of IVIG and cryoprecipitate.
- Symptoms of TRALI typically develop during, or within 6 hours of a transfusion. Patients present with the rapid onset of dyspnea and tachypnea. There may be associated fever, cyanosis, and hypotension and clinical exam reveals non-cardiogenic pulmonary edema.

55. Ans. (a) Iron deficiency anemia

(Ref: Harrison 20th edition, p 685, 687; Table 93-4)

Disease	Serum iron	Serum ferritin	TIBC
Iron deficiency anemia	Decreased	Decreased	Increased
Chronic kidney disease (anemia is due to deficiency of erythropoietin)	Normal	Normal/decreased if lost in urine due to kidney pathology	Normal
Sideroblastic anemia	Increased	Increased	Decreased
Fanconi anemia (anemia is due to congenital aplastic anemia)	Normal	Normal	Normal

56. Ans. (c) Donor serum is tested against recipient packed cells

(Ref: Harrison 20th edition, p 811; Harrison 19th ed. / 138e-2)

Cross-matching blood is performed prior to a blood transfusion in order to determine if the donor's blood is compatible with the blood of an intended recipient, or to identify matches for organ transplantation.

57. Ans. (a) Acanthocyte

(Ref: Harrison 20th edition, p 382 Fig. 58-16; Harrison 19th edition, p 445, 81e-1,)

Acathocyte	Spiculated thorny RBC (*irregularly placed*)	
Schistocyte	Irregular jagged and have two pointed ends	
Echinocyte	Abnormal cell membrane with small evenly spaced(*regularly placed*) thorny projections	
Stomatocyte	Slit or mouth like opening replacing the central pallor	

58. Ans. (b) Folic acid alone causes improvement of anemic symptoms but neurological dysfunction continues

(Ref: Katzung 10th/532; KDT 6th /591)

- Vitamin B_{12} is required for conversion of methionine to homocysteine and for formation of succinyl CoA from meth-ylmalonyl CoA.
- Deficiency of vitamin B_{12} results in megaloblastic anemia, GI manifestations and neurological abnormalities (due to demyelination).
- Folic acid alone will correct the symptoms of megaloblastic anemia but it does not prevent neurological abnormalities, which continue to proceed.
- Neurological abnormalities manifests initially in the form of loss of posterior column sensations (vibration, proprioception etc.), but later on can result in subacute combined degeneration of spinal cord.

59. Ans. (d) Decreased total iron-binding capacity (TIBC)

(Ref: Harrison 20th edition, p 684-86; Harrison 19th edition, p 627)

- Iron-deficiency Anemia is one of the most prevalent forms of malnutrition.
- Initially, a state of negative iron balance occurs during which iron stores become slowly depleted.
- Serum ferritin may decrease, and the presence of stainable iron on bone marrow preparation decreases. When iron stores are depleted (serum iron begins to fall Total iron-binding capacity (TIBC) starts to increase, reflecting the presence of circulating unbound transferrin. When the transferrin saturation falls to 15% to 20%, hemoglobin synthesis is impaired. The peripheral blood smear reveals the presence of microcytic and hypochromic red blood cells.
- Clinically, these patients exhibit the usual signs of anemia, which are fatigue, pallor, and reduced exercise capacity
- Cheilosis and koilonychia are signs of advanced tissue iron deficiency. Some patients may experience pica, a desire to ingest certain materials, such as ice (pagophagia) and clay (geophagia).
- Reticulocytes may also become hypochromic. Reticulocyte numbers are reduced relative to the level of anemia, reflecting a hypoproduction anemia secondary to iron deficiency.

60. Ans. (d) Increased fecal urobilinogen

(Ref: Harrison 19th edition, p 658/1649)

- Haptoglobin is an α-globin which binds specifically to globin of hemoglobin. Hemolytic anemia leads to intravascular hemolysis that leads to hemoglobinuria.
- Haemolytic anemia is characterized by hemoglobinuria, hemosiderinuria, increased reticulocyte count, unconjugated hyper-bilirubinaemia, increased plasma haemoglobin and LDH, polychromatophilia and bone marrow erythroid hyperplasia.

61. Ans. (a) Atransferrinemia

(Ref: Manual of clinical hematology 3rd edition, p 33)

Interpretation of values given:
Low serum iron = Normal (50-170 g/dl)
High serum ferritin = Normal (30-400 ng/ml)
High transferrin saturation = Normal (30-50%)

Iron deficiency anemia
- Can be easily ruled out as serum ferritin is low in Iron deficiency anemia.

Hemochromatosis
- Can be easily ruled out as hemochromatosis is characterized by increased serum iron level.

Atransferrinemia
- Transferrin is an iron carrying protein that transmits iron to the erythroblasts.
- Atransferrinemia or hypotransferrinemia results in reduced delivery of iron to erythroblasts and development of iron deficient anemia. This explains low serum iron.
- This leads to massive but futile iron absorption and whatever LITTLE transferrin is there is saturated. This explains High serum transferrin. The difference from DMT 1 mutation is that since the iron absorption is defective transferrin saturation is low.
- Iron is deposited in the visceral organs rather than in the bone marrow.

DMT 1 mutation
- DMT 1 is a transmembrane protein involved in dietary non heme iron uptake at the brush border of duodenal

enterocytes and also plays crucial role in iron utilization at the endosomal membrane of the erythroid precursors. Divalent metal transporter 1 (DMT1) is a duodenal apical iron transporter encoded by the SLC11A2 gene.
- In DMT 1 mutation the iron absorption in the duodenum continues because the absorption of heme iron is not affected.
- The mutation primarily affects iron utilization and not absorption. Iron utilization in erythroid precursors is disturbed leading to severe iron deficiency anemia.

	DMT1 mutation	Atransferrinemia
Age of diagnosis	At birth	Late onset
Anemia	Microcytic Hypochromic	Microcytic hypochromic
Serum iron	High	Low
Transferrin saturation	High	High
Ringed sideroblasts	No	No
Liver iron overload	Yes	Yes
Brain damage	No	No
Hepcidin levels	Low	Not yet measured

Genetic forms of Iron deficiency anemia
- Iron deficiency anemia is an acquired disease. It is generally associated with low cost diet and bleeding.
- Recent advances in iron metabolism led to the recognition of new entities of iron deficiency anemia in nonbleeding and "high cost diet" nourished individuals. These are known as genetic forms of iron deficiency anemia.
- Apparently rare these genetic forms of iron deficiency anemia should be recognized by hematologists as they are refractory to classical oral or intravenous iron administration.

These includes:
1. Mutations in gene encoding DMT1
2. Mutations in gene encoding glutaredoxin 5.
3. Hypotransferrinemia or Atransferriemia
4. Deficiency of ceruloplasmin
5. IRIDA (Iron Refractory, Iron Deficiency Anemia)

62. Ans. (a) Serum iron ↓ S. ferritin ↑ and transferrin ↓

(Ref: Harrison's 18th edition, p 849, 850)
1. In anemia of chronic disease, a product liberated by liver hepicidin, inhibits release of iron from the stores.
2. Hence the stores will get increased while serum iron will fall.
3. TIBC always shows an inverse relation to serum ferritin.

63. Ans. (d) 2.5%

(Ref: Harrison's 18th edition, ch. 57)

Normally, reticulocytes are red cells that have been recently released from the bone marrow. They are identified by staining with a supravital dye that precipitates the ribosomal RNA. These precipitates appear as blue or black punctate spots. This residual RNA is metabolized over the first 24–36 h of the reticulocyte's life span in circulation.

Normally, the reticulocyte count ranges from 1 to 2% and reflects the daily replacement of 0.8–1.0% of the circulating red cell population. A corrected reticulocyte count provides a reliable measure of red cell production.

64. Ans. (a) Microangiopathic hemolytic anemia

(Ref: Harrison 19th edition, p 658)

65. Ans. (c) SLE

(Ref: API, 18th/ed. 810, Harrison 19th edition, p 658/138e-4)

Connective tissue disorders associated with autoimmune hemolytic anemia
(Associated with IgG autoantibody warm autoantibody)

Common
- Systemic lupus Erythematosus

Rare
- Polyarteritis nodosa
- Rheumatoid arthritis
- Sjogrens syndrome
- Scleroderma

66. Ans. (c) High Packed cell volume

(Ref: Harrison's 18th edition, p 885, 886)

- In acute blood loss, the platelets and circulating granulocytes increase within few hours. Immature WBC's may also be seen. Increase leucocytes and platelets are normal body response to stress. The body continuously strives to maintain homeostasis.

Packed Cell Volume
- The body adjusts to severe hemorrhage by expanding the circulating volume at the expense of the extravascular fluid leading to low PCV
- A hematocrit that is done immediately after a haemorrhage usually does not show the extent of RBC loss because at the time of haemorrhage plasma and red blood cells are lost in equal proportions.
- However, within several hours after haemorrhage, plasma volume begins to increase due to shift of interstitial fluid into the vascular space.
- Red blood cells, however, cannot be replaced quickly as the bone marrow takes approximately ten days to produce mature red blood cells.
- As a result PCV done several hours after bleeding episode will show a more accurate picture of the hematocrit which is a DECREASED PACKED CELL VOLUME.

67. Ans. (b) Hepatocellular disease

(Ref: Harrison 19th edition, p 396 f)

A mild hypoproliferative anemia may develop in patients with chronic liver disease from nearly any cause. The peripheral blood smear may show spur cells and stomatocytes from the accumulation of excess cholesterol in the membrane from a deficiency of lecithin-cholesterol acyltransferase.

68. Ans. (c) Bile duct obstruction

(Ref: Hematology in clinical practice. 4th edition ch. 11)

- Haptoglobin binding of free haemoglobin results in removal of the complex from the circulation.
- Reduced levels occur in haemolysis (particularly intravascular), megaloblastic anaemia (red cell turnover in marrow) following blood transfusion, massive tissue haemorrhage, and hepatocellular disease.
- Congenital absence of haptoglobin has also been recognised.
- High levels may be seen in pregnancy, with steroid or oestrogen therapy, in conditions associated with an acute phase response, and in biliary obstruction.
- Pre-existent high levels may mask haemolysis

69. Ans. (d) EBV

(Ref: Harrison 19th edition, p 667)

Viruses leading to aplestic anemia
1. EBV
2. Hepatitis (non-A, non-B, non-C)
3. HIV–I
4. Parvovirus B_{19} (aplastic CRISIS)

70. Ans. (d) Anemia of chronic infection

(Ref: Harrison 19th edition, p 637)

Interpretation of parameters provided in question

MCV	Decreased	(N 80-100 fl)
Serum iron	Lower range of normal	(N 50-150 g/dl)
Serum ferritin	Normal	(N 50-300 g/dl)
Hemoglobin	Decreased	(N 14-16 g/dl)

- Thalassemia trait is not diagnosed on the basis of serum iron indices, instead, definitive diagnosis of thalassemia trait is based on hemoglobin electrophoresis." HbA2 levels > 3.6-8% are considered diagnostic for thalassemia trait." Serum iron level is increased in thalassemia trait because of increased intestinal absorption of iron. Choice A is ruled out
- Due to low iron but normal ferritin iron deficiency is ruled out as serum ferritin is first to reduce in iron deficiency anemia. Choice B is ruled out.
- Since MCV is low it is a microcytic anemia. Choice C is ruled out
- This is likely a case of anemia of chronic disease in which serum ferritin is normal to increased while the serum iron level is usually on the lower side.

71. Ans. (d) Infectious mononucleosis

(Ref: Harrison 19th edition, p 658)

Warm antibody hemolytic anemia is the most common form of autoimmune hemolytic anemia (AIHA); it is more common among women. Autoantibodies in warm antibody hemolytic anemia generally react at temperatures > 37° C. The autoantibodies may occur.
- Spontaneously
- In association with certain disorders (SLE, lymphoma, chronic lymphocytic leukemia)
- After use of certain drugs which stimulate production of autoantibodies against Rh antigens (α-methyldopa-type of AIHA). Other drugs stimulate production of autoantibodies against the antibiotic–RBC-membrane complex as part of a transient hapten mechanism; the hapten may be stable (e.g., high-dose penicillin, cephalosporins)
- In warm antibody hemolytic anemia, hemolysis occurs primarily in the spleen. It is often severe andcan be fatal. Most of the autoantibodies in warm antibody hemolytic anemia are IgG. Most are pan-agglutinins and have limited specificity.

72. Ans. (b) Decreased Fe, decreased transferrin, increased Ferritin

(Ref: Harrison 19th edition, p 393)

Condition	Iron deficiency anemia	Sideroblastic anemia	Anemia of chronic disease
Serum iron	Decreased	Increased	Decreased
Serum ferritin	Decreased	Increased	Increased
TIBC	increased	decreased	Decreased

73. Ans. (a) Fanconi's Anemia

(Ref: Harrison 20th edition, p 724, Table 98-1; Harrison 19th edition, p 434/664)

Pancytopenia with hypo-cellular marrow
1. Acquired aplastic anemia
2. Constitutional aplastic anemia (Fanconi's anemia, dyskeratosis congenita)
3. Some myelodysplasia
4. Rare aleukemic leukemia
5. Acute lymphoid leukemia
6. Lymphomas originating from the bone marrow

74. Ans. (d) Increased reticulocyte count

(Ref: Harrison 19th edition, p 2346 t)

In a setting of vitamin B_{12} deficiency, DNA synthesis is impaired. Hence increased reticulocyte count is not seen with pernicious anemia.

75. Ans. (b) Hemolytic anemia

(Ref: Harrison 20th edition, p 708. Table 96-2; Harrison 19th edition, p 658)

In a setting of Reticulocytosis with splenomegaly, hemolytic anemia is seen.Skull and skeletal deformities can occur in childhood due to a marked increase in hematopoiesis and resultant bone marrow expansion in disorders such as thalassemia.

76. Ans. (a) 2.3 x wt (kg) x Hb deficit (g/dl) + 500

(Ref: Harrison 20th edition, p 687; Harrison 19th edition, p 628)

Total iron requirement can be calculated by the formula:
- Parenteral iron is used in two ways: One is to administer the total dose of iron required to correct the hemoglobin deficit and provide the patient with at least 500 mg of iron stores;

the second is to give repeated small doses of parenteral iron over a protracted period.
- The amount of iron needed by an individual patient is calculated by the following formula:
  - Body weight (kg) × 2.3 × (15–patient's hemoglobin, g/dL) + 500 or 1000 mg (for stores).

77. Ans. (c) **Liver disease**

(Ref: Harrison's 18th edition, p 845, 846 table (103-2)

Ferritin levels are increased in the following:
- Acute and chronic liver disease
- Infection
- Inflammation
- Alcoholism
- Malignancies
- Hyperthyroidism
- Gaucher disease
- Myocardial infection
- Iron overload (hemochromatosis)
- End-stage renal disease
- Renal cell cancer
- Anemia other than iron deficiency

Ferritin levels are decreased in the following:
- Iron deficiency
- Hemodialysis

78. Ans. (b) **Vitamin B_{12} and Folic acid deficiency**

(Ref: Hematology in clinical practice. 4th ed. ch. 8, Harrison 19th edition, p 643)

Differential diagnosis of anemia in the adult
Low mean corpuscular volume (microcytic anemia: MCV< 80 fL)
- Sideroblastic anemia (eg, congenital, lead, alcohol, drugs; uncommon)
- Iron deficiency anemia
- Thalassemic disorders
- Anemia of inflammation/anemia of chronic disease (late; uncommon)
- Copper deficiency, zinc poisoning (rare)

Normal mean corpuscular volumes (normocytic anemia: MCV 80 to 100 fL)
- Acute blood loss
- Anemia of inflammation/anemia of chronic disease (e.g., infection, inflammation, malignancy)
- Bone marrow suppression (may also be macrocytic)
  - Bone marrow invasion (e.g., leukoery-throblastic blood picture)
  - Acquired pure red blood cell aplasia
  - Aplastic anemia
  - Chronic renal insufficiency
  - Endocrine dysfunction
  - Hypothyroidism
  - Hypopituitarism

Increased mean corpuscular volume (macrocytic anemia: MCV > 100 fL)
- Ethanol abuse
- Folate deficiency
- Vitamin B_{12} deficiency
- Myelo-dysplastic syndromes
- Acute myeloid leukemias (e.g., erythroleukemia)
- Reticulocytosis
- Hemolytic anemia
- Response to blood loss
- Response to appropriate hematinic (e.g., iron, B_{12}, folic acid)
- Drug-induced anemia (e.g., Hydroxyurea, Chemotherapeutic agents)
- Liver disease

79. Ans. (d) **Lead poisoning**

(Ref: Harrison 19th edition, p 643)

Microcytic Anaemia	Megalocytic Anaemia
Fe def.	Vit B12 deficiency
	Cobalamin deficiency
Lead poisoning	Folate deficiency
Sideroblatic Anaemia	Goat milk ingestion
Thalassemia	Type-A gastrites
	Anti metabolits (Methotrexate)

80. Ans. (b) **Duodenum**

(Ref: Harrison 19th edition, p 643)

81. Ans. (c) **Coomb's test**

(Ref: Nelson 17th/pg. 1620, Harrison 19th edition, p 658)
- Presence of spherocytes alone is not sufficient for the diagnosis of hereditary spherocytosis. Evidence of hereditary nature of the disease is also required.C.M.D.T. 2013 states
- "Increased osmotic fragility merely reflects the presence of spherocytes and does not distinguish hereditary spherocytosis from other spherocytic hemolytic disorders".
- Spherocytes are also associated with autoimmune hemolytic anemias.
- Hereditary spherocytosis should be distinguished from spherocytic hemolytic anemias associated with RBC autoantibodies,
- Increased osmotic fragility does not establish the diagnosis of hereditary spherocytosis.
- Increased osmotic fragility only indicates the presence of spherocytes and spherocytes are associated with both hereditary spherocytosis and autoimmune hemolytic anemia.

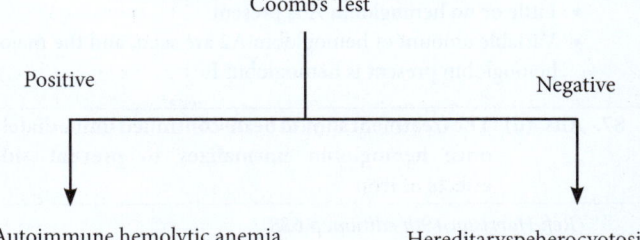

Presence of Spherocytes in young adult → Coomb's Test → Positive: Autoimmune hemolytic anemia / Negative: Hereditary spherocytosis

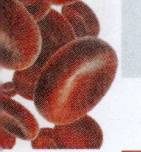

82. **Ans. (a) Hypothyroidism**

(Ref: Harrison 19th edition, p 643)

83. **Ans. (a) Tolerable dose will deliver 40 to 60 mg of iron per day**

(Ref: Katzung 10th/530; KDT 6th/585-86, Harrison 19th edition, p 398)
- Tolerable dose of elemental iron is 200 mg per day in three divided doses i.e. app. 60 mg per dose.
- Mass of elemental iron is more important in determining daily dose rather than mass of total salt, because different salts provide different amount of elemental iron.
- Treatment with oral iron should be continued even after reaching the desired hemoglobin level to replenish the stores.
- Desired rate of hemoglobin improvement is 0.5 to 1 mg per week.

84. **Ans. (c) Carpal tunnel syndrome**

(Ref: Harrison 19th edition, p 643)
- Vitamin B12 deficiency, as can occur in pernicious anemia, causes a macrocytic anemia and may also damage the nervous system affecting the posterior columns (loss of position and vibratory sense) and cortico-spinal tracts (hyperactive tendon reflexes with Babinski responses); it also damages peripheral nerves, resulting in sensory loss with depressed tendon reflexes.
- The two close answers are carpal tunnel syndrome and infertility.
- Multiple medical journals mention regarding vitamin B12 deficiency to be associated with Hyper-homocystinemia lead to hypercoagul-ability and resultant abortions. Plus vitamin B12 is required for DNA synthesis and hence recurrent abortions will develop.

85. **Ans. (d) Positive direct Coomb's test**

(Ref: Harrison's 18th ed. ch. 106)

Positive coombs test is indicative of autoimmune hemolytic anemia.

86. **Ans. (b) Enlargement of medullary cavity**

(Ref: Harrison 19th edition, p 633, 637)

Beta thalassemia major produces severe anemia, and without transfusion the hematocrit may fall to less than 10%.
- The peripheral blood smear is bizarre, showing severe Poikilocytosis, Hypochromia, Micro-cytosis, target cells, basophilic stippling, and nucleated red blood cells.
- Little or no hemoglobin A is present.
- Variable amount of hemoglobin A2 are seen, and the major hemoglobin present is hemoglobin F.

87. **Ans. (d) The treatment should be discontinued immediately once hemoglobin normalizes to prevent side effects of iron**

(Ref: Harrison 19th edition, p 628)
- The response to iron therapy varies, depending on the erythropoietin stimulus and the rate of absorption. Typically, the reticulocyte count should begin to increase within 4–7 days after initiation of therapy and peak at 1–1 1/2 weeks. The absence of a response may be due to poor absorption, noncompliance (which is common), or a confounding diagnosis.
- A normal individual without iron deficiency absorbs 5-10% of this iron, or about 0.5-1 mg daily. Iron absorption increases in response to low iron stores or increased iron requirementshi an iron deficient individual, about 50-100 mg of iron can be incorporated into hemoglobin daily, and about 25% of oral iron given as ferrous salt can be absorbed. Therefore, 200-400 mg of elemental iron should be given daily to correct iron deficiency most rapidly.
- However, as the hemoglobin level rises, erythropoietin stimulation decreases, and the amount of iron absorbed is reduced.
- The goal of therapy in individuals with iron-deficiency anemia is not only to repair the anemia, but also to provide stores of at least 0.5–1 g of iron. Sustained treatment for a period of 6–12 months after correction of the anemia will be necessary to achieve

88. **Ans. (d) Fanconi's Anemia**

(Ref: Harrison 18th edition, p 847, 848)

89. **Ans. (b) ↓ TIBC; (c) ↑ S. ferritin**

(Ref: Harrison 18th edition, p 848)

90. **Ans. (b) Iron deficiency anemia**

(Ref: Harrison 18th edition, p 847–848)

91. **Ans. (c) Haemochromatosis**

(Ref: Harrisons 17th edition, p /2432, 2433, 631)

92. **Ans. (c) Decreased TIBC**

(Ref: Harrisons 18th edition, p Ch. 109)

93. **Ans. (b) Decrease in serum ferritin level**

(Ref: Harrison 18th edition, p Chapter 109)

94. **Ans. (b) Serum ferritin levels**

(Ref: Harrison 18th edition, p 846)

95. **Ans. (c) Polycythemia vera**

(Ref: Harrison 18th edition, p 846, 900, 3162)

96. **Ans. (a) Serum iron ↓, S. ferritin ↑ and transferrin ↓**

(Ref: Harrison 18th edition, p 849)

97. **Ans. (b) Increased total iron binding capacity (ITBC)**

(Ref: Harrison 18th edition, p 849)

98. Ans. (a) **Decreased erythropetin production**

(Ref: Harrison 18th edition, p 850)

99. Ans. (b) **Decreased transferrin saturation**

(Ref: Harrison 18th edition, p 848)

100. Ans. (b) **Copper deficiency**

(Ref: Harrison 18th edition, p 862)

101. Ans. (b) **Bacterial overgrowth**

(Ref: Love & Bailey 23rd/1031)

102. Ans. (d) **All of the above**

(Ref: Harrison 18th edition, ch. 106)

103. Ans. (d) **Increased Haptoglobin**

(Ref: Harrison 18th edition, p 873)

104. Ans. (a) **Thrombocytopenia**

(Ref: Harrison 18th edition, p ch. 106)

105. Ans. (d) **Anemia of chronic renal failure**

(Ref: Harrison 18th edition, p ch. 106)

106. Ans. (a) **IgM**

(Ref: Harrison 18th edition, p 882)

107. Ans. (b) **Chronic lymphatic leukemia (CLL)**

(Ref: Harrison 18th edition, p 882)

108. Ans. (a) **Alcoholic cirrhosis**

(Ref: Harrison 18th edition, p ch. 106)

Coomb's positive hemolytic anemia may be seen in autoimmune conditions. All options other than alcoholic cirrhosis may have autoimmune etiologies and hence, may very well have coomb's positive haemolytic anemia as a feature.

109. Ans. **None or (b) Metallic heart valve**

(Ref: Rubin's Pathology 8th edition, p ch 12/p471)

110. Ans. (a) **Autosomal dominant inheritance**

(Ref: Harrison's 18th edition, p ch. 107)

Thalassemia and Sickle Cell Anemia

111. Ans. (b) **Alpha thalassemia trait**

(Ref: Wintrobe's Hematology: 12th edition, Chapter 38)

Hb-electrophoresis can estimate the elvel of the HbA2 and HbF fractions. In hemoglobin H disease 20–40% of total hemoglobin is of hemoglobin bart. However, in the silent carrier alpha thalassemia condition, the percentage is only 1–2% with low or normal amounts of hemoglobin. Hemoglobin electrophoresis is generally not sufficiently sensitive to diagnose silent carrier alpha thalassemia.

Currently, genetic testing is used to establish the diagnosis in patients with a suggestive family history and/or hematologic findings suggestive of alpha thalassemia.

1. Recombinant DNA technology can be diagnostic but is still a research tool.
2. Gene mapping
3. Polymerase chain reaction (PCR)
4. Restriction endonucleases
5. Anti-L globin monoclonal antibodies

112. Ans. (b) **HbH disease**

(Ref: Page 338: Essentials in Haematology and clinical practice by Nayak; 1st edition

Golf ball inclusion bodies are called as HbH bodies and are seen in alpha thalassemia. The peripheral smear stained with supravital stain brilliant cresyl blue shows *multiple inclusions in an evenly distributed panel.*

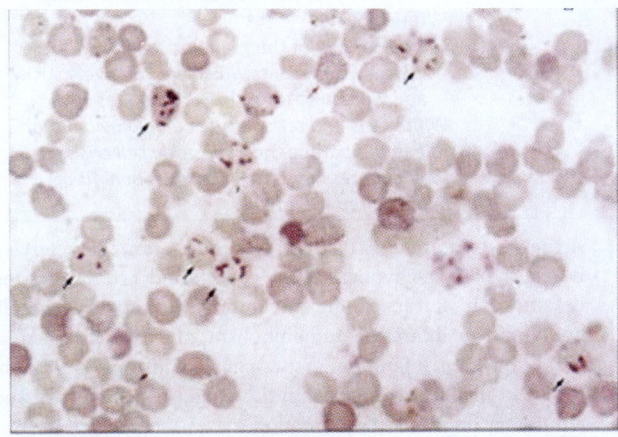

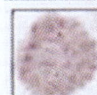 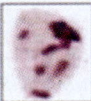

HbH inclusion body   Reticulocyte

Reticulocytes are differentiated from these RBCs with inclusions as they have uneven reticulin deposits.

Heinz bodies are larger, single inclusions and not so numerous as Howell jolly bodies.

113. Ans. (c) **She can present with pulmonary bleeds**

(Ref: Harrison 20th edition, p 692-93. Harrison 19th edition, p 634-35)

- Anemia with jaundice points to hemolytic anemia and presence of joint pain indicates sickling leading to vaso-occlusive crisis.
- Bone pain occurs as gnawing, progressive pain, most commonly in the humerus, tibia, and femur and less commonly in the facial bones.
- Periarticular pain and joint effusion, often associated with a sickle cell crisis, are considered a result of ischemia and infarction of the synovium and adjacent bone and bone marrow

- Patients can present with acute chest syndrome and not pulmonary syndrome.
- *Acute chest syndrome* is a distinctive manifestation characterized by chest pain, tachypnea, fever, cough, and arterial oxygen desaturation. It can *mimic* pneumonia, pulmonary emboli, bone marrow infarction and embolism, myocardial ischemia, or in situ lung infarction.

Choice A HbF and HbA2 will be undetectable	The major hemoglobin in sickle cell anemia is HbS
Choice B she may have retinopathy	Non-proliferative or background sickle retinopathy includes the following manifestations: • Venous tortuosity • Salmon-patch hemorrhage • Schisis cavity • The black sunburst Proliferative sickle retinopathy (PSR) is the most severe ocular change in SCD. This is a peripheral retinal change most frequent in patients with hemoglobin SC but also can be present in patients with hemoglobin S-thalassemia disease.
Choice D Hydroxyurea will help her	Mechanism of action of hydroxyurea: 1. Increases fetal hemoglobin and reducing sickling 2. Beneficial effects on RBC hydration 3. Reduces Vascular wall adherence of sticky reticulocytes 4. Suppression of the granulocyte and reticulocyte counts which are relatively sticky and worsen vaso-occlusive episodes *White cells and reticulocytes may play a major role in the pathogenesis of sickle cell crisis, and their suppression is an important benefit of hydroxyurea therapy.*

Acute chest syndrome is a distinctive manifestation characterized by chest pain, tachypnea, fever, cough, and arterial oxygen desaturation. It can mimic pneumonia, pulmonary emboli, bone marrow infarction and embolism, myocardial ischemia, or in situ lung infarction. Acute chest syndrome is thought to reflect in situ sickling within the lung, producing pain and temporary pulmonary dysfunction.

114. Ans. (b) **Paget's disease**

(Ref: Neuro-radiology, 3rd edition, p 383)

The X- Skull shows presence of Lytic lesions

Differential diagnosis of lytic lesion on X ray Skull:
1. Multiple myeloma
2. Hyperparathyroidism
3. Histiocytosis-X
4. Metastasis(breast, thyroid, lung and kidney cancer)
5. TB
6. Osteomyelitis
7. CNS Epidermoid cyst
8. Hemangioma
9. Fibrous dysplasia

115. Ans. (a) **Sickle cell anemia**

(Ref: Harrison 20th edition, p 693; Harrison 19th edition, p 635)

Acute vaso-occlusion may also cause stroke due to sinus thrombosis in priapism.

Priapism is defined as erection lasting for > 4 hours. Low-flow priapism may be due to any of the following:
- An excessive release of neurotransmitters
- Blockage of draining venules (e.g., mechanical interference in sickle cell crisis, leukemia, or excessive use of intravenous parenteral lipids)
- Paralysis of the intrinsic detumescence mechanism
- Prolonged relaxation of the intracavernous smooth muscles (most often caused by the use of exogenous smooth-muscle relaxants such as injectable intra-cavernosal prostaglandin E1)

Prolonged low-flow priapism leads to a painful ischemic state, which can cause fibrosis of the corporeal smooth muscle and cavernosal artery thrombosis. The degree of ischemia is a function of the number of emissary veins involved and the duration of occlusion. Light-microscopy studies conducted early on demonstrated that corporeal tissue becomes thickened, edematous, and fibrotic after days of priapism.

116. Ans. (c) **Severe anemia**

(Ref: Harrison 20th edition, p 697; Harrison 19th edition, p 638)

- Beta thalassemia minor: Is a thalassemia trait, these patients have a modest anemia with hematocrit between 28% and 40%.
- The *MCV* ranges from 55 to 75 fL, and the red blood cell count is *normal or increased*.
- The peripheral blood smear is mildly abnormal, with hypochromia, microcytosis, and target cells. In contrast to alpha thalassemia, basophilic stippling slightly elevated.
- Hemoglobin electrophoresis (using quantitative techniques) may show an elevation of hemoglobin A2 to 4-8% & occasional elevations of hemoglobin present is hemoglobin.

117. Ans. (b) **Altered solubility**

(Ref: Harrison 20th edition, p 692)

- When HbS is deoxygenated the sticky patch present on its surface binds to the complementary patch on another deoxygenated HbS molecule.
- "Binding of a number of deoxygenated HbS in this way leads to formation of long fibrous polymers of HbS."
- This stiffens and distort the red cells producing rigid misshaped erythrocytes.
- A molecule of hemoglobin S (HbS) contains two normal á globin chains and two mutant â globin chains in which glutamate at position 6 has been substituted with valine.
- This substitution replaces the polar glutamine residue with a nonpolar valine.
- This change decreases the solubility of the hemoglobin when deoxygenated.
- The replacement of glutamate by valine generates a sticky patch on the surface of HbS.
- The sticky patch is present on both oxygenated and deoxygenated HbS but deoxygenated HbS also contains a complementary site for the sticky patch.
- Such sickle cells frequently block the flow of blood in the narrow capillaries. (The mean diameter of red blood

cells is 7.5 m while that of micro vasculature is 3-4 m so instead of squeezing through the microvasculature like HbA containing RBCs, sickled RBCs have decreased ability to deform and so have difficulty moving through small vessels).

118. Ans. (a) Intron 1 inversion

(Ref: Harrison 19th edition, p 637)

The most common mutation causing â thalassemia is intron /inversion

- Thalassemias are autosomal recessive disorder.
- β thalassemias are caused due to reduced synthesis of beta chain of hemoglobin.
- β thalassemias are the consequence of various point mutations on the globin gene clusters.
- Most of the β thalassemias are caused by point mutations affecting one or few bases.
- Five or six specific mutations usually accounts for more than 90% of cases of β thalassemias.

The most common mutation causing b thalassemia is intron / inversion

Also know:

Synthesis of alpha chain is controlled by 2 gene clusters on → chromosome 16

Synthesis of beta chain is controlled by 2 gene clusters on → chromosome 11

Thalassemia mutations in India

Mutations	Frequency
IVS1-5 (G→C)	48%
619 bp deletion	18%
IVS-1 (G→T)	9%
FR41/42(TCTT)	9%
FR8/9 (+G)	5%
Codonl5 (G→A)	5%
Others	6%
Total	100%

119. Ans. (a) 6 months of age

(Ref: Wintrobe Hematology 11th ed. pg. 442)

- At approximately 20 weeks of fetal development, the site of erythropoiesis begins to switch from the liver and spleen to the bone marrow, where progenitors show increased expression of adult globins, a and ß.
- Hemoglobin A may constitute 5% of ß-family globin expression during this time. Beginning at the thirtieth week and proceeding to the time of birth, a significant switch from fetal to adult erythropoiesis takes place, such that at the time of birth, fetal hemoglobin constitutes approximately 80% of the total hemoglobin.
- Over the next 25 to 30 weeks after birth, fetal hemoglobin concentration decreases by approximately 10% every 2 weeks until it reaches its normal adult level of less than 2% by 30 weeks of age

120. Ans. (b) Normal reticulocyte count

(Ref: Harrison 20th edition, p 692-3; Harrison 19th edition, p 635)

- Reticulocytosis is a feature of all hemolytic anemia. The reticulocyte count is used to estimate the degree of effective erythro-poiesis,which can be reported as absolute reticulocyte count or as a reticulocyte percent-age. The (Ref: range of the reticulocyte percentage in adults is 0.5%-1.5%
- Sickle cell anemia is an autosomal recessive disorder in which an abnormal hemoglobin leads to chronic hemolytic anemia with numerous clinical consequences.
  - A single DNA base change leads to an amino acid substitution of valine for glutamine in the sixth position on the â-globin chain.
  - The abnormal beta chain is designated as p and the tetramer of á2â2 is designated hemoglobin S.
  - When in the deoxy-form, hemoglobin S forms polymers that damage the red blood cell membrane. Both polymer formation & early membrane damage are reversible.
  - However, red blood cells that have undergone repeated sickling are damaged beyond repair & become irreversibly sickled.
  - The rate of sickling is influenced by a number of factors, most importantly by the concentration of hemoglobin S in the individual red blood cell. Red cell dehydration makes the cell quite vulnerable to sickling.
  - Sickling is also strongly influenced by the presence of other hemoglobins within the cell.
  - Hemoglobin F cannot participate in polymer formation.

121. Ans. (c) Thalassemia major

(Ref: Harrison 19th edition, p 638)

The hair on end sign refers to a radiographic appearance on a skull which results from a periosteal reaction manifesting as perpendicular trabeculations interspersed by radiolucent marrow hyperplasia along the skull vault. It is classically described with plain skull radiographs although can also be appreciated on CT or MRI.

Mnemonic: H.I -N.E.S.T

- Herditary spherocytosis
- Iron deficiency Anemia
- Neuroblastoma
- Enzyme deficiency (e.g. G-6-P deficiency causing Hemolytic Anemia)
- Sickle cell disease
- Thalassemia major

122. Ans. (a) Systemic Lupus erythematosus

(Ref: Rosen Emergency Medicine Concepts and Clinical Practice, 2-Volume Set-edited by John A. Marx, Robert S. Hockberger, Harrison 19th edition, p 2134)

- SLE patients with thrombocytosis and anti-phospholipid antibody syndrome are at risk of developing auto-splenectomy. Patients with sickle cell disease often suffer from autosplenectomy as a result of splenic destruction by the numerous infarcts associated with sickle cell crises during childhood. Indeed, the presence of a palpable spleen in a patient with sickle cell disease after age five suggests a coexisting hemoglobinopathy, e.g., thalassemia or hemoglobin C. In addition, patients who receive splenic irradiation for a neoplastic or autoimmune disease are also functionally hyposplenia.

123. Ans. (a) Deletion of three alpha chain genes

(Ref: Harrison 20th edition, p 697; Harrison 19th edition, p 638)

Alpha-Thalassemia		
Silent carrier state	1 gene deletion	$-\alpha\alpha\alpha$
α thalassemia trait	2 gene deletion	$-\alpha-\alpha$
HbH disease	3 gene deletion	$---\alpha$
Hydrops fetalis	4 gene deletion	$----$

124. Ans. (b) Severe iron-deficiency anemia

(Ref: Harrison 20th edition, p 724, Table 98-1; Harrison 19th edition, p 662)

CAUSES OF PANCYTOPENIA

Decreased bone marrow function
1. Aplasia
2. Acute leukaemia, myelodysplasia, myeloma
3. Infiltration with lymphoma, solid tumours,
4. tuberculosis
5. Megaloblastic anaemia
6. Paroxysmal nocturnal haemoglobinuria
7. Myelofibrosis
8. Haemophagocytic syndrome

125. Ans. (c) Portland

(Ref: Harrison 20th edition, p 690; Harrison 19th edition, p 632)

Gower 1	$Z_2\varepsilon_2$	Zeta 2 Epsilon 2
Gower 2	$\alpha^2\varepsilon_2$	Alpha 2 Epsilon 2
Portland	$Z_2\gamma_2$	Zeta 2 Gamma 2
Fetal Hb	$\alpha_2\gamma_2$	Alpha 2 Gamma 2

126. Ans. (b) Oral Deferiprone

(Ref: Harrison 20th edition, p 698; KDT's 6th/868, Harrison 19th edition, p 638)

- Drug of choice for acute iron poisoning is desferrioxamine, however it has to be administered parenterally. It is not effective by oral route.
- In beta thalassemia major, iron excess can result due to repeated blood transfusions and massive hemolysis. The chelating agent has to be administered for long time in this case. Therefore, oral Deferiprone is preferred in this case.

127. Ans. (d) Splenomegaly

(Ref: Harrison 20th edition, p 692-93)

"Sickle cell anemia is characterized by Hyposplenism/ Autosplenectomy (not Splenomegaly)".

128. Ans. (c) Leukopenia

(Ref: Harrison 20th edition, p 692-93)

"Sickle cell anemia is associated with granulocytosis (leukocytosis) and not leukopenia".

129. Ans. (b) Bone pain

(Ref: Harrison 20th edition, p 693)

130. Ans. (a) 0 and 100%

(Ref: Harrison 18th/p 855)

131. Ans. (d) Sickle cell Anemia

(Ref: Robbins 8th edn. ch. 12/p428; Outlines in pathology (2005)/80,82,199)

132. Ans. (d) Patient requires blood transfusion

(Ref: Harrison 20th edition, p 696)

133. Ans. (c) Microcytosis

(Ref: Harrison 20th edition, p 696)

134. Ans. (d) Hb-electrophoresis

(Ref: Harrison 18th/p 854, 859)

G6PD Deficiency and Hereditary Spherocytosis

135. Ans. (d) Bite cells of G-6-PD deficiency

(Ref: Harrison 20th edition, p 717, Fig. 96-7; chapter 12: Robbin's Pathology, 8th edition)

The image shows presence of Bite cells characteristic of G6PD deficiency

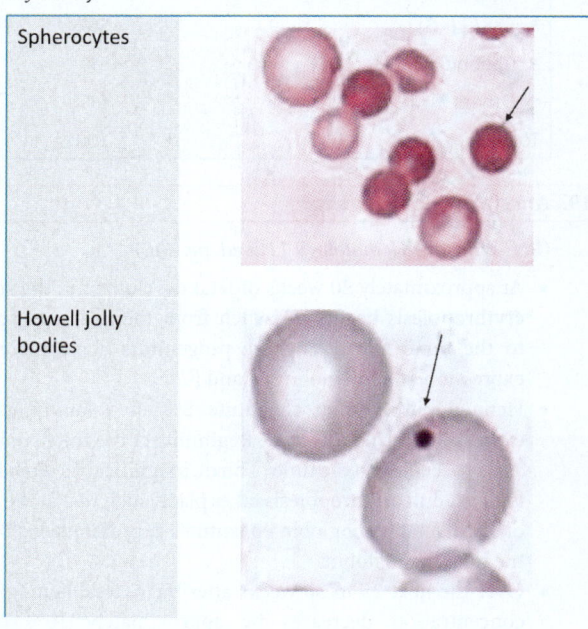

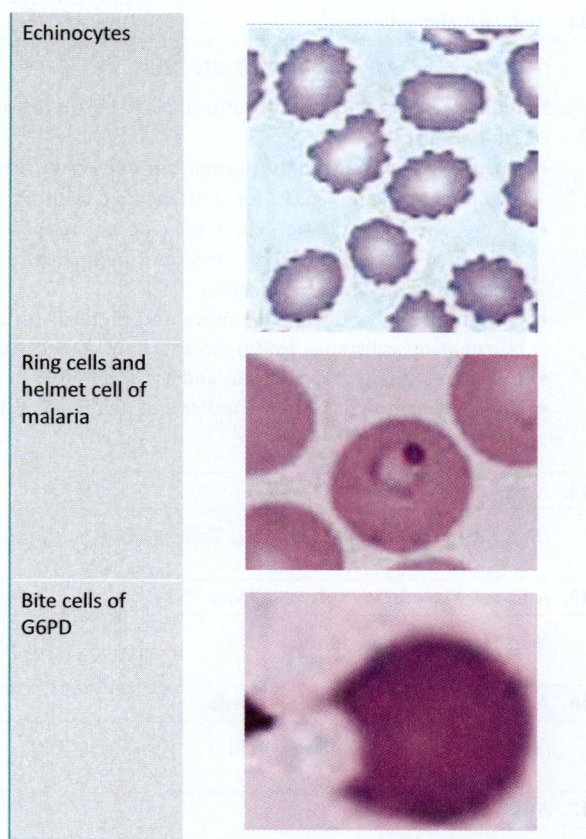

Echinocytes	
Ring cells and helmet cell of malaria	
Bite cells of G6PD	

136. Ans. (d) Penicillin

(Ref: Harrison 20th edition, p 716, Table 96-5; Harrison 19th edition, p 656)

Common oxidative stresses that have been associated with hemolytic crises in patients with G6PD deficiency include the following:

Antibacterial	Antimalarials	Misc. Agents/foods	Misc. Drugs
Dapsone	Primaquine	Fava beans	Doxorubicin
Nalidixic acid	Pamaquine	Naphthalene (mothballs)	Methylene blue
Nitrofurantoin		Toluene	Pyridium
Sulfamethoxazole			Phenylhydrazine
Sulfapyridine			Probenecid

137. Ans. (d) Hemolysis from G6PD enzyme deficiency

(Ref: Harrison 20th edition, p 715-16; Harrison 19th edition, p 662)

- The vast majority of people with G6PD deficiency remain clinically asymptomatic throughout their lifetime
- However, all of them have an increased risk of developing neonatal jaundice, and a risk of developing acute hemolytic anemia (AHA) when challenged by a number of oxidative agents.
- NNJ related to G6PD deficiency is very rarely present at birth. The peak incidence of clinical onset is between day 2 and day 3, and in most cases the anemia is not severe

Hypersplenism	Pancytopenia due to increased destruction in the spleen with splenomegaly and compensatory increase in bone marrow precursors.
Aplastic anemia	Bone marrow damage
Cancer infiltrating the marrow	Bone marrow damage

138. Ans. (d) Common cause of neonatal jaundice

(Ref: Harrison 20th edition, p 714-15; Harrison 19th edition, p 656)

Clinical features of G6PD
1. G6PD confers a relative resistance against falciparum malaria and is XLR in inheritance.
2. Majority of people with G6PD deficiency remain clinically asymptomatic throughout their lifetime.
3. On the contrary, *all of them have an increased risk of developing neonatal jaundice*, with peak incidence of clinical onset is between day 2 and day 3.
4. Increased Risk of developing acute hemolyticanemiaas a result of three types of triggers: (1) fava beans, (2) infections, and (3) drugs

139. Ans. (a) Howell Jolly Bodies

(Ref: Harrison 20th edition, p 379, 383 [Fig. 58-17]; Harrison 19th edition, 81e, 2105)

The image shows presence of basophilic inclusions in pink cytoplasm of RBC diagnostic of Howell jolly bodies.
Heinz bodies are seen only with supravital stain
Pappenhiemer bodies are iron inclusions and are multiple. They are visible with a Wright and/or Giemsa stain but *confirmation of non-heme iron in the granules is made with a Perls' Prussian blue stain.*
Cabot rings are red-violet staining, threadlike strands in the shape of a loop

Red blood cell inclusions

Name of Inclusions	Content
• Howell-Jolly body	DNA
• Basophilic stippling	RNA
• Pappenheimer body	Iron
• HbH body (supravital only)	β-Globin tetramers(β^4)
• Heinz body (supravital only)	Denatured haemoglobin
• Fessus body (supravital only)	α-Globin tetramers(α^4)
• Crystals	Hemoglobin-C
• Cabot rings	Mitotic spindle remnants
• Nucleus	DNA

140. Ans. (c) Howell Jolly bodies

(Ref: Harrison 20th edition, p 379; Harrison's ch. e17. Atlas of Hematology Fig. e17-17)

Howell-Jolly bodies, small nuclear remnants normally removed by the intact spleen, are seen in RBCs in patients after splenectomy and with maturation or dysplastic disorders characterized by excess production.

141. Ans. (d) Confers protection against plasmodium vivax

(Ref: Harrison 20th edition, p 714-16; Harrison 19th edition, p 656)

- About 400 million people have a G6PD deficiency gene.
- In several of these areas the frequency of a G6PD deficiency gene may be as high as 20% or more.
- Indeed, G6PD is one of the best characterized examples of genetic polymorphisms in the human species.
- There is strong evidence that G6PD deficiency has been selected by Plasmodium falciparum malaria, by virtue of the fact that it confers a relative resistance against this highly lethal infection
- There are three types of triggers: (1) fava beans, (2) infections, and (3) drugs.
- Typically, a hemolytic attack starts with malaise, weakness, and abdominal or lumbar pain. After an interval of several hours to 2–3 days, the patient develops jaundice and often dark urine, due to hemoglobinuria.
- The blood film shows anisocytosis, polychro-masia, and spherocytes.
- The most typical feature is the presence of bizarre poikilocytes, with red cells that appear to have unevenly distributed hemoglobin ("hemighosts") and red cells that appear to have had parts of them bitten away ("bite cells" or "blister cells").

142. Ans. (c) Hemolysis on exposure to hypertonic saline environment

(Ref: Harrison 20th edition, p 711; Hematology in clinical practice 4th ed. ch. 11)

The osmotic fragility test (OFT) is used to measure erythrocyte resistance to hemolysis while being exposed to varying levels of dilution of a saline solution. *When erythrocytes are exposed to a hypotonic environment, water enters the cell and causes swelling and eventual lysis. The susceptibility of osmotic lysis of erythrocytes is a function of surface area to volume ratio.*
In a disease such as hereditary spherocytosis, erythrocytes have a smaller ratio of surface area to volume and are thus more susceptible to osmotic stress, as opposed to the increased resistance characteristic of thalassemia, iron deficiency anemia, or any other condition that would cause an increased surface area–to–volume ratio.

Conditions associated with increased osmotic fragility include the following:
Hereditary spherocytosis
Poisoning
Severe burns

The following conditions are associated with decreased fragility:
Thalassemia
Iron deficiency anemia
Sickle cell anemia

143. Ans. (b) Hyperkalaemia

(Ref: Harrison 19th edition, p 281, 81e-3f)

Hereditary spherocytosis is an autosomal dominant disease of variable severity.

- Anemia may or may not be present, since the bone marrow may be able to compensate for shortened red cell survival
- Severe anemia (aplastic crisis) may occur in folic acid deficiency or when bone marrow compensation is temporarily impaired by infection.
- Chronic hemolysis causes jaundice and pigment (calcium bilirubinate) gallstones, leading to attacks of cholecystitis
- Examination may reveal icterus and a palpable spleen.
- Chronic haemolysis causes jaundice and pigment gall stone and hyperkalemia.

144. Ans. (c) Glycophorin C

(Ref: Harrison 20th edition, p 711, Table 96-3)

145. Ans. (c) Hereditary spherocytosis

(Ref: Harrison 20th edition, p 711)

146. Ans. (b) Hereditary spherocytosis

(Ref: Harrison 20th edition, p 712)

147. Ans. (a) Oestrogen

(Ref: Harrison 18th/p 879)

PNH and PCH

148. Ans. (b) Thalassemia major

(Ref: Harrison 19th edition, p 637, 660)

Celiac disease	It is a disease of small intestine where villous atrophy is seen. Since duodenum is involved it would lead to decreased iron absorption. *Hence iron deficiency anemia and low serum ferritin is seen in celiac disease.*
PNH	The complement mediated hemolysis occurs intravascularly and leads to hemoglobinuria and hemosiderinuria. Since hemosiderin is being lost, loss of iron will result in ferritin stores will be consumed at a faster rate leading to low ferritin.
Nutritional anemia	Due to dietary deficiency iron and ferritin both would be low.

Ferritin is increased in several chronic hemolytic conditions:
1. Congenital membrane defects
2. Enzymopathies
3. Chronic cold agglutinin disease
4. Congenital dyserythropoietic anemia.

The iron produced by ineffective erythropoiesis and extravascular hemolysis is not easily eliminated and that anemia itself is a powerful stimulus for iron absorption in the gut.

149. Ans. (a) Fanconi's anemia

(Ref: Harrison 20th edition, p 724, Table 98-1; Harrison 19th edition Chapter 107, p 664)

Pancytopenia with Hypocellular Bone Marrow
Acquired aplastic anemia
Constitutional aplastic anemia (*Fanconi's anem*ia, dyskeratosiscongenita)
Some myelodysplasia
Rare aleukemicleukemia
Some acute lymphoid leukemia
Some lymphomas of bone marrow

150. Ans. (d) G6PD deficiency

(Ref: Harrison 20th edition, p 724, Table 98-1; Harrison 19th edition, p 654, and Chapter 107)

Pancytopenia with Cellular Bone Marrow	
Primary bone marrow diseases	Secondary to systemic diseases
Myelodysplasia	Systemic lupus erythematosus
Paroxysmal nocturnalhemoglobinuria	Hypersplenism
	B_{12}, folate deficiency
Myelofibrosis	Overwhelming infection
Some aleukemicleukemia	Alcohol
Myelophthisis	Brucellosis
Bone marrow lymphoma	Sarcoidosis
Hairy cell leukemia	Tuberculosis
	Leishmaniasis

151. Ans. (a) Flow cytometry

(Ref: Harrison 20th edition, p 721; Harrison, 19th edition, p 660)

The image shows dark coloured urine in first sample with progressive change to normal straw colour with subsequent samples. This is suggestive of diagnosis of paroxysmal nocturnal hemoglobinuria.
The investigation of choice for PNH is Flow cytometry.
In alklaptonuria, urine turns black on air exposure and hence all samples should have been uniformly black.
In myoglobinuria urine is of colour *red* and occurs with crush injury.

152. Ans. (d) G6PD deficiency

(Ref: Harrison 20th edition, p 724, Table 98-1; Harrison 19th edition, p 656)

Pancytopenia with Cellular Bone Marrow

Primary bone marrow diseases	Secondary to systemic diseases
Myelodysplasia syndromes	
• Hypersplenism	• Systemic lupus erythematosus
	• Paroxysmal nocturnal hemoglobinuria
• Myelofibrosis	• B_{12} folate deficiency (Megaloblastic anemia)
• Aleukemic leukemia	• Overwhelming infection
• Myelophthisis	• Alcohol
• Bone marrow lymphoma	• Brucellosis
• Hairy cell leukemia	• Sarcoidosis
	• Tuberculosis
	• Leishmaniasis

153. Ans. (b) Increased LAP scores

(Ref: Harrison 20th edition, p 720-21; Harrison 19th edition, p 662)

- Since in PNH there is loss of hemoglobin and iron in urine, the negative iron deficit will lead to iron deficiency anemia.
- The hypercoagulable state in PNH leads to Budd Chiari syndrome and this disorder, being an acquired stem cell defect can lead to aplastic anemia.
- The clinical syndrome can present in 3 types of symptoms including (1) an acquired intracorpuscular hemolytic anemia due to the abnormal susceptibility of the RBC membrane to the hemolytic activity of complement; (2) thromboses in large vessels, such as hepatic, abdominal, cerebral, and subdermal veins; and (3) a deficiency in hematopoiesis that may be mild or severe, such as pancytopenia in an aplastic anemia state

154. Ans. (c) Nutritional anemia

(Ref: Harrison's 18th edition, p 449, 450, 452)

Choices A and B are ruled out on being hemolytic anemias

Congential Dyserythropoietic anemia

- It represents a family of inherited refractory anemias characterized by ineffective erythropoiesis.
- Clinically it is characterized by varying degrees of anemia inspite of increased marrow erythroid activity.
- There is reticulocytosis but it is less than expected far the degree of anemia.
- Dyserythropoietic anemia could be suspected in the presence of symptoms and signs of increased hemoglobin (Hb) turnover, such as mild jaundice, and low or absent haptoglobin, as in hemolytic anemias, with a reticulocytosis that does not correspond to the degree of anemia. The bone marrow is always hypercellular, exclusively due to a pronounced increase of erythroblasts, with increased erythropoietic/granulopoietic ratio. Extra-medullary hematopoiesis presenting as paravertebral bulks may be observed in all types of CDAs

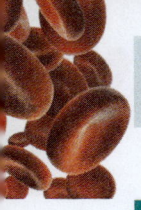

Reticulocyte count		
Decreased		**Increased**
Hypoproliferative Disorder Marrow damage • Infiltration/fibrosis • Aplasia Decreased stimulation • Inflammation • Metabolic defect • Renal disease	Maturation disorder Cytoplasmic defects Iron deficiency • Thalassemia • Sideroblastic anemia Nuclear defects • Folate deficiency • Vitamin B12 deficiency • Drug toxicity • Refractory anemia	Hemolysis/hemorrhage • Blood loss • Intravascular hemolysis • Metabolic defect • Membrane abnormality • Hemoglobinopathy • Autoimmune defect • Fragmentation hemolysis PNH

155. Ans. (a) Chronic autoimmune form responds well to splenectomy

(Ref: Harrison 20th edition, p 719; Harrison 19th edition, p 662)

- PCH is a rather rare form of AIHA occurring mostly in children, usually triggered by a viral infection, usually self-limited, and characterized by the involvement of the so-called Donath-Landsteiner antibody.
- In vitro this antibody has unique serologic features: it has anti-P specificity and it binds to red cells only at a low temperature (optimally at 4°C), but when the temperature is shifted to 37°C, lysis of red cells takes place in the presence of complement. Consequently, in vivo there is intravascular hemolysis, resulting in hemoglo-binuria.
- Clinically, the differential diagnosis must include other causes of hemoglobinuria, but the presence of the Donath-Landsteiner antibody will prove PCH
- Once strongly linked with syphilis, paroxysmal cold hemoglobinuria is now associated with numerous infectious agents. Identified pathogens have included the following: measles, mumps, influenza, varicella-zoster virus (VZV), cytomegalovirus (CMV), Epstein-Barr virus (EBV), adenovirus, parvovirus B19, Coxsackie A9, Haemophilus influenzae, Mycoplasma pneumoniae, and Klebsiella pneumoniae. The development of the D-L antibody has also been reported following measles immunization. Other associations include solid organ and hematopoietic neoplasms. The mainstay of treatment for paroxysmal cold hemoglobinuria is supportive care and the avoidance of cold exposure.

Management
1. Once hemolysis is suspected, folic acid 1 mg/d orally should be instituted to help with erythropoiesis. Folic acid is lost via the hemolytic process and hence needs to be replenished.
2. Administer warmed, packed RBC transfusions for life-threatening hemolysis and symptomatic anemia. Utilizing washed RBC units has not been proven to improve transfusion safety, but this can be performed if patient's condition remains refractory to standard warmed products.
3. As most of the blood supply is P-antigen positive, finding phenotypic p, also called Tj(a-), blood may not be feasible. However, the antibody should not interfere with donor cell survival, nor should it be problematic with pretransfusion and compatibility testing, as the pathogenic immunoresponse does not occur at normal body temperatures.
4. Treat the uncommon chronic form with RBC transfusions only when severe exacerbation occurs.
5. Plasma exchange therapy with 5% albumin fluid replacement has been successfully employed

156. Ans. (a) Flow cytometry

(Ref: Harrison 20th edition, p 721; Harrison 19th edition, p 660)

- Flow cytometry is used to detect CD59 (MIRL), a glycoprotein, and CD55 (DAF) in regulation of complement action. Absence or reduced expression of both CD59 and CD55 on PNH RBCs is diagnostic.
- The Ham test (acidified serum lysis) establishes the diagnosis of paroxysmal nocturnal hemoglobinuria (PNH), demonstrating a characteristic abnormality of PNH red blood cells by acidified fresh normal serum. Here is a PNH patient's (Pt) red blood cells lysed by normal serum at room temperature (RT) and at 37°C compared with normal red cells (no hemolysis) (control [C]). Heated serum at 56°C inactivates complement and prevents hemolysis in PNH cells.

157. Ans. (b) Increased LAP scores

(Ref: Harrison 20th edition, p 720-21)

158. Ans. (a) Hypocellular marrow

(Ref: PNH is associated with a normocellular or hypercellular marrow and not with a hypocellular marrow. Rubin's 8th edn/p 432)

159. Ans. (c) Decreased LDH

(Ref: Harrison 20th edition, p 721)

160. Ans. (a) Diabetes Mellitus

(Ref: Harrison 20th edition, p 720, 1910)

161. Ans. (d) Thrombosis of hepatic veins

(Ref: Harrison 20th edition, p 837)

Disorders of WBC & Leukemias

162. Ans. (a) Chemoport

(Ref: Internet)

The image shows a chemoport which allows the patient to deliver drugs into a central line by himself/herself. It avoids the hassles and pain associated with repeated peripheral line insertion. The schematic diagram depicting the tip of the catheter in the Superior vena cava is shown below. The diagram on left shows insertion of a needle into the port by the patient himself.

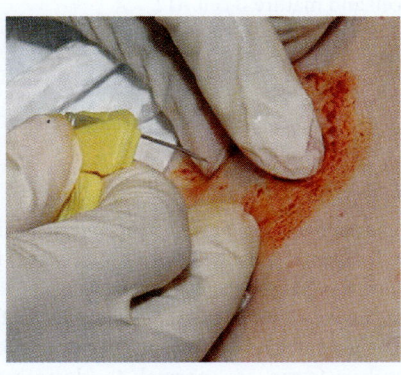
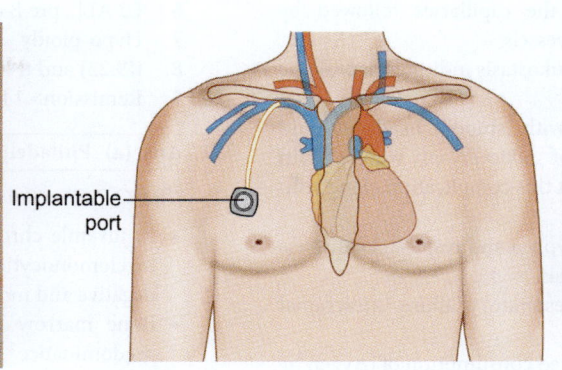
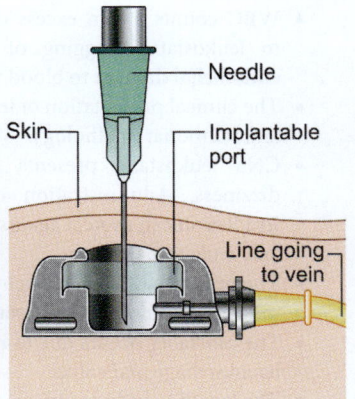

163. Ans. (d) Adult T-cell Leukemia

(*Ref: Harrison 20th edition, p 1391*)

- Adult T-cell leukemia is caused by HTLV-1 whereas the remaining diseases are caused by HHV-8.
- Diseases caused by HHV-8 infection include Kaposi sarcoma, multicentric Castleman disease (MCD), and primary effusion lymphoma (PEL), which occur primarily in patients with HIV infection.

164. Ans. (a) Dexamethasone

(*Ref: Harrison 20th edition, p 748; Harrison 19th edition, p 686*)

- The DOC for management of APML is ATRA (Al Trans Retinoic acid)
- Use of tretinoin decreases the frequency of DIC but produces another complication known as *APL differentiation syndrome*.
- On administration of tretinoin the immature cells will mature. However due to adhesion of these differentiated neoplastic cells to pulmonary vasculature endothelium, the *microcirculation of lungs is affected*. Hence the features of respiratory distress develop in the patient.
- It occurs within 3 weeks of treatment and is characterised by fever, fluid retention, dyspnea, chest pain and pulmonary infiltrates.
- The mortality rate for APL Differentiation syndrome can approach 10% due to development of severe hypoxia and pericardial/pleural effusions.
- The best management for APL differentiation syndrome is administration of steroids.

165. Ans. (a) ALL; (b) CLL; (c) CML; (d) AML

(*Ref: Page 603: O.P. Ghai: 8th edition*)

The drug regimen for induction in ALL is Vincristine, Adriamycin, L-Asparaginase and Prednisolone. Remission is achieved in 95-98% of cases.

Chemotherapy protocol for ALL

Cycle	Chemotherapy
Induction 1(I1)	Prednisone Vincristine Daunorubicin L-asparaginase
Induction 2 (I2)	Methotrexate 6-mercaptopurine Cyclophosphamide Methotrexate Cranial irradiation
Repeat induction 1 (RI 1) Consolidation (C)	Same as induction 1 Cyclophosphamide Vincristine Cytosine arabinoside
Maintenance (M): 6 cycles	6-mercaptopurine Prednisone Vincristine Daunorubicin L-asparaginase 6-mercaptopurine

Acute Lymphoblastic leukaemia is the most common cancer seen in children.
Most common benign tumour in children is hemangioma.

166. Ans. (c) Blast Crisis in CML

(*Ref: Harrison: 19th edition, p 139-e3*)

5 year Survival rate after bone marrow transplantation
SCID, Aplastic Anaemia, Thalassemia	90%
A.M.L	40-60%
A.L.L	40-50%
C.M.L Chronic phase	70%
C.M.L Blast crisis	15%
C.L.L	50%
N.H.L	40%

167. Ans. (b) AML

(*Ref: Harrison 20th edition, p 517; Harrison: 19th edition, p 1793*)

Leukostasis is common with Acute Myeloid leukemia followed by ALL. It is rare in case of CLL or CML.

168. Ans. (d) Lung

(*Ref: Harrison 20th edition, p 517; Harrison 19th edition, p 1793*)

Contd...

- WBC counts are in excess of >100,000/cu.mm and leads to leukostatic plugging of the capillaries followed by endothelial damage to blood vessels.
- The clinical presentation of leukostasis indicates neurologic and pulmonary pathology.
- CNS leukostasis presents with stupor, headache and dizziness. Administration of 600cGY of whole brain irradiation can protect against this complication along with anti-leukemic therapy
- The presence of dyspnea, tachypnea and respiratory distress indicates pulmonary leukostasis.
- The mortality occurs due to respiratory failure, intracranial haemorrhage and coma.
- The low PO2 is due to increased consumption of oxygen by leucocytes.
- It is common with Acute leukemia subtypes like Acute promyelocytic leukemia, acute monocytic leukemia and T cell type of ALL

169. Ans. (a) Kaposi sarcoma

(Ref: Harrison 20th edition, p 768, 775, 799; Harrison 19th edition, p 716)

Hodgkin lymphoma	The most popular chemotherapy regimens used in Hodgkin's disease include doxorubicin, bleomycin, vinblastine, and dacarbazine (ABVD) and mechlorethamine, vincristine, procarbazine, and prednisone (MOPP). ABVD is preferred but for solving the question MOPP is what needs to be considered.
CLL	Treatment for CLL/ SLL is RCHOP incorporating rituximab, Cyclophosphamide, vincristine and prednisolone.
Multiple myeloma	Lenalidomide, *dexamethasone* and Bortezomib.

170. Ans. (c) Response to treatment

(Ref: Robbins 9th edition, p 590-592)

Leucocyte count> 50000/ul	Poor prognosis TLC> 10,000/ul has good prognosis
Hyperploidy	Favourable prognostic factor
Response to treatment	Remission status at 14 days of chemotherapy is best guide to prognosis.
Organomegaly	poor prognosis Lymph node, liver, spleen and testis enlargement indicate spread of cancer

Unfavourable prognostic factors for ALL
1. Extreme age group: <1 year or >10 years
2. Black males
3. TLC>2 lac/cu.mm
4. Organomegaly
5. CNS Leukemia
6. L2 ALL, pre B cell and mature B cell ALL
7. Hypo-ploidy
8. t(9;22) and t(4;11)
9. Remission> 14 days

171. Ans. (a) Philadelphia chromosome is negative

(Ref: O.P. Ghai 8th edition, p 308)

- In juvenile chronic myeloid leukemia or juvenile chronic myelomonocytic leukemia, Philadelphia chromosome is negative and monosomy 7 is seen in 30% cases.
- Bone marrow aspirates show increased cellularity with predominance of granulocytic cells in all stages of maturation, megakaryocytes are normal to decreased. Hence low platelets are seen and need platelet transfusions.
- The disease has a fulminant, rapidly progressive course. Even with transplant there is 50% event free survival at 3 years.
- Management is supportive and needs packed RBC, platelet transfusions, infection management and allogenic stem cell transplantation.

172. Ans. (b) Cladiribine

(Ref: Harrison 20th edition, p 784; 706; Harrison 19th edition, p 412)

Cell leukemia is responsive to chemotherapy with interferon alpha, pentostatin, or cladribine, with the latter being the usually preferred treatment.

Cell leukemia presents predominantly in older males. Typical presentation involves pancytopenia, although occasional patients will have a leukemic presentation. Splenomegaly is usual.

- The malignant cells appear to have "hairy" projections on light and electron microscopy and show a characteristic staining pattern with tartrate-resistant acid phosphatase.
- Bone marrow is typically not able to be aspirated, and biopsy shows a pattern of fibrosis with diffuse infiltration by the malignant cells. Patients with this disorder are prone to unusual infections, including infection by *Mycobacterium aviumintracellulare*, and to vasculitic syndromes.

173. Ans. (a) Age between 1-10 years

(Ref: Harrison 19th edition, p 699-700)

Prognostic factor in acute lymphoblastic leukemia

Excellent prognosis	t(12;21) and TEL-AML1 fusion Hyperdiploidy and trisomy of specific chromosomes (4, 10 and 17) is associated with an excellent prognosis. Age > 1 years and < 10 years
Dismal prognosis	t(9;22) or Philadelphia chromosome and BCR-ABL fusion Hypodiploidy with chromosome number <45 is associated with a poor prognosis Age > 10 years WBC> 50,000/cu.mm^3 CNS leukemia at presentation

174. Ans. (a) Long arm of chromosome 9 and long arm of chromosome 22

(Ref: Harrison 20th edition, p 748; Harrison 19th edition, p 101e-3)

- The exact chromosomal defect in Philadelphia chromosome is a translocation, in which parts of two chromosomes, 9 and 22, swap places. The result is that a fusion gene is created by juxta positioning the *Abl1* gene on chromosome 9 (region q34) to a part of the BCR ("breakpoint cluster region") gene on chromosome 22 (region q11). This is a reciprocal translocation, creating an elongated chromosome 9, and a truncated chromosome 22 (the Philadelphia chromosome).
- The significance of knowing this information is that this chromosome defect causes activation of an enzyme by the name of tyrosine kinase which provides energy to the cancer cells to divide uncontrollably.

175. Ans. (a) Elevated

(Ref: Harrison 20th edition, p 751; Harrison 19th edition, p 687)

In CML there will be rise in
1. B12 level
2. LDH level

And decreased levels of ALP.

176. Ans. (a) 100/μL

(Ref: Harrison 20th edition, p 398; Harrison 19th edition, p 237)

The term agranulocytosis is used to communicate a more severe subset of neutropenia. Agranulocytosis refers to a virtual absence of neutrophils in peripheral blood. It is usually applied to cases in which the ANC is lower than 100/μL.

177. Ans. (a) Allogeneic bone marrow transplantation

(Ref: Harrison 20th edition, p 755; Harrison 19th edition, p 694)

Allogeneic Stem Cell transplantation is currently the only curative therapy for CML and, when feasible, is the treatment of choice.
- Interferons when allogeneic SCT is not feasible, IFN-a therapy used to be the treatment of choice before Imatinib Mesylate became available.
- Only longer follow-up of patients treated with imatinib will prove whether IFN-a will still have a role in the treatment of CML.
- Hydroxyurea, a ribonucleotide reductase inhibitor, induces rapid disease control.
- Allogenic bone marrow transplantation is treatment of choice for patients of CML.

178. Ans. (b) 500-1000/mm³

(Ref: Hematology in clinical practice. 4th ed. ch. 16)

Neutropenia is classified as mild, moderate, or severe, based on the ANC. Mild neutropenia is present when the ANC is 1000-1500 cells/μL, moderate neutropenia is present with an ANC of 500-1000/μL, and severe neutropenia refers to an ANC lower than 500 cells/μL. The risk of bacterial infection is related to both the severity and duration of the neutropenia.

179. Ans. (d) CLL

(Ref: Harrison 20th edition, p 763; Harrison 19th edition, p 701)

Radiation has been mentioned as risk factor for both the myeloid cancers as well as ALL.

180. Ans. (a) Neutropenia

(Ref: Harrison 20th edition, p 403-4; Katzung's 11th 580-581, Harrison 19th edition, p 103e-24)

- Filgrastim (G-CSF) and sargramostim (GM-CSF) are used to prevent or treat chemotherapy induced neutropenia.
- Erythropoietin is used to treat anemia associated with chronic renal failure and cancer chemo-therapy.
- Oprelvekin (1L-11) is used to prevent and treat thrombocytopenia.

181. Ans. (a) Acute promyelocytic leukemia

(Ref: Harrison 20th edition, p 748; Harrison 19th edition, p 686)

- Arsenic trioxide has significant anti-leukemic activity and is being explored as part of initial treatment in clinical trials of APL.
- In a randomized trial, arsenic trioxide improved outcome if utilized after achievement of Complete Remission and before consolidation therapy with anthracycline-based chemotherapy.
- Patients receiving arsenic trioxide are at risk of APL differentiation syndrome, especially when it is administered during induction or salvage treatment after disease relapse. In addition, arsenic trioxide may prolong the QT interval, increasing the risk of cardiac arrhythmias

182. Ans. (a) M2

(Ref: Harrison 19th edition, p 678)

- M2- AML with maturation is characterized by 20% or more myeloblasts in the blood or bone marrow and 10% or more neutrophils at different stages of maturation. Monocytes constitute less than 20% of bone marrow cells
- M2- AML comprises approximately 30% to 45% of cases of AML. While it occurs in all age groups, 20% of patients are younger than 25 years and 40% of patients are aged 60 years or older. Patients frequently present with anemia, thrombocytopenia, and neutropenia.
- Morphologic features include the following:
  1. Myeloblasts with and without azurophilic granules.
  2. Auer rods.
  3. Promyelocytes, myelocytes, and neutrophils 10% or more of the bone marrow cells.
  4. Abnormal nuclear segmentation in neutrophils.
  5. Increased eosinophil precursors (frequently).
  6. Hypercellular marrow (usually).
  7. Blasts and maturing neutrophils reactive with antibodies to MPO and lysozyme

183. Ans. (a) LAP (leukocyte alkaline phosphatase)

(Ref: Harrison's 18th edition, p 477)

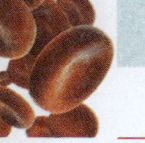

184. Ans. (a) M3

(Ref: Harrison 19th edition, p 678)

- In acute promyelocytic leukemia (APL), TF is secreted directly into the bloodstream by the membranes of the promyelocyte blast cells, which initiates the coagulation cascade causing DIC.
- An estimated 85% of patients diagnosed with APL will develop DIC.
- Although DIC is common in APL, APL itself is a rare form of acute myelogenous leukemia (AML), subtype M3. APL accounts for approximately 10%-15% of adult patients diagnosed with AML
- Cytogenetically, APL is identified by a translocation between chromosomes 15 and 17 (t[15, 17]), which results in the formation of promyelocytic leukemia gene and retinoic acid receptor.
- Significant gastrointestinal bleeding, intrapulmo-nary hemorrhage, or intracranialhemorrhage occurs most often in M3 AML.
- Bleeding associated with coagulopathies may also occur in M5 AML and with extreme degrees of leukocytosis or thrombocytopenia in other FAB subtypes.
- Retinal hemorrhages are detected in 15% of patients.
- Infiltration of the gingivae, skin, soft tissues, or the meninges with leukemic blasts at diagnosis is characteristic of the monocytic subtypes (M4 and M5)

185. Ans. (c) Lagherhan's cell histiocytosis

(Ref: O.P. Ghai 7th edition, p 595, Harrison 19th edition, p 135e-9/1713)

Seborrheic dermatitis, polyuria, hepatosplenomegaly and ear discharge suggests the diagnosis of Langerhan 's cell histiocytosis.

186. Ans. (b) Myelomonocytic leukaemia

(Ref: Harrison 19th edition, p 682)

- Significant gastrointestinal bleeding, intra-pulmonary hemorrhage, or intracranial hemorrhage occur most often in M3 AML.
- Bleeding associated with coagulopathies may also occur in M5 aML and with extreme degrees of leukocytosis or throm-bocytopenia in other FAB subtypes.
- Retinal hemorrhages are detected in 15% of patients.
- Infiltration of the gingivae, skin, soft tissues, or the meninges with leukemic blasts at diagnosis is characteristic of the monocytic subtypes (M4 and M5)
- **Note:** *Gum hypertrophy (leukemia infiltration) is most common in Monocytic Leukemia*

187. Ans. (c) CLL

(Ref: Harrison 19th edition, p 703)

- B cell CLL represents the most common lymphoid leukemia
- Median age of presentation is 65 years with 53% male presentation
- The diagnosis of typical B cell CLL is made when an increased number of circulating lymphocytes (i.e. >4 x 109/L and usually >10 x 109/L) is found that are monoclonal B cells expressing the CD5 antigen. Finding bone marrow infiltration by the same cells confirms the diagnosis.
- The peripheral blood smear in such patients typically shows many "smudge" or "basket" cells, nuclear remnants of cells damaged by the physical shear stress of making the blood smear. If cytogenetic studies are performed, trisomy 12 is found in 25–30% of patients. Abnormalities in chromosome 13 are also seen
- CML presents insidiously with massive splenomegaly Elevated white blood (cell) counts (WBCs), with increases in both immature and mature granulocytes, are present at diagnosis. Usually <5% circulating blasts and <10% blasts and promyelocytes are noted, with the majority of cells being myelocytes, metamyelocytes, and band forms NONE OF WHICH ARE MENTIONED IN QUESTION.At diagnosis, bone marrow cellularity is increased, with an increased myeloid-to-erythroid ratio. The marrow blast percentage is generally normal or slightly elevated. Marrow or blood basophilia, eosinophilia, and monocytosis may be present.
- TB presents with symptoms while presentation of patient is asymptomatic

188. Ans. (a) Intrathecal methotrexate

(Ref: Ghai 7th edition, p 590)

To prevent C.N.S. Relapse intra-thecal triple, therapy of methotrexate, cytosine arabinoside and hydrocortisone is preferable to intracranial irradiation/methotrexate alone.

189. Ans. (d) M3

(Ref: Harrison 19th edition, p 683)

Ref: FAB = French-Americal-British system

Acute Myeloid Leukemia

Categorized on basis of Morphology & Histochemistry

M1	Acute myeloblastic leukemia
M2	Acute myeloblastic leukemia with differentiation
M3	Acute promyelocyte leukemia
M4	Acute myelomonocytic leukemia
M5	Acute monoblastic leukemia
M6	Erythroleukemia
M7	Megakaryoblastic leukemia.

Acute myeloid: FAB1 Classification; MO un-differentiated; M1 minimal differentiation; M2 differentiated; M3 promyelocytic; M4 myelomono-cytic; M5 monocytic; M6 erythrocytic; M7 megakar-yocytic

190. Ans. (a) JMML

(Ref : Nelson's 18th edition, p 495.5)

- JMML (also known as juvenile chronic myelomonocytic leukemia) is a rare hematopoietic malignancy of childhood accounting for 2% of all childhood leukemias.
- Definitive treatment is bone marrow transplantation and medical treatment with 13-cis retinoic acid provides an improvement. Do not confuse with A.T.R.A (al-trans-retinoic acid) used for acute meloid leukemia.

- A number of clinical and laboratory features distinguish JMML from adult-type chronic myeloid leukemia, a disease noted only occasionally in children. In children presenting with clinical features suggestive of JMML, a definitive diagnosis requires the following

Major criteria (all three required)
- No Philadelphia chromosome or BCR/ABL fusion gene.
- Peripheral blood monocytosis is greater than $1 \times 10^9/L$.
- Fewer than 20% blasts (including promonocytes) in the blood and bone marrow.

Minor criteria (two or more required)
- Fetal hemoglobin (Hb F) increased for age.
- Immature granulocytes in the peripheral blood.
- White blood cell count is greater than $1 \times 10^9/L$.
- Clonal chromosomal abnormality (e.g., monosomy 7).
- Granulocyte-macrophage colony-stimulating factor (GM-CSF) hypersensitivity of myeloid progenitors in vitro.

The clinical features of JMML at the time of initial presentation may include the following:
- Constitutional symptoms (e.g., malaise, pallor, and fever) or evidence of an infection.
- Symptoms of bronchitis or tonsillitis (in approximately 50% of cases).
- Bleeding diathesis.
- Maculopapular skin rashes (in 40%–50% of cases).
- Lymphadenopathy (in approximately 75% of cases).
- Hepatosplenomegaly (in most cases).

191. Ans. (c) Philadelphia chromosome is positive

(Ref: Nelson 18th ed. ch. 495.5 and Ghai 5th edition, p 465, Harrison 19th edition, p 687)

- Juvenile myelomonocytic leukemia is a variant of chronic myeloid leukemia.

It differs from CML in following features:
- Affects children <4 years of age
- Philadelphia chromosome negative
- HbF level is increased
- The main cells involved are monocytes instead of granulocytes
- Thrombocytopenia instead of thrombocytosis
- Poorer prognosis

Diagnostic criteria for Juvenile myelomonocytic myeloid leukemia (JMML)

Clinical Features
- Hepatosplenomegaly
- Lymphadenopathy
- Rash
- Pallor

Laboratory Features

Essential	Atleast two of the following
• No bcr-abl fusion gene	• Increased HbF
• Monocytes>$1.0 \times 10^9/L$	• Circulating myeloid precursors
• Marrow blasts < 20%	• WBC>$10 \times 10^9/L$
	• Clonal cytogenetic abnormality
	• Hypersensitivity of myeloid precursors to GM-CSF in vitro

192. Ans. (c) Chronic Myelogenous leukemia

(Ref: Harrison 19th edition, p 687)

Chronic myeloid leukemia is characterized by proliferation of multi-potent progenitor cell that is capable of giving rise to mature erythrocytes, platelets, granulocytes, monocytes (and in some cases) lymphocyte

Findings in Peripheral smear in CML
1. In contrast to normal bone marrow, which is usually about 50% cellular and 50% fat, CML marrow are usually 100% cellular, with maturing granulocytic precursors comprising most of the increased cellularity.
2. Marked myeloid hyperplasia
3. M.E. ratio increased to 20:1
4. Increase in granulocytic precursors i.e. increase in basophil, eosinophil and their precursor
5. Erythroid precursors normal decreased (d/t increased myeloid precursors)
6. Megakaryocytes normal or increased

193. Ans. (a) Juvenile Chronic myelogenous leukemia (CML)

(Ref: Ghai 6th edition, p 569)

194. Ans. (a) Steroid

(Ref: Harrison 18th edition, p 931, 932)

195. Ans. (d) All of the above

(Ref: Wintrobe's Atlas of Clinical Hematology (2007)/138)

196. Ans. (c) Philadelphia chromosome is positive

(Ref: Ghai 5th edition, p 465)

197. Ans. (d) MPO

(Ref: Harrison's 18th edition, Ch 109)

198. Ans. (d) Hyperdiploidy

(Ref: Wintrobe's 11th edition, p 2145, 2142)

199. Ans. (a) Intrathecal methotrexate

(Ref: Cancer Chemotherapy: Medicine outlinr series 2nd/167; Ghai 6th edition, p 564)

200. Ans. (b) White cell infusion

(Ref: Harrison 18th edition, p 476 Read text below)

While all might be used, the best to be eliminated here is a 'white cell transfusion' as its exact role is yet to be established. White cell infusion (transfusion) as a measure is still controversial- Harriso

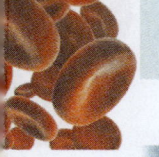

Lymphomas

201. Ans. (a) Nodular lymphocytic predominant

(Ref: Harrison 20th edition, p 783; Harrison 19th edition, p 709)

- The key words are cells in enlarged lymph nodes being CD20 positive and CD15 and CD30 negative which is seen exclusively in nodular lymphocytic predominant Hodgkin's disease.
- This subtype is also called Atypical Hodgkin's disease. The RS cell variant is called popcorn cell/LH cell variant.
- This subtype exhibits number of characteristics which suggest its relationship to non-Hodgkin lymphoma. They are

1. Expression of J chain
2. CD45 positivity
3. Epithelial membrane antigen expression
4. Absence of CD15 and CD 30 expression

202. Ans. (d) Lymphocyte predominant Hodgkin's disease

(Ref: Harrison 20th edition, p 783; Robbins 7th edition, p 686-68)

Variants of Reed-Sternberg Cells	Subtypes of Hodgkins Associated
Mononuclear variant = Variant of R.S. cell which has the same characteristic but is mononucleated.	Mixed cellularity
Lacunar Variant = Large cells with hyper-lobated nucleus, multiple small nuclei and eosinophilic cytoplasm around the nucleus creating an empty space called lacunae	Nodular sclerosis
Lympho-histiocytic variant (popcorn cell variant) = Cell with multiple folded or convoluted nuclear contour resembling a "popcorn kernel"	Lymphocytic predominant

203. Ans. (d) In general follicular NHL has worse prognosis compared to diffuse NHL

(Ref: Harrison 20th edition, p 776; Harrison 19th edition, p 701)

The prognosis of Non-Hodgkin's lymphoma varies markedly with various histological types of Non Hodgkin's lymphoma. In general lymphomas with a follicular histological pattern are of lower grade (longer survival than those of diffuse pattern)

Clinical Difference between Hodgkins and Non Hodgkins Lymphoma

Hodgkins lymphoma	Non Hodgkins lymphoma
• More often localized to a single axial group of cervical, mediastinal, para-aortic nodes.	• More frequent involvement of multiple peripheral nodes
• Orderly spread by contiguity	• Waldeyer ring and mesenteric nodes commonly involved
• Mesenteric nodes and Waldeyerring rarely involved	• Extranodal involvement common
• Extra-nodal involvement uncommon	

204. Ans. (a) Large B cell lymphoma

(Ref: Harrison 20th edition, p 767; Hematology in clinical practice. 4th ed. ch. 21, Harrison 19th edition, p 703)

Richter syndrome or Richter transformation refers to the transformation of CLL into an aggressive large B-cell lymphoma (diffuse Histocytic lymphoma) and is seen in approximately 3-10% of cases. Patients will often present with symptoms of weight loss, fevers, night sweats, muscle wasting, (i.e, B symptoms) and increasing Hepatospleno-megaly and lymphadenopathy.

205. Ans. (a) B Cells

(Ref: Harrison 19th edition, p 709f)

The hallmark of Hodgkin lymphoma (HL) is the presence of large, mono-nucleated Hodgkin and multinucleated Reed/Sternberg cells.

- These cells represent the tumor cells, but usually comprise less than 1% of the cellular infiltrate in the lymphoma tissue. Due to the rarity of the Hodgkin and Reed/Sternberg (HRS) cells and their unusual phenotype, the origin of these cells from germinal center B cells in both the lymphocyte predominant (LP) and the classical subtype of HL could be clarified only recently.
- Only in very rare cases, HRS cells of classical HL represent transformed T cells. In classical HL, which accounts for 95% of the cases, the pattern of somatic mutations in the rearranged Ig genes suggests that the cells derive from GC B cells that normally would have undergone apoptosis as they acquired unfavorable somatic mutations.
- Despite their GC B cell origin, HRS cells have lost expression of many B cell marker. Moreover, expression of markers typical for other hematopoietic lineages is often observed, such as the myelocytic antigen CD15, the cytotoxic T cell/NK cell marker granzyme B, and the dendritic cell–specific chemokine TARC

206. Ans. (d) Hodgkin's disease

(Ref: Harrison 20th edition, p 782; Harrison 19th edition, p 697)

Hematological malignancy	Chemotherapy used
Acute lymphoblastic leukemia	V.A.L.P plus intra-thecal methotrexate
Acute myeloid leukemia	Cytarabine and Dacarbazine
Acute promyelocytic leukemia	Al trans retinoic Acid
Chronic myeloid leukemia	Imatinib mesylate
Chronic lymphocytic leukemia	Fludarabine
Hodgkin disease	ABVD
Non-Hodgkin lymphoma	R-CHOP

207. Ans. (d) IgM

(Ref: Harrison 20th edition, p 777-78; Harrison 19th edition, p 706)

- The other name for lymphoplasmacytoid lymphoma is Waldenstrom's Macroglobulinemia.
- The majority of patients in this disease have monoclonal IgM serum para-protein. In contrast to myeloma, the disease was associated with lymphadenopathy and hepatosplenomegaly, but the major clinical manifestation was the hyperviscosity syndrome

208. Ans. (a) Nodular sclerosis

(Ref: Harrison 20th edition, p 780)

209. Ans. (a) CD15 and CD30

(Ref: Harrison 20th edition, p 780)

210. Ans. (c) Absolute lymphocyte count < 600/μL

(Ref: Robbins 8th edition, ch. 12)

211. Ans. (b) REAL Classification

(Ref: Robbins 7th edition, p 668)

212. Ans. (a) t (8:14)

(Ref: Harrison 20th edition, p 775)

Platelet and Bleeding Disorders

213. Ans. (a) Left lower lobe consolidation

(Ref: Wintrobe's Hematology 12th edition chapter 69; Bailey and love 26th edition, p 1096)

Complications of splenectomy	
1.	Intra operative — a. Hemorrhage from slipped ligature: (MC intra-operative complication) b. Organ injury
2.	Early post-operative — a. Pulmonary: Left lower lobe atelecasis (MC) b. Sub phrenic abscess c. Wound problems- Hematoma, seromas, infections. d. Splenic/portal vein thrombosis e. Ileus
3.	Late post-operative— a. OPSI (Overwhelming post-splenectomy infection) — presents with non-specific flu like symptoms, bacteremia due to ENCAPSULATED bacteria like Streptococcus pneumonia, H. Influenza type B and Neisseria meningitidis. b. Splenosis- presence of disseminated intra-abdominal splenic tissue.

214. Ans. (d) 11

(Ref: Wintrobe Hematology 12th edition, Chapter 20)

215. Ans. (b) Increased D dimer

(Ref: Harrison 20th edition, p 835-36; Harrison 19th edition, p 737)

Laboratory findings in disseminated intravascular coagulation
1. Prolongation of PT and or APTT
2. Platelet counts <100,000/cu.mm or a rapid decline in platelet numbers
3. Presence of schistocytes fragmented red cells in the blood smear an
4. Elevated levels of FDP
5. The most sensitive test for DIC is the FDP level
   - DIC is an unlikely diagnosis in the presence of normal levels of FDP
   - The D dimer test is more specific for detection of fibrin.
   - Fibrinogen degradation products indicates that the cross linked fibrin has been digested by plasmin
   - Because fibrinogen has a prolonged half-life plasma levels diminish acutely only in severe cases of DIC
   - High grade DIC is also associated with levels of antithrombin III or plasminogen activity <60% of normal

216. Ans. (a) Platelet elevation

(Ref: Harrison 20th edition, p 737-38)

Essential thrombocytosis (primary thrombocythemia) is a nonreactive, chronic myeloproliferative disorder in which sustained megakaryocyte proliferation leads to an increase in the number of circulating platelets.

217. Ans. (b) Bleeding into the joints

(Ref: Harrison 20th edition, p 825-26)

Possible diagnosis of patient is acute/chronic ITP. Bleeding into the joints is a feature of clotting factor deficiency.

Features of Acute and Chronic Idiopathic Thrombocytopenic Purpura

Feature	Acute ITP	Chronic ITP
Peak age of incidence	Children 2-6 year	Adults, 20-40 year
Sex predilection	None	3:1 female to male
Antecedent infection	Common 1-2 week	Unusual
Onset of bleeding	Abrupt	Insidious
Hemorrhagic bullae in mouth	Present in severe cases	Usually absent
Platelet count	<20000/μL	3000-80000/μL
Eosinophilia and lymphocytosis	Common	Rare
Spontaneous remission	Occurs in 80% cases	Months or years Uncommon

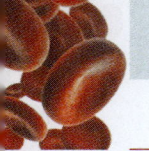

218. Ans. (b) Oprelvekin

(Ref: Harrison 19th edition, p 103e-24)

Oprelvekin (1L-11) is used to prevent and treat thrombocytopenia.

219. Ans. (d) 4 hours

(Ref: Wintrobe's Hematology 12th edition, p 1683)

- Platelet concentrates may be provided by the blood bank in their individual plastic bags or pooled before transfusion. Once the blood bag is opened by puncturing one of the sealed ports, the platelets must be administered within 4 hours.
- Platelets must be administered through a filter approved for platelet use, either a standard 170-μm filter or a leukoreduction platelet filter

220. Ans. (a) Hyperfibrinogenimia

(Ref: Harrison 20th edition, p 834-36; Harrison 19th edition, p 736)

- Common findings include the prolongation of PT and/or aPTT; platelet counts <100,000/μL^3, or a rapid decline in platelet numbers
- The presence of schistocytes (fragmented red cells) in the blood smear elevated levels of FDP.
- The most sensitive test for DIC is the FDP level.
- DIC is an unlikely diagnosis in the presence of normal levels of FDP.
- The D-dimer test is more specific for detection of fibrin— but not fibrinogen—degradation products and indicates that the cross-linked fibrin has been digested by plasmin.
- Because fibrinogen has a prolonged half-life, plasma levels diminish acutely only in severe cases of DIC.
- Hence the conclusion is that Fibrinogen can be decreased or normal but NEVER increased in cases of DIC.

221. Ans. (d) I.V. fluids

(Ref: Harrison 20th edition, p 836; Harrison 19th edition, p 736)

- Massive fresh whole blood transfusion is the sheet anchor to replenish not only the fibrinogen but also the other procoagulants.; This is mostly indicated in obstetrics and can be used safely without any biochemical guidance.
- About 500 ml of fresh blood rises the fibrinogen level approximately by 12.5 mg/100 ml & adding 10,000-15,000 platelet per cumm.
- The PT (>1.5 times the normal) provides a good indicator of the severity of the clotting factor consumption. Replacement with FFP is indicated (1 unit of FFP increases most coagulation factors by 3% in an adult without DIC).
- Cryoprecipitate which is rich in fibrinogen and factor VIM contains 250 gm of fibrinogen per bag. There is less chance of hepatitis. 10-20 units are quite effective. It lacks AT III.
- Platelet concentrates may be given to a patient with very low platelet count (< 50,000/ml.) & persistent bleeding
- Low levels of fibrinogen (<100 mg/dL) or brisk hyperfibrinolysis will require infusion of cryoprecipitate (plasma fraction enriched for fibrinogen, FVIII, and vWF). The replacement of 10 U of cryoprecipitate for every 2–3 U of FFP is sufficient to correct the hemostasis.

- Clotting factor concentrates are not recommended for control of bleeding in DIC because of the limited efficacy afforded by replacement of single factors (FVIII or FIX concentrates), and the high risk of products containing traces of aPCCs that further aggravate the disease
- The use of antifibrinolytic drugs, EACA, or tranexamic acid, to prevent fibrin degradation by plasmin may reduce bleeding episodes in patients with DIC and confirmed hyper-fibrinolysis. However, these drugs can increase the risk of thrombosis and concomitant use of heparin is indicated. Patients with acute promyelocytic leukemia or those with chronic DIC associated with giant hemangiomas are among the few patients who may benefit from this therapy

222. Ans. (c) 72 hours

(Ref: Wintrobe 13th ed. pg. 552 and Manual of Perioperative Care in Adult Cardiac Surgery: Robert M. Bojar 5th ed., Harrison 19th edition, p 138e-4)

- Platelets are provided as a pooled preparation from one or several donors, usually as a 6-unit bag, which is the usual amount given to an average-sized adult.
- Each unit contains approximately 8x10^{10} platelets and should increase the platelet count by about 7000-10,000/μL in a 75 kg adult. One unit of platelets contains 70% of the platelets in a unit of fresh blood, but platelets lose some of their functional capacity during storage.
- Platelets stored at room temperature can be used for up to 5 days and have a life span of 8 days.
- Those stored at 4°C are useful for only 24 hours (only 50-70% of total platelet activity is present at 6 hours) and have a life span of only 2-3 days.
- Platelet function is impaired in patients with hypofibrinogenemia and when the hematocrit is less than 30%. Thus, use of cryoprecipitate and red cell transfusion to raise the hematocrit towards 30% can be considered to improve platelet function
- Transfused platelets will be less effective when given within 6 hours of a loading dose of 4 hours of a maintenance dose of clopidogrel or prasugrel, because the active compound may still be present in the bloodstream.
- ABO compatibility should be observed for platelets, but is not essential. For each donor used, there is a similar risk of transmitting hepatitis and HIV as for one unit of blood.
- Platelet should be administered through a 170μm filter.

223. Ans. (c) Decrease aPTT

(Ref: Harrison 20th edition, p 835-36)

In case of D.I.C fibrinogen level decreased, leading to excessive bleeding.

224. Ans. (a) Lepirudin

(Ref: Harrison 20th edition, p 852; Harrison 19th edition, p 749)

225. Ans. (d) Hemophilia

(Ref: Harrison 20th edition, p 835, Table 112-2; Harrison 19th edition, p 736)

Etiologic Factors and Disorders Causing Disseminated Intravascular Coagulation:
1. Obstetric syndrome — abruptio placentae, amniotic fluid embolism, retained dead fetus, second trimester abortion.
2. Neoplasms, particularly mucinous adenocarcinomas, acute promyelocytic leukemia.
3. Intravascular hemolysis; Fat embolism; Tissue damage — burns, frostbite, head.
4. Endothelial damage: Aortic aneurysm; Hemolytic uremic syndrome Acute glomerulonephritis; Rocky Mountain spotted fever
5. Vascular malformation, decreased blood flow: Kasabach. Merritt syndrome
6. Infections: Bacterial: Staphylococci, streptococci, pneumococci, meningococci, gram -ve bacilli
   - Viral: arboviruses, varicella, variola, rubella
   - Parasites: malaria, kala-azar
   - Rickettsial: Rocky Mountains spotted fever
   - Mycotic: Acute histoplasmosis

226. Ans. (d) Clopidogrel

(Ref: Harrison 20th edition, p 845, 847; KDT 6th 610, Harrison 19th edition, p 747)

Clopidogrel inhibits ADP receptors whereas abciximab, tirofiban and eptifibatide are GP IIb/IIIa antagonists.

227. Ans. (c) Dilute russel viper venom time

(Ref: Harrison 20th edition, p 838; Harrison 19th edition, p 740)

Criteria for Anti-phosphotipid syndrome (Sapporo criteria)

A. Clinical criteria
1. Vascular thrombosis; >1 Clinical finding of arterial/ venous/ small thrombosis confirmed by imaging/ histopathology
2. Pregnancy morbidity
   a. > 1 unexplained death of a morphologically normal fetus > 10 weeks gestation
   b. > 1 premature birth of a morphologically normal neonate < 34th week
   c. > 3 unexplained consecutive spontaneous abortions < 34th week of gestation

B. Lab criteria
1. Anticardiolipin antibody IgG/IgM +ve on >2 occasions at least 6 weeks apart, tested by ELISA.
2. Lupus anticoagulant positive on at least 2 occasions, at least 6 weeks apart.
   a. Prolonged phospholipid dependent coagulation e.g. APTT, KCT, (Kaolin clotting time), dilute Russel viper venom time.
   b. Failure to correct the above test by mixing with normal platelet poor plasma.
   c. Correction of the time with addition of excess phospholipid
   d. Exclusion of other coagulopathies

Obstetrical complication of lupus anticoagulant
- Recurrent spontaneous abortion
- Abruptio placenta
- Intrauterine growth restriction
- Preeclampsia
- Prematurity

228. Ans. (c) ITP

(Ref: Harrison 20th edition, p 825; Harrison 19th edition, p 728)

- Idiopathic thrombocytopenic purpura is not associated with thrombosis. Its main clinical manifestation is bleeding which occurs due to thrombocytopenia.
- Heparin induced thrombocytopenia (HIT) is the most important and most frequent drug induced immune mediated type of thrombocytopenia.
  1. It is seen in about 1-5% of patients on heparin.
  2. In patients receiving heparin for the first time, the onset of thrombocytopenia usually occurs 5-10 days after the administration of heparin.
  3. The thrombocytopenia in HIT is usually moderate in severity with a median platelet count being between 50 and 80 × 10^9/L. Despite thrombocytopenia bleeding is rare. On the other hand heparin induced thrombocytopenia is strongly associated with thrombosis which frequently leads to diagnosis of heparin induced thrombo-cytopenia.
  4. Thrombosis in heparin induced thrombo-cytopenia is associated with a mortality of approximately 20-30% with an equal per-centage of patients becoming permanently disabled by amputation/stroke or other causes.
  5. Thromboembolic complications can be venous, arterial both and include deep venous thrombosis, pulmonary embolism myocardial infarction, thrombotic stroke and occlusion of limb arteries.
  6. The mechanism underlying heparin induced thrombo-cytopenia is an immune response.
  7. The principal antigen is a complex of heparin and platelet factor 4 (PF4).
  8. Patients who develop HIT produce anti-bodies against Heparin platelet F4 complex.
  9. Thrombocytopenia in HIT is largely due to the clearance of activated platelets and antibody coated platelets by the reticulo-endothelial system.

229. Ans. (a) Protein C deficiency

(Ref: Harrison 20th edition, p 834; Harrison 19th edition, p 737)

- Purpura fulminans is a severe form of DIC resulting from thrombosis of extensive areas of the skin; it affects predominantly young children following viral or bacterial infection, particularly those with inherited or acquired hypercoagulability due to deficiencies of the components of the protein C pathway.
- Neonates homozygous for protein C deficiency also present high risk for purpura fulminans with or without thrombosis of large vessels.

230. Ans. (a) Prolonged prothrombin time

(Ref: Harrison 20th edition, p 836)

Normal new horns are moderately deficient in vitamin K. This deficiency increases on 3rd to 5th day when, vitamin K level falls further.

The serum level of vitamin K starts increasing from 13th to 15thQ day of life and achieves adult level at 3 months.

This is normal, and does not produce any bleeding.

In hemorrhagic disease of the newborn there is delay in achieving the normal vitamin K level further.

The serum level of vitamin K starts increasing from 13th to 15thQ day of life and achieves adult level at 3 months.

This is normal, and does not produce any bleeding.

In hemorrhagic disease of the newborn there is delay in achieving the normal vitamin K level.

231. Ans. (b) Non palpable purpura

(Ref: Harrison 20th edition, p 825; Harrison 19th edition, p 728)

Acute ITP exhibits the following physical findings:
1. Nonpalpable petechiae, which mostly occur in dependent regions
2. Hemorrhagic bullae on mucous membranes
3. Purpura
4. Gingival bleeding
5. Signs of GI bleeding
6. Menometrorrhagia, menorrhagia
7. Retinal hemorrhages
8. Evidence of intracranial hemorrhage, with possible neurologic symptoms
9. Nonpalpable spleen: The prevalence of palpable spleen in patients with ITP is approximately the same as that in the non-ITP population (i.e, 3% in adults, 12% in children
   - Palpable purpura is a clinical finding that represents antigen-antibody deposition along small cutaneous vessels, resulting in extravasation of blood cells into the interstitium. The most common cause of palpable purpura is leukocytoclastic vasculitis, a disease involving cutaneous postcapillary venules. Although often idiopathic, leukocytoclastic vasculitis has been associated with numerous infections, drugs, rheumatic diseases and malignancies
   - Evan syndrome is characterized by overall pathology resembling a combination of autoimmune hemolytic anemia and idiopathic thrombocytopenic purpura.

Non palpable	Palpable
1. Trauma	1. Vasculitis
2. Solar (actinic, senile) purpura	a. Cutaneous smallvessel vasculitis
3. Steroid purpura	b. Polyarteritis nodosa
4. Capillaritis	2. Emboli
5. Livedoid vasculopathy in the setting of venous hypertension	a. Acute meningococcemia
6. Thrombocytopenia (including ITP)	b. Disseminated gonococcal infection
7. Abnormal platelet function	c. Rocky Mountain spotted fever
8. Clotting factor defects	d. Ecthyma
9. Amyloidosis	
10. Ehlers-Danlos syndrome	
11. Scurvy	
12. Antiphospholipid antibody syndrome	

232. Ans. (d) Eltrombopag

(Ref: Harrison 20th edition, p 826; Harrison 19th edition, p 728)

- Glucocorticoids and IVIg are the mainstays of medical therapy for acute ITP.
- Bleeding crisis requires administration of High - dose I.V. immunoglobulin 1 g/kg for 1 or 2 days
- Currently IV RhIG in acute ITP in children and adults show platelet count increases at 24 hours faster than medicating with steroids and at 72 hours similar to IVIg. Although generally less toxic than IV steroids, IV RhIG is more expensive than IV steroids.
- Studies in children with chronic ITP show that escalating or elevated doses of IV RhIG have comparable responses to those of high-dose IVIg therapy in children. This therapy is not appropriate for patients who have undergone splenectomy
- Thrombopoietin (TPO) receptor agonist eltrombopag interacts with transmembrane domain of human TPO receptor and induces megakaryocyte proliferation and differentiation from bone marrow progenitor cells. Indicated for thrombocytopenia associated with chronic idiopathic thrombocytopenic purpura in patients experiencing inadequate response to corticosteroids, immunoglobulins, or splenectomy

233. Ans. (c) Effective for 9-10 days

(Ref: Harrison 20th edition, p 812; Harrison 19th edition, p 138e-1)

234. Ans. (a) 5 days

(Ref: Harrison 20th edition, p 812; Wintrobe's Hematology 11th edition, p 1681, Harrison 19th edition, p 138e-5)

- Platelets are kept in blood bank for 5 days because of risk of bacterial contamination, though platelets are viable for 7days in new plastic containers.
- Viability is enhanced if gentle agitation of platelets is kept and sufficient plasma is kept to maintain pH>6.2.

235. Ans. (c) Acute monocytic leukaemia

(Ref: https://www.orpha.net/data/patho/GB/uk-AMLM5.pdf)

236. Ans. (c) It's effect is monitored by observing the clotting time

(Ref: Harrison 20th edition, p 853; Harrison 19th edition, p 756)

Warfarin monitoring is done by testing for INR/prothrombin time.

237. Ans. (d) + 20-24 degrees Celsius

(Ref: Harrison 20th edition, p 812; Wintrobe's Hematology 11th ed. 1681, Harrison 19th edition, p 138e-4)

Refer to explanation of Question no. 42

238. Ans. (a) Normal platelet counts and prolonged Bleeding time

(Ref: Harrison 19th edition, p 138e-4)

239. Ans. (a) Myelodysplastic syndrome

(Ref: Hematology in clinical practice. 4th ed. ch. 9, Harrison 19th edition, p 669)

240. Ans. (d) Acquired hemophilia

(Ref: Harrison 19th edition, p 138e-3)

- aPTT is increased in acquired hemophilia
- Glanzmann's Thrombasthenia: It is a autosomal recessive condition where Platelets are unable to aggregate because of lack of receptors (containing glycoproteins IIb and IIIa) for fibrinogen, which form the bridges between platelets during aggregation. Clinically, it is manifested chiefly as mucosal (epistaxis, gingival bleeding, menorrhagia) and postoperative bleeding. The defect is of variable severity but may be severe. Platelet numbers and morphology are normal, but the bleeding time is markedly prolonged.
- It is likely that multiple factors are responsible for the plateletdysfunction in uremia. Three of the factors that may contribute are the retention of uremic toxins, anemia, and nitric oxide. Platelet dysfunction is observed mainly in advanced uremia before starting dialysis treatment. It is probably related to uremic toxins present in the circulation. The importance of circulating toxins is suggested by commonly seen a beneficial effect of acute dialysis on platelet dysfunction, although the bleeding time israrely normalized

241. Ans. (d) Less than 20,000 mm^3

(Ref: Harrison 20th edition, p 825)

242. Ans. (d) Wiskott Aldrich syndrome

(Ref: Harrison 20th edition, p 2494; Harrison 19th edition, p 2110)

Wiskott Aldrich Syndrome
- Wiskott Aldrich syndrome is an X-linked disorder that usually present in infancy.
- Monocytes and macrophages from patient with Wiskott Aldrich syndrome have reduced capacity for phagocytosis. The other cells affected are B, NK and T lymphocytes.
- There is loss of cellular immunity with depletion of T lymphocytes.Humoral immunity, too, is affected. Patient with Wiskott Aldrich syndrome do not make antibodies to polysaccharide antigen and the response to protein antigen is poor.
- The most severe complication of Wiskott Aldrich syndrome arises from failure to clear bacterial infections and to protect from Epstein Barr virus associated lymphomas.
- Serum immunoglobulins level in Wiskott Aldrich dyndrome has been asked frequently.
  - IgE and IgA = Often high
  - IgG = usually normal
  - IgM =Usually decreased
- Thrombocytopenia and abnormally small platelets that fail to aggregate effectively. IN CONTRAST BERNARD SOULIER IS CHARACTERISED BY LARGE PLATELETS WITH DEFICIENCY OF GLYCOPROTEIN 1B.

Wiskott-Aldrich syndrome
Think "WAX TIE"
WA: Wiskott-Aldritch
X: X-linked Recessive
T: Thrombocytopenia
I: Infections
E: Eczema
Also, this helps with the immunoglobulins present:
WAX TIE... decreased IgM (think of the W as an upside down M, suggesting a decreased IgM), Increased IgA, Increased IgE

243. Ans. (c) Decreased coagulation factor levels

(Ref: Harrison 20th edition, p 834-35; Harrison 19th edition, p 736)

- While D.I.C. and thrombotic microangiopathies share features such as microvascular occlusion and micro-angiopathic hemolvtic anemia, they are patho-geneticallv distinct. In T.T.P and HUS (unlike DIC), activation of the coagulation cascade is not of primary important, and hence results of laboratory tests of coagulation such as PT and PTT are usually normal."
- DIC is characterized by excessive activation of the coagulation system. That leads to formation of microthrombi throughout the microcirculation of the body, often in a quixotically even distribution.
- As a consequence of the thrombotic diathesis, there is consumption of platelets, fibrin and coagulation factors and secondary activation of fibrinolytic mechanism
- DIC can also lead to hemolytic anemia. It occurs due to fragmentation of red cells as they try to squeeze through the narrowed microvasculature. Schistocytes, the cells characteristic ofmicroangiopathic hemolytic anemia are quiet common in patients with D.I C (seen in 50 %) of cause.

244. Ans. (a) Prolonged bleeding time (BT)

(Ref: Robbins 8th ch. 12)

245. Ans. (c) Autosomal dominant

(Ref: Harrison 18th/p 971)

246. Ans. (d) Wiskott Aldrich syndrome

(Ref: Harrison 20th edition, p 2494)

247. Ans. (a) Henoch schonlein purpura

(Ref: Harrison 18th/p 2797)

248. Ans. (a) SLE

(Ref: Harrison 20th edition, p 825)

249. Ans. (c) Henoch Sconlein Purpura

(Ref: Harrison 20th edition, p 2586)

250. Ans. (a) Splenomegaly

(Ref: Harrison 20th edition, p 825; Robbins 7th/651,652; Ghai 6th/324)

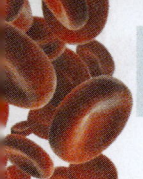

251. Ans. (b) **Immunogenic thrombocytopenia**

(Ref: Harrison 20th edition, p 826)

252. Ans. (d) **Grossly abnormal coagulation tests**

(Ref: Harrison 20th edition, p 826)

Von Willebrand Disease and Clotting Factor Defects

253. Ans. (d) **Increased Fibrin degradation products**

(Ref: Harrison 20th edition, p 834)

The most sensitive test for DIC is FDP. Others findings in DIC are:

- Prolongation of PT/aPTT
- Rapid decline in platelets
- Presence of schistocytes in peripheral smear

254. Ans. (a) **Desmopressin**

(Ref: Harrison 20th edition, p 829; Harrison 19th edition, p 731-32)

- *In patients of von wilebrand disease, DDAVP can be given intra-nasally 2 hours before a procedure like dental extraction which is associated with mild to moderate risk of bleeding and can be repeated 12-24 hours.*
- In *vWD type 3* for major procedures requiring longer periods of normal hemostasis VWF replacement can be given and DDAVP is *not effective*
- Amino-caproic acid or Tranexamic acid is an important therapy either alone or in an adjunctive capacity particularly for the prevention or treatment of mucosal bleeding.
- These agents are particularly useful in prophylaxis for dental procedures with DDAVP for dental extraction and tonsillectomy menorrhagia and prostate procedures.

255. Ans. (a) **Epsilon aminocaproic acid**

(Ref: Harrison 20th edition, p 829; Harrison 19th edition, p 731/732)

- Antifibrinolytic therapy using either epsilon-aminocaproic acid or tranexamic acid is an important therapy, either alone or in an adjunctive capacity, particularly for the prevention or treatment of mucosal bleeding.
- These agents are particularly useful in prophylaxis for dental procedures, with DDAVP for dental extractions and tonsillectomy, menorrhagia, and prostate procedures. It is contraindicated in the setting of upper urinary tract bleeding, due to the risk of ureteral obstruction.

256. Ans. (d) **vWD type 3**

(Ref: Harrison 20th edition, p 828-29; Harrison 19th edition, p 732)

- Patients with vWD type III, a severe, quantitative deficiency associated with very little or no detectable plasma or platelet vWF, have a profound bleeding disorder. vWD type III appears to result from the inheritance of a mutant vWF gene from both parents. In the most straightforward model, vWD type I would simply represent the heterozygous form of vWD type III; however, inheritance patterns indicate greater complexity.
- vWD type III is much rarer having a frequency closer to 1 case per 1 million persons.

Condition	Defect[a]
vWD type 1	Mild to moderate quantitative deficiency of vWF (i.e., about 20-50% of normal levels).
vWD type 2A	The most common qualitative abnormality of vWF, is associated with selective loss of large and medium-sized multimers
vWD type 2B	Loss of only large multimers as mutant vWF spontaneously binds to GpIb in the absence of subendothelial contact.
vWD type 2N	Characterized by a defect residing within the patient's plasma vWF that interferes with its ability to bind FVIII.
vWD type 2M	Involves qualitative variants with decreased platelet-dependent function not resulting from absence of high–molecular weight multimers
vWD type 3	A severe, quantitative deficiency associated with very little or no detectable plasma or platelet vWF, have a profound bleeding disorder

257. Ans. (a) **Sepsis**

(Ref: Harrison 20th edition, p 834-35, Table 112-2; **Harrison 19th edition, p 736**)

- The most common causes are bacterial sepsis, malignant disorders such as solid tumors or acute promyelocytic leukemia, and obstetric causes.
- DIC is diagnosed in almost one-half of pregnant women with abruptio placentae, or with amniotic fluid embolism. Trauma, particularly to the brain, can also result in DIC.
- The exposure of blood to phospholipids from damaged tissue, hemolysis, and endothelial damage are all contributing factors to the development of DIC in this setting.

258. Ans. (b) **Dilute russel viper venom assay**

(Ref: Harrison 20th edition, p 2522; Harrison 19th edition, p 2131)

- Choice A is ruled out as hemophilia presents in males and presents with bleeding
- Choice C is ruled out as platelet aggregation test is used for platelet disorders which lead to bleeding.
- Ristocetin co-factor assays are used to detect Von wilebrand's disease. Von wilebrands disease cause prolongation of PTT but it is also associated with clinical bleeding so choice D can be ruled out.
- *Causes of isolated prolongation of PT*
  1. Heparin
  2. Lupus anticoagulant-
  3. Coagulation factor deficiency (factor VIII, IX and XI, XII, prekallikrein, high molecular weight kininogen (HMWK)

4. Specific coagulation factor inhibitors (antibodies against factor VIII or IX)

Russel viper venom test (Dilute Russel viper venom test) (dRVVT)
- Dilute Russel viper venom test is one of the test to detect lupus anticoagulant.
- Lupus anticoagulant is associated with prolongation in PTT and thrombosis but no bleeding.
- Russell's viper initiates plasma clotting activating factor X in the presence of calcium. The activated factor X then activates prothrombin (factor II) in the presence of factor V and phospholipid. If lupus anticoagulant (LA) antibodies are present in the patient and interfere with phospholipid required for coagulation, then the dRWT will be prolonged.
- If this test is prolonged, a confirmatory test is performed using a high concentration of a phospholipids. The excess phospholipid will neutralize the LA antibody present in the patient's plasma and shorten the clotting time. The final result is a ratio of the two clotting times, which is compared with the values of a Ref population. A lupus anticoagulant is defined by inhibition of a phospholipid-dependent clotting assay, such as the aPTT or dRWT, which corrects with excess phospholipid. The dRWT is more specific for LA than the aPTT since it is not influenced by deficiencies of the contact intrinsic pathway factors or antibodies to factors VIII or IX.

259. Ans. (a) Von Wilebrand disease

(Ref: Harrison 20th edition, p 828; Harrison 19th edition, p 731)
- von Willebrand disease (vWD) is the most common inherited bleeding disorder. It is autosomal dominant, and its prevalence is estimated to be as high as 1 case per 1000 population.
- The hallmark of von Willebrand disease is defective platelet adhesion to subendothelial components caused by a deficiency of the plasma protein vWf. This factor is a large, multimeric glycoprotein that is synthesized, processed, and stored in the Weibel-Palade bodies of the endothelial cells, and secreted constitutively and following stimulation

260. Ans. (a) Hemorrhage

(Ref: Harrison 19th edition, p 733)
- Hemophilia B/Factor IX deficiency is one-seventh as common as factor VIIIdeficiency hemophilia but is otherwise clinically & genetically identical.
- Hemophilia B is an inherited, X-linked, recessive disorder resulting in deficiency of functional plasma coagulation factor IX. Spontaneous mutation and acquired immunologic processes can result in this disorder as well. Hemophilia B comprises approximately 20% of hemophilia cases, approximately 50% of whom have factor IX levels of greater than 1%.
- Morbidity and death are primarily the result of hemorrhage, although infectious diseases (e.g., HIV, hepatitis) became prominent

261. Ans. (c) Both A & B

(Ref: Hematology in clinical practice. 4th ed. ch. 32)

Factor VIII antibodies also occur in 15% of patients with hemophilia A who have received infusion of plasma concentrates.
1. The most common associated illnesses are autoimmune, with the two largest series showing an autoimmune association in 17–18%. This subset of patients is most commonly diagnosed with systemic lupus erythematosus, rheumatoid arthritis or Sjögren's syndrome.
2. Cancer or precancerous states including both solid tumors and lymphoproliferative malignancies.
3. In addition, skin disorders (such as pemphigus and epidermolysis bullosa), drugs (including penicillin and interferon), infections and even chronic graft-versus-host disease have been reported.
4. The postpartum state is one of the more frequent settings in which acquired hemophilia may occur and acquired hemophilia should be considered early in the evaluation of cases of abnormal bleeding in the postpartum setting. Most commonly the inhibitor develops after parturition but sometimes can be found during labor, leading to severe blood loss and even hysterectomy. When the inhibitor does develop during pregnancy, there is a risk of trans-placental transfer of the antibody and neonatal hemorrhage.

262. Ans. (a) Isolated prolonged PTT with a normal PT

(Ref: Harrison 20th edition, p 828-29; Harrison 19th edition, p 732)

In Vonwilebrand's disease coagulation defect occurs due to deficiency in factor VIII

Factor VIII is a part of intrinsic coagulation pathway. So PTT is increased.

263. Ans. (a) Autosomal dominant

(Ref: Harrison 20th edition, p 828; Hematology in clinical practice. 4th ed. ch. 31, Harrison 19th edition, p 731)

vWD is inherited either autosomal dominant or antosomal recessive trait

Von Willbrand's Disease: Most common hereditary coagulation disorder. Characterized by qualitative and quantitate defect in VW factor.
- Gene: Located on Chromosome XII
- Inherited: Autosomal dominant (most commonly)
- In the most common form of von Willebrand's disease (type I), vWF levels in plasma are reduced.
- This may be measured by factor VIII antigen, which measures the immunologic presence of vWF, or by ristocetin cofactor activity, which measures functional properties of vWF in mediating platelet adhesion.

264. Ans. (b) Cryoprecipitate

(Ref: Harrison 20th edition, p 832; Harrison 19th edition, p 733, 450t)
- Various FIX concentrates are now available to treat hemophilia B.
- Fresh frozen plasma is no longer used in hemophilia because of the lack of safe viral elimination and concerns regarding volume overload.

- Cryoprecipitate contains no factor IX and is not appropriate for factor IX therapy.
- Various purification techniques are used in plasma-based FIX concentrates to reduce or eliminate the risk of viral transmission, including heat treatment, cryoprecipitation, and chemical precipitation. These techniques inactivate viruses such as hepatitis B virus, hepatitis C virus, and HIV. However, the transmission of nonenveloped viruses (e.g., parvovirus and hepatitis A virus) and poorly characterized agents (e.g, prions) is still a potential problem.
- Recombinant FIX products are now commercially available and have a lower risk of viral contamination. These products are FDA-approved for control and prevention of bleeding episodes, and for perioperative management and approved for use in children

265. Ans. (a) Increased bleeding time (BT)

(Ref: Harrison 20th edition, p 830-31)

266. Ans. (c) Decreased PTT

(Ref: Harrison 20th edition, p 835; Harrison 19th edition, p 736)

267. Ans. (b) Serum levels of FDP

(Ref: Harrison 20th edition, p 835)

268. Ans. (d) Homocystenemia

(Ref: Harrison 20th edition, p 841, Table 113-2A)

Multiple Myeloma

269. Ans. (a) Unifocal Langerhans cell histiocytosis

(Ref: Harrison 20th edition, p 792; Lever's Histopathology and synopsis, p 209)

- The slide shows large number of histiocytes with excessively pink cytoplasm in all quadrants of the slide. The nucleus of cells looks irregular like a coffee bean. The clinical history of a single lytic bone lesion and histopathology points to the aetiology as Langerhans cell histiocytosis.
- Choice B is ruled as it will show M spike on urine electrophoresis
- Choice C is ruled out as it will have multiple lytic lesions in skull in raindrop configuration.
- Choice D is ruled out as it will have change in shape of skull with histology showing mosaic pattern of lamellar bone, resembling a jigsaw puzzle with prominent irregular cement lines

270. Ans. (a) Vertebral column

(Ref: Harrison 20th edition, p 795-96; Wintrobe's hematology 12th edition, chapter 99)

- Approximately 75% of patients have punched-out lytic lesions, osteoporosis, or fractures on conventional radiography. The vertebrae, skull, ribs, sternum, proximal humeri, and femora are involved most frequently
- Myeloma bone disease is a major source of morbidity and may present as an area of persistent pain or as a vague migratory bone pain, often in the lower back and pelvis

271. Ans. (d) Cold spot

(Ref: Pathophysiological basis of nuclear medicine: 3rd edition, p 236)

Scintigraphy with radioactive technetium for finding bone lesions is dependent on:
1. Osteoblastic activity
2. Increased blood flow to involved areas which generally occur as a result of a reparative process in reaction to bone destruction.

Cold spots	Hot spots
Cold spots may be caused by Malignant tumors Lung (2-4%), breast (5%), renal(10%), neuroblastoma, thyroid, *multiple myeloma* Bone abscess Bone ischemia: AVN, sickle cell anemia Hemangioma: Normal or decreased activity	Breast carcinoma Prostatic carcinoma Healing fracture Bone cancer Osteomyelitis Arthritis Paget's disease

- Bone scans are particularly sensitive in the diagnosis of bony metastases, especially osteoblastic metastases, as often seen in cases of breast and prostatic carcinoma. The scan findings are generally abnormal before there is sufficient bone loss to be noticed on conventional radiographs.
- Bone scintigraphy is much less sensitive than radiography in the diagnosis of multiple myeloma, which is usually an almost purely osteoclastic disease process, except when fractures occur.
- Nuclear scintigraphy of the bone commonly utilizes the radionuclides
  1. Technetium-99m usually attached to Medronic acid (Tc-99m MDP)
  2. Fluoride-18 incorporated into sodium fluoride (F-18 NaF)

272. Ans. (d) Hyperviscosity syndrome

(Ref: Harrison 20th edition, p 795-97; Harrison 19th edition, p 721)

Hyperviscosity syndrome is a rare complication of multiple myeloma.

Frequency of symptoms and signs in multiple myeloma:

Anemia	73%
Bone pain	58%
Elevated creatinine	48%
Fatigue/generalized weakness	32%
Hypercalcemia	28%
Weight loss	24%

273. Ans. (b) Seligmann Disease (Alpha heavy chain disease)

(Ref: Harrison 20th edition, p 803; Harrison 19th edition, p 718)

Most common heavy chain disease is alpha chain disease called as seligmann disease.

274. Ans. (c) Tubular proteinuria

(Ref: Harrison 20th edition, p 796; Wintrobe Hematology: p 5184, Harrison 19th edition, p 721)

The pathologic lesion of myeloma kidney consists of monoclonal light chains in the tubules in the form of dense, often laminated, tubular casts. These casts contain albumin and Tamm-Horsfall protein. Light chains are normally filtered by the glomeruli and are reabsorbed and catabolized in the nephron's proximal tubules. It is postulated that these systems become overwhelmed, and casts result.

Controversy occurs because Harrison 18th ed. mentions hypercalcemia and tubular damage simultaneously.

275. Ans. (c) Sickle cell anaemia

(Ref: Harrison 19th edition, p 635)
Lower-than-normal E.S.R levels occur with:
1. Congestive heart failure
2. Hyperviscosity
3. Hypofibrinogenemia
4. Low plasma protein (due to liver or kidney disease)
5. Polycythemia
6. Sickle cell anemia

276. Ans. (c) λ chain disease

(Ref: Harrison 19th edition, p 721)

Light chain disease (LCD) is a variant of multiple myeloma in which the malignant population of marrow cells produces free monoclonal light chains but not associated heavy chains. The monoclonal light chains are small enough to be freely filtered by the kidneys and become Bence-Jones protein. LCD comprises about 18% of multiple myeloma patients.

Laboratory Features:
The laboratory features of LCD show distinction from classical myeloma.
- The serum total protein is normal to low.
- Hypogammaglobyulinemia is common.
- 100% of the patients show evidence of Bence-Jones proteins in the urine.
- Many patients do not have a serum M (monoclonal) component on electrophoresis as most light chains are quickly filtered by the kidneys Urine electrophoresis becomes an important test in such cases.
- Using Immuno Fixation Electrophoresis the ratio of kappa, to lamda chains in the disease population is about 2:1.

Clinical Features:
1. More malignant course as compared to classic myeloma.
2. Extremely rapid doubling time.
3. Tendency for more osteolytic lesions.
4. Increased hypercalcemia.
5. Higher incidence of renal failure (including azotemia at presentation) as compared to other patients with multiple myeloma.
6. Higher incidence of amyloidosis and plasma cell leukemia in the terminal stages of the disease. Renal failure is the principle cause of death in these patients.

7. Light chains can cause a rapid decline of renal function and early onset of clinical deterioration in LCD. Renal damage caused by the freely filtered light chains affects every segment of the nephron.

All other options are seen in heavy chain diseases.

277. Ans. (c) IgM

(Ref: Harrison 20th edition, p 797; Harrison 19th edition, p 715)

Presence of monoclonal (M) protein in the serum or urine is a major criterion for the diagnosis of multiple myeloma. *The serum M component will be IgG in 53% of patients, IgA in 25%, and IgD in 1%; 20% of patients will have only light chains in serum and urine.*

278. Ans. (c) Polycythemia

(Ref: Harrison 20th edition, p 795-96; Harrison 19th edition, p 721)

279. Ans. (a) Infection

(Ref: Harrison 20th edition, p 795; Wintrobe Hematology 11th edition, p 5185, Harrison 19th edition, p 721)

- Besides progressive disease, the most frequent causes of death are infection in 24 to 52% and renal failure in approximately 20% of patients.
- Most common organism leading to death in multiple myeloma is gram negative bacilli >staph aureus >capsulated organisms.

280. Ans. (c) Multiple Myeloma

(Ref: Clinical Medicine 7th edition, by Bradley 2012 edition, p 323: Hematology, Harrison 19th edition, p 721)

E.S.R >100/hr tends to be markedly elevated in:

1. Monoclonal blood protein disorders such as multiple myeloma.
2. Temporal arteritis
3. Polymyalgia rheumatic
4. SLE

Moderate elevation of E.S.R is seen in:
- Active inflammatory disease such as rheumatoid arthritis
- Chronic infections, collagen disease and neoplastic diseases.
- Neoplastic disease.

Low ESR is seen in sickle cell anemia and polycythemia vera ESR = 0 in afibrinogenemia/agammaglobulinemia/extreme polycyathemia Hct > 65%

281. Ans. (a) Mu chain disease

(Ref: Harrison 20th edition, p 803; Hematology in clinical practice. 4th edition, ch. 25)

- The secretion of isolated mu heavy chains into the serum appears to occur in a very rare subset of patients with chronic lymphocytic leukemia.
- The only features that may distinguish patients with mu heavy chain disease are the presence of vacuoles in the malignant lymphocytes and the excretion of kappa light chains in the urine.

- The diagnosis requires ultracentrifugation or gel filtration to confirm the nonreactivity of the paraprotein with the light chain reagents, because some intact macroglobulins fail to interact with these serums.
- The tumor cells seem to have a defect in the assembly of light and heavy chains, because they appear to contain both in their cytoplasm

282. Ans. (b) Anemia

(Ref: Harrison 20th edition, p 796; Wintrobe's hematology 11th edition, p 5180, Harrison 19th edition, p 721)

- The most common *clinical feature* of multiple myeloma is anemia. A haemoglobin concentration of less than 120 g/L occurs in 40 to 73% of patients at presentation and contributes to the weakness and fatigue observed in as much as 82% of patients.
- The *anemia is normochromic, normocytic* in most patients.
- When there are high concentrations of serum Ig, rouleaux formation may be observed. The combination of anemia and Hyper-proteinemia leads to a marked increase of the erythrocyte sedimentation rate in more than 90% of cases.
- Bone pain is the second most common symptom. The pain usually involves the back and ribs, and unlike the pain of metastatic carcinoma, which often is worse at night, the pain of myeloma is precipitated by movement. Persistent localized pain in a patient with myeloma usually signifies a pathologic fracture. The bone lesions of myeloma are caused by the proliferation of tumor cells, activation of osteoclasts that destroy bone, and suppression of osteoblasts that form new bone
- The next most common clinical problem in patients with myeloma is susceptibility to bacterial infections. The most common infections are pneumonias and pyelonephritis, and the most frequent pathogens are Streptococcus pneumoniae, Staphylococcus aureus, and Klebsiella pneumoniae in the lungs and Escherichia coli and other gram-negative organisms in the urinary tract.

283. Ans. (c) Multiple myeloma

(Ref: Understanding X-Rays: A Synopsis of Radiology by Fred van Gelderen pg. 291, Harrison 19th edition, p 72)

The appearance of multiple, well-defined lytic lesions (punched out lesions) of various size scattered throughout the skull constitutes the raindrop skull appearance of multiple myeloma. This term is applied as an analogy to rain hitting a surface and splashing, where it leaves a random pattern of dark spots.

284. Ans. (a) Vertebral column

(Ref: Harrison 20th edition, p 795; Harrison 19th edition, p 721)

In case of multiple mycloma.
Bone lesions are most common in vertebral column. The pain usually involves the back and ribs, and unlike the pain of metastatic carcinoma, which often is worse at night, the pain of myeloma is precipitated by movement. Persistent localized pain in a patient with myeloma usually signifies a pathologic fracture.

The most common site of lytic lesion in multiple myeloma is vertebra > Skull> ribs. Distal to elbow and knee lesions are not seen.

285. Ans. (d) Hyperviscosity syndrome

(Ref: Harrison 20th edition, p 797)

286. Ans. (c) Plasmacytoma on tissue biopsy

(Ref: William's Hematology 7th/1507)

287. Ans. (a) Vertebral column

(Ref: Harrison 20th edition, p 795; Robbins 8th edn/p 455)

288. Ans. (b) Multiple myeloma

(Ref: Harrison 18th/p 940, 2529)

289. Ans. (c) Monoclonal gammopathy of unknown significance

(Ref: Harrison 20th edition, p 793)

290. Ans. (a) Gamma heavy chain disease

(Ref: Harrison 20th edition, p 803)

Myeloproliferative and Other Bone Marrow Disorders

291. Ans. (d) PQR = ZXY

(Ref: Harrison 20th edition, p 729, 731, 733; Harrison 19th edition, p 667, 669-670)

Myelodysplastic anaemia: Look for B12/folate/B6 deficiency	For evaluation of refractory anemia in MDS, vitamin B6 and folic acid levels should be checked.
Myelophthisicanemia: Look for tuberculosis infection.	Myelophthisic anemia is a form of fibrosis, which occurs secondary to injury by non-hematopoietic cells or pathogens. This fibrosis destroys the normal hematopoietic cells and their supportive stromal cells and bone marrow becomes infiltrated by collagen, reticulin, and other forms of fibrosis. Causes include 1. Inflammatory cells, *miliary tuberculosis*, and fungal infections 2. Sarcoidosis 3. Macrophage proliferation in storage diseases, such as Gaucher disease 4. Necrosis in sickle cell disease and septicemia 5. Bone disease in congenital osteopetrosis
Pure red cell aplasia: Human Parvo Virus B19	Persistent pure red cell aplasia can be a manifestation of parvovirus B19 infection in immunocompromised hosts. Failure of the humoral immune response to clear parvovirus B19 in such patients results in persistent pure red cell aplasia

292. Ans. (c) Chronic corpulmonale

(Ref: Harrison 20th edition, p 393)

Polycythemia is often present in cor pulmonale secondary to COPD. The chronic hypoxia leads to increase release of erythropoietin from peri-tubular cells of the kidney.

293. Ans. (b) 55%

(Ref: Harrison 20th edition, p 734; Harrison 19th edition, p 674)

Diagnosis of polycythemia

Hematocrit

Polycythemia in the adult patient is suspected when the hematocrit is:
- > 48% in women
- >52% in men

Hemoglobin concentration:
- Polycythemia in the adult is suspected when the hemoglobin is:
  - >16.5% in women
  - >18.5% in men

Red Blood Cell Count
- It is least often used to suggest polycythemia since patients with thalassemia minor may have an elevated RBC count but a normal or reduced hematocrit or hemoglobin due to presence of small (microcytic) poorly hemoglobinized cells.
- The most common cause of polycythemia is hypoxia secondary to pulmonary disease as a result pertaining eliciting symptoms pertaining to altered lung function.

294. Ans. (a) Polycyathemia vera

(Ref: Harrison 20th edition, p 733; Harrison 19th edition, p 673)

The most common of the chronic myeloproliferative disorders, PV occurs in 2 per 100,000 persons, sparing no adult age group and increasing with age to rates as high as 18/100,000. Familial transmission occurs but is infrequent and women predominate among sporadic cases.

295. Ans. (d) Spontaneous severe infection

(Ref: Harrison 20th edition, p 734; Harrison 19th edition, p 673)

296. Ans. (d) Absent spleen

(Ref: Harrison 20th edition, p 735; Harrison 19th edition, p 675)

Myelofibrosis
- Striking splenomegaly
- Dacryocytes (teardrop-shaped red blood cells) are common. Nucleated red blood cells and aniso-poikilocytosis are also frequently seen. Myelocytes and Promyelocytes are present in small proportions in most patients; blasts may also be seen. Platelets may be large or unusually shaped. In rare cases, the platelet count may be elevated
- Tear drop poikilocytosis on peripheral smear
- Leukoerythroblastic blood picture
- Giant abnormal platelets.

297. Ans. (d) Increased erythropoietin

(Ref: Harrison 20th edition, p 734; Harrison 19th edition, p 678)

- An important parodox in polycythemia vera is that it is associated with both bleeding and thrombosis, Polycythemia vera is characterized by arterial and venous thrombosis. Bleeding occurs due to abnormality in platelets (In 80% patients of polycythemia functional platelet abnormalities can be detected by aggregation studies).
- Since the neutrophil level and function remain normal in polycythemia vera, it is not associated with increased infection.
- In polycythemia E.S.R. is reduced due to hyperviscosity. If E.S.R. is abnormal another diagnosis or complication should be considered.

298. Ans. (c) Acute myeloid leukemia (AML)

(Ref: Harrison 20th edition, p 733, Table 99-1; Harrison 19th edition, p 672)

Chronic myeloproliferative disorders are:
1. Chronic myelogenous leukemia, bcr-abl–positive
2. Chronic neutrophilic leukemia
3. Chronic eosinophilic leukemia, not otherwise specified
4. Polycythemia vera
5. Primary myelofibrosis
6. Essential thrombocytosis
7. Mastocytosis
8. Myeloproliferative neoplasms, unclassifiable

299. Ans. (d) Decreased platelet count

(Ref: Harrison 20th edition, p 733-34; Harrison 19th edition, p 674)

PV is a clonal disorder involving a multipotent hematopoietic progenitor cell in which phenotypically normal red cells, granulocytes, and platelets accumulate in the absence of a recognizable physiologic stimulus.

However, a mutation in the autoinhibitory, pseudokinase domain of the tyrosine kinase JAK2—that replaces valine with phenylalanine (V617F), causing constitutive activation of the kinase—appears to have a central role in the pathogenesis of PV.

300. Ans. (d) Infections

(Ref: Harrison 20th edition, p 734; Harrison 19th edition, p 672)

Clinical features of Polycythemia Vera
1. Although splenomegaly may be the initial presenting sign in PV, most often the disorder is first recognized by the incidental discovery of a high hemoglobin or hematocrit.
2. With the exception of aquagenic pruritus, no symptoms distinguish PV from other causes of erythrocytosis.
3. Uncontrolled erythrocytosis causes hyper-viscosity, leading to neurologic symptoms such as vertigo, tinnitus, headache, visual disturbances, and transient ischemic attacks (TIAs).
4. Systolic hypertension is also a feature of the red cell mass elevation. In some patients, venous or arterial thrombosis may be the presenting manifestation of PV. Any vessel can be affected; but cerebral, cardiac, or mesenteric vessels are most commonly involved.
5. Intraabdominal venous thrombosis is particularly common in young women and may be catastrophic if a sudden and complete obstruction of the hepatic vein occurs. Indeed, PV should be suspected in any patient who develops hepatic vein thrombosis.

6. Digital ischemia, easy bruising, epistaxis, acid-peptic disease, or gastrointestinal hemorrhage may occur due to vascular stasis or thrombocytosis.
7. Given the large turnover of hematopoietic cells, hyperuricemia with secondary gout, uric acid stones, and symptoms due to hypermetabolism can also complicate the disorder
8. Erythema, burning, and pain in the extremities, a symptom complex known as erythromelalgia, is another complication of the thrombocytosis of PV due to increased platelet stickiness.

301. Ans. (a) Tyrosine kinase JAK2 mutations

(Ref: Harrison 20th edition, p 734; Harrison 19th edition, p 672)

Major WHO criteria are as follows:
- Hemoglobin > 18.5 g/dL in men and > 16.5 g/dL in women, or other evidence of increased red blood cell volume
- Presence of JAK2 617VF or other functionally similar mutation, such as JAK2 exon 12 mutation

Minor WHO criteria are as follows:
- Bone marrow biopsy showing hypercellularity for age with trilineage growth (panmyelosis) with prominent erythroid, granulocytic, and megakaryocytic proliferation
- Serum erythropoietin level below the Ref range for normal
- Endogenous erythroid colony formation in vitro

302. Ans. (c) Red cell mass

(Ref: Harrison 20th edition, p 734)

303. Ans. (d) Spontaneous severe infection

(Ref: Harrison 20th edition, p 734)

304. Ans. (a) Thrombocytopenia

(Ref: Harrison 20th edition, p 734)

305. Ans. (b) Increased erythropoietin level

(Ref: Harrison 20th edition, p 734)

306. Ans. (c) Myelofibrosis

(Ref: Harrison 20th edition, p 736, F: 99-1)

Miscellaneous

307. Ans. (c) FISH

(Ref: Harrison 20th edition, p 3367)
- FISH is used to identify chromosomal translocation. It uses fluorescent probes that bind to only those parts of the chromosome that are swapped between two chromosomes.
- Next generation sequencing can sequence the entire human genome in a single day. Contrast that to the Sanger sequence technology that took a decade to decipher human genome.
- Karyotyping can identify variation in number of chromosomes.
- PCR is used to amplify a single copy or few copies of segment of DNA.

308. Ans. (c) Platelet count of 40,000/cu.mm is a contraindication

(Ref: Washington manual of hemato-oncology: 3rd edition, p 7)
- The image shows a bone marrow biopsy needle called Jamshidi needle.
- The procedure can be done in prone or lateral position for posterior superior iliac spine or iliac crest.
- Adequate local anaesthesia should be administered below the periosteum since it is the pain sensitive structure in the bone. The patient does not need to hold breath during the procedure since only bone marrow is being assessed.
- The main purpose is to diagnose infiltrative disorders of the bone marrow that result in pancytopenia.
- Thrombocytopenia is not a contraindication for the procedure. Only patients with coagulopathy need replacement with clotting factors before the procedure.

Indications for trephine biopsy

1. Marrow fibrosis
2. Granulomatous disorders
3. Aplastic Anaemia
4. AML or MDS
5. Lymphoma
6. P.U.O
7. Multiple Myeloma
8. To assess mineralization front and appositional growth after tetracycline labelling.

309. Ans. (a) GVHD

(Ref: Atlas of Immunology: 3rd edition, p 340)

Runt disease is a graft verus host reaction. It was first observed in mice following administration of allogenic spleen cells into the new-born animals. It develops due to complex interaction between donor and recipient adaptive immunity.

310. Ans. (d) Nephritis

(Ref: Harrison 20th edition, p 819-20; Harrison: 19th edition, p 139e-4)

GVHD is a distinctive syndrome developing within 100 days after allogeneic hematopoietic-cell transplantation (HCT) and shows-
- Dermatitis-pruritic painful rash
- Hepatitis-pruritus and hepatic coma
- Enteritis-secretory diarrhea

Clinical Staging and Grading of Acute Graft-versus-host disease

Clinical stage	Skin	Liver—Bilirubin, mmol/L (mg/dL)	Gut
1.	Rash <25% body surface	34–51 (2–3)	Diarrhea 500–1000 mL/d
2.	Rash <25–50% body surface	51–103 (3–6)	Diarrhea 1000–1500 mL/d
3.	Generalized erythroderma	103–257 (6–15)	Diarrhea >1500 mL/d
4.	Desquamation and bullae	>257 (>15)	ileus

Chronic GVHD describes a more diverse syndrome developing after day 100.

311. Ans. (d) Rhabdomyolysis

(Ref: Harrison 20th edition, p 2166; Harrison 19th edition, p 1865)

- HELLP syndrome has haemolysis, elevated liver enzymes and low platelets. It is a dangerous complication of pregnancy associated with microvascular injury.
- Renal failure occurs in 50% patients of HELLP Syndrome due to thrombotic microangiopathy secondary to pre-eclampsia.
- The liver involvement defines this syndrome due to formation of sub-capsular hematomas. They can rupture spontaneously and can be life threatening.
- Neurological complications are like cerebral infarction or brain stem haemorrhage. Permanent vision loss like purtschner retinopathy may occur.
- HELLP syndrome has low serum levels of ADAMTS13 activity which is reduced to 30-60% of normal. In contrast ADAMTS13 activity is reduced to <5% in TTP.
- Treatment is glucorticoids and Plasma exchange if hemolyisis is refractory to steroids.

312. Ans. (c) ALS is a homologous antiserum raised against lymphocytes

(Ref: Harrison 19th edition, p 1828)

- Anti-lymphocyte globulin has action on only lymphocytes while new agents like alemtuzumab are directed against the CD52 protein act on B and T cells, natural killer cells, macrophages and some granulocytes.
- It acts only on circulating lymphocytes and not on cells in lymphoid organs.
- Anti-lymphocyte globulin is a *heterologous serum raised against lymphocytes in horses.*
- It has an *immune-regulatory action by stimulating the T cells* and making them go into proliferative phase. These cells then will release lymphokines that will regulate immune response and reduce the incidence of transplant rejection.
- Repeated injection will lead to production of low avidity antibodies that will reduce the efficacy.

313. Ans. (c) Low serum levels of IgA

(Ref: O.P. Ghai 8th edition, p 186)

- Wiskottaldich syndrome occurs due to mutations at X chromosome, Xp11.22-23 which encodes for WAS protein present in cytoplasm of platelets and lymphocytes
- There is profound IgM deficiency and defective T cell signaling due to deficient expression of CD43 in lymphocytes.
- Clinical presentation is in form of eczema (mimicking atopic dermatitis) with repeated illness of child due to infection with Strep. Pneumoniae, H. influenza, N. meningitidis.
- Thrombocytopenia is associated with small platelets. (Large platelets are seen in Bernard Soulier syndrome).
- Most children die of overwhelming infections and even if they survive can bleed to death.

314. Ans. (d) All of the above

(Ref: Harrison's 17th ed. Ch. 109)

- Schistocytes are fragmented part of a red blood cells which are typically irregularly shaped, jagged, and have two pointed ends. A true schistocyte does not have central pallor. *They are sometimes referred to as* **"helmet cells".**
- The presence of schistocytes on the peripheral blood smear suggests red blood cell injury from damaged endothelium *and is a characteristic feature of microangiopathic hemolytic anemia.*

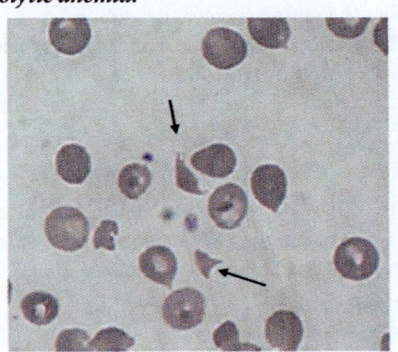

- Microangiopathic hemolytic anemia is an infrequent cause of Coombs-negative intravascular hemolytic anemia, and its causes include:

Thrombotic thrombocytopenic purpura
Hemolytic uremic syndrome
Disseminated intravascular coagulation
Defective valvular prosthesis.

315. Ans. (a) Associated thrombocytopenia with prolonged bleeding

(Ref: Harrison 20th edition, p 836; Harrison 19th ed./96e-8)

- Vitamin-K is a fat soluble compound. It promotes blood clotting by increasing hepatic biosynthesis of prothrombin and other coagulation factors.
- The best sources are green leafy vegetables, liver, cheese, butter and egg yolk. Deficiency, usually seen only in neonates, in disorders of absorption or during antibiotic therapy is characterized by hemorrhage.
- Warfarin acts by inhibiting Vitamin K, and does not causes deficiency of the same.

316. Ans. (c) Meth-hemoglobinaemia

(Ref: Harrison 20th edition, p 695; Harrison 19th ed./636)

- Sickle cell anemia has a pediatric presentation.
- Hemolytic anemia will cause pallor and not brown discoloration of blood.
- *In G6PD in event of intravascular hemolysis the hemoglobin-uria will cause a black urine. Therefore by exclusion also the answer is meth-hemoglobinaemia.*

317. Ans. (a) H. Influenza

(Ref: Harrison 20th edition, p 502; Harrison 19th ed./484, 652)

- Spleen protects from capsulated organisms and hence protects from infection from organisms like pneumococcus, meningococcus, hemophilus influenza.
- *Vaccination against these organisms must be done 4 weeks before planned splenectomy.*

318. Ans. (d) Cirrhosis

(Ref: Harrison 20th edition, p 837; Harrison 19th ed./739)

- In cirrhosis of the liver the production of all clotting factors will be reduced and therefore in these patients bleeding diathesis is seen.
- In pregnancy the elevated fibrinogen levels will lead to hyper-coagulable state.
- In abruption placentae the retro-placental clot formation implies the same hypercoagualability.
- In MI the preceding plaque fissure results in development of increased clotting tendency.

319. Ans. (a) C.M.L

(Ref: Harrison 20th edition, p 751; Harrison 19th ed. / 324, 634)

Priapism is characterized by prolonged, painful and irreducible erection, not resulting in ejaculation. It is an emergency with a poor prognosis, as the risk of impotence is 50%.

Causes of Priapism
- Sickle cell anemia
- Chronic myelogenous leukemia, Chronic lymphocytic leukemia, and acute lymphoblastic leukemia
- Drugs

320. Ans. (a) B cell tumor

(Ref: Harrison 20th edition, p 784; Harrison 19th ed./706)

- Hairy cell leukemia is a B cell tumor disease that presents in older males.
- Usual presentation involves pancytopenia with splenomegaly.
- The malignant cells appear to have "hairy" projections on light and electron microscopy and show a characteristic staining pattern with tartrate-resistant acid phosphatase.
- Bone marrow is typically not able to be aspirated, and biopsy shows a pattern of fibrosis.
- Patients with this disorder are prone to unusual infections, including infection by Mycobacterium avium intracellulare, and to vasculitic syndromes.
- Hairy cell leukemia is responsive to chemotherapy with interferon, pentostatin, or cladribine, with the latter being the usually preferred treatment.

321. Ans. (b) Acanthocyte

(Ref: Harrison 20th edition, p 382, Fig. 58-16; Harrison's. Atlas of Hematology Fig. e17-16)

Acanthocytes are contracted dense RBCs with irregular membrane projections that vary in width and length. They are seen in patients with severe liver disease and abetalipoproteinemia and in patients with McLeod blood group

322. Ans. (a) Schistocyte

(Ref: Harrison 20th edition, p 382, Fig. 58-11)

Fragmented red cells, or schistocytes, are helmet-shaped cells that reflect microangiopathichemolyticanemia (e.g., thrombotic thrombocytopenic purpura, disseminated intravascular coagulation, hemolytic uremic syndrome, scleroderma crisis) or shear damage from a prosthetic heart valve.

323. Ans. (a) Hemolytic uremic syndrome (HUS)

(Ref: Harrison 20th edition, p 824, Fig. 111-1D)

The peripheral smear shows fragmented RBC with abnormal shapes secondary to micro-angiopathichemolyticanemia. In setting of Acute Renal failure with thrombocytopenic and anemia the clinical diagnosis for this patient is H.U.S

324. Ans. (d) Observation and calf pain report ASAP

(Ref: Harrison's 18th edition, Chapter 262)

- Factor V Leiden, or factor V G1691A, is a single-point mutation in the gene that codes for coagulation factor V. It involves a G (guanine)-to-A (adenine) substitution at nucleotide 1691 (G1691A) in exon 10, which predicts the replacement of arginine at amino acid residue 506 by glutamine (Arg506Gln). The mutation, transmitted through autosomal dominant inheritance, renders factor V resistant to inactivation by APC (a natural anticoagulant protein)
- *Initiation of oral anticoagulation for primary VTE prophylaxis in asymptomatic carriers of any hypercoagulable state has not been advised, mainly because the annual absolute risk of idiopathic VTE is low or not high enough to be favorably balanced against the annual risk of oral anticoagulation-related major and fatal hemorrhage.*
- Since most VTEs (50%-70%) in patients with a predisposition to hypercoagulability occur following a situational risk factor, such as major or orthopedic surgery, aggressive VTE prophylaxis should be prescribed to asymptomatic carriers of hyper-coagulable states during high-risk situations
- Reasons for considering long-term anticoagulation therapy for conditions known to be associated with increased rates of VTE recurrence.
    1. Patients with documented, persistent lupus anticoagulants
    2. homozygous factor V Leiden
    3. deficiency of protein C or protein S
    4. Double heterozygosity for factor V Leiden
    5. Prothrombin G20210A mutation.

325. Ans. (d) Thalassemia

(Ref: Harrison 20th edition, p 732-33; Harrison 19th edition, p 638)

Leucoerythroblastosis refers to the presence of a variable number of immature erythroid and myeloid cells in circulation. The blood film shows the presence of erythroblasts and granulocyte precursors (e.g. myelocytes and myeloblasts). It is seen in primary myelofibrosis and is frequent when there is marrow infiltration by tumour. This disturbs the marrow infrastructure and allows early release of the precursor.

Causes of Leuco-erythroblastosis

Infections	Fungal, HIV etc.
Tumors	Metastastic carcinomas Lymphomas e.g. Hodgkins Leukaemias e.g. CML, AML, Hairy cell leukemia Plasma cell disorders: Multiple Myeloma Polycythemia vera
Lipid deposition	Gaucher's disease

326. Ans. (a) Dabigatran

(Ref: Harrison 20th edition, p 855)

Ximelagatran was the first oral direct thrombin inhibitor approved; however it was later withdrawn because of hepatotoxicity. Recently a new direct thrombin inhibitor dabigatran has been approved for the prophylaxis of stroke and systemic embolism in nonvalvular atrial fibrillation. It is administered as a prodrug; dabigatran etexilate. It is not metabolized by CYP enzymes however dose adjustment is required in renal failure.

327. Ans. (a) Erythrocytosis

(Ref: Harrison 20th edition, p 2759, 2490; Harrison 19th edition, p 668)

- About 40% of patients with thymoma have another systemic autoimmune illness related to the thymoma.
- About 30% of patients with thymoma have myasthenia gravis, 5% to 8% have pure red blood cell aplasia, and about 5% have hypogammaglobulinemia.
- Thymectomy results in the resolution of pure RBC aplasia in about 30% of patients but rarely benefits patients with hypogammaglobulinemia.
- Among patients with myasthenia gravis, about 10% to 15% have a thymoma. Thymectomy produces at least some symptomatic improvement in about 65% of patients with myasthenia gravis.
- Thymoma more rarely may be associated with polymyositis systemic lupus erythematosus, thyroiditis, Sjogren's syndrome, ulcerative colitis, pernicious anemia. Addison's disease, scleroderma, and panhypopituitarism.

328. Ans. (b) 5q

(Ref: Harrison 20th edition, p 730-31, Table 98-5; Harrison 19th edition, p 670)

- Unbalanced recurrent aberrations, most commonly -5, 5q-, -7, 7q-, +8, 11q-, 13q-, and 20q-, suggest that genes within these regions have a role in the pathogenesis of MDS or myeloproliferative disorder (MPD), which is based on loss of tumor suppressor genes or haploinsufficiency of genes necessary for normal myelopoiesis.
- Approximately 80% of patients with MDS do not have an obvious exposure or cause for MDS. In these cases, the disorder is classified as primary or idiopathic MDS.
- Secondary MDS describes the development of MDS or acute leukemia years after known exposure to sources of chromosomal damage. Patients who survive cancer treatment with alkylating agents, with or without radiotherapy, have a high risk of developing MDS or secondary acute leukemia 5-7 years after the exposure. These drugs are associated with a high prevalence of chromosomal abnormalities in bone marrow [-5, del(5q), -7, del(q) and complex karyotype

329. Ans. (a) Anti-thymocyte globulin followed by cyclosporine

(Ref: Harrison 20th edition, p 727, 728; Harrison 19th edition, p 667)

- Immunosupressive therapy using ATG plus CSA is being used as first-line therapy for patients older than 40 years and as second-line therapy in younger patients if a matched sibling donor is not available. Central venous catheter placement is required before the administration of IST. Patients also require intense platelet support during ATG therapy
- The standard regimen of ATG in combination with cyclosporine induces hematologic recovery (independence from transfusion and a leukocyte count adequate to prevent infection) in majority of patients.
- Children do especially well, while older adult patients often suffer complications due to the presence of comorbidities. An early robust hematologic response correlates with long-term survival.
- Improvement in granulocyte number is generally apparent within 2 months of treatment. Most recovered patients continue to have some degree of blood count depression, the MCV remains elevated, and the bone marrow cellularity returns toward normal very slowly if at all.

330. Ans. (a) Trisodium citrate 3.2%

(Ref: Wintrobe 11th edition, p 28; Harrison 19th edition, p 749)

331. Ans. (d) Electrophoresis

(Ref: Harrison 20th edition, p 797; Harrison 19th edition, p 721)

Bence Jones proteins are seen in multiple myeloma.
- Urinary protein electrophoresis will exhibit a discrete protein peak.
- In myeloma plasma cells produce immuno-globulin of a single heavy and light chain, a monoclonal protein commonly referred to as a paraprotein.
- Heat test is false negative in 50% of patients with light chain myeloma.
- Dipstick detects albumin and not paraproteins.

332. Ans. (a) Anti-thymocyte globulin + cyclosporine

(Ref: Harrison 20th edition, p 727, 728; Harrison 19th edition, p 667)

- The standard regimen of ATG in combination with cyclosporine induces hematologic recovery (independence from transfusion and a leukocyte count adequate to prevent infection) in 60–80% of patients of aplastic anemia.
- Children do especially well, while older adult patients often suffer complications due to the presence of comorbidities.
- Improvement in granulocyte number is generally apparent within 2 months of treatment.
- Development of MDS, with typical marrow morphologic or cytogenetic abnormalities, occurs in approximately 15% of treated patients, usually but not invariably associated with a return of pancytopenia, and some patients develop leukemia.

333. Ans. (d) Hemolytic disease of newborn

(Ref: Harrison 19th edition, p 649)

Hemorrhagic disease of newborn occurs due to vitamin K deficiency

334. Ans. (a) Selective separation of components of blood

(Ref: Harrison 20th edition, p 811; Harrison 19th edition, p 138e-2)

Apheresis technology is used for the collection of multipleunits of platelets from a single donor.

These single-donor apheresis platelets (SDAP) contain the have fever contaminating leukocytes than pooled RD platelets. Plasma may also be collected from apheresis and subsequently other blood products are also collected. There are large categories of component collections:

- **Plasmapheresis**- Plasmapheresis is useful in collecting FFP (fresh frozen plasma) of a particular ABO group. Commercial uses aside from FFP for this procedure include immune globulin products, plasma derivatives, and collection of rare WBC and RBC antibodies.
- **Erythrocytapheresis**- Erythrocytapheresis is the separation of erythrocytes from whole blood. It is most commonly accomplished using the method of centrifugal sedimentation. This process is used for red blood cell diseases such as sickle cell crises or severe malaria. The automated red blood cell collection procedure for donating erythrocytes is referred to as 'Double Reds' or 'Double Red Cell Apheresis.
- **Plateletpheresis** (thrombapheresis, thrombo-cytapheresis) - blood platelets. Plateletpheresis, like it sounds, is the collection of platelets by apheresis; while returning the RBCs, WBCs, and component plasma. The yield is normally the equivalent of between six and ten random platelet concentrates. Quality control demands the platelets from apheresis be equal to or greater than 3.0×10^{11} in number and have a pH of equal to or greater than 6.2 in 90% of the products tested and must be used within five days.
- **Leukapheresis**- Leukopheresis is the removal of PMNs, basophils, eosinophils for transfusion into patients whose PMNs are ineffective or where traditional therapy has failed. There is limited data to suggest the benefit of granulocyte infusion. The complications of this procedure are the difficulty in collection and short shelf life (24 hours at 20 to 24°C). Since the "buffy coat" layer sits directly atop the RBC layer, HES, a sedimenting agent, is employed to improve yield while minimizing RBC collection. Quality control demands the resultant concentrate be 1.0×10^{10} granulocytes in 75% of the units tested and that the product be irradiated to avoid graft-versus-host disease (inactivate lymphocytes). Irradiation does not affect PMN function. Since there is usually a small amount of RBCs collected, ABO compatibility should be employed when feasible.
- **Stem cell harvesting**- circulating bone marrow cells are harvested to use in bone marrow transplantation

335. Ans. (c) Bone marrow

(Ref: Harrison's 18th edition, Table 81.2)

- The cause of cancer death differs across the life span.
- In women who are younger than 20 years of age, the largest cause of cancer death is leukemia.
- Between the ages of 20 and 59 years, breast cancer becomes the leading cause of any of the disorders mentioned above. Biopsy is clearly the most important diagnostic procedure.

336. Ans. (c) Hemochromatosis

(Ref: Harrison 20th edition, p 820-22; Harrison 19th edition, p 139e-1)

Conditions for Bone Marrow Transplantation

- Inherited metabolic disorders - Adrenoleuko-dystrophy, Hurler syndrome, metachromatic leukodystrophy, osteopetrosis, and others
- Inherited red cell disorders - Pure red cell aplasia, sickle cell disease, beta-thalassemia, and others
- Marrow failure states - Severe aplastic anemia, Fanconi anemia
- Inherited immune disorders -Severe combined immunodeficiency, Wiskott-Aldrich syndrome, and others

337. Ans. (b) Inhibiting coagulation factor Xa

(Ref: Harrison 20th edition, p 854; Harrison 19th edition, p 756)

Rivaroxaban and Apixaban are newer oral anticoagulants that act by inhibiting factor Xa.

Newer oral anticoagulants that are currently being asked in the exams are:

- Dabigatran (Direct thrombin inhibitor)
- Rivaroxaban
- Apixaban

338. Ans. (b) It results in decrease in reticulocyte count

(Ref: Katzung 10th/537-538; KDT's 6th/592)

- Erythropoietin is a hematopoietic growth factor that is normally produced by the kidneys.
- Normally, there is an inverse relationship between serum erythropoietin levels and hemoglobin levels. When Hb decreases and anemia becomes more severe, serum erythropoietin level increases exponentially. But, anemia due to chronic renal failure is an exception to this inverse relationship. In CRF, erythropoietin is not produced, that results in anemia. So, exogenous erythropoietin will markedly improve anemia in CRF patients whereas there is less likelihood of response in other anemias.
- Erythropoietin consistently improves the hematocrit and Hb levels and usually eliminates the need of blood transfusions in CRF patients.
- An increase in reticulocyte count is usually observed in 10 days and increase in hematocrit and Hb levels in about 2-6 weeks.

339. Ans. (a) CML

(Ref: Harrison 20th edition, p 730, Table 98.5; Harrison 19th edition, p 693)

2008 WHO classification of MDS is as follows:

1. Refractory cytopenia with unilineage dysplasia – this includes refractory anemia, refractory neutropenia, or refractory thrombocytopenia
2. RARS (Refractory Anemia with singed sideroblasts)
3. RAEB (Refractory Anemia with excess Blasts)
4. Refractory cytopenia with multilineage dysplasia
5. MDS with isolated deletion of 5q
6. MDS, unclassifiable
7. Childhood MDS

340. Ans. (c) Bleeding episodes in patients with Las may be severe and life threatening

(Ref: Harrison 20th edition, p 838; Harrison 19th edition, p 740)

- Lupus anticoagulants (Las) cause prolongation of coagulation tests by binding to phospholipids. Although most often encountered in patients with systemic lupus erythematosus, they may also develop in normal individuals.
- The diagnosis is first suggested by prolongation of coagulation tests. Failure to correct with incubation with normal plasma confirms the presence of a circulating inhibitor. Contrary to the name, patients with LA activity have normal hemostasis and are not predisposed to bleeding. Instead, they are at risk for venous and arterial thromboembolisms.
- Patients with a history of recurrent unplanned abortions or thrombosis should undergo lifelong anticoagulation. The presence of LAs or anticardiolipin antibodies without a history of thrombosis may be observed because many of these patients will not go on to develop a thrombotic event.

341. Ans. (d) Its dose is increased in liver disease

(Ref: Harrison 20th edition, p 852, 853; Katzung 11th/595-596, Harrison 19th edition, p 7E)

- Warfarin is an oral anticoagulant that acts by inhibiting the y- carboxylation of glutamate residues in vitamin-K dependent clotting factors (II, VII, IX and X).
- It has 99% binding to albumin that result in
  1. Long half life (t1/2 = 36 hours)
  2. Small volume or distribution
  3. Lack of urinary excretion of unchanged drug
- It readily crosses the placenta. If given during pregnancy, it can result in 'Conradi syndrome' in the fetus.
- Liver disease reduces the synthesis of clotting factors, thus increases the effect of warfarin. The dose of this drug therefore, needs to be reduced in liver disease

342. Ans. (c) SLE

(Ref: Harrison 20th edition, p 2522; Harrison 19th edition, p 2132)

Hematological features of SLE
- Antibody mediated destruction of peripheral blood cells may cause neutropenia, lympho-penia, thrombocytopenia or hemolytic anemia (Pancytopenia).
- The degree of leucopenia, most commonly lymphopenia, is often a good guide to disease activity.
- Although the ESR is usually elevated, CRP is often normal unless there is serositis or infection.

343. Ans. (d) Pancreatic carcinoma

(Ref: Harrison 20th edition, p 394)

- Ectopic production of erythropoietin by cancer cells cause most paraneoplastic erythrocytosis
- Cancers typically associated with this syndrome include Renal cancer, Hepatocarcinoma and cerebellar Hemangioblastoma.

344. Ans. (d) Rituximab

(Ref: Harrison 20th edition, p 2049-52)

- Septic shock is managed by maintaining the cardiovascular system with the help of i.v. fluids particularly normal saline along with antibiotics.
- Adrenal insufficiency has been noted in many cases of septic shock that can be treated by steroids.
- Activated protein C available as drotrecogin alpha is also approved for septic shock.
- Rituximab has no role in treatment of septic shock.

345. Ans. (d) 70%

(Ref: Harrison 20th edition, p 702)

- Folic acid supplements at the time of conception and in the first 12 weeks of pregnancy reduce by <70% the incidence of neural tube defects (NTDs) (anencephaly, meningomyelocele, encephalocele, and spina bifida) in the fetus. Most of this protective effect can be achieved by taking folic acid, 0.4 mg daily at the time of conception.
- The incidence of cleft palate and harelip also can be reduced by prophylactic folic acid. There is no clear simple relationship between maternal folate status and these fetal abnormalities, although overall the lower the maternal folate, the greater the risk to the fetus. NTDs also can be caused by antifolate and antiepileptic drugs

346. Ans. (b) Anti-human globulin antiserum

(Ref: Harrison 20th edition, p 718; Harrison 19th edition, p 138e-4, 138e-4f)

- Coomb's antiglobulin test is the major tool for diagnosing autoimmune hemolysis.
- This test relies on the ability of antibodies specific for immunoglobulins (especially IgG) or complement components (especially C3) to agglutinate RBC coated with these proteins.
- With specific anti-IgG and anti-C3, the direct Coomb's test detects IgG or C3 on the patient's RBC, which indicates the presence of immune hemolysis and may help define its cause.
- Rarely, neither IgG nor complement may be found on the RBC of the patient (Coomb's -negative immune hemolytic anemia).
- Antibodies in the serum of the patient that recognize RBC antigens can be detected by reacting the serum with normal RBC bearing the antigen. With the exception of cold reacting antibodies and some drug related antibodies this is of value primarily in compatibility testing for transfusion.

347. Ans. (b) Homocystinemia

(Ref: Harrison 20th edition, p 2310, Table 326-1)

348. Ans. (d) High altitude

(Ref: Harrison 18th edition, p 456, 898)

349. Ans. (a) Prolonged prothrombin time

(Ref: Ghai 6th edition, p 31)

10
Fluids and Electrolytes

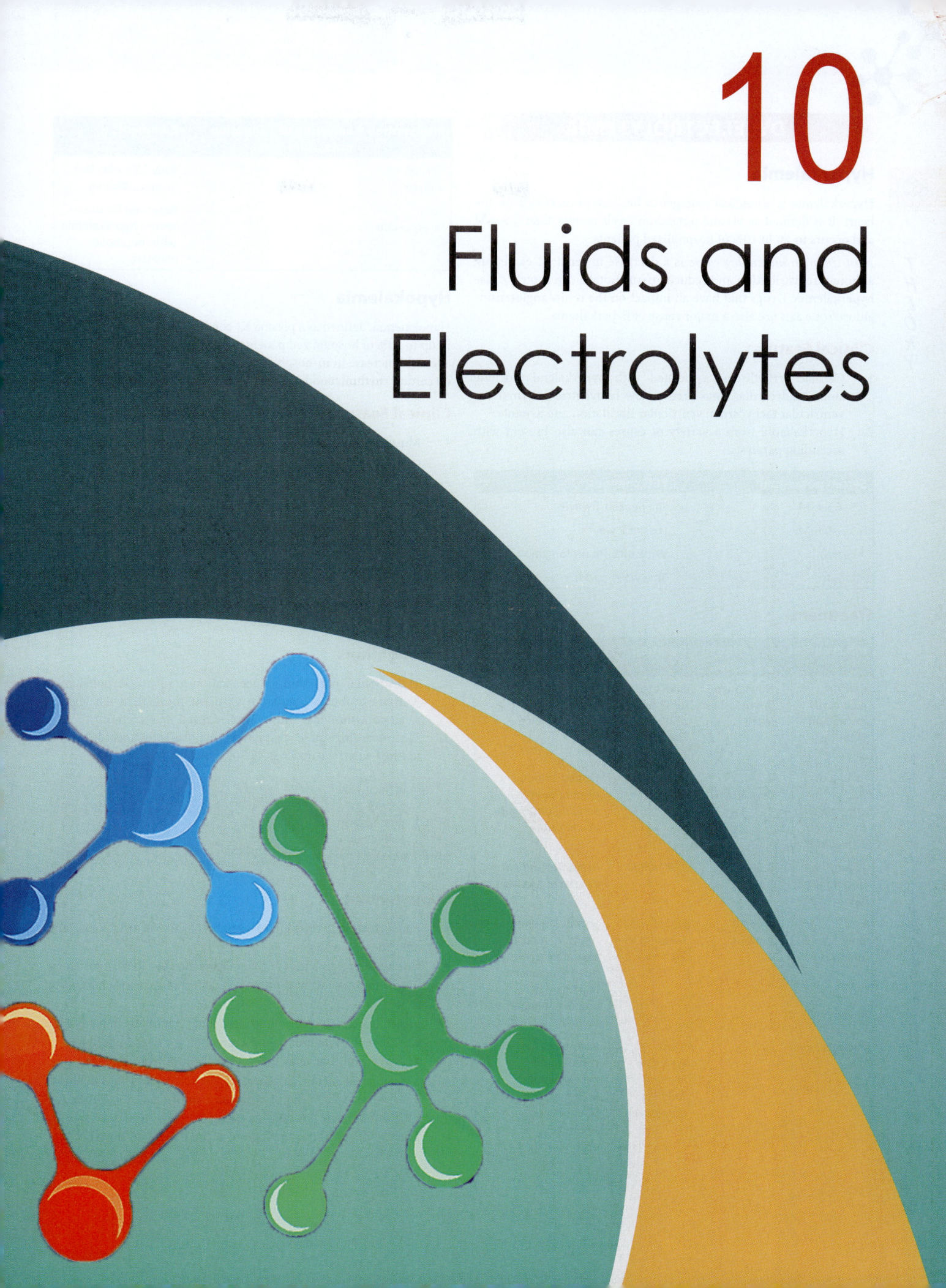

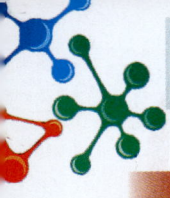

DYSELECTROLYTEMIA

Hyperkalemia

Hyperkalemia is a medical emergency because of its effects on the heart. It is defined as plasma potassium levels greater than 5.5 mM and occurs in up to 10% of hospitalized patients.

Most common underlying cause is a decrease in renal K^+ excretion, although redistribution and reduced tissue uptake can acutely cause hyperkalemia. Drugs that have an impact on the renin-angiotensin-aldosterone axis are also a major cause of hyperkalemia.

Clinical Features

1. Cardiac arrhythmias associated with hyperkalemia include sinus bradycardia, sinus arrest, slow idioventricular rhythms, ventricular tachycardia, ventricular fibrillation and asystole.
2. Hyperkalemia from a variety of causes can also present with ascending paralysis.

Serum potassium	ECG changes
5.5–6.5 mM	Tall peaked T waves
6.5–7.5 mM	Loss of P waves
7–8 mM	Wide qRS, PR prolongation
>8 mM	Sine wave pattern

Treatment

Intervention	Lowering of potassium	Duration	Comments
Calcium gluconate or calcium chloride	No change in potassium levels	Effect starts 1–3 minutes and lasts for 30–60 minutes	Reduces excitability of heart and is the drug of choice
Insulin drip (most effective drug to lower K^+ concentration)	0.5–1.5 mmol/L	4–6 hours	Redistribution of potassium by sending potassium inside cells
Parenteral or nebulized salbutamol	0.5–1.5 mmol/L	2–4 hours	Promotes cellular uptake of potassium
Sodium polystyrene sulfonate	0.5–1.0 mmol/L	Full effect takes up to 24 hours	Sorbitol in enema omitted in post-operative patients due to increased incidence of sorbitol-induced colonic necrosis
Hemodialysis		Most effective method to lower potassium	Refractory life-threatening hyperkalemia failing to respond to conventional measures
Peritoneal dialysis			Only 15% effective as hemodialysis
Soda bicarbonate			Reserved for use in severe hyperkalemia with metabolic acidosis

Contd...

Hypokalemia

Hypokalemia, defined as a plasma K^+ concentration <3.6 mM, occurs in up to 20% of hospitalized patients. Hypokalemia is associated with a tenfold increase in in-hospital mortality rates due to adverse effects on cardiac rhythm, blood pressure, and cardiovascular morbidity rate.

Clinical Features

1. Muscle cramps and weakness as hypokalemia has prominent effects on cardiac, skeletal, and intestinal muscle cells.
2. The hyperpolarization of skeletal muscle, thus impairing the capacity to depolarize and contract; weakness and even paralysis may ensue.
3. In particular, it is a major risk factor for both ventricular and atrial arrhythmias.
4. It also causes a skeletal myopathy and predisposes to rhabdomyolysis.
5. The paralytic effects of hypokalemia on intestinal smooth muscle leads to intestinal ileus.

Investigations

1. Transtubular potassium concentration gradient: Hypokalemia with transtubular potassium gradient more than 4 suggests renal potassium loss with increased distal K^+ secretion.
2. Electrocardiographic changes in hypokalemia include (most marked when serum K^+ is <2.7 mmol/L):

- Broad flat T wave
- ST depression
- QT prolongation
- PR prolongation
- *Pseudo P–Pulmonale*

Management

- For correction to raise blood levels by 1 mM, 200 mEq potassium chloride is to be given.
- Correction up to 3 mM is given intravenously. To upgrade from 3 mM to 3.5 mM, oral potassium chloride supplementation is used.
- Example, patient on amphotericin B has potassium value of 2.3. Calculate the total potassium correction for next 24 hours?
  - We would have to increase potassium from current value of 2.3 to 3.0 mM. Mathematically, to correct 1 mM in blood we need 200 mEq of potassium chloride. For 0.7 mEq, we would need 140 mEq/24 hours.
- The peripheral intravenous dose is usually 20–40 mmol of K^+-

Cl⁻ per liter; higher concentrations can cause localized pain from chemical phlebitis, irritation, and sclerosis.
- If hypokalemia is severe (<2.5 mmol/L) and/or critically symptomatic, intravenous K⁺Cl⁻ can be administered through a central vein with cardiac monitoring in an intensive care setting at rates of 10–20 mmol/h; higher rates should be reserved for acutely life-threatening complications

Hyponatremia

Hyponatremia, which is defined as a plasma Na⁺ concentration <135 mEq is a very common disorder, and is the *most common electrolyte abnormality in hospitalized patients*. Hyponatremia, thus is subdivided diagnostically into three groups, depending on clinical history and volume status.

Hypovolemic Hyponatremia

Hypovolemia causes a marked neurohumoral activation, increasing circulating levels of AVP and activation of V_2 receptors that can lead to hyponatremia in the setting of increased free-water intake.
- *Non-renal* causes of hypovolemic hyponatremia are gastrointestinal loss (vomiting, diarrhea, tube drainage, etc.) and insensible loss (sweating, burns) of Na⁺Cl⁻ and water in the absence of adequate oral replacement.
- The *renal* causes of hypovolemic hyponatremia share an inappropriate loss of Na⁺Cl⁻ in the urine, leading to volume depletion and an increase in circulating AVP; urine Na⁺ concentration is typically >20 mM. The renal causes are
  - Primary adrenal insufficiency
  - Salt-losing nephropathies
  - Thiazide diuretics cause hyponatremia via a number of mechanisms, including polydipsia and diuretic-induced volume depletion.
  - Cerebral salt wasting is a rare cause of hypovolemic hyponatremia, encompassing hyponatremia with clinical hypovolemia and inappropriate natriuresis in association with intracranial disease; associated disorders include subarachnoid hemorrhage, traumatic brain injury, craniotomy, encephalitis, and meningitis.

Hypervolemic Hyponatremia

The pathophysiology of hypervolemic hyponatremia in the sodium-avid edematous disorders (congestive heart failure, cirrhosis, and nephrotic syndrome) is similar to that in hypovolemic hyponatremia except that arterial filling and circulatory integrity are decreased due to the specific etiologic factors, e.g. cardiac dysfunction in CHF and peripheral vasodilation in cirrhosis.

Euvolemic Hyponatremia

- The syndrome of inappropriate antidiuresis is the most common cause of euvolemic hyponatremia
- Moderate to severe hypothyroidism, with correction after the achievement of a euthyroid state.
- Secondary adrenal insufficiency due to pituitary disease; whereas the deficit in circulating aldosterone in primary adrenal insufficiency causes *hypovolemic* hyponatremia, the predominant glucocorticoid deficiency in secondary adrenal failure is associated with *euvolemic* hyponatremia.

Glucocorticoids exert a negative feedback on AVP release by the posterior pituitary so that hydrocortisone replacement in these patients will rapidly normalize the AVP response to osmolality, reducing circulating AVP.

Clinical Symptoms
1. Seizures reflecting the development of cerebral edema.
2. Acute hyponatremic encephalopathy ensues when these volume regulatory mechanisms are overwhelmed by a rapid decrease in tonicity, resulting in acute cerebral edema.
3. Early symptoms can include nausea, headache, and vomiting.
4. A key complication of acute hyponatremia is normocapnic or hypercapnic respiratory failure.

Treatment
- Restriction of free water and hypotonic fluid intake. Free water intake to be less than 1–1.5 L/day.
- Symptomatic hyponatremia is managed with 4–6 mEq/L increment to reverse neurological deficit.
- Acute hyponatremia with severe neurological features is managed with 100 mL of 3% hypertonic saline over 10 minutes.
- Correct chronic hyponatremia at 4-8 mEq/L every 24 hours
- For severe symptomatic patients, deliver 3% hypertonic saline and formula for correcting deficit is:

> Deficit = Total body water deficit × (Desired serum Na – actual serum Na)

Total body water = 0.6 × weight (for males)
0.5 × weight (for females)

Hypernatremia

Hypernatremia is defined as an increase in the plasma Na⁺ concentration to >145 mM.

Causes
1. Elderly individuals with reduced thirst and/or diminished access to fluids are at the highest risk of developing hypernatremia.
2. Central defect in hypothalamic osmoreceptor function, with a mixture of both decreased thirst and reduced AVP secretion. Causes of this adipsic diabetes insipidus include primary or metastatic tumor, occlusion or ligation of the anterior communicating artery, trauma, hydrocephalus, and inflammation.
3. Hypernatremia can develop after the loss of water via both renal and nonrenal routes. Insensible losses of water may increase in the setting of fever, exercise, heat exposure, severe burns, or mechanical ventilation.
4. Diarrhea is the most common gastrointestinal cause of hypernatremia.
5. Common causes of renal water loss include osmotic diuresis secondary to hyperglycemia, excess urea, postobstructive diuresis, and mannitol.
6. Nephrogenic DI is characterized by renal resistance to AVP, which can be partial or complete.

Clinical Features
1. Altered mental status is the most common manifestation, ranging from mild confusion and lethargy to deep coma. The sudden shrinkage of brain cells in acute hypernatremia may lead

to parenchymal or subarachnoid hemorrhage and/or subdural hematomas.
2. Patients with *chronic* hypernatremia are less likely to develop severe neurologic compromise. However, the cellular response to chronic hypernatremia predisposes these patients to the development of cerebral edema and seizures during overly rapid hydration (overcorrection of plasma Na⁺ concentration by >10 mM/d.)

Treatment
- Severe hypernatremic is defined as sodium > 158 meq/L
- Perform urine osmolality to determine etiology

Choice of fluid for replacement
- Hypernatremia with hypovolemia: Isotonic 0.9% normal saline
- Hypernatremia with euvolemia: Water ingestion or intravenous 5% dextrose
- Hypernatremia with hypervolemia: 5% dextrose ± loop diuretics

Calculation of water deficit
- Acute hypernatremia: Start with 5% dextrose and as correction progresses, therapy should continue with 0.45% saline with dextrose

$$\text{Volume to be replaced} = TBW \times \frac{(Na^+) - 140}{140}$$

DISORDERS OF PHOSPHATE METABOLISM

Hypophosphatemia
- The most important regulator of phosphate metabolism is kidney.
- PTH and FGF 23 (fibroblast growth factor 23) have phosphaturic action
- GH augments proximal renal tubular reabsorption of phosphate.
- Cell phosphate uptake is stimulated by insulin, epinephrine, feeding, accelerated cell metabolism and alkalemia.
- Severe hypophosphatemia is defined as value less than 1 mg/dL or 0.32 mmol/L. This leads to increased affinity of hemoglobin and oxygen. Hence the oxygen availability to cells is lesser leading to tissue anoxia and rhabdomyolysis.
- Respiratory alkalosis and metabolic alkalosis lead to cell shift of phosphorus leading to hypophosphatemia.
- During treatment of DKA insulin administration leads to intracellular phosphate uptake leading to hypophosphatemia.

Causes of Hypophosphatemia

Increased loss of phosphate
- Phosphaturic drugs like theophylline, diuretics and bronchodilators
- Hyperparathyroidism
- Fanconi syndrome and renal tubular defects
- Hypophosphatemic rickets due to PHEX gene
- Oncogenic osteomalacia due to production of FGF-23

Cellular shift of phosphate
- Respiratory alkalosis
- Hungry bones syndrome
- Glucose administration
- Anabolic steroids

Electrolyte imbalance
- Metabolic alkalosis
- Hypomagnesemia

Low supply/ absorption
- Starvation
- Parenteral nutrition with low phosphate supply
- Malabsorption
- Antacids blocking absorption
- Vitamin D deficient osteomalacia

Abnormal losses followed by insufficient repletion
- DKA correction
- Recovery from starvation
- Recovery from severe burns
- Chronic alcoholism

Clinical features: They are explained by tissue anoxia leading to compromise of all organs including RBC, WBC and platelets
1. Rhabdomyolysis
2. Encephalopathy
3. Respiratory failure or inability to wean off ventilator
4. CHF
5. Hemolytic anemia
6. Petechiae
7. Increased susceptibility to infections (impaired chemotaxis)

Work up
1. Urine phosphate level
2. Serum PTH
3. Serum PTHrP
4. Serum FGF
5. Urine for aminoacids
6. Urine anion gap

Management
- Oral replacement preferred as parenteral delivery leads to concomitant hypocalcemia
- Infusion in severe hypophosphatemia (<1 mg/dL) with sodium or potassium phosphate
- Switch to oral therapy and keep a watch on hypotension during parenteral delivery.

Hyperphosphatemia

Most common cause of Hyperphosphatemia is advanced chronic kidney disease.

Causes of Hyperphosphatemia

Decreased excretion of phosphate into the urine
- CKD/ AKI
- Hypoparathyroidism
- Pseudohypoparathyroidism
- Acromegaly

Addition of phosphate load to extracellular fluid
- Hypervitaminosis D
- Laxative or enema with high phosphate content
- Tumor lysis syndrome
- Rhabdomyolysis
- Metabolic and respiratory acidosis

Contd...

Clinical features of the underlying disorder will predominate and lab work shows greatly elevated phosphate

Treatment

- *Oral phosphate binders:* Calcium acetate, sevelamer carbonate, lanthanum carbonate and aluminium hydroxide.
- In setting of co-existent hypercalcemia calcium salts are avoided.
- In case of AKI or severe CKD, dialysis will lower phosphate to normal limits.

ANION GAP

The anion gap is estimated by subtracting the sum of Cl^- and HCO_3^- concentrations from the plasma Na^+ concentration.

Anion gap = $[Na^+] - ([Cl^-] + [HCO_3^-])$

The reference range of the anion gap is 3–11 mEq/L

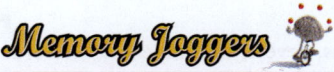

*Causes of elevated Anion gap acidosis is best remembered by the mnemonic **MUDPILES** or a shorter version called K.U.L.T*

M	=	Methanol
U	=	Uremia
D	=	DKA (also AKA and starvation)
P	=	Paraldehyde
I	=	INH
L	=	Lactic acidosis
E	=	Ethylene glycol poisoning
S	=	Salicylates

or

K	=	Ketoacidosis (DKA, alcoholic ketoacidosis, starvation)
U	=	Uremia (Renal failure)
L	=	Lactic acidosis
T	=	Toxins (Ethylene glycol, methanol, paraldehyde, salicylate)

A decreased anion gap (< 6 mEq/L) may suggest the following:
- Hypoalbuminemia
- Plasma cell dyscrasia
- Monoclonal protein
- Bromide intoxication
- Normal variant.

A normal anion gap (6–12 mEq/L) may indicate the following:
- Loss of bicarbonate (i.e. diarrhea)
- Recovery from diabetic ketoacidosis
- Ileostomy fluid loss
- Carbonic anhydrase inhibitors (acetazolamide, dorzolamide, topiramate)
- Renal tubular acidosis
- Arginine and lysine in parenteral nutrition
- Normal variant.

ACID-BASE REGULATION AND DISORDERS

To maintain cellular function, the body has elaborate mechanisms that maintain blood H^+ concentration within a narrow range—typically 35 – 45 nmol/L (pH 7.45 – 7.35, where pH = –log $[H^+]$).

Acid-Base Physiology

- Most acid comes from carbohydrate and fat metabolism, which generates 15,000 – 20,000 mmol of CO_2 daily.
- CO_2 is not an acid itself but combines with water (H_2O) in the blood to create carbonic acid (H_2CO_3), which in the presence of the enzyme carbonic anhydrase dissociates into H^+ and HCO_3^-.
- The H^+ binds with Hb in RBCs and is released with oxygenation in the alveoli, at which time the reaction is reversed, creating H_2O and CO_2, which is exhaled in each breath.
- Most bases come from metabolism of anionic amino acids (glutamate and aspartate) and from oxidation and consumption of organic anions such as lactate and citrate, which produces HCO_3^-.

Acid-Base Balance

Acid-base balance is maintained by mainly three systems, chemical buffering, pulmonary elimination and renal elimination.

Chemical Buffering

The most important extracellular buffer is the HCO_3^-/CO_2 system, described by the equation:

$$H^+ + HCO_3^- \rightarrow H_2CO_3 \rightarrow CO_2 + H_2O$$

An increase in H^+ drives the equation to the right and generates CO_2. This important buffer system is highly regulated; CO_2 concentrations can be finely controlled by alveolar ventilation, and H^+ and HCO_3^- concentrations can be finely regulated by renal excretion.

Other important physiologic buffers include intracellular organic and inorganic phosphates and proteins, including Hb in RBCs. Less important are extracellular phosphate and plasma proteins.

Pulmonary Regulation

CO_2 concentration is finely regulated by changes in tidal volume and respiratory rate (minute ventilation). A decrease in pH is sensed by arterial chemoreceptors and leads to an increase in tidal volume or respiratory rate; CO_2 is exhaled and blood pH increases. *In contrast to chemical buffering, which is immediate, pulmonary regulation occurs over minutes to hours. It is about 50 – 75% effective; it does not completely normalizes pH.*

Renal Regulation

The kidneys control pH by adjusting the amount of HCO_3^- that is reabsorbed and the amount of H^+ that is excreted; increase in HCO_3^- is equivalent to removing free H^+. **Changes in renal acid-base handling occur hours to days after changes in acid-base status.**

HCO_3^- reabsorption occurs mostly in the proximal tubule and to a lesser degree, in the collecting tubule.

The Delta Gap

The difference between the patient's anion gap and the normal anion gap is termed the delta gap. This amount is considered an HCO_3^- equivalent, because for every unit rise in the anion gap, the HCO_3^- should lower by 1 (by buffering).

Compensations in Simple Acid-Base Disorders

Primary disturbance	pH	HCO_3^-	pCO_2	Compensation calculation
Metabolic acidosis	< 7.35	Primary decrease	Compensatory decrease	$pCO_2 = (1.5 \times HCO_3^-) + 8 (\pm 2)$
Metabolic alkalosis	> 7.45	Primary increase	Compensatory increase	pCO_2 should not rise above 55 mm Hg in compensation $pCO_2 = (0.7 \times HCO_3^-) + 21$
Respiratory acidosis	< 7.35	Compensatory increase	Primary increase	**Acute:** 1–2 mmol/L increase in HCO_3^- for every 10 mm Hg increase in pCO_2 **Chronic:** 3–4 mmol/L increase in HCO_3^- for every 10 mm Hg increase in pCO_2
Respiratory alkalosis	> 7.45	Compensatory decrease	Primary decrease	**Acute:** 1–2 mmol/L decrease in HCO_3^- for every 10 mm Hg decrease in pCO_2 **Chronic:** 4–5 mmol/L decrease in HCO_3^- for every 10 mm Hg decrease in pCO_2

Symptoms and Signs of Acid-Base Derangements

Compensated or mild acid-base disorders cause few symptoms or signs. Severe, uncompensated disorders have multiple cardiovascular, respiratory, neurologic, and metabolic consequences described below

System-wise consequences of acid-base disorders		
System	**Acidemia**	**Alkalemia**
Cardiovascular	• Impaired cardiac contractility • Arteriolar dilatation • Venoconstriction • Centralization of blood volume	• Arteriolar constriction • Reduced coronary blood flow • Reduced anginal threshold • Decreased threshold for cardiac arrhythmias
Metabolic	• Insulin resistance • Inhibition of anaerobic glycolysis • Hyperkalemia • Bone demineralization	• Stimulation of anaerobic glycolysis and decreased oxyhemoglobin dissociation • Decreased ionized Ca • Hypokalemia • Hypomagnesemia • Hypophosphatemia
Neurologic	• Inhibition of metabolism and cell-volume regulation • Obtundation and coma	• Tetany • Seizures • Delirium
Respiratory	Compensatory hyperventilation with possible respiratory muscle fatigue	Compensatory hypoventilation with hypercapnia and hypoxemia

Metabolic Acidosis

Metabolic acidosis is primary reduction in HCO_3^-, typically with compensatory reduction in pCO_2. Metabolic acidoses are categorized as high or normal anion gap based on the presence or absence of unmeasured anions in serum.

Causes of metabolic acidosis	
Cause	**Examples**
High anion gap	
Ketoacidosis	• Diabetes • Chronic alcoholism • Undernutrition • Fasting
Lactic acidosis (from physiologic processes)	• Shock • Primary hypoxia due to lung disorders • Seizures

Causes of metabolic acidosis	
Cause	**Examples**
Lactic acidosis (from exogenous toxins)	• Carbon monoxide • Cyanide • Iron • Isoniazid • Toluene (initially high gap; subsequent excretion of metabolites normalizes gap)
Renal failure	—
Toxins metabolized to acids	• Alcohol • Methanol • Ethylene glycol (oxalate) • Paraldehyde (acetate, chloracetate) • Salicylates
Rhabdomyolysis	—

Contd...

Causes of metabolic acidosis	
Cause	Examples
Normal anion gap (hyperchloremic acidosis)	
GI HCO_3^- loss	• Colostomy • Diarrhea • Enteric fistulas • Ileostomy • Use of ion-exchange resins
Urologic procedures	• Ureterosigmoidostomy • Ureteroileal conduit
Renal HCO_3^- loss	• Tubulointerstitial renal disease • Renal tubular acidosis, types 1, 2, and 4 • Hyperparathyroidism
Ingestions	• $CaCl_2$ • Mg sulfate ($MgSO_4$)
Parenteral infusion	• Arginine lysine • Ammonium chloride (NH_4Cl) • Rapid NaCl infusion
Other	• Hypoaldosteronism • Hyperkalemia • Toluene (late)

Symptoms and Signs

Symptoms and signs are primarily those of the cause. Mild acidemia is itself asymptomatic. More severe acidemia (pH < 7.10) may cause nausea, vomiting, and malaise. Symptoms may appear at higher pH, if acidosis develops rapidly. The most characteristic sign is hyperpnea (long, deep breaths at a normal rate), reflecting a compensatory increase in alveolar ventilation.

Severe, acute acidemia predisposes to cardiac dysfunction with hypotension and shock, ventricular arrhythmias; and coma. Chronic acidemia causes bone demineralization disorders (rickets, osteomalacia and osteopenia).

Diagnosis

1. ABG and serum electrolytes
2. Anion gap and delta gap calculated
3. Winter's formula for calculating compensatory changes
4. Testing for cause.

Blood testing should include glucose, BUN, creatinine, lactate, and tests for possible toxins. Salicylate methanol and ethylene glycol levels should be measured.

Calculated serum osmolarity (2 [Na] + [glucose]/18 + BUN/2.8 + blood alcohol/5) is subtracted from measured osmolarity. A difference >10 implies the presence of an osmotically active substance, which in the case of a high anion gap acidosis is methanol or ethylene glycol.

If the anion gap is normal and no cause is obvious (e.g., marked diarrhea), urinary electrolytes are measured and the urinary anion gap is calculated as [Na] + [K] − [Cl]. *A negative urinary anion gap indicates GIT cause, while positive urinary anion gap is seen with renal tubular acidoisis.*

Treatment

- Treat the cause.
- $NaHCO_3$ is rarely indicated.

Treatment is directed at the underlying cause. Hemodialysis is required for renal failure and sometimes for ethylene glycol, methanol, and salicylate poisoning.

The usual initial target is to increase bicarbonate to 10–12 mEq/L over 3–4 hours.

Subsequently the goal is to increase bicarbonate to 15 mEq/L over the next 24 hours. Once the pH is 7.2 – 7.25, serum HCO_3^- should not be increased to more than 4–8 mEq/dL over 6–12 hrs. This is to avoid risks of over alkalization like paradoxical CNS acidosis, sodium overload, tissue hypoxia. Replace only 50% over 3–4 hours and remainder over 24 hours.

Calculation of base deficit = $0.5 \times$ weight $\times$ [15 − serum HCO_3^-] (mEq/L)]

Example, calculate base deficit in a 75 kg man with pH = 6.96, pCO_2 = 30 mm Hg and HCO_3^- = 6 mEq/L.
Total base deficit = $[15 − 6] \times 75 \times 0.5 = 337$ mEq.
Second method of calculation of base deficit in MCQ section.

Lactic Acidosis

Lactate is a normal byproduct of glucose and amino acid metabolism.
- **Type A lactic acidosis** occurs due to tissue hypoxia when lactic acid is overproduced in ischemic tissue to generate ATP during O_2 deficit. This is the most serious form of lactic acidosis
  - *Tissue hypoperfusion:* Abnormal vascular tone or permeability, left ventricular failure, decreased cardiac output and hypovolemic, cardiac, or septic shock
  - *Reduced arterial oxygen content:* Asphyxia, primary hypoxia from lung disease, hypoxemia (PaO_2 <35 mm Hg), carbon monoxide poisoning and life-threatening anemia
- **Type B lactic acidosis** occurs in states of normal global tissue perfusion (and hence ATP production) and is less ominous. Lactate production may be increased from local relative hypoxia as with vigorous muscle use (e.g., exertion, seizures, hypothermic shivering) and with cancer and ingestion of certain drugs or toxins.
  - *B1 (common disorders):* Hepatic failure, Renal failure, diabetes mellitus, cancer, malaria and cholera
  - *B2 (drugs or toxins):* Biguanides, acetaminophen, ethanol, nalidixic acid, salicylates, isoniazid, methanol, streptozotocin, ethylene glycol, sorbitol, cyanide, parenteral nutrition, nitroprusside, lactulose, niacin, theophylline, catecholamines, cocaine, diethyl ether, vitamin deficiency, papaverine, paraldehyde
  - *B3 (other conditions):* Strenuous muscular exercise, grand-mal seizures.

D-lactic Acidosis

It is an *unusual form of lactic acidosis in which d-lactic acid, the product of bacterial carbohydrate metabolism in the colon of patients with jejunoileal bypass or intestinal resection, is systemically absorbed.* It persists in circulation because human lactate dehydrogenase can metabolize only l-lactate.

Metabolic Alkalosis

Metabolic alkalosis is primary increase in HCO_3^- with or without compensatory increase in pCO_2.

Causes of metabolic alkalosis	
Cause	Comments
GI acid loss	
Due to vomiting or nasogastric suction	Loss of HCl and acid coupled with contraction alkalosis from release of aldosterone and subsequent resorption of HCO_3^-
Congenital chloridorrhea	Fecal Cl loss and HCO_3^- retention
Villous adenoma	Probably secondary to K^+ depletion
Renal acid loss	
1° hyperaldosteronism	Conn syndrome, Congenital adrenal hyperplasia
2° hyperaldosteronism	Occurs with volume depletion, Heart failure, cirrhosis with ascites, nephrotic syndrome, Cushing's syndrome or disease, renal artery stenosis, renin-secreting tumor
Bartter syndrome	Disease of TAL in kidney causing hyperaldosteronism and hypokalemic metabolic alkalosis that manifests in early childhood with renal salt wasting and volume depletion
Gitelman's syndrome	Defect in DCT of kidney leading to same manifestation as Bartter syndrome. Additional features are hypomagnesemia and hypocalciuria
Diuretics (thiazide and loop)	Multiple mechanisms: secondary hyperaldosteronism due to volume depletion, or contraction alkalosis
Hypokalemia and hypomagnesemia	Low K^+ causes H^+ to shift into cells raising extracellular pH
HCO_3^- excess	
Fast breathing	Persistent elevation of compensatory HCO_3^- levels, often with volume, K^+ and Cl^- depletion
$NaHCO_3$ loading	Occurs with overzealous loading or loading in patients with hypokalemia; as H^+ shifts back into cells, the serum becomes more alkalotic
Milk-alkali syndrome	Chronic ingestion of Ca carbonate antacids provides Ca^{2+} and HCO_3^- load; hypercalcemia decreases and GFR prevents elimination of the excess HCO_3^- load
Contraction alkalosis	
Diuretics (all types) Sweat loss in cystic fibrosis	NaCl loss concentrates a fixed amount of HCO_3^- in a smaller total body volume
Others	
Carbohydrate refeeding after starvation	Resolution of starvation ketosis or acidosis with improved cellular function
Laxative abuse	Unclear mechanism
Some antibiotics (carbenicillin, penicillin, ticarcillin)	Contain nonabsorbable anion, which increases K^+ and H^+ excretion

Symptoms and Signs

Symptoms and signs of mild alkalemia are usually related to the underlying disorder. More severe alkalemia increases protein binding of ionized Ca^{++}, leading to hypocalcemia and subsequent headache, lethargy, and neuromuscular excitability, sometimes with delirium, tetany, and seizures. Alkalemia also lowers threshold for anginal symptoms and arrhythmias. Concomitant hypokalemia may cause weakness.

Diagnosis

1. ABG and serum electrolytes
2. Measurement of urinary Cl^- and K^+.

Treatment

- Treat the underlying cause
- IV 0.9% saline solution for Cl^--responsive metabolic alkalosis.

Respiratory Acidosis

Respiratory acidosis is CO_2 accumulation from a decrease in respiratory rate, respiratory volume (hypoventilation), or both with or without compensatory increase in HCO_3^-; pH is usually low but may be near normal. Cause is a decrease in respiratory rate, volume (hypoventilation), or both from CNS, pulmonary, or iatrogenic conditions. Respiratory acidosis can be acute or chronic; the chronic form is asymptomatic, but the acute, or worsening form causes headache, confusion, and drowsiness. Signs include tremor, myoclonic jerks, and asterixis.

Causes

1. Conditions that impair CNS respiratory drive
2. Conditions that impair neuromuscular transmission and other conditions that cause muscular weakness
3. Obstructive, restrictive, and parenchymal pulmonary disorders
Hypoxia typically accompanies hypoventilation.

Symptoms and Signs

Symptoms and signs are a result of high CNS CO_2 concentrations and any accompanying hypoxemia.

Acute (or acutely worsening chronic) respiratory acidosis causes headache, confusion, anxiety, drowsiness and stupor (CO_2 narcosis). Slowly developing, stable respiratory acidosis (as in COPD) may be well tolerated, but patients may have memory loss, sleep disturbances, excessive daytime sleepiness, and personality changes. Signs include gait disturbance, tremor, blunted deep tendon reflexes, myoclonic jerks, *asterixis* and papilledema.

Diagnosis

- ABG and serum electrolytes
- Diagnosis of cause: usually clinical.

Treatment

- Adequate ventilation will washout carbon dioxide
- $NaHCO_3$ almost always contraindicated (one exception may be

in cases of severe bronchospasm, in which HCO_3^- may improve responsiveness of bronchial smooth muscle to β-agonists).

Respiratory Alkalosis

Respiratory alkalosis is a primary decrease in pCO_2 with or without compensatory decrease in HCO_3^-; pH may be high or near normal. Cause is an increase in respiratory rate or volume (hyperventilation) or both. Respiratory alkalosis can be acute or chronic. The chronic form is asymptomatic, but the acute form causes light-headedness, confusion, paresthesias, cramps, and syncope.

Etiology

Respiratory alkalosis is a primary decrease in pCO_2 from an increase in respiratory rate or volume (hyperventilation), or both. Ventilation increase occurs most often as a physiologic response to hypoxia, metabolic acidosis, and increased metabolic demands (e.g., fever), and as such is present in many serious conditions. In addition, pain and anxiety and some CNS disorders can increase respiratory rate without a physiologic need.

Symptoms and Signs

Symptoms and signs depend on the rate and degree of fall in pCO_2. Acute respiratory alkalosis causes light-headedness, confusion, peripheral and circumoral paresthesias, cramps, and syncope. Mechanism is thought to be changed in cerebral blood flow and pH. Tachypnea or hyperpnea is often the only sign; *carpopedal spasm* may occur in severe cases. Chronic respiratory alkalosis is usually asymptomatic and has no distinctive signs.

Diagnosis

- ABG and serum electrolytes
- If hypoxia present, cause vigorously pursued.

Treatment

Treatment is directed at the underlying cause. Respiratory alkalosis is not life threatening, so no interventions to lower pH are necessary. *Increasing inspired CO_2 through rebreathing (such as from a paper bag) is common practice)* but may be dangerous in some patients with CNS disorders in whom CSF pH may already be below normal.

Image-Based Question

1. A child with villous adenoma complains of muscle cramps. The given ECG shows which electrolyte abnormality?

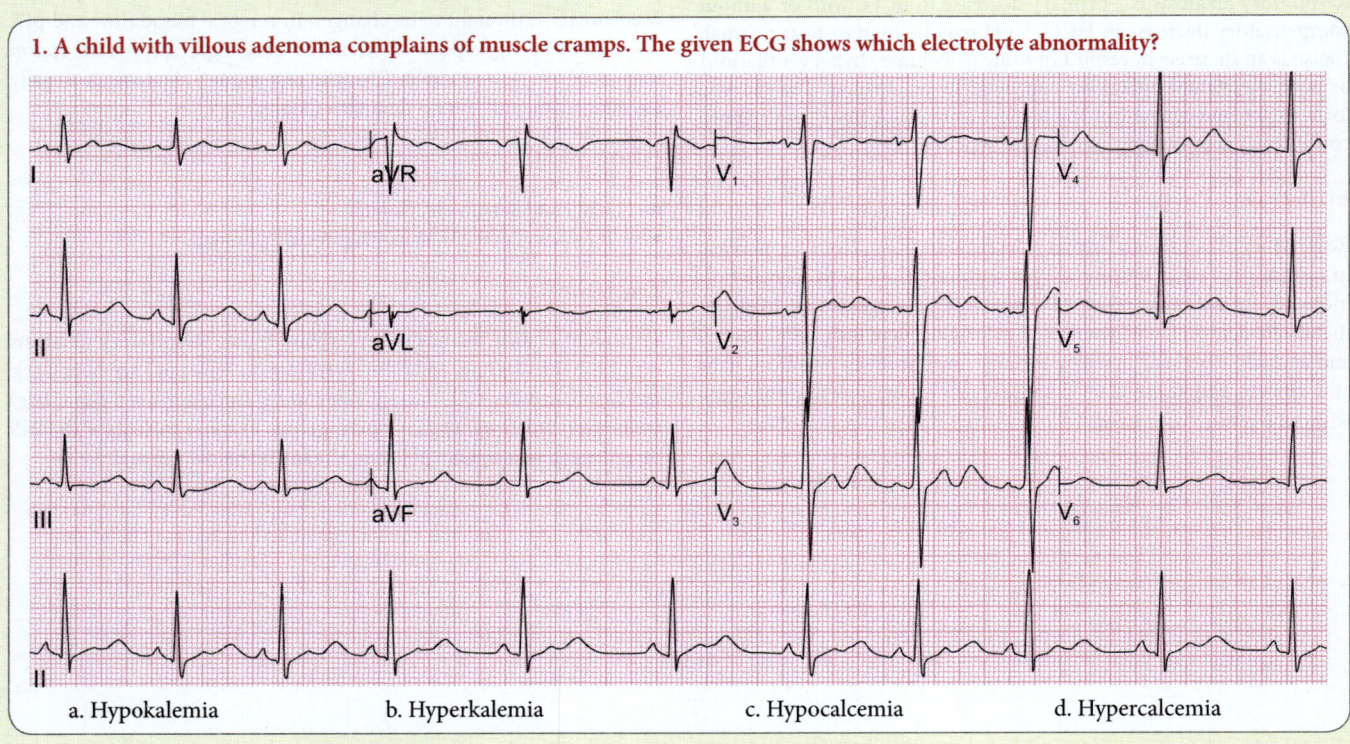

a. Hypokalemia b. Hyperkalemia c. Hypocalcemia d. Hypercalcemia

Answer of Image-Based Question

1. Ans. (a) **Hypokalemia**
   The ECG shows presence of U waves (see the long lead II at inferior most strip) where they are merging with T wave.

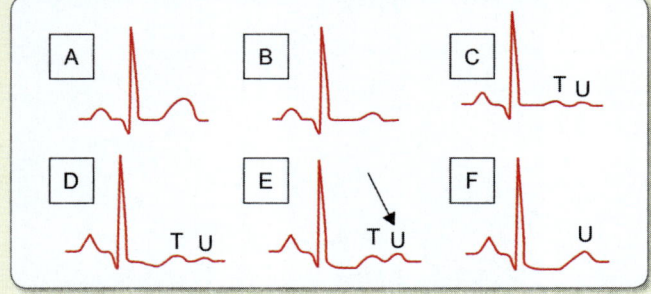

Conceptual Diagnostic Algorithm

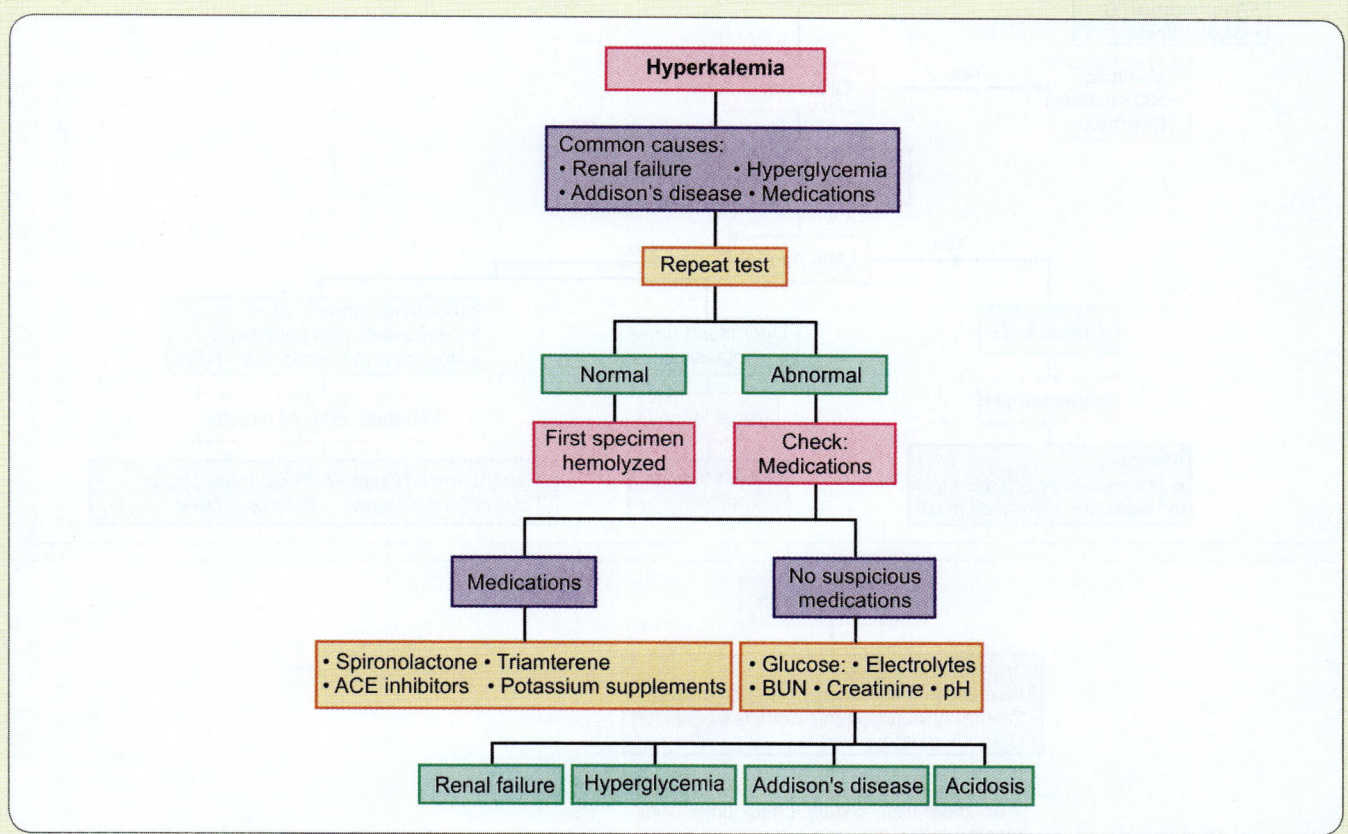

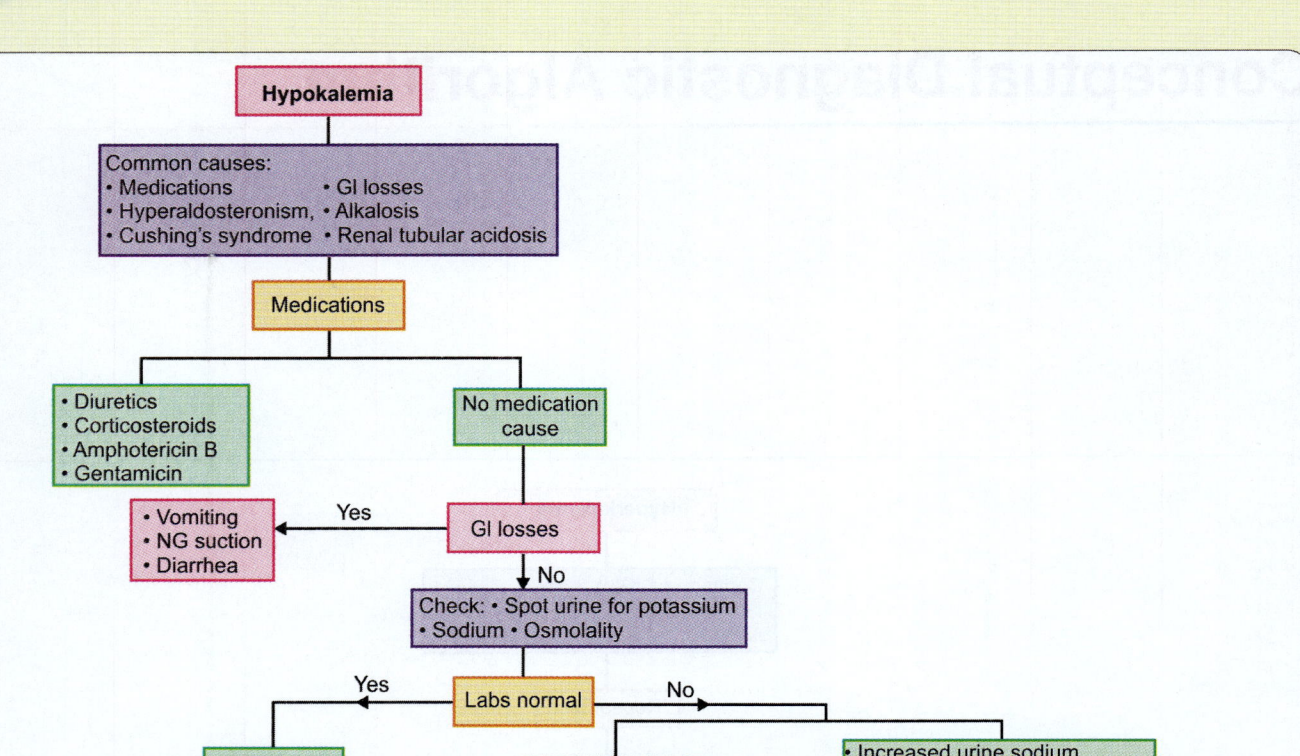

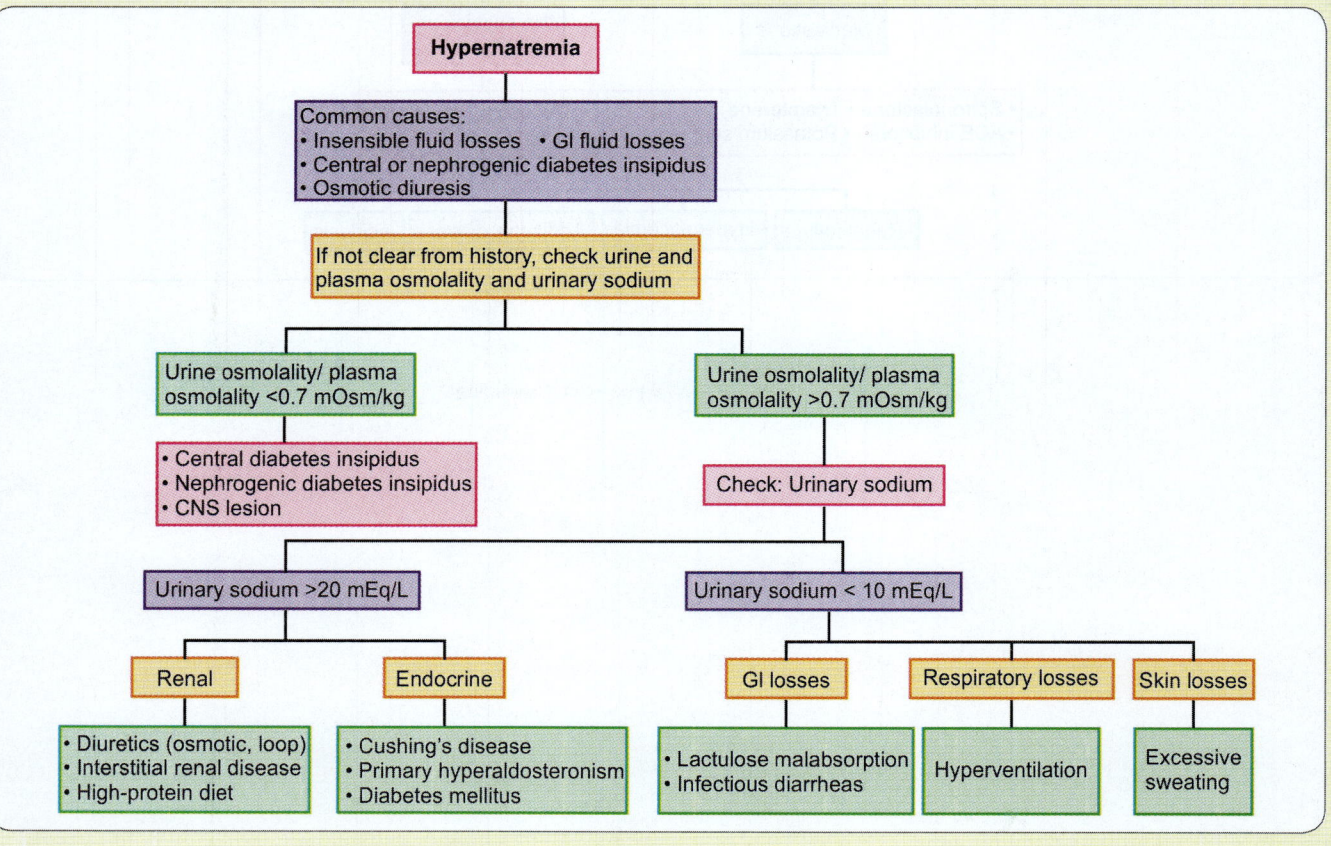

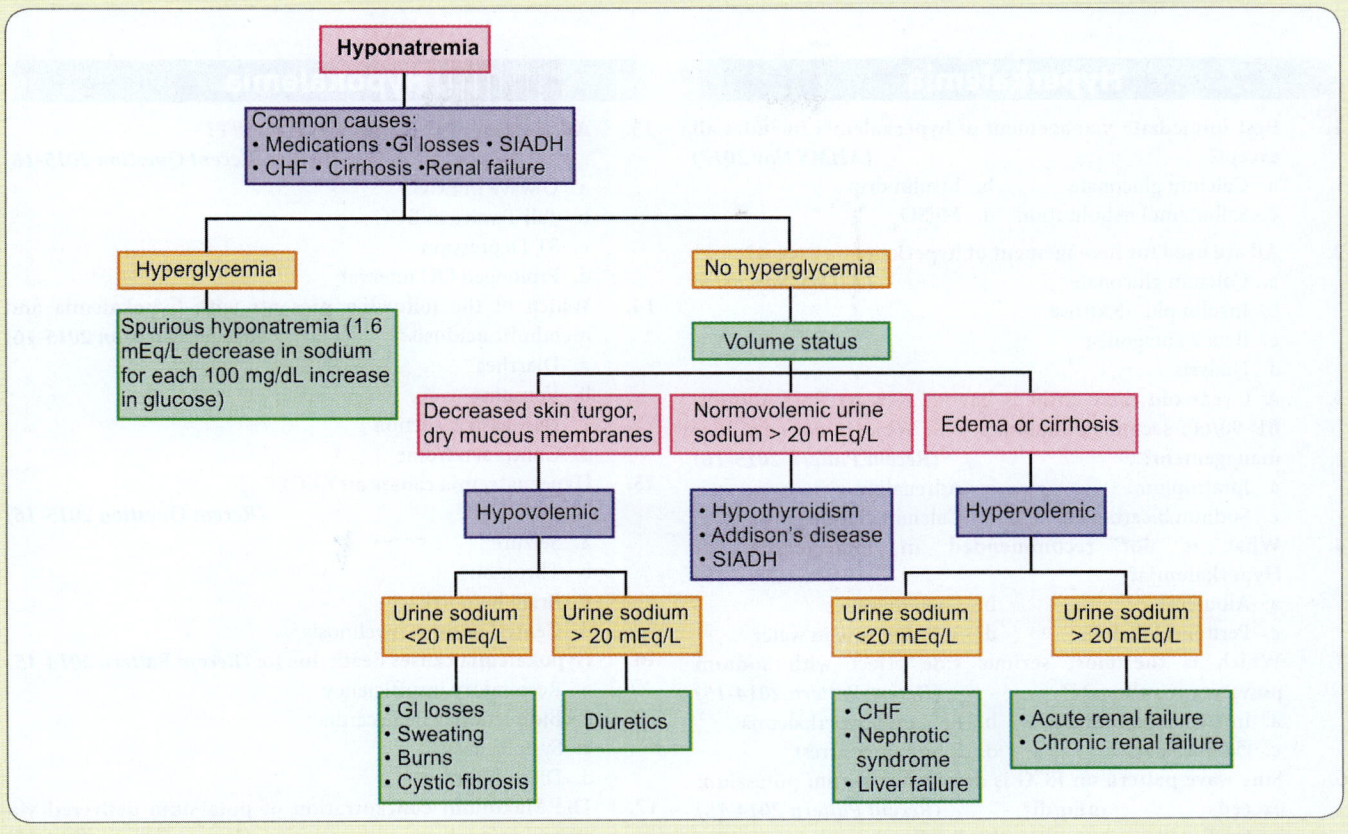

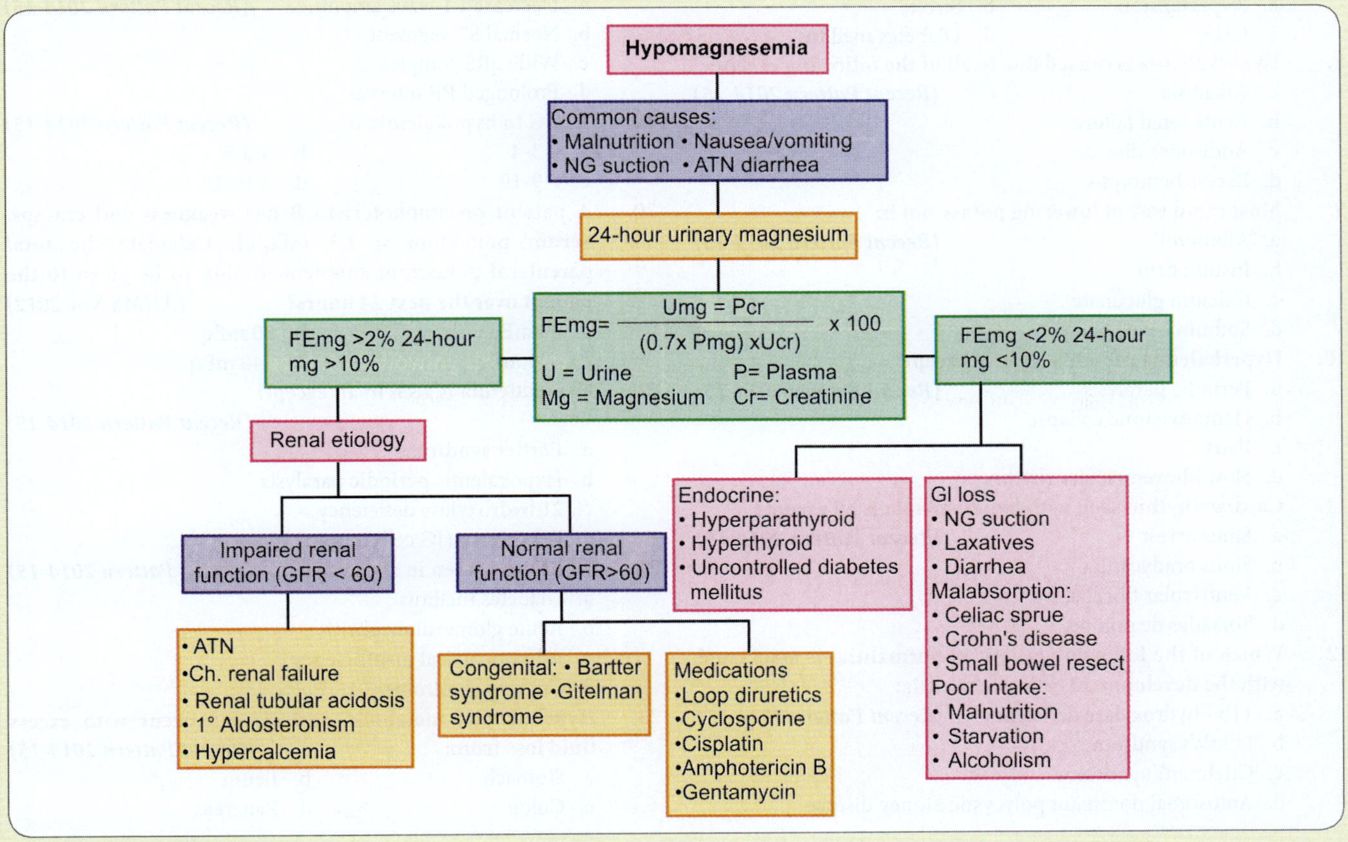

Multiple Choice Questions

Hyperkalemia

1. **Best immediate management of hyperkalemia includes all except?** *(AIIMS Nov 2017)*
   a. Calcium gluconate b. Insulin drip
   c. Salbutamol nebulization d. $MgSO_4$

2. **All are used for management of hyperkalemia except?**
   a. Calcium gluconate *(AIIMS Nov 2014)*
   b. Insulin plus dextrose
   c. Beta 2 antagonist
   d. Dialysis

3. **A 1 year old male child is having a Heart Rate 40/min, BP 90/60, serum Potassium = 6.5. What is the next best management?** *(Recent Pattern 2015-16)*
   a. Ipratropium b. Adrenaline
   c. Sodium bicarbonate d. Calcium chloride

4. **What is not recommended in management of Hyperkalemia?** *(PGI 2014-15)*
   a. Albuterol b. Loop diuretics
   c. Peritoneal dialysis d. 50% dextrose in water

5. **Which is the most serious side effect with sodium polystyrene sulfonate?** *(Recent Pattern 2014-15)*
   a. Intestinal perforation b. Rebound hyperkalemia
   c. Cardiac arrest d. Respiratory arrest

6. **Sine wave pattern on ECG is done when serum potassium exceeds_____ mEq/dl?** *(Recent Pattern 2014-15)*
   a. 6 mEq/dl b. 7 mEq/dl
   c. 8 mEq/dl d. 10 mEq>dl

7. **Decreased dietary intake of potassium is incriminated in leading to all except?** *(Recent Pattern 2014-15)*
   a. Hypertension b. Stroke
   c. CHF d. Diabetes mellitus

8. **Hyperkalemia is caused due to all of the following except:**
   a. Alkalosis *(Recent Pattern 2014-15)*
   b. Acute renal failure
   c. Addisons's disease
   d. Excess hemolysis

9. **Most rapid way of lowering potassium is:**
   a. Albuterol *(Recent Pattern 2014-15)*
   b. Insulin drip
   c. Calcium gluconate
   d. Sodium bicarbonate

10. **Hyperkalemia presents with all except?**
    a. Periodic paralysis *(Recent Pattern 2014-15)*
    b. Hemodynamic collapse
    c. Ileus
    d. Slow idioventricular rhythms

11. **Cardiac rhythm seen with hyperkalemia is all except?**
    a. Sinus arrest *(Recent Pattern 2014-15)*
    b. Sinus bradycardia
    c. Ventricular fibrillation
    d. Torsades de pointes

12. **Which of the following genetic abnormalities is associated with the development of hyperkalemia:**
    a. 11b - hydroxylase deficiency *(Recent Pattern 2014-15)*
    b. Liddle's syndrome
    c. Gitelman's syndrome
    d. Autosomal dominant polycystic kidney disease

Hypokalemia

13. **All are seen in Hypokalemia EXCEPT?** *(Recent Question 2015-16)*
    a. U wave in ECG
    b. Tall T wave in ECG
    c. ST Depression
    d. Prolonged QU interval

14. **Which of the following presents with hypokalemia and metabolic acidosis?** *(Recent Question 2015-16)*
    a. Diarrhea
    b. Vomiting
    c. Nasogastric suction
    d. Conn's syndrome

15. **Hypernatremia causes all EXCEPT:** *(Recent Question 2015-16)*
    a. Seizure
    b. Thrombus
    c. Brain hemorrhage
    d. Central pontine myelinosis

16. **Hypokalemia causes death due to:** *(Recent Pattern 2014-15)*
    a. Respiratory insufficiency
    b. Bidirectional Tachycardia
    c. Systolic arrest
    d. Diastolic arrest

17. **The Maximum concentration of potassium delivered via central vein is?** *(Recent Pattern 2014-15)*
    a. 20 mmol/L b. 40 mmol/L
    c. 60 mmol/L d. 100 mmol/L

18. **In hypokalemia all ECG changes are seen except:**
    a. Decreased T wave amplitude *(Recent Pattern 2014-15)*
    b. Normal ST segment
    c. Wide qRS complex
    d. Prolonged PR interval

19. **TTKG in hypokalemia is:** *(Recent Pattern 2014-15)*
    a. < 3-4 b. > 6-7
    c. > 9-10 d. > 10-15

20. **A patient on amphotericin B has weakness and cramps. Serum potassium = 2.3 mEq/dl. Calculate the total parenteral potassium supplementation to be given to the patient over the next 24 hours?** *(AIIMS Nov 2012)*
    a. 40 mEq b. 80 mEq
    c. 100 mEq d. 140 mEq

21. **Hypokalemia is seen in all except?** *(Recent Pattern 2014-15)*
    a. Bartter syndrome
    b. Hypokalemic periodic paralysis
    c. 21 hydroxylase deficiency
    d. Reninoma (JG cell tumour)

22. **TTKG >8 is seen in all except:** *(Recent Pattern 2014-15)*
    a. Diabetes mellitus
    b. Acute glomerulonephritis
    c. Adrenocortical insufficiency
    d. Cushing syndrome

23. **Hypokalemic, metabolic acidosis can occur with excess fluid loss from:** *(Recent Pattern 2014-15)*
    a. Stomach b. Ileum
    c. Colon d. Pancreas

Hyponatremia

24. Hypertonic hyponatremia is seen in? *(JIPMER May 2018)*
    a. CRF
    b. Mannitol
    c. Thiazide diuretics
    d. Vomiting

25. An alcoholic developed intractable vomiting for 2 days with loose motions. Since he had decreased food intake and altered sensorium, he was brought to the hospital, where the fluid loss and dyselectrolytemia was aggressively corrected with fluid infusion. Post treatment, the patient started having quadriplegia and mutism. What is the diagnosis?
    a. Osmotic demyelination syndrome *(AIIMS May 2018)*
    b. Syndrome of inappropriate ADH production
    c. Brain stem infarct
    d. Acute disseminated encephalomyelitis

26. Consider the following statements and choose the correct answer.
    Statement 1: Fluid restriction and not medication is the best for management of asymptomatic hyponatremia with serum Sodium less than 120 mEq/L, in patients of cirrhosis with oedema
    Statement 2: Conivaptan decreases B.P. and increases risk of variceal bleeding and so relatively contraindicated in cirrhotics with hyponatremia. *(AP PG 2016)*
    a. Statement 1 is wrong and Statement 2 is correct
    b. Both Statements 1 & 2 are correct
    c. Both Statements 1 & 2 are wrong
    d. Statement 1 is correct and Statement 2 is wrong

27. Poorly controlled diabetes with blood sugar of 450 mg% is associated with: *(Recent Pattern 2014-15)*
    a. Hyponatremia
    b. Hypernatremia
    c. Hypokalemia
    d. Hypomagnesemia

28. What is the of correction of sodium deficit? *(Recent Pattern 2014-15)*
    a. 0.5 mmol/hour
    b. 1 mmol/hour
    c. 1.5 mmol/hour
    d. 2.0 mmol/hour

29. Most common electrolyte abnormality in hospitalised patient? *(Recent Pattern 2014-15)*
    a. Hyponatremia
    b. Hypernatremia
    c. Hypokalemia
    d. Hyperkalemia

30. Maximum loss of sodium in a child occurs in: *(Recent Pattern 2014-15)*
    a. Gastric juice
    b. Ileal fluid
    c. Non cholera Diarrhoea
    d. Cholera

31. Acute hyponatremia becomes symptomatic at: *(Recent Pattern 2014-15)*
    a. <135 mEq
    b. <125 mEq
    c. <120 mEq
    d. <110 mEq

32. Hyponatremia is seen in: *(Recent Pattern 2014-15)*
    a. Hyperthyroidism
    b. Hypothyroidism
    c. Diabetes insipidus
    d. Increased insensible losses

33. Incorrect about cerebral salt wasting syndrome?
    a. Urine sodium >20 mEq/dl *(Recent Pattern 2014-15)*
    b. Hyponatremia
    c. Fludrocortisone is used
    d. Expansion of plasma volume

34. A 70 kg adult male presents with serum sodium of 110 mEq/dl. Calculate correction required in 24 hours?
    a. 100 mEq *(Recent Pattern 2014-15)*
    b. 200 mEq
    c. 300 mEq
    d. 400 mEq

35. Which one of the following is the major determinant of plasma osmolality: *(Recent Pattern 2014-15)*
    a. Serum sodium
    b. Serum potassium
    c. Serum Creatinine
    d. Blood urea nitrogen

36. Which of the following leads to hyponatremia and low osmolality: *(Recent Pattern 2014-15)*
    a. Hyperlipedemia
    b. Hyperproteinemia
    c. IVIG therapy
    d. CHF

37. Pseudohyponatremia is seen in? *(Recent Pattern 2014-15)*
    a. Hyperlipidemia
    b. SIADH
    c. CHF
    d. CKD

38. Correct about osmotic demyelination syndrome? *(Recent Pattern 2014-15)*
    a. More common with acute hyponatremia
    b. Characterised by focal seizures
    c. Seen due to slow correction of hyponatremia
    d. Lesions occur in pontine and extrapontine areas

39. Neonate is posted for Congenital Hypertrophic Pyloric Stenosis, Pre-op work up shows serum calcium = 6 mg%. What should be done next? *(Recent Pattern 2014-15)*
    a. Serum protein
    b. Oxygen saturation
    c. USG abdomen
    d. Serum bilirubin

40. All are included in diagnostic criteria for SIADH in children except? *(Recent Pattern 2014-15)*
    a. Normal creatinine clearance
    b. Urine osmolality > 100 mEq/dl
    c. Serum osmolality < 280 mOsm
    d. Urine sodium < 25 mEq/dl

41. A 30 years old HIV positive man is admitted with confusion. Physical examination shows a blood pressure of 140/70 with no orthostasis, normal jugular venous pressure, and no edema. Serum chemistries are notable for sodium 120 mmol/L, K+ = 4.2 mmol/L, bicarbonate = 24 mmol/L, and uric acid 1.5 mg/dL. The most likely diagnosis is:
    a. Hepatic cirrhosis *(Recent Pattern 2014-15)*
    b. Cerebral toxoplasmosis with SIADH
    c. Addison's disease
    d. Significant gastrointestinal fluid loss

42. Which one of the following statements about electrolytes in colon is correct: *(Recent Pattern 2014-15)*
    a. Absorption of Na+ in the colon is under hormonal (aldosterone) control
    b. Bile acids enhance absorption of water from the colon
    c. Net absorption of HCO_3^- occurs in the colon
    d. Net absorption of K+ occurs in the colon

Hypernatremia

43. All are used for management for hypernatremia except? *(Recent Pattern 2014-15)*
    a. 5% dextrose in water
    b. N/2 in 5% dextrose
    c. Nil by mouth
    d. Indomethacin

44. **Most common cause of hypernatremia?**
    (Recent Pattern 2014-15)
    a. Primary hypodipsia   b. Carcinoid syndrome
    c. Renal losses   d. Sweating
45. **Doughy skin and woody induration of tongue is seen in?**
    (Recent Pattern 2014-15)
    a. Hypernatremia   b. Hyponatremia
    c. Hypokalemia   d. Hyperkalemia
46. **All are features of hypernatremia except?**
    a. Convulsions   *(Recent Pattern 2014-15)*
    b. Elevated intracranial tension
    c. Periodic paralysis
    d. Doughy skin
47. **Hypernatremia causes all EXCEPT:**
    (Recent Pattern 2014-15)
    a. Seizure   b. Paralysis
    c. Brain hemorrhage d. Cerebral edema
48. **Not a cause of hypernatremia:** *(Recent Pattern 2014-15)*
    a. Primary hypodipsia
    b. Decreased insensible losses
    c. Nephrogenic diabetes insipidus
    d. Carcinoid syndrome
49. **Calculate water deficit for 50 kg male with Na = 160 mEq:**
    a. 2.9 L hypertonic saline *(Recent Pattern 2014-15)*
    b. 2.9L half normal saline
    c. 1.5 L 5% dextrose in water
    d. 1.5 L 10% dextrose in water
50. **Brain tumour causing hypernatremia in children?**
    a. Medulloblastoma *(Recent Pattern 2014-15)*
    b. Cerebellar astrocytoma
    c. Craniopharyngioma
    d. Brain stem glioma
51. **Tolvaptan is useful for?**   *(Recent Pattern 2014-15)*
    a. Hyponatremia
    b. Hypernatremia
    c. Nephrogenic diabetes insipidus
    d. Decreased water clearance

Disorders of Calcium Metabolism

52. **Chvostek's sign is elicited by:**   *(Recent Question 2015-16)*
    a. Facial nerve stimulation by tapping over the parotid
    b. BP cuff in arm for 5 minutes
    c. Tapping over extensor pollicis brevis
    d. Tapping over flexor retinaculum
53. **Fever increases water losses by _____ ml/day per degree Celsius:**   *(Recent Pattern 2014-15)*
    a. 100   b. 200
    c. 400   d. 800
54. **Prolonged immobilization leads to?**
    (Recent Pattern 2014-15)
    a. Hypercalcemia   b. Hypocalcemia
    c. Hyperkalemia   d. Hypokalemia
55. **Tetany may be a feature of the following except:**
    a. Hyperventilation   *(Recent Pattern 2014-15)*
    b. Hypokalaemic alkalosis
    c. Thyroid surgery
    d. Hyponatremia
56. **Not useful for acute Hypercalcemia?**
    (Recent Pattern 2014-15)
    a. Normal saline   b. Calcitonin
    c. Thiazide   d. Bisphosphonates
57. **Incorrect about hypocalcemia:**   *(Recent Pattern 2014-15)*
    a. Shortening of QT interval
    b. Seizures
    c. Larygospasm
    d. Di George syndrome
58. **Why is tetany seen with hyperventilation:**
    a. Metabolic alkalosis   *(Recent Pattern 2014-15)*
    b. Respiratory alkalosis
    c. Metabolic acidosis
    d. Respiratory acidosis
59. **Tumor induced osteomalacia is caused due to?**
    (Recent Pattern 2014-15)
    a. FGF-23   b. PTH
    c. Calcitonin d. All of above

Disorders of Magnesium Metabolism

60. **All are features of hypermagnesemia except?**
    (Recent Pattern 2014-15)
    a. Hypotension   b. Ileus
    c. Tetany   d. Decreased DTR
61. **Heart block is seen in:**   *(Recent Pattern 2014-15)*
    a. Hypermagnesemia   b. Hyperphosphatemia
    c. Both   d. None
62. **Not a cause of Hypomagnesemia:**   *(Recent Pattern 2014-15)*
    a. Gitelman syndrome   b. Re-feeding syndrome
    c. Hyperaldosteronism d. Rhabdomyolysis
63. **All are indicators of hypermagnesemia except?**
    (Recent Pattern 2014-15)
    a. Decreased DTR   b. Decreased BP
    c. Heart block   d. 'Main d'accoucheur'
64. **Not seen in Hypermagnesemia:**   *(Recent Pattern 2014-15)*
    a. Bradycardia
    b. QT prolongation
    c. Dilated pupils
    d. T wave inversion
65. **Percentage of magnesium absorbed in TAL?**
    (Recent Pattern 2014-15)
    a. 20%   b. 40%
    c. 60%   d. 80%
66. **All are useful for management of Hypermagnesemia except?**   *(Recent Pattern 2014-15)*
    a. Magnesium free enema   b. IVF
    c. Calcium gluconate   d. Amiloride
67. **Incorrect about Hypomagnesemia?**
    a. Tetany   *(Recent Pattern 2014-15)*
    b. Causes resistance to PTH
    c. Arrhythmia
    d. Intramuscular magnesium sulphate
68. **Heart block is seen in:**   *(Recent Pattern 2014-15)*
    a. Hypermagensemia
    b. Hypomagnesemia
    c. Hypernatremia
    d. Hypocalcemia

Acidosis and Alkalosis

69. A patient has pH = 7.21, HCO_3 = 28mEq and pCO_2 = 50 mm Hg. What is the acid base disorder in this patient?
    (AIIMS May 2018)
    a. Metabolic acidosis with respiratory compensation
    b. Metabolic alkalosis with respiratory compensation
    c. Respiratory acidosis with renal compensation
    d. Respiratory alkalosis with renal compensation

70. A patient of Chronic Kidney disease is having protracted vomiting. ABG report is pH = 7.4, pCO_2 = 40 mm Hg, HCO_3 = 25 mEq, Na = 145 mEq and Chloride s 100 mEq. Diagnosis is? *(AIIMS Nov 2018)*
    a. Normal anion gap metabolic acidosis
    b. High anion gap metabolic acidosis
    c. No acid base abnormality
    d. High anion gap metabolic acidosis and metabolic alkalosis

71. Which of the following is not done before ABG?
    a. Allen test *(AIIMS Nov 2018)*
    b. Heparin to rinse the syringe
    c. Flexion of wrist
    d. Poking the artery at 45 degrees angle

72. Interpret the following ABG values: $PaCO_2$ – 50, HCO_3 – 27, pH – 7.2: *(JIPMER May 2018)*
    a. Uncompensated metabolic alkalosis
    b. Mixed respiratory and metabolic acidosis
    c. Combined respiratory and metabolic acidosis
    d. Compensated respiratory acidosis

73. Interpret the following ABG values: $PaCO_2$ – 40, HCO_3 – 55 mEq/L and pH – 7.7. *(JIPMER May 2018)*
    a. Uncompensated metabolic alkalosis
    b. Mixed respiratory and metabolic acidosis
    c. Combined respiratory and metabolic acidosis
    d. Compensated respiratory alkalosis

74. Interpret the following ABG values: $PaCO_2$ – 65, HCO_3 -15 mEq/L and pH – 7.21. *(JIPMER May 2018)*
    a. Uncompensated metabolic alkalosis
    b. Mixed respiratory and metabolic acidosis
    c. Combined respiratory and metabolic acidosis
    d. Compensated respiratory acidosis

75. 25-year-old construction is admitted with severe breathlessness. He is drowsy and speaks in monosyllables. SaO_2 is 90% on 15 L high flow mask and salbutamol nebulization. ABG is done. Which of the following is of most concern in ABG report of this patient?
    (Recent Question 2019)
    a. Raised Lactate   b. Low bicarbonate
    c. Low pH   d. Positive base excess

76. A 40 year old man comes with complaints of vomiting for last 3 days. ABG report shows a pH = 7.22, pCO_2 = 21 mmHg and HCO_3 = 9 mEq/dl. Diagnosis is? *(AIIMS Nov 2016)*
    a. Mixed metabolic acidosis and respiratory alkalosis
    b. Metabolic acidosis
    c. Respiratory alkalosis
    d. Mixed respiratory acidosis and metabolic alkalosis

77. A 75 kg man has an ABG report of pH= 6.96, pCO_2 = 30 mm Hg and pO_2 = 90 mmHg and HCO_3 = 6 mEq/dl. Calculate the immediate HCO_3 deficit to be corrected in the individual?
    a. 200 mEq   b. 300 mEq *(AIIMS Nov 2016)*
    c. 400 mEq   d. 500 mEq

78. All are true about performing an ABG except?
    a. Radial artery is the preferred site *(AIIMS May 2016)*
    b. Syringe is filled with 0.3 ml heparin prior to drawing blood
    c. Normal levels of HCO_3, pCO_2 and pH does not exclude acid base disturbance
    d. Different site is chosen if Modified Allen's test is positive on the side

79. ABG report shows pH= 7.30 and pCO_2 = 35 mmHg. Diagnosis is? *(AIIMS May 2016)*
    a. Metabolic acidosis   b. Metabolic alkalosis
    c. Respiratory acidosis   d. Respiratory alkalosis

80. ABG of a patient shows decreased pH, increased pCO_2 and high bicarbonate. Diagnosis: *(JIPMER May 2015)*
    a. Respiratory alkalosis, compensated
    b. Respiratory acidosis, compensated
    c. Respiratory acidosis not fully compensated
    d. Metabolic alkalosis, uncompensated

81. Which metabolic derangement is seen in pregnancy?
    (Recent Pattern 2015-16)
    a. Metabolic acidosis   b. Metabolic alkalosis
    c. Respiratory acidosis   d. Respiratory alkalosis

82. Type B lactic acidosis occurs due to?
    (Recent Pattern 2014-15)
    a. CHF   b. Cyanide poisoning
    c. Short gut syndrome   d. Diabetes mellitus

83. Fomepizole is used for: *(Recent Pattern 2014-15)*
    a. Ethylene glycol poisoning b. Ethyl alcohol poisoning
    c. Ether poisoning   d. Type A Lactic acidosis

84. pH = 7.31 pCO_2 = 33 mm Hg and HCO_3 = 16 mEq/dl:
    (Recent Pattern 2014-15)
    a. Metabolic acidosis   b. Metabolic alkalosis
    c. Respiratory acidosis   d. Respiratory alkalosis

85. pH = 7.55, pCO_2 = 38, HCO_3 = 33, what is the primary abnormality: *(Recent Pattern 2014-15)*
    a. Metabolic acidosis   b. Metabolic alkalosis
    c. Respiratory acidosis   d. Respiratory alkalosis

86. Hyperchloremic metabolic acidosis is seen in all except?
    a. RTA 1 *(Recent Pattern 2014-15)*
    b. Diarrhea
    c. Uraemia
    d. Gitelman syndrome

87. Best for management of respiratory alkalosis?
    a. Rebreathing in paper bag *(Recent Pattern 2014-15)*
    b. IPPV
    c. Normal saline
    d. Acetazolamide

88. A 70 year old man with history of CHF presents with increased shortness of breath and leg swelling. ABG: pH 7.24, pCO_2 = 60 mmHg, PO_2 = 52, HCO_3^- = 27
    a. Metabolic acidosis *(Recent Pattern 2014-15)*
    b. Metabolic alkalosis
    c. Respiratory acidosis
    d. Respiratory alkalosis

89. A plasma HCO_3^- concentration of 15 mEq/L and a plasma pCO_2 of 30 mmHg with a pH of 7.5 represents:
    a. Simple metabolic acidosis *(Recent Pattern 2014-15)*
    b. Compensated metabolic acidosis
    c. Simple respiratory alkalosis
    d. Compensated respiratory alkalosis

90. pH = 7.30, pCO₂ = 38, HCO₃ = 18:
    (Recent Pattern 2014-15)
    a. Metabolic acidosis with compensatory respiratory alkalosis
    b. Respiratory acidosis with compensatory metabolic alkalosis
    c. Respiratory alkalosis with compensatory metabolic acidosis
    d. Metabolic acidosis with respiratory acidosis

91. **All are useful for treatment of metabolic alkalosis except**
    a. Sodium chloride   *(Recent Pattern 2014-15)*
    b. Potassium chloride
    c. Hydrochloric acid
    d. Ammonium chloride

92. **Most common acid base disturbance in critically ill patients?**   *(Recent Pattern 2014-15)*
    a. Chronic respiratory alkalosis
    b. Chronic respiratory acidosis
    c. Metabolic acidosis
    d. Metabolic alkalosis

93. **pH = 7.46, pCO₂ = 57 mm Hg and HCO₃ = 42 mEq:**
    (Recent Pattern 2014-15)
    a. Metabolic alkalosis with compensatory respiratory acidosis
    b. Metabolic acidosis with compensatory respiratory alkalosis
    c. Respiratory acidosis with compensatory metabolic alkalosis
    d. Respiratory alkalosis with compensatory metabolic acidosis

94. **29 year old female with history of Sjogren's syndrome presents with a 2 day episode of watery diarrhea 2 days ago. Physical examination is unremarkable. Because of her history, the physician decides to check her urine electrolytes. Urine chemistry:**
    K = 31, Na = 100, Cl = 105. Her current diagnosis is?
    a. Renal tubular acidosis   *(Recent Pattern 2014-15)*
    b. Hypochloremic Metabolic alkalosis
    c. Malignant hypertension
    d. Respiratory alkalosis

95. **pH = 7.27, HCO₃⁻ = 10 mEq/dl pCO₂ = 23 mm Hg:**
    a. Metabolic acidosis   *(Recent Pattern 2014-15)*
    b. Metabolic alkalosis
    c. Respiratory acidosis
    d. Respiratory alkalosis

96. **In metabolic acidosis caused by diabetic ketoacidosis, which of the following would be greater than normal:**
    (Recent Pattern 2014-15)
    a. Concentration of plasma HCO₃⁻
    b. Anion gap
    c. Arterial pCO₂
    d. All of the above

97. **A patient presents with following parameters pH 7.5, pCO₂ 30 mmHg, pO₂ 102 mmHg and HCO₃ 16 mEq/l. Which of the following correctly describes the compensatory mechanism:**   *(AI 2010)*
    a. Respiratory Alkalosis
    b. Metabolic Alkalosis
    c. Respiratory Acidosis
    d. Metabolic Acidosis

Anion gap

98. **All of the following are causes of metabolic acidosis with normal anion Gap except:**   *(AIIMS Nov 2017)*
    a. Proximal renal tubular acidosis
    b. Salicylate poisoning
    c. Diarrhea
    d. Pancreatitis

99. **A normal anion gap metabolic acidosis is seen in?**
    a. Methanol poisoning   b. Salicylate poisoning
    c. Diarrhea   d. Diabetic ketoacidosis

100. **Normal anion gap is seen in:**   *(Recent Question 2015-16)*
     a. Diabetic ketoacidosis   b. Chronic renal failure
     c. Renal tubular acidosis   d. Methanol toxicity

101. **Normal anion gap is seen in:**   *(Recent Question 2015-16)*
     a. Diabetic ketoacidosis   b. Lactic acidosis
     c. Starvation ketoacidosis   d. Renal tubular acidosis

102. **Widened anion gap is caused by all EXCEPT :**
     a. Lactic acidosis   b. Diarrhea
     c. Diabetic keto-acidosis   d. Methanol poisoning

103. **All are causes of increased anion gap except?**
     (Recent Pattern 2014-15)
     a. Diabetic ketoacidosis   b. Renal tubular acidosis
     c. Diabetic nephropathy   d. Starvation

104. **Reduced anion gap is seen in?**   *(Recent Pattern 2014-15)*
     a. Nephrotic syndrome
     b. Fistula
     c. Fanconi syndrome
     d. Renal tubular acidosis Type 4

105. **Increased anion gap is seen in all except?**
     a. Fistula   *(Recent Pattern 2014-15)*
     b. Starvation
     c. Ethylene glycol poisoning
     d. Phenformin

106. **Metabolic acidosis with a normal anion gap is found in a patient with:**   *(Recent Pattern 2014-15)*
     a. Alcohol intoxication   b. Aspirin ingestion
     c. Shock   d. Small bowel fistula

107. **Urinary anion gap is increased in:** *(Recent Pattern 2014-15)*
     a. Diarrhea   b. Renal tubular acidosis
     c. Ureterosigmoidostomy   d. Water intoxication

Disorders of Phosphate Metabolism

108. **A 60 year man presents to the emergency department in shock. Vasopressors are initiated@10 mcg/Kg/min. Patient weighs 80 kg and you take 2 vials of drug each containing 200 mg and dilute it in 250 ml of normal saline. The standard is 16 drops/ml. In that case what will be the drop rate to give the desired concentration of the drug?**   *(AIIMS Nov 2016)*
     a. 8   b. 12
     c. 16   d. 24

109. **Calculate plasma osmolality with Na = 141 mEq and K = 4 mEq and blood glucose of 18 mmol/L and urea of 10 mmol/L.**   *(JIPMER Nov 2015)*
     a. 310 mosm   b. 320 mosm
     c. 330 mosm   d. 340 mosm

110. **Blast crisis leads to:** *(Recent Pattern 2014-15)*
    a. Hyperphosphatemia
    b. Hypophosphatemia
    c. Hyperkalemia
    d. Hypokalemia

111. **Hyperphosphatemia is treated by?**
    (Recent Pattern 2014-15)
    a. Calcitonin
    b. Sevelamer
    c. Magnesium hydroxide
    d. Diuretics

112. **Hypophosphatemia is seen in:** *(Recent Pattern 2014-15)*
    a. Blast crisis
    b. Tumor lysis syndrome
    c. Addisonian crisis
    d. Myxedema coma

Miscellaneous

113. **In a patient who was brought to casualty after RTA with pulse rate 108, SBP 80. Which fluid is to be given ideally?**
    (Recent Question 2015-16)
    a. Plasma
    b. Normal Saline
    c. Blood
    d. 5% dextrose

114. **Which can be given in hemorrhagic stroke?**
    (Recent Question 2015-16)
    a. Packed RBC
    b. Colloids
    c. Blood transfusion
    d. Hypertonic fluids

115. **Man working in hot environment & drinking lots of water without intake of salts is liable to develop?**
    (Recent Question 2015-16)
    a. Heat hyperpyrexia
    b. Heat cramps
    c. Heat stroke
    d. Heat encephalopathy

116. **After Road traffic accident a patient presented to casualty with vitals showing BP of 90/60 mm Hg with heart of 56 bpm. Which kind of shock occurs?**
    (Recent Question 2015-16)
    a. Cardiogenic
    b. Neurogenic
    c. Distributive
    d. Hypovolemic shock

117. **Jansen disease is?** *(Recent Pattern 2014-15)*
    a. Defect of PTH receptor
    b. Defect of GH receptor
    c. Defect of GHRH receptor
    d. Defect of ADH receptor

118. **Insensible losses of water per day are:**
    (Recent Pattern 2014-15)
    a. 400 ml per day
    b. 600 ml per day
    c. 800 ml per day
    d. 1500 ml per day

119. **What is the minimum fluid urine output for neutral solute balance?** *(Recent Pattern 2014-15)*
    a. 300 ml
    b. 400 ml
    c. 500 ml
    d. 750 ml

120. **Shohl's solution is:** *(Recent Pattern 2014-15)*
    a. Sodium citrate
    b. Potassium binding resin
    c. Lugol iodine
    d. Radio-iodine

121. **The enteric fluid with an electrolyte (Na+, K+, Cl) content similar to that of Ringer's lactate is:**
    a. Saliva *(Recent Pattern 2014-15)*
    b. Contents of small intestine
    c. Contents of right colon
    d. Pancreatic secretions

122. **High urinary chloride is seen in all except?**
    a. Barter syndrome *(Recent Pattern 2014-15)*
    b. Gitelman syndrome
    c. Vomiting
    d. Thiazide

123. **Extracellular bicarbonate ions serve as an effective buffer for all of the following EXCEPT:** *(Recent Pattern 2014-15)*
    a. Sulphuric acid
    b. Phosphoric acid
    c. Lactic acid
    d. Carbonic acid

Answers with Explanations

Hyperkalemia

1. Ans. (d) MgSO₄

(Ref: Harrison 19th edition pg. 312)

- Calcium gluconate will antagonize the depressive effects of potassium on cardiac myocytes.
- Insulin drip and salbutamol nebulization will reduce actual serum levels of potassium by sending potassium inside the cells.
- Magnesium sulfate has no role in management of hyperkalemia.

2. Ans. (c) Beta 2 antagonist

(Ref: Harrison 19th p 312)

Management of Hyperkalemia

- *Antagonism of the cardiac effects of hyperkalemia* with intravenous calcium gluconate/ chloride
- *Rapid reduction in plasma K⁺ concentration by redistribution into cells.* Insulin lowers plasma K⁺ concentration by shifting K⁺ into cells.
- Beta 2 agonists, most commonly albuterol, are effective but underutilized agents for the acute management of hyperkalemia.
- Intravenous bicarbonate has no role in the routine treatment of hyperkalemia. It should be reserved for patients with hyperkalemia and concomitant metabolic acidosis, and only if judged appropriate for management of the acidosis.
- *Removal of potassium* by using cation exchange resins, diuretics, and/or dialysis. Sodium polystyrene sulfonate (SPS) exchanges Na⁺ for K⁺ in the gastrointestinal tract and increases the fecal excretion of K⁺

3. Ans. (d) Calcium chloride

(Ref: Harrison 19th p 312)

- In a clinical setting of hyperkalemia in 1 year old child, cardiac arrhythmias associated with *hyperkalemia include sinus bradycardia, sinus arrest, slow idioventricular rhythms, ventricular tachycardia, ventricular fibrillation, and asystole*
- Intravenous calcium serves to protect the heart while measures are taken to correct hyperkalemia.
- Calcium raises the action potential threshold and reduces excitability without changing the resting membrane potential. By restoring the difference between the resting and threshold potentials, calcium reverses the depolarization blockade caused by hyperkalemia.
- *The recommended dose of treatment of hyperkalemia is 10 mL of 10% calcium gluconate (3–4 mL of calcium chloride), infused intravenously over 2 to 3 min with cardiac monitoring.*
- The effect of the infusion starts in 1–3 min and lasts 30–60 min; the dose should be repeated if there is no change in ECG findings or if they recur after initial improvement.

4. Ans. (d) 50% dextrose in water

(Ref: Harrison 19th p 312)

- Bolus D50W without insulin is never appropriate because of the risk of acutely worsening hyperkalemia due to the osmotic effect of hypertonic glucose.
- Intravenous bicarbonate has no role in the routine treatment of hyperkalemia. It should be reserved for patients with hyperkalemia and concomitant metabolic acidosis, and only if judged appropriate for management of the acidosis.

5. Ans. (a) Intestinal perforation

(Ref: Harrison 19th p 312)

- Sodium polystyrene sulfonate (SPS) exchanges Na⁺ for K⁺ in the gastrointestinal tract and increases the fecal excretion of K⁺.
- The recommended dose of SPS is 15-30 g, typically given in a premade suspension with 33% sorbitol to avoid constipation.
- The effect of SPS on plasma K⁺ concentration is slow; the full effect may take up to 24 hours and usually requires repeated doses every 4–6 hours. Intestinal necrosis is the most serious complication of SPS.

6. Ans.(c) >8 mEq/dl

(Ref: Harrison 19th p 310)

Severe hyperkalemia results in loss of the P wave and a progressive widening of the qRS complex; development of a sine-wave sinoventricular rhythm suggests impending ventricular fibrillation or asystole.

Classically, the electrocardiographic manifestations in hyperkalemia progress from

Tall peaked T waves	5.5 – 6.5 mEq/dl
Loss of P waves	6.5 – 7.5 mEq/dl
Widened qRS complex	7 – 8mEq/dl
Sine wave pattern	>8 mEq/dl

7. Ans. (d) Diabetes mellitus

(Ref: Harrison 19th p 304)

Reduced dietary K⁺ are implicated in the pathophysiology and progression of hypertension, heart failure, and stroke. For example, short-term K⁺ restriction in healthy humans and patients with essential hypertension induces Na⁺-Cl⁻ retention and hypertension. Correction of hypokalemia is particularly important in hypertensive patients treated with diuretics, in whom blood pressure improves with the establishment of normokalemia.

8. Ans. (a) Alkalosis

(Ref: Harrison 19th p 309-310)

- Alkalosis causes extracellular to intracellular shift of potassium leading to hypokalemia
- In acute kidney injury the kidneys lose their ability to excrete potassium.
- In Addison disease, aldosterone deficiency, protons and potassium can be excreted via the distal tubule leading to hyperkalemia. Conns syndrome will have opposite effect and lead to hypokalemia.
- Excess hemolysis like in mismatched Blood transfusion will lead to hyperkalemia as RBCs are loaded with potassium.

9. Ans. (b) Insulin drip

(Ref: Harrison 19th p 312)

Intervention	Lowering of potassium	Duration	M.O.A
Calcium gluconate	No change in potassium levels	Effect starts 1–3 minutes and lasts for 30–60 minutes	Reduces excitability of heart
Insulin drip	0.5-1.5 mmol/L	4–6 hours	Redistribution of potassium by sending potassium inside cells
Parenteral or nebulised salbutamol	0.5-1.5 mmol/L	2–4 hours	Promotes cellular uptake of potassium
Sodium polystyrene sulfonate	0.5-1.0 mmol/L	Full effect takes up to 24 hours	Sorbitol in enema omitted in post-operative patients due to increased incidence of sorbitol induced colonic necrosis
Hemodialysis		Most effective method to lower potassium	Refractory life-threatening hyperkalemia failing to respond to conventional measures.
Peritoneal dialysis			Only 15% effective as hemodialysis
Soda bicarbonate			Reserved for use in severe hyperkale with metabolic acidosis

10. Ans. (c) Ileus

(Ref: 45, Harrison 19th p 310)

- Hyperkalemia from a variety of causes can also present with ascending paralysis; this is known as secondary hyperkalemic paralysis to differentiate it from familial hyperkalemic periodic paralysis (HYPP). The presentation may include diaphragmatic paralysis and respiratory failure.
- Cardiac rhythm disorder with hyperkalemia includes slow idioventricular rhythm.
- Hypokalemia results in slow repolarization of skeletal muscle, impairing the capacity to contract; weakness and even paralysis may ensue. The paralytic effects of hypokalemia on intestinal smooth muscle may cause intestinal ileus.

11. Ans. (d) Torsades de pointes

(Ref: Harrison 19th p 310)

Cardiac arrhythmias associated with hyperkalemia are:
1. Asystole
2. Sinus bradycardia
3. Sinus arrest
4. Slow idioventricular rhythms
5. Ventricular tachycardia
6. Ventricular fibrillation

12. Ans. (d) Autosomal dominant polycystic kidney disease

(Ref: Harrison 19th Table 63-5, p 309)

11 beta hydroxylase deficiency	• Patients with 11-beta-hydroxylase deficiency present with features of androgen excess, including masculinization of female newborns and precocious puberty in male children. • Approximately two thirds of patients also have hypertension, which may or may not be associated with mineralocorticoid excess, *hypokalemia*, and *metabolic alkalosis*.
Liddle syndrome	• An autosomal dominant disorder characterized by early, and frequently severe, hypertension associated with low plasma renin activity, metabolic alkalosis, *hypokalemia*, and normal to low levels of aldosterone
Gitelman syndrome	• Gitelman syndrome is an autosomal recessive kidney disorder characterized by *hypokalemic* metabolic alkalosis with hypocalciuria, and hypomagnesemia. • It is caused by loss of function mutations of the thiazide sensitive sodium-chloride symporter (also known as NCC, NCCT, or TSC) located in the distal convoluted tubule
Autosomal dominant polycystic kidney disease	• Since ESRD will ensue in these patients, hyperkalemia will always be a feature of ADPKD. • A definite diagnosis of ADPKD relies on imaging or molecular genetic testing. The sensitivity of testing is nearly 100% for all patients with ADPKD who are age 30 years or older and for younger patients with PKD1 mutations; these criteria are only 67% sensitive for patients with PKD2 mutations who are younger than age 30 years. • Large echogenic kidneys without distinct macroscopic cysts in an infant/child at 50% risk for ADPKD are diagnostic.

Contd...

Hypokalemia

13. Ans. (b) Tall T waves in ECG

(Ref: Harrison 19th ed./307, 310)

- *The earliest electrocardiogram (ECG) change associated with hypokalemia is a decrease in the T-wave amplitude.*
- As potassium levels decline further, ST-segment depression and T-wave inversions are seen, while the PR interval can be prolonged along with an increase in the amplitude of the P wave.
- The U wave is described as a positive deflection after the T wave, often best seen in the mid-precordial leads (eg, V2

and V3). When the U wave exceeds the T-wave amplitude, the serum potassium level is < 3 mEq/L.
- In severe hypokalemia, T- and U-wave fusion with giant U waves masking the smaller preceding T waves becomes apparent on the ECG.
- A pseudo-prolonged QT interval may be seen, which is actually the QU interval with an absent T wave.

Severe hypokalemia can also cause a variety of tachyarrhythmias, including ventricular tachycardia/ fibrillation and rarely atrioventricular block.

14. Ans. (a) Diarrhea

(Ref: Harrison 19th ed.)

Diarrhea	Loss of potassium in stool and hypoperfusion of tissues explains the presence of lactic acid leading to metabolic acidosis
Vomiting	Loss of acid in vomiting leads to metabolic alkalosis
Nasogastric suction	Same as above
Conn syndrome	Hyperaldosteronism will promote acid loss leading to metabolic alkalosis

Must Know

Must know causes of metabolic acidosis= K.U.L.T
K= ketoacidosis due to starvation or diabetic complications
U= uremia
L= Lactic acidosis
T= Toxins (methyl alcohol, ethylene glycol)

15. Ans. (d) Central pontine myelinosis

(Ref: Harrison's 19th ed. page 301-302)

- Normal serum sodium concentration: 135-145mEq/L. Hypernatremia is defined as a sodium concentration > 145 mEq/L.
- All patients with hypernatremia have hyperosmolality, unlike hyponatremic patients who can have a low, normal, or high serum osmolality.
- *Altered mental status is the most common manifestation, ranging from mild confusion and lethargy to deep coma.*
- Hyperthermia, delirium, *seizures,* and coma may be seen with severe hypernatremia (ie, sodium > 158 mEq/L). Symptoms in the elderly may not be specific; a recent change in consciousness is associated with a poor prognosis.
- The sudden shrinkage of brain cells in acute hypernatremia may lead to **parenchymal or subarachnoid hemorrhages and/ or subdural hematomas**; however, these vascular complications are encountered primarily in pediatric and neonatal patients.
- Central pontine myelinolysis *presents most commonly as a complication of treatment of patients with profound, life threatening* **hyponatremia** *(if hypertonic saline is given too rapidly in a patient in whom hyponatremia has been present for >24–48 h).*
- It is characterized by quadriparesis, ataxia, and abnormal extraocular movements.

Hyponatremia should be corrected at a rate of no more than 12-20mmol/L of sodium per day.

16. Ans. (a) Respiratory insufficiency

(Ref: Harrison 19th p 307)

17. Ans. (c) 60 mmol/L

(Ref: Harrison 19th p 307)

Maximum concentration possible delivered via central vein = 60 mmol/L
Maximum concentration possible delivered via peripheral vein= 40 mmol/L

18. Ans. (b) Normal ST segment

(Ref: Harrison 19th p 307)

ST segment depression is seen in hypokalemia.

19. Ans. (a) < 3-4

(Ref: Harrison 19th p 311)

The expected values of the Transtubular potassium gradient (T.T.K.G) are <3–4 in the presence of hypokalemia and >6-7 in the presence of hyperkalemia. TTKG is measured as follows:

$$\frac{\text{Urine potassium} \times \text{serum osmolality}}{\text{Serum potassium} \times \text{urine osmolality}}$$

20. Ans. (d) 140 mEq

(Ref: Harrison 19th p 307)

- For causing a rise of potassium in blood by 1mEq/dl, 200 mEq of potassium supplementation is required.
- Since symptoms develop with serum potassium less than 3 mEq/dl, the clinician should give sufficient potassium to rise up to 3 mEq/dl via intravenous route. Following this oral potassium supplement will suffice
- Hence mathematically speaking this patient requires approximately 0.7 mEq /dl of potassium to rise in the blood leading to a requirement of $0.7 \times 200 = 140$ mEq over 24 hours

21. Ans. (c) 21 hydroxylase deficiency

(Ref: Harrison 19th p 307)

Choices a and d have increased aldosterone, leading to hypokalemia. 21 hydroxylase deficiency has deficiency of aldosterone leading to hyperkalemia.

22. Ans. (d) Cushing syndrome

(Ref: Harrison 19th p 311)

- Transtubular potassium gradient > 8 is associated with hyperkalemia. Choices a, b, c lead to hyperkalemia
- *Cushing syndrome* has excess of cortisol, which stimulates the mineralocorticoid receptors to cause *hypokalemic metabolic alkalosis.*

23. Ans. (c) Colon

(Ref: Harrison 19th p 305)

Excessive loss of fluid from the gastrointestinal tract can lead to dehydration and, depending upon the origin of the fluid loss, electrolyte and acid-base disturbances. *Because the pancreas, liver, ileum, and colon secrete bicarbonate as part of their electrolyte solution, excessive loss leads to metabolic acidosis. In addition, the colon secretes potassium and loss of colonic fluid can lead to hypokalemia.* Loss of gastric juice results in hypokalemic metabolic alkalosis

Hyponatremia

24. Ans. (b) Mannitol

(Ref: CMDT 2019, page 899)

- If high doses of mannitol are administered or if it is given to patients with preexisting renal insufficiency, the drug may be retained in the circulation.
- The resulting elevation in plasma osmolality results in the passage of water out of cells into intravascular compartment and leads to dilutional hyponatremia.
- The hyponatremia is usually transient and sometimes resolves in a short period of time with adequate hydration and diuresis.
- *Do not confuse hypertonic hyponatremia with Hypervolemic Hyponatremia.*

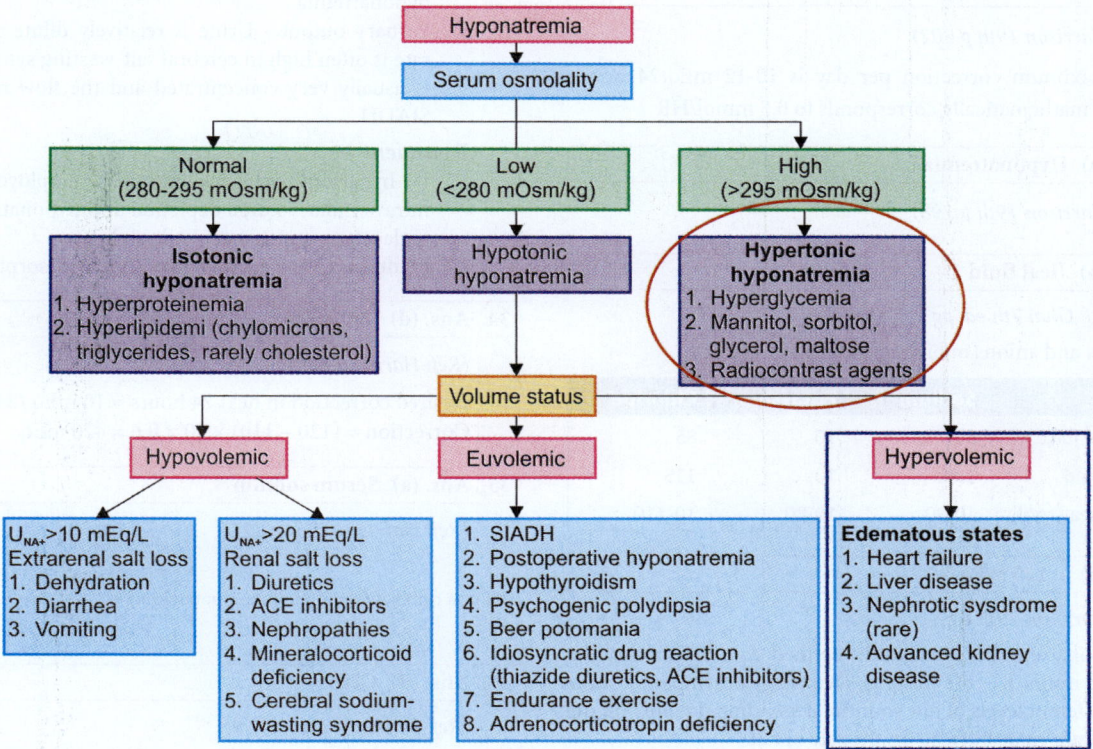

25. Ans. (a) Osmotic demyelination syndrome

(Ref: Harrison 20th edition, page 301)

- Rapid correction of hyponatremia with fluids can result in development of osmotic demyelination syndrome. It is more common in alcoholics or people suffering from malnutrition.
- The most consistent examination findings are those of pseudobulbar palsy and spastic quadriplegia caused by demyelination of corticospinal and corticobulbar tracts within the pons.
- It occurs 48-72 hours after the correction of electrolyte deficit.

26. Ans. (b) Both Statements 1 & 2 are correct

(Ref: CMDT 2016, page 874)

Fluid restriction and not medication is the best for management of asymptomatic hyponatremia with serum Sodium less than 120 mEq/L, in patients of cirrhosis with oedema	Asymptomatic hyponatremia will respond to fluid restriction. Symptomatic hyponatremia with neurological implications must be corrected at a rate of 4-8mEq/L over 24hours with 3% Hypertonic saline
Conivaptan decreases B.P. and increases risk of variceal bleeding and so relatively contraindicated in cirrhotics with hyponatremia	Conivaptan acts on V1A and V2 receptors. V1A stimulation is associated with vasoconstrictive, mitogenic, and possibly platelet aggregative effects. *Conivaptan causes inhibition of V1A receptors* and is beneficial for patients with CHF with concomitant hypertension and atherosclerotic disease. In contrast, the very same effects derived from V1A inhibition can be harmful for hypotensive patients or cirrhotic patients with dilated splanchnic beds and variceal bleeds. Further dilatation of the splanchnic bed and interference with platelet aggregation by V1A inhibition could exacerbate variceal bleeding.

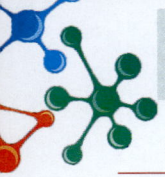

27. Ans. (a) Hyponatremia

(Ref: Harrison 19th p 299)

- Poorly controlled diabetes draws water out of cells resulting in hyponatremia.
- Plasma concentration falls by 1.4 mmol/L for every 100mg/dl rise in plasma glucose concentration of sodium.

28. Ans. (a) 0.5 mmol/Hr

(Ref: Harrison 19th p 302)

The maximum correction per day is 10-12 mEq/24 hours. Which mathematically corresponds to 0.5 mmol/HR

29. Ans. (a) Hyponatremia

(Ref: Harrison 19th p 298)

30. Ans. (b) Ileal fluid

(Ref: OP Ghai 7th ed. pg. 48: table 4.1)

Cations and anions in biological fluids in meq/dl

Fluid	Sodium	Potassium	Chloride
Gastric juice	60	10	85
Ileal fluid	130	10	115
Diarrhea stool	10-90	10-80	10-110

31. Ans. (b) < 125 mEq

(Ref: Harrison 19th ed.)

- Hyponatremia is commonly defined as a serum sodium <135 mmol/L (<135 mEq/L). Neurological symptoms occur at different levels of low sodium, depending not only on the absolute value but also on the rate of fall.
- In patients with hyponatremia that develops over hours, life-threatening seizures and cerebral edema may occur at values as high as 125 mmol/L.
- In contrast, some patients with more chronic hyponatremia that has slowly developed over months to years may be asymptomatic even with serum levels <110 mmol

32. Ans. (b) Hypothyroidism

(Ref: Harrison 19th p 300)

- *Hypothyroidism is characterised by low cardiac output leading to increased AVP production and resultant hyponatremia.*
- Addison disease must be ruled out in chronic cases of hyponatremia.

33. Ans. (d) Expansion of plasma volume

(Ref: Harrison 19th p 299)

Cerebral salt-wasting syndrome, or renal salt wasting, occurs in the setting of acute central nervous system disease. Conditions leading to cerebral salt-wasting syndrome include the following:
- Brain tumor
- Intracranial surgery
- Stroke
- Intracerebral hemorrhage
- Tuberculous meningitis
- Craniosynostosis repair

The following lab studies are indicated in patients with cerebral salt-wasting syndrome:
1. Serum sodium concentration - Patients with untreated cerebral salt-wasting syndrome are often hyponatremic
2. Serum osmolality - If measured serum osmolality exceeds twice the serum sodium concentration and azotemia is not present, suspect hyperglycemia or mannitol as the cause of hyponatremia
3. Urinary output - Urine is relatively dilute and the flow rate is often high in cerebral salt-wasting syndrome; urine is usually very concentrated and the flow rate is low in SIADH

Treatment
1. IV hypertonic saline solutions are employed to correct intravascular volume depletion and hyponatremia and to replace ongoing urinary sodium loss
2. Fludrocortisone promotes sodium re-absorption.

34. Ans. (d) 400 mEq

(Ref: Harrison 19th p 302)

Desired correction in next 24 hours = 10 mEq /24 hours
Correction = (120 – 110) × 70 × 0.6 = 420 mEq

35. Ans. (a) Serum sodium

(Ref: Harrison 19th p 294)

$$\text{Plasma osmolality} = 2(\text{sodium} + \text{potassium}) + \frac{\text{BUN}}{2.8} + \frac{\text{Blood sugar}}{18}$$

36. Ans. (d) CHF

(Ref: Harrison 19th p 299)

- CHF is characterised by low perfusion of kidneys stimulating R.A.A.S and resultant absorption of salt and disproportionate amount of water would lead to hyponatremia with decreased osmolality.
- Isotonic hyponatremia is seen with hyperlipidemia and hyperproteinemia like in paraproteinemia.
- Intravenous immunoglobulin therapy also interferes with measurement of serum sodium leading to pseudo-hyponatremia.

37. Ans. (a) Hyperlipidemia

(Ref: Harrison 19th p 299)

38. Ans. (d) Lesions occur in pontine and extra-pontine areas

(Ref: Harrison 19th p 301)

- *The term osmotic myelinolysis is more appropriate than central pontine myelinolysis for demyelination occurring in extrapontine regions after the correction of hyponatremia.*
- Other regions of the brain can also be involved in ODS, most commonly in association with lesions of the pons but occasionally in isolation; in order of frequency, the lesions of extrapontine myelinolysis can occur in the cerebellum, lateral geniculate body, thalamus, putamen, and cerebral cortex or subcortex.

- *Patients with chronic hyponatremia are more at risk for ODS if plasma Na⁺ concentration is corrected by >8–10 mM within the first 24 h and/or by >18 mM within the first 48 hours.*
- As osmolality increases after correction of hyponatremia, sometimes resulting in degenerative loss of oligodendrocytes and an osmotic demyelination syndrome
- The lesions of ODS classically affect the pons, a structure in which the delay in the re-accumulation of osmotic osmolytes is particularly pronounced
- Clinically, patients can present one or more days after overcorrection of hyponatremia with
    1. Para- or quadraparesis
    2. Dysphagia
    3. Dysarthria
    4. Diplopia, a "locked-in" syndrome
    5. Loss of consciousness.
- The clinical presentation of ODS therefore can vary as a function of the extent and localization of extrapontine myelinolysis, with the reported development of ataxia, mutism, Parkinsonism, dystonia, and catatonia.
- **Management of ODS**: Relowering of plasma Na⁺ concentration after overly rapid correction can prevent or attenuate ODS. However, even appropriately slow correction can be associated with ODS, particularly in patients with additional risk factors; these factors include alcoholism, malnutrition, hypokalemia, and liver transplantation

39. Ans. (a) Serum protein

(Ref: Harrison 19th p 314)

It is imperative to know whether this low calcium is due to albumin deficiency or due to metabolic alkalosis seen in C.H.P.S.

Corrected Calcium (mg/dL) = Measured total Ca (mg/dL) + 0.8 (4.0 - serum albumin [g/dL])

Where 4.0 represents the average albumin level in g/dL.

40. Ans. (d) Urine sodium < 25 mEq/dl

(Ref: Nelson 18th ed. Table 52.3, Harrison 19th p 301)

Diagnostic Criteria for Syndrome of Inappropriate Antidiuretic Hormone

Absence of:
1. Renal, adrenal, or thyroid insufficiency
2. Congestive heart failure, nephrotic syndrome, or cirrhosis
3. Diuretic ingestion
4. Dehydration

Presence of
1. Urine osmolality > 100 (usually > plasma)
2. Serum osmolality < 280 and serum sodium < 135
3. Urine sodium > 25 mEq/dl

41. Ans. (b) Cerebral toxoplasmosis with SIADH

(Ref: Harrison 19th p 1401-2)

- Hepatic cirrhosis in this case is unlikely because of the absence of edema. Hence choice A is ruled out.
- Gastrointestinal fluid (Choice B) loss is unlikely because of normal blood pressure without orthostasis. Furthermore, depending on whether the fluid loss is upper (vomiting with resultant alkalosis) or lower (diarrhea with resultant acidosis), it often is accompanied by a disturbance in acid – base balance.
- Addison's disease is associated with metabolic acidosis, but in the question bicarbonate is normal with value of 24 meq.
- Uric acid can be very helpful in the differential diagnosis of hyponatremia. It is typically elevated in patients with congestive heart failure and renal failure, two other important causes of hyponatremia, and tends to be quite low in patient with SIADH. In setting of HIV infection cerebral toxoplamosis with SIADH is best answer.

42. Ans. (a) Absorption of Na⁺ in the colon is under hormonal (aldosterone) control

(Ref: NMS physiology by john bullock: ch. 44, pg. 550)

- The major route of absorption of sodium in the colon is electrogenic transport. Because of the "tight" nature of the tight junctions that connect cells in the colon, a relatively large potential difference exists between the mucosal (negative) and serosal (positive) surfaces of the absorptive cells. This electrical difference favours the net secretion of K⁺ into the lumen.
- The amounts of absorption of Na⁺ and secretion of K⁺ can be affected by changes in levels of aldosterone. Secretion of HCO_3^- occurs in exchange for absorption of Cl⁻. No counter-balancing cation exchange pumps are present in the colon

Hypernatremia

43. Ans. (c) Nil by mouth

(Ref: Harrison 19th p 304)

- *Hypernatremia is treated with free water intake by mouth or NG tube if patient is not obtunded.* Dilute hypotonic fluids like 5% dextrose in water and N/2 in 5% water are given to decrease serum sodium @0.5mmol/hour or 12 mmol/ 24 hour.
- Drug that stimulate vasopressin stimulation like chlorpropamide/indomethacin/ carbamazepine and clofibrate will also increase water absorbtion from collecting duct and reduce serum sodium

44. Ans. (c) Renal losses

(Ref: Harrison 19th p 303)

Renal losses are more important cause of hypernatremia as compared to other choices.

45. Ans. (a) Hypernatremia

(Ref: OP ghai 7th ed. pg. 52, Harrison 19th p 303)

46. Ans. (c) Periodic paralysis

(Ref: Harrison 19th p 303)

- The fluid shift in hypernatremia leads to convulsions and intracranial hemorrhage would lead to raised ICP.
- In pediatric patients with hypernatremia, extracellular and plasma volumes tend to be maintained in hypernatremic

dehydration until dehydration is severe (i.e., when the patient loses >10% of body weight). When dehydration is severe, skin turgor is reduced, and the skin develops a characteristic doughy appearance

47. Ans. (b) Thrombosis Paralysis

(Ref: Harrison 19th p 303)

Hypernatremia increases osmolality of the ECF, generating an osmotic gradient between the ECF and the ICF, an efflux of intracellular water, and cellular shrinkage.
- Altered mental status is the most common manifestation, ranging from mild confusion and lethargy to deep coma.
- *The sudden shrinkage of brain cells in acute hypernatremia may lead to parenchymal or subarachnoid hemorrhages and/or subdural hematomas; however, these vascular complications are encountered primarily in pediatric and neonatal patients.*
- Osmotic damage to muscle membranes also can lead to hypernatremic rhabdomyolysis. Brain cells accommodate to a chronic increase in ECF osmolality (>48 h) by activating membrane transporters that mediate influx and intracellular accumulation of organic osmolytes (creatine, betaine, glutamate, myo-inositol, and taurine); this results in an increase in ICF water and normalization of brain parenchymal volume.
- In consequence, patients with chronic hypernatremia are less likely to develop severe neurologic compromise. However, the cellular response to chronic hypernatremia predisposes these patients to the development of *cerebral edema and seizures* during overly rapid hydration (overcorrection of plasma Na+ concentration by >10 mM/d).

48. Ans. (b) Decreased insensible losses

(Ref: Harrison 19th p 303)

- Decreased thirst in primary hypodipisia will lead to hypernatremia. It occurs due to damage to osmo-receptors by malignancy, trauma.
- Nephrogenic diabetes insipidus due to V2 receptor insensitivity will lead to loss of water.
- Carcinoid syndrome leads to secretory diarrhea with more water loss as compared to sodium.

49. Ans. (b) 2.9 L half normal saline

(Ref: Harrison 19th Table 63-3, p 302)

Formula for calculation of water deficit =
$$\frac{\text{Plasma Na- 140} \times \text{Total Body water}}{140}$$

Total body water for males = weight × 0.6
Total body water for females = weight × 0.5
Mathematically = 160 – 140/140 × 0.6 × 50kg = 2.9 Liters over 48 – 72 hours

50. Ans. (c) Craniopharyngioma

(Ref: O.P Ghai 7th ed. pg. 52)

Craniopharyngioma leads to central diabetes mellitus and resultant loss of water leads to hypernatremia.

51. Ans. (a) Hyponatremia

(Ref: Harrison 19th p 302)

- Selective vasopressin V2-receptor antagonist is indicated for Hypervolemic and euvolemic hyponatremia (i.e., serum sodium level < 125 mEq/L) or less marked hyponatremia that is symptomatic and has resisted correction with fluid restriction.
- It is used for hyponatremia associated with congestive heart failure, liver cirrhosis, and syndrome of inappropriate antidiuretic hormone secretion. Initiate or reinitiate in hospital environment only.
- Selective vasopressin V2-receptor antagonist that causes an increase in urine water excretion results in an increase in free water clearance (aquaresis), a decrease in urine osmolality, and an increase in serum sodium concentration

Disorders of Calcium Metabolism

52. Ans.(a) Facial nerve stimulation by tapping over the parotid

(Ref: Harrison 19th ed. / 315)

Hypocalcemia /Tetany is characterized by irritability of nerves. This can be elicited by tapping over the facial nerve when it is entering into the parotid gland. This will cause twitching of facial musculature. The sign is referred to as Chvostek sign.

53. Ans. (b) 200 ml/day per degree Celsius

(Ref: Harrison's 17th ed. pg. 437)

54. Ans. (a) Hypercalcemia

(Ref: William endocrinology 12th ed., 1268, Harrison 19th p 313)

- Immobilization can lead to bone resorption sufficient to cause hypercalcemia.
- The immobilization is usually caused by spinal cord injury or extensive casting after fractures, although it can occur in settings such as Parkinson's disease.
- Hypercalcemia of immobilization occurs predominantly in the young and in patients with other reasons for a high rate of bone turnover, such as Paget's disease or extensive fractures.
- After spinal cord injury, the hypercalciuria is maximal at 4 months and can persist for longer than 1 year.
- Bisphosphonates have been used to reverse the hypercalcemia and hypercalciuria of spinal cord injury.

55. Ans. (d) Hyponatremia

(Ref: Harrison 19th p 314 Table 65-2)

Hyperventilation leads to Respiratory alkalosis and alkalosis is associated with low ionized calcium. Inadvertent removal of parathyroid glands during Thyroid surgery leads to Tetany.

56. Ans. (c) Thiazide

(Ref: William textbook of endocrinology 12th ed./pg. 1272)

Treatment of acute Hypercalcemia:
1. *Volume expansion*, because hypercalcemia invariably leads to dehydration; 4–6 L of intravenous saline may be required over the first 24 h, keeping in mind that underlying comorbidities (e.g., congestive heart failure) may require the use of loop diuretics to enhance sodium and calcium excretion. Loop diuretics should be initiated in drip and added to bottle of normal saline. Diuretics, particularly thiazides, should be discontinued as they reduce urinary excretion of calcium.
2. *Zoledronic acid /pamidronate and etidronate.* Onset of action is within 1–3 days, with normalization of serum calcium levels occurring in 60–90% of patients.
3. *Calcitonin*, which directly inhibits osteoclast function, may be used with other antiresorptive agents to achieve more rapid control of severe hypercalcemia. However, calcitonin rarely produces a decline in serum calcium of more than 1 to 2 mg/dL, and its efficacy typically is limited to a few days at most, possibly because of receptor downregulation in target cells of bone and kidney. Its major advantages are a more rapid onset of action than bisphosphonates
4. *In patients with 1, 25(OH)2D-mediated hypercalcemia, glucocorticoids are the preferred therapy,* as they decrease 1, 25(OH)2D production.

57. Ans. (a) Shortening of QT interval

(Ref: Harrison 19th p 314-15)

- Moderate to severe hypocalcemia is associated with paresthesias, usually of the fingers, toes, and circumoral regions, and is caused by increased neuromuscular irritability. On physical examination, a Chvostek's sign (twitching of the circumoral muscles in response to gentle tapping of the facial nerve just anterior to the ear) may be elicited. Carpal spasm may be induced by inflation of a blood pressure cuff to 20 mmHg above the patient's systolic blood pressure for 3 min (Trousseau's sign). *Severe hypocalcemia can induce seizures, carpopedal spasm, bronchospasm, laryngospasm, and prolongation of the QT interval.*
- A rare form of hypoparathyroidism associated with defective development of both the thymus and the parathyroid glands is termed the DiGeorge syndrome, or the velocardiofacial syndrome. Congenital cardiovascular, facial, and other developmental defects are present, and patients may die in early childhood with severe infections, hypocalcemia and seizures, or cardiovascular complications.

58. Ans. (b) Respiratory alkalosis

(Ref: Harrison 19th p 323-324)

- Carbon dioxide washout in hyperventilation will lead to alkalosis. Hence to compensate for this alkalosis, some protons will be released from the proteins. This will lead to vacant space on proteins which will be occupied by calcium ions.
- Since ionic calcium will migrate to fill in the vacant space left by protons on the protein, the total ionised calcium will fall leading to tetany.

59. Ans. (a) FGF-23

(Ref: Harrison 19th p 2459, 2460)

- Tumour induced osteomalacia is seen with mesenchymal origin tumours that liberate FGF-23. This molecule acts on PCT and causes phosphate wasting.
- This condition exhibits resolution within days of successful resection of tumour.

Disorders of Magnesium Metabolism

60. Ans. (c) Tetany

(Ref: Harrison 19th p 2462)

- Hypermagnesemia leads to inhibition of PTH release as well as inhibits Calcium absorbtion from Calcium sensitive receptor.
- The resultant calcium depletion leads to Vasodilation and Neuromuscular blockade.
- Comparison of clinical findings of hypermagnesemia and hypomagenesemia

	Hypermagnesemia	Hypomagnesemia
Mechanism of action	Inhibits PTH release. Inhibits Calcium re-absorbtion from TAL	Resistance to PTH Decreased Production of vitamin D3
Clinical features	Vasodilation : Hypotension Neuromuscular blockade: D.T.R inhibited Respiratory failure: Decreased Respiratory rate. Bowel sounds reduced/ileus Pupils dilated Heart rate decreased	Tetany Vertigo/ataxia/nystagmus Depression Psychosis *Heart rate increased*
ECG findings	ECG: PR, qRS and QT Prolongation	PR and QT prolongation with T wave inversion

Note: QT prolongation is seen with both of them

61. Ans. (c) Both

(Ref: Harrison 19th p 2463)

- Hypermagnesemia slows the heart and leads to heart block.
- Hyperphosphatemia will lead to deposition of calcium phosphate in cardiac conduction tissue leading to heart block.
- When multiplication product of (phosphate) × (calcium) > 55, the complex deposits in tissue like kidney leading to nephrocalcinosis and in basal ganglia leading to Parkinsonism like features.

62. Ans. (d) Rhabdomyolysis

(Ref: Harrison 19th Table 423-4, 2462)

- Gitelman is a defect of DCT where TRPM6 receptor for magnesium reabsorption is present and is defective leading to Hypomagenesemia
- In Re-feeding syndrome seen with starvation, provision of nutrition in form of substrates will lead to cellular consumption leading to rapid shift of magnesium from extracellular fluid to intracellular compartments.
- Hyperaldosteronism will lead to expansion of plasma volume and resultant fall of magnesium.
- In Rhabdomyolysis cell destruction will lead to Hypermagnesemia.

63. Ans. (d) 'Main d'accoucheur'

(Ref: Harrison 19th p 2463)

Normal Magnesium: 1.5-2.0 meq/dl or 1.7-2.4 mg/dl

Magnesium levels	Clinical features
3.5–5 mEq/L	Disappearance of DTR and muscle weakness
5–6 mEq/L	Hypotension and vasodilation
8–10 mEq/L	Arrhythmia (atrial fibrillation) and muscle paralysis
>10 mEq/L	Conduction block and death

64. Ans. (d) T wave inversion

(Ref: Harrison 19th p 2463)

65. Ans. (c) 60%

(Ref: Harrison 19th p 2461)

Site of phosphate reabsorption	% of total reabsorbed
PCT	20%
TAL	60%
DCT	5–10%

66. Ans. (d) Amiloride

(Ref: Harrison 19th p 2463)

- Hypermagnesemia is seen rarely seen in the absence of renal insufficiency as kidneys can excrete a large load of magnesium.

Management of Hypermagnesemia
1. Use of magnesium free cathartics may clear ingested magnesium from the gut.
2. Intravenous hydration will reduce chances of cardiac toxicity.
3. Temporary improvement will be provided by calcium gluconate.
4. Amiloride is a diuretic and by causing loss of water from body will worsen the pre-existing hypermagnesemia.

67. Ans. (d) Intramuscular magnesium sulphate

(Ref: Harrison 19th p 2462)

Hypomagnesemia may cause generalized alterations in neuromuscular function, including:
1. Tetany
2. Tremor
3. Seizures
4. Muscle weakness, ataxia, nystagmus, vertigo,
5. Apathy, depression, irritability, delirium, and psychosis.
6. Cardiac arrhythmias may occur, including sinus tachycardia, other supraventricular tachycardias, and ventricular arrhythmias.

Investigations:
1. Electrocardiographic abnormalities may include prolonged PR or QT intervals, T-wave flattening or inversion, and ST straightening.
2. Serum magnesium levels (Normal =1.7-2.4 mg%)
   The hypocalcemia may be a result of concurrent vitamin D deficiency, although hypomagnesemia can cause impaired synthesis of 1, 25(OH)2D, cellular resistance to PTH, and, at very low serum magnesium [<0.4 mmol/L (<0.8 meq/L; <1 mg/dL)], a defect in PTH secretion; these abnormalities are reversible with therapy

Treatment:
1. Use of IM $MgSO_4$ is discouraged; the injections are painful and provide relatively little magnesium (2 mL of 50% $MgSO_4$ supplies only 4 mmol). $MgSO_4$ may be given IV instead of $MgCl_2$, although the sulfate anions may bind calcium in serum and urine and aggravate hypocalcemia.
2. Mild, asymptomatic hypomagnesemia may be treated with oral magnesium salts [$MgCl_2$, MgO, $Mg(OH)_2$] in divided dosages
3. More severe hypomagnesemia should be treated parenterally, preferably with IV $MgCl_2$, which can be administered safely as a continuous infusion of 50 mmol/d (100 mEq Mg_2^+/day).

68. Ans. (a) Hypermagnesemia

(Ref: Harrison 19th edition, p 2463)

- Hypermagnesemia slows the heart and leads to heart block
- Hypomagesemia leads to cardiac arrhythmias like SVT and VT

Acidosis and Alkalosis

69. Ans. (c) Respiratory acidosis with renal compensation

(Ref: Harrison 20th edition, page 316)

The patient has presented with acidosis. Elevated pCO_2 indicates respiratory component. For neutralizing the protons generated due to respiratory acidosis, bicarbonate reabsorption from the proximal tubule of the kidney is increased. Hence the patient is having partially compensated respiratory acidosis.

70. Ans. (d) High anion gap metabolic acidosis and metabolic alkalosis

(Ref: Harrison 20th edition, page 316)

- The first two choices are eliminated as pH is normal.
- CKD leads to metabolic acidosis while vomiting leads to metabolic alkalosis.
- The key to the answer is anion gap which is elevated to 45 implying unmeasured anions. (Normal average of 10 meq).
- It points to mixed etiology of metabolic acidosis and alkalosis.
- Normal values of pH, pCO_2 and HCO_3 does not ensure absence of acid base imbalance.

71. Ans. (c) Flexion of wrist

(Ref: WHO guidelines on drawing Blood sample)

During poking of radial artery at 45 degrees, the wrist of the patient should be kept *extended to make the radial artery taut and straight*.

Procedure for performing ABG

- Feel the arterial pulse with non-dominant hand.
- Both fingers should be proximal to the desired puncture site and site is prepared.
- The prefilled heparin expelled, and the vented plunger repositioned to the 2 mL mark.
- Extend the wrist and poke the artery at an angle of 45 degrees.
- Arterial blood samples should be obtained in strict anaerobic conditions and should be placed on ice and held at 0°C until analysis.
- Any air bubbles introduced during the sampling procedure will lead to overestimation of arterial oxygen tension (PaO_2) and underestimation of arterial carbon dioxide tension ($PaCO_2$).

72. Ans. (d) Compensated respiratory acidosis

(Ref: Harrison 20th edition, page 316)

The patient has acidosis. The increase in value of $PaCO_2$ implies respiratory component. The patient has primary change of respiratory acidosis. The increase in bicarbonate is due to increased reabsorption from proximal tubule of kidney. Hence the patient is having compensated respiratory acidosis.

73. Ans. (a) Uncompensated metabolic alkalosis

(Ref: Harrison 20th edition, page 316)

- The patient has alkalosis. The increased bicarbonate points to metabolic etiology. The primary change is metabolic alkalosis. For compensation hypoventilation will occur as it will increase CO_2 and generate protons to neutralize the excess bicarbonate.
- Since CO_2 is normal in the question, it implies the compensation process has not started. The answer is uncompensated metabolic alkalosis.

74. Ans. (c) Combined respiratory and metabolic acidosis

(Ref: Harrison 20th edition, page 316)

- The patient has acidosis. The decreased bicarbonate points to metabolic etiology. For compensation in metabolic acidosis, patient will hyperventilate and carbon dioxide washout will occur. But in this patient CO_2 values are elevated pointing to a concomitant etiology of respiratory acidosis in the patient.

- There is a linear relationship between $PaCO_2$ and serum HCO_3 in metabolic acidosis.
- Winter's formula: Expected $PaCO_2 = [1.5 \times (\text{serum } HCO_3)] + [8 \pm 2]$
- Expected $PaCO_2 = (1.5 \times 15) + 8 \pm 2 = 22.5 + 8 \pm 2 = 28 - 32$

Interpretation from Winter's formula

- If $PaCO_2$ is lower than normal, there is a concomitant primary respiratory alkalosis
- If $PaCO_2$ is higher than normal, there is a concomitant primary respiratory acidosis

75. Ans. (c) Low pH

(Ref: Harrison 20th edition, page 1968)

- The clinical profile of patient is of *severe acute asthma exacerbation*. Worrisome is that he is not maintaining normal oxygen saturation even on high flow oxygen with continuous salbutamol nebulization. Since he might *progress to imminent respiratory failure*, an urgent ABG should be performed. High CO_2 levels and low pH will help in decision making of elective intubation for this patient.
- Choice A and B are seen in metabolic acidosis, while positive base excess is a feature of metabolic alkalosis.

76. Ans. (b) Metabolic Acidosis

(Ref: Harrison 19th edition, page 317)

- The pH shows acidosis and HCO_3 is low indicating the primary derangement as metabolic acidosis. The patient will compensate with respiratory alkalosis.
- To check for compensation, winter's formula is applied $= 1.5 \times (HCO_3) + 8 \pm 2 = 1.5 \times 9 + 8 \pm 2 = 21.5 \pm 2$
- Since the value of pCO_2 of the patient is as per the calculation, patient is having partially compensated metabolic acidosis.
- If the value of pCO_2 was less than 19.5 or more than 23.5, then mixed disorder would have been present.

77. Ans. (c) 400 mEq

(Ref: Washington Manual of critical Care, page 185)

- Formula for calculation of bicarbonate deficit

Step 1 = Body weight × [0.4 + 2.4 / HCO_3] = Apparent volume of distribution
Step 2 = Apparent volume of distribution × Target change in HCO_3

The following mathematical calculations are
Step 1 = 75 × [0.4 + 2.4/6] = 75 × 0.8 = 60 L
Step 2 = 60 × [12-6] = 360 mEq.

- The primary goal in metabolic acidosis is correction of acidosis. In life threating acidosis with pH of <7.1, serum bicarbonate is <10-12 mEq/dl. At this time the pCO_2 is about 20mmHg and the respiratory compensation fails. When respiratory compensation fails, the pCO_2 rises suddenly to beyond 55mm Hg and leads to CO_2 narcosis.
- Hence the objective is to increase the value of bicarbonate up to 12 mEq/dl.
- For Soda bicarbonate administration, it is recommended that 50% of total deficit be given over 3 to 4 hours, and the remainder replaced over 8–24 hours. The **usual initial**

target (desired HCO$_3$- concentration): 10 - 12 mEq/L, which should bring the blood pH to ~7.20. The subsequent goal is to increase the bicarbonate level to 15 meq/L over the next 24 hours.
- Avoid the risks of Over-alkalinization like paradoxical CNS acidosis, decreased affinity of haemoglobin for oxygen leading to tissue hypoxia, lactic acid production and sodium overload.

78. Ans. (b) Syringe filled with 0.ml heparin prior to filling with blood

(Ref: Oxford Handbook of clinical medicine: 9th edition, page 785)

Don'ts of ABG sampling

1. DON'T Forget to perform modified Allen's test before taking the sample
2. DON'T Ever leave air bubbles in syringe or draw air before de-airing
3. DON'T fail to adequately heparinise a sample to prevent clotting. Ideally use a pre-heparinised syringe.

Due to compensatory processes the values of ABG can be normal in early phase of illness.

79. Ans. (a) Metabolic acidosis

(Ref: Harrison: 19th edition, page 317)

- The patient has acidosis. The low CO_2 is not a primary change but a response to metabolic acidosis.
- The compensation process of metabolic acidosis is respiratory alkalosis which is achieved by hyperventilation and carbon dioxide washout. This explains the pCO_2 on the lower side of normal.
- The easiest way to understand this is diabetic ketoacidosis state where the metabolic acidosis component leads to kussmual breathing. The hyperventilation will lead to pCO_2 to be on the lower side.

80. Ans. (b) Respiratory acidosis, compensated

(Ref: CMDT 2015, page 889)

- Increased pCO_2 indicates generation of protons in the body leading to acidosis.
- Since increase in CO_2 occurs due to respiratory pathology patient has respiratory acidosis.
- For compensation HCO_3 increases and neutralizes the pH.

81. Ans. (d) Respiratory Alkalosis

(Ref: Harrison 19th p 323)

Hyperventilation in pregnancy will lead to respiratory alkalosis.

82. Ans. (d) Diabetes mellitus

(Ref: Harrison 19th p 318)

- **Type A lactic acidosis:** An increase in plasma l-lactate may be secondary to poor tissue perfusion—circulatory insufficiency (shock, cardiac failure), severe anemia, mitochondrial enzyme defects, and inhibitors (carbon monoxide, cyanide)—or to aerobic disorders

- **Type B Lactic acidosis:** malignancies, nucleoside analogue reverse transcriptase inhibitors in HIV, diabetes mellitus, renal or hepatic failure, thiamine deficiency, severe infections (cholera, malaria), seizures, or drugs/toxins (biguanides, ethanol, methanol, propylene glycol, isoniazid, and fructose).
- **Type D Lactic Acid Acidosis:** which may be associated with jejunoileal bypass, short bowel syndrome, or intestinal obstruction, is due to formation of d-lactate by gut bacteria

83. Ans. (a) Ethylene glycol poisoning

(Ref: Harrison 19th p 319)

- For management of ethylene glycol poisoning, prompt institution of a saline or osmotic diuresis, thiamine and pyridoxine supplements, fomepizole or ethanol, and hemodialysis.
- The IV administration of the alcohol dehydrogenase inhibitor fomepizole (4-methylpyrazole; 15 mg/kg as a loading dose) or ethanol IV to achieve a level of 22 mmol/L (100 mg/dL) serves to lessen toxicity because they compete with ethylene glycol for metabolism by alcohol dehydrogenase. Fomepizole, although expensive, is the agent of choice and offers the advantages of a predictable decline in ethylene glycol levels without excessive obtundation during ethyl alcohol infusion.
- Hemodialysis is indicated when the arterial pH is <7.3, or the osmolar gap exceeds 20 mOsm/kg.

84. Ans. (a) Metabolic acidosis

(Ref: Harrison 19th p 317)

Using Winter's formula; $PCO_2 = 1.5 \times [HCO_3^-]) + 8 \pm 2 = 1.5 \times 16 + 8 \pm 2 = 30–34$

Since the actual PCO_2 falls within the estimated range, we can deduce that the compensation is adequate and there is no separate respiratory disorder present

	pH	PCO$_2$	HCO$_3$
Respiratory acidosis	Decreased	Increased	Increased
Metabolic acidosis	Decreased	Decreased	Decreased
Prediction of compensation			

For every 10 mm Hg rise in CO_2
- HCO_3 increased by 1 mmol/L in acute
- HCO_3 increases by 4 mmol/L in chronic

$pCO_2 = HCO_3 + 15$

85. Ans. (b) Metabolic alkalosis

(Ref: Harrison 19th p 322)

- Since pH = 7.55, and since the direction of change of pH and HCO_3 is same, it implies primary change is metabolic change.
- Prediction of compensation: $pCO_2 = HCO_3 + 15 = 33 + 15 = 48$ mm Hg.
- However the value of pCO_2 given is normal and not increased, it implies a mixed disorder.
- Conclusion metabolic alkalosis with secondary respiratory alkalosis

- Now if you are wondering how is it possible? Then an example is a COPD patient on diuretics for cor pulmonale.
- The diuretics will leads to metabolic alkalosis while the patient's lung disease will lead to hyperventilation leading to respiratory alkalosis

86. Ans. (d) Gitelman syndrome

(Ref: Harrison 19th p 321)

- In kidney tubules H^+ is lost as NH_4 (positive charges) in 1:1 ratio with chloride (negative charges) in urine. To maintain electroneutrality positive and negative charges are lost equally.
- In all renal disorders (tubular or glomerular) metabolic acidosis ensues because loss of protons as NH_4^+ is impaired. Hence Chloride which is lost with NH_4^+ to maintain electroneutrality is also less lost.
- The build of H^+ explains acidosis and Chloride build-up explains Hyperchloremia.
- In diarrhea HCO_3 loss in stool leads to loss of negative charges from body. Hence the kidney preserves the negative charges leading to hyperchloremic metabolic acidosis
- Gitelman syndrome leads to salt loss and water loss from the body. The resultant dehydration triggers the R.A.S system leading secondary aldosteronism and development of metabolic alkalosis.

87. Ans. (a) Rebreathing in a paper bag

(Ref: Harrison 19th p 324)

88. Ans. (c) Respiratory acidosis

(Ref: Harrison 19th p 323)

Method 1: Estimation of expected extent of compensation for respiratory acidosis

1. If there is acute respiratory acidosis, expected compensation is rise of $[HCO_3^-]$ by 1 mEq/L for every 10 mm Hg rise of pCO_2.
2. In this question change in pCO_2 = 60 – 40 = 20 mm Hg.
3. Therefore expected elevation in $[HCO_3^-]$ = 2 mEq.
4. Since the actual HCO_3^- is close to the calculated HCO_3, the diagnosis is respiratory acidosis.

Method 2 for Estimation of expected extent of compensation for respiratory acidosis

1. Based on the pCO_2, we may also calculate the expected pH in acute respiratory acidosis.
2. $\Delta pH = 0.008 \times pCO_2 = 0.008 \times (60 - 40) = 0.16$
3. Therefore expected pH = 7.4 - 0.16 = 7.24.
4. Since the actual pH is consistent with expected value, acid base disorder is likely due to acute respiratory acidosis and other acid base disorders are most likely not present.

89. Ans. (d) Compensated respiratory alkalosis

(Ref: Harrison 19th p 323)

90. Ans. (d) Metabolic acidosis with respiratory acidosis

(Ref: Harrison 19th Table 66-2, p 316)

- Since pH is less, and HCO_3 is less, it implies metabolic acidosis (see table in Q. 60)
- Now for compensation $pCO_2 = HCO_3 + 15 = 18 + 15 = 33$.
- The value predicted is not matching with given pCO_2 of 38 mm Hg.
- It implies compensation is not there and it is a mixed disorder
- Conclusion metabolic acidosis with respiratory acidosis

91. Ans. (d) Ammonium chloride

(Ref: Harrison 19th p 322)

- Normal saline is useful if volume contraction is present
- PPI is given if H^+ is lost from stomach or kidney
- Dilute HCL (0.1N HCL) can be effective but can lead to hemolysis and hence should be given slowly via a central line
- KCL will correct K^+ deficits due to hyperaldosteronism.

92. Ans. (a) Chronic respiratory alkalosis

(Ref: Harrison 19th p 323)

93. Ans. (a) Metabolic alkalosis with compensatory respiratory acidosis

(Ref: Harrison 19th p 316, Table 66-2)

- Since in both pH and PCO_2 direction of change is same, it implies metabolic problem
- Prediction of compensation: $pCO_2 = HCO_3 + 15 = 42 + 15 = 57$ mm Hg.
- Conclusion metabolic alkalosis with compensatory respiratory alkalosis

Following table for ABG questions on alkalosis

	pH	pCO$_2$	HCO$_3$
Respiratory alkalosis	Increased	Decreased	Decreased
Metabolic alkalosis	Increased	Increased	Increased

Prediction of compensation

For every mm Hg fall in CO_2
- HCO_3 decreases by 0.2 mmol/L in acute compensation.
- HCO_3 Decreases by 0.4 mmol/L in chronic compensation.

$PaCO_2 = [HCO_3^-] + 15$

94. Ans. (a) Renal tubular acidosis

(Ref: Harrison 19th p 323, 320, 64e-6)

- The urine electrolytes are used to distinguish between RTA and diarrhea,
- Remember that the UAG is an indirect measure of ammonium excretion, which should be very high in the presence of acidosis if renal function is not impaired.
- UAG = (Na + K) – Cl
- UAG = 100 + 31 – 105 = 26.

- A positive UAG suggest RTA because in the setting of diarrhea, ammonium chloride concentration in the urine would be high and the UAG would be negative.
- A postive value suggests that the kidney is unable to adequately excrete ammonium, leading to a reduction in net acid excretion and thus metabolic acidosis.

95. Ans. (a) Metabolic acidosis

(Ref: Harrison 19th p 317)

Applying Winter's formula
Estimated pCO_2 = $\{HCO_3 \times 1.5\} + 8 \pm 2$
= $\{10 \times 1.5\} + 8 \pm 2$
= 21–25

Since the actual pCO_2 falls within the estimated range, we can deduce that the compensation is adequate and there is no separate respiratory disorder present

96. Ans. (b) Anion gap

(Ref: Harrison 19th p 317)

In diabetic ketoacidosis there is an increased production of acetoacetic and b-hydroxybutyric acids, which leads to an increase in plasma concentration of hydrogen ions. These fixed acids are buffered by all body buffers but mainly by bicarbonate. The concentration of plasma HCO_3^- is therefore below normal. The consumption of bicarbonate and the addition of the anions of the fixed acids to the plasma cause an elevation of the anion gap. The anion gap is equal to plasma (Na^+) – (plasma $[HCO_3^-]$ + plasma $[Cl^-]$), and is normally about 12 to 15 mEq/L. The acidosis would stimulate the carotid body chemoreceptors (and eventually the central chemoreceptors) to cause an increase in ventilation, which decreases arterial pCO_2.

97. Ans. (d) Metabolic Acidosis

(Ref: Oxford Hand book of Medicine 5th/684, Harrison 19th p 317)

Anion Gap

98. Ans. (b) Salicylate poisoning

(Ref: Harrison 19th edition, page 318)

High anion gap metabolic acidosis	Normal anion gap metabolic acidosis
Ketoacidosis: diabetic/ alcohol/ starvation	Diarrhea
Uremia	RTA 1, 2 and 4
Lactic acidosis	External pancreatic or small bowel drainage
Toxins: Salicylates, ethylene glycol, methanol, propylene glycol	Ureterosigmoidostomy

99. Ans. (c) Diarrhea

(Ref: Harrison 19th edition, Table 66.4, page 318)

Increased anion gap metabolic acidosis is seen in K.U.L.T
K = Ketoacidosis
U = Uremia
L = Lactic Acidosis
T = Toxins (Methanol poisoning, Ethylene Glycol poisoning)
Normal anion Gap acidosis = DR FUSE
D = Diarrhea
R = RTA
F = Fistula
Use = Uretero-sigmoidostomy

100. Ans. (c) Renal tubular acidosis

(Ref: Harrison's 17th ed. Ch. 48)

- **Anion gap:** The anion gap is the difference between primary measured cations (sodium Na^+ and potassium K^+) and the primary measured anions (chloride Cl^- and bicarbonate HCO_3^-) in serum.
- So we take value of sodium and from it subtract the value of chloride and bicarbonate.
- Value of Normal anion gap = 10 to 12 mmol/L

AG calculated as follows: AG = $Na^+ - (Cl^- + HCO_3^-)$

Normal anion gap (Mn: FUSED CAR)	Increased anion gap (Mn: MUDPILES)	Decreased anion gap (Mn: BPH-M)
F- Fistula pancreatic U- Ureterosigmoido-stomy S- Small bowel fistula E- Extra chloride D- Diarrhea C- Carbonic anhydrase Inhibitor *(acetazolamide)* A- Adrenal insufficiency R- Renal tubular acidosis	M - Methanol U - Uremia D - DKA/AKA/SKA *(diabetic/alcoholic/ starvation)* P - Paraldehyde / phenformin I - Iron / INH L - Lactic acidosis E - Ethylene glycol S - Salicylates	Bromide intoxication Plasma cell dyscrasia Hypoalbuminemia Monoclonal protein

101. Ans. (d) Renal tubular acidosis

Please refer to above question.

102. Ans.(b) Diarrhea

Please refer to above question.

103. Ans. (b) Renal Tubular acidosis

(Ref: Harrison 19th p 317)

104. Ans. (a) Nephrotic syndrome

(Ref: Harrison 19th p 317)

105. Ans. (a) Fistula

(Ref: Harrison 19th p 317)

Causes of increased anion gap is K.U.L.T

Anion gap = $[Na^+] - ([Cl^-] + [HCO_3^-])$

The reference range of the anion gap is 3 -11 mEq/L

Causes of elevated Anion gap acidosis is best remembered by the mnemonic KULT or the popular MUDPILES

M	=	Methanol
U	=	Uremia
D	=	DKA (also AKA and starvation)
P	=	Paraldehyde
I	=	INH
L	=	Lactic acidosis
E	=	Ethylene Glycol
S	=	Salycilate
K	=	Ketoacidosis (DKA, alcoholic ketoacidosis, starvation)
U	=	Uremia (Renal Failure)
L	=	Lactic acidosis
T	=	Toxins (Ethylene glycol, methanol, paraldehyde, salicylate

Decreased anion gap (< 6 mEq/L) may suggest the following:

- Hypoalbuminemia
- Plasma cell dyscaria
- Monoclonal protein
- Bromide intoxication
- Normal variant

Normal anion gap (6-12 mEq/L) may indicate the following

- Loss of bicarbonate (i.e., diarrhea)
- Recovery from diabetic ketoacidosis
- Ileostomy fluid loss
- Carbonic anhydrase inhibitors (acetazolamide, dorzolamide, topiramate)
- Renal tubular acidosis
- Arginine and lysine in parenteral nutrition
- Normal variant

106. Ans. (d) Small bowel fistula

(Ref: Harrison 19th p 317)

Refer to question 80)

107. Ans. (b) Renal tubular acidosis

(Ref: Oski essential pediatrics, 2nd ed. pg. 504)

UAG = Urinary (sodium) –Urinary (potassium + chloride)

In kidney H^+ are excreted in DCT along with ammonia as NH_4^+ ions

Now to maintain Electro-neutrality, Chloride is also excreted with both being secreted in 1:1 ratio.

- In Diarrhoea since metabolic acidosis will ensue, the kidney will secrete this extra H^+ in urine in large amounts in an effort to maintain pH.
- This will lead to increase in secretion of chloride ions in urine to maintain the Electro-neutrality of urine
- Now mathematically speaking if urinary chloride will increase it will lead to decrease of urinary anion gap.
- Now let us Consider choice B, in Renal tubular acidosis the tubules are damaged and cannot secrete H^+, and hence NH_4^+ in urine is less.
- This means chloride loss in urine will also decrease correspondingly.
- Now mathematically speaking if urinary chloride is less then urinary anion gap will increase.
- UAG becomes NEGATIVE in GIT causes and INCREASES in Tubular defects of the kidney

Disorders of Phosphate Metabolism

108. Ans. (a) 8 drops/min

(Ref: Clinical pharmacology by Edmunds: 8th edition, page 76)

The vasopressor to be given to the patient at the rate of 10 mcg × 80 kg per minute = 800 mcg/min or 0.8 mg/min

- You have diluted 400 mg of drug (2 ampoules) in 250 ml which works out a concentration of 400 mg/250 ml = 1.6 mg/mL
- Since 1 mL = 16 drops per minute, 1.6 mg of drug can be delivered per minute.
- The patient's requirement is 0.8 mg/min which would be at 8 drops/min

Common drop factors are

Blood set	10 drops/min
Regular set	16 drops/min
Micro-drops	60 drops/min

Formula for drops per minute

$$\frac{\text{Rate of drug to be infused} \times \text{Weight} \times \text{Volume of Infusate} \times 60}{1000 \times \text{amount of drug added to Infusate}} \times \frac{\text{Drop factor}}{60}$$

109. Ans. (c) 330 mosm

(Ref: CMDT 2016, page 869)

The concentration of blood glucose and urea is given in mmol/L and needs to be converted into mg%.

1 mmol/L of glucose = 30 mg%

1 mmol/L of urea = 2.8 mg%

Serum Osmolality = (2 x (Na + K)) + (BUN / 2.8) + (glucose / 18)
= 2 × (141 + 4) + 28/2.8 + 540/18
= 330 mosm

110. Ans. (b) Hypophosphatemia

(Ref: Harrison's 18th ed. table 346-1)

Rapid cellular proliferation in blast crisis will lead to consumption of phosphate, thereby leading to shift of extracellular phosphate into the cells. Another such example is intensive erythropoietin therapy or CSF therapy. Do not confuse with tumor lysis syndrome where increased phosphate levels are seen.

111. Ans. (b) Sevalemer

(Ref: Harrison 19th p 2461)

Sevalemer is a Polymeric phosphate binder; decreases serum phosphate concentrations without changing calcium, aluminum, or bicarbonate concentrations.

112. Ans. (a) Blast crisis

(Ref: Harrison 19th p 2462)

Miscellaneous

113. Ans. (b) Normal Saline

(Ref: Harrison 19th ed. / 1749-50)

- *In controlled hemorrhagic shock (CHS), where the source of bleeding has been occluded, fluid replacement is aimed toward normalization of hemodynamic parameters.*
- *In uncontrolled hemorrhagic shock (UCHS), in which the bleeding has temporarily stopped because of hypotension, vasoconstriction, and clot formation, fluid treatment is aimed at restoration of radial pulse or restoration of sensorium or obtaining a blood pressure of 80 mm Hg by aliquots of 250 mL of normal saline (hypotensive resuscitation).*
- *Crystalloid is the first fluid of choice for resuscitation. Immediately administer 2 L of isotonic sodium chloride solution or lactated Ringer's solution in response to shock from blood loss.* Fluid administration should continue until the patient's hemodynamics become stabilized. Because crystalloids quickly leak from the vascular space, each liter of fluid expands the blood volume by 20-30%; therefore, 3 L of fluid needs to be administered to raise the intravascular volume by 1 L.
- Alternatively, colloids restore volume in a 1:1 ratio. Currently available colloids include human albumin, hydroxy-ethyl starch products (mixed in either 0.9% isotonic sodium chloride solution or lactated Ringer's solution), or hypertonic saline-dextran combinations.

114. Ans.(d) Hypertonic fluids

(Ref: Harrison 19th ed. / 1779)

Hypertonic 3% saline can be used in Raised ICT
- Osmotic therapy (i.e, mannitol, hypertonic saline), barbiturate, anesthesia, and neuromuscular blockage, along with concomitant monitoring of intracranial pressure with intracranial pressure monitor is generally required in order to maintain adequate cerebral perfusion pressure of greater than 70 mm Hg.

115. Ans.(b) Heat cramps

(Ref: Harrison 19th ed. / 479e-2)

Heavy sweating causes heat cramps, especially when the water is replaced without also replacing salt or potassium.

116. Ans.(b) Neurogenic

(Ref: Harrison 19th ed. / 1750)

- In road traffic accident case there can be poly-trauma which can damage the spine as well. The damage to thoracic spine can destroy the sympatho-mimetic outflow to the heart causing bradycardia with hypotension.

In this question if *tachycardia was given with hypotension, the answer would be hypovolemic shock* **secondary to damage to organs like liver and spleen.**

117. Ans. (a) Defect of PTH receptor

(Ref: Harrison 19th p 2475)

- Jansen syndrome occurs due to activating mutations in the PTH/PTHrP receptor (PTH1R) have been identified as the cause of this rare autosomal dominant syndrome. Because the mutations lead to constitutive receptor function, one abnormal copy of the mutant receptor is sufficient to cause the disease, thereby accounting for its dominant mode of transmission.
- The disorder leads to short-limbed dwarfism due to abnormal regulation of chondrocyte maturation in the growth plates of the bone that are formed through an endochondral process.
- In adult life, there are numerous abnormalities in bone, including multiple cystic resorptive areas resembling those seen in severe hyperparathyroidism. Hypercalcemia and hypophosphatemia with undetectable or low PTH levels are typically seen.

118. Ans. (c) 800 ml per day

(Ref: Harrison 19th p 298)

- Water loss in stool = 50–100 ml per day in faeces
- Insensible loss from the skin cannot be eliminated. Daily loss is about 400 ml in an adult.
- Insensible loss from the respiratory tract is also about 400 ml/day in an unstressed adult. The water loss here is variable: it is increased if minute ventilation increases and can be decreased if inspired gas is fully humidified at a temperature of 37°C (e.g. as in a ventilated ICU patient).
- The minimal insensible loss in an adult is about 800 ml. This is equivalent to a heat loss of about 480 kcals/day which is about 25% of basal heat production. On an 'average' day, activity will increase insensible respiratory water losses so that the overall insensible loss is more than the minimum: an estimate of 50 ml/hr has been suggested for use in unstressed hospitalised patients

119. Ans. (c) 500 ml

(Ref: Harrison's 17th ed. pg. 275)

Normally about 600 mosm must be excreted per day and since the maximal urine osmolality 1200 mosm/kg: a urine output of 500 ml day is required for neutral solute balance.

120. Ans. (a) Sodium citrate

(Ref: Harrison 19th p 318, 320)

Sodium citrate (Shohl's solution) or $NaHCO_3$ tablets (650-mg tablets contain 7.8 mEq) are equally effective alkalinizing salts. Citrate enhances the absorption of aluminum from the gastrointestinal tract and should never be given together with aluminum-containing antacids because of the risk of aluminum intoxication.

121. Ans. (b) Contents of small intestine

(Ref: Harrison 19th p 305)

Ringer's lactate is isotonic solution with blood. Its contents in one litre are:

Na   =   130 mmol/L
Chloride =   109 mmol/L
Lactate   =   28 mmol/L
K   =   4 mmol/L
Ca   =   1.5 mmol/L

- *Bile and the fluids found in the duodenum, jejunum, and ileum all have an electrolyte content similar to that of Ringer's lactate.*
- Saliva, gastric juice, and right colon fluids have high K^+ and low Na^+ content.
- Pancreatic secretions are high in bicarbonate.

122. Ans. (c) Vomiting

(Ref: Harrison 19th p 306, 307)

- In vomiting since the patient is developing dehydration the resultant R.A.A.S stimulation leads to increase of aldosterone and metabolic alkalosis ensues.
- Loss of hydrochloric acid in vomiting leads to kidney to conserve chloride leading to low urinary chloride.
- In Bartter syndrome, TAL is defective and promotes chloride loss. In Gitelman DCT is defective and promotes chloride loss. Since thiazides act on DCT, they have same effect as Gitelman syndrome.

123. Ans. (d) Carbonic acid

(Ref: Guyton, 9th ed. Pg. 387-389)

The bicarbonate buffer system is of major importance in the buffering of fixed acids produced in the body, such as sulfuric acid, phosphoric acid, lactic acid, and ketone acids (e.g., b-hydroxybutyric acid). The reaction is $H^+ + HCO_3^- \leftrightarrows H_2CO_3 \leftrightarrows CO_2 + H_2O$.

Bicarbonate is ineffective in buffering acid produced from CO_2. e.g., carbonic acid (H_2CO_3), because CO_2 is a product of the buffering reaction.

11
Nutrition

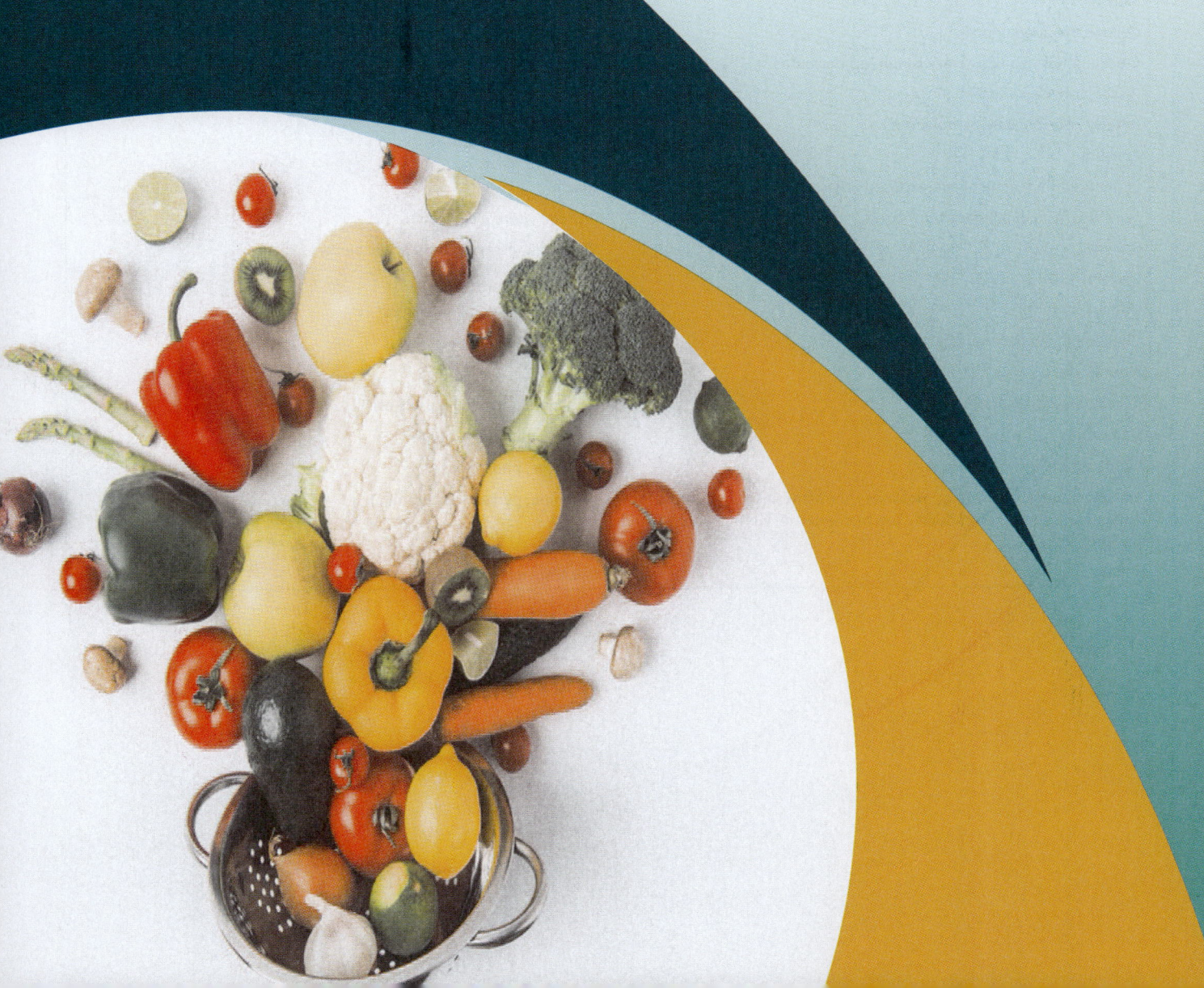

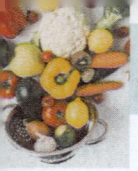

BODY MASS INDEX, MUSCLE MASS AND PEM

BMI (Kg/m^2)	Skeletal muscle mass	Nutritional status
20–24.9	Normal	Normal
18.5–20	Decreased	PEM
<18.5	Decreased	Moderate PEM
<16	Decreased	Severe PEM
<13	Decreased	Lethal in men
<11	Decreased	Lethal in women

NUTRITIONAL DEFICIENCIES AND THEIR FINDINGS

Findings in nutritional deficiencies	Possible Deficiency
Oral	
Atrophic lingual papillae (slick tongue)	Riboflavin, niacin, folate, vitamin B$_{12}$, protein, iron
Glossitis (scarlet, raw tongue)	Riboflavin, niacin, pyridoxine, folate, vitamin B$_{12}$
Hypogeusia, hyposmia	Zinc
Swollen, retracted, bleeding gums	Vitamin C
Skin	
Cellophane appearance	*Protein*
Cracking (flaky paint or crazy pavement dermatosis)	Protein
Follicular hyperkeratosis	Vitamins A, C
Petechiae (especially perifollicular)	Vitamin C
Purpura	Vitamins C, K
Pigmentation, scaling of sun-exposed areas	Niacin
Poor wound healing, decubitus ulcers	*Protein, vitamin C, zinc*
Scaling	Vitamin A, essential fatty acids, biotin
Perioral	
Angular stomatitis	Riboflavin, pyridoxine, niacin
Cheilosis (dry, cracking, ulcerated lips)	Riboflavin, pyridoxine, niacin
Neurologic	
Confabulation, disorientation	Thiamine (Korsakoff's psychosis)
Dementia	Niacin, vitamin B$_{12}$, folate
Ophthalmoplegia	Thiamine, phosphorus
Peripheral neuropathy (e.g., weakness, paresthesias, ataxia, footdrop, and decreased tendon reflexes, fine tactile sense, vibratory sense, and position sense)	Thiamine, pyridoxine, vitamin B$_{12}$
Tetany	Calcium, magnesium

MANIFESTATIONS OF DEFICIENCY AND TOXICITY OF ELEMENTS

Element	Deficiency	Toxicity
Calcium	Reduced bone mass, osteoporosis	Renal insufficiency (milk-alkali syndrome), nephrolithiasis, impaired iron absorption
Copper	Anemia, growth retardation, defective keratinization and pigmentation of hair, hypothermia, degenerative changes in aortic elastin, osteopenia, mental deterioration	Nausea, vomiting, diarrhea, hepatic failure, tremor, mental deterioration, hemolytic anemia, renal dysfunction
Chromium	Impaired glucose tolerance[Q]	*Occupational:* renal failure, dermatitis, pulmonary cancer
Iron	Muscle abnormalities, koilonychia, PICA, anemia, poor work performance, impaired cognitive development, premature labor, perinatal maternal mortality	Gastrointestinal effects (nausea, vomiting, diarrhea, constipation), iron overload with organ damage, acute systemic toxicity
Manganese	Impaired growth and skeletal development, reproduction, lipid and carbohydrate metabolism; upper body rash	*General:* Neurotoxicity, Parkinson-like symptoms; *Occupational:* Encephalitis-like syndrome, Parkinson-like syndrome, psychosis, pneumoconiosis
Molybdenum	Severe neurologic abnormalities	Reproductive and fetal abnormalities
Selenium	Cardiomyopathy, heart failure, striated muscle degeneration	*General:* Alopecia, nausea, vomiting, abnormal nails, emotional lability, peripheral neuropathy, lassitude, garlic odor in breath, dermatitis; *Occupational:* Lung and nasal carcinomas, liver necrosis, pulmonary inflammation
Zinc	Growth retardation, taste and smell, alopecia, dermatitis, diarrhea, immune dysfunction, failure to thrive, gonadal atrophy, congenital malformations	*General:* Reduced copper absorption, gastritis, sweating, fever, nausea, vomiting; *Occupational:* Respiratory distress, pulmonary fibrosis

VITAMIN TOXICITY

Vitamin A (First seen in Arctic explorers who ate polar bear liver)	• Increased intracranial pressure • Dry skin, cheilosis, glossitis, vomiting, alopecia • Bone demineralization and pain and hypercalcemia
Vitamin C	• Taking >2 g of vitamin C in a single dose may result in abdominal pain, diarrhea, and nausea • Increased prevalence of kidney stones • Promote iron overload in patients taking supplemental iron • Induce hemolysis in patients with glucose-6-phosphate dehydrogenase deficiency
Vitamin D	• Acute vitamin D intoxication is rare and usually is caused by excessive ingestion of supplements and leads to hypercalcemia
Vitamin E	• High doses of vitamin E (>800 mg/d) may reduce platelet aggregation and interfere with vitamin K metabolism • Nausea, flatulence, and diarrhea have been reported at doses >1 g/d
Vitamin K	• *Toxicity from dietary phylloquinones and menaquinones* has not been described • High doses of vitamin K can impair the actions of oral anticoagulants

Must Know Points About Vitamin B-Complex

- *Anaphylaxis has been reported after high doses of thiamine,* no adverse effects have been recorded from either food or supplements at high doses.
- *When B6 toxicity occurs, it causes a severe sensory neuropathy,* leaving patients unable to walk.
- *Prostaglandin-mediated flushing due to binding to a G protein–coupled receptor has been observe*d at daily doses as low as 50 mg of niacin when taken as a supplement or as therapy for dyslipidemia.
- Human pantothenic acid deficiency has been demonstrated only in experimental feeding of diets low in pantothenic acid.
- *No toxicity of riboflavin, pantothenic acid and biotin has ever been reported.*

Multiple Choice Questions

1. **Identify the lethal BMI in males?** *(Recent Pattern 2018)*
   a. 11 b. 13
   c. 14 d. 15

2. **A 2 year old child with failure to thrive and growth retardation presents to the outpatient department. On examination kinky hair are seen. What could be the possible disease?** *(AIIMS Nov 2017)*
   a. Menke's Disease b. Leigh's Disease
   c. Wilson disease d. Phenylketonuria

3. **Which of the following is not a clinical feature of Kwashiorkor?** *(UPSC 2015)*
   a. Bipedal oedema b. Muscle wasting
   c. Low serum albumin d. Moon face

4. **Match List I with List II and select the correct answer using the code given below the lists:** *(UPSC 2015)*

List I (Clinical features)	List II (Deficiency of)
A. Peri-orificial rashes	1. Niacin
B. Goose-hump skin lesion	2. Thiamine
C. Confabulation	3. Zinc
D. Dementia	4. Vitamin A

   Code:
       A B C D
   a. 1 2 4 3   b. 1 4 2 3
   c. 3 4 2 1   d. 3 2 4 1

5. **A 2 year old boy is being evaluated for severity of malnutrition. The child weighs 7 kg and measures 72 cm in length. Expected (median) weight for height, and height for age for this child are 9 kg and 86 cm respectively. According to WHO classification of undernutrition, which of the following is the correct category for this child?** *(UPSC 2015)*
   a. Wasted, Stunted
   b. Wasted, Severely Stunted
   c. Severely wasted, Stunted
   d. Severely wasted, Severely stunted

6. **A chronic alcoholic presenting with bleeding gums and petechiae is more likely to have deficiency of?** *(JIPMER Nov 2014)*
   a. Vitamin B_{12} b. Vitamin C
   c. Thiamine d. Pyridoxine

7. **Which vitamin is not associated with toxicity:** *(Recent Pattern 2014-15)*
   a. Pantothenic acid b. Pyridoxine
   c. Vitamin A d. Vitamin C

8. **Most specific screening test for vitamin D deficiency rickets:** *(Recent Pattern 2014-15)*
   a. Serum vitamin vitamin D_3 levels
   b. X-ray wrist joint
   c. Serum calcium levels
   d. Serum alkaline phosphatase

9. **Manifestations of Vitamin E deficiency are all except:** *(Recent Pattern 2014-15)*
   a. Hemolytic anemia
   b. Posterior column abnormalities
   c. Cerebellar ataxia
   d. Autonomic dysfunction

10. **Vitamin E toxicity is associated with:** *(Recent Pattern 2014-15)*
    a. Ataxia b. Peripheral neuritis
    c. Loss of vibrations d. Exfoliative dermatitis

11. **Hyperhomocystenemia can be treated with:** *(Recent Pattern 2014-15)*
    a. Vitamin B_6 b. Vitamin B_{12}
    c. Folic acid d. All of the above

12. **Calculate resting energy expenditure for a 70 kg sedentary man:** *(Recent Pattern 2014-15)*
    a. 1900 Kcal b. 2200 Kcal
    c. 2500 Kcal d. 2900 Kcal

13. **Vitamin D resistant rickets has all the following characteristics except:** *(Recent Pattern 2014-15)*
    a. Hypophosphatemia
    b. X-linked inheritance
    c. Reduced calcium absorption from gut
    d. Renal stones

14. **Mineral which activates action of insulin:** *(Recent Pattern 2014-15)*
    a. Selenium b. Chromium
    c. Zinc d. Copper

15. **Not improving with thiamine replacement:** *(Recent Pattern 2014-15)*
    a. Pulmonary edema b. Psychosis
    c. Peripheral neuritis d. Opthalmoplegia

16. **Which is not a cause of vitamin E deficiency?** *(Recent Pattern 2014-15)*
    a. Dietary deficiency b. Celiac disease
    c. Abetalipoproteinemia d. Cholestasis

17. **Significant weight loss is** *(Recent Pattern 2014-15)*
    a. 5% over 6-12 months b. 10% over 6-12 months
    c. 5 % over 6 weeks d. 10% over 6 weeks

18. **Calcium requirement of a growing school age child is about:** *(Recent Pattern 2014-15)*
    a. 10 gm/day b. 0.1 gm/day
    c. 1.0 gm/day d. 2.0 gm/day

19. **Flushing with niacin is reduced by:** *(Recent Pattern 2014-15)*
    a. Laropiprant b. Premedication with aspirin
    c. Tachyphylaxis d. All of the above

20. **Not recommended in coronary artery disease patients:** *(Recent Pattern 2014-15)*
    a. Daily exercise b. Potassium
    c. Vitamin E d. Statins

21. **Which vitamin's deficiency can cause lactic acidosis?** *(Recent Pattern 2014-15)*
    a. Niacin b. Pantothenic acid
    c. Thiamine d. Riboflavin

22. **Dietary deficiency of which vitamin usually does not exist?** *(Recent Pattern 2014-15)*
    a. Vitamin B_6 b. Thiamine
    c. Vitamin E d. Vitamin D

23. **Severe malnutrition in adults is defined as BMI less than:** *(Recent Pattern 2014-15)*
    a. 18.5 b. 16
    c. 13 d. 11

24. **Deficiency of which vitamin can lead to Methyl malonic aciduria:** *(Recent Pattern 2014-15)*
    a. Pyridoxal Phosphate b. Vitamin C
    c. Vitamin B_{12} d. Folic acid

25. **All are diagnostic criteria for Kwashiorkor except:**
    a. Easily pluckable hair *(Recent Pattern 2014-15)*
    b. Decubitus ulcers
    c. Serum albumin < 2.8 g/dl
    d. Triceps fold thickness < 3mm

26. **Which is not a cause of obesity associated hypertension**
    a. Insulin mediated salt retention *(Recent Pattern 2014-15)*
    b. Increased peripheral resistance
    c. Non-alcoholic hepatic steatosis
    d. Obesity hypoventilation syndrome

27. **The Vitamin which has inhibitory effect on wound healing is:** *(Recent Pattern 2014-15)*
    a. Vitamin-A b. Vitamin-E
    c. Vitamin-C d. Vitamin B-complex

28. **Kwashiorkor is characterized by all except:**
    a. Wound dehiscence *(Recent Pattern 2014-15)*
    b. Lymphopenia
    c. Anergy
    d. Low creatinine height index

29. **All are associated with development of obesity except:**
    a. Carpenter syndrome *(Recent Pattern 2014-15)*
    b. Ahlstrom syndrome
    c. Laurence moon Biedl syndrome
    d. Turner syndrome

30. **All are features of scurvy except:** *(Recent Pattern 2014-15)*
    a. Cork screw hair b. Follicular hyperkeratosis
    c. Cellophane skin d. Sub periosteal bleeding

31. **Maximum half-life is of:** *(Recent Pattern 2014-15)*
    a. Albumin b. Transthyretin
    c. Retinol binding protein d. Transferrin

32. **Death in PEM is due to all exept:** *(Recent Pattern 2014-15)*
    a. Hypothermia b. CCF
    c. Worm infestation d. Electrolyte imbalance

33. **Vitamin deficiency associated with coronary artery disease?** *(Recent Pattern 2014-15)*
    a. Vitamin A b. Vitamin D
    c. Vitamin E d. Vitamin K

34. **Main clinical distinction between anorexia nervosa and bulimia nervosa:** *(Recent Pattern 2014-15)*
    a. Binge eating
    b. Electrolyte abnormalities
    c. Self-induced vomiting
    d. Underweight

35. **Which vitamin toxicity is associated with excessive sweating:** *(Recent Pattern 2014-15)*
    a. Choline b. Biotin
    c. Folic acid d. Vitamin B

36. **Dermatitis may be a clinical manifestation of deficiency states of all of following nutrients except:** *(Recent Pattern 2014-15)*
    a. Biotin b. Niacin
    c. Pyridoxine d. Thiamine

37. **All are false statement about pyridoxine except:** *(Recent Pattern 2014-15)*
    a. Deficiency can cause hemolytic anemia
    b. Deficiency can cause normochromic anemia
    c. RDA for pyridoxine 5 mg.
    d. Can cause burning foot syndrome

38. **Low serum copper is seen in all except?** *(Recent Pattern 2014-15)*
    a. Aceruloplasminemia b. Menke's disease
    c. Wilson disease d. Primary biliary cirrhosis

39. **One of the following is not reported to be a clinical manifestation of zinc deficiency state in children:**
    a. Dwarfism and hypogonadism *(Recent Pattern 2014-15)*
    b. Liver and spleen enlargement
    c. Impaired cell mediated immunity
    d. Macrocytic anemia

40. **Vitamin D resistant rickets occurs due to all except:** *(Recent Pattern 2014-15)*
    a. 1 alpha hydroxylase deficiency
    b. Renal tubular acidosis
    c. Fanconi syndrome
    d. Drugs

41. **Not seen with vitamin C toxicity:** *(Recent Pattern 2014-15)*
    a. Abdominal pain b. Kidney stones
    c. Hemolysis d. Thrombosis

42. **Most common problem with parenteral nutrition is:** *(Recent Pattern 2014-15)*
    a. Fluid overload b. Hyerinsulinemia
    c. Hyperglycemia d. Hypertriglyceridemia

43. **Poor prognostic factors in a child with Kwashiorkor include all of the following except:** *(Recent Pattern 2014-15)*
    a. Hypothermia b. Hepatomegaly
    c. Purpura d. Dermatosis

44. **Not a component of involuntary weight loss** *(Recent Pattern 2014-15)*
    a. Osteopenia b. Sarcopenia
    c. Cachexia d. Anorexia

45. **Vitamin E deficiency presents with all except?** *(Recent Pattern 2014-15)*
    a. Ataxic gait b. Peripheral neuropathy
    c. Opthalmoplegia d. Peri-follicular rash

46. **Cause of recent onset genu valgum and metaphyseal widening in a child with serum calcium 11.0 mEq/L serum parathormone increased and phosphate 2.8 mEq/L is:**
    a. Nutritional rickets *(Recent Pattern 2014-15)*
    b. Azotemic osteodystrophy
    c. Hypophosphatemic rickets
    d. Primary hyper-parathyroidism

47. **Maximum dose of vitamin A in pregnancy:** *(Recent Pattern 2014-15)*
    a. 30µg b. 300µg
    c. 3mg d. 30mg

48. **Photosensitivity is seen with deficiency of which vitamin:** *(Recent Pattern 2014-15)*
    a. Niacin b. Pyridoxine
    c. Folic acid d. Vitamin B_{12}

49. **Not a treatment for porphyria:** *(Recent Pattern 2014-15)*
    a. Hemin
    b. Beta carotene
    c. Hydroxychloroquine
    d. Insulin

50. **Vitamin D deficiency rickets is confirmed by demonstration of:** *(Recent Pattern 2014-15)*
    a. Epiphyseal changes in X-ray
    b. Hypocalcaemia and hypo-phosphatemia
    c. Raised serum alkaline phosphatase
    d. Healing with physiologic doses of vitamin D_3

51. **Most common cause of death in Menke's disease is?** *(Recent Pattern 2014-15)*
    a. Cardiac rupture
    b. Diaphragmatic paralysis
    c. Laryngospasm
    d. Cyano-methemoglobinemia

52. **Cobalt is a part of which vitamin:** *(Recent Pattern 2014-15)*
    a. Retinol
    b. Pyridoxine
    c. Cyanocobalamin
    d. Vitamin C

53. **Not a cause of Beri-Beri:** *(Recent Pattern 2014-15)*
    a. Malignancy
    b. Diuretic use
    c. Dietary deficiency
    d. ATT

Answers with Explanations

1. **Ans. (b)** 13

   (Ref: Harrison 19th edition, Table 98e-1)

   TABLE: Body Mass Index (BMI), Muscle Mass, and Protein Energy Malnutrition (PEM)

BMI (kg/m²)	Skeletal Muscle Mass	Nutritional Status
>30	Normal	Obese
25–29.9	Normal	Overweight
20–24.9	Normal	Normal
>18.5	Decreased	PEM despite adequate or excessive adipose tissue store
<18.5	Decreased	Moderate PEM
<16	Decreased	Severe PEM
<13	Decreased	Lethal in men
<11	Decreased	Lethal in women

2. **Ans. (a)** Menke's Disease

   (Ref: Harpers illustrated biochemistry, 30th edition page 281-2)
   - Kinky hair is a clinical feature of Menke' disease.
   - It is an X linked multi-system lethal disorder of copper metabolism dominated by neurodegenerative symptoms.
   - The gene is on long arm of X chromosome and the defective gene is ATP7A.
   - The defective gene product is P type Adenosine triphosphatase.
   - It leads to defective cellular copper transport affecting the gut. Hence copper accumulates in gut and leads to growth retardation, abnormal hair and cerebellar degeneration. Vasculopathy with fractures and early death is common.
   - Choice B Leighs' disease is mainly autosomal recessive disorder. It also shows mitochondrial inheritance mtDNA, including *MT-ATP6* and leads to neurodegeneration.
   - Choice C and D are easily ruled out.

3. **Ans. (d)** Moon Face

   (Ref: OP Ghai 8th edition, page 99)
   - The child with kwashiorkor will have a *fat sugar baby appearance*, with characteristic edema representing upto 5-20% of the body weight.
   - The presence of pitting edema is a characteristic sign of kwashiorkor and initially the parents of these children might view them as well fed as the edema masks the wasting.
   - *Muscle wasting is present and made out by the fact that the child is weak, hypotonic and unable to stand.*
   - Due to insufficient protein intake, serum albumin is low.
   - The skin shows flaky paint dermatosis and hair shows Flag sign with easily pluck able hair
   - Smooth tongue with cheliosisand child shows apathy with no signs of hunger and it is difficult to feed them.

4. **Ans. (c)** 3 4 2 1

   (Ref: Harrison 20th edition, Chap 326; Harrison 19th edition 96e-9)

Peri-orificial rashes	Seen around genitilia in children with zinc deficiency.
Goose hump lesion	Implies hyperkeratosis seen with vitamin A deficiency.
Confabulation	Seen in Korsakoff psychosis which is related to thiamine deficiency.
Dementia	Seen as reversible dementia with niacin deficiency. 4D= Diarrhea, Dementia, Dermatitis, Death.

5. **Ans. (b)** Wasted, Severely Stunted

   (Ref: IAP Textbook of Pediatrics, 3rd edition, p 126)

Severity of Malnutrition: Stunting and Wasting			
Grade of Malnutrition	Weight for Age* (Wasting)	Height for Age+ (Stunting)	Weight for Height ++)
0, Normal	>90	>95	>90
1, mild	75–90	90–95	81–90
2, moderate	60–74	85–89	70–80
3, severe	<60	<85	<70

Actual weight	Expected median weight for height	Grading of malnutrition)
7 kg	9 kg	77% (mild Wasting)
Actual height	Expected height for age	
72cm	86 cm	83% (severe stunting)

6. **Ans. (b)** Vitamin C

   (Ref: Harrison 20th edition, p 2313; Harrison 19th edition, 96e-5:)

7. **Ans. (a)** Pantothenic acid

   (Ref: Harrison 20th edition, p 2314; Harrison 19th p 96e-5)
   - Pantothenic acid deficiency is believed to have caused the burning feet syndrome seen in prisoners of war during World War II.
   - No toxicity of this vitamin has been reported.
   - No toxicity of pantothenate and biotin has been reported

8. **Ans. (a)** Serum vitamin vitamin D_3 levels

   (Ref: Harrison 20th edition, p 2920; Harrison 19th p 2465, 2485)
   - The most specific screening test for vitamin D deficiency in otherwise healthy individuals is a serum D_3 level.
   - Although the normal ranges vary, levels of 25(OH)D <15 ng/mL are associated with increasing PTH levels and lower bone density; optimal vitamin D levels are >32 ng/mL.
   - Vitamin D deficiency leads to impaired intestinal absorption of calcium, resulting in decreased serum total and ionized calcium values. This hypocalcemia results in secondary hyperparathyroidism, a homeostatic response that initially maintains serum calcium levels at the expense of the skeleton.

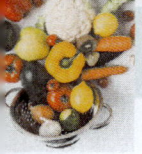

9. Ans. (d) Autonomic dysfunction

(Ref: Harrison 20th edition, p 2316-7; Harrison 19th p 96e-1t, 96e-8, 462e-19)

- Vitamin E deficiency causes axonal degeneration of the large myelinated axons and results in posterior column and spino-cerebellar symptoms.
- Peripheral neuropathy is initially characterized by areflexia, with progression to an ataxic gait, and by decreased vibration and position sensations.
- Ophthalmoplegia, skeletal myopathy, and pigmented retinopathy may also be features of vitamin E deficiency.

10. Ans. (d) Exfoliative dermatitis

(Ref: Harrison 19th p 96e-8)

Vitamin E deficiency causes axonal degeneration of the large myelinated axons and results in posterior column and spinocerebellar symptoms. Peripheral neuropathy is initially characterized by areflexia.
1. Ataxic gait
2. Decreased vibration and position sensations
3. Ophthalmoplegia
4. Skeletal myopathy
5. Pigmented retinopathy

- In contrast Acute toxicity of vitamin A is manifested by increased intracranial pressure, vertigo, diplopia, bulging fontanels in children, seizures, and exfoliative dermatitis

11. Ans. (d) All of the above

(Ref: Harrison 20th edition, p 3018; Harrison 19th p 434e-4)

12. Ans. (a) 1900 Kcal

(Ref: Harrison 20th edition, p 2303; Harrison 19th p 95e-1, 415e-2, 415e-5)

Resting Energy Expenditure = 900 + 10w where w is weight in Kg

Multiply by following for different lifestyle

Sedentary	1.2
Moderately active	1.4
Very active	1.8

13. Ans. (c) Reduced calcium absorption from gut

(Ref: Harrison 20th edition, p 2913-14; Harrison 19th p 2465)

14. Ans. (b) Chromium

(Ref: Harrison 20th edition, p 2319; Harrison 19th p 96e-10)

15. Ans. (b) Psychosis

(Ref: Harrison 20th edition, p 2310; Harrison 19th p 96e-3)

- In acute thiamine deficiency with either cardiovascular or neurologic signs, 100 mg/d of thiamine should be given parenterally for 7 days, followed by 10 mg/d orally until there is complete recovery.
- Cardiovascular and ophthalmoplegic improvement occurs within 24 h.
- Other manifestations gradually clear, although psychosis in Wernicke-Korsakoff syndrome may be permanent or persist for several months

16. Ans. (a) Dietary deficiency

(Ref: Harrison 20th edition, p 2316; Harrison 19th p 96e-1t)

- Vitamin E deficiency is not seen after dietary deficiency
- It is pronounced after small intestinal malabsorbtion, celiac sprue, cystic fibrosis and prolonged cholestasis
- In abetalipoproteinemia, the absorption and transport of vitamin E is defective

17. Ans. (a) 5% over 6-12 months

(Ref: Harrison 20th edition, p 270; Harrison 19th p 274)

Clinically important weight loss is defined as the loss of 10 pounds (4.5 kg) or >5% of one's body weight over a period of 6–12 months.

18. Ans. (c) 1.0 gm/day

(Ref: Harrison 20th edition, Table 325-2, p 2306; Nutrient Requirements and Recommended Dietary Allowances for Indians - A Report of the Expert Group of Indian Council of Medical Research, 2009, page 162, Harrison 19th p 95e-3t, 2496-97)

19. Ans. (d) All of the above

(Ref: Harrison 20th edition, p 2312; Harrison 19th p 96e-4)

- Flushing always starts in the face and may be accompanied by skin dryness, itching, paresthesia, and headache.
- Pharmaceutical preparations of nicotinic acid combined with laropiprant, a selective prostaglandin D2 receptor antagonist, or premedication with aspirin may alleviate these symptoms.
- Flushing is subject to tachyphylaxis and often improves with time.

20. Ans. (c) Vitamin E

(Ref: Harrison 20th edition, p 2317; Harrison 19th p 96e-3f, 96e-8)

- Intervention studies using vitamin E to prevent cardiovascular disease or cancer have not shown efficacy.
  - Infact dosages > 400 mg/day may even increase all cause morbidity
  - Vitamin E has been shown to protect in:
    1. Oxygen induced retrolental dysplasia
    2. Broncho-pulmonary dysplasia
    3. Intra-ventricular haemorrhage of prematurity

21. Ans. (c) Thiamine

(Ref: Harrison 20th edition, p 2309; Harrison 19th p 96e-1)

- Due to defective glucose metabolism in setting of thiamine deficiency, lactic acidosis ensues.

- Type A is lactic acidosis occurring in association with clinical evidence of poor tissue perfusion or oxygenation of blood (e.g, hypotension, cyanosis, cool and mottled extremities). It can be caused by the overproduction of lactate or the underutilization of lactate. In cases of overproduction, circulatory, pulmonary, and hemoglobin transfer disorders are commonly responsible.
- In cases of underutilization of lactate, liver disease, gluconeogenesis inhibition, thiamine deficiency, and uncoupled oxidative phosphorylation can be responsible.
- Type B lactic acidosis occurs when no clinical evidence of poor tissue perfusion or oxygenation exists. However, in many cases of type B lactic acidosis, occult tissue hypoperfusion is now recognized to accompany the primary etiology.
  - Type B1 occurs in association with systemic disease, such as renal and hepatic failure, diabetes and malignancy.
  - Type B2 is caused by several classes of drugs and toxins, including biguanides, alcohols, iron, isoniazid, zidovudine, and salicylates.
  - Type B3 is due to inborn errors of metabolism

22. Ans. (c) Vitamin E

(Ref: Harrison 20th edition, p 2316; Harrison 19th p 96e-1t)

Dietary deficiency of vitamin E does not exist. Vitamin E deficiency is seen in only severe and prolonged malabsorptive diseases, such as celiac disease, or after small-intestinal resection.

23. Ans. (b) 16

(Ref: Harrison 20th edition, p 2326; Harrison 19th p 459)

BMI	Nutritional Status
>30 kg/m^2	Obese
>25–30 kg/m^2	Overweight
20–25 kg/m^2	Normal
<18.5 kg/m^2	Moderate malnutrition
<16 kg/m^2	Severe malnutrition
<13 kg/m^2	Lethal in males
<11 kg/m^2	Lethal in females

24. Ans. (c) Vitamin B$_{12}$

(Ref: Harrison 20th edition, p 705; Harrison 19th p 96e-1t, 96e-8, 462e-19)

25. Ans. (d) Triceps fold thickness < 3mm

(Ref: Harrison 19th p 460, 463t)

Triceps fold thickness< 3mm and mid arm circumference< 15 cm are diagnostic features of marasmus.

Signs that support the diagnosis of Kwashiorkor
1. Easy hair pluckability
2. Edema
3. Skin breakdown
4. Poor wound healing.

5. Major sine qua non is severe reduction of levels of serum proteins such as albumin (<2.8 g/dL) and transferrin (<150 mg/dL) or iron-binding capacity (<200 ug/dL).
6. Cellular immune function is depressed, reflected by lymphopenia (<1500 lymphocytes/dL in adults and older children)
7. Lack of response to skin test antigens (anergy).

The prognosis of adult patients with full-blown Kwashiorkor is not good even with aggressive nutritional support.

26. Ans. (c) Non-alcoholic hepatic steatosis

(Ref: Harrison 19th p 415e-6, 1612, 1622)

- Obesity-induced hypertension is associated with increased peripheral resistance and cardiac output, increased sympathetic nervous system tone, increased salt sensitivity, and insulin-mediated salt retention; it is often responsive to modest weight loss
- Severe obesity may be associated with obstructive sleep apnea and the "obesity hypoventilation syndrome" with attenuated hypoxic and hypercapnic ventilatory responses. Sleep apnea can be obstructive (most common), central, or mixed and is associated with hypertension.

27. Ans. (b) Vitamin E

(Ref: Facial and plastic reconstruction surgery pg. 23: 3rd ed., Ira D Papel, Harrison 19th p 96e-8)

Factors affecting wound healing:
1. Cortisone/Corticosteroids markedly inhibit capillary budding, fibroblast proliferation, and the rate of epithelialization.
2. Similar to cortisone, vitamin E adversely affects wound healing by slowing collagen production. This effect may be reversed with vitamin A. Additional vitamin A will not improve wound healing in the absence of vitamin E or cortisone.
3. Excessive zinc delays wound healing by inhibiting macrophage function.
4. Radiation is detrimental to wound healing. Given 7 days before wound creation, healing is impaired.
5. Hypo-proteinemia
6. Uremia
7. Diabetes mellitus
8. Obesity contributes to poor wound healing, primarily as a consequence of poor suture holding in the subcutaneous fat layers
9. Cytotoxic drugs may also delay wound healing.
10. Alkylating agents (e.g, cyclophosphamide, melphalan) slow wound healing by blocking DNA synthesis.

28. Ans. (d) Low creatinine height index

(Ref: Harrison 19th p 460, 463t)

- Signs that support the diagnosis of Kwashiorkor include easy hair pluckability, edema, skin breakdown, and poor wound healing.
- The major sine qua non is severe reduction of levels of serum proteins such as
- Albumin (<2.8 g/dL)

- Transferrin (<150 mg/dL) or iron-binding capacity (<200 ug/dL).
- Lymphopenia (<1500 lymphocytes/uL in adults and older children
- Lack of response to skin test antigens (anergy).

Creatinine height index <60% is a diagnostic criteria for marasmus in adults.

29. Ans. (d) Turner syndrome

(Ref: Harrison 20th edition, p 2842 Table 394-2; Nelson'18th ed. ch. 80)

Feature	Prader-Willi	Laurence-Moon-Biedl	Ahlstrom's	Cohen's	Carpenter's
Inheritance	Sporadic; two-thirds have defect	Autosomal recessive	Autosomal recessive	Probably autosomal recessive	Autosomal recessive
Stature	Short	Normal; infrequently short	Normal; infrequently short	Short or tall	Normal
Obesity	Generalized	Truncal	Truncal, gluteal	Truncal	Truncal

30. Ans. (c) Cellophane skin

(Ref: Harrison 19th p 96e-1t, 461, 732)

- Scurvy causes impaired formation of mature connective tissue and include bleeding into skin (petechiae, ecchymoses, perifollicular hemorrhages); inflamed and bleeding gums; and manifestations of bleeding into joints, the peritoneal cavity, the pericardium, and the adrenal glands.
- Corkscrew hair
- In children, vitamin C deficiency may cause impaired bone growth and present with pseudoparalysis due to sub-periosteal bleeding.
- Laboratory diagnosis of vitamin C deficiency is made on the basis of low plasma or leukocyte levels.
- Administration of vitamin C (200 mg/d) improves the symptoms of scurvy within a matter of several days.
  - Cellophane skin is seen with protein deficiency.

31. Ans. (a) Albumin

(Ref: Harrison 20th edition, p 2340; Harrison 19th p 464t)

The serum proteins most commonly used to assess nutritional status include:
1. Albumin with half-life of 21days
2. Transferrin with half-life of 8-10 days
3. Thyroxine-binding pre-albumin (or transthyretin) with half- life of 2 days
4. Retinol-binding protein with half-life of 12 hours.

32. Ans. (c) Worm infestation

(Ref: Nelson 18th ed. ch. 43)

33. Ans. (b) Vitamin D

(Ref: Harrison 20th edition, p 2316; Harrison 19th p 96e-7, 2463)

Vitamin D insufficiency may increase the risk of:
1. Type 1 diabetes mellitus
2. Cardiovascular disease (Hypertension)
3. Brain Dysfunction (e.g., depression).

34. Ans. (d) Underweight

(Ref: Harrison 20th edition, p 3274; Harrison 19th p 2719-20)

The main clinical distinction between the two depends on bodyweight. Patients with Anorexia nervosa are underweight while patients with bulimia are overweight or normal weight. The presence of electrolyte imbalances confers and increased morbidity for both disorders.

Clinical features	Anorexia nervosa	Bulimia nervosa	Binge eating disorder
Onset	Mid-adolescence	Late adolescence/early adulthood	Late adolescence/early adulthood
Female:male	10:1	10:1	2:1
Weight	Markedly decreased	Usually normal	Usually obese
Menstruation	Absent	Usually normal	Usually normal
Binge eating	25–50%	Required for diagnosis	Required for diagnosis

35. Ans. (a) Choline

(Ref: Harrison 20th edition, p 2314; Harrison 19th p 95e-2t, 96e-5)

- Choline is a precursor for acetylcholine, phospholipids, and betaine.
- Choline is necessary for the structural integrity of cell membranes, cholinergic neurotrans-mission, lipid and cholesterol metabolism, methyl-group metabolism, and transmembrane signaling.
- Toxicity from choline results in hypotension, cholinergic sweating, diarrhea, salivation, and a fishy body odour. The upper limit for choline has been set at 3.5 g/d.

36. Ans. (d) Thiamine

(Ref: Harrison 19th p 96e-1t, 373)

37. Ans. (b) Deficiency can cause normochromic anemia

(Ref: Harrison 20th edition, p 2313; Harrison 19th p 96e-1t, 360)

Symptoms of vitamin B$_6$ deficiency
1. Include epithelial changes, as seen frequently with other B vitamin deficiencies.
2. Peripheral neuropathy
3. Abnormal electroencephalograms
4. Personality changes, Depression and confusion.
5. Microcytic hypochromic anemia is due to diminished hemoglobin synthesis, since the first enzyme involved in heme biosynthesis (Amino-levulinate synthase) requires PLP as a cofactor
6. Increased risk of cardiovascular disease.

38. Ans. (d) **Primary biliary cirrhosis**

(Ref: Harrison 20th edition, p 2318; Harrison 19th p 96e-10, 2690-91)

- Low ceruloplasmin in all the three choices a,b,c explains the presence of low serum copper.
- Menke is due to defect of ATP7A gene leading to low ceruloplasmin
- Serum copper is paradoxically low in Wilson as it is deposited in tissues and lost in urine. The gene defective is ATP 7B gene on chromosome 13.

39. Ans. (d) **Macrocytic anemia**

(Ref: Harrison 20th edition, p 2317; Nelson 18th ed. ch 670, Harrison 19th p 96e-9, 461)

- Autosomal recessive disorder caused by an inability to absorb sufficient zinc from the diet.
- The genetic defect is in the intestinal zinc specific transporter gene SLC39A4.

Clinical findings include:
1. The cutaneous eruption consists of eczematous skin lesions symmetrically distributed in the perioral, acral, and perineal areas and on the cheeks, knees, and elbows.
2. Chronic diarrhea, stomatitis, glossitis, paronychia, nail dystrophy, growth retardation
3. Delayed wound healing,
4. Intercurrent bacterial infections,and super-infection with Candida albicans.
5. Growth retardation and delayed development may be apparent.
6. Hair often has a peculiar reddish tint, and alopecia.
7. Ocular manifestations include photophobia, conjunctivitis, blepharitis, and corneal dystrophy detectable by slit-lamp examination.

40. Ans. (d) **Drugs**

(Ref: Harrison 19th p 2465)

41. Ans. (d) **Thrombosis**

(Ref: Harrison 20th edition, p 2313; Harrison 19th p 96e-5)

- Taking >2 g of vitamin C in a single dose may result in abdominal pain, diarrhea, and nausea.
- Since vitamin C may be metabolized to oxalate, it could result in an increased prevalence of kidney stones.
- High doses of vitamin C could promote iron overload in patients taking supplemental iron.
- High doses of vitamin C can induce hemolysis in patients with glucose-6-phosphate dehydrogenase deficiency.

42. Ans. (a) **Fluid overload**

(Ref: Harrison 20th edition, p 2330; Harrison 19th p 98e-6-8, 98e-7t)

- The most common problems related to PN are fluid overload and hyperglycemia.
- Hypertonic dextrose stimulates a much higher insulin level than meal feeding. Because insulin is a potent anti-natriuretic and antidiuretic hormone, hyper-insulinemia leads to sodium and fluid retention.
- In the absence of gastrointestinal losses or renal dysfunction, net fluid retention is likely when total fluid intake exceeds 2000 mL/d.
- Close monitoring of body mass, as well as fluid intake and output, is necessary to prevent this complication.

43. Ans. (b) **Hepatomegaly**

(Ref: Harrison 19th p 460t)

44. Ans. (a) **Osteopenia**

(Ref: Harrison 20th edition, p 271; Harrison 19th p 275-76)

The four major manifestations of Involuntary Weight Loss are:
1. Anorexia
2. Sarcopenia (loss of muscle mass)
3. Cachexia (a syndrome that combines weight loss, loss of muscle and adipose tissue, anorexia, and weakness)
4. Dehydration

45. Ans. (d) **Peri-follicular rash**

(Ref: Harrison 20th edition, p 2316; Harrison 19th p 96e-1t, 96e-8)

- Vitamin E deficiency is associated with axonal degeneration of spino-cerebellar and dorsal column tracts.
- Hence most patients present with peripheral neuropathy with arreflexia and later with ataxic gait
- Opthalmoplegia, skeletal myopathy and pigmentary retinopathy are also seen

46. Ans. (c) **Hypophosphatemic rickets**

(Ref: Nelson 18th ed. ch. 48, Harrison 19th p 332e-7t, 2458)

- Choices a and b have low serum calcium and are ruled out due to normal serum calcium level of the patient.
- Choice D has elevated serum calcium and ruled out

Detail given	Normal value	Interpretation
Serum calcium 11 mEq/dl	9-11mEq/dl	Normal
Phosphate 2.8mEq/dl	Serum phosphate levels in the children (5.0-7.5 mg/dL) is high compared with that for adults (2.7-4.5 mg/dL)	Low
PTH increased	10-55pg/ml	Numerical value mentioned increased

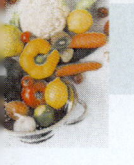

- PHEX gene on chromosome X leads to Hypo-phosphatemic rickets and expression of a substance known as fibroblast growth factor-23 (FGF23).
- FGF23 acts on the kidney to cause increased phosphate excretion and decreased alpha-1 hydroxylase activity.

47. Ans. (c)   3 mg

(Ref: Harrison 20th edition, p 2315; Harrison 19th p 256e-12, 96e-7)

When vitamin A is provided in excess to pregnant women, congenital malformations have included spontaneous abortions, craniofacial abnormalities, and valvular heart disease. In pregnancy, the daily dose of vitamin A should not exceed 3 mg.

48. Ans. (a)   Niacin

(Ref: Harrison 19th p 96e-4)

Physical appearance	Deficiency state
Cellophane appearance	Protein
Cracking (flaky paint or crazy pavementdermatosis)	Protein
Follicular hyperkeratosis	Vitamins A,C
Petechiae (especially perifollicular)	Vitamin C
Purpura	Vitamins C, K
Pigmentation, scaling of sun-exposed areas	Niacin
Poor wound healing, decubitus ulcers	Protein, Vitamin C, zinc
Scaling	Vitamin A, essential fatty acids, biotin Zinc (hyperpigmented)

49. Ans. (d)   Insulin

(Ref: Harrison 20th edition, p 2993-2994; Nelson 18th ed. ch. 91, Harrison 19th p 367e-3, 2530-31)

	Presenting Symptoms	Exacerbating Factors	Most important screening tests	Treatment
Acute intermittent porphyria	Neurologic	Drugs (mostly P450-inducers), progesterone, dietary restriction	Urinary porphobilinogen	Hemin, glucose
Porphyria cutanea tarda	Skin blistering and fragility	Iron, alcohol, smoking estrogens, hepatitis C, HIV,	Plasma or urine porphyrins	Phlebotomy, low – dose hydroxychloroquine or chloroquine
Erythropoietic protoporphyria	Skin pain and swelling		Erythrocyte (or plasma) porphyrins	β- Carotene

50. Ans. (d)   Healing with physiologic doses of vitamin D_3

(Ref: Nelson 18th ed. ch. 48, Harrison 19th p 2465-66, 2485)

51. Ans. (a)   Cardiac rupture

(Ref. Harrison 19th p 96e-10)

- Menke is XLR defect caused by ATP 7A gene
- It is characterised by mental retardation and kinky hair and copper deficiency anemia.
- Most children die within 5 years of diagnosis because of dissecting aneurysm or cardiac rupture.
- Diagnosis is based on low serum copper levels with low ceruloplasmin levels.
- Serum copper can be elevated in pregnancy or stress conditions since ceruloplasmin is an acute phase reactant.

52. Ans. (c)   Cyanacobalamin

(Ref: Harrison 19th p 1691, 263e-3t)

53. Ans. (d)   ATT

(Ref: Harrison 20th edition, p 2309; Harrison 19th p 96e-1t, 2690)

Causes of thiamine deficiency:

1. Poor dietary intake.
2. In Western countries, the primary causes of thiamine deficiency are alcoholism and chronic illnesses such as cancer.
3. Hyperemesis gravidarum
4. Bariatric bypass surgery
5. Chronic diuretic therapy due to increased urinary thiamine losses.

12
Tumors

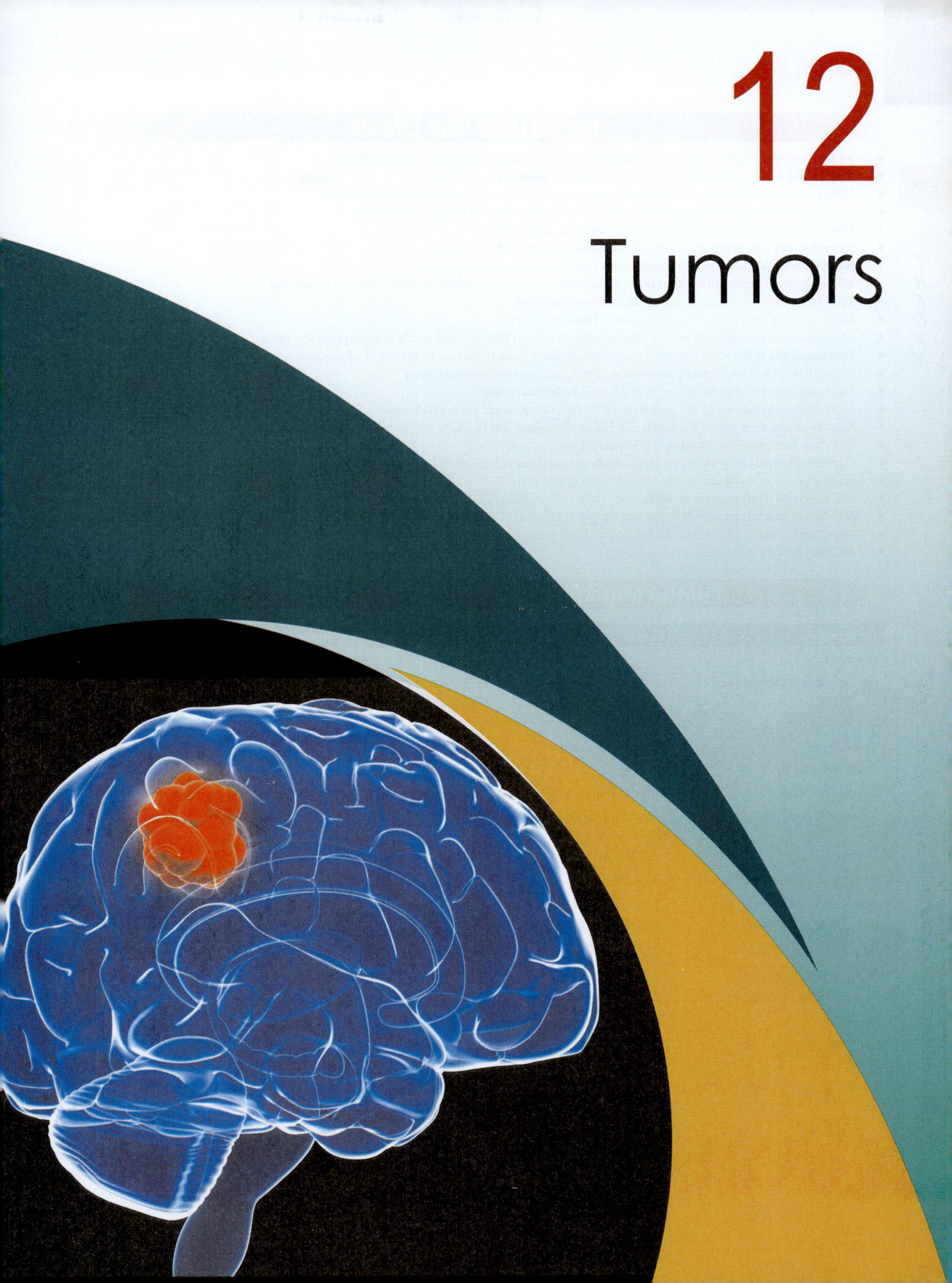

IMPORTANT ONE-LINERS

- **ALL** accounts for 77% of childhood leukemia and is the most common cancer in children.
- **Childhood ALL** was the first disseminated cancer shown to be curable.
- Most common malignancy in adolescents age group (15–16 years) is **Hodgkin's lymphoma**.
- Second most common malignancy in children and adolescents: **Primary CNS tumors**.
- Most common brain tumor in children is **pilocytic astrocytoma**.
- **Neuroblastoma** is the most commonly diagnosed malignancy in infancy.
- **Neuroblastoma** is the most common extracranial solid tumor in children.
- **Wilm's tumor (nephroblastoma)** is the most common primary malignant renal tumor of childhood.
- Most common sarcoma in children: **Rhabdomyosarcoma**.
- Most common sites of rhabdomyosarcoma: **Head and neck**.
- Most common presentation of soft tissue sarcomas in both children and adults is **asymptomatic mass**.
- **Osteosarcoma** is the most common primary malignant bone tumor in children and adolescents followed by **Ewing's sarcoma**.
- In children <10 years, **Ewing's sarcoma** is more common than **osteosarcoma**.
- Most common intraocular tumor in children is **retinoblastoma**.
- Most malignant tumors of the gonads in children and adults are **germ cell tumors**.
- Most common liver tumor in children in **hepatoblastoma** and in adults it is **hepatocellular carcinoma**.
- The most benign tumor of infancy is **hemangioma**.
- Cancers preventable by vaccines: **Hepatocellular carcinoma** (Hepatitis B vaccine) and **cervical cancer** (HPV) vaccine.
- Cancer preventable by antibiotics is MALToma (*H. pylori*)
- MC cancer in adult males is prostate cancer (pg 1608, CMDT 2017)
- MC cancer in adult females is breast cancer (pg 1608, CMDT 2017)
- MC cancer in adult males/females leading to death is lung cancer
- MC preventable cause of cancer is Tobacco

TUMOR MARKERS AND ASSOCIATED CONDITIONS

Tumor markers	Cancer	Non-neoplastic conditions
Hormones		
Human chorionic gonadotropin	Gestational trophoblastic disease, gonadal germ cell tumor	Pregnancy
Calcitonin	Medullary cancer of the thyroid	
Catecholamine	Pheochromocytoma	
Oncofetal antigens		
Alpha fetoprotein	Hepatocellular carcinoma, gonadal germ cell tumor	Cirrhosis, hepatitis
Carcinoembryonic antigen	Adenocarcinomas of the colon, pancreas, lung, breast, ovary	Pancreatitis, hepatitis, inflammatory bowel disease, smoking
Enzymes		
Prostatic acid phosphatase	Prostate cancer	Prostatitis, prostatic hypertrophy
Neuron–specific enolase	Small cell cancer of the lung, neuroblastoma	
Lactate dehydrogenase	Lymphoma, Ewing's sarcoma	Hepatitis, hemolytic anemia, many others
Tumor-associated proteins		
Prostate–specific antigen	Prostate cancer	Prostatitis, prostatic hypertrophy
Monoclonal immunoglobulin	Myeloma	Infection, MGUS
CA-125	Ovarian cancer, some lymphomas	Menstruation, peritonitis, pregnancy
CA-19-9	Colon, pancreatic, breast cancer	Pancreatitis, ulcerative colitis
CD30	Hodgkin's disease, anaplastic large cell lymphoma	-
CD 25	Hairy cell leukemia, adult T cell leukemia/lymphoma	-

COMMON ONCOGENES ALTERED IN HUMAN CANCERS

Oncogene	Alteration in cancer	Neoplasm
AKT1	Amplification	Stomach
AKT2	Amplification	Ovarian, breast, pancreatic cancer
CTNNB1	Point mutation	Colon, prostate, melanoma, skin, others
FOS	Overexpression	Osteosarcomas
ERBB2	Point mutation, amplification	Breast, ovary, stomach, neuroblastoma
JUN	Overexpression	Lung
MET	Point mutations, rearrangement	Osteocarcinoma, kidney, glioma
MYB	Amplification	AML, CML, colorectal, melanoma
C-MYC	Amplification	Breast, colon, gastric, lung
L-MYC	Amplification	Lung, bladder
N-MYC	Amplification	Neuroblastoma, lung
HRAS	Point mutation	Colon, lung, pancreas
KRAS	Point mutation	Melanoma, colorectal, AML
NRAS	Point mutation	Various carcinomas, melanoma
REL	Rearrangement, amplification	Lymphomas
WNT1	Amplification	Retinoblastoma

CANCER PREDISPOSITION SYNDROMES AND ASSOCIATED GENES

Syndrome	Gene	Chromosome	Inheritance	Tumors
Ataxia telangiectasia	ATM	11q22–q23	AR	Breast
Autoimmune lymphoproliferative syndrome	FAS	10qq24–1q23	AD	Lymphomas
Bloom's syndrome	BLM	15q26.1	AR	Several types
Cowden's syndrome	PTEN	10q23	AD	Breast, thyroid
Familial adenomatous polyposis	APC	5q21	AD	Intestinal adenoma, colorectal
Familial melanoma	p16INK4	9q21	AD	Melanoma, pancreatic carcinoma
Familial Wilm's tumor	WT1	11q13	AD	Kidney
Hereditary breast (ovarian) cancer	BRCA1	17q21, 13q12.3	AD	Breast, ovarian, colon, prostate
Hereditary diffuse gastric cancer	CDH1	16q21	AD	Stomach
Hereditary multiple exostoses	EXT1 EXT2	8q24, 11p11–12	AD	Exostoses, chondrosarcoma
Hereditary prostate cancer	HPC1	1q24–25	AD	Prostate
Hereditary retinoblastoma	RB1	13q14.2	AD	Retinoblastoma, osteosarcoma
Hereditary nonpolyposis colon cancer (HNPCC)	MSH2 MLH1 MSH6 PMS2	2p16 3p21.3 2p16 7p22	AD	Colon, endometrial, ovarian, stomach, small bowel, ureter carcinoma
Hereditary papillary renal carcinoma	MET	7q31	AD	Papillary kidney
Juvenile polyposis	SMAD4	18q21	AD	Gastrointestinal, pancreatic
Li-Fraumeni	TP53	17p13.1	AD	Sarcoma, breast
Multiple endocrine neoplasia type-1	MEN1	11q13	AD	Parathyroid, endocrine, pancreas and pituitary

Contd...

Syndrome	Gene	Chromosome	Inheritance	Tumors
Multiple endocrine neoplasia type 2a	RET	10q11.2	AD	Medullary thyroid carcinoma, pheochromocytoma
Neurofibromatosis type-1	NF1	17q11.2	AD	Neurofibroma, neurofibrosarcoma, brain
Neurofibromatosis type-2	FF2	22q12.2	AD	Vestibular schwannoma, meningioma, spine
Nevoid basal cell carcinoma syndrome (Gorlin's syndrome)	PTCH	9q22.3	AD	Basal cell carcinoma, medulloblastoma, jaw cysts
Tuberous sclerosis	TSC1 TSC2	9q34 16p13.3	AD	Angiofibroma, renal angiomyolipoma
Von Hippel-Lindau	VHL	3p25–26	AD	Kidney, cerebellum, pheochromocytoma

AR-Autosomal recessive; AD-Autosomal dominant

SUSPECTED CARCINOGENIC AGENTS THOUGHT TO ACT AS CANCER INITIATORS

Carcinogens	Associated cancer or neoplasm
Alkylating agents	Acute myeloid leukemia, bladder cancer
Androgens	Prostate cancer
Aromatic amines (dyes)	Bladder cancer
Arsenic	Cancer of the lung, skin
Asbestos	Cancer of the lung, pleura, peritoneum
Benzene	Acute myelocytic leukemia
Chromium	Lung cancer
Diethylstilbestrol (prenatal)	Vaginal cancer (clear cell)
Epstein – Barr virus	Burkitt's lymphoma, nasal T cell lymphoma, Hodgkins lymphoma, leiomyosarcoma in immunosuppressed persons
Epipodophyllotoxins	AML
Estrogens	Cancer of the endometrium, liver, breast
Ethyl alcohol	Cancer of the liver, esophagus, head and neck
Helicobacter pylori	Gastric cancer, gastric MALT lymphoma
Human immunodeficiency virus	Non – Hodgkin's lymphoma, Kaposi's sarcoma, squamous cell carcinomas (especially of the urogenital tract)
Human papilloma virus	Cervix cancer, head and neck cancer
Human T cell lymphotropic virus type I (HTLV – I)	Adult T cell leukemia/lymphoma
Immunosuppressive agents (azathioprine, cyclosporine, glucocorticoids)	Non – Hogkin's lymphoma
Ionizing radiation (therapeutic or diagnostic)	Breast, bladder, thyroid, soft tissue, bone, hematopoietic, and many more
Nitrogen mustard gas	Cancer of the lung, head and neck, nasal sinuses
Nickel dust	Cancer of the lung, nasal sinuses
Phenacetin	Cancer of the renal pelvis and bladder
Polycyclic hydrocarbons	Cancer of the lung, skin (especially squamous cell carcinoma of scrotal skin)
Polyoma virus (BK, JC, SV 40) (N – 19, 1725)	Brain cancer
Schistosomiasis	Bladder cancer (squamous cell)
Sunlight (ultraviolet)	Skin cancer (squamous cell and melanoma)
Tobacco (including smokeless)	Cancer of the upper digestive tract, bladder
Vinyl chloride	Liver cancer (angiosarcoma)

CONGENITAL ANOMALIES AND MALIGNANCIES

Aniridia, Beckwith Wiedemann syndrome	Wilms tumor
Cryptorchidism	Testicular germ cell tumors
Major birth defects	Rhabdomyosarcoma

NEUROBLASTOMA

- Neuroblastoma are malignant embryonal tumors of precursor cells of the sympathetic ganglia and adrenal medulla. Half of the tumors arise from adrenal glands and the remainder largely from paraspinal sympathetic ganglia.
- Most common malignancy in infancy and most common extracranial solid tumor in children.
- Median age of diagnosis is 22 months and 90% are diagnosed by 5 years of age.

Clinical Features

1. Abdominal mass incidentally discovered crossing the midline (differentiates it from Wilm's tumor)
2. Hepatomegaly: Pepper liver
3. Paroxysmal attacks of sweating, pallor, flushing, headache, palpitations and hypertension (due to increased catecholamine secretion)
4. Paraneoplastic: Opsoclonus myoclonus syndrome or VIP syndrome (diarrhea, hypokalemia).
5. Raccoons eyes: Periorbital edema and ecchymosis
6. Dumb bell tumor: Infiltration into the intervertebral spaces
7. Horner's syndrome
8. Lytic lesions in X ray in skull and long bones. Most common sites of metastases: regional or distant lymph nodes, long bones and skull, bone marrow, liver and skin.

Investigations

1. **Biopsy**: Small round blue cell tumor, Homer Wright pseudorosettes.
2. CT shows hemorrhage and calcification.
3. Vanillylmandelic acid (VMA): 3-methoxy-4-hydroxy phenylglycol (MHP) and homovanilic acid (HVA) are positive in urine.
4. **MIBG scan**: Very sensitive method for primary evaluation and follow up of primary and metastatic disease.
5. **Staging system**: INSS – International Neuroblastoma Staging System, pathologic classification system – SHIMADA, clinical staging system – EVAN's
6. **Stage 4 S**: Localized primary tumor, with dissemination limited to skin, liver and bone marrow (limited to infants < 1 yrs), very good prognosis; survival at 5 yrs is 80%.

Treatment

- **For low risk neuroblastoma**: Surgery for stages 1 and 2 and observation for 4S.
- **Treatment of intermediate risk neuroblastoma**: Surgery, chemotherapy (cisplatin or carboplatin, cyclophosphamide, etoposide and doxorubicin) and radiation therapy.
- **Treatment of high risk neuroblastoma**: Intensive chemotherapy, autologous stem cell transplantation, surgery, irradiation and 13 cis retinoic acid.

INTESTINAL CARCINOID TUMORS

- MC site is small intestine > Rectum
- Can produce 5 HT derivatives like serotonin and histamine
- Can also produce somatostatin, gastrin and substance P.
- They have an indolent course and risk of metastasis increases when tumor is > 1 cm.

Clinical Features

1. Abdominal pain, bowel obstruction/infarction due to loco-regional spread.
2. *Carcinoid syndrome incidence is highest with midgut carcinoid.*
3. Bronchial carcinoid mainly presents with flushing
4. Abdominal cramps and secretory diarrhea
5. Tricuspid and pulmonic stenosis/regurgitation.

Investigations

1. Serum chromogranin A (more sensitive than below mentioned 2 tests)
2. *Urinary 5-HIAA (Hydroxyindole acetic acid)*
3. Plalelet serotonin levels
4. Somatostatin receptor scintigraphy is positive in 90% patients with metastatic carcinoid. It helps in tumor localization with staging.

Treatment

DOC is octreotide for carcinoid syndrome. Resection of hepatic metastasis also helps in reduction of symptoms.

Multiple Choice Questions

1. **Which of the following is not a feature of tumor lysis syndrome?** *(AIIMS Nov 2017)*
   a. Hyperkalemia
   b. Hyperphosphatemia
   c. Hypercalcemia
   d. Hyperuricemia

2. **Most common histology in Cancer of unknown primary is?** *(Recent Question 2016-17)*
   a. Squamous cell cancer
   b. Well to moderately differentiated adenocarcinoma
   c. Poorly differentiated adenocarcinoma
   d. Neuroendocrine tumours

3. **All tumours are CK7+ and CK 20+ except?** *(Recent Question 2016-17)*
   a. Urothelial tumours
   b. Ovarian mucinous adenocarcinoma
   c. Cholangiocarcinoma
   d. Renal cell carcinoma

4. **Vanishing tumour is seen with?** *(Recent Question 2016-17)*
   a. Chloroma
   b. Inter-lobar effusion
   c. Tumour lysis syndrome
   d. Malignant biliary obstruction

5. **Winking owl sign is seen in?** *(Recent Question 2016-17)*
   a. Vertebral metastasis
   b. Subacute combined demyelination of spinal cord
   c. Burkitt's lymphoma
   d. Ependymoma

6. **All of the following cancers are linked with HIV except:** *(Recent Pattern 2014-15)*
   a. Kaposi sarcoma
   b. Urogenital cancer
   c. Non Hodgkin lymphoma
   d. Adult T cell leukemia

7. **Most common cause of death in cancer is?** *(Recent Pattern 2014-15)*
   a. Bleeding
   b. Infection
   c. Respiratory failure
   d. Renal failure

8. **Which is the most common tumor leading to death in adults?** *(Recent Pattern 2014-15)*
   a. Lung cancer
   b. Prostate cancer
   c. Colorectal cancer
   d. Leukemia

9. **Streptococcus bovis infection is associated with:** *(Recent Pattern 2014-15)*
   a. CLL
   b. Hairy cell leukemia
   c. Colorectal cancer
   d. Multiple myeloma

10. **Most significant risk factor for cancer is:** *(Recent Pattern 2014-15)*
    a. Age
    b. Smoking
    c. Viruses
    d. Physical inactivity

11. **Most common malignant tumor of heart in adults?** *(Recent Pattern 2014-15)*
    a. Angiosarcoma
    b. Rhabdomyoma
    c. Lipoma
    d. Paraganglioma

12. **All are seen in Carney's triad except?** *(Recent Pattern 2014-15)*
    a. Atrial myxoma
    b. GIST
    c. Pulmonary chordoma
    d. Paraganglioma

13. **Incorrect about LAMB syndrome:** *(Recent Pattern 2014-15)*
    a. Lentigines
    b. Atrial Myxoma
    c. Myaesthenic syndrome
    d. Blue Nevi

14. **Most common MALIGNANT tumor of heart in children is:** *(Recent Pattern 2014-15)*
    a. Rhabdomyoma
    b. Rhabdomyosarcoma
    c. Angiosarcoma
    d. Lipoma

15. **All of the following statements about atrial myxomas are true, except:** *(Recent Pattern 2014-15)*
    a. Most common site is left atrium
    b. More common in females
    c. Tumor plop in systole
    d. Raynaud phenomenon

16. **Most common tumor of heart valves:** *(Recent Pattern 2014-15)*
    a. Papillary fibroelastoma
    b. Malignant fibrous histiocytoma
    c. Angiosarcoma
    d. Rhabdomyosarcoma

17. **Most common benign tumor of heart in children is:** *(Recent Pattern 2014-15)*
    a. Rhabdomyoma
    b. Rhabdomyosarcoma
    c. Angiosarcoma
    d. Lipoma

18. **Most common site of atrial myxoma is:** *(Recent Pattern 2014-15)*
    a. Inter-atrial septum
    b. Right atrium
    c. Inter-ventricular septum
    d. Left Ventricle

19. **Clubbing is least common in:** *(Recent Pattern 2014-15)*
    a. Squamous cell carcinoma
    b. Adenocarcinoma
    c. Small cell carcinoma of lung
    d. Mesothelioma

20. **Pancoast tumour causes:** *(Recent Pattern 2014-15)*
    a. Increased sweating
    b. Wasting of muscles of hand
    c. Destruction of lower ribs
    d. Bony metastasis

21. **Most common primary lung cancer in children:** *(Recent Pattern 2014-15)*
    a. Metastasis
    b. Bronchial adenoma
    c. Adenocarcinoma
    d. Pulmonary blastoma

22. **Which of the following statement about lung carcinoma is true?** *(Recent Pattern 2014-15)*
    a. Squamous cell variant accounts for 70% of all lung cancers
    b. Oat cell variant typically present with cavitation
    c. Oat cell variant presents an endobronchial growth
    d. Adenocarcinoma variant is typically central in location

23. **Ectopic ACTH syndrome is seen most commonly with:** *(Recent Pattern 2014-15)*
    a. Renal cell carcinoma
    b. Lymphoma
    c. Bronchogenic carcinoma
    d. Pituitary adenoma

24. Which one of the following statements is true of systemic treatment of NSCLC? *(Recent Pattern 2014-15)*
    a. Chemotherapy has no effect on survival in advanced NSCLC
    b. Adjuvant platinum-based chemotherapy confers no survival benefit
    c. Epidermal Growth Factor Receptor Tyrosine Kinase Inhibitors (EGFR-TKI) such as Erlotinib have proven active in previously treated patients with advanced NSCLC
    d. EGFR-TKI have a higher chance of response in male smokers

25. All of the following Para-neoplastic syndrome are seen in Ca lung except: *(Recent Pattern 2014-15)*
    a. Hypertrophic osteodystrophy
    b. Myasthenia gravis
    c. Cushing's syndrome
    d. Hypoglycemia

26. Which one of the following is true regarding lung cancer? *(Recent Pattern 2014-15)*
    a. Adenocarcinomas tend to grow quickly
    b. 5% of patients with lung cancer present with, or develop complications of non-metastatic paraneoplastic syndromes
    c. Syndrome of Inappropriate Anti Diuretic Hormone (SIADH) is associated with hypernatraemia
    d. 80-90% of small cell carcinomas have spread beyond the thorax at the time of diagnosis

27. A young male presented with asymptomatic lymph node enlargement in supraclavicular region. The biopsy shows squamous cells, the likely site of carcinoma will be:
    (Recent Pattern 2014-15)
    a. CA stomach   b. CA colon
    c. CA Breast   d. CA Lung

28. Hyperglycaemia is seen in which type of bronchogenic carcinoma: *(Recent Pattern 2014-15)*
    a. Squamous cell carcinoma
    b. Oat cell carcinoma
    c. Adenocarcinoma
    d. Large cell carcinoma

29. The most radiosensitive lung cancer is:
    a. Squamous cell carcinoma *(Recent Pattern 2014-15)*
    b. Small cell carcinoma
    c. Adenocarcinoma
    d. Giant cell carcinoma

30. The most common type of lung carcinoma in non-smokers is: *(Recent Pattern 2014-15)*
    a. Squamous cell carcinoma
    b. Adenocarcinoma
    c. Small cell carcinoma
    d. Large cell carcinoma

31. Most common cancer associated with asbestosis:
    (Recent Pattern 2014-15)
    a. Adenocarcinoma   b. Mesothelioma
    c. Squamous cell carcinoma d. Bronchial adenoma

32. Which one of the following types of bronchogenic carcinoma is most likely to cavitate:
    a. Adenocarcinoma *(Recent Pattern 2014-15)*
    b. Bronchoalveolar carcinoma
    c. Oat-cell carcinoma
    d. Squamous cell carcinoma

33. Following are increased in small cell carcinoma of lung except *(Recent Pattern 2014-15)*
    a. ACTH   b. Growth hormone
    c. ANF   d. AVP

34. A 70-year-old smoker male presents with breathlessness, facial swelling. Incorrect is? *(Recent Pattern 2014-15)*
    a. Dilated veins have blood flow away from umbilicus
    b. Worse on bending forward
    c. Non-pulsatile elevated JVP
    d. Glossal edema

35. A 55-year-old man, a chronic smoker is brought to emergency with history of polyuria, polydipsia, nausea and altered sensorium for last two days. He had been diagnosed as having squamous cell carcinoma of lung two months prior to this. On examination, he was lethargic and confused. An ECG was normal except for a narrowed QT interval. Which one of the following is the most likely metabolic abnormality? *(Recent Pattern 2014-15)*
    a. Hypernatremia   b. Hypercalcemia
    c. Hypokalemia   d. Hyponatremia

36. Popcorn calcification is seen in: *(Recent Pattern 2014-15)*
    a. Pulmonary hamartoma   b. Pulmonary hemorrhage
    c. Pulmonary teratoma   d. Pulmonary embolism

37. Eaten Lambert syndrome is associated with?
    (Recent Pattern 2014-15)
    a. Anti P/Q antibodies   b. Anti – HU antibodies
    c. Anti – Jo-1 antibody   d. Anti GQ_{1B} antiboy

38. ANF is produced by: *(Recent Pattern 2014-15)*
    a. Squamous cell carcinoma
    b. Adenocarcinoma
    c. Alveolar cell carcinoma
    d. Oat cell carcinoma

39. True statement about pancoast tumour is:
    a. Affects left lower lobe *(Recent Pattern 2014-15)*
    b. Causes radicular pain in upper limb
    c. Produces recurrent laryngeal nerve palsy
    d. Exclusively associated with adenocarcinoma

40. 5 year survival rate for small cell cancer lung is:
    (Recent Pattern 2014-15)
    a. 1%   b. 5%
    c. 10%   d. 25%

41. All are paraneoplastic syndromes except:
    a. Cerebellar degeneration *(Recent Pattern 2014-15)*
    b. Progressive multifocal leukoencephalopathy
    c. Amyotropic lateral sclerosis
    d. Opsoclonus myoclonus

42. Most common carcinoma of lung is:
    (Recent Pattern 2014-15)
    a. Squamous cell carcinoma b. Adenocarcinoma
    c. Small cell carcinoma   d. Large cell carcinoma

43. Bronchial adenoma commonly present as:
    (Recent Pattern 2014-15)
    a. Recurrent hemoptysis   b. Chronic Cough
    c. Dyspnea   d. Chest pain

44. Well-defined rounded opacity in the lung with coarse irregular calcification is a feature of:
    (Recent Pattern 2014-15)
    a. Hamartoma   b. Hydatid cyst
    c. Amoebic abscess d. Ca lung

45. **Most common symptom of lung cancer?**
    (Recent Pattern 2014-15)
    a. Weight loss b. Hemoptysis
    c. Chest pain   d. Clubbing

46. **Horner's syndrome is associated with long standing pain in shoulder and arm. This presentation is mimicked by all except?** *(Recent Pattern 2014-15)*
    a. Chronic stable angina b. Coronary ostial occlusion
    c. Cervical spondylosis   d. Cervical rib

47. **Ampiphysin antibodies are seen in?**
    a. Stiff person syndrome *(Recent Pattern 2014-15)*
    b. Opsoclonus
    c. Paraneoplastic cerebellar degeneration
    d. Lambert Eaton syndrome

48. **Most aggressive kidney tumour is?** *(Recent Pattern 2014-15)*
    a. Bellini tumor   b. Clear cell tumor
    c. Chromophobe adenoma   d. Papillary carcinoma

49. **Most common type of renal cell cancer in dialysis patient is?**
    (Recent Pattern 2014-15)
    a. Clear cell carcinoma   b. Papillary carcinoma
    c. Bellini tumour   d. Oncocytoma

50. **Which of the following is effective against both HCC and RCC :** *(Recent Pattern 2014-15)*
    a. Erlotinib   b. Sorafenib
    c. Bortezomib   d. Cetuxtimab

51. **Triad of renal cell carcinoma includes all except?**
    a. Hematuria   *(Recent Pattern 2014-15)*
    b. Abdominal pain
    c. Abdominal mass
    d. Fever

52. **Papillary carcinoma of kidney is associated with defect on:**
    (Recent Pattern 2014-15)
    a. Chromosome 3   b. Chromosome 7
    c. Chromosome 11   d. Chromosome 21

53. **Polychronotropism is seen with:** *(Recent Pattern 2014-15)*
    a. Urothelial tumors   b. G.I.S.T
    c. Pancreatic cancer   d. Hepatocellular cancer

54. **Incorrect about Wilm's tumor:** *(Recent Pattern 2014-15)*
    a. Associated with hemi-hypertrophy
    b. Hematuria
    c. Embolise to lungs and heart
    d. Most common malignant tumor of abdomen of childhood

55. **Most common intra-abdominal mass in neonates is?**
    a. Multi-cystic dysplastic kidney *(Recent Pattern 2014-15)*
    b. Wilm's tumor
    c. Hydronephrosis
    d. Rhabdomyosarcoma

56. **The most common presenting feature of bladder carcinoma is:** *(Recent Pattern 2014-15)*
    a. Painless profuse intermittent haematuria
    b. Clot colic
    c. Dysuria
    d. Sterile acid pyuria

57. **Most common benign solid tumor of kidney is:**
    a. Oncocytoma   *(Recent Pattern 2014-15)*
    b. Bellini tumor
    c. Chromophobe adenoma
    d. Papillary carcinoma

58. **Interleukin involved in pathogenesis of Stauffer syndrome?**
    (Recent Pattern 2014-15)
    a. IL-1   b. IL-2
    c. IL-6   d. IL-11

59. **Paraneoplastic syndrome associated with RCC are all of the following except:** *(Recent Pattern 2014-15)*
    a. Polycythemia   b. Hypercalcemia
    c. Malignant hypertension d. Cushing syndrome

60. **Aflatoxin causes:** *(Recent Pattern 2014-15)*
    a. Lathyrism   b. Hepato cellular carcinoma
    c. Cholangiocarcinoma d. Botulism

61. **Most common liver tumour:** *(Recent Pattern 2014-15)*
    a. Metastasis
    b. Hemangioma
    c. Hepatocellular carcinoma
    d. Focal nodular hyperplasia

62. **The most common cause of hepatocellular carcinoma in India is:** *(Recent Pattern 2014-15)*
    a. Hepatitis A   b. Hepatitis B
    c. Non A Non B hepatitis d. Alcoholic cirrhosis

63. **Hypoglycemia is seen with:** *(Recent Pattern 2014-15)*
    a. RCC   b. HCC
    c. Glucagonoma   d. Breast cancer

64. **Best prognosis in H.C.C is seen in:** *(Recent Pattern 2014-15)*
    a. Fibrolamellar hepatoma b. Hepatoblastoma
    c. Angiosarcoma   d. Cholangiosarcoma

65. **Which is a hormone dependent liver tumor:**
    a. Hepatoma   *(Recent Pattern 2014-15)*
    b. Hemangioma
    c. Hepatocellular carcinoma
    d. Hemangiopericytoma

66. **Opsoclonus is seen with all except?**
    (Recent Pattern 2014-15)
    a. Neuroblastoma   b. Lung cancer
    c. Brain cancer   d. Breast cancer

67. **Isaac syndrome is characterised by?**
    a. Peripheral nerve excitability *(Recent Pattern 2014-15)*
    b. Opsoclonus
    c. Encephalomyelitis
    d. Limbic encephalitis

68. **Most common soft tissue tumor in children?**
    (Recent Pattern 2014-15)
    a. Rhabdo-myosarcoma b. Lipoma
    c. Hemangioma   d. Fibrous histiocytoma

69. **Most common malignant soft tissue tumor in adults:**
    a. Rhabdo-myosarcoma *(Recent Pattern 2014-15)*
    b. Lipoma
    c. Hemangioma
    d. Fibrous histiocytoma

70. **Rhabdomyosarcoma with the worst prognosis is:**
    a. Alveolar type   *(Recent Pattern 2014-15)*
    b. Botyroid type
    c. Pleomorphic type
    d. Embryonal type

71. **Rhabdomyosarcoma in children is most commonly present at which site:** *(Recent Pattern 2014-15)*
    a. Head and neck   b. Extremities
    c. Genitourinary   d. Sacral area

72. Which is rarest site of spread of colorectal cancer?
 (Recent Pattern 2014-15)
    a. Liver
    b. Lung
    c. Mesentary
    d. Peritoneum
73. Aspirin decreases the risk of development of which of the following: (Recent Pattern 2014-15)
    a. Colorectal cancer
    b. Stomach cancer
    c. Carcinoid
    d. MALToma
74. Most common extra-nodal site for lymphoma is?
 (Recent Pattern 2014-15)
    a. Stomach
    b. Colon
    c. Intestine
    d. Waldeyer ring
75. Lynch syndrome is characterized by:
 (Recent Pattern 2014-15)
    a. One or more case in family of colorectal cancer < 50 years
    b. 2 or more cases in family of polyps
    c. Cancer arising in recto-sigmoid junction
    d. Defect on chromosome 10
76. Most common site of spread of colorectal cancer is?
 (Recent Pattern 2014-15)
    a. Liver
    b. Lung
    c. Brain
    d. Peritoneum
77. Peutz Jehgers syndrome is associated with:
 (Recent Pattern 2014-15)
    a. Ovarian tumor
    b. Brain tumor
    c. Osteoma
    d. Lung cancer
78. Not seen with stomach cancer? (Recent Pattern 2014-15)
    a. Acanthosis Nigricans
    b. Superficial migratory thrombophlebitis
    c. Microangiopathic hemolytic anemia
    d. Polycythemia
79. Most common site of spread of gastric tumor?
 (Recent Pattern 2014-15)
    a. Liver
    b. Ovary
    c. Peritoneum
    d. Blumer shelf
80. Enteropathy type T cell lymphoma is associated with:
 (Recent Pattern 2014-15)
    a. M.A.L.Toma
    b. Celiac Sprue
    c. Menetrier disease
    d. Crohn's disease
81. All are risk factors for development of colorectal cancers except? (Recent Pattern 2014-15)
    a. Intake of vegetable fat
    b. Polyposis coli
    c. IBD
    d. Lynch syndrome
    e. All
82. Tumor exhibiting regression to anti-microbials?
    a. Kaposi sarcoma (Recent Pattern 2014-15)
    b. M.A.L.T.oma
    c. G.I.S.T
    d. Zollinger Ellison syndrome
83. Incorrect about colorectal cancer? (Recent Pattern 2014-15)
    a. Right sided lesions associated with occult bleeding
    b. Left sided lesions associated with tenesmus
    c. Apple core appearance on barium study
    d. Haem-occult is best screening tool
84. Complications of esophageal cancer are all except?
    a. Trachea-esophageal fistula (Recent Pattern 2014-15)
    b. Hypercalcemia
    c. Aspiration pneumonia
    d. Gastric tetany
85. Percentage of blockage of esophagus by cancer to cause symptoms: (Recent Pattern 2014-15)
    a. 30%
    b. 40%
    c. 50%
    d. 60%
86. Not seen with carcinoid is? (Recent Pattern 2014-15)
    a. Peyronie disease
    b. Mitral valve involvement
    c. Cushing disease
    d. Hypertension
87. Flushing is most common seen with?
 (Recent Pattern 2014-15)
    a. Appendiceal carinoid
    b. Midgut carcinoid
    c. Hindgut carcinoid
    d. Gastric carcinoid
88. Most common cardiac lesion in carcinoid syndrome is?
 (Recent Pattern 2014-15)
    a. Tricuspid regurgitation
    b. Pulmonic stenosis
    c. Mitral regurgitation
    d. Aortic stenosis
89. Not used for diagnosis of carcinoid syndrome ?
 (Recent Pattern 2014-15)
    a. Somatostatin receptor scintigraphy
    b. Chromogranin A
    c. Neuron specific enolase
    d. Synaptophysin
90. Most common site of carcinoid tumor leading to carcinoid syndrome? (Recent Pattern 2014-15)
    a. Appendicular carcinoid
    b. Metastatic Midgut carcinoid
    c. Midgut carcinoid
    d. Bronchial carcinoid
91. Drug of choice for carcinoid crisis?
 (Recent Pattern 2014-15)
    a. Methysergide
    b. Cyproheptadine
    c. Octreotide
    d. Kentaserin
92. Most common symptom of carcinoid syndrome is:
 (Recent Pattern 2014-15)
    a. Diarrhea
    b. Flushing
    c. Pellagra
    d. Bronchospasm
93. All are correct about atypical carcinoid except?
 (Recent Pattern 2014-15)
    a. High urinary 5HTP
    b. Seen with foregut carcinoid
    c. Absent dopa decarboxylase
    d. High urinary 5-HIAA
94. Pellagra is seen with: (Recent Pattern 2014-15)
    a. Carcinoid
    b. Phaeochromocytoma
    c. Peutz Jegher syndrome
    d. Cronhkhite Canada syndrome
95. Most common cause of dry tap on bone marrow examination is: (Recent Pattern 2014-15)
    a. Myelofibrosis
    b. Hairy cell leukemia
    c. Cancer infiltration into bone marrow
    d. Chronic myeloid leukemia
96. Most common site of metastasis of Neuro-blastoma?
 (Recent Pattern 2014-15)
    a. Lung
    b. Liver
    c. Bones
    d. Bone marrow
97. Not a clinical feature of Neuroblastoma:
    a. Paraplegia (Recent Pattern 2014-15)
    b. Raccoon eyes
    c. Opsoclonus
    d. Recurrent syncopal attacks

98. **A 2 year old baby with hypertension and increased urinary Homovanillic acid is suggestive of:**
    (Recent Pattern 2014-15)
    a. 11 hydroxylase deficiency
    b. Neuroblastoma
    c. Wilms tumor
    d. Phaeochromocytoma

99. **Gold standard test for neuroblastoma:**
    (Recent Pattern 2014-15)
    a. Immunohistochemistry b. N-myc oncogene
    c. Serum ferritin d. MIBG scan

100. **Most common site of Neuroblastoma?**
    (Recent Pattern 2014-15)
    a. Adrenal gland b. Retroperitoneum
    c. Pelvis d. Cervical area

101. **Not associated with neuroblastoma:**
    (Recent Pattern 2014-15)
    a. Neurofibromatosis b. Hischsprung's disease
    c. Heterochromia d. Defect on chromosome 2

102. **Most common symptom of Wilm's tumour?**
    (Recent Pattern 2014-15)
    a. Abdominal pain b. Hypertension
    c. Hematuria d. Fever

103. **Most common involvement in Histiocytosis?**
    a. Bones *(Recent Pattern 2014-15)*
    b. Skin
    c. Lymph nodes
    d. Liver skin

104. **All of the following are features of tumor lysis syndrome except:**
    (Recent Pattern 2014-15)
    a. Hyperuricemia b. Hyperkalemia
    c. Hyperphosphatemia d. Hypercalcemia

105. **Most common cause of tumor lysis syndrome in children?**
    (Recent Pattern 2014-15)
    a. Burkitt lymphoma b. Acute leukemia
    c. CLL d. Neuroblastoma

106. **Hemangioblastoma associated with VHL are most commonly seen in:** *(Recent Pattern 2014-15)*
    a. Cerebellum b. Liver
    c. Kidney d. Pancreas

107. **Brain tumor showing diffuse infiltration of brain without focal mass:** *(Recent Pattern 2014-15)*
    a. Glioblastoma multiforme
    b. Gliomatosis cerebri
    c. PNET
    d. Meningioma

108. **Cowden syndrome is associated with:**
    a. Medulloblastoma *(Recent Pattern 2014-15)*
    b. Astrocytoma
    c. Dysplastic gangliocytoma
    d. PNET

109. **Most common part of spine involved in malignant spinal cord compression:** *(Recent Pattern 2014-15)*
    a. Cervical b. Thoracic
    c. Lumbar d. Sacral

110. **Chang classification is used for?** *(Recent Pattern 2014-15)*
    a. PNET
    b. Astrocytoma
    c. Pinealoma
    d. Craniopharyngioma

111. **Most common cause of Carcinomatous meningitis:**
    (Recent Pattern 2014-15; Bihar PG 2015)
    a. Carcinoma breast b. Carcinoma lung
    c. Carcinoma gut d. Malignant melanoma

Answers with Explanations

1. Ans. (c) Hypercalcemia

(Ref: Harrison 20th edition, p 519; Harrison 19th edition page 1795)

Tumor lysis syndrome is characterized by:

1. Hyperkalemia (Potassium is a major intracellular cation)
2. Hyperphosphatemia due to release of intracellular phosphate pools
3. *Hypocalcemia* due to reciprocal depression
4. Hyperuricemia (Can lead to urate nephropathy)

In *laboratory tumor lysis syndrome*, two or more metabolic abnormalities must be present during the same 24-hour period within 3 days before the start of therapy or up to 7 days afterward. *Clinical tumor lysis syndrome* requires the presence of laboratory tumor lysis syndrome plus an increased creatinine level, seizures, cardiac dysrhythmia, or death.

Metabolic abnormality	Criteria for classification of laboratory tumor lysis syndrome
Hyperuricemia	Uric acid >8.0 mg/dl (475.8 µmol/liter) in adults or above the upper limit of the normal range for age in children
Hyperphosphatemia	Phosphorus >4.5 mg/dl (1.5 mmol/liter) in adults or >6.5 mg/dl (2.1 mmol/liter) in children

Contd...

Metabolic abnormality	Criteria for classification of laboratory tumor lysis syndrome
Hyperkalemia	Potassium >6.0 mmol/liter
Hypocalcemia	Corrected calcium <7.0 mg/dl (1.75 mmol/liter) or ionized calcium <1.12 (0.3 mmol/liter)
Acute kidney injury	Not applicable

2. Ans. (b) Well to moderately differentiated adenocarcinoma

(Ref: Harrison 20th edition, p 658; Harrison 19th edition, page 120-e:)

Major Histologies in Cancer of unknown primary

Histology	Percentage %
Well to moderately differentiated adenocarcinoma	60
Squamous cell cancer	5
Poorly differentiated adenocarcinoma, poorly differentiated carcinoma	30
Neuroendocrine	2
Undifferentiated malignancy	3

3. Ans. (d) Renal cell carcinoma

(Ref: Harrison 20th edition, p 659; Figure : 88-1; Harrison 19th edition, page 120e-2)

Cytokeratin markers used for assessment of adenocarcinoma of unknown primary

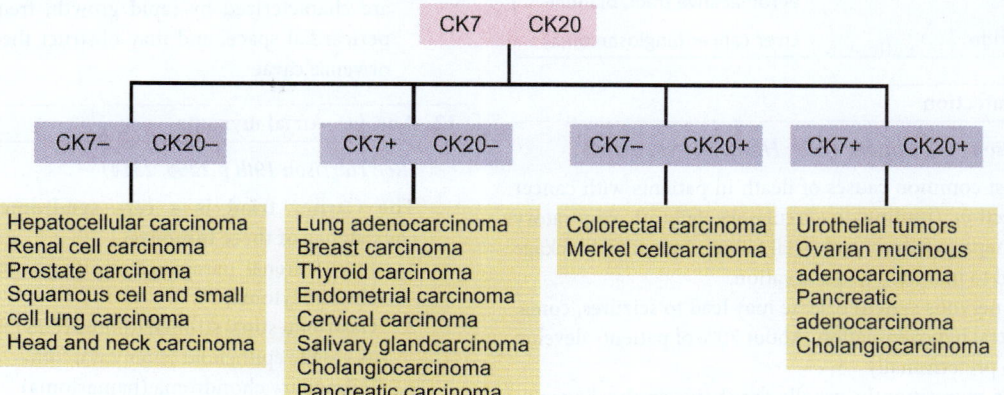

4. Ans. (b) Inter-lobar effusion

(Ref: Harrison 20th edition, p 514; Felson's principles of Radiology: 4th edition, page 205)

- Phantom/ vanishing tumour is a term used for a localized transudative inter-lobar pleural fluid collection in congestive heart failure.
- The name originates from its frequent resemblance to a tumour on the CXR and from its tendency to vanish after appropriate management of heart failure.

5. Ans. (a) Vertebral metastasis

(Ref: Harrison 20th edition, p 514; Harrison 19th, page 1791)

- Malignant spinal cord compression is characterised by compression of spinal cord and/or cauda equina by extra-dural tumour mass.
- The erosion of pedicles is the earliest radiological finding of vertebral tumour and is called winking owl sign. This can lead to development of Cauda Equina Syndrome.

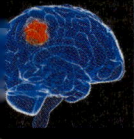

6. Ans. (d) Adult T cell leukemia

(Ref: Harrison 19th p 1268, 70)

Viruses/Agents	Associated Cancer
Human immunodeficiency virus	Non-Hodgkin's lymphoma, Kaposi's sarcoma, squamous cell carcinomas (especially of the urogenital tract)
Human papilloma virus	Cervix cancer, head and neck cancer
Human T cell lymphotropic virus type I (HTLV-I)	Adult T cell leukemia/lymphoma
Immunosuppressive agents (azathioprine, cyclosporine, glucocorticoids)	Non-Hodgkin's lymphoma
Ionizing radiation	Breast, bladder, thyroid, soft tissue, bone, hematopoietic
Nitrogen mustard gas	Cancer of the lung, head and neck, nasal sinuses
Nickel dust	Cancer of the lung, nasal sinuses
Phenacetin	Cancer of the renal pelvis and bladder
Polycyclic hydrocarbons	Cancer of the lung, skin (especially squamous cell carcinoma of scrotal skin)
Schistosomiasis	Bladder cancer (squamous cell)
Sunlight (ultraviolet)	Skin cancer (squamous cell and melanoma)
Tobacco	Cancer of the upper aerodigestive tract, bladder
Vinyl chloride	Liver cancer (angiosarcoma)

7. Ans. (b) Infection

(Ref: Harrison 20th edition, p 502; Harrison 19th p 484)

- The most common causes of death in patients with cancer are infection (leading to circulatory failure), respiratory failure, hepatic failure, and renal failure. Intestinal blockage may lead to inanition and starvation.
- Central nervous system disease may lead to seizures, coma, and central hypoventilation. About 70% of patients develop dyspnea preterminally.
- However, many months usually pass between the diagnosis of cancer and the occurrence of these complications, and during this period the patient is severely affected by the possibility of death

8. Ans. (a) Lung cancer

(Ref: Harrison 20th edition, p 435, Table 65-1; Harrison 19th p 470, 471; Table 99-2)

- Lung cancer constitutes upto 29% of all cancer related deaths in males and 26% of all cancer related death in women.

9. Ans. (c) Colorectal cancer

(Ref: Harrison 20th edition, p 574; Harrison 19th p 104-3, 486)

Cancer	Organisms Causing Infection related mortality
Chronic lymphocytic leukemia	S. pneumoniae, H. influenzae, N. meningitidis
Hairy cell leukemia	Intracellular pathogens (M. tuberculosis, Listeria, Cryptococcus, M. avium
Multiple myeloma	Streptococcus pneumoniae
Colon and rectal tumors	Streptococcus bovis (bacteremia)

10. Ans. (a) Age

(Ref: Harrison 20th edition, p 435; Harrison 19th p 467)

The most significant risk factor for cancer overall is age; two-thirds of all cases were in those older than age 65 years. Cancer incidence increases as the third, fourth, or fifth power of age in different sites

11. Ans. (a) Angiosarcoma

(Ref: Harrison 20th edition, p 1849; Harrison 19th p 289e)

- Almost all primary cardiac malignancies are sarcomas, which may be of several histologic types.
- In general, these tumors are characterized by rapid progression that culminates in the patient's death within weeks to months from the time of presentation as a result of hemodynamic compromise, local invasion, or distant metastases.
- Sarcomas commonly involve the right side of the heart, are characterized by rapid growth, frequently invade the pericardial space, and may obstruct the cardiac chambers or venae cavae

12. Ans. (a) Atrial myxoma

(Ref: Harrison 19th p 2266, 2314)

The Carney triad is a rare syndrome defined by the coexistence of three tumours:
1. Extra-adrenal paraganglioma (e.g. extra adrenal phaeochromocytoma)
2. Gastrointestinal stromal tumors (GIST): previously known as gastric epithelioid leiomyosarcoma
3. Pulmonary chondroma (hamartoma)

In most cases, only 2 of the 3 tumours are present at the time of diagnosis. It typically affects young people.

Carney complex is an autosomal dominant syndrome associated with spotty pigmentation of the skin, endocrinopathy, and endocrine and nonendocrine tumors, including the following:
1. Myxomas of the skin, heart, breast, and other sites
2. Primary pigmented nodular adrenocortical disease
3. Psammomatous melanotic schwannomas
4. Growth hormone–producing pituitary adenomas
5. Testicular Sertoli-cell tumors

6. Possibly, other benign and malignant neoplasms and conditions, including tumors of the thyroid gland and ductal adenomas of the breast, as well as acromegaly due to somatomammotroph hyperplasia and adenomas not dependent on growth hormone–releasing hormone.

13. Ans. (c) Myasthenic syndrome

(Ref: Harrison 20th edition, p 1847; Harrison 19th p 2265t)

- The LAMB syndrome is characterized by presence of Lentigines, Atrial Myxoma, and Blue nevi.
- Certain constellations of findings have been referred to as the NAME syndrome (Nevi, Atrial myxoma, Myxoid neurofibroma, and Ephelides).

14. Ans. (b) Rhabdomyosarcoma

(Ref: Harrison 20th edition, p 1849; Nelson 18th ed., ch. 441)

Primary malignant cardiac tumors in children are almost exclusively sarcomas. These tumors are usually located in the right side of the heart, atrial septum, right atrial wall, or root of the pulmonary artery. They may extend either into the adjacent chamber and cause obstruction to blood flow or into the pericardial cavity and produce effusion or tamponade

15. Ans. (c) Tumour plop in systole

(Ref: Harrison 20th edition, p 1847-8; Harrison 19th p 289e)

- Tumour plop sound is a low pitch sound heard in diastole when the tumour impacts against the opening mitral valve.
- The characteristic low-pitched sound, a "tumor plop," may be appreciated on auscultation during early or mid-diastole and is thought to result from the impact of the tumor against the mitral valve or ventricular wall.
- Myxomas may also present with peripheral or pulmonary emboli or with constitutional signs and symptoms, including fever, weight loss, cachexia, malaise, arthralgias, rash, digital clubbing, Raynaud's phenomenon, hypergammaglobulinemia, anemia, polycythemia, leukocytosis, elevated erythrocyte sedimentation rate, thrombocytopenia, and thrombocytosis.
- It is more common in females.

16. Ans. (a) Papillary fibroelastoma

(Ref: Harrison 20th edition, p 1848; Harrison 19th p 289e)

- Most common tumor of heart valves in papillary fibroelastoma.
- PF are generally small and single, occur most often on valvular surfaces, and may be mobile, resulting in embolization. Because of the potential for embolic events, symptomatic patients, patients undergoing cardiac surgery for other lesions, and those with highly mobile and large PF should be considered for surgical excision.

17. Ans. (a) Rhabdomyoma

(Ref: Harrison 20th edition, p 1848; Nelson 18th ed., ch. 441)

The most common benign cardiac tumors in children are rhabdomyomas, fibromas, and myxomas. Rhabdomyomas occur as single or, usually, multiple nodules embedded in chamber walls. They often remain clinically unimportant and regress with age, but they may cause mechanical obstruction, heart failure, or arrhythmias. They may be familial and are often found in association with Gorlin syndrome or tuberous sclerosis

18. Ans. (a) Inter-atrial septum

(Ref: Harrison 20th edition, p 1847; Harrison 19th p 289e)

- Most atrial myxomas are solitary, are located in the atria (particularly the left atrium, where they usually arise from the interatrial septum in the vicinity of the fossa ovalis), and are often pedunculated on a fibrovascular stalk.
- In contrast to sporadic tumors, familial or syndromic tumors tend to occur in younger individuals, are often multiple, may be ventricular in location, and are more likely to recur after initial resection

19. Ans. (c) Small cell carcinoma of lung

(Ref: Harrison 20th edition, p 542; Harrison 19th p 511)

- Skeletal–connective tissue syndromes include clubbing in 30% of cases (usually NSCLCs) and hypertrophic primary osteoarthropathy in 1–10% of cases (usually adenocarcinomas).
- Clubbing is not seen with the most aggressive lung cancer i.e. small cell lung cancer.

20. Ans. (b) Wasting of muscles of hand

(Ref: Harrison 20th edition, p 541, 3223; Harrison 19th p 510-11)

Pancoast syndrome is characterized by a malignant neoplasm of the superior sulcus of the lung with destructive lesions of the thoracic inlet and involvement of the brachial plexus and cervical sympathetic nerves (stellate ganglion). This is accompanied by the following:

1. Severe pain in the shoulder region radiating toward the axilla and scapula along the ulnar aspect of the muscles of the hand. This is due to involvement of the eighth cervical and first and second thoracic nerves, with shoulder pain that characteristically radiates in the ulnar distribution of the arm,
2. Radiologic destruction of the first and second ribs
3. Atrophy of hand and arm muscles
4. Horner syndrome (ptosis, miosis, hemianhidrosis, enophthalmos)
5. Compression of the blood vessels with edema

- Most Pancoast tumors are adenocarcinomas >> squamous cell carcinomas.
- Involvement of the phrenic or recurrent laryngeal nerve or superior vena cava obstruction is not representative of the classic Pancoast tumor

21. Ans. (b) Bronchial adenoma

(Ref: Nelson 18th ed., ch. 408)

- Bronchial adenoma and carcinoid are the most common primary tumors.

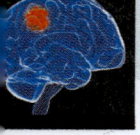

- Metastatic lesions are overall the most common forms of pulmonary malignancy in children; primary processes include Wilm's tumor, osteogenic sarcoma, and hepatoblastoma. Adenocarcinoma and undifferentiated histology are the most common pathologic findings in primary lung cancer; pulmonary blastoma is rarer and frequently occurs in the setting of cystic lung disease

22. Ans. (c) Oat cell variant presents as an endobronchial growth

(Ref: Harrison 19th p 508)

- Small cell carcinoma is a poorly differentiated neuroendocrine tumor that tends to occur as a central mass with endo-bronchial growth and is strongly associated with smoking. Small cell carcinoma cells have scant cytoplasm, small hyperchromatic nuclei with a fine ("salt and pepper") chromatin pattern and prominent nucleoli
- Cavitation is associated with squamous cell cancer. The pathogenesis of cavitary malignancies has not been fully elucidated. It has been postulated that cavity formation in tumors is a consequence of rapid tumor growth which exceeds the supporting blood supply resulting in tumor necrosis and cavitation.
- Most common lung cancer on global basis is adenocarcinoma and it presents as a peripheral growth.

23. Ans. (c) Bronchogenic carcinoma

(Ref: Harrison 19th p 511/609)

- Ectopic ACTH production is predominantly caused by occult carcinoid tumors, most frequently in the lung, but also in thymus or pancreas.
- Advanced small cell lung cancer can cause ectopic ACTH production. In rare cases, ectopic ACTH production has been found to originate from medullary thyroid carcinoma or pheochromocytoma, the latter co-secreting catecholamines and ACTH.

24. Ans. (c) Epidermal Growth Factor Receptor Tyrosine Kinase Inhibitors (EGFR-TKI) such as erlotinib have proven active in previously treated patients with advanced NSCLC

(Ref: Harrison 20th edition, p 548-552; Harrison 19th p 516-17)

- Erlotinib and gefitinib are oral small-molecule kinase inhibitors that inhibit signaling via EGFR. These were the first EGFR inhibitors to be approved for the treatment of patients with NSCLC
- Clinical features that have been shown to correlate with responsiveness to EGFR TKI treatment include female sex, never smoking status, adenocarcinoma histology, and Asian ethnicity. Somatic mutations in the kinase domain of EGFR and high EGFR copy number have also been shown to correlate with response and improved survival with oral EGFR inhibitors.
- NSCLC had an improved survival when treated with cisplatin and pemetrexed compared to cisplatin and gemcitabine, while patients with squamous carcinoma had an improved survival when treated with cisplatin and gemcitabine

25. Ans. (d) Hypoglycemia

(Ref: Harrison 19th p 511/609)

- Paraneoplastic syndromes are common in patients with lung cancer, especially those with SCLC, and may be the presenting finding or the first sign of recurrence.

Endocrinological Profiles of Lung Cancer Patients
1. Hypercalcemia resulting from ectopic production of parathyroid hormone (PTH)
2. Hyponatremia may be caused by the Syndrome of Inappropriate Secretion of Anti Diuretic Hormone (SIADH) or possibly Atrial Natriuretic Peptide (ANP).
3. Ectopic secretion of ACTH by SCLC and pulmonary carcinoids usually results in additional electrolyte disturbances, especially hypokalemia, rather than the changes in body habitus that occur in Cushing's syndrome from a pituitary adenoma.
4. Clubbing in 30% of cases (usually NSCLCs)
5. Hypertrophic primary osteoarthropathy (usually adenocarcinomas).

Neurologic–Myopathic Syndromes Include
1. Myasthenic Eaton-Lambert syndrome
2. Retinal blindness with SCLC
3. Peripheral neuropathies
4. Subacute cerebellar degeneration
5. Cortical degeneration
6. Polymyositis
7. Paraneoplastic encephalomyelitis and sensory neuropathies, cerebellar degeneration, limbic encephalitis, and brainstem encephalitis occur in SCLC

Coagulation, Thrombotic, or other Hematologic Manifestations
1. Migratory venous thrombophlebitis (Trousseau's syndrome)
2. Nonbacterial thrombotic (marantic) endocarditis with arterial emboli
3. Disseminated intravascular coagulation with hemorrhage
4. Anemia
5. Granulocytosis

Cutaneous Manifestations such as
1. Dermatomyositis
2. Acanthosis nigricans

Renal Manifestations
1. Nephrotic syndrome
2. Glomerulonephritis

26. Ans. (d) 80-90% of small cell carcinomas have spread beyond the thorax at the time of diagnosis

(Ref: Harrison 19th p 508, 11)

Since small cell cancer exhibits micro-metastasis it can disseminate to multiple organs like adrenal> Brain> bones> liver

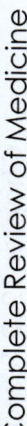

27. Ans. (d) CA Lung

(Ref: CMDT-2014, ch. 39, pg. 1597)

Diagnosis of lung cancer rests on examination of a tissue or cytology specimen
1. Sputum cytology is highly specific but insensitive; the yield is highest when there are lesions in the central airways.
2. Thoracocentesis (sensitivity 50–65%) can be used to establish a diagnosis of lung cancer in patients with malignant pleural effusions. If cytologic examination of an adequate sample (50–100 mL) of pleural fluid is nondiagnostic, the procedure should be repeated; approximately 30% of second samples are positive when the first sample is negative.
3. If results remain negative, thoracoscopy is preferred to blind pleural biopsy.
4. Fine-needle aspiration (FNA) of palpable supraclavicular or cervical lymph nodes is frequently diagnostic.
5. Serum tumor markers are neither sensitive nor specific enough to aid in diagnosis.

28. Ans. (b) Oat cell carcinoma

(Ref: Harrison 19th p 511)

- Para-neoplastic syndromes are common in patients with lung cancer, especially those with SCLC, and may be the presenting finding or the first sign of recurrence.
- The ectopic ACTH production can lead to development of Cushing syndrome and resultant hyperglycemia.
- In addition, paraneoplastic syndromes may mimic metastatic disease and, unless detected, lead to inappropriate palliative rather than curative treatment

29. Ans. (b) Small cell carcinoma

(Ref: Harrison 19th p 522)

- There is currently no role for adjuvant radiation therapy in patients following resection of stage I or II NSCLC.
- Patients with SCLC are treated with combined modality therapy with cisplatin and etoposide chemotherapy and radiation therapy. Small cell cancer of lung is both chemosensitive and radiosensitive.

30. Ans. (b) Adenocarcinoma

(Ref: Harrison 19th p 522)

- Adenocarcinomas often occur in more peripheral lung locations and may be associated with a history of smoking.
- However, adenocarcinomas are the most common type of lung cancer occurring in never smokers.
- Bronchioloalveolar carcinoma (BAC) is a subtype of adenocarcinoma that grows along the alveoli without invasion and can present radiographically as a single mass, as a diffuse multinodular lesion, as a fluffy infiltrate, and on CT scans as a "ground-glass" opacity

31. Ans. (a) Adenocarcinoma

(Ref: Harrison 19th p 1689)

- Lung cancer is the most common cancer associated with asbestos exposure. The excess frequency of lung cancer (all histologic types) in asbestos workers is associated with a minimum latency of 15–20 years between first exposure and development of the disease. Adenocarcinoma of lung is most common cancer seen in asbestosis, while mesothelioma is seen but is less common.
- Mesotheliomas both pleural and peritoneal, are also associated with asbestos exposure. In contrast to lung cancers, these tumors are less common.

32. Ans. (d) Squamous cell carcinoma

(Ref: BAILEY AND LOVE 26th ed., pg. 861 and DeVita 8th ed.,ch. 37)

33. Ans. (b) Growth hormone

(Ref: Harrison 19th p 511)

34. Ans. (a) Dilated veins have blood flow away from umbilicus

(Ref: Harrison 20th edition, p 511; Harrison 19th p 1787-88)

Patients with SVCS usually Present with
1. Neck and facial swelling (especially around the eyes)
2. Dyspnea, and cough.
3. Hoarseness, tongue swelling, headaches, nasal congestion, epistaxis, hemoptysis, dysphagia, pain, dizziness, syncope, and lethargy.
4. The characteristic physical findings are dilated neck veins; an increased number of collateral veins covering the anterior chest wall; cyanosis; and edema of the face, arms, and chest. More severe cases include proptosis, glossal and laryngeal edema, and obtundation.
5. Dilated veins have blood flow towards the umbilicus. (dilated veins around umbilicus with flow away is seen in portal hypertension.)
6. Bending forward or lying down may aggravate the symptoms.
7. The clinical picture is milder if the obstruction is located above the azygos vein. Symptoms are usually progressive, but in some cases they may improve as collateral circulation develops.

35. Ans. (b) Hypercalcemia

(Ref: Harrison 20th edition, p 2924-5; 2930 Harrison 19th p 2469/247)

- Squamous cell carcinoma is associated with release of PTH-rp leading to hypercalcemia.
- Acute hypercalcemia crisis can present with delirium
- QT interval in ECG is inversely related to calcium values.
- Endocrine syndromes are seen in 12% of patients; Hypercalcemia resulting from ectopic production of parathyroid hormone (PTH), or more commonly, PTH-related peptide, is the most common life-threatening metabolic complication of malignancy.
  - Hyponatremia is ruled out as ECG findings are not seen with it.

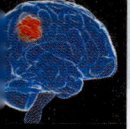

36. Ans. (a) Pulmonary hamartoma

(Ref: Harrison 19th p 515)

- Lung hamartomas are usually peripheral lung masses composed of normal pulmonary tissue components such as smooth muscle and collagen.
- They are more common in men than in women and have a peak incidence in the 60s.
- They are often incidental radiographic findings as solitary nodules. They have a pathognomonic "popcorn" pattern of calcification in some cases; however, without such a finding, resection is necessary to rule out malignancy, especially in smokers

37. Ans. (a) Anti P/Q antibodies

(Ref: Harrison 20th edition, p 3235; Harrison 19th p 2703)

- Anti Hu antibody is seen with SCLC leading to encephalomyelitis
- Anti– Jo-1 antibody is seen with dermatomyositis
- Anti–GQ1 antibody is seen with Miller Fisher syndrome

38. Ans. (d) Oat cell carcinoma

(Ref: Harrison's 18th ed., ch. 100, pg. 738)

Small cell carcinomas, more often than non-small cell carcinomas, may produce specific peptide hormones such as
1. Adrenocorticotrophic hormone (ACTH)
2. Arginine vasopressin (AVP)
3. Atrial natriuretic factor (ANF)
4. Gastrin-releasing peptide (GRP).

39. Ans. (b) Causes radicular pain in upper limb

(Ref: Harrison 20th edition, p 541; Harrison 19th p 510-511)

Pancoast Syndrome Results from
1. Local extension of a tumor growing in the apex of the lung
2. Involvement of the eighth cervical and first and second thoracic nerves, with shoulder pain that characteristically radiates in the ulnar distribution of the arm
3. Radiologic destruction of the first and second ribs.
   - Pancoast tumors typically present as an insidious onset of pain in the upper arm, sensory disturbance in the medial aspect of the forearm and hand, and weakness and atrophy of the intrinsic hand muscles along with an ipsilateral Horner syndrome.
   - Chest CT scans or MRI can demonstrate extension of the tumor into the plexus. Metastatic involvement of the brachial plexus may occur with spread of breast cancer into the axillary lymph nodes with local spread into the nearby nerves.

40. Ans. (b) 5%

(Ref: Bailey and Love 26th ed., pg. 861)

Five-year Survival According to Cell Type	
Squamous cell carcinoma	35–50%
Adenocarcinoma	25–45%
Adenosquamous carcinoma	20–35%
Undifferentiated carcinoma	15–25%
Small cell carcinoma	0–5%

41. Ans. (b) Progressive multifocal leukoencephalopathy

(Ref: Harrison 20th edition, p 668, Table 90-1; Harrison 19th p 614)

Paraneoplastic Syndromes of the Nervous System
Classic Syndromes: Usually Occur with Cancer Association
1. Encephalomyelitis
2. Limbic encephalitis
3. Cerebellar degeneration
4. Opsoclonus – myoclonus
5. Subacute sensory neuronopathy
6. Gastrointestinal paresis or pseudo – obstruction Dermatomyositis (adults) Lambert – Eaton myasthenic syndrome

Nonclassic Syndromes: May Occur with/or without Cancer Association
1. Brainstem encephalitis
2. Stiff – person syndrome
3. Necrotizing myelopathy
4. Motor neuron disease
5. Guillain – Barre syndrome
6. Subacute and chronic mixed sensory – motor neuropathies
7. Neuropathy associated with plasma cell dyscarias and lymphoma

42. Ans. (b) Adenocarcinoma

(Ref: Harrison's 18th ed., ch. 89, pg 738)

- Squamous carcinoma was the most commonly diagnosed form of NSCLC; however, with the steady decline in cigarette consumption over the past four decades and changes in cigarette manufacturing (including use of different types of filters), adenocarcinoma has replaced squamous cell carcinoma as the most frequent histologic subtype
- The incidence of small cell carcinoma is also on the decline. In lifetime never smokers, all histologic forms of lung cancer can be found, although adenocarcinoma tends to predominate. Among women and young adults (<60 years), adenocarcinoma tends to be the most common form of lung cancer.

43. Ans. (b) Chronic cough

(Ref: Harrison's 18th ed., ch. 89)

- Bronchial adenoma is a centrally located slow-growing endobronchial lesions that are generally carcinoid tumors. Most common presentation is asymptomatic.
- Mean age at presentation is 45 years.
- Patients often give a history of chronic cough, intermittent hemoptysis, or repeated episodes of airway obstruction with atelectasis, or pneumonias with abscess formation due to endobronchial lesions obstructing the airway.
- In all textbooks cough is mentioned first and pubmed search also mentioned cough as 18% and hemoptysis as 17%.
- They are usually visible at bronchoscopy but are highly vascular and may bleed profusely after a bronchoscopic biopsy. They are largely curable by surgical resection (local excision), but they may recur locally or become invasive and metastasize

44. Ans. (a) Hamartoma

(Ref: Harrison's 18th ed., ch. 89)

Pulmonary hamartomas are usually asymptomatic and are typically discovered as an incidental coin lesion on a routine chest radiograph. On chest radiographs, pulmonary hamartomas characteristically appear as well-defined, solitary pulmonary nodules; they may show varying patterns of calcification, including an irregular popcorn, stippled, or curvilinear pattern, or even a combination of all 3 patterns. Calcification that is detectable on plain radiography is reported to occur in 10-15% of patients.

45. Ans. (a) Weight loss

(Ref: Harrison 20th edition, p 541, Table 74-4; Harrison 19th p 510; Table 107-4)

- Most common symptom of lung cancer is cough (not given in choices) followed by weight loss.
- Symptoms of lung cancer (incidence wise) cough> weight loss > dysnea> chest pain> hemoptysis.

46. Ans. (b) Coronary ostial occlusion

(Ref: Harrison's 18th ed., ch. 89, pg. 750, 3471)

- The pain in Horner syndrome is chronic and is present in arm and shoulder. In coronary ostial occlusion, myocardial infarction will ensue and the resultant pain will be acute in onset.
- Cervical spondylosis will cause neurogenic claudication while cervical rib can cause vascular claudication leading to arm pain on chronic basis
- Chronic stable angina presents with chronic chest pain radiating to medial left arm.

47. Ans. (a) Stiff person syndrome

(Ref: Harrison 20th edition, p 668, Table 90-2; Harrison 19th p 614; Table 122-2)

- Antibodies associated with the stiff-person syndrome target proteins (GAD, amphiphysin) involved in the function of inhibitory synapses utilizing gamma-aminobutyric acid (GABA) or glycine as neurotransmitters.
- Paraneoplastic stiff-person syndrome and amphiphysin antibodies are often related to SCLC and breast cancer.
- This disorder is characterized by progressive muscle rigidity, stiffness, and painful spasms triggered by auditory, sensory, or emotional stimuli. Rigidity mainly involves the lower trunk and legs, but it can affect the upper extremities and neck.
- Symptoms improve with sleep and general anesthetics.
- Electro-physiological studies demonstrate continuous motor unit activity.

48. Ans. (a) Bellini tumor

(Ref: Harrison 20th edition, p 616)

49. Ans. (b) Papillary carcinoma

(Ref: Devita, Hellman & Rosenberg's Cancer: Principles & Practice of Oncology, 8th ed., ch. 40 - Cancers of the Genitourinary System, Section 3: Cancer of the Kidney)

The risk of developing kidney cancer has been estimated to be greater than 30 times higher in dialysis patients with cystic changes in their kidney than in the general population.

- The second most common histopathological subtype (Papillary carcinoma) has been found to be the commonest one in patients on kidney dialysis.
- It is estimated that 35% to 47% of patients on long-term dialysis will develop acquired cystic disease, and that about 5.8% of the patients with acquired cystic disease will develop renal cancer.
- Kidney cancer can develop at any time in patients with end-stage renal disease, and it can also occur in kidney transplant recipients. Kidney cancer can occur in patients with end-stage renal disease who are undergoing either hemodialysis or chronic ambulatory dialysis

50. Ans. (b) Sorafenib

(Ref: Harrison 20th edition, p 494, Table 69-5)

Drug	Acts against	Mechanism of action
Sorafenib	RCC; hepatocellular carcinoma	Targets VEGFR pathways in RCC. Possible activity against BRAF in melanoma, colon cancer, and others

- Erlotinib is used in GIST and CML
- Bortezomib is used in multiple myeloma
- Cetuximab is used in colon cancer

51. Ans. (d) Fever

(Ref: Harrison 20th edition, p 617; Harrison 19th p 578)

- The classic triad in RCC is seen in 10-20% cases only and consists of hematuria, abdominal pain and abdominal mass
- Fever weight loss and anemia are associated features but not included in triad
- Anemia is more common than eythrocytosis as paraneoplastic manifestation.

52. Ans. (b) Chromosome 7

(Ref: Harrison 20th edition, p 617; Harrison 19th p 578)

53. Ans. (a) Urothelial tumor

(Ref: Harrison 20th edition, p 620)

Polychronotropism is seen in urothelial tumors as tendency to recur over time and in new locations along the urothelial tract

54. Ans. (d) Most common malignant tumor of abdomen of childhood

(Ref: Nelson 18th ed., ch. 499)

Wilm's Tumour accounts for approximately 6% of pediatric cancers and is the second most common malignant abdominal tumor in childhood.

(Ref: Harrison 20th edition, p 616)

- Beckwith-Wiedemann syndrome is characterized by hemihypertrophy, macroglossia, and visceromegaly, with a 3–5% risk of developing Wilm's tumor
- Wilm's tumor usually presents as an abdominal mass. It generally is discovered while bathing the infant. Some patients may present with abdominal pain and vomiting, and hematuria is seen in 12–25% of patients. Hypertension is also seen and is probably is due to renal ischemia

55. Ans. (a) Multi-cystic dysplastic kidney

(*Ref: Nelson textbook 18 th ed., ch. 537*)

- Multicystic dysplastic kidney is the most common cause of an abdominal mass in the newborn.
- In most cases it is discovered incidentally during prenatal sonography. In some individuals, the cysts are identified prenatally or postnatally, but no renal tissue is identified because of cyst regression in utero.
- Contralateral hydronephrosis is present in 5–10% of patients.
- Sonography shows the characteristic appearance of a kidney replaced by multiple cysts of varying sizes that do not communicate, and no identifiable parenchyma is present; the diagnosis should be confirmed with a renal scan, which should demonstrate nonfunction. Obtaining a voiding cystourethrogram also is advisable, because 15% of patients have contralateral reflux. Management is controversial

56. Ans. (a) Painless profuse intermittent haematuria

(*Ref: Harrison 20th edition, p 617; Harrison 19th p 576*)

- Hematuria occurs in 80–90% of patients of bladder cancer and often reflects exophytic tumors. The bladder is the most common source of gross hematuria (40%), but benign cystitis (22%) is a more common cause than bladder cancer (15%).
- Microscopic hematuria is more commonly of prostate origin (25%); only 2% of bladder cancers produce microscopic hematuria

57. Ans. (a) Oncocytoma

(*Ref: Devita, Hellman & Rosenberg's Cancer: Principles & Practice of Oncology, 8th ed., ch. 40 - Cancers of the Genitourinary System, Section 3: Cancer of the Kidney, Harrison 19th p 578*)

Renal oncocytoma, which consists predominantly of eosinophilic cells in a characteristic nested or organoid pattern, is considered to be predominantly a benign lesion.

Tumor of kidney	Origin	Remarks
Clear cell carcinoma	PCT	Most common kidney tumour
Papillary carcinoma	DCT	Most common kidney tumour in dialysis patients
Chromophobe adenoma	Intercalcating cells CD	Must be differentiated from oncocytoma
Bellini tumour	Collecting duct	Most aggressive though 1-3% of all kidney tumours
Oncocytoma	Intercalcating cells CD. An oncocytoma is an epithelial tumor composed of oncocytes, large eosinophilic cells having small, round, benign-appearing nuclei with large nucleoli with excessive amounts of mitochondria	Benign

58. Ans. (c) IL-6

(*Ref: Practical Urology: Essential Principles and Practice: Essential Principles By Christopher R. Chapple, William D. Steers: page 234.*)

Stauffer syndrome is a transient hepatic dysfunction of obstructive variety linked to renal cell carcinoma and IL-6 plays a pathological role.

59. Ans. None

(*Ref: Harrison 20th edition, p 617; Harrison 19th p 578/614*)

- Most cases of RCC are diagnosed incidentally on radiographic investigation done for other reasons.
- The classic triad of hematuria, abdominal pain, and a palpable mass is present in 10% of cases
- A spectrum of paraneoplastic syndromes has been associated with these malignancies, including erythrocytosis, hypercalcemia, nonmetastatic hepatic dysfunction (Stauffer syndrome), and acquired dysfibrinogenemia. Erythrocytosis is noted at presentation in only about 3% of patients. Anemia, a sign of advanced disease, is more common.
- Renal cancers have been called "the internist's tumor" and are among the great mimics in medicine because they present with systemic symptoms unrelated to the kidney cancer, such as hypertension (renin), hypercalcemia (PTHrP), polycythemia (erythropoietin), eosinophilia, leukemoid reactions, Cushing's syndrome (ACTH), fever or wasting syndromes, and Stauffer's syndrome (reversible hepatic dysfunction after primary tumor removal). Some books wrongly answer as Cushing Syndrome.

60. Ans. (b) Hepato cellular carcinoma

(*Ref: Harrison 20th edition, p 579f, 580*)

Factors Associated with an Increased Risk of Developing HCC

Common	Unusual
Cirrhosis from any cause	Primary biliary cirrhosis
Hepatitis B or C chronic infection	Hemochromatosis

Contd...

Common	Unusual
Ethanol chronic consumption	α1 Antitrypsin deficiency
NASH/NAFL	Glycogen storage diseases
Aflatoxin B1 or other mycotoxins	Citrullinemia, Porphyria cutanea tarda, Hereditary tyrosinemia, Wilson's disease

61. Ans. (a) Metastasis

(Ref: Robbins 8th ed., pg 663-666)

62. Ans. (b) Hepatitis B

(Ref: Harrison 20th edition, p 578; Harrison 19th p 544)

63. Ans. (b) HCC

(Ref: Harrison's 18th ed., ch. 100)

Hepatic Tumors have been reported to produce excessive amounts of insulin-like growth factor type II (IGF-II) precursor, which binds weakly to insulin receptors and strongly to IGF-I receptors, leading to insulin-like actions.

Tumors showing similiar actions are
1. Mesenchymal tumors
2. Hemangiopericytomas
3. Hepatocellular tumors
4. Adrenal carcinomas

64. Ans. (a) Fibrolamellar hepatoma

(Ref: Harrison 20th edition, p 590)

The fibrolamellar variant of HCC has a quite different biology than adult-type HCC.
- It is multifocal in the liver, and therefore not resectable, metastases are common, especially to lungs and locoregional lymph nodes, but survival is often much better than with adult-type HCC. Resectable tumors are associated with 5-year survival >50%

65. Ans. (a) Hepatoma

(Ref: Harrison's 18th ed., ch. 92)

Adenomas are associated with contraceptive hormone use.
- They can cause pain and can bleed or rupture, causing acute problems.
- Their main interest for the physician is a low potential for malignant change and a 30% risk of bleeding.
- On discovery of a liver mass, patients are usually advised to stop taking sex steroids, as adenoma regression may then occasionally occur.
- Adenomas can often be large masses ranging from 8–15 cm. Due to their size and definite, but low, malignant potential and potential for bleeding, adenomas are typically resected.

Three common benign tumors occur and all are found predominantly in women. They are hemangiomas, adenomas, and focal nodular hyperplasia (F.N.H). F.N.H is typically benign, and usually no treatment is needed. Hemangiomas are the most common and are entirely benign. Treatment is unnecessary unless their expansion causes symptoms. The most useful diagnostic differentiating tool is a triphasic CT scan performed with H.C.C fast bolus protocol for arterial-phase imaging, together with subsequent delayed venous-phase imaging.

66. Ans. (c) Brain cancer

(Ref: Harrison 20th edition, p 193, 672; Harrison 19th p 618)

- Opsoclonus is a disorder of eye movement characterized by involuntary, chaotic saccades that occur in all directions of gaze; it is frequently associated with myoclonus and ataxia.
- Opsoclonus-myoclonus may be cancer-related or idiopathic.
- When the cause is paraneoplastic, the tumors involved are usually cancer of the lung and breast in adults and neuroblastoma in children

67. Ans. (a) Peripheral nerve excitability

(Ref: Harrison 20th edition, p 673-674; Harrison 19th p 619)

- Peripheral nerve hyperexcitability (neuromyotonia, or Isaacs' syndrome) is characterized by spontaneous and continuous muscle fiber activity of peripheral nerve origin. Clinical features include cramps, muscle twitching (fasciculations or myokymia), stiffness, delayed muscle relaxation (pseudomyotonia), and spontaneous or evoked carpal or pedal spasms.
- The electromyogram (EMG) shows fibrillations; fasciculations; and doublet, triplet, or multiplet single-unit (myokymic) discharges that have a high intraburst frequency.
- Approximately 20% of patients have serum antibodies to Caspr2-related proteins.

68. Ans. (a) Rhabdo-myosarcoma

(Ref: Nelson 18th ed., ch. 500)

- Most common soft tissue tumour of childhood = Rhabdomyosarcoma
- Most common soft tissue tumour of Adolescence = Rhabdomyosarcoma
- Most common soft tissue tumour of Adults = Lipoma
- Most common malignant soft tissue tumour of adults = malignant fibrous histiocytoma

69. Ans. (d) Fibrous histiocytoma

(Ref: Harrison 20th edition, p 654)

70. Ans. (a) Alveolar type

(Ref: Nelson 18th ed., ch. 500)

There are four recognized histologic subtypes of Rhabdomyosarcoma.
1. The embryonal type accounts for about 60% of all cases and has an intermediate prognosis.

2. The botryoid type, a variant of the embryonal form in which tumor cells and an edematous stroma project into a body cavity like a bunch of grapes, is found most often in the vagina, uterus, bladder, nasopharynx, and middle ear.
3. The alveolar type accounts for about 15% of cases and often is characterized by 2;13 or 1;13 chromosomal translocations. The tumor cells tend to grow in cores that often have cleft-like spaces resembling alveoli. Alveolar tumors occur most often in the trunk and extremities and carry the poorest prognosis.
4. The pleomorphic type (adult form) is rare in childhood and accounts for only 1% of cases.

71. Ans. (a) Head and neck

(Ref: Harrison's 18th ed., ch. 500)

Rhabdomyosarcoma may occur at virtually any anatomic site but usually are found in the head and neck (25%), genitourinary tract (22%), extremities (18%); retroperitoneal and other sites account for the remainder of primary sites.

72. Ans. (b) Lung

(Ref: Harrison 20th edition, p576; Harrison 19th p 541)

In general, colorectal cancer rarely spreads to the lungs, supraclavicular lymph nodes, bone, or brain without prior spread to the liver.
A major exception to this rule occurs in patients having primary tumors in the distal rectum, from which tumor cells may spread through the paravertebral venous plexus, escaping the portal venous system and thereby reaching the lungs or supraclavicular lymph nodes without hepatic involvement

73. Ans. (a) Colorectal cancer

(Ref: Harrison 20th edition, p 574)

- The most effective class of chemo-preventive agents for colorectal cancer is aspirin and other NSAIDs, which are thought to suppress cell proliferation by inhibiting prostaglandin synthesis.
- Regular aspirin use reduces the risk of colon adenomas and carcinomas as well as death from large-bowel cancer; such use also appears to diminish the likelihood for developing additional premalignant adenomas following treatment for a prior colon carcinoma. This effect of aspirin on colon carcinogenesis increases with the duration and dosage of drug use.
- Oral folic acid supplements and oral calcium supplements reduce the risk of adenomatous polyps and colorectal cancers in case-controlled studies

74. Ans. (a) Stomach

(Ref: Harrison 20th edition, p 570)

- Primary lymphoma of the stomach is relatively uncommon, accounting for <15% of gastric malignancies and < 2% of all lymphomas.
- The stomach is, however, the most frequent extranodal site for lymphoma, and gastric lymphoma has increased in frequency during the past 30 years

75. Ans. (a) One or more case in family of colorectal cancer < 50 year

(Ref: Harrison 20th edition, p 573; Harrison 19th p 538t)

Hereditary nonpolyposis colon cancer (HNPCC), also known as Lynch syndrome, is another autosomal dominant trait with defects related to chromosome 2 and 3.
1. It is characterized by the presence of three or more relatives with histologically documented colorectal cancer, one of whom is a first-degree relative of the other two
2. One or more cases of colorectal cancer diagnosed before age 50 in the family
3. Colo-rectal cancer involving at least two generations.
   - In contrast to polyposis coli, HNPCC is associated with an unusually high frequency of cancer arising in the proximal large bowel.
   - The median age for the appearance of an adenocarcinoma is <50 years, 10–15 years younger than the median age for the general population.
   - Families with HNPCC often include individuals with multiple primary cancers; the association of colorectal cancer with either ovarian or endometrial carcinomas is especially strong in women.

76. Ans. (a) Liver

(Ref: Harrison 20th edition, p 576)

Cancers of the large bowel generally spread to regional lymph nodes or to the liver via the portal venous circulation. The liver represents the most frequent visceral site of metastasis; it is the initial site of distant spread in one-third of recurring colorectal cancers and is involved in more than two-thirds of such patients at the time of death.

77. Ans. (a) Ovarian tumor

(Ref: Harrison 20th edition, p 573t; Harrison 19th p 538t)

Syndrome	Malignant Potential	Associated Lesions
Familial adenomatous polyposis	Common	None
Gardner's syndrome	Common	Osteomas, fibromas, lipomas, epidermoid cysts, ampullary cancers, congenital hypertrophy of retinal pigment epithelium
Turcot's syndrome	Common	Brain tumors
Nonpolyposis syndrome (Lynch syndrome)	Common	Endometrial and ovarian tumors
Peutz-Jeghers syndrome	Rare	Mucocutaneous pigmentation; tumors of the ovary, breast, pancreas, endometrium
Juvenile polyposis	Rare	Various congenital abnormalities

78. Ans. (d) Polycythemia

(Ref: Harrison 20th edition, p 569; Harrison 19th p 534)

Unusual clinical features associated with gastric adenocarcinomas include
1. Migratory thrombophlebitis
2. Microangiopathic hemolytic anemia
3. Diffuse seborrheic keratoses (Leser-Trélat sign)
4. Acanthosis nigricans

79. Ans. (a) Liver

(Ref: Harrison 20th edition, p 569; Harrison 19th p 534)

- The liver is the most common site for hematogenous spread of gastric tumor.
- Gastric carcinomas spread by direct extension through the gastric wall to the peri-gastric tissues, occasionally adhering to adjacent organs such as the pancreas, colon, or liver. The disease also spreads via lymphatics or by seeding of peritoneal surfaces.
- Metastases occur to
  1. Intra-abdominal and supraclavicular lymph nodes.
  2. Metastatic nodules to the ovary (Krukenberg's tumor)
  3. Peri-umbilical region ("Sister Mary Joseph node")
  4. Peritoneal cul-de-sac (Blumer's shelf palpable on rectal or vaginal examination)
  5. Malignant ascites

80. Ans. (b) Celiac sprue

(Ref: Harrison 20th edition, p 779, 786)

- Enteropathy-type T cell lymphoma is a rare complication of long-standing Celiac disease. It most commonly occurs in the jejunum or the ileum.
- In adults, the lymphoma may be diagnosed at the same time as celiac disease, but the suspicion is that the celiac disease was a longstanding precursor to the development of lymphoma.
- The tumor usually presents as multiple ulcerating mucosal masses, and expresses CD3 and CD7 nearly always and may or may not express CD8.
- The normal-appearing lymphocytes in the adjacent mucosa often have a similar phenotype to the tumor.
- Most patients have the HLA genotype associated with celiac disease, HLA DQA1*0501 or DQB1*0201.
- The prognosis of this form of lymphoma is typically (median survival is 7 months) poor but some patients have a good response to CHOP chemotherapy.

81. Ans. (a) Intake of vegetable fat

(Ref: Harrison 20th edition, p 572t; Harrison 19th p 538)

Risk Factors for the Development of Colorectal Cancer

| Diet: Animal fat |
| Hereditary syndromes (autosomal dominant inheritance) |
| Nonpolyposis syndrome (Lynch syndrome) |
| Polyposis coli |
| I.B.D |
| Streptococcus bovis bacteremia |
| Ureterosigmoidostomy |

82. Ans. (b) M.A.L.T oma

(Ref: Harrison's 18th ed., ch. 91)

- Antibiotic treatment to eradicate H. pylori infection has led to regression of about 75% of gastric MALT lymphomas and should be considered before surgery, radiation therapy, or chemotherapy are undertaken in patients having such tumors.
- A lack of response to such antimicrobial treatment has been linked to a specific chromosomal abnormality, i.e., t(11;18).
- Responding patients should undergo periodic endoscopic surveillance because it remains unclear whether the neoplastic clone is eliminated or merely suppressed, although the response to antimicrobial treatment is quite durable

83. Ans. (d) Haem-occult is best screening tool

(Ref: Harrison 20th edition, p 574; Harrison 19th p 541)

- The development of the Hemocult test has greatly facilitated the detection of occult fecal blood.
- Unfortunately, even when performed optimally, the Hemoccult test has major limitations as a screening technique for colorectal cancer.
- About 50% of patients with documented colorectal cancers have a negative fecal Hemoccult test, consistent with the intermittent bleeding pattern of these tumors

84. Ans. (d) Gastric tetany

(Ref: Harrison 20th edition, p 567; Harrison 19th p 583)

- Dysphagia may be associated with pain on swallowing, pain radiating to the chest and/or back, regurgitation or vomiting, and aspiration pneumonia.
- The disease most commonly spreads to adjacent and supraclavicular lymph nodes, liver, lungs, pleura, and bone.
- Tracheoesophageal fistulas may develop as the disease advances, leading to extreme suffering.
- As with other squamous cell carcinomas, hypercalcemia may occur in the absence of osseous metastases, probably from parathormone-related peptide secreted by tumor cells

85. Ans. (d) 60%

(Ref: Harrison 20th edition, p 567)

- Dysphagia initially occurs with solid foods and gradually progresses to include semisolids and liquids. By the time these symptoms develop, the disease is usually incurable, since difficulty in swallowing does not occur until >60% of the esophageal circumference is infiltrated with cancer.
- About 10% of esophageal cancers occur in the upper third of the esophagus (cervical esophagus), 35% in the middle third, and 55% in the lower third. Squamous cell carcinomas and adenocarcinomas cannot be distinguished radiographically or endoscopically.
- Progressive dysphagia and weight loss of short duration are the initial symptoms in the vast majority of patients

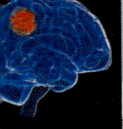

86. Ans. (d) Hypertension

(Ref: Harrison 20th edition, p 603; Harrison 19th p 564)

- During a flushing episode color changes from red to violet are associated with lacrimation, diaphoresis, diarrhea and hypotension.
- Lesions of right side of heart are more common but mitral valve involvement is also seen
- Foregut carcinoids are associated with ectopic ACTH production leading to Cushing syndrome.
- Most common systemic syndrome with carcinoid tumor is carcinoid syndrome
- Non cardiac lesions in carcinoid occur due to increased fibrous tissue leading to retroperitoneal fibrosis and ureter obstruction, Peyronie disease of penis and occlusive disease of mesenteric arteries or veins.

87. Ans. (b) Midgut carcinoid

(Ref: Harrison 20th edition, p 603; Harrison 19th p 563)

- Flushing episodes are characterized by red to violet discoloration of face and neck with feeling of warmth and associated with pruritus, lacrimation, Diarrhea.
- It is mostly seen with midgut carcinoids and foregut carcinoids.
- Diarrhea and flushing occur together in 85 % of cases

88. Ans. (a) Tricuspid regurgitation

(Ref: Harrison 20th edition, p 603; Harrison 19th p 564)

- Cardiac disease is due to the formation of fibrotic plaques involving the endocardium, primarily on the right side, although lesions on the left side also occur occasionally, especially if a patent foramen ovale exists.
- The dense fibrous deposits are most commonly on the ventricular aspect of the tricuspid valve and less commonly on the pulmonary valve cusps. They can result in constriction of the valves, and pulmonic stenosis is usually predominant, whereas the tricuspid valve is often fixed open, resulting in regurgitation predominating.
- Overall, in patients with carcinoid heart disease, 97% have tricuspid insufficiency, 59% tricuspid stenosis, 50% pulmonary insufficiency, 25% pulmonary stenosis, and 11% (0–25%) left-side lesions

89. Ans. (d) Synaptophysin

(Ref: Harrison 19th p 566)

- The most accurate imaging technique is somatostatin receptor scintigraphy.
- The technique can aid diagnosis by localizing primary and metastatic sites of gastro-enteropancreatic endocrine tumors. The degree of radionuclide uptake is related to somatostatin receptor density. In gastrointestinal carcinoids, the concentration at the receptor sites is high (90%).
- Chromogranin A levels correlate with tumour bulk
- Neuron specific enolase is less sensitive than chromogranin A.

90. Ans. (b) Metastatic midgut carcinoid

(Ref: Harrison's 18th ed., ch. 350)

- Most common site of carcinoid tumor is bronchus BUT most common site of carcinoid tumor leading to syndrome manifestation is midgut mentioned in Harrison's as 78-87%.
- Syndrome manifestations occur only after the secreted products of the tumour reach systemic circulation and this occurs after distant metastasis to the liver.

91. Ans. (c) Octreotide

(Ref: Harrison 20th edition, p 604, 606; Harrison 19th p 566)

- Carcinoid crisis is more common in patients who have intense symptoms or have greatly increased urinary 5-HIAA levels (i.e., >200 mg/d).
- The crises may occur spontaneously or be provoked by stress, anesthesia, chemotherapy, or a biopsy.
- Patients develop intense flushing, diarrhea, abdominal pain, cardiac abnormalities including tachycardia, hypertension, or hypotension.
- If not adequately treated, this can be a terminal event
- Drug of choice to treat and prevent carcinoid crisis is octreotide given injectable sub-cutaneously 8 hourly before and during surgery

92. Ans. (a) Diarrhea

(Harrison 20th edition, p 603, 601, Table 80-6; Harrison 19th p 564)

Diarrhea is seen in 73% patients of carcinoid as 5HT3 receptors are stimulated to cause secretory diarrhea. Though both diarrhea and flushing occur together, flushing is found in 65% of all patients.

Pellagra is seen in only 2% of patients while asthma in 4-8%.

93. Ans. (d) High urinary 5HIAA

(Ref: Harrison 20th edition, p 604; Harrison 19th p 566)

- Atypical carcinoid syndrome that is thought to be due to a deficiency in the enzyme dopa decarboxylase; thus, 5-HTP cannot be converted to 5-HT (serotonin), and 5-HTP is secreted into the bloodstream.
- In these patients, plasma serotonin levels are normal but urinary levels may be increased because some 5-HTP is converted to 5-HT in the kidney.
- Characteristically, urinary 5-HTP and 5-HT are increased, but urinary 5-HIAA levels are only slightly elevated.
- Foregut carcinoids are the most likely to cause an atypical carcinoid syndrome.

94. Ans. (a) Carcinoid

(Ref: Harrison 20th edition, p 603)

Since in carcinoid syndrome, 5HT is produced in large amounts tryptophan is consumed and hence less of it is available to synthesize niacin. This leads to niacin deficiency and resultant pellagra.

95. Ans. (c) Cancer infiltration into bone marrow

(Ref: Harrison 20th edition, p 784, Table 106-3)

Differential Diagnosis of "Dry Tap"—Inability to Aspirate Bone Marrow

Dry taps occur in about 4% of attempts and are associated with:	
Metastatic carcinoma infiltration	17%
Chronic myeloid leukemia	15%
Myelofibrosis	14%
Hairy cell leukemia	10%
Acute leukemia	10%
Lymphomas, Hodgkin's disease	9%
Normal marrow	Rare

96. Ans. (c) Bones

(Ref: Nelson 18th ed., ch. 498: Neuroblastoma)

The most common sites of metastasis of neuroblastoma are the long bones and skull, bone marrow, liver, lymph nodes, and skin. Lung metastases are rare, occurring in <3% of cases. Prenatal diagnosis of NB sometimes is possible on maternal ultrasound scans.

97. Ans. (d) Recurrent syncopal attacks

(Ref: OP Ghai 7th ed., pg 590-91, Harrison 19th p 618)

- Neuroblastoma can present as asymptomatic abdominal lump to an extreme of sick febrile child with bone pain periorbital ecchymosis
- The dumb bell tumor can grow through the intervertebral foramen and form a intraspinal mass crushing corticospinal pathways leading to paraplegia.
- Opsoclonus is dancing eyes due to inhibition of parapontine reticular formation by cytokines.
- The child presents with sweating, diarrhea, hypertension and cerebellar signs

98. Ans. (b) Neuroblastoma

(Ref: Nelson 18th ed., ch. 498, Neuroblastoma)

Tumor markers, including homovanillic acid (HVA) and vanillylmandelic acid (VMA) in urine, are elevated in 95% of neuroblastoma cases and help to confirm the diagnosis. A pathologic diagnosis is established from tumor tissue obtained by biopsy. NB can be diagnosed in a typical presentation without a primary tumor biopsy if the patient has neuroblasts observed in bone marrow and elevated VMA or HVA in the urine

99. Ans. (a) Immunohistochemistry

(Ref: OP ghai 7th ed., pg 570, Neslon 19th p 1754)

A pathologic diagnosis is established from tumor tissue obtained by biopsy. NB can be diagnosed in a typical presentation without a primary tumor biopsy if the patient has neuroblasts observed in bone marrow.

100. Ans. (a) Adrenal gland

(Ref: OP Ghai 7th ed., pg 590, Neslon 19th p 1754)

Sites of origin of Neuroblastoma
1. Adrenal gland = 30%
2. Paravertebral Retro-peritoneum = 28%
3. Posterior mediastinum = 15%
4. Pelvis = 5%

101. Ans. (d) Defect on chromosome 2

(Ref: OP Ghai 7th ed., pg. 90)

Neuroblastoma is associated with
1. Re-arrangment or deletion on short arm of chromosome no 1
2. Neurofibromatosis
3. Hischsprung disease
4. Fetal hydantoin syndrome
5. Fetal alcohol syndrome

102. Ans. (a) Abdominal pain

(Ref: OP ghai 7th ed., pg 570, Neslon 19th p 1758)

O.P. Ghai mentions the symtoms in wilm's tumour as
1. Abdominal pain = 30%
2. Hypertension = 25%
3. Hematuria = 25%
4. Fever = 20%

103. Ans. (a) Bones

(Ref: OP ghai 7th ed., pg 571-2)

Most common involvement in histiocytosis is bones (80%) followed by seborrheic skin rash (60%) and Lymphadenopathy, Hepato-splenomegaly and exophthalmos.

104. Ans. (d) Hypercalcemia

(Ref: Harrison 20th edition, p 519; Harrison 19th p 1795)

Tumor lysis syndrome is characterized by hyperuricemia, hyperkalemia, hyperphosphatemia, and hypocalcemia.
- It is caused by the destruction of a large number of rapidly proliferating neoplastic cells. Acidosis may also develop.
- Acute renal failure occurs frequently.
- TLS is most often associated with the treatment of Burkitt's lymphoma, acute lymphoblastic leukemia, and other rapidly proliferating lymphomas, but it also may be seen with chronic leukemias and, rarely, with solid tumors.
- TLS usually occurs during or shortly (1–5 days) after chemotherapy

105. Ans. (a) Burkitt lymphoma

(Ref: Harrison 20th edition, p 519; O.P Ghai, 7th ed., pg. 597, Harrison 19th p 1795)

The most common cause of tumor lysis syndrome in children is Burkitt lymphoma> T cell lymphoblastic lymphoma.

106. **Ans. (a) Cerebellum**

 (*Ref: Harrison 20th edition, p 2754*)

107. **Ans. (b) Gliomatosis Cerebri**

 (*Ref: Harrison's 17th ed., pg 2604*)

 Gliomatosis cerebri is a rare form of astrocytoma in which there is a diffuse infiltration of brain by malignant astrocytes without focal enchancing mass.
 - It presents with dementia, seizures and personality changes
 - CT/MRI are not useful and biopsy is used to confirm diagnosis
 - Management is by whole brain radiation and Temozolomide

108. **Ans. (c) Dysplastic gangliocytomas**

 (*Ref: Nelson 18th ed., pg 2129, table 497-1, Harrison 19th p 2344*)

 Familial syndrome associated with pediatric brain tumour

NF-1	Optic glioma
NF-2	Acoustic vestibular schwannoma
Von hippel landau	Hemangioblastoma
Tuberous sclerosis	Subependymal giant cell astrocytoma
Li fraumeni	Astrocytoma
Turcot syndrome	Medulloblastoma
Cowden syndrome	Dysplastic gangliocytoma of the cerebellum (lhermite –duclos disease)

109. **Ans. (b) Thoracic**

 (*Ref: Harrison 20th edition, p 514*)

 Thoracic cord is most commonly affected presenting with weakness, sensory loss, Autonomic insufficiency with urinary incontinence and sexual impotence in men.

110. **Ans. (a) PNET**

 (*Ref: Nelson textbook of pediatrics: 18th ed., pg. 2134-35*)

111. **Ans. (a) Carcinoma breast**

 (*Ref: Harrison 20th edition, p 650*)

 For leptomeningeal/ carcinomatous meningitis the most common cause is breast cancer

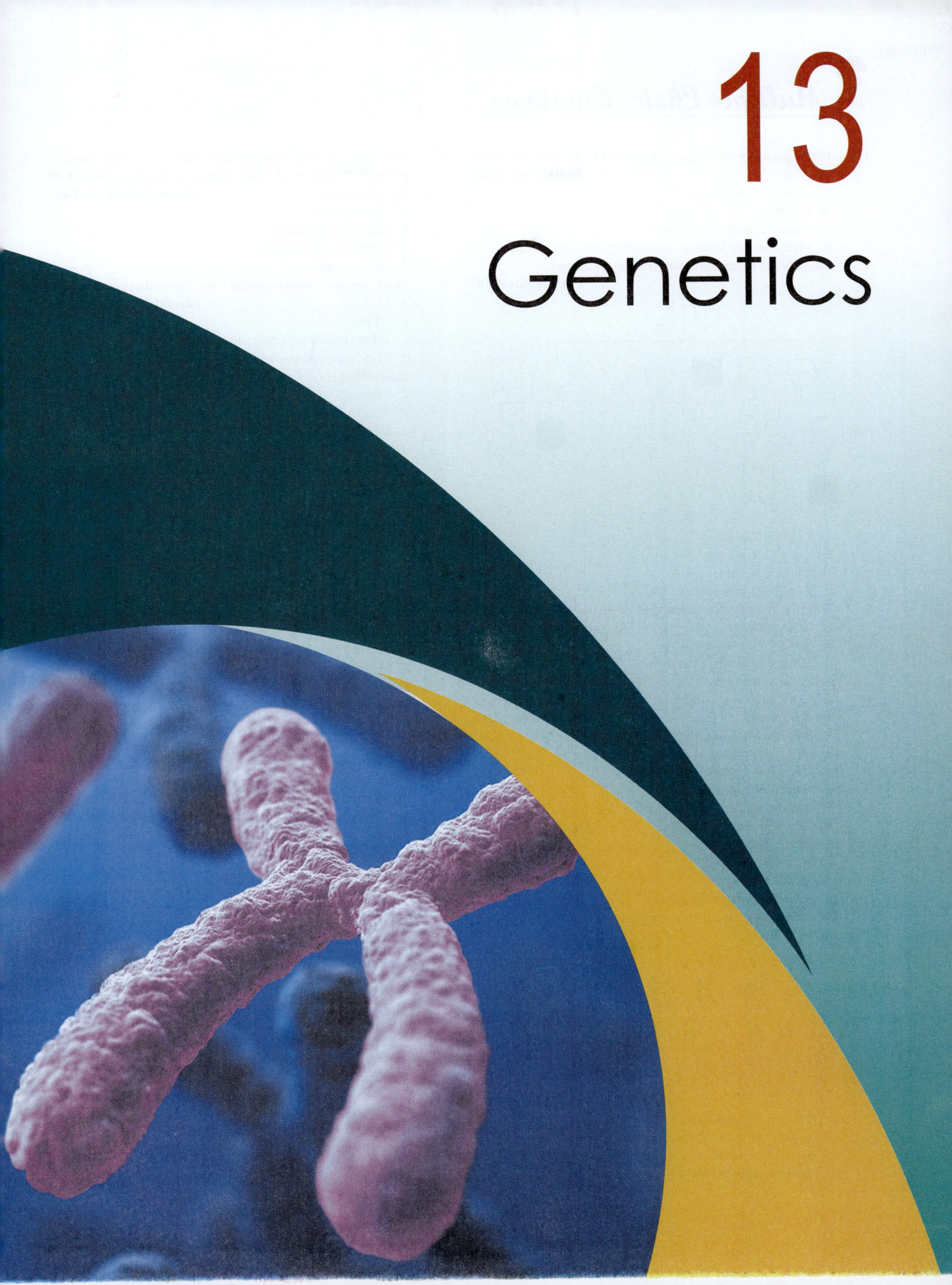
13
Genetics

Multiple Choice Questions

1. Nobel prize for medicine / physiology in 2018 for discovery of? *(AIIMS Nov 2018)*
   a. Apoptotic pathway
   b. Crispr
   c. Negative immune regulation
   d. Molecular mechanisms controlling circadian rhythm

2. Identify the inheritance pattern shown below? *(AIIMS Nov 2018)*

   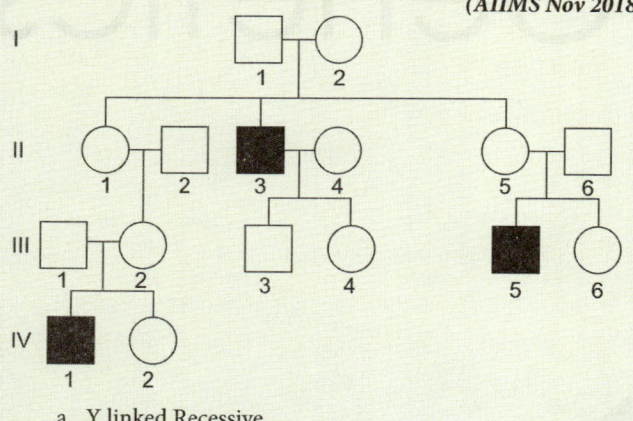

   a. Y linked Recessive
   b. X linked Recessive
   c. X linked Dominant
   d. Y linked Dominant

3. Which is the most common genetic disorder in the world? *(Recent Question 2016-17)*
   a. Thalassemia
   b. HOCM
   c. Familial hypercholesterolemia
   d. Sickle cell anaemia

4. Select the incorrect combination of chromosomal pattern & the syndrome? *(APPG 2016)*
   a. Turner's syndrome-45XO
   b. Swyer's syndrome-46XY
   c. Klinefelter syndrome-47XXY
   d. Mayer Rokitansky-46XY

5. In a patient of Turner syndrome, search for Y chromosome is done for detection of? *(JIPMER Nov 2015)*
   a. Gonadoblasotma
   b. Neuroblastoma
   c. Uterine myoma
   d. Autoimmune thyroid disease

6. Identify the genetic disease and heart disease associated?

   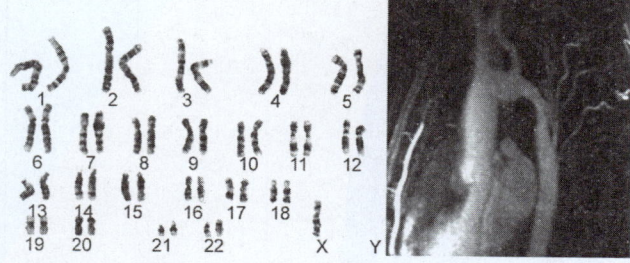

   a. Turner syndrome, Coarctation of aorta
   b. Turner syndrome, left ventricular hypertrophy
   c. Marfan Syndrome, Aortic Root dilatation
   d. Marfan syndrome, left atrial appendage dilatation

7. Two siblings with Osteogenesis Imperfecta have normal parents. The mode of inheritance is explained by which of the following? *(Recent Pattern 2014-15)*
   a. Anticipation
   b. Genomic imprinting
   c. Germ-line Mosaicism
   d. New mutation

8. Most common mitochondrial inheritance disease? *(Recent Pattern 2014-15)*
   a. MELAS
   b. CPEO
   c. Lebers hereditary optic neuropathy
   d. Myoclonic epilepsy and ragged red fibers

9. True statements regarding the mitochondrial genes are: *(Recent Pattern 2014-15)*
   a. Paternal transmission
   b. Maternal transmission
   c. Mendelian inheritance
   d. Mitochondrial myopathy

10. All of the following are chromosomal breakage syndromes except: *(Recent Pattern 2014-15)*
    a. Fanconi's anemia
    b. Ehler-Danlos syndrome
    c. Bloom's syndrome
    d. Ataxia telangiectasia

11. The mother has sickle cell disease; Father is normal; Chances of children having sickle cell disease and sickle cell trait respectively are: *(Recent Pattern 2014-15)*
    a. 0 and 100%
    b. 25 and 25%
    c. 50 and 50%
    d. 10 and 50%

12. The genetics involved in Down syndrome is: *(Recent Pattern 2014-15)*
    a. Mitotic non-disjunction
    b. Meiotic non-disjunction
    c. Mosacism
    d. Monosomy

13. Most common type of MODY is associated with defect on *(Recent Pattern 2014-15)*
    a. Chromosome 12
    b. Chromosome 13
    c. Chromosome 17
    d. Chromosome 22

14. All are true about Mitochondrial DNA (mt-DNA) except: *(Recent Pattern 2014-15)*
    a. Maternal inheritance
    b. Heteroplasmy
    c. Leber hereditary optic neuropathy is the prototype
    d. Nemaline myopathy results due to mutations in mt-DNA

15. The chances of having an unaffected baby, when both parents have achondroplasia, are: *(Recent Pattern 2014-15)*
    a. 0%   b. 25%
    c. 50%   d. 100%

16. All of the following are characterized by 'trinucleotide repeats' affecting the non-coding regions except *(Recent Pattern 2014-15)*
    a. Friedreich's ataxia
    b. Fragile X syndrome
    c. Huntington's disease
    d. Myotonic dystrophy

17. **The gene that regulates normal morphogenesis during development is:** *(Recent Pattern 2014-15)*
    a. FMR-1 gene
    b. Homeobox gene
    c. P-16
    d. PTEN
18. **Father has a blood group B; Mother has AB; Children are not likely to have the following blood group:** *(Recent Pattern 2014-15)*
    a. O
    b. A
    c. B
    d. AB
19. **Incorrectly matched is:** *(Recent Pattern 2014-15)*
    a. SCA type 3: CAG repeats
    b. Myotonic dystrophy: CTG
    c. Fragile X syndrome: CGG
    d. Frederich ataxia: GAC
20. **Karyotyping is done for:** *(Recent Pattern 2014-15)*
    a. Chromosomal disorders
    b. Autosomal recessive disorders
    c. Autosomal dominant disorders
    d. Linkage disorders
21. **A Phenylketonuric girl gets married to a normal boy, what are the chances of their having an affected child and what are the chances of their children being carriers?**
    a. None affected, all carriers *(Recent Pattern 2014-15)*
    b. All normal
    c. 50% carriers
    d. 50% affected, 50% carriers
22. **Interaction of gene with environment is known as**
    a. Epistasis *(Recent Pattern 2014-15)*
    b. Phenocopy
    c. Transmission Dys-equilibrium effect
    d. Polymorphism
23. **The following diseases have defect in DNA repair mechanism except for:** *(Recent Pattern 2014-15)*
    a. Xeroderma Pigmentosum
    b. Fanconi syndrome
    c. Huntington's disease
    d. Hereditary non polyposis colon cancer
24. **Most common sex chromosomal aneuploidy in males?** *(Recent Pattern 2014-15)*
    a. XX males
    b. Praderwili syndrome
    c. Klinefelter syndrome
    d. Fragile X syndrome
25. **Gene for folate carrier protein is located on?** *(Recent Pattern 2014-15)*
    a. Chromosome 10
    b. Chromosomes 5
    c. Chromosome 21
    d. Chromosome 9
26. **The approximate number of genes contained in the human genome is:** *(Recent Pattern 2014-15)*
    a. 20,000
    b. 25,000
    c. 40,000
    d. 1,00,000
27. **In Prader Willi syndrome, which of the following leads to obesity?** *(Recent Pattern 2014-15)*
    a. Neuropeptide Y increase
    b. Neuropeptide Y decrease
    c. Ghrelin decrease
    d. Ghrelin increase
28. **Thalassemia occurs due to which mutation?** *(Recent Pattern 2014-15)*
    a. Missense
    b. Splicing
    c. Transition
    d. Frame-shift
29. **In Marfan's syndrome there is defect in protein** *(Recent Pattern 2014-15)*
    a. Collagen
    b. Elastin
    c. Fibrillin
    d. All of the above
30. **Maternal disomy of chromosome 15 is seen in** *(Recent Pattern 2014-15)*
    a. Prader-Willi syndrome
    b. Klinefelter's syndrome
    c. Angelman syndrome
    d. Turner's syndrome
31. **Dominant negative inheritance is seen in:** *(Recent Pattern 2014-15)*
    a. EhlerDanlos syndrome
    b. Marfan's syndrome
    c. Hunter syndrome
    d. Osteogenesis imperfecta
32. **Gene therapy is used for:** *(Recent Pattern 2014-15)*
    a. Cystic fibrosis
    b. Sickle cell anemia
    c. Thalassemia
    d. All of the above
33. **NARP syndrome is seen in:** *(Recent Pattern 2014-15)*
    a. Mitochondrial diseases
    b. Glycogen storage diseases
    c. Lysosomal storage diseases
    d. Lipid storage diseases
34. **Which of the following is an autosomal dominant metabolic disorder?** *(Recent Pattern 2014-15)*
    a. Cystic fibrosis
    b. Phenylketonuria
    c. α-1 antitrypsin deficiency
    d. Familial hypercholesterolemia
35. **Males are more commonly affected than females in which of the following genetic disorders?** *(Recent Pattern 2014-15)*
    a. Autosomal Recessive Disorder
    b. Autosomal Dominant Disorder
    c. X-linked Recessive Disorder
    d. X-linked Dominant Disorder
36. **Which of the following is an autosomal recessive condition?** *(Recent Pattern 2014-15)*
    a. Ataxia telangectasia
    b. PeutzJeghers syndrome
    c. Neurofibromatosis
    d. Tuberous sclerosis

37. Which of the following is not associated with Down's syndrome? *(Recent Pattern 2014-15)*
   a. Trisomy 21
   b. Mosaic 21
   c. Translocation t (14, 21), t (21, 21)
   d. Deletion of 21

38. Increasing severity of mental retardation in male members over generations is a result of: *(Recent Pattern 2014-15)*
   a. Mitochondrial DNA mutation
   b. Frameshift mutation
   c. Y linked disorder
   d. Trinucleotide repeat mutation

39. True statements about α-1 anti-trypsin deficiency are all except: *(Recent Pattern 2014-15)*
   a. Autosomal dominant disease
   b. Emphysema
   c. Fibrosis of portal tract
   d. Diastase resistant positive hepatocytes

40. Catastrophic variant of EhlerDanlos syndrome is: *(Recent Pattern 2014-15)*
   a. I
   b. II
   c. III
   d. IV

41. BRCA1 gene is located on? *(Recent Pattern 2014-15)*
   a. Chromosome 13
   b. Chromosome 11
   c. Chromosome 17
   d. Chromosome 22

42. Match List-I with List-II and select the correct answer using the code given below the lists: *(UPSC 2015)*

   List-I (disease state)
   A. Pemphigus vulgaris
   B. Psoriasis
   C. 45XO
   D. Primary hyperparathyroidism

   List-II (clinical feature)
   1. Acro-osteolysis
   2. Brachydactyly
   3. Koebner phenomenon
   4. Nikolsky sign

   Code:
	A	B	C	D
a.	1	2	3	4
b.	1	3	2	4
c.	4	2	3	1
d.	4	3	2	1

Answers with Explanations

1. Ans. (c) Negative immune regulation

(Ref: Nobelprize.org)

- Nobel prize on physiology/ medicine was based on a paper on cancer immunotherapy by James P. Allison and Tasuka Honjo. It describes their discovery of cancer therapy by inhibition of negative immune regulation.

2. Ans. (b) X linked Recessive

(Ref: Robbins pathology: 9th edition p 142)

- The pedigree chart shows only males getting affected which is a feature of X- Linked recessive. Females can be affected whenever there is random X inactivation.

Autosomal recessive

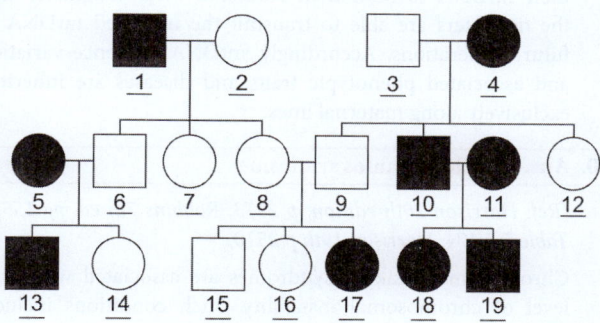

Autosomal dominant

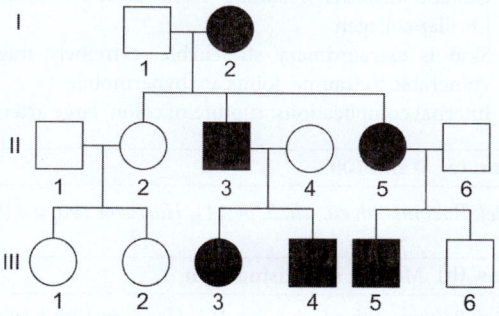

X linked recessive

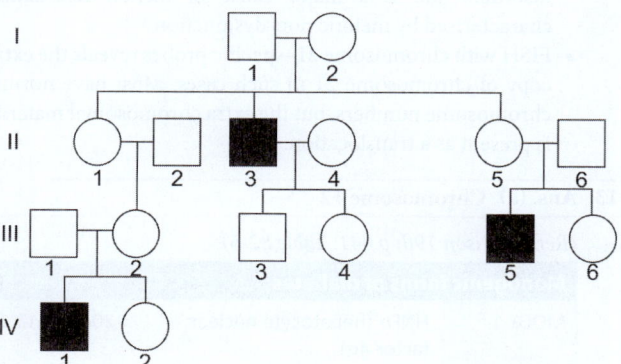

X linked dominant

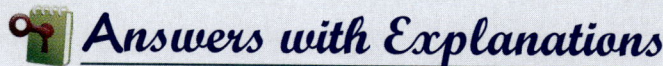

3. Ans. (a) Thalassemia

(Ref: Harrison 19th and who.int p 633)

The question is replicated verbatim from Harrison, "Thalassemias are the most common genetic disorders in the world, affecting nearly 200 million people worldwide"

4. Ans. (d) Mayer Rokitansky-46XY

(Ref: Harrison 20th edition, p 2769; Harrison 19th edition p 2350, 2357:)

Mayer Rokintansy syndrome is **46XX**	The genotype is 46XX with • *Vagina and uterus are underdeveloped or absent.* Thus women develop primary amenorrhea. • Normally functioning ovaries. • Normal female external genitalia • Normal breast and pubic hair development
Swyer syndrome	46 XY, Complete gonadal dysgenesis • Uterus and fallopian tubes are normally-formed, but the *gonads (ovaries or testes) are not functional* • Affected individuals have undeveloped clumps of tissue called streak gonads. The residual gonadal tissue often becomes cancerous, so it is usually removed surgically early in life. • People with Swyer syndrome are typically raised as girls and have a female gender identity. • Hormone replacement therapy is started during adolescence to induce menstruation and development of female secondary sex characteristics such as breast enlargement and uterine growth.
Klinefelter syndrome	47XXY tall male with gynaecomastia, cryptorchidism. They have higher incidence of autoimmune disorders like SLE and develop osteoporosis.
Turner syndrome	45 XO, Short stature female with neck webbing, regression of secondary sexual characteristics, broad shield chest with infantile uterus.

5. Ans. (a) Gonadoblastoma

(Ref: Rudolph paediatrics 22nd edition p 2070)

- Mosaicism involving the Y chromosome occurs in 5%.
- Gonadoblastoma among Y-positive patients occurred in 7–10%.
- The current recommendation that prophylactic gonadectomy should be performed even in the absence of MRI or CT evidence of tumors
- The gonadoblastoma locus on the Y chromosome (GBY) maps close to the Y centromere.

6. Ans. (a) Turner syndrome, Coarctation of aorta

(Ref: Harrison 20th edition, p 2764; Harrison 19th edition p 2351)

The image shows Karyotype of XO, with Coarctation of aorta. You can see the flow in collateral vessels.

7. Ans. (c) Germ line mosaicism

(Ref: Harrison 20th edition, p 2972; Robbins 8th ed. p. 173, Harrison 19th p 439)

- Gonadal mosaicism results from a mutation that occurs postzygotically during early (embryonic) development if the mutation affects only cells destined to form the gonads, the gametes carry the mutations, but the somatic cells of the individual are completely normal. Such an individual is said to exhibit germ line or gonadal mosaicism.
- A phenotypically normal parent who has germ line mosaicism can transmit the disease-causing mutation to the offspring though the mutant gamete.
- Since the progenitor cells of the gametes carry the mutations, there is a definite possibility that more than one child of such a parent would be affected. It is seen with tuberous sclerosis and osteogenesis imperfecta.

8. Ans. (a) MELAS

(Ref: Harrison 20th edition, p 3479-81; Harrison 19th p 85e-4)

Mitochondrial Encephalomyopathy, Lactic Acidosis, and Stroke like episodes (MELAS) is the most common mtDNA disease, consisting of a progressive encephalomyopathy characterized by repeated stroke like events involving mainly posterior cerebral areas. Recurrent migraine-like headache and vomiting, exercise intolerance, seizures, short stature, and lactic acidosis are other common clinical features

Leber Hereditary Optic Neuropathy (LHON)	Bilateral subacute or acute painless optic atrophy
N.A.R.P. (Neurogenic weakness, ataxia and retinitis zigmentosa)/Leigh disease	Loss of central vision leading to blindness in young adult life
MELAS	Mitochondrial encephalomyopathy, lactic acidosis, and stroke like episodes; may manifest only as diabetes

Contd...

MERRF	Myoclonic epilepsy, ragged red fibers in muscle, ataxia, increased CSF protein, sensorineural deafness, dementia

9. Ans. (b) Maternal transmission

(Ref: Harrison 20th edition, p 3478; Harrison 19th p 437, 85e)

In contrast to the homologous pair recombination that takes place in the nucleus, mtDNA molecules do not undergo recombination, and so mutational events represent the only source of mtDNA genetic diversification. Moreover, with very rare exceptions, it is only the maternal DNA that is transmitted to the offspring. The fertilized oocyte degrades mtDNA carried from the sperm in a complex process that involves the ubiquitin proteasome system. Thus, whereas mothers transmit their mtDNA to both their sons and their daughters, only the daughters are able to transmit the inherited mtDNA to future generations. Accordingly, mtDNA sequence variation and associated phenotypic traits and diseases are inherited exclusively along maternal lines.

10. Ans. (b) Ehler-Danlos syndrome

(Ref: Harrison 20th edition, p 2973; Robbins 7th ed. pg. 155-6, Table 5.5 174, Harrison 19th p 2510)

Chromosome breakage syndromes are associated with high level of chromosomal instability. Such conditions include. Fanconi anemia, Bloom syndrome, Ataxia telangiectasia. Ehlers-Danlos syndrome (EDS):
- Genetic disorder resulting from defective synthesis of fibrillar collagen
- Skin is extraordinary stretchable, extremely fragile and vulnerable to trauma, joints are hypermobile
- Internal complications: rupture of colon, large arteries

11. Ans. (a) 0 and 100%

(Ref: Robbins-9th ed., ch. 5, pg:141, Harrison 19th p 438)

12. Ans. (b) Meiotic non disjunction

(Ref: Robbins: 9th ed, ch 5, pg, 161, Harrison 19th p 83e-1)

- Down's syndrome is the most common of the chromosomal disorders and is a major cause of mental retardation characterised by meiotic non-dysjunction.
- FISH with chromosome 21–specific probes reveals the extra copy of chromosome 21 in such cases. Most have normal chromosome numbers, but the extra chromosomal material is present as a translocation.

13. Ans. (a) Chromosome 12

(Ref: Harrison 19th p 441, Table 82-5)

Monogenic forms of diabetes		
MODY 1	HNFα (hepatocyte nuclear factor 4α)	20q12-q13.1
MODY 2	GCK (glucosekinase)	7p15-p13

Contd...

Monogenic forms of diabetes		
MODY 3	HNF1 α (hepatocyte nuclear factor 1 α)	12q24.2
MODY 4	IPF1 (insulin receptor substrate)	13q12.1
MODY 5 (renal cysts, diabetes)	HNF1β (hepatocyte nuclear factor 1β)	17cen-q21.3
MODY 6	NeuroD1 (neurogenic differention factor 1)	2q32

14. Ans. (d) Nemaline myopathy results due to mutations in mt-DNA

(Ref: Robbins 8th 171, Harrison 19th p 451, 85e)

Nemaline myopathy is inherited as autosomal recessive disorder. It is a clinical heterogeneous condition and not a mitochondrial disease. Five genes have been associated with this myopathy. All code for thin filament-associated proteins, suggesting disturbed assembly or interplay of these structures as a pivotal mechanism, mutations of the nebulin (NEB) gene account for most cases, including both severe neonatal and early childhood forms.

15. Ans. (b) 25%

(Ref: Harrison 19th p 437)

Achondroplasia is an autosomal dominant condition, where only one mutant allele is enough to cause disease. Thus, AA and Aa will be affected whereas aa will be unaffected. ['A' is mutant allele whereas 'a' is normal].

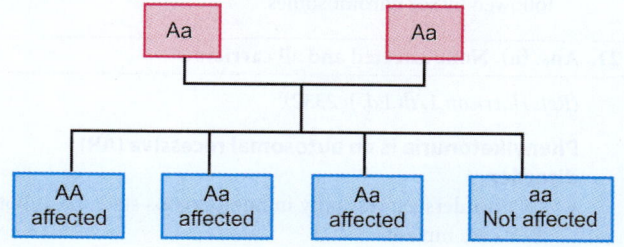

16. Ans. (c) Huntington's disease

(Ref: Robbins: 9th ed. ch., 5, p 168, Harrison 19th p 434, 444e-9)

Examples of Trinucleotide-Repeat Disorder

Disease	Gene	Locus	Protein	Repeat
Expansions Affecting Noncoding Regions				
Fragile X syndrome	FMRI (FRAXA)	Xq27.3	FMR-1 protein (FMRP)	CGG
Friedreich ataxia	FXN	9q21.1	Frataxin	GAA
Myotonic dystrophy	DMPK	19q13.3	Myotonic dystrophy protein kinase (DMPK)	CTG
Expansions Affecting Coding Regions				
Spinobulbar muscular atrophy (Kennedy disease)	AR	Xq12	Adrogen receptor (AR)	CAG
Huntington's disease	HTT	4p16.3	Huntingtin	CAG
Dentatorubral-pallidoluysian atrophy (Haw River syndrome)	ATNL	12p13.31	Atrophin-1	CAG

17. Ans. (b) Homeo-box gene

(Ref: Robbins 9 ed., p 456)

In vertebrates, HOX (homeobox) proteins have been implicated in the patterning of limbs, vertebrae, and craniofacial structures.

18. Ans. (a) O

(Ref: Harrisons 18th ed., ch 61, p 500)

19. Ans. (d) Friedreich's ataxia: GAC

(Ref: Nelson 18th ed., ch. 80 and table 373-2 Harrison 19th p 451e-2t)

Myotonic dystrophy (DMI: chromosome 19)	Muscle loss, cardiac arrhythmia, cataracts, frontal balding	CTG
Myotonic dystrophy (DM2: chromosome 3)	Muscle loss, cardiac arrhythmia, cataracts, frontal balding	CCTG
Friedreich ataxia (FXN gene chromosome 9)	Progressive limb ataxia, dysarthria, hypertrophic cardiomyopathy, pyramidal weakness in legs	GAA
Fragile X syndrome	Mental retardation, large ears and jaws, macroorchidism in males	CGG
SCA 1 (Ataxin-1, 6p 22-p23)	Ataxia with Opthalamoparesis	CAG

* Most common SCA in India is SCA 2.

20. Ans. (a) Chromosomal disorders

(Ref: Robbin's 9th ed, p 158 ch, 5)

- Karyotyping is the basic tool of the cytogeneticist. The usual procedure to examine chromosomes is to arrest dividing cells in metaphase with mitotic spindle inhibitors (e.g., N-diacetyl-N-methylcolchicine [Colcemid]) and then to stain the chromosomes. In a metaphase spread, the individual chromosomes take the form of two chromatids connected at the centromere. A karyotype is obtained by arranging each pair of autosomes according to length, followed by sex chromosomes.

21. Ans. (a) None affected and all carriers

(Ref: Harrison 17th Ed. p 2332)

Phenylketonuria is an autosomal recessive (AR) disorder

- AR disorders express only in homozygous state, i.e. if both alleles are mutant
- If 'P' is normal allele and 'p' is mutant, then the given cross in the question can be made as follows

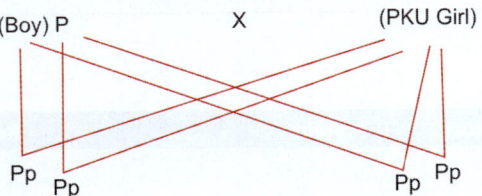

- Therefore genotypically all offsprings are carriers and phenotypically, all of them will be normal

22. Ans. (a) Epistasis

(Ref: Nelson 18th edition, chapter 82)

- The interaction between genes and the environment is called epistasis. Epistatic effects could affect the expressivity of a trait as well as the penetrance.
- An example of this is G6PD deficiency where an individual could carry the altered gene and be deficient in the enzyme, yet would never have a hemolytic crisis unless exposed to an oxidative stress.

23. Ans. (c) Huntington's disease

(Ref: Harrison 19th p 2621-22)

Because mutations caused by defects in DNA repair accumulate as somatic cells divide, these types of mutations are particularly important in the context of neoplastic disorders

- Xeroderma pigmentosum has defects in DNA damage recognition or in the nucleotide excision and repair pathway.
- Ataxia telangiectasia causes large telangiectatic lesions of the face, cerebellar ataxia, immunologic defects, and hypersensitivity to ionizing radiation. The discovery of the ataxia telangiectasia mutated (ATM) gene reveals that it is homologous to genes involved in DNA repair and control of cell cycle checkpoints.
- Fanconi's anemia is also associated with an increased risk of multiple acquired genetic abnormalities. It is characterized by diverse congenital anomalies and a strong predisposition to develop aplastic anemia and acute myelogenous leukemia.
- HNPCC (Lynch's syndrome) is characterized by autosomal dominant transmission of colon cancer, young age (<50 years) of presentation, predisposition to lesions in the proximal large bowel, and associated malignancies such as uterine cancer and ovarian cancer. Germline mutations in these genes lead to microsatellite instability and a high mutation rate in colon cancer.

Nucleotide repeat expansion disorders are associated with an increase in the number of nucleotide repeats above a certain threshold. The repeats are sometimes located within the coding region of the genes, as in Huntington's disease or the X-linked form of spinal and bulbar muscular atrophy (SBMA, Kennedy's syndrome).

24. Ans. (c) Klinefelter syndrome

(Ref: Harrison 19th p 2350)

- Approximately 1/500 newborn males has a 47, XXY chromosome complement, representing the most common sex chromosomal aneuploidy in males. The incidence approximates 1% among the mentally retarded, clustering among patients with IQs greater than 50 and in infertile males.
- The chromosomal aberration most often results from meiotic nondisjunction of an X chromosome during parental gametogenesis; the extra X chromosome is maternal in origin in 54% and paternal in origin in 46% of patients.
- XX male is thought to occur in 1 in 20, 000 newborn males. Affected individuals have a male phenotype, small testes, a small phallus, and no evidence of ovarian or müllerian duct tissue; they appear, therefore, to be distinct from the ovotesticular disorder of sexual development. This disorder resembles Klinefelter syndrome, but stature is greater in the latter. Undescended testes and hypospadias occur in a minority of patients. The histologic features of the testes are essentially the same as in Klinefelter syndrome. Patients with the condition usually come to medical attention in adult life because of hypogonadism, gynecomastia, or infertility. Hypergonadotropic hypogonadism occurs secondary to testicular failure.

25. Ans. (c) Chromosome 21

(Ref: Nelson 19th edn.)

Folate cofactors are one-carbon donors essential for the biosynthesis of purines and thymidylate. Mammalian cells are devoid of folate biosynthesis and are therefore folate auxotroph that takes up folate vitamins primarily via the reduced folate carrier (RFC). The gene for RFC is located on chromosome 21.

26. Ans. (b) 25000

(Ref: Nelson 18th ed., ch., 79 and Robbins-9ed/p 1)

The human genome has approximately 25, 000 genes, which are the individual units of heredity of all traits The human genome contains roughly 3.2 billion DNA base pairs. These proteins variously function as enzymes, structural components, and signalling molecules and are used to assemble and maintain all of the cells in the body.

27. Ans. (d) Ghrelin increase

(Ref: Robbins &cotran: 9th, ch. 9, p 446, Nelson 19th Ch-74)

- Prader-Willi syndrome (PWS) is associated with failure to thrive in infancy and progressive hyperphagia and obesity in childhood. This progressive weight gain is associated with hyper-ghrelinaemia and increased insulin sensitivity.
- Ghrelin is produced in the stomach and in the arcuate nucleus of the hypothalamus. It is the only known gut hormone that increases food intake (orexigenic effect).
- Gut peptides act as short-term meal initiators and terminators. They include ghrelin, PYY, pancreatic polypeptide, insulin, and amylin among others.
- Ghrelin levels rise before meals and fall between 1 and 2 hours after eating. In obese individuals the postprandial suppression of ghrelin is attenuated and may contribute to overeating.
- Rare genetic disorder with defect on chromosome 15
- The variety of symptoms can range from poor muscle tone during infancy to behavioral problems in early childhood.
- In Childhood: Delayed milestones/intellectual delay, Excessive sleeping, Strabismus, Scoliosis, Cryptorchidism, Speech delay, Poor physical coordination.
- Hyperphagia begins between the age of 2 and 8, and continues on throughout adulthood leading to obesity.

28. Ans. (d) Frame shift

(Ref: Robbins 9th ed., ch 5, p 140)

Structural Alterations of the Globin Gene

Alteration	Function	Affected Disease
Point mutations	Protein folding Transcriptional control Frameshift and nonsense mutations	Sickle cell disease Thalassemia Thalassemia
Deletion	RNA processing mRNA production	Alpha-Thalassemia Hemoglobin Lepore
Rearrangement	mRNA production	Thalassemia

29. Ans. (c) Fibrillin

(Ref: Robbins: 9th ed. ch., 5, p 144, Harrison 19th p 2513)

- Marfan syndrome results from an inherited defect in an extracellular glycoprotein called fibrillin-
- There are two fundamental mechanisms by which loss of fibrillin leads to the clinical manifestations of Marfan syndrome: loss of structural support in microfibril rich connective tissue and excessive activation of TGF-β signaling.

30. Ans. (a) Prader-Wili syndrome

(Ref: Robbins: 9th ed, ch. 5, p 172, Nelson 19th p Table 76-13, p 409)

- Prader-Willi syndrome is characterized by mental retardation, short stature, hypotonia, profound hyperphagia, obesity, small hands and feet, and hypogonadism.
- In 65% to 70% of cases, an interstitial deletion of band q12 in the long arm of chromosome 15, del (15)(q11.2q13), can be detected.
- In most cases the breakpoints are the same, causing a 5-Mb deletion. It is striking that in all cases the deletion affects the paternally derived chromosome 15.

31. Ans. (c) Hunter syndrome

(Ref: Robbins 7th ed. p 151, Harrison 19th p 432e-2t)

Dominant negative affects occurs when a mutant polypeptide not only loses its own function but also interferes with the product of normal allele in a heterozygote, thus causing more severe effects than deletion or non-sense mutations in the same gene. Structure proteins that contribute to multimeric structures are vulnerable to dominant negative affect e.g. collagen. Seen in: Osteogenesis imperfecta, Ehler Danlos syndrome, Marfan's syndrome

32. Ans. (d) All of the above

(Ref: Harrison: 18th, 547-551)

Gene transfer is a novel area of therapeutics in which the active agent is a nucleic acid sequence rather than a protein or small molecule. Most gene transfers are carried out using a vector or gene delivery vehicle because delivery of naked DNA or RNA to a cell is an inefficient process. More clear-cut success has been achieved in a gene therapy trial for another form of SCID, adenosine deaminase (ADA) deficiency. Other diseases likely to be amenable to transduction of haemopoietic stem cells (HSCs) include:

- Wiskott-Aldrich syndrome
- Chronic granulomatous disease
- Sickle cell disease
- Thalassemia

33. Ans. (a) Mitochondrial disease

(Ref: Harrison 19th p 85e-6)

34. Ans. (d) Familial hypercholesterolemia

(Ref: Robbins Basic pathology 8th ed., ch. 7, Harrison 19th p 2440)

35. Ans. (c) X linked recessive disorder

(Ref: Robbins: 9th ed, p169)

36. Ans. (a) Ataxia Telengiectasia

(Ref: Robbins Basic pathology 8th Ed. chap-6, Harrison 19th p 2109)

37. Ans. (d) Deletion of 21

(Ref: Nelson 18th edition, chapter 81, Nelson p 400-401)

38. Ans. (d) Trinucleotide repeat mutation

(Ref: Robbins-9th ed., ch 5, p 168, Nelson p 391)

39. **Ans. (a) Autosomal dominant disease**

   (Ref: Robbins -9th ed/p 850, Harrison 19th p 367e-2)

40. **Ans. (d) Type IV**

   (Ref: Robbins: 9th ed., ch. 5, p 145, Harrison 19th p 2510)

41. **Ans. (c) Chromosome 17**

   (Ref: Robbins 9th ed. p 1054, Harrison 19th p 523)

42. **Ans. (d) 4 3 2 1**

   (Ref: Harrison 19th edition, page 372, 374)

Choice	Correct match	Reasoning
Pemphigus vulgaris	Nikolsky sign	It is dislodgement of intact superficial epidermis by a shearing force, indicating a plane of cleavage in the skin. Seen in: • Toxic epidermal necrolysis • Pemphigus vulgaris • Staphylococcal scalded skin syndrome It is useful in differentiating between pemphigus vulgaris or mucous membrane pemphigoid (where it is present) and bullous pemphigoid (where it is absent).
Psoriasis	Koebner phenomenon	Characterized by lesions occurring along the lines of trauma
45XO	Brachydactyly	Short 4th metacarpal
Primary hyperparathyroidism	Acro-osteolysis	Sub-periosteal resorption of phalanges

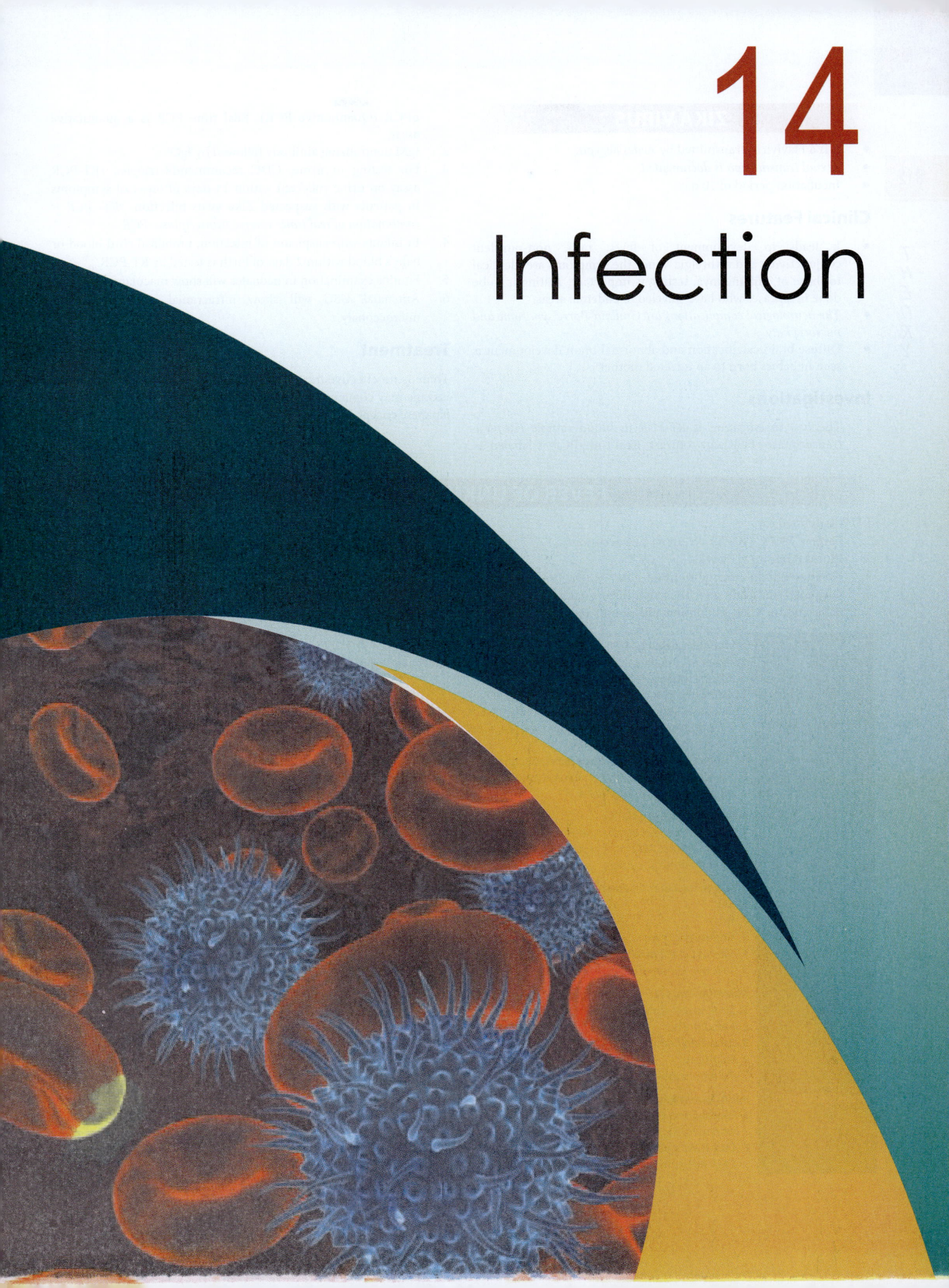

14 Infection

ZIKA VIRUS

- It is a Flavivirus transmitted by *Aedes aegypti*.
- *Sexual transmission is documented.*
- Incubation period of 10 days

Clinical Features

- It leads to development of fever, rash, non-purulent conjunctivitis and arthralgia. Since the symptoms are identical to those of chikungunya, testing is important. Testing is to be done in all cases who have traveled to endemic areas.
- *The neurological complications are Guillain-Barré syndrome and microcephaly.*
- Diffuse brain calcification and abnormal brain development is seen in babies born to an infected mother.

Investigations

1. The *best investigation is RT-PCR* in blood sample (Reverse transcriptase- PCR). In contrast, Real time PCR is labeled as qPCR (Quantitative PCR). Real time PCR is a quantitative assay.
2. IgM neutralizing antibody followed by IgG.
3. For testing in urine, CDC recommends trioplex rRT-PCR assay on urine collected within 14 days of onset of symptoms in patients with suspected Zika virus infection. *rRT- PCR is combination of real time- reverse transcriptase- PCR.*
4. In infants with suspicion of infection, umbilical cord blood or baby's blood within 2 days of birth is tested by RT-PCR.
5. Fundus examination in neonates will show macular atrophy.
6. Antenatal USG will show intracranial calcification and microcephaly.

Treatment

There is no effective treatment or vaccine available currently, but a vaccine may come up soon since vaccines for other flaviviruses like Japanese encephalitis and dengue virus vaccine are available.

FEVER OF UNKNOWN ORIGIN

F.U.O is defined as
1. Fever > 38.3°C (101°F) on atleast two occasions
2. Illness duration ≥ 3 weeks
3. No known immunocompromised state
4. Diagnosis uncertain after thorough history taking, physical examination and obligatory investigations, including blood culture (n=3), urine culture, CXR, abdominal ultrasound and tuberculin skin test.

Etiology	
	Infectious cause (15–25%)
	1. Abscess- usually in abdomen or pelvis due to risk factors like cirrhosis, steroid or immunosuppressive medications, recent surgery, diabetes
	2. Osteomyelitis
	3. Bacterial endocarditis-culture negative in 2–5 %, especially in *Coxiella burnettii, Tropheryma whipplei, Brucella, Mycoplasma, Chlamydia, Histoplasma, Legionella, Bartonella,* HACEK organisms which required either special media or longer than usual incubation
	4. Prostatitis, dental abscesses, sinusitis, and cholangitis are sources of occult fever
	5. TB, HIV/AIDS, CMV, EBV, malaria, typhoid fever, dengue fever, hepatitis A, Lyme disease, syphilis, psittacosis (bird exposure) and rat-bite fever
	Neoplastic causes (<20%)
	1. Lymphomas (especially non-Hodgkin's lymphoma, most common cause)
	2. Solid tumors: RCC most common, also breast, liver, colon, pancreas or liver metastases
	3. Malignant histiocytosis
	Collagen vascular disease (15–25% of cases):
	1. SLE
	2. RA
	3. Rheumatic fever
	4. Vasculitis, especially temporal (giant cell) arteritis
	5. Juvenile rheumatoid arthritis (JRA), Still's disease
	Miscellaneous (15–20% of cases)
	1. Drug fever: commonly antibiotics, antihistamines, antiarrhythmics, methyldopa, phenytoin, dilatin and NSAIDs
	2. Sarcoidosis
	3. Inherited Familial Mediterranean Fever
	4. Factitious
	5. Pulmonary embolism
Investigations	**Initial Investigations**
	1. **Bloodwork:** CBC with differential and smear, electrolytes, BUN, Creatinine, calcium profile, LFTs, ESR, CRP, muscle enzymes, RF, ANA, serum protein electrophoresis, Fe, transferrin, TIBC, B_{12}
	2. **Cultures:** blood (x 2 sets), urine, sputum, stool C&S, other fluids as appropriate VDRL, heterophile Ab (mononucleosis), CMV antigenemia tests, HIV serology, PPD and CXR.

Contd...

	If no diagnostic clues from the above, proceed with further investigations including: 1. CT chest, abdomen and pelvis with contrast 2. Colonoscopy *If no diagnostic clue from the above, proceed with further investigations including-* 1. 67-Gallium scan 2. 111 Indium PMN scan 3. FDG PET scan
Management	• Treatment is directed at the specific cause found from the above investigations • If no diagnosis with the above consider empiric therapy vs. watchful waiting • Prognosis for most patients with FUO persisting without a diagnosis is very good without intervention • **Empirical therapies may include:** anti-TB therapy, broad –spectrum antibiotics, colchicine, NSAIDS, steroids

HIV/AIDS

- CDC case definition states HIV positive patients with *CD4 counts <200 cells/mcl or CD4 lymphocyte percentage below 14%*.
- AIDS develops within 10 years of acquiring HIV infection and within 3 years of 80% of total patients with CD4 count <200.
- HIV-1 occurs predominantly in India and takes 10 years to convert to AIDS.

Chance of Acquiring HIV Infection

- Receptive anal intercourse = 1:30
- Intravenous drug abuser (needle sharing) = 1:150
- *Infected needle stick injury = 1:300*
- Receptive vaginal intercourse = 1:1000
- Receptive fellatio with ejaculation = 1:10000
- Blood transfusion = 95% chances of transmission
- *Perinatal transmission risk = 15–40%*

CDC AIDS Case Definition for Surveillance of Adults and Adolescents

1. Candidiasis of esophagus, trachea, bronchus and lungs
2. Cryptococcosis, extrapulmonary
3. Cryptosporidium diarrhea
4. CMV retinitis
5. Herpes simplex ulcer persisting for >1 month or bronchitis
6. Kaposi Sarcoma
7. Primary CNS lymphoma
8. Mycobacterium avium intercellulare disease
9. Pneumocystis jiroveci pneumonia
10. Progressive multi-focal lymphadenopathy
11. Toxoplasmosis

Laboratory Findings with HIV Infection

ELISA for HIV	Screening test 50% turn positive within 22 days after HIV transmission 95% turn positive within 6 weeks Sensitivity >99.9%
Western blot	Confirmatory test Indeterminate results with early HIV infection, HIV-2 infection, influenza vaccine, pregnancy, recent tetanus toxoid administration

Contd...

HIV rapid antibody test	Produces result in 10-20 minutes and can be done by semi-trained personnel
Absolute CD4 count	Predictor of HIV progression
CD4 lymphocyte percentage	Predictor of HIV progression
HIV viral load	Correlates with disease progression and response to anti-viral medication

False positive ELISA
1. Biological variant
2. Influenza
3. Connective tissue diseases

Complications

1. Weight loss and wasting
2. **Pulmonary disease**
   a. Most common *pulmonary disease in HIV infected* patients is community acquired pneumonia.
   b. Most common *opportunistic infection in AIDS patients* is TB followed by P. jiroveci pneumonia.
   c. Non-infectious cause of lung disease is *Kaposi sarcoma*. It presents as *pleural effusion*.
   d. P. jiroveci pneumonia is an interstitial pneumonia with CXR showing diffuse or perihilar infiltrates. Hypoxia is severe with pO_2 <60 mmHg. Diagnosis is confirmed with direct fluorescent antibody test on Bronchoalveolar lavage or induced sputum. *Serum beta (1,3) Glucan test* is also a non-invasive test that aids in diagnosis. It is usually seen when CD4 count decreases to less than 200 cells/mcL.
3. **CNS disease**
   a. *Toxoplasmosis is the most common space occupying lesion* in HIV infected patients. It presents with headache, focal deficit and altered sensorium. CT head shows sinel contrast enhancing lesion with predilection for basal ganglia.
   b. 2nd most common ICSOL in AIDS patient is *Primary CNS lymphoma*. Diagnosis is confirmed with stereotactic brain biopsy.
   c. HIV associated dementia is a diagnosis of exclusion.
   d. *Cryptococcal meningitis* presents with fever and headache.

Diagnosis is based on *CRAG test* (Cryptococcal reactive antigen test) done by latex agglutination.
    e. HIV myelopathy presents with paraparesis.
    f. Progressive multifocal leukoencephalopathy presents with cortical blindness, aphasia, hemiparesis with imaging showing non-enhancing white matter lesions without mass effect.
    g. Inflammatory demyelinating neuropathy similar to GBS.
4. **Retinitis**
    a. CMV retinitis develops in AIDS and leads to pizza pie retinopathy. It can lead to blindness and seen when CD4 count is less than 50 cells/mcl.
    b. Cotton wool spots are seen in *early* HIV infection.
5. **Oral lesions** in form of aphthous ulcers and hairy leukoplakia. EBV is incriminated in causing these corrugated hairy projections.
6. **Hepatic disease**
    a. Co-infection with hepatitis B is managed with tenofovir, emtricitabine and lamivudine
    b. Co-infection with hepatitis C is managed with ledipsavir and sofosbuvir.
7. **GIT disease**
    a. Cryptosporidium is the most common cause of diarrhea in AIDS positive patients and most effective treatment is to improve immune function with use of ART.
8. **Endocrine manifestation**
    a. Most common endocrine manifestation in AIDS positive patients is *hypogonadism*.
9. **Skin disease**
    a. Viral dermatides: HSV and HZV
    b. Bacterial dermatides: Staphylococcus aureus
    c. Bacillary angiomatosis: Bartonella henslae/quintana. It is transmitted via fleas of infected domestic cats. Most common manifestation is raised, reddish and highly vascular lesions that mimic lesions of Kaposi sarcoma. Treatment is doxycycline or erythromycin.
10. **HIV-related malignancies**

    a. *Kaposi sarcoma*: 5000 times increased risk purple blanching lesions in all organs especially shins. The causative organism is HHV8 which is transmitted via saliva.
    b. *Non Hodgkin lymphoma*: 10 times increased risk and *most common subtype seen in immunoblastic type*.
    c. *Primary CNS lymphoma*
    d. *Invasive cervical cancer*

    Hodgkin's disease is also increased in cases of HIV infection. However it has not been included in CDC definition. HIV positive patients are more likely to have mixed cellularity and lymphocyte depletion subtypes.
11. **IRIS**: (immune reconstitution inflammatory syndrome)– cART leads to spike in CD4 counts and causes sudden worsening of patient with development of fever, sweating, malaise, new pulmonary infiltrates and lymphadenopathy.

Preventive Aspects

Post exposure prophylaxis:
- Initiate within 4 hours
- Not effective after 72 hours
- Initiate Tenofovir (300 mg) + Emtricitabine (200 mg) + Raltegravir (300 mg)

Perinatal transmission:
- Zidovudine plus lamivudine and ritonavir boosted lopinavir
- C-section is must if viral load > 1000 copies/dL

Latent TB:
- INH daily with pyridoxine for 9 months

Immunization:
Yellow fever vaccine is contraindicated
1. Hepatitis B
2. Diphtheria plus tetanus booster
3. Measles

Prevention of infections in AIDS

P. Jiroveci	Co-trimoxazole
M.A.I	Azithromycin
M.TB	INH + pyridoxine
Toxoplasma	TMP-SMX

Treatment

WHO Clinical Staging	Recommendations
HIV Infected Adults and Adolescents	
• Clinical stage I and II • Clinical stage III and IV	• Start ART if CD4 ≤ 500 • **Start ART irrespective of CD4 count**
All Pregnant/Breast Feeding Women	
• All clinical stages	• Start ART irrespective of CD4 count
HIV-TB Co-infected Patients	
• Patients with HIV and TB co-infection (Pulmonary or extra pulmonary)	• Start ART irrespective of CD4 count • Start ATT first, initiate ART as early as possible between 2 weeks and 2 months. • For patients with CD4 below 50, ART might be initiated simultaneously with ATT with strict clinical and laboratory monitoring
HIV-Hepatitis B/C Co-infected Patient	

Contd...

WHO Clinical Staging	Recommendations
• HIV and HBV/HCV co-Infection-without any evidence of severe chronic liver disease	• Start ART if CD4 ≤ 500
• HIV and HBV/HCV co-infection-with evidence of severe chronic liver disease	• Start ART irrespective of CD4 count
HIV-Visceral Leishmaniasis (Kala Azar) Co-infecion Patient	
• Patient with HIV-Visceral Leishmaniasis co-infected	• Start ART irrespective of CD4 count

*Earlier guidelines were to start ART at <350 cells/mm^3

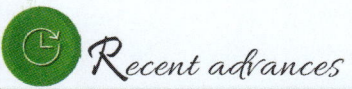

Recommended Regimen as per CMDT 2017
- Dolutegravir + Abacavir + Lamivudine (single pill once a day)
- Dolutegravir + Emtricitabine/Tenofovir Desoproxil (Single pill once a day)
- Emtricitabine + Tenofovir Alafenamide + Elvitegravir with cobicistat boosting (Single pill once a day)
- Emtricitabine + Tenofovir Desoproxil + Elvitegravir with cobicistat boosting (Single pill once a day)
- Raltegravir + Emtricitabine/Tenofovir Desoproxil
- Darunavir + Ritonavir + Emtricitabine

*According to older guidelines for ART remember that zidovudine is not used in anemic patients and nevirapine in case of coexistent TB.

Antiretroviral Regimens or Components that should not be Offered at Any Time

	Rationale	Exception
Antiretroviral regimens Not recommended		
Monotherapy with NRTI (AII)	• Rapid development of resistance • Inferior ARV activity when compared to combination of three or more ARV agents	• No exception
Dual-NRTI regimens (AI)	• Rapid development of resistance • Inferior ARV activity when compared to combination of three or more ARV agents	• No exception
Triple-NRTI regimens (AI) except for ABC/ZDV/3TC (BI) or possibly TDF + ZDV/3TC (BII)	• High rate of early virologic nonresponse seen when triple-NRTI combination, including ABC/TDF/3TC/ and TDF/ddI/3TC, were used as initial regimen in ART-naive patients • Other triple-NRTI regimens have not been evaluated	• ABC/ZDV/3TC (BI) and possibly TDF + ZDV/3TC (BII) in patient in whom other combinations are not desirable

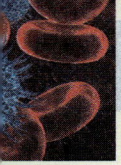

Conceptual Diagnostic Algorithm

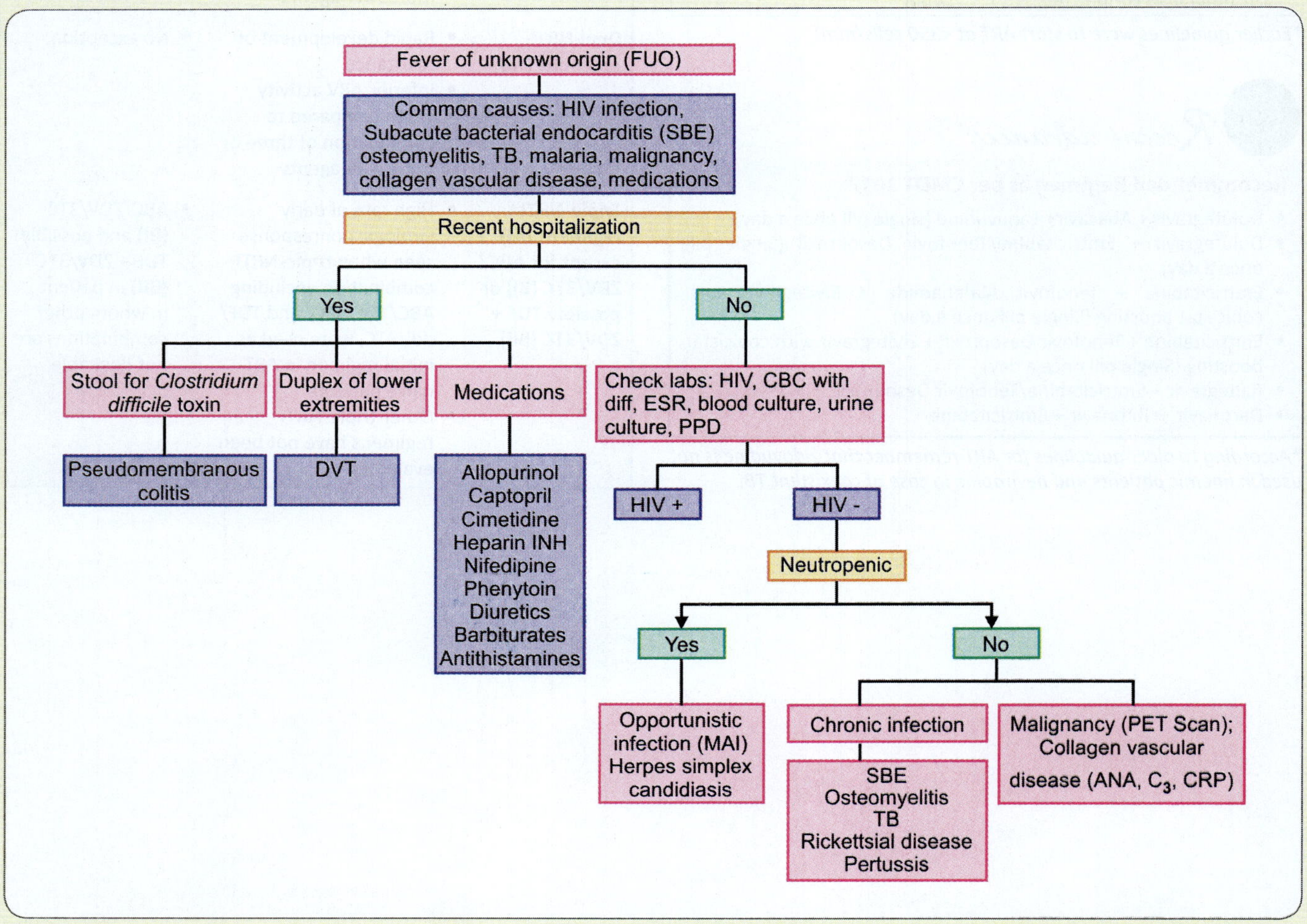

```
Fever of unknown origin (FUO)
            │
Common causes: HIV infection,
Subacute bacterial endocarditis (SBE)
osteomyelitis, TB, malaria, malignancy,
collagen vascular disease, medications
            │
   Recent hospitalization
      ┌─────┴─────┐
     Yes          No
```

Yes branch:
- Stool for *Clostridium difficile* toxin → Pseudomembranous colitis
- Duplex of lower extremities → DVT
- Medications: Allopurinol, Captopril, Cimetidine, Heparin INH, Nifedipine, Phenytoin, Diuretics, Barbiturates, Antihistamines

No branch:
- Check labs: HIV, CBC with diff, ESR, blood culture, urine culture, PPD
  - HIV +
  - HIV − → Neutropenic
    - Yes → Opportunistic infection (MAI), Herpes simplex, candidiasis
    - No →
      - Chronic infection: SBE, Osteomyelitis, TB, Rickettsial disease, Pertussis
      - Malignancy (PET Scan); Collagen vascular disease (ANA, C_3, CRP)

Multiple Choice Questions

1. A 12-year-old boy develops multiple lumps in the skin. Biopsy of the lumps is shown below. What is the probable causative agent? *(Recent Pattern Question 2019)*

   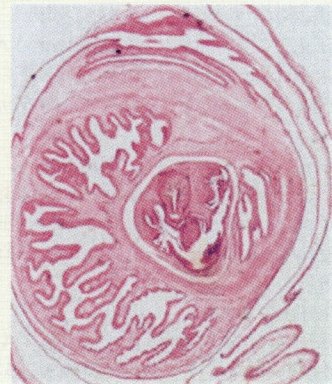

   a. Cysticercus cellulosae b. Cysticercus bovis
   c. Echinococcus granulosus d. Hymenolepis Nana

2. Which is not correct about the lesion shown?
   (Recent Pattern Question 2019)

   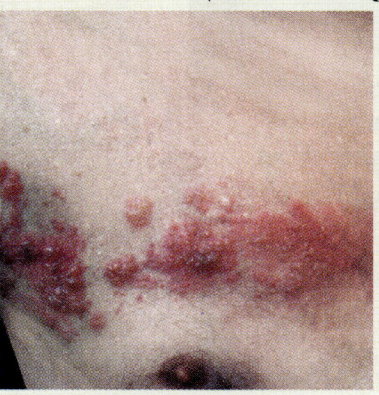

   a. The lesions are infectious to seronegative individuals
   b. Can be associated with meningoencephalitis
   c. Bilaterally symmetrical dermatomal vesicular eruption
   d. Geniculate ganglion is involved in Ramsay hunt syndrome

3. Identify the parasite shown in the image.
   (Recent Pattern Question 2019)

   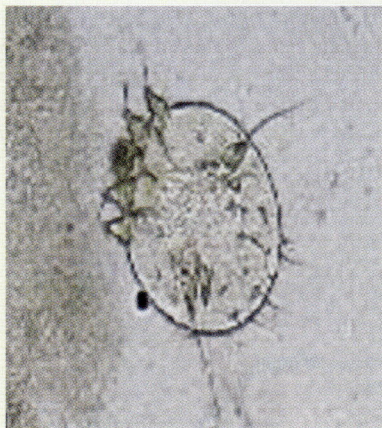

   a. Sarcoptes scabiei b. Pediculus humanus capitis
   c. Pthirus Pubis d. Dermatobia hominis

4. A child presents with the following lesion in the neck folds. The gram stain from the lesion is shown below. Comment on the diagnosis. *(Recent Pattern Question 2019)*

   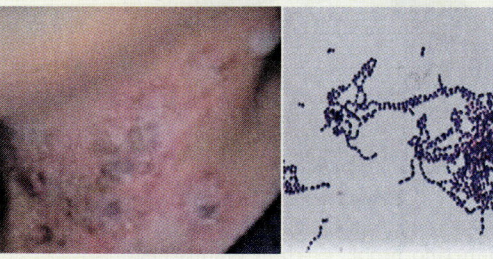

   a. Impetigo contagiosa b. Erythrasma
   c. Scrofuloderma d. Scrum pox

5. What is the diagnosis of the lesion visible in neck folds of this child? *(Recent Pattern Question 2019)*

   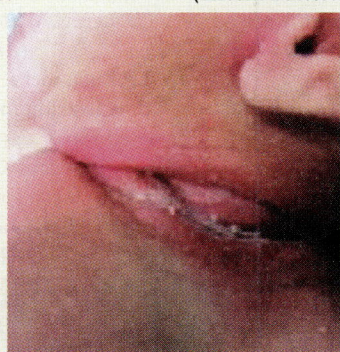

   a. SSSS b. Intertriginous candida
   c. Impetigo d. Ecthyma

6. Which of the following is not an AIDS defining illness?
   a. Tertiary syphilis *(Recent Pattern Question 2019)*
   b. Lymphoma of brain < 60 years of age
   c. Progressive multifocal leukoencephalopathy
   d. Extra-pulmonary cryptococcosis

7. Relative bradycardia is not seen in? *(AIIMS Nov 2018)*
   a. Malaria b. Brucella
   c. Toxoplasma d. Factitious fever

8. What is the best management of the case shown?
   (AIIMS Nov 2018)

   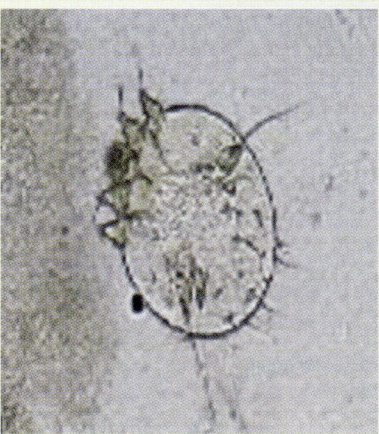

   a. Dapsone plus steroids
   b. Stop smoking and screen for cancer
   c. Vitamin supplements
   d. Antifungals for oral candidiasis

9. Which of the following is shown below? *(AIIMS Nov 2018)*

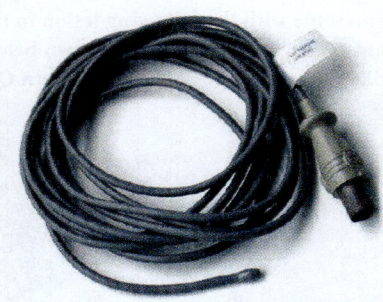

   a. Rectal thermo-probe   b. Colonoscope
   c. Hickman catheter   d. Cautery pencil

10. Patient presents with complaints of lower abdominal pain, fever and repeated stools with little faecal matter and blood and mucus. On stool microscopy paucity of WBCs in stool is noted with positive test for heme. Which is the likely organism? *(AIIMS Nov 2018)*
    a. Giardia   b. Entamoeba
    c. Staphylococcus   d. Clostridium perfringens

11. A patient presented with fever for 8 days with nausea, vomiting and abdominal pain for two days. On examination there is a red painless rash and a lesion found on the left side of the posterior chest. Treatment will be? *(AIIMS May 2018)*

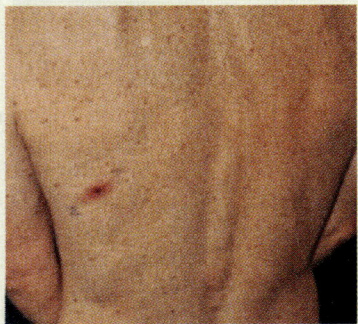

    a. Oseltamivir   b. Streptomycin
    c. Doxycycline   d. Ceftriaxone

12. A patient was suffering from hepatorenal syndrome. Urine sample was obtained from the patient and was examined under microscope. Which technique is used to make the organism visible? *(AIIMS May 2018)*

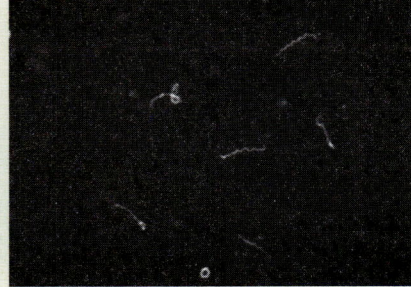

    a. Dark field microscopy
    b. Routine microscopy with negatively stained background
    c. Phase contrast microscopy
    d. Compound light microscopy

13. A 50-year-old male is having fever for last 1 week with abdominal distention and loss of appetite. The fever is not responding to antibiotics and anti-malarials. Widal test is negative but RK39 dipstick test is positive. Which of the following can be used in the above patient? *(AIIMS May 2018)*
    a. Bedaquiline   b. Linezolid
    c. Fluconazole   d. Liposomal Amphotericin B

14. Approximate time interval between HIV infection and manifestations of AIDS is? *(Recent Pattern 2018)*
    a. 7.5 years   b. 10 years
    c. 12 years   d. 15 years

15. What is the correct order of blood sampling?
    a. Verification of patient profile from case file
    b. Labeling by bedside   *(AIIMS Nov 2017)*
    c. Sampling
    d. Ask patient his name

16. 1, 3 beta D –glucan is helpful for identification of?
    a. Invasive candidiasis   b. Rhizopus *(AIIMS Nov 2017)*
    c. Cryptococcus   d. Mucormycosis

17. Which causative organism is responsible for this disease? *(AIIMS Nov 2017)*

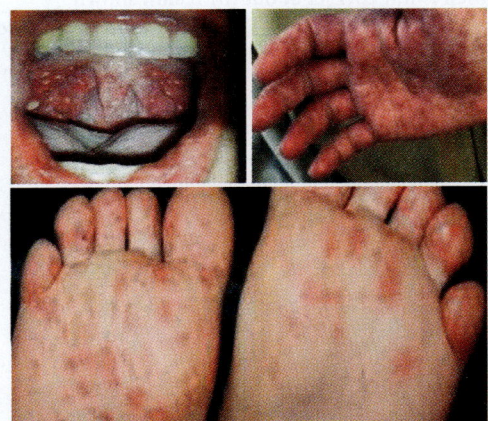

    a. Coxsackie virus   b. Human herpes virus 7
    c. Pox virus   d. Molluscum Contagiosum

18. Urine LAM is used for diagnosis of?
    a. Mycobacterium tuberculosis   *(AIIMS Nov 2017)*
    b. Mycobacterium leprae
    c. Mycoplasma Pneumoniae
    d. Listeria monocytogenes

19. A female from Himachal Pradesh presented with history of thorn prick, a year back. She now has verrucous lesions in the skin with following microscopic findings. Identify the agent. *(AIIMS Nov 2017)*

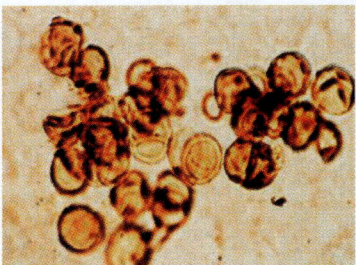

    a. Blastomycosis   b. Chromoblastomycosis
    c. Phaeohyphomycosis   d. Sporotrichosis

20. A patient with HIV develops fever weight loss and diarrhea. Fecal examination shows isospora belli. He was given treatment with TMP – SMX. Diarrhea subsided but fever persisted. Bone marrow examination showed the following picture with intracellular fungi. Which of the following statements is wrong? *(AIIMS Nov 2017)*

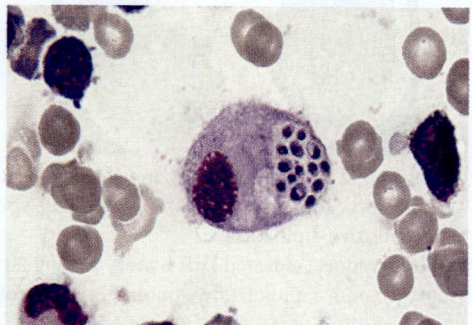

   a. It cannot be grown in SDA
   b. Spores are infective form
   c. It is intracellular budding yeast
   d. It can cause systemic disease

21. Hutchinson's triad consists of all except? *(AIIMS Nov 2017)*
   a. Interstitial keratitis
   b. Eight cranial nerve deafness
   c. Hutchinson teeth
   d. Mulberry teeth

22. Which of the following drug can be given in a case of combined gonococcal and non-gonococcal cervicitis? *(AIIMS Nov 2017)*
   a. Ceftriaxone
   b. Azithromycin
   c. Ciprofloxacin
   d. Cefixime

23. What is the drug of choice for scrub typhus? *(AIIMS Nov 2017)*
   a. Erythromycin   b. Doxycycline
   c. Ciprofloxacin   d. Linezolid

24. All of the following clinical features are seen in Zika Fever except? *(AIIMS May 2017)*
   a. Guillain Barre Syndrome
   b. Petechial Rash
   c. Fever with polyarthralgia
   d. Conjunctivitis

25. The definition of pyrexia of unknown origin includes all except? *(AIIMS May 2017)*
   a. Illness persisting for more than 3 weeks
   b. Undiagnosed fever after 1 week of inpatient work up
   c. Absence of immunocompromised state
   d. Temperature of >38.3 degree C or more

26. A young male is admitted with history of altered sensorium and hydrophobia. A clinical diagnosis of rabies was made and corneal scrapings were taken. Which is the best test to confirm his diagnosis? *(AIIMS May 2017)*
   a. Seller's stain for Negri bodies
   b. Indirect immunofluorescence
   c. Real time PCR
   d. Viral culture

27. 1,3 β-glucan test can be used for all of the following infections except? *(AIIMS May 2017)*
   a. Invasive Aspergillosis
   b. Invasive Candidiasis and Candidemia
   c. Pneumocystis Jiroveci pneumonia
   d. Invasive cryptococcosis

28. A patient with suspected rabies encephalitis is admitted in your hospital. Corneal scraping was taken from the patient. Which of the following test will be performed on the patient to confirm the diagnosis? *(AIIMS Nov 2016)*
   a. Indirect immune-fluroscence
   b. Real Time PCR
   c. Viral culture
   d. Stain for negri bodies

29. A 12-year-old patient presents with fever for 3 days. You have clinical suspicion of dengue and have to investigate him. Which test will not be helpful at this point of time? *(AIIMS Nov 2016)*
   a. Real time PCR   b. NS1 antigen
   c. Viral culture   d. Anti- IgM dengue antibody

30. All of the following patients should be tested for respiratory tuberculosis except? *(AIIMS Nov 2016)*
   a. HIV positive patients with persistent cough
   b. Diabetic patients with persistent cough
   c. Known case of extra-pulmonary TB with persistent cough
   d. Contact with sputum positive patient of TB with persistent cough

31. A young male came with complaints of high grade fever and malaise. His peripheral smear was prepared and is shown below. Diagnosis is? *(AIIMS Nov 2016)*

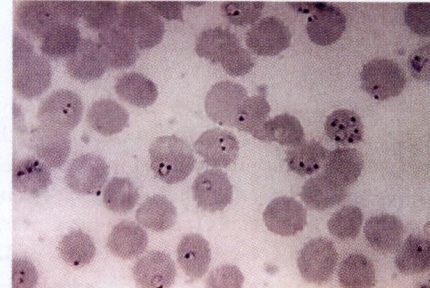

   a. Plasmodium vivax   b. Plasmodium falciparum
   c. Babesiosis   d. Plasmodium malariae

32. Tourniquet test is used for monitoring patients with? *(AIIMS May 2016)*
   a. Infectious mononucleosis
   b. Zika Virus infection
   c. Dengue fever
   d. Chikungunya

33. The most important parameter to monitor dengue haemorrhagic fever is? *(AIIMS May 2016)*
   a. Platelet count   b. Haemoglobin
   c. Total leucocyte count d. Haematocrit

34. A 26-year-old presents with history suggestive of tuberculosis. On examination he has pleural effusion. All of the following parameters will be used for analysis of pleural fluid except? *(AIIMS May 2016)*
   a. Gene XPERT   b. LDH
   c. Albumin   d. ADA

35. A 26-year-old male presents with fever and headache for 3 days. On the 3rd day of illness, BP=90/60 mmHg and examination reveals rashes on the legs as shown. What is the likely diagnosis? (AIIMS May 2016)

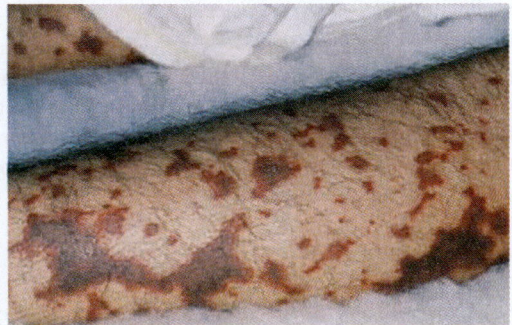

   a. Meningococcus
   b. Dengue Hemorrhagic fever
   c. Enteric Fever
   d. Scrub Typhus

36. All are true about whip worm except?
   a. Worms in jejunal mucosa (Recent Question 2016-17)
   b. No pulmonary passage of Larva
   c. Incubation period is 90 days
   d. Lemon shaped eggs on stool examination

37. Purpura fulminans is a feature of which of the following?
   A. Scarlet fever (APPG 2016)
   B. Acute meningococcemia
   C. Pseudomonas infection
   D. Staphylococcus aureus infection in splenectomised patients
   a. B & D only
   b. A & D only
   c. A & B only
   d. C & D only

38. A 30-year-old farmer is admitted with fever, myalgias and cough. He has conjunctival suffusion and headache; his liver & spleen are palpable. BP=80/60. Blood cultures negative. TLC=14,000. Platelet count is 1 lakh. Liver enzymes are elevated. These are pictures related to his illness. Which of the following statements is TRUE? (APPG 2016)

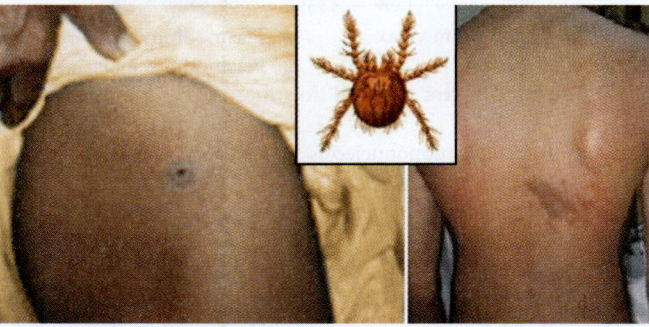

   a. Picture C shows the causative organism Oriental tsutsugamushi
   b. Picture B shows a maculopapular rash which confirms the diagnosis of Lyme disease in this patient
   c. Picture A shows an eschar which confirms the diagnosis of anthrax in this patient
   d. Infected chiggers inoculate organisms into the skin

39. Which one of the following is most likely to be associated with this image? (APPG 2016)

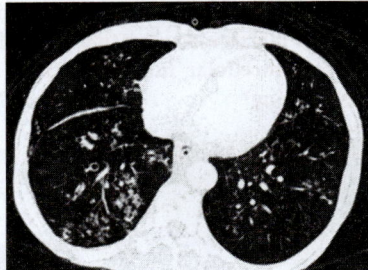

   a. Fever, weight loss, night sweats and elevated ESR
   b. Community acquired infection with rusty sputum and Gram positive diplococci
   c. Acute dyspnoea, elevated JVP, history of long air travel
   d. Acute dyspnoea, pink frothy sputum, mid diastolic rumble at apex

40. A nursing staff while putting IV line to a severely ill patient of HIV accidentally got a needle stick injury. Which of the following investigations will be most appropriate for her?
   a. P24 antigen capture assay (APPG 2016)
   b. ELISA test
   c. Western blot
   d. Blood culture

41. In which of the following diseases, primary skin lesions are not seen? (UPSC 2015)
   a. Leptospirosis   b. S.L.E
   c. Hepatitis-B   d. Infectious mononucleosis

42. Which of the following is least suggestive of poliovirus infection? (UPSC 2015)
   a. Low grade fever and malaise with complete resolution in 2 to 3 days
   b. Biphasic illness with several days of fever, then meningeal symptoms and asymmetric flaccid paralysis 5 to 10 days later
   c. Descending motor paralysis with preservation of tendon reflexes and absent sensation
   d. Failure to isolate a virus from the CSF in the presence of marked meningismus

43. The most common microorganism known to cause tropical pyomyositis is? (UPSC 2015)
   a. Streptococcus viridans   b. Staphylococcus albus
   c. Klebseilla pneumonia   d. Staphylococcus aureus

44. A farmer presents with history of fever and chills, severe bodyache, headache, conjuctival suffusion and jaundice. He has severe muscle tenderness, leukocytosis and mild uremia. The most likely diagnosis would be: (UPSC 2015)
   a. Leptospirosis   b. Typhoid fever
   c. Typhus   d. Viral hepatitis

45. Consider the following statements regarding falciparum malaria? (UPSC 2015)
   A. The mortality rises steeply when the proportion of infected erythrocytes increases above 3 percent.
   B. The patient may develop hypoglycemia even when not treated with quinine.
   Which of the statements given above is/are correct?
   a. A only   b. B only
   c. Both A and B   d. Neither A nor B

46. The cutaneous viral infection which is commonly seen in children and characterized by single or multiple pearly-white skin colored smooth dome shaped papules with central pitting is: *(UPSC 2015)*
    a. Chicken pox   b. Herpes zoster
    c. Molluscum Contagiosum d. Verruca vulgaris

47. Which one of the following tests has the highest chance of detecting HIV infection in a blood donor during the window period? *(Recent Pattern 2015-16)*
    a. Demonstration of antibody to HIV by ELISA
    b. CD4 count
    c. P24 antigen detection
    d. Western blot test

48. The following are exotoxin-mediated infections except: *(UPSC 2015)*
    a. Cholera   b. Typhoid
    c. Botulism   d. Tetanus

49. A child presents with moderate fever for two months. On examination, she had moderate anemia and a few petechiae. All the following can be the diagnosis except? *(UPSC 2015)*
    a. Acute leukemia   b. Tuberculosis
    c. Typhoid   d. Juvenile rheumatoid arthritis

50. An 8-year-old boy presented to the Emergency Department on the fourth day of fever during a dengue epidemic. He had a mild erythematous rash on his body and no bleeding from any site. His BP was 110/70 mmHg and pulse was 104/minute. Hess test was positive. Dengue serology report is awaited. Platelet count is 30,000/cm^3 and PCV: 36%. What is the treatment of choice? *(UPSC 2015)*
    a. Plenty of oral/ IV fluids and observation
    b. Emergency platelet transfusion to raise platelets above 50,000/cm^3
    c. IV anti-D immune globulin
    d. Give antipyretic and wait for dengue serology report

51. Which one of the following is the most likely diagnosis from the picture depicted below? *(APPG 2015)*

    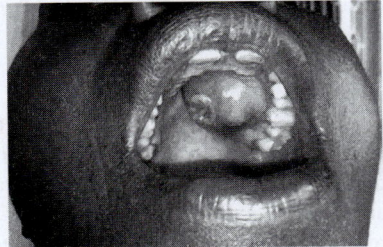

    a. Syphilitic gumma   b. Aphthous ulcer
    c. Dentigenous ulcer d. Leukoplakia

52. Which of the following is true regarding tuberculosis: *(APPG 2015)*
    a. Primary tuberculosis usually involves the mid and lower zones
    b. Primary tuberculosis carries a high level of transmissibility
    c. 90% of inhaled bacilli from droplet nuclei reach the alveoli
    d. Hilar/paratracheal lymphadenopathy is characteristically absent in primary tuberculosis

53. Post exposure prophylaxis of HIV is? *(JIPMER Nov 2015)*
    a. Raltregavir + Emtricitabine + Tenofovir
    b. Zidovudine + Lamivudine + Indinavir
    c. Zidovudine + lamivudine + abacavir
    d. Raltregavir + Emtricitabine + Maraviroc

54. Membrane over tonsil with atypical lymphocytes 12%. Treatment is? *(JIPMER Nov 2015)*
    a. Acyclovir   b. Prednisolone
    c. IVIG   d. Acetaminophen

55. A 16 years boy had urethral discharge 1 week after having unprotected intercourse gram staining of the discharge reveals diplococci he was treated with few intracellular gram negative diplococci He was treated with 250 mg intramuscular injection of ceftriaxone 7 days later he present with same complains, what is the most probable cause? *(JIPMER Nov 2014)*
    a. Reinfection with gonorrhea
    b. Resistance to Penicillin
    c. Infection with Chlamydia
    d. Ureaplasma Urealyticum Infection

56. A young male with history of diarrhea for month and fever was suspected to have HIV blood tests positive for HIV. A diagnosis of AIDS will be made by the presence of which of the following? *(JIPMER Nov 2014)*
    a. Oral candidiasis   b. Pulmonary tuberculosis
    c. Lyme's disease   d. Hemolytic uremic syndrome

57. Which of the following lesion represent tertiary syphilis: *(PGI May 2015)*
    a. Condylomata lata   b. Matted lymph nodes
    c. Condylomata acuminata d. Tabes dorsalis
    e. Gumma formation

58. True about Kaposi sarcoma: *(PGI May 2015)*
    a. Vascular tumor
    b. Associated with HIV
    c. Involves visceral organs
    d. Associated with Human herpes virus-8
    e. Radiotherapy may be used in treatment

59. Which parasite is shown in the peripheral smear?
    a. Plasmodium falciparum b. Plasmodium vivax
    c. Plasmodium ovale   d. Plasmodium malariae

60. All are true about Dengue hemorrhagic fever except? *(AIIMS Nov 2014)*
    a. Lamivudine is drug of choice
    b. Malnutrition is protective
    c. Transmitted by Aedes
    d. Causative agent belongs to Flaviviradae group

61. Typhoid is treated by all except? *(Recent Pattern 2015-16)*
    a. Erythromycin   b. Ceftriaxone
    c. Amikacin   d. Ciprofloxacin

62. Drug treatment is given for how many days in pneumococcal meningitis? *(Recent Pattern 2015-16)*
    a. 5 days   b. 7 days
    c. 14 days   d. 21 days

63. Most common pulmonary manifestation in AIDS: *(Recent Pattern 2014-15)*
    a. TB
    b. Pneumonia
    c. Bronchiectasis
    d. Mycobacterial avium intercellulare

64. Most common presentation of extra-pulmonary TB: *(Recent Pattern 2014-15)*
    a. Tubercular lymphadenitis
    b. Peritoneal TB
    c. Pericardial TB
    d. Tubercular meningitis

65. **Kaposi sarcoma is commonly seen in:**
    (Recent Pattern 2014-15)
    a. Upper limbs   b. Lower limbs
    c. Head and neck   d. Trunk

66. **Site of Gohn focus in congenital TB:**
    (Recent Pattern 2014-15)
    a. Lung   b. Liver
    c. Git   d. Brain

67. **Pathognomonic of miliary TB:** *(Recent Pattern 2014-15)*
    a. Snow storm appearance in CXR
    b. Choroid tubercles on fundus examination
    c. Pericardial TB
    d. Peritoneal TB

68. **In AIDS patient presenting with fever, cough a diagnosis of pneumocystis pneumonia is best established by:**
    a. CT scan chest   *(Recent Pattern 2014-15)*
    b. Bronchoalveolar lavage
    c. Staining of intra-nuclear inclusion with Silver staining
    d. Aspiration and Culture

69. **The most common cause of seizures in a patient of AIDS is:**
    a. Toxoplasmosis   *(Recent Pattern 2014-15)*
    b. Cryptococcal meningitis
    c. Progressive multifocal leucoencephalopathy
    d. CNS lymphoma

70. **Incorrect about Tuberculous meningitis:**
    a. Normal CSF sugar   *(Recent Pattern 2014-15)*
    b. Cerebral infarction
    c. Communicating hydrocephalus
    d. Tuberculoma resolves after treatment

71. **Gene responsible for resistance to rifampicin:**
    (Recent Pattern 2014-15)
    a. Rpo B gene   b. Kat G gene
    c. Rpm B gene   d. Emb B gene

72. **All are indications for stopping offending ATT drug permanently except?**
    (Recent Pattern 2014-15)
    a. Gout
    b. Autoimmune Thrombocytopenia
    c. Optic neuritis
    d. Hepatitis

73. **Side-effect of zidovidine in AIDS patient is:**
    a. Megaloblastic anemia   *(Recent Pattern 2014-15)*
    b. Hyperuricaemia
    c. Nephrocalcinosis
    d. Pancreatitis

74. **Consider the following statements regarding HIV.**
    (UPSC 2014)
    1. The risk of infection is 10 times more with solid needle than hollow needle.
    2. The mode of transmission is through infected blood
    3. CD 4 cell amount is directly related to viral load
    4. Post exposure prophylaxis should start within one hour of contamination
    Which of these statements are correct?
    a. 1 & 2   b. 2 only
    c. 3 & 4   d. 2,3 & 4

75. **Interferon gamma release assay measures IFN release against which M.TB antigen:** *(Recent Pattern 2014-15)*
    a. ESAT 6   b. ESAT 7
    c. CF 11   d. CF 12

76. **MDR TB must be treated for at least:**
    (Recent Pattern 2014-15)
    a. 12 months   b. 18 months
    c. 20 months   d. 36 months

77. **All are seen with Pneumocystis carini in AIDS except:**
    a. Pneumonia   *(Recent Pattern 2014-15)*
    b. Otic polypoid mass
    c. Ophthalmic choroid lesion
    d. Meningitis

78. **Earliest and often the only presentation of TB kidneys is:**
    (Recent Pattern 2014-15)
    a. Increased frequency   b. Colicky pain
    c. Hematuria   d. Renal calculi

79. **Most common cause of diarrhea in AIDS patients:**
    (Recent Pattern 2014-15)
    a. Salmonella typhimurium b. Cryptosporidium
    c. Candida   d. Isophora

80. **Relative risk of developing TB in patients already infected with TB bacillus is highest in:** *(Recent Pattern 2014-15)*
    a. Diabetes   b. Recent infection
    c. Post transplantation   d. Malnutrition

81. **I.R.I.S is:**   *(Recent Pattern 2014-15)*
    a. Immune reconstitution idiopathic syndrome
    b. Immune reconstitution immunological syndrome
    c. Immune reconstitution inflammatory syndrome
    d. Inflammatory reconstitution immune syndrome

82. **Incorrect about HIV associated nephropathy?**
    a. Proteinuria   *(Recent Pattern 2014-15)*
    b. Shrunken kidneys
    c. 15% cases show mesangial proliferation
    d. Develops when CD4 < 200 cells/cu.mm

83. **All are seen in acute HIV syndrome except:**
    (Recent Pattern 2014-15)
    a. Diarrhoea   b. Pneumonia
    c. Weight loss   d. Myelopathy

84. **HIV RNA by PCR can detect as low as:**
    a. 30 copies viral RNA/ml of blood *(Recent Pattern 2014-15)*
    b. 40 copies viral RNA/ml of blood
    c. 50 copies of viral RNA/ml of blood
    d. 60 copies of viral RNA/ml of blood

85. **Most common cause of pleural effusion in AIDS patients?**
    (Recent Pattern 2014-15)
    a. Kaposi Sarcoma   b. TB
    c. Pneumocystis Jiroveci d. mycoplasma

86. **Interferon is not used in:** *(Recent Pattern 2014-15)*
    a. CML
    b. Polymyositis
    c. Hairy cell leukaemia
    d. Chronic hepatitis c infection

87. **Treatment of Latent TB infection in Tuberculin positive, HIV positive patients:** *(Recent Pattern 2014-15)*
    a. INH biweekly for 9 months
    b. $2(HRZ)_3 + 4(HR)_3$
    c. Rifampicin biweekly for 6 months
    d. Pyrazinamide daily for 6 months

88. **Latex agglutination test in CSF is done for detection of:**
    (Recent Pattern 2014-15)
    a. Cryptococcus   b. E.Coli
    c. Tuberculosis   d. Coxsackie

89. **Which among the following statements is true about toxoplasma:** *(Recent Pattern 2014-15)*
    a. In adults it is mostly asymptomatic
    b. IgG antibodies in the newborn is confirmatory of diagnosis
    c. Toxoplasmic encephalitis can occur in immunocompetent
    d. Most infections are transmitted by blood products

90. **There is no correlation between X-ray appearance and clinical state of the patient in, pneumonia:** *(Recent Pattern 2014-15)*
    a. Mycoplasma   b. Freidlanders
    c. Pneumococcal   d. Staphylococcal

91. **Best test for determining eradication of H.Pylori infection:** *(Recent Pattern 2014-15)*
    a. Urease test   b. Breath urea test
    c. Tissue biopsy   d. Serum ELISA

92. **True about Cryptococcus Neoformans is A/E:** *(Recent Pattern 2014-15)*
    a. Capsule excludes India ink particles
    b. Common in immunocompromised patient
    c. Anti-capsular antibody prevents recurrence
    d. Strongly positive Mucicarmine stain of the organism in tissue is useful

93. **CLO test is used for:** *(Recent Pattern 2014-15)*
    a. H.pylori   b. Brucella
    c. Gonorrhoea   d. EBOLA

94. **An 8-year old patient presents with fever, sore throat and lymphadenopathy. On examination hepatosplenomegaly was found. Peripheral blood film shows 20% atypical lymphoctytosis, the most likely diagnosis is:** *(Recent Pattern 2014-15)*
    a. CLL   b. Infectious mononucleosis
    c. ALL   d. CML

95. **While discharging a patient of meningitis due to H. influenzae the essential step you will do:** *(Recent Pattern 2014-15)*
    a. EEG
    b. Assess developmental milestones
    c. Bilateral evoked auditory response
    d. Refer for physiotherapy

96. **Valve affected in infective endocarditis due to septic abortion?** *(Recent Pattern 2014-15)*
    a. Mitral   b. Tricuspid
    c. Pulmonary   d. Aortic

97. **Best management after human bite:** *(Recent Pattern 2014-15)*
    a. Ampicillin plus sulbactam
    b. Clindamycin plus TMP-SMX
    c. Fluroquinolone
    d. Doxycycline

98. **All of the following are morphological neurological complication of measles except:** *(Recent Pattern 2014-15)*
    a. Transverse myelitis   b. Encephalitis
    c. Optic neuritis   d. SSPE

99. **Which is not a feature of cerebral malaria?** *(Recent Pattern 2014-15)*
    a. Bloody CSF   b. Retinal haemorrhages
    c. Extensor plantar reflex   d. Absent abdominal reflex

100. **Healing with calcification is a feature of:** *(Recent Pattern 2014-15)*
    a. Cryptococcosis   b. Mucormycosis
    c. Aspergillosis   d. Histoplasmosis

101. **Bacterial endocarditis is most commonly seen in:** *(Recent Pattern 2014-15)*
    a. VSD   b. PDA
    c. ASD   d. AS

102. **All are useful for management of severe clostridium difficile treatment except:** *(Recent Pattern 2014-15)*
    a. Intravenous Metronidazole
    b. Neomycin enema
    c. Fecal transplant
    d. Tigecycline

103. **Faget sign is:** *(Recent Pattern 2014-15)*
    a. Tachycardia with hypertension
    b. Bradycardia with hyperthermia
    c. Tachycardia with hyperthermia
    d. Bradycardia with hypothermia

104. **Which of the following is not associated with Streptococcus?** *(Recent Pattern 2014-15)*
    a. Rheumatic fever
    b. Scarlet fever
    c. Acute GN
    d. Scalded skin syndrome

105. **Best test for mycoplasma infection is?** *(Recent Pattern 2014-15)*
    a. PCR of respiratory secretions
    b. Gram stain of transtracheal aspirate
    c. Culture of transtracheal aspirate
    d. CXR

106. **All can be seen as Post-Diarrhoea complications except:** *(Recent Pattern 2014-15)*
    a. HUS   b. Nephritic syndrome
    c. Reactive arthritis d. Guillain Barre syndrome

107. **Most common cause of death in diphtheria is due to?** *(Recent Pattern 2014-15)*
    a. Airway compromise
    b. Toxic cardiomyopathy
    c. Sepsis
    d. Descending polyneuropathy

108. **Aspergilloma is commonly a complication of:** *(Recent Pattern 2014-15)*
    a. TB   b. Bronchogenic carcinoma
    c. Cystic fibrosis   d. Wegener's granulomatiosis

109. **Lucio phenomenon is treated with:** *(Recent Pattern 2014-15)*
    a. Steroids   b. Lenalidomide
    c. Clofazimine   d. Exchange transfusion

110. **Among the toxins produced by Clostridium botulinum, the most potent is:** *(Recent Pattern 2014-15)*
    a. A   b. C
    c. D   d. F

111. **Drug of choice in type I lepra reaction with severe neuritis is:** *(Recent Pattern 2014-15)*
    a. Systemic steroid   b. Clofazimine
    c. Thalidomide   d. Chloroquine

112. **Correct about CURB 65 score:** *(Recent Pattern 2014-15)*
    a. Patient with score of 0 has 1.5% chances of dying
    b. Urea < 7mmol/L
    c. BP > 90/60 mm Hg
    d. Coma

113. A 15-year-old boy presents to you with history of fever, altered sensorium and purpuric rash for two days. On examination, the patient is found stuporous. He has BP of 90/60 mm Hg and extensive palpable purpura over the legs. Which of the following would be the most appropriate initial choice of antibiotic? *(Recent Pattern 2014-15)*
    a. Vancomycin
    b. Penicillin G
    c. Ciprofloxacin
    d. Ceftriaxone

114. The statements regarding falciparum malaria are all except:
    a. Haemoglobinuria and renal failure
    b. Hypoglycemia *(Recent Pattern 2014-15)*
    c. Cerebral malaria
    d. Adequately prevented with chloroquine therapy

115. Most common cause of death in measles? *(Recent Pattern 2014-15)*
    a. Encephalitis
    b. Meningitis
    c. Dehydration
    d. Pneumonia

116. Most common extra-cutaneous manifestation of chicken pox is: *(Recent Pattern 2014-15)*
    a. CNS involvement
    b. Varicella pneumonia
    c. Congenital varicella
    d. Reye syndrome

117. EB virus is associated with all except: *(Recent Pattern 2014-15)*
    a. Bell's palsy
    b. Hepatitis
    c. Guillain-Barre syndrome
    d. Laennec's cirrhosis

118. Changing character of a murmur in a patient with joint pain and embolic phenomenon indicates the diagnosis of: *(Recent Pattern 2014-15)*
    a. Mitral stenosis
    b. SABE
    c. Rheumatiod arthritis
    d. Aortic regurgitation

119. Romana's sign is seen in: *(Recent Pattern 2014-15)*
    a. Toxoplasma
    b. Trypanosoma cruzi
    c. Loa loa
    d. Wuchereria

120. Incorrect about prosthetic valve endocarditis is:
    a. Embolism *(Recent Pattern 2014-15)*
    b. Mitral valve mostly involved
    c. C.O.N.S < 1 year of operation
    d. Strept. Viridans > 1 year of operation

121. Skeleton changes in syphilis are all except? *(Recent Pattern 2014-15)*
    a. Saber shin
    b. Olympian brow
    c. Scaphoid scapula
    d. Thickening of acromio-clavicular joint

122. Which of the following is not a finding in kala azar?
    a. Pancytopenia *(Recent Pattern 2014-15)*
    b. Oral miltefosine
    c. Hyperpigmentation
    d. Tropical splenomegaly syndrome

123. Most common presentation of gonorrhoeal infections is: *(Recent Pattern 2014-15)*
    a. Urethritis
    b. Prostatitis
    c. Orchitis
    d. Epididymitis

124. The following is true about malaria: *(Recent Pattern 2014-15)*
    a. P. falciparum can cause relapse
    b. P. vivax can be detected by HRP-2 Dipstick
    c. P. vivax causes enlargement of affected RBC
    d. LDH card test quantitates the falciparum parasitemia

125. Bull neck in diphtheria is due to: *(Recent Pattern 2014-15)*
    a. Retropharyngial abscess
    b. Laryngeal oedema
    c. Cellulitis
    d. Lymphadenopathy

126. DOC for treatment of SSPE: *(Recent Pattern 2014-15)*
    a. Abacavir
    b. Isoprinosine
    c. Glatiramer
    d. Interferon

127. True statement about Neuro-cysticercosis is:
    a. Usually presents with seizures *(Recent Pattern 2014-15)*
    b. Albendazole is more effective than praziquantel
    c. Usually presents with 6th nerve palsy and hemiparesis
    d. High does steroid are given for hydrocephalus

128. Which about Legionnaires pneumonia is not true: *(Recent Pattern 2014-15)*
    a. Erythromycin is the drug of choice
    b. Seen mainly in immune-suppressed patients
    c. Smoking and alcohol are risk factors
    d. Common in children and adults

129. Rademecker complex in EEG is seen in: *(Recent Pattern 2014-15)*
    a. SSPE
    b. vCJD
    c. cCJD
    d. Kuru

130. Regarding amoebic liver abscess which of the following is true: *(Recent Pattern 2014-15)*
    a. Multiple abscess are more common
    b. Most of the patients have a history of dysentery at the time of presentation
    c. May rupture into the pleural cavity
    d. For asymptomatic luminal carriers parmomycin is the drug of choice

131. A 60-year-old man has developed atypical pneumonia. Which of the following statements regarding pneumonia is correct: *(Recent Pattern 2014-15)*
    a. Urine test for legionella antigen is 90% sensitive
    b. A negative blood culture would rule out the diagnosis of infecting organism
    c. Absence of rigors excludes a diagnosis of pneumococcal pneumonia
    d. Drug of choice is levofloxacin

132. All of the following are associated with HUS except:
    a. Thrombocytopenia *(Recent Pattern 2014-15)*
    b. Oliguria
    c. Pain
    d. Purpura

133. The following statements are correct for Helicobacter pylori except: *(Recent Pattern 2014-15)*
    a. It shows positive urease test
    b. It is spiral gram negative flagellate
    c. It can invade tissue to a great depth
    d. It is linked with duodenal ulcer

134. Eosinophilic meningo-encephalitis is caused by: *(Recent Pattern 2014-15)*
    a. Acanthamoeba
    b. Naegleria
    c. Angiostrongylus
    d. Toxoplasma

135. Left sided endocarditis is associated with: *(Recent Pattern 2014-15)*
    a. Endocardial cushion defect
    b. O. Secondum ASD
    c. O. Primum ASD
    d. Patent Fossa Ovalis

136. **Stage III of Lyme's disease is characterized by:**
    (Recent Pattern 2014-15)
    a. Meningoencephalitis   b. Myocarditis
    c. Arthritis   d. Nephritis
137. **Differential diagnosis of Botulism are all except?**
    a. GB syndrome   *(Recent Pattern 2014-15)*
    b. Myasthenia gravis
    c. Lambert Eaton syndrome
    d. Clostridial myonecrosis
138. **Not major criteria for diagnosis of neurocysticercosis?**
    (Recent Pattern 2014-15)
    a. Detection of cysticerci antigen by immunoblot
    b. Detection of cysticerci antigen by ELISA
    c. Cystic lesion in brain parenchyma by MRI
    d. Calcified lesion in brain parenchyma by CT
139. **Prophylactic antibiotic therapy not given for infective endocarditis are A/E:**   *(Recent Pattern 2014-15)*
    a. Permanent transvenous pacemaker
    b. Atrial septal defect
    c. Ventricle septal defect
    d. Coronary artery bypass graft
140. **A 30-year-old man, presented with subcutaneous itchy nodules over the left iliac crest. On examination, they are firm, non-tender and mobile. Skin snips contain microfilaria and adult worms of:** *(Recent Pattern 2014-15)*
    a. Loa Loa   b. Onchocerca volvulus
    c. Brugia malayi   d. Mansonella perstans
141. **"In pseudomembranous colitis" the investigation of choice is?**
    a. Stool microscopy   *(Recent Pattern 2014-15)*
    b. CT scan abdomen
    c. Glutamate dehydrogenase immunoassay
    d. Sigmoidoscopy
142. **Treponema pallidum crosses placenta:**
    a. After 36 weeks   *(Recent Pattern 2014-15)*
    b. After 28 weeks
    c. After 2nd trimester
    d. At any stage of pregnancy
143. **Neisseria infection is characteristic of deficiency of:**
    (Recent Pattern 2014-15)
    a. C2   b. C3
    c. C4   d. C5
144. **Dawson disease is:**   *(Recent Pattern 2014-15)*
    a. SSPE
    b. Acute disseminated encephalomyelitis
    c. Neuromyelitis optica
    d. Paralysis agitans
145. **Volcano ulcers in esophagus are seen in:**
    a. Herpetic esophagitis   *(Recent Pattern 2014-15)*
    b. Candida esophagitis
    c. Apthous ulcer in crohn
    d. HIV esophagitis
146. **Neurological manifestation of Whipple's disease is:**
    a. Seizures   *(Recent Pattern 2014-15)*
    b. Cerebellar ataxia
    c. Focal neurological deficits
    d. Encephalopathy
147. **Rhinocerebral mucormycosis is present with:**
    a. Broad spectrum antibiotic use   *(Recent Pattern 2014-15)*
    b. Pregnancy
    c. Diabetic ketoacidosis
    d. Renal tubular acidosis
148. **Most common cause of death in EBV?**
    a. Splenic abscess   *(Recent Pattern 2014-15)*
    b. Meningo-encephalitis
    c. Fulminant hepatitis
    d. Auto-immune haemolytic anemia
149. **Pontiac fever is caused by:**   *(Recent Pattern 2014-15)*
    a. Marbug virus
    b. Legionella
    c. Tuberculosis bacilli
    d. Sindbis virus
150. **In giardiasis malabsorption is due to all except:**
    a. Mucosal injury   *(Recent Pattern 2014-15)*
    b. Bacterial overgrowth
    c. Lactose intolerance
    d. Hypogammaglobulinaemia
151. **Indications to eradicate H. pylori:** *(Recent Pattern 2014-15)*
    a. Low grade B cell lymphoma
    b. Gastric outlet obstruction
    c. Duodenal ulcer
    d. Family history of gastric cancer
152. **All of the following are true regarding snake bite management in India except?**   *(AIIMS Nov 2015)*
    a. Atropine and neostigmine play a major role in management of snake bite
    b. Hump nosed pit viper (Hypnale hypnale) is not covered under the ASV provided in India
    c. ASV is the mainstay of treatment
    d. Neostigmine and Atropine can be used in the treatment of Bungarus cerulas (Common Krait) poisoning
153. **Hutchinson sign is a feature of ocular involvement by which of the following viruses?**   *(UPSC 2015)*
    a. Herpes simplex   b. Epstein-Barr virus
    c. Cytomegalovirus   d. Herpes zoster
154. **Scorpion sting may present with the following except?**
    a. Salivation and lacrimation   *(APPG 2015)*
    b. Arrhythmias
    c. Hypothermia
    d. Hypertension and pulmonary edema

Answers with Explanations

1. Ans. (a) Cysticercus cellulosae

(Ref: cdc.gov)

The image shows a globular scolex with suction cups and a circular row of rostellum that gives a solar appearance. This is a feature of cysticercosis.

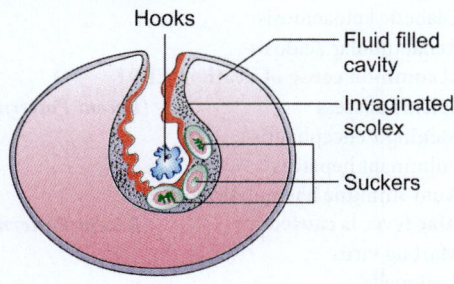

2. Ans. (c) Bilaterally symmetrical dermatomal vesicular eruption

(Ref: Harrison 20th edition, page 1355:)

- The image shows lesions of herpes zoster that develop unilaterally in a single dermatome.
- Choice A is correct since seronegative individuals on contact with these patients can develop chicken pox.
- Choice B is correct since neurological complication can develop in form meningoencephalitis.
- Choice D is correct since Ramsay hunt syndrome leads to eruption in external auditory canal and the geniculate ganglion of sensory division of facial nerve is involved.

3. Ans. (a) Sarcoptes scabiei

(Ref: Fitzpatrick Colour Atlas: 8th edition, page 732)

- The image shows Sarcoptes scabiei (itch mite) which burrows into the skin and causes scabies.
- Choice B is an obligate ectoparasite that leads to head lice infestation.
- Choice C is an obligate ectoparasite that feeds on human blood and is found in pubic hair and eye lashes
- Choice D is the human bot fly, the larva of which parasitize humans.

4. Ans. (a) Impetigo contagiosa

(Ref: Harrison 20th edition, page 1084)

The image shows impetigo contagiosa which is the most common bacterial infection in children. It is a highly contagious infection of the superficial layers of the epidermis that is primarily caused by *Streptococcus pyogenes* or *Staphylococcus aureus*.

The first image shows partially healed lesion in the area of neck and hence the classical honey crusting is not seen. The second image show streptococcus bacteria in chains.

5. Ans. (b) Intertriginous candida

(Ref: Fitzpatrick Colour Atlas: 8th edition, page 598)

- The image shows intertriginous dermatitis which can be induced or aggravated by heat, moisture, maceration, friction, and lack of air circulation.
- Intertrigo is frequently worsened by infection, which most commonly is with *Candida* species. Bacterial, viral, or other fungal infections may also occur.
- Intertrigo commonly affects the axilla, perineum, inframammary creases, and abdominal folds. In infants it can also affect the neck creases and interdigital areas.
- Choice A will lead to extensive desquamation all over the body. Choice C presents as honey crust lesions. Choice D is an ulcerative form of impetigo characterised by small punched out ulcer with thick crusting and surrounding erythema.

6. Ans. (a) Tertiary syphilis

(Ref: CMDT 2019, page 1139)

Definitive AIDS diagnoses (with or without laboratory evidence of HIV infection)

• Candidiasis of the esophagus, trachea, bronchi, or lungs
• Cryptoccoccosis, extrapulmonary
• Crytosporidiosis with diarrhea persisting longer than 1 month
• Cytomegalovirus disease of an organ other than liver, spleen, or lymph nodes
• Herpes simplex virus infection causing a mucocutaneous ulcer that persists longer than 1 month; or bronchitis, pneumonitis or esophagitis of any duration
• Kaposi sarcoma in a patient younger than 60 years of age
• Lymphoma of the brain (primary) in a pattient younger than 60 years of age.
• *Mycobacterium avium* complex or *Mycobacterium kansasii* disease, disseminated (at a site other than or in addition to lungs, skin or cervical or hilar lymph nodes).
• Peneumocystis jirovecii pneumonia
• Progessive multifocal leukoencephalopathy
• Toxoplasmoss of the brain.

7. Ans. (c) Toxoplasma

(Ref: Harrison 20th edition, page 862)

Normally For every 1 degree Celsius rise of body temperature, heart rate increases by 15-20 beats/min. But the same is not seen in Toxoplasmosis. Both malaria and babesia are causes of relative bradycardia.

Causes of Relative Bradycardia

Infectious	Non-infectious
Legionella	b-blockers
Psittacosis	CNS lesion
Q fever	Lymphomas
Typhoid fever	Factitious fever
Typhus	Drug fever
Babesiosis	
Malaria	
Leptospirosis	
Yellow fever	
Dengue fever	
Viral hemorrhagic fevers	
Rocky mountain spotted fever	

8. Ans. (d) Antifungals for oral candidiasis

(Ref: Harrison 20th edition, page 1529)

The image shows cheesy white confluent adherent plaques on hard palate, uvula and tonsils. These are a feature of oropharyngeal candidiasis.

9. Ans. (a) Rectal thermo-probe

(Ref: Internet)

The image shows a rectal thermo-probe which is used to evaluate core temperature.

10. Ans. (b) Entamoeba

(Ref: Harrison 20th edition, page 1571)

- The presentation is of amoebic colitis which presents with scanty fecal matter and mainly blood and mucus in stools. The definitive diagnosis is made by demonstration of hematophagous trophozoites of E. Histiolytica. Stool tests positive for heme with few WBC seen. Fever can be seen in 40% cases of E. Histiolytica infection.
- Choice A leads to watery diarrhoea and malabsorption but does not have blood in the stool.
- Choice C presents mainly with nausea and vomiting.
- Choice D presents with profuse watery diarrhoea.

11. Ans. (c) Doxycycline

(Ref: Harrison 20th edition, page 1307)

- The image shows an eschar with a rash on the trunk of the patient. In setting of fever with the cutaneous findings, the diagnosis is Rickettsial pox. The drug of choice is doxycycline.
- It is caused by R. akari and is transmitted via the bite of a mite. The bite goes unnoticed till patient develops fever with chills, rash and regional lymphadenopathy. Some patients develop GI Symptoms like nausea, vomiting and abdominal pain.
- Eschar formation is also a feature of scrub typhus transmitted by bite of chiggers (larval mites). This infection is re-emerging in India.
- The eschar of Rickettsial pox should not be confused with that of anthrax.

12. Ans. (a) Dark field microscopy

(Ref: Harrison 20th edition, page 1293-94)

The presentation of hepatorenal syndrome with dark field microscopy tight spiral appearance of organisms with hooked ends is a feature of Leptospirosis.

Definitive diagnosis of leptospirosis is based on following methods:
- Positive PCR
- Seroconversion or rise in antibody titer (Four times elevation by convalescence)
- Microscopy agglutination test

13. Ans. (d) Liposomal Amphotericin B

(Ref: Harrison 20th edition pg. 1597; Katzung 13th edition pg. 901)

RK 39 dipstick test is a rapid immunochromatographic test being widely used in diagnosis of Visceral Leishmaniasis. The test requires a drop of finger prick blood and the result can be read in 15 minutes. Liposomal amphotericin B is the drug of choice for management of Leishmaniasis.

14. Ans. (b) 10 years

(Ref: Harrison 20th edition, p 1406; Harrison 19th edition, p 1429)

Harrison states *"the length of time from initial infection to development of clinical infection varies, the median time for untreated patients is approximately 10 years"*

15. Ans. (b) 4,1,3,2,

(Ref: WHO Guidelines on drawing blood and page 3, Dacie and lewis practical hematology 11th edition)

16. Ans. (a) Invasive candidiasis

(Ref: Harrison 20th edition, p 1531; Harrison 19th edition, page 1330 and 1360)

Non-invasive methods for the detection of *invasive fungal infections*:
1. Galactomannan *Aspergillus* antigen
2. Fungal wall component (1–3)-β-D-glucan
   - Glucan is the most important and abundant polysaccharide component of the cell wall of most fungi with the exceptions of *Mucor, Rhizopus, Blastomyces dermatitidis*, and *Cryptococcus* species.
   - The current guidelines of the Infectious Diseases Society of America for the management of candidiasis

and aspergillosis recommend serum (1–3)-β-D-glucan testing to assist in the assessment of patients with suspected deep-seated fungal infections.
- For diagnosis of Cryptococcus infection, Cryptococcal antigen (CRAg) test in CSF and blood is used.

17. Ans. (a) Coxsackie virus

(Ref: Harrison 19th edition, page 238 and Ananthanarayan Microbiology – 10th ed. – page 497)

- The image shows vesicular eruptions on the palms and undersurface of the tongue. Involvement of palms, soles, oral mucosa and oropharynx is a feature of hand foot and mouth disease. The organism responsible is Coxsackie virus A 16.
- The lesions are infectious and painful. Healing occurs in 2–4 weeks.
- HHV 7 has been found to be associated with Pityriasis Rosea.
- Molluscum Contagiosum virus causes characteristic skin lesions consisting of single or multiple, rounded, dome-shaped, pink, waxy papules which are 2-5 mm (rarely up to 1.5 cm in the case of a giant molluscus) in diameter. The papules are umbilicated and contain a caseous plug.

18. Ans. (a) Mycobacterium tuberculosis

(Ref: Manson's Tropical diseases 23rd edition, page 491)

- Urinary Lipoarabinomannan allows for detection of MTB, including extra-pulmonary or disseminated forms of disease. The WHO has recently advocated the use of lateral flow LAM assay for HIV infected hospitalized individuals with CD4<100.
- Lipoarabinomannan is involved in pathogen host interaction and facilitates the survival of M. Tuberculosis.
- This test is in addition to XPERT MTB/ RIF, a rapid nucleic acid amplification test for extra-pulmonary TB diagnosis.

19. Ans. (b) Chromoblastomycosis

(Ref: Ananthanarayan and Panikar T.B. of microbiology – 10th ed. – page 605)

The image shows KOH mount showing *copper penny cells/ muriform cells* diagnostic of chromoblastomycosis. They are thick walled round cells with muriform septation.

Choice A Blastomycosis is ruled out as it is a *systemic* fungal infection involving lungs, CNS and renal system.
Budding round thick walled yeast cells are seen.

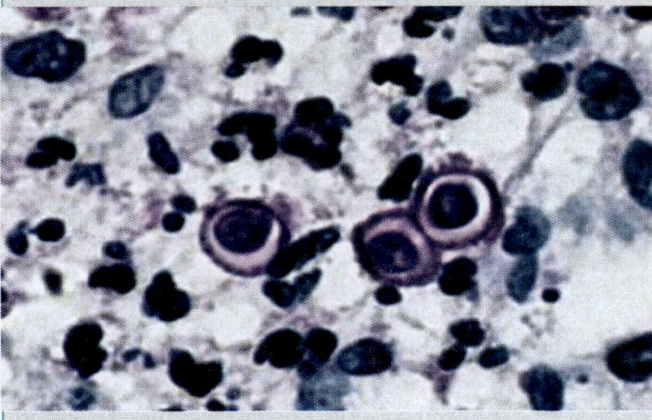

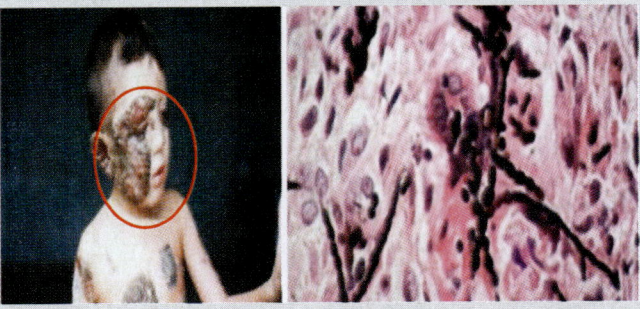

Choice C Phaeohyphomycosis is a subcutaneous *and* systemic fungal infection and is *not locally restricted* like chromoblastomycosis.

Choice D Sporotrichosis is caused by trauma mostly thorn pricks. The tissue section will show *cigar shaped yeast* cells and exhibit Splendore Hoeppli phenomenon.

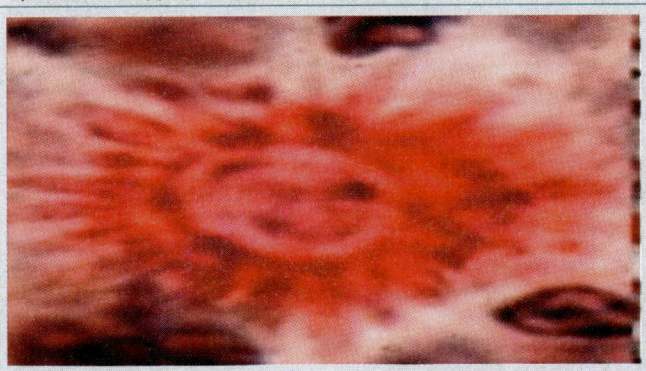

20. Ans. (a) It cannot be grown in SDA

(Ref: Ananthanarayan 10th edition, page 610)

The image shows intracellular yeast inside a macrophage with a peripheral nucleus.

The nucleus is dark purple and crescent shaped. This is a feature of Histoplasma capsulatum.

Notice the retraction of cell wall of yeast (red mark) giving it a capsule like appearance

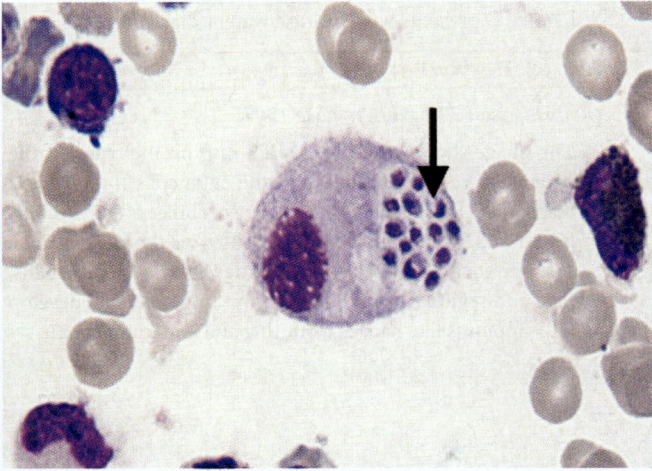

The fungus enters via the lungs and due to immuno-compromised state can cause disseminated disease. The fungus can be cultured on *Sabouraud's dextrose agar* but takes 15-20 days to grow.

21. Ans. (d) Mulberry teeth

(Ref: Harrison 20th edition, p 1283; Rook's textbook of Dermatology, page 29; Harrison 19th edition page no. 1134)

Hutchinson Triad

Interstitial keratitis	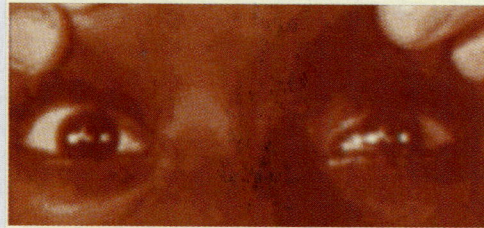
Hutchinson teeth	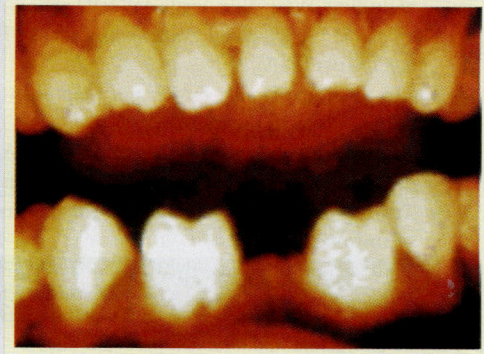
Deafness (Sensorineural)	

- *Hutchinson pupil*: Ipsilateral mid dilated pupil with sluggish reaction to light in raised ICP
- *Hutchinson sign*: Ocular symptoms are more common when vesicles form on the nose during reactivation of latent varicella infection.
- *Hutchinson Gilford progeria syndrome*: Accelerated aging leading to atherosclerosis, cataracts and kidney malfunction.

22. Ans. (b) Azithromycin

(Ref: Harrison 20th edition, p 1128; Harrison 19th edition, page 1008)

- Currently ceftriaxone is the mainstay of therapy for uncomplicated gonococcal infection of the urethra, cervix, rectum or pharynx.
- Alternative regimens for uncomplicated gonococcal infection are:
  1. Gemifloxacin plus Azithromycin
  2. Gentamycin plus Azithromycin
- Because of co-infection with C. Trachomatis initial treatment regimen must incorporate azithromycin (extended release microsphere formulation) or doxycycline.
- Rising MIC of *cefixime* has resulted in CDC to *discontinue* its recommendation.

23. Ans. (b) Doxycycline

(Ref: Harrison 20th edition, p 1306, 1309; Harrison 19th edition page no. 1159)

Serological assays like indirect fluorescent antibody test, indirect immune-peroxidase are used for diagnosis. Patients are treated with:
1. Doxycycline 100mg BD for 2 weeks
2. Azithromycin 500 mg OD for 3 days
3. Chloramphenicol 500mg QID for 2 weeks

24. Ans. (b) Petechial Rash

(Ref: Harrison 20th edition, p 1499; CMDT 2018, page 1422-23)

- Zika fever presents with acute onset fever with pruritic maculopapular rash.
- Concomitant non-purulent conjunctivitis and arthralgia occurs and mimics chikungunya infection.
- Symptoms last for about 7 days
- Though it does not cause haemorrhagic complications, NSAIDS are avoided.
- Two neurological complications are seen
  1. Microcephaly with brain calcification due to transplacental passage
  2. Guillain Barre Syndrome

Work up in Zika

1. Zika Mac ELISA IgM neutralizing antibody detectable, 4 days after symptom onset.
2. Ig G antibody to Zika virus, 7 days after symptom onset.
3. Trioplex real time RT-PCR assay on blood/ urine/ amniotic fluid/CSF. Negative test does rule out infection in other tissues. In case of negative test further antibody testing should be done.

25. Ans. (b) Undiagnosed fever after 1 week of inpatient work up

(Ref: Harrison 20th edition, p 115; Harrison 19th edition, page 135)

Fever of unknown origin is defined as:

1. Fever >38.3 degrees Celsius on at least 2 occasions
2. Illness duration > 3weeks
3. No known immunocompromised state
4. Diagnosis is uncertain after thorough history taking, physical examination, and lab investigations including 3 blood culture samples, urine culture

This is a modification over the original definition given by Petersdorf and Beeson which was being used since 1960, as per which "uncertain diagnosis after one week of inpatient evaluation" was a diagnostic criteria.

The latest definition is mentioned in the box in this explanation. The next point is also to be noted and remembered. **CMDT 2018 states "diagnosis of fever not made inspite of three outpatient visits or 3 days of hospitalization" is essential for diagnosis of FUO.**

26. Ans. (d) Viral culture

(Ref: Harrison 20th edition, p 1487; Manson textbook of tropical diseases, page 201; Harrison 19th edition, E- Book and page 1302)

- Diagnosis of rabies is made usually using skin biopsy from hairy skin over the nape of the neck.
- The rabies virus antigen is found in cutaneous nerves at the base of hair follicles.
- Corneal impression smears are low diagnostic yield and hence not performed.
- Choice A is ruled out as it used in post mortem. Negri bodies are eosinophilic inclusions seen in Purkinje cells of cerebellum, pyramidal neurons of hippocampus.
- Choice B is ruled out as many vaccinated individuals are positive for antibodies in serum. Infact it is direct fluorescent antibody test that is used for skin biopsies and brain tissue and not indirect immunofluorescence.
- Choice C and D are very close choices in this question.
- *Manson text book of tropical diseases* on page 201 mentions viral culture for corneal impression smears. Real time PCR is mentioned for saliva, CSF and skin biopsy only.

27. Ans. (d) Invasive cryptococcosis

(Ref: Harrison 20th edition, p 1527, 1531; CMDT 2018: page 1564 and Harrison 19th edition, page 1330 and 1360)

- The current guidelines of the Infectious Diseases Society of America for the management of candidiasis and aspergillosis recommend serum (1–3)-β-D-glucan testing to assist in the assessment of patients with suspected deep-seated fungal infections.
- It is also useful for diagnosis of P. Jiroveci infection.
- This test is **not useful** for diagnosis of *Mucor, Rhizopus, Blastomyces dermatitidis,* and *Cryptococcus* species.
- For diagnosis of Cryptococcus infection, Cryptococcal antigen (CRAg) test in CSF and blood is used.

28. Ans. (c) Viral culture

(Ref: Harrison 20th edition, p 1487; Manson's Tropical diseases: 23rd edition, page 201)

- The ante-mortem test for diagnosis of rabies is *direct fluorescent antibody on skin sample* taken from hairy area like the nape of the neck. Hence choice A is ruled out.
- *Real time PCR is not routinely available* and is done on saliva, CSF and skin biopsy and not corneal impression smears. Hence choice B is ruled out.
- *Stain for Negri Bodies is done for brain tissue* where the negri bodies are found in the hippocampus (Ammon horn), cerebellar purkinje fibres and cortical neurons. Hence choice D is ruled out.
- *Culture of virus is most successful in the first week of illness.* Viral culture is *done on brain tissue, saliva, tracheal, CSF, corneal impression smears and centrifuged urine.* Inoculation in sucking mice yields results in 1-3 weeks but tissue culture isolation in murine neuroblastoma cells takes about 2 days.
- Indirect immunofluorescence test is not useful for diagnosis since many vaccinated individuals remain positive for antibodies.
- Manson text book of tropical medicine states that corneal impression smears are too insensitive to be useful and false positives have occurred.

29. Ans. (d) Anti-IgM dengue antibody

(Ref: Harrison 20th edition, p 1504)

- In the first 3-5 days of dengue infection RT-PCR is useful to detect dengue RNA and is the most sensitive and specific test. After defervesce it becomes less useful.
- Serological detection by IgM- anti- dengue by ELISA can be used to differentiate primary and secondary infection but lacks the sensitivity in early stages.
- *According to C.D.C guidelines "IgM antibodies for dengue may remain elevated for 2 to 3 months after the illness. The elevated IgM observed in a sample could be the result of an infection that occurred 2 to 3 months ago"*
- In addition, there is cross reactivity with other flaviviruses including West Nile virus (WNV), St. Louis encephalitis virus (SLE), Japanese encephalitis virus (JEV) and yellow fever virus (YFV).
- Hence choice D anti-IgM is not helpful in diagnosis of the patient given in the question.
- IgM antibody capture (MAC) – ELISA is specific in distinguishing dengue from other flavivirus infections.
- **Timing of collection of sample for dengue after onset of symptoms**

Sample	Time of Collection after symptom onset
RT-PCR nucleic acid detection	1-5 days
NS1 antigen	1-6 days
IgM ELISA IgM Rapid test	After 5th day
IgG paired by ELISA	1-5 days for acute sera Convalescent after 15 days

30. Ans. (c) Known case of Extra-pulmonary TB with persistent cough

(Ref: TB control programme 2016 update)

Screening for TB is done in cases of –

1. Contact with a case of TB with microbiological confirmation
2. People living with HIV
3. Diabetics
4. Patients on Immunosupression
5. Malnourished patients
6. Patients on Steroids
7. Malignancy

- Extra-pulmonary TB is defined as microbiologically confirmed case of TB involving organs like lymph nodes, pleura, intestine, genitourinary tract, meninges.
- If a patient has both extra-pulmonary and pulmonary TB he is defined as having pulmonary TB and same treatment is given.

31. Ans. (b) Plasmodium falciparum

(Ref: Harrison 20th edition, p 158, 82-83; Harrison: 19th edition, Page 1368 and 245-e2)

- The peripheral smear shows multiple rings inside RBC. In some RBC's only chromatin dots are visible. The clinical diagnosis is falciparum malaria.

- In vivax malaria the infected RBC are larger and may show an amoeboid trophozoite with Schuffner dots.

Comparison of ring stages in vivax and falciparum malaria

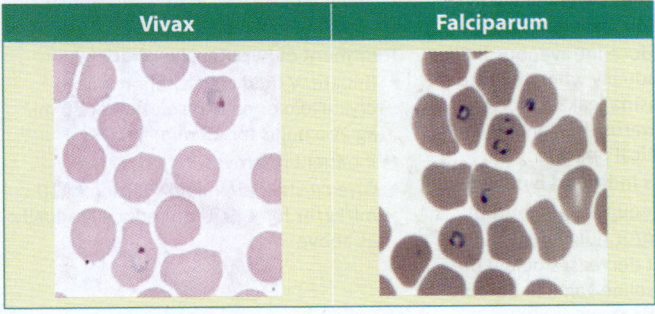

32. Ans. (c) Dengue fever

(Ref: CDC guidelines 2016 for dengue)

- The Tourniquet test is a part of WHO case definition for dengue. It is a marker for capillary fragility and can be used as triage tool. It can be done even in cases of dengue minus bleeding manifestation.

Procedure of Tourniquet test

1. Take the BP, example 120/80
2. Inflate cuff to midway between SBP and DBP (120+80/2)=100mm Hg and maintain for 5 minutes.
3. Reduce the cuff pressure and wait for 2 minutes.
4. Count the petechiae below antecubital fossa. A positive test is >10 or more petechiae per square inch.

33. Ans. (d) Hematocrit

(Ref: WHO handbook for management of Dengue fever)

- For monitoring patients of severe dengue haematocrit is performed.
- A rising haematocrit indicates development of dengue shock syndrome
- A falling haematocrit indicates bleeding and need for platelet transfusion in case the platelets are less than 10,000/cu.mm.
- Haematocrit values can be used to monitor fluid resuscitation in patients of dengue.

	Dengue without Warning	Dengue with Warning Signs		Severe Dengue
	Group A May be sent home	**Group B Referred for in-hospital care**	**Or**	**Group C**
	Group criteria	**Group criteria**		**Group criteria**
Management	Patients who do not have warning signs AND Who are able: • To tolerate adequate volumes of oral fluids • To pass urine at least once every 6 hours	Patients with any of the following features: • Co-existing conditions such as pregnancy, infancy, old age, diabetes mellitus • Social circumstances such as living alone, living far from hospital	Existing warning signs: • Abdominal pain or tenderness • Persistent vomiting • Clinical fluid accumulation • Mucosal bleeding • Lethargy/restlessness • Liver enlargement > 2 cm • Laboratory increase in HCT	Patients with any of the following features. • Severe plasma leakage with shock and/or fluid accumulation with respiratory distress • Severe bleeding • Severe organ impairment
	Laboratory tests • Full blood Count (FBC) • Haematocrit (Hct)	**Laboratory tests** • Full blood Count (FBC) • Haematocrit Hct)		**Laboratory tests** • Full blood Count (FBC) • Other organ function tests as • Haematocrit (Hat) • Other organ function tests as indicated
	Treatment Advice for: • Adequate bed rest • Adequate fluid intake • Paracetamol 4 gram max. per day in adults and accordingly in children Patients with stable Hct can be sent home	**Treatment** • Encouragement for oral fluids • If not tolerated, start intravenous fluid therapy 0.9% saline or Ringer lactate at maintenance rate	**Treatment** • Obtain reference Hct before fluid therapy • Give isotonic solution such as 0.9% saline, Ringer lactate, start with 5–7 ml/kg/hr for 1–2 hours, then reduce to 3–5 ml/kg/hr or less according to clinical response • Reassess clinical status and repeat Hct • If Hct remains the same or rise only minimally > continue with 2–3 ml/kg/hr for another 2–4 hours • If worsening of vital signs and rapidly rising Hct > increase rate to 5–10 ml/kg/hr for 1–2 hours	**Treatment of compensated shock:** • Start IV resuscitation with isotonic crystalloid solutions at 5–10 ml/kg/hr over 1 hr • Reassess patient's condition **If patient improves:** • IV fluids should be reduced gradually to 5–7 ml/kg/hr for 1–2 hr, then to 3–5 ml/kg/hr for 2–4 hr, then to 2–3 ml/kg/hr for 2–4 hr and then reduced further depending on haemodynamic status • IV fluids can be maintained for up to 24–48 hours • If patient still unstable: • Check Hct after first bolus • **If Hct increases**/still high (> 50%), repeat a second bolus of crystalloid solution at 10–20 ml/kg/hr for 1 hr. • If improvement after second bolus, reduce rate to 7–10 ml/kg/hr for 1–2 hr, continue to reduce as above.

Contd...

	Dengue without Warning	Dengue with Warning Signs		Severe Dengue
Management			**Reassess clinical status, repeat Hct and review fluid infusion rates accordingly** • Reduce intravenous fluids gradually when the rate of plasma leakage decreases towards then end of the critical phase. **This is indicated by:** • Adequate urine output and/or fluid intake • Hct decreases below the baseline value in a stable patient	• **If Hct decreases**, this indicates bleeding and need to cross-match and transfuse blood as soon as possible **Treatment of hypotensive shock** • Initiate IV fluid resuscitation with crystalloid or colloid solution at 20 ml/kg as a bolus for 15 min • If patient improves • Give crystalloid/colloid solution of 10 ml/kg/hr for 1 hr, then reduce gradually as above
	Monitoring • Daily review disease progression • Decreasing WBC • Defervescence • Warning signs (unit out of critical period) • Advice for immediate return to hospital if development of any warming signs • Written advice of management (e.g. home care card for dengue)	**Monitoring** • Temperature pattern • Volume of fluid intake and losses • Urine output-volume and frequency • Warning signs • Hct, white blood cell and platelet counts	**Monitoring** • Vital signs and peripheral perfusion (1–4 hourly until patient is out of critical phase • Urine output (4–6 hourly) • Hct (before and after fluid replacement, then 6–12 hourly) • Blood glucose • Other organ functions (renal profile, liver profile, coagulation profile, as indicated)	**If patient still unstable** • Review the Hct taken before the first bolus • **If Hct was low** (<40% in children and adult females, < 45% in adult males) this indicates bleeding the need to cross-match and transfuse (see above) • **If HCT was high** compared to the baseline value, change to IV colloids at 10–20 ml/kg as a second bolus over to hour, reassess after second bolus • **If improving** reduce the rate to 7–10 ml/kg/hr for 1–2 hours, then back to IV crystalloids and reduce rates as above • If condition still unstable repeat Hct after second bolus • **If Hct decreases** this indicates bleeding see above • **If Hct increases** remains high (>50%) continue colloid infusion at 10–20 ml/kg as athird bolus over 1 hr, then reduce to 7–10 ml/kg/hr for 1–2 hours, then change back to crystalloid solution and reduce rate as above

34. **Ans. (c) Albumin**

(Ref: Harrison 19th edition, page 1110)
- Pleural effusion in TB could be a presentation of primary TB due to sub-pleural location of Gohn's focus or can present as extra-pulmonary TB.
- Gene XPERT is a nucleic acid amplification based test which in matter of few hours can tell if MTB is present and can also determine resistance.
- The values of LDH are taken in light's criteria for pleural effusion to determine exudative nature of the fluid
- Adenosine deaminase has 90% sensitivity and 92 % specificity for determining the tubercular nature of fluid.
- The question is based on common sense that albumin values in serum and ascitic fluid are evaluated in patients of ascites.

35. **Ans. (a) Meningococcus**

(Ref: Harrison 20th edition, p 1118-9 and 327; Harrison: 19th edition, page 1401 and page 1464)
- Scrub typhus is ruled out due to absence of eschar. Choice C is ruled out to absence of hepatomegaly and step ladder pattern of fever.
- The main feature of dengue is that it has biphasic fever. When the fever goes down after 3-4 days, rash sparing palms and soles will appear with cluster of petechiae.
- In the question the fever is persisting and the images shows stellate purpura, which favours diagnosis of meningococcus.

Points in favour of diagnosis of meningococcus	Points against diagnosis of dengue haemorrhagic fever

Fulminant meningococcemia can present in a dramatic fashion with short history Stellate purpura with central dusky or gray hue is seen. The central discoloration is called gun metal gray. 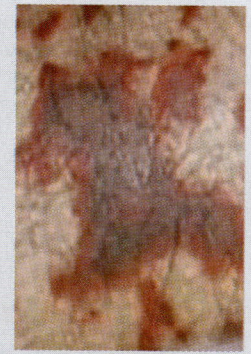 Notice the *gray hue* in the lesions shown in the picture	I. Dengue hemorrhagic fever has a biphasic fever curve
	II. Minimal criteria for the diagnosis of dengue are as follows:
	The clinical description of dengue fever is an acute febrile illness of 2–7 days duration associated with 2 or more of the following:
	  A. Severe and generalized headache
	  B. Retro-orbital pain
	  C. Severe myalgia, especially of the lower back, ams, and legs
	  D. Arthralgia, usually of the knees and shoulders
	  E. Characteristic rash
	  F. Hemorrhagic manifestations
	  G. Leukopenia

36. Ans. (a) Worms in jejunal mucosa

(Ref: Harrison 20th edition, p 1628; Harrison 19th edn, page 1416)

Features of trichuris trichura

The characteristic 50- by 20 μm lemon-shaped Trichuris eggs are readily detected on stool examination. Adult worms, which are 3–5 cm long, are occasionally seen on proctoscopy. The adult worms are located in caecum and colonic mucosa.

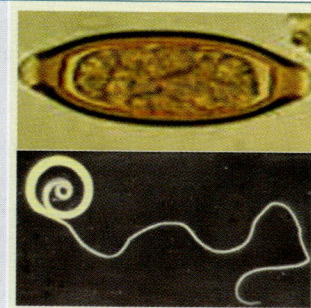

Feature	Ascaris lumbricoides (Roundworm)	Necator americanus, Ancylostoma duodenale (Hookworm)	Strongyloides stercoralis (Thread worm)	Trichuris trichlura (whipworm)	Enterobius vermicularis (Pinworm)
Infective stage	Egg	Filariform larva	Filariform larva	Egg	Egg
Route of infection	Oral	Percutaneous	Percutaneous or autoinfection	Oral	Oral
Gastrointestinal location of worms	Jejunal lumen	Jejunal mucosa	Small-bowel mucosa	Cecum, colonic mucosa	Cecum, appendix
Adult worm size	15–40 cm	7–12 mm	2 mm	30–50 mm	8–13 mm (Female)
Pulmonary passage of larvae	Yes	Yes	Yes	No	No
Longevity	1 years	N. americanus: 2–5 year A. duodenale: 6–8 year	Decades (owing to autoinfection)	5 years	2 months
Fecundity (eggs/day/worm)	240,000	N. americanus: 4000–10,000 A. duodenale: 10,000–25,000	5000–10,000	3000–7000	2000

37. Ans. (a) B and D only

(Ref: Harrison 20th edition, p 113t-114, 879t, 881; Harrison 19th edition, page 780t and 782)

Purpura fulminans presents with intravascular thrombosis and hemorrhagic infarction of the skin that is rapidly progressive and is accompanied by vascular collapse and disseminated intravascular coagulation.

The two most important causes of purpura fulminans are meningococcus and varicella Zoster.

Options B, C and D are correct but since it is not given in the choices, hence B and D is the best answer

Purpura fulminans is caused by
- Neisseria meningitidis
- Streptococcus pneumoniae
- Hemophilus influenzae and H. Aegypti
- Staphylococcus aureus
- Group A and other Beta hemolytic streptococci
- Pseudomonas aeruginosa
- Rickettsiae and candida albicans

38. Ans. (d) Infected chiggers inoculate organisms into the skin

(Ref: Harrison 20th edition, p 1309; Harrison 19th edition, page 128t, 1155)

- Choice A is wrong since the image shows not the organism but the vector chigger.
- Choice B is wrong since rash shows scrub typhus and not Lyme's disease.
- Choice C is wrong since the picture shows an eschar but clinical presentation is not of anthrax.
- Choice D is correct as scrub typhus is transmitted by chiggers.

Scrub typhus
- Causative organism is *O. tsutsugamushi*
- Differs from *Rickettsia* species in terms of cell wall composition as it lacks lipopolysaccharide.
- Infection is maintained by trans-ovarian transmission in trombiculid mites.
- After hatching, infected larval mites (chiggers, the only stage that feeds on a host) inoculate organisms into the skin.
- Infected chiggers are found in areas of heavy scrub vegetation.
- *Presentation includes an eschar where the chigger has fed, regional lymphadenopathy, and a maculopapular rash.*
- Investigations done are Serologic assays (IFA, indirect immunoperoxidase, and enzyme immunoassays)
- Patients are treated with Doxycycline, Azithromycin, or chloramphenicol.

39. Ans. (a) Fever, weight loss, night sweats and elevated ESR

(Ref: Harrison 19th edition, page 1112-1113)

The image shows a CT chest with mild bronchiectasis (notice the right lung at 8'o clock) along with parenchymal disruption in the right lung. The remaining pulmonary parenchyma demonstrated scattered tree-in-bud. This is diagnostic of pulmonary tuberculosis. It will present with fever, weight loss, night sweats and elevated ESR.

Community acquired infection with rusty sputum and Gram positive iplococcic	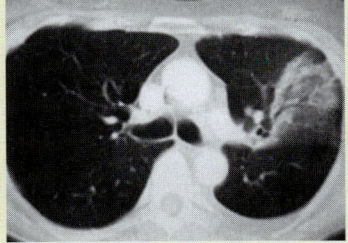
	CT scan showing Lobar pneumonia
Acute dyspnoea, elevated JVP, history of long air travel	Pulmonary embolism will show a normal CT scan
Acute dyspnoea, pink frothy sputum, mid diastolic rumble at apex	Mitral stenosis with decompensated CHF will show pulmonary oedema

40. Ans. (a) P 24 antigen capture assay

(Ref: Harrison 20th edition, p 1425, 26, 27; Harrison 19th edition, page 1246-47)

After accidental needle stick injury the chances of developing HIV infection are 0.3%. S. ELISA test can become positive any time after 6 weeks to 6 months of actual infection. Hence p24 antigen is favoured for early detection.

41. Ans. (c) Hepatitis B

(Ref: Harrison 19th edition, page 353)

Leptospirosis	Skin rash is seen is more common in anicteric leptospirosis. Petechial and purpura are seen in icteric leptospirosis where multi-organ dysfunction ensues.
SLE	Malar rash, discoid rash and Petechiae due to autoimmune thrombocytopenia
Infectious mononucleosis	A morbilliform or papular erythematous eruption of the upper extremities or trunk accompanies infectious mononucleosis in approximately 5% of cases. A macular erythematous rash may occur in patients with infectious mononucleosis who are treated with ampicillin. This usually occurs after 5-9 days of antibiotic treatment, and typically this rash is tan or brownish in color.

Extrahepatic skin manifestations of chronic hepatitis B

There are several cutaneous disorders associated with HBV infection, typically related to immune complex deposition. **These present later and *not* as primary skin lesions.**
- Bullous Pemphigoid
- Lichen Planus
- Gianotti-Crosti Syndrome Also known as papular acrodermatitis of childhood, this syndrome is characterized by small, flat, erythematous, papular eruptions that appear on the face and extremities.
- Rashes associated with chronic HBV infection are more likely to have palpable purpura, which is associated with neutrophil infiltration that leads to small vessel necrosis.

42. Ans. (c) Descending motor paralysis with preservation of tendon reflexes and absent sensation

(Ref: Harrison 20th edition, p 1469; Harrison 19th edition, page 1290-91)

Polio is a pure motor paralysis disorder characterized by descending paralysis and arreflexia. Sensations are usually preserved in polio.

Only febrile illness (5%)	After an incubation period of 3–6 days, 5% of patients present with a minor illness (abortive poliomyelitis) manifested by fever, malaise, sore throat, anorexia, myalgias. This condition usually resolves in 3 days.
Aseptic (1%) meningitis	About 1% of patients present with aseptic meningitis (non-paralytic poliomyelitis). Examination of CSF reveals lymphocytic pleocytosis, a normal glucose level, and a normal or slightly elevated protein level.
Paralysis	The disease appears to be biphasic, with aseptic meningitis followed first by apparent recovery but then (1–2 days later) by the return of fever and the development of paralysis; this form is more common among children than among adults. Examination reveals weakness, fasciculations, decreased muscle tone, and reduced or absent reflexes in affected areas

43. Ans. (d) Staphylococcus Aureus

(Ref: Harrison 20th edition, 142 p 937, 1075; Harrison 19th edition, page 831, 935)

Organisms causing muscle and deep tissue infections

Necrotizing fasciitis	
Streptococcal gangrene	S. pyogenes
Fournier's gangrene	Mixed aerobic and anaerobic bacteria
Staphylococcal necrotizing fasciitis	Methicillin-resistant S. aureus
Myositis and myonecrosis	
Pyomyositis	S. aureus
Streptococcal necrotizing myositis	S. pyogenes
Gas gangrene	Clostridium spp.
Nonclostridial (crepitant) myositis	Mixed aerobic and anaerobic bactgeria
Synergristic nonclostridial anaerobic myonecrosis	Mixed aerobic and anaerobic bacteria

44. Ans. (a) Leptospirosis

(Ref: Harrison 20th edition, p 1292-93; Harrison 19th edition, page 1140)

Leptospirosis	*Features in favor of diagnosis* • Occupation since Leptospires infect humans through the mucosa or through macerated, punctured, or abraded skin, farmer can be exposed. • Conjunctival suffusion • Muscle tenderness • Jaundice • Concomitant renal malfunction • Weil's disease presents with combination of jaundice, acute kidney injury, hypotension, and pulmonary hemorrhage.
Typhoid fever	Points *against the diagnosis*: • Absence of rash –"rose spots" • Absence of Hepatosplenomegaly • Absence of Epistaxis • Absence of relative bradycardia at the peak of high fever
Typhus	Absence of history of exposure to louse feces, tick feces, mite bite Absence of history of fever with rash or eschar
Viral hepatitis	Uremia is not seen in viral hepatitis unless it is fulminant hepatitis leading to hepato-renal syndrome. Absence of tender hepatomegaly negates the diagnosis of viral hepatitis.

45. Ans. (c) Both A and B

(Ref: Harrison 20th edition, p 1578; Harrison 19th edition, page 1368)

Hypoglycemia in malaria results from
- Failure of hepatic gluconeogenesis
- Increase in the consumption of glucose by both host and, to a much lesser extent, the malaria parasites.

Quinine used in both severe and uncomplicated falciparum malaria, is a powerful stimulant of pancreatic insulin secretion Mortality total proportion of erythrocytes infected increases to >2% (a level corresponding to >10^{12} parasites in an adult), mortality risk rises steeply

Parameters increasing mortality in falciparum malaria are:

Impaired consciousness/ unarousable	Unable to sit or stand without support
Extreme weakness	Prostration: inability to sit in bed
Hyperparasitemia	Parasitemia level of >5% in nonimmune patients (>20% in any patient)
Jaundice	Serum bilirubin level of >50 mmol/L (>3 mg/dL) if combined with other evidence of vital-organ dysfunction

Complications of falciparum malaria
- Coma unarousable
- Acidosis
- Severe normochromic, normocytic anemia
- Renal failure
- Pulmonary edema/adult respiratory distress syndrome
- Hypoglycemia
- Hypotension /shock
- Bleeding /disseminated intravascular coagulation
- Convulsions
- Hemoglobinuria

46. Ans. (c) Molluscum Contagiosum

(Ref: Harrison 20th edition, p 1366; Harrison 19th edition, page 220e-1)

Molluscumcontagiosum	Verruca vulgaris
It is caused by DNA virus producing characteristic skin lesions consisting of single or, more often, multiple, rounded, dome-shaped, pink, waxy papules that are 2-5 mm	Verruca vulgaris is a flesh-colored, firm papule or nodule due to infection of epidermal cells with human papillomaviruses.
Lesions are discrete, nontender, flesh-colored, dome-shaped papules that show a central umbilication (which is more apparent when the lesion is frosted with liquid nitrogen)	On close inspection, normal skin lines over the surface of the lesion are typically disrupted. The dome-shaped lesions can also be studded with black puncta. The growth is characterized by hypertrophy of dermal papillae and thickening of the keratin layers of the epidermis.

47. Ans. (c) p24 antigen

(Ref: Harrison 20th edition, p 1424-27; Harrison 19th, page 770, 1246-47)

- The "window period" refers to the maximum amount of time it may take for a person's body to create HIV antibodies after HIV infection. Usually ELISA test turns positive after 3-6 months of infection.
- The p24 antigen test can detect the p24 protein on average 10 to 14 days after infection with HIV.
- One drawback of this test is that levels of the p24 protein peak at around three to four weeks after exposure to HIV and are usually not detectable after five to six weeks (and sometimes even earlier). A positive p24 test means that someone is HIV-positive.
- However, a negative p24 test can mean three things:
  - The person is HIV-negative
  - The person is HIV-positive but that the test could not detect the p24 protein because the person was infected more than four to six weeks earlier
  - The levels of p24 antigen are too low to be detectable with current technologies.
- The HIV NAAT test is a very sensitive test designed to detect HIV RNA in blood. The NAAT test is able to detect HIV RNA as early as seven to 14 days after infection with HIV. Unlike the p24 test, the NAT test will always give a positive result as long as there is HIV in someone's blood.

48. Ans. (b) Typhoid

(Ref: Harrison 19th, page 1051)

Classification of exotoxins based on action:

A. Toxins that Aid in spreading by acting on the extracellular matrix of connective tissue breaking down extracellular matrix. Examples include;
1. Collagenases produced by clostridium perfringens
2. Hyaluronidase produced by S. aureus and S. pygenes
3. DNAse produced by S. aureus and S. pyogenes, which thins out pus
4. Collageneses and elastases produced by clostridium perfirngens
5. Exfoliative toxin produced by S. aureus

B. Toxins that block nerve function: interfere in neurotransmission and thereby result in spastic or flaccid paralysis. Examples include:
1. Tetanus toxin (tetanospasmin) produced by clostridium tetani
2. Botulinum toxin produced by clostridium botulinum

C. Enterotoxin: Most of the toxins have effect on the gut resulting in diarrhea or dysentery. Examples include:
1. Cholera toxin produced by vibrio cholera
2. Shiga toxin produced by shigella dysenteriae
3. LT and ST produced by Enterotoxigenic E. coli
4. Shiga-like toxins produced by Entero-hemorraghic E.coli
5. Others: other toxins that have different effects include Anthrax toxin produced by Bacillus anthracis, which in turn is three components namely, edema factor, protective antigen and lethal factor.

49. Ans. (c) Typhoid

(Ref: Harrison 19th edition, page 699, 2136)

Acute leukemia	Fever for 2 months can be explained by immature white (pre-B or Pre-T) cells in circulation in leukemia. These immature cells in circulation will not be able to launch an offensive and hence repeated infection occurs in acute leukemia inspite of high TLC Clonal expansion of pre cells leads to thrombocytopenia and petechiae due to less megakaryoblast proliferation.
Tuberculosis	Disseminated TB occurs in immunocompromised patients and leads to fever with anemia. Various hematologic abnormalities may be seen, including: • Anemia with leukopenia • Lymphopenia • Neutrophilic leukocytosis (leukemoid reactions) • Polycythemia. • Disseminated intravascular coagulation leading to thrombocytopenia.
Juvenile rheumatoid arthritis	JRA is an immunologically mediated disease presenting with fever. Systemic onset JIA presents with quotidian fever(peaks twice daily) Anemia of chronic disease can occur. Usually thrombocytosis occurs but immune mediated thrombocytopenia is described in Harrison.

Typhoid will present with the most prominent symptom which is prolonged fever (38.8°–40.5°C; 101.8°–104.9°F), which can continue for up to 4 weeks if untreated.

Early physical findings of enteric fever include hepatosplenomegaly, epistaxis, and relative bradycardia at the peak of high fever. Rose spots are usually not seen in Indian patients.

50. Ans. (a) Plenty of oral/iv fluids and observation

(Ref: OP Ghai 8th edition, page 226)

Consider the details of the patient:
Heart rate = increased
Blood pressure = Normal
Hess's test = positive
Platelet count = Low
Hematocrit = low to normal

Since patient is having presence of fever with rash with positive tourniquet test with tachycardia with normal BP he is fitting in *grade 1 DHF* by 7th edition of OP Ghai and *Dengue without warning signs* by 8th edition of OP Ghai.

For management of DHF1/ Dengue without warning signs the following guidelines are recommended:

- All children without hypotension should be given ringer lactate infusions at rate of 7 ml/kg over 1 hour. After one hour if hematocrit decreases and vital parameters improve, fluid infusion rate should be 5 ml/kg over next hour and 3ml/kg/hour for 24-48 hours.
- When the patient is stable as indicated by normal Blood pressure and satisfactory oral intake and urine output the patient can be discharged.

For management purposes dengue is classified as:

Undifferentiated fever	Non-specific symptoms
Dengue without warning signs	Fever, body aches, rashes or minor bleeding.
Dengue with warning signs	Suspected dengue with any one of the following • Persistent vomiting • Abdominal pain or tenderness • Clinical fluid accumulation • Mucosal bleeding • Lethargy • Liver enlargement > 2 cm • Lab features like increase in hematocrit with concurrent rapid decrease in platelets
Severe dengue infection	Severe plasma leakage leading to shock /fluid accumulation with shock Severe bleeding Severe organ involvement Liver: AST or ALT >1000IU/L CNS : impaired consciousness Heart or other organ involvement

51. Ans (a) Syphilitic gumma

(Ref: Harrison 20th edition, p 1281, 1283; Harrison 19th edition, page 1134 and 1136)

- The image shows presence of mass with ulceration on hard palate which could be a malignancy. However the since it is not in choice the infective process can be a gumma.
- Apthous ulcers don't have a mass associated. Dentigerous cysts are located related to mainly molar teeth. Leukoplakia presents as a whitish lesion on oral cavity and is ruled out.

Syphilitic gumma	Gummas tend to arise on the hard palate and tongue, although very rarely they may occur on the soft palate, lower alveolus, and parotid gland. A gumma manifests initially as 1 or more painless swelling. There may be eventual bone destruction, palatal perforation, and oro-nasal fistula formation. Gumma manifests radiologically as ill-defined radiolucencies that may resemble malignancy. The areas of ulceration eventually heal, although the resultant scarring can, at least on the tongue, cause fissuring.
Apthous ulcer	Features of apthous ulcers Small round or ovoid ulcers 2-4 mm in diameter They have an ulcer floor that is initially yellowish but assumes a gray hue as healing and epithelialization proceeds. They are surrounded by an erythematous halo and some edema. Found on non-keratinized mobile mucosa of the lips, cheeks, floor of the mouth, sulci, or ventrum of the tongue Uncommon on the keratinized mucosa of the palate or dorsum of the tongue.

Dentigerous ulcer	The most common location of dentigerous cysts are the Mandibular 3rd Molars and the Maxillary Canines, and they rarely involve deciduous teeth. *In this picture the location of swelling is on hard palate.*
Leukoplakia	Is focal area of keratosis appear as firmly attached white patches on the mucous membranes of the oral cavity.

52. Ans. (a) Primary tuberculosis usually involves the mid and lower zones

(Ref: Harrison 20th edition, p 1241-2; Harrison 19th edition, page 1112-13)

Since most inspired air is distributed to the middle and lower lung zones, these areas of the lungs are most commonly involved in primary TB. The lesion forming after initial infection (the Ghon focus) is usually peripheral and accompanied by transient hilar or paratracheal lymphadenopathy, which may not be visible on standard chest radiography

Primary tuberculosis carries a high level of transmissibility	Wrong statement	Cavity is must for transmission
90% of inhaled bacilli from droplet nuclei reach the alveoli	Wrong statement as coughing will produce droplets of varying sizes.	Large droplets (>5 μm) do not reach the alveolar space because they land on the ciliated epithelium of the airways and are carried up by the mucociliary escalator, swallowed, and rendered harmless. While the majority of inhaled bacilli are trapped in the upper airways and expelled by ciliated mucosal cells, a fraction (usually <10%) reach the alveoli The diameter of an infectious droplet nucleus is approximately 1 to 3 μm, and its content is one to three bacilli
Hilar/paratracheal lymphadenopathy is characteristically absent in primary tuberculosis	Wrong statement	Gohn's complex is characterized by presence of hilar lymphadenopathy.

53. Ans. (a) Raltregavir + Emtricitabine + Tenofovir

(Ref: CDC Guidelines for PEP in HIV)

- The preferred PEP regimen is tenofovir + emtricitabine plus raltegravir.
- Zidovudine is no longer recommended in the preferred PEP regimen.
- The first dose should be given as soon as possible after exposure, ideally *within 2 hours*.
- The recommended *duration of PEP is 28 days*.

Contd...

54. Ans. (d) Acetaminophen

- The clinical diagnosis is infectious mononucleosis with atypical lymphocyte count >10%.
- Diagnosis can be confirmed with IgM antibody to viral capsid antigen along with Mono-spot test.
- 95% cases recover without any specific anti-viral therapy. Acetaminophen and saline gargles will reduce symptoms.
- Acyclovir decreases viral shedding but does not show any clinical benefit.
- Steroids are recommended for cases where
  - Impending airway compromise is present
  - Haemolytic anaemia
  - Severe thrombocytopenia

If throat swab shows presence of beta haemolytic streptococcus then 10day course of penicillin or azithromycin is recommended. *Ampicillin is to be avoided because of frequent association with rash.*

55. Ans. (a) Reinfection with gonorrhea

(Ref: Harrison 20th edition, p 1125, 1128; Harrison 19th edition, page 1003)

A teenager has come back with same symptoms which implies that he may be continuing with same high sexual behavior with same or different partner. His Partner should always be treated otherwise there is an increased chance of re infection from further sexual contact

Gonococcal urethritis

- Treat with ceftriaxone 250 mg IM+azithromycin 1g PO or Doxycycline 100 mg BD for 7 days
- Cefixime 400 mg single dose is alternative for ceftriaxone
- Strains of gonococci are resistant to penicillin cephalosporin tetracycline or ciprofloxacin
- The partners should be treated and tested for HIV and syphilis

56. Ans. (b) Pulmonary tuberculosis

(Ref: Harrison 20th edition, p 1394; Harrison 19th edition, page 1215)

AIDS defining opportunistic illnesses

Multiple recurrent Bacterial infections
Candidiasis of bronchi trachea or lungs
Esophageal Candidiasis
Invasive cervical cancer
Coccidioidomycosis disseminated or extra-pulmonary
Cryptococcosis extra-pulmonary
Cytomegalovirus disease other than liver spleen or nodes onset at age>1 month
Cytomegalovirus retinitis with loss of vision
Encephalopathy HIV related
Herpes simplex chronic ulcers >1months durations or bronchitis pneumonitis or esophagitis onset at age >1 months
Histoplasmosis disseminated or extra-pulmonary
Isosporiasis chronic intestinal >1month duration
Kaposi sarcoma
Lymphoid interstitial pneumonia or pulmonary lymphoid hyperplasia complex
Lymphoma burkitt
Lymphoma immunoblastic or equivalent term
Lymphoma primary of brain
Mycobacterium avium complex or mycobacterium kansaii disseminated
Mycobacterium other species or unidentified species disseminated or extra-pulmonary
Pneumocystis jirovecii pneumonia
Pneumonia recurrent
Progressive multifocal leukoencephalopathy
Salmonella septicemia recurrent
Toxoplasmosis of brain onset at age>1 month
Wasting syndrome attributed to HIV

57. Ans. (d) Tabes dorsalis; (e) Gumma formation

(Ref: Harrison 20th edition, p 1282-3; Harrison 19th/1134-38; Robbins 9th/379)

- Condyloma Lata is seen in secondary syphilis while condyloma acuminata is caused by HPV.
- Matted lymph nodes are seen with TB while in syphilis shotty (lead shot) lymph nodes are seen.

Tabes dorsalis is seen in tertiary syphilis and leads to:
• Sensory ataxia   • Lhermitte sign   • Urinary incontinence   • High steppage gait

- IOC for Tabes dorsalis is CSF VDRL and TOC is Penicillin G iv for 2 weeks
- Gumma formation can leads to bulbar and pseudobulbar palsy due to gumma affecting cranial nerve nuclei or corticobulbar fibers.

58. Ans. (a) Vascular tumor (b) Associated with HIV (c) Involves visceral organs (d) Associated with Human herpes virus-8 (e) Radiotherapy may be used in treatment

(Ref: Harrison 20th edition, p 1448-49; Harrison 19th/1268-70; Robbins 9th/ 253- 54)

For management of Kaposi Sarcoma radiation is given to shrink the vascular tumor.

59. Ans. (a) Plasmodium Falciparum

- The image shows *banana shaped gametocyte of plasmodium falciparum.*

60. Ans. (a) Lamivudine is drug of choice

(Ref: K. Park, 22ndEdn/, Pg 225; Infectious Diseases and Arthropods by J. Goddard, 2nd Edn., Pg 62)

- Moderate to severe protein energy malnutrition reduces risk of DHF/DSS in dengue-infected children.

61. Ans. (a) Erythromycin

(Ref: Harrison 20th edition, Table 160-1, p 1176; Harrison 19th p 1052, Table 190-1)

62. Ans. (c) 14 days

(Ref: Harrison 20th edition, p 1002; Chapter 602, Nelson 18th edition, Harrison 19th p 889)

- Therapy for uncomplicated penicillin-sensitive S. *pneumoniae meningitis* should be completed with 10 to 14 days with a 3rd-generation cephalosporin or intravenous penicillin (400,000 U/kg/24 hr, given every 4–6 hr). If the isolate is resistant to penicillin and the 3rd-generation cephalosporin, therapy should be completed with vancomycin.

63. Ans. (b) Pneumonia

(Ref: Harrison 20th edition, p 1430; Harrison 19th p 1250)

- Pulmonary disease is one of the most frequent complications of HIV infection.
- The most common manifestation of pulmonary disease is pneumonia.
- Three of the 10 most common AIDS-defining illnesses are recurrent bacterial pneumonia, tuberculosis, and pneumonia due to the unicellular fungus *P. jiroveci*. Other major causes of pulmonary infiltrates include other mycobacterial infections, other fungal infections, nonspecific interstitial pneumonitis, KS, and lymphoma.

64. Ans. (a) Tubercular Lymphadenitis

(Ref: Harrison 20th edition, p 1243; Harrison 19th p 1109)

The most common presentation of extra-pulmonary TB in both HIV sero-negative and HIV-infected patients is lymph node disease and is particularly frequent in children.

Lymph node TB presents as painless swelling of the lymph nodes, most commonly at posterior cervical and supraclavicular sites. Lymph nodes are usually discrete in early disease but develop into a matted non tender mass over time and may result in a fistulous tract draining caseous material.

Type of TB	Incidence
TB lymphadenitis	40%
Genitourinary TB	10-15%
Skeletal TB	10%
CNS TB	5%
Gastrointestinal TB	3.5%
Pericardial TB	0.5% (mainly in HIV positive patients with Case fatality of 40%)

65. Ans. (b) Lower limbs

(Ref: Harrison 20th edition, p 1448; Harrison 19th p 1268)

- *Cutaneous lesions may occur at any location but typically are concentrated on the lower extremities and the head and neck region.*
- Lesions often appear in sun-exposed areas, particularly the tip of the nose, and have a propensity to occur in areas of trauma (Koebner phenomenon).
- Lesions may have macular, papular, nodular, or plaque like appearances.
- Nearly all lesions are palpable and nonpruritic.
- Lesions may range in size from several millimeters to several centimeters in diameter

66. Ans. (b) Liver

(Ref: Nelson 18th ed. ch. 212)

- Congenital transmission usually occurs from a lesion in the placenta through the umbilical vein. Primary infection in the mother just before or during pregnancy is more likely to cause congenital infection than is reactivation of a previous infection. *The tubercle bacilli first reach the fetal liver, where a primary focus with periportal lymph node involvement may occur. Organisms pass through the liver into the main fetal circulation and infect many organs.*
- The bacilli in the lung usually remain dormant until after birth, when oxygenation and pulmonary circulation increase significantly. Congenital tuberculosis may also be caused by aspiration or ingestion of infected amniotic fluid.

67. Ans. (b) Choroid tubercles on fundus examination

(Ref: Harrison 20th edition, p 1245; Harrison 19th p 1112)

- Fundus examination may reveal choroidal tubercles, which are pathognomonic of miliary TB, in up to 30% of cases.
- Meningismus occurs in <10% of cases.
- A high index of suspicion is required for the diagnosis of miliary TB. Frequently, chest radiography reveals a miliary reticulo-nodular pattern (more easily seen on underpenetrated film), although no radiographic abnormality may be evident early in the course and among HIV-infected patients. Other radiologic findings include large infiltrates, interstitial infiltrates (especially in HIV-infected patients), and pleural effusion.

68. Ans. (b) Bronchoalveolar lavage

(Ref: Harrison 20th edition, p 1430; Harrison 19th p 1253)

Definitive diagnosis of PCP requires demonstration of the organism in samples obtained from induced sputum, bronchoalveolar lavage, transbronchial biopsy, or open-lung biopsy. PCR has been used to detect specific DNA sequences for P. jiroveci in clinical specimens where histologic examinations have failed to make a diagnosis.

69. Ans. (a) Toxoplasmosis

(Ref: Harrison 20th edition, p 1445; Harrison 19th p 1265)

Among the more frequent opportunistic diseases that involve the CNS are toxoplasmosis, cryptococcosis, progressive multifocal leukoencephalopathy, and primary CNS lymphoma.

Disease	Overall Contribution to First Seizure, %
HIV encephalopathy	24-47
Cerebral toxoplasmosis	28
Cryptococcal meningitis	13
Primary central nervous system lymphoma	4
Progressive multifocal leukoencephalopathy	1

70. Ans. (d) Tuberculoma resolves after treatment

(Ref: Nelson 18th ed. ch. 212, Harrison 19th p 1111)

- During early stage I, the CSF may resemble that of viral aseptic meningitis only to progress to the more severe CSF profile over several weeks. Hence normal CSF sugar may be seen and choice A is correct.
- Since the advent of CT, *the paradoxical development of tuberculomas in patients with tuberculous meningitis who are receiving ultimately effective chemotherapy has been recognized. The cause and nature of these tuberculomas are poorly understood, and do not represent failure of drug treatment. This phenomenon should be considered whenever a child with tuberculous meningitis deteriorates or develops focal neurologic findings while on treatment.*
- Corticosteroids may help alleviate the occasionally severe clinical signs and symptoms that occur. These lesions may persist for months or even years.
- As disease progresses, basilar enhancement and communicating hydrocephalus with signs of cerebral edema or early focal ischemia are the most common findings. Some small children with tuberculous meningitis may have 1 or several clinically silent tuberculomas, occurring most often in the cerebral cortex or thalamic regions.

71. Ans. (a) Rpo B gene

(Ref: icmr.nic.in/ijmr/2003/0204.pdf)

Multidrug resistant (MDR) tuberculosis (TB) is a problem of increasing importance in the world due to limited treatment options. Resistance to rifampicin results from nucleotide changes in the gene encoding the b subunit of the RNA polymerase (rpoB) of Mycobacterium tuberculosis. Rifampicin resistance is considered as a marker for MDR TB.

ATT DRUG	Gene responsible for drug resistance
Rifampicin	rpoB gene
INH	inhA and Kat G gene
Pyrazinamide	pncA gene
Ethambutol	emb B gene

72. Ans. (d) Hepatitis

(Ref: Harrison 20th edition, p 1252; Harrison 19th p 1117)

- Hyper-uricemia and arthralgia caused by pyrazinamide can usually be managed by the administration of acetylsalicylic acid; however, pyrazinamide treatment should be stopped if the patient develops gouty arthritis.
- Individuals who develop autoimmune thrombo-cytopenia secondary to rifampicin therapy should not receive the drug thereafter.
- Similarly, the occurrence of optic neuritis with ethambutol is an indication for permanent discontinuation of this drug.
- For patients with symptomatic hepatitis and those with marked (five- to six fold) elevations in serum levels of aspartate aminotransferase, treatment should be stopped and drugs reintroduced one at a time after liver function has returned to normal.

73. Ans. (a) Megaloblastic anemia

(Ref: Harrison 20th edition, p 1453; Harrison 19th p 1273)

Side effects of zidovudine is Anemia, granulocytopenia, myopathy, lactic acidosis, hepatomegaly with steatosis, headache, nausea, nail pigmentation, lipid abnormalities, lipoatrophy, hyperglycemia.

74. Ans. (b) 2 only

(Ref: Harrison 20th edition, p 1399-1402; Harrison 19th p 1222)

- Greater volume of blood is transmitted by hollow needle.
- HIV is transmitted primarily by sexual contact (both heterosexual and male to male); by blood and blood products; and by infected mothers to infants intrapartum, perinatally, or via breast milk. Parenteral transmission of HIV during injection drug use does not require IV puncture; SC ("skin popping") or IM ("muscling") injections can transmit HIV as well.
- CD4 count is inversely related to viral load. Low CD4 count indicate oppurtunistic infections with high viral load.
- PEP must begin within 72 hours of exposure before the virus has time to make too many copies.

75. Ans. (a) ESAT 6

(Ref: Harrison 20th edition, p 1249; Harrison 19th p 1115)

Interferon gamma release assay (IGRA) measure T cell release of gamma interferon against TB antigen ESAT 6 and CF 10. This test also called as Quantiferon – TB Gold test is more specific than Tuberculin skin testing as a result of less cross reactivity due to BCG vaccination and sensitization by non-tuberculosis mycobacteria.

It is also logistically convenient as it reduces patient visits and gives an ability to perform serial testing without the hassle of boosting phenomenon caused by Tuberculin skin testing.

76. Ans. (c) 20 months

(Ref: Harrison 20th edition, p 1253-54; Harrison 19th p 1116)

- MDR-TB is more difficult to manage than is disease caused by drug-susceptible organisms, especially because resistance to other first-line drugs besides isoniazid and rifampin is common.
- For treatment of TB due to strains resistant to isoniazid and rifampin, combinations of a fluoroquinolone, ethambutol, pyrazinamide, and streptomycin or, for strains resistant to streptomycin as well, another injectable agent (amikacin, kanamycin, or capreomycin) should be used.
- For patients with bacilli resistant to all of the first-line agents, cure may be attained with a combination of four second-line drugs, including one injectable agent.

Resistance (or intolerance) to H	Throughout (6)	RZE
Resistance (or intolerance) to R	Throughout (12-18)	HZEQ
Resistance to H + R	Throughout (at least 20 months)	ZEQ + S (or another injectable agents)
Resistance to all first-line drugs	Throughout (at least 20 months)	1 injectable agent + 3 of these 4: ethionamide, cycloserine, Q, PAS
Intolerance to Z	2	HRE

77. Ans. (d) Meningitis

(Ref: Harrison 20th edition, p 1430, 1433; Harrison 19th p 1253)

- In addition to pneumonia, a number of other clinical problems have been reported in HIV-infected patients as a result of infection with *P. jiroveci*.
- Otic involvement may be seen as a primary infection, presenting as a polypoid mass involving the external auditory canal.
- In patients receiving aerosolized pentamidine for prophylaxis against PCP, one may see a variety of extrapulmonary manifestations of *P. jiroveci*. These include ophthalmic lesions of the choroid, a necrotizing vasculitis that resembles Burger's disease, bone marrow hypoplasia, and intestinal obstruction.
- Other organs that have been involved include lymph nodes, spleen, liver, kidney, pancreas, pericardium, heart, thyroid, and adrenals.

78. Ans. (a) Increased frequency

(Ref: Harrison 20th edition, p 1244; Harrison 19th p 1110)

- Genitourinary TB, which accounts for 10–15% of all extra-pulmonary cases, may involve any portion of the genitourinary tract.
- Local symptoms predominate, and up to 75% of patients have chest radiographic abnormalities suggesting previous or concomitant pulmonary disease.
- *Urinary frequency, dysuria, nocturia, hematuria, and flank or abdominal pain is common presentations. However, patients may be asymptomatic and the disease discovered only after severe destructive lesions of the kidneys have developed.* Urinalysis gives abnormal results in 90% of cases, revealing pyuria and hematuria.
- The documentation of culture-negative pyuria in acidic urine raises the suspicion of TB. IV pyelography, abdominal CT, or MRI may show deformities and obstructions, and calcifications and ureteral strictures are suggestive findings.
- Culture of three morning urine specimens yields a definitive diagnosis in nearly 90% of cases.

79. Ans. (b) Cryptosporidium

(Ref: Harrison 20th edition, p 1435-36; Harrison 19th p 1257)

- Cryptosporidia, microsporidia, and Isospora belli are the most common opportunistic protozoa that infect the GI tract and cause diarrhea in HIV-infected patients.
- In 75% of cases the diarrhea is accompanied by crampy abdominal pain, and 25% of patients have nausea and/or vomiting.
- The diagnosis of cryptosporidial diarrhea is made by stool examination or biopsy of the small intestine. The diarrhea is noninflammatory, and the characteristic finding is the presence of oocysts that stain with acid-fast dyes.
- Therapy is predominantly supportive, and marked improvements have been reported in the setting of effective cART. Treatment with up to 2000 mg/d of nitazoxanide (NTZ) is associated with improvement in symptoms or a decrease in shedding of organisms in about half of patients.

80. Ans. (c) Post transplantation

(Ref: Harrison 20th edition, p 1239, Table 173-1; Harrison 19th p 1105)

Condition	Relative risk of developing TB in decreasing order
Post transplantation	20-70
HIV	30
Silicosis	30
Recent infection	12
Diabetes	3-4
Malnutrition	2-3

81. Ans. (c) Immune reconstitution inflammatory syndrome

(Ref: Harrison 20th edition, p 1441; Harrison 19th p 1261)

- Immune reconstitution inflammatory syndrome (IRIS)— has been associated with the administration of ART. Usually occurring 1–3 months after initiation of ART, IRIS is more common among patients with advanced immunosuppression and extra-pulmonary TB.
- "Unmasking IRIS" may also develop after the initiation of ART in patients with undiagnosed subclinical TB.
- The presumed pathogenesis of IRIS is an immune response that is elicited by antigens released when bacilli are killed during effective chemotherapy and that is temporally associated with improving immune function.
- The first priority in the management of a possible case of IRIS is to ensure that the clinical syndrome does not represent a failure of TB treatment or the development of another infection.

82. Ans. (b) Shrunken kidneys

(Ref: Harrison 20th edition, p 1438; Harrison 19th p 1259)

- HIV associated nephropathy : Proteinuria is the hallmark of this disorder. Edema and hypertension are rare. Ultrasound examination reveals enlarged, hyperechogenic kidneys.
- A definitive diagnosis is obtained through renal biopsy. Histologically, focal segmental glomerulosclerosis is present in 80%, and mesangial proliferation in 10–15% of cases.
- Prior to effective antiretroviral therapy, this disease was characterized by relatively rapid progression to end-stage

renal disease. Patients with HIV-associated nephropathy should be treated for their HIV infection regardless of CD4+ T cell count.
- Treatment with angiotensin-converting enzyme (ACE) inhibitors and/or prednisone, 60 mg/d, has also been reported to be of benefit in some case.

83. Ans. (b) Pneumonia

(Ref: Harrison 20th edition, p 1429, Table 197-10; Harrison 19th p 1249)

Findings in Acute HIV syndrome is:
1. Fever
2. Lymphadenopathy
3. Pharyngitis
4. Headache
5. Arthralgias
6. Myalgias
7. *Weight loss*
8. *Nausea/vomiting/diarrhea*
9. Meningitis
10. Encephalitis
11. Peripheral neuropathy
12. Myelopathy
13. Erythematous maculo-papular rash
14. *Mucocutaneous ulceration*

84. Ans. (b) 40 copies of viral RNA/ml of blood

(Ref: Harrison 20th edition, p 1426, Table 197-8; Harrison 19th p 1248)

85. Ans. (a) Kaposi sarcoma

(Ref: Harrison 20th edition, p 1448; Harrison 19th p 1269)

- Pulmonary involvement with KS generally presents with shortness of breath. The chest X-ray characteristically shows bilateral lower lobe infiltrates that obscure the margins of the mediastinum and diaphragm. *Pleural effusions are seen in 70% of cases of pulmonary KS.*
- Pneumocystis carini which apparently looks like the answer is negated by the following text of Harrison "The most common finding on chest X-ray is either a normal film, if the disease is suspected early, or a faint bilateral interstitial infiltrate. The classic finding of a dense perihilar infiltrate is unusual in patients with AIDS".
- In patients with PCP who have been receiving aerosolized pentamidine for prophylaxis, one may see an X-ray picture of upper lobe cavitary disease, reminiscent of TB. Other less common findings on chest X-ray include lobar infiltrates and pleural effusions

86. Ans. (b) Polymyositis

(Ref: Harrison 20th edition, p 1343; Harrison 19th p 2200)

Uses of Interferon
1. Interferon beta-1a and interferon beta-1b are used to treat and control multiple sclerosis, and for reducing attacks in relapsing-remitting multiple sclerosis and slowing disease progression and activity in secondary progressive multiple sclerosis.
2. It is also used in Hairy cell leukemia, chronic myeloid leukemia, nodular lymphoma, cutaneous T-cell lymphoma.
3. Patients with recurrent melanomas receive recombinant IFN-α2b.
4. Hepatitis B and hepatitis C are treated with IFN-α, often in combination with other antiviral drugs. Some of those treated with interferon have a sustained virological response and can eliminate hepatitis virus. The most harmful strain—hepatitis C genotype I virus—can be treated with a 60-80% success rate with the current standard-of-care treatment of interferon-α, ribavirin and recently approved protease inhibitors such as Telaprevir. *Polymyositis respond to corticosteroids.* Often a daily dose of 40–60 mg or more of oral prednisone is required initially. The dose is then adjusted downward while monitoring muscle strength and serum levels of muscle enzymes. In patients resistant or intolerant to corticosteroids, therapy with methotrexate or azathioprine may be helpful. Intravenous immune globulin is effective for dermatomyositis resistant to prednisone.

87. Ans. (a) INH biweekly for 9 months

(Ref: Harrison 20th edition, p 1257, Table 173-6; Harrison 19th Table 202-3, p 1116)

- Treatment of HIV positive persons with latent TB infection (LTBI) aims at preventing active disease. This intervention (also called preventive chemotherapy or chemoprophylaxis) is based on the results of a large number of randomized, placebo-controlled clinical trials demonstrating that a 6- to 12-month course of isoniazid reduces the risk of active TB in infected people by up to 90%.
- Isoniazid is administered at a daily dose of 5 mg/kg (up to 300 mg/d) for 9 months.

88. Ans. (a) Cryptococcus

(Ref: Harrison 20th edition, p 1001; Harrison 19th p 1339)

- Latex agglutination tests can detect antigens of encapsulated organisms (S pneumoniae, H influenzae, N.meningitidis, and Cryptococcus neoformans) but are rarely used except for detection of Cryptococcus or in partially treated patients.
- Polymerase chain reaction (PCR) testing of cerebrospinal fluid has been used to detect bacteria (S pneumoniae, H influenzae, N meningitidis, M tuberculosis, B burgdorferi, and Tropheryma whippelii) and viruses (herpes simplex, varicella-zoster, CMV, Epstein-Barr virus, and enteroviruses) in patients with meningitis.

89. Ans. (a) In adults it is mostly asymptomatic

(Ref: Harrison 20th edition, p 1609, 1611; Harrison 19th p 1401)

- T. gondii rapidly induces detectable levels of both IgM and IgG serum antibodies. Monoclonal gammopathy of the IgG class can occur in congenitally infected infants.
- IgM levels may be increased in newborns with congenital infection.

- *In persons whose immune systems are intact, acute toxoplasmosis is usually asymptomatic and self-limited. This condition can go unrecognized in 80–90% of Cases.*

90. Ans. (a) Mycoplasma

(Ref: Harrison 20th edition, p 1314; Harrison 19th p 1163)

- Mycoplasma infection may begin with a sore throat and the most common presenting symptom is cough. The possibility of M. Pneumoniae infection needs particular consideration when community-acquired pneumonia fails to respond to treatment with a penicillin or a cephalosporin—antibiotics that are ineffective against mycoplasmas.
- Clinical findings, non-microbiologic laboratory tests, and chest radiography are not useful for differentiating M. pneumonia pneumonia from other types of community-acquired pneumonia. In addition, since M. pneumoniae lacks a cell wall, it is not visible on gram's stain.

91. Ans. (b) Breath urea test

(Ref: Harrison 20th edition, p 1164, Table 158-1; Harrison 19th p 1040)

Tests Commonly Used to Detect Helicobacter pylori. Advantages and Disadvantages :

Invasive (Based on Endoscopic Biopsy)
1. Biopsy urease: Test Quick, simple
2. Histology: May give additional histologic information. Sensitivity dependent on experience and use of special stains.
3. Culture: Permits determination of antibiotic susceptibility. Sensitivity dependent on experience.

Non-invasive
1. Serology: Inexpensive and convenient; not affected by recent antibiotics or proton pump inhibitors to the same extent as breath and stool tests. Cannot be used for early follow-up after treatment
2. 13-C urea breath test. Inexpensive and simpler than endoscopy; useful for follow-up after treatment
3. Stool antigen test: Inexpensive and convenient; useful for screening

92. Ans. (c) Anticapsular antibody prevents recurrence

(Ref: Harrison 19th p 1340)

- Cryptococcal gelatanious capsule stains bright pink with mucicarmine stain and discriminates the organism from histoplasma and blastomycosis.
- India ink stain particles are extruded by the gelatanious capsule and hence only the background is stained.
- In cryptococcal meningitis, CSF examination usually reveals evidence of chronic meningitis with mononuclear cell pleocytosis and increased protein levels.
- A particularly useful test is cryptococcal antigen (CRAg) detection in CSF and blood. The assay is based on serologic detection of cryptococcal polysaccharide and is both sensitive and specific. A positive cryptococcal antigen test provides strong presumptive evidence for cryptococcosis

93. Ans. (a) H.Pylori

(Ref: Harrison 19th p 1040)

- Rapid urease test, also known as the CLO test (Campylobacter-like organism test), is a rapid diagnostic test for diagnosis of Helicobacter pylori. The basis of the test is the ability of H. pylori to secrete the urease enzyme, which catalyzes the conversion of urea to ammonia and carbon dioxide
- The urease produced by H. pylori hydrolyzes urea to ammonia, which raises the pH of the medium, and changes the color of the specimen from yellow (NEGATIVE) to red (POSITIVE)

94. Ans. (b) Infectious mononucleosis

(Ref: Harrison 20th edition, p 1358; Harrison 19th p 1187)

- CLL is seen in adults and CML presents with massive splenomegaly and are hence ruled out. ALL has a stormy onset but a peripheral smear finding negates the possibility.
- Infectious mononucleosis presents with Fever, sore throat, fatigue, malaise, anorexia, and myalgia and below mentioned findings.

Physical findings
1. Lymphadenopathy (discrete, non-Suppurative, slightly painful, especially along the posterior cervical chain)
2. Transient bilateral upper lid Edema (Hoagland sign),
3. Splenomegaly (in up to 50% of patients).
4. Maculo-papular or occasionally petechial rash occurs in < 15% of patients unless ampicillin is given.
5. Conjuctival Hemorrhage, exudative pharyngitis, uvular edema, tonsillitis, or gingivitis may occur and soft palatal petechiae may be seen

Investigations: The white blood cell count is usually elevated and peaks at 10,000–20,000/μL during the second or third week of illness. Lymphocytosis is usually demonstrable, with >10% atypical lymphocytes. The latter cells are enlarged lymphocytes that have abundant cytoplasm, vacuoles, and indentations of the cell membrane

95. Ans. (c) Bilateral evoked auditory response

(Ref: Nelson 18th ed., Harrison 19th p 1011)

- Nontypable H. influenzae is one of the three most common causes of childhood otitis media (the other two being Streptococcus pneumoniae and Moraxella catarrhalis).
- The diagnosis is made by pneumatic otoscopy. An etiologic diagnosis, although not routinely sought, can be established by tympanocentesis and culture of middle-ear fluid.
- A diagnosis of otitis media is based on the detection by pneumatic otoscopy of fluid in the middle ear and bilateral evoked auditory response. An etiologic diagnosis requires tympanocentesis but is not routinely sought.

96. Ans. (b) Tricuspid

(Ref: Harrison 19th p 819)

In septic states the bacteria will enter into right side of heart and can bust the tricuspid valve.

97. Ans. (a) Ampicillin plus Sulbactam

(Ref: Harrison 20th edition, Table 136-1, p 1021)

The organisms incriminated are Streptococcus viridans, S.Aureus, H.influenzae, Anaerobes, Eikinella corrodens, H. influenzae, Eikinella corrodens. Preferred antibiotics are ampicillin/sulbactam or imipenem. In penicillin allergic patients cefoxitin is used.

98. Ans. (c) Optic neuritis

(Ref: Harrison 20th edition, p 1477; Harrison 19th p 1298)

Encephalomyelitis occurs within 2 weeks of rash onset and is characterized by fever, seizures, and a variety of neurologic abnormalities. The finding of periventricular demyelination, the induction of immune responses to myelin basic protein, and the absence of *measles virus in the brain suggest that post measles encephalomyelitis is an autoimmune disorder triggered by measles virus infection.*

Other CNS complications that occur months to years after acute infection are measles inclusion body encephalitis (MIBE) and sub-acute sclerosing pan-encephalitis (SSPE).

99. Ans. (a) Bloody CSF

(Ref: Harrison 20th edition, p 1578-79; Harrison 19th p 1372)

- Cerebral malaria manifests as diffuse symmetric encephalopathy; focal neurologic signs are unusual.
- Although some passive resistance to head flexion may be detected, signs of meningeal irritation are absent.
- Bloody CSF is seen in SAH and herpes encephalitis.
- Convulsions, usually generalized and often repeated, occur in ~10% of adults and up to 50% of children with cerebral malaria.
- Whereas adults rarely (i.e., in <3% of cases) suffer neurologic sequelae, ~5% of children surviving cerebral malaria especially those with hypoglycemia, severe anemia, repeated seizures, and deep coma—have residual neurologic deficit when they regain consciousness; hemiplegia, cerebral palsy, cortical blindness, deafness, and impaired cognition and learning
- The eyes may be divergent and a pout reflex is common, but other primitive reflexes are usually absent.
- On routine funduscopy
  - Discrete spots of retinal opacification (30–60%)
  - 15% of patients have retinal hemorrhage
  - Papilledema (8% among children, rare among adults)
  - Cotton wool spots (<5%)

100. Ans. (d) Histoplasmosis

(Ref: Harrison 20th edition, p 1520; Harrison 19th p 1333)

In case of histoplasma infection in the immunocompetent host, macrophages, lymphocytes, and epithelial cells eventually organize and form granulomas that contain the histoplasma organisms. These granulomas typically fibrose and calcify; calcified mediastinal lymph nodes and hepatosplenic calcifications are frequently found in healthy individuals from endemic areas.

101. Ans. (a) VSD

(Ref: CMDT-14/ch:33/pg: 1435)

- Valvular disease alters blood flow and produces jet effects that disrupt the endothelial surface, providing a nidus for attachment and infection of microorganisms that enter the bloodstream.
- Predisposing valvular abnormalities include rheumatic involvement of any valve, bicuspid aortic valves, calcific or sclerotic aortic valves, hypertrophic subaortic stenosis, mitral valve prolapse, and a variety of congenital disorders such as ventricular septal defect, tetralogy of Fallot, coarctation of the aorta, or patent ductus arteriosus. Rheumatic disease is no longer the major predisposing factor in developed countries. Regurgitation lesions are more susceptible than stenotic ones.
- Though PDA is a close answer, since VSD is more common a lesion and pressure gradient between LV and RV is ,more than pressure gradient between aorta and pulmonary artery, VSD should be answered for the above question

102. Ans. (b) Neomycin enema

(Ref: Harrison 20th edition, p 967, Table 129-2; Harrison 19th p 860, Table 161-2)

- Fecal transplantation is recommended for multiple recurrent CDI.
- Severe complicated or fulminant CDI is defined as severe CDI with the addition of hypotension, shock, ileus, or toxic megacolon. The duration of treatment may need to be >2 weeks and is dictated by response. Consider using IV tigecycline in place of metronidazole
- Vancomycin PO plus metronidazole IV and Rectal instillation of vancomycin (500 mg in 100 mL of normal saline as a retention enema q6–8h)
- For mild/moderate disease, oral metronidazole (500 mg 3 times daily for 10 days) is recommended as initial treatment
- In patients for whom oral treatment is inappropriate, fidaxomicin may be used; specific indications include first-line treatment in patients with recurrence or at risk for recurrence
- For patients with colonic perforation and/or systemic inflammation and deteriorating clinical condition despite antibiotic treatment, total abdominal colectomy or diverting loop ileostomy combined with colonic lavage is recommended.

103. Ans. (b) Bradycardia with hyperthermia

(Ref: Harrison 20th edition, p 861; Family Medicine Board Review 2014, A. Baltimore, pg. 6)

The Faget sign (sphygmothermic dissociation) is the unusual pairing of fever and bradycardia (slow pulse). It is often seen in:

1. Yellow fever
2. Typhoid Fever
3. Tularaemia
4. Brucellosis
5. Colorado tick fever

6. Some pneumonias - Legionella pneumonia and Mycoplasma pneumonia
7. Drug Fever (e.g. Beta-Blockers, known as the Beta-Faget sign)

Notably, Faget sign in bacterial infections is associated with bacteria that have an intracellular life cycle

104. Ans. (d) Scalded skin syndrome

(Ref: Harrison 19th p 959)

Non-Suppurative complications of streptococcus are rheumatic fever and glomerulonephritis.
1. Rheumatic fever may follow recurrent episodes of pharyngitis beginning 1–4 weeks after the onset of symptoms.
2. Glomerulonephritis follows a single infection with a nephritogenic strain of streptococcus group A (eg, types 4, 12, 2, 49, and 60), more commonly on the skin than in the throat, and begins 1–3 weeks after the onset of the infection.

Suppurative complications of streptococcus: include sinusitis, otitis media, mastoiditis, peritonsillar abscess, and suppuration of cervical lymph nodes.

105. Ans. (a) PCR of respiratory secretions

(Ref: Harrison 20th edition, p 1314; Harrison 19th p 1164)

- Acute M. pneumoniae infection can be diagnosed by polymerase chain reaction detection of the organism in respiratory tract secretions.
- Oropharyngeal, nasopharyngeal, and pulmonary specimens are all acceptable for diagnosing M. pneumoniae pneumonia.
- M. pneumoniae culture requiring special media is not recommended for routine diagnosis because the organism may take weeks to grow and is often difficult to isolate from clinical specimens. In contrast, PCR allows rapid, specific diagnosis earlier in the course of clinical illness

106. Ans. (b) Nephritic syndrome

(Ref: Harrison 19th p 855, Table 160-2)

Complications of Chronic diarrhea
- Lactase deficiency
- Small-bowel bacterial overgrowth
- Malabsorption syndromes (tropical and celiac sprue)
- Initial presentation or exacerbation of inflammatory bowel disease
- Irritable bowel syndrome
- Reactive arthritis (formerly known as Reiter's syndrome)
- Hemolytic-uremic syndrome (hemolytic anemia, thrombocytopenia, and renal failure)
- Guillain-Barré syndrome

107. Ans. (b) Toxic cardiomyopathy

(Ref: Harrison 20th edition, p 1097, 1786; Harrison 19th p 978)

Toxic cardiomyopathy occurs in 10–25% of patients with respiratory diphtheria and is responsible for 50–60% of deaths. Subtle signs of myocarditis can be detected in most patients, especially the elderly, but the risk for significant complications correlates directly with the extent and severity of exudative local oropharyngeal disease and delay in administration of antitoxin.

108. Ans. (d) Wegener's granulomatiosis

(Ref: Harrison 20th edition, p 1535)

- Aspergillosis is seen to be angio-invasive in neutropenia, non-angioinvasive in granulomatous lesions of the lung and the one that is granulomatous lesion of the four choices is the choice D: Wegner Granulomatosis.
- Aspergillomas of the lung occur when pre-existing lung cavities become secondarily colonized with Aspergillus species. These may be found by incidental radiographic studies but may also present with significant hemoptysis.
- These include chronic sinusitis, colonization of preexisting pulmonary cavities (aspergilloma), and chronic necrotizing pulmonary aspergillosis.

109. Ans. (d) Exchange transfusion

(Ref: Harrison 20th edition, p 1266; Harrison 19th p 1125)

- Lucio phenomenon seen in leprosy is not seen in Indian settings, but patients with this reaction develop recurrent crops of large, sharply marginated, ulcerative lesions—particularly on the lower extremities. These are frequently fatal as a result of secondary infection and consequent septic bacteremia
- Neither glucocorticoids nor thalidomide is effective against this syndrome. Optimal wound care and therapy for bacteremia are indicated. Ulcers tend to be chronic and heal poorly.
- In severe cases exchange transfusion is indicated.

110. Ans. (a) A

(Ref: Harrison 20th edition, p 1106; Harrison 19th p 987)

- Eight antigenically distinct C botulinum toxins are known, including A, B, C (alpha), C (beta), D, E, F, and G. Each strain of C botulinum can produce only a single toxin type. Types A, B, E, and, rarely, F cause human disease.
- Toxins A and B are the most potent, and the consumption of small amounts of food contaminated with these types has resulted in full-blown disease. During the last 20 years, toxin A has been the most common cause of foodborne outbreaks; toxins B and E follow in frequency.
- In 15% of C botulinum infection outbreaks, the toxin type is not determined.
- Toxins C and D cause disease in various animals

111. Ans. (a) Systemic steroids

(Ref: Harrison 20th edition, p 1265; Harrison 19th p 1125)

Therapy for Reactions
- Type 1 lepra reactions are best treated with glucocorticoids (e.g., prednisone, initially at doses of 40–60 mg/d). As the inflammation subsides, the glucocorticoid dose can be tapered, but steroid therapy must be continued for at least 3–6 months lest recurrence supervenes.

- Thalidomide is ineffective against type 1 lepra reactions. Clofazimine is of questionable benefit but in any event is far less efficacious than glucocorticoids.
- Type 2 Lepra reaction: Treatment of ENL must be individualized. If ENL is mild (i.e., without fever or other organ involvement, with occasional crops of only a few skin papules), it may be treated with antipyretics alone. However, in cases with many skin lesions, fever, malaise, and other tissue involvement, brief courses (1–2 weeks) of glucocorticoids are effective.
- If, despite two courses of glucocorticoid therapy, ENL appears to be recurring and persisting, treatment with thalidomide should be initiated, with the dose depending on the initial severity of the reaction.

112. Ans. (a) Patient with score of 0 has 1.5% chances of dying

(Ref: Harrison 20th edition, p 912; Harrison 19th p 807)

The CURB-65 criteria include five variables:

C = Confusion (C)
U = Urea >7 mmol/L (U)
R = Respiratory rate >30/min (R)
B = Blood pressure=systolic <90 mmHg or diastolic <60 mmHg
  Age>65 years

- Patients with a score of 0, among whom the 30-day mortality rate is 1.5%, can be treated outside the hospital.
- With a score of 2, the 30-day mortality rate is 9.2%, and patients should be admitted to the hospital.
- Among patients with scores of >3, mortality rates are 22% overall; these patients may require admission to an ICU.

113. Ans. (d) Ceftriaxone

(Ref: Harrison 20th edition, p 999-1001)

- The clinical pointers are in favour of meningoccal sepsis. Early symptoms are nonspecific and suggest an influenza-like illness with fever, headache, and myalgia accompanied by vomiting and abdominal pain. As discussed above, the rash, if present, may appear to be viral early in the course until petechiae or purpuric lesions develop. Purpura fulminans occurs in severe cases, with multiple large purpuric lesions and signs of peripheral ischemia
- Empirical antibiotic therapy for suspected meningococcal disease consists of a third-generation cephalosporin such as ceftriaxone or cefotaxime to cover the various other (potentially penicillin-resistant) bacteria that may produce an indistinguishable clinical syndrome

114. Ans. (d) Adequately prevented with chloroquine therapy

(Ref: Harrison 20th edition, p 1578; Table 219-2, p 1588; Harrison 19th p 1378)

1. Severe falciparum malaria can include dysfunction of any organ system, Neurologic abnormalities progressing to alterations in consciousness
2. Repeated seizures, and coma (cerebral malaria)
3. Severe anemia
4. Hypotension and shock
5. Non-cardiogenic pulmonary edema
6. Acute kidney injury due to acute tubular necrosis or, less commonly, severe Hemolysis
7. Hypoglycemia
8. Acidosis
9. Hemolysis with jaundice; hepatic dysfunction; retinal hemorrhages.

115. Ans. (d) Pneumonia

(Ref: Harrison 20th edition, p 1475)

- The intense immune responses induced by measles virus infection are paradoxically associated with depressed responses to unrelated (non measles virus) antigens, which persist for several weeks to months beyond resolution of the acute illness.
- This state of immune suppression enhances susceptibility to secondary infections with bacteria and viruses that cause pneumonia and diarrhea and is responsible for a substantial proportion of measles-related morbidity and deaths.

116. Ans. (a) CNS involvement

(Ref: Harrison 20th edition, p 1355)

- The most common extracutaneous site of involvement in chicken pox in children is the CNS.
- The cerebrospinal fluid (CSF) contains lymphocytes and elevated levels of protein. CNS involvement is a benign complication of VZV infection in children and generally does not require hospitalization.
- Aseptic meningitis, encephalitis, transverse myelitis, and Guillain-Barré syndrome can also occur.

117. Ans. (d) Laennec's cirrhosis

(Ref: Harrison 20th edition, p 1359; Harrison 19th p 1188)

Explanation: EB virus

Complications with EBV infection

1. Meningitis and encephalitis are the most common neurologic abnormalities. Acute EBV infection has also been associated with cranial nerve palsies (cranial nerve VII), Guillain-Barré syndrome, acute transverse myelitis, and peripheral neuritis.
2. Autoimmune hemolytic anemia, Red cell aplasia, severe granulocytopenia, thrombocytopenia, pancytopenia, and hemophagocytic lympho-histiocytosis.
3. The spleen ruptures in <0.5% of cases. Splenic rupture may manifest as abdominal pain, referred shoulder pain, or hemodynamic compromise.
4. Hypertrophy of lymphoid tissue in the tonsils or adenoids can result in upper airway obstruction, as can inflammation and edema of the epiglottis, pharynx, or uvula.
5. Other rare complications associated with acute EBV infection include hepatitis (which can be fulminant), myocarditis or pericarditis pneumonia with pleural effusion, interstitial nephritis, genital ulcerations, and vasculitis.

118. Ans. (b) SABE

(Ref: Harrison 19th p 819)

The initial symptoms and signs of endocarditis may be caused by direct arterial, valvular, or cardiac damage. Although a changing Regurgitant murmur is significant diagnostically, it is the exception rather than the rule.

The damage to valve may cause a perforation of develop in a valve cusp, that explains the manifestation of development of new onset murmur.

119. Ans. (b) Trypanosoma Cruzi

(Ref: Harrison 20th edition, Table 222-1, p 1603; Harrison 19th p 1395)

- Romaña's sign —the classic finding in acute Chagas' disease, which consists of unilateral painless edema of the palpebrae and periocular tissues—can result when the conjunctiva is the portal of entry.
- These initial local signs may be followed by malaise, fever, anorexia, and edema of the face and lower extremities. Generalized lymphadenopathy and hepatosplenomegaly may develop.

120. Ans. (b) Mitral valve mostly involved

(Ref: Harrison 19th p 817)

- N.V.E (Native valve endocarditis)= mitral valve MC involved.
- P.V.E (Prosthetic valve endocarditis)= Aortic valve MC involved.
- Early infections (i.e., those occurring within 2 months after valve implantation) are commonly caused by staphylococci—both coagulase-positive and coagulase negative—gram-negative organisms, and fungi.
- In late prosthetic valve endocarditis, streptococci are commonly identified, although coagulase-negative and coagulase positive Staphylococci still cause many cases.

121. Ans. (d) Thickening of acromio-clavicular joint

(Ref: Harrison 20th edition, p 1283; and ch. 215, Nelson 18th ed.)

Classic stigmata of syphilis include
1. Hutchinson's teeth (centrally notched, widely spaced, peg-shaped upper central incisors)
2. "Mulberry"molars (sixth-year molars with multiple, poorly developed cusps)
3. Saddle nose
4. Skeletal changes due to persistent or recurrent periostitis and associated thickening of bone include frontal bossing, a bony prominence of the forehead (**Olympian brow**)
5. Unilateral or bilateral thickening of the sternoclavicular third of the clavicle (**Clavicular or Higouménaki sign**)
6. An anterior bowing of the midportion of the tibia (**Saber shins**)
7. Convexity along the medial border of the scapula (**Scaphoid scapula**)

122. Ans. (d) Tropical splenomegaly syndrome

(Ref: Harrison 20th edition, p 1580-1581; Harrison 19th p 1374-75)

- Tropical splenomegaly syndrome is now known as Hyperreactive malarial syndrome (HMS) is prevalent in native residents of regions where malaria is endemic. Patients with HMS have high levels of antibody for Plasmodium falciparum, Plasmodium vivax, or Plasmodium ovale.
- Presentation of kala Azar includes include fever, chills and spleen progressively becomes greatly enlarged, and bone marrow damage leads to pancytopenia.
- The liver is somewhat enlarged, and generalized lymphadenopathy may occur. Hyperpig-mentation of skin can be seen, leading to the name kala azar. Oral miltefosine is used as a new drug.

123. Ans. (a) Urethritis

(Ref: Harrison 20th edition, p 1125; Harrison 19th p 870)

Gonococcal infections in males

Acute urethritis is the most common clinical manifestation of gonorrhea in males. The usual incubation period after exposure is 2–7 days, although the interval can be longer and some men remain asymptomatic. The discharge initially is scant and mucoid but becomes profuse and purulent within a day or two. Gram's stain of the urethral discharge may reveal PMNs and gram-negative intracellular monococci and diplococci

- Before the antibiotic era, symptoms of urethritis persisted for <8 weeks.
- Epididymitis is now an uncommon complication, and gonococcal prostatitis occurs rarely.
- Other unusual local complications of gonococcal urethritis include edema of the penis due to dorsal lymphangitis or thrombophlebitis
- Sub-mucous inflammatory "soft" infiltration of the urethral wall
- Peri-urethral abscess or fistula, inflammation or abscess of Cowper's gland, and seminal vesiculitis.
- Balanitis may develop in uncircumcised men.

124. Ans. (c) P. vivax causes enlargement of affected RBC

(Ref: Harrison 20th edition, Table 219-5, p 1583; Harrison 19th p 1376)

Method	Procedure	Advantages	Disadvantages
PfHRP2 dipstick or card test	A drop of blood is placed on the stick or card, which is then immersed in washing solutions. Monoclonal antibody captures the parasite antigen and reads out as a colored band.	Inexpensive; rapid; sensitivity similar to or slightly lower than that of thick films (-0.001% parasitemia)	Detects only Plasmodium falciparum; remains positive for weeks after infection; does not quantitate P. falciparum parasitemia
Plasmodium LDH dipstick or card test	Drop of blood is placed on the stick of card, which is then immersed in washing solutions. Monoclonal antibodies capture the parasite antigens and read out as colored bands.	Rapid; sensitivity similar to or slightly lower than that of thick films for P. falciparum (-0.001% parasitemia)	Slightly more difficult preparation than PfHRP2 tests; may miss low-level parsitemia with P. vivax, P. ovale, and P. malariae and does not speciate these organisms; does not quantitate P. falciparum

* Falciparum and malariae do not cause enlargement of infected RBC whereas vivax and ovale cause infected RBC to enlarge.

125. Ans. (d) Lymphadenopathy

(Ref: Harrison 20th edition, p 1096; Harrison 19th p 978)

- A few patients of diptheria develop massive swelling of the tonsils and present with "bull-neck" diphtheria, which results from massive edema of the submandibular and paratracheal region and characterized by foul breath, thick speech, and stridorous breathing.
- The systemic manifestations of diphtheria stem from the effects of diphtheria toxin and include weakness as a result of neurotoxicity and cardiac arrhythmias or congestive heart failure due to myocarditis.

126. Ans. (b) Isoprinosine

(Ref: Harrison 20th edition, p 997; Nelson 18th ed. ch. 243)

Isoprinosine is used as an immune-modulator for the management of patients with:
1. Immune-depression suffering from viral infections such as SSPE, varicella, herpes simplex Type 1 & 2.
2. In the management of recurrent herpes simplex Type 1 & 2.
3. As an adjunct in the treatment of genital warts

127. Ans. (b) Albendazole is more effective than praziquantel

(Ref: Harrison 20th edition, p 1015; Harrison 19th p 1432)

- When treatment is deemed appropriate, standard therapy consists of Albendazole (10–15 mg/kg/d orally) or praziquantel (50 mg/kg/d orally). Albendazole is preferred, since it has shown better efficacy in some comparisons and since corticosteroids appear to lower circulating praziquantel levels but increase albendazole levels.
- The medical management of neurocysticercosis is controversial, as the benefits of cyst clearance must be weighed against potential harm of an inflammatory response to dying worms.
- Anti-helminthic therapy hastens radiologic improvement in parenchymal cysticercosis.
- However, some randomized trials have shown that corticosteroids alone are as effective as specific therapy plus corticosteroids for controlling seizures and some reports have shown exacerbation of disease after anti-helminthic therapy. Active lesions with a high likelihood of progression, such as intra-ventricular cysts, may benefit from therapy.
- At the other end of the spectrum, inactive calcified lesions probably do not benefit from therapy. Overall, it remains difficult to determine when treatment is indicated.

128. Ans. (a) Erythromycin drug of choice

(Ref: Harrison 20th edition, p 1138, 1141; Harrison 19th p 1017)

- Azithromycin (500 mg orally once daily), clarithromycin (500 mg orally twice daily), or a fluoroquinolone (eg, levofloxacin 500 mg orally once daily), and not erythromycin, are the drugs of choice for treatment of legionellosis because of their excellent intracellular penetration and in vitro activity, as well as desirable pharma-cokinetic properties that permit oral administration and once or twice daily dosing. Duration of therapy is 10–14 days, although a 21-day course of therapy is recommended for immunocompromised patients.
- Patients are often immunocompromised, smokers, or have chronic lung disease. Scant sputum production, pleuritic chest pain, toxic appearance. Chest radiograph: focal patchy infiltrates or consolidation.

129. Ans. (a) SSPE

(Ref: Nelson 18th ed. ch. 283)

- Characteristic periodic activity (Rademecker complex) is seen on EEG showing widespread cortical dysfunction in SSPE. It is characterised by high voltage spike occurring at high frequency of 0.5 -1.5 seconds.
- Pathologically, the white matter of both the hemispheres and brainstem are affected, as well as the cerebral cortex, and eosinophilic inclusion bodies are present in the nuclei of neurons and oligodendrocytes.

130. Ans. (c) May rupture into the pleural cavity

(Ref: Harrison 20th edition, p 1571; Harrison 19th p 1365)

- The most common extra intestinal manifestation of amoebic dysentery is amoebic liver abscess.
- This frequently presents without history of prior intestinal symptoms.

- Physical examination shows intercostal tenderness. *Abscesses are most commonly single and in the right lobe of the liver, and they are much more common in men. Without prompt treatment, amoebic abscesses may rupture into the pleural, peritoneal, or pericardial space, which is often fatal.*

131. Ans. (a) Urine test for legionella antigen is 90% sensitive

(Ref: Harrison 20th edition, p 911-12; Harrison 19th p 1017)

- The test for L. pneumophila detects only serogroup 1, but this serogroup accounts for most community-acquired cases of Legionnaires' disease.
- The sensitivity and specificity of the *Legionella* urine antigen test are as high as 90% and 99%, respectively.
- The pneumococcal urine antigen test is sensitive and specific (80% and >90%, respectively). Although false-positive results can be obtained with samples from pneumococcus-colonized children, the test is generally reliable. Both tests can detect antigen even after the initiation of appropriate antibiotic therapy.

132. Ans. (c) Pain

(Ref: Harrison 19th p 1863)

- *Hemolytic-uremic syndrome (HUS) and, less commonly, thrombotic thrombocytopenic purpura (TTP) may rarely occur after treatment with antineoplastic drugs including mitomycin, cisplatin, bleomycin, and gemcitabine. It occurs most often in patients with gastric, lung, colorectal, pancreatic, and breast Carcinoma.*
- HUS usually has its onset 4–8 weeks after the last dose of chemotherapy, but it is not rare to detect it several months later.
- HUS is characterized by:
  - Microangiopathic hemolytic anemia and thrombocytopenia
  - Renal failure
  - Dyspnea, weakness, fatigue
  - Oliguria
  - Purpura is also common initial symptoms and findings.
  - Systemic hypertension and pulmonary edema frequently occur. Severe hyper-tension, pulmonary edema, and rapid worsening of hemolysis and renal function may occur after a blood or blood product transfusion.
  - Cardiac findings include atrial arrhythmias, pericardial friction rub, and pericardial effusion.
  - Raynaud's phenomenon is part of the syndrome in patients treated with bleomycin.

133. Ans. (c) It can invade tissue to a great depth

(Ref: Harrison 20th edition, p 1162-64; Harrison 19th p 1039)

H pylori is a spiral gram-negative rod that resides beneath the gastric mucous layer adjacent to gastric epithelial cells.

- Although not invasive, it causes gastric mucosal inflammation with PMNs and lymphocytes.
- About 15% of infected people have inflammation that predominates in the gastric antrum but spares the gastric body (where acid is secreted). People with this phenotype tend to have increased gastrin; increased acid production; and increased risk of developing peptic ulcers, especially duodenal ulcers

134. Ans.(c) Angiostrongylus

(Ref: Harrison 20th edition, p 1623-24; Harrison 19th Table 165-2, p 908)

- Angiostrongylus cantonensis, the rat lungworm, is the most common cause of human *eosinophilic meningitis*
- Humans acquire the infection by ingesting raw infected mollusks; vegetables contaminated by mollusk slime; or crabs, freshwater shrimp, and certain marine fish that have eaten infected mollusks.
- Clinical symptoms develop 2–35 days after the ingestion of larvae. Patients usually present with an insidious or abrupt excruciating frontal, occipital, or bitemporal headache. Neck stiffness, nausea and vomiting, and paresthesias are also common.
- Management consists of supportive measures, including the administration of analgesics, sedatives, and—in severe cases— glucocorticoids. Repeated lumbar punctures with removal of CSF can relieve symptoms.
- **Causes of eosinophilic meningitis:**
  1. The most common cause is human infection with the rat lungworm, Angiostrongylus cantonensis
  2. Gnathostoma spinigerum (dog and cat roundworm)
  3. Baylisascaris procyonis (raccoon roundworm)
  4. Ascaris lumbricoides (human roundworm), Trichinella spiralis, Toxocara canis, Toxoplasma gondii,
  5. Paragonimus westermani, Echinococcus granulosus, Schistosoma japonicum, Onchocerca volvulus, and T. solium.
  6. Eosinophilic meningitis may also occur as an unusual manifestation of more common viral, bacterial, or fungal infections of the CNS.
  7. Noninfectious causes of eosinophilic meningitis include multiple sclerosis, malignancy, hypereosinophilic syndrome, or a reaction to medications or a ventriculoperitoneal shunt

135. Ans. (d) Patent Fossa Ovalis (P.F.O.)

(Ref: CMDT-14/ch:33/pg:143)

- The course of infective endocarditis is determined by the degree of damage to the heart, by the site of infection (right-sided versus left-sided, aortic versus mitral valve), by the presence of metastatic foci of infection, by the occurrence of embolization, and by immuno-logically mediated processes.
- In setting of Patent Fossa Ovalis paradoxical embolism ensues and can cause left sided endocarditis.

Other septic complications seen with infective endocarditis

1. The infection can also extend into the myocardium, resulting in abscesses leading to conduction disturbances, and involving the wall of the aorta, creating sinus of Valsalva aneurysms.
2. Peripheral embolization to the brain and myocardium may result in infarctions. Embolization to the spleen and kidneys is also common.
3. Peripheral emboli may initiate metastatic infections or may become established in vessel walls, leading to mycotic aneurysms.

4. Right-sided endocarditis, which usually involves the tricuspid valve, causes septic pulmonary emboli, occasionally with infarction and lung abscesses.

136. Ans. (c) Arthritis

(Ref: Harrison 19th p 1151)

Lyme disease is the most common tick-borne disease in western countries and is caused by spirochete B. Burgdorferi.

Essentials of Diagnosis
1. Erythema migrans, a flat or slightly raised red lesion that expands with central clearing.
2. Headache or stiff neck.
3. Arthralgias, arthritis, and myalgias; arthritis is often chronic and recurrent
4. Wide geographic distribution in U.S

- **Stage 1 infection** is characterized by erythema migrans. About 1 week after the tick bite (range, 3–30 days; median 7–10 days), a flat or slightly raised red lesion appears at the site, which is commonly seen in areas such as the groin, thigh, or axilla.
- **Stage 2, early disseminated infection:**
- Up to 50–60% of patients with erythema migrans are bacteremic. Within days to weeks of the original infection, secondary skin lesions that are not associated with a tick bite develop in about 50% of patients. These lesions are similar in appearance to the primary lesion but are usually smaller.
  - Malaise, fatigue, fever, headache, neck pain, and generalized achiness are common with the skin lesions.
  - Cardiac involvement includes myo-pericarditis, with atrial or ventricular arrhythmias and heart block.
  - Neurologic manifestations include both the central and peripheral nervous systems. The most common central nervous system manifestation is an aseptic meningitis with mild headache and neck stiffness. The most common peripheral manifestation is a cranial neuropathy, i.e, facial palsy.
- **Stage 3, late persistent infection:**
  - Stage 3 infection occurs months to years after the initial infection and again primarily manifests itself as musculoskeletal, neurologic, and skin disease. The classic manifestation of late disease is a monarticular or oligoarticular arthritis most commonly affecting the knee or other large weight bearing joints.

137. Ans. (d) Clostridial myonecrosis

(Ref: Harrison 19th p 988)

- The differential diagnosis of botulism includes:
  1. Guillain-Barre syndrome
  2. Myasthenia gravis
  3. Stroke syndromes
  4. Eaton-Lambert syndrome
  5. Tick paralysis.
  6. Less likely are poisoning by tetrodotoxin, shellfish, or a host of rarer agents and antimicrobial drug–associated paralysis.

138. Ans. (b) Detection of cysticerci antigen by ELISA

(Ref: Harrison 19th p 1431)

- Neuroimaging findings suggestive of neuro-cysticercosis constitute the primary major diagnostic criterion. These findings include cystic lesions with or without enhancement (e.g., ring enhancement), one or more nodular calcifications (which may also have associated enhancement), or focal enhancing lesions.
- The second major diagnostic criterion is detection of specific antibodies to cysticerci. While most tests employing unfractionated antigen have high rates of false-positive and false-negative results, this problem can be overcome by using the more specific immunoblot assay. ELISA for cysticerosis antigen is a minor diagnostic criteria.
- Cysticerci in the brain parenchyma are usually 5–20 mm in diameter and rounded. Cystic lesions in the subarachnoid space or fissures may enlarge up to 6 cm in diameter and may be lobulated. For cysticerci within the subarachnoid space or ventricles, the walls may be very thin and the cyst fluid is often iso-dense with CSF. Thus, obstructive hydrocephalus or enhancement of the basilar meninges may be the only finding on CT in extra-parenchymal neuro-cysticercosis.
- CT is more sensitive than MRI in identifying calcified lesions, whereas MRI is better for identifying cystic lesions, scolices, and enhancement.
- Clinical manifestations of neuro-cysticercosis like seizures are minor diagnostic criteria for the same.

139. Ans. (d) Coronary artery bypass graft

(Ref: Harrison 19th p 826)

Cardiac conditions with high risk of adverse outcomes from endocarditis for which prophylaxis with dental procedures is recommended.
1. Prosthetic cardiac valve
2. Previous infective endocarditis
3. Congenital heart disease
4. Unrepaired cyanotic CHD, including palliative shunts and conduits
5. Completely repaired congenital heart defect with prosthetic material or device, whether placed by surgery or by catheter intervention, during the first 6 months after the procedure
6. Repaired CHD with residual defects at the site or adjacent to the site of a prosthetic patch or prosthetic device
7. Cardiac transplantation recipients in whom cardiac valvulopathy develops.

140. Ans. (b) Onchocerca volvulus

(Ref: Harrison 19th 1421)

- Onchocerciasis primarily affects the skin, eyes, and lymph nodes. In contrast to the pathology in lymphatic filariasis, the damage in onchocerciasis is elicited by microfilariae and not by adult parasites
- Definitive diagnosis depends on the detection of an adult worm in an excised nodule or, more commonly, of microfilariae in a skin snip. Skin snips are obtained with a corneal-scleral punch, which collects a blood-free skin

biopsy sample extending to just below the epidermis, or by lifting of the skin with the tip of a needle and excision of a small (1 to 3 mm) piece with a sterile scalpel blade

141. Ans. (c) Glutamate dehydrogenase Enzyme immunoassay

(Ref: Harrison 19th p 859)

- The pseudo-membranes of PMC are confined to the colonic mucosa and initially appear as 1 to 2 mm whitish-yellow plaques. The intervening mucosa appears unremarkable, but, as the disease progresses, the pseudo-membranes coalesce to form larger plaques and become confluent over the entire colon wall.
- The whole colon is usually involved, but 10% of patients have rectal sparing.
- *Abdominal computed tomography (CT) scanning is the imaging modality of choice for C difficile colitis.*
- *Sigmoidoscopy alone may not reveal any abnormality if the disease is confined to the right colon. Typical pseudo-membranes are beyond the limit of flexible sigmoidoscopy in 10% of patients. Therefore, colonoscopy is more useful.*
- In Colonoscopy Pseudomembranes are observed in 14-25% of patients with mild C difficile disease and 87% of patients with fulminant disease
- Stool assays for C difficile, from the most to the least sensitive, include the following:
    1. **Stool Culture:** The most sensitive test (sensitivity, 90-100%; specificity, 84-100%), but the results are slow and may lead to a delay in the diagnosis if used alone
    2. **Glutamate Dehydrogenase Enzyme Immunoassay (EIA):** This is a very sensitive test (sensitivity, 85-100%; specificity, 87-98%); it detects the presence of glutamate dehydrogenase produced by C difficile
    3. **Stool Cytotoxin Test:** A positive test result is the demonstration of a cytopathic effect that is neutralized by a specific antiserum (sensitivity, 70-100%; specificity, 90-100%)
    4. **EIA for detecting toxins A and B:** This test is used in most laboratories (moderate sensitivity, 79-80%; excellent specificity, 98%).

142. Ans. (d) At any stage of pregnancy

(Ref: Harrison's-18e/ch: Infectious diseases/pg: 1384)

- Transmission of T. pallidum across the placenta from a syphilitic woman to her fetus may occur at any stage of pregnancy, but fetal damage generally does not occur until after the fourth month of gestation, when fetal immunologic competence begins to develop.
- The risk of fetal infection during untreated early maternal syphilis is 75–95%. Adequate treatment of the woman before the 16th week of pregnancy should prevent fetal damage, and treatment before the third trimester should adequately treat the infected fetus. Untreated maternal infection may result in a rate of fetal loss of up to 40%.

143. Ans. (d) C5

(Ref: Harrison's-18e/ch:144/pg:1501)

- The best-documented genetic association with meningococcal disease is complement deficiency, chiefly of the terminal complement components (C5–9), properdin, or factor D; such a deficiency increases the risk of disease by up to 600-fold and may result in recurrent attacks.
- Complement components are believed to be important for the bactericidal activity of serum, which is considered the principal mechanism of immunity against invasive meningococcal disease.

144. Ans. (a) SSPE

(Ref: Nelson 18th ed. ch. 283)

SSPE is also known as **Dawson encephalitis** and **measles encephalitis**.

145. Ans. (a) Herpetic esophagitis

(Ref: Mayo clinic gastroenterology and Hepatology Board review-5th ed. by Stephen C. Hauser)

- The ulcers of herpes esophagitis can have a punctate, linear, stellate, or volcano-like appearance, often with a thin halo of edema at the margins. The ulcers may be clustered together or widely separated with normal intervening mucosa.
- The most common cause of infectious esophagitis is candida esophagitis.

146. Ans. (a) Seizures

(Ref: Harrison 19th p 1945)

- Whipple is a Multi-systemic disease caused by Tropheryma Whippelli and is characterised by Fever, lymphadenopathy, arthralgias Weight loss, malabsorption, chronic diarrhoea.
- Diagnosis is made with Duodenal biopsy with periodic acid-Schiff (PAS), showing intracellular macrophages with characteristic bacillus.
- *Central nervous system involvement is manifested by a variety of findings such as dementia, lethargy, coma, seizures, myoclonus, or hypothalamic signs. Cranial nerve findings include ophthalmoplegia or nystagmus in adults and children with acquired infection.*

147. Ans. (c) Diabetic ketoacidosis

(Ref: Harrison 19th p 2429)

- Patients with diabetes or immunocompromising conditions are at risk for invasive rhinocerebral mucormycosis.
- *The acidosis causes dissociation of iron from sequestering proteins in serum, resulting in enhanced fungal survival and virulence. It is likely that hyperglycemia during DKA also contributes to the risk of mucormycosis through its association with poorly characterized defects in phagocytic function.*
- Patients present with low-grade fever, dull sinus pain, diplopia, decreased mental status, decreased ocular motion, chemosis, proptosis, dusky or necrotic nasal turbinates, and necrotic hard-palate lesions that respect the midline.
- Without rapid recognition and intervention, the process continues on an inexorable invasive course, with high mortality.

148. Ans. (b) Meningo-encephalitis

(Ref: Harrison 20th edition, p 1359)

Most cases of Infectious Mononucleosis are self-limited. Deaths are very rare and most often are due to central nervous system (CNS) complications, splenic rupture, upper airway obstruction, or bacterial superinfection.

149. Ans. (b) Legionella

(Ref: Harrison 20th edition, p 1137; Harrison 19th p 1015)

Legionellosis refers to the two clinical syndromes caused by bacterium of the genus Legionella. Pontiac fever is an acute, febrile, self-limited illness that has been serologically linked to Legionella species, whereas Legionnaires' disease is the designation for pneumonia caused by these species.

150. Ans. (a) Mucosal injury

(Ref: Harrison 20th edition, p 1617-18; Harrison 19th p 1406)

- The reasons that some, but not all, infected patients develop clinical manifestations and the mechanisms by which Giardia causes alterations in small-bowel function are largely unknown. *Although trophozoites adhere to the epithelium, they do not cause invasive or locally destructive alterations.*
- The lactose intolerance and, in a minority of infected adults and children, significant malabsorption that develop are clinical signs of the loss of brush-border enzyme activities. *In most infections, the morphology of the bowel is unaltered; however, in a few cases (usually in chronically infected, symptomatic patients), the histopathologic findings (including flattened villi) and the clinical manifestations resemble those of tropical sprue and gluten-sensitive enteropathy.*
- The natural history of Giardia infection varies markedly. Infections may be aborted, transient, recurrent, or chronic. Parasite as well as host factors may be important in determining the course of infection and disease.

151. Ans. (b) Gastric outlet obatruction

(Ref: Harrison 20th edition, p 1165; Harrison 19th p 1041)

- The most clear-cut indications for treatment are *H. pylori*–related duodenal or gastric ulceration or low-grade gastric B cell lymphoma.
- H. pylori should be eradicated in patients with documented ulcer disease, whether or not the ulcers are currently active, to reduce the likelihood of relapse
- Individuals with a strong family history of gastric cancer should be treated to eradicate *H. pylori* in the hope that their cancer risk will be reduced

152. Ans. (d) Neostigmine and Atropine can be used in the treatment of Bungarus cerulas (Common Krait) poisoning

(Ref: http://www.apiindia.org/medicine_update_2013/chap 94.pdf)

- Anti-snake venom (ASV) is the mainstay of treatment. In India, polyvalent ASV, i.e. effective against all the four common species; Russell's viper, common cobra, common Krait and saw-scaled viper and no monovalent ASVs are available.
- There are known species such as the humpnosed pit viper (Hypnale hypnale) where polyvalent ASV is ineffective.
- In addition, region specific species such as Sochurek's saw-scaled viper (*Echis carinatus sochureki*) in Rajasthan, where the effectiveness of polyvalent ASV is questionable.

- *Neostigmine is an anticholinesterase, which is particularly effective in postsynaptic neurotoxins such as those of cobra and is not useful against presynaptic neurotoxin i.e. common Krait and the Russell's viper.*
- Neostigmine test should be performed by administering 0.5–2 mg IV and if neurological improvement occurs, it should be continued 1/2 hourly over next 8 hours.

153. Ans. (d) Herpes Zoster

(Ref: Harrison 20th edition, p 182; Harrison 19th, page 1184)

- *Classically, involvement of the tip of the nose (Hutchinson's sign) has been thought to be a clinical predictor of ocular involvement in herpes zoster opthalmicus.*
- The skin manifestations of herpes zoster ophthalmicus strictly obey the midline with involvement of one or more branches of the ophthalmic division of the trigeminal nerve, namely the supraorbital, lacrimal, and naso-ciliary branches.
- Because the naso-ciliary branch innervates the globe, the most serious ocular involvement develops if this branch is affected.

154. Ans. (a) Salivation and lacrimation

(Ref: Harrison 20th edition, p 3328-29; Harrison 19th edition, Page 2748)

- The primary targets of scorpion venom are voltage-dependent ion channels. Venom toxins alter these channels, leading to prolonged neuronal activity. Many end-organ effects are secondary to this excessive excitation.
- *Autonomic excitation leads to cardiopulmonary effects* observed after some scorpion envenomations.
- Somatic and cranial nerve hyperactivity results from neuromuscular overstimulation.
- Additionally, *serotonin* may be found in scorpion venom and is thought to contribute to the *pain* associated with scorpion envenomation.

Physical Findings in Scorpion Bite

- Local tissue effects vary among species. Tapping over the injury site (ie, tap test) may cause severe pain after a sting by C exilicauda.
- Sympathetic overdrive symptoms predominate, causing tachycardia, hypertension, hyperthermia, and pulmonary edema.
- Arrhythmias
- Respiratory arrest and loss of protective airway reflexes are common causes of mortality.
- Pulmonary edema has been described and may be secondary to cardiogenic causes and to increased capillary permeability.
- Parasympathetic symptoms include hypotension, bradycardia, salivation, lacrimation, urination, defecation, and gastric emptying.
- Cranial nerve effects include the following:
- Classic roving or rotary eye movements, blurred vision, tongue fasciculations, and loss of pharyngeal muscle control may be observed.
- Difficulty swallowing combined with excessive salivary secretions may lead to respiratory difficulty.
- Somatic effects include the following: Restlessness and involuntary muscle jerking that can be mistaken for seizures have been described.

The "wow" factor of the book is the brief explanation of each section and innumerable diagrams for quick revision. Overall the book is very good, the content is precise. Recent questions given chapterwise are enough for practice. Book covers all the important point according to latest exam pattern. Overall layout and presentation is outstanding.
Vidhya Bhat
Gulbarga Inst. of Medical Sciences, Kalaburgi

The pictorial and lucid presentation is the WOW Factor here. Anatomy isn't brought or confusing anymore, with such extra ordinary color and pictures the book is gripping, the charts are so Good!!
Rajkumar Patel, AMCMET Medical College, Ahmedabad

Extensive coverage of contents, colored images, to the point text, high yield facts makes the book interesting. The clinical aspects helps us to correlate and reading is much Easy. Anatomy reading is very hard but the hard work of the authors have made our job much easier.
Mainak Mandal, KIMS, Bhubaneshwar

Synopsis is amongst the best. Putting the entire anatomy, Embryology and histology so concisely shows the knowledge, endeavour and talent of the authors
Shivam Sabharval Dr SN Medical College, Jodhpur

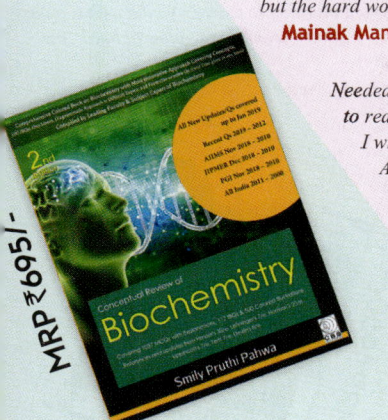

Needed information for PGMEE are given in well arranged. Easy to read format. If anyone want to read and revise the only book I will advise to buy this CBS Anatomy book. All the regional Anatomy is given superb with Images, clinical boxes and remember boxes
Sandeep P S, Tagore Medical College, Chennai

A must buy to ease your anatomy preparation. I have always found reading anatomy difficult, in 1st mbbs and even for preparing for pg exams but when I studies this book it made my FRICTION of DIFFICULTY into CLEAR AND SMOOTH knowledge of easiness. It is so easy to read and understand that you will LOVE anatomy as a subject after giving it a look. Nicely and crisply penned down by one of the best subject experts.
I will love to consult it to my juniors for preparing for pg entrance exams and even for 1st mbbs students to get *their thoughts clear.*
Syed A.

The book focuses on "to know everything about something & something about everything" by giving a comprehensive approach to Anatomy which is a strategy to clear exams like NEET, AIIMS, PGI, JIPMER. The book contains simplified, fully colored diagrams with meticulous labeling along with authentic content
Alish R Mehta
SBH Govt. Medical College, Dhule

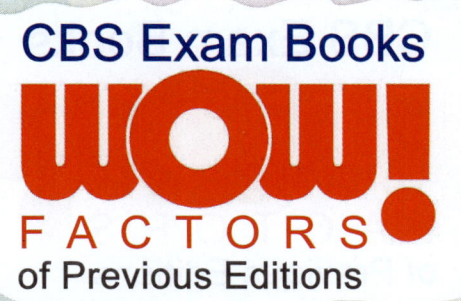

CBS Exam Books
WOW! FACTORS
of Previous Editions

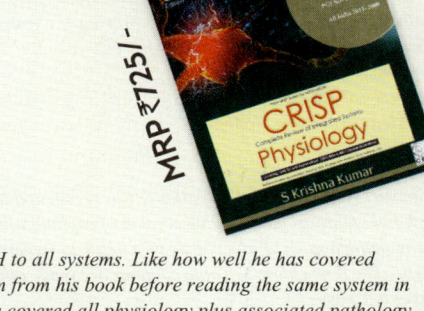

Each and everything is covered in well explained manner, colorful book, Interesting to read, hard topics covered in very easy manner, Recent questions updated, overall the best book of biochemistry so far.
Prabal Singh, SGRD Medical College, Amritsar

The colourful pages of the book doesn't make a reader sleep with a subject like biochemistry. I feel someone cannot get a simpler version of biochemistry than this book. The author has excellently simplified every topic.
P Harish
Kaminei Inst. Of Medical Sciences, Hyderabad

Its concept making skills can be illustrated from 1st chapter itself. She doesn't just state a fact but gives a reason behind it as well. Each line and sentence is through provoking and also contains one liner, and post each concept a small diagram for easy review is present. Reading text is sufficient to answer any question. Synopsis as a whole is sufficient for attempting all the questions and the question and answers are good for concept building and should be attempted after synopsis.
Saranya Mohan, Lady Hardinge Medical College, Delhi

Book contains the entire Biochemistry in the most concise and conceptual ways. The division of the syllabus in the various understandable units and chapter is quite adorable. The various high yielding boxes like additional edge, fundamental box, etc. is a major boost. In synopsis, the division of syllabus into the various different heading is done exceptionally well. It appears to be the most applauding feature. The number of questions and their explanation appears suitable and exact
Shivam Sabharwal, SN Medical College, Jodhpur

It's a good book as it is concise, biochemistry is a nightmare for everyone the point based manner of the book makes it easy to study and remember the overall layout is good and everything is covered. Practice questions are up to date and many are there so its very useful.
Apeksha, ESI Medical College, Bengaluru

Difficult topics are supplemented by Diagrams. Easy to understand. Awesome creation of High Return box, Fundamental Box & MCQ are clearly explained. This book is enough for PGMEE
Cheeran R, GMC, Villupuram

The best thing is INTEGRATED APROACH to all systems. Like how well he has covered Endocnology, just wow. If you read a system from his book before reading the same system in medicine it saves you a hell lot of time. He is covered all physiology plus associated pathology and pharmacology wherever needed plus many syndromes.
Aditya Gudheniya, Lokmanya Tilak Municipal Medical College, Mumbai

Really the wow factor is its appearance, colourful, high quality smooth colour papers, clinical importance tables are high yielding as well as conceptual. Nice layouts and presentations for diagrams. Two column concept is excellent. Concise Content and concept oriented. Lots of new question patterns added
Prithvi Raj, Govt Thiruvarur Medical College, Thiruvarur

Well presented in student friendly manner, CRISP content with integration from all subjects with detailed explanations with proper references, good page quality. IBQ'S and well-illustrated graphs are the strong features of the book
Rachit Singhania, North Bengal Medical College, Darjeeling

Well this no doubt the best book in the market in physiology. Integration of different systems as the name suggests is the key part of the book. And what's more interesting is the integrated view sir possess which includes mentioning about the subjects like medicine, pathology, pharmacology.
Vatsal Sampat, PDU, Rajkot

Remember & high yield points in between the chapters thus helping students understand what is focus on. Clubbing of pharmacology with physiology that's the best thing done. I don't think author has left any topic untouched with make it unique and apt to clear any exams physiology questions.
Alish R Mehta, SBH Govt Medical College, Dhule

The clinical correlation of every subject in this book is the best thing that makes every student to read this book. I never read such a book in my past, the final hard work of author is truly visible. Everything- the explanation, clinical correlation, IBQs synopsis all are better. No book will beat this book in the future.
Sandeep PS, Tagore Medical College, Chennai

 **Scan the QR Code to View Sample Pages of the Books**

It is very presentable than any other review books on this subject, Conceptual box makes learning of pharmacology a pleasant experience, The brilliant use of colors and explanation of concept makes this book a Go-to-reference for all the doubts that went unasked.

Balasaranya S
Coimbatore Medical College, Coimbatore

Excellent book, concept oriented, presentation is good with lot of flow charts that add to the beauty. Only review of pharma with maximum image based questions and numerical in general pharma. BIGGEST ADVANTAGE "ALL LATEST DRUGS COVERED". Practice questions in this book are much much better. I really appreciate the quality of MCQs (as well as IBQs)

Ch Idrees Rashid, GMC, Srinagar

The book is concise version of so vast PATHOLOGY which makes it best book for PG preparation. Since I am a final year student this book really needed to revise through pathology with recent updates which form base of medicine. The best feature of book is to the point info in tables. This really aids the learning. The concept maps to images are really good which are easy to understand. Everything is good but the synopsis is really best. The theory is aided with question answer and every MCQ is explained which has enhanced the learning level.

Shubha Singh
Malda Medical College, Malda

Wow factor is concept explanation, Orientation; I think quality of MCQs and image based questions is best. Also the best thing of book is all latest drugs are covered. Mechanism of action is explained in easy way with this book, we can also write theory exams also well. Pharmacology is very difficult to remember, but this book has made it easy by giving mnemonics. This is the best book for those who are preparing for PG entrance exams.

Bhuvana N
ESIC Medical College, Gulbarga

The 'wow' factor of the book is the question coverage. There are so many questions that brushes up every aspect of concept. The book has included all the contents required efficiently. Other best part is the conceptual box and mnemonics box. It is colourful and really interesting presentation. The explanation is really relevant and given in a simple manner which makes it easy to grasp. The questions are really very good – from simple ones to hard ones.

Shivani Singh
Kathmandu School of Medical Sciences, Nepal

The overall presentation of the context put the book far ahead of other competitors. Makes the concepts clear and understandable Covers the entire pharmacology. Numerous "Small- small" things that other book lack; make one to love this book and say "WOW". Synopsis covers the entire syllabus in the text. All the major points of the subjects are covered in the form of table; boxes; prose; etc. Practice Questions are at par with AIIMS and NEET level.

Shivam Sabharwal
SN Medical College, Jodhpur

A carol of Pathology books, a concise review of the entire pathology, A great collection of MCQs and image based questions, Apt diagram, illustrations and flow chart, Annexures in the initial pages are the major boost; provide a through, quick and concise review. Synopsis in the book is concise, conceptual and an excellent guide to Pathology, the number of MCQ's covering the previous year's questions, practice questions, etc. are apt. their explanation doubtfully correct.

Shivam Sabharwal
SN Medical College, Jodhpur

Annexures are superb....Key points & Key recent updates & high field facts are nice...Table content of explanations for many major topics...Flow charts that helps to understand easily. The flow charts & Table contents are made difficult topics into easy.

Theeran R
GMC, Villupuram

"Everything is WOW" let it be Annexures, high yield boxes, recent update sections or authentic images in a lucid language. Layout and presentation, makes the reader truly hooked up to the book. Absolute Book for Pathology.

Rajkumar Patel
AMCMET Medical College, Ahmedabad

This is one of the best books of Pathology in the market. The concepts are dilating with proper & logical thinking and are to the point. The tables in the book are high-yielding. The "high –yielding facts" are very much helpful and are an extra- edge to the book. The updates from robins 10th edition are really of great help too. The answers to the questions are well-dealt in most of the questions and are well explained. The IBQs also according to latest NEET exam pattern and are really explained.

Sayan Banerjee
Malda Medical College, Malda

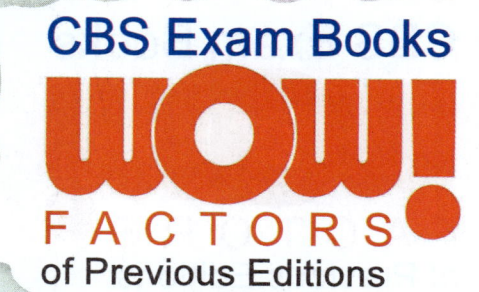

CBS Exam Books
WOW!
FACTORS
of Previous Editions

Image based questions are covered just after the end of chapter review which cover a good portion of papers. Only Recent years questions are included as we know the pattern of paper is quite variable so it's useless to practice old paper questions. Though every author provides very good explanation of mcq answers but in this book, the relevant information is also mentioned in box. The pages of book are coloured and of good quality. Overall representation of chapter review content is awesome with tables, graph.

Rashi

Covered and included all the recent updates req for the ongoing and upcoming next meet. Better explanations for the difficult portions of Park text. Given all recent MCQs. Minimum no. Of very old questions. Considering present NEET pattern new questions are framed.

Abhijeet Hiremath

PSM is a boring subject in MBBS, but Mukhmohit singh sir **ex**plained the subject very interestingly in the book. High Yielding **po**ints are reader friendly, boxes are very useful. All recent **que**stions are covered in this book. The pages are of good quality **and** nice presentation.

Siva Subramanian
Madurai Medical College, Madurai

All the latest updates are covered till date. The national programs and policies are given topic wise in each chapter instead of keeping all the programs at one place which is a good thing by the way. Best thing about this book is that all the chapters are given equal justice. The chapter of immunization and vaccine is one to mention here. Well the epidemiology section was literally amazing, all the tables, the diagrams ,charts made everything so easy. One of the nightmares is biostatistics for many students, well guys this book has covered that too in a proper way I must say. Lastly the 'good to remember', 'must remember' and 'high yield points' makes us differentiate the importance of the data in a way what to remember first. Must must buy book. This book is best for the subject instead of memorizing the data from the same old updated edition of the named book which was the only option until now.

Vatsal Sampat, PDU, Rajkot

Scan the QR Code to View Sample Pages of the Books

Best book available in the market for Forensic Medicine not only in terms of latest MCQs with explanation but also in terms of chapter summary, mnemonics, flow chart. It's not fanatically & haphazdly written like other guide books available in the market. It is a must read book.
Amazon Customer

This review book is the new gold standard for NEET pg preparation!!!! The images and the illustrative case study is what makes this book stand out from other books. Every important topics covered with latest questions and potential questions.
Amazon Customer

Wow factors are:- Tab columns are the best, Intro of the topics, Annexures & examples, Diagrams & explanations, To remember points, Synopsis & q2a are the best, Recent Advances are given in a clear way.
Melbin James
Sri Manaukula Vinayagar Medical College, Puducherry

The best part about the book is its illustrations. It's impossible to retail FMT if one has not seen pictures. It is not only good for AIPG preparing students but also second year students. "How to decode this book" mentioned next to acknowledgements is the best study tip for FMT I have ever received.
Amazon Customer

Finally a book for FMT with images and clinicals which helps to cover all aspects in NEET PG , AIIMS & JIPMER. As compared to other books in market which are without clinical a**nd boring to read.**
Shubham Jain
NSCB Medical College, Jabalpur

"Flowcharts in Forensic Medicine" this steals the show entirely, totally innovative style to teach this neglected subject and making it interesting!! the mnemonics and last minute FAQs are just awesome, made me fall in love with the subject!. Crisp and much adequate details on each topic and the images are so helpful as even in the textbooks there are no images. The mechanism and flowchart presentation definitely makes this book much friendlier
Rajkumar Patel
AMC MET Medical College, Ahmedabad

Pictorial representation, colorful, full of charts, pictorial representation of biochemical test, colourful lifecycle, Synopsis everything which required for a vast elaborated subject like Microbiology. I most likes the chart, High Yield facts, concise theory. For the vast subject like Microbiology this book is far away from other books in market because of it approach, colorful diagrams and charts and now concepts, No other books in the market has such system wise approach.Nice Tables for better understanding. Easy Simplified Language.
Vedanth Gowda
Vydehi Institute of Medical Sciences, Bangalore

Amazing book.. for PG prep..easy understandabale. Important p**oint well** illustrated. All the important MCQs covered. Lots of image inc**luded,** highly recommended. Highly modified
Ganaie Ishtiyaq
ASCOMS, Jammu

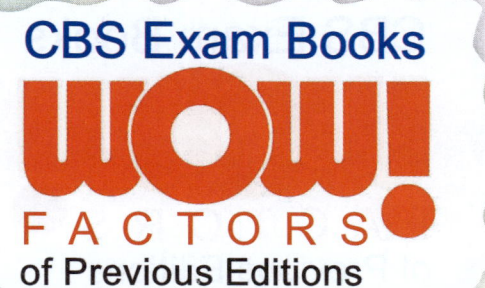

"The best book for ophthalmology for PGMEE"". No one make ophthal concepts so simple like this.....every concepts are explained neatly with suitable diagrams and flow charts...There are separate boxes for high yielding points, concepts and flowcharts....If anyone wants to take seat in AIIMS, don't ever miss to read this book as it covers the most of the AIIMS imp topics to attend all ophthal MCQs...
Sandeep (Amazon Customer)

Such a simplified book of microbiology that you can read in 10 days. Easy to revise. Images are very helpful to retain the microbiology for long time. Concise but compact very good book for NEET pg aspirant.
Pawan

Feedbacks Recd on CBS Exam Books FB Page

Mind blowing book of Micro really looking forward for it. - **Raj Patolia**
These books are more competent with enough that presently books in the market - **Shivaganesh Chellappa**
It will be masterpiece of Malti madam academic work - **Baba Kolhal**

Waited for this book for years. Best book available in market. Not only helps you to retain microbiology
Also colourful presentation helps in better learning.
Shubham Jain

The book has been beautifully compiled with all the necessary data. Photographs has been taken with the permission of CDC and other very reliable sources. So no need to doubt the accuracy as well as quality. Photographs are the key ingredient to the micro prep so I would say that this book is running first in that aspect. The formatting of the TWO COLUMN style is quite good considering the previous books from the publisher. I quite like it how the data and the photos have been placed in the page, Very concise and very easy to read and learn.
Ronak Javia
PDFU, Rajkot

I read 1st edition of this book, I am reviewing after 1 year of study (prefinal). This book is complete ophthalmology book for UG and PGMEE in every aspect, be it images, MCQs or latest updates /procedures. It's really a must buy book! Far far superior than other books available. Moreover, in 2nd edition I saw size (length *breadth wise) has been increased, that even makes it more wonderful to read. Thank u CBS Publishers.
Syed Aijaz

The most perfect book for ophthalmology preparation. It covers almost all important topics, presentation is superb, this is the first CBS book i thought of giving a try when everybody recommended Ruchi Rai. I am reviewing after 1 year of studying this book (1 edition). I must say i am a fan of this book now and has recommended this book already to all my juniors & seniors. Everything, be it theory, images, MCQs, i loved every single aspect of the book.
Idrees Rashid, GMC, Srinagar

WOW factor of the book is the picturistic correlation of the content and the content given in simplified box format. Overall the book is easy to comprehend and understand. Coverage is extensive. The book is very colorful and fun to read. The Presentation is good. The book has the text in a box format which makes it easier to read and revise. The author has covered all the important topics without being too lengthy. IBQs are very helpful and the explanation is also well given.
Vidhya Bhat
Gulbarga Inst of Medical Sciences – Kalaburgi

 **Scan the QR Code to View Sample Pages of the Books**

Vast and concise coverage of all important topics for proff exams as well a pg entrance exams. Presentation of topics are so arranged that are easy to remember via help of flowcharts and colourful diagrams. Detailed description of difficult questions helps to understand the concept. Topic wise practice questions helps to establish grip over the chapter topic by topic. IBQs are like cherry over the cake because IBQs are increasing in recent exam trends
Ankit Tiwari
Bundelkhand Medical College, Sagar

Question bank available for practice is good n enough comparing other books. Crisp concepts and brief explanations are given for quick revision to topics while solving questions. The volume of the book is tried to be kept as its minimum without compromising the quality. Language is student friendly even for hindi medium students and proper use of highlighting fonts n colours.
Naman Tiwari, GMC, Kota

SURGERY SIXER very nice book for PG preparation it contains all important points in all standard books like Sabiston, Bailey, Schwartz etc. Surgery Sixer book is very easy to prepare during last preparation & during last time revision best book is surgery sixer, high yield one liners in all chapters was very nice clear image in all chapters with brief explanations, this book is apt for all exam preparations, image based questions was nice
Karthick Raja, GMC, Vilupuram

Excellent book written by one of the top faculty of Medicine. Fully – colored layouts and it is reader – friendly. Synopsis is given in the form of bullet points which help in easy revision. MCQs are explained in a way to eliminate the options and opt for the best choice.
Liyakat Ahmed
Navodaya Medical College, Raichur

WOW factor for me is Dr Deepak Marwah Sir. A must have book for every medical student due to its excellent content which is covered in a beautiful layout and presentation of colourful pages (best quality), soothing to eyes and conceptual boxes. Excellent presentation of theory part, way too many MCQs with logical references, not too much length to make it difficult to revise
Syed Aijaz Ahmad, GMC, Srinagar

Wow factors are point wise description of content, uses of tables and diagrams, all updates included, conceptual diagnostic algorithm.
Rashi Jain
JLN Medical College, Ajmer

Tables, Harrison updates and practice questions are the best part of the book. The number of practice questions are plenty for better preparation
P Harish
Kamineni Inst. Of Medical Sciences, Hyderabad

Surgery Sixer book's One line creation is awesome to revise easily in last time. Recent advances, Bailey's update is correctly mentioned in this book... Image based questions with explanations are excellent. Surgery Sixer book is simplified book of Bailey & Love... The synopsis of this book are easily understood than any other book... It's easy to prepare
Theeran R, GMC, Villupuram

Wow is its concise appearance, colorful, high quality smooth colour papers, Reading monotonous papers are really tiring. Nice layout and presentation. Two column concept is excellent. Concise content. IBQs are given sufficiently. Clear Radiology images. Above All, CRYSTAL CLEAR CONCEPTS.
Prithvi Raj, GMC, Thiruvarur

Surgery Sixer for NBE by R Rajamahendran is the most reffered MCQ book for surgery and so I got a copy of it. The book gives us a 15 day plan to complete it plus 5 days for revision just before the exam. The PGI section is sorted separately towards the end and the students not aspiring for that can skip that part. It also has MCQs on Instruments and image based questions which is the recent pattern in the entrance exams. Quick tables for last minute revision are also there making revision even more easy!!
Shivani Desai
(Feedback on CBS Exam Books FB Page)

CBS Exam Books
WOW! FACTORS
of Previous Editions

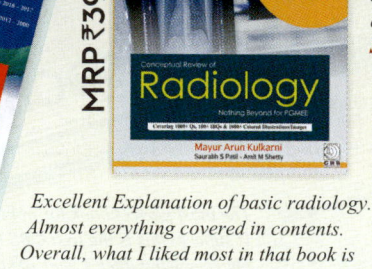

I should say whole book itself is a wow factor. The book is one of its kind so well explained, this is concise and adequate for undergraduates to prepare for entrance as well as for practical knowledge. I liked every bit of it the X Ray, CT Scan, USG all are so well explained in starting and here by disease wise. I think this is the best book for Radiology I have ever seen.
Shubhda Singh, Malda Medical College, Malda

Absolutely Stunning Book ..!! Surgery Presented in Easiest Way Possible. Colorful Presentations High Quality Paper, Seperate Boxes for Controversies, Bailey 27e Updates ..! Everything is Top Notch . No Second Thoughts . Go For it !!
Prithvi Raj
(Feedback on CBS Exam Books FB Page)

The book by Dr MAK is the best book in the subject for PG Aspirants. It covers many radiological images which have made understanding easy not only radiology but also related subjects. Extensive content and topic wise distribution of chapters have given the book an extra edge with such a great presentation. Radiology learning will be fun and interesting in SIR's way. The text in each chapter is very helpful to know the subject and then solving the practice questions is very helpful.
Mainak Mandal
KIMS, Bhubaneshwar

Concise matter that plays a vital role during revision. Centre of attraction in this book is separate column of bailley updates. Controversy desk as a column is a nice concept. I like it diagrammatic representation is best part of this book, practice questions by author are best selected questions from surgery. Helps in proff exams too. Hence, Undoubtedly best book for surgery in market. separate theory part is better for learning in comparison to other available surgery books in market.GIT in this book is so well presented that it made me fall for it. Correlated images favours it as best book of surgery. Instrument images and controversy desk leaves no stone unturned.
Shubham Jain, NSCB, Jabalpur

Excellent Explanation of basic radiology. Almost everything covered in contents. Overall, what I liked most in that book is interactive at many places (in many concept boxes). I liked the images of the book, which I don't think any other review has, and also the way these images has been explained with arrows, that makes concept more clear.
Ishtiyaq Ahmad Ganaie, ACOMS Jammu

The wow factor of the book is the content and the detailed explanation of the physics involved in each including the explanation of electromagnetic spectrum. Image based MCQs are amazing. All that is required for PG NEET is present in the book. Students need not refer to any additional source. The layout is presented well.
Apeksha, ESI Medical College, Bangaluru

Scan the QR Code to View Sample Pages of the Books

CBS Exam Books WOW! FACTORS of Previous Editions

All the 20 subjects are covered. Best book for last minute revision and for also the beginners who wants orientation about PG Preparation. Well organized Notes with Images for each topics. Most of the important topics are covered. One of the best book in the market for PG Aspirants. Everything is given in a condensed manner what the things needed is beautifully given. Like an extract from the so many fruits. This book provides the high yielding topics in condensed manner.
P S Sandeep
Tagore Medical College, Chennai

"Everything is given in an condensed format" best book for revise in last minute. All the important points are summarized in easy to read format. Synopsis is best in this book. Like the name saying one can complete the four subjects in 10 days a short span of time. Particularly in Psychiatry all the terminologies are explained with proper meaning.
Sandeep PS
Tagore Medical College, Chennai

The wow factory of the book is that it is a comprehensive compilation of 4 short subjects which is holding much importance in PG entrance and Professional Exam and I really liked the skin and anesthesia part. The book is well updated. Crisp contest and filled with lot of latest questions.
Shubhda Singh
Malda Medical College, Malda

There's hardly any good book for short subjects in market but this being written by 4 authors for 4 subjects is going to be the new gold standard for Short subjects preparation. There are lots of images in Derma, new guidelines in anesthesia are present. No need to buy any other subject specific book for these short subjects now.
Aditya (Amazon Customer)

WOW, each subject is written by the subject specialist it itself a big PLUS. Its concise appearance, colorful, high quality smooth colour papers, Reading Multicolor pages gives some sense of pleasure to eyes. Nice layout and presentation. Two column concepts is excellent, concise content. IBQs are given sufficiently. Above all, Crystal Clear Concepts. Content of 4 individual speciality subjects is nicely compated. Synopsis of content is excellent concept oriented is superb.
Prithivi Raj
GMC, Thiruvarur

This book is an innovative pedagogical method to approach PGME exams in the subjects of Dermatology, Anesthesia, Radiology & Psychiatry by condensing complex material for easier retention. The book contains numerous figures, tables, flowcharts, simple texts and mnemonics to make things easy. Authentic content with extensive explanations, Q&A framed according to the latest trend of examinations, Quick revision segment at the end of chapter for last minute revision. "LAST-AID" as is the most amazing part, "SKIN"- CONTENT IS SUFFICE TO TACKLE ANY QUESTION (INCLUDING IMAGE BASED)
Alish R Mehta
SBH Medical College, Dhule

WOW Factor: Everything about something and something about everything. Perfect for "Read, Revise & retain" as it is a concise book especially for DNB Exams. Mnemonics & tricks included to let things remember is nice. Anti Dyslipidemic table – great help to remember, Parasitology – section perfect, ENT & Ophthalmology – everything needed is covered
Alish R Mehta
SBH Govt Medical College, Dhule

WOW FACTOR- comparison tables, This is a "must have book not only during PG Preparation (internship) but also in prof years it gives crisp, concise concept, in tabular form with which pictures, easy to read & remember. Concepts based short & Crisp information, Radiological, Pathological slide, any other relevant images for the topic, are given at same place. All subjects in 1 book, which helps in easy reference plus SAVES TIME, Best Mnemonics.
Ekta Mishra
GMC, Chandigarh

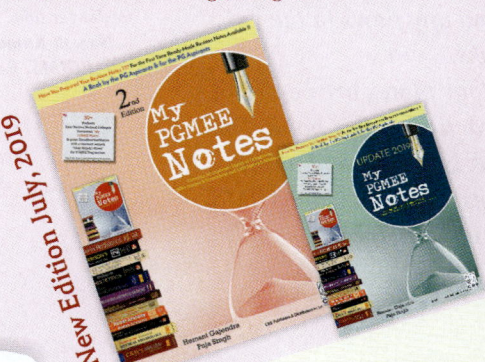
New Edition July, 2019

2019 Edition (June End)
MRP ₹895/-

Presentation is very good with flow charts which are easily understandable and covered all concepts very neatly. Image based question are good. I feel all contents and topics which are important and asked in previous entrance exams are covered within point wise. Highlighting of important points and mention of (Q) at previously asked questions is best. Synopsis is very good because 10-15 pages of topic is covered in 2 or 2 pages which will be easy to memorize.
Bhuvana N
ESIC Medical College, Kalaburgi

"My PGMEE notes" book itself is not a conventional book this is a note that's the good thing I like it and the plus point that the front of this book the front is amazing and the new step to make the book more close to the students. It is a bold step on the part of CBS to take to compile all that it subject in a single book internal Mnemonics and illustrations. I salute Dr. Hemanth and Puja for this unique idea. All in one complete concise to revise at last time, Eye catchy font, Mnemonics are coloured, Updates are marked with blue colour, All related points in a single picture, Cranial nerve and nuclei chart is useful.
Debjyoti Halder (Amazon Customer)

The wow factor is that all subjects are covered in such a small book. Each chapter is filled with such important topics, I thank CBS for giving me such a wonderful book. It is absolutely the best for revision and contains all high yield stuff. All topics has been covered and layout with that of a diary background is amazing
Apeksha, ESI Medical College, Bangalore

Undoubtedly the best book in pediatrics for PGMEE preparation. A comprehensive book with regards to theory and MCQ questions. The presentation of the book is lucid and easy for revision. The Image based questions are the best part of this book. Esp. neonatology section is a wow factor. (has > 40 image based qs in newborn chapter). Icing on the cake is latest exam question (upto may 2018) which no other books have. Just One line - "Do think anything beyond this book for pediatrics"
PG Aspirants

Complete Review of Pediatrics by Dr.Deepak Marwah is a nice book for MCQ preparation. The book has most recent questions of 2017-18 with solved answers. The theory about the topics is given in short in the start and then the image based questions and 100+ MCQs for each topic with answers and explanation along with the referred book. The images are very clear. The written matter is simple and the print is not monotonous. Colourful and glossy pages attract the interest of the reader.
Shivani Desai (Feedback on CBS Exam Books FB Page)

Book is easy to read with relavant images along with the theory. Even most recent may 18 questions are covered.
Utkarsh N (Amazon Customer)

A book you need to have for making you understand and complete pediatrics in 3 odd days. Well compiled and written by the great Deepak Marwah sir
Syed Aijaz

The best part of the book is tables / facts / data have been taken from Nelson's 20/e and very well illustrated. Facts are genuine, suitable diagrams and Recent Advances with Image based questions and sufficient number of questions (MCQs) at the end of every chapter. Explanation has been given apt. from reference of international books.
Anand Tiwari, GMC, Amritsar

Scan the QR Code to View Sample Pages of the Books

This book is a complete package with all genuine questions with wonderful explanation. Didn't found any flaws in the books.
Colour plates are centre of attraction in this book. This book is a complete package for aiims. Must buy for AIIMS.
-Shubham Jain

Well the most eye-catching feature of the book is definitely the inclusion of all the MBBS subjects in single text. One can go through all these quickly during the PG Exam revision. Even different various sub domains are also included into the book eg. Genetics, Immunology etc are provided as different indices. This definitely helps in easy understanding. Test is presented in the most concise way possible. This is highly appreciable. A large number of diagrams and easy to go through tables are provided. High yield points are like sugar coating. Some picture based questions also find into the text.
Shivam Sabharwal
SN Medical College, Jodhpur

ROAMS is the best book for final revision of all subjects at a single place. Best part of this by which I like most table and flowchart to memorise something. By flowcharts we can learn easily and for longer time.
Naresh Kumar
PGIMS, Rohtak

ROAMS is really so good and makes the base for any entrance exam. The theory provided and illustrations make the concept last longer!
Abhimanyu Agrawal
GR Medical College, Gwalior

I like the way how similar sounding terms are clubbed together in one place for the ease of the ease of the reader. The important tables have also been included in this book which is helpful since we don't have to refer other bulky books. The mnemonics provided are very helpful for retention of facts.
Reuben Toi
MGMCRI, Puducherry

Its comprehensive very useful for last minute preparation. It contain all facts, tables for PGMEE. Very helpful for revision and make me feel mentally strong when ROAMS is giving to revise in a short term.
Siva Subramanian
Madurai Medical College, Madurai

This book is very much balanced and covers all the topics which is important for NEET PG as well as proff exams. Flowcharts, image based questions and tabulated content make it a MUST BUY.
Ankit Tiwari
Buldelkhand Medical College, Sagar

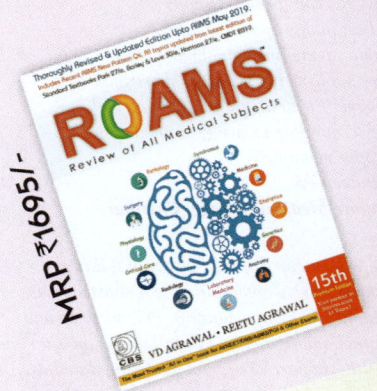

Highest collection of COLOR PLATES...Controversial Questions are clearly explained... New boxes of RECALL BIAS are superb... High Yield tables & Mnemonics More explanations for MCQ that helps easy to understand
Theeran R

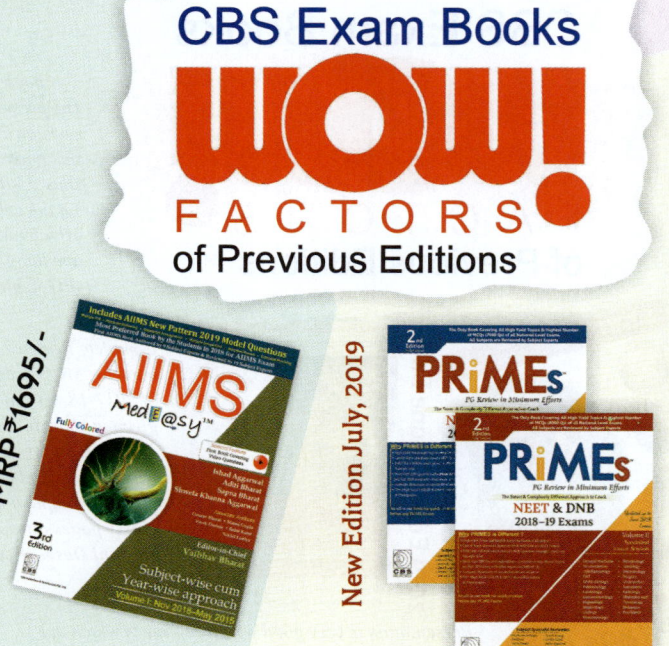

CBS Exam Books
WOW!
FACTORS
of Previous Editions

This books definitely gives you the edge to get through the middle ranks and go on to the top ranks, owing to its latest updates section. Highlighted points which are crucial for scoring marks. High yield facts section which is also amazing as it gives a condensed form of the topic.
Manish Khichar

A perfect book for AIIMS Preparation. It contains all AIIMS Questions, nice to read all questions.
It contains all type of questions, optional questions, image based questions with nice explanations
-Karthick Raja

This is a good book for quick revision before NEET PG. Its presented as 2 volumes. Basic sciences and clinical sciences. It has 15,000 MCQs from last 10 yrs including recent pattern questions, all questions are organized subject wise, topic wise and subtopic wise..answers to MCQs are given with reference books and their page number..theory is presented as facts, most common, important topics and tables..theory is reviewed by individual subject specialists..
Dr Anirudha (Amazon Customer)

 Scan the QR Code to View Sample Pages of the Books

CBS Exam Books 2019

Exam Wise Books

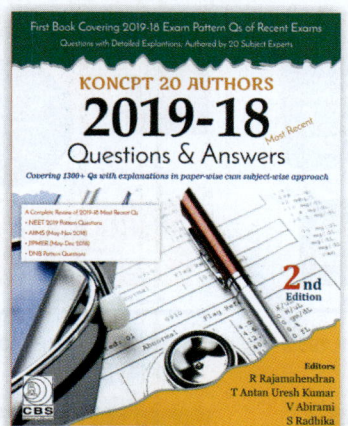
2/e, 2019 — MRP ₹595/-

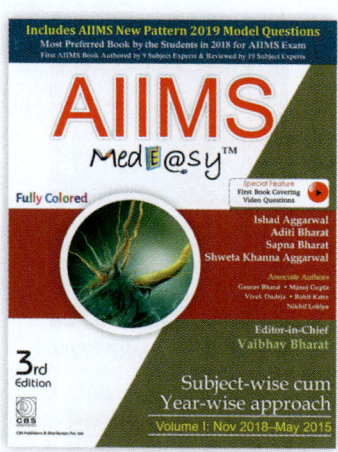
3/e, 2019 — MRP ₹1695/-

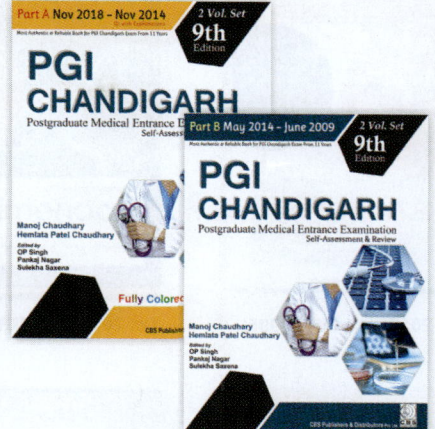
9/e, 2019 — MRP ₹1895/-

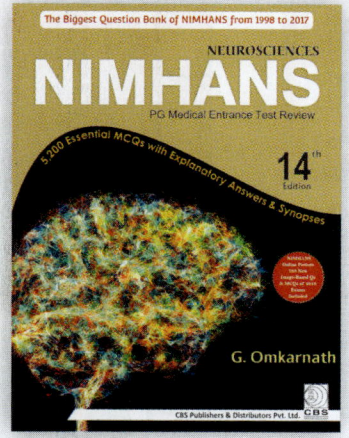
14/e, 2019 — MRP ₹1495/-

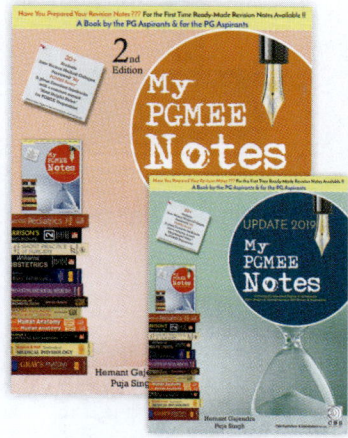
1/e, 2018 — MRP ₹1155/-

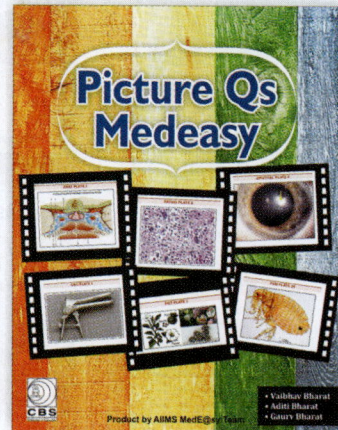
1/e, 2019 — Releasing in June

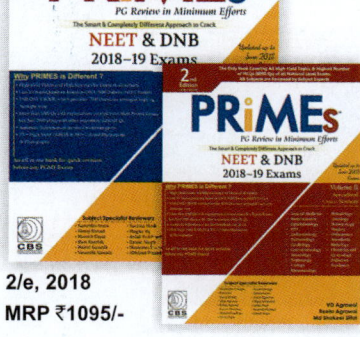
2/e, 2018 — MRP ₹1095/-
2/e, 2018 — MRP ₹1195/-

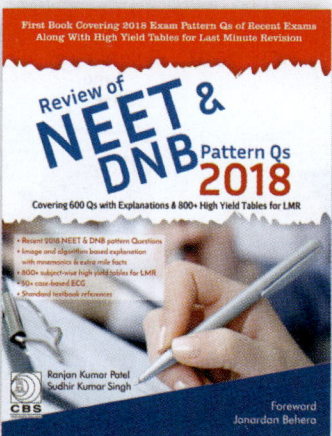
1/e, 2018 — MRP ₹695/-

4/e, 2019 — Releasing in June

CBS Publishers & Distributors Pvt. Ltd.
New Delhi • Bengaluru • Chennai • Kochi • Kolkata • Mumbai • Pune • Hyderabad • Nagpur • Patna • Vijaywada

Above books available at **All Medical Book Stores of India**

Buy online: PrepLadder | cbspd.co.in | amazon.in | Parasredkart.com | flipkart

For any availability issue please contact: +91-9555559901

CBS Exam Books 2019
Subject Wise Books

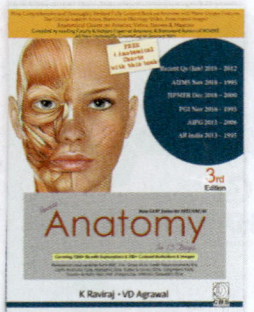
Anatomy — K Raviraj - VD Agrawal
3/e, 2019 — MRP ₹995/-

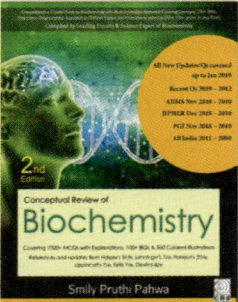
Conceptual Review of Biochemistry — Smily Pruthi Pahwa
2/e, 2019 — MRP ₹695/-

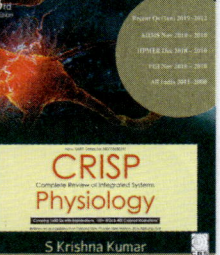
CRISP — Complete Review of Integrated Systems Physiology — S Krishna Kumar
3/e, 2019 — MRP ₹725/-

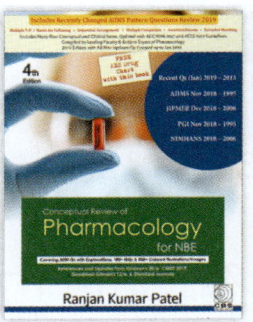
Conceptual Review of Pharmacology for NBE — Ranjan Kumar Patel
4/e, 2019 — MRP ₹950/-

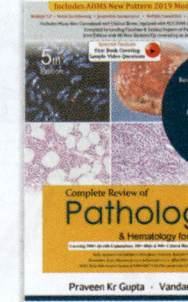
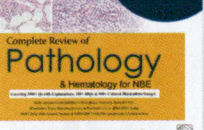
Complete Review of Pathology & Hematology for NBE — Praveen Kr Gupta • Vandana Puri
5/e, 2019 — MRP ₹995/-

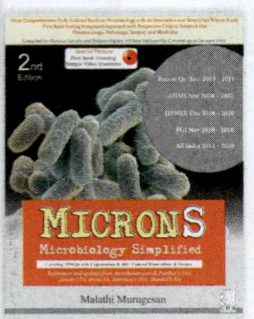
MICRONS — Microbiology Simplified — Malathi Murugesan
2/e, 2019 — MRP ₹895/-

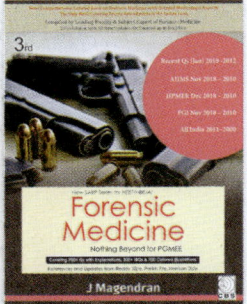
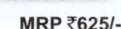
Forensic Medicine — Nothing Beyond for PGMEE — J Magendran
3/e, 2019 — MRP ₹625/-

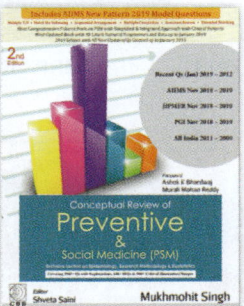
Conceptual Review of Preventive & Social Medicine (PSM) — Shveta Saini, Mukhmohit Singh
2/e, 2019 — MRP ₹1195/-

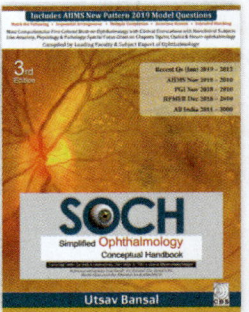
SOCH — Simplified Ophthalmology Conceptual Handbook — Utsav Bansal
3/e, 2019 — MRP ₹695/-

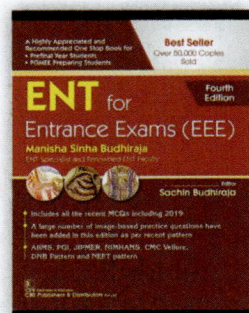
ENT for Entrance Exams (EEE) — Manisha Sinha Budhiraja
4/e, 2019 — MRP ₹795/-

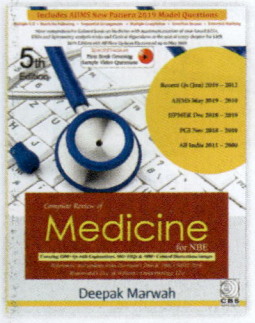
Conceptual Review of Medicine for NBE — Deepak Marwah
5/e, 2019 — Releasing in June

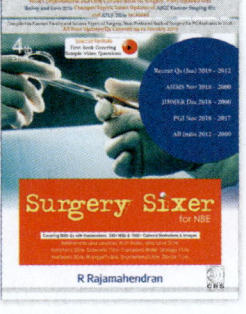
Surgery Sixer for NBE — R Rajamahendran
4/e, 2019 — MRP ₹1395/-

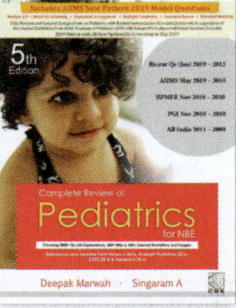
Complete Review of Pediatrics for NBE — Deepak Marwah, Singaram A
5/e, 2019 — Releasing in June

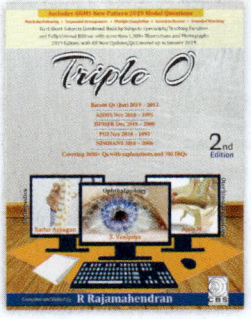
Triple O — R Rajamahendran
2/e, 2019 — MRP ₹1095/-

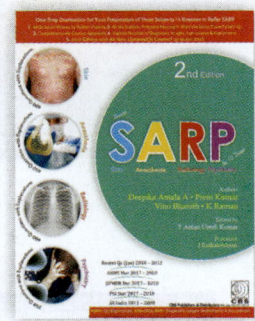
SARP — Anatomy — Deepak Antala A • Prem Kumar, Vibu Bharath • K Raman
2/e, 2018 — MRP ₹895/-

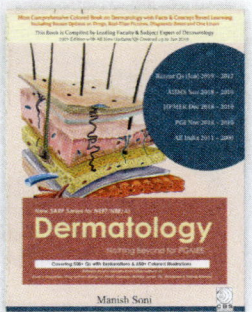
Dermatology — Nothing Beyond for PGMEE — Manish Soni
1/e, 2019 — MRP ₹495/-

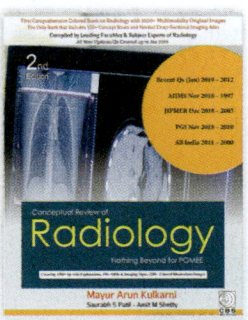
Conceptual Review of Radiology — Nothing Beyond for PGME — Mayur Arun Kulkarni, Saurabh S Patil - Amit M Shetty
2/e, 2019 — MRP ₹395/-

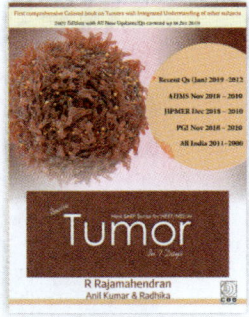
Tumor in 7 Days — R Rajamahendran, Anil Kumar & Radhika
1/e, 2019 — Releasing in June

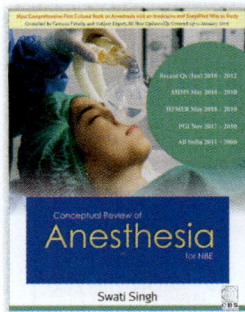
Conceptual Review of Anesthesia for NBE — Swati Singh
1/e, 2019 — Releasing in June

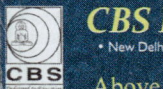
CBS Publishers & Distributors Pvt. Ltd.
New Delhi • Bengaluru • Chennai • Kochi • Kolkata • Mumbai • Pune • Hyderabad • Nagpur • Patna • Vijayawada

Above books available at **All Medical Book Stores of India**

Buy online: PrepLadder | CBS cbspd.co.in | 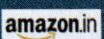 amazon.in | Parasredkart.com | 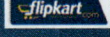 flipkart

For any availability issue please contact : +91-9555590180